Nursing and Midwifery
A Practical Approach

Sally Huband

Pam Hamilton-Brown

Gillian Barber

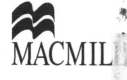

MACMILLAN

Macmillan Education
Between Towns Road, Oxford OX4 3PP
A division of Macmillan Publishers Limited
Companies and representatives throughout the world

www.macmillan-africa.com

ISBN: 978-14050-973-7

ISBN 10 - 140500973X

Text © Sally Huband, Pam Hamilton-Brown, Gillian Barber 2006
Design © Macmillan Publishers Limited 2006
Illustrations © Tina Gardiner 2006

First published 2006

Designed by Amanda Easter
Typeset by EXPO Holdings, Malaysia
Illustrated by Tina Gardiner with additional artwork by
David Gifford Appendix A, page 392
Cover design by Charles Design Associates
Cover photographs by Sally Huband

Photographs by Sally Huband

The publisher and authors wish to thank the following rights holders
for the use of copyright material:
Oxford University Press for the image Fig 14-36 from *Nutrition for
Developing Countries* 2/e by Savage King, Felicity and Burgess, Ann
(1993) on page 341.
TALC for the growth assessment chart on p. 393.

If any copyright holders have been omitted, please contact the
publishers who will make the necessary arrangements at the first
opportunity.

Printed and bound in Malaysia

2010 2009 2008 2007
10 9 8 7 6 5 4 3 2

Contents

Practical procedures

The symbol **Pp** indicates a practical procedure.
These are found throughout the book.

Tables

Contents

Preface

The three editors of this book have each worked in different countries in Africa. They became aware that there was a significant lack of appropriate textbooks for nurses and midwives. Many countries lack funds to buy texts and many of the books available are designed for use by nurses and midwives in western countries and working in very different circumstances. Diseases and patterns of ill health prevalent in Africa and other areas of the world may not be seen in the West and those seen in the West may be rare elsewhere.

The text is intended to be a useful reference tool for staff working in rural clinics and health centres and also student nurses and midwives undertaking basic training. It is not in sufficient depth for those doing a degree course. Qualified staff supporting students will find information that will assist them in their role. The emphasis of the book is on practical care, supported by theoretical information where necessary. Clinical skills form the basis for all nursing and midwifery practice.

The book is not intended to cover the whole range of health problems or the variety of courses people undertake. Reasons for ill health are often complex and solutions vary according to the context in which the practitioner is working. The book will need to be supported by other appropriate and more specialist resources. A list of sources and suggested further reading is therefore included at the end of the book. As access to the internet is becoming more common, details of useful websites are also given.

Each chapter starts with a short introduction which indicates its contents. Some chapters have a short section on anatomy and physiology where it was felt that this would aid understanding. Most chapters have activities comprising questions to test understanding of material found in the text or activities aimed at encouraging readers to think about what they have read. To avoid unnecessary repetition, cross referencing helps the reader find additional information in other chapters.

As health promotion is an essential part of nursing and midwifery practice, most chapters have a short section at the end identifying relevant aspects of health promotion.

The glossary is intended to help readers who may be unfamiliar with some of the medical terms. The first time a word that may be unfamiliar is used in a chapter, it appears in bold italics. This means that the word is explained in the glossary.

The editors appreciate that there is a wide variation across the world in the prevalence of diseases and the resources available to treat them. We are indebted to our colleagues from Botswana, Uganda, Kenya and South Africa who have contributed to the text and advised on content. We hope that this text will be of use to nurses and midwives who are often working in areas that lack resources.

Foreword

During a unique experience working with Yoruba mothers in the Nigerian village of Imesi Ile, I tried to help them improve the health of their children. I came to realise that the demands put on the nurse or midwife in Africa are different to the demands made in the North. Often she is the only health worker available. She has to make the diagnosis, organise the treatment, and give advice on nutrition and rehabilitation. Even when she is working in a hospital she has more responsibility than colleagues trained in countries of the North. For example in many cultures the patient expects relatives to be present at all times. Nurses and midwives can help these relatives to be responsible for part of the care and at the same time give important health education. Lecturing to post graduate doctors I emphasised that in many countries in the South the nurses and midwives provide more primary health care than the doctors but look to the doctor to provide support and guidance.

I was delighted to hear that Sally Huband and her team were undertaking the formidable task of writing a book to help in the training and practice of the thousands of nurses and midwives that countries in Africa need if they are to play their part in the reduction of an unacceptably high mortality and bring the level of health care up to acceptable standards.

This welcome addition to the Macmillan and TALC literature is the result of collaboration between the editors and nursing and midwifery writers from a variety of countries. They all know from personal experience what it is like to work where health care facilities and resources are often limited and medical support may be at a minimum. The contents of the book have been read and approved by a number of nurses and doctors with experience in different countries.

In most resource-poor countries there is a lack of personnel. Nurses and midwives are often the only contact many people have with health care and prevention. They are in the forefront in providing information and care, and in preventing ill health.

A strength of the book is that contributors were asked to consider the reality of these working situations. They were asked to focus on the essentials that readers need to know in order to provide the best possible care at both hospital and community level, and when modern technology is limited or not available. At the same time psychological, social and cultural aspects and also health promotion were to be included to help readers to provide the care people need.

It is hoped that the book will be used in a wide variety of environments to train and support nurses and midwives to achieve the skills so badly needed.

David Morley

List of editors and contributors

Editors

Gillian Barber MA(Ed) RM RN PhD, Midwife teacher, nurse, anthropologist and reproductive health specialist

Pam Hamilton-Brown MA RGN RM MTD DN DMS Public Administration, Formerly Principal Lecturer, Midwifery, University of Brighton

Sally Huband BA RGN RSCN RM RNT, Formerly Senior Lecturer, Paediatrics, University of Brighton

Illustrator: Tina Gardiner BA RM, Labour Ward Co-ordinator, Pembury Hospital, Kent

Contributors to sections

Introduction
Gillian Barber

Principles of care
Gillian Barber
Pam Hamilton-Brown
Sally Huband

Patient care
Professor H.S. Adala MB ChB Med-Ophth (Nbi) DORCS (London) Associate Professor Department of Ophthalmology, College of Health Sciences, Nairobi
Gillian Barber

Sara Burr RN BN(Hons) FETC ENB N18 Dip Trop Nurse, Freelance Dermatology Speciality Nurse

Kathy Dennill RN RM Dip Nursing Education B Cur Health Management and Community Health, Nursing Leadership Programme, Foundation for Professional Development, South Africa

Kefalotse Dithole RN RM MSc, Lecturer, Department of Nursing Education, University of Botswana

Pam Hamilton-Brown

Sally Huband

Lilian Sera Moremi RN RM MNS HIV and AIDS Coordinator, Ministry of Lands and Housing, Botswana

Ephraim Ncube RN RM BEd MNS, Lecturer, Department of Nursing Education, University of Botswana

Esther Ntsayagae MCur RM RN, Lecturer, Department of Nursing Education, University of Botswana

Theresa Odero MSc Health Promotion and Education, PGDip KRN KRM Ophthalmic Nurse Aga Khan University, Kenya

Rebecca Penzer RN BSc(Hons) PGDip Professional Education MSc, Independent Nurse Consultant in Skin Health; Member of International Skin Care Nursing Group

Nthabiseng A Phaladze PhD RN RM, Lecturer, Department of Nursing Education, University of Botswana

Cynthia Nkhumisang Pilane RN CM BSc Nursing MNS/FNP D Litt et Phil, Lecturer, Department of Nursing Education, University of Botswana

Ivy Poodhun RGN RNT BEd(Hons), Senior Lecturer, Institute of Nursing and Midwifery, University of Brighton

Motshedisi B. Sabone RN RM PhD, Lecturer, Department of Nursing Education. University of Botswana

Naomi Mmapelo Seboni RN PhD, Senior Lecturer, Department of Nursing Education, University of Botswana

Sheila Shaibu PhD RN, Lecturer, Department of Nursing Education, University of Botswana

Terry Stubbings RGN DN (London) PGCEA, Senior Lecturer, Institute of Nursing and Midwifery, University of Brighton

Wananani B Tshiamo MSN RN RM, Lecturer, Department of Nursing Education, University of Botswana

Reproductive and sexual health
Gillian Barber

Sam Bassett BSc RGN RM, Lecturer, University of Brighton

Sian Edwards RGN RNT BSc MSc, Senior Lecturer in HIV and Sexual Health, Institute of Nursing and

Midwifery, University of Brighton; Member of the Executive Committee for the National HIV Nurses Association UK

Pam Hamilton-Brown

Kamya M.M. Kabanga RN RM Dip Nurse Tutor Diploma Medical Education MA(Ed), Principal, Mulago School of Nursing and Midwifery Training, Kampala, Uganda

Eileen Nixon RGN MSc, Nurse Consultant Brighton and Sussex University Hospitals; Honorary Lecturer at Brighton University; Member of the Executive Committee for the National HIV Nurses Association UK

Esther S. Seloilwe PhD RN RM, Senior Lecturer and Head of Department Nursing Education, Director of WHOCC for Nursing and Midwifery Development, University of Botswana

Maternity care
Gillian Barber
Pam Hamilton-Brown
Sally Huband

Care of children
Sally Huband

Mental health
Gillian Barber
Esther S. Seloilwe

Gloria B Tshweneagae RN RM MSc, Lecturer and Head of Community Mental Health Programme, Institute of Sciences, Lobatswe, Botswana

Promoting good health
Gillian Barber

Acknowledgements

Professor David Morley for his encouragement and support throughout, without which this book would never have been completed

Liz Paren for her enthusiasm and advice, which enabled the book to reach the publishers

The following people for reading scripts and giving constructive advice:

Gwen Barber, Senior Clinical Training Scholar in Veterinary Anaesthesia, University of Bristol

Dr Nynke van den Broek, Obstetrician and Gynaecologist, Course Director, Diploma in Reproductive Health, Liverpool School of Tropical Medicine

Ann Burgess, Nutrition Consultant

David Cannon, Retired from General Practice in Watford, previously Obstetrician Wesley Guild Hospital, Nigeria

William Cutting, Retired, Reader in International Child Health, Edinburgh, previously London School of Hygiene and Tropical Medicine, and many years as missionary doctor in India

Maureen Duggan, formerly paediatrician in Nigeria and Malawi

Prof John Guillebaud, Emeritus Professor of Family Planning and Reproductive Health, University College, London

Linda Hodgson, formerly Senior Nursing Adviser, Kiwoko Hospital, Uganda

Pat Hughes, International Council of Nurses

Sebalda Leshabari, Faculty of Nursing, Muhimbili University College of Health Sciences, Dar Es Salaam, Tanzania

Edwin Mapara, formerly Chief Medical Officer, National Antiretroviral Therapy Project, Gaborone, Botswana

Nester Moyo, International Confederation of Midwives

Dr Vikram Patel, Reader in International Mental Health, London School of Hygiene and Tropical Medicine

Sister Isabelle Smyth and others, Medical Missionaries of Mary

Professor Sheila Tlou RN PhD, Professor of Nursing, University of Botswana

Introduction

1

Issues in nursing and midwifery care

Nurses and midwives care for people in many different environments, from rural clinics to referral hospitals, from high-rise apartment blocks to one-room dwellings. They work in prisons, expensive clinics, mission and government hospitals. Their work is often carried out in situations of poverty and deprivation. This chapter aims to raise some of the questions that arise. Generalising is difficult but there are some common themes.

Introduction

Nurses and midwives are taking increasing responsibility and advancing their education. At the same time they encounter staff shortages and lack of resources and their work load increases, particularly as HIV infection and AIDS take their toll. After some improvements in the health of populations through the twentieth century, statistics indicate that this is now deteriorating.

There are, of course, shining examples of individual initiatives that make a difference. In Lusaka, Zambia, the HIV infection rate of teenage girls has been significantly reduced. Malawi has improved access to family spacing services and increased primary school enrolment of girl children. Many countries are making efforts to provide clean water supplies. These are all factors known to have a long-lasting influence on the health of whole communities. In fact, education of girl children is thought to be more important than almost anything else as children born to uneducated mothers are known to be twice as likely to die early as others whose mothers have been to school.

In contrast, the gap between rich and poor continues to widen. Here are some examples from countries classified as 'least developed':

- One in 20 women from poor backgrounds die in childbirth, perhaps 100 times more than women in industrialised nations.
- Population growth is nearly double the world average. Half the population will soon be under 18 years old. Many will be orphans who may have to fend for themselves from an early age because of lack of adult support.
- Governments may spend little of their income on health, and some have to put large sums (including aid given to them) into paying back debts. Many people are campaigning to reduce this burden by cancelling debt.
- Children are much less likely to be immunised, fed adequately, receive education (especially if female), or live as long.
- One child in six dies before its fifth birthday in these countries, one in 14 elsewhere in Africa and one in 167 in industrialised nations. The figure may reach one in three in conflict situations.

Nurses and midwives have obvious roles in providing care for those who need help and this is well described in the following chapters. However, there is more we can contribute. This chapter does not attempt to address practical aspects of caring. Instead it aims to help you consider the background issues that make a difference to the effectiveness of what you do. For those who work in the community, the issues may be more obvious than for hospital based nurses and midwives, but they apply to both.

The issues

You may encounter some or all of these problems during your career:
- Poverty and lack of essential services
- Lack of education, illiteracy, and ignorance about health and nutrition
- Sickness. Do we all look at sickness in the same way?

- Access to care. What are the barriers?
- Urban–rural divide. Do rural communities get fair shares?

■ Activity

The issues above are just a selection. Can you think of any more in your area?
- List barriers in your area:
  - to deciding to seek care
  - to actually getting to care facilities
  - to receiving treatment on arrival.
- Suggest ways in which you might make a difference.

(To give you some examples, common barriers to getting care might range from flooded roads to poor attitudes of staff.)

What can nurses and midwives do?

Maybe you feel you cannot do much about poverty. Remember, however, that healthy people can look after themselves more easily, so you have important contributions to make to the alleviation of poverty. Quality of care is a different matter; health care teams can make a real difference by considering the quality of services they provide, and trying to identify sticking points that need special attention.

■ Activity

- Are there any common health problems directly related to poverty in your area?
- What are they?

You will surely be involved in critical incidents, emergencies and accidents as well as seeing longer-term ill health. The very sick will come to you – or maybe they won't. Do you feel frustrated when you hear that an old lady has been sick in her house for days before coming to you? How do you feel when you hear of the death of a child whose parents have not sought your help, or left it too late? There are all sorts of reasons why people do not seek help and these are often related to lack of knowledge, or even to different ways of seeing the world. They may seem ignorant but this is a complex issue that will be considered again later.

■ Activity

What types of sickness do you see in your area?

In richer nations, most people who are sick can take a bus, use the family car, or call an emergency ambulance. How do people in your area get help if they are sick?

■ Activity

- Note down any specific cases that you can think of where people had difficulty getting to health care.
- Think about what the difficulties were and why those people had problems.
- What could you do to encourage the community to improve the situation?

Rural areas are often last in the line for resource allocation. For example, health spending may be put into visible projects and high technology equipment. A scanner unit may be opened with great ceremony, whilst elsewhere rubber gloves and medicines run out. This can make carers feel powerless, hopeless, frustrated and unwilling to keep trying.

■ Activity

Do you have associations of nurses and midwives that can influence the decision makers more than you can alone? Locally, too, you are stronger together than you are alone.
- Suggest some ways in which you could support each other better.

Prioritising

What matters most? What actions will have most impact? It might be to provide mother and baby clinic services to distant villages or a cluster of houses in a township. It might be to act as an *advocate* for a community to persuade the local authorities to repair a water pump. Many nurses and midwives feel confused in the face of so much need and find it hard to prioritise.

■ Activity

Do you want to try to do something really useful but find it hard to work out what this might be when there is so much to be done? Try this:

1. Write down on separate pieces of card or paper:
   - A: five health problems that cause concern
   - B: five local community difficulties
   - C: five difficulties that you experience as a nurse or midwife.

(Some examples of the types of items you might write down are A: tuberculosis, diarrhoea; B: very low income, no transport; C: erratic medical supplies in the wet season, failure of people to return for follow-up treatment.)

2. Re-arrange the lists in order of importance, laying them side by side.
You will soon see which issues are the most urgent ones, and any connections between them. Does this give you ideas of which issues should have highest priority? For example, in the suggestions provided, there could be a connection between tuberculosis, failure to turn up for treatment, and poor transport.

Ways of thinking about health

Many nurses and midwives suffer acute frustration at the way in which people misuse services, or do not use them at all. Asking for injections to cure minor ills might be one of them.

■ Activity

Suggest three ways services are used that disturb you?

This might be caused just by lack of knowledge and understanding of the body. For example, people who do not understand the effects of food contamination are less likely to realise how important hand washing is following *defaecation*. Health promotion and education are well-known aspects of nursing and midwifery work but problems may be deeper than just lack of knowledge. People think about their bodies, and what causes illness and disease, in different ways. You may find yourself working with people who have different ideas about how illness, and life changes such as pregnancy, should be treated. They may think differently about what causes problems too. Some examples are:

- getting wet in the rain
- breaking taboos
- upsetting the ancestors
- eating particular foods in pregnancy
- being bewitched.

They may also consult a diviner before seeking treatment to find out what (or who) caused a particular problem.

■ Activity

Think of examples that are given in your area of how illness is caused?

The way people think about health and illness, their bodies, minds and spirits depends largely on their view of life.

- Western-style health care concentrates mainly on the physical. It is based on the idea that body and mind are separate, and that the spirit (or spiritual needs) are less significant to health.
- Another view is that mind, body and spirit cannot be separated and they all influence health.

The reality is that patients will probably use only local, familiar help unless they are confident of the benefits of hospital treatment and can get it easily. Many people use the services of traditional healers, herbalists, diviners or witch doctors first. They may return to them if modern medicine does not bring about satisfactory cures. They may use the two types of treatment at the same time. There is increasing interest worldwide in what traditional knowledge has to offer. Also, herbalists' knowledge is gaining respect in some areas as they form associations and make their treatments available to study by others. Modern pharmacology is itself founded on herbalist traditions of centuries past.

■ Activity

Describe two or three instances when you have been aware that patients have combined 'treatments' or tried local and modern medicine. Do you believe these combinations are dangerous, helpful or of no importance? Can you explain why you think this?

Sometimes local ideas seem to have no reason to them. Others seem to have some sense if you are prepared to be open-minded. Listening to people will always help you to see how local culture affects people's actions and choices. Open attitudes can also help to find a way around dangerous ideas, or allow use of harmless treatments alongside modern ones. Listening does not mean you have to agree! Two examples might help here:

- You know that men are reluctant to carry sick women to hospital on the stretcher the community has made for emergencies. You find out that they believe they too will get sick if they touch a bleeding woman or a woman in labour.

- You hear that a family delayed taking a pregnant woman to hospital until she had laboured for two days. They expected her adulterous husband to confess his sexual partners before seeking help. They believe that confession is necessary to allow the birth to happen naturally. It seemed sensible to them to find out what they saw as the cause. They did not realise that delay is deadly.

■ Activity

- Think of ways around these difficulties without making actual criticisms of local beliefs.
- Try to describe one or two situations you have encountered where ideas and beliefs have made it difficult to provide the necessary care.
- Suggest two or three local practices that are probably harmless.
- Suggest two or three local practices that may be useful.

Education alone may not be enough to change people's ideas and practices. An example of this is when traditional birth attendants (TBAs) continue to give herbal medicines to speed up women's labours despite being told how dangerous this is. They may have been influenced by two completely different ways of thinking, the modern ideas taught in TBA training, and ideas learnt when apprenticed to another TBA. Old ideas can be very influential and may not always be completely wrong.

This shows how important carers can be as advocates. When you know an area well you have a valuable role in acting as mediator between the local population and health service personnel and influencing both. Health service personnel may be ignorant and dismissive of local ideas, which can lead to people concealing their actions or being less willing to seek skilled help. Nurses and midwives are more likely to understand local cultures. They may see more clearly how western medicine and traditional values, customs and practices can meet. They may be able to help to make use of the best from both worlds; there may

indeed be simple herbal remedies that can be as effective as more expensive manufactured medications when used in controlled ways. Local knowledge may be important in other ways. Understanding local power structures is important and you may know to whom planners should go to obtain cooperation for community health initiatives. However 'junior' they may be, those who are prepared to speak up can influence the success of projects.

The wider nursing role

Culture can be defined as a shared system of ideas and ways of living, often passed through generations. Nursing, midwifery and medicine have their own cultures, so do the communities from which patients come. Often they misunderstand and mistrust each other. Providing effective care, as described in the following chapters, can only be done properly if this is realised. There are obvious areas that are culturally sensitive, such as practices that are required when someone dies, or knowing when it is inappropriate for a man to provide a woman's care. There are, however, many other areas in which nurses and midwives can use their knowledge of the community to act as intermediary, advocate, educator (of both patients and colleagues alike) and as skilled listener and adviser.

■ Activities

1. Talk to the local community and its leaders to find out what they see as their main needs:
   - What solutions do they see?
   - What barriers may hamper their (and your) success?
   - How can you support them in achieving a solution?
   - What support or training do you need to achieve this?
   - And how might you get it?

2. Go back through this section and review what you have written. Identify at least one issue and create an action plan. Remember to include in your action plan what resources you need, whose help you need to enlist, and a time line, as well as your specific aim.

Part 1

Principles of care

2

Organisation and provision of care

This chapter introduces the concepts of organisation and planning for care. It introduces the importance of communication and record keeping and a short discussion on task allocation and patient allocation. The Nursing Process and Nursing Models are briefly covered together with some of the basic assessment skills required by the nurse to give care.

Introduction

Resources in most countries are scarce and nurses are responsible for ensuring that best use is made of them. It is worth remembering that preventing illness costs less than curing illness. It is cheaper to provide safe, clean water than to treat thousands of people with cholera or other forms of gut infection. It is cheaper to immunise a child against measles than it is to care for a child with measles. It is cheaper to ensure that a baby is born safely, than to care for a handicapped person for the rest of their life. Nurses and midwives should therefore always see themselves as promoters of health as well as carers of sick people. Health education should underpin all care that is given.

When faced with a sick person, the nurse should ask herself:

- Could this illness have been prevented? Was it caused by dirty water, poor food, dirty surroundings, lack of immunisation, or risky lifestyle?
- If it could have been prevented, how could it have been done?
- Who is responsible for the failure to prevent it?
- Can I prevent this person getting sick again, by giving some health education?

Environment of care

Sick people are cared for in many different environments. They may be cared for at home with supervision from a local clinic. They may be cared for in a clinic or in a small hospital with much of the care given by relatives. They may be in a large hospital with highly trained doctors and nurses and up-to-date equipment. Nurses may be involved in making decisions about where the sick person should be cared for. If they are working in a clinic, they need to decide whether they have the resources to care for the patient there, or whether they should refer the patient to a larger hospital for more intensive care. Sometimes there is no choice, because the clinic is far from the nearest hospital and there is no transport to take the patient to the hospital.

Working as a member of a team

The team includes all of the following: doctors, nurses/midwives, patients and relatives; and sometimes some of these: physiotherapists, occupational therapists, speech therapists, traditional birth attendants and village health workers.

All members of the team are important. They are involved in keeping people healthy and treating and caring for sick people. To use resources properly, the skills of each person in the team need to be recognised and used in the most effective way. Nurses and midwives are crucial people in this team, as they are the only people who are likely to be around every hour of the day and night.

Communication is essential in ensuring that every member of the team is aware of the responsibilities and actions of the other members of the team. Nurses need to be told the results of the doctor's examination and the treatment ordered. The doctor needs to know from the nurses the results of the initial assessment, and how they feel the patient is responding to the treatment. The physiotherapist needs to know what treatment she is to give the patient and she needs to communicate with the nurses so that they can help the patient continue with any exercises when the physiotherapist is not there.

Skill mix

The senior nurse in the hospital or clinic needs to decide how to allocate nurses to different departments or areas. Some departments need several highly trained nurses. Others may function well with one trained nurse and several auxiliary or assistant nurses. It is a waste of scarce resources to use trained nurses or midwives to give care that can be given by someone less well trained. However, it is dangerous to allocate a nurse or midwife in training to care for patients, if she has not yet been taught the skills to give that care. In children's wards, in particular, most of the basic care is given by parents or guardians. However, this does not mean that a children's ward needs fewer nurses. Children can deteriorate very quickly and they respond to illness in a different way to adults. Ideally the team on the children's ward should be led by nurses experienced in the care of sick children.

Communication and record keeping

Nurses and midwives need to be good communicators. First of all they communicate with the patients and their relatives, they also communicate with each other and with other professionals regarding the care of their patients.

Verbal communication

We need to consider what we say and how we say it. Patients are not used to medical terms that may be commonly used in hospitals and clinics. Nurses need to be sure that the patient can understand what has been said and what it means. Sometimes the patient speaks a different language or dialect to the nurse. Wherever possible, the nurse needs to find an interpreter who can translate what is being said into the patient's language to prevent misunderstandings, for example:

Nurse: *Has anyone in your family ever had a cardiac arrest?*
Patient: *No, we have never been in trouble with the police.*

Using unfamiliar language can be frightening and also cause misunderstanding. If patients are anxious, they may be unable to hear what is being said, or may only hear part of what is said, for example:

Doctor: *I am afraid your wife is seriously ill, but if we operate there is a slight chance she may be cured.*

The relative **may** have heard the first part, 'I am afraid your wife is seriously ill'. Because he is anxious and is very much hoping the operation will cure his wife, he may think he has heard the doctor say, 'If we operate, your wife will get better'. It is always worth asking the patient to repeat what they think you have told them, so that misunderstandings can be quickly sorted out.

Some patients may be unable to speak because of their illness. The nurse still needs to talk to them and explain what is happening. It may be possible for her to teach the patients some signs that he can make to indicate his wishes. He may be able to write things down.

If patients are unconscious it is important to remember that hearing is the last sense to be lost. So nurses must be very careful of what they say when near the patient.

Non verbal communication

When we speak, we may emphasise different words and also can alter the meaning of a phrase by the tone of voice we use. For example:

*What **are** you doing?*

This can suggest that the person is doing something they should not be. However, the nurse may just be asking a straightforward question and may have been about to offer help.

Our facial expression and body language will also alter the way in which what we say will be understood. If we are trying to make patients feel welcome and less afraid, then what we say should be accompanied by a friendly smile and perhaps a gentle touch on the arm or shoulder. Children who are frightened will need to be cuddled and comforted.

Written communication and record keeping

Because doctors and nurses are looking after many different patients at any one time, it is important that there are written records that are easily read and understood. The use of abbreviations can be confusing. For example, PID can mean 'Prolapsed

Intravertebral Disc', or it can mean 'Pelvic Inflammatory Disease'.

Most hospitals and clinics will have their own rules about what is written and by whom. The nurse should have access to the doctor's notes, and the doctor should have access to the nurses' written records.

Patients should have a written record of their condition and progress written each day by the nurse who is caring for them. Nurses who are coming on duty then have both the verbal handover and a written record.

It is important to record on charts observations that have been taken on patients, and the time that they were taken. One recording of a temperature, pulse, respiratory rate and blood pressure is not much use on its own. The patient may have been frightened when it was taken, and the readings may be raised by the fear. It is the comparison of the observations at different times that gives an indication as to whether the patient is improving or deteriorating.

Fluid balance charts will need to be kept on patients who are dehydrated, or are in danger of becoming dehydrated. They will also need to be kept on patients who are having difficulty eating and drinking, or who are vomiting or have diarrhoea. The fluid chart needs to record all fluid the patient is having, oral and intravenous. It also needs to record all output – urine, gastric aspirate, vomit or bowel actions.

Organisation on the ward

It is usually the responsibility of the most senior member of the nursing team to decide the roles of each nurse working on that shift. There are different ways of organising the care.

Task Allocation

This method is still used in many hospitals and clinics but does have disadvantages.
- Each nurse is given a list of tasks to perform.
- They may be asked to do all the injections and give out the medicines.
- They may be asked to record the temperature, pulse and respiratory rates on all the patients.
- They may be asked to do all the dressings.

Disadvantages of Task Allocation
- Many different nurses give different aspects of care to the patients, increasing the risk of cross-infection.

- No one nurse knows all the details about any one patient.
- It is very confusing for the patients, who come into contact with many different nurses during the course of the day and do not know who they should contact in an emergency.
- There is little job satisfaction for the nurse.

Patient Allocation

The senior nurse allocates a number of patients to each nurse to care for. This nurse is then responsible for all care given to that patient.

The senior nurse is able to allocate the sickest patients to the next most senior nurse, and the junior nurse can care for the patients who do not require high levels of nursing intervention.

Advantages of Patient Allocation
- The patients know which nurse is caring for them.
- One nurse will be able to make an assessment of the progress of each patient. This leads to better patient care.
- There is less risk of cross-infection.
- Care can be carried out in a planned way with fewer disturbances to the patient.
- The care is *holistic*. It looks at the patient as a whole and does not break the care down into small portions.

Team nursing

If there are many patients on a ward, it is sometimes helpful to split the ward into areas and allocate a team of nurses to a group of patients. Nurses can be allocated to care for specific patients within their area. The patients in a specific area will get to know all the nurses within the team, so that when their special nurse is off duty, they can be cared for by another nurse within the team.

Care given by relatives/guardians

Whichever method is used for organising the care on the ward, it is important to include relatives and guardians in the giving of the care whenever it is possible. Patients will often prefer to be washed by someone they know, rather than by a strange nurse, which can cause embarrassment. Relatives can also help give patients food and drink and can provide comfort and reassurance. Nurses must remember that they are still responsible for the patient, so they must ensure that all relatives know what care they may give and how to give it. It is especially important to involve relatives when caring for children.

The nursing process

This is the term given to the way in which nurses structure their care of patients. It is divided into four main components.

Assessment and identification of problems

Nurses assess the patient, taking a history, familiarising themselves with any medical notes or previous nursing notes and recording observations. From this, they are able to identify the problems that the patient is having.

Planning the care

Before carrying out the care, the nurse:
- makes a plan of the care required by the patient now and decides whether any health education in the future will help prevent further illness
- identifies the priorities within the plan
- decides when and how she will carry out the plan and whether she needs to involve other personnel.

Implementing the care

The nurse needs to ensure that she carries out the care she has planned. Sometimes nurses spend so much time planning their care that they do not leave themselves enough time to implement it.

CASE STUDY A:
The Nursing Process in use

Musa, aged four years, is brought to the clinic by a young friend. He has fallen out of a mango tree and hurt his leg. He is in pain and very frightened. There is some bleeding from the wound on his leg and he is reluctant to move it.

Assessment

The nurse needs to assess the amount of pain that Musa is in. She also needs to assess the damage to his leg and decide whether it can be treated in the clinic or whether he needs to be referred for further treatment. She also needs to assess whether there is any dirt in the wound and whether he has had his tetanus immunisation. She needs to find out whether he hit his head when he fell and whether there was any loss of consciousness.

Identification of problems

- Musa's fear
- His pain
- The damage to his leg – possible fracture, the amount of bleeding, the contamination of the wound
- Possible head injury

Planning his care

- See if his mother is able to come to the clinic to reduce his fear.

- Give him analgesia to reduce pain.
- Examine the leg carefully, clean the wound. Assess the amount of bleeding. If a fracture is suspected, plan for transfer unless it is a simple fracture and a plaster of Paris can be applied.
- Decide whether Musa should have anti-tetanus toxoid.
- If there is any danger that he could have a compound fracture, consider giving antibiotics.
- If there is a possibility that Musa hit his head or lost consciousness, record neurological observations which will need to be repeated, possibly every half hour.

Implementation

Carry out the care which has been planned. Control any bleeding and continue neurological observations for as long as is necessary.

Evaluation

At each step of the care, the nurse needs to be evaluating.
- Is Musa less frightened when his mother arrives?
- Is his pain controlled by the analgesia?
- Has the bleeding stopped?
- Is the nurse satisfied with the care given to the possible fracture of the leg?

Musa's future care will depend on the result of this evaluation.

Evaluation

Evaluating the care given is a very important part of the whole process and the part that gets left out on occasions. A patient's condition changes over time and the care that was right at one time may no longer be appropriate. It may be that the patient has a dirty wound that is being dressed with Savlon (chlorhexidine).

CASE STUDY B:
Task v Patient Allocation

Task Allocation

Musa is frightened and in pain.
- Nurse A sees him when he first gets to the clinic and asks Nurse B to carry out the assessment while she sends for his mother.
- Nurse B reports to Nurse A who asks Nurse C to give him analgesia and Nurse D to do the dressing.
- Unfortunately Nurse D starts to do the dressing before the analgesia has had time to work and before his mother has arrived. Musa screams and cries in fear and pain. He does not understand what is happening to him.
- Nurse A is called back to discuss whether Musa should have anti-tetanus toxoid.
- Nurse C comes to give anti-tetanus and an antibiotic.

Musa's mother arrives after all this care has been given.

Musa has been cared for by four different nurses.

Patient Allocation

The nurse who sees Musa when he first comes to clinic assesses him and plans his care. She then gives him analgesia and sends a message to his mother.

In one hour, his mother has arrived and the analgesia is working. Musa is reassured by his mother and is no longer crying.

His nurse is now able to do his dressing, while his mother explains to him what is happening. He is also given his anti-tetanus and antibiotic by the same nurse. Musa now trusts this nurse and, as his mother is there, is able to cooperate.

Musa has been cared for by one nurse.

The nurse needs to evaluate the wound and decide whether it is improving. Following her evaluation, it may be necessary to change the solution that the wound is being treated with.

Consider case study A on page 11 which shows how the Nursing Process might look in use.

Now consider how Musa might see his care when nurses practise Task Allocation and when Patient Allocation is used (see case study B).

Nursing models

A nursing model is a way in which a patient can be assessed according to a set of beliefs and values and tries to define what nursing is.

Virginia Henderson's nursing model

Henderson defined nursing as 'The unique function of the nurse is to assist the individual, sick or well, in the performance of those activities contributing to health or its recovery (or to a peaceful death) that he would perform unaided if he had the necessary strength, will or knowledge, and to do this in such a way as to help him gain independence as quickly as possible.

She then lists 14 activities of daily living:

1. Breathe normally.
2. Eat and drink adequately.
3. Eliminate body wastes.
4. Move and maintain desirable postures.
5. Sleep and rest.
6. Select suitable clothes. Dress and undress.
7. Maintain body temperature within normal range by adjusting clothing and modifying the environment.
8. Keep the body clean and well groomed and protect the integument, that is the skin.
9. Avoid dangers in the environment and avoid injuring others.
10. Communicate with others expressing emotions, needs, fears or opinions.
11. Worship according to one's faith.
12. Work in such a way that there is a sense of accomplishment.
13. Play or participate in various forms of recreation.
14. Learn, discover, or satisfy the curiosity that leads to normal development and health, and use the available health facilities.

Roper, Tierney and Logan's nursing model

Henderson's ideas about nursing were further developed considering the lifespan of the patient, and the degree of dependence/ independence.

The authors list 12 activities of living:

1. Maintaining a safe environment
2. Breathing
3. Eliminating
4. Controlling body temperature
5. Working and playing
6. Sleeping
7. Communicating
8. Eating and drinking
9. Personal cleansing and dressing
10. Mobilising
11. Expressing sexuality
12. Dying

In Roper, Tierney and Logan's nursing model, initially the baby is very dependent, but if he is well he can breathe, eliminate and sleep on his own, with no difficulty. He cannot keep himself safe, nor is he good at controlling his body temperature and his ability to communicate is limited. However, a healthy adult can perform all the activities for himself. If he is ill, he may find that he is unable to perform all the activities. A very elderly person may also become more dependent, even when well.

Each activity has three parts:
- physical or physiological
- social
- psychological.

For example, when we eat, there is obviously a physical/ physiological strand. The food has to be chewed, swallowed, digested and absorbed. However, eating is also a social function. Families or friends will usually eat together. There is also a psychological strand. If someone is very upset they may not feel like eating.

Roper, Tierney and Logan also identify three other activities: 'preventing, comforting and seeking'. These three will overlap with the 12 other activities. For example, if someone feels ill, they may not be able to eat properly.
- They may ask for help (seeking).
- They may eat more easily digestible food (comforting).
- They will try to get over the illness and prevent it recurring (preventing).

This model then sees the goals of nursing as:
- helping the individual to acquire, maintain, or restore maximum independence in the activities of daily living, or enabling them to cope with dependence on others if circumstances make this necessary
- helping the individual to carry out activities to prevent ill health (encouraging the mother to take the children for immunisation)
- providing comforting strategies to help the individual to recover and eventually regain full independence
- providing treatments to overcome illness or its symptoms, leading to recovery and eventual independence.

These 12 activities of living are then used in the assessment of the patient.

There are other models of nursing that may be used to plan patient care, for example Orem described a 'Self-care model', Roy an 'Adaptation model' and Neumann a 'Health Care systems model'.

Do models help us in nursing?

Models cannot improve nursing care on their own. They can help nurses think about their roles and what nursing is. Is nursing just carrying out tasks, such as feeding patients, giving medicines and doing dressings? Or is it more about seeing each patient as an individual, with individual needs and problems which the nurse will seek to alleviate and prevent recurring?

Models can provide a structure for nurses to assess patients and plan their care.

There is no easy answer about which model to use. Some models seem more suited to different patients. Orem's model is often used in children's wards; Roy's model is perhaps more suited to psychiatric patients. The problem is that on one ward there is a mixture of patients, many of whom would benefit from the use of different models. This is not practicable, as it would be too confusing for the nurses working on the wards.

Models can work if a group of nurses sit down and devise their own model to suit their particular circumstances. Their own model may be based on one of the ones written up, or it can be entirely new.

Nursing assessment

Basic skills required for assessment

Taking the temperature: The normal range of temperature is between 36° and 38° C. Individuals will have their own normal temperature. Some people may usually have a low reading, others a higher reading. This is why it is important to record observations as a baseline so that the nurse can come to some conclusion as to whether this patient has a higher than normal temperature for them.

Temperature is altered according to hormonal changes, exposure to heat or cold, infection and exercise. The temperature is most commonly taken using a glass mercury thermometer (see Figure 2.1) or digital thermometer. The digital thermometer needs batteries which are not always available.

Pp Taking the temperature

There are different methods used for measuring a person's temperature depending on the circumstances. If glass thermometers are used, each patient should have their own glass thermometer so that there is less risk of cross-infection. If this is not possible, the glass thermometer should be disinfected after each use before it is used on another patient. The thermometer should be shaken down, holding by the upper end, to ensure that the reading is below the patient's normal reading. It should then be wiped with an alcohol wipe before being used.

Axillary temperature: This is the most common method of taking the temperature. The thermometer can be placed under the axilla, the forearm is placed over the chest and held in place for 5 minutes. The patient must hold their arm still during this time.

Oral temperature: This method is not often used now. It should not be used in children under the age of five years, anyone who may have a fit, unconscious patients, or those who are having problems in breathing.

The nurse should first check that the patient has not just had a hot or cold drink. She should then place the thermometer under the patient's tongue for 3 minutes, asking the patient to keep their mouth closed during this time. The thermometer is then removed, the reading is taken and recorded on the patient's chart.

Rectal temperature: This method should not be used in very young children as perforation of the rectum has been recorded. Nor should it be used for patients who have any bowel disorder or rectal surgery.

The thermometer is prepared as before and then lubricated with petroleum jelly. Lay the patient on their side, with the upper leg flexed and insert the thermometer gently into the rectum. The thermometer should be held in place for 2 minutes. Withdraw the thermometer, take the recording and clean thoroughly.

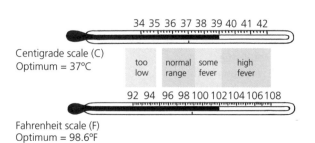

Centigrade scale (C)
Optimum = 37°C

| too low | normal range | some fever | high fever |

Fahrenheit scale (F)
Optimum = 98.6°F

Figure 2.1 *Thermometer reading*

Pp Recording the pulse

The pulse can be taken at a number of points in the body (see Figure 2.2). A pulse point is where an artery lies just below the skin, so it is possible to feel the expansion and recoil of the artery with each left ventricular beat. The easiest and most common place to take the pulse is at the radial site as it does not disturb the patient. In young babies, it is sometimes easier to take the temporal pulse or listen to the apex beat.

When taking a pulse rate, the nurse will need to count the rate, note the volume and also whether the pulse is regular. The patient should be resting quietly, and the nurse then places her fingers in the groove of one of the wrists and feels for the pulse. When she is sure that she is in the correct place, using a watch with a second hand, she counts the pulse for $\frac{1}{2}$ a minute, then doubles this rate for recording. For instance, if the pulse beats 35 times in $\frac{1}{2}$ a minute, the pulse rate is 70. If the pulse is very irregular, it is necessary to take the pulse for a full minute. The nurse should note whether the pulse feels normal, or whether it is weak or thready, and whether it is regular or irregular.

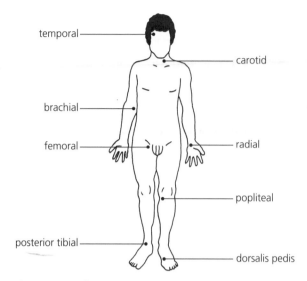

Figure 2.2 *Pulse points*

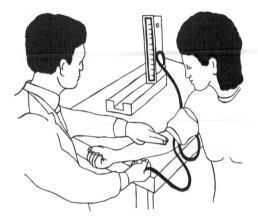

Figure 2.3 *Palpating the brachial artery while taking the blood pressure*

Pp Counting respirations

The nurse counts the rate at which the patient is breathing for 1 minute. The patient should be sitting or lying down, and if possible should not realise that the nurse is counting. Some patients' rate of breathing will be affected by the fact that they know the nurse is watching. It is easy to pretend that you are waiting to remove the thermometer from the patient's axilla, at the same time as you count the respirations. The nurse needs to observe the rate of respirations, the depth, whether the patient is using the accessory muscles of respiration to breathe (see Chapter 10), and whether there is any noise, for instance a wheeze or *stridor*. The rate is then noted on the chart and any abnormality reported to the senior nurse.

Pp Measuring the blood pressure

The blood pressure is a useful measurement in assessing patients and the nurse needs to be skilled at taking the blood pressure. There are electronic devices that will measure blood pressure, but they are not available in many hospitals. The instrument that is commonly used is a sphygmomanometer (see Figure 2.3). The cuff should cover two-thirds of the upper arm, so that when recording blood pressures in children, a variety of different sized cuffs are required to enable an accurate

recording to be made. Obese patients also need a larger cuff to ensure an accurate reading. The patient should be resting quietly, the cuff is placed round the left upper arm, and secured by tucking in the end of the cuff, or if fastened with Velcro, ensuring that it is closed securely. The nurse then places the stethoscope over the brachial artery (see Figure 2.2) and listens to the pulse. The cuff is then pumped up and the nurse records the point on the sphygmomanometer at which the pulse disappears. The nurse then gradually deflates the cuff, watching the level of mercury in the sphygmomanometer. The point at which the pulse reappears is known as *systole* and is a measurement of the force at which the blood is pumped against the arterial walls during the contractions of the left ventricle of the heart. The cuff is deflated still further, until the pulse disappears. This is known as the *diastolic* pressure and measures the force of the blood in the arteries during the resting phase of the ventricle. In a fit adult man, the blood pressure is usually around 120 systolic and 80 diastolic. This will be recorded as 120/80.

Nutritional assessment

Good nutrition is essential for good health. The nurse should always notice whether the patient is well nourished. It is useful to ask the patient about their normal diet and whether they have been eating well recently. Ask them whether they have noticed if they have lost or gained weight recently.

It may be helpful to weigh the patient to see whether the weight is about right for their height.

Observe the amount of body fat and whether this is normal. If a patient has lost weight recently, the skin may be hanging in folds and there may be muscle wasting. Check to see that the skin, hair and teeth are healthy. Obesity can also cause problems for a patient's health and it may be possible to give some advice concerning their diet while they are in hospital.

■ Activities

1. If the ward you are working on uses Task Allocation as a way of organising care, count the number of different patients you have contact with during one working shift. How many times have you had to wash your hands during this shift?

2. Use a nursing model of your choice to plan the nursing care for one patient.

3

Ethical issues

This chapter describes what ethics are and what the word means to nurses and midwives. Some ethical theories will be outlined and applied to clinical situations. The activities are intended to help nurses to think the issues through and apply them to caring for their patients.

What is ethics?

The terms *morals* and *ethics* mean almost the same thing. 'Moral' means the standard of behaviour that groups or individuals believe to be right, whilst 'ethics' refers to the science or study of morals. In nursing and midwifery the words are used in particular ways, for example 'ethics' often means the code of behaviour that guides how nurses should act with patients and their relatives.

Everybody is faced with choices relating to what they should or should not do. There are some issues on which there is no doubt, such as telling the truth. There are other situations in which it is clear what should not be done, for example someone should not inflict pain on another person unnecessarily. Ethics is involved with deciding between right and wrong and how to make decisions relating to what we should or should not do. It is about how to decide which actions are good and which are bad.

Saving life is good but lack of money and staff means that it is not always possible to do this. Choices have to be made about who should be treated and whose life will be saved when there are not enough resources to treat everyone. In many situations there is not one right answer to a problem and a moral choice has to be made. It is essential that health professionals have a plan that they can easily use to make decisions that are morally appropriate.

Moral dilemmas are faced in everyday life as well as in health care. Consider the situation in the activity that follows.

As you walk to market there is a person sitting on the roadside begging for money to feed her children. You have money to buy food in the market and to buy some cooking pots that you have been saving for. You do not need them to survive but you have worked hard to get them and it would make life easier if you had them. You wonder why this person asking you for money is not working to earn the money to feed her children. Would you give her some of your money or would you pass on feeling that it is your right to use your money as you had planned to?

Ethical decision making

There are two basic ethical theories that can be used to help make moral decisions:

Utilitarianism: In this theory the decision should be made according to the good that results from the decision. The outcome of the decision should be the greatest good for the greatest number of people. The more good that results from the decision the more right the decision is.

Deontology: The rightness of the action does not depend solely on its consequences. There are rules and codes that must be followed. Telling the truth is one such situation. It is right to tell the truth even when telling the truth may cause unhappiness or more harm. This theory considers it right always to obey the law of the land even if it does not result in the 'most good'.

■ Activity

It is a very busy day in the health centre; three new patients have arrived:
- an elderly gentleman with bowel obstruction needing surgery immediately
- a 20 year old man who has been shot in the leg and needs to have the bullet removed by surgery as soon as possible

- a 22 year old lady, the mother of two children, who has had an abortion and is bleeding profusely. She needs an evacuation of the uterus as quickly as possible to remove retained products of conception.

It is not possible to treat them all at the same time. How will you decide who to treat first, using the principles of utilitarianism and deontology?

It is difficult to be clear about what to do using only these two theories. There are four principles which can be applied too. These are justice, beneficence, non-maleficence and autonomy. Put simply these mean acting fairly, doing good, doing no harm and a person having the right to decide what happens to them.

Justice: To act justly is to treat people equally and fairly. The status of the person should not influence the amount of good that is done to them. However, people have differing needs so it would seem appropriate to help those with the greatest need. It is also difficult sometimes to decide between a need and a want.

Beneficence: Everyone should receive only that which is good for them. This causes some problems as some treatments are unpleasant and may be seen as anything but good. An example is the administration of chemotherapy for cancer which may cause great suffering to the patient at the beginning, but may bring about a cure or at least a lengthening of life. However, it may lead to an unpleasant death. The important issue here is that the intention was to bring about good.

Non-maleficence: This is the principle of causing no harm. Again this is not straightforward as many treatments cause some harm, for example when children are immunised a very small number may be harmed by the injections. It is important always to cause as little harm as possible.

Autonomy: It is easy to believe that, as professionals, nurses always know what is best for patients. It is important to remember that people have choices and that they must be given enough information on which to base their choices. They have the right to refuse treatment. Autonomy is a person's right to make choices about their own life.

■ Activity

A woman has two children, both of whom are girls. She tells you that tomorrow the two girls are going to her mother's village to have the operation 'that girls have'. You know that this means they are going to have female genital 'cutting'. Given the information in Chapter 28:

- What would you say to her?
- Would you tell anyone that she is going to send the girls for the operation? If so, who would you inform?
- Should she be allowed to make this decision for her own daughters? Consider this in the light of beneficence, non-maleficence, autonomy and justice.

Apply the principles of deontology and utilitarianism to your thinking.

A model for ethical decision making

There are many ways to approach decision making but one simple model can be applied and is easy to remember. M O R A L spells out the word.

- **M**ake a thorough enquiry into all the possible difficulties
- **O**utline the options
- **R**eview the alternatives
- **A**ct
- **L**ook back and evaluate

Information gathering is vital.

- Look at the facts, attitudes, beliefs and external factors that affect the situation.
- Consider the clinical issues, such as the patient's condition, the prognosis, available treatment choices and the outcomes for each treatment option.
- Consider patient preferences. Is there a family member who should be involved in helping the patient come to a decision?
- External factors and the resources available need to be assessed. What is it possible to do and what factors may affect the choices, for example are there enough resources available?
- How competent are the carers?
- Policies of the hospital or care group need to be taken into account.

The questions that need to be asked are:

- What can be done?
- What are all the options available?
- What are the benefits and bad effects of each of the options?

Action should be taken only when all these things have been considered and the four principles of autonomy, beneficence, non-maleficence and justice have been applied. Evaluation of the decision should take place when actions have been taken.

Codes of ethics

The nursing and midwifery professions have codes of ethics on which to base practice. These consist of a number of moral standards set by a group of experienced nurses and midwives. Codes of ethics help nurses to carry out their work in ways which are best for patients. It is important to know the code of ethics which the regulatory body of your country has produced. If there is no code of ethics in place there are international ones that contain basic principles. Your professional association may consider helping to prepare a code for your area.

■ Activity

Read the code of ethics relating to the country and profession in which you are working. What difference does this make to the way you provide care? You could talk about this with your colleagues.

It is essential that you are able to give a reasoned account of your decisions and actions. You need to be able to set out the key facts of the case and the relevant principles you have used in reaching a decision. You will then be able to justify any action you take.

Rights

A basic issue for a nurse is the concept that every person has rights. There is a fundamental principle of respect for a person. This involves:

- Respecting autonomy and dignity
- Promoting well being and autonomy

- Being sincere and honest
- Having a duty to protect the weak, vulnerable and incompetent and to advocate for them. *Advocacy* involves defending people's rights and speaking on their behalf when they are unable to do so adequately. It also includes trying to restore autonomy to those who have lost it due to illness, injury or mental disorder.

Respecting a person involves remembering the patient's right to know, the right to privacy and confidentiality and the right to receive treatment and care. Some people may express a desire not to know; this too should be that person's right. It is often difficult to provide this respect in the care settings where nurses and midwives work. However, it is necessary for health professionals to work towards establishing respect for everyone.

■ Activity

Consider the following situations that you may find yourself in and think of the moral dilemmas that might arise:

- Assisting with birth
- Dealing with neonatal death and abortion
- Advising parents on the care of their child in relation to immunisation
- Helping people cope with mental disorder
- Helping parents who have a child with a serious congenital disorder
- Coping with ageing and chronic dependency
- Care of the dying and bereaved
- Administering a blood transfusion.

Consider what you might do and discuss your thoughts with a colleague. You might find that you have differing opinions about the right thing to do.

4

Research in nursing and midwifery

This chapter considers the place of research in nursing and midwifery practice, introduces some of the processes and language of research and ways of presenting information. Activities are included to help readers to understand how research is carried out.

Why is research important?

Research is about discovering new information and finding out how accurate our old ideas are. Many of the ways in which we provide care are very effective and are accepted as good practice. Others are the result of tradition and because 'we have always done it that way'. Some can be more harmful than we realise. We can find better ways of providing care through carrying out research. It is important that we can justify what we do, and are confident that we are providing care in the best possible way. To achieve this we need to use a systematic approach to answering questions. Then others may examine the work and be convinced that this evidence is reliable enough to be acted on.

There are five reasons why nurses and midwives do not use research findings:
- Lack of knowledge. Nurses and midwives have poor access to information through libraries or the Internet.
- Lack of skills. They do not know how to evaluate and apply the results.
- Disbelief. They remain unconvinced by research that challenges traditional practice.
- Lack of permission. Practitioners may not be allowed to introduce change. Confidence is needed to justify changes to colleagues and managers.

- Lack of incentive. Nurses and midwives are rarely rewarded for introducing change. Praise, promotion or extra money are encouraging but improving patient care can be a reward and good enough reason in itself.

Evaluating research

Not all of us have the opportunity to carry out our own research. Some do take part, however, in research that colleagues are doing, for example by collecting *data* for them. It is also important that we are able to read and understand research that other people have carried out. We need to be able to decide whether research is reliable enough to make us change what we do. Evaluating published research is an important skill to develop. As we read we must decide whether the conclusions are reasonable to make on the evidence presented. There are some key questions that need to be asked to help with this:
- What was the study about?
- Why was the study carried out?
- How was it done? Was the research designed in a way that seems appropriate to the research question? For example, if you wanted to know whether a new type of dressing helped burns to heal better than one that is being used at the present time then you would need to test the dressings on a large number of patients who were being treated for burns. It would not be helpful to try one on burns patients and the other on surgical wounds.
- Does the researcher convince you that the findings are reasonable and relevant?

The research process

Most research follows a general pathway:
1. Seeing a problem or being curious about something – formulating the question

2. Finding out what is already known – reviewing the literature
3. Planning ways to discover new information – choosing the method
4. Collecting the information
5. Analysing the results, deciding what they mean and what the implications are, and presenting them
6. Sharing the information with others and changing practice.

These points are expanded in the sections that follow.

Figure 4.1 shows a summary of this research process.

1. Formulating the question

Research starts with a question in someone's mind. Maybe the researcher has noticed something whilst working with patients but is not sure if she is right. An example of the kind of question that may form the basis of the research is 'should the umbilical cord be treated at birth or left alone?' This has been the subject of much research in different parts of the world. You may have questions in your mind about your own practice that could become the subject of a small research project. It is important that the subject is not too big or too complex. Questions need to be broken down into parts which are reasonable to study. It might be necessary to do more than one piece of research.

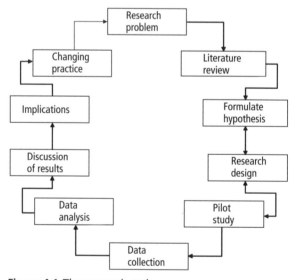

Figure 4.1 *The research cycle*

The question is often turned into a statement to be tested. This statement is called the **hypothesis** which can be proved or disproved, for example 'The umbilical cord should be kept clean and dry in the neonate for the best healing'. Some types of research focus on finding the answer to a simple question or describe a situation, for example 'What types of cord treatment do local traditional birth attendants use?'

It is always helpful to discuss the question with colleagues and note down issues and ideas they raise. This helps you to focus and put aside aspects of the problem which are less important. It is also wise to seek help early on from an experienced researcher. Some of the questions which are useful to ask yourself are:

- Is it really a problem? Do others see it as a problem or is it only me?
- How important is the issue? Will it make a difference? It is only going to be of use if it will be of benefit to people, if it will increase knowledge, or if practice will get better as a result.
- Is the problem researchable? Are there ethical problems that might arise? For example, nobody must be given substandard care in order to carry out the research.
- How possible is it to do it? Is there time? Is it possible to finance the project? Is it worth the cost involved both in terms of manpower and money? Do people have the skills and knowledge they need?
- Will people participate and help? Is there enough enthusiasm to keep going when progress is slow and difficulties arise? Do you care enough?

2. Reviewing the literature

Research is time-consuming and can be expensive so it is important that the work and even the mistakes of others are not repeated. Reading the literature helps in specifying the hypothesis more precisely. Looking at how others have tackled similar topics will help with choosing the **method** of research to use. It is also possible to use these same methods that others have tried. You might want to discover what questions were asked in interviews and how well they worked, or what difficulties were encountered. To undertake a literature search the research question needs to be precisely stated, then the key words in the question identified. Bibliographies, abstracts, indexes and encyclopaedias may be searched. The Internet is a very important source of information if you have access to it. Librarians are usually very willing to assist you in finding the information you need. Two useful resources are the TALC CD-ROMs and the Cochrane Library of Evidence-Based Medicine (see resource list on page 397).

3. Choosing the method

There are different methods of research, which are appropriate for different types of problems. The two main types are known as *quantitative* and *qualitative research*. Quantitative research measures and counts. It is useful for proving and disproving ideas and telling us how important a result is. Using the example of burn dressings, you need quantitative methods to discover how quickly burns heal with different types of dressing. If you wanted to know what it is like to undergo treatment for a burn you might use qualitative methods. These are about feelings, emotions and experiences instead of numbers.

Quantitative methods

Quantitative methods might be *experimental*, *observation* or *survey* (see below). They all produce numerical results or statistics.

Whichever type of research is chosen, the researcher has to identify the *population* from which the *sample* will be taken. The population is the large group which may be available (such as all people admitted to hospital). The population is usually too large for all to take part in the research so a sample is selected, such as every tenth person admitted.

Experimental methods: In an experiment a change is made and the outcome measured. There are different kinds of experimental design but a simple one would be when a set of measurements are made before a change, and then a new set of measurements are made afterwards. Here is an example:

> You want to know how much respiratory rate increases with specific amounts of exercise. The respiratory rate of a number of people is measured after they have sat in a chair for five minutes. You ask them to climb ten steps and come down again, and then measure the respiratory rate a second time. You could work out the effect that this amount of exercise has had from the difference between the two respiratory rates for each person.

You might have people of different ages or fitness levels in the group, or some who are heavy smokers or have respiratory problems or heart disease. Such differences are known as *variables*. It is often important that the groups are as similar as possible in every way except for the thing you are testing. This is known as controlling the variables. Examples of other variables are sex, weight, income group, education level, whether they live in towns or villages and whether they have a particular condition such as heart disease.

A common way of doing research is to use more than one group. In one group the change is made (known as the *experimental* or *intervention group*). In the other the usual care is given (known as the *control* group). But it would be very easy to give a false impression by selecting people with particular characteristics to each group. This can happen accidentally. For example, if you select people using a telephone directory, you will select people wealthy enough to afford a phone. Introducing *bias* in this way makes research unreliable and untrustworthy.

Randomised controlled trials: Probably the experimental method that best avoids these problems is the *randomised controlled trial* (RCT). In an RCT people are given an equal chance of being allocated to either the intervention group or the control group. *Random allocation* also makes sure there are no differences between the groups. An example of this randomisation is the research carried out by Jenny Sleep and her colleagues in 1984 on the use of episiotomy during birth. They were looking for the effect on the newborn, on perineal tears and on urinary symptoms and pain levels of women. The two groups were:

- those who should have an episiotomy to prevent perineal tears
- those who should have it only if the foetus was distressed.

A sample of 1000 women was allocated randomly to the two groups. To do this, their midwives were instructed to open a sealed envelope during the second stage of labour. Neither she nor the woman herself had any influence on the choice. Taking these precautions means that the findings are relevant to a far wider population than just the sample involved. The RCT is now thought to be the best type of research for comparing alternative forms of care, provided it is carried out properly.

Research can be made even more trustworthy by ensuring that the subjects of the research do not know to which group they have been allocated. It is even better if the person giving the treatment does not know either. This is called a *blind* trial but is not always possible to do. For example, the midwives and women in the episiotomy trial obviously knew what had happened to them. Those assessing the after effects did not need to know so this made their judgements more believable.

Quantitative observation methods: You may want to find out what happens in a setting like a hospital ward during a typical day. This can be achieved by simple observation. At first people may change what they do because an observer is present, but they soon get used to it. An example of this type of research would be to investigate how often, and how well, nurses or doctors wash their hands. Perhaps the researcher will count the number of times staff members wash before touching patients. Perhaps she will watch for the way in which they do it. These are quantitative methods because they involve counting and produce statistical results just as RCTs do.

Survey methods: *Surveys* are good methods for collecting information very quickly from large numbers of people. *Questionnaires* will be used to make sure that the same questions are put to everyone. Some questionnaires are designed to be completed by people without any help. These have the disadvantage that people may be unable to read well, or may misunderstand the questions. Other questionnaires are designed to be completed with the help of an interviewer. These avoid the problems that have just been described but interviewers can influence the answers. Also some people may not wish to answer questions on sensitive topics face-to-face. The questions that are asked will be designed to obtain particular answers so everyone will be asked exactly the same. These are called *structured* questionnaires or interviews.

Although quick to do, surveys like this can be superficial. There are other ways of carrying out research that examine what is happening in more depth. These are called qualitative or *interpretative* methods.

Qualitative (interpretative) methods

The main ways in which researchers can probe into people's ideas, experiences and feelings more deeply are through observation and *unstructured interviews*. These methods are very time-consuming and the

results may be very specific to the area studied. However, the richness of the information gathered can make it very worthwhile. Also the information obtained can help us to be more aware of the issues that matter to people even if we practise in a different situation. This is called sensitisation.

Qualitative observation: There are different ways of carrying out qualitative observation. These are *participant* and *non-participant observation*. In the first the researcher observes while taking part in what is happening, such as working in a clinic. In the second she stands back and takes no part in activities.

Interviewing: There are also different ways of interviewing. Often the researcher will have a list of questions but encourages the person to talk about the topic. This is *semi-structured interviewing*. Alternatively there may just be a checklist of topics to cover. The final type of interview is very informal and *unstructured*. The researcher starts by explaining what she is interested in and leaves the person to talk without doing any more than encourage.

These types of research are much more personal than quantitative methods. It is important that the researcher understands how she may be influencing what happens or is said, and takes this into account. This research produces words and examples from which we can find out what matters to people. It does not produce statistics.

4. Collecting the information

The information will be collected in whatever way is appropriate for the planned research (see previous section on choosing the method). It is important to decide exactly what is needed to carry it out, for example a questionnaire or a counting sheet may have to be designed. The researcher may need to train people to help with collecting the information. She will need to think through any ethical issues and wait for permission to continue from the Research Ethics Committee (see the final section). Obtaining permission to proceed from managers is also important. The most important people who need to give permission are the subjects of the research. Normally they will need to sign consent forms after having the research explained.

Once the plans are ready they are tried out using a *pilot study*. This is a small preparatory study that tests data collection methods. It is a good opportunity to test things such as questionnaires or interview schedules to see whether they achieve what is intended. Trying them out often shows up questions that are difficult to understand or do not produce the type of answers needed. This avoids wasting the time and effort of the researcher and those taking part. Questionnaires that are difficult to understand usually end up in the waste bin.

5. Analysing and presenting the results

Analysis is a stage that needs to be carried out methodically and is very time-consuming. The way in which information is analysed and presented depends on the type of data collected. It is a very complex subject so many researchers need to seek help and advice on it.

Analysing quantitative data

Analysing quantitative data can be a simple thing to do or can be much more complicated. This depends on what the researcher is trying to achieve. If she wants to describe a situation, it can be simple. If, however, she wants to find out how much better one form of treatment is than other, data analysis can be much more complicated. Here are two examples where more complicated analysis is needed:

- The researcher has tested two types of burn dressing. One appears to help wounds to heal faster than the other but is more expensive. Is the difference great enough to be worth the extra cost? This is called significance. Statistical tests are needed to make this analysis.

- It is now known that the more expensive dressing is definitely more effective and is worth the extra cost because people can leave hospital faster. However, the researcher has noted that the patients were of very different ages and some were diabetics. Does this make a difference? To analyse this, other tests are needed that look at the differences or variables. Experienced advice is essential for doing these tests.

Simpler methods could be used in these three examples of descriptive research:

- The researcher has counted the number of women and men who are admitted to the hospital after car accidents because she wishes to find out if there is a difference.

- Information is collected on the ages of all the women who have come this year for antenatal care in their first pregnancy because there appear to be many pregnant adolescents in the area.

- The blood pressures (BPs) of the first 25 women to attend antenatal clinic over one day have been measured and recorded. One woman felt unwell so you admitted her and recorded her BP over six hours (see later Activity).

This simple process can be used for each of these:

- Organise the collected data into a *table*.
- Make a graph or chart to represent the data.
- Work out useful *values* from the results: the *mean*, the *mode*, the *median* and the *range*.

These terms stand for the average (*mean*), the commonest (*mode*), the mid-way point (*median*) and the top and bottom results (*range*). To find out about pregnant adolescents, the mode is probably the most useful. You may just need actual numbers of men and women for the accident victims. The range or mean might be useful for the pregnant women's blood pressure readings. Each could be illustrated by a chart.

■ Activity

This activity is about the BP readings of the group of pregnant women. Trying it will make these ideas clearer. More detail is given in the next section headed 'Presenting data' to help you.

1. Write down the blood pressure recordings of the first 25 women attending the antenatal clinic on one day.
2. Count how many are of the same age and put them in groups.
3. Work out what the mean is. (Add together the value of all observations, and divide them by the number of observations you made).
4. Decide what the mode is (the value that occurs most often).
5. Draw a graph to show all the readings for the woman who felt unwell so you can see the variations. (This will look like a normal blood pressure chart.)
6. Look at the examples in the next section to see other ways of displaying the data.

Presenting quantitative data

How data is communicated is important. Confusing data is quickly ignored. Quantitative data are numbers and the simplest way of presenting them is as a list, but the results do not mean much this way. A table (see Table 4.1) provides more information.

Note: These examples use the blood pressure collected from the 25 women in the antenatal clinic. There were six different BP levels noted and each occurred several times as can be seen in Table 4.1. Only the systolic readings are used here.

Table 4.1 Systolic BP readings from 25 women

Blood pressure group	Numbers of women
BP 105	3
BP 110	4
BP 115	2
BP 120	5
BP 125	6
BP 130	5

It is fairly easy to see here that the systolic reading 125 was the most common. It is difficult, though, to build up a clear understanding of results from tables, so graphs and charts are often used (see Figures 4.2, 4.3 and 4.4).

Figure 4.2 is a *histogram*. (The chart could be produced horizontally and that would be called a *bar chart*.) This shows the same information in a different format. It is much easier to pick out the most and least common BP readings.

Figure 4.3 is a pie chart showing the same information. It is a very clear way of presenting information especially when colour is used. It is particularly good for showing up the largest and smallest groups or values.

Blood pressure averages

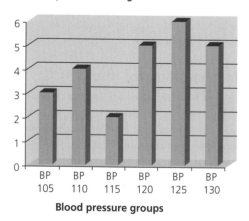

- Numbers of women

Figure 4.2 *Histogram to show average blood pressure among 25 women*

Blood pressure averages

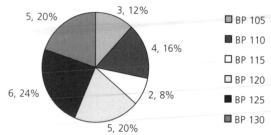

Figure 4.3 *Pie chart showing average blood pressure among 25 women*

Note: Here the first figure shows the groups 1–6 which each consist of women who share a particular BP measurement. The second figure is the percentage of women that it represents.

Lastly, one woman had her BP taken every hour for six hours. The systolic readings are shown below as a table (Table 4.2), then as a line graph. The line graph shows clearly how her BP changed over time. This graph will be familiar to you as it is the same type as seen on patient observation charts. This type of graph could show more than one series of readings in separate lines.

Table 4.2 Blood pressure (systolic) for one woman over six hours

Blood pressure	Hours elapsed
110	1
115	2
105	3
120	4
125	5
120	6

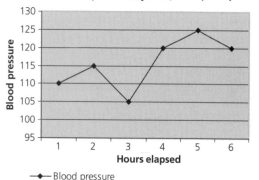

- Blood pressure

Figure 4.4 *Line graph to show a woman's rise in blood pressure over six hours*

Analysing qualitative data

Qualitative research uses different ways of analysing data compared with the statistical methods used for numerical data. However, the analysis needs to be carried out just as rigorously. The data will consist of people's words, or the researcher's words written in observation notes. Many qualitative researchers also keep a journal or notes called 'field notes'. Here they write down anything that might become important. They may note everything that happens as it is difficult to predict what might later prove to be important. Other types of records that may need to be examined are items such as minutes of meetings or reports produced by a hospital but we will concentrate here on observation and interviews.

Qualitative interviews and observations: No matter what kind of interview has been carried out, preparation work is important for analysis. Firstly notes have to be sorted and written up, audiotapes of interviews transcribed into a written form (known as transcripts), questionnaires perhaps divided into topics. Copies of notes, interviews and tape recordings are made and the originals stored safely to safeguard the data from loss. Extra copies are useful to allow for sorting methods like cutting up the data and moving it around.

All the data has to be read and important ideas identified. A common way of doing this is to look for similar responses and put codes against them. Using this method, researchers can quickly start to identify common responses and make them into categories. Returning to the example of someone who has received burns, common responses might be about fear of pain, anxiety about the cost of care, concern about being able to work in the future, or about disfigurement from scarring.

If there is a lot of data to be analysed it may be possible to use one of the special computer software packages that have been produced. These do some of the tedious and time-consuming work very quickly.

Here are some ideas researchers use to help with sorting and identifying common themes and categories:

- Does anything stand out?
- Do some phrases, actions or attitudes show up several times?
- Can they be grouped and classified?
- Do some of the responses or events seem to express certain feelings or attitudes, for example fear, guilt, frustration, impatience?

Categories are marked on the portions of the transcript. All sections that refer to one category are highlighted, for example frustration. It helps to use colour coding. The transcript can be scrutinised for categories and sub-categories. The original always remains unmarked. Parts of a transcript which refer to a particular concept can be cut out. They are then stuck on to blank sheets and filed in envelopes or sorted into piles. This can be done on a computer. It is always important to record the source of comments on each portion. Usually researchers find that some sections can be classified in more than one way so having spare transcripts can be useful. The purpose of all this is to get at the meaning of the situation, to see what concepts are behind the given answers. If there are statements and ideas that contradict each other researchers need to work out why this is happening. Ideas and cases which are different from others are not disregarded as these may give a better understanding of the situation.

As categories are sorted, particular themes usually become obvious. The researcher can then start to build a broader picture of the chosen topic. The information can now be looked at in relation to the original research question and the researcher can start to consider how to explain what has been found. The literature search often helps to find similarities and differences from other work.

Presenting qualitative data

Qualitative data is usually presented as words describing what the researcher found. She will give examples of the data in the form of anonymous quotations and details of events that have been observed. In this way she can build up a word picture for readers.

6. Communicating the results

Only by writing up and publishing studies which nurses and midwives undertake can we build up a body of professional knowledge. It is important that work is opened up to comment and criticism. The first step is to write the research report. This is often required by employers or the organisation that has contributed funds. Researchers then have to consider submitting articles for publication in journals.

Reports include:

- An *abstract* that outlines the research in a few words
- Why the study was undertaken

- Differences between this and other similar studies
- How the study was carried out, including why particular methods were used
- The results
- A discussion of the results and their implications
- Recommended next steps such as changes in practice and further research
- List of references to other publications used, often called a *bibliography*.

Ethical issues in research

Research is a very important part of improving care but people must never be harmed. People who agree to take part in research have rights, which can be summed up as follows:
- Not to be harmed
- Self-determination. Individuals need to give consent without pressure or coercion. They need enough information to know what is involved and to make a free choice but without undermining the research process.
- Privacy
- Confidentiality and anonymity. Others should not know what has happened with individuals and they should not be named without permission.

- Dignity. Participants should never be made to look foolish or be embarrassed.
- To be able to refuse to participate at any stage of the research without being pressurised
- Their care should not be dependent on agreeing to take part in the research.

There are some vulnerable people who must be given special consideration. These include the following:
- Children
- The elderly especially if they are confused
- Those with learning difficulties
- Mentally ill people
- Those who are dying
- Unconscious persons
- Sedated persons
- Captive persons
- Those who feel very dependent such as the very poor.

Research plans always need to be checked for ways in which they may intrude on people's rights. If health care patients are involved then this should be done by people who understand the issues and have some knowledge of research. They should meet to discuss the implications and ensure that the researchers are acting in an ethical manner. Such a group is called a Research Ethics Committee. It usually has the power to prevent research from being carried out or to ask for changes to be made.

Research definitions

Abstract: A summary of a piece of research

Bar chart: A way of displaying *data* in which horizontal bars on a chart show values

Bias: A situation where something causes results to be untrustworthy

Bibliography: List of published material which the researcher used; may also mean a list of publications on a particular topic

Blind: Not knowing what *interventions* are being used for a particular *subject*

Control group: People in an experiment who do not have any deliberate changes (known as interventions) made to what happens to them

Data: The facts and information collected during a project

Experimental group: People in an experiment who have deliberate changes (interventions) made to what happens to them

Experimental research: Research that tests a *hypothesis* by means of making changes in a deliberate way

Histogram: A way of displaying data in which vertical columns on a chart show values

Hypothesis: A statement predicting a situation that will be found or what will happen if a particular action is taken

Interpretative research: Research that tries to understand the question from the viewpoint of those taking part in the study, also called *qualitative* research

Intervention: An action taken to test what happens in an experiment

Mean: The average of a set of numbers, calculated by adding them all together and dividing by the number of items or people

Median: The middle value in a *range* of numbers

Method: The way evidence is collected; often called methodology

Mode: The value that occurs most often in a set of numbers

Non-participant observation: A data collection method in which the researcher takes no active part in the situation being observed

Participant observation: A data collection method in which the researcher is actively engaged in the situation being observed

Pilot study: A small preparatory study conducted to test the research methods

Population: The whole group of people from among whom the *sample* is selected to take part in the research

Qualitative research: Research that tries to identify feelings, experiences, ideas and common themes. The data are in the form of words

Quantitative research: Research in which the data collected is in the form of numbers

Questionnaire: A written list of questions that is put to *respondents* aimed at discovering facts, attitudes, opinions or experiences

Random allocation: Selecting research subjects in such a way that each one has an equal chance of being chosen

Randomised controlled trial: Research in which *random allocation* is used for selection to either *control* or *experimental* groups

Range: The lowest and highest results in a set of numbers

Reliability: Research findings that would be the same if tried in another setting using the same methods

Respondents: People taking part in research, also called subjects and informants (in qualitative research)

Sample: The group of people or items chosen from which data will be collected

Semi-structured interview: An interview in which questions or topics are provided but the interviewer uses them flexibly

Structured interview: An interview with a set pattern of questions that cannot be changed

Subject: Someone who takes part in research; a topic or theme

Survey: A way of researching that tries to describe and analyse the present situation using questionnaires or interviews with a *sample* of the *population*

Table: Representation of data in orderly columns for easier reference

Unstructured interview: Topics are put in such a way as to allow free expression

Value: A particular amount or number

Variable: A difference between one group or person and another, for example smokers or age

Part 2

Patient care

5

Introduction to illness, disability and care

This chapter covers the basic concepts of illness and disability. It considers differences between caring for patients with acute illness, chronic illness and those with disabilities.

Introduction

It has been said that an acute illness is like a visitor who comes unexpectedly and stays only a short while. Chronic illness is like a visitor who stays a long time and becomes part of the household. Disability can be caused by problems before or after birth, or can result from an acute or chronic illness.

Factors affecting illness and disability

Age: Very old and very young people are likely to get sicker more quickly and will need faster treatment. Some illnesses affect all age groups. Some are more likely to affect specific age groups. Children may die of an illness before they become adults, for instance in congenital heart disease or leukaemia. Other diseases may start in childhood and continue into adulthood, for example diabetes and asthma. As people get older, *degenerative* processes may start to affect them as in arthritis and *hypertension*. As a population's life expectancy increases, diseases such as cancer become more common.

Gender: In many cultures, men are supposed to demonstrate their manhood by not complaining of pain. This may mean that they do not come to the clinic until late in the illness. Women have been found to be more interested in preventing illness and men may rely on their wives for information on health matters. Education of women has been found to have a very large effect in reducing child mortality and

Definition of terms

The terms disease, illness and sickness are often used as if they mean the same thing but they can mean different things to different people.

Disease is the term used by doctors to suggest a diagnosis or condition.

Illness is the way people experience disease, including the way in which they feel about the disease and the effect it has on their lives.

Sickness is the word used by other people to explain that people are ill. Sick people may be expected to behave in a certain way. They may be expected to do things that will make them healthy again or to stop spreading the disease to other people. In some cultures, such as Botswana, those people whose husbands/wives or children have died are thought to be sick. They have to follow rituals in order to get better themselves and to contain the effects of the death to prevent other people being harmed.

Disability is a restriction or lack of ability to perform an activity in the normal manner.

Impairment is loss or abnormality of psychological, physiological or anatomical structure or function.

improving the health of all the family. However, when resources are scarce, women may be the last to get treatment. Men may come first, then the children and lastly the women.

Education: People who have been educated may have more information about disease so come for help more quickly. They can understand what doctors and nurses are telling them and can follow advice to minimise the effects of the illness. Those who are not educated may not realise when symptoms are serious or that they can be helped.

Socio-economic status: The amount of money

people have can change the way they live their lives. People with money can afford good housing and food. They can make choices which can protect them from some illnesses. People who have little money do not have much choice. They may be forced to live in poor housing, with a dirty water supply and food may be in short supply. Buying medicines may be difficult and they may decide that they cannot afford to go to the clinic. Getting help may be delayed until the illness is more serious. Transport may be very difficult and they may have to walk to get help which may make their condition worse.

Ethnicity, race and cultural background: Cultural background and ethnicity of an individual influences the way in which health is valued. Studies show that Africans take illness as part of life and may not come for help early. Westerners and Asians are more likely to come for help as soon as they realise they are ill.

Family functioning: This has a great effect on how a person is affected by illness or disability. Where there are close family relationships, the family plays a major role in supporting the sick person. They may provide direct care and also help to pay for expenses and support the person emotionally.

Occupation: Some occupations may increase the risk of illness or disability occurring. For instance people who work in dusty conditions have an increased risk of respiratory illness and chronic lung disease. Occupations that involve dangerous machinery increase the risk of injuries occurring and may lead to permanent or long-term disability. If the work place is not supportive, a person with diabetes may not be able to eat at the right time or may exercise too much without taking the extra glucose that they need, leading to a risk of a *hypoglycaemic* attack.

Lifestyles: Some social habits can make the onset of illness more likely or make the condition worse. Tobacco smoking can cause lung cancer and also make chest problems worse. Children who live in families who smoke are more likely to get respiratory problems. Alcohol can cause liver disease and make the symptoms of diabetes worse.

Life satisfaction: This is how people see their lives and how they feel about themselves, whether they feel they are worthwhile people with good relationships with other people. If their illness or disability limits what they can do, they may have a negative view of themselves, with a low self-esteem. Depression is then more likely and they may not get help for their illness.

Acute illness
Phases of illness

Early signs and symptoms: There may be complaints of discomfort or pain, fever, bleeding, swelling or cough. These may be treated with remedies bought at the market or in the drug store. Symptoms may disappear and no further action be taken or they may get more serious.

Assumption of the sick role: People may realise they are sick and ask a friend about the symptoms. They may stay away from work or school. If there is no improvement they may then seek help.

Seeking medical help: A variety of people may be consulted. They may go to a clinic, a doctor or a traditional healer. If they do not agree with the diagnosis or do not get better, different people may be consulted. They may be given different treatments by different people and may buy a variety of medicines to treat themselves.

Assumption of a dependent role: Sick people may become dependent on members of the family to help care for them either in the health clinic or at home.

Recovery or rehabilitation: This is the last phase of the acute illness. People are helped to resume normal functioning. How long this takes depends on the severity of the illness and the motivation to get better. Some people may not recover and the illness may lead to chronic illness, disability or death.

The impact of acute illness on the client and the family: Behavioural and emotional changes affect both the people who are ill and their families. The individual's role in the family may be threatened and there may be anxiety and fear of the unknown. There may be a financial loss due to loss of wages or costs of treatment.

Causes of acute illness

There are many causes of acute illness, the following identify a few:
* Trauma from an accident or violence
* Acute infections by bacteria, viruses or fungi
* Hypersensitive response as in asthma, or reaction to a substance
* Acute surgical emergencies as in strangulated hernia or perforated ulcer
* *Ischaemic* damage such as in myocardial infarction, or damage from a blood clot as in a cerebrovascular accident.

Shock in acute illness

Shock is life-threatening and can develop as a result of different problems but all will give similar symptoms. Not enough oxygen is available to meet all the demands of the body. The pulse rate rises and becomes weak, the blood pressure falls, the skin becomes cool and damp and the patient may become cyanosed.

Hypovolaemic shock: This happens when there is not enough fluid in the *intravascular* system. Common causes are haemorrhage and dehydration. Sometimes the fluid loss can be seen for example in burns and scalds, diarrhoea, obvious external haemorrhage or the vomiting of blood. Sometimes the fluid loss cannot be seen, as in a ruptured spleen, fracture of a long bone or internal haemorrhage. Pain and swelling may be the only symptoms.

Cardiogenic shock: This happens as a result of a problem with the heart, or pump failure. The heart is not able to pump the blood round the body sufficiently well to meet all the demands.

Septic shock: When there is an overwhelming bacterial infection, the toxins produced by the bacteria can cause an increased *permeability* of the capillary walls of the blood vessels. This means that plasma leaks out of the circulation into the surrounding tissues and the patient becomes hypovolaemic.

Anaphylactic shock: When the body is introduced to an *antigen* for the first time, an *antibody* is produced. Meeting the same antigen again can result in the antibody releasing large amounts of *histamine*. This can lead to narrowing (constriction) of the bronchi and increased permeability of the walls of the capillaries. There can be sudden problems with the patient having difficulty in breathing, the leakage of plasma leads to oedema and hypovolaemia. Common causes of anaphylactic shock are bee stings, some drugs, especially antibiotics such as penicillin, and some foods such as peanuts. The patient needs to be given an injection of adrenaline quickly to reduce the amount of histamine being produced. People who develop severe allergic reactions should avoid coming into contact with the substance wherever possible and seek emergency medical help.

Management of shock

Nurses must always stay with patients as they may become unconscious, collapse quickly and die.
- Make sure the patient has a good airway. Give oxygen if necessary.
- Raise the feet of the patient above the head as this allows more blood to flow to the brain.

- Control any bleeding.
- Replace fluid intravenously as soon as possible, using blood, plasma or plasma expanders such as Haemocell or Dextran 40. If none of these are available, give a solution of sodium chloride with glucose.
- Monitor the pulse rate and blood pressure every 15 minutes.
- Get medical assistance and treat the cause of the shock.
- Give pain relief, as pain increases shock.

Role of the nurse

The nurse is usually the first person to meet the patient in the clinic or hospital. Nurses have an important role in deciding which patients need urgent treatment to avoid a life-threatening episode, and which patients can wait a little longer. Some departments will have a system in place known as *triage*. This means that patients will be quickly assessed and those who are most seriously ill will be seen first.

Nurses working in isolated or small clinics will have to make decisions about transferring patients with serious illness to a larger hospital (see Chapter 2). You need to:
- Take a comprehensive history of the present illness and other problems
- Make a thorough assessment which includes:
  - Respiratory status: respiratory rate, *dyspnoea*, cough, cyanosis
  - Cardiovascular status: blood pressure, pulse rate, any signs of shock, history or signs of bleeding
  - Temperature: high or low
  - Skin condition; rashes or bruising
  - Gastro-intestinal: history of constipation or diarrhoea, abdominal distension, nausea or vomiting
  - Renal: frequency or *dysuria*; hydration, whether dehydrated or signs of oedema
  - Neurological: fits, paralysis, severe headaches, visual disturbances
  - Emotional state: anxiety or distress
  - Pain: location, severity and type.

Once a full assessment has been made, you may refer the patient to a doctor if there is one available. You may need to decide which laboratory investigations are necessary and organise them.

Diagnosis

The diagnosis must be made as quickly as possible, from the history, assessment and results of investigations. Nursing diagnosis is different from a medical diagnosis, though often nurses have to make both.

Medical diagnosis

This decides what illness the patient is suffering from and what treatment is necessary. For instance:

- Patient A may be diagnosed with malaria and need anti malarials.
- Patient B may have meningitis and need a lumbar puncture to confirm the diagnosis and then the correct antibiotics.

Nursing diagnosis

This is more concerned with how the illness is affecting the patient and what can be done for the symptoms.

- Patient A is feverish and needs to be kept cool. He also needs plenty of fluids to keep him well hydrated. He needs bed rest until he is feeling better. Anti malarial drugs must be given at the correct time.
- Patient B is complaining of a severe headache and *photophobia*. She needs to be nursed away from bright lights and noise kept to a minimum. She may need to have an intravenous line inserted to give the antibiotics ordered and to keep her hydrated, though she must not be over hydrated. She will need pain relief for her headache and regular assessment of her vital signs.

Care of the patient with a life-threatening condition

Where possible the patients should be cared for in a hospital with facilities for carrying out investigations and with adequate medical staff to ensure the best possible treatment. They may be nursed in an intensive care unit or high dependency area of a ward. These areas should have a higher number of nurses available so that patients can be carefully monitored at all times.

Pain/discomfort

Assess the patient's pain and give relief (see Chapter 7).

Respiratory status

Assess the respiratory status (see Chapter 10 and 47). Record and report any deterioration.

- Sit the patient up to help expand the lungs if there is difficulty in breathing.
- Keep well hydrated so that sputum can be coughed up.
- Give oxygen if necessary. This must be humidified.
- Turn the patient 2 hourly to help expand all areas of the lungs.
- Give medication as ordered, such as antibiotics, expectorants.
- In severe cases the patient may need assisted ventilation or a tracheostomy.
- Suction may be required.

Cardiovascular status

Assess the cardiovascular status (see Chapter 11). Record and report any deterioration.

- Encourage rest.
- Monitor oedema or breathlessness which could be due to cardiac failure.
- Report chest pain which could be due to angina, myocardial infarction, pulmonary embolism or pneumonia.
- Watch for confusion which can be a sign of *hypoxia*.
- In some centres, the patient may be attached to cardiac monitors to show abnormal heart rhythms.
- Make sure resuscitation equipment is nearby and is in working order. It may be needed if the patient has a cardiopulmonary arrest.

Fluid balance

- Keep a record of all fluid intake, both intravenous and oral.
- Make sure that intravenous fluids are given at the correct rate.
- If oral fluids are allowed, help the patient to drink. They may need to be supported.
- Record all fluid output: urinary output, gastric aspiration or vomiting, diarrhoea.
- Monitor the hydration level of the patient and report dehydration or oedema.

Temperature control

- If the temperature is raised (*hyperthermic*), keep cool. Nurse near open windows or fans. Tepid sponging may help reduce the temperature. Ensure patients are well hydrated.
- If the patient is cold (*hypothermic*), keep away from draughts, and cover with warm blankets.

Level of consciousness and neurological status

(see Chapter 14)

- Monitor and report any alteration in level of consciousness, and fits.
- Note signs of paralysis or difficulty in moving.

Skin care

Patients who are seriously ill are unable to care for their own hygiene. They are also at risk from developing pressure sores. Pressure sores are more likely to occur when patients cannot move around so that the circulation can be restored to the pressure points.

- Ensure good skin hygiene (see Chapter 17).
- Alter the patient's position every 2 hours, so that all pressure points are protected from damage.

Mouth care

If patients are unable to take oral fluids, they may need to have their mouths cleaned or be helped to clean their teeth.

Anxiety

Seriously ill patients and their relatives are likely to be very frightened and worried that they are going to die. The nurse must be honest and tell the truth about what is happening. Patients who are kept well informed are likely to be less frightened than those who are not told what is happening to them.

Fatigue

It is important to see that patients get enough sleep. They may be disturbed frequently by nurses and doctors who are monitoring their condition and giving care. The nurse should plan the care so that patients are left undisturbed for periods. They may need sedatives to help them sleep.

Recovery and rehabilitation

As the condition improves, patients can be moved to a different part of the ward and encouraged to start looking after themselves. A good diet is necessary after an acute illness, to replace nutrients that have been lost. Help may be needed to start mobilising again and plans should be made for future care. Some patients will be completely cured, others may be left with lasting problems. For instance, a patient who has had cerebral malaria may be left with some paralysis. Relatives will need help to adjust to the new situation before discharge. Information must be given about any drugs that are needed to take home and appointments made for return visits to the clinic or hospital.

Chronic illness

People who develop chronic illnesses have to learn to live with them. Some people live almost normal lives; others have to make alterations in the way they live. They may be disabled by their illness or the illness may be a continuing threat to their lives.

Some chronic illnesses, such as diabetes and cancer tend to run in families. If this is known, it may be possible for the person to make changes that will reduce the chances of them developing the disease.

Some illnesses have acute *exacerbations*. People with asthma may be able to live a normal life most of the time, but when they suffer an asthmatic attack, they become acutely ill and need immediate treatment.

The nursing role in chronic illness

The nurse will need to make an assessment of the patient and decide what help can be given to overcome problems that they may be facing.

Pain

This may be a particular problem. Chronic pain can interfere with all aspects of a person's life (see Chapter 7).

Mobility

Many people with chronic illness have problems with mobility. They may have stiff joints and find walking difficult. They may get breathless when they are active. If people limit their activities because they have difficulty, their mobility gets worse and muscles get weak when not used. Nurses need to assess mobility and think of ways people may be helped.

Fatigue/tiredness

Many people complain that they are tired and have no energy. Chronic pain is tiring so it is important to control the pain. Sleeping may be difficult. They may get very breathless when lying down or stiff from lying in one position. The nurse needs to find out what is causing the problem and try to find a solution. They may need to have frequent rests. They can be advised to do more strenuous tasks when they have more energy and less energetic tasks when they are tired. The nurse can also check the diet as they may be anaemic or lacking in vitamins or minerals. A healthy diet can improve the well being of the person.

Patient and family education

This is the most important part of helping the patient with a chronic illness. Education needs to cover the illness itself, the way it may progress, the symptoms and how the symptoms can be treated and further problems prevented.

Patients who know about their illnesses feel more in control of their lives. When a chronic illness is first diagnosed, the nurse needs to make out a teaching plan to cover all the information that will be needed. Teaching needs to begin at once so that the patient and the family start being partners in the management of the illness right away. Education should cover both negative and positive sides of the illness. Patients may be told that they should stop doing some things. The nurse needs to think of things they can still do and try to give a positive view of their future.

Often there is so much new information that patients and their families will not be able to take it all in at once. The nurse needs to remember this when writing her plan. She should decide what she will teach in each session and following sessions should go back over previous information to see that it has been fully understood. Sometimes patients may not want to know everything or may not seem to understand the seriousness of the illness. Nurses have to respect the right of patients both to know and not to know.

Sometimes friends and neighbours have given wrong information, some of which may be very worrying. Patients must feel able to share any worries or concerns without being made to feel foolish.

Stigmatisation

Some diseases are associated with stigmas. Patients with AIDS may be stigmatised because in the early days it was associated with socially unacceptable behaviour such as homosexuality. Mental illness is often stigmatised and the patient may be thought to be possessed by the devil or affected by witchcraft. Nurses are in a good position to teach the community about illnesses and help to reduce stigmatisation.

Patients with chronic illness listed five areas that are important to them:

Information: They want to be given information on the illness, its causes, treatment and whether they are likely to recover.

Psychological: Patients wanted to be encouraged and reassured, respected as individuals and to feel safe.

They wanted hospital staff to show caring attitudes.

Physical: Patients wanted their needs to be met in the areas of elimination, nutrition, hygiene, sleep, rest, mobility and comfort.

Social: They wanted to be helped with transport and finances when needed. They also wanted to be able to join in social activities.

Spiritual: Patients wanted to be supported in their spiritual lives.

Disability

People with disabilities have impairments which restrict them in some part of their everyday life. The type and number of impairments and the level of restriction they cause determine the effect on their lives.

Disability can occur at any stage as a result of illness or accident. Some people are born with disabilities, either as a result of an injury occurring during birth or as a congenital defect.

Nurses will care for a variety of disabled people during the course of their work. They may have to help patients accept that they have become disabled, for example people who develop paralysis following a severe illness or accident and children who become blind. Nurses will also care for people who are already disabled but may have developed new problems.

The nurse's role is to work with other professionals to try to ensure that people can lead as independent lives as possible and achieve their full potential.

Health promotion

- Patients who have a history of anaphylactic shock should be taught to avoid the cause (food, drug, bees). They can be taught to inject themselves with adrenaline if they come in contact with the problem. A special pen/syringe makes this easier.

■ Activities

1. Write a nursing care plan for a patient admitted to your ward following a road traffic accident. He is suffering from shock and may have internal bleeding.
2. Plan a teaching programme for a patient who has just been diagnosed as having epilepsy.

6

Infection prevention and control

This chapter will cover issues around causes of infection, prevention of infection and international precautions.

Introduction

People expect health care to improve their lives. Unfortunately it is very common for them to be infected by the organisms that other people have in situations like hospitals. People are more likely to become ill from this cross-infection when their resistance is already lowered by the condition for which they are seeking help. This is a problem everywhere, with new or changed organisms threatening people's lives as they become resistant to commonly-used drugs such as penicillin.

Causes of infection

Infection is caused mainly by the micro-organisms bacteria, viruses and fungi. These pass from one person to another by a 'chain of infection'. The chain is made up of the source of the infection, the way in which it is spread (transmission) and the person who becomes infected.

Sources of infection

- Patients
- Visitors
- Medical, nursing, domestic staff
- Infected clinical waste
- Dirty equipment
- Insects or animals
- Dust
- Contaminated food or water

Transmission

Infections are passed in many ways in hospitals and one of the main routes is on the hands of health care staff. Other routes are by ingestion of infected material, contact with dirty equipment or unsterilised instruments, and spread through the air via droplets of moisture, known as airborne infection. The patient with active tuberculosis who coughs spreads infection this way. Infection can be spread by skin contact and, more rarely, in other ways, for example by tears.

Common causes of spread of infection in hospital

- Staff who do not apply basic precautions of hand washing before and after making contact with patients
- Soap and soap dishes that are contaminated
- Gloves worn incorrectly or re-used without adequate cleaning
- Careless disposal of used needles and sharp instruments
- Poorly cleaned and sterilised equipment
- Unsafe disposal of clinical waste and dirty linen
- Poor handling of specimens
- Poor care of patients with indwelling catheters or other invasive procedures
- Overcrowding, beds too close together, patients sharing beds or sleeping on the floor
- Inadequate ventilation resulting in reduced air flow
- Badly maintained equipment such as torn chairs or cracked and broken tiles
- Dirty environment – floors, walls, and door handles; latrines and toilets that are dirty and unhygienic
- Uncontrolled pests such as flies, mice, rats, cockroaches and mosquitoes
- Poor hygiene when preparing food; contaminated food or water

- Failure to isolate those patients who have highly infectious diseases such as measles or active pulmonary tuberculosis
- Failure to protect those who have low levels of immunity, such as premature babies, the elderly, those with HIV and those who have had chemotherapy for malignant disease

Prevention of infection

Hand washing

This is a vital part of preventing infection. All medical staff have a responsibility to make sure that their hands are not the way in which infection passes from one patient to another. The hands should be cleansed by rubbing all surfaces (including between the fingers and the backs of the hand) with a cleansing agent such as soap and then rinsed, preferably under running water (see Figure 6.1). This will remove most micro-organisms. Adequate water must be available for hand washing. If running water is not available, water can be poured from a jug over the hands, or bowls of clean water must be provided. This water ought to be changed after every use.

Prior to surgical procedures, the hands must be vigorously rubbed under running water using an antiseptic solution. Elbow taps should be provided for hand washing, if possible, as handling the taps may contaminate the hands again after washing. Soap dishes must be clean and should have holes in, so that water can drain away. Sometimes, when patients are highly infectious, it is better to cut soap into small pieces so that it can be discarded after use.

Principles of hand washing

- Remove all rings as organisms may live around them and will be difficult to remove. Nurses undertaking clinical duties should not wear nail polish.
- Ensure that there is a bin for towel disposal with a lid that can be lifted without touching with the hands, as this will contaminate the clean hands.
- Very hot water is best for washing hands as it opens up the pores of the skin to remove more organisms.
- Cuts, abrasions and skin lesions such as paronychia or eczema may be an infection risk. There is a danger of both getting and giving infection.

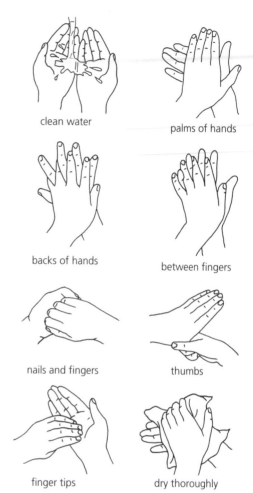

clean water   palms of hands

backs of hands   between fingers

nails and fingers   thumbs

finger tips   dry thoroughly

Figure 6.1 *The technique for hand washing to reduce cross-infection*

Gloves

Gloves reduce the risk of contamination when handling blood or body fluids or if there is broken skin. They help to protect both patients and staff. These should be discarded after handling contaminated material and between patients. After removing the gloves, the hands should be washed thoroughly. There can be leakage through gloves so double gloves should be worn when handling very contaminated material. Disposable gloves are much safer than re-usable ones. However, when there is a shortage of disposable gloves, they may have to be re-used. They should be thoroughly washed and dried, and then examined for any splits before re-using.

Protecting clothing from contamination

If available, disposable plastic aprons should be used for patient care. All clothes have microbes living on them and those worn by the nurse whilst caring for patients become contaminated. Nurses should take care to reduce the contamination of their clothes, for example by holding dirty linen away from the body. Aprons should be changed between dirty and clean tasks and disposed of carefully. Hands should be washed again after removing the apron. Disposable aprons are not always available and nurses must use whatever they can. A clean cloth wrapped around the clothing can take the place of an apron. Pieces of clean polythene could also be used.

Aprons should be worn for all patient care but especially when:
- undertaking aseptic procedures
- serving meals and feeding patients
- making beds
- performing dirty tasks, such as emptying bedpans
- caring for patients with diarrhoeal diseases.

Face masks

During surgical procedures, nursing and medical staff should wear face masks to prevent droplet infection. When removing the masks they should be handled carefully, using the tapes. They are then placed in a bin and the hands washed. Masks should be changed frequently.

Face protection

Spectacles or goggles can be worn to protect the eyes when there is a risk of blood or body fluid being splashed, for example in theatre or during childbirth.

Waste disposal

Sharps

Blades, needles, amnihooks and any sharp equipment (sharps) that needs to be disposed of should be put into a rigid, puncture-proof container immediately after use. The container should never be filled more than two-thirds of its capacity and it should be firmly closed before being taken for disposal. Injection needles should not be re-sheathed before being put into the container as this increases the risk of needle stick injury. Sharps should be incinerated and never handled without good protection.

If needles and syringes have to be re-used, they should be washed thoroughly in soapy water. Full strength bleach should then be drawn through the needle into the barrel of the syringe. Discard the bleach, and refill again with full strength bleach. The needle and syringe should then be allowed to dry in the air and stored in a clean jar.

Contaminated waste

All contaminated waste should be placed in properly labelled bags and then taken for incineration.

Infected linen

All patient linen is contaminated but some will be more dangerous. Dirty linen must be held away from the body when handled and put into linen carriers. Infected linen must be put into special bags and taken to the laundry for washing. The water must be hot enough to destroy micro-organisms. Disinfectant may be used.

Care of eating utensils

Dirty feeding utensils should be washed immediately and not left around for insects and animals. Disposable utensils should be used for infectious patients if possible. Babies who are not able to breast feed should be fed using cups and spoons that can be sterilised. Bottles and teats are dangerous as they are difficult to clean.

Equipment

It is important that equipment is well maintained. It is dangerous to use tape to repair equipment as it cannot be sterilised properly. Trolleys, chairs or mattresses that are torn are also an infection risk as they allow organisms to enter and are difficult to clean.

Equipment which comes into contact with blood or body fluids must be particularly well cleaned. The HIV virus can survive in a dirty syringe at room temperature for four weeks. Syringes and needles that have to be re-used are therefore a particular risk. Intravenous giving sets should not be re-used. Suction apparatus, breast pumps, vacuum extractors and all mechanical equipment must be cleaned well. All surgical instruments should be well maintained and thoroughly cleaned after use before they are sterilised. Infant incubators are particularly dangerous, as micro-organisms thrive in a warm humid atmosphere.

Health of hospital staff

Nursing staff that have an infection should be aware that they can pass it to patients easily, so they should not work until they have recovered. This applies to others who come into contact with patients. Staff are continually exposed to infection in hospital, so should be offered any immunisations that are available.

Universal precautions

Health care professionals are exposed to many micro-organisms. HIV, Hepatitis B and C and other blood-borne diseases have increased the need for protecting nurses, midwives and patients from infection. For this reason Universal precautions have been designed to protect health care workers from infection and to prevent cross-infection to other patients. Since it is impossible to know who is infected and who is not, it is important to use these precautions with everyone. Universal precautions should be used when there is contact with:

- blood
- cerebrospinal fluid
- saliva
- breast milk
- vaginal and seminal secretions
- amniotic fluid
- any other body fluid or where there is doubt about what is being handled.

The following principles should be followed:

- Cuts and abrasions on hands and arms of staff should be covered with waterproof plasters that will provide a barrier to bacteria and viruses.
- Latex or vinyl gloves should be worn in any situation where the hands may be contaminated with body fluids. Sterile gloves should be worn for sterile procedures. Gauntlet gloves that cover the arms as well as the hands may be worn for particular procedures. for example manual removal of the placenta.
- Hand washing should be practised routinely, even when gloves are to be worn.
- Plastic aprons should be worn. Gowns may be worn in some circumstances over a plastic apron.
- Eye protection is necessary if there is danger of body fluids being splashed, for example childbirth, or particles sprayed into the air, for example orthopaedic surgery.
- Sharps must be disposed of in a recognised sharps disposal container.

Midwives need to be particularly careful in the following situations since all of their patients have had unprotected sex:

- Specimen collection
- Injections
- Vaginal examination, use of amnihook and fetal scalp electrodes
- Cannulation and venepuncture
- Disposal of IV and blood transfusion administration sets and all sharps
- Theatre work, including suction and aspiration of body fluids
- Birth
- Perineal repair
- Newborn babies prior to bathing
- Postnatal observation of *lochia* and perineum.

Particular care should be taken when accidents occur and body fluids are spilt. Skin that has been exposed should be washed with soap and water. If the eyes have been splashed then they should be irrigated with large amounts of a sodium chloride (salt) solution. In the event of a needle stick injury, the area should be encouraged to bleed. The area should then be washed vigorously with soap and water and then covered with a waterproof dressing. In some situations, staff who have suffered a needle stick injury should be immediately started on a short course of anti-retroviral drugs. Spillages should be cleared up wearing apron and gloves and then the area cleansed with a hypochlorite solution or household bleach. The soiled area should be left to soak in the bleach for a few minutes to be most effective.

Health promotion

The nurse has a unique opportunity to help prevent infection by teaching local communities about the importance of good hygiene and general cleanliness so that cross-infection is minimised if patients are ever admitted. Particularly important is to give teaching and guidance to relatives involved with the care of patients in hospital.

■ Activity

Many patients in hospital are infected with the HIV virus. Think of all of the ways in which it is possible for the virus to be passed to other patients or members of staff while they are having treatment. What are your responsibilities as a health care worker in reducing the risk?

7

Management of pain

This chapter will explore the concept of pain, suggest how to assess it and discuss methods of relieving it.

Introduction

Pain is an unpleasant sensation which is often associated with disease or injury. Pain is also protective, as children learn to avoid things that cause them pain, such as hot fires or sharp objects. Sometimes damage to the nerves can lead to a loss of the sensation of pain, for example in leprosy or after a spinal injury. As the person no longer feels pain in the part of the body affected, they may injure themselves without knowing and extensive tissue damage can result.

Only the person who feels the pain can know how much pain they have and nurses have to believe what their patients are telling them and learn to assess how much pain the person has and how to relieve it.

Pain is made worse by certain factors:

- Anxiety
- Fatigue or lack of sleep
- Muscle spasm
- Memory of a previous painful experience
- Fear.

Types of pain

Pain may be acute, usually occurring suddenly and due to a definite cause, for instance a broken limb or the headache suffered by someone with meningitis. It is useful as it warns that there is a problem.

Chronic pain is pain lasting longer than six months. The cause may be known, for instance the person may have cancer, or it may not be known. The pain is not useful and can affect the person's lifestyle.

Assessment of pain

The nurse must learn to assess each person's pain, taking into account their culture, gender, age and previous response to pain. For example men may not want to say that they have pain because in their culture it may be seen as weak to admit to pain. In some countries women are expected to stay silent during child birth to show how brave they are. In other countries, boys and girls are expected to undergo circumcision without showing pain. It is difficult to assess pain in children who may not have the language to explain that they have pain. Patients who have had bad experiences of pain and not had it relieved may be very frightened and therefore the pain may seem to be more acute.

- Ask the patient to describe their pain. Is it a stabbing pain, a dull ache, a cramping pain? Is it there all the time or are there times when there is no pain?
- Where is the pain? Ask them to point to the place where they feel pain. Remember some pain is referred. It is felt in a different place. For example when a patient has angina, the pain is felt across the chest but may also pass down the left arm to the fingers. A patient who has had a limb amputated may complain of pain in the limb that has been removed. This is known as phantom pain.
- Are they frightened by the pain? Ask them whether they are worried about what is going to happen. Explaining what will happen at an operation and afterwards has been shown to reduce the amount of pain felt by the patient in the post-operative period.
- Are they very tired? Did they have a good night's sleep the previous night or did the pain prevent them from sleeping?
- Do they have any muscle spasm? When someone fractures his femur, there is usually a great deal of muscle spasm which makes the pain worse.
- Is the pain worse if they move?

- Is the pain associated with taking food? Do they have pain before a meal or after a meal?
- Observe the position of their body. They may be holding themselves very stiffly to try to reduce the amount of pain. Or they may be lying with their legs drawn up. In meningitis, bright light can cause a worse headache and more pain (*photophobia*), so the patient may lie under the blanket to try to reduce the amount of light.
- Does the patient say that there is anything that helps the pain? Some patients may get relief from moving around or getting into a different position.
- Observe the expression on their faces. Sometimes it is obvious from looking at a patient that they are in pain.
- Are they making any noise, for instance groaning or crying?
- Pain can cause physiological changes. There may be a rise in the pulse and respiratory rates. Pain can increase shock so there may be a fall in the blood pressure, or the blood pressure may rise.

Pain in babies and young children

It is difficult to assess the pain in young children who are unable to describe their pain. Some people will say that babies do not have pain. This is not true. Sometimes people will say that a child who is asleep cannot have pain. This is also not true. The nurse must learn how to assess pain in a young child. The most important point is to ask the mothers whether they think their children are in pain. They are the people who know them best and will be able to tell if they are behaving in a different way. The nurse must also observe the following:

- Crying; there may be a particular cry which may be very high pitched or the children may moan.
- A special look on the child's face; the mother may be able to describe this.
- Children who withdraw, become less active and do not want to play or respond to other people, except for their mothers.
- They may grind their teeth or be sweating.
- The pulse and respiratory rates may rise.
- They may lie in a particular position, for example with their legs drawn up.
- They may say they have a headache when they mean they have a stomach ache.
- Always believe mothers who tell you that their children are in pain.

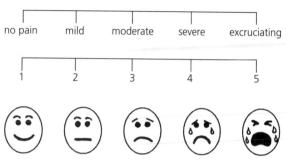

Figure 7.1 *Pain scales*

The use of pain scales may be useful (see Figure 7.1). Children can sometimes show how much pain they have by pointing to the picture which describes how they are feeling.

Pain relief

The type of pain relief that will be necessary will depend on the cause and severity of the pain. There are many drugs available but most have some side effects so must be used with caution. There are also other ways of helping to relieve pain. The patient may use home remedies. The nurse should ask them about these so that they can be used as part of the management, rather than forbidding them to use them. Pain relief should be given so that it gives maximum relief with the fewest side effects. The timing of the relief is therefore very important. The nurse must know how long the drug takes to work and how long it lasts for and also the maximum dose that can be given. Pain relief may be given to prevent pain so it is given on a regular basis or given as necessary (*prn*). It has been found that lower doses are needed if it is given preventively and this also keeps the patient out of pain for most of the time. The nurse should watch for the following:

- Very sleepy or depression of the respirations — Too much medication
- Pain occurs too soon after drug given with little relief — Too little medication
- Relief is poor but the patient is sedated — Wrong medication
- Relief is adequate but does not last long — Medication not given often enough

Medication

This depends on what is available and the type of pain. There are many possible drugs to use and sometimes

Table 7.1 Examples of drugs used for pain relief

Drug	Adult dosage	Interval	Potential side effect
Aspirin	300–900 mg (Maximum daily dose 4 g)	4–6 hourly	Gastric irritation Bleeding Heartburn, nausea
Paracetamol	500 mg–1 g (Maximum daily dose 4 g)	4 hourly	Liver damage following over dosage
Ibuprofen	1.2–1.8 g daily in 3–4 divided doses (Maximum daily dose 2.4 g)		Nausea, diarrhoea, dizziness Gastric irritation

combinations of drugs work best. Some drugs can be given orally, others work better if given intravenously or intramuscularly. A child who is frightened of injections will often pretend he does not have any pain if he thinks he will get an injection. Commonly used drugs include aspirin (not for children under 12 if possible as it may cause **Reye's syndrome**), and paracetamol. These both reduce temperature as well as relieving pain. There is a group of non steroid anti-inflammatory drugs (NSAID), such as ibuprofen, which should be given after food and are useful for joint or muscular pain. Opiates, like morphine, are very good for severe pain and are often used in terminally ill patients. They can cause addiction so need to be used carefully.

It is important to time the giving of the drug so that it has the most effect when most is needed. For instance if you were asked to do the dressings of a patient with major burns, the medication would need to be given at least an hour before starting the dressings.

Other methods of relieving pain

- Find out if patients are anxious and see that they get good explanations of any treatment.

- Make sure the patient is not tired. See that they get a good night's sleep.
- Make sure they are comfortable in the bed, alter the position as necessary.
- Massage may help, or rubbing an area, as it releases endorphins which are natural pain killing hormones.
- Applying heat or cold to an area.
- Sometimes exercise gives some relief.
- Distraction. If a patient can be involved in something else, they may find the pain is not so bad. Music helps some patients.

Remember to assess the pain, plan the care, give the care and evaluate (see if it has worked).

■ Activity

Umaru, aged 40 years, is admitted to your ward with a fractured femur. He has never been in hospital before, has had to travel on a lorry for six hours before reaching the hospital and is in severe pain. Think of all the things that will be making Umaru's pain worse and things that you can do to help him.

8

Bereavement and loss

This chapter will explore some of the concepts of bereavement and loss, identify some of the effects and suggest ways that nurses can help those who are suffering.

Introduction

Bereavement is the process of grieving following the death of a loved one. Loss can also be used to describe the death of a loved one, or can be associated with the loss of an object, a job, or part of a person's ability to function as before.

Case histories

Bereavement and loss are such large subjects that it may be useful to consider some of the following case studies:

CASE STUDY A

Fatima is 18 months old and has recently had severe measles. Her mother noticed that her eyes looked cloudy and she did not appear to be able to see. When she takes her to the doctor, he says that Fatima is now blind and there is nothing that can be done.

Areas of loss: Fatima's mother has lost the child she had who could see and now has a blind child who will have very different needs. Fatima has lost her sight and will be handicapped for the rest of her life. Fatima's mother may feel guilty that she did not get help earlier and she may be angry that she will now have to cope with a blind child.

CASE STUDY B

Ibrahim is a 7 year old boy who fell out of a tree and broke his leg. He lived far away from a health clinic and was treated by a traditional healer, who put a splint on his leg. Unfortunately the splint was too tight, the leg became gangrenous and the doctor who has just seen him, says that he will need to have the leg amputated.

Areas of loss: Ibrahim has lost his leg. He will be able to get a *prosthesis* at the hospital many miles away but it will cost the family money. Ibrahim loved playing football which he can no longer do. His family face the extra expense of dealing with his disability and also the loss of a fit son who was beginning to help with the family finances by looking after the goats and cattle. His ability to help look after them when they get old is now more limited. They are angry with the hospital doctor who is telling them that Ibrahim has to have his leg amputated.

CASE STUDY C

Amina is 35 years old. She has had 12 pregnancies but has no live children. She has had several miscarriages (spontaneous abortions) and the other three children died at a very young age. She has just had a stillborn boy and has been told by the doctor that she cannot have any more children as she has had a hysterectomy. Her husband is threatening to divorce her as she has not given him any live children. If this happens she will have to return to the village and live with her parents who have little money and may be unable to support her.

Areas of loss: Amina has lost the chance of having any live children and may lose her husband. She has lived with him for 15 years so has many friends in the area. If her husband divorces her, she will lose her house and her friends. She may be blamed for having brought misfortune on the family.

CASE STUDY D

Yusuf is 40 years old and is dying of AIDS. His wife is HIV positive and they have eight children. Yusuf's brother and his wife died of AIDS last year, leaving their elderly mother to look after their six children. Yusuf is being cared for at home by his wife and other members of the family. There is very little money as Yusuf can no longer work on the coffee plantation. Six of the children were going to school but all but the eldest two boys have had to leave as there is no money for uniforms or books.

Areas of loss: Yusuf has lost his job. He is losing his position as head of the family as he is now too sick and his eldest son has had to take on the responsibility. He also knows that he is dying and is worried about the future of his family. His wife is shortly to lose her husband. She is also feeling very tired and is wondering if she is developing full blown AIDS. There is very little money and finding food for the family is getting increasingly difficult. The four children who have had to leave school have lost the chance of gaining an education and now stay at home, helping their parents. They may soon be orphans and will be left to look after themselves. The eldest son has lost his childhood as he is now the head of the family and has to take on extra responsibilities. He had hoped to go to university and become a doctor but knows this is now unlikely to happen as he will be responsible for providing for his younger brothers and sisters.

CASE STUDY E

Solomon is 8 years old and is the only survivor of his family. He lived with his parents and four siblings in a remote part of the country. His grandparents and other members of his family lived in the same village. One day rebel soldiers came to the area and tortured members of his family before killing them. Solomon was taken into the forest by the soldiers but managed to escape after several weeks and is now being looked after in an orphanage.

Areas of loss: Solomon has lost his entire family and way of life. He has seen things that no child should have to see. He is now being brought up by strangers who do not even speak the same language and have different customs. He is expected to sleep in a large hut with 15 other children and is given strange food to eat.

Stages of grieving

In all the above case studies the people involved are likely to be grieving for what they are going to lose or have lost. Grieving has different stages and not everyone will go through the same stages in the same order. There is no time limit on grief. Some people will take a long time to come to terms with their loss, others may seem to adapt more quickly.

Shock, disbelief and denial: In the early stages people may not be able to believe what is happening and may pretend that it has not and will not happen. They may experience physical symptoms of numbness, choking, shortness of breath, loss of appetite and not being able to sleep.

Anger, rage and frustration: They may then become very angry. Sometimes they are angry with the person who is dying or has died, or they are angry with the doctor or the nurse who has had to give them bad news.

Bargaining: Sometimes people will try to find a way out. They may promise to do something or try to find a witch doctor who can help if the traditional doctor is giving the bad news.

Depression, sorrow and sadness: Once people realise that there is no way out, they may have intense feelings of grief and sometimes become depressed (see Chapter 49).

Acceptance and resolution: Most people learn to live with their loss. It does not mean that they are no longer sad or have forgotten, but they are able to return to some sort of normal living.

Sometimes people cannot come to terms with their loss and may be left with a long-term mental illness.

Ways in which nurses can help

- The nurse should be available to listen to people who are grieving. Sometimes there is a need to repeat the story again and again. The nurse needs to realise that this is normal behaviour. It is very important to always be truthful. Never pretend that things are better than they are. If someone is dying, it is necessary to tell the family that this is happening. The nurse will need to take into account the culture and tradition of the area when giving the news.
- Some cultures are very noisy about their grieving, others grieve more quietly. People who are quiet

and withdrawn may be just as sad as those making a great noise.

• Make sure that physical needs are met. Ensure people get regular meals and enough rest.
• Funerals and mourning rituals are important in acknowledging the loss by the community.

Conclusion

Nurses are often in a position where they can help other people who are suffering a loss or bereavement.

They need to be aware of all the different emotions that can be aroused.

■ Activity

Discuss the different case studies with your friends and think of ways in which you might be able to help the people involved.

9

Pre- and post-operative care

> This chapter covers the basic care needed by patients before and after an operation. Care required for specific operations is covered in the chapters where they are discussed.

Pre-operative care

Some patients are admitted for surgery as an emergency and the amount of care that is able to be given will be partly determined by the time available. Other patients are admitted for routine surgery and it is then possible to give more thorough explanations and care. This will help the patient recover following surgery.

Communicating

Some patients will never have been in hospital before and it is important that they are welcomed by the nurse and given good explanations as to what will happen. The nurse should check that the patient knows why they have come into hospital, when they are likely to go to theatre, what operation will be performed, how they will feel after surgery and how long they are likely to be in hospital.

Baseline observations

A full nursing assessment of the patient should be made. It is important to record the temperature, pulse, respirations and blood pressure before theatre, so that any alteration following surgery can be noted. The nutritional status should be assessed. Malnourished patients will need extra food following surgery to help with wound healing. Obese patients may have respiratory problems and will need help to mobilise after surgery. If available, these patients should wear support stockings during surgery to reduce the risk of deep vein thrombosis. The urine should be tested and any abnormality noted. The state of the skin should be noted. The patient should be clean before going to theatre to reduce the risk of infection. Some surgeons will request that the patient is shaved prior to theatre, depending on the type of surgery.

Eating and drinking

The nurse should find out what the patient normally eats and when. In some cases the relatives will be expected to bring food into the hospital for the patient and they need to be told where they can prepare food and what the patient is allowed to eat. Usually patients going to theatre are not allowed to eat or drink for 2-4 hours before going to theatre. This is to ensure that the stomach is empty and there is less likelihood of the patient vomiting and aspirating the vomit after an anaesthetic. The exact length of time may be determined by the anaesthetist. In emergency cases, it is important to ask the patient when they last ate or drank. It may be necessary to delay the surgery until the stomach is empty or if surgery is very urgent, the stomach may need to be aspirated using a nasogastric tube.

Specific preparation

There may be specific preparation required. If the bowel is to be operated on, it is often necessary for an enema or rectal washout to be given pre-operatively, so that the bowel is as clear as possible. If the surgery is major, it may be necessary for the patient to have a blood transfusion during or after the operation. The patient will then need to have their blood grouped and cross-matched and the nurse must check that there will be blood available. In some areas it is necessary for relatives to donate blood; this will need to be arranged before admission of the patient. Any donor must be tested for HIV and only virus-free blood given. The nurse must check to see if any X-rays are required prior to theatre, and if so arrange for these to be done and the X-rays available to go to theatre with the patient.

Immediate pre-operative care

- Check the theatre list and tell the patient when they are likely to go to theatre. Ensure that they understand the operation that they are to have and have signed a consent form, or made a mark if they are unable to write their name.
- Ensure that any jewellery is removed and the patient is clean and wearing an operation gown or clean cloth.
- Ask the patient to pass urine, so that the bladder is empty when they go to theatre.
- Check the drug sheet and ensure that any premedication is given at the right time. Often a sedative is given to relax the patient and also atropine or scopolamine to dry up the secretions. Once the premedication has been given, the patient should be left quietly to rest, and warned not to get up.
- When the theatre is ready to take the patient, check the identity of the patient to ensure that the right patient goes for the right operation. Sometimes the surgeon will make a mark on the skin of the patient, to identify the site of the operation. Reassure the patient as they are taken to theatre. If it is a child going to theatre, it is sometimes possible for the mother to carry the child to the door of the theatre or even stay with the child until the anaesthetic is started. This is less frightening for the child and should be encouraged.

Post-operative care

The nurse should be aware of the problems that may face patients following surgery and take steps to avoid or minimise them. To care for the patient well, the nurse needs to know exactly what surgery has been done, the site of any drains, any instructions concerning intravenous fluids, pain relief, commencement of oral fluids or any other specific instructions. Always check the written instructions.

Maintenance of airway

If the patient is still unconscious, then the nurse needs to ensure that the airway is patent. The patient should be nursed on their side, so that the tongue cannot fall back and obstruct the airway and any secretions can drain out of the mouth. If available, a suction machine should be close at hand to remove secretions. The nurse should check the patient's colour and the respiratory rate. Any deterioration should be reported immediately. Sometimes the patient will have an airway in position. This can be removed once the patient is regaining consciousness and they can be encouraged to spit it out. Oxygen should be available in case of deterioration.

Observation for *haemorrhage*

Bleeding may occur at different times after surgery. It may occur immediately, or it may occur as the patient's blood pressure rises and this can be several hours after surgery. It can also occur as a result of wound infection and it then occurs several days following surgery. Bleeding may be easily seen at the site of the operation, or via drainage tubes, but the bleeding may be internal and there may be no sign of it externally. There may be a vaginal or rectal loss.

The nurse must therefore monitor the patient carefully following surgery. The pulse rate and volume should be recorded, the blood pressure taken, the wound site and any drains checked for obvious bleeding, and the skin of the patient checked for warmth, indicating good circulation. Immediately after surgery, it may be necessary to take observations every $1/4$ hour, until the patient is stable. As the condition improves, the observations can be done less frequently.

Signs of haemorrhage are a rising pulse rate with a poor volume, a falling blood pressure and signs of shock. If left unchecked, the respirations may become deep, rapid and sighing, known as air hunger. If haemorrhage is suspected, the doctor must be informed as it may be necessary for the patient to return to theatre. If there is obvious bleeding from the wound site, direct pressure should be applied.

Observation for shock

Following surgery, there are several reasons why the patient may become shocked. If there has been major surgery, this can result in shock. Haemorrhage can cause shock; severe pain or infection can also cause shock (see Chapter 5). Shock is a serious complication, so the nurse must watch the patient carefully. Early signs are a fall in blood pressure, a rise in pulse rate, cold clammy skin and restlessness. The cause of the shock will need to be found and immediate action taken to rectify it. Intravenous fluids will need to be given to the patient immediately to increase the circulating volume. If possible, blood or a plasma expander such as Dextran should be given, or normal saline. The foot of the bed should be raised so that blood flow to the brain and heart are increased.

Observation for pain

As the patient recovers consciousness, they will become aware of pain from the operation site. Analgesia should be given before they have complained of pain. Some operations are more painful than others and some patients have a higher pain threshold than others. It is important that pain relief is given, as pain can lead to shock, it stops the patient from moving around after surgery and this can cause further problems and it is frightening. The type of pain relief given will depend on the surgery that has been done and the pain relief available. The nurse should always monitor the effect of pain relief and increase the amount given if it does not appear to be effective (see Chapter 7).

Vomiting

Many patients vomit following surgery as a result of the anaesthesia. In most cases this is not serious, and the nurse should ensure that there is a vomit bowl near the bedside and support the patient whilst they are vomiting.

Fluids and diet

Unless the surgery has been on the gastro-intestinal tract, the patient is usually allowed to drink once they have regained consciousness. Small sips of water are given initially to prevent vomiting. The amounts can be increased once the sips are tolerated. Unless the surgeon has stated otherwise, food can be given once the patient feels like eating. Usually a light diet is tolerated better initially.

Paralytic ileus

If the gut has been handled during surgery, *peristalsis* of the bowel stops initially. The patient will often have a nasogastric tube in place when they return from theatre. This will need to be aspirated regularly and the amount measured. The nasogastric tube helps prevent the patient from vomiting by keeping the stomach empty. Intravenous fluids will need to be given, to ensure that the patient does not become dehydrated. If large amounts of fluid are aspirated from the nasogastric tube, increased amounts of fluid will need to be given intravenously. It is important to keep an accurate fluid chart, so that the amount of fluid given and the amount eliminated (gastric aspiration, urine and any drainage) can be monitored.

The nurse should check the patient's abdomen, which may be distended at first. The return of bowel sounds will be shown by a decrease in the amount of gastric aspiration, lessening of distension and the passing of flatus. Listening to the patient's abdomen with a stethoscope, the nurse will be able to hear the bowel sounds. As peristalsis recommences, fluids can be started slowly. As oral fluids are introduced, the intravenous infusion can be decreased.

Elimination

Check that the patient is passing urine after surgery. If there is a delay, it may be because the patient is dehydrated, or, in spite of a full bladder, they may have difficulty in passing urine. Sometimes this is due to being in an awkward position or it may be because they are afraid that it will be painful. Often patients complain of being constipated after surgery. There are many reasons why this may occur. The patient is likely to be less mobile than usual, they may have a lower fluid intake than before, they may not be eating well and many of the drugs given for pain relief cause constipation as a side effect. Usually this problem resolves once the patient becomes more mobile and starts to eat and drink well. Occasionally it may be necessary for a laxative to be given. However, if there has been gastro-intestinal surgery, no laxatives should be given without authorisation from the surgeon.

Mobilisation

It is important that the patient is encouraged to move as soon after surgery as possible. Moving the legs and turning from one side to the other is valuable. There are various complications that can arise if the patient remains immobile. Deep vein thrombosis can occur, where a clot forms in the leg. This can be serious as the clot can move to the lungs, causing a *pulmonary embolism*, which can be fatal. Some patients are also at risk from developing pressure sores if they do not move well. These include the elderly, the immobile, those who are overweight, the severely malnourished and those who are incontinent.

The patient may also develop a chest infection if they are not encouraged to move around. Following surgery, unless there is a specific reason, the patient should be sat up, well supported with pillows. They should be encouraged to take deep breaths to expand the lungs fully. Following abdominal surgery, they may be afraid to cough as it will hurt. The nurse can help by supporting the wound area with her hand and then encouraging the patient to cough to remove secretions. As soon as possible, the patient should be sat in a chair beside the bed and then encouraged to walk around.

Care of drains

If the patient returns from theatre with drains in place, the nurse will need to find out the purpose of the drains and what care is required. Some drains may need to be attached to bottles, so that the fluid can drain out. Sometimes a vacuum suction drain is used. The purpose of the drain is to remove any serous fluid or blood that collects around the site of the operation so that wound healing is encouraged. The amount of drainage needs to be checked and large amounts should be reported.

Some drains will be covered with dressings, and these dressings will need to be changed as they become wet, to prevent infection. Many drains need to be shortened before being removed. It is necessary to ask the surgeon for specific instructions. No drains should be left long in situ, as they can cause irritation.

Wound care

The aim is to obtain healing by primary intention. With any wound, there is initially inflammation. This is a normal process. The release of histamine due to the tissue damage causes dilatation of the capillary blood vessels and an increased permeability of the vessel walls. The blood supply to the area is increased, and white cells invade the area to fight off infection. The wound edges become swollen, red and warm. Sometimes there may be a slight rise in the patient's temperature at this time.

The wound may be held together with sutures or clips, and a dressing placed over the wound. This dressing should be left undisturbed unless it becomes soaked with blood or serous fluid, or there is concern that the wound has become infected. Clips or sutures are removed 5–10 days after surgery, depending on the area of the body and the surgeon's wishes. Check that the wound is well healed before removing sutures or clips.

Wounds do not heal well if the patient has AIDS or is malnourished. The hospital may know whether the patient is HIV positive, but if there is no record of testing having been carried out, HIV should be suspected in a patient with delayed wound healing. Infected wounds need to be cleaned daily with a solution that is non-toxic. Normal saline is available, cheap and as effective as many other more expensive ones. If the patient is showing general signs of infection, it is necessary to take a wound swab to test for organisms and antibiotic sensitivity. Antibiotics may be needed. Wounds that have become infected do not heal as well and do not leave neat scars.

■ Activity

When a patient has fully recovered from their operation, ask them whether they understand what treatment has been given. Ask whether they would have liked more explanation.

10

Nursing care of adults with breathing problems

This chapter will cover the basic anatomy and physiology of the respiratory system. It will give an overview of the common respiratory problems and outline the nursing care required by patients. It will also cover the clinical skills of tracheal suction and care of a patient with a chest drain.

The respiratory system

The respiratory system has the role of getting oxygen from the air into the blood. Once in the blood, oxygen is sent by the heart and circulatory system to all the cells of the body. The respiratory system also has the role of getting rid of carbon dioxide from the blood (see Figure 10.1).

Much of the respiratory system is a series of passages through which air moves. Such passageways include the rigid tubes of the pharynx, larynx, left and right bronchi. The lining tissues of these passageways warm and moisten air. Some lining cells produce sticky mucus that traps dust and micro-organisms to stop them from passing deep into the lungs. Tiny projections called *cilia*, from the cells lining the tubes, continuously push tiny amounts of mucus up towards the back of the throat, where they are swallowed or coughed up.

The lower passageways of the respiratory system are not rigid tubes. They have circular muscle in their walls and therefore can dilate (get wider), such as when exercising, or constrict (narrow). The dilation/constriction of the tubes (*bronchioles*) is under the control of the autonomic nervous system.

These bronchioles are branches off the bigger passageways and the whole network of branches means that there are several hundred bronchioles in total in the two lungs.

Each bronchiole ends in what can be thought of as a collection of tiny balloons. Each balloon is an *alveolus*. Healthy adults have about 300 million alveoli. These alveoli are the functional units of the lungs, where oxygen diffuses into the blood and carbon dioxide diffuses out of the blood (see Figure 10.2).

These fine air passages and the millions of alveoli make up the two lungs. Surrounding each lung is a double layer of membrane (*pleura*). The outer pleura is attached to the chest wall and the inner pleura sticks

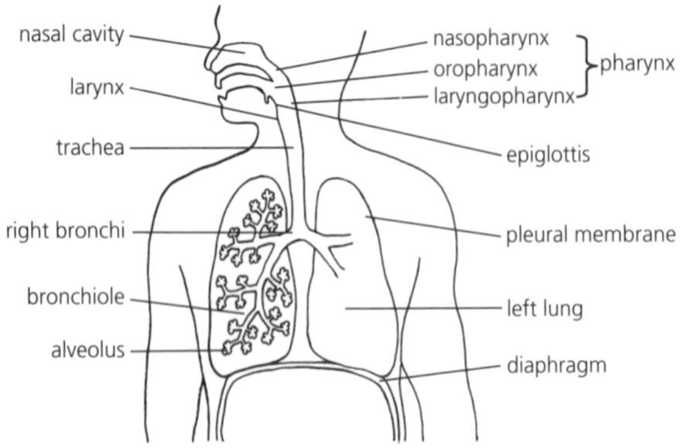

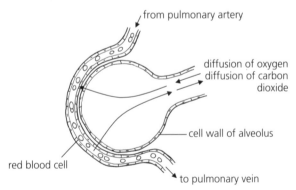

Figure 10.1 *The respiratory system*

nasal cavity
larynx
trachea
right bronchi
bronchiole
alveolus

nasopharynx
oropharynx — pharynx
laryngopharynx
epiglottis
pleural membrane
left lung
diaphragm

from pulmonary artery

diffusion of oxygen
diffusion of carbon dioxide

cell wall of alveolus

red blood cell

to pulmonary vein

Figure 10.2 *Gaseous exchange at the site of an alveolus*

to it because a small amount of pleural fluid creates a surface tension. This is what keeps each lung inflated and attached to the chest wall.

Ventilation

For the blood to be oxygenated, oxygen-rich air must be drawn into the alveoli. All gases, including air, behave in the same way. They move towards an area of lower pressure. Breathing in (*inspiration*) and breathing out (*expiration*) requires air to move in two different directions. The body achieves this by changing the size of the chest cavity, which contains the lungs.

Inspiration occurs because the chest cavity is made bigger, which makes the pressure inside it fall. This allows air to move through the passageways to the alveoli from a high pressure to a lower pressure. The size of the chest cavity is mainly enlarged by the contraction of the diaphragm. Also, the contraction of the internal intercostals, the muscles between the ribs, lifts the chest wall up and out. The chest wall can be further lifted by contraction of shoulder and neck muscles. These are called the accessory muscles of respiration but for healthy people these are only used during or after exercise.

Expiration occurs because the chest cavity is made smaller by the elastic recoil of the diaphragm and the fall of the chest wall. This makes the pressure inside the cavity rise. The result of this is that gas with carbon dioxide in it moves from the alveoli and out through the air passages. In exercise, contraction of external intercostal muscles actively pulls the chest wall down.

Contraction of muscles occurs because of nerve activity. The nerves of breathing run from respiratory control areas in the brain stem. These nerve centres control rhythm and rate, allowing the body to adapt to different situations, for example rest and exercise. This is because these nerve centres can respond to rising blood levels of carbon dioxide (the primary respiratory stimulus) and falling blood oxygen (the secondary respiratory stimulus).

Gaseous exchange

The process of ventilation draws oxygen-rich air into the alveoli of the lungs. Capillary blood vessels cover the surface of the thin-walled alveoli. These thin walls allow oxygen to diffuse directly from alveoli to capillaries. Carbon dioxide moves in the opposite direction from the blood capillaries into the air in the alveoli. Blood only flows through the alveolar capillaries because it is pumped by the right side of heart. Therefore heart function is essential for this process of oxygenating the blood and getting rid of carbon dioxide from the blood.

Alteration in respiratory function

Normal respiratory function requires:
* movement of the diaphragm and chest wall
* nerve control of movement of the diaphragm and chest wall, from brain-stem nerve centres
* expansion and contraction of the lungs within the chest
* unobstructed large airways
* unobstructed small airways
* normal alveoli and alveolar capillaries, each with thin walls
* normal perfusion of the lungs with blood that flows through alveolar capillaries.

Alteration in respiratory function occurs as a result of failure of one or more of these normal requirements. Usually, the response of the patient is to breathe deeper and faster. This response causes the patient to complain of breathlessness.

Obstruction of large airways

This is usually the result of foreign objects. In adults this is most likely to be food, including stones from fruit or large pieces of meat.
* The obstruction needs to be removed rapidly.
* First, briefly inspect the mouth removing any visible foreign body.
* Bend person forward and give up to 5 sharp slaps between shoulder blades.
* If this doesn't work, try abdominal thrusts: standing behind the person, interlock your hands in front of them and pull sharply inwards and upwards, below the person's ribs.
* If necessary continue to alternate 5 slaps on the back with 5 abdominal thrusts.

Another cause of obstruction may be the person's tongue falling back. This can happen if the person's level of consciousness is lowered, as a result of accident, illness or anaesthesia. It is important to turn unconscious people onto their side, in the recovery position.

Obstruction of small airways

Many disease processes can affect small air passageways. They can become obstructed by mucus, by their lining tissue becoming swollen (mucosal oedema) or because the muscle of their walls goes into a constricting spasm (*bronchospasm*). Often these effects are associated with inflammation. This may happen in medical conditions such as asthma, bronchitis and pneumonia. Cancers can obstruct airways, directly or through stimulating mucus production.

Note: It is important to recognise that many of the conditions where excess mucus is produced are infectious. Separating these patients from others with as much space as possible (if possible in a separate, closed room) is important. Patients should cough into pots with lids which are later burned.

Alteration in alveolar structure

Long-term lung diseases usually cause some changes to the structure of alveoli, decreasing gaseous exchange. *Emphysema* is when there is an abnormal enlargement of terminal bronchioles accompanied by destruction of alveolar walls. Pulmonary fibrosis is usually secondary to healing processes after infections and affects the alveolar-capillary membranes. Patients with these conditions suffer from breathlessness.

Alteration in pleurae and pleural fluid

If the pleurae are damaged by trauma (road traffic injury, stabbing, shooting) or sometimes just tear spontaneously, the lung on the affected side will collapse (*pneumothorax*). Severe lung infections, including tuberculosis and lung cancers, can cause the pleurae to produce large amounts of pleural fluid (*pleural effusion*). This can badly restrict lung expansion and affect breathing.

Impaired perfusion of the lungs with blood

Poor blood flow to lungs is associated with right sided heart failure or the obstruction of the lungs' blood vessels with a blood clot or pulmonary embolism.

Impaired movement of the diaphragm and chest wall

A range of uncommon neurological disorders and muscular disorders may affect the muscles of breathing. Drugs used during anaesthetics may be used deliberately to paralyse the muscles of breathing. Damage to the respiratory centres in the brain stem, through head injury or stroke, may affect the nerve control of ventilation.

Nursing observations

Observation of patients with breathing problems is important in assessing how serious things are.

When the body needs more oxygen than is getting into the blood, it responds by trying to improve things. Such changes can be seen in normal people during exercise. There is an increase in the respiratory rate, depth and effort and an increase in the heart rate. The same changes happen in those with acute or chronic respiratory disease, to compensate for impairment in oxygenation of their blood. Therefore it is important to observe changes to breathing rate, depth and effort to estimate the degree of *impairment* that there is in oxygenating the blood.

Respiratory rate

At rest a normal rate is about 10 to 16 breaths per minute. Patients with acute problems may have a rate of 40 or 50 breaths per minute at rest. However, it is important to recognise that obstruction of airways through bronchospasm may lengthen the time to breath out and the overall respiratory rate per minute may not be particularly high.

Respiratory effort

The use of the neck and shoulder (accessory) muscles during inspiration and the external intercostal muscles during expiration makes breathing look much more laboured. Laboured breathing is, therefore, a sign that the body is compensating for difficulties oxygenating the blood. Restriction to movement of the chest wall results in shallow breaths but a very rapid rate.

Nurses who are observing those with acute shortness of breath must be aware that **reduction of respiratory effort may be a danger sign**, rather than a sign of improvement. Exhaustion from the effort of breathing will cause respiratory failure. Signs of this are irregular breathing, reduced depth of ventilation, *tachycardia*, drowsiness and disorientation.

Noisy respiration

Breathing through obstructed airways causes abnormal noises. Wheezing on expiration is heard in those with asthma or other causes of bronchospasm. *Stridor* is noisy breathing on inspiration and is usually due to narrowing of the larynx. These patients struggle to breathe. Sometimes breathing moves mucus in the airways and creates rattling sounds.

Cyanosis is blueness of the lips and mucus membranes when the lungs are not able to exchange enough oxygen into the blood.

Heart rate

An increased heart rate helps to circulate blood with some oxygen more rapidly to compensate for difficulties oxygenating the blood. The faster the pulse rate, the more serious the impairment in oxygenating blood. However, when the heart works at a faster rate, its own heart muscle cells need more oxygen and these cells get less of a rest period. Therefore, very fast pulse rates (110 beats or more a minute), over a long period, should not only be seen as a serious sign but also a problem, since the heart may fail secondary to the respiration problem. An increased heart rate can also be caused by other factors and diseases as well as respiratory disease.

Body temperature

A respiratory infection is one of many causes of a raised body temperature.

Patient activity

The amount of activity that patients can do helps to show the degree of respiratory problem. In acute situations they may be able to do very little. Speaking, eating and drinking may be too much for them. In less acute situations, respiratory impairment could be assessed in terms of how much it affects walking and carrying out usual self-care activities. Resting will reduce the need for oxygen and all those with breathing problems should be advised and helped to rest.

Other aspects of assessment

Increased respiratory rate will be associated with increased loss of fluid through breathing and may prevent patients drinking. Therefore, assessment of the patient's hydration and mouth are important.

Where the patient is able to speak (or has friends/relatives), it may be possible to question them about the history of the person's breathing problem: its onset or any triggering factors.

Increased respiratory effort over a long time will increase the person's need for food as energy is being used up. Someone who is very thin will need to have their nutrition improved.

Cough and sputum

Persistent cough is associated with respiratory disease. Where a cough is productive, nurses should encourage patients to spit it out into a sputum mug. Observe the sputum that is produced. Infected sputum will have a thick consistency and be creamy. Sputum which has a distinctive colour or smell may indicate infection by a specific organism. Brown/red colour may indicate blood-staining. Sometimes bright red blood or blood mixed with sputum may be coughed up (*haemoptysis*). Observation of the amount and nature of sputum helps doctors to make an accurate diagnosis.

Pain

Assessment of pain associated with respiratory disease is important. Inflammation in the pleura of the lungs is a common cause of pain, which is usually worse on inspiration and localised to one area of the chest. Pleural pain may make patients take shallow, rapid respirations.

Planning and implementing nursing care

Nursing an individual requires individual assessment of the nature and extent of the breathing problem. In planning nursing care, the following interventions will need to be considered.

Positioning

Sitting upright in bed or a chair usually helps patients to ventilate their lungs. Leaning forward slightly, with forearms on a table or holding the arms of a chair, will make use of accessory muscles more effective.

Oxygen

Giving oxygen through a mask may improve the situation. The nurse needs to be sure to which of two categories the patient belongs: those needing high percentage of oxygen or those requiring controlled oxygen therapy. Those requiring controlled oxygen therapy are those with a long history of respiratory disease. Since those with long-term disease cannot eliminate carbon dioxide from their blood very well, the control of their breathing no longer relies upon the brain-stem respiratory centres responding to rising carbon dioxide but relies upon low oxygen in the blood to stimulate breathing (hypoxic respiratory drive). If nurses give higher than 24 per cent oxygen, they may suppress this hypoxic respiratory drive and so cause respiratory failure.

For those with long-term conditions, such as chronic bronchitis and emphysema, oxygen should therefore only be given through a Venturi type mask (see Figure 10.3). For those without long-term respiratory disease, high percentage (40–60 per cent) oxygen should be given through a standard oxygen mask (see Figure 10.4).

Helping clear the airways of mucus

- Assisting to cough (frequent drinks; sitting upright; controlling pain; supporting wounds or sore areas with a pillow)
- Postural drainage (for those who are not too breathless to tolerate it, positioning for 20 minutes at a time, in tipped positions, will allow drainage of mucus into the main bronchi and trachea). The position needs to be changed to allow drainage of all five lobes of the lungs.
- Percussion (rhythmic striking of the chest wall, with cupped hands, for 3 to 5 minutes, with the patient lying in tipped position, may dislodge secretions in small airways)
- Vibration (as the patient breathes out, the nurse can vibrate her hands, positioned flat against the chest wall, to loosen secretions)
- Tracheal suctioning

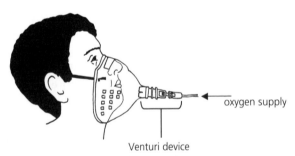

Venturi device

Figure 10.3 *A mask with Venturi system*

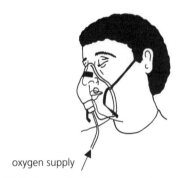

oxygen supply

Figure 10.4 *A standard oxygen mask*

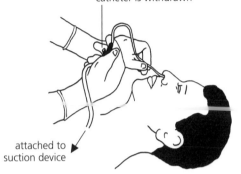

The airvent is left open when inserting the catheter, and covered (to close it) as the catheter is withdrawn

attached to suction device

Figure 10.5 *Applying suction via the nose*

Pp **Tracheal suction** (see Figure 10.5)

- Prepare the equipment required.
- If possible this should be treated as an aseptic technique. Use a sterile suction catheter to prevent cross-infection.
- Give oxygen prior to the suctioning to increase the oxygen in the blood.
- Attach suction catheter to suction machine and switch on. Set at recommended pressure (10–15 mm Hg for adults for portable suction machines; 100–140 mm Hg for wall suction systems).
- Moisten the tip of suction catheter by dipping it into a bowl of sterile saline or boiled water.
- Insert the catheter along the floor of the nose, **without applying suction** (leave the air vent open, or pinch the tubing).
- Wait until the patient takes a breath, before pushing the tubing forward 20–25 cm.
- If the patient does not cough, encourage them to do so.
- Apply suction by closing air vent, or releasing the pinch. Withdraw the catheter, twisting as you do so. This should take about 10 seconds.
- Rinse catheter by sucking up some boiled water or saline.
- Allow patient to rest for 2–3 minutes, breathing oxygen if possible, before repeating the procedure.

Suctioning can also be used to clear secretions from the mouth or through a tracheostomy (see Chapter 20).

Care of patient with a chest drain

Chest drains are used for two different purposes:
- To remove air and/or blood from the pleural space, following collapse of a lung (*pneumo/haemo-thorax*)
- To drain an effusion or pus from the pleural cavity, secondary to lung cancer or infection.

In each case, a thoracic cannula will have been introduced by a doctor and stitched with a purse string suture.

Pp Care of chest drains

Pneumothorax
- Check the connections between thoracic cannula and drainage tube.
- Loop drainage tube and attach it to the chest, so that any traction on the tubing will not pull directly on the thoracic cannula.
- Attach end of the drainage tube to water-seal drainage bottle; fill with just enough water to cover the end of the tube (ideally sterile water).
- Only air should come out: look to see that water in tube rises and falls with each inspiration(shows tube is not obstructed).
- Keep drainage bottle always below chest level.
- Encourage deep breathing and coughing to encourage lung expansion.
- Clamp tubing as little as possible; then only briefly.

Pleural effusion
- Check the connections between thoracic cannula and drainage tube.
- Loop drainage tube and attach it to the chest, so that any traction on the tubing will not pull directly on the thoracic cannula.
- Attach end of the drainage tube to water-seal drainage bottle; fill with just enough water to cover the end of the tube (ideally sterile water).
- The bottle will fill with pleural fluid: empty it (and record) when bottle is half to three-quarters full. Tubing must be clamped above the drainage bottle before disconnecting (don't use toothed clamps which may damage tubing).
- Keep drainage bottle always below chest level.
- Clamp tubing as little as possible; then only briefly.

Health promotion

Nurses should teach patients that cigarette smoking can cause respiratory disease. Smoky and dusty atmospheres can also cause problems. People with productive coughs should not spit in public places as this can spread infection.

■ Activity

Plan the care of a 35 year old man who is admitted to the ward with an acute lower respiratory tract infection.

11

Care of adults with cardiovascular problems

This chapter is about care for the most common problems affecting hypertension and heart failure.

Introduction

The cardiovascular system has the principal role of circulating blood. This is essential for distributing oxygen from the lungs and carbon dioxide from the tissues. It also transports nutrients absorbed from the intestine to meet the metabolic needs of all the cells and organs of the body. It transports cellular wastes to the lungs and kidneys for elimination.

The heart

The diagram (Figure 11.1) shows the chambers of the heart and the layers of its walls.

There are two circulation systems of the heart:

The pulmonary circulation: Blood from the body is pumped by the right chambers of the heart to the lungs.

The systemic circulation: Blood from the lungs is pumped by the left heart chambers to all other organs and systems of the body.

The heart is a muscular pump. Mechanical pumping occurs because electrical activity triggers contraction of the muscle layer (*myocardium*). This contraction happens in a coordinated way because impulses travel from the *sino-atrial* node via the atrio-ventricular

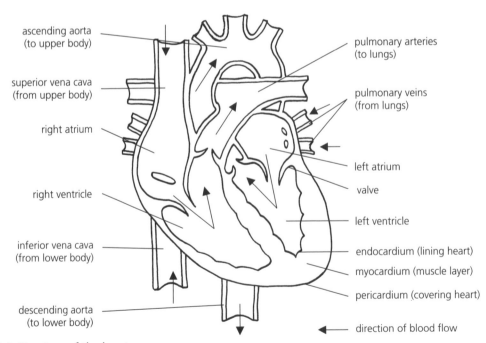

Figure 11.1 *Structure of the heart*

ascending aorta (to upper body)

superior vena cava (from upper body)

right atrium

right ventricle

inferior vena cava (from lower body)

descending aorta (to lower body)

pulmonary arteries (to lungs)

pulmonary veins (from lungs)

left atrium

valve

left ventricle

endocardium (lining heart)

myocardium (muscle layer)

pericardium (covering heart)

direction of blood flow

node in the right atrium. The impulse then travels across both atria, triggering a contraction, via the atrio-ventricular node and down the central septum of the heart before spreading through the walls of both ventricles. This triggers a contraction from the base of the ventricles, which ejects blood into the pulmonary artery for distribution to the lungs, and to the aorta for distribution to the cells and tissues. Blood can only flow in one direction because of the valves.

- The tricuspid valve between the right atrium and ventricle
- The mitral valve between the left atrium and ventricle
- The pulmonary valve which separates the pulmonary artery from the right ventricle
- The aortic valve which separates the aorta from the left ventricle.

These valves prevent a backflow of blood when the ventricles contract.

External nerves influence impulses in the sino-atrial node so that the heart can adapt to different circumstances by beating faster or slower.

The heart itself requires a blood supply so that its cells can function and this reaches heart muscle through the coronary arteries. These are the first branches off the aorta, the main artery leaving the left side of the heart.

As well as contracting to pump blood (called *systole*), it is important that between contractions there is enough time for the ventricles to fill with blood (*diastole*). BlooD flows through the coronary arteries during diastole. It is a normal response of the heart to increase its rate if there are problems in oxygenating the blood. However, very rapid or irregular heart rates may reduce the overall function of the heart in pumping blood if there is insufficient time for the ventricles to fill with blood between contractions. This will mean an increased demand on heart muscle cells that are already short of oxygen.

Irregular heart rates (*arrhythmias*) may be associated with disruption of the electrical activity of the heart: some arrhythmias are therefore life-threatening.

To function properly the heart muscle must both contract and stretch. A good blood flow through the arteries is also essential. Disease may occur as a result of coronary artery narrowing or from disease of the heart muscle itself.

Blood vessels

The role of the heart is to pump blood into the network of blood vessels that take oxygen and nutrients to the cells, tissues and organs. The vessels that leave the heart are arteries. They have thick muscular and elastic walls. Smaller branches off arteries are called *arterioles*. The structure of blood vessels prevents oxygen and nutrients from leaving the circulation until the blood leaves the arterioles and flows into the thin-walled *capillaries*.

All tissues are fed by a large capillary network. The capillary network is drained by *venules*; blood flows then into veins and so back to the heart via the vena cava.

- Deoxygenated blood from the general circulation to the vena cava and the right side of the heart
- Oxygenated blood from the lungs to the pulmonary veins and to the left side of the heart

Blood pressure

Oxygen and nutrients leave the circulation dissolved in fluid. It is therefore important that there is enough pressure against the walls of the capillaries to force this fluid out of the circulation, so that it can wash around the cells of the tissues. This force, which is measured in the large arteries, is called blood pressure.

There are two main components of blood pressure:

Cardiac output: That is the amount of blood pumped out of either side of the heart every minute.

Vascular resistance: Blood flowing through the vessels creates a friction against the wall of the blood vessels. If flow is through narrow vessels there is more resistance to flow. This raises the blood pressure.

Since many blood vessels have muscle in their walls and a *sympathetic nerve* supply to this muscle, the body can adjust blood pressure according to circumstances by contracting these muscular walls (increasing blood pressure) or relaxing them (decreasing blood pressure). Hormones also influence this muscle and therefore influence control of blood pressure. Increasing vascular resistance may be a compensation for difficulties in maintaining cardiac output, for example when a person is bleeding.

Abnormal function of cardiovascular system

Hypertension

Arterial blood pressure that is above the normal level is called *hypertension*. It can damage many blood vessels and organs causing, for example, strokes, kidney damage, heart failure or blindness due to damage to the eye's retina. Hypertension is often without symptoms and may only be picked up by screening.

Factors that may lead to hypertension include a family history of hypertension, cigarette smoking, heavy alcohol intake, high sodium diet, obesity and diabetes mellitus.

Heart failure

Heart failure is the inability of the heart to supply the body and the heart muscle with an adequate circulation of oxygen and nutrients to meet the needs of cells and tissues. Such failure may result from damage to heart muscle, damage to valves of the heart or from disturbed heart rhythm.

There are a large number of underlying factors contributing to heart failure. Rheumatic fever is a complication of a Group A streptococcal infection that can damage heart muscle and also heart valves, as can other infections including tuberculosis. Once heart valves are damaged, their *endocardial* covering layer may later be colonised by infection (bacterial endocarditis). Heart muscle is also affected by poor nutrition. Lack of vitamin B6 is especially associated with heart failure (Beriberi). Changes to blood vessels, resulting in narrowing (*sclerosis*), will affect the coronary arteries and therefore the function of the myocardium. Heart failure may be more severe in *anaemia* or

respiratory disease because oxygenation of the blood will be impaired.

Childbirth makes a lot of demands of the mother's heart and so prolonged labour may bring on heart failure, especially where there are local practices of heating the mother after childbirth or if her heart was damaged previously by rheumatic fever.

Effects of heart failure

If the heart is failing to pump enough blood, the main effects will be enlargement and overfilling of the chambers of the heart. This causes congestion of the veins draining into those chambers and of the capillary beds drained by those veins/venules. Congestion in these vessels will raise the blood pressure in them and this increased pressure will force out more fluid into the tissues. This excess tissue fluid is called *oedema*.

In some cases just one side of the heart will fail and this often leads to the other side failing at a later date.

Table 11.1 below shows some of the effects on the body.

Caring for a patient with heart failure
Left sided pulmonary oedema: Acute emergency

- Report the patient's condition so that diuretics and other drugs can be given quickly.
- Sit person up in a comfortable position, so clearing the lungs of fluid and aiding oxygenation of the blood.
- Give oxygen via a mask.
- Keep person at complete rest, to reduce oxygen demands.
- Monitor urine output, since kidney function may deteriorate; keep a fluid balance chart.

Table 11.1 Effects of heart failure on the body

Heart failure	Congestion (excessive collection of blood)	Subsequent effects
Left sided	In circulation to the lungs Pulmonary oedema	Severe shortness of breath, *dyspnoea*, cough
Right sided	In veins of legs and abdomen Congestion of the liver; kidneys	Oedema of the legs and ankles, abdominal discomfort, loss of appetite, tiredness
Both sides (Congestive)	In the pulmonary and systemic circulation	Effects of right sided failure with breathlessness on exertion

Table 11.2 Drug treatment for a patient with heart failure

Drug type	Examples	Common side effects
Diuretic drugs		
These act on the kidneys to produce more urine so reducing the blood volume and congestion.	Frusemide 20 mg to 80 mg daily	Can lower blood potassium levels leading to arrhythmias.
	Amiloride 5 mg to 20 mg daily	Drowsiness, nausea, dizziness. Can exacerbate gout or diabetes.
Vasodilating drugs		
These act on blood vessels to reduce return of blood to the congested heart and reduce resistance to the heart's pumping.	Isosorbide mononitrate 30 mg to 60 mg daily in divided doses	Headache, flushing, dizziness, postural hypotension
Inotropic drugs		
These increase the force of cardiac contraction.	Digoxin 0.625 mg to 0.25 mg daily Introduce gradually, observing the effects	Loss of appetite, nausea, arrhythmias, visual disturbance
Opiate analgesic drugs		
These reduce pain and anxiety but also dilate blood vessels to reduce return of blood to the congested heart.	Morphine 5–10 mg or Diamorphine 2.5–5 mg Can be given orally or by injection	Nausea, hypotension, constipation

Right sided pulmonary oedema

- Plan care recognising that activity will increase demands on the heart and will be exhausting. Monitor for fast pulse rate and breathlessness when exercising.
- Encourage to take plenty of rest; recognise risk of pressure sores is high because of oedema.
- Weigh patient every day (weight loss will be due to loss of oedema – one litre of fluid weighs one kilogram).
- Encourage small, frequent meals of high energy/high protein foods that are low in sodium – no added salt.
- Give prescribed drug treatment and monitor the effects.

Cardiac resuscitation

Cardiac arrest is when the heart suddenly stops beating. This can occur in patients with heart problems as a result of arrhythmias. Basic life support is needed to maintain adequate ventilation and circulation until skilled medical help arrives. It is important for nurses to practise this on a model so that when an emergency occurs, the nurse knows what to do. (See page 60.)

■ Activities

1. Why may anaemia make the effects of heart disease worse?
2. What is the reason for weighing someone with heart failure regularly?

Cardiac resuscitation

Always send for help as soon as possible.

- **Assess the situation:** Check for a response by gently shaking the shoulders. Turn on to back and tilt the head back. Clear any visible obstruction from the patient's mouth. Lift the chin to open the airway. Look, listen and feel for breathing.
- **If breathing:** Turn into the recovery position and go or send for help.
- **If not breathing:** Send someone for help, or if alone leave the patient and go for help. Return and start rescue breathing. Ensuring that the head is tilted and the chin is lifted, pinch the nose and open the mouth a little. Take a deep breath and place your lips around the mouth making sure you have a good seal. Give 2 slow effective breaths/inflations, each of which makes the chest rise and fall.

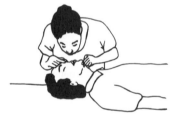

Figure 11.2 Position for ventilations

- **Assess patient for signs of circulation:** Check the carotid pulse.
- **If signs of circulation:** Continue rescue breathing. About every 10 breaths, recheck for circulation, taking no more than 10 seconds each time. Continue until the patient starts breathing on his own. Then if not fully conscious, turn into the recovery position.

- **If no signs of circulation:** Start chest compressions. Place the heel of the hand over the lower half of the sternum. Place the heel of the other hand on top of the first and interlock the fingers of both hands. Position yourself vertically above the patient's chest and with your arms straight, press down on the sternum with the heel of the hand only, to depress it 4–5 cm. Without losing contact between the hand and the sternum, release the pressure and repeat at a rate of about 100 times a minute.

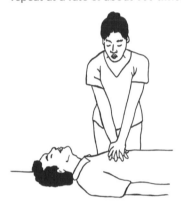

Figure 11.3 Position for cardiac compressions

- **Combine rescue breathing and chest compression:** After 15 chest compressions, tilt the head and lift the chin and give 2 effective breaths. Continue compressions and breaths in a ratio of 15:2. Continue resuscitation until qualified help arrives and takes over or the patient shows signs of life.

  If two people are available, work from opposite sides of the patient. A ratio of 15 compressions to 2 inflations should be used. Ventilations should take 2 seconds each, during which chest compressions should cease.

Health promotion

For the health of the heart and circulation it is important to do the following:

- Eat a good mixed diet, including food with a high fibre content: whole grain cereals and rice, whole grain bread, fruit and vegetables. Avoid foods high in fat and do not add too much salt to the diet.
- Check weight regularly and do not let yourself get obese.
- Take regular exercise, for example walking, running, cycling, swimming, football.
- Do not smoke tobacco.

12

Care of patients with blood disorders

Blood is the essential transport system of the body. The fluid of the blood maintains blood pressure. This chapter looks at some problems that occur in this system: principally *anaemia* and *haemorrhage*. It also covers the care of a patient requiring a blood transfusion.

Blood has a role in protection:
- White blood cells (WBCs) have an important role in destroying bacteria and viruses.
- Blood contains platelets and clotting factors that help to protect against blood loss.
- Proteins in the blood contribute to the balance of fluid in the blood and tissues.
- Special proteins called *antibodies* protect from many infections.

The blood

Blood is the transport medium of the body (see Figure 12.1).
- It carries oxygen, mainly combined with haemoglobin in the red blood cells (RBCs), from the lungs to the tissues.
- It transports nutrients absorbed from the intestine, to the liver and then to the tissues.
- It transports cell wastes to the lungs and kidneys for elimination.
- It distributes chemicals, such as hormones, that regulate cell functions.

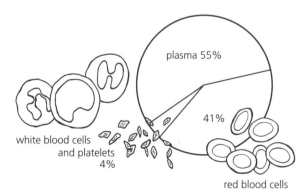

Figure 12.1 *Composition of blood*

white blood cells and platelets 4%

plasma 55%

41%

red blood cells

Haemorrhage

Loss of blood through haemorrhage will interfere with the function of the blood in delivering oxygen to the cells, since RBCs will be lost. Loss of the fluid part of the blood threatens to cause low blood pressure since cardiac output will fall. The more blood that is lost, the greater will be the effects. Sometimes bleeding can be seen but often it is happening inside the body and nurses need to know the signs of haemorrhage.

The body will try to compensate for the loss of blood by circulating the blood that remains more rapidly (*tachycardia*) and by increasing the rate of breathing (*tachypnoea*). Some blood vessels will close down, for example those to the skin. This will direct blood flow to the vital areas of the brain, heart, lungs and kidneys. The effects of these responses means that the signs of haemorrhage are:
- Cold, clammy, pale skin
- Tachycardia
- Tachypnoea
- Falling blood pressure.

When blood loss is severe there may be confusion and changes in consciousness as the brain is not getting enough oxygen.

Haemorrhage may occur as a result of trauma or as a complication of surgery. Internal bleeding is often due to ulcers or liver disease.

Table 12.1 Cells in the blood

(All of these are made in the bone marrow from stem cells)

Type	Function	Usual number per litre
Erythrocytes RBCs with haemoglobin	Transport of oxygen and carbon dioxide in combination to	4,200,000,000,000 5,800,000,000,000
Leucocytes WBCs	Protection against micro-organisms and parasites	5,000,000,000 to
a) Neutrophils	a) Destroy micro-organisms by intra-cellular enzymes (*phagocytosis*)	9,000,000,000 (increases in response to infection)
b) Basophils	b) Involved in inflammation	
c) Eosinophils	c) Involved in defence against parasites	
d) B Lymphocytes	d) Produce antibodies as part of acquired immunity	
e) T Lymphocytes	e) Also involved in acquired immunity (can directly destroy specific virus-infected or cancerous cells)	
f) Monocytes	f) Also involved in phagocytosis. Monocytes leave the blood to become tissue *macrophages*	
Thrombocytes (platelets)	A key role (along with plasma clotting factors) in the process of blood clotting	150,000,000,000 to 400,000,000,000

Nursing actions in haemorrhage

- If the bleeding can be seen, apply direct pressure to the bleeding site.
- If possible, raise the bleeding site (arm, leg) above the level of the person's heart.
- Always keep the person at rest, so the body needs less oxygen.
- Give oxygen via a mask.
- Get medical help, as the person may need to go for surgery to stop the bleeding.
- Monitor pulse and blood pressure every 15 minutes, to detect deterioration.
- Intravenous fluids are important in restoring the blood volume. This involves putting in a venous cannula and giving the following:
  - Clear crystalline fluids. Sodium chloride 0.9% will increase the volume in the blood vessels; glucose 5% will help to correct tissue cell dehydration; Ringer's lactate will help to reverse the acidosis that occurs with blood loss.
  - Blood transfusion. This is essential in severe haemorrhage in order to restore blood cells and increase the volume in the blood vessels.

- Platelets or Fresh Frozen Plasma. These will be used where there are blood clotting problems.

Anaemia

Haemorrhage reduces the oxygen-carrying capacity of the blood but so do conditions where there is a lack or abnormality of RBCs. The mucous membranes, for example the tongue and palms, become abnormally pale.

Anaemia is a lack of RBCs or a reduction in their oxygen-carrying capacity. Common causes are:
- Nutrient deficiency. This causes the commonest type of anaemia, which will occur if diet is poor or important nutrients are not absorbed from the intestine. Iron, vitamin C, vitamin B_{12} and folic acid are all important for making RBCs.
- Chronic blood loss from hookworms or excessive menstrual flow
- Bleeding from the gastro-intestinal tract
- *Haemolytic* anaemias. RBCs are destroyed sooner than normal.
- *Aplastic* anaemias. RBCs are not made in sufficient numbers.

Table 12.2 Haemoglobinopathies

Inherited disorders of haemoglobin structure or production

	Sickle cell disease	Sickle cell trait	Thalassaemia
Hb	Structure of haemoglobin is abnormal (haemoglobin S)	Haemoglobin is largely normal but some abnormal haemoglobin S exists	Abnormal haemoglobin results in fragile RBCs that break down easily. Several genes are responsible for the production of haemoglobin; the more genes affected the worse the effects (Thalassaemia Major and Thalassaemia Minor)
Health problems	RBCs will become unstable and form sickle shape, when blood oxygen is low. This can happen when someone has an infection, is stressed or cold (sickle cell crisis). Sickled cells break down easily, leading to anaemia and jaundice. Sickled cells clump together, *thrombosis*, blocking small blood vessels which can cause severe pain; *haematuria*; organ damage, cerebral thrombosis. **A sickle cell crisis can be life-threatening.**	No problems except if subjected to severe infection, stress or cold.	Profound anaemia; jaundice; swelling of bones, including bones of head, as bone marrow enlarges to increase production. Iron from breakdown of red blood cells can collect in the tissues
Treatment	**To prevent crisis** Protection from cold, dehydration and risk of infection; vaccination against infectious diseases; malaria protection (although sickle cell trait gives some protection against malaria). Oxygen must be given for several hours before and after any anaesthetic that a patient has. Planned supervised pregnancy and delivery **Care during a crisis** Pain relief; I.V. fluids to encourage blood flow and reduce risk of thrombosis; rest; reassurance; oxygen. Folic acid to help new red cell production but iron **must not** be given and blood transfusion **only if** severe anaemia. Excessive iron from breakdown of RBCs builds up in the body, damaging organs.		Repeated blood transfusion. Iron chelating agent (e.g. Desferrioxamine) to help excretion of iron from the body if this is available.
Support for family	Parents and relatives will need to know how to keep their child as healthy as possible. They will want explanation of the risks of their other children being affected. Parents may need support to cope with the death of a child or young adult as thalassaemia major and sickle cell disease are difficult to manage even if the child lives near the hospital.		

One of the main causes of haemolytic anaemia is that the cells have abnormal haemoglobin (Hb) in them, due to genetic factors (haemoglobinopathies, such as sickle cell disease and thalassaemia, see Table 12.2). Haemolysis also occurs in malaria and in severe infections.

As well as deficiency anaemias resulting from poor diet, or poor absorption, iron deficiency anaemia can happen where there is chronic bleeding. Most of the iron used in making RBCs comes from the breakdown of old, worn out RBCs.

Aplastic anaemia is usually due to bone marrow failure. Complete failure is extremely serious and only treatable with bone marrow or Stem cell transplants. This can only be done in major specialist centres.

Kidney disease often causes slight anaemia because the diseased kidneys do not release a hormone (*erythropoietin*) that stimulates the production of RBCs.

General care of a patient with anaemia

Finding the cause of the anaemia is important. A good clinical history will be needed:

- Do they or anyone else in the family have a history of anaemia?
- What does the person usually eat?
- Do they have bowel disease or symptoms that suggest they may have absorption problems?
- Have they noticed any blood loss, for example *menorrhagia*, red urine or black stools.
- Have they had fever or malaria?
- Do they have any cough or wheezing that might be due to hookworms?

Since the person will have reduced oxygen-carrying capacity they may need help with personal tasks, to prevent breathlessness or *angina* pains. Rest will be important but complete bed rest is not necessary unless the anaemia has led to heart failure.

In many cases, improving diet will help. Meat, especially liver, fish, green leafy vegetables, beans, peas and lentils contain important nutrients for RBC production. In deficiency anaemia it may be necessary to give iron, vitamin C, vitamin B_{12}, or folic acid by tablet or injection. Blood transfusion may be necessary in severe cases.

Care of a patient having blood transfusion

Blood transfusion is safe only if the blood of the patient has been cross-matched with the donated blood and screened for infections. In a laboratory blood must be observed for any incompatibility. Nurses must take great care to check that they have the right unit of blood for the right patient. Only in a real emergency, when a person has lost a great deal of blood and their life is threatened, should blood be given without it being cross-matched first. Then giving Group O, Rhesus negative blood may be justified and life-saving.

Before a blood transfusion is given, the donor blood should be tested for syphilis, hepatitis B and C and HIV.

Table 12.3 shows that those with AB+ blood can receive any blood (universal recipient) and O- can be given to anyone (universal donor).

Ideally a hospital will have a blood bank, where blood can be kept for emergencies.

Table 12.3 Compatibility of blood groups

Patient's blood group	Can receive	Must not be given	Best avoided (especially women of childbearing age)
A Rhesus Positive (A+)	A+. A-. O+. O-	B+.B-. AB+. AB-	
A Rhesus Negative (A-)	A-. O-	B+. B-. AB+. AB-	A+. O+
B Rhesus Positive (B+)	B+. B-. O+. O-	A+. A-. AB+. AB-.	
B Rhesus Negative (B-)	B-. O-	A+. A-. AB+. AB-	O+. B+
AB Rhesus Positive (AB+)	AB+. AB-. O+. O- B+. B-. A+. A-		
AB Rh Negative (AB-)	AB-. O-. B-. A-		A+.O+.B+. AB+
O Rhesus Positive (O+)	O+. O-	A+. A-. B+. B- .AB+. AB-	
O Rhesus Negative (O-)	O-	A+. A-. B+. B- .AB+. AB-.	O+

Blood must be stored at around 4°C and can be kept in these conditions for up to 36 days. Always check the expiry date before giving the blood.

If a hospital does not have a blood bank, relatives can donate blood in advance before a patient has an operation. They should be the right group, well themselves and between the ages of 17 and 65. Women having frequent pregnancies should **not** give blood.

Pp Procedure for giving a blood transfusion

- Collect the blood from the blood bank.
- Check (by two people, one of whom is a registered nurse or doctor): the patient's name; identification number; blood group; blood bag number; expiry date to ensure it is the right blood for the right person.
- Prepare for transfusion: insert intravenous cannula; run normal saline through the blood administration set (never use solutions containing dextrose, as it causes RBCs to clump together).
- If a diuretic drug, such as frusemide, has been prescribed give this just before the transfusion starts. Record the patient's output of urine.
- Begin the transfusion, running the blood at a steady rate. It must not be too fast to put the patient's heart under strain but should run fast enough to be finished within about four hours, since bL/od will begin to deteriorate after this time.
- For giving sets that have 15 drops per ml, a rate of 30 drops per minute will take about 3 hours 45 minutes (whole blood) or just less than 3 hours for packed cells.
- Keep a careful record of the amount of blood given.
- Observe the patient frequently, for signs of reaction to the blood. Temperature, pulse, respiration should be recorded every 15 minutes for the first hour and then, if no problems, every 30 minutes. Hourly blood pressure recordings (or more frequent if patient has heart disease).
- Speak to the patient to see how they are. What they say may make you aware that they are having a reaction to the blood.
- If any of the following reactions occur, stop the blood and call a doctor: high temperature; fast pulse rate; breathlessness; wheeziness; chest pain; pain in the lower back (from the kidneys); blood in the urine; rash; sudden collapse.

Health promotion

- Give extra iron and folic acid for women during the childbearing years.
- Encourage a good mixed diet, including nuts and pulses, meat, whole grain cereals, fruit and vegetables.
- Prevention and early treatment of malaria.
- Good hygiene to reduce the risk of hookworm and schistosomiasis.
- Genetic counselling and testing for haemaglobinopathies if available.
- Planned pregnancy will reduce risks to women with many children. Remember they have an increased need for food during pregnancy and breastfeeding.
- Those with sickle cell disease should learn to avoid situations that bring on a crisis.

■ Activities

1. Why might anaemia bring on chest pains in someone with heart disease?
2. Which blood type can be called the 'universal donor'?
3. What observations would you make on a patient having a blood transfusion?

13

Care of patients with orthopaedic problems

This chapter will cover the major problems affecting the musculoskeletal system, including joint injuries, fractures and their management, tuberculosis of the bone and osteomyelitis.

Introduction

The skeleton is a framework of bones and cartilage that protects organs and allows movement. There are 206 bones in the human body.

Bones are made up of two types of tissue. Compact tissue is hard bone and cancellous tissue is a spongy bone. These tissues are made up of two types of cells: *osteoblasts* for building up bone and *osteoclasts* for bone shaping. Bones are in different shapes, long, short, irregular or flat, depending on their function.

Bone contains red bone marrow which produces blood cells. Ninety-nine per cent of the body's calcium is found in the bones.

Joints or articulations

Bones are hard and therefore they have soft tissue between them to form joints. All joints have some movement ranging from immovable to freely movable.
- Immovable joints as in skull bones
- Slightly movable as in the spine
- Freely movable as in the hip joint
    Joints give movement and stability to the body.

Muscles

Muscles are made up of bundles of fibres. These shorten, contract and relax when stimulated by nerve impulses. Muscles make up 40–50 per cent of the body weight. Muscles are always in a state of slight contraction, ready for action. This is called muscle tone.

Muscles are attached to bones by the tendons and give strength and movement to the body.

Care of patients with joint injuries

Strain of the muscles occurs through injury to the ligaments around the joint which then causes swelling and pain. Dislocation can occur when the joint surfaces move apart through injury or disease. Babies may be born with a deformity, for example congenital dislocation of the hip. Dislocation causes pain and sometimes loss of function of the joint.

Nursing care of patients with a joint injury
- Rest the limb and raise it if there is swelling. A cold compress may be applied.
- The doctor will move the bones into their normal position under anaesthetic if there is a dislocation.
- Pain control should be given. The limb should be supported by a sling or bandages to help reduce the pain.
- A sterile dressing should be applied if there is a wound to the skin.

Care of patients with fractures

A fracture is a break in the bone, caused through injury.
- A closed fracture has a broken bone and no open wound.
- An open fracture has a broken bone and a wound. This means that bacteria can enter the body and therefore the wounds should be covered with sterile dressings.
- A greenstick fracture is when one side of the bone is broken and the other side bends. This is seen in children as their bones are soft.

- Pathological fractures occur in bones weakened by disease, for example *osteomyelitis* and cancers.
- Depressed fractures are when the bone is pressed down on other organs, for example in head injuries. This can cause neurological problems.

Key aspects of nursing care of patients with a fracture

- Do not move a patient with a fracture until a splint has been applied as movement may cause further injury.
- Give pain relief as necessary.
- Cover open wounds with sterile dressings and give antibiotics.
- Patients with deep penetrating wounds should have the wound irrigated and be given tetanus antitoxin.
- Patients with severe blood loss should be given intravenous fluids. Observe the patient for further loss of blood and shock (see Chapters 5 and 12).
- X-rays are taken to show the extent of the fracture.
- Some patients will need to go to theatre for surgical repair. Bones are sometime fixed with screws, nails, plates, tractions or plaster of Paris.
- The patient should be nursed on a firm mattress.
- The diet should include protein and calcium to help healing of the wound.

Most of the complications that can arise are due to immobility and can also happen with other orthopaedic conditions.

Potential complications of immobility

Pressure sores and lack of cleanliness: Check that all splints, plasters and other aids are not causing any redness of the skin. Help the patient to move around the bed. They may not be able to wash themselves so should be given help with all aspects of personal hygiene.

Urinary retention/infection: Poor fluid intake and lack of movement can cause infection. Make sure that the patient has a high fluid intake and observe the urine for smell.

Hypostatic pneumonia: This is due to lack of movement. Teach and encourage deep breathing exercises. This will also make sure that there is a good supply of oxygen to the tissues to help with healing.

Deep vein thrombosis: This is also due to lack of movement. The patient should be taught exercises to reduce the risk. If the patient is unable to move they may need to be given *anticoagulants*.

Specific potential problems with fractures

Confusion: This can occur in elderly patients particularly if they are moved away from their home. It can also be caused by dehydration or infection.

Fat embolism: This is a serious complication that may occur if there have been multiple fractures of the long bones. The patient may become restless, tachycardic and confused.

Pp Nursing care of patient with a plaster of Paris

The aim of a plaster is to give support and keep the bone in a good position for healing. Plaster does not gain its full strength until it is completely dry and this takes 24 hours for a small arm cast and as much as 96 hours for a full body cast.

- A fracture board should be placed under the mattress to give support.
- Rest the limb on a pillow covered with a plastic cover and a towel, which will help absorb the moisture, to prevent swelling and pressure. The towel needs to be changed as it gets wet to help the plaster dry quickly.
- The plaster must not rest on a hard surface while it is drying as this can cause uneven pressure.
- Wet plasters should not be covered but have plenty of air circulating to help with the drying.
- Limbs which have plasters on them should be raised to help the venous return and prevent oedema.
- Make sure that the plaster dries completely.
- Check the warmth, colour, movement and feeling in the extremity every 2 to 4 hours. If the patient has a plaster on the forearm, they should be able to move their fingers freely. If they have a plaster on the lower leg, they should be able to move all their toes. If the plaster is too tight, the circulation can be restricted leading to *gangrene* (see Figure 13.1). Equipment should always be ready so that a plaster can be removed urgently, if there are signs that the circulation has become restricted.
- Each day, the toes or fingers should be carefully washed and dried. This gives the nurse the opportunity to see that the circulation is satisfactory. If the toes or fingers are cold, oedematous, blue or painful, it may be necessary to split the plaster immediately.

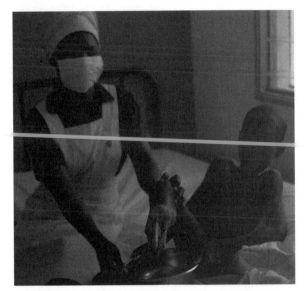

Figure 13.1 *Gangrene resulting from a splint that was too tight*

- After a few days, the swelling around the fracture will get less and the plaster may become too loose. This can lead to sores due to rubbing.
- Sometimes a sore can form under the plaster and there may be a burning pain and offensive smell. This is more likely to happen when the plaster is covering a bony prominence. A window can be cut in the plaster over the area and a dressing applied. Sometimes it is necessary to remove the whole plaster.
- Pain in a patient who has a plaster must not be ignored. It may be due to the development of a plaster sore, or lack of blood circulating to the area causing tissue damage.
- Before the patient goes home they will need to be taught how to care for the plaster. The plaster must be kept dry.

Pp **Care of the skin and limb following removal of the plaster**

- The patient should be warned that the skin underneath the plaster will be dry and flaky.
- The limb can be soaked in warm oil and then gently washed and dried. It must not be scrubbed.
- The limb must be handled gently, as it will feel weak and may ache. It may be supported on a pillow.

- Exercises should be encouraged so that the limb gains in movement and strength, but this must be done gradually.

Traction

When a long bone is fractured, for example the femur, the strength of the muscles can lead to an overlapping of the bone ends, so that if nothing is done, the bone will heal in such a way that there is permanent shortening of the limb. To avoid this, traction is applied to provide a counter pull to the muscle. Sometimes traction is used to immobilise inflamed joints or to correct deformities.

Types of traction

Traction may be:

Fixed: A pulling force is applied between two fixed points, for example Gallows traction which can be used in young children with fractured femurs (see Figure 13.2).

Balanced: The pulling force is applied between two mobile points which can allow the patient to move about the bed. In this type of traction, weights and pulleys are involved (see Figure 13.3).

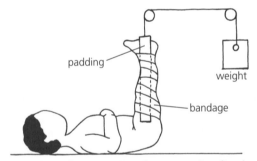

Figure 13.2 *Gallows traction demonstrating fixed and skin traction*

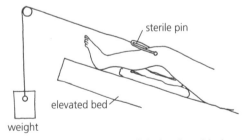

Figure 13.3 *Demonstration of skeletal and balanced traction*

Skin: This can either be fixed or balanced. Special sticking plaster that does not stretch is applied to both sides of the limb (usually the leg), which is then bandaged carefully leaving the knee free. Cords are attached to the plaster and weights applied. The foot of the bed is raised. Only limited weights can be applied, so it is usually used in the case of children.

Skeletal: For adults, or where the fracture is severe, or the skin damaged, skeletal traction is more usual. The patient has to go to theatre for the insertion of a sterile pin. A metal stirrup is then attached to the pin ends and cord fastened to it. Weights are then attached to the cord and the foot of the bed elevated.

Pp Specific nursing care of a patient on traction

- Check that any splints are in the correct position and that the skin under the ring is clean and dry.
- Check that all cords are taut and weights are hanging freely.
- Remove any bandages daily to check for rashes or pressure sores.
- If skeletal traction has been used, check the site of the pin daily for any signs of infection. The sites should be cleaned and dressed with an iodine preparation.

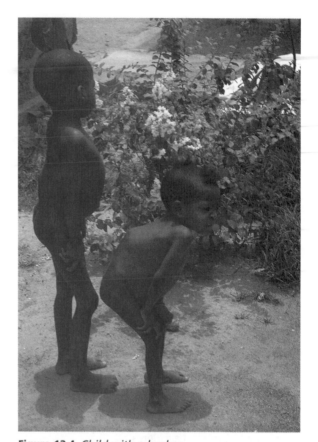

Figure 13.4 *Child with a kyphos*

Nursing care of patients with tuberculosis of the spine (Pott's disease) See Chapter 25

The vertebral column may be affected by the tubercle bacillus at any point throughout its length. The most commonly affected areas are the vertebrae in the thoraco-lumbar regions. Children are particularly susceptible to the disease in this region. Collapse of the vertebral bodies may produce a swelling of the spinous processes and this causes an acute 'hump' on the patient's back called a *kyphos* (see Figure 13.4). The swelling may put pressure on the spinal cord and this can cause a paralysis of the lower limb called a Pott's paraplegia.

Management of Pott's disease

- It may be necessary for the patient to go to theatre for decompression of the spinal cord.

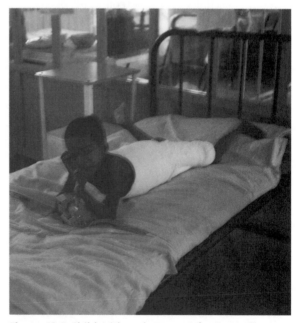

Figure 13.5 *Child with a plaster cast for Pott's disease*

- Anti-tubercular drugs must be given (see Chapter 25).
- Rest is necessary to allow healing of the bone. This is best achieved by either using a plaster bed or a plaster cast (see Figure 13.5).
- The patient will need a good diet with plenty of calcium to aid healing, and a high fluid intake to prevent urinary infections.

Nursing care of a patient following an amputation

Amputation is loss of part or all of a limb. It is a mutilation of the body and so the nurse must be very understanding when she is caring for the patient. If the amputation is due to trauma there is little time to prepare the patient and the family but if it is planned then careful physical and mental preparation of the patient is possible.

Reasons for amputations

- Peripheral vascular disease. Caused by poor circulation leading to irreversible death of tissue
- Trauma. Where there has been excessive damage to tissue due to bomb blast, land mines, burns, crush injury or road accidents
- Cancers of the bone
- Severe infections such as osteomyelitis or gas gangrene
- Deformity which cannot be corrected. An amputation may help the patient to lead a more active life.

Key aspects of nursing a patient with an amputation of a limb

The aim of surgery is to provide a well moulded stump that is able to take a *prosthesis*.

Pp Physical preparation for amputation of lower limb

- The toe nails should be cut and cleaned and the skin washed well.
- The patient is taught exercises to strengthen the good leg and helped to practise lifting their buttocks from the bed. It is also helpful if they practise lying on their front for part of each day as this position will be necessary following surgery.

- The patient is taught to walk with crutches. They will need to strengthen the muscles of their upper body.

Psychological care

The patient will need time to get used to the idea of an amputation and they must be given good explanations of why it is necessary and what will happen afterwards (see Chapter 8). They may be warned that following an amputation they may feel as if they have pain in the limb that has been amputated (phantom pain). It may help them if they can talk to a patient who has had the same operation done. They may be worrying about:

- Loss of function. They will wonder how the loss of a limb will affect their life and whether they will be able to work and look after themselves.
- Body image. Their body has been altered and they may worry about the effect this will have on their friends and relatives.

Pp Specific post-operative care for amputation of lower limb

- Observe the stump carefully for haemorrhage. The top bedclothes should be divided so that the stump can be easily seen, and the bandages watched for staining.
- The stump should be carefully positioned, flat on the bed and lying close to the good leg. A towel can be placed over the stump and fixed with sandbags.
- Pain relief must be given.
- The patient should be encouraged to lie prone twice each day for at least an hour to prevent flexure contractures.
- Drains may be removed at 48 hours if there is no more drainage. The stump should be carefully bandaged to help it keep a good shape. Sutures will be removed at 10–14 days if the wound is well healed.
- The patient will need to be encouraged to do deep breathing exercises and to exercise the good leg. They will be encouraged to move around and may sit out of bed for short periods after 3 days. After 10 days they can be helped to walk with crutches. To begin with they may find it difficult to get their balance.

- A prosthesis may be fitted after 28 days if the stump has healed well. It is important to see that the prosthesis does not cause any rubbing or sores to the stump.
- Before they are discharged the nurse should check that they will be able to manage to care for themselves at home.

Amputation of upper limb

Preparation and post-operative care will be similar, but the patient will have different problems following surgery. If the limb (hand/arm) that has been amputated is the one that they use most, they will have to get used to using their other hand. They will also find there are many things they can no longer do, as they only have one hand.

Osteomyelitis

This is a bacterial infection of bone tissue. It is usually caused by the **Staphylococcus aureus**, but can be caused by **Streptococcus, Pneumococcus** or other strains of **Staphylococcus**.

Causes

- From an open fracture
- From infected tissue near the bone
- Blood borne from other parts of the body where there is an infection, for example from a boil, tooth abscess or infected tonsils

Bone which is growing is more commonly affected, so it is usually seen in children and adolescents. Patients with sickle cell anaemia are also more likely to get the infection.

The infection starts in the bone marrow, pus is formed and collects in the bone tissue. Pressure builds up inside the bone and the exudate breaks through to the space under the *periosteum*. Eventually the periosteum will be stripped away from the bone interrupting the blood supply and leading to the death of that part of the bone. This is called a *sequestrum*.

Nursing care of the patient with osteomyelitis

- Intravenous antibiotics are given in large doses once the causative organism has been isolated. Antibiotics will be needed for several weeks but may be changed to oral once the infection begins to respond.
- Pain control. This is a very painful condition, so in the early stages large doses of intramuscular or oral analgesia will be required (see Chapter 7).
- The affected limb should be immobilised with sandbags, or in splints or traction.
- Sometimes the patient will need to go to theatre for the removal of dead bone or drainage of pus.

Once the acute phase is over, the patient can be helped to mobilise again. With osteomyelitis of the lower limb, they should not be allowed to weight bear for several weeks as the bone will be weak. Crutches will be necessary until new bone has had time to form.

■ Activities

1. Why are open fractures more serious than closed fractures?
2. What observations should be made on a patient who has just had a plaster of Paris applied?
3. Which patients are more likely to get osteomyelitis and why?

14

Care of patients with neurological conditions

This chapter covers important aspects of the nervous system's function. It considers the care of patients who have fits, head injuries, reduced level of consciousness, paralysis, meningitis, and those having lumbar punctures.

Introduction

The nervous system is the body's control centre. It is involved in how we see the world around us, control of physical activity, vital functions such as breathing and heart rate, thought, speech, memory and intellectual activities. Neurological problems cause many different difficulties.

The nervous system

The nervous system consists of brain, spinal cord and nerves distributed throughout the body (*peripheral* nerves). It is responsible for movement, sensory stimuli, behaviour, and regulation of internal systems and organs. Nerve fibres are bundles of elongated cells – *neurons* and *neuroglia*.

- Neurons carry electrical signals through the body.
- Neuroglia provide support, nutrition and electrical insulation for neurons. They are important as primary tumours of the nervous system usually start in neuroglia tissue.

The brain and spinal cord are covered by three protective layers of connective tissue known as *meninges*. They are surrounded by cerebrospinal fluid which also protects the delicate tissue.

Coordinating and transmitting neuron activity

The billions of neurons that make up the nervous system must work in coordination. Activity in neurons

spreads to receptors on others across minute gaps between them called *synapses* (see Figure 14.1). Impulses cross the synapses one way using neurotransmitters – chemical messengers. Some diseases are associated with disturbance of these (for example Parkinson's disease, myasthenia gravis, depression, schizophrenia). Many drug treatments are aimed at blocking, stimulating or replacing them. Some drug side effects occur as a result of unintended effects on neurotransmitters and receptors.

Functions can be broadly divided into motor and sensory:

- Sensory neurons supply information to the brain about what is happening to the body.
- Motor neurons send instructions from the brain to the body to perform tasks.

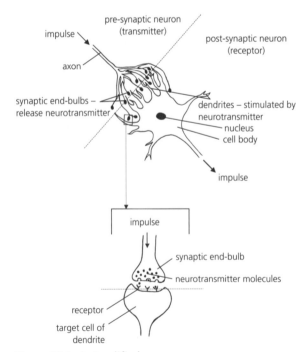

Figure 14.1 *A simplified synapse*

The central nervous system (CNS)

The central nervous system includes the brain and spinal cord. The brain can be divided into two broad areas, the upper or fore brain, and lower or mid and hind brain (see Figure 14.2).

The upper or fore brain (cerebrum)

The cerebrum consists of white and grey matter. The grey matter lies on the outside (cerebral cortex) and is made up of the cell bodies of the neurons. The white matter is made up of the axons coming from these cell bodies and their supporting glial cells; so much of the brain is made up of neuron pathways.

The cerebrum can be thought of as the conscious brain, since it is here that the main sensory messages (touch, pressure, pain, hearing, sight) are processed and from where movement of joints and muscles is coordinated (motor functions). The cerebrum is also responsible for language, memory and mood. Specific areas of the brain have specific functions so disease or injury to one area will have a different result from problems in another. Symptoms such as loss of vision can themselves suggest where problems lie.

The cerebrum is divided into two halves (hemispheres) connected by a bridge of neurons. Each has specialised functions:

- Language, reasoning and right hand dominance (left hemisphere)
- Left hand control, creativity, imagination and sensory awareness (right hemisphere).

The pathways between the cerebrum and the spinal cord cross over. Stroke occurring in the left hemisphere can be used as an example of how this affects a person. Right sided paralysis often results

and may be accompanied by speech problems as both areas are usually controlled from the left brain.

The lower, or mid and hind brain (cerebellum and brain stem)

The lower brain consists of the cerebellum and brain stem:

The cerebellum: This is positioned under the back of the cerebrum and also consists of grey and white matter. It is connected to many other areas of the nervous system. It is responsible for balance and posture and uses messages from the inner ear to help with this.

The brain stem: This lies in front of the cerebellum and connects it and the cerebrum to the spinal cord. It acts as a neuron pathway and coordination centre. It contains the 'vital centres' for survival and maintaining essential processes. Body temperature, heart rate, breathing and blood pressure are controlled here so injury can rapidly lead to death. Sleep, hormone activity, sexual behaviour and some aspects of digestion such as hunger and blood sugar levels are also coordinated here.

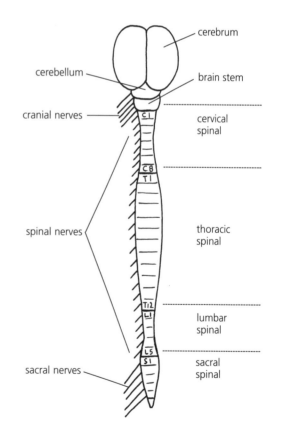

Figure 14.3 *The nerves of the central nervous system*

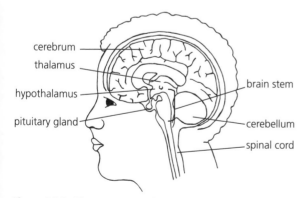

Figure14.2 *The structure of the brain*

The spinal cord

The spinal cord is an essential part of the central nervous system and carries two-way communications for both sensory and motor functions (see Figure 14.3).

- Many of the sensory messages from the skin, muscles and organs such as the bladder and intestine have to travel through central sensory neurons in the spinal cord to reach the sensory areas of the brain.
- Instructions from the brain to muscles of limbs and internal organs pass through the upper motor neurons of the spinal cord. This includes much of the non-conscious coordination of vital functions.

Spinal reflexes

Some other responses happen directly within the spinal cord without involving the brain. It takes time for sensory impulses to travel to the brain and motor impulses to travel back. The body may need a more rapid response than this and this is achieved via a spinal reflex which does not require involvement by the brain (see Figure 14.4). These spinal reflexes are important to a lot of functions, especially maintaining muscle tone. They are also very important for protecting against injury, for example from heat or sharp objects. Even a person with a severed spinal cord may still be able to withdraw a limb in response to a painful stimulus, but not be aware of it.

The peripheral nervous system (PNS)

This includes all of the nerves not classified as CNS. The spinal cord is a key area for two-way communication between the CNS and PNS:

Peripheral sensory neurons: These carry impulses in from the body to synapses with central sensory neurons in the spinal cord.

Lower motor neurons: These carry impulses via synapses from upper motor neurons out to the body to carry out functions.

Cranial, sacral and spinal nerves have important roles:

Cranial nerves: These are bundles of sensory and motor neurons serving areas such as the face, mouth, eyes and ears. They bypass the spinal cord as messages are carried directly between them and the brain stem and perform many unconscious functions (see the autonomic nervous system below). The largest cranial nerve, the vagus, has wider importance as it serves organs and glands such as the heart, lungs, gastro-intestinal tract, liver and pancreas.

Sacral nerves: These are bundles of sensory and motor neurons which synapse with the sacral segments of the spinal cord, and serve organs such as the bladder and anus.

Spinal nerves: These contain peripheral sensory and lower motor neurons, including neurons of the sympathetic nervous system (see below).

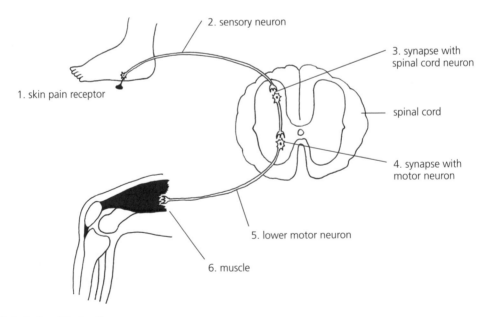

Figure 14.4 *A simplified reflex arc*

The autonomic nervous system

This is a functional term often used to describe those peripheral nerves and groups of cells (ganglia) that are also involved in controlling involuntary functions, for example heart and blood vessels, salivary glands, stomach and intestines. It works together with the CNS and allows the body to remain stable but respond to emergencies and stress, then to return to normal afterwards. Two opposing but balancing systems take care of these responses:

The sympathetic nervous system: Stimulation provides the emergency response, for example increased heart rate, breathing and blood supply to muscles to allow for escape, and decreased urine production and bowel activity during the stress period. It produces its effects:

- via spinal nerves supplied directly to target organs
- to the adrenal gland which secretes hormones such as adrenaline into the bloodstream.

The parasympathetic nervous system: Stimulation returns heart rate and breathing to normal and allows functions such as digestion and urinary output to recommence. It consists of the:

- cranial nerves
- sacral nerves which connect to the sacral segments of the spinal cord.

Care of patients with neurological problems

Seizures (fits)

Seizures occur as a result of unchecked electrical activity spreading between neurons to involve large parts of the brain. There are many different causes including:

- tumours and diseases that cause an increase in the intracranial pressure, for example cerebral

bleeding or oedema, and inflammation, for example meningitis and encephalitis
- alteration in blood chemistry, for example *hypocalcaemia, hypoglycaemia, hyponatraemia* or *hypernatraemia, hyperbilirubinaemia*
- *idiopathic* epilepsy or epilepsy as a result of previous brain injury.

The symptoms that an individual experiences will depend on what areas of the brain are involved. If sensory areas only are affected then seizures may only involve the person experiencing strange feelings, sights or sounds. If motor control areas are affected, the seizure will involve muscle movement, often with violent thrashing about of the arms and legs (tonic-clonic or grand-mal seizure).

Care of patients having seizures

- Observe the seizure. Note:
  - how it begins and which areas of the body are affected – one sided or the whole body (this may give a clue to which part of the brain is affected)
  - whether or not the person loses consciousness
  - how long the seizure lasts.
- Do not attempt to restrain or move the person, unless in a very dangerous situation. Do not try to put anything into the mouth.
- If seizures come in an uninterrupted series, the person urgently needs drugs to stop them.
- After the seizure, put the person in the recovery position until recovered completely.
- If the person has never had seizures before, reassure them that this may be a single incident and does not necessarily mean a diagnosis of epilepsy.
- If the person has had seizures before, check and report:
  - drug treatment
  - the frequency of seizures
  - whether this frequency has changed recently.

Table 14.1 Drugs for use in epilepsy

Situation	Drug	Dosage
Emergencies e.g. repeated seizures	Intravenous diazepam	10–20 mg
	Intravenous clonazepam	1 mg
	Rectal diazepam	0.5 mg/kg
Long-term control of epilepsy (grand-mal)	Therapy is best with a single drug:	
	• phenytoin	150–300 mg daily
	• sodium valproate	600 mg daily (in 2 divided doses), increasing if necessary up to 2500 mg daily (in 3 divided doses)
	• phenobarbitone	90–360 mg daily (in 3 divided doses)

Head injury

Road traffic and other accidents may result in trauma to the head and neck. This may interfere with the function of nerve tissue of the brain or spinal cord. Accurate assessment is vital.

Assessment tools

Scales are useful tools for standardising assessment. They make it easier to recognise improvement or deterioration when different nurses care for the same patient over a period of time. The Glasgow coma scale reflects alterations of nerve function as a result of rising intracranial pressure from bleeding or *oedema*. It is composed of three parameters (see Table 14.2) and is scored between 3 and 14.

- 3 is most serious response indicating severe injury.
- 14 is the best response indicating minor damage.

A change from a low to a high score shows that there is improvement. A downward change may indicate rising intracranial pressure and should be reported.

When assessing children, it is easier to use the Blantyre coma scale (see Chapter 46).

Other assessment tools are:

- Pupil size. Pupils should constrict rapidly in response to bright light. First observe the size of each pupil, noting if they are not equal and test them by shining a small torch into each eye. A rise in the intracranial pressure results in pupils that are slow to respond to light and unequal in size.
- Pulse rate. Rising intracranial pressure causes the pulse rate to fall.

Table 14.2 The Glasgow coma scale

Eyes open	Best verbal response	Best motor response
Spontaneously 4	Orientated 5	Obeys commands 5
To speech 3	Confused 4	Localises pain 4
To pain 2	Inappropriate words 3	Flexion to pain 3
Never 1	Incomprehensible 2	Extension to pain 2
1	None 1	None 1

- Blood pressure. Rising intracranial pressure causes a rise in blood pressure.

It is important to make regular assessments, usually every 15 minutes. Patients may arrive with a slightly reduced Glasgow coma scale and rapidly deteriorate. This may be due to bleeding inside the skull compressing brain tissue or to the brain swelling. Pupils may be normal at first and then dilate as intracranial pressure rises.

Other nursing care

As well as frequent observation, it is important to try to protect brain tissue from further injury. Since it is living tissue any reduction in oxygen supply will cause further damage. Blood loss or swelling will reduce the delivery of oxygen to brain tissue. A normal response to low oxygen in tissues is that blood vessels dilate. If this occurs in the head it will cause some fluid to leak out adding to brain swelling. **Therefore, giving oxygen, controlling bleeding and keeping the person quiet and at rest are vital.** If intracranial pressure is thought to be rising, the situation must be reported to the doctor or nurse in charge immediately. The patient may need to go to theatre, or need drugs to reduce the brain swelling. Fluid intake should be restricted.

Reduced level of consciousness

Patients with head injuries and those having convulsions are likely to have a reduced level of consciousness. Many other neurological conditions, for example stroke, meningitis/encephalitis, cerebral malaria, drug overdose are also likely to affect consciousness with special care being necessary (see below).

Key aspects of nursing individuals with impaired consciousness

- Check the safety of the airway and assess breathing: If necessary use the recovery position to aid breathing.
- Use coma scale to assess degree of neurological impairment.
- Ensure limbs are well-supported with pillows with joints slightly extended to prevent joint contractures (particularly if there is weakness of one side of the body as in stroke). Put joints through a range of movements several times daily.
- Unless turning themselves, turn the patient every 2–4 hours to prevent pressure sore and reduce risks of chest infection.

- Talk to the patient whenever you are with them, explaining anything you are about to do. This stimulates the sensory nervous system. Consider playing tape-recorded music as stimulation.
- Keep patient's eyelids closed to prevent dry eyes and surface ulceration.
- Attend to the patient's oral care and general hygiene.
- If impaired consciousness continues, give attention to the patient's fluid and food intake. **It is unsafe to give drinks by mouth** but alternatives are:
  - intravenous fluid
  - liquid food through a nasogastric tube.
- Contain incontinence using urinary catheter, sheath or incontinence pads. Record bowel actions, assess and treat for constipation.

Role of relatives and friends in the care of patients with reduced consciousness

Some of the care can be given to patients' relatives and friends to do if the ward is busy, as they are able to remain with patients constantly. They can observe for any change in their breathing, their behaviour, any fits and their response to pain. They should be taught what to look for and who to report to if problems occur. Family and friends can take a special role in talking to patients to stimulate them.

Spinal cord injury

Spinal cord injury and paralysis can occur through motor accidents, sports injuries, falls, stabbings, beatings and shootings. It is often associated with damage to bones of the vertebral column and with interruption to blood supply. Tumours and tuberculosis of the spine can also result in cord damage and *paraplegia*. Since the spinal cord is the route for most sensory and motor impulses, including sympathetic and some parasympathetic activity (see above), spinal cord damage potentially disrupts many nerve functions. Paralysis is common (*quadriplegia* if cervical spine, or paraplegia if thoracic spine). See information box below for key aspects of nursing care.

Autonomic hyperreflexia

This is a **life-threatening** syndrome that can occur weeks or months after upper spinal cord injury. It is usually triggered by a full bladder or rectum. Massive sympathetic nerve stimulation causes blood vessels in

Key aspects of nursing individuals after spinal cord injury	
Problem and cause	**Nursing care/prevention**
Hypotension because of impaired sympathetic nerve function	Monitor blood pressure and circulation.
Poor function of cooling mechanisms because of impaired autonomic nervous system	Monitor temperature for rise.
Reduced nerve stimulation to bladder and bowel	Monitor bladder size for retention of urine and constipation. Treat if necessary.
High risk of pressure sores because of immobility, impaired circulation and sensory awareness	Turn every 2 hours, preventing further spinal damage by using a spinal board or pillows to support the vertebral column.
Joint contractures	Ensure limbs are well-supported with pillows, with joints slightly extended. Put joints through a range of movements several times daily.
Emotional distress and anxiety about the future	Acknowledge the distress of the patient and family and try to give psychological support.
Increased nutritional needs and inability to feed	Encourage good nutritional intake. Give help with feeding if quadriplegic.
Impaired spinal reflexes	Observe for the gradual return of spinal reflexes: indicated by joint flexion in toes, feet, legs and emptying of bowel and bladder.

the trunk and limbs to constrict (unopposed by any input from the brain-stem control centres). Therefore, extreme hypertension occurs. Medical staff should be informed immediately.

Rehabilitation following spinal cord injury

The aim of rehabilitation is to promote the activity of the individual, especially through the development of upper body strength (unless quadriplegic) and self-care. This applies to feeding, attending to personal hygiene, dressing, managing elimination and mobilising with the aid of a wheelchair. Different members of the health care team should be involved where possible. Physiotherapists have a vital role with mobilisation; local workshops may be able to make mobility aids. Family members should be included in the planning, as they will be involved in the long-term care. Each individual will experience a period of psychological adjustment and will need support. Another patient with a similar injury may be willing to give advice and practical help.

Meningitis

Meningitis is the inflammation of the meninges, which cover the brain and spinal cord, usually caused by viruses, or bacteria such as Meningococci. Bacterial meningitis is generally more serious. Cryptococcal meningitis is seen in patients with AIDS and is very difficult to treat. Tuberculous meningitis is slower to develop. See Chapters 25, 32 and 46.

Symptoms of meningitis
- Fever
- Vomiting
- Drowsiness and reduced consciousness
- Severe headache
- Neck stiffness
- Dislike of bright light (*photophobia*)

Meningococcal septicaemia may also occur as a complication of meningococcal meningitis. Bacteria release toxins into the blood which break down the walls of blood vessels allowing blood to leak out under the skin. This causes a rash of red or brownish pin-prick spots which develop into purple bruises and blood blisters. Septicaemia is a threat to major organs like the liver (see Chapter 16) and kidneys.

It is important to differentiate between cerebral malaria and meningitis, especially in children. The neck stiffness is worse in meningitis. Cerebral malaria can cause continuous fitting and coma.

Effective antibiotic treatment can be given if symptoms are identified early. Diagnosis may be helped by a lumbar puncture. Lumbar puncture may also be done to investigate other neurological conditions. Nurses need to know how to assist in doing a lumbar puncture.

Pp Assisting at lumbar puncture

- The individual needs to understand what will happen and why. If they are restless, some mild sedation may be necessary.
- Aseptic technique is vital.
- Prepare equipment: sterile gloves, skin cleanser e.g. iodine, local anaesthetic e.g. lignocaine, lumbar puncture needle, manometer (to measure spinal fluid pressure if required), specimen bottles, dressing to cover the puncture site.
- Help the patient into position: on the left side, knees drawn up towards chest, with neck and spine flexed to allow entry of the lumbar puncture needle between the spines of the lumbar vertebrae. Keeping the patient in the correct position whilst the procedure is performed is extremely important. It may be necessary for the nurse to kneel on the far side of the bed to hold the patient steady.
- There is a risk of 'coning' especially if intracranial pressure is high or more than a few ml of spinal fluid is removed. (Coning is a complication where pressure around the brain pushes nerve tissue through the hole in the base of the skull causing death.) The doctor should examine the *fundi* of the eyes prior to the procedure to give some indication of the intracranial pressure. A lumbar puncture should **not** be performed if the pressure is high.
- Label specimens accurately and send to the laboratory.
- Advise the patient to lie flat in bed for at least 6 hours following lumbar puncture.
- Offer drinks. Check the needle entry site for bleeding or discharge.

Health promotion

- Encourage good nutrition. All B vitamins are needed for healthy nerves: good sources are green vegetables, grains, liver, red meat. Overcooking vegetables destroys these water soluble vitamins.
- Avoid overcrowding and sleeping close together during a meningitis epidemic. Close contacts can be given rifampicin. Immunisation against some meningococcal strains is now available (see Chapter 24 and 46).
- Prevention of malaria (see Chapter 46).
- Diabetes can damage the nervous system, so develop screening programmes by testing urine for glucose and give advice to control the condition (see Chapter 19).
- Hypertension can lead to strokes, so monitor patient's blood pressure (see Chapter 11).
- Avoid obesity.
- Encourage the use of seat belts to reduce head injuries in car accidents.
- Encourage good practice on industrial sites, for example wearing protective hats, and safe environments to reduce the risk of falls.

■ Activities

1. How would you assess someone's level of consciousness?
2. After an upper spinal cord injury, why would it be important to measure the patient's blood pressure regularly?

15

Care of patients with gastro-intestinal problems

This chapter looks at some problems that occur in the gastro-intestinal system, principally diarrhoea, constipation, intestinal obstruction and disease of the liver and biliary tract.

Introduction

The gastro-intestinal tract enables us to break down complex foods into nutrients that can be absorbed into the bloodstream. These nutrients include *polypeptides*, *amino acids* and simple sugars. The blood transports these nutrients to the liver and from there to the tissues so that they can be used for cell growth, cell activity and the functions of the body. The intestines are also important to fluid balance, through the absorption of fluid.

The digestive system

The digestive system is a long muscular tube that begins at the mouth and ends at the anus (see Figure 15.1). It consists of the oesophagus, the stomach, the small and large intestines, the rectum plus accessory organs such as the liver and pancreas. These release large amounts of fluid containing chemicals into the system to digest food.

The system works in two ways to digest food: mechanically and chemically.
- There is mechanical grinding activity from the teeth.
- There is churning and mixing activity from the tongue, cheeks and the muscles built into the wall of the oesophagus, stomach and the intestines.

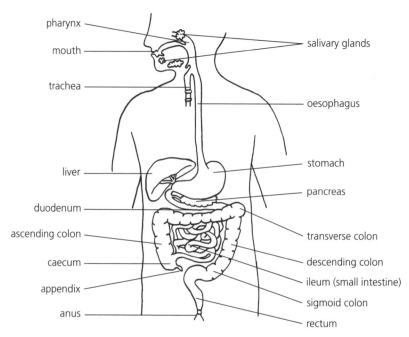

pharynx
mouth
trachea
salivary glands
oesophagus
liver
stomach
pancreas
duodenum
ascending colon
transverse colon
caecum
descending colon
appendix
ileum (small intestine)
anus
sigmoid colon
rectum

Figure 15.1 *Structure of the gastro-intestinal tract*

- Chemical activity is through *enzymes* produced by cells in different parts of the system and through other chemicals such as hydrochloric acid in gastric juice and bile. Bile is made in the liver, it is stored in the gall bladder and released into the intestines.

The function of the digestive system is to break down complex, insoluble foods into simple, soluble foods that can be absorbed into the circulation and used by the body. Carbohydrate foods like maize, millet, cassava and rice are broken down into glucose which is absorbed into the bloodstream. Protein foods like meat, fish, nuts, eggs and cereals are broken down into amino acids and absorbed. Fat from foods like ground nuts, cooking oil, meat and milk are digested to fatty acids and absorbed. Fluid, and both water soluble and fat soluble vitamins and minerals are also absorbed. Fibre in the food is not absorbed but is important for the functioning of the intestines as it provides the roughage.

The veins that drain the small intestine take these nutrients straight to the liver, which manufactures important proteins such as blood clotting factors from them. The liver stores glucose and other nutrients for future use. Other important functions of the liver include turning toxic ammonia into urea.

Disease in the gastro-intestinal system

Disease will affect the system's important role in providing the body with fluid and nutrients.

Diarrhoea

Diarrhoea, the frequent passing of watery or mucousy stools, is an important symptom with many different causes. It may be due to infections with bacteria such as Vibrio cholerae (cholera). These produce *entero-toxins* which stimulate the lining cells of the intestine to secrete large amounts of fluid. This usually happens because infected food or water has been taken in.

The most important aspects of dealing with a person with diarrhoea are infection control (see Chapters 6 and 24) and assessment of the person's state of hydration. Very large amounts of fluid can be lost and severe persistent diarrhoea can be life-threatening. (See Chapter 45 for diarrhoea in children.)

Assessing fluid balance

- Is the person thirsty? Look at the tongue, is it dry and coated?

- Has less urine been passed recently and is it dark and concentrated?
- Look at the veins at the back of the hands to see if they are collapsed. Are the hands and feet cold?
- Is the skin hot and dry?
- Pinch the skin on the abdominal wall. Does it stay pinched rather than springing back to normal?
- Record the pulse rate and volume. Is it rapid and thin in volume?

If the answer to many of the questions above is 'Yes', then the dehydration is serious. Fluid and electrolyte replacement is necessary. It is dangerous to give plain water as it will not be absorbed from the intestine very well. A salt and sugar solution will be absorbed a lot better. A preparation of oral rehydration solution can be used, but if this is not available, add one 5 ml teaspoon of salt and four 5 ml teaspoons of sugar to a litre of clean, boiled and cooled water. Alternatively a thin porridge can be given, as salt is usually added for cooking and the starches will be digested to simple sugars.

Nurses must be able to estimate the amount of fluid needed to rehydrate the patient. An adult needs about 3 litres per day of fluid normally. When there is excess loss, as in the case of diarrhoea, vomiting or excess sweating, the fluid intake needs to be increased. Nurses must keep an intake and output chart and give extra fluid each time the patient passes a watery stool. If oral fluids cause vomiting, intravenous fluids will need to be given.

The cause of the diarrhoea should be found and treated if necessary. Antibiotics are not indicated unless there is a specific infection (see Chapter 45). Good patient hygiene is very important so that other patients do not become infected. Nurses must dispose of all waste safely and wash their hands after attending to the patient.

Obstruction of the gastro-intestinal tract

Oesophageal obstruction

There are various reasons why the oesophagus may become obstructed. A large amount of food can become lodged in the *lumen*, there can be a tumour or a caustic substance may have been ingested causing fibrosis. A careful history will usually give some indication. If food is causing the obstruction, an oesophagoscopy may need to be done urgently to remove the food. If a caustic substance has been ingested, oesophageal dilatations may need to be done once the area has healed. It may be necessary for the patient to have a gastrostomy initially. If there is a tumour, surgery is likely to be necessary (see Chapter 22).

Intestinal obstruction

The intestine is said to be obstructed when it fails to move its contents onward either due to a physical blockage of the lumen or to cessation of *peristalsis*. Large amounts of fluid and chemicals are normally released into the gastro-intestinal tract, but fluid is also constantly reabsorbed. When the peristalsis ceases, this does not happen. The fluid is not reabsorbed into the blood and it is lost from the circulation and body tissues. The intestine may become obstructed because it has twisted, blocked or become paralysed.

Causes of intestinal obstruction

- Volvulus. The gut becomes twisted.
- Intussusception. The gut prolapses into itself.
- Strangulated hernia (usually an inguinal hernia). The gut herniates through a small opening and becomes oedematous and trapped.
- Cancer causing a blockage
- Paralytic ileus. The gut becomes paralysed either due to handling during surgery or to peritonitis. Both may stop peristalsis. Peritonitis (infection of the peritoneum) may be caused by a perforated ulcer or perforated appendix.

Signs and symptoms

- Pain, often colicky in nature from bowel spasms. If due to paralytic ileus, the pain is more constant and is due to the abdominal distension.
- Vomiting. This is an early sign if the obstruction is in the stomach or first part of the small intestine; a late sign if lower down in the tract. The vomit may become bile stained or brown (faecal) if the obstruction is low.
- Abdominal distension. This is due to the build up of fluids and gases in the intestines. Abdominal distension is more marked where the obstruction is lower down in the tract.
- Bowel sounds. If the lumen of the gut is blocked, peristalsis becomes more active, bowel sounds increase and are high pitched and tinkling. In paralytic ileus, there is absence of bowel sounds.

As fluid is not absorbed, it accumulates in the gut lumen. So the person becomes dehydrated and shocked even though there may not be any signs of excessive loss of fluid from the body. The effects on fluid balance are the same as in severe diarrhoea and fluid replacement is vital. As oral fluids cannot be absorbed, intravenous or subcutaneous fluids should be given. A nasogastric tube should be passed and aspirated regularly to prevent vomiting and to help relieve the distension. The amount aspirated must be measured and taken into account when calculating fluid replacement. Rest is also very important. The cause of the obstruction will need to be treated, often by surgery.

Constipation

Constipation is when faeces are hard and difficult to pass. It happens when food waste stays in the large intestine too long, and therefore a lot of water is reabsorbed from the lower bowel. This condition often occurs when diet does not contain enough fibre, or it could be as a result of not taking enough fluids. Mild aperients should be used in the short-term only and the main approach should come from health education. Absolute constipation occurs in intestinal obstruction.

Enemas and bowel washouts may be used when constipation is severe or when surgery on the gut is planned.

Hepatitis

Hepatitis is inflammation of the liver. There may be flu-like symptoms, pain and tenderness under the right ribs, nausea and vomiting, lack of appetite, dark urine, pale faeces, jaundice, dry itchy skin, and fever. It can lead to liver failure and death.

Causes of hepatitis

Many types are caused by viruses:
- Hepatitis A. This is the most common type; it occurs in epidemics and is spread through the oral–faecal route (see Chapter 24).
- Hepatitis B, C and E. These are most commonly spread in blood and blood products, and also through body fluids and sexual contact (see Chapter 24).

Other causes include drugs, aflatoxins from mouldy maize, groundnuts, other starchy foods and legumes.

Management

- Observe for deterioration: low blood sugar, nerve tremors and poor coordination of movement, confusion, disorientation and loss of consciousness.
- Strict infection control. Take care with body fluids and their disposal. Many patients can still pass on the infection even after recovery (see Chapter 6).
- Rest and treatment of symptoms.
- If signs of liver failure occur, lactulose can be given. This causes the person to open their bowels three to four times daily. This means that less of the toxic ammonia is absorbed into the bloodstream. During the infection, the failing liver is unable to convert toxic ammonia into urea.

Biliary disease

When the liver is inflamed, jaundice is common because the fine bile channels inside the liver become obstructed. If obstruction occurs outside of the liver, in the gall bladder or the biliary tract, through which bile flows to reach the intestine, then jaundice will also occur. This obstruction is usually caused by gallstones or by a cancer at the head of the pancreas. The effects on the patient are likely to be: pain towards the right shoulder, often after meals (especially fatty meals); nausea; lack of appetite; dark urine; pale faeces.

Surgery will usually be needed.

Nursing care of patients with gastro-intestinal problems

Pp Using a nasogastric tube

- Select a tube wide enough for the purpose: fine-bore tubes for feeding only; medium size (about 10–12 FG) for aspirating stomach fluid; wide-bore if tube is to wash substances (such as drug tablets) out of the stomach. See information on page 84.
- Explain the procedure to the patient and obtain agreement to it. Ask the patient to clear the nose and remove dentures.
- Estimate the length of the tube to be inserted: measure the tube against the distance from nostril to earlobe and earlobe to lower margin of ribs in middle of chest (*xiphisternum*), noting the length (see Figure 15.2).
- Lubricate the tip of the tube with clean water.
- Pass the tube gently into the nostril and then backwards into the nasopharynx. Stop if an obstruction is felt, remove and try again.
- Ask the patient to breathe through the mouth and swallow; sips of water may help this. Gently push the tube onward during swallowing. Stop when it has reached the right length.
- Check that the tube is in the stomach: attach a 10 ml syringe and pull gently to aspirate some fluid. Squirt this onto blue litmus paper: if it turns red you know the tube tip is in the right place as you have withdrawn acid stomach contents. Alternatively, test by pushing 5 ml of air into the tube from a syringe while another person listens through a stethoscope over the stomach. If the tube is in the right place, air will be heard entering as a strong gurgling sound.
- Put a spigot into the end of the tube, or attach the tube to a drainage bag or feeding system.
- Tape the tube carefully to the nose to stop it moving.

Using nasogastric tubes for different purposes

For gastric lavage (washout of drug overdose)
- Prepare 2 litres of tepid water.
- Attach a funnel to tube.
- Introduce 100–200 ml of fluid at a time into funnel, with funnel lower than patient's head.
- Gradually raise funnel, allowing most but not all fluid to run in.
- Lower funnel below the level of the patient's stomach, observing the fluid flowing back for tablets or blood.
- Empty drainage into bucket and repeat as necessary, ensuring similar amount returns to that introduced.

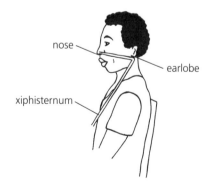

Figure 15.2 *Measuring the length of a nasogastric tube*

For aspiration of stomach fluid
- Attach a 20 ml or 50 ml syringe.
- Pull gently on piston of syringe.
- Observe the fluid flowing out.
- Empty drainage into jug and repeat, until little or no fluid is obtained.
- Record amount aspirated on a fluid balance chart.

For feeding
- Use an aseptic technique in preparing or handling any liquid food.
- Check position of tube in stomach.
- If possible use a continuous feeding system, which must be sterilised before use. Fill and attach to tube, allow to drip in slowly (100 ml/hour).
- If a continuous feeding bottle is not available, use a 50 ml syringe, fill with fluid, gradually raise it, allowing most but not all fluid to run in. Repeat to total 200 ml.
- Total intake of liquid food must be planned for 24 hour period, allowing rest periods for full absorption of food.
- Record amount given on a fluid balance chart.

Enemas and bowel washouts

An enema may be needed to treat severe constipation or before some surgical procedures. Muscle activity in the walls of the rectum can be stimulated by giving an enema. Disposable phosphate or other small volume enemas are effective. If these are not available, it will be necessary to introduce a large volume of fluid into the rectum, to stretch its walls and trigger the muscle contraction that causes *defaecation*.

Pp To give an enema

- Prepare 600–1000 ml of fluid by dissolving a small piece of soft soap in water (smaller quantities of water for children).

- Check the temperature is about 37°C using a thermometer, or it should feel tepid if you dip your elbow into the water.
- Lie the patient on the left side with the buttocks on the edge of the bed and a protective sheet underneath.
- Pass a lubricated rectal tube about 10 cm long into the patient's rectum. Attach tubing and funnel.
- Run the fluid in steadily. If the patient becomes uncomfortable, wait for a few moments then continue until all of solution has run in.
- Encourage the patient to wait a little before emptying the bowels. If a disposable enema has been used, the patient should be able to wait longer.

Note: The rectum has a good blood supply and it is possible for fluids to be absorbed through the rectal wall. Patients with heart or circulatory problems should not be given large volume enemas.

Bowel washouts are different from enemas. They are used to clean out the bowel before surgery on the large intestine.

Pp To give a bowel washout

- Prepare 1000 ml of normal saline (0.9 per cent sodium chloride) at 37°C. Normal saline cannot be absorbed into the bloodstream from the bowel, whereas water can.
- Position the patient as for an enema.
- Fluid should be run in about 100 ml at a time and then the funnel lowered to allow the same fluid to run back.
- Repeat this several times until the fluid that runs back is clear.

■ **Activities**

1. A person is admitted with diarrhoea. How would you assess him and deal with his dehydration?

2. Intestinal obstruction will only cause dehydration if the person is vomiting. Is this true or false?

Health promotion

Normal functioning of the bowel and effective nutrition are more likely if individuals:

- Drink at least two litres a day of water or other non-alcoholic drinks, more when it is hot
- Eat a good mixed diet, including food with a high fibre content: whole grain cereals, roots and root vegetables, legumes, fruits and leafy vegetables.

16

Care of patients with urinary problems

This chapter looks at common problems that occur in the urinary system: infections, inflammation due to other factors (nephritis), stones, chronic loss of protein in the urine (nephrotic syndrome) and the failure of the kidneys to function normally (renal failure).

Structure and function of the urinary system

The urinary system is essential to eliminating waste products produced by cell activity in the body and keeping a balance of fluid in the blood and tissues.

The kidneys produce urine which leaves the body through the ureters, the bladder (which stores urine) and the urethra (see Figure 16.1). Inside each kidney are the structures that actually make the urine, the nephrons. Nephrons are tiny organs which filter the blood and remove unwanted metabolic products like urea and excess ions (particles in the blood holding electric charges, for example sodium and potassium). Many drugs are excreted via the kidney and it is also responsible for controlling water loss and maintaining water *homeostasis*. In healthy young people, there are about a million of these nephrons in each kidney. If they become damaged, the kidneys do not function properly.

As the diagram shows (Figure 16.2), each nephron is a long tubule, lined with cells. The functions of filtration, reabsorption and secretion all occur within the nephrons.

Glomerular filtration

Blood is carried via the renal artery to tangled blood vessels in the kidneys called glomeruli. The walls of these blood vessels have tiny holes and slits in them. This allows small particles to pass through under the force of the blood pressure into the capsule surrounding the glomerulus (glomerular capsule). The capsule leads to the tubule, the start of the collection system. Water, waste products from cell activity (such as urea and creatinine), glucose and *ions* (for example sodium, potassium, hydrogen, chloride and calcium) are small enough to be forced out of the blood into the tubule. In health, the small size of the holes prevents larger particles in the blood (blood cells and plasma proteins) being forced into the tubule. The fluid in the first part of the nephron tubule is called glomerular filtrate.

Since this filtration is influenced by blood pressure, any condition where blood pressure is low or high could affect kidney function.

Tubular reabsorption and secretion

In a healthy person, about 120 ml of glomerular filtrate is formed every minute but only about 1 ml of urine leaves the kidney. This is because reabsorption of water takes place through the cells that line the remaining length of the tubule. The water passes into the blood vessels surrounding the tubule. Many other substances

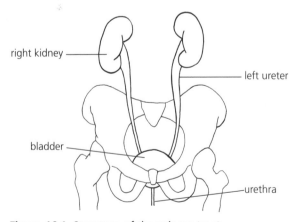

right kidney

left ureter

bladder

urethra

Figure 16.1 *Structure of the urinary tract*

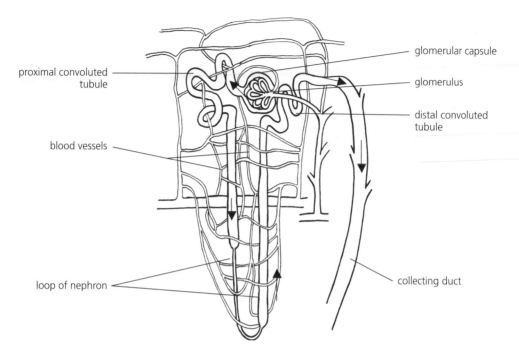

proximal convoluted tubule

glomerular capsule

glomerulus

distal convoluted tubule

blood vessels

loop of nephron

collecting duct

Figure 16.2 *Structure of a nephron*

are reabsorbed to prevent them being lost from the body. Some substances are also secreted into the filtrate in the tubule from these blood vessels. Some of the reabsorption and secretion is under the control of hormones. These control what is lost in the urine and retained in the blood as part of maintaining homeostasis.

Overall functions of the kidney

What happens in the nephrons of the kidney is relevant to the overall kidney function:

- Control of fluid balance in the body
- Clearing the blood of wastes, for example urea and creatinine (nitrogen wastes from protein breakdown in the liver), hormones, many drugs
- Control of the *electrolyte balance* of blood
- Control of the pH balance of blood at around 7.38–7.42

  Also, the kidney:
- releases the enzyme rennin, which helps to raise blood pressure
- releases the hormone erythropoetin, which stimulates production of red blood cells (erythrocytes) in the bone marrow
- activates vitamin D, which helps maintain calcium balance in bones.

Micturition

The kidneys make urine that then flows down the ureters into the bladder where it is stored. As the amount of urine in the bladder increases, nerve endings in the bladder wall are stimulated and send a message to the spinal cord that results in nerve impulses travelling to the bladder, causing the muscle in its wall to contract, so that urine is voided (*micturition*).

Young children empty their bladders through this spinal reflex. However, as we grow our brains learn to inhibit this reflex by blocking it with impulses down the spinal cord. So we gain control over the process of micturition and become continent of urine.

Urinary tract infection (UTI)

Infection may occur anywhere within the urinary system. It is usually caused by multiplication of bacteria such as Escherichia coli that have spread up the urethra into the bladder. These bacteria live in the lower bowel, so can spread from there or from another person, often during sexual intercourse.

Common causes of urinary tract infection

- It is more common in women because the urethra is shorter and the entrance (meatus) closer to the anus than in men.

- Changes in the woman's body during pregnancy make UTI a common problem (see Chapter 34).
- Stagnation of urine. Causes might include blockage of the urethra by an enlarged prostate or kidney stones.
- Ureteric reflux can occur in children. During micturition, some of the urine refluxes back up the ureter. This urine then stagnates in the bladder. Children can be taught double micturition – empty the bladder once, wait a few minutes and then empty the bladder again.
- Indwelling urinary catheters.
- Infection is common in menopausal and newly sexually active women.

Symptoms of urinary tract infection

- Frequency of micturition and an urgency to empty the bladder. This can lead to incontinence.
- Burning pain when passing urine. This may be severe.
- Pain in the lower back or loins
- Fever and shivering
- Nausea and vomiting
- The urine may smell offensive, look dark or cloudy and contain blood.
- Confusion, fever and frequent falls in elderly people may indicate infection.

Note: Bacteria may be present in the urine (bacteriuria) without any signs or symptoms, especially if infection is recurrent. The bacteria may still spread to the kidneys.

Management of urinary tract infections

Management	Aim
■ Encourage a high fluid intake (about 1500 ml per day). Patients may be reluctant to drink, fearing this will worsen frequency.	To flush bacteria out of the urinary tract, dilute the urine and reduce pain
■ Avoid citrus juices and caffeine drinks such as cola and coffee.	These irritate bladder lining
■ Give analgesia e.g. paracetamol, and anti-inflammatory drugs e.g. ibuprofen.	Reduce pain and inflammation in bladder wall
■ Give anti-spasmodic drugs e.g. Flavoxate if available.	Reduce painful muscle spasm in bladder or ureters
■ Give antibiotic or urinary antiseptic medication, preferably after laboratory has identified the bacteria, e.g. nitrofurantoin, cefalexin, amoxicillin, trimethoprim (not in pregnancy). Women need treatment 3–5 days, children 5–10 and men for 14 days.	To destroy bacteria or prevent them multiplying
■ Advise on the importance of finishing the course of antibiotics, even if symptoms improve.	Reduce incidence of resistance to antibiotics and/or re-infection
■ Warn about/observe for thrush (candidiasis): • Oral: soreness and creamy white patches on the tongue or membranes of mouth (may spread to throat) • Vaginal: white or yellow discharge, severe itchiness and dryness, pain during sexual intercourse	Common fungal infections that result from a change in balance of natural bacteria following antibiotic treatment
■ Warm bath may be helpful (and warmth over the lower abdomen).	Warmth soothes pain

Management of urinary tract infections *continued*	
Management	**Aim**
■ Provide information on how to avoid future problems: • high fluid intake • good hygiene (wipe bottom from front to back after using the toilet, wash if possible). ■ If sexually active advise: • avoiding injury to the woman's urethra during sexual intercourse • lubrication – especially for menopausal women • washing hands and genitalia before and after • avoiding touching the anus • women should pass urine after.	To prevent recurrence
■ Teach the symptoms of UTI.	Prompt recognition and earlier help-seeking

Urinary stones

Stones (calculi) form from crystals of substances in the urine. There are different types of stone caused by different crystals. They can block the pelvis of the kidney or the ureter. Blockage results in waves of muscle contraction in the ureter, resulting in severe gripey pain called colic. Other common symptoms of stones are those that happen in UTI; sometimes they can cause kidney failure (see below).

Management of urinary stones

*   Control severe pain with narcotic analgesia such as pethidine and apply warmth to the side.
*   Observe for and treat urine infection.
*   Encourage high fluid intake, more than 3 litres a day unless kidney failure is suspected.

Patients may pass stones by themselves but surgery may be needed to remove them. In specialist centres patients can be given controlled doses of shock waves under anaesthetic. These break up stones into small parts so they can then be passed.

Teaching patients is important in order to reduce the growth of more stones:

*   Encourage high fluid intake, mainly clear fluids.
*   Avoid too much alcohol, since it has a dehydrating effect.
*   Provide information about the symptoms of UTI so help can be sought early.
*   Provide information about drug treatments for specific types of stone if available, for example

sodium citrate to treat calcium stones. Other possible medications are D-Penicillamine, allopurinol and pyridoxine.

Nephrotic syndrome

Nephrotic syndrome is the abnormal loss of proteins from the body via the kidneys in the urine. The structure of the glomerulus normally prevents the large proteins of the blood becoming part of the glomerular filtrate. These proteins are albumin, globulin and fibrinogen. However, kidney infections and long-term high blood pressure can damage the glomeruli and protein will then be lost from the blood and appear in the urine. The effects of this are called nephrotic syndrome:

*   Plasma proteins, especially albumin, have an important role in maintaining the balance of fluid between the blood and the tissues. They maintain the *oncotic* pressure. The effect of a chronic loss of protein in the urine is that fluid leaks into the tissues. This results in generalised *oedema*, including swelling of the face, and *ascites*.
*   The loss of **immunoglobulins** can make the person more at risk of infection.
*   Proteins of the blood normally combine with fat molecules. When protein is lost, the person is more at risk from blood vessel disease caused by fatty deposits in blood vessel walls (*atherosclerosis*). *Haematuria* can also occur and is evidence of a more complicated cause.

Causes of nephrotic syndrome

Nephrotic syndrome can be caused by a variety of other conditions, such as malaria, tuberculosis, hepatitis C, or typhoid. It is a more complex condition in adults and often associated with progressive renal disease, leading to chronic renal failure. In children it is usually *idiopathic* and may respond to steroids.

Management of nephrotic syndrome

In major centres, a renal biopsy may be done to identify the type and indicate the best course of management.

- Maintain the serum albumin. This will increase the amount of fluid retained in the circulation. This can be done by encouraging a high protein diet (meat, fish, eggs, groundnuts, beans). The source of the protein should be low in fat. In some centres it may be possible to give intravenous albumin.
- Follow a low salt diet as sodium causes fluid to be retained.
- Diuretic drugs may be used but often have no effect.
- Prevent infection; infection is more likely because of low levels of immunoglobulin.

Inflammatory conditions (nephritis or nephritic syndrome, glomerulonephritis)

Nephritis is a condition in which the kidney is damaged by inflammation. The glomeruli may be damaged, so may the tubules and spaces between them depending on the cause. This means that filtering and excretion becomes inefficient. Nephritis may be temporary, or worsen progressively and become chronic.

Causes

- An immune response following an infection, for example with Haemolytic Streptococcus Group A.
- Medications
- Autoimmune disorders where antibodies are produced that damage the patient's own tissues

Symptoms

- Increased or decreased urinary output
- High blood pressure
- Nausea and vomiting
- Feeling generally unwell, aches and pains
- Headache, blurred vision

- Oedema and weight gain
- Blood in the urine
- Drowsiness, confusion, coma

Management

Diagnosis of the type of nephritis and its cause is important. Bed rest may be needed, antibiotics given, and treatment as for renal failure if necessary. Permanent kidney damage may occur.

Renal failure

Renal failure is the failure of the kidneys to carry out their normal functions properly. They no longer clear waste products properly or retain electrolytes and other essential substances. Waste products accumulate in the blood (azotaemia) and eventually cause symptoms. This is uraemia.

The term renal insufficiency may be used for some loss of function. When less than 10 per cent of kidney function is left the term end-stage renal failure is used. The effects of renal failure will depend on how much of normal function is lost. Renal failure is often labelled as acute or chronic. Acute renal failure is the sudden interruption of kidney function. It is usually a complication of another disorder and is reversible but can lead to death even with prompt treatment. Chronic renal failure is due to progressive disease of the kidneys and is not reversible. Severe damage may already be present by the time renal failure becomes obvious. The first sign of chronic disease may be high blood pressure.

Acute renal failure
Causes of acute renal failure

- Poor blood pressure in the glomerulus. This can be due to cardiac problems, severe haemorrhage, dehydration and lack of salt, shock, burns, renal thrombosis.
- Hypoxia
- Acute inflammation of the glomerulus of the kidney (see nephritis or nephritic syndrome above)
- Acute tubular necrosis (ATN): the tubules of the nephrons are damaged by restriction to the blood supply, drugs or poisons.
- Infections, for example pyelonephritis or septicaemia
- Crush injury to muscles; muscle proteins in the blood reach the urine

- Acute obstruction of the urinary tract, for example by tumours, stones, prostate enlargement
- Blood transfusion reaction
- Inherited blood disorders causing *haemolysis*

The signs, symptoms, diagnostic tests and management of acute renal failure are included in Table 16.1.

Chronic renal failure

Causes of chronic renal failure

Long-term damage to the kidneys has many causes and is normally secondary to an existing condition, for example:

- Acute renal failure
- Diabetes mellitus
- Hypertension
- Long-term blockage of the kidneys and urinary tract
- Inherited conditions such as polycystic kidney disease
- Recurrent kidney infections.

Finding out the cause of renal failure and monitoring progress is vital. Common diagnostic tests are used:

- Blood levels – serum creatinine and creatinine clearance, serum potassium
- Blood gas analysis if possible to identify *acidosis*
- Test urine for infection
- Monitor blood pressure and urine output volume
- Abdominal X-ray, CT or MRI scans and ultrasound if available.

The signs, symptoms and management of chronic renal failure are included in Table 16.1.

Nursing care will include the general care of a patient who may be feeling very ill and frightened and may be agitated or confused.

Overall management aims:

- Acute renal failure: to maintain life and manage symptoms until renal function recovers, treat the cause and reversible changes
- Chronic renal failure: to maintain life, manage symptoms, slow down deterioration and improve function where possible.

Note: Signs and symptoms will include those of the underlying cause of the renal failure, for example low blood pressure in acute failure if bleeding has occurred.

Table 16.1 Acute and chronic renal failure: main problems and management

Normal kidney function	Acute renal failure			Chronic renal failure	
	Problems, signs and symptoms	Management		Problems, signs and symptoms	Management
Controls the body's fluid balance	*Oliguria* (only 100–400 ml urine passed per 24 hours) or none (*anuria*)	Fluid restriction. Intake should be equivalent to output plus allowance for hidden loss through skin, breath, faeces etc. (500–1500 ml per day depending on climate and altitude)		As acute renal failure	As acute renal failure
	Tissue oedema, especially in lower limbs and face e.g. eyes may be puffy in the morning				
	During recovery *polyuria* may occur (3–4 litres daily)	High fluid replacement levels and potassium supplements needed if polyuria occurs.		*Nocturia* is common Either oliguria or polyuria are possible	
Removes waste products from the blood including hormones and some drugs	High levels of urea and creatinine (nitrogen wastes from protein breakdown)	High carbohydrate/low protein diet helps to reduce urea. Rest may lower creatinine.		As acute renal failure	As acute renal failure
	Nausea and vomiting due to retention of toxic wastes	Care needed with drug administration.			
	Infections such as UTI are common because high urea levels interfere with immune system.	Prevention of infection			

Table 16.1 Acute and chronic renal failure: main problems and management *continued*

	Acute renal failure		Chronic renal failure	
Normal kidney function	Problems, signs and symptoms	Management	Problems, signs and symptoms	Management
Controls the body's electrolyte balance	High blood potassium (*hyperkalaemia*)	Low potassium foods (avoid bananas, legumes, spinach)	As acute renal failure	As acute renal failure
	Heart rhythm problems	Give ion-exchange resins by mouth or enema	High blood pressure occurs if rennin levels are high (caused by sodium being lost). This can cause seizures.	Medication to lower blood pressure
	Fatigue, weakness, headache, agitation, confusion, delirium, coma			Ensure rest
				Low salt diet and protein restriction
			Calcium deficiency can lead to fractures.	
			Low calcium and high phosphates lead to nerve tingling, numbness, *tetany*, and severe *pruritis*.	Emollient skin products for pruritis
Controls the pH balance of the blood	*Acidosis:* Body responds with deep, fast breathing	Dialysis if pH falls excessively (see below). Patient feels better, may be life-saving.	As acute renal failure	As acute renal failure
Prevents loss of large molecules such as blood cells			Lack of erythropoietin causes anaemia.	Iron and erythropoietin supplements, blood transfusion if safe
Manufactures hormones such as rennin and erythropoietin				Ensure rest

Renal dialysis

Dialysis is necessary if measures to control fluid balance, urea, creatinine and rising blood potassium are not successful. During dialysis, toxic substances are removed from a patient's blood by *diffusion* and *osmosis* (and sometimes by exerting pressure). This is carried out through a *semi-permeable* membrane into a specially prepared fluid (dialysate). A special diet has to be followed to reduce the build-up of toxins.

There are two types of dialysis: both must be carried out in specialist centres, or with their support (some centres have facilities for home dialysis):

Haemodialysis: The semi-permeable membrane and the dialysate are inside a dialysis machine. The blood passes through the dialysis machine via a large venous catheter. This is the most effective but most expensive option and must be done every 2–3 days.

Peritoneal dialysis: The patient's own peritoneum is used as the semi-permeable membrane so acting as a filter. Toxins are washed into the dialysate which is run into and out of the peritoneal cavity through a catheter and cannula inserted in the abdominal wall. This is clamped to allow the dialysate to absorb urea, fluid and electrolytes, and then released. Daily dialysis is necessary.

Nursing care of patients with urinary problems

Urinary catheterisation

There are four main reasons for using urinary catheters:

- The passage of urine from the bladder is blocked (for example by enlargement of the prostate gland at the bladder neck in men, constipation or tumours in women).
- The nerve control of bladder emptying is upset (for example by anaesthetics or other drugs).
- To assess the function of the kidney in producing urine. Hourly measurements are important where acute kidney failure is suspected.
- Management of some types of urinary incontinence.

Urinary tract infection is more common following catheterisation, so it should only be used if necessary.

Pp Urinary catheterisation

- Daily review of the need for a catheter is important with removal as early as possible.
- Catheterisation must be carried out using an aseptic technique after thorough cleaning of the genital area, including under the male foreskin.
- Catheters should be lubricated before being inserted. Use sterile anaesthetic gel if possible, or alternatively use sterile fluid. Non-sterile lubricants may introduce infection.
- For continuous drainage, attach it to a urine collection bag (being careful not to introduce bacteria by touching the area of the connection). Bags with a tap are best so that the connection to the catheter is not opened and the drainage system remains closed. When necessary empty the bag carefully into a clean container to reduce the infection risk.

Choosing a catheter

It is important to consider the reason for catheterisation, how long it needs to remain in place, and the person being catheterised.

Type:
- Balloon Foley two-way for bladder drainage over a short- to long-term period
- Balloon Foley three-way for bladder irrigation and drainage after prostate operations

- Non-balloon for one-off or intermittent bladder drainage.

Diameter:
Use the smallest size possible that maintains adequate drainage:
- Size 12 for adults with clear urine
- Larger where blood or other debris is draining.

Length:
- Short catheters (20–25 cm) for women except if very obese
- Longer catheters for men (40–45 cm).

Material:
- PVC for short-term use only (up to 10 days)
- Latex for short-term use only (up to 14 days). Must not be used if allergy is known to exist
- Silicone-coated latex for medium-term use only (up to 6 weeks)
- Teflon-coated latex for medium-term use only (up to 6 weeks)
- All-silicone catheters for long-term use only (up to 3 months). Check inflation of balloon weekly as the catheter will fall out if it deflates.
- Hydrogel-coated catheters (the most recent) last very well and are suitable for long-term use (up to 6 months).

Pp Bladder washout

Catheters may become blocked with debris and blood clots. Bladder washout may be used to clear the debris. If this is inadequate then continuous irrigation may be needed (see next procedure).
- Explain what you wish to do.
- Use an aseptic technique.
- Use a 50 ml bladder-tip syringe.
- Introduce sterile saline that has been warmed to body temperature.
- Draw the saline back gently, in the hope that the obstruction is freed.
- If unsuccessful, use special solutions for reducing encrustation inside catheters (if available).
- Remove and replace if necessary.

Pp Bladder irrigation

Irrigation may be performed continuously to prevent catheter blockage especially following prostate surgery when a lot of bleeding occurs. It will also allow the bladder to rest. Explain what you wish to do.

• Use an aseptic technique and gloves.
• A balloon Foley three-way catheter is used for continuous bladder irrigation, together with a bag of normal saline and urine collection bag (see Figure 16.3).
• Run fluid into the bladder continuously and then out again into the collection bag. Set the normal saline to run in at about 500 ml an hour at first. Slow this gradually as the blood-staining reduces until the urine runs clear (usually 2–3 days).
• Watch for complications caused by absorption of the fluid through the bladder wall. This causes *haemodilution* and is known as post-prostatectomy syndrome. The signs are neurological: confusion, weakness, twitching and seizures. If suspected, the irrigation should be stopped and medical help be sought urgently.

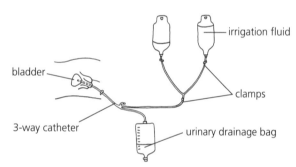

Figure 16.3 *Bladder irrigation*

Urine testing

Urine testing is needed for detecting and monitoring disorders in the body.

Testing urine can reveal and monitor problems in the bladder, the kidney and wider metabolic problems such as diabetes. Table 16.2 below shows the possible meaning of positive results.

Testing is easiest using chemical reagent strips if they are available and following the manufacturer's instructions.

If reagent strips are not available:

• Urine can be boiled in a glass container and observed. Albumin will solidify.
• Sulphosalycylic acid can be added to urine. Albumin will make the urine cloudy.

• Benedicts solution can be used for testing for glucose.

Table 16.2 Urine testing and conditions indicated by positive results

Urine test for	Positive result usually means
Protein: Large amounts	Kidney disease, pre-eclampsia of pregnancy
Protein: Small amounts	Urinary tract infection (or early sign of kidney disease)
Glucose	Diabetes mellitus (however in pregnancy trace amounts of glucose are normal)
Haemoglobin or red blood cells	Haemoglobin may be present because of haemolysis due to G6PD or blackwater fever. Red cells may suggest infection, schistosomiasis, malignancy or trauma to the urinary tract.
Ketones	Indicate incomplete breakdown of fat in starvation, or poorly controlled diabetes mellitus (if glucose is also present)
Bilirubin	Obstructive jaundice, or incompatible blood transfusion

Health promotion

Healthy kidneys are important. To keep them healthy:

• Drink at least three litres a day of water or other non-alcoholic drinks, more during hot, dry weather. It is important to carry water when travelling. During Ramadan, there may be restrictions on drinking fluids. Women who are pregnant or breastfeeding need to continue to drink and postpone their fasts.
• Eat a good mixed diet, with a low or moderate amount of salt.
• Good hygiene is important, including before and after sexual activity.
• Seek treatment for symptoms that suggest you may have urinary tract infection.

■ **Activities**

1. Why is the level of blood pressure important to the function of the kidney?
2. How may the kidneys be affected if a patient suffers from a severe haemorrhage?
3. Why is oedema a symptom of nephrotic syndrome?
4. How would you make sure a person in renal failure has the right amount to drink?

17

Care of people with skin problems

In this chapter information is provided about how to manage common skin conditions. The structure and functions of the skin are reviewed and the fundamentals of keeping the skin healthy are described. Common skin conditions and their management outlined.

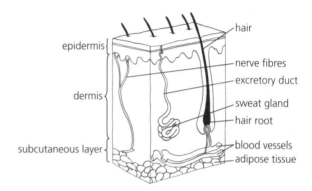

Figure 17.1 *Structure of the skin*

Introduction

The skin is the largest organ of the body, vital for physical and psychological well being. It has a number of functions which allow humans to exist within a hostile environment.

Functions of the skin

- Protection (both a physical barrier and as a location for immunological response)
- Psychological well being and social acceptance
- Temperature control
- Manufacture of vitamin D
- Sensation (both pain and pleasure)

These functions mean that humans can successfully interact with one another and with the world around them. When any of them fail (but most particularly the protective function) there can be a serious risk to health. Skin disease is rarely life-threatening, but it can cause serious discomfort and affect the quality of life of sufferers. Their ability to earn a living may also be affected. Therefore nurses and other health care practitioners need to take skin health seriously. They can have a significant impact on the lives of the patients who they look after using minimal resources and a knowledge of some simple concepts.

Structure of the skin

To perform its functions the skin has to be flexible yet tough. Its complex structure and ability to renew itself

constantly allows it to fulfil these two criteria. The skin is made up of three layers: the epidermis, dermis and subcutaneous tissue (see Figure 17.1).

Epidermis: This is the outer layer of the skin, made up of four distinct layers of different skin cells. Cells move from the basal layer to the top layer (stratum corneum) where they are gradually shed. This allows the skin's protective properties to be maintained.

Dermis: This is the layer containing blood vessels, nerve endings and lymphatics that provide nutrition for the epidermis.

Subcutaneous tissue: This is the cushion for the skin providing structural support. Adipose tissue found here is important for temperature regulation.

What's in a centimetre of skin?

- ■ Almost a metre of blood vessels
- ■ 100 sweat glands
- ■ 300,000 epidermal cells
- ■ 200 nerve endings
- ■ 10 hairs

Fundamentals of skin care and promoting skin health

There are some important messages to remember when looking after the skin. Perhaps the most important is ensuring that the skin remains healthy and unbroken with no abrasions, lesions or wounds. To do this there are five steps to follow which are described in the information box below.

All the points made in the box are strategies that will help maintain a healthy skin. However, they can also be used to improve the condition of the skin when there is a disease present. For example in *lymphoedema* (often caused by lymphatic filariasis) looking after the skin on the limbs can limit the progression of the disease. The same is true of leprosy. In patients with HIV and AIDS it is vital to maintain good skin hygiene as they are particularly prone to infection. These strategies alone are often helpful for some of the common yet simple cases of fungal infections and bacterial skin infections. They can be effective by themselves and even more so when used in conjunction with other treatments, for example antibiotics and anti-fungal medication.

Five steps to healthy skin

Action	Why?
1. Wash with clean water at room temperature with a gentle soap when available. Avoid harsh soap (e.g. soap for washing clothes) and use a soap substitute cleanser when possible. If no soap is available washing with clean water is still worth doing. Individuals can wash using their hands but a clean wash cloth is useful. Rinse soap and dirt away with clean fresh water.	Washing helps to remove pathogenic bacteria which may result in infection. Skin has its own *commensal* bacteria which are vital for its health; this is why washing is best carried out with gentle soap which will not kill the commensal bacteria. A wash cloth helps to wash more effectively but it must be clean; a dirty wash cloth will harbour pathogenic bacteria.
2. Dry with a clean towel or similar cloth. The drying motion should be gentle, vigorous rubbing should be avoided. *Flexures* and *interdigital* spaces should be dried with extra care.	A moist warm environment occurs if the body is not dried properly (especially in flexures and interdigital spaces). This is an ideal place for fungal infections to develop.
3. Prevent dryness by using an emollient (often known as a moisturiser). This can be smoothed on after washing. Petroleum jelly or home made coconut oil can be used.	A dry skin is more likely to crack which allows penetration of pathogenic bacteria. Skin that is well moisturised is generally more comfortable and less itchy, so less likely to be scratched.
4. Manage wounds using appropriate medicaments, wound dressings and analgesics when needed (see Chapter 9).	Wounds are breeches in the skin barrier and so provide ideal entry points for bacteria. They also cause pain and suffering for the individual.
5. Protection from the sun is vitally important for albino people. Wearing long sleeved clothes, a wide brimmed hat and sun glasses are all important. Where available sun screen should be used. Albino people must learn to avoid the sun whenever possible. The psychological and social impact of albinism is significant and must be taken into account. Education is important so the genetic factors are understood.	Exposure to the sun leads to skin tumours and eye problems. Albino people lack the *melanin* which protects from the sun. Children are at special risk so need to be taught early in life how to protect themselves and reduce the likelihood of serious skin tumours. Some mothers, for example, may be accused of adultery with a white man. The impact of being 'different' may be important.

Common skin conditions

This section will consider bacterial infections (see Chapter 26 for parasitic and fungal infections).

Bacterial skin infection (also known as *pyoderma*)

The skin can become infected by a number of pathogenic bacteria. Table 17.1 lists the main ones:

Good skin hygiene and maintenance of the skin as an unbroken barrier will reduce the incidence of bacterial infection. In addition soaking the affected area (often a limb) in a solution of potassium permanganate can be helpful. Potassium permanganate acts as an antiseptic and is particularly useful for drying up excessive *exudate*. Potassium permanganate should be diluted in clean water to form a light pink solution.

Other treatment such as oral antibiotics may be necessary as well as these actions. Topical antibiotics may be helpful in superficial infections; however care should be taken when using them because of the risk of sensitisation and life-threatening allergic reaction.

Some symptoms are common to most infections:

- Erythema (redness)
- Swelling
- *Pyrexia* and heat
- Pain
- Exudate

Table 17.1 Types of bacterial infection

Causative bacteria	Disease/symptoms
Staphylococcus aureus	Impetigo – vesicles containing honey coloured fluid, often occurs on the face
	Ecthyma – multiple round shallow ulcers sometimes progressing to deeper ulcers
	Folliculitis – pustule around a hair follicle
Streptococcus	Erysipelas – dermal infection leading to well defined erythematous swollen areas
	Cellulitis – a deeper infection causing darker red lesions and more significant oedema

Eczema or dermatitis

Either of these terms may be used. Eczema can be subdivided into two types:

Exogenous eczema: This has an external cause, that is the skin has come into contact with something that causes an eczematous reaction.

Endogenous eczema: (also known as atopic eczema). This is part of a picture of *atopy*, that is there is a genetic reason for developing an eczematous reaction.

Eczema of either type is characterised by severe, often constant itch. It occurs in acute, subacute and chronic stages:

- The acute phase is characterised by redness, swelling, papules, vesicles, exudate and crusting.
- In the subacute phase these characteristics may be present but to a lesser extent, however the skin is thickened and excoriations (scratch marks) are obvious.
- The chronic phase is marked by dryness, fissuring and exaggerated skin markings (know as lichenification).

Special points about the management of exogenous eczema

- Identify the substance that is causing the eczema and remove it where possible. It may be difficult to identify and impossible to remove, for example if the offending substance occurs in a person's workplace.
- Protect the dry skin, for example through wearing gloves and maintaining the skin integrity (prevent injury and use skin moisturisers at least twice a day).
- Topical steroids used up to twice daily might be necessary for short periods to control acute flare ups.

Special points about the management of endogenous eczema

Endogenous eczema is a chronic complaint, particularly common in children. Although many grow out of eczema, some will continue to experience it as a problem throughout their lives. Key strategies are to keep the number of acute flare ups to a minimum through good skin hygiene and avoidance of substances which irritate the skin, extensive and constant use of emollients and careful use of topical steroids when needed:

- Use emollients at least twice daily on the very dry skin.

- Use twice daily topical steroids during flare ups.
- People with atopic eczema are prone to bacterial (especially Staphylococcus aureus) and viral infections (herpes) and may need treatment with the appropriate antibiotics or antivirals.
- **Note:** If a potent topical steroid is used, for example betamethasone valerate, it is wise to wean the individual off the steroid by reducing use to once daily and then alternate days before stopping completely.

Tropical ulcers

Tropical ulcers usually affect young adults and older children. They occur mainly on the lower limbs and can be distressing, painful and also very disabling.

A tropical ulcer starts with an acute and localised *necrosis* of the skin and subcutaneous tissues. The ulcer may heal spontaneously leaving a slightly depressed scar. However, the individual may be left with a chronic, non specific ulcer which is difficult to heal. The ulcer can grow to cover the full circumference of the leg. Erosion of the deeper tissues, muscle and bone may occur, possibly leading to osteomyelitis and gangrene.

Tropical ulcers are caused by infective bacterial agents. The specific bacteria involved are fusiform bacilli and treponemes. There may also be secondary infection by bacteria such as Staphylococcus aureus. A form of tropical ulcer may also result from infection by parasites (protozoa) after a sandfly bite. This is known as cutaneous leishmaniasis and is commonest in North Africa. There are several factors that contribute to a tropical ulcer forming:

- Malnutrition
- Poor hygiene and living conditions
- Contact with raw sewage through contaminated water and mud
- Poor immunity
- Minor injuries and insect bites.

Special points about management of tropical ulcers

- The wound should be kept clean, protected from flies and covered with a dressing.
- Oral antibiotics, for example penicillin V may be given.
- Nutritional advice or support may be needed.
- Sometimes the area is so large that skin grafts may be necessary.

Health promotion

- Keep the skin clean and dry well after washing.
- Make sure the skin does not become dry and cracked. Apply vaseline or coconut oil.
- Avoid injuring the skin. Prevent infection in any wounds.
- Protect albino people from the effects of the sun.

■ Activity

Count the number of people on your ward or who come to the clinic who have some problem with their skin? Is this their main complaint?

18

Burns and scalds

This chapter outlines the common causes and types of burns and scald injuries. It lists the characteristics of burns injuries and how you as a nurse can help the patient. It states the different grades of wounds that may result from a burn and the simple ways nurses can manage them from first aid to hospital nursing. Ways of teaching people prevention and health promotion are outlined at the end.

Causes of burns and scalds

Burns refer to injuries caused by:
- Dry heat, often a fire or a very hot object; smoke
- Chemicals, acids and alkalis; often substances found in the home, such as caustic soda or bleach
- Friction from a moving rope or wire
- Electricity from a live wire or lightning
- Radiation from X-rays or sunburn. Albinos are at particular risk from sunburn.

Scalds refer to injuries caused by hot water or fluids, cooking oil, or steam.

Risk factors

Some people are more likely to suffer burns and scalds and may be more badly affected.
- Young children are at particular risk as they have not yet learnt by experience that burns are painful and that hot objects and fires should be avoided.
- The elderly are also more at risk. Their balance may not be good and they may fall into open fires or spill hot fluids over themselves.
- People who have fits may fall or roll into a fire.
- Those who are paralysed or have a lowered conscious level may not move away from danger quickly enough.

- Those with reduced sensation, for instance people with leprosy.

Effects of burns and scalds

- Pain. The skin is richly supplied with nerve endings, so any burn is painful.
- Fluid loss. Fluid is lost from the skin as *exudate* and into the tissues as *oedema*. The greater the surface area affected, the greater the fluid loss.
- Anaemia. If a large surface area is affected, there will be *haemolysis*. Red cells in the area will be broken down.
- Infection. The skin provides a protective barrier. When there is a large skin loss, there is very likely to be infection. This can lead to a generalised *septicaemia*.
- Disfigurement. Deep injuries will form scar tissue.
- Loss of function. Muscle tissue can be lost and scar tissue is less flexible than normal skin. Sometimes two skin surfaces will fuse together causing a web.

Severity of the injury

This will depend on the surface area involved, the part of the body and the depth of the burn.

Surface area

If the person is over 15 years old then the surface area affected can be estimated by using the 'Rule of Nines'. The body is divided into areas, each representing 9 per cent as shown in Figure 18.1.

If the burns are scattered and don't fit into these body areas then the palm of the patient's hand may be taken to represent 1 per cent of the total body surface area. This second method is the way surface area can be estimated for children under 15 years of age. It is important to remember that a child's surface area is different to that of an adult, for example the surface area of the head of a young child is about 15 per

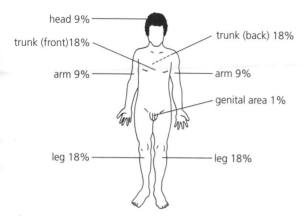

Figure 18.1 *Rule of nines*

Table 18.1 Tissue damage and healing times

Depth of tissue damage	Length of time to heal	Type of tissue damaged
Superficial partial thickness (first degree)	7–10 days	Total destruction of top layer of skin (epidermis), minor damage to the dermis
Deep partial thickness (second degree)	14–21 days	Total destruction of the epidermis plus major damage to the dermis which will result in some scarring
Full thickness (third degree)	Will vary	Full destruction to epidermis and dermis with fat, muscle, tendon and bone damage too. This results in more severe scarring.

cent of the total area. If a child sustains more than 10 per cent surface area burns or an adult more than 15 per cent then the injury is considered to be a major burn. They will require hospitalisation and fluid replacement to prevent shock.

The part of the body affected

Inhaled smoke or fumes from chemicals are particularly dangerous, as they damage the respiratory tract. Fires in houses are more likely to result in death from smoke inhalation than from the fire. The skin on the face is thinner than the skin on the feet, so the damage is greater. Burns affecting the face are disfiguring and cause psychological trauma.

Depth of tissue damage and healing times

The depth of skin affected will depend on the intensity of the heat and the length of the exposure. Hot oil on clothes keeps the heat for longer, and the depth of the damage will be greater.

The general state of an individual's health will also determine how well the injuries will heal. Those who are poorly nourished, have diabetes or a lowered immunity will have a slower rate of healing.

Nursing management of patients with burns and scalds
First aid

The immediate priority is to stop the burning process. If there are still flames, the person must lie on the ground and be rolled in cloths to help put them out. Cooling of the burn wound is the next priority. Hold the burned area under cold running water from a tap or water vessel. If running water is not available, put wet towels or cloths on the skin. Blisters should be left as they will help protect the area from bacteria.

Oils, ointments, lotions, or any other preparations should not be applied to burns and any clothes covering the skin should be left on if they appear to be sticking.

An assessment of the patient is vital to decide the management.

- Airway and breathing. Has the patient inhaled smoke?
- Circulation. Assess for hypovolaemic shock. Use the rule of nines and if more than 15 per cent of the surface area is affected, then fluid replacement is a priority.
- Pain. Give pain relief as soon as possible as pain will increase the shock.
- Extent of the burn/scald
- Any other injuries

If the patient is conscious during this time then it is important that simple explanations of what is happening are given frequently. This will considerably reduce the fear that the patient may be feeling.

Pain relief

Burns are very painful, so pain relief must be given regularly and always before doing any dressings allowing enough time for it to take effect (see Chapter 7).

Fluid replacement

The amount of fluid needing to be replaced will depend on the area that has been burnt. Intravenous fluids will be needed for any person who has burns covering more than 15 per cent or 10 per cent in the child. Oral fluids should be encouraged but in severe cases are not likely to be tolerated.

Prevention of infection

The patient should be nursed in a very clean environment. Protect from flies and all contamination. Those who have a large surface area affected may be given antibiotics immediately to help prevent infection. Observe carefully for any infection and start antibiotics if suspected. Dressings and bed linen will need frequent changing.

Burns that do not form blisters (1st degree)

These burns may be painful but are not serious. Cool the area and give aspirin or other analgesia.

Burns that cause blisters (2nd degree)

- Do not break the blisters.
- If the blisters are already broken clean gently. Gentian violet may be applied and the area left uncovered. The area will form a dry scab, and the skin will heal underneath in 10–14 days.
- If the burn is over a moving joint, like the elbow, Vaseline gauze should be applied and covered with a dry dressing. Flamazine cream can also used for dressing burns. It is an antiseptic which is active against the Pseudomonas aeruginosa, a common bacterial infection that causes sepsis in burns.
- Burned surfaces should be kept separate so that they do not grow together during healing.
- Fingers, arms and legs should be straightened every day whilst healing to prevent stiff scars developing which could limit movement in the future. Although this is painful it is important for future independence.

- The use of moisturisers on the healing scars can also reduce the stiffness of them once they have healed. Vaseline or cooking oil can be used for this.

Deep burns (3rd degree)

Burns that destroy the skin and expose raw or charred flesh are always serious and may need extensive surgery and skin grafts. If possible, transfer the patient to a major hospital for treatment.

Diet

The patient will need a high carbohydrate diet as the metabolic rate is increased, a high protein diet to help repair the damaged tissue and also one high in iron and folic acid to prevent anaemia.

Health promotion

- Warn people about cooking on open fires.
- Don't let young children and babies play or sleep near open fires.
- Turn pan handles away so that they don't hang over the top of inside cookers.
- Keep lamps and matches out of reach of children.
- Be careful when children are wearing clothes made with flammable material, for example party dresses for girls.
- Encourage patients with epilepsy to tell other people so they can help keep them away from fires if they have a fit.

■ Activity

When a patient is admitted with burns or scalds, work out what percentage of surface area you think is affected. Get a colleague to check this with you.

19

Care of patients with disorders of the endocrine system

The *endocrine* and nervous systems together help to control functions of the body. Endocrine tissues make *hormones* and release them into the blood which carries them to cells throughout the body. These hormones affect what cells do. This chapter covers the care of patients with diabetes mellitus and thyroid problems, both endocrine disorders.

- regulate *metabolic* activities
- maintain *homeostasis*
- regulate growth and development
- regulate the reproductive system.

Hormones are released in short bursts. There are three different controls over hormone release (see Table 19.1).

Fine control of blood hormone levels is essential for the system to work efficiently. Control is mostly through negative feedback. A rise in hormones in the blood acts as a switch to turn off further release once the required level has been reached. A fall switches the release back on.

The endocrine system

Different endocrine tissues exist throughout the body in glands and organs and produce many hormones (see Figure 19.1). The overall effect is to:

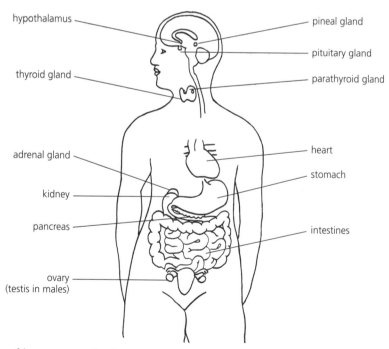

Figure 19.1 *Sources of hormone production*

Table 19.1 Control effects of hormones

Control effect	Examples
Nerves directly stimulate hormone release.	Adrenaline: sympathetic nerves (see Chapter 14) cause release of adrenaline (a hormone also known as epinephrine) as part of the fight or flight reaction.
Hormones stimulate the release of other hormones.	Thyroid hormones (control metabolism): • Thyrotrophin releasing hormone (TRH) is produced by the hypothalamus of the brain. • TRH stimulates release of thyroid stimulating hormone (TSH) from the pituitary gland. • TSH stimulates release of thyroid hormones from the thyroid gland.
The level of a substance in the blood directly stimulates hormone release.	Insulin: • When blood glucose levels rise, the pancreas is stimulated to release the hormone insulin so glucose enters the cells. • When blood glucose falls, the pancreas is stimulated to release the hormone, glucagon.

Endocrine problems are usually due to:
• failure of the gland that produces the hormone (primary failure)
• failure of the method of stimulating that gland (secondary failure), or
• resistance to the hormone's effect on the target cells.

Diabetes mellitus and thyroid gland problems are common endocrine disorders, and occasionally occur together.

Diabetes mellitus

People with diabetes are unable to control blood glucose properly. They may have too little insulin produced by the pancreas, or reduced sensitivity to it, or both.

As shown in Table 19.1, insulin and glucagon are involved in the control of blood glucose. Insulin is important because it allows glucose to be transported from the blood into cells where it is essential for energy.

• When blood glucose is high following a meal, beta-cells in the islets of Langerhans of the pancreas secrete insulin. Glucose is then transported into cells, or stored in the liver in the form of glycogen.
• When blood glucose is low, alpha-cells in the islets of Langerhans secrete glucagon. Glucagon causes the glycogen in the liver cells to be turned back to glucose and released into the bloodstream which raises blood glucose levels.

There are different forms of diabetes:

Type 1: failure to produce insulin. This usually occurs first in children and young people up to about age 35 years. The person becomes ill quite suddenly. There is a complete lack of insulin being made, so patients are dependent on insulin injections throughout their lives (insulin dependent diabetes mellitus IDDM).

Type 2: cells become less responsive to insulin or there is insufficient produced. This usually occurs over age 35, often in people who are obese, lack exercise, or have a family history. However, it is happening now among very obese younger people. It is seen in some young women who are expected to gain weight before marriage by overeating and remaining inactive. (Remember they may be pregnant also.) Onset can be gradual and it is usually controlled by diet, exercise and/or tablets (some need insulin). Weight loss often allows pancreatic function to improve.

Gestational diabetes: may occur during pregnancy as a result of insulin resistance. Problems may arise for the fetus and newborn (see Chapter 36). It usually disappears following the birth, but Type 2 diabetes may develop later especially with obesity and inactivity.

All types of diabetes cause high blood glucose (*hyperglycaemia*). This occurs when people do not take enough insulin or tablets, are very inactive, eat the wrong foods or gain excess weight.

Other effects occur as a result of cells being unable to get the glucose they need.

• The body reacts to the lack of glucose inside cells by breaking down muscle protein to form glucose. Fats are broken down to provide a source of energy. This causes weight loss and *ketonuria*.
• Hyperglycaemia results in *polyuria*. The kidneys respond to the increased concentration of glucose in the *glomerular* filtrate. This extra fluid loss leads to thirst and sometimes dehydration (see diabetic ketoacidosis below). Potassium and sodium balance are also affected (see Chapter 16).

The degree to which these effects happen depends on whether there is still some insulin having effect (Type 2), or complete lack of it (Type 1).

The onset of diabetes

The onset of Type 1 diabetes may be very obvious with weight loss in spite of increased appetite or as an emergency diabetic ketoacidosis (DKA).

Type 2 and gestational diabetes may show no signs or symptoms but still cause damage (see below). Type 2 may be discovered by accident as hyperglycaemia or *glycosuria*, or when problems such as *hypertension* or heart attack occur. Some problems act as warnings of Type 2 although usually less acutely than in Type 1:

- Thirst and polyuria (bedwetting in children)
- Fatigue
- Blurred vision
- Frequent infections (for example urinary and vaginal) and slow wound healing.

Diabetes may occur in relation to other disorders or drug treatment, for example HIV and AIDS.

Control of diabetes

All diabetics need to control their diet and weight, and take exercise. Dietary advice is included in the information box on page 107. Type 1 diabetics must have daily insulin injections. Type 2 may require tablets and/or insulin. These may, of course, be difficult to obtain or afford.

- Tablets (for example glibenclamide) help the pancreas make more insulin, or the body to use it more effectively. These must not be used in pregnancy.
- Insulin cannot be given by mouth. It is supplied as fast (for example Actrapid) and slower-acting (lente) forms which are sometimes mixed. A regular supply is vital for Type 1 diabetics to avoid coma and death. *Subcutaneous* injection and rotation of sites is important to avoid fatty lumps that cause erratic absorption.

Diabetic ketoacidosis (DKA)

In Type 1 diabetes there can be huge breakdown of body fat into fatty acids from which the liver makes large amounts of *ketones*. Some cells can use ketones for energy, but large amounts are toxic and can disturb the blood pH causing reduced brain function, even coma. DKA is often the emergency event that leads to diagnosis of Type 1 diabetes.

DKA can also occur in people known to have diabetes following:

- Emotional or physical stress
- Serious injury
- Illness including infection
- Receipt of too little insulin.

Signs and symptoms of DKA

- Hyperglycaemia
- Polyuria with glycosuria and ketonuria
- Extreme thirst and dehydration, dry skin and mouth
- Feeling nervous and dizzy
- Shaking and sweating
- Nausea and vomiting
- Breath smells fruity
- Blurred vision
- Over-breathing from trying to correct acidosis
- Alteration in consciousness level, possibly coma

Nursing care of people with DKA

The main aims of care are to correct dehydration and return the blood glucose level to normal, so correcting ketoacidosis. These people need immediate hospital admission. Nursing care begins with assessment of the person's condition, including baseline observations, and finding out what has already happened. The information box below shows a typical care plan.

Care plan for patients with DKA

Problem	Nursing care	Rationale
Dehydration due to polyuria – usually severe	IV saline infusion according to local protocol Careful monitoring of fluid balance, BP, pulse and respiration	Correct dehydration. **Note**: *Hypotension* and *tachycardia* are due to reduced fluid volume in the blood.

Care plan for patients with DKA *continued*

Problem	Nursing care	Rationale
Metabolic imbalance due to lack of insulin	IV insulin according to sliding scale/local protocol Hourly tests: ▪ blood sugar ▪ urine for ketones and glucose ▪ blood for low potassium	Insulin promotes glucose uptake and reduces breakdown of fats and proteins.
Respiratory rate increased in an attempt to correct the acidosis	Monitor respiratory rate and rhythm.	Acidosis can lead to *hyperventilation*. Steady reduction in breathing rate suggests blood pH is returning to normal.
Changed level of consciousness	Assess consciousness levels. Put in recovery position if consciousness is affected.	Acidosis can cause brain *dysfunction* and coma.
Risk of vomiting in a person with reduced consciousness	If unconscious, insert a nasogastric tube and aspirate to keep the stomach empty.	Bowel movements may stop: there is a risk of vomiting and inhaling stomach contents.
Reduced mobility due to weakness and fatigue and treatment requirements	Encourage leg movement and deep breathing. Perform passive leg movements if unconscious.	At risk of deep leg vein *thrombosis* from dehydration and inactivity
Infection or other cause	Diagnose e.g. culture blood and urine. Treat as necessary.	Infection may have caused the ketoacidosis.

Hyperglycaemic hyperosmolar non-ketotic coma (HONK)

People who have had undiagnosed Type 2 diabetes for many years can suffer from severe hyperglycaemia and dehydration, acidosis and coma, but without ketones. They can be treated as DKA but using weaker IV saline. They are often old and many die in places where resources are limited.

Hypoglycaemia

Blood sugar levels can become too low if people miss meals or exercise vigorously having taken insulin or tablets, or if dosage and needs are out of balance. Symptoms will include dizziness, pallor and sweating. Sometimes there is a change in mood. Children can become naughty and disobedient. It is important to immediately take sugar followed by a proper meal. Seizures and coma can follow on rapidly. Immediate treatment is necessary:

- IV dextrose infusion given rapidly followed by saline
- Sugary drinks once conscious
- Monitoring of vital signs and blood levels

Long-term problems

Long-term hyperglycaemia and lack of glucose in cells are associated with:

- eye disease (diabetic retinopathy, retinal detachment, glaucoma, cataracts)
- kidney damage (diabetic nephropathy)
- narrowing of arteries (atherosclerosis), high cholesterol levels, hypertension, coronary artery disease, heart attack
- male impotence
- nerve damage (diabetic neuropathy) – injuries, especially to feet, may not be noticed
- *peripheral* blood vessel damage (the cause of most problems)

- reduced function of the immune system.

These last three factors mean that minor injury can become serious, for example foot sores can become gangrenous.

The nursing role and educating for self-care

The nursing role includes monitoring and teaching self-care (see information box below), as well as emergency assistance. Helping people and their families to manage their diabetes, look after themselves, and understand that it is for life is very important. People need to understand about what is happening to them, why it causes problems and why treatment and lifestyle change must continue. Vital messages are:

For those with Type 1 diabetes: Since natural insulin is not being produced in response to eating, eating must respond to regular doses of injected insulin.

For those with Type 1 and 2 diabetes: Good diet, exercise and weight control are key to preventing long-term damage.

Regular monitoring is needed of:

- insulin and other medication dosage (peoples' needs change, especially in the young)
- blood glucose and ketone levels
- eyes with an ophthalmoscope
- urine albumin
- peripheral nerves and blood vessels (foot pulses).

Regular monitoring of symptoms is important too. This becomes even more important when supplies of self-testing equipment are unreliable or unaffordable. Finding out what has happened to people, for example 'hypos' or hyperglycaemic symptoms, and linking that with activities and food intake, may be the only means of gaining some idea of their diabetic status.

Suggestions for a teaching plan	
Topic	**Content**
Diet	Eat regularly, especially if taking tablets or insulin injections. Include: ■ starchy food in each meal (maize porridge, rice, Irish potatoes, plantains, cereals – whole grain where possible). These are broken down more slowly leading to more stable blood glucose levels. Small amounts only of sweet potato, yams, cassava, sweet bread. ■ protein (fish, eggs, beans, peas, groundnuts, soya, lean meat) ■ vegetables, green leaves and fruit (care with sweet bananas) ■ reduce fat, sugar and salt intake (cooking oils, meat fat, sweet tea, alcoholic drinks, soda, cola, sugar cane). Eat enough to keep your weight steady: if overweight cut down, especially fatty foods. Eat more when extra active as this uses glucose up quickly. If you feel ill and unable to eat, you must continue to drink (add some sugar). Drink only a little alcohol – and never on an empty stomach. This may lower your blood sugar suddenly and too much (see *hypoglycaemia* below).
Medication	Learn how your tablets or insulin work, especially how long they work for. If on insulin: ■ Learn how to look after syringes and needles, calculate the dose and draw it up, and inject beneath a pinch of skin as taught. Change the sites (upper legs, belly or upper arms). ■ Refrigerate insulin if possible (never freeze). It is damaged by heat and strong light. Otherwise, keep it cool by suspending the vial in a clay pot kept damp with wet cloths. Will last one month only. If you feel unwell, even if you don't want to eat, **you must always take your tablets or insulin to avoid hyperglycaemia. Try to take something** e.g. milk, thin porridge, sugary drinks. Often you need extra insulin when ill, so see a doctor or nurse if you can.

Suggestions for a teaching plan *continued*	
Topic	**Content**
Skin care	Your skin may not heal well: ■ Try to keep it clean and avoid damage. ■ Protect your feet (avoid walking barefoot or wearing shoes that cause blisters), inspect daily. ■ If your skin is damaged and slow to heal, (especially feet) see a doctor or nurse if you can.
Monitoring urine or blood glucose	You will be taught to check how well your diabetes is being controlled by testing your urine or blood. See a doctor or nurse if signs appear of your diabetes not being well controlled: ■ urine contains more than a trace of glucose and/or ketones ■ blood glucose level is above 12 mmol/l. Because you will need extra insulin, see a doctor or nurse urgently if urine tests show: ■ glucose +++ or more ■ ketones ++ or more ■ blood glucose level is above 20 mmol/l.
Identifying hypoglycaemia	People on insulin or tablets are at risk of lowering their blood glucose too much (hypoglycaemia or 'hypo'), especially if they have missed a meal or been very active. Warning signs of a 'hypo' attack are sudden: ■ Feeling strange and dizzy ■ People see your behaviour change ■ Paleness and sweating. Eat some sugar immediately, you should then get back to normal; if you don't you might become unconscious. Always carry sugar or glucose sweets with you for immediate use. Carry a card to say you have diabetes, in case you collapse and need help. Eat a proper meal following a 'hypo' as soon as possible. Tell your nurse or doctor about what happened next time you see them.
Diabetic complications	You need to control your diabetes well to avoid serious health problems. Long-term high blood glucose damages blood vessels throughout the body. Possible problems include blindness, kidney damage, gangrenous feet, heart attack and stroke. **Good control of your blood glucose makes these complications much less likely, so follow advice about managing your diabetes properly. This includes stopping or reducing smoking tobacco.**

Thyroid dysfunction

The main function of thyroid hormones and others that stimulate their production (see page 104) is to control metabolic reactions within the body's cells. Two common conditions are related to these hormones. Secretion of too much hormone is known as hyperthyroidism (thyrotoxicosis), too little leads to hypothyroidism (myxoedema). This condition rarely occurs in young people but babies can be born with it (congenital hypothyroidism or cretinism).

Hyperthyroidism

Hyperthyroidism is an overproduction of thyroid hormones (thyroxin, T_3 and T_4). This raises the metabolic rate, causing a higher demand by cells for oxygen and nutrients.

Effects of hyperthyroidism

- Raised body temperature and feeling hot
- Tachycardia
- Raised respiratory rate and feeling short of breath
- Insomnia and becoming easily tired

- Nervousness, irritability, agitation and restlessness
- Muscle weakness and shaking when holding hands out
- Increased appetite
- Gastro-intestinal disturbances
- Weight loss
- Hair loss
- Enlarged thyroid gland
- Protruding eyeballs (exophthalmia)

Hyperthyroidism is more common in women than men. Blood tests can confirm the diagnosis. Hyperthyroidism is usually treated with oral medication, for example carbimazole, but surgery or radiation treatment may be required.

Nursing care of patients with hyperthyroidism

Nursing care must start with an assessment and current history which can be used to write a care plan (see information box below). Admission to hospital may be unnecessary. Education is important so that patients will:

- understand the nature of the disease

Care plan for patients with hyperthyroidism

Problem	Nursing care	Rationale
Tachycardia, raised temperature and respiratory rate	4-hourly observations Record pulse while sleeping	To monitor signs of an increase in hyperthyroidism The fast pulse rate puts a strain on the heart.
Weight loss	Daily weighing Balanced diet Good fluid intake	To ensure that food intake provides enough calories to meet metabolic needs and gain weight High fluid loss through sweating
Tiredness because of general agitation and raised activity levels	Encourage rest. Suggest activities that require less physical effort.	Activity increases metabolic rate and the goal is to reduce it.
Reduced ability to regulate temperature	Keep the environment cool and well ventilated. Keep clothing light.	More body heat generated because of increased metabolic rate.
Skin care	Daily bathing and general hygiene Observe for breaks in skin integrity.	Sweating is excessive Reduced mobility, restlessness and weight loss may cause pressure area damage.
Eye care	If exophthalmos is present, instill drops to prevent drying of cornea and conjunctiva. Sunglasses protect the eyes. Test vision	Change in the shape of the eye affects vision; can be corrected with prescription glasses.
Change in sexual function and body image	Provide opportunities for the expression of anxieties. Explain the causes and that sexual function improves as hormone balance is achieved.	Hyperthyroidism can cause changes to the menstrual cycle, loss of sex drive and impotence.
Thyroid hormone imbalance	Regular blood tests	To assess hormone levels so that adjustments to dosage of medication can be made.

- manage lifestyle changes
- manage their own medication.

Nursing care following thyroidectomy

If medical treatment fails, surgical removal/reduction of the thyroid gland may be necessary. Sometimes thyroidectomy is done for malignancy or because of pressure. The thyroid lies close to important structures including the larynx, and parathyroid glands which control calcium levels. If the patient is thyrotoxic, medical treatment must be given before surgery to reduce the gland's function. The information box below gives care needed following surgery.

Nursing care of patients following thyroidectomy

Problem	Nursing care	Rationale
Difficulty in clearing airway	Support in semi-recumbent position. Suction to clear the airway. Make sure wound drains are functioning.	Patients may find clearing their airways difficult because of pain and/or pressure from the operation and reduced head and neck mobility.
Pain	Give analgesics as prescribed.	Surgery will cause pain which should be controlled.
Problems may include: ■ haemorrhage and collection of blood (*haematoma*) ■ laryngeal nerve damage	Observe: ■ pulse and blood pressure ■ wound area for swelling ■ respiratory function	*Tachycardia* and hypotension may indicate haemorrhage. Difficult or noisy breathing may indicate pressure from haematoma backwards onto trachea. Emergency removal of stitches or clips may be necessary if haematoma is obstructing breathing. Laryngeal nerve damage causes hoarseness (unilateral) or obstruction (bilateral). Tracheostomy may be needed.
■ low blood calcium (*hypocalcaemia*) from damage to parathyroid glands	■ for muscle twitching and spasm (tetany)	Muscle twitching may indicate damage to the parathyroid glands. Emergency injection of 10 ml calcium gluconate 10% may be necessary to increase blood calcium.

Hypothyroidism (myxoedema)

More women than men are affected by hypothyroidism, and the incidence increases with age. It occurs when too little thyroid hormone is secreted from the thyroid gland. It may happen because of iodine lack in the diet, known as IDD (iodine deficiency disorder). This occurs more commonly in some geographic areas, for example in the mountain areas bordering the African Rift valley in Ethiopia and Malawi. Limited access to sea fish or salt with added iodine also causes problems.

Characteristics of hypothyroidism

- Slowing of mental and physical abilities and responses
- Enlarged thyroid gland (goitre)

- Slow monotonous speech
- Swelling of ankles
- Apathy, tiredness, general weakness
- Constipation
- Loss of interest in sex
- Reduced appetite, but general weight gain
- Menstrual disorders
- Feeling cold even on hot days
- Low blood pressure, pulse and temperature
- Dry, thickened skin, puffy eyes, lips and tongue

Nursing care of patients with hypothyroidism

Assessment of the patient is important. Hospital admission is unlikely but education is important, and remembering that patients are individuals with personal needs that must be identified. For advice you may give see the information box below. Patients need to be able to:

- understand the nature of the disease
- plan their own care in relation to lifestyle
- understand the need to take medication (thyroxin tablets) regularly and probably forever.

Once treatment is started, improvement is usually quick. Constipation will improve and the pulse rate rise. Patients must be reminded to continue treatment, even if they feel better, or the condition will recur.

Care plan for patients with hypothyroidism

Problem	Nursing care	Rationale
Feeling cold	Wear adequate clothing. Avoid draughts	Reduced metabolic activities lower the amount of heat generated.
Weight gain	Low calorie and fat diet	Reduced metabolic rate may lead to weight gain. Blood cholesterol rises.
Constipation	High fibre diet Plenty to drink	Reduced cellular metabolism also slows physical processes such as digestion.
Possible side effects of thyroxin tablets	Take medication as prescribed: low dose to start (50 micrograms daily), increasing gradually, as advised. Report tachycardia, chest pains, restlessness or diarrhoea.	Thyroxin raises the metabolic rate. This must be gradual, since rapid change may stimulate the heart too much and trigger problems, such as angina, myocardial infarction or heart failure.

Health promotion

- Endocrine disorders cannot really be avoided, although good diet and exercise help to prevent obesity and Type 2 diabetes, and reduce or delay complications.
- Those with diabetes should follow the advice in the information box on page 107, including having regular check ups.
- Nurses can help diabetics by encouraging them to form support groups, for example those living close could save together to buy shared blood monitoring equipment.

■ Activities

1. Someone with diabetes suddenly starts behaving in strange ways, is pale and sweating profusely. What would you do and why?
2. Why should someone who has started treatment with thyroxin for hypothyroidism be told to report palpitations or chest pain?
3. Your patient is having difficulty breathing following thyroidectomy. What should be done urgently?

20

Care of patients with problems of the ear, nose and throat

Anatomically, the ear, nose and throat are connected, so often a problem that affects one will affect one of the others. This chapter will cover some of the more basic problems that are met and suggest ways of managing them.

The ear

The ear is the organ which enables us to hear and also part of the mechanism that controls balance. Some problems that affect the ear can therefore lead to deafness if not properly managed and can also lead to dizzy spells by affecting balance.

The outer ear

This consists of the pinna which is made of cartilage covered with skin and the external auditory canal. The canal is S-shaped and about 2.5 cm long. The tympanic membrane, also called the ear drum, separates the outer ear from the middle ear. It is a membrane which transmits sound waves from the outer ear to the middle ear.

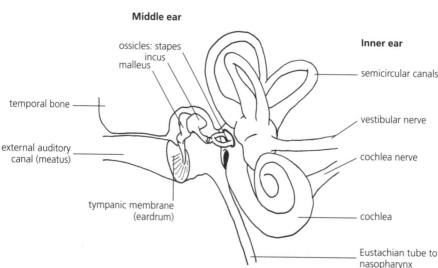

right ear lobe

Middle ear

ossicles: stapes
incus
malleus

temporal bone

external auditory
canal (meatus)

tympanic membrane
(eardrum)

Inner ear

semicircular canals

vestibular nerve

cochlea nerve

cochlea

Eustachian tube to
nasopharynx

Figure 20.1 *The structure of the ear*

The middle ear

This is a small air filled cavity. It contains three tiny bones (auditory ossicles), the malleus, the incus and the stapes. It is separated from the inner ear by a bony partition which contains two openings, the round and oval windows. The middle ear is connected to the nasopharynx by the Eustachian tube. This tube helps keep the pressure equal on both sides of the tympanic membrane. Sound waves are transmitted from the tympanic membrane through the ossicles to the inner ear.

The inner ear

This contains the bony and membranous labyrinth. The bony labyrinth is divided into three parts, the cochlea, the vestibule and the semicircular canals. The inner part of the cochlea contains the organ of Corti which is the organ of hearing. Within the vestibule and semicircular canals are sensory receptors which sense position and the movement of the head and help us to maintain balance.

The structure of the ear is shown in Figure 20.1.

Problems of the middle ear (otitis media)

As the mucous membranes of the middle ear are continuous with those of the respiratory tract, viral and bacterial infections can easily pass from the throat to the ear. This is more common in children as the Eustachian tube is short, wide and straight.

Acute otitis media

This usually follows an upper respiratory infection. Common symptoms include pain, fever and discharge if the ear drum perforates. As it is so common in children, all sick children should have their ears examined. Antibiotics should be given if the infection is bacterial.

Chronic otitis media

This can be the result of recurrent or badly treated acute otitis media. It is common in both adults and children and is characterised by a purulent discharge and a perforated ear drum. Long-term antibiotics may be needed and the ears should be cleaned and antibiotic drops instilled. Treatment must continue until the discharge stops as otherwise there may be permanent loss of hearing.

Pp Instilling ear drops

- Warm ear drops to body temperature, by placing the bottle in a bowl of warm water.
- Tilt the head to the unaffected side.
- Straighten the canal by pulling the ear up and back.
- Instil the drops as instructed.

Mastoiditis

This is a secondary infection resulting from poorly treated otitis media. The mastoid is a sinus containing air cells. It lies just behind the ear and immediately above the venous sinus which receives blood from the brain. Infection can pass easily from the mastoid to the meninges or the brain. In mastoiditis, the area behind the ear becomes swollen and inflamed. Any infection must be treated quickly to prevent meningitis or brain abscesses occurring.

Signs and symptoms

- Acute, sharp pain behind the ear
- Swelling behind the ear which may cause the pinna to be pushed forward
- Fever and loss of appetite. Vomiting may occur.
- The ear drum instead of being shiny and semi transparent may appear thick and dull.

Management

- *Systemic* antibiotics
- Analgesia
- Encourage fluids

If the infection becomes chronic, surgery may become necessary. The infected bone has to be scraped away.

Deafness (loss of hearing)

There are two main types of deafness:
- Conductive deafness when sound waves fail to reach the inner ear
- Sensorineural deafness which is due to problems with the organ of Corti or damage to the nerve supplying the ear.

Congenital deafness

Some babies are born deaf which can be due to the mother having problems during the antenatal period, for example if she develops rubella (German measles) or poor development of the ear. These children will grow up with problems in learning to speak, as they have never heard sound. They can be helped through early diagnosis, the fitting of hearing aids and special schools. They can learn to communicate by learning sign language. Some can be taught to speak with the use of special equipment and teachers trained to help the deaf.

Acquired deafness

This is more common and may be partial or total. It is important to see that there are no obstructions in the auditory canal, for example foreign bodies, growths or an accumulation of wax. Deafness can result from meningitis or as a complication of drug therapy, for example gentamicin. In adults the hearing can deteriorate gradually through continuous exposure to loud noise. Hearing aids will help many people but they are not always available. Deafness is a major disability because it can lead to isolation and loss of self-esteem. Some people are unable to do the jobs that they used to do because of their difficulty in communicating with others.

The nose

The nose has two major functions. It is the organ of smell and it also warms, filters and moistens the air as we breathe in. The nose connects with the ear through the Eustachian tube and is also connected to eight cavities in the skull which are called sinuses. The sinuses are thought to help with the warming and moistening of the air which is inhaled, and also make the skull lighter than it would be if the bones were solid. Behind the nose on the wall of the nasopharynx are two small patches of lymphoid tissue called the adenoids. The adenoids help to prevent infection reaching the lower respiratory tract. They are larger in childhood but usually begin to shrink once the child reaches five years and will eventually disappear.

Problems affecting the nose
The common cold (rhinitis)

This is a common viral infection especially in children who may have as many as five to ten a year. There may be coughing and sneezing and a watery discharge. This may cause babies problems as they can only breathe through their noses until they are three months old. No treatment is necessary in most cases but if completely blocked the nose must be cleaned immediately as the condition is life-threatening. It also helps to clean the noses of babies before they feed if they are having difficulty.

Foreign bodies

Some children will poke foreign bodies up their noses and they can become wedged. The child may come to clinic with a persistent purulent nasal discharge. Careful examination of the nose, using an auriscope, may show the problem. The foreign body will need to be removed. If it cannot be easily seen, it may be necessary for the child to have an anaesthetic.

Sinusitis

The sinuses may become inflamed following a cold. There is acute pain over the cheekbones and sometimes headaches. It may be necessary to give ephedrine nasal drops to shrink the swollen mucous membranes which block the passages and if bacterial infection is suspected, give systemic antibiotics.

Nosebleeds (epistaxis)

Nosebleeds are caused by bleeding from the small vessels. They can occur after a blow to the nose or as a result of foreign bodies or blowing the nose too vigorously. Sit the person up and pinch the nostrils together until the bleeding stops. Heavy or frequent nosebleeds will need further investigation as they may be a sign that there is a problem with clotting. This can occur in leukaemia, Ebola and Rift Valley fever.

The throat

The throat is made up of the pharynx and larynx and forms part of the upper respiratory system and gastro-intestinal tract. The pharynx is a muscular tube lined with mucous membrane and is a common pathway for air to enter the larynx and food to enter the oesophagus. Food is prevented from entering the larynx by the epiglottis, a small structure which closes off the larynx when food or fluid reaches the pharyngeal tube.

The larynx is made up of muscle and cartilage and is lined with mucous membrane. It is the passageway for air to pass from the pharynx to the trachea and it also contains the vocal cords. The tonsils are patches of lymphoid tissue found in the pharyngeal cavity. They help to filter out infection and are larger in children than in adults.

Problems affecting the throat

Sore throats

People who have colds will often also complain of a sore throat. There may be inflammation of the pharynx and larynx leading to a troublesome cough and sometimes a husky voice. As the infection is usually viral, no treatment is necessary except for making sure that the fluid intake is kept high.

Tonsillitis

The tonsils may become acutely inflamed leading to:
- a very sore throat
- difficulty in swallowing
- high temperature
- earache sometimes.

Tonsillitis is often caused by the Haemolytic Streptcoccus Group A. This organism can also cause rheumatic fever which can damage the heart valves. Antibiotics must be given as soon as throat swabs have been taken. Penicillin is very effective. Children may get as many as five attacks of tonsillitis a year and the tonsils can become chronically enlarged.

Carcinoma of the larynx

This is more common in males who smoke and drink alcohol excessively. The patient may complain of:
- an increasingly hoarse voice
- difficulty in swallowing and speaking
- earache
- lump in the neck.

The patient should be referred to a major centre, if possible, for further investigation. Treatment is either by laryngectomy, or in some cases radiotherapy. Once a laryngectomy has been performed, the patient is not able to speak as the vocal cords have been removed. A permanent tracheostomy is performed and the patient can sometimes learn to make sound by controlling their breathing.

Tracheostomy

This is an artificial opening into the trachea and may need to be done for many reasons:
- Following laryngectomy
- To enable patients to be ventilated if this is likely to be needed for some time
- For children with diphtheria, epiglottitis, laryngo tracheo bronchitis (see Chapter 47).

An incision is made in the trachea and a tube inserted into the hole. The type of tube used will depend on what is available. Sometimes it may be a plastic tube, sometimes a silver tube which will have an inner tube to make it easier for cleaning. Both types must have introducers to make them easier to insert.

Nursing care of a patient with a tracheostomy

Patients with tracheostomies are unable to speak, so remember to talk to them. They may be able to communicate by writing down what they want to say.

Equipment to keep at the bedside

- Suction apparatus with catheters of a suitable size
- Box of 5 ml ampoules of normal saline
- 2 or 5 ml syringes depending on whether it is for a child or adult
- Sachets of sterile normal saline
- Disposable gloves. These should not be powdered and need not be sterile.
- Spare tracheostomy tube of the same size as the one inserted in the patient
- Tracheal dilators
- Spare set of tapes

Pp Tracheal suction

If the secretions are very thick it may be necessary to apply suction to prevent the tube blocking with secretions.
- 0.5–1 ml of normal saline should be instilled into the tube, immediately before suction.
- Wash your hands.
- Use a suction catheter of a suitable size. If it is too big it will cause blockage of the tube, if it is too small it will not remove the secretions.
- The suction apparatus should not be set at too high a pressure as it can damage the mucous lining of the trachea.
- The suction catheter should be introduced into the tracheostomy and inserted to the length of the tube + 0.5 cm. It is important not to introduce it too far as it will cause damage.

Suction should be applied as the catheter is withdrawn, turning it slightly. The length of time that suction is applied should not be more than 15 seconds as this can cause the patient to become short of oxygen. If the nurse feels that there are secretions that have not been removed, the procedure can be repeated.

Pp Cleaning a silver tracheostomy tube

You will need:
- 2 gallipots
- Gloves
- Sodium bicarbonate

This should be done 3–4 hourly, depending on the patient's condition. If there are a lot of secretions, it needs to be done more frequently. If few, it can be done less frequently. The aim is to keep the tube from blocking.
- Wash your hands and put on gloves.
- The inner tube is removed and placed in one of the gallipots.
- Put some sodium bicarbonate and water in the gallipot containing the dirty tube.
- Take to the sink and clean thoroughly, removing all secretions. Pipe cleaners or cotton wool can be used.
- Rinse thoroughly and place in the clean gallipot.
- Replace the clean inner tube into the tracheostomy.

Caring for the tracheostomy

The area around the tracheostomy can become sore, especially if the tapes securing the tube are wet. Clean around the area, using an aseptic technique, removing the crusted secretions. The neck should be dried and a barrier cream applied. Tapes should be changed as necessary. Always secure new tapes before removing the old tapes.

Pp Changing the tracheostomy tube

- This should always be done with two nurses.
- Prepare the clean tube, inserting the introducer first.
- Insert tapes into the new tube.
- Place a rolled towel under the patient's neck and see that the neck is extended.

- Cut the old tapes and remove the old tube, immediately replacing with the new tube. **Remove the introducer at once as it will be blocking the airway**.
- Fasten the tapes securely.

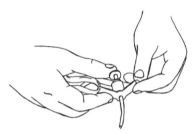

Figure 20.2 *Tracheostomy tube is prepared for insertion: tapes are threaded and introducer is inserted*

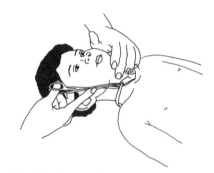

Figure 20.3 *Existing tracheostomy tape is cut*

It is always important to watch patients, especially children, carefully to see that the tube does not come out. If the tube comes out accidentally, a new tube must be inserted immediately and the patient's respiratory function watched carefully.

The patient also needs careful watching once the tube has been finally removed. A nurse should stay with the patient for the first few hours, monitoring their colour and respirations carefully. Tracheal dilators and a tracheostomy tube should be beside the bed, as sometimes the tube needs to be replaced quickly. It may be helpful to nurse the patient in a humid environment during this time.

Health promotion

- Treat all ear infections quickly and effectively.
- Teach parents to keep objects which can be pushed into the nose or ear away from small children.
- Avoid drinking too much alcohol.
- Help people to give up cigarette smoking.

■ Activity

What would make you suspect that the tracheostomy tube of a patient was becoming blocked with secretions and what action would you take?

21

Care of patients with problems affecting the eyes

The eye is a delicate organ and serious cases which are not well handled can lead to people becoming blind. Blindness is more common in Africa than elsewhere but is often preventable. This chapter covers the main eye problems and suggests ways in which you can help prevent patients from developing long-term problems (see Figure 21.1).

The structure of the eye

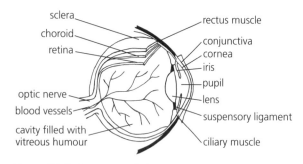

Figure 21.1 *Structure of the eye*

History and examination

Before examining the eye, it is important to take a careful history from the patient.

- When did they first notice signs or symptoms? Sudden onset of loss of vision could be a result of acute glaucoma or retinal detachment.
- Blurred vision could be a result of cataract, glaucoma or high blood sugar.
- Was the loss of vision associated with pain or was it painless?
- Has there been any recent injury or irritation and pain? There may be a foreign body.
- Has the patient had any infections recently?

- Are there problems with reading or distance work? These patients may benefit from spectacles.
- Are there problems with the whole visual field or just part of it?
  - Central blurred vision is found in cataract.
  - Peripheral vision and central loss is seen in glaucoma.
  - Are there specks or strands seen in the field of vision? These suggest lesions in the front of or on the retina. These patients should be referred.
- Is there a family history of problems?

The examination of the eye should include an inspection to see if there is any inflammation, irritation, watering or other obvious signs of problems.

Pp Eye examination

Visual acuity: This can be tested using a Snellen's chart. Normal vision is expressed at 6/6. If even the biggest letters cannot be read, see if the patient can count your fingers at different distances or whether they can only see a light shone into their eyes (perception of light).

Torch: Use a torch with good batteries that can be focused to a small beam. Darken the room and then shine the torch in the eye to examine eyes and eyelids. It can also be used to test whether the pupils constrict normally.

Local anaesthesia: Certain procedures may need local anaesthetic drops, usually methocaine or benoxinate drops. They may sting at first.

Fluorescein: This is a dye which can be used to show corneal abrasion, ulceration or foreign bodies. The dye is orange but looks green when instilled in the eyes. It is best to use it dry on tips of soft paper. This is first touched inside the lower eyelid (not the eye), till the stain flows into the tears.

Lid eversion: Ask the patient to look down, then catch the upper lashes in your fingers and pull them down and out. With your finger or pen against the outside of the eyelid, flick the eyelid inside out and examine its inner surface. This should not be done if the eyelid is inflamed.

Visual field: This is to test the extent of the person's field of vision. There are special pieces of equipment for testing this.

Colour vision: Some people have problems with seeing colours. Red and green are the ones that often cause problems. The person is said to be colour-blind.

Injuries to the eye

Injuries to the eye can arise from physical objects or chemicals. The eyelids and the bony orbit of the eye can protect from physical injuries but not from chemicals. Once you have asked what happened, inspect the eye for obvious injury, tiny punctures, visible objects or objects protruding.

Sub-conjunctival haemorrhage

There can be leakage of blood from the blood vessels into the conjunctiva. The 'white' of the eye looks very bloodstained, but there is no pain (unless associated with trauma) or discharge. This common condition can occur spontaneously, usually in an older person or after trauma or coughing. No treatment is necessary if the sub-conjunctival haemorrhage is the only problem, and the patient should be reassured. However if the bleeding persists, it may be a sign of HIV and AIDS.

Foreign bodies

Small foreign bodies are often found embedded in the conjunctiva or cornea. Examples of these are dust, insect wings, pieces of metal, glass or wood.

The patient will complain of feeling something in the eye, watering and blurring of vision if the foreign body is in the cornea. Metal and other foreign bodies can scratch the cornea causing severe pain and irritation. Sharp objects can penetrate the eye and result in *hyphaema* (blood in the anterior chamber) or *hypopyon* (pus in the anterior chamber). Corneal ulcers resulting from a foreign body can be diagnosed by staining the eye with fluorescein 1% and then examining it with a blue light.

Treatment

If the foreign body is superficial:
- Instil local anaesthetic drops.
- Remove the foreign body using a clean swab. *Evert* the eyelid if necessary.

If the foreign body is embedded in the cornea:
- Instil local anaesthetic drops.
- Remove using a small sterile needle.
- If possible, refer the patient for checking by an eye-care health worker. Never try to remove a deeply embedded foreign body, always refer the patient.

Blunt, non penetrating injuries

Common injuries are:

Corneal abrasion: This will be revealed by fluorescein stain. Use antibiotic ointment and cover with a pad for a few days.

Traumatic iritis: The eye will be red, watering and painful, especially in a bright light. There may be a tear in the iris. Instil atropine until the redness subsides.

Hyphaema: If less than half the anterior chamber is full of blood, keep the patient quiet and instil atropine ointment. If more than half the anterior chamber is full, the pressure inside the eye will rise which can lead to blindness. The patient should be treated with Diamox and kept quiet. It may be necessary for the blood to be washed out of the chamber. The patient should be referred to a specialist centre if possible.

Penetrating injuries

Severe ones should be referred at once. A torn conjuctiva will heal well, but if there are deeper wounds they need specialist treatment. Do not instil any ointment or drops but cover the eye with a pad and send to the eye-care health worker.

Burns and chemical injuries

Acids or alkalis can enter the eye either by accident or by assault. Steam, hot water or ashes can cause damage. The patient presents with inflammation, a feeling of foreign bodies in the eye, *lacrimation*, pain and visual disturbances. This is an emergency and treatment must begin immediately.

Treatment

- The eyes should be washed out with water, continuing for 10–15 minutes if necessary. Milk is an alternative, particularly if the irritant is known to be an acid.
- The patient should then be referred urgently to a specialist centre.

Cataracts

Cataracts are opacities of the lens inside the eye. They may be congenital or acquired. Cataracts are responsible for 20 million cases of blindness worldwide.

Congenital cataracts

These are often seen when the mother has had a viral infection, commonly rubella, especially between the 9th and 12th week of pregnancy.

Acquired cataracts

These may be due to:

Old age: This is the commonest form of cataract and the main cause of blindness around the world. It is not often seen before the age of 40 but then becomes increasingly common.

Diabetes: Constantly high blood sugar can damage the lens. Diabetes that is not well controlled will make this more likely. It may be seen in younger patients.

Trauma: A cataract can develop following an injury.

Signs and symptoms

There is no pain. Patients with age-related cataract will complain of poor vision that is slowly getting worse.

Treatment

- The patient is referred for surgical removal of the lens under local or general anaesthetic. The best method of surgery is to have an artificial lens placed inside the eye. Alternatively, spectacles will have to be worn after the operation.
- Following surgery, steroid/antibiotic drops are instilled for about 2 weeks.
- Patients should be advised not to lift heavy objects which could increase pressure within the eye.
- They should return in 6–8 weeks (or when the surgeon advises) to have their eyes tested and collect spectacles if necessary.

Eye infections and inflammation

Conjunctivitis

The conjunctiva can become inflamed, sometimes as a result of an allergy, sometimes due to an infection, most often bacterial. If due to a bacterial infection, antibiotic drops or ointment should be instilled.

Gonococcal conjunctivitis

This is common in newborn babies who are infected during birth from a maternal genital infection. It can rapidly progress to corneal ulceration and blindness, so treatment should be started quickly. In many areas it is routine to wipe the babies eyes immediately after birth, and instil tetracycline eye ointment or silver nitrate 1% drops.

Signs and symptoms

These will be seen within the first 48 hours following birth:
- The eyes are swollen and there is a heavy purulent discharge.
- An eye swab will grow the gram negative organism Neisseria gonorrhoea.

Treatment

- The baby should be nursed away from other newborns if possible.
- Nurses must wash their hands carefully before and after giving treatment.
- Take a swab if there are laboratory facilities available.
- Wipe the eyes (not the cornea) carefully from the inside to the outside, to prevent infection spreading into the other eye. Wipe away the pus.
- Start treatment at once. Put in penicillin drops or tetracycline ointment every $\frac{1}{2}$ hour for 24 hours, then 2 hourly for 7 days. Mothers can be taught to do this, to save nurses' time and make sure the treatment is continuous.
- Systemic antibiotics are needed, such as penicillin, gentamycin or kanamycin if there is no improvement after 24 hours.
- Both parents must be treated for gonorrhoea.

Chlamydia infection

These babies present with a less severe infection occurring a few days after birth. They can be treated with tetracycline eye ointment or, sometimes, erythromycin by mouth for children.

Trachoma

Trachoma is the commonest infective cause of blindness in adults, affecting 150 million worldwide and causing $5\frac{1}{2}$ million cases of blindness. It is caused by Chlamydia trachomatis, carried by flies and is highly contagious. It causes a chronic infection in children whose faces are not well washed and whose hygiene is poor. Flies feed on faeces and also discharge from the eyes. Repeated inflammation of the eye lids causes scarring. This pulls the eye lashes inwards which is called *trichiasis*. The continuous scratching of the cornea by the lashes causes scarring and eventually blindness.

Signs and symptoms

- Red inflamed eyes and a sticky discharge affecting several children in the family or school friends
- The tarsal conjunctiva under the eyelids is thick and red.
- Follicles, tiny raised spots, may be seen on the tarsal conjunctiva.

Treatment

- Tetracycline eye ointment should be given twice daily to the whole family for 6 weeks.
- If the eye lashes are scratching the eye, the child or adult should be referred for surgery before the cornea is damaged.
- Children's faces should be washed thoroughly every day.
- The family should be taught about good hygiene in the home, to reduce the number of flies. Fly traps made from plastic bottles can be very effective. See Appendix A on page 392.
- Latrines should be kept clean and placed away from living areas.

Remember the five 'Fs' in providing trachoma control in a community:

1. **F**lies
2. **F**aeces
3. **F**aces
4. **F**ingers
5. **F**omites (for example towels and face cloths).

Onchocerciasis (River blindness)

Eighteen million people are affected by this disease, 270,000 of whom are blind. Most of these people live in sub-Saharan or West Africa. In some villages, 100 per cent of the population is affected, 10 per cent of whom will be blind. The disease is spread by a black fly that lives in well oxygenated water, usually fast running rivers. The fly spreads the worm, Onchocerca volvulus,

which releases microfilaria. It is these microfilaria which are responsible for the skin and eye problems. In areas which are heavily infested, populations are forced to leave some of the most fertile land to avoid problems.

The microfilaria cause an inflammatory reaction in the eye, leading to sclerosing keratitis. It can also lead to secondary glaucoma, cataract and changes at the back of the eye affecting the retina and optic nerve.

Treatment

- Ivermectin (mectizan) does not cure, but can control the disease. It should not be given to pregnant women, women during the first month of breastfeeding, or children under the age of five years. It is necessary to give ivermectin once a year for some years as the worm lives for 10–12 years.
- Control of the black fly by the use of larvicides.

Xerophthalmia: Vitamin A deficiency

Vitamin A deficiency is a major cause of blindness in some areas, yet it is easily avoidable. It mainly affects children under the age of five years, particularly those aged one to two years who are no longer breast-feeding. Vitamin A is found in:

- Milk, meat such as liver and chicken, oily fish and eggs
- Margarine, dried skimmed milk and other foods that have had vitamin A added
- Dark/medium green and orange vegetables: carrots, tomatoes, spinach and pumpkin
- Orange fruits such as mangoes and pawpaw
- Red palm oil.

These should form part of the diet from the time of weaning to prevent the deficiency.

Vitamin A deficiency is particularly high in children, because they are growing quickly so have an increased need. Some mothers are low in vitamin A during pregnancy and their babies are therefore at risk. Colostrum and breast milk are good sources. Infections increase the demand for vitamin A and children with diarrhoea do not absorb the vitamin well. The severe blinding form of vitamin A deficiency, affecting the cornea (keratomalacia), may develop acutely during a measles epidemic. Those most at risk include:

- Babies whose mothers stop breastfeeding early
- Children who are malnourished

- Children who have measles
- People with persistent diarrhoea
- People suffering from recurrent infections.

Signs and symptoms

- Night blindness. Children have difficulty in walking around in the dark and may fall over a lot. Mothers are quick to notice this, although very young children will not complain of night blindness.
- Dryness of the conjunctiva and Bitot's spots. The conjunctiva appears thickened, dry and wrinkled. Bitot's spots are 'foam-like' cream or white patches (sometimes pigmented) on the conjunctiva close to the cornea.
- The cornea becomes dry and rough (xerosis).
- Corneal ulcers (keratomalacia). These can occur suddenly and be full thickness. The contents of the eye can protrude and sight in the eye is lost. As this often happens to both eyes at the same time, the child becomes blind. This is an eye emergency.

Treatment

If you suspect that children are at risk of vitamin A deficiency, they should be treated immediately with high dose vitamin A capsules. These contain 100,000–200,000 units each. The amount of vitamin A in ordinary multivitamin capsules is not enough.

- Give vitamin A 200,000 units immediately to children over one year; 100,000 units to children under one year.
- Repeat the following day and 1–4 weeks later.
- Make sure that the child's diet contains plenty of vitamin A. Cooking oil will help with absorption.
- If there is a secondary infection of the eye, use local antibiotics.
- Give vitamin A to every child at risk.

The most important thing to remember about vitamin A deficiency is that it is preventable but when it occurs it can cause blindness.

Glaucoma

Glaucoma causes more than 10 per cent of all cases of blindness worldwide. A rise in the pressure inside the eye damages the optic disc and leads to loss in the visual field. It usually affects people over the age of 40 years; occasionally it can be congenital. In Africa and many other parts of the world, the loss of sight is usually gradual so often patients do not come for help until the condition is well advanced, when there is loss of central vision.

Treatment

- Patients should be referred to a centre where the intraocular pressure can be measured and their visual field tested.
- Early treatment is often with pilocarpine 2% eye drops and in some cases Diamox tablets. This will lower the intraocular pressure but is usually a short-term measure.
- In many cases surgery will be needed to reduce the pressure.
- Early treatment can prevent blindness. It is best to refer patients who have:
  - gradual loss of vision for no obvious cause
  - both eyes affected (usually one eye is worse than the other)
  - occasional pain and headache.

HIV and AIDS

Herpes zoster ophthalmicus

In Africa, this is often the first sign that the person has HIV or AIDS. It affects the area supplied by the ophthalmic nerve. The person usually complains of severe pain and a few days later there is a vesicular rash. When the vesicles burst, bacterial infection can occur.

Treatment

- Give Acyclovir by mouth, if available.
- Give pain relief.
- Treat secondary bacterial infection.

Kaposi's sarcoma

This rare skin tumour may involve eyelids, conjunctiva and orbit. The vascular tumour appears as a red or purple nodule on the skin of the eyelid or the conjunctiva. There may be a persistent sub-conjunctival haemorrhage. If the tumour causes problems it can be surgically removed or treated with radiotherapy.

HIV associated retinopathy

Ischaemic changes may be seen in the retina and can lead to blindness. These are caused by opportunistic infections such as cytomegalovirus (CMV). These are usually late signs and therefore not seen often, as patients usually die from other infections first. CMV can be treated with antiviral drugs (see Chapter 32).

Conclusion

Nurses have an important role to play in preventing blindness. They must be aware of danger signs and know which patients they should refer to specialist centres and which ones they can treat themselves.

■ Activity

What questions do you need to ask and what investigations can you do if a patient comes to the clinic complaining that they have difficulty in seeing clearly?

Health promotion

- Refer any patient with eye injury, unless the trauma is superficial.
- Chemical eye injury needs immediate washing with water.
- Treat a bacterial conjunctivitis with antibiotic eye drops. If the cause of a red eye is uncertain (or does not respond to antibiotics within 24–48 hours) refer to a specialist centre.
- Ensure that mothers are not deficient in vitamin A and treat during pregnancy if there is a risk (but seek advice about dosage).
- Encourage breastfeeding which is a good source of vitamin A.
- Give advice about foods which are good sources of vitamin A.
- Give vitamin A capsules to all children at risk.
- Teach people how to reduce flies around the home.
- Wash children's faces thoroughly at least once a day.
- Teach about the importance of clean water in both the village and the home. Wells, springs and bore holes should be protected. Utensils used for carrying water should be clean.
- Teach people about sexually transmitted infections and prevention of neonatal conjunctivitis.

22

Nursing care of patients with malignancy

This chapter starts with an introduction to cancer and some of the causes, signs and symptoms. Possible treatments and nursing management of patients with malignant disease then follows.

Introduction

Cancer is a disease of the cell resulting in multiplication of abnormal cells. This produces a growing mass of disorganised tissue known as a tumour. A tumour can either be benign or malignant. It can develop anywhere in the body where there is an abnormal cell multiplication. Tumours have different causes, start in different tissues, develop in different ways and need different kinds of treatment and management.

Incidence of cancer

Cancer is a widespread problem in all countries in the world. However, there is a difference in types of cancer and this is thought to be mainly due to variations in the way people live and their environments. The incidence of cancer increases with age, with certain types of cancers being common in children while others affect mostly adults. People who live a long time are more likely to get cancer than those who die at a young age, so long lived populations will inevitably see more cancer.

Causes of cancer

There are many different factors involved in the development of cancers and no single cause has been found. In many cases, it probably results from a combination of factors. A great deal of research is continuing around the world. Important factors are listed below:

- Genetic and familial factors
- Viruses and bacteria
- Chemical and physical agents
- Dietary factors

Genetic and familial factors

Cancer has been shown to run in families. This may be because families live in similar environments and have similar diets and lifestyles. Breast cancer and leukaemia are examples of this. However, the cause of cancer may be genetic and about 15 per cent of all human cancers have a hereditary component. Familial *carcinogenesis* is based on a group of genes which prevent cancer when working normally. If they *mutate* they seem to cause cancer by their absence.

Viruses and bacteria

Viruses work themselves into genetic structures, altering the growth of new cells and this can lead to cancer. Examples of cancers caused by viruses or bacteria:
- Hepatitis B and cancer of the liver
- Helicobacter pylori and gastric lymphoma
- Epstein Barr virus and Burkitt's lymphoma
- HIV and Kaposi's sarcoma and lymphomas

Physical and chemical agents

Many agents have been associated with the development of cancer if individuals have a long contact with them.
- Cigarette and pipe smoking causing lung cancer
- Asbestos causing mesothelioma
- Exposure to the ultra violet rays of sunlight causing skin cancers, especially in albino and light skinned groups
- Radiation from X-rays or nuclear leakages
- Industrial dyes and chemicals

Dietary factors
- High fat diets are linked with breast cancer.

- Low fibre diets are linked with bowel cancer because of the slow passage of faeces.
- Dietary carcinogens from smoked and pickled foods are linked with oesophageal cancer.
- *Oxidants* and toxins, for example aflatoxin in mouldy pulses and grains.

Other causes

Other factors that predispose individuals to the development of cancer include the following: age, sex, geographic distribution, familial susceptibility and previous history of cancer. For example:

- Burkitt's lymphoma is usually found in Central Africa and is most common between the ages of 2 and 15 years (see Figure 22.1).
- Breast cancer is more common in females than in males and there may be a family history.

Pathogenesis

Normal cells have a distinct size, shape and appearance depending on their maturity. In malignancy, cells lose most of the characteristic features of normal cell appearance, so that it can become difficult to decide the origin. The nucleus of a cancer cell is frequently larger than that of a normal cell and there may be more than one. These cells may not be able to perform their usual function.

Normal cells multiply in an orderly manner, so that the number remains constant. They remain with the tissue of origin. But malignant cells are changed. They continue to divide uncontrollably and are capable of moving from the tumour site to distant organs or systems, usually via the bloodstream or lymphatic system. This is called *metastasis*. They can also spread into tissues near them. Some cancers seem to spread to particular parts of the body. For instance breast cancer often spreads to the lungs, the liver or the bones.

Tumours can occur in any tissue of the body and are given names according to tissue and cell type, as shown in Table 22.1.

Table 22.1 Types of cancer

Type of cancer	Tissue/organ
Carcinoma	Epithelial tissues. Skin or lining of cavities of the body
Adenocarcinoma	Glandular tissue. Breast or prostate gland
Sarcomas	Connective tissue. Bone, cartilage, nerves or fat
Lymphomas	Lymphatic system
Leukaemias	Bone marrow

Signs and symptoms

Cancers show up as various signs and symptoms. Changes that require medical attention if they persist for two weeks or more include:

- A change in bowel or bladder habits
- A sore that does not heal
- Unusual bleeding or discharge from vagina or rectum
- A thickening or lump, especially in the breast or testicle
- Indigestion or difficulty in swallowing
- Unexplained weight loss and *anorexia*
- Unexplained anaemia
- Unexplained and persistent bone pain
- Bony swelling, for example jaw or cranium;
- Changes in a wart or mole
- Nagging cough or hoarseness or voice loss.

Diagnostic measures

The nurse plays an important role in the prevention and detection of cancer. Early detection and prompt treatment are responsible for increased survival rates.

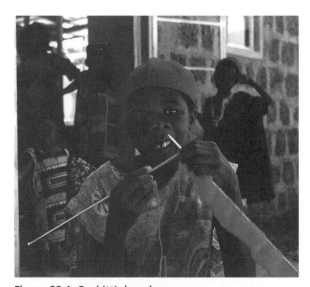

Figure 22.1 *Burkitt's lymphoma*

Diagnostic studies to be performed will depend on the suspected primary or metastatic sites of cancer and also whether the tests are available in the local area. Sometimes it may be possible for patients to be transferred to major hospitals for tests. If cancer is suspected because the patient has complained of one of the above signs, it may be possible to do some of the following tests:

- Examination of the breasts for lumps
- Examination of the testicles for lumps
- Rectal examination and testing stools for occult blood
- X-rays, for example intravenous pyelogram, barium studies
- Full blood screen including liver function tests, differential white cell count, bone marrow aspiration
- Biopsies and cytology studies
- CT scan (computerised tomography)
- Endoscopy (the introduction of a tube with a light into a body passage or organ so that the area can be directly inspected), for example cystoscopy (bladder), laparoscopy (abdomen), oesophagoscopy (oesophagus)

Types of treatment

The type of treatment chosen will depend on what is available as well as the site of the cancer, the age of the patient and the size and extent of the tumour. Cancers are often described as being at a certain stage. This is a term used to grade the cancer according to certain principles. Roman numbers are used to show the stage of the cancer, ranging from I – IV. Stage I is the least serious, stage IV the most serious. Staging helps with giving a prognosis but this also depends on other factors such as the general condition of the patient, the nutritional state and the care available. The system takes into account:

- The size of the primary tumour
- The involvement of local and regional lymph nodes
- Metastasis – whether there is any evidence of the cancer having spread and if so how extensive it is.

So stage I may be localised and curable with treatment. Stage IV will be advanced and incurable. In major centres this staging will decide what type of treatment is likely to be given. However in many areas, there is little choice and the treatment given will depend on what is available.

Surgery

This is the oldest form of cancer therapy still in use. Most individuals with cancer will have some sort of surgery. This may be removal of the tumour, or reduction in the size of large primary tumours. The role of surgery is being questioned and modified as current understanding of cancer improves. However, surgery is still the best option for many tumours, for example breast cancer. It is sometimes combined with chemotherapy and radiation therapy, or can be used as the only treatment.

Radiation therapy

Radiation is the emission of invisible particles or waves of energy from radioactive sources. Radiation works by destroying the ability of cancer cells to reproduce themselves. Its use can be curative (for example in skin cancer, carcinoma of the cervix) or can be for control as in recurrent breast cancer. Lastly radiation therapy can be palliative, that is used in relief of pain. Sometimes large doses of radiation are given over a short period of time or smaller doses given over a longer period. Radiation is not effective in all cases, so the patient will need to be assessed to see if their tumour is likely to respond to this treatment.

The patient will first be seen to decide the dose, length of treatment and method of administration. Most radiation is given externally and the area that will be treated is marked out on the skin. Sometimes it is given internally. Radioactive needles or wires can be placed near the tumour, or radiation can be given in a liquid form, for example Iodine 131 for cancer of the thyroid.

Side effects of radiation

Unfortunately radiation affects normal cells as well as malignant cells, especially those that are dividing and growing rapidly.

- Skin. The skin can become inflamed and sore. It should be kept dry. Soaps, powders or lotions should be avoided. The patient should be told to keep the area out of direct sunlight.
- Depression of the bone marrow. There may be a fall in the blood count, leading to anaemia and increased susceptibility to infection. The patient will need to take extra precautions to avoid infection by avoiding other people with infections, giving attention to personal cleanliness and avoiding contaminated water or food.

- Gastro-intestinal tract. The mouth may become sore, there may be difficulty in swallowing, loss of appetite, nausea and vomiting, or diarrhoea. The patient may need to be given anti-emetics or treatment for diarrhoea. Meal times may need to be altered so that the patient can eat when he feels more like it.
- General effects. Patients often complain of feeling extremely tired. They may become depressed or irritable. The nurse will need to assess the effect of the treatment and adjust the care of the patient accordingly.

Chemotherapy

This is the use of drugs to destroy cancer cells without causing too much harm to normal, healthy cells. Chemotherapy may be used to cure the disease, to help with metastatic disease or to prolong survival and improve the quality of a person's life. However, all chemotherapy drugs will cause side effects and the patient may not be able to tolerate the treatment. Drugs are expensive, often have to be given intravenously and must be given at the right time. Patients are usually allocated to a combined drug protocol. This means that the drugs that they are given are chosen taking into account the latest research, the type and stage of the tumour, the drugs that are available and the age and general health of the patient. Nurses must ensure that:

- The dosage of the drug is correct.
- The drug is given at the right time.
- If given intravenously, the intravenous does not run into the tissues, as this can cause extensive tissue damage.
- They know the side effects of the drugs they are giving.

Side effects of chemotherapy

The side effects will depend on the drugs used. These may include:

- Depression of the bone marrow, in particular the white blood cells and platelets. The patient becomes susceptible to infection and may have bruising or episodes of bleeding.
- Hair loss
- Nausea and vomiting
- Sore mouth
- Diarrhoea
- Sterility. The patient may become infertile.

- Neurological problems. They may suffer loss of sensation in their fingers or toes.
- Kidney problems. Increased fluid intake and a forced *diuresis* are necessary when some drugs are being used.
- Eye problems. There can be *photophobia*, excessive watering of the eye, conjunctivitis or formation of cataracts.

Nursing management

Care of cancer patients must include the principles of nursing care for the general surgical patient as well as specific care for people with malignant disorders. Nursing care will vary according to the specific operative site, the surgical procedure that has been used and the nature of the cancer.

Principles of care

Anxiety about diagnosis and treatment

Most people are very anxious when they are told they may have cancer. While they are being diagnosed they are likely to be very afraid as they do not know what is likely to happen. They may be afraid of pain, changes in their body and the possibility that they may die. Other members of the family may also be very frightened. Patients and families need good explanations, information and support. This will include follow up after discharge.

Pain

Most cancer patients will experience pain and some of it may be severe. It is essential that this pain is correctly assessed, treated and the success of the treatment evaluated (see Chapter 7). Patients should be informed of what is happening so that they can follow treatment prescribed by the doctor and keep pain to a minimum.

Altered body image

Cancer and the treatment involved may change the way patients look and also alter the way in which they see themselves. This can affect their self-esteem and cause a sense of loss (see Chapter 8). They may lose their hair after chemotherapy, or they may become very thin. Nurses need to be aware of the feelings of their patients and help them to accept any changes.

Nutrition

People with cancer and their families must be given good nutritional advice. Cancer cells can use up nutrients because they reproduce so quickly. Cancer also alters the metabolism so that food is used less efficiently. Patients may also have sore mouths or difficulty in swallowing. They may have nausea and vomiting and in some cases diarrhoea. The nurse needs to assess each patient. It may be necessary to give anti-emetics to stop the nausea. Small, high energy meals should be given. Vitamin and mineral supplements (for example zinc) may improve the quality of life. A good fluid intake will help keep the mouth moist. Mouth care and special mouthwashes may be needed.

Skin care

Drugs and radiotherapy can cause soreness of the skin. Also if patients are not able to move around and are losing weight, they are likely to get pressure sores. Care of the skin is therefore very important (see Chapter 17).

Conclusion

The nursing care of a patient with malignancy presents many challenges and new types of treatment and drugs are being introduced all the time. Nurses need to continue to update their knowledge and remain well informed so that they can give the best possible care to their patients. Nurses often need to become involved with supporting patients and families emotionally as they deal with the future (see Chapter 23).

Health promotion

- Discourage young people from starting to smoke tobacco and other substances and help adults who smoke to give up.
- Discourage young people from drinking too much alcohol which can cause oesophageal cancer if continued.
- High fibre diets help to protect against cancer of the colon.
- Teach albino and fair-skinned people how to protect themselves against the sun rays by wearing long sleeved shirts, sunhats and dark glasses.
- Avoid carcinogens that are known, for example asbestos.
- Avoid eating mouldy pulses.

■ Activity

What would make you suspect that a patient who comes to the clinic may have cancer of the bowel? What questions would you ask and what investigations would you do?

23

Care of terminally ill patients

This chapter discusses issues around caring for terminally ill patients. The focus is on culture, cultural practices and care giving, gender roles and power dynamics. The concept of palliative care is introduced and the needs of terminally ill people and their relatives are considered.

Culture and nursing

Culture refers to the beliefs, values and behaviours which are passed between generations.

Patients' beliefs and value systems should be respected and taken into consideration at all times while providing care. The needs, feelings, attitudes and beliefs of the living should also be considered. It should not be taken for granted that terminally ill people lose contact with their own culture or interest in it as there are always meanings attached to whatever is done. This applies wherever care is provided and includes what nurses and other carers do. If the patient is unable to explain beliefs and values, families and significant others should be asked. For example, in many African cultures, patients are expected to bear pain so nurses should recognise that they may be hiding or denying it.

People's ways of viewing culture must not be taken for granted as they do not necessarily depend on education and status. People may marry those from other groups, or move away, and cultural ideas change anyway.

It is important to people's dignity and sense of identity that cultural practices are respected. Neglecting this may leave relatives feeling shamed or criticised. All cultures have rituals that centre around dying, such as the ones from the Setswana of Botswana given below. Rituals are called 'rites of passage' when they mark changes in the stage of life.

Cultural practices and care giving

Many differences exist across areas such as Africa, but also similarities. Nurses should find out from patients or relatives which practices are important. The case studies outline practices from the Setswana.

These examples show the importance of understanding local practices, for example:

> **CASE STUDY:**
> **Gender roles in Botswana**
>
> The sex of carers decides what they can do. For instance patients must be bathed by carers of the same sex. Female carers are responsible for the cleanliness of the environment, cooking meals, feeding patients, and preparing herbs.
>
> Primary carers of terminally ill people are expected to behave in certain ways. They must refrain from sexual activities or attending ceremonies like weddings and funerals. This is to avoid getting 'hot feet' caused, the Setswana believe, by mixing with many people. When carers have 'hot feet' they can make patients' conditions worse.
>
> Based on these ideas of 'hot' and 'cold', visitors may be limited or sick people may be isolated. A log of wood (mopakwana in Setswana) is placed immediately outside the house where the sick person is being cared for. Visitors know they should not enter to see the patient when they see the log. Terminally ill people may not share utensils, linen, blankets, towels and other household materials with other family members.

CASE STUDY:
Power dynamics

Power dynamics become obvious when families decide who to inform about the condition of sick relatives and when critical decisions are made regarding treatment. Male relatives usually have the most authority in families in Botswana. However, maternal uncles play central roles in making decisions that affect their sisters' children, so must be informed of events such as marriage and serious illness by the paternal uncles. These maternal uncles then influence decisions about types of treatment. The paternal uncles will help to pay for these. Often patients will be seen by both modern and traditional doctors and will take both western and traditional medicine.

- Sick people may secretly use herbs, roots or animal parts alongside western medicine. Mixing medicines can be dangerous.
- Relationships can be upset when power dynamics are misunderstood. Often, the right people must be consulted and informed, in the right order. Such people might be individuals, 'therapy groups', family councils, or older women. Waiting for decisions can delay treatment.
- People may be new to caring tasks. For example men may need guidance about washing male relatives.
- Carers may refuse help to dying relatives. They may fear disease, or perhaps fear carrying harm to others, for example newly delivered mothers and babies, because of 'hot/cold' beliefs.
- Some religious groups expect dead bodies to be touched only by their members, or to be washed and laid out in special ways.

Note: Carrying out traditional practices such as washing bodies may be impossible when death is caused by dangerously infective conditions.

Palliative care

The World Health Organisation (WHO) defines palliative care as 'an approach that improves the quality of life of patients and their families facing the problems associated with life-threatening illness, through the prevention and relief of suffering by means of early identification and impeccable assessment and treatment of pain and other problems, physical, psycho-social and spiritual'.

As the AIDS pandemic sweeps across Africa, with increasing numbers of young people affected, new initiatives have sprung up. It is recommended that palliative care for HIV patients begins as soon as they are diagnosed. When people become aware that help may be available, they are more likely to come forward for testing. The number of people with cancer is also increasing and the health services face an enormous problem. Hospices are opening across the continent and providing essential training for health professionals as well as training courses for carers.

Choice of place of death

Terminally ill people should be given the opportunity to choose where they would like to die. Studies of patients with AIDS in Zambia, and anecdotal evidence from Botswana, have demonstrated that most people with AIDS prefer to die at home instead of in health facilities. There they can be surrounded by the people who are most important to them. Sometimes sick people are neglected or feared, or made to feel a burden; then hospital may be seen as preferable. Often, however, there is no choice because of lack of money. Home based care is an important part of palliative care. Relatives and others in the community can be taught to give the basic care that is needed, supported by health professionals.

Palliative care is effective and appropriate because it:

- Improves the quality of life for the patient
- Is suited to home based care
- Controls pain and suffering
- Enables patients to get treatment for acute problems
- Makes the best use of cheap drugs
- Helps the families to provide care for their relatives
- Supports the patient both physically and emotionally so that carers have more time to go out to work
- Enables people to prepare for death and to die with dignity
- Is concerned with supporting families and carers as well as the patient
- Helps the community respond to the HIV and AIDS crisis and the increasing incidence of cancer.

Patients and families need:

- Practical care
- Pain and symptom control
- Counselling/emotional/psychological support
- Income generation
- Financial support for food, shelter, funeral costs and school fees
- Respite (a break from caring, when others take over the role)
- Spiritual support
- Orphan care.

A wide range of care is needed during night and day. As the condition becomes more serious, care becomes more demanding and is needed more frequently.

Physical needs

Pain: Pain control is one of the most important aspects of palliative care. WHO describes a three step ladder:

- *Step one.* Non-opioids such as aspirin, paracetamol or a non-steroidal anti-inflammatory drug such as ibuprofen.
- *Step two.* Weak opiods such as codeine or dihydrocodeine with or without step one drugs.
- *Step three.* Strong opioids such as morphine with or without step one drugs. Step two drugs must never be given at the same time as step three drugs. Oral morphine solutions are becoming more widely available. However, some countries still have problems in importing the morphine powder that can then be made up into the oral solution. For them to be available to all patients, regulations governing the prescribing of drugs may need to be changed. Nurse prescribing will have to become more widespread.

The aim of pain relief is for the patient to be free of pain. Nurses need to develop pain assessment skills (see Chapter 7). Remember that patients may deny they are in pain.

Treatment of opportunist infections in patients with AIDS: (see Chapter 32) Opportunist infections increase discomfort and should be treated. Many patients with AIDS also have tuberculosis, and cough and dyspnoea are distressing symptoms (see Chapter 25).

Touch: Patients need to be touched, as it provides comfort and reassurance. It also helps carers to decide whether patients are stiff and would feel better if helped to exercise.

Nutrition and fluids: Fluids help keep the mouth moist. This makes eating easier, may make patients feel better and helps to keep them active. Good nutrition helps patients with HIV fight infections.

Hygiene needs: Patients need help with bathing and, if they become incontinent, diapers or cloths will need to be changed. Nurses or carers need to be sensitive to patients' feelings as they will be touching parts of their body which are normally private.

Change of position: Patients need help to change their position to try to prevent breakdown of the skin.

Elimination: They may need help to urinate and *defaecate*. Often patients become constipated through lack of movement and fluids, or as a side effect of pain relieving drugs.

Psychological

Anxiety: Patients often feel angry. They may feel it is unfair that they are going to die and may try to blame their condition on others, or believe they have been bewitched or cursed.

Denial: Many people try to deny their illness and pretend that they are not going to die. This makes it hard for the family.

Hopelessness: Some people may feel very depressed and hopeless. They may go through a period when they are unable to sleep or eat and will not talk about what is happening.

Loneliness: People may feel lonely if friends and relatives stop visiting, either because of cultural beliefs, or because they are afraid or ashamed of them. Where possible family and friends should be encouraged to visit and spend time with them.

Fear: Some people may be very afraid of dying and of what will happen to their family after their deaths, especially when they have children. They need a lot of reassurance, and perhaps practical assistance to ensure their affairs are in order. Planning for the family's future can reduce their fear.

Guilt: People may feel guilty because they are no longer able to do things as usual and take their usual responsibilities. This is particularly so for heads of families or parents. Guilt may accompany some illnesses that are stigmatised. This is especially so with problems like alcoholism or AIDS. Even staff can make this worse by poor attitudes.

In some cultures it is unacceptable to talk about death. People with terminal illnesses are not told of their condition and this can make the psychological problems worse. Health professionals may be frightened of death and feel unable to discuss the subject with their patients. Families may try to protect the patient and pretend that they are not going to die. These attitudes can increase the fear and anxiety felt by the patient. Alternatively the patients may know they are dying, but pretend they are not. Nurses need to be able to talk honestly with patients and families and help them to come to terms with their fears and anxieties.

Spiritual needs

Spiritual needs should be accepted even if different from the person giving the care. Different religions have varying ideas about death and what happens afterwards. Some will believe in an after life, others in reincarnation. Terminally ill people may find comfort in talking with a priest or imam about their approaching death.

Financial needs

Care giving can exhaust family financial resources as they need money for nutritious food, and items such as medicines and diapers if they are not free. Visiting can be expensive, as can transporting the patient if needed. The patient may have been the person in the family who provided the financial support and is no longer able to do so. Carers may also be unable to do the farming or other work. Transporting the body following death can leave families in debt. Big funerals may be expected, which can cause hardship. Knowing all this can cause sick people great anxiety and they may wish to make wills before they die. This should be done according to local laws and include what the dying person wants to happen to personal possessions, and perhaps instructions concerning the funeral.

The family and terminal illness

Families coping with terminal illness experience a variety of concerns, threats and challenges, some of which are related to their own stage in life. Changes in family roles and relationship problems can be major issues for those coping with terminal illness:

- Caring for sick elderly parents might overwhelm newly married couples.
- Children may have to take on the new role of main carers to ill parents. They may face the demands of sick parents and also looking after others in the

family, sometimes several young children. This can mean that child carers have neither the time nor resources to attend school themselves.
- Grandparents may find themselves caring for sick adult sons or daughters, while having to provide for grandchildren who may be losing one or both parents.

Communication within the family

Care giving to terminally ill patients may cause problems if families are not honest about the health status of patients. They may know that patients are going to die but may not admit it to the patient or their friends. This can prevent families talking honestly and planning for the future. They may continue to spend money on traditional healers or diviners, perhaps to find out the cause of the illness or who has bewitched the patient. Talking about death is unacceptable in some cultures while in others it may be more acceptable.

Needs of families

The families of patients may experience feelings similar to those of their relative. At the same time patients require their comfort, strength and support. Even when relationships have been good, and family members have a good basis for meeting relatives' needs, they too require comfort and emotional support. Involving them in the care and decision making will help to lessen the feelings of hopelessness.

Families need to feel that they are not alone. Nurses can help them fulfill their role by accepting their behaviour even when it seems unreasonable. They can show respect for their feelings by listening, and treating family members with courtesy and kindness.

When a patient dies unexpectedly, families may need help in accepting the death. Reactions may be different when illnesses are prolonged and death is expected, as families may have already started to grieve. Reactions can also be different when relationships with the dying person have been difficult. Relatives may feel both relief and guilt.

Family deaths can bring great fear and relatives may need practical help and support. Widows, for example, may fear for their future. They may be HIV positive themselves and fear their children will be left as orphans. They may fear destitution, seizure of property and children, or expectations of marriage to husbands' brothers. Nurses can help by identifying sources of advice and support.

The impact of caring for the terminally ill on the family

Caring can affect families in different ways depending on the family history.

Social value

This is often defined by the position held by the terminally ill person in the family. If the sick person is the parent, breadwinner, the eldest child, or the only child, the burden can be very heavy. The entire family socio-economic welfare can be destroyed. The age of patients can also affect the level of grief and stress in families. When terminally ill people are young, older relatives may wish that they could die in their place.

Conflict or collaboration

Some families come together when people are very ill, and even mend old hurts. Others may fall to pieces through arguments, jealousies and old problems. Failure to inform close relatives about the condition of the terminally ill may create conflict in the extended family.

Families are often expected to consult traditional doctors even though this may be expensive. However, later they may explain the cause of the disease as witchcraft or the result of offended ancestors. Close relatives are the most likely to be accused of witchcraft, for example sisters, aunts, uncles and grandmothers. Blaming illness on others can create conflict between families.

Following the death

When people die in hospital or clinics, families may need help in transporting the body for burial. Nurses should find out what families wish to happen and try to help them achieve this. Many hospitals have inadequate mortuary facilities so this usually needs to be done quickly. Quick burial is often considered to be important, especially for Muslims. Particular difficulties and delays may arise when relatives have to travel to obtain money or permission to act.

Medical staff may wish to carry out a post-mortem examination of the body. The authorities may require it, especially if the cause of death is uncertain. Sensitivity and tact are essential when relatives are approached about this and, in some cultures, permission is unlikely to be granted willingly.

Families may wish the body to be handled in a specific way, perhaps to be embalmed. They may require a place where they can carry out their rites. Nurses may be able to act as *advocates* in pressing for improvements such as having chapels of rest.

Funerals and mourning

Most societies have their own ways of arranging for the disposal of bodies, usually by burial or cremation. Special sites or family graves may be important. Mourning rites and periods differ across cultures and nurses need sensitivity in observing family wishes.

Conclusion

The criteria that should be met in the care of the terminally ill are that patients should be:

- Cared for with dignity, respect and humanity whatever the cause of the illness
- Given the opportunity to recall the love and benefits of a lifetime of sharing by being visited by family and friends
- Able to express their wishes and share feelings
- Cared for in familiar surroundings, or in ones made as homelike as possible
- Free from pain and distressing symptoms as much as possible.

■ Activities

1. Think about your own beliefs and culture concerning death and the rituals that follow. How does this differ from someone you are caring for from another culture?
2. Does the death of some patients affect you more than others? Try to talk this through with a group of colleagues. Does the age of the person who is dying make a difference? Is the cause of death a factor?

24

Care of people with communicable diseases

This chapter will discuss the way in which infectious diseases are spread and consider why some people are more likely to be infected than others. The nursing care required by patients with a communicable disease will be covered. A table outlines the main diseases and nursing care required.

The balance between host, agent and the environment

The three factors, host, agent and environment, interact and cannot be considered separately in both the spread and control of communicable diseases. Many books refer to these three factors as a *triad* and the balance between them determines whether disease occurs in the individual or is prevented. The three parts of the triad are the:

Host

The successful invasion of the body of the host by a micro-organism depends on the host's susceptibility to that particular micro-organism. This is dependant on a number of factors:

- The genetic makeup of a person can make them more susceptible to some organisms than others, for example in leprosy.
- Age affects susceptibility. Children are more likely to get certain diseases, such as measles, while the elderly are more sensitive to other infections such as influenza.
- Gender has an influence on susceptibility and a good example of this is that polio affects women more frequently than men. Infections such as malaria and chickenpox are more common during pregnancy.

- Immune response. Malnutrition, pregnancy and HIV all reduce the competence of the immune system and make infection more likely to occur.

Agent

An agent can be biological in the form of a micro-organism, or can be physical or chemical in nature. A micro-organism is an organism that is usually microscopically small. The micro-organism can be a:

Pathogen: This is an infective agent that causes a specific communicable disease. It can be a bacterium, virus, parasite, spirochaete, rickettsia, protozoa or fungus.

Non-pathogen: This term refers to micro-organisms that are a normal part of the body and of bodily functions and are referred to as *flora*.

In order for a micro-organism to cause an infection it has to be pathogenic and must:

- Gain entry into the host's body, via the appropriate route for that specific organism, and in large enough numbers to cause the infection
- Overwhelm the host's defence mechanisms
- Cause an infective reaction in the host.

Environment

The environment usually refers to the physical environment but can also refer to the socio-economic and the socio-cultural environment. In Africa many people still do not have access to safe drinking water and effective sewage and garbage management. This allows for the fast spread of diseases not only through the water and sewage but also through *vectors* that live in such an environment. *Endemic* diseases such as cholera and typhoid are spread in this manner. Mosquitoes breed in this environment causing malaria, which is a major public health problem in Africa.

Poverty leads to poor environments. Squatter or slum dwellings lead to the spread of disease because of overcrowding, poor access to uncontaminated water, poor personal hygiene and poor environmental

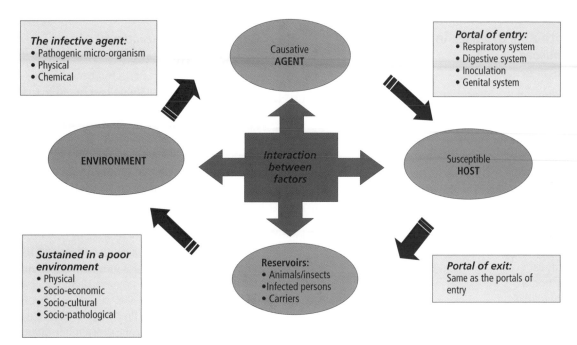

Figure 24.1 *The communicable disease cycle*

hygiene. Measles is more severe in overcrowded envir-onments because children may be sharing beds and the dose of virus is likely to be high. Tuberculosis, a disease that appeared to be under control two decades ago, is again on the increase across Africa in these environments.

The communicable disease cycle

All communicable diseases occur due to a cycle of events that involves these three components (see Figure 24.1).

Prevention of spread of communicable diseases

Early diagnosis and treatment

Patients are at their most infectious before the specific signs and symptoms are obvious. The quicker the person is diagnosed and effective treatment started, the less likely they are to infect other people.

Legislation and notifiable diseases

Most countries make it compulsory for certain diseases, referred to as a notifiable disease, to be reported to the authority. The lists differ from country to country. It is important that nurses know which diseases are notifiable in their specific country and the methods of

notification required. Notification is important in the control of communicable diseases as it allows the health department to start an investigation. This will identify the source of infection and implement a plan to prevent the spread of the disease. Identification of outbreaks of measles and polio are now of international importance as attempts are being made to eradicate them.†

Notifiable diseases in South Africa
(other countries in the region have similar lists, most of the diseases listed will be common throughout southern Africa)

Acute rheumatic fever
Anthrax
Brucellosis
CHOLERA*
Diphtheria
Encephalitis
Food poisoning (more than four persons)
HAEMORRHAGIC FEVERS OF AFRICA*
(Congo, Dengue, Ebola, Lassa, Marburg and
    Rift Valley fevers)
Lead poisoning
Legionellosis
Leprosy

Notifiable diseases in South Africa
continued

Malaria
Measles[†]
Paratyphoid fever
PLAGUE*
Poisoning from any agricultural or stock remedy
   (insecticides or fertilisers)
Poliomyelitis[†]
Rabies (human cases and contacts)
Rheumatic heart disease (first diagnosis)
SLEEPING SICKNESS*
SMALLPOX* and smallpox-like diseases
   (not chickenpox)
Tetanus
Trachoma
Tuberculosis
Typhoid fever
TYPHUS FEVER*
Viral hepatitis (all kinds)
Meningococcal infections
YELLOW FEVER*

The seven diseases in bold capitals are known as
the **FORMIDABLE EPIDEMIC DISEASES***: When
outbreaks occur, the government concerned is
required to notify the World Health Organisation
(WHO). The WHO has the technical support
available to help stop the spread of the disease
within the country or region.
* Formidable diseases
[†] Formidable diseases that it is hoped will be
eradicated

Common terms

Carrier: A person who has got and passes on the
agent or pathogenic micro-organism of a disease.
They do not show any of the symptoms of the
disease. A carrier can be temporary during the
convalescent period when they are recovering
from the disease. They can be permanent when
they live with the micro-organism in their bodies,
without symptoms, for a number of years.

Contact: A person who has been near a sick
person or animal, or has been exposed to an
object and has become infected by the agent

Common terms   *continued*

Endemic disease: A disease that is always
present within an area or region because the
causative microbes are being harboured in that
region. TB is a good example.

Epidemic: An outbreak or increase in the
number of cases of a disease during a specific
time period

Fomites: Objects such as eating utensils, books,
toys that have been in contact with the
infectious person. They could therefore be
contaminated by the infective micro-organism.

Incidence: The number of new cases that occur
in a specific population within an identified time
period. This can be a day, a month or a year. It is
normally expressed as a rate per 1000 or 10,000
population.

Incubation period: The first stage of the
disease, which extends from contamination until
the first signs of the infection occur

Isolation period: The length of time that a
person with a communicable disease must be
kept away from other people as they may infect
them

Pandemic: An outbreak of a worldwide
epidemic. Influenza can sometimes occur in
pandemic proportions. Recently the term has
been used to describe HIV and AIDS.

Prevalence: The number of cases of a disease at
any one time. Prevalence is affected by two
factors: the incidence and the duration of the
disease. In epidemics both the incidence and the
prevalence can be high as with HIV and AIDS. In
acute infections, there will usually be a low
prevalence rate, as the infection remains for a
limited time only. Prevalence is also usually
expressed as a rate per 1000 or 10,000 cases.

Quarantine: The time that contacts need to be
isolated to make sure they do not contract or get
the disease and infect other people. The
quarantine period is usually a day more than the
incubation period.

Sporadic: Occasional or scattered instances of a
disease within a given area or region

Zoonoses: Infections which humans and
vertebrate animals have in common, for example
rabies, anthrax and brucellosis

Immunity and immunisation

Immunity refers to the body's resistance to infection. The healthy well nourished person has a natural resistance to infection. Their healthy skin and mucous membrane form a barrier to the entrance of micro-organisms to the body. These micro-organisms may enter the body through the alimentary or respiratory tracts or by other means. The healthy body has sufficient defence in the appropriate *leucocytes* to resist the infection.

Individuals can acquire specific immunity to a specific disease. They will have the specific antibodies in their blood. These antibodies are acquired in two ways:

Active acquired immunity: This is acquired through the infected person's body forming its own *antibodies* against a specific micro-organism. It takes a few days or weeks to develop and lasts for many years. It can be artificially stimulated through vaccination. Vaccines contain weakened forms of the micro-organism which stimulate the body to form antibodies. They are not strong enough to give the person the disease. Childhood immunisation is perhaps the most important form of communicable disease control. It is inexpensive and usually effective.

Passive acquired immunity: This is temporary and can be acquired in two ways. The newborn baby acquires these antibodies from the mother through the placenta, and to a lesser extent, through breast milk. A person can also obtain antibodies through a serum that is given as an injection. The serum is given to people who have been exposed to the infection or have a disease. It gives short-term resistance while the body makes its own antibodies, for example for Hepatitis B.

WHO Expanded Programme of Immunisation:

- ▨ In 1975 the WHO introduced the Expanded Programme of Immunisation (EPI). Its introduction was based on the belief that it was one of the most cost-effective measures to improve the health of children. Targets were set to achieve high coverage of the target populations. Within a few years of the programme's introduction, smallpox was eradicated from the world. This achievement led to increased trust in vaccination.

- ▨ By 1988 it was established that 60 per cent of the children worldwide were vaccinated against polio, diphtheria, whooping cough, tetanus, measles and tuberculosis. It was believed that polio would be eradicated from the world by the year 2000. This was not achieved but the global distribution was reduced drastically. Cases are found in only two regions of the world, Africa and the Middle East as far as India.

- ▨ Trends have indicated that immunisation gains of the 1970s and 1980s began to fall in the 1990s. Immunisation against Hepatitis B started in the 1990s. Although the programme is successful, there are strains of the micro-organism developing already which are resistant to the vaccine.

- ▨ The immunisation schedule they advocate is adapted by different countries according to the specific situation. The EPI proposed schedule for childhood immunisations is as follows:

Age	Vaccine
Birth	OPV (1), HBV (1) BCG*
6 weeks	OPV (2), DPT (1) HBV (2)
10 weeks	OPV (3), DPT (2) HBV (3)
14 weeks	OPV (4), DPT (3)
9 months	Measles (1) Yellow Fever**
	Vitamin A 200,000 units

Notes:

- • * Only recommended in countries with a high incidence of TB. Repeat BCG once at next visit if no scar is visible.
- • Figures in brackets identify which dose e.g. 1st, 2nd, 3rd, 4th
- • OPV = Poliomyelitis vaccine
- • DPT = Diphtheria, pertusis, tetanus vaccine
- • HBV = Hepatitis B vaccine
- • BCG = Tuberculosis vaccine
- • ** Yellow fever is only offered in countries where the disease is a risk.
- ▨ Vitamin A deficiency is a major contributing factor in childhood deaths from communicable diseases. It is the single most important

cause of childhood blindness. A deficiency exists in 75 countries – affecting an estimated 3 million children under five. Most of these countries (43 per cent) are in Africa. Therefore vitamin A should be offered with immunisation programmes.

The role of nurses in the success of EPI programmes includes:

Maintaining the cold chain: Vaccines have to be kept at *optimal* temperatures from manufacture to administration. The biggest breakdown occurs at clinics where fridges and iceboxes are not maintained to keep the optimal temperature for each vaccine. It is important that nurses are aware of the policy and procedures necessary to ensure vaccines maintain their effectiveness.

Accurate record keeping: The failure of some programmes is due to poor records and the inability to follow up on *defaulters*. Good records allow programmes to be evaluated and adapted to meet the needs of specific regions. Accurate data is essential to evaluate plans and to make informed decisions regarding the future immunisation and disease control.

Vaccinator failure: For vaccines to be effective they need to be administered in a specific manner. Nurses must be aware of the local process as it can differ according to the types of vaccines used.

Involving the community: Community involvement at all stages of the programme is important to its success. Nurses can help develop an alliance between government, local elected authorities and the community.

Other factors to be considered: The effectiveness of immunisation is compromised in HIV infected children. In children with full blown AIDS, administration of BCG can result in TB infection.

Displacement of populations: At any one time there are approximately a million displaced people in Africa. Refugee camps are usually overcrowded, so measles, diarrhoeal diseases, malaria and acute respiratory infections increase. Measles causes approximately 500,000 deaths in Africa each year

Poverty

Poor nutrition, lack of hygiene, lack of clean water, poor sewage disposal and overcrowding are all breeding grounds for pathogenic micro-organisms. Poor people have little opportunity to develop resistance to infection as they may be undernourished.

Healthy environment

Rapid urbanisation and unemployment have led to increasing numbers of homeless people and the mushrooming of informal housing or squatter areas in most countries in Africa.

Medication

The sensible use of appropriate medicines to treat communicable diseases is part of a preventive programme. However, medication must be given and taken for the full period. In Africa the resistance of micro-organisms to available medication has developed to alarming proportions. This makes the treatment of some conditions difficult and very expensive in health systems already over extended and under resourced.

Disinfection

Disinfection of fomites is important. Disposable cups and plates should be used, where possible, so that they can be burned along with materials contaminated with secretions from noses, throats and wounds. Articles that are not disposable should be disinfected in a chemical solution that must be replaced regularly. These eating utensils should be kept separate for the use of the infected person only.

Infected linen should be kept separate and soaked in a disinfectant before washing. Mattresses and pillows used in hospitals should have washable covers to protect them.

Flush toilets can be washed down with a disinfectant but the sewage need not be disinfected. When other types of sewerage system are used, waste will require disinfection before disposal. Advice will be given about the chemical to be used, according to the system used. Incorrect chemicals used in a septic tank can cause more harm than good. Any waste that needs to be disposed of should be buried away from and below the water source at a depth of approximately one metre.

- Terminal disinfection is carried out when the person is discharged from hospital or is no longer regarded as being infectious. This involves normal routine cleaning and ventilation.
- If the medical health officer thinks that specific buildings are likely to give rise to the development of a communicable disease, he can inform the owner or occupier and then evacuate and disinfect or disinfest the premises.

Control of insect vectors

See Chapter 26.

Control of contacts and carriers

Contacts must be traced. If they are not infected or are immune, they may return to work or school. Anyone who is susceptible to the infection is medically examined. If necessary they are immunised, placed in quarantine and given prophylactic medication. Most countries have regulations, which order carriers to have treatment and to cooperate with health officials.

Dissemination of health information

Members of the family and staff, including porters, cleaners, laboratory, nursing and medical staff, must all be aware of the type of communicable disease and the way in which it is spread. This will enable them to use measures to prevent the transmission of the disease.

Nursing strategies

Every nurse should be able to identify and respond to patients who present with a communicable disease.
Note: Essential nursing care plans for a patient suffering from a communicable disease should include prevention of the spread of the disease and barrier nursing.

Prevention of the spread of the disease

- Notification if legally required
- Identification and treatment of contacts and carriers where applicable
- Protection of the nurse using barrier nursing (see information box)
- Continuous and terminal disinfection
- Identifying and managing environmental issues that can affect the transmission of the disease

General nursing care plan
Physical care

- Personal hygiene. Care of the skin (including rashes), eyes, ears, and mouth
- Monitoring of vital signs is important. Pyrexia is common in communicable diseases. The temperature should be kept below 39°C. A high fluid intake, cool bedclothes, antipyretic drugs and tepid sponging are some of the measures

---

Barrier nursing

This is a term given to isolation procedures that can be implemented by the nurse to prevent the spread of infection. It is only applied when the disease rapidly spreads from patient to patient. The form of isolation is determined by the disease:

Strict isolation: This is implemented for highly infectious diseases transmitted through contact of droplet/airborne routes. A private room is required with an independent air supply. Gowns, masks and gloves are worn by all entering the room. Hand washing is required on entering and leaving. All fomites, waste and other materials being removed require special disinfection or burning.

Respiratory isolation: A private room is required and all entering must wear masks. Hands must be washed on entering and leaving the room. All articles directly contaminated with secretions must be disinfected or burnt.

Enteric precautions: This prevents the spread of diseases that occur due to direct or indirect contact with faeces, vomitus, heavily contaminated articles or fomites. A private room is not required but high standards of personal hygiene must be kept. Gloves are worn when handling and disinfecting faeces and vomitus. Hands must be washed.

Blood/body fluid precautions: Maintaining good hygienic standards is important. Gloves must be worn when dealing with blood or other body secretions. Goggles are advisable is some situations.

that can be used to lower the patient's temperature.

- Patients who are *hypoxic* should be given oxygen.
- During an infection, the *metabolic* rate increases and more calories are required. The patient will therefore need a good diet, high in energy. During the acute stage, the patient may not have an appetite. He can be given fluids with a high carbohydrate value. As he improves, a high protein diet can be introduced. Frequent, small meals may be needed (6-8 times per day).
- Monitor elimination and ensure adequate fluid intake to prevent dehydration and constipation.
- Ensure rest and adequate sleep. Complete bed rest is usually recommended during the acute stage of the disease.
- Recognise, identify and report complications. Prevent secondary infections that may occur due to lowered resistance. Complications that may occur due to bed rest, such as deep vein thrombosis and pulmonary embolism can be avoided by encouraging movement of the legs.
- Administer medication as ordered and monitor reactions.
- Collect specimens for tests as required.

Pp **Guidelines for the collection of a specimen**

- Wash hands.
- Prepare site aseptically.
- Wear mask, goggles and gloves as appropriate.
- Obtain an adequate amount of the specimen.
- Collect and transport in a closed sterile container.
- Label sample with the name, type of specimen, date and time collected.
- Store properly and transport promptly.
- Keep records.

Psychological support

Barrier nursing, and placing patients in isolation, can be frightening. The process must be explained to the patient and the family to relieve anxiety. Time must be spent with the patient to allow them time to talk.

Nursing care of patients with specific communicable diseases

A full nursing assessment is required. See Chapter 2.

History taking of patients suffering from a communicable disease

The normal process of taking a history from a patient will apply but specific attention will be given to the following:

- Has the patient had any previous communicable disease, and when?
- Contacts – Has there been contact with another person or host with a communicable disease?
- Has the patient recently travelled to an area where there is an endemic or epidemic disease such as cholera or malaria?
- What is the immunisation history?
- Tests – Have tests such as Tuberculin, Schick, Widal been done recently?
- Carriers – Has the patient been in contact with known carriers?
- Previous illnesses – What previous illnesses has the patient had?
- Allergies – Are there any known allergies that may influence the treatment?
- Medication – What medication is the patient taking, from the doctor, self medication or the traditional healer?
- Nutrition – What are the patient's eating habits and how is the food prepared? This may highlight unhygienic practices that could be responsible for enteric diseases.
- General – Any *malaise*? Headaches, *nausea*, *coryza*, *anorexia* and pyrexia are common to most communicable diseases and usually decrease when the rash occurs.
- Skin rashes – When skin lesions appear, the presentation and distribution across the body will help diagnose the communicable disease.
  - Erythema: a general redness of the skin
  - Macule: a discoloured or red spot that is not raised above the level of the skin
  - Papule: a solid spot or lesion which is raised above the level of the skin
  - Pustule: a small raised skin lesion that contains pus
  - Vesicle: a raised skin lesion that contains a clear fluid and resembles a blister

Nursing care

Specific nursing care will be discussed according to the routes of transmission and the portal of entry. The special delivery of nursing care to patients with specific communicable diseases will be dealt with under the affected system.

Some diseases can cause specific problems for those who are immune deficient and for pregnant women whose fetus' may be damaged by the infection. **Note:** In Tables 24.1–24.4, the following symbols have been used:

* Those diseases marked with one star require strict isolation.

*** Haemorrhagic fevers of Africa (Congo, Dengue, Ebola, Lassa, Marburg and Rift Valley fevers) are marked with three stars.

N Identifies the notifiable diseases.

Respiratory tract

Mode of spread: Droplet infection or inhalation.
Disinfection: Secretions from the nose and throat and fomites.

Alimentary system

Mode of spread: Ingestion of infected water, milk and food.
Specific nursing care required:
- Rehydration is the basis of successful treatment. A combination of IV and oral rehydration is given. Ringer's lactate IV and Darrow's solution or oral rehydration fluid (1 litre of boiled water, 6 teaspoons of sugar and $\frac{1}{2}$ salt).
- Plastic aprons and gloves to be worn when handling faeces, vomitus and other body fluids.
- Use disposable drinking cups and eating utensils. If not disposable, keep separate and use disinfectant for washing.
- Chlorination of water and boiling of water /milk where required
- Food well cooked and protected from flies
- Hand washing before and after dealing with patients
- Sanitary precautions

Disinfection: Special attention to the handling and disinfection of faeces and vomitus; disinfection of fomites.

Genital tract

See Chapter 31.

Mode of spread: Sexual intercourse, infected blood and blood products including the placenta, also needles and sharp instruments through inoculation.
Specific nursing care required:
- Patients are often sensitive about sexually transmitted infections (STI) and therefore must be treated with respect and confidentiality must be guaranteed.
- The importance of treating partners as well as patients is important to prevent re-infection.
- General education on sexuality and healthy safe sexual activities must be given. All sexually active people are at risk. Use of condoms should be explained. Some groups, such as sex workers, migrant workers and convicts are at particular risk. They should seek assistance if symptoms are present.
- Syndromic management of STIs as advocated by the WHO is used extensively in Africa. Access to laboratory facilities is limited and diagnoses made on clinical symptoms often incorrect. Common signs and symptoms are grouped into syndromes and treatment based on that syndrome. Drug protocols have been developed according to each syndrome rather than each infection. Gloves and goggles should be worn when handling blood and other body secretions.

Disinfection: Blood products, body fluids and any matter contaminated by these products should be burnt or disinfected.

Skin

Mode of spread: Bite of an infected interim host or inoculation through a prick with infected fomites. Once the patient is infected most of these conditions are transmitted by droplet infection, direct contact or through fomites.
Specific nursing care required:
- Strict isolation of those marked with *
- Control of interim host, rodents, fleas, ticks, mosquitoes

Disinfection: Secretion from the nose and throat and fomites.

Table 24.1 Diseases of the respiratory tract

Disease	Causative organism	Incubation period	Clinical picture	Specific prevention	Drugs
Anthrax * (Zoonoses) N	Bacillus anthraces (Spore forming and extremely resistant to all conditions)	2–7 days	Cough, pyrexia with pneumonia and toxaemia that is often fatal. Direct contact with infected animals or animal products such as meat hides or bone meal can result in Cutaneous anthrax. Results in lesions known as malignant pustules with a central black area surrounded by inflammation.	Vaccine for those at risk	Penicillin Tetracycline Streptomycin All in high doses
Chickenpox (Varicella)	Varicella zoster virus	14–21 days	Sudden onset with mild pyrexia. Rigors and joint pain can occur. Rash appears in crops that pass through stages from macules, to papules, to vesicles and result in scab formation. Scabs do not transmit the virus. Rash starts on the trunk and then the arms, legs and face. Can appear in mucous membrane in severe cases.	High-risk people can be given immunoglobulin within 96 hours of exposure.	Antibiotics for secondary infections
Ebola Virus* (Haemorrhagic fever ***) N	Ebola virus	14–16 days	Flu-like symptoms with muscle and joint pain. Followed by nausea, vomiting, laryngitis and chest pains. Maculopapular rash occurs over the whole body followed by haemorrhages in skin, liver, and kidneys causing necrosis. Destroys lymphocytes. High death rate	No specific measures	Blood transfusions and platelets Antibiotics for secondary infections
Influenza	Various viruses (Viruses *mutate* continuously)	2–3 days	Rigors, sore throat, coryza	Active immunisation by means of a vaccine	Antibiotics for secondary infections
Lassa Fever * (Haemorrhagic fever ***) N	Lassa virus Endemic in rodent population in West Africa	3–21 days	Transmitted through food or fomites contaminated with rodent excreta. Highly contagious between people. 80% of those affected will have no symptoms. 20% have multisystem failure with high death rate. General malaise, anorexia, diarrhoea, pyrexia. This is followed by oedema of the face, pharyngitis and conjunctivitis. Progresses to kidney failure with proteinuria. Haemorrhages occur in body tissues.	Control of rodents	Blood transfusions and platelets. Ribavirin given in early days may help. Antibiotics for secondary infections

Table 24.1 Diseases of the respiratory tract   *continued*

Disease	Causative organism	Incubation period	Clinical picture	Specific prevention	Drugs
Leprosy (Hansen's disease) N	Mycobacterium leprae	2–10 years in susceptible persons	Manifestation is slow. First presents as skin lesions which change colour and are painless. Muscle weakness and loss of sensation in the feet and hands usually results in accidents and patients present with burns or other injuries. Nodules appear on the peripheral nerves and are palpable. Paralysis is a late sign and is usually accompanied by bone changes in the hands and feet.	No specific measures	Rifampicin Clofazimine Dapsone
Measles** (Morbilli) See Chapter 48 N	Morbilli virus	8–14 days	Pyrexia, conjunctivitis, coryza and Koplik's spots (white spots resembling a grain of salt on a red base found on the mucosa of the lateral walls of the mouth). Rash is maculopapular and appears on the face and neck on the third day of the infection and then disperses over the rest of the body. Complications can result in respiratory infections including laryngeal strydor and broncho pneumonia. **More than 50% of all global deaths from measles occur in sub-Saharan Africa (500,000 per annum).**	Active immunisation by means of vaccine	Vitamin A Antibiotics for secondary infections or if persons state of health is poor
Marburg Fever * (Haemorrhagic fever***) N	Virus	4–16 days	Onset is sudden with pyrexia, muscle pain, and arthritis. Abdominal pain is followed by vomiting and acute diarrhoea for about 3 days. A maculopapular rash appears over the whole body and desquamation occurs. Patient also presents with a dry cough. Encephalitis can occur. Haemorrhages start from the sixth day due to *thrombocytopaenia*.	No specific measures	Blood transfusions and platelets Antibiotics for secondary infections

Table 24.1 Diseases of the respiratory tract *continued*

Disease	Causative organism	Incubation period	Clinical picture	Specific prevention	Drugs
Meningitis* (Meningococcal cerebrospinal fever) See Chapter 46	Neisseria meningitidis (Meningococcus)	2–10 days	Sudden onset, severe headache, pyrexia, vomiting, neck rigidity and photophobia. A varying level of consciousness can occur from drowsiness to delirium, stupor and coma.	Prophylactic drugs (Contacts)	IV Cefataxime or Ceftriaxone or Ampicillin **plus** Chloramphenicol
N	Other bacteria and viruses can cause meningitis, but they are not usually spread from person to person.	2–4 days	A maculopapular rash is common but if septicaemia occurs, a petechial rash is often present. Look for the petechiae in the sclera of the eyes as a quick way to pick out those patients needing very urgent treatment.	HIB vaccine available to prevent meningitis caused by Haemophilus Influenzae in a few countries.	Rifampicin/ Sulphonamides
Mumps (Infective parotitis)	Parayxoviridae	14–21 days	Pyrexia, anorexia, malaise and headaches. Within 24 hours pain is experienced near the ear lobe and on swallowing. Swelling of the parotid or other salivary glands occurs. May only affect one side, but can spread to other side a few days later. Complications can result and *orchitis* may occur in males and occasionally *oophoritis* in females	Active immunisation by means of a vaccine is available but effectiveness is questionable.	Antibiotics for secondary infections
Poliomyelitis * (Can also be transmitted through the faecal-oral route) N	Three Polio enteroviruses – Brunhilda – Lansing – Leon	7–21 days	Can present as a subclinical, non-paralytic or a paralytic disease. All present with pyrexia, headache, vomiting, sore throat and nausea. Followed in a minority of cases by *flaccid* paralysis of certain muscles, most commonly the legs. All flaccid paralysis is notifiable to eliminate the possibility of it being poliomyelitis.	Active immunisation by means of an oral vaccine	No specific treatment
Rubella (German measles)	Rubella virus	14–21 days	Mild pyrexia, malaise, enlarged cervical and often occipital glands. An irregular pink and red macular rash appears on the first day on the face and body, spreads to the limbs on the second day and disappears within 3–5 days. (Serious risks for the fetus if the mother contracts rubella during the first trimester.)	Vaccine, which confers active immunity. Human gamma globulin for pregnant contacts	Antibiotics for secondary infections

Table 24.1 Diseases of the respiratory tract *continued*

Disease	Causative organism	Incubation period	Clinical picture	Specific prevention	Drugs
Scarlet Fever (Streptococcal sore throat)	Streptococcal Pyogenes (Group A)	2–5 days	Onset is sudden with a severe sore throat, tonsils are red, swollen with an *exudate*, tongue is coated white and temperature is high 39–40 °C. A red papular rash appears on the second day starting on the neck and chest and then spreads to the rest of the body. After 2–3 days the tongue peels and a red raw tongue known as strawberry tongue occurs. A pale circle around the mouth also appears. Skin peels after 3–4 weeks. Can progress to rheumatic fever and damage the heart valves.	No specific measures	Benzyl-penicillin IV or Phenoxymethyl-penicillin oral
Tuberculosis Pulmonary See Chapter 25 The prevalence rate in some parts of South Africa is the highest in the world at about 600:100,000.	Mycobacterium tuberculosis	4–6 weeks	Chronic infection characterised in the later stages by a cough. There may be haemoptysis, night sweats, and loss of weight. NB Rising rates of multi-drug resistant TB occur in Africa. Protocols for treatment will vary according to this resistance. Good management and the use of Directly Observed Treatment Short course (DOTS) ensure that the full 6-month course of treatment is taken and ensures a better cure rate. TB can affect other organs but the rate of infection is low.	BCG vaccination of infants and tuberculin-negative individuals, use of antimicrobial drugs prophylactically for close contacts	Combination of rifampicin, isoniazid, pyrazinamaide. Ethambutol. Streptomycin for retreatment is advocated but not in pregnancy or in patients over 65.
Whooping cough (Pertussis) See Chapter 47	Bordetella pertussis	7–12 days	Disease occurs in 3 stages: • Catarrhal stage: 1–2 weeks with malaise, anorexia and coryza • Paroxysmal stage: Lasts about 3 weeks and consists of bouts of coughing which become severe, spasmodic, repetitious coughing attacks which are followed by a 'whoop', as the patient sucks in air, and vomiting. • Recovery stage: Lasts 3–4 weeks during which the bouts of coughing get less.	Vaccine available	Antibiotics for secondary infections. Cough suppressant and *mucolytic* can be given to children over 2.

145

Table 24.2 Diseases of the alimentary system

Disease	Causative organism	Incubation period	Clinical picture	Specific prevention	Drugs
Bacillary Dysentery	Shigella dysenterae, S. flexneri, S. boydii or S. sonnei	2–3 days	Often related to large gatherings and unhygienic environments. Abdominal pain and cramps with pyrexia. Vomiting precedes diarrhoea that can last for a week or more.	Hygienic environment	No drugs
Cholera (Formidable epidemic disease) N	Vibrio cholerae (Specific bio-types are responsible for the disease in different areas in Africa)	2–5 days Contacts to be observed for 5 days – no quarantine necessary	Sudden onset of abdominal cramps with severe diarrhoea (rice water stools), vomiting and results in very rapid dehydration. Patient can lose 15 litres or more in 24 hours, which can lead to renal failure, vascular collapse and shock.	Vaccine (Not very effective) Doxycycline can be used as chemoprophylaxis for close contacts.	Ringers Lactate IV Doxycycline/ Tetracycline
Hepatitis Epidemic jaundice N	Type A or B virus. (There are also less common forms of viruses responsible for infections. They include Types C, D, E, F, G and other undifferentiated types)	Type A: 2–7 weeks Type B: 6–25 weeks	Anorexia, nausea, pyrexia, malaise. Pain in upper right quadrant of abdomen. Pale fatty stools and dark urine containing bilirubin. Jaundice occurs after a few days. May result in liver damage. Other viruses, bacteria and parasites can also cause hepatitis.	Immune serum globulin for passive immunity of people at risk Carriers of Type B are responsible for the transmission of hepatitis. They may not donate blood.	No specific treatment Multivitamins, phospholipids and anti-inflammatory drugs may be prescribed.
Typhoid Fever N	Salmonella typhi	7–14 days	**First week.** Infection starts in the biliary tract, inflammation of the small intestine follows, with diarrhoea (pea soup stools) at the end of the week. **Second week.** Pyrexia with a slow pulse. Abdomen distended, liver and spleen enlarged. A pink maculopapular rash on the abdomen. This is hard to see on a pigmented skin. Widal test becomes positive. **Third week.** Toxaemia. Patient may become delirious or semi-comatosed. Bowel haemorrhages can occur.	Hygienic environment Carriers are responsible for keeping the disease endemic.	Chloramphenicol, Ampicillin or Ceftriaxone

Table 24.2 Diseases of the alimentary system *continued*

Disease	Causative organism	Incubation period	Clinical picture	Specific prevention	Drugs
Brucellosis (Zoonoses)	Brucellosis melitensis	5–30 days	Slow onset with malaise and intermittent pyrexia and rigors. The patient may present with an enlarged spleen, liver and lymph nodes (cervical and axillary) that are not painful. However, muscle and joint pain can occur.	Immunisation of animals Wearing of protective clothing when working with animals or animal products	Antimicrobials
	Sheep Goats Pigs Cattle		Bacteraemia can occur, causing *endocarditis, osteomyelitis, hepatitis, meningo-encephalilitis, nephritis* and renal failure.	Pasteurisation or boiling of milk	
N			If it is not diagnosed, it can lead to a chronic condition with recurring symptoms.		

Table 24.3 Diseases of the genital tract

Disease	Causative organism	Incubation period	Clinical picture	Specific prevention	Drugs
HIV and AIDS See Chapter 33	HIV Virus: Types a, b and c	Unknown, but from 1–8 years	Asymptomatic for some time, then fatigue, loss of weight, recurrent infections, most commonly respiratory such as pneumonia, occur. Affects the autoimmune system and results in those infected being subject to secondary infections which result in death.	Avoid sexual contact with multiple or anonymous partners. Use of condoms. Screening blood donors. Heat treatment of blood products	Anti-retroviral drugs are available for some patients with a CD4 cell count of less than 200. Expensive but becoming more available in Africa.

Table 24.4 Diseases of the skin

Disease	Causative organism	Incubation period	Clinical picture	Specific prevention	Drugs
Rabies (Hydrophobia) (Zoonoses)	Rabies virus Transmitted in the saliva of infected domestic or wild animal through a bite	2 weeks to 2 months	First stage lasts 2–10 days and is non specific with the person complaining of flu-like symptoms and irritability. The infected person becomes more sensitive to light, noise and produces excess saliva, perspiration and tears. Pupils become dilated, pulse and respirations rapid. The site of the bite becomes very sensitive, may be painful or itchy. The acute neurological stage follows with a period of excitability. Double vision and involuntary movements of the eyeball occur. There are spasms when oral fluids are taken and the choking that follows can lead to *apnoea, cyanosis* and death. This can be followed by paralysis of the respiratory muscle and those controlling chewing and swallowing. The patient becomes confused and comatosed. Death follows.	Compulsory immunisation of domestic animals Control of animals known as vectors Destroying animals that show aggressive behaviour and have a record of biting people Vaccination of humans working with animals Wearing of gloves and other protective clothing when working with sick animals Animal bites to be thoroughly cleaned with a strong disinfectant, alcohol or hydrogen peroxide The wound may be surgically treated.	Rabies vaccine and rabies immune human globulin This is given even if the animal is not caught or tested. Other treatment is given according to the symptoms.
N Bubonic plague* (Zoonoses) (Formidable epidemic disease) N	Yersinia pestis Transmitted by an infected flea from an infected animal. Can be spread by droplet infection when the lungs are infected.	2–7 days Contacts are isolated for 6 days. If necessary whole communities are isolated.	Enlarged and painful lymph glands, usually in the groin (bubo) and pyrexia. Bacteraemia occurs resulting in purulent, necrotic and haemorrhagic lesions in the lymph nodes. Results in toxaemia and septicaemia and spreads to all organs resulting in purulent, necrotic and haemorrhagic lesions in all affected organs and skin. Gives rise to the name of 'black death'. Death can occur in over 60% of cases when treatment is not given or is commenced 12 hours or more after symptoms have been noticed.	Active immunisation by vaccine Prophylactic antibiotics and Plague antiserum Control of fleas and rodents	Plague antiserum and antibiotics for 10 days

Table 24.4 Diseases of the skin *continued*

Disease	Causative organism	Incubation period	Clinical picture	Specific prevention	Drugs
Congo-Crimea fever* (Haemorrhagic fever***) N	Nairo and arbovirus Transmitted by an infected tick	3–5 days	Sudden onset with rigors, acute headaches and epigastric pain. Viraemia results with pyrexia that can last for 3 to 16 days. Haemorrhages occur in the tissue and organs that can result in organ failure, shock and death.	Preventive measures to prevent tick bites	Blood transfusions and platelets Antibiotics for secondary infections
Dengue fever * (Haemorrhagic fever***) N	Caused by four closely related viruses and transmitted by the infected Aedes female mosquito	5–8 days	Endemic in many African countries. Presents as a flu-like illness that affects infants and often this is all the disease consists of. Dengue haemorrhagic fever is a potentially deadly complication that is characterised by high fever, haemorrhagic symptoms, often with enlargement of the liver, and in severe cases circulatory failure. The illness usually begins with a sudden rise in temperature accompanied by facial flush. The fever usually continues for 2 to 7 days and can be as high as 40–41°C, often with febrile convulsions. Can result in shock and death.	Vaccine being developed	Blood transfusions and platelets Antibiotics for secondary infections
Rift Valley fever * (Zoonoses) (Haemorrhagic fever***) N	Virus transmitted by the mosquito or contact with infected animal material or milk Infected animals include game, sheep and cattle	3–7 days	*Viraemia* and pyrexia with *rigors* develop followed by capillary damage. This results in the loss of plasma and *erythrocytes*. During the acute stage that lasts for up to 2 weeks, headaches, diarrhoea, vomiting and muscle weakness occur. This stage can last for 2 weeks and organ failure and haemorrhages can result in shock and death. Nose bleeds may be the main clue to the diagnosis.	Control mosquitoes	Blood transfusions and platelets Antibiotics for secondary infections

Health promotion

Nurses and health care workers have a responsibility to give advice on:

- Clean water, safe preparation of food and disposal of sewage
- Controlling of insects and other vectors
- Keeping houses and environments clean
- Preventing overcrowding where possible
- Implementing immunisation programmes.

They should keep records of patients presenting with communicable diseases. Contacts should be traced and treated if necessary.

Early notification of dangerous diseases can limit the spread.

■ Activity

Find out which diseases are notifiable in your country. You should know how to notify the authorities if a patient presents with one of these diseases.

25

Care of patients
with tuberculosis

This chapter outlines the scale of the problem of tuberculosis and describes the causes and disease process, transmission, prevention, risk factors, diagnosis, management and nursing care in a variety of settings. Drug resistance, HIV, health promotion and community involvement are included.

Scale of the problem

Tuberculosis (TB) is a serious public health problem worldwide. It is caused by infection with the myco-bacterium tuberculosis (the tubercle bacillus). Some strains of TB are now resistant to the usual drugs and this is causing great concern.

The number of people with TB is increasing worldwide and faster where HIV and AIDS are common. TB is the leading cause of death in people with AIDS. The situation is made worse by poverty, poor housing and sanitation, conflict and migration. These are some facts about TB:

- About 2 million deaths due to TB occur annually throughout the world.
- About one-third of the world population is infected, half of which are in sub-Saharan Africa.
- 5–10 per cent of these will show symptoms and become sick or infectious at some point, more if they are HIV positive. That is about 7–8 million people per year.
- Untreated people with active TB can infect 10–15 others per year.
- TB cases have doubled or trebled in the past 10 years in several African countries owing to the HIV epidemic.
- TB is responsible for about 13 per cent of all AIDS deaths worldwide.

Note: Someone can be infected, but not suffer symptoms and become sick provided the immune system can resist the bacteria. Meanwhile it lies dormant.

Tuberculosis is a *notifiable* disease, so statistics are collected by the WHO from most countries. People making or suspecting a diagnosis of TB are usually legally responsible for notifying this through their national reporting systems. Most countries have specific agencies for this and publish their own statistics. Notification is necessary for contact tracing, so that those in close contact with the case may be screened. This forms part of Tuberculosis Control Programmes which countries are recommended by the WHO to develop.

Transmission and risk factors

TB is an infectious disease spread by people with active pulmonary disease. It is spread by droplet infection as is the common cold. Coughing, sneezing, talking, singing and spitting cause bacilli to be forcibly propelled through the air. In the case of bovine TB, infection can also be caused by drinking contaminated milk. Bacilli can remain inactive for many years. Once a person's immunity is damaged or suppressed, dormant bacilli can become active and multiply, so causing tuberculosis.

People may have other ideas about how TB is caused, such as through supernatural powers. They may also seek alternative methods of treatment that they believe to be appropriate, such as from traditional healers. Understanding such beliefs is important for the development of appropriate public health policies and for planning appropriate nursing care.

Risk factors

People at highest risk for acquiring the infection are those:
- With lowered resistance due to:
  - HIV infection and AIDS (see below)

- being on steroids or immunosuppressive therapy (for example drugs and radiation for treating cancer)
- malnutrition, starvation, smoking or alcoholism
- being stressed
- young children recovering from measles or whooping cough
- other medical conditions, for example diabetes, malignancy, chronic renal failure patients on haemodialysis.
- In overcrowded situations, for example prisons, refugee camps and shelters.

Disease processes and immunity

Becoming infected happens in two stages: infection of the person, then progression to disease.

1. Tubercle bacilli are transmitted through inhalation or ingesting contaminated milk or food, occasionally through broken skin (see Chapter 17). Inside the body they are engulfed by *phagocytes* and carried to regional lymph nodes. They may pass into the bloodstream and to any organ. At first they cause little or no reaction in the host tissues. Then the body develops antibodies within 3 to 8 weeks and some degree of acquired immunity. The organisms may lay dormant for many years. People in good health do not develop active disease but those in poor health may do.

2. The disease can develop in three ways:
- The primary lung lesion may cause a tuberculous pneumonia or it can spread into the pleura causing pleurisy.
- The pressure of glands on the bronchi can cause lobes of the lung to collapse, or a gland can rupture into a bronchus and the disease spreads through the bronchi.
- Spread via the bloodstream or lymphatic system. This can lead to many different problems, for example miliary tuberculosis, TB meningitis, abdominal tuberculosis or tuberculosis of the bone (see below).

Prevention of TB

An important part of prevention is improvements to socio-economic conditions and health education (see below) but also includes immunisation and drug prevention. Prevention is considered again in the Directly Observed Treatment Shortcourse (DOTS) section.

DOTS itself is important as prevention because fewer people will transmit TB.

Immunisation

Routine immunisation with Bacille Calmette-Guerin (BCG) vaccine is important in areas where TB is common. BCG is a live *attenuated* strain of bovine tuberculosis. It produces immunity for up to 15 years and reduces the risk of pulmonary TB. Immunisation does not give life-long immunity and infection is still possible. People who need BCG are:

- Neonates at birth, or infants (only those without active AIDS)
- Contacts of TB patients who have tuberculin-negative skin tests (see below)
- Tuberculin-negative health care workers.

Isoniazid preventive therapy

The drug isoniazid is very effective when given for 6–12 months. It may be used for people who are susceptible to tuberculosis to eliminate the tubercle bacilli before they become established. They may be people who are:

- Negative to skin tests but live with someone who has TB
- Positive to skin test and in a high-risk group.

Note: Babies born to sputum-positive mothers may be given isoniazid. Breastfeeding should be continued.

Diagnosis of TB

The main methods used to diagnose TB are:
- History taking
- Clinical examination
- Chest X-ray
- Tuberculin skin test
- Examination of sputum
- Lumbar puncture if meningitis is suspected.

Clinical examination and symptoms of lung TB

A person with lung TB will have all or some of the following symptoms:
- Persistent cough
- Weight loss
- Night sweats
- Loss of appetite (*anorexia*)
- Coughing up blood (*haemoptysis*)
- Feeling tired all the time
- Low grade fever.

Tuberculin skin test

A small amount of protein taken from tuberculosis bacteria is injected between the layers of the skin, usually on the forearm. About 2 days later, the injection site is inspected. Swelling and redness indicate a positive result. However, negative tuberculin results may occur in immuno-suppressed and malnourished individuals, (and after measles in children) so giving inaccurate false-negative results. A positive result does not mean that the patient has clinical TB. They may have had the infection and recovered.

Sputum testing

To confirm a diagnosis of tuberculosis, a sample of sputum must be collected and examined for Acid-Fast Bacilli (AFB) on 3 consecutive days. For patients with a productive cough, an early morning freshly expectorated sputum is recommended. Mycobacterial culture, if available, is a more sensitive test for diagnosing tuberculosis in patients with negative results on direct sputum examination.

Special points about different forms of TB

(See also Chapters 10, 13, 14, 46 and 47.)
Pulmonary tuberculosis: Chest X-ray, sputum examination and the tuberculin skin test are used.
Tuberculosis of the cervical glands: The lymph glands in the cervical region become large and infected especially in children. A biopsy of the gland may be necessary.
Abdominal tuberculosis: The mesenteric glands may be infected from drinking contaminated milk. There is likely to be abdominal pain and wasting. A *scites* may develop.
Tuberculous meningitis: The symptoms are slower to develop than in the more common bacterial meningitis. Diagnosis is confirmed by lumbar puncture.
Bone and joint tuberculosis: The most commonly affected bones are the vertebrae (Pott's disease). Hip and knee joints may be affected.
Miliary tuberculosis: TB spreads throughout the body. Chest X-rays show a mottled appearance. Fever and wasting is likely. Signs of meningitis may develop and the person is very ill.

Nursing care of patients

The objectives of tuberculosis treatment and management are to:
• provide lasting cures with few treatment failures and relapses
• treat symptoms quickly
• render highly infectious patients non-infectious
• prevent drug resistance from developing.

Community-based services

Treatment must be easily accessible. The WHO recommends that services should be flexible and integrated with other health services so people can gain access to them near their homes or workplace. This is especially important where HIV is common. (See also Chapters 31 and 32.)

The therapy that is most universally used and strongly recommended by the WHO is Directly Observed Treatment Shortcourse (DOTS) (see below).

The nursing role in TB programmes

Nurses are taking increasing responsibilities in many areas, becoming involved in programme management as well as TB case management with medical support. They have important roles in following up patients and training and supervising community care workers.

Nurses and assistants must know:
• how to administer and record TB drugs
• how to keep TB registers
• procedures for tracing contacts
• when and how to collect sputum for microscopy.

Standardised treatment regimes

Several drugs are now commonly used in combination for TB chemotherapy. Often four drugs are given for the first 2 months, then two drugs after that. Specific regimes vary between countries. They are used for 6-8 months in sputum smear-positive cases and include:
• Rifampicin
• Isoniazid
• Ethambutol
• Streptomycin
• Pyrazinamide.
Sputum is tested again after 2 months to check progress, and at the end of the regime. The end result must be negative.

Directly Observed Treatment Shortcourse (DOTS)

DOTS is the most effective treatment for TB and for controlling the epidemic. Ninety-five per cent of people who receive DOTS therapy survive TB provided they do not have HIV. DOTS involves nurses, other health workers or trained volunteers giving patients the prescribed drugs and watching them being swallowed. Patients may be hospitalised, attending outpatients or community units, or other selected sites. Patients can then share responsibility for the complicated long-term treatment.

DOTS is a combination of a therapy that works, and good management. Very importantly, it is expected by the WHO that DOTS treatment is given free of charge although this often does not happen.

The WHO describes five key components to DOTS:

■ Government commitment to sustainable TB programmes
■ Case detection by sputum microscopy examination

■ Standardised treatment for 6–8 months, directly observed for at least the first 2 months to ensure maximum bacilli are killed
■ Regular uninterrupted drug supplies
■ Effective monitoring with standardised recording and reporting:
  • Individual treatment cards
  • Laboratory registers
  • TB registers to monitor patient details and progress
  • Reporting systems up to national level to allow programme evaluation.

A vital part of DOTS is ensuring that people take medications regularly and correctly to prevent drug resistance (see below) which is becoming an increasing worldwide problem. It is essential that they complete their treatment courses despite often feeling better after a few weeks. Drug regimes vary. Some use daily administration. Others administer drugs 3 times per week but observation is then even more important. Patients who fail to attend should be followed up.

Infection control

Admission to hospital is unnecessary unless patients are obviously unwell or if it is considered that starting treatment will be difficult at home. Most patients with TB can be treated at home or in care homes. As family members have already been exposed to the risk of infection, isolation is unnecessary. However, patients should be encouraged to stay within their homes until 2 weeks of treatment have been completed. Visitors should be restricted at first, especially young children who are more susceptible.

Good infection control techniques will help in preventing the spread of infection. Important factors are:
• Only those who test positive for AFB in the sputum are infectious:
  • Sputum-negative patients are unlikely to infect others.
  • Those with positive sputum cultures are usually regarded as non-infectious after 2 weeks of treatment or once sputum cultures are negative.

  • People who are not infectious may become so if regular and adequate drug treatment is not given.
• Patients living at home should keep their rooms well-ventilated, and open to sunlight if possible. Darkness allows bacilli to survive for long periods.
• Bacilli in, for example, sputum or bedding are killed by:
  • direct sunlight for 5 minutes
  • heat at 60°C for 20 minutes or 70°C for 5 minutes
  • 1% hypochlorite solution.
• Patients admitted to hospital with suspected pulmonary tuberculosis should, if possible, only be nursed in the same wards as others with TB. Only close family members should visit; babies and young children must be kept away. HIV positive patients must not come into contact with infectious TB patients.
• Rooms that have been used by sputum-positive patients should be left empty and ventilated for 24 hours, then cleaned well.

- Preventing the spread of disease involves:
  - making sure patients are well fed
  - sticking to drug regimes
  - quick recognition and treatment of further symptoms
  - tracing and testing contacts.
- Inform patients about taking precautions such as:
  - covering the mouth and looking away to prevent spreading infection through coughing
  - using tissues, newspaper or sputum pots for spitting, and disposing of them safely. Where garbage disposal is a problem, burning is best.
  - not spitting. If patients must spit, they must cover sputum with soil.
- Consider those at risk: those who are HIV positive, other vulnerable people such as the malnourished and immuno-suppressed, prisoners, street children, the homeless and those with alcohol, tobacco and drug dependency.

Protecting yourself and other staff:
- When caring for patients who are considered to have multi-drug resistant tuberculosis you should protect yourself with filter masks, such as high efficiency particulate air (HEPA) masks (if available).
- Known HIV positive staff should not care for TB patients.
- Important points about safe sputum collection:
  - Collection in the open air or special room
  - Standing behind patients while they cough up sputum
  - Secure closure of leak-proof containers
  - Hand washing (see Chapter 6)
- Immunisation (see Prevention above).
- Remember universal precautions against HIV (see Chapters 6 and 32).

Multi-drug resistant tuberculosis (MDR-TB)

Multi-drug resistant tuberculosis (MDR-TB) is a very dangerous form of TB that is threatening to make TB incurable. The bacilli become resistant to the effects of some TB drugs, particularly the two most powerful ones, isoniazid and rifampicin. MDR-TB results from mismanagement when treatment is not properly controlled. Incorrect regimes may be prescribed and direct observation of patients may be lacking. Some patients are given single drugs and are not referred for DOTS. This is worse than giving no treatment at all.

MDR-TB is becoming an increasing problem in Eastern Europe, Africa and South-East Asia. Some strains of the bacillus are resistant to one drug only, others are resistant to all major drugs. Those who have MDR-TB will pass the same resistant strains on to others they infect.

MDR-TB treatment uses second-line drugs and can take up to two years to be effective. This is very expensive whereas DOTS is cheap and cost-effective. Treatment is also more toxic. The WHO and its partners are developing a strategy for badly affected areas called DOTS-Plus.

HIV, AIDS and TB

(See also Chapter 32.)

HIV and AIDS are thought to be the main cause of the increased number of TB deaths. People living with HIV and AIDS are much more likely to develop TB and less likely to survive it. TB may cause HIV to progress faster to AIDS.

TB may appear differently in HIV positive people:
- Sputum and skin tests may remain negative.
- There is more fever and weight loss, less cough and blood-spitting.
- TB can appear in unusual places and miliary TB is common.
- X-ray changes may be different.

Often services for HIV and AIDS, and TB are separate but efforts are being made to integrate them more. People living with HIV and AIDS can then get the help they need. They may have a range of conditions and treatment needs to be available in one place. Nurses can help to ensure this happens. The recommended focus of joint programmes is towards:
- improving prevention and DOTS
- national coordination
- HIV counselling and testing for TB patients
- TB screening for those using HIV services.

Community involvement

Community involvement is very important to provide support to TB patients and their families, mobilise resources and assist professional carers. Church groups and other societies can help. Support clubs can be formed that help with education and motivation. Traditional healers have also been used.

Conclusion

Although the incidence of tuberculosis varies significantly in different parts of the world, there is major concern about its potential spread to the general population. Preventing the spread of TB and MDR-TB in all settings is a major challenge for nurses. Furthermore, a global effort is required to prevent and control its spread effectively. Factors contributing to the epidemic have to be addressed, such as poverty, homelessness and migration of refugees, political and ethnic conflicts, HIV infection and lack of access to health care.

Health care providers, and in particular nurses, must intensify their health promotion and education efforts and instruct clients and care givers about infectious diseases, modes of transmission, and specific control procedures if the battle against TB is to be won.

Health promotion

Nurses and midwives have important roles in preventing the spread of TB through health promotion:

- Inform people about the importance of covering their mouths when coughing, and the danger of spitting in public places. They should provide good examples themselves.
- Provide information about the signs of pulmonary tuberculosis.
- Ask people who have signs of active pulmonary tuberculosis to attend a clinic for diagnosis and treatment.
- Where people have active pulmonary tuberculosis, protect those who are vulnerable from infection.
- Make sure that those receiving treatment take the drugs correctly and complete the treatment.

■ Activity

Write a plan of the information you would provide for a family who have come to a clinic. One adult has active pulmonary tuberculosis. There are three young children in the family and another adult is HIV positive.

Care of people with parasitic diseases

This chapter covers the main parasitic infections found in Africa. It identifies the way in which these infections are transmitted and covers the management of people with the infections.

Common terms

Dysentery: Diarrhoea containing blood and mucus

Infestation: A place or an individual that is inhabited by harmful vermin

Parasite: An organism living in or on another and benefiting at the expense of the other

Vermin: Mammals, birds, rodents, insects or parasites that are harmful. They, or the micro-organisms that they carry, cause problems for the individual that they come into contact with.

Vector: A person or other living animal or insect that is a carrier of disease

Introduction

Most parasitic conditions occur in places where standards of hygiene are poor. Poor environmental sanitation, the accumulation of refuse and the unsatisfactory disposal of human excreta and other waste, offer ideal breeding grounds for parasites. The situation is made worse by the lack of safe water for drinking and personal hygiene. Over 60 per cent of Africa's communities do not have the services necessary to provide a healthy environment. Poverty makes the situation worse. The control of these parasitic conditions is therefore difficult. It is vital that any plan to reduce these diseases is done together with development programmes. People need access to safe water, the management of sanitation, better housing and education.

Types of parasite

External parasites

Infestation with external parasites is usually associated with overcrowding and poor environmental hygiene.

Lice (Pediculosis): The sexually mature female lays her eggs (nits) on the body, usually in hair, or in the clothing. The eggs hatch and reach maturity in 2–3 weeks.

There are three types:

- Head louse
- Body louse
- Pubic or crab louse.

Body lice can be the vectors of typhus, the formidable epidemic disease and relapsing fever. A secondary infection often occurs as a result of scratching, which is known as impetigo (see Chapter 17).

Fleas: There are three important types of fleas: the rat, the dog or cat and the human flea. The rat flea is the most feared as it is responsible for the transmission of plague to humans. The adult flea lays her eggs in dust and cracks and these eggs can remain *dormant* for long periods of time. This can result in recurring infestations.

Flies: The housefly is not parasitic and is not the vector of a specific disease. It does, however, carry *pathogenic* micro-organisms from one source to another. This can lead to diseases such as trachoma (see Chapter 21) and gastro-intestinal infections. The fly lays eggs in decaying matter where they hatch into larvae/maggots in about 24 hours. These bury themselves in *organic* matter and hatch into flies within 3–10 days depending on conditions. The tumbu fly lays eggs on dirty ground or clothes and the maggots develop under the skin.

Internal parasites and vectors

Tsetse flies: In some areas of Africa there are biting flies that can carry protozoan parasites causing a serious disease known as trypanosomiasis or sleeping sickness.

Blackflies: These occur near fast flowing rivers, mainly in Africa. The flies spread the worm Onchocerca volvulus. The microfilariae affect the skin and eye, causing river blindness (see Chapter 21). Weekly applications of larvicides to the breeding areas of the flies have helped control the condition.

Mites (Scabies): The mite (Sarcoptes or scabei) burrows into the skin and reproduces in 3–4 days causing a skin irritation known as scabies. The infection is characterised by small raised pink lines on the skin. They are very itchy and usually occur in areas where the skin is moist (behind the knee, in the groin and under the elastic or waistbands of clothes). Scratching leads to secondary infections. This can be common in communities with poor sanitation.

Mosquitoes: There are a number of species of mosquito and the females of specific species are responsible for the transfer of diseases such as filariasis and malaria.

Nurses' role in the prevention and treatment of parasite infestations

Preventive care

- Health education aimed at improving standards of personal hygiene and the eradication of the vector
- Prevention of overcrowding
- Development programmes leading to better access to a safe adequate water supply and appropriate sewage and refuse management, better housing and nutrition

Treatment

Mites (Scabies) and lice (Pediculosis):

- Bath using 5% monosulfiram medicated soap (Tetmosol).
- Dry the skin.
- Apply a 25% benzyl benzoate preparation (Ascabiol), or any other 1% gamma hexachloride preparation.
- In severe cases the preparation can be left on overnight before being washed off.

Septic skin lesions: These should be treated with antimicrobial ointment.

Note: The lotion is toxic and should not be taken internally. Avoid contact with eyes or broken skin.

Bedding and clothing: These should be treated, washed and ironed. Alternatively place in direct sunlight for as long as possible.

Malaria

Malaria is one of Africa's most serious public health problems. Efforts implemented by the WHO to eradicate the disease have not been successful as yet. This is due mainly to the failure to control the vector. More than 90 per cent of the world's total malaria incidence, and the great majority of malaria deaths, occur in tropical African countries. Most of these deaths occur in young children. Political instability, wars and the movement of refugees have made the problem worse. They have led to environments where the mosquito is able to breed and people are unable to protect themselves.

What is malaria?

Malaria is a parasitic disease which is spread by the female anopheles mosquito. There are four main types of the parasite, plasmodium:

- Plasmodium malariae
- Plasmodium vivax
- Plasmodium ovale
- Plasmodium falciparum. This is the most common in Africa and the type that causes the most deaths.

Where does malaria occur?

The anopheles mosquito breeds in areas of high humidity and where there is stagnant water. The parasites do not develop in the mosquito in temperatures less than 15°C. They like a temperature between 20 and 30°C. This means that in some areas of Africa, there will be many cases of malaria during the wet season and few in the dry season. In mountainous areas, the temperature may be too low for the parasite to develop.

Transmission

The female anopheles mosquito needs blood to feed her eggs. She feeds mainly at night. She sucks up blood from an infected person and the parasite is stored in her saliva. The next time she bites a human, the parasites are injected into that person.

Effects of the parasite on the host

The parasites develop first in the host's liver and then invade the *erythrocytes*. They multiply very quickly in the erythrocytes which then burst and the parasites are then able to invade more red cells.

There is an incubation period of 10–14 days before symptoms develop.

Immunity to malaria

People who live in areas where malaria is endemic develop some immunity. Mothers will pass **antibodies** on to their babies, if their immunity is high, so these babies do not usually develop malaria until they are 6 months old.

People most at risk are those who have not been in contact with malaria before or have a reduced immunity. These include:
- Children from the age of 6 months until they develop their own immunity, usually by the age of 4 or 5 years. This depends on the frequency of attacks.
- People travelling from a malaria-free area to an area of high incidence
- People who move away from a malarial area for some time and then return. They lose some of their immunity.
- Pregnant women.

Some genetic conditions reduce the susceptibility to malaria. These include the sickle cell gene, thalassaemia and G6PD deficiency.

Effects of infection with the Plasmodium falciparum parasite

Not all of these will occur.
- The erythrocytes break down and there can be widespread haemolysis leading to anaemia and jaundice.
- Periodic fever as the parasites release their toxins. This can lead to a misdiagnosis of typhoid or influenza.
- Enlarged liver and spleen
- Heart failure from the anaemia
- Kidney damage, with a low urine output. Renal failure may occur in severe cases, usually in adults.
- Abdominal pain and diarrhoea caused by the capillaries of the gut being blocked by the sticky red cells carrying the parasite
- Convulsions and coma from blockage of the capillaries in the brain (cerebral malaria)
- Death can be rapid, especially in young children.

Management

Anti malarial drugs are used. There are several available, including:
- Chloroquine. This is the cheapest and most widely available. Unfortunately, in many areas the parasite has become resistant. However, it is usually the first choice. Change to another drug if there are still symptoms after 72 hours.
- Halofantrine. Effective against falciparum which is resistant to other drugs, but it is expensive.
- Mefloquine. Resistance is occurring in some areas of the world.
- Fansidar. Resistance is occurring in some areas. It has become the first line drug in some countries.
- Quinine. Useful for cerebral malaria.
- Artemisin. Based on a herbal treatment used in Thailand and China. Becoming more widely available.

Nursing care

As the majority of severe cases occur in children, this is discussed in Chapter 46.

Prevention and control

The WHO Division of the Control of Tropical Diseases (WHO/CTD) have been involved in giving technical assistance and support to malaria control in selected health districts in Africa and on a national level. The control efforts have focused on six areas of activities.
- Effective drug policies
- Case management through the availability of well trained teams of health workers
- Effective vector control
- Community based involvement in activities
- Epidemic prevention and control
- Health information systems for monitoring and evaluation

This initiative is part of the WHO Global Roll Back Malaria Partnership.

To prevent malaria a control programme needs to be implemented. The programme consists of the following components:

The eradication of the mosquito: The larvae must be eradicated through the draining of stagnant water which offers breeding grounds for the mosquito. Where this is not possible, spray the water with oil containing an insecticide. Mosquitoes are eradicated by the spraying of insecticide on the walls and under the eaves of houses.

WHO Global Roll Back Malaria (RBM) Partnership

The WHO RBM initiative draws on global political interest in more effective and coordinated action, the potential for existing interventions to be used more effectively, and the growing commitment, among the research community and private sector, to discovering new products and cost-effective control tools (WHO, 1999).

The RBM objective is to halve the malarial burden and, specifically, malaria mortality. This is to be done by adapting to local needs and strengthening the health sector. Vector control, along with rapid case detection and effective treatment, form the basis of any successful malaria control programme. By changing the environment, the transmission of a disease can be reduced significantly.

There is an urgent need for the introduction of new, effective and affordable drugs to treat people who are suffering from malaria, as well as the development of an effective vaccine and safe insecticides. There are clear links between malaria, human development and poverty. Therefore development programmes must be run together with programmes introduced to combat malaria. The main thrust of the RBM efforts are being focused in Africa.

One of the goals of the RBM Partnership is to reduce malaria-related deaths by at least 50 per cent by the year 2010. The strategy adopted to achieve this goal is based on:

- early detection
- rapid treatment
- multiple means of prevention
- well coordinated action
- dynamic global movement
- focused research.

One of the exciting outcomes of this project is that a vaccine has been developed and is ready for testing. It is hoped it will be available for use soon.

Protection of individuals from mosquito bites: In places where malaria is endemic windows should have insect screens. Those who are most susceptible should sleep under insecticide treated mosquito nets. Covering the body as much as possible during the evening and night will protect from bites as the mosquitoes are night biting. Insect repellents can be applied to any exposed skin.

Chemoprophylaxis: The use of appropriate malarial drugs to prevent getting malaria. These are mainly used by visitors or people returning to an endemic area.

Note: This vector control programme for malaria can be adapted to the control of other vectors and the prevention of the potential diseases that they carry. Success of the control programme is dependant on community participation and acceptance of the activities. It is important therefore that community members are involved from the planning stage of disease control programmes.

Parasites that cause specific communicable diseases

N denotes notifiable disease in Tables 26.1–26.4.

Fungi

The form of fungi that causes disease in humans is mostly mycelia, such as Candida albicans that causes thrush. The other group causes conditions of the skin, such as ringworm and athletes' foot and is known as dermatomycosis. Fungi thrive in warm, moist environments. See Table 26.1.

Helminthic infections

Worm infestation is very common and widespread in Africa. Infestation is mainly intestinal but can affect other organs. Children are principally affected and the condition contributes to malnourishment in children who are already vulnerable as the result of poverty and poor environmental hygiene. See Table 26.2.

Rickettsia

Transmitted to humans by the bite of blood-sucking insects such as fleas, ticks and lice. See Table 26.3.

Protozoa

These single cells exist in a variety of shapes, size and structure. See Table 26.4.

Table 26.1 Fungal infections

Disease	Causative organism	Clinical picture	Specific prevention	Drugs
Ringworm (Tinea) Also known as dermatomycosis	Trichophyton This is a dermophyte that invades the skin, hair and nails.	Tinea capitis. Ringworm of the scalp. Mostly seen in children. Round or oval patches of scaling *alopecia* in the scalp Tinea corporis. Ringworm of the body. Presents as red scaly patches which are very itchy and tend to appear in non-hairy environments. Transmission can be from animals. Tinea pedis. Ringworm of the foot. (Athletes' foot) Commonly presents as cracks and softening of skin, mostly between the 4th and 5th toes. It can be sore and itchy.	Avoid sharing clothes, towels and other toiletry articles	6% Benzoic and 3% salicylic. (Whitfield's) ointment twice daily. If not successful use Imidazole or Cicloprirox cream Selsun shampoo Griseofulvins orally for chronic infections especially where nail beds and hair are infected. NB Griseofulvin can influence the effectiveness of oral contraception
Thrush (Candida)	Candida albicans Oral Vagina	Most commonly seen in infants as a creamy white to grey membrane on the tongue and inside the cheeks. It can be easily removed showing a red oozing base. Occurs mostly in malnourished and bottle fed babies. In adults indicates a suppressed immune system, frequently seen in patients with AIDS. Vaginal thrush is common in pregnant women and diabetic women. It is the most common opportunistic infection associated with diseases that suppress the autoimmune system such as AIDS. Irritation is severe and there may be a watery or profuse cheesy discharge.	Good infant nutrition Breastfeeding	**Oral** *Infants:* – Paint mouth with 5% Gentian violet – Nystatin suspension orally *Adults:* – Nystatin lozenges – Miconazole oral gel if other does not work **Vagina** Nystatin or Miconazole pessaries or vaginal cream

Table 26.1 Fungal infections *continued*

Disease	Causative organism	Clinical picture	Specific prevention	Drugs
	Skin	Common sites are skin creases, on vulva and penis. Skin has red patchy areas with white scaly edges to the lesions. Small pustules may be found in the infected areas.	Keep skin clean and dry. Avoid sharing clothes and towels.	**Skin** Nystatin ointment Miconazole cream
	Candida interigo	Common in infants with nappy rash	Good personal hygiene, especially of infants' nappy areas	
	Nail infection	Often seen in those who have their hands in water frequently and diabetics		
	Candida paronychia	Usually a chronic infection, with redness and pain in tissues round the nail. Nail may become discoloured and have ridges		
Pityriasis versicolor	Normal commensals that become pathogenic	Most commonly seen superficial infection. Normally asymptomatic Pale, irregular lesions usually on the trunk		Whifield's ointment Selsun shampoo

Table 26.2 Helminthic infections

Disease	Causative organism	Clinical picture	Specific prevention	Drugs
Bilharzia	Schistosoma haematobium (veins of the bladder) Schistosoma mansoni (veins of the large intestine) (Spread by a fresh water snail)	The human host becomes infected when the skin comes into contact with cercariae in infected water. See lifecycle, Figure 26.1. The only symptoms may be tiredness. However, other symptoms can occur within 4 to 6 weeks. At the site of the bite there is an itchy papular rash for 24 hours. Within 4 to 8 weeks there may be pyrexia, rigors, headaches, joint pains and a rash. Haematuria or melaena stools follow and can result in anaemia. Urinary tract infections occur. Often the only symptom is lethargy. Pulmonary, liver and cerebral complications can be fatal.	Educate to discourage passing urine and faeces into rivers, lakes and dams. Mass chemotherapy campaigns. Discourage washing and swimming in infected water. Control snails by removing vegetation along the shores of rivers and dams. Kill the snails. Provide latrines.	Praziquantel orally. (Not for children under 2 or breastfeeding mothers)
Tapeworm	Taenia saginata (cattle) and Taenia solium (pork) (small intestine)	Cysts are present in the muscle of the infected animal. The human host ingests the cyst through eating infected meat. The worm emerges from the cyst in the small intestine and attaches itself to the wall. It develops new, flat, white segments and the worm grows through this process. The Taenia saginata reaches 5–10 metres while the T. solium reaches 2–4 metres. Within 3 months the terminal segments are mature and pass out of the body in the faeces sometimes. Cysts of T. solium can lodge in the brain and cause neurological problems if the eggs are ingested.	Improve sanitation and environmental hygiene where animals graze. Meat inspection and adequate cooking.	Single dose purgative – Sodium sulphate Followed by a single dose of Niclosamide. Single dose of prazinguanel or albendazole. Dosage is determined by the weight of the patient.

Table 26.2 Helminthic infections *continued*

Disease	Causative organism	Clinical picture	Specific prevention	Drugs
Hookworm	Ancylostoma duodenale (small intestine)	The host is the human carrier who produces eggs that are found in the faeces. Eggs hatch in the soil and larvae penetrate the skin of the new host, usually between the toes. The larvae are taken to the lungs and move to the larynx and pharynx where they are swallowed and develop into worms in the small intestine. They fix themselves to the wall where they feed off the blood of the host. See lifecycle, Figure 26.2.

Patient may have iron deficiency anaemia and distended abdomen. The host is continuously hungry and may have an appetite for soil and salt. No pain is experienced. | Improve sanitation. Stop children playing in sand that may be contaminated by faeces. Avoid walking barefoot in long grass contaminated by larvae. | Mebendazole for 3 days. Albendazole in a single dose. Dosage is determined by the weight of the patient. |
| Roundworm (Ascariasis) | Ascaris lumbricoides (small intestine) | Long whitish/pink worms often found in stools. Grows to approximately 35 cm in length. Infestation is often associated with a cough and a painful distended abdomen. Intestinal obstruction can occur. | Improve sanitation, environmental and personal hygiene. | Mebendazole for 3 days. Albendazole in a single dose. Dosage is determined by the weight of the patient. |
| Threadworm | Enterobius vermicularis | White thread-like worms often seen in the stools. Anal itching occurs especially at night. Spread by hand to mouth and through contaminated *fomites*. | Improve environmental and personal hygiene. | Mebendazole for 3 days. Albendazole in single dose. Dosage is determined by the weight of the patient. |

Table 26.3 Rickettsia infections

Disease	Causative organism	Clinical picture	Specific prevention	Drugs
Relapsing fever	Borrelia duttonii (spread by lice) Borrelia recurrentus (spread by ticks)	Onset is sudden with *rigors*, pyrexia, muscular and joint pain, *photophobia* and a cough. A pink rash appears on the trunk and bleeding can be present as an *epistaxis*, *haemoptysis*, *haematemesis* or as *haematuria*. Meningitis with neurological symptoms can occur. After the 3–6 day period the symptoms disappear for about 6 to 10 days and then recur but with less severity.	Disinfestations of body lice. Improve environmental and personal hygiene. Protection from tick bites.	Doxycycline Antipyretics
Tickbite fever	Rickettsia conorii	Incubation period can be 10 to 18 days. Bite is characterised by a black centre that may form pus. Patient may present with a cold, pyrexia and headaches. Lymph glands near the site of the bite may enlarge. The patient will develop a *maculopapular* skin rash that appears over the whole body. Symptoms will get better in about 14 days.	Protection from tick bites.	Doxycycline Antipyretics
Typhus (Formidable epidemic disease)	Rickettsia prowazekii (spread by body lice)	The micro-organisms enter and multiply in the small blood vessels causing vessels to leak and *thrombi* to form. The patient will present with headaches and a dry cough. There will be a maculopapular rash over the whole body except on the palms of the hands and the soles of the feet. Pneumonia, toxaemia and gangrene of the limbs can occur. Hypotension can lead to renal failure.	Disinfestations of body lice.	Doxycycline Antipyretics

Table 26.4 Protozoan infections

Disease	Causative organism	Clinical picture	Specific prevention	Drugs
Amoebic dysentery	Entamoeba histolytica (large intestine)	Occurs mostly in tropical areas through the contamination of vegetables by cysts of the parasite. The disease can be asymptomatic but can cause abdominal pain and discomfort with intermittent diarrhoea that contains mucus and blood. General malaise and anorexia occurs. Dangerous if in the liver.	Good environmental and personal hygiene. Avoid contamination of vegetables and food with faeces.	IV or oral fluids for rehydration. Metronidazole orally.
Giardiasis	Giardia lamblia (small intestine)	There may be no symptoms, or there may be acute or chronic diarrhoea with bulky, greasy offensive stools. Tiredness and weight loss can occur.	Good environmental and personal hygiene. Avoid contamination of vegetables and food with faeces.	IV or oral fluids for rehydration. Metronidazole orally for 5 days.
Toxoplasmosis	Toxoplasma gondii (white cells) (Spread by domestic pets, infected meat and rodents)	Transmitted via the oral-faecal route. Can cause spontaneous abortion, stillbirths and congenital abnormalities in pregnant women There may be no symptoms, or the person presents with enlarged cervical glands, pyrexia, muscle pain, headache, sore throat and a maculopapular rash. *Myocarditis*, pneumonia and *meningo-encephalitis* may present occasionally and can be fatal.	Maintain healthy domestic animals. Wash hands after handling pets especially cats and cat sand boxes. Cook meat properly.	Sulphonomides and Pyrimethamine (Pregnant women must be referred for advice.)
Trypanosomiasis Sleeping sickness (Formidable epidemic disease)	Trypanosoma rhodesiense or T. gambiense (spread by the bite of an infected tsetse fly)	The site of the bite is characterised by oedema and enlarged lymph glands. The spleen and the liver may be enlarged and palpable. This phase can last for 2 to 6 months. If untreated, results in neurological symptoms. This includes meningo-encephalitis, *apathy* with slow speech. Later a shuffling gait and tremor affecting the tongue. The patient eventually becomes difficult to rouse and death follows.	IV or oral fluids.	Suramin has been used with some success in the early stages.

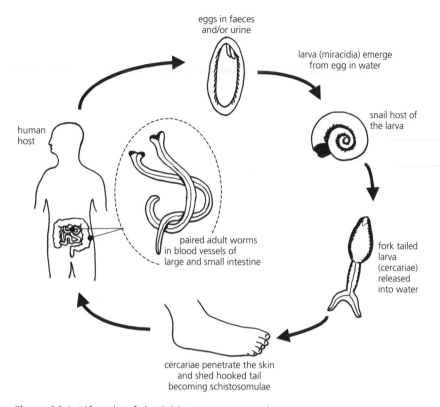

Figure 26.1 *Lifecycle of the Schistosoma mansoni*

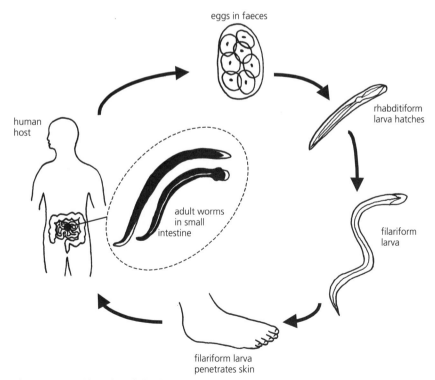

Figure 26.2 *Lifecycle of the hookworm*

Conclusion

Communicable diseases can be controlled and yet they are still responsible for the most morbidity and mortality in Africa. There is a need to improve the ability of health workers to identify outbreaks and to respond appropriately. This has to be done at global, national and local levels. The experts suggest that it is the control methods at community level that will make the biggest contribution to the control of communicable diseases. The nurse is the most prominent health practitioner at this level.

■ Activities

1. What is the incidence of malaria in your area?
2. Does it occur at certain times of the year?
3. Find out what drugs are most effective in your area and whether there are any contraindications.
4. Discuss with colleagues whether there are any measures you could take to reduce the incidence in your area.

Part 3

Reproductive and sexual health

27

Sexual and reproductive health care for adolescents

This chapter concentrates on sexual and reproductive health in adolescence and ways in which nurses and midwives can assist in making services available to young people.

Introduction

'Adolescence' describes the period between about 10 and 19 years when young people move from childhood toward becoming adult. Like all transition stages in life it can be confusing to experience and difficult for those around. It involves physical, psychological and biological changes.

The physical and mental health needs of adolescents include those important throughout life with some additional special needs (for example see Chapter 49). Adolescents are learning independence and how to look after themselves and this is not easy. Many young people find it hard to understand that things like poor nutrition and smoking may cause them serious problems eventually. They often say they don't want to become old anyway! Adolescents need to learn to take adult roles without damaging their health. They are vulnerable and may be subject to pressures that are difficult to handle especially regarding sexual activity and reproductive health.

Reproductive health care

Health services for adolescents address several issues that are relevant to those who are entering their reproductive years and are sexually active or may become so. Some issues may be relevant to much younger children who may be abused. Possible issues may be:
- Puberty and the onset of menstruation
- Early commencement of sexual activity
- Choosing not to have sex before stable partnerships are established

- Avoiding multiple sexual partners
- Unprotected sex
- Sexually transmitted infections (STIs), including HIV and AIDS
- Unplanned and unwanted pregnancy
- Unsafe abortions
- Sexuality: heterosexuality and homosexuality
- Substance and drug abuse including alcohol.

Drug and alcohol abuse, and practices such as glue sniffing, have direct health effects on young people and may endanger them in other ways. For example adolescents may be less able to control what happens to them when drunk or under the influence of drugs. Drug and alcohol addiction or dependency can also lead to sex for money, or for the drugs themselves.

Young people are at special risk from early sexual activity. They may not have the knowledge and maturity to negotiate whether they have intercourse or not, and to make sure they are safe if they do. Girls may find this particularly difficult and boys may become sexually active just because they think it is manly. Both girls and boys may have friends who boast about their sexual exploits. Most young people do not use condoms or practise safe sex. This means that they are at risk of both pregnancy and HIV and other STIs.

These issues are of concern at all ages but adolescents are especially vulnerable. They may lack confidence and be unsure of themselves. Relationships with their families may be difficult but they do not know how to get help from other people. Particularly difficult areas are:
- Limited access to information and education, particularly on sex, sexuality and life skills. Older people may be unwilling to talk about these issues and laws may make this impossible.
- Experimentation and risk-taking behaviour due to peer pressure, for example unsafe sex and drug abuse. Even uncertainty about the future can lead to risky behaviour.

- No access to money for buying things like clothes, and even food and school fees. This can lead to malnutrition, school drop-out and sex for money, often with older 'sugar daddies'.
- Harmful traditional practices such as genital cutting and food taboos
- Socio-cultural beliefs that influence giving information about the use of modern contraceptives and reproductive health services
- Homelessness and being orphaned
- Family pressures for early marriage
- Restrictions on rights of choice of partner.

Young people who have received a good education may find some issues especially difficult to deal with if their choices are restricted. They may believe they should have a right to decide for themselves what happens to them, but feel unable to do anything about it. Examples of issues they may feel unable to control are early arranged marriage, having to leave school early, and genital cutting.

What services do adolescents need?

Firstly, adolescents need understanding from their families. They also need:

- Services provided by local authorities and government officials that are:
  - appropriate to their needs
  - accessible
  - acceptable to both young women and young men
  - provided in environments that young people are willing to use
  - staffed by people who have approachable, non-judgmental and understanding attitudes, and are prepared to listen – and be friendly.
- To feel they can trust providers to maintain confidentiality. This is particularly difficult in small communities where carers and parents may know each other and information can so easily be spread accidentally.
- Providers who are realistic. For example, withdrawal is known to have very limited effectiveness as a contraception, but is better than nothing when sex is taking place with no condoms available.

You may need to make difficult choices about using resources when they are limited. Some young people may already be exposed to high-risk activities and need urgent help. Other vulnerable individuals who need special attention are listed below:

- People with mental and physical disabilities
- Displaced adolescents, for example refugees, orphans and the homeless who may be exploited by older people, be living on the street or recruited into military or criminal activity
- Unsupported pregnant and newly delivered teenagers
- HIV positive adolescents.

Other adolescents may be vulnerable too. Young people with disorders of normal development may be given very low priority in countries with few resources. They may just get forgotten. Such problems include menstrual disorders in girls and delayed puberty in either sex. Young people may need emergency physical and psychological help if raped or abused, including HIV and STI testing (see Chapters 31 and 32). They may need treatment for injuries, and emergency contraception (see Chapter 29), anti-retrovirals and antibiotics. Also important to treat adequately are complications of genital cutting, for example sepsis or HIV infection following unhygienic cutting, and obstruction to urination and menstrual flow from scarring (see Chapter 28).

You will need to refer adolescents with such disorders to appropriate specialists or medical care and may need to become involved with supporting them and intervening with families and authorities.

Cultural practices that are considered important in a locality may also provide challenges for nurses and midwives. Examples of harmful practices are early marriage and ritual sexual initiation of girls by older men. In some areas people believe common myths about sex, such as the belief that having sex with a virgin will cure a man of AIDS. Men may also seek out young girls for sex just because they are thought to be less likely to carry HIV.

Such issues can be difficult ones for nurses and midwives to address. They also demonstrate how their roles may extend beyond the clinical ones into advocacy and community mobilisation.

How can nurses and midwives be involved?

You have an important role in ensuring appropriate services are available:

- Family planning and contraceptive advice, and supplies such as condoms and contraceptive pills. Counselling for unwanted pregnancy and emergency contraception are important also (see Chapter 29)
- Cervical screening
- STI screening and voluntary counselling and testing for HIV (see Chapters 31 and 32)
- Post abortion care (see Chapter 30)
- Maternal health care: very young pregnant women are at special risk
- Support services for young and single mothers and their babies whether they are with their families or are homeless, and for very young couples who are parents
- **Advocacy**, information and advisory services. Special areas include rights to protection from harmful practices, drug abuse, rape, violence, sexual and other exploitation, pregnancy and homelessness, early marriage.

Nurses and midwives are in a unique position to talk with adolescents when they need health care. This may be the only opportunity young people have to talk without people in authority being involved. They have clear roles in providing information that young people are often not given by parents and from schools.

■ Activity

Young people can be very difficult to reach even for people who have not long left adolescence behind themselves. Select a hard-to-reach group of adolescents in your locality. Discuss with your colleagues what their particular reproductive health problems are likely to be. Then suggest some ways you might be able to reach out to them and meet some of their service needs.

You could also discuss the obstacles that get in the way of helping these young people, and who might be able to help you overcome them.

Health promotion

Those who do not have reason to seek health care may be much more difficult to reach. You may need to work with communities and those who are in regular contact with young people on health promotion activities. They can assist parents and teachers in helping young people to say 'no' to sex by teaching them the necessary skills. Nurses and midwives have well established roles in clinical and health advisory services for adolescents but other areas can benefit from your special knowledge and understanding of teenagers and their needs. Some people with whom you could collaborate are:

- School teachers
- Parents
- Community leaders at all levels
- Young people's groups and clubs
- NGOs and development partners
- Religious bodies and leaders
- Women's groups and societies, for example Mothers' Unions, and traditional groups such as the Sande of Sierra Leone and Dimba of Senegal
- Police
- Shop and bar owners or clubs where young people may gather
- High-risk groups, for example taxi and truck drivers, discos, night club workers, informal film shows, sex worker groups and drug addicts.

Working with such groups can bring fresh approaches to adolescent reproductive health care and encourage others to consider young people's needs. Counselling services can be provided, for example to help with psycho-social difficulties and relationships. Helping parents and their children to improve their communication can help to resolve family conflict. Young people may also need help to sort out confusion over sexual identity. This can be difficult to talk about when heterosexual relationships are the only acceptable ones. The existence of homosexuality is often unacknowledged and subject to taboo and stigma.

28

Female and male genital cutting

This chapter concerns genital cutting of both females and males. The different types, problems that can occur and ways of caring for women and male babies are described. Some of the issues around genital cutting are outlined.

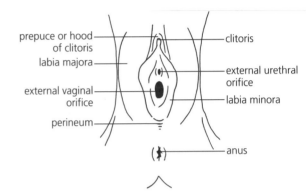

Figure 28.1 *Unaltered female genitalia*

Introduction

Many of the issues concerning genital cutting raised in this chapter are relevant to both male and female but significant differences also arise. Female genital cutting is generally considered to have more serious consequences and is illegal in many countries. This is considered first.

Note: Female genital cutting (FGC) is also known as female genital mutilation (FGM) and as female circumcision. Male genital cutting is commonly known as male circumcision. All refer to a range of traditional practices that involve cutting the genitalia in different ways.

Female genital cutting

What is female genital cutting?

The WHO (2001) defines FGM as all procedures involving partial or total removal of the external genitalia or other injury to the female genital organs whether for cultural or for other non-therapeutic reasons. It is a medical and human rights issue as well as cultural practice.

Four main types of FGM can be identified according to the WHO (2001). These are shown below, together with a drawing of the unaltered female genitalia (see Figure 28.1).

Type 1: Excision of the prepuce (the covering or hood) of the clitoris perhaps with excision of part or the whole of the clitoris itself (see Figure 28.2).

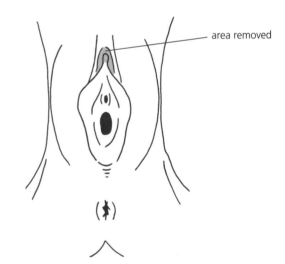

Figure 28.2 *Type 1: Excision of the prepuce*

Type 2: Excision of the clitoris with partial or total excision of the labia minora. The raw edges may be held together with stitches or something sharp like a thorn to make them heal together (see Figure 28.3).

Type 3: Excision of part or all of the external genitalia and narrowing of the vaginal opening by stitching. This is known as infibulation and involves cutting away both the labia minora and labia majora

173

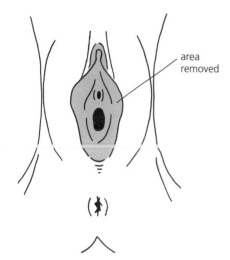

Figure 28.3 *Type 2: Excision of the clitoris*

and holding the raw edges together as with type 2 (see Figure 28.4).

Type 4: Pricking, piercing or incising of the clitoris and/or labia. It can involve stretching of the labia or clitoris, cauterisation (burning) of the clitoris and surrounding tissue. It can also involve scraping of the tissue surrounding the vaginal orifice or cutting of the vagina. Sometimes herbs or corrosive substances are put into the vagina to cause inflammation and bleeding so narrowing the vaginal orifice.

These procedures are all irreversible and their effects last a lifetime. FGC is often carried out by traditional practitioners in dirty surroundings or using crude and unsterilised instruments and with dirty hands. The procedure is usually carried out by force and with no pain relief. The risk of cross-infection and bleeding is very high and there are many later consequences. Even cutting performed, usually illegally, by health care professionals has serious consequences. New concerns have arisen about the possible transmission of HIV through re-using instruments without sterilisation. HIV transmission is also a risk for women whose scarring may lead to damage during intercourse.

FGC is practised in about 30 African countries and in the Middle East. According to WHO (2001), approximately 2 million girls and women are at risk of cutting in one form or other every year. This means 5000–6000 each day are at risk. Some live outside these countries but return there for FGC. It may be performed in infancy, during childhood or adole-

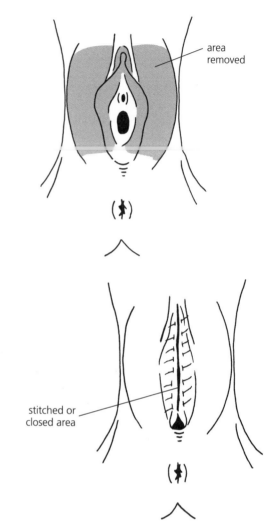

Figure 28.4 *Type 3: Excision of part or all of the external genitalia and narrowing of the vaginal opening by stitching*

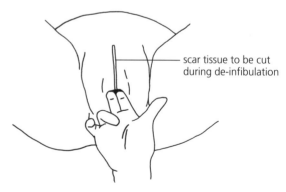

Figure 28.5

scence, or to adult women and is commonly performed as part of initiation rites or just before marriage. The timing depends on the community. It is practised in many religious groups including Muslims, Christians and animists. Although claims are made that it is a religious necessity, many religious leaders deny that it has any such significance according to their holy books. FGC is older than all the major faiths.

Most importantly FGC doubles the chance of the mother's death in childbirth and increases the risk of the baby being born dead by three to four times. In Somalia, where over 90 per cent of women are infibulated, one in every hundred women giving birth die in the process, simply as a result of such practices (WHO 1993).

FGC is a particularly difficult issue. It is illegal now in most countries, most of which have pledged to abolish such practices. Protection from FGC is a human right. It is so difficult because many see FGC as an important tradition. Traditions are the customs, beliefs and values of a community which govern and influence people's behaviour. Traditions are made up of learnt habits which are passed on from generation to generation. They are often guided by taboos and they are not easy to change. Many traditions are linked to rites such as initiation. Sometimes traditions are beneficial to health, or are thought to be helpful. Some are extremely damaging as is FGC. People may believe the female genitalia are 'dirty', shameful or 'too male'. Others believe that young women become sexually promiscuous if not cut and that it protects their virginity. It is also performed to discourage infidelity in marriage. FGC is a form of control of women. Many mothers fear that it will be difficult to find a husband for daughters without FGC. Those who are specialists in cutting may fear losing their incomes and the power they hold, so wish to continue the practice.

The nursing and midwifery role

Nurses and midwives have a duty of *advocacy* and should do all they can to convince women that FGC is harmful and dangerous. It may be possible to work with community and religious leaders or women's organisations to find ways of changing practices. Replacement rites need to be started to mark important occasions such as the transition to womanhood. This is more effective than just banning FGC.

Education on the physical and human rights issues is important. Women need to know that it has no advantages and that cut genitalia are not more hygienic than uncut. FGC is now considered to be deliberate damage to healthy organs for non-therapeutic reasons, even when carried out by health care professionals in clean surroundings. FGC violates the ethical requirement to do no harm and can never be permissible for nurses and midwives to do. One issue that makes FGC especially difficult is that it may cause differences of opinion between the women you care for, their families and you as a professional person. You and your colleagues may also have different ideas. You still have a moral obligation to do the most good possible for these women. In the end you may have to take action to protect young girls if the laws in your country expect this. You should know what action is expected of you.

Complications of FGC
Immediate complications

- Haemorrhage from severed arteries
- Severe pain
- Shock
- Infection, for example tetanus, bacterial infection, septicaemia, and HIV introduced by dirty or shared instruments and poor hand hygiene (see Chapter 32)
- Urine retention
- Injury to surrounding tissue
- Death

Longer term complications

- Delayed wound healing and localised infection
- Excessive scarring which may be keloid
- Pelvic infection
- Cyst and abscess formation
- Neuromata. Cut and trapped nerve endings can cause severe pain.
- Psychological trauma, such as flashbacks, anxiety and depression (see Chapter 49) and lack of trust in the family
- Vaginal narrowing or closure that can lead to the impaired or totally obstructed flow of menstrual blood and so result in pain and serious infection over months
- Recurrent urinary tract infection and kidney disease
- Lack of sensation and inability to enjoy sex
- Painful *coitus*. A man may be unable to penetrate the introitus on first intercourse and may use a

knife to open scarred tissue. Severed nerves can cause severe pain over the whole vulva. Relationship problems are likely especially if pregnancy is impossible to achieve.

- Delay and obstruction in the second stage of labour from scarring of the perineum and vagina. This can lead to uterine inertia or rupture and maternal death. Prolonged pressure of the fetal head on the vagina can cause gangrene and vesico-vaginal or recto-vaginal fistula.
- Stillbirth or death of the newborn infant because of obstructed labour (see Chapter 39).

Care of the pregnant woman who has undergone FGC

- Find out in the antenatal period whether the woman has had FGC performed and how extensive this is.
- Surgical *defibulation* can be carried out mid-pregnancy so that it is healed before labour begins. Some women prefer to have this done in labour so that they experience one painful episode instead of two (see Figure 28.5).
- Care at the birth. Make an anterior midline incision if scarring is extensive or tight. This exposes the urethra and clitoris which is sometimes difficult to locate under the scar tissue. It may be necessary to do a mediolateral incision of the perineum also.
- Excised external genitalia should not be returned to their pre-labour (and post FGC) state when perineal repairs are carried out. This is known as re-infibulation. The anterior incision, or any tears that occur, should be 'over-sewn' so that the edges of the wound do not fuse together again during the healing process. Women or their husbands or mothers may request re-infibulation. It is important to explain the consequences sensitively. You should be guided by national policy. In many countries re-infibulation is illegal and carries punishments for both women and the people who perform it.

Male genital cutting

What is male genital cutting?

Cutting the penis may be carried out for non-therapeutic cultural or religious reasons. It is occasionally performed for local therapeutic reasons – a true tight or scarred foreskin that cannot be retracted – but this is very rare.

The commonest form of MGC is cutting away of the foreskin or prepuce (circumcision). Other rarer types of MGC are piercing or cutting the shaft of the penis, or cutting open the urethra (subincision).

MGC is practised in many countries. It is most often performed in infancy but may be done later, especially before puberty. The timing depends on the community, for example it is done at 8 days old in Jewish communities. It is a key feature of Islam and Judaism but may be practised for traditional reasons by others. Although generally seen as less controversial than FGC, there are now serious debates about MGC even within some groups where it is usually considered important. It is both opposed and promoted on medical grounds, and opposed by some for human rights reasons. One issue is that of children's rights being in opposition to parental rights to bring up children according to their own traditions and culture. Unlike FGC, laws do not currently protect male children from permanent modification of their genitals without their consent.

The reasons given for performing MGC are varied and similar to FGC:

- An important reason is religious decree but some scholars disagree about this.
- Reasons of cleanliness and preventing a tight foreskin (phimosis) are commonly used. Parents worry about being unable to pull back the infant's foreskin for cleaning. However, these reasons have mainly been disproved. It is now understood that the infant's foreskin is normally attached until two or even three years and damage results from forcing it back.
- As with FGC, the prepuce may be considered 'too female' and MGC may be considered as part of becoming a man.
- Other commonly quoted reasons for MGC are to prevent urinary tract and sexually transmitted infections. These have mostly been disproved. The apparent link between MGC and reduced prevalence of HIV infection in countries where many men are circumcised is the subject of intense scientific debate. It is complicated by socio-cultural issues such as differences in ways of behaving, and it is not yet known whether the link is coincidental or whether there is a true cause and effect.

Complications of MGC

MGC is irreversible but complications are relatively unusual when it is carried out in a safe manner and many circumcisers are very skilled. However, both immediate and longer term difficulties can occur:

Immediate complications

- Haemorrhage and infection as for FGC although less common
- Pain. The nerve supply to the prepuce (foreskin) is extensive and MGC is usually carried out with no pain relief. Even analgesics and local anaesthetics do not remove pain sensations adequately. Very young babies may be severely stressed and breastfeeding may be impaired.

Longer term complications

- Scarring and skin adhesions can occur and cause difficulties in passing urine.
- The unprotected glans (head) of a baby's penis can become sore if it remains in contact with wet napkins (wraps or diapers) for long periods.
- Stress reactions such as prolonged crying, and difficulties with bonding between mother and baby, sometimes follow. Some men report experiencing psychological trauma such as flashbacks, distrust, anxiety and depression when MGC has been performed without consent. Physical force or coercion may have been used, often as part of initiation rites.
- Some people report experiencing reduced sensation during intercourse.

Care following MGC

Babies may need extra attention after MGC because of stress-related crying and feeding difficulties. The mother may then need encouragement to keep going with breastfeeding.

- Watch the baby for bleeding and teach the mother how to do this, keep the wound clean, and watch for infection.
- The family will need to return to have the wound inspected after two or three days.
- Soak off any dressing instead of pulling.
- Instruct older boys and men about danger signs and wound care.
- Boys who have infected wounds need antibiotics and may need surgical intervention.

The nursing and midwifery role

This concerns understanding the human rights issues discussed above, and ethical ones concerning the expectation that health care workers will do no harm. The minimum expectation is that you will make the possible complications clear to parents so they make an informed choice. The advocacy role is the same as for FGC.

■ Activities

1. Mrs X is a primigravid woman who is admitted in labour at 40 weeks gestation. She has been infibulated.
   - What are your responsibilities to her regarding the infibulation?
   - How would you make sure the risk of complications caused by the infibulation is reduced during this labour and any she may have in the future?
2. The following case studies are adapted from ones provided by the WHO (2001). What do you believe is the responsibility of the nurse or midwife in each situation? Discuss the issues that arise with colleagues.

CASE STUDY A

Amouna has not yet conceived after four years of marriage without using contraception. She had a type 2 excision of her genitalia when she was eight years old. The wound on her vulva smelled badly before it healed and she was very ill afterwards. The doctor finds that her fallopian tubes have become blocked due to the infection. What advice and support could you give her?

CASE STUDY B

Yasmin and John are health workers who are refusing to have their young son and daughter circumcised. Their families are very unhappy about this and the grandparents are pressurising them to change their minds. What information and advice would you give them to help them make their decisions?

CASE STUDY C

Elisa was excised when she was a child. She gave birth at home helped by her mother's friend when she was 17 years old. She laboured for two days and finally delivered a stillborn baby. She now leaks urine constantly from a vesico-vaginal fistula and her husband is threatening to send her away from home. How would you advise her?

29

Family planning
and contraception

This chapter reviews the current contraceptive methods available. It provides information about their use, how they work, their advantages and disadvantages. There are also sections on special circumstances – following birth, older women, adolescents and those with medical disorders.

Introduction

Family planning protects women and their families. When children are born close together, they all have less chance of health and survival to adulthood. It also helps to ensure women are not harmed by becoming mothers too often, too young, or too old. Family planning is about saving lives.

No method has yet been discovered that gives complete protection against unplanned pregnancy without some unwanted aspects. They all have something that causes difficulty. The perfect contraceptive would:

- Be 100 per cent effective
- Not rely on memory or on people making efforts before or after intercourse
- Be free, easily available, cheap to produce and not involve health services
- Be free of health risks and side effects
- Be completely reversible so women can get pregnant easily when they wish
- Prevent the transmission of HIV and other sexually transmitted infections (STIs) (see Chapters 31 and 32).

Couples need to talk about how to control their fertility. This can be difficult. Nurses and midwives can provide information, help people to identify their needs, and provide contraceptive items. They may help people to learn to communicate with each other. They can educate others who supply contraceptives, such as village health workers, traditional midwives and shopkeepers.

An effective family planning service gives people confidence that their privacy and confidentiality are protected, and that professionals have appropriate knowledge, skills and attitudes. A completely reliable contraceptive supply and easy access to friendly, competent advice is vital. Many people need repeat visits to clinics when deciding what to use. Individual clients' needs must be identified and guidance given on methods according to their health, lifestyle and the risk factors. They then can make choices and decisions with which they feel happy and confident. Services need to be closely linked to those for maternal health, STIs and HIV.

The main methods can be classed in groups:

- Barrier methods that stop sperm and egg from meeting
- Natural methods that make use of women's own rhythms
- Intrauterine devices that prevent pregnancy from starting
- Hormonal methods that affect ovulation and the uterus
- Surgical methods that prevent eggs from reaching the uterus or make sure men produce no sperm at intercourse.

A note about effectiveness: Percentages are often provided for individual contraceptive methods to indicate how effective they are (see below). These percentages refer to the number of women who do **not** conceive out of a hundred using the method and having regular sex for one year. So 98 per cent effective means that 98 do not conceive, but two will, in a year of use. Failure rates may also be used, for example two per cent failure rate is equivalent to 98 per cent effective.

The information given here aims to reflect current WHO advice when written (see Resource list on page 397), but may change.

Dual protection against pregnancy and sexually transmitted infections

Sexual intercourse involving penetration always carries risks of both pregnancy and STIs. The ideal contraceptive provides good protection against both (called dual protection). Condoms give good protection from HIV and other STIs. The ideal combination is a condom and hormonal or intrauterine contraception at the same time, as some pregnancies still occur with condom use.

Considering dual protection can cause difficulties within a relationship when one partner does not see the need. Trust issues arise and can lead to gender-based violence. Some women may choose not to inform partners that they are using hormonal or intrauterine methods in order to ensure condom use continues. This needs to be considered when giving advice. Condoms may be more acceptable, as their pregnancy protection is fairly good as well as their protection against STIs and HIV.

Barrier methods

Barrier methods include male and female condoms, diaphragms and cervical caps. They provide a physical barrier, preventing sperm from meeting the ovum. Failure rates are high without consistent and correct use. Only male and female condoms protect against STIs and HIV.

Male condoms

Male condoms are thin latex-rubber or polyurethane bags that roll onto the penis. They have a small teat at the end to collect fluid and sperm (see Figure 29.1). Condoms are known by many different names and

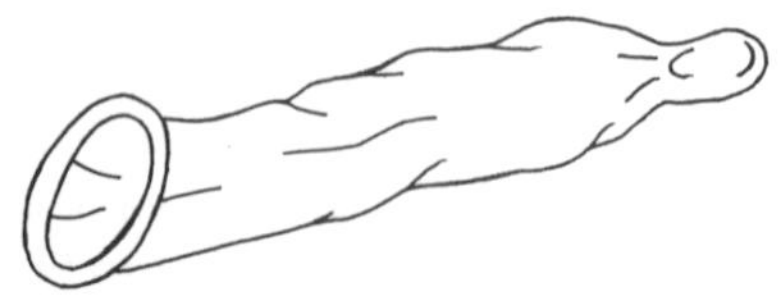

Figure 29.1 *Male condom unrolled*

have been used in some form or other for many years. They are probably the most widely available contraceptive. They prevent pregnancy by stopping sperm from being released into the vagina.

Condoms should be lubricated, but not with a spermicide containing nonoxynol-9 because of increased risk of HIV transmission (see Spermicides below). However, these are better than none. Condoms must be put on the penis before it has any contact with the female genitalia. Many men put them on only halfway through intercourse. This can lead to pregnancy as some sperm are passed before ejaculating, and permits infection transmission.

Advantages

- 85–98 per cent effective depending on how correctly and consistently they are used
- Easy to use, no supervision required once the method is understood
- No side effects
- Involve the male in sharing contraceptive responsibility
- Offer visible evidence of contraceptive use
- Protect against most STIs including HIV and pelvic inflammatory disease (PID)
- May protect against cervical cancer
- May increase pleasure for both partners

Disadvantages

- They may be viewed as interrupting sexual intercourse. Thinking of them as part of foreplay can change this.
- Motivation is needed to use them properly. Young people, and those new to using them, have higher failure rates.
- Occasional allergy to rubber or spermicide (see Spermicides below)
- Condoms occasionally slip off or split (see Emergency Contraception below).
- Some men report reduced sensitivity.
- There may be cultural taboos against using them, such as believing skin-to-skin contact is essential during intercourse.
- False stories are spread, for example that condoms contain tiny holes.
- Disposing of used condoms can be difficult. They should be wrapped and destroyed or put in household waste if good collection facilities exist. They should not be flushed into sewage systems.

- There is *stigma* attached to using condoms in some areas, for example when condom use is associated with promiscuity or infidelity. People may then believe they are not appropriate for married couples.

Common problems

People have many reasons for refusal or failures, for example:

- 'It came off': condoms can be left in the vagina if men do not hold them at the base of the penis when losing erections and withdrawing.
- 'It burst': this is caused by putting them on wrongly, using them inside out, biting them, or opening packets with the teeth. Oil-based lubricants, for example petroleum jelly, baby and body oil or cooking fats can damage rubber condoms, as can sharp nails. Silicone and water-based lubricants are safe.
- 'He says he can't feel anything': ribbed or thinner condoms may be available.

- 'Condoms are too small for him': condoms accommodate any penis size.

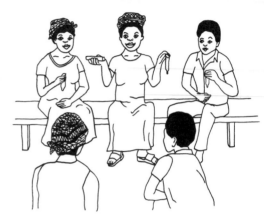

Figure 29.2 *Nurses can change attitudes towards using condoms by discussing their use in a relaxed and open way*

Step by step guide to condom use

- Store away from direct sunlight and heat.
- Check the quality mark and expiry date on the package.
- Open the wrapper carefully without tearing the condom.
- Check which way the condom will unroll; the rolled rim should face outwards.
- Vaginal secretion is good and important. Taking time for foreplay helps to ensure both partners are wet. Sex becomes more pleasurable for the woman and prevents damage to the vagina. Herbal preparations or cloths that remove this secretion can increase the risk of infection transmission. 'Dry' sex can also damage the penis.
- Additional lubrication may be required but must be water-based (for example KY Jelly), never oil-based such as petroleum jelly (Vaseline) or cooking oil, as they will damage the condom. Many condoms are lubricated.
- Place the condom on the erect penis before any contact with the partner's genitals, as contact with sexual parts and body fluids can transmit infections and pregnancy sometimes occurs.

- The tip of the condom will collect the fluid and sperm, so squeeze air out of it, and keep squeezing while rolling the condom down the penis (see Figure 29.3).
- After ejaculation remove the penis before it goes soft and while the condom is still on. Hold the condom at the base of the penis as it comes out so that the condom does not slip off and sperm do not leak out.
- Do not re-use the condom as the sperm and vaginal secretions on it may contain infections.
- Wrap the used condom and discard safely where children will not be able be find it and play with it!

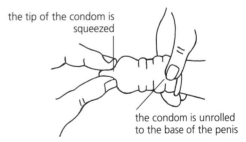

the tip of the condom is squeezed

the condom is unrolled to the base of the penis

Figure 29.3 Putting on a male condom

Learning how to put a condom on properly is essential for both men and women.

Guidelines for discussing condom use

Talking about condoms can be difficult and embarrassing. Demonstrating on a penis-shaped object makes sessions easier, more real and often funny! (See Figure 29.2.)

Female condoms

Condoms for women prevent unwanted pregnancies and the spread of STIs/HIV reliably when properly used. The effectiveness rate for preventing pregnancy is 80–95 per cent depending on how well they are used. They protect the vagina and cervix from contact with the penis, seminal fluid and sperm. Female condoms protect both the female external genital area and the base of the penis to some extent. Viruses, bacteria and sperm cannot penetrate it. The woman's body fluids cannot pass through to the man.

It is a soft polyurethane sheath long enough to line the whole vagina and cover the cervix. It has an open flexible ring at one end, and a small closed ring at the other (see Figure 29.4).

The closed ring is held between the fingers and inserted into the vagina; the large open ring fits over the labia. One size fits all women. It should be inserted before intercourse and can be removed at any

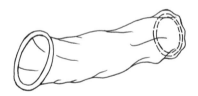

Figure 29.4 *Female condom*

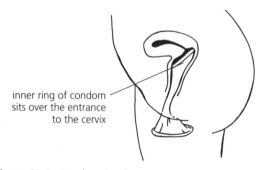

inner ring of condom sits over the entrance to the cervix

Figure 29.5 *Condom in place*

time afterwards. It remains flat over the vulva as well as lining the vagina (see Figure 29.5).

Advantages

- Stronger than male condoms
- No waiting for a male erection; can be inserted before intercourse
- Men report more freedom of penile movement during intercourse
- The woman controls its use. This is a real advantage when women cannot influence male condom use.
- They cause no irritation.
- Any lubricant may be used, including oil-based ones.
- Protects against pregnancy and infections
- Protects the vulva from infection to some extent and the cervix and vagina. It may protect against PID.

Disadvantages

- It is visible over the vulva.
- Some people dislike the rustling sound it can make.
- Female condoms cost more than male condoms.

Re-using female condoms

Female condoms are designed to be thrown away after each use but many women re-use them because of the expense. The safety and effectiveness of their re-use is currently being investigated. A safe handling and re-use protocol has been developed because women risk infecting themselves by washing and re-using them. This involves disinfection for 2 minutes in a 1 in 40 bleach solution, washing, drying and re-lubricating. Full details of the protocol are given on the WHO website (see Resource list).

Diaphragm and cervical cap

These are latex dome-shaped devices that are inserted before intercourse to cover the cervix. Both are normally used with spermicide (see below) applied over the cervical surface.

Diaphragms and caps work by:
- Keeping sperm away from the cervical mucus long enough for them to die in the acid vagina
- Preventing aspiration of sperm into the cervix and uterus
- Possibly holding spermicide against the external cervical os.

Effectiveness and use

The effectiveness rate is very low at 82–96 per cent depending on how correctly and consistently women use them. *Parous* women have particularly high failure rates. It is not considered to be a good contraceptive method even for consistent users. Caps, diaphragms and spermicide may be impossible to obtain in some areas.

Diaphragms have flexible flat rims and are inserted high in the vagina by squeezing the ring flat, and checking that the cervix is covered (see Figures 29.6 and 29.7). Caps are smaller and just cover the cervix (see Figures 29.8 and 29.9). Insertion is more difficult, especially in some situations. They should be left in for at least 6 hours after intercourse (up to 24), washed

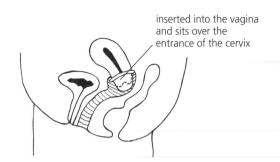

Figure 29.9 *Cap over the cervix*

with warm water and mild soap, dried, checked for holes and stored in the case in a cool, dry place.

A trained provider must examine the woman to choose the best size, teach her how and when to use it and provide the opportunity to practise in private. She should be asked to return with the diaphragm or cap in place so proper placement can be checked.

Advantages

- Controlled by the woman
- No *systemic* side effects
- May help to protect the cervix against STIs and cancer
- Can be inserted in advance of intercourse
- Can be used during menstruation
- Can provide acceptable contraception for older, less fertile women who perhaps have less frequent intercourse, and when pregnancy would be accepted

Disadvantages

- Effectiveness is poor. This is partly because sperm can 'swim' around the edge especially when the vagina enlarges with sexual arousal.
- Spermicide is used which can increase HIV transmission rates, as can irritation caused by latex.
- Obesity can make correct insertion difficult.
- Women with weak pelvic floor muscles may find diaphragms difficult to keep in place. Caps are more suitable for these women.
- Diaphragms can cause urinary tract infections by pressing on the bladder and urethra.
- Some woman dislike touching their genitalia.
- Need for planning reduces spontaneity.
- Must be fitted for size by trained personnel, refitted following childbirth and weight alteration of 3 kg or more.

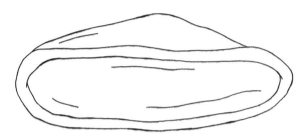

Figure 29.6 *Diaphragm*

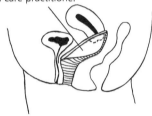

the vaginal diaphragm sits diagonally across the vagina, the correct size is determined by a health care practitioner

Figure 29.7 *Diaphragm in position*

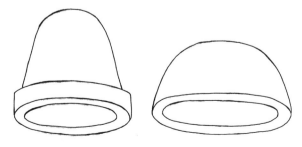

Figure 29.8 *Cervical caps*

Spermicides

These chemicals that kill sperm or make them inactive are sold as pessaries, gel, film, and foam. They give some protection against pregnancy. However, the failure rate is high (6–36 per cent) when used without a barrier method and they are expensive. Vaginal and cervical irritation and ulceration, candidiasis and urinary tract infection can occur, especially with frequent use. This increases the risk of HIV transmission. The WHO now advises that nonoxynol-9 spermicides should not be used with male condoms.

The intrauterine device (IUD)

The IUD is known also as the IUCD (intrauterine contraceptive device), loop or coil and is a tiny polypropylene device which is inserted into the uterus through the cervical canal. Contemporary IUDs are T shaped, about 3.5 cm long and 2.5 cm wide with threads hanging down through the cervix into the vagina. These threads enable

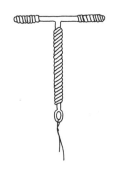

Figure 29.10 *IUD*

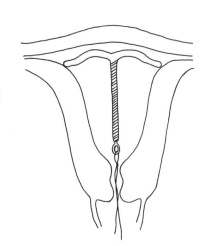

Figure 29.11 *IUD in position*

women to check IUDs are still in place. They need no attention once inserted (see Figures 29.10 and 29.11).

IUDs can remain in place for several years depending on the type. Women who have them fitted when they are over 40 can keep them until after the menopause when they must be removed.

IUDs work mainly by:
- Causing an inflammatory response which increases the number of white blood cells
  - The movement of sperm in the cervix and uterus is prevented so stopping them reaching the ovum in the fallopian tube to fertilise it.
  - Sperm are destroyed.
  - The ovum may be destroyed once in the uterus.
- Stimulating prostaglandin production causing the uterus to contract and bleed
- Making the endometrium unsuitable for pregnancy.

There are three main types of IUD, only two now being recommended. Each works slightly differently.

Copper-bearing IUD

The IUD is wrapped in fine copper wire and has bands on its side arms (see Figure 29.10). It is called the copper T because of its shape. The copper affects the sperm and ova directly so they do not survive. The failure rate is very low at less than one per cent in the first year of use. It can stay in for 10 years before replacement. It is probably still effective up to 12 years.

Lippes loop

This is no longer recommended as it is less effective than the others. Women who have had one for some time do not need to change until it is removed after the menopause.

Hormone-releasing IUD

This is the newest, most effective but most expensive type of IUD, often called the intrauterine system (IUS). (The effectiveness of the banded copper T is now known to be similar.) The IUS is shaped similarly to a copper T. The vertical shaft contains a reservoir that releases the hormone levonorgestrel slowly. This:
- slows down the sperm entering the uterus by making the cervical mucus thick
- changes the endometrium (uterine lining)
- makes menstruation lighter and less painful so is useful for women with anaemia or heavy painful periods.

Devices need replacement at 1 or 5 year intervals depending on type.

The copper T and hormone-releasing IUS have particular advantages and disadvantages. These are compared in Table 29.1.

Women who can use an IUD

IUDs are used most by women who have already given birth. They do not cause infection by themselves but no protection is given from STIs including HIV. Women who are at significant risk should use a barrier method as well (see Dual Protection above). IUDs are most suitable for:

- Women who are breastfeeding and need contraception
- Women who are not breastfeeding after the birth
- Women who have completed their family

Nulliparous women who are in mutually loyal relationships can use IUDs. They may occasionally expel them so follow-up checks are important.

Note: IUDs can be inserted immediately after the birth or an abortion provided there are no signs of infection or PID.

IUDs are especially useful for women who experience problems with other forms of contraception such as:

- forgetting to take oral contraceptives
- being unable to influence the use of condoms
- being unable to reveal their use of contraception (however some men do find them).

Women who should not use an IUD

- Suspected pregnancy
- Active or recent pelvic infection
- Reduced immune response, for example known HIV or AIDS
- Deformed uterus
- Severe menstrual cramping or heavy bleeding, and unexplained bleeding
- Rheumatic heart disease or history of bacterial endocarditis

Pp Fitting the IUD

IUDs must not be inserted if there is any possibility of pregnancy or infection. The woman should be tested for STIs first. Otherwise the banded copper T can be fitted at any time.

The insertion procedure should be performed by nurses, midwives, doctors or other health care workers, all having received proper training. Practice is essential. It is important to continue to fit IUDs regularly to stay proficient. Proper technique and good hygiene are essential to prevent PID and expulsion of the IUD.

The procedure is uncomfortable and may be painful, especially stretching the cervix. It is highly recommended that a non-steroidal anti-inflammatory such as ibuprofen 400 mg be given $1/2$ hour before inserting an IUD.

Table 29.1 Comparison of benefits and disadvantages of copper T and hormone-releasing IUS

Banded Copper T	Hormone-releasing IUS
Advantages and benefits	
Under woman's control	
Both are very effective at preventing conception	
Contraceptive effect quickly reversible by removal	
Independent of intercourse, no planning needed	
Fairly cheap and available	Very low ectopic
No systemic effects	pregnancy rate
Very long-term – 10 years	Lighter menstrual periods
Can be used until the	Periods less painful
menopause if fitted over	May prevent infection by
the age of 40	thickening cervical
	mucus
	Helps to prevent fibroids
Disadvantages and side effects	
Can be expelled	
Uterus can be perforated during insertion	
Threads may be withdrawn into the cervix making it necessary to get medical help to check the placement.	
Pain and menstrual cramps	Very expensive and not
Abnormal bleeding	available everywhere
Ectopic pregnancy can still	Broader than copper T
occur although the rate	because of the reservoir
is reduced	so insertion is more
Increased risk of abortion	uncomfortable
if conception still occurs	Irregular and prolonged
	bleeding in first
	3 months is common
	(nearly always settles if
	the woman perseveres)
	Short term hormonal
	changes e.g. breast
	tenderness
	Ovarian cysts may occur

- A vaginal examination is performed to check for tenderness and the position of the uterus.
- A speculum is inserted, the cervix cleaned and gripped with long handled toothed or Allis-type forceps. Injection of 2 ml of lignocaine into the site of application of the forceps 2 minutes beforehand is recommended.
- The IUD is introduced through the cervical canal using a disposable introducer (supplied with the IUD).
- The threads are trimmed so they can be reached by the woman's fingers.
- She is taught how to feel the strings and instructed to do so every month to ensure the IUD remains in place.
- The woman should rest for 10 minutes and be warned that she may have some vaginal bleeding and cramping sensations for a day or two.
- A follow-up appointment is made, usually after one month and then annually. It is important to ensure the woman understands she can return at any time without delay if she gets pain, heavy bleeding or vaginal discharge.

Problems in fitting

- Perforation of the uterus with poor technique
- Abnormal uterine anatomy causing failed insertion
- *Vasovagal* attack or persistent *bradycardia*
- Persistent uterine cramps which do not settle in 29 minutes

Some unusual complications can include:

- Asthmatic or other allergic attack
- Convulsion

Equipment should be available and another person present who can assist with resuscitation. If complications do occur, symptoms should be treated and the IUD removed if the symptoms do not improve after 30 minutes.

Pelvic inflammatory disease and prevention of infection with antibiotics

IUDs do not themselves cause PID. It is always caused by a sexually transmitted infection, whether or not an IUD is used. The only time an IUD can increase the risk is at insertion if a *pathogen* is already in the cervix, such as clamydia or gonococcus. Ideally, antibiotics should be given before a first IUD insertion in areas of high STI prevalence (especially gonorrhoea and chlamydia). The highest risk of PID is in the first four weeks after insertion. There is no evidence of antibiotic *prophylaxis* being helpful otherwise.

Natural family planning – fertility awareness

Women may prefer natural methods for spacing pregnancies or they may be used for a variety of reasons such as poor contraceptive supplies. For most natural methods, women need to get to know their menstrual cycles and learn the signs and symptoms of the fertile and infertile phases. The woman and her partner have to agree to avoid intercourse when she is fertile, and to understand that there is a high failure rate, especially when not used consistently and correctly. It is unsuitable for women whose cycles are irregular, or who will be having penetrative sex whenever they or their partners wish to. Barrier methods can be used at fertile times. The effectiveness rate is poor. Although they may be told otherwise, about 20 per cent of women become pregnant. They are not therefore suitable for women for whom avoiding pregnancy is essential.

The methods all work on the principle that the woman conceives within 24 hours of the ovum being released from her ovary. Sperm can live 3 days on average inside the woman's body, but some can live and remain fertile for up to 7 days. Therefore she should not have intercourse for the required time before ovulating, during that day, and as recommended after. For some methods she must get to know when she is ovulating or can expect to do so. It takes about 6 months to work this out reliably.

There are several methods:
- Standard Days
- Cervical mucus
- Changes in the cervix (This has been used as a method on its own but should only be used with the cervical mucus method.)
- Temperature changes.

Standard Days Method

This modern method is effective if used consistently and correctly (about 95 per cent). Unprotected intercourse must be avoided during days 8–19 of the menstrual cycle. The method takes account of variations in cycles and the survival periods of sperm. It has the big advantage that women do not have to work out the usual day of ovulation (as with the old calendar method) so it much easier to use provided both man and woman collaborate. It is less effective for women who have cycles of more than 32 or less than 26 days.

Changes in the cervical mucus (the Billings Method)

The woman observes the cervical mucus every time she passes urine to learn how it looks and feels. She examines it between two fingers and looks for the quantity, colour, how fluid and glossy it is, and its transparency and stretchiness (see Table 29.2).

The woman must not have unprotected intercourse:
- after her period from when any mucus is first detected
- thereafter while the mucus is slippery and stringy.

She should wait four days after the 'peak day' of slippery stretchy mucus and recommence unprotected intercourse only after that time.

Table 29.2 Changes in the cervical mucus

Name	Type / time	Characteristics
Moist and sticky	Early mucus, soon after the menstrual period ends	Small quantity, thick white, sticky, holds its shape
Wet	Transitional mucus Becoming fertile	Increasing amounts, thin, cloudy or transparent, watery
Slippery	Highly fertile mucus	Profuse, transparent, stretchy or stringy (like raw egg white)

Changes in the cervix itself

This should only be used to confirm the findings of the cervical mucus method.
- Before ovulation: easy to reach, firm, dry and closed
- At ovulation: difficult to reach, soft, open, straight and feels wet or slippery (as Table 29.2)
- After ovulation: easy to reach, tilted, firm, dry and closed

Changes in Basal Body (waking) Temperature (BBT)

The woman measures her temperature with a thermometer when waking, without getting out of bed, having a drink or smoking. These are known as 'basal' conditions. The temperature can be taken in the mouth, vagina or rectum for at least 3 minutes, using the same place for any one cycle. She should chart the temperatures. Her temperature rises slightly when she ovulates (0.2–0.6° C, or 1–2° F). The couple should then wait another 3 days after the shift in temperature before having unprotected intercourse, that is 3 temperatures all higher than the preceding 6 readings.

Sympto-thermal Method

This is a combination of the three methods used together to improve their reliability at predicting ovulation and fertility:
- Changes in the cervical mucus
- Confirmatory cervical changes
- Changes in waking body temperature.

All three results are charted giving a graph which indicates fertility (see Figure 29.12). (A blank chart is provided for copying, see Appendix C.) Some women will just use the cervical changes and mucus only.

Advantages of natural family planning

- Free from known physical side effects
- Acceptable as family spacing through abstinence amongst many religious and cultural groups
- Under the couple's control
- Costs nothing once training has been received, no follow up needed
- Can be combined with other methods: a barrier method could be used when the woman is fertile although this increases the failure rate compared with abstinence.
- Understanding the methods can help couples to achieve a pregnancy.

Disadvantages of natural family planning

- Can cause conflict and frustration. Great motivation is needed.
- Pregnancy can occur with unprotected intercourse during the fertile time.
- Barrier methods must be used while the woman is preparing for natural contraception. These do not change the normal cervical mucus.
- Signs are all affected by recent childbirth and breastfeeding.
- No protection against HIV and other STIs

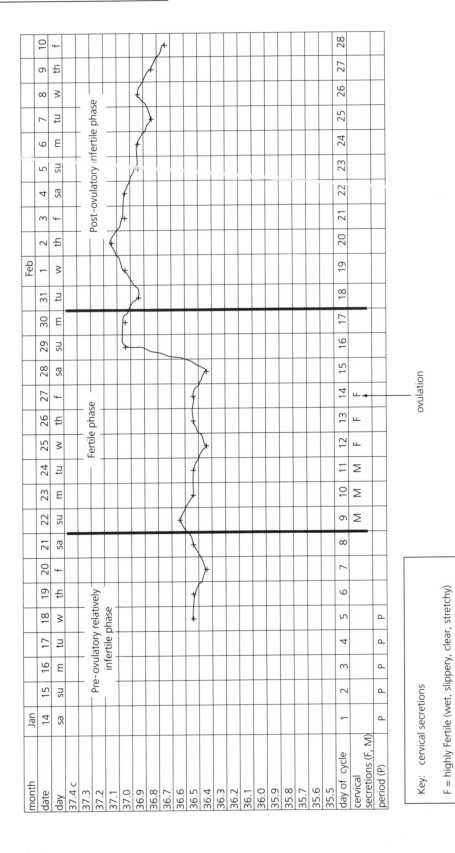

Key: cervical secretions

F = highly Fertile (wet, slippery, clear, stretchy)
M = Mucus (moist, thick, white, cloudy, sticky)

Figure 29.12 *Example of sympto-thermal chart*

Hormonal contraception

There are a variety of ways of using hormones to prevent conception. Hormone releasing IUDs have been discussed above. Other methods are contraceptive implants, injections, skin patches or taking by mouth. These methods are changing all the time.

The hormones used as contraceptives are changing constantly as new combinations and dosages are developed. These changes are aimed at increasing the safety and acceptability to women.

Hormones used in contraception

Two main groups of hormones are used, progestogens and oestrogens. These are synthetic steroid hormones. A variety of methods are used to deliver them (see below). The hormones affect women in different ways, each having advantages and disadvantages (see Table 29.3).

Progestogen: This may be given in combination or alone. It works in three ways:

- Stops the body from releasing an ovum from the ovary (ovulating) every month. This is its main action.
- Thickens the cervical mucus so sperm cannot pass through
- Changes the lining of the uterus and alters the pattern of bleeding.

Adding oestrogen to progesterone:

- Strengthens the action and prevents egg release (oestrogen's main contraceptive effect)
- Makes it possible to achieve a more regular bleeding pattern.

Oestrogen: This is given only in combination with progestogen.

Table 29.3 Advantages and disadvantages of hormones used in contraceptives

	Advantages	Disadvantages and side effects
General features of using progestogen only	Suitable for lactating women PID protection May reduce symptoms of pre-menstrual tension Fewer effects on metabolism so suitable for women who cannot tolerate oestrogen	Irregular bleeding patterns, breakthrough bleeding There may be amenorrhoea, especially with long-term use. (Increased risk of ovarian cysts)
Progestogen implants, injections and skin patches	Very effective for 3 years (more than 99%) Light periods or none	Weight gain, acne, breast discomfort Some women experience mood swings, abdominal pain, painful periods, headaches and hair loss. Unacceptably prolonged or frequent bleeds can occur.
Progestogen only pill (POP)	Effectiveness 99% if taken correctly, stronger during lactation There appears to be no increased risk of circulatory or malignant disease. Avoidance of all side effects where artificial oestrogen is implicated, including thrombosis (as with all progestogen-only methods) Most minor symptoms of COC not a problem Return to fertility more rapid than after COC No harmful effects from overdose	Timing of pill-taking is vitally important. Higher risk of any pregnancy being ectopic Younger women have higher pregnancy rates. Affected by diarrhoea and vomiting – see below

Table 29.3 Advantages and disadvantages of hormones used in contraceptives *continued*

	Advantages	Disadvantages and side effects
Combined oral contraceptive pill (COC)	More than 99% effective if taken correctly Regular cycles with less pain, lighter bleeding, no mid-cycle pain, pre-menstrual tension reduces Fewer fibroids, ovarian cysts, less endometriosis Protection against ovarian and endometrial cancer Protection against ectopic pregnancy Some protection against PID	Break through bleeding (change to a pill with increased progestogen) Headaches in pill-free weeks, mood swings (try changing the dose), weight gain, acne Very rarely – risk of thrombosis. Not suitable for smokers over 35 years or those seriously overweight

Note: All hormone methods can be weakened by rifampicin and some anti-convulsants. Antibiotics need no special precautions.

Methods of administering hormonal contraceptives

Contraceptive implants

Progestogen can be delivered to the body through small plastic rods about the size of matchsticks and inserted under the skin, usually inside the upper arm. Rods are flexible and unlikely to be visible. Progestogen is released slowly into the bloodstream over three years. Two types are Implanon (1 rod), Norplant (6 rods) and Jadelle (2 rods). Implants are highly effective at preventing pregnancy. Almost no pregnancies occur.

Implants are suitable for most women looking for reliable long-term contraception.

The method is particularly useful for women who cannot tolerate oestrogen and those who forget to take daily contraception. Note, however, that they can usually be felt through the skin.

Insertion and removal

Implants may be inserted at any time during the menstrual cycle if it is reasonably certain that the woman is not pregnant and will not have unprotected sex for the next 7 days. Day 1–7 is recommended. Contraception is then immediate. Insertion is very quick:

- Local anaesthetic is given to numb the skin.
- The rod(s) is inserted through a small incision.
- No stitches are required.
- A pressure bandage is placed on the arm to reduce bruising.

Some tenderness and bruising may be felt for a few days once the anaesthetic wears off. Movement should be normal. A layer of tissue forms around the implant which should keep it in place. It is recommended that it be removed and replaced with a new one after 3 years (sometimes 5). This can be done any time by a trained person.

Contraceptive injections

The same protocol is used as for implants:

- No extra precautions are needed if given during days 1–7.
- Extra precautions are needed for next 7 days if given from day 8 onward. (This applies to first injections only.)

The hormone is absorbed over two or three months after which another injection is needed. Commonly used injections are progestogen only Depo-provera and Noristerat. Combined injectable contraceptives are becoming available in some areas.

Characteristics of implants and injections

See Table 29.4 for summaries of hormone related characteristics and Table 29.5 for methods.

Table 29.4 Characteristics of implant and injection methods

Implants	Injections
Prevents pregnancy for 3 years or more	Injection every 2 (Noristerat) or 3 (Depo-provera) months
Can be removed at any time but minor surgery is needed	If side effects occur, they last for the time of the injection
Ovulation returns rapidly within 29 days	Fertility returns slowly (about 5–7 months) but always returns eventually.
No protection against HIV and other STIs Irregular bleeding and weight gain may occur, especially with injections	

Absolute contraindications to progesterone only injections, implants (and pills)

(For pills, see Progesterone only pills section below)
- Very severe arterial and cardiac disease
- Liver tumour
- Breast cancer (can be used if in remission for 5 years)
- Abnormal vaginal bleeding until an unimportant cause has been established
- Previous ectopic pregnancy
- Women who insist on having regular bleeds
- Women whose lifestyle is very irregular and may forget pills

Oral contraceptives

'Pills' are of different types, their main differences being related to when they should be taken and whether they use progestogen only, or combine this with oestrogen.

Combined oral contraception (COC)

The COC pill is taken by mouth. It is a combination of oestrogen and progestogen that prevents pregnancy, mainly by preventing ovulation and thickening the cervical mucus. Pills are supplied in two forms:
- 28 day packets marked with days of the week. A pill is taken every day. 21 contain hormones (active pills), 7 contain no hormones (inactive pills).
- 21 day packets of hormone (active) pills, their use to be followed by 7 pill-free days.

Instructions for taking the COC: These must be followed carefully:
- Start first day of period.
- Take for 21 days around the same time each day, followed by 7 pill-free days, or straight through for 28 day packs.
- If 1 active pill is missed, take it as soon as possible and continue with remainder. Extra precautions are unnecessary. (Missing an inactive pill – discard it and continue as usual.)
- If 2 active pills are missed, a pack is started 2 or more days late, or vomiting or severe diarrhoea occurs for 2 days or more:
  - Take an active pill as soon as possible and continue with remainder.
  - Use extra precautions, for example condom until 7 active pills have been taken.
  - Very important – 7 active pills are needed to suppress ovulation. Start the next pack immediately if the 7 days run into the pill free (or inactive pill) week.

- Severe diarrhoea, and vomiting within 2 hours of taking an active pill – take another active pill.

Contraindications: Caution is needed with smokers, especially older ones because of increased risk of stroke and heart attack, (more cigarettes = higher risk). COC is usually stopped by women over 50 (can use POP). Other contraindications are:
- High blood pressure
- Circulatory or cardiac disease, for example cardiac defects like rheumatic or congenital heart disease, sickle cell anaemia, past thrombosis or embolism, major surgery, prolonged immobilisation
- Current liver disease, for example hepatitis, tumours
- Steroid dependant cancer (breast)
- Severe diabetes with effects on eyes, arteries or kidneys
- Grossly overweight
- Migraine headaches with aura (for example visual and nerve disturbances)
- Undiagnosed genital tract bleeding
- Actual or possible pregnancy.

Advantages and disadvantages: See Table 29.3.

Progestogen only pill (POP)

This works in the same way as progestogen only implants and injections (see above). However it is less effective (99 per cent) except during breastfeeding and above age 40.

Instructions for taking the POP: The exact timing is very important:
- Start first day of period
- Take every day without a break
- Must be the same time every day, or within 3 hours (if longer take extra precaution for 48 hours)
- If there is diarrhoea and vomiting – use extra precautions, for example condom for 7 days after last vomiting.

Women weighing over 70 kg may be advised to take two pills a day.

Indications for POP: This is suitable for women who cannot use oestrogen:
- Lactating mothers – the combination is nearly 100 per cent effective
- Older women (50+ or 35+ for smokers)
- Diabetic
- Hypertensive
- History of thrombosis
- History of migraine with aura
- Sickle cell anaemia
- Women's choice.

Advantages and disadvantages: See Table 29.3.
Contraindications: These are the same as for POP injections and implants (see above).

Sterilisation

Sterilisation prevents pregnancy by preventing sperm from being ejaculated, or preventing the ovum from reaching the uterus. There is no effect on hormones or on sexual interest and arousal. Couples may find these improve when they are not worrying about pregnancy. Male sterilisation is easier and has fewer possible complications than female. These surgical procedures must be seen as permanent, as reversal is very expensive and often unsuccessful, so careful counselling of clients is essential.

Male vasectomy

The vas deferens is cut and the ends sealed with diathermy, by tying or clips. Local anaesthesia and a very small incision are used. Other precautions must be used until at least one specimen (taken after at least 8 weeks) shows no sperm present. (Some places without testing facilities recommend 20 ejaculations to clear sperm before unprotected sex is commenced.) Reforming of the vas is very rare so the failure rate is very low (less than 1 in 2000).

Contraindications: There are no long-term ones. Prior treatment is needed for STIs and problems of the scrotum. Care is needed with previous surgery to the area – (especially for undescended testicle) trauma, hernia, hydrocele and varicocele.

Female sterilisation

The fallopian tubes are cut and tied or sealed with diathermy, clips or rings. The ends may be buried away from each other. A mini-*laparotomy* can be done (by specially trained nurses and midwives) using light sedation and local anaesthesia. *Laparoscopy* needs a surgeon. Contraception is immediate although ova could already be in the fallopian tube or uterus. Other methods are advised until the next menstruation.

The lifetime failure rate is about 1 in 290 (1 in 1000 using Filshie clips). Ectopic pregnancy is more likely if sterilisation fails. Some women have sterilisation performed immediately after childbirth, especially with planned caesarean section. This increases the risk of thrombosis but is useful for women anticipating prob-

lems in returning. Counselling should be done in late pregnancy, preferably one week or more before delivery (not just before caesarean section). It is safer 6–12 weeks after the birth.
Contraindications:

- Normal surgery and anaesthesia warnings
- Survival of baby in doubt
- Postnatal mental health problems
- Pregnancy or birth problems, for example haemorrhage, severe anaemia, pre-eclampsia if BP still high, infection and trauma
- Other health problems may make sterilisation more important but must be controlled first (see below).

Contraception following birth

Women may be keen to accept contraception soon after birth. Such discussions are better in pregnancy to avoid feelings of pressure or later regret. However, many women receive no postnatal care and may not be seen again until the next pregnancy. It is important to discuss contraception before they leave midwifery care. Concerns women may have often relate particularly to the effect on lactation and the infant. The use of various methods by breastfeeding and non-breastfeeding women is summarised in Table 29.5.

Table 29.5 Postnatal contraception methods

	Breastfeeding	Bottle feeding
First possible ovulation	Day 43	Day 28
Breastfeeding (see LAM below)	98% effective in first 6 months if fully breastfeeding with amenorrhoea. Breastfeeding + other methods = even better contraception	Not applicable
Combined pill (COC)	Not advisable, reduces milk production. Can change from POC to COC at weaning.	Appropriate at day 21, no need to wait for period. If later than day 2 use added precautions for 7 days.

Table 29.5 Postnatal contraception methods *continued*

	Breastfeeding	Bottle feeding
Progestogen only pill (POP)	Recommended, effectiveness of POP + breastfeeding is 100%. Start after 6 weeks to avoid irregular bleeding, but can supply POP before discharge.	As for COC – day 21. If later, added precautions for 7 days.
Barrier methods	Condoms very effective used with breastfeeding. Diaphragm fitted 4–6 weeks postnatal. Refit in previous user.	Usual (limited) effectiveness
Emergency contraception	Progestogen emergency contraception suitable but not usually necessary in first 6 months of lactational amenorrhoea.	All suitable
Intrauterine device IUD	Generally fitted 6 weeks postpartum. Take extra care to avoid infection or uterine perforation. Can be fitted immediately postpartum. Retention more likely if fitted within 10 minutes of placental expulsion.	
Progestogen implants and injections	Suitable 6 weeks postpartum. Day 21 with added precautions if later (as for COC and POP).	
Female sterilisation	Sterilisation possible within one week of birth or, with pre-counselling, at caesarean section. Leaving to 6–12 weeks preferable.	
Natural family planning	Cervical mucus change observation unreliable.	Start when regular menstruation returns.

Lactational amenorrhea method (LAM)

Full breastfeeding suppresses ovulation and is a very effective temporary method of contraception (about 98 per cent) provided these conditions are met:

- Breastfeeding on demand day and night, with no other foods or liquids given to the baby to replace suckling. Occasional tastes are acceptable.
- The menstrual period has not returned since the birth. (Menstruation acts as a marker for ovulation but after 6 months may be preceded by one fertile ovulation.)
- The baby is under 6 months.

LAM works because suckling stimulates hormone release from the woman's hypothalamus. This suppresses ovulation. The effectiveness of LAM depends on suckling. More frequent suckling day and night gives better protection. LAM does not work well when:

- some breastfeeds are replaced with drink or weaning foods
- mother expresses milk for others to give the baby in her absence
- other women suckle her baby for her
- the baby stops night feeds.

Bleeding before 56 days following the birth is not menstruation. After that, a 2 day bleed or spotting should be counted as a period.

Note: After 6 months women can ovulate before a period.

Women should be advised to consider long-term contraception choices early on. All progestogen only methods can be started during breastfeeding without impairing it. They then continue working at, and after, weaning.

Contraception for older women

Older women need contraception until one year after the last menstrual period. IUDs should be removed then. Except for the POP, which is safe into the 50s, hormonal contraception is not advisable after 50. Women should consider using POP or barrier methods until they can safely stop. Women may need counselling as they may fear pregnancy, or be upset at the passing of their fertile years.

Contraception for women with medical disorders

Effective contraception may be vital for these women as pregnancy can be life-threatening. Sterilisation may be chosen. If this is unsafe for the woman, vasectomy is the ideal solution for *monogamous* women. IUDs have no systemic side effects. The hormone-releasing IUS can be ideal if available. Barrier methods have no systemic effects but are less effective.

Emergency contraception (EC)

This can reduce the chance of pregnancy following unprotected intercourse at fertile times from 33 per cent to one or two per cent of all of those seeking help. Among those who would have conceived, the levonorgestrel (LNG) method has five per cent failure rate when used in the first 24 hours after a single sexual exposure. EC works in the same way as other contraception, affecting sperm and ova to prevent conception occurring, and making the uterus unsuitable for pregnancy. It does not remove an embryo from the endometrium of the uterus, that is it does not abort a pregnancy or harm an existing one.

Oral contraceptives

- POP may be used but at higher doses than usual, for example 50 tablets of Norgeston (each levonorgestrel 30 mcg) taken preferably as a single dose within 72 hours of intercourse (24 hours if possible).
- COC use is possible but less effective than POP and has more side effects. If used, the dose is 4 tablets of, for example, Microgynon at once, repeated 12 hours later.

Copper T IUDs

- Must be inserted within 5 days of unprotected intercourse or 5 days after earliest calculated ovulation (before implantation can occur)
- The most effective EC method (failure rate 1 in 1000)
- Can be kept for continuing protection

Counselling should be provided to help women avoid unprotected intercourse and to organise sustained contraception following EC use. Community information is important so people know about EC and understand it (for example by radio). The possibility of women seeking unsafe abortion is high if unwanted pregnancy occurs. Unwanted pregnancy and unsafe abortion also increases maternal ill-health and death (see Chapters 30 and 33).

Adolescent contraception

Contraceptive services are vital for sexually active adolescents (see Chapters 27 and 33). Individual lifestyle needs to be considered when helping them to make choices. The ideal choice for those who will not remain *celibate* may be condoms to protect against HIV and other STIs, and a more effective method for contraception. Oral contraceptives are very suitable for those who will take them regularly. COCs are less time-dependant than POPs. They can be commenced even if the menstrual cycle is not yet regular. IUDs, implants and injectables are also suitable. Natural methods are only suitable for highly motivated adolescents who accept the risk of pregnancy sufficiently that they would keep a baby. Withdrawal is better than nothing when condoms etc. are unavailable.

■ Activities

1. Your clinic cleaner's daughter Mary is about to be married aged 16. You are worried she may become pregnant too young. What would you do and how would you advise her?
2. Sarah is about to leave the hospital after the birth of her son. She asks you about contraception. How would you advise her?

30

Miscarriage and post-abortion care (PAC)

This chapter deals with the care of women following miscarriage or abortion. It reviews the signs and symptoms and complications, and provides details of the emergency management and aftercare needed to save lives. It also considers follow up, counselling, family planning and what communities can do to refer women with complications in a timely way and, above all, help prevent unsafe abortions.

Introduction

The information in this chapter applies to all women who have had an abortion or miscarriage. The word 'abortion' is often used for both miscarriage and intentional ending of a pregnancy. However, many people prefer to use 'miscarriage' for spontaneous loss of the fetus. They then use 'abortion' for the deliberate termination of pregnancy either legally or illegally.

Miscarriage and abortion, especially unsafe abortion, are very serious threats to women's lives and health. It is estimated that about 80,000 women around the world die every year from the complications out of about 50 million carried out. All of these would have been better prevented by contraception or sterilisation. 'Unsafe abortion' refers to those carried out in unsuitable environments, using non-sterile or dangerous implements, or with limited skills and knowledge. Unsafe abortions are often illegal ones although not all 'legal' abortions are safe either.

Abortion and miscarriage are classified in different ways:

Spontaneous abortion or miscarriage: This happens without deliberate intervention. It is common (it happens to about one in four women), and the cause is often unknown. It may be associated with maternal ill health but usually happens because the fetus is not well formed. If it happens more than three times it is called recurrent. This is very distressing for women.

Induced abortion: This is the intentional termination of pregnancy before the fetus is able to survive. This is defined as 22 or 24 weeks gestation. Some countries allow abortion to be carried out for clearly defined reasons, such as to save the mother. In others it is always illegal.

Unsafe abortion: This is one which is performed in an inadequate environment or by unskilled persons (or both). Facilities may be dirty and instruments unsterile so risking cross-infection with bacteria or HIV. There may be no electricity or clean water, no blood supplies or drugs, and no assistance available when things go wrong.

The management of PAC: basic components

PAC involves:

- Treatment that is needed to save life when complications such as bleeding and infection occur
- Help in coming to terms with losing a wanted baby and reassurance about trying again
- Provision of the longer term support needed to prevent unwanted pregnancy
- An effective referral system for preventing and managing complications if the local facilities, resources and skill levels are not appropriate.

The involvement of management and policy makers in PAC is important to ensure adequate resources and legislation exist. Community involvement helps to make PAC programmes successful.

Emergency management

Emergency management consists of resuscitation, assessment and diagnosis, and treatment of complications.

Assessment and diagnosis

A woman who arrives with signs and symptoms of complicated abortion must receive priority treatment and should be assessed immediately. She may already be very sick on arrival and must be referred rapidly if the help required is not locally available. Her temperature, pulse and blood pressure must be measured and general condition assessed. She will be frightened and in pain so kindly and non-judgmental reassurance is important.

Abortion or miscarriage is classified as threatened, inevitable, complete and incomplete. Signs and symptoms will depend upon the type of abortion as shown in Table 30.1.

Note:

- Products of conception consist of the embryo or fetus, placenta and membranes. Blood, clots and some fluid will also be expelled.
- Complications are very common especially with unsafe abortion.

The most common complications and common signs and symptoms of complicated abortion or miscarriage are listed in the information boxes below.

Common complications of miscarriage or abortion

Bleeding: Heavy or prolonged bleeding:
- **Primary**. Immediate from a uterus that is not contracted and/or still contains retained products of conception
- **Secondary**. Several days after the miscarriage or abortion has taken place and is caused by infection

Infection:
- Retained products of conception will always become infected if not removed. This may lead to generalised septicaemia.
- Septicaemia can occur even without evidence of retained products (known as septic abortion) and is often a complication of unsafe or illegal abortion.
- Prolonged or chronic pelvic infection, pelvic abscess and infertility

Shock: From heavy bleeding, pain, injury, severe infection (septicaemia)

Anaemia and infertility: Long-term complications

Common signs and symptoms of complicated miscarriage or abortion

Symptoms reported by woman	Signs noticed on examination
History of bleeding	May look pale
Feeling unwell	Low blood pressure
History of partial (or complete) expulsion of products of conception	High temperature and rapid pulse rate
Lower abdominal pain, cramping	Bleeding
	Foul-smelling or purulent vaginal discharge
	Cervix open
	Products protruding through cervix or in vagina
	Tender abdomen may be noted

Table 30.1 Signs and symptoms of miscarriage or abortion

	Threatened	Inevitable	Incomplete	Complete
Uterus	Size as dates May be tender May be soft	Size as dates May be tender	Smaller than dates May be tender	Smaller than dates and soft May be tender
Cervix	Closed	Open	Open	Closed (open initially)
Pain	Lower abdomen, often described as 'cramping', may be light or severe			
Bleeding	May be light or heavy			
Products of conception	No	No	Partly expelled	Expelled fully
Shock	No	May be present	May be present	Depends on previous events

Note:

- The woman's uterus may still be the right size for her dates (especially in early pregnancy) even if products of conception have been expelled.
- Pregnancy tests are usually positive. They may stay positive for up to one week after both complete and incomplete abortion.
- Observe for signs of injury such as lacerations of the vulva and vagina. Watch for substances inserted into the cervix and uterus especially when unsafe abortion is suspected. Refer as necessary. Laparotomy may be needed.
- In cases of attempted illegal abortion the woman may also have drunk or eaten local medicines such as quinine or other substances such as washing powders. These can cause signs and symptoms of general poisoning. If a woman has obtained and taken drugs such as misoprostol or Cytotec, she will show the gynaecological signs and symptoms of abortion in Table 30.2.
- A woman may have signs of abortion without immediate visible bleeding if her pregnancy is *ectopic*. She may complain of irregular bleeding, lower abdominal pain which is mainly one-sided, shoulder tip pain and dizziness. If during bimanual examination of the cervix the cervix is moved very gently to one side, it causes much more pain toward the side of the ectopic than to the other. This very useful clinical sign can be learnt by those who are not gynaecologists.
- If ectopic pregnancy is suspected she must be given an IV infusion and be referred immediately for proper diagnosis and possibly a laparotomy.

Resuscitation

Assess, then if the woman's condition requires it:
- Treat for shock (see Chapter 5).
- Commence intravenous infusion of fluids.
- Organise referral to a centre where evacuation of the uterus, cross-matching and blood transfusion are possible.

Prevention and treatment of infection

Bacterial infection: Women who have had an incomplete abortion are extremely likely to sustain a life-threatening bacterial infection of the reproductive tract. This is even more likely if she has had an unsafe abortion. To prevent infection, it is essential to empty the uterus of all retained products of conception and give antibiotics. This is especially important when un-

safe foreign bodies, instruments, substances or hands have been inserted into the vagina and uterus.

A good broad spectrum antibiotic should be given as soon as possible. If there are signs of infection, it is best to give them intravenously for 24–48 hours, then by mouth until the end of the course. Examples are Metronidazole, Azithromycin, Ampicillin with Gentamicin, Chloramphenicol. These may be given as follows:

- Metronidazole 500mg IV every 8 hours. Rectal administration is a useful alternative if IV not possible. Give 1g (2 suppositories) every 8 hours.
- Ampicillin 2 g IV every 6 hours
- Gentamicin 5 mg per kg of body weight IV every 24 hours (**Note:** Gentamicin may cause anaphylactic shock, see Chapter 5.)

Tetanus infection: Women who have undergone unsafe abortion are at high risk of tetanus infection. The WHO (2000) recommends that women who have:

- not been immunised in this pregnancy should receive a booster of tetanus toxoid 0.5 ml IM.
- never been immunised should receive anti-tetanus serum 1500 units IM followed by a tetanus toxoid 0.5 ml IM booster dose after 4 weeks.

Administering oxytocin and evacuating the uterus

Oxytocin: You may need to give oxytocin if emptying of the uterus cannot be performed at once. Table 30.2 shows the regime recommended by the WHO (2000).

Table 30.2 WHO recommended drug regime for evacuating the uterus

	Inevitable abortion	Incomplete abortion
Less than 16 weeks gestation	Ergometrine 0.2 mg IM, repeated after 15 minutes if evacuation of the uterus is delayed, OR Misoprostol 400 mcg given by mouth, repeated once after 4 hours if necessary	
More than 16 weeks gestation	Oxytocin 40 units infusion in 1 litre IV fluid (normal saline or Ringer's lactate) at a speed of 40 drops per minute (if needed to help achieve expulsion of products of conception)	
		Misoprostol 200 mcg administered vaginally every 4 hours until the products are expelled (maximum total dose of 800 mcg) if needed

Surgical evacuation of the uterus

This may be needed if products of conception remain within the uterus, cervix or vagina. It is usually done as a D and C (dilatation and curettage) but some places now can perform Manual Vacuum Aspiration (MVA). MVA is preferable to surgical evacuation as injury is less likely to occur and paracetamol may be the only analgesia needed. It is performed using a device that sucks out the remaining products of conception. It can be performed after miscarriage if gestation is 16 weeks and below. MVA can be performed by midwives and nurses but special training is essential (see WHO 2000 for a detailed description). Some countries have appropriate policies and protocols so that midwives and nurses can perform MVA.

Rhesus incompatibility

If anti-D and blood testing are available, women with rhesus negative blood group should be offered this following miscarriage and abortion. This prevents rhesus incompatibility and haemolytic anaemia in future babies.

Referral

If facilities for transfusion and evacuation of the uterus are not available on site you must send any woman who has complications to a larger centre which has them. All clinics should have referral, communication and emergency transport plans made, and staff should be familiar with them to avoid delays.

Information-giving and consent

Women and their partners must have information about what is happening and the possible consequences. This is important for long-term health but also for immediate confidence and giving consent for PAC services. Written consent must be obtained for operative procedures. If a woman is too ill to give written consent, life-saving measures may have to be taken without waiting.

Counselling and follow up

Post treatment expectations and self-care

Before a woman leaves hospital, it is important to explain again what has happened. She may be very disappointed that she has miscarried so needs to know that it is common and most women can become pregnant again. She may need to talk about her feelings and her home situation, such as the reaction of her husband and family. She should be advised to delay pregnancy until she is well. She needs to be guided about care and hygiene as she recovers. She is likely to be anaemic so should be provided with iron and folic acid tablets. Advice should also be given about how to get help and the danger signs to look for:

- Pain continuing past a few days or becoming severe
- Continued bleeding, or heavier than a menstrual bleed
- Bad odour from the vagina or a vaginal discharge
- Feeling feverish or ill
- Dizziness or fainting
- Shoulder tip pain and abdominal pain.

A follow-up appointment should be given before the woman leaves hospital and the opportunity taken to link her to other services she may need. A booster dose of tetanus toxoid may be needed. She should be advised to attend antenatal clinic early in her next pregnancy. This is a good opportunity to offer counselling and treatment for sexually transmitted infections and HIV. Good links with other services are vital, and so is record keeping, to make sure the care needed is delivered after she leaves hospital. Most important is to provide contraception advice.

Family planning and contraception

It is important to make sure the woman understands that pregnancy can be prevented. You should encourage her to attend a family planning clinic. You should also explain the dangers of unsafe induced abortion. She may need immediate contraception as ovulation can take place as early as 10 days after the abortion. This may be in the form of hormonal pills or injections, intrauterine devices (provided no infection is suspected), tubal ligation, or advice on condom use. Many women do not return despite advice so it is better to commence family planning methods before they leave hospital or at least provide for later use (see Chapter 29).

Note: In some places, emergency contraception may be provided in advance to be taken following the first intercourse after the abortion if condoms are not used (see Chapter 29).

Health promotion

Mobilising health care workers

All health care workers have a role in saving lives, including managers, administrators and support workers. Security guards can help or hinder saving women's lives. Storekeepers are essential people in the supply of equipment, and cleaners are vital to infection prevention. All need to understand:

- the dangers of miscarriage and unsafe abortion
- early recognition and reporting that a woman needs urgent help
- where to seek assistance.

Those caring for women and advising communities and village health workers also need to understand:

- common causes of abortion and their prevention
- self-care after abortion
- importance of emergency contraception after abortion
- the importance of continuing contraception using proper techniques.

Attitudes

The attitudes of health care providers toward women who have had an abortion are crucial if PAC is to be successful. Women may respond to bad experiences and unhelpful attitudes by not making use of follow-up services or not reporting to a health care facility in another similar situation. News of bad treatment can cause other women to risk their lives by delaying seeking help for abortion. Women who feel that their dignity has been respected will pass on good reports and also be more willing to return. Service 'with a smile' is very important.

Staff training – life-saving skills

All staff likely to need to care for women post-abortion must receive appropriate life-saving skills training, such as how to resuscitate women who are in shock and, preferably, how to carry out MVA. They must also know how to refer women who need more help than can be provided locally, and where to send them. They need supervision, follow up and continuing education. This is a major resource issue.

Supportive legislation for nurses and midwives

Appropriate policies, protocols and legislation are important to ensure nurses and midwives are able to practise to the full extent of their knowledge. Examples are policies that specify that they can give oxytocics, start IV antibiotics and learn to do MVA. They need to know that supportive policies exist for PAC so they can work confidently and without fear of disciplinary action.

Mobilising communities

Whole communities need to understand how to prevent and deal with emergencies. They have a strong role to play in reacting quickly and appropriately when abortion or miscarriage occurs. They can help to prevent unwanted pregnancy by supporting efforts to encourage family planning. Some groups may be more difficult to reach and need special attention (see Chapter 50).

Nurses and midwives have equally important roles in helping to mobilise and guide communities in these activities.

Emergency preparedness

Some activities are especially important so that women get help very quickly. The public must be aware of the dangers of unsafe abortions and also how to react quickly and appropriately. This applies whether a woman aborts accidentally or intentionally. Some activities that communities and health care workers can do together are:

- Increase public awareness of the dangers of miscarriage and unsafe abortion
- Learn and teach about the complications and danger signs
- Identify well equipped health facilities in advance and how to get there day and night
- Devise plans for emergency evacuation of women and communicating with the facilities
- Develop community credit systems to help women who cannot afford emergency care. An example of a credit system is when people get together to contribute to central funds from which members can borrow in emergencies.
- Actively support family planning initiatives.

■ Activities

1. Find out and list the local procedures that are in place to make sure women receive the emergency treatment they need without delay.
2. A woman arrives at the hospital gate suffering from an incomplete abortion. List the people she will meet and the actions they might take as she receives the help she needs. Draw a diagram of the pathway she takes through the care process. What are the possible points where she may encounter life-threatening delay?

31

Care of patients with sexually transmitted infections

This chapter presents a five-step approach to caring for patients with STIs. This includes and explains *syndromic* management:
- Step 1 – taking a sexual history
- Step 2 – physical examination
- Step 3 – assessment and treatment of STIs by syndromic management
- Step 4 – health promotion to prevent further infection
- Step 5 – follow-up assessment.

Introduction

Sexually transmitted infections (STIs) cause major health problems everywhere, especially where resources are limited. Untreated STIs are distressing and unpleasant and can result in major complications including chronic pain, infertility, miscarriage, ectopic pregnancy, cancer and death. They can also have damaging effects on babies and young children through mother to child transmission.

The chapter should be read alongside Chapters 29 and 32.

STIs and HIV

STIs have become an even more serious issue since HIV became common. STI patients should always be offered testing for HIV. It is now clear that there is a strong relationship between them:
- HIV infection is more easily transmitted:
  - to men and women who have STIs, especially with genital ulceration
  - from people who have STIs, especially genital infection.
- STIs can be more severe and difficult to treat in those who are HIV positive and immuno-suppressed. Failure is common.

- People at risk of STIs are at risk of HIV transmission.

The nursing role

Research has shown that effective community care strategies for patients with STIs can reduce the rates of both STIs and HIV. Nurses need to be central to these strategies in the following ways:
- By establishing nurse-led clinics to diagnose and treat patients with STIs and their sexual partners.
- By treating individuals with respect, listening to their concerns and advising and educating them while reassuring them of confidentiality. Individuals will then be much more likely to come for assistance and follow the advice given.
- By changing negative attitudes towards people with STIs and challenging the unpleasant way that patients with STIs are often treated.
- By giving appropriate health promotion advice on a community level to increase awareness and prevent further infection.

Caring for patients with STIs using syndromic management

Syndromic management means that the common signs and symptoms of infections are grouped into *syndromes* and treatment is based on that syndrome, for example 'genital ulceration' or 'vaginal discharge'. This is different to the traditional approach of taking a swab or specimen from the patient and diagnosing a specific infection. There are limitations to using syndromic management and it can cost more in medications but there are also clear advantages:
- No need to wait for laboratory test results. Treatment can be started immediately, patients are more *compliant* and cure rates are higher. (Many patients do not return for test results anyway.)
- Costs of laboratory services are reduced.

- Can be delivered by non-medical personnel and integrated into other established services such as mother and child health, primary health care and family planning. These can be delivered easily in urban and rural settings.
- People often have mixed infections anyway.

Step 1: Taking a sexual history

Reasons

A sexual history is taken to:
- discover the concerns of individuals
- assess their likely contact with STIs and other sexual health related problems
- assess their clinical condition in order to prescribe appropriate treatment
- check their knowledge and understanding of sexual health issues in order to give information to help prevent further STIs
- discover their sexual contacts who may also require assessment and treatment.

Symptoms

Ask about the symptoms that patients are experiencing in order to assess the clinical condition. Ask how long they have had the symptoms, to describe what they see and what they are feeling. This should include:
- Ulcers. Where? How many? What they look like? Painful or non-painful?
- Rashes. Where? Colour? Itchy?
- Discharge. From where? Colour? Smell? Amount?
- Pain. Where? On passing urine? On having sex?
- Abnormal bleeding. Changes in menstrual bleeding pattern? After sex? Between periods?

Note: Women often have STIs without having symptoms but still suffer damage and are at increased risk of HIV transmission.

Sexual partners and behaviour

It is useful to know patients' sexual histories in order to assess their risk and know what information may be useful for them. This needs to be explained clearly before questioning so that they understand why they are being asked such personal information and do not feel the questions are intrusive. If possible, discover:
- When they last had sex, who with and whether that person was a new or regular sexual partner
- What type of sex – vaginal, oral and/or anal sex

- Whether any herbal or western medicines have been used to tighten or 'clean' the vagina, or increase sexual pleasure
- Whether condoms were used successfully. If not, what prevented condom use or what problems were experienced?
- Was the start of the symptoms associated with a particular sexual contact?
- Information about all recent sexual partners in the last three months, and whether those sexual partners have any symptoms
- When was the last time they examined their own genitalia for ulcers, rashes or discharges?

STIs and sexual behaviour are often very difficult to discuss and questions should be asked in private and in a respectful manner. Explain that the information will help to decide on treatment and will stay confidential. Obtaining this information requires asking open questions such as 'tell me about your symptoms' or 'tell me why you do not use condoms when you have sex'. Asking a list of questions which can be answered with 'yes' or 'no' provides more limited information. Respond to the information in a non-judgemental manner and without criticism.

Step 2: Physical examination

Examine the patient if appropriate, explaining that examining the genital area enables you to make a better assessment. It is important to provide privacy and comfort, find ways to lessen patients' embarrassment and continue to give reassurance. Examine the lower abdomen, groin, genitals and anal area looking for signs which might suggest a STI as discussed in step 1.

It is very important to perform a vaginal speculum examination on women to:
- identify cervical erosions caused by chlamydia
- perform cervical smear tests to detect changes and prevent cancer.

Note: Always consider HIV infection in a patient with other STIs and look for signs of immune suppression (see Chapter 32).

Step 3: Assessment and treatment of STIs by syndromic management

From the sexual history and the examination decide which of the following four syndromes are present:
- Genital ulceration (men and women)
- Urethral discharge (men)

- Vaginal discharge (includes female urethral discharge)
- Lower abdominal pain (women).

People may also report:

- Swollen lymph glands
- Burning when passing urine.

Note: Urethral discharge may be reported as vaginal in women.

Genital ulceration syndrome in men and women

It is usually syphilis and chancroid that cause open sores. In syphilis these sores are likely to be painless; in chancroid they are painful. Patients should be treated for both because it is often difficult to distinguish between them by clinical examination, and infection with both is common.

Genital herpes can be distinguished from chancroid and syphilis if the patient describes the presence of fluid-filled blisters before the ulcers appeared. Herpes is painful, usually settles in 10–14 days but often occurs again. Severe or frequently recurring herpes needs treatment.

Urethral discharge syndrome in men

When men describe discharge from the penis and/or pain on urination, it is usually caused by gonorrhoea or chlamydia. Gonorrhoeal discharge is often thick yellow-green, chlamydia is thin and watery, but sometimes symptoms are similar. Having both infections is common so treatment for both is recommended.

Vaginal discharge syndrome

Note that discharge may not actually be from the vagina but from the urethral opening. Urethritis in women is caused by gonorrhoea and chlamydia as in men.

Identifying the cause of vaginal discharge can be difficult. Increase or changes in the normal vaginal discharge may be caused by candidiasis or bacterial vaginosis. Although these do cause inflammation of the vagina, they are **not** sexually transmitted. Vaginal discharge may be caused by trichomoniasis (an infection of the vagina), gonorrhoea or chlamydia (infections of the cervix), all of which **are** sexually transmitted.

It is not sensible to treat all women who have vaginal discharge as if they have STIs such as gonorrhoea and chlamydia as this would lead to over-treatment. Instead do an assessment based on the sexual history to identify those women who might be at greater risk:

- Treat for gonorrhoea and/or chlamydia if:
  - her male partner has discharge from his penis or genital sores, OR

- she has had sex with more than one partner in the last three months, OR
  - she has had a new partner in the past three months.
- Treat as a vaginal infection alone (candidiasis or bacterial vaginosis) if:
  - the sexual history indicates that none of the above statements are true
  - there is severe itching and thick white vaginal discharge which is difficult to remove (candidiasis)
  - discharge has a strong fish-like smell (bacterial vaginosis).

Remember that all women have a natural, clear, whitish non-irritant vaginal discharge. Not all women know this so examination is required rather than treating on women's reports of discharge alone.

Women can transmit infections to their babies during birth, especially causing conjunctivitis (ophthalmia neonatorum) which can cause blindness if untreated. Babies develop red, swollen and 'sticky' eyelids, and may have a *purulent* discharge. It can be treated by cleaning the eyes at birth and applying 1% silver nitrate solution or 1% tetracycline ointment immediately. Gonorrhoea is the most common cause but treatment for chlamydia is also advised (see Table 31.1).

Lower abdominal pain syndrome in women

Lower abdominal pain might indicate pelvic inflammatory disease (PID) in which infections have spread from the cervix to the uterus, fallopian tubes, ovaries and lining of the pelvic cavity. PID may also be associated with heavy and irregular menstrual bleeding, painful periods, pain on passing urine, pain during sex or vaginal examination, fever, diarrhoea and vomiting. The most common causes of PID are gonorrhoea and chlamydia, which may be complicated by *anaerobic* bacterial infection.

PID can cause damage to the fallopian tubes leading to infertility and *ectopic pregnancy*. Ectopic pregnancy may be life-threatening and should be considered if lower abdominal pain and tenderness is associated with a missed period. If possible perform a pregnancy test. Refer to hospital immediately (see Chapter 35).

No symptoms

It is important to remember that many women and some men who have STIs do not have any symptoms at all. Even without symptoms the infections can cause

Table 31.1 Treatment for the syndromic management of STIs

Syndrome	Management	Suggested treatment
Genital ulceration in men and women	Treat for both syphilis and chancroid	**Syphilis – use one of:** • (First line treatment) Benzathine penicillin G: 2.4 million units IM injection as single dose (inject half into each buttock) • Aqueous procaine penicillin G: 1.2 million units IM injection daily for 10 days • (If penicillin allergic): Doxycycline: 200 mg by mouth daily for 15 days (**not** if pregnant) • Erythromycin: 500 mg by mouth 4 times a day for 15 days • Tetracycline: 500 mg orally 4 times a day for 15 days **Chancroid – use one of:** • Ceftriaxone: 250 mg IM injection single dose (ineffective if HIV positive) • Ciprofloxacin: 500 mg by mouth 2 times a day for 3 days (not if pregnant, ineffective if HIV positive) • Erythromycin: 500 mg by mouth 4 times a day for 7 days • Azithromycin: 1 g orally as a single dose • Trimethoprim: 80 mg / sulphamethoxazole 400 mg: 2 tablets 2 times a day for 7 days (NB resistance is very high in many areas so use only if known to be effective locally) **Genital herpes – use one of:** • Acyclovir: 200 mg orally 5 times day for 7 days • Famciclovir: 250 mg 3 times a day for 5 days • Valaciclovir: 500 mg 2 times a day for 5 days
Urethral discharge in men	Treat for both gonorrhoea and chlamydia	**Gonorrhoea – use one of:** (NB Penicillin is no longer effective in many areas) • Cefixime: 400 mg as a single dose by mouth • Ciprofloxacin: 500 mg as a single dose by mouth • Ceftriaxone: 125 mg IM injection as single dose • Spectinomycin: 2 g IM injection as a single dose • Trimethoprim: 80 mg / sulphamethoxazole 400 mg: 10 tablets once daily for 3 days (NB resistance is very high in many areas so use only if known to be effective locally) • Kanamycin: 2 g IM injection as single dose **Chlamydia – use one of:** • Doxycycline: 200 mg by mouth once a day for 7 days • Tetracycline: 500 mg by mouth 4 times a day for 7 days • Erythromycin: 500 mg by mouth 4 times a day for 7 days • Azithromycin: 1 g orally in a single dose • Amoxycillin: 500 mg orally 3 times a day for 7 days • Ofloxacin: 300 mg orally 2 times a day for 7 days

Table 31.1 Treatment for the syndromic management of STIs *continued*

Syndrome	Management	Suggested treatment
Vaginal discharge in women. Undertake a risk assessment to decide whether cervical or vaginal infection exists.	Cervical infection: treat for both gonorrhoea and chlamydia	Gonorrhoea and chlamydia: Same treatment as for urethral discharge in men BUT ciprofloxacin, doxycycline and tetracycline should not be prescribed to pregnant women.
	Vaginal infection: treat for candidiasis, trichomoniasis and bacterial vaginosis	Candidiasis – use one of: • Miconazole/clotrimazole: 200mg in vagina once a day for 3 days • Nystatin: 100,000 units (1 pessary) in vagina for 14 days • Fluconazole: 150 mg orally as a single dose • Gentian violet: 1% aqueous solution applied to vulva and vagina each night for 5 nights Trichomoniasis and bacterial vaginosis – use one of: • Metronidazole: 2 g by mouth as single dose • Metronidazole: 400 mg by mouth 2 times a day for 7 days • Clindamycin: 300 mg orally 2 times a day for 7 days • Metronidazole gel 0.75%: 5 g into the vagina for 7 days • Clindamycin vaginal cream 2%: 5 g at night for 7 nights
Newborn eye infection	Treat for both gonorrhoea and chlamydia	Gonorrhoea – use one of these as a single dose IM: • Ceftriaxone: 50 mg/kg IM (maximum 125 mg) • Kanamycin: 25 mg/kg IM (maximum 75 mg) • Spectinomycin: 25 mg/kg (maximum 75 mg) Chlamydia – use one of: • Erythromycin syrup: 50 mg/kg by mouth divided into 4 doses a day for 14 days • Trimethoprim: 40 mg and sulfamethoxazole: 200 mg by mouth 2 times a day for 14 days

Drugs should be given orally as single doses where possible. If the same drug is needed to treat two infections (e.g. erythromycin for syphilis and chancroid) do **not** give two doses, give whichever is the longer and higher dose.

serious problems such as PID, infertility, ectopic pregnancy, and they increase the risk of transmitting and acquiring HIV. It is therefore important to treat the sexual partner of someone who has an infection **even** when the sexual partner has no symptoms. Contacting sexual partners may be a difficult and sensitive issue and should **only** be undertaken with the permission and help of the patient.

Principles of treatment

The specific recommended drugs for each syndrome are listed in Table 31.1. Choices are made depending on what is locally available and effective. It is important to stress:

- The prescribed course of tablets must be completed; take all tablets until they are finished even if the symptoms improve before the end of the course.
- All recent sexual partners should be contacted and treated if possible even if they have no symptoms.
- Not to have sex until the treatment is finished, the symptoms have gone and sexual partners have also been treated.

Genital and anal warts

Warts are commonly seen around the genitalia and anus caused by the human papilloma virus (HPV). Although they are painless they can cause obstruction to urinary flow and during birth. They are also highly infectious and cervical warts are linked with cancer of the cervix. Warts can be treated by surgery, cautery (burning), cryotherapy (freezing) if available or by applying podophyllin. Traditional methods are used in some areas.

Step 4: Health promotion to prevent further infection

- Give patients information on how infections are passed on and how they can be prevented.
- Discuss with them the options they have to prevent passing on the infection to their sexual partners.
- Use a wooden penis model to demonstrate how to use condoms (see Chapter 29).
- Encourage them to demonstrate on the model themselves.

- Advise where to get condoms locally. If possible give them some.
- Listen to their questions and concerns.

They should ask all sexual partners to come for treatment, even if they have no symptoms, otherwise infection can pass between them again. It may be easier for the patients to give contact slips to their sexual partners. These contain information about the clinic and why they should attend. They also include information about the disease (in code) for the clinics the contacts attend. Contacting sexual partners may be a sensitive and difficult issue. Although it is very important to contact sexual partners for treatment, this should not be done without the permission and assistance of patients. No information about patients or their partners should be given to anyone who is not directly involved in their care.

Step 5: Follow-up assessment

Ask patients to return after seven days for a follow-up appointment. At this visit ask:
- Do they still have symptoms?
- Have they had sex whilst on treatment?
- Have sexual partners been treated?
- Has treatment been completed?
- Have any other treatments, such as herbal or spiritual ones, been used?

Note: Medical treatment such as antibiotics may be stopped by traditional healers.

Refer them for further investigations and treatment if:
- symptoms are still present **but**
- treatment **was** taken correctly **and**
- they have not had sexual contact.

Further treatment may be needed if:
- symptoms are still present **and**
- the treatment **was not** taken correctly or
- they **have** had sexual contact and so possibly have become infected again.

It is important at this point not to be critical but to allow patients time to explain why treatments were not taken correctly and/or why they were unable to avoid sexual contact. Then help them find a way to deal with the difficulty.

Remember the 5 Cs

Complete treatment as prescribed

Counsel patients about sexual practices and reducing risk

Condoms must be used, if having sex, until STIs are healed and treatment finished, and afterwards for prevention – show how to use condoms

Contacts should be treated as well

Consider possibility of HIV at all times

Conclusion

This chapter has included how to care for people with STIs, how to make health care services more accessible and welcoming, and how to deal with patients' needs and anxieties in relation to STIs.

People avoid STI clinics. They fear being judged and fear the negative attitudes and behaviour of many health care workers. A good supply of effective drugs makes little difference if people are too frightened to approach health care workers for help and are unable to have trusting and honest discussions.

It must be acknowledged that even the most effective health care services will make only a limited difference to the spread of STIs and HIV. The reasons for their rapid spread are complex. It is fuelled by poverty, desperation, unequal relationships between men and women and low educational opportunities. Reliance on traditional customs is common; these may be dangerous or at least delay seeking effective treatment. To make a real difference, improving services needs to go hand in hand with addressing the desperate economic conditions that people often face, and challenging individual sexual behaviour that increases the risk of infection. This requires community solidarity and determination and involvement at national and international levels.

■ Activities

1. Sexual history taking

It is important to discover ways you can ask about sexual history, sexual behaviour and symptoms so that you feel comfortable and relaxed. This makes patients feel more relaxed and able to talk openly and will mean they are more likely to return for help and assistance in the future.

Read Step 1. Write down a list of open questions that you could use to find out the details of patients' symptoms and sexual behaviour. Practise using your questions on a colleague and discuss how they can be improved.

2.

CASE STUDY

A young man comes to see you and tells you that he has a 'big spot' on his penis. You talk with him and examine him and discover that there is an open sore in the middle of his penis that has appeared in the last few days but is not painful. The man had sex with two new girlfriends recently and did not use condoms.

- How would you treat the infection and why? What advice would you give about the treatment?
- What would you discuss with this man about his sexual behaviour?
- In what way do you think that your manner might make a difference?

32

Care of patients with
HIV and AIDS related conditions

This chapter provides information and guidance to enable you to provide safe nursing care for people infected with HIV. It will help you to contribute to fighting the spread of HIV within the community. The chapter includes:
- The difference between HIV and AIDS
- Testing for HIV infection
- The role of nurses and midwives in challenging stigma and discrimination
- How HIV is transmitted and how nurses and midwives can help to reduce transmission including preventing Mother to Child Transmission (MTCT)
- The nursing role in the treatment and care of patients with HIV and AIDS related symptoms
- Anti-retroviral therapy (ART) and the nursing role

Introduction

The global impact is enormous and massive efforts are needed to slow the spread of the disease, reduce ill health and death, and develop new effective and accessible treatments and prevention strategies.

The connection between HIV, sexually transmitted infections (STIs) and tuberculosis, is very significant. Because of this, this chapter needs to be read with Chapters 25 and 31.

The scale of the epidemic

The WHO estimated that over 40 million people were living with HIV in 2005 (see Figure 32.1).

The problems are much worse where resources are limited and where access to effective treatment is poor. Rates are also much higher where STIs are common (see Chapter 31). In some areas there is more infection among women and infections occur at a younger age.

When this book was passed for press, more than half of those infected were from sub-Saharan Africa, although only one tenth of the world's population live there. Of those, nearly half were young people between 15 and 24 years and very many were children. Millions of children have been orphaned.

The overall infection rates for sub-Sarahan Africa continue to rise. In a few countries, rates are as high as one third of adults being infected. However, rates are reducing in some countries.

Recent world trends show increasing infection everywhere. This includes the northern hemisphere and South and South-east Asia. The only exception is the Caribbean where infection rates are falling. Not all countries worldwide collect reliable data.

HIV and AIDS cause immense suffering for individuals and families and devastate communities and national economies. HIV infection affects young healthy men and women who have vital roles to play. They care for and educate children, provide for the elderly, produce and manufacture food and manage businesses, the economy and governments. As increasing numbers of people become sick and die, or are required to care for sick family members, the stability of communities is seriously threatened. In some places, young people have to care for older relatives or take responsibility alone for younger children. Health services themselves are severely affected by losing staff.

Nurses and midwives have significant contributions to make in:
- caring for people with HIV infection and those who are sick with HIV related conditions
- educating friends and family, work colleagues and communities about spread, treatment and care

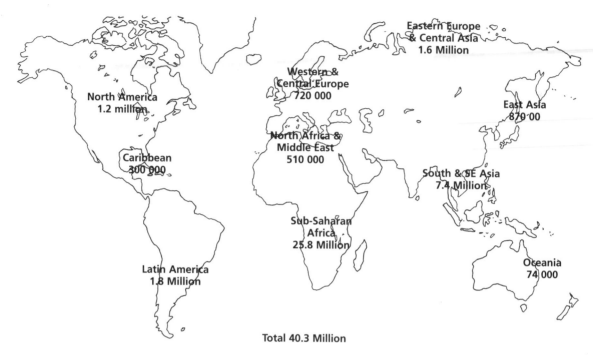

Figure 32.1 *Population estimated to be living with HIV in 2005*

• challenging negative attitudes and behaviours towards people living with HIV.

The difference between HIV and AIDS

HIV

HIV stands for Human Immunodeficiency **V**irus. As the name indicates, it only affects **H**umans, it causes a deficiency in the **I**mmune system and is a **V**irus. HIV survives only if it can make copies of itself, by multiplying in very specific cells of the human body – namely the T4 cells (also known as CD4 cells or T4 lymphocytes). The role of T4 cells is vital in controlling and supporting the immune system to fight infections. The virus uses T4 cells to make copies of itself and then destroys the cells, resulting in a weakened immune system.

HIV and the immune system

The immune system protects the body from many different viruses, bacteria, fungi and cancers that could cause serious illness. When the immune system is strong and there are enough T4 cells present, these organisms remain in small quantities in the body and are harmless, never causing illness. For this reason someone infected with HIV is unlikely to know for many years.

Progressing from HIV to AIDS

Over time, the virus multiplies in the T4 cells and destroys them. The immune system becomes weakened and unable to provide effective protection. This can happen more quickly when people's general health and nutrition are poor or they have other physical or emotional illnesses. People with HIV then become vulnerable to a variety of conditions. At first these can be quite minor (see Figure 32.2) but as the immune system becomes increasingly weak, people can then develop serious infections and cancers. These may result in death if not treated quickly and effectively.

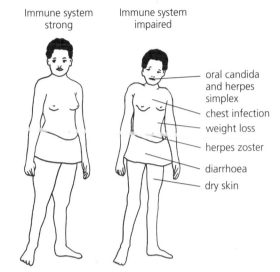

Immune system strong   Immune system impaired

oral candida and herpes simplex

chest infection

weight loss

herpes zoster

diarrhoea

dry skin

Figure 32.2 *The effect of an impaired immune system*

AIDS

This progression to life-threatening conditions is known as AIDS – **A**cquired **I**mmune **D**eficiency **S**yndrome. A *syndrome* is a collection of conditions that can affect different parts of the body (see Figure 32.3 for adults

WHO case definition for AIDS	
Major signs	Weight loss more than 10% of body weight over a short period of time
	Diarrhoea for more than one month
	Fever for more than one month
Minor signs	Cough for more than one month (for people with TB this cough would not be considered a minor sign for AIDS)
	Generalised itching skin rash
	Recurrent herpes zoster (shingles) in last two years
	Candida of mouth and/or throat
	Chronic and aggressive herpes simplex infection
	Generalised enlarged lymph nodes
The presence of either generalised Kaposi's sarcoma or cryptococcal meningitis is sufficient for a case definition of AIDS	

and Figure 32.4 for children). The infections are referred to as 'opportunistic'. This means that relatively harmless organisms in the body can cause illness when the immune system is very weak. Specific infections are more common in some communities than others depending on the *prevalence* of those infections in the region.

AIDS is diagnosed in the western world by identifying the specific opportunistic infection or cancers that are causing symptoms, but diagnosis can require sophisticated testing facilities, which are unavailable in many areas. In the absence of testing for opportunistic infections and cancers or for HIV, an AIDS diagnosis can be based on clinical signs and symptoms. The information box shows the WHO case definition for AIDS. The patient must have at least two of the 'major' signs and at least one of the 'minor' signs to be classified as having AIDS.

Testing for HIV infection

People infected with HIV may feel well at first and are often unaware that they are infected. They may, however, suffer some flu-like symptoms – known as sero-conversion illness:

- Tiredness and feeling unwell
- Fever, headache, sore throat
- Skin rash
- Gastro-intestinal problems
- Painful joints and muscles.

There is a test that can detect if HIV *antibodies* are present. The body of someone infected with HIV will react by making antibodies to try to destroy the virus. The HIV test looks for these antibodies in the blood. If the test is 'positive' this indicates that HIV is present in the blood and also other parts of the body and bodily fluids. Antibodies can take up to 12 weeks after infection to show up on the blood test but may show by 4–6 weeks. This is called the 'window period'.

In many areas the 'rapid test' for HIV is now available and results can be given to people within one visit. This test is very simple and can be undertaken by health care workers after short training.

HIV testing is best undertaken where voluntary counselling and testing facilities (VCT), with trained health care workers, are available.

Testing babies for HIV

Testing babies born to mothers who are HIV positive is more complicated. Pregnant woman automatically

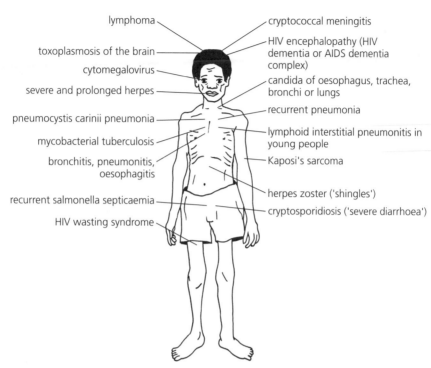

Figure 32.3 *HIV related conditions indicating severe weakness of the immune system in adults*

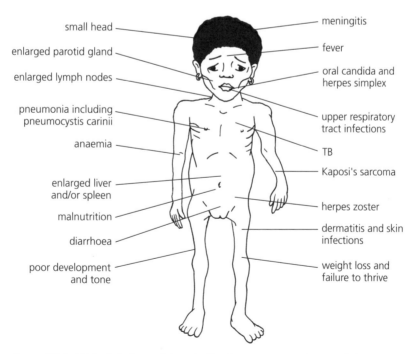

Figure 32.4 *HIV related conditions indicating severe weakness of the immune system in growing children*

pass HIV antibodies to their children, so all babies are born with their mothers' HIV antibodies. These antibodies, passed from mothers to babies naturally, can remain for up to 18 months. HIV antibody tests on young babies are therefore not reliable. If antibodies are present in a baby, it does not necessarily mean that the virus is present. However, if at 18 months children still have antibodies to HIV, this will be because they are actually infected with the virus and are producing their own antibody response.

Testing adults for HIV

In spite of fears about testing there are many advantages for people in knowing they are infected with HIV:

- People who know they are infected may consider changing their behaviour to ensure that the virus is not passed on to others.
- Health care workers can more easily identify the signs and symptoms of HIV and AIDS related conditions and start appropriate treatment to prolong life.
- People who know they are infected may be able to change to healthier lifestyles to keep the immune system as strong as possible. Good nutrition is particularly important.
- Drug treatment for HIV and AIDS, if available, can be used to prevent serious HIV and AIDS related illness.
- Pregnant women who know they are infected with HIV may be able to reduce the chances of their babies becoming infected.

The nursing role in challenging stigma and discrimination

In spite of the advantages of being aware of HIV infection, diagnosis can be extremely distressing. Families, friends and whole communities can react badly towards people who are infected with HIV. Many people refuse to have tests or keep the information secret because they fear these negative responses.

Nurses and midwives are in an excellent position to address discrimination against people with HIV and AIDS. They can educate colleagues, friends and families and challenge negative attitudes. Most importantly, they can lead by example and treat people with HIV infection with care, kindness, compassion and respect.

■ Activity

To explore this issue, undertake the following activity:

Discuss in a small group or write down your thoughts on the following questions:

- If you were diagnosed with HIV, how would you want your family and community to treat you?
- How would you feel if you were not able to talk to your closest friend about being HIV positive?
- Describe how you would want doctors and nurses to behave towards you if they were the only people you could talk to about being HIV positive. What skills do you think they should have?

Now discuss or write down your thoughts on the following questions about your role:

- Why do people in the community react negatively towards people who are infected with HIV? What could you do to change this reaction?
- Who are the local leaders in your community who might be able to change these attitudes?
- How do your colleagues behave towards people with HIV and AIDS? What changes, if any, do you think are required?

Consent and confidentiality

HIV testing should only be undertaken with the agreement of the person being tested. This consent should be obtained only after the person has had the opportunity to consider the advantages and disadvantages of finding out they are infected. The help and support of trained health care workers is important. For many people there are more disadvantages, especially where no treatment is available. No-one should be pressurised into being tested.

People who decide to undertake testing must be assured that all information discussed, and test results, will remain confidential between them and the health care worker. This information should only be shared with those involved in that person's care and with that person's permission.

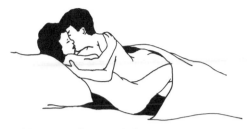

Figure 32.5 *Sexual transmission*

How is HIV transmitted?

HIV can be transmitted or passed on from one person to another sexually, blood to blood, or mother to baby.

Sexual transmission

HIV is present in the vaginal fluids of women and the semen of men. If these body fluids pass from one person to another during vaginal or anal sex, HIV may also be passed. Transmission is much more likely when people have STIs. Vaginal and urethral discharges, open sores in the genital and anal areas (such as chancroid and syphilis), or damage to the vagina from drying out with cloths or herbs (or from using spermicides) all can increase transmission rates (see Chapter 31).

Blood to blood transmission

HIV is present in blood and can be passed from one person's blood to another person's blood by:

- Using the same needle to inject or vaccinate several people without sterilising it between each injection. This includes the sharing of needles by injecting drug users.
- Any form of cutting, for example ritual circumcision or tattooing, which uses instruments on different people without sterilisation between them.

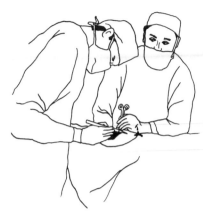

Figure 32.7 *Blood to blood transmission – accidental injury from a scalpel or a needle during a clinical procedure*

- The transfusion of blood or blood products in places where donated blood is not tested and screened for HIV.
- Accidental HIV exposure in the health care setting. This rarely happens because large quantities of HIV must be passed, or it must enter via a deep cut or large blood vessel. Studies indicate that 3 in every 1000 exposures result in transmission. The following can allow transmission:
  - a sharp instrument or needle that has just been used on an HIV positive person injures a health care worker
  - infected blood or birth fluid is spilled into an open wound of a health care worker
  - blood of an HIV infected health care worker passes into a patient's open wound or blood circulation.

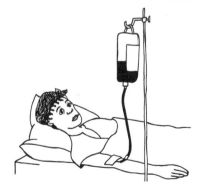

Figure 32.6 *Blood to blood transmission – blood transfusion*

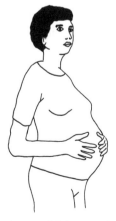

Figure 32.8 *Mother to child transmission*

Mother to child transmission (MTCT)

HIV positive women can pass HIV on to their babies during pregnancy, at delivery and through breastfeeding. There is a 20–40 per cent chance that this will happen. The risk is greater when women are unwell with HIV and AIDS as they then have high quantities of virus within their bodies (known as a high viral load) and will be more infectious. MTCT is often known as 'vertical transmission'.

Important note on HIV transmission

HIV is **not** transmitted through day-to-day contact with people with HIV or AIDS (see Fig. 32.9) and it is **not** transmitted by caring for patients. There is no reason to fear becoming infected with HIV

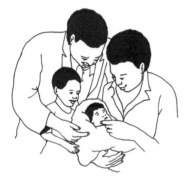

Figure 32.9 *HIV is not transmitted through day to day contact*

The role of nurses and midwives in reducing HIV transmission

Nurses and midwives have important responsibilities in reducing transmission through the three ways described above:

Sexual transmission

- Talk about sex. Many people find it difficult to talk about sexual practices or behaviour but this will become easier if health workers start the discussion and feel relaxed and confident. This helps people to discuss their concerns more openly and they will be more likely to come for care and treatment. Additional training offered in VCT centres might be needed to develop confidence and sensitivity in discussing sexual behaviour.
- Give clear accurate information about how HIV and other STIs are passed from one person to another and how people can change their behaviour.
- Explain sexual practices that increase the risk of passing HIV from one person to another, such as dry sex, having many sexual partners and having penetrative sex without condoms.
- Challenge the myths and traditional practices that may increase the risk of HIV transmission, such as:
  - having sex with virgins to 'cleanse' someone with HIV
  - penetrating the woman's anus with the belief that the lack of vaginal fluids means there is no virus (people may be reluctant to discuss this as it is often illegal)
  - condoms have HIV put in them to reduce the population.

Note: Some people are teaching that condoms are porous to HIV. This is not true and must be challenged.

- Demonstrate how to use condoms properly and advise people how to obtain cheap or free condoms locally (see Chapter 32).
- Provide information about:
  - signs and symptoms that may indicate STIs and encouraging people to go for treatment as soon as possible
  - where treatment for STIs is available in the local community.
- Talk about the advantages of having HIV tests and about where they can be done.
- Provide information to assist people in deciding what action might be best rather than telling them what to do.

Blood to blood contact

- Use infection control precautions in the health care setting for **all** patients and staff members. This avoids the need to know whether particular individuals are infected with HIV (see Chapter 6).
  - Train other health care workers in infection control precautions.
  - Inform carers such as family members and friends about precautions.

- Use disposable needles and equipment and use them on only one patient. Where these are not available, sterilise re-usable equipment by boiling or steaming between using on each individual.
- Never place used disposable needles back into their plastic sheaths after use as this increases the risk of needle injury and infection.
- Dispose of sharp instruments/needles in specially designed boxes or other strong containers such as drink cans or bottles.
- Wear gloves when having contact with all patients' blood and body fluids.
- Wear facial protection when exposure to large volumes of blood/body fluids is likely, for example during surgery or childbirth. Consider applying for additional funding if protection is not easily available.
- Cover all open wounds with plasters or dressings.
- Where accidental exposure to blood or body fluids does occur, rinse and bleed the wound thoroughly under running water for 5 minutes.
- Obtain information about the local availability of anti-retroviral therapy (ART) for health care workers who know they have been accidentally exposed to HIV.
- Reduce the chance of HIV positive health care workers passing HIV to patients by avoiding procedures which involve sharp instruments and open wounds.
- Educate community leaders to ensure that traditional procedures which involve blood-letting or cutting are undertaken in the safest possible way if they wish to continue them.
- Find out if blood donations are tested for HIV. In areas where blood donations are not tested, transfusions should be avoided except in life-threatening situations that require blood.

Mother to child transmission

- Give contraceptive advice to prevent unplanned pregnancies.
- Give information and advice on HIV transmission to reduce the risk for women who are pregnant.
- Discuss with all women the advantages of being tested for HIV before becoming pregnant. Choices about the pregnancy could then be informed by knowledge of HIV infection. Giving ART to HIV infected women before they become pregnant can

reduce the likelihood of passing HIV to the baby (see ART section below).
- Discuss what women can do to reduce the transmission of HIV to their babies including:
  - Use condoms to prevent re-infection in pregnancy and during breastfeeding
  - Seek help rapidly if they suspect STIs
  - Follow ART instructions carefully if it is provided for pregnancy or to take in early labour and for 6 weeks (baby and possibly mother)
  - Caesarean section rather than vaginal delivery for women with very high viral loads
  - Exclusive breastfeeding for 6 months then abrupt weaning on to locally available nutritious foods (see below)
  - Formula feeding during first 3 months (only if safe) and then solid foods as soon as possible (see below and Chapter 43).

For many women ART will not be available, caesarean section may be unsafe or too expensive, and formula feeding may be expensive, unacceptable and be dangerous for the baby if water supplies and sterilising procedures are inadequate.

- Encourage women to attend for antenatal care early in pregnancy.
- Avoid unnecessary procedures during labour, especially artificial rupture of membranes and episiotomy. (Prolonged membrane rupture also increases transmission.)
- Protect the baby from injury during birth including from suction equipment.
- Ensure rapid treatment of breast infections.
- Advocate for integrated care programmes: mother and child programmes that include antenatal care, HIV testing for mothers, and regular monitoring of the health and development of babies born to infected mothers.

HIV positive women require a lot of support and advice during this time; maybe because little can be done to reduce HIV transmission to their babies, or because they are faced with difficult choices, such as whether to breastfeed or not.

■ Activity

Try to identify with colleagues any areas described above that need to be improved in your work area. Discuss with them how you could make a difference to this situation.

The nursing role in the treatment and care of patients with HIV and AIDS related symptoms

Extreme poverty and food shortage, widespread malaria, TB, STIs and other infections are common in areas of high HIV prevalence. Patients frequently suffer weight loss, fever, diarrhoea and skin problems. It is easy to misjudge such symptoms and fail to recognise HIV and AIDS related conditions. When they are persistent and unexplained and not responding to usual treatment, you should always consider the possibility of HIV. In such circumstances a history of the risk factors for HIV infection could be taken (see Chapter 31) and a HIV test suggested. This is best taken in a VCT centre or clinic where counselling resources are available.

Patients with HIV and AIDS related conditions often experience more severe symptoms, and require prompt and prolonged treatment to prevent further deterioration. Many conditions are life-threatening without treatment. If it is not possible to make an accurate diagnosis of specific infections, recognition of the signs and symptoms that are likely to be related to HIV and AIDS is important. The section below presents these more serious signs and symptoms and includes appropriate care and treatment.

Suggested drug treatments for specific infections are suggested below. Trained staff should prescribe these drugs using local guidelines and protocols. For correct dosages and methods of administration refer to nationally adapted WHO Essential Drugs Lists.

Diarrhoea

People with HIV and AIDS commonly have diarrhoea, especially children. There are many possible causes – bacterial, viral and fungal infections including:

- Shigella
- Salmonella
- Campylobacter
- Cryptosporidium
- Isospora
- Giardia
- Microsporidia
- Cytomegalovirus.

Severe diarrhoea is commonly caused by crypto-sporidium and patients have profuse, watery, prolonged and debilitating diarrhoea.

Table 32.1 Recommended adult drugs for gastro-intestinal problems

Problem	Recommended drugs
Bacterial infections	Co-trimoxazole, ampicillin, chloramphenicol, erythromycin, ciprofloxacin
Campylobacter	Erythromycin
Giardia	Metronidazole
Cytomegalovirus	Ganciclovir

Treatment and care (see Chapters 15 and 45)

Diarrhoea may indicate an extremely serious condition in people with HIV. Rapid recognition and treatment is essential, particularly in children where dehydration due to diarrhoea can be fatal. The main priorities are to:

- Treat the cause of the diarrhoea, if known or suspected, with available and appropriate drugs (see Table 32.1).
- Prevent and treat dehydration with intravenous fluids or oral fluids such as oral rehydration salts (ORS) or home-made equivalents.
- Monitor food and fluid intake and weight loss, particularly in small children as diarrhoea can be critical and cause very rapid deterioration.
- Give dietary advice regarding high calorie, high energy, high protein foods if possible and about food supplements such as Complan, Ensure or protein, vitamin and mineral mixtures (PVM).
- Give anti-diarrhoeal treatments such as loperamide, codeine phosphate, diphenoxylate kaolin and pectin to adults, but avoid in children under five years old. Monitor the effects and alter treatment as necessary.

Remember that diarrhoea can be extremely severe, distressing and particularly difficult and undignified for adults. Patients may need help to find practical and convenient ways in which they can cope, for example being near a toilet, access to washing facilities, using pads and barrier creams. Nursing and family support is essential.

Weight loss

Weight loss is common in patients with HIV and AIDS and 'failure to thrive' is a significant sign of deterioration in children who need to have growth monitored every three months (more often if ill). Weight loss is usually the result of:

- infections such as TB, Pneumocystis carinii pneumonia (PCP) and lymphoma
- other conditions causing severe diarrhoea, such as cryptosporidium
- the direct effect of the virus on the gastro-intestinal tract
- poor nutritional intake.

Treatment and care (see also Chapter 43)

Severe weight loss associated with HIV and AIDS conditions indicates a weakened immune system. Among children in particular, weight loss affects their immune system still further, making them vulnerable to opportunistic infections. Weight gain is often difficult to achieve, particularly in children, and preventing further weight loss is a high priority:

- Treat the cause of the weight loss, if known, with available drugs.
- Encourage frequent small meals and snacks. Dietary advice should suggest high energy foods such as maize, potato and rice, and high protein foods such as eggs, milk, beans, fish and meat.
- Assess food intake and consider food supplements such as Ensure, Complan and PVM where intake is insufficient. Vitamin deficiency is common in children and should be treated with regular vitamin supplements.
- Monitor weight and height in children, also head circumference, growth and developmental progress.

Weight loss has always been associated with HIV and AIDS which was commonly called 'Slim disease'. Consider the effect that such rapid weight loss is having on patients and their families, and what support and practical assistance may be required.

Sore mouth

Soreness of the mouth can be caused by a number of conditions including:

- Oral candida (thrush). This shows as a white coating or patches around the mouth and tongue. It can spread to the throat and oesophagus and cause chest pain and severe difficulty swallowing. It is particularly common in children.
- Herpes simplex. Blistering sores on the outside of the lips also seen frequently in children.
- Kaposi's sarcoma. A cancer of the blood vessel walls, often first seen as purple patches on the roof of the mouth.

- Other less serious conditions of the mouth including gingivitis, glossitis and dental problems.

Treatment and care

A sore mouth can have serious consequences due to the effect on eating and further loss of weight. The presence of candida, particularly oesophageal candida, indicates the patient already has a weakened immune system and may be feeling extremely unwell. Nurses should:

- Examine patients' mouths regularly and treat conditions promptly with the most appropriate drugs available (see Table 32.2).
- Advise about treatments such as saltwater rinses, mouthwashes and lozenges to relieve pain and discomfort. For external infected lesions treat with antibiotics, gentian violet or potassium permanganate.
- Prevent weight loss with nutritious and high energy and protein foods (see above). Meals should be soft and frequent, not spicy, and include plenty of fluids.
- Monitor dietary intake and weight loss to detect serious complications.
- Advise patients with herpes that it can be passed to others by contact, especially to others who may have weakened immune systems.

Table 32.2 Recommended adult drugs for mouth problems

Problem	Recommended drugs
Oral or oesophageal candida	Gentian violet, chlorhexidine mouthwash, nystatin, miconazole, clotrimazole, ketaconazole, itraconazole, fluconazole, amphotericin B (depending on severity)
Herpes	Acyclovir
Kaposi's sarcoma	Main option is chemotherapy
Glossitis and gingivitis	Common antibiotics

Nausea and vomiting

There are many causes of nausea and vomiting but the following are of particular concern:

- Lymphoma. Cancer of the lymph tissue which may occur anywhere in the body. In the gastro-intestinal tract it will present with gastric symptoms such as nausea and vomiting.

- Space occupying lesions such as cerebral lymphoma or toxoplasmosis can cause nausea and vomiting due to increased pressure in the brain.
- Side effects of drugs, particularly co-trimoxazole
- Infections of the gastro-intestinal system as discussed under Diarrhoea.

Treatment and care

The presence of nausea and vomiting in patients with HIV and AIDS can indicate the presence of very serious HIV and AIDS related infections. Rapid recognition of the problem and appropriate treatment is important. Nausea and vomiting can result in poor nutritional intake, weight loss, dehydration and the inability to take oral medication. Priority must be given to the following:

- The cause of the nausea and vomiting, if known or suspected, should be treated with the most appropriate and available drugs.
- Prevent dehydration by using oral hydration fluids. Nasogastric administration or intravenous fluids may be necessary.
- Use anti-sickness tablets such as metoclopromide and prochlorperizine, especially before food.
- Prevent weight loss with very small, frequent meals of high energy and protein foods (see above) eaten when patients are able to eat.
- Monitor overall effect of the nausea and vomiting. If vital medication cannot be tolerated consider other routes of administration.

Respiratory conditions

Respiratory symptoms are common. Patients are likely to present with a number of symptoms including coughing, difficult or rapid breathing, fever and night sweats. All these indicate respiratory infection and may be caused by:

- Bacterial infections. Pneumococcal and streptococcal haemophilus influenza. Patients have a cough producing sputum which may become serious and develop into pneumonia. Bacterial infections are common in children.
- TB. People with HIV are very susceptible to TB even when their immune systems are relatively strong. Fifty per cent of people with TB have acquired it because they have HIV (see Chapter 25).
- Pneumocyctis carinii pneumonia (PCP). This infection is not as common among adults in Africa as in the West but it does exist. Patients have a characteristic dry non-productive cough. PCP is,

however, one of the more common HIV and AIDS infections among children, and presents with sudden fever, fast breathing, and cyanosis. PCP in children has a very poor prognosis.

- Lymphoid interstitial pneumonitis (LIP). An unusual disease found mostly in children. Children have an ongoing cough and mild wheezing. Symptoms are not usually serious and prognosis is good.

Treatment and care (see Chapters 10, 25 and 47)

It is very important that respiratory problems are recognised and treated as quickly as possible. TB may present with an unusually acute episode when people have HIV. PCP, often not recognised, can progress extremely rapidly and is life-threatening without treatment:

- The cause of the respiratory problem, if known or suspected, should be treated with the most appropriate drugs available (see Table 32.3).
- Treat the symptoms of the respiratory distress:
  - oxygen therapy for severe breathlessness (if available)
  - strong pain relief for chest pain
  - low dose morphine to relieve distress.
- Monitor for respiratory deterioration and consider prompt and urgent treatment for PCP and TB where the patient is not responding to usual antibiotic treatments.
- Hospital admission is often needed for patients with severe respiratory symptoms as they may require intravenous treatment and close observation for further respiratory deterioration.
- Encourage patients to report respiratory symptoms urgently so that treatment can be commenced.

Table 32.3 Recommended adult drugs for respiratory problems

Problem	Recommended drugs
Bacterial infections	Penicillin, ampicillin, co-trimoxazole
TB	Ethambutol, isoniazid, rifampicin, pyrazinamid, streptomycin (DOTS) (see Chapter 25)
PCP	Co-trimoxazole, clindamycin, primaquine
LIP	Prednisolone

Patients with respiratory symptoms require a lot of support; difficulty in breathing can be very frightening for them and for families. If patients are not able or willing to come to hospital, home care may assist with practical and emotional support.

Neurological conditions

There are many symptoms of neurological conditions associated with HIV and AIDS that can be roughly summarised as four categories (see also Chapter 14):

- Fever headache, fits, decreased mobility, poor coordination, confusion, raised blood pressure, slow pulse, vomiting and loss of consciousness. These signs and symptoms of increased intracranial pressure indicate a space occupying lesion in the brain caused by toxoplasmosis or lymphoma.
- High fevers, headaches, *photophobia*, neck stiffness, confusion and loss of consciousness are most likely to indicate cryptococcal meningitis, but may also indicate TB meningitis.
- Lethargy, loss of memory and social withdrawal might indicate a direct effect of HIV on the brain due to AIDS encephalopathy /AIDS dementia. In children this shows as developmental delay, behavioural abnormalities and fits (see Chapter 49).
- Peripheral tingling, 'pins and needles', pain and loss of feeling in the hands and feet may be caused by the effects of:
  - anti-retroviral drugs
  - the virus on the central nervous system
  - dietary deficiencies.

Treatment and care (see Chapters 14, 46 and 49)

Symptoms that appear to be mild such as headache and fever may indicate the start of serious HIV related neurological conditions. To prevent any further deterioration in the condition the following care and treatment should be a priority:

- Treat the cause of the symptoms, where known or suspected, as quickly as possible with the most appropriate and available drugs (see Table 32.4).
- Administer pain relief medication, and treatment such as aspirin or paracetamol to reduce fevers as necessary.
- Observe for deterioration in neurological status as HIV and AIDS neurological conditions can result in permanent brain damage.
- Advise patients and families to report changes in

patients' behaviour or coordination and any other neurological symptoms.

Neurological problems can be very distressing for patients and their families. Patients may require assistance with all aspects of daily life and home care programmes can offer valuable support. Treatment may reduce the symptoms, but in many cases ongoing medical problems may continue.

Table 32.4 Recommended adult drugs for neurological problems

Problem	Recommended drugs
Toxoplasmosis	Co-trimoxazole Pyremethamine and sulfadiazine Pyremethamine and dapsone Pyremethamine and clindamycin Pyremethamine and sulfadoxine Calcium folinate must be used with pyremethamine drugs to prevent serious toxic side effects
Lymphoma	Extremely difficult to treat, poor prognosis even with treatment
Cryptococcal meningitis	Amphotericin, fluconazole, flucytosine
TB meningitis	Ethambutol, isoniazid, rifampicin, pyrazinamide, streptomycin (DOTS)
Encephalopathy/ Dementia	There is no specific treatment but reducing viral activity with the use of ART (see below) that crosses the blood brain barrier is of value.
Peripheral neuropathy	Vitamin B supplements. Pain relief with analgesia and amytriptiline. Refer to doctor for review.

Skin problems

Skin problems are common throughout the course of HIV infection. Dry itchy skin, seborrhoeic dermatitis, psoriasis, folliculitis and rashes can occur early when people are relatively well. In children severe nappy rash is common. The more serious skin conditions associated with HIV and AIDS are:

- Herpes zoster (shingles) presents as pain with burning and tingling sensation. It follows nerve pathways but may involve wide areas around nerves. Blisters appear which are more common, prolonged and severe than in those who are not HIV infected.

- Kaposi's sarcoma is a relatively common condition in Africa but is far more aggressive with HIV and AIDS. It is a tumour of the capillary walls appearing as purple/brown nodules on skin and mucous membranes. KS is not usually painful and when limited to the skin is not particularly serious. It may occur in patients with relatively healthy immune systems.
- Severe rash all over the body caused by an allergic reaction to medication used to treat other infections, for example co-trimoxazole, amoxicillin, penicillin, INH, dapsone, fansidar and some anti-retroviral treatments.
- Severe rash all over the body may indicate secondary syphilis.

Treatment and care (see Chapters 17 and 26)

This varies enormously depending on the particular skin condition and its severity. Skin problems associated with HIV are often more severe and treatment needs to reflect this:

- Examine and identify cause of symptoms and treat with the most appropriate drugs available (see Table 32.5).
- If an allergic reaction is identified stop the drug immediately. It may be life-threatening in the case of co-trimoxazole reaction (Stevens-Johnson's syndrome).
- To reduce pain, discomfort and itching give anti-histamines and cooling ointments such as calamine lotion, emollient cream (for example E45) and analgesia.
- Advise people with herpes that the infection

Table 32.5 Recommended adult drugs for skin problems

Problem	Recommended drugs
Bacterial infections	Flucloxacillin, clindamycin
Folliculitis	Antiseptic lotions
Herpes zoster	Acyclovir
Kaposi's sarcoma	If severe – local injections with vinblastin or interferon. If affecting internal organs, only available treatment is radiotherapy or chemotherapy with vincristine

could be easily passed to others by direct contact, particularly to those that are immune suppressed.

- Treat lesions with topical treatment such as gentian violet, betadine, potassium permanganate and hydrogen peroxide, especially if they become infected.

Eye problems

These may be some of the first problems to be noticed (see Chapter 21).

Preventative therapy

All the symptoms that have been discussed indicate a severely weakened immune system and patients will be vulnerable to other opportunistic infections, many of which occur at the same time. *Prophylactic* treatment should be commenced at this point, if possible, to prevent such infections (see information box below). ART should also be considered if available.

Childhood immunisations

Many children, particularly those who have HIV and AIDS, die of diseases which can be prevented by immunisation in areas such as Africa. Full immunisation should be encouraged according to national programmes. Immunisation programmes now includes HiB (haemophilus influenza type B). Children born to HIV infected mothers can be given BCG at birth (also see Chapter 24).

Anti-retroviral therapy (ART)

There have been many important developments in producing drugs that directly attack HIV in the body and prevent them from multiplying rapidly. Anti-retroviral (ARV) drugs are now widely distributed in most of the western world and are making a great difference to people's lives. Efforts are being made to make these drugs available everywhere but progress has been slow especially in poorer countries. These drugs are often referred to as anti-retroviral therapy (ART) or combination therapy.

The aim of ART is to stop:

- virus multiplying in the T4 cells of the immune system
- T4 cells from being destroyed and so improve the immune system.

Patients on ART will still be infected with HIV and can still pass the virus on. However, if the drugs work well, there will only be a small amount of virus in the body.

Conditions for which preventative treatment is available

Condition	Treatment	Guidance
Candidiasis oral and oesophageal	Nystatin Amphotericin B lozenges Ketaconazole Fluconazole Itraconazol	Intermittently or continuous after first appearance of candida
PCP	Co-trimoxazole	After first episode of PCP or when signs and symptoms of severely weakened immune system For children born to HIV positive women start co-trimoxazole at 6 weeks and continue for 1 year (unless advanced testing proves baby uninfected).
TB	Isoniazid (INH)	To prevent re-activation of TB (see Chapter 25) Do not give when active TB present For all children in contact with TB
Toxoplasmosis	Co-trimoxazole Sulfadiazine + pyrimethamine Clindamycin + pyrimethamine (Give calcium folinate with pyrimethamine)	When there are signs and symptoms of severely weakened immune system
Cryptococcal meningitis	Fluconazole	After first episode of cryptococcal meningitis
Herpes	Acyclovir	For severe and recurrent herpes
Recurrent bacterial infection	Co-trimoxazole H influenza B Pneumococcal vaccine (for children over 2)	Particularly valuable in children
Measles, chickenpox in children	Immunoglobulin. Zoster immune globulin	If exposed

The immune system then remains more effective and protects the patient against HIV related conditions.

Despite the success of these drugs in many parts of the world there are problems and concerns that need to be considered carefully before ART is started, particularly in low resourced areas.

HIV testing

To start anti-retroviral treatment, HIV testing is required. It is therefore necessary to have a reliable HIV test, and appropriately trained workers to undertake the testing and necessary counselling.

Expense

ART is extremely expensive. Although efforts are being made to reduce these costs, long-term financial plan-ning is required to ensure that drugs are available on a regular and long-term basis. This may be very difficult for individuals and for national health care systems. The cost also includes the availability of staff to monitor and support patients.

Side effects

ART is very effective in stopping the virus multiplying in the body but the drugs can cause many side effects and are potentially toxic. Patients need access to trained health care workers who can monitor and identify harmful side effects and deal with them appropriately. Drugs should not be stopped because of side effects without review by a doctor. Mild side effects are to be expected in the first few weeks of treatment but usually improve.

Taking HIV treatment

In order for ART to be effective a patient needs to take all the drugs and must not miss a tablet or take it late. If a drug is not taken, even for a very short time, the virus is able to multiply again very quickly and can change its structure. This is called resistance and dramatically reduces the effectiveness of that drug and other similar drugs.

Checking the drugs are working; checking the immune system.

Patients must be monitored to see if ART is working properly. This requires tests that can monitor the amount of virus in the blood (viral load test) and tests to measure the progress of the immune system and the increase in T4 cells (CD4 cell count). These tests require skilled technicians and appropriate equipment. Less complicated testing methods are being designed.

The nursing role when patients are on ART

Knowledgeable and well-trained nurses are central to ensuring the success of ART programmes for people living with HIV. Their role is likely to include:

- Assessing whether the long-term supply of particular drugs is secure
- Explaining the costs of drugs to patients and planning how they will be paid for and what implications this may have
- Explaining the importance of taking drugs exactly as they are prescribed and the consequences if this does not happen
- Discussing the best time for taking drugs, establishing a routine, writing or drawing charts to help patients take their drugs at the correct time each day, and working out what will be the best way to help them remember their drug routine
- Ensuring patients have regular appointments to monitor their progress on treatment and that they have access to health care workers to sort out concerns
- Explaining about the common less serious side effects, emphasising those that are potentially serious and require immediate intervention

- Observing and monitoring patients for side effects, apparent treatment failure and clinical deterioration
- Treating patients for HIV related conditions and advising them on taking prophylactic treatment to prevent such conditions occurring
- Giving support and listening to patients' concerns and difficulties. A patient may, for example, be worried about not having told anyone else about being HIV positive and taking drug treatment. Nurses can offer valuable support and encouragement.

Established community projects such as Home Based Care can make major contributions in introducing and maintaining ART in the community. There are a number of guidelines available to assist such projects and some of these can be found in the resource list on page 397.

All health care workers should be encouraged to participate in discussions relating to the introduction of ART in their own communities. They will be very involved once ART is established. However, ART is not the only answer and does not yet reflect the reality of care and treatment for people with HIV and AIDS in many communities.

Conclusion

This chapter focuses only on the role of nurses and midwives in preventing and treating HIV and AIDS. Many complex and interrelated factors fuel the rapid spread of HIV but these are beyond the scope of this chapter. Such issues include social deprivation, poverty, inequality between men and women, limited educational opportunities and the influence of some traditional customs, all of which contribute to HIV's devastating impact. These central issues need to be addressed at all levels, community, national and international.

Nurses and health care workers are faced with an enormous task in reducing the devastation caused by HIV and AIDS alongside those who influence areas such as policy and funding. If a nurse is able to prevent one person becoming infected with HIV, or assist one person to live longer and have a better quality of life, then that nurse has made a difference.

Health promotion

Many aspects of this chapter address health promotion, such as avoiding the spread of HIV, nutrition and the use of prophylactic drugs. There are some general things that people living with HIV can do to keep themselves healthy and nurses and midwives have important roles in encouraging this:

- Eating as well as money and food availability allows, and taking supplements if possible
- Keeping fit and active but avoiding overdoing exercise if unwell
- Getting plenty of rest and sleep, and avoiding stress if possible
- Reducing exposure to new HIV infection – safer sex protects patients as well as partners. Condoms can be used or non-penetrative sex.
- Avoiding alcohol, tobacco, drugs (for example marijuana or ganja), and unnecessary medication as the liver and kidneys may be damaged
- Taking local advice about non-western therapies as some can be harmful.

■ Activity

1. Find out the support services that are available in your area to assist people living with HIV or who have AIDS. Gather the information together into a pack that can be used by you and your colleagues when you have a patient who is known to be HIV positive or has AIDS. Arrange to update it at regular intervals.
2. You realise that support services in your area for people living with HIV and AIDS are inadequate. What do you believe is needed and how could the situation be improved?

Part 4

Maternity care

33

Introduction to midwifery

This chapter deals with the importance of maternity care and how it is provided. There is also guidance on how to work with others to improve women's chances of having a safe pregnancy and birth and also of having a healthy baby.

Introduction

Pregnancy and birth are very important events for womEn everywhere. Childbirth has physical, social and emotional aspects. Becoming a mother will change the life of a woman. For many, it is considered to be an essential part of being a woman. However, some mothers and babies die during the process, others may become disabled or suffer long-term illness.

The importance of maternity care

Avoiding ill health and saving lives

Nobody knows exactly how many women die each year from becoming pregnant. We have even less idea about how many babies die before and soon after the birth. Many of these deaths are never recorded. Some things we do know. We know even more women are left permanently disabled than those who actually die. We know most of the women who die are poor, or come from inaccessible areas of the world, or have limited access to skilled help. Deaths of mothers and even their long-term ill health have terrible results for families and few babies survive infancy when their mothers die. Access to good care can prevent many of these deaths and disabilities. However, health problems cannot always be predicted so all women need care although it can be provided in different ways.

The main causes of death and ill health

The main causes of problems vary around the world but there are five that are considered to be most important when resources for women are limited. These are:

- *Hypertensive* disorders (mainly pre-eclampsia and eclampsia)
- *Haemorrhage*
- Obstructed labour and ruptured uterus
- Infection
- Unsafe *abortion*.

Other factors are also linked with death and disability such as a history of heart disease, malaria, infection with Human Immunodeficiency Virus (HIV), thrombo-embolic conditions and viral hepatitis. Women are also more likely to be injured or killed by abusive partners in pregnancy than at other times. This applies to wealthier women as well as to poorer ones.

Pre-eclampsia and eclampsia: These disorders that occur only in pregnant and newly delivered women are responsible for many maternal deaths (see Chapter 35). Women may remain symptom free until the situation is so serious that it becomes life-threatening. Antenatal care improves the chances of diagnosing the condition in time to refer the woman to hospital so that the mother and baby can be saved.

Haemorrhage: Women die from haemorrhage. This can happen in pregnancy, during labour or the birth and after the birth (see Chapters 35, 39 and 40). Some women are at special risk of bleeding. These women can be advised to give birth in hospital. However, the possibility of bleeding cannot be predicted reliably so good access to emergency support is vital for all women. Many poorer women are *anaemic*. This is a major factor in causing deaths of women and their babies that should be possible to identify in good time. Bleeding is also linked to infection (see next page).

Prolonged labour: This happens when progress is hindered by a problem with the contractions, the woman's pelvis or the position of the fetus.

Obstructed labour: The passage of the *fetus* through the woman's pelvis is stopped and no further progress can be made (see Chapter 39). If contractions continue, the woman's uterus may tear. This is known as uterine rupture. Death from obstructed labour is avoidable with good care. Both mother and baby may die if skilled help is not obtained in time.

Infection: *Sepsis* causes women to die from infection of the genital tract and eventually, *septicaemia*. Dirty hands, dirty instruments, poor aseptic technique and cross-infection in hospital are all linked with maternal mortality. Sepsis, when it has been present for some days, also causes haemorrhage to occur. Damaged immune systems also increase the threat of infection.

Unsafe abortion: This is a major cause of death worldwide. Deliberate attempts to cause an abortion using dangerous and unclean techniques may lead to the death of a woman. Death may also follow badly treated or untreated accidental abortion (miscarriage).

Deaths in childbearing women can be avoided in most instances. It is important that midwives consider what could have been done to prevent such a death.

■ Activity

Think of a situation in which you have been involved where a woman has either died or been very seriously ill due to childbirth. Consider the factors that could have been avoided and list them. Then list steps you would take to help prevent the same thing happening another time. You could talk to colleagues about changes you might make together, and people you would need to talk to about them.

Social and economic issues

Mortality is highest in areas where there is no knowledge of asepsis, no means of dealing with life-threatening complications of childbirth, and no access to antibiotics or blood transfusions. Poor nutrition and hard physical work, large families and pregnancies which are too close together, all make death from childbirth more likely.

Where rates of maternal death and ill health are high the social status of women is usually low. A woman's status is often described in terms of her income, employment, education, health and fertility.

Social customs and cultural traditions may also put women at a disadvantage if they harm their health. A woman may be in danger simply from being born female. Any attempt to improve the health of women, if it is to succeed, must deal firstly with these issues.

One of the most important factors is the age at which a woman has her first baby. The safest time to have a baby is between 20 and 30 years when the pelvis has developed properly. However, a very high number of babies are born to teenagers. This may be because marriage happens very early, even before puberty in some places. Teenagers are often malnourished and anaemic. Both these factors affect their physical development and their ability to give birth safely. The pelvis will still be small or may be malformed. Obstructed labour is then much more likely. This can lead to terrible consequences for the woman's later health, even if she survives, because of the damage that may have been done.

The prevention of problems such as obstructed labour and their consequences requires action from all members of society, including health care workers. This involves ensuring girls and young women have the same access to services as do boys and men. It also involves feeding girl children and adolescents well. Better nutrition helps to make sure that girls do not grow abnormally small pelves and avoids pelvic deformities caused by *rickets*. Delaying marriage, or at least pregnancy, until women have reached full physical maturity is important. Compulsory education of girls may help to prepare them to make more appropriate choices. These changes can be difficult to introduce as they mean that people have to be prepared to change long-held traditions.

In some societies women are valued mostly for their childbearing. Indeed it may be seen as their main role and they may suffer the disapproval of families and even be sent away if they do not have children. It is important for people to recognise that women can more easily bear healthy children if their own health and welfare is cared for. They have the right to be healthy and not to be put at risk by childbearing. Communities, politicians and health service personnel need to work together to make a difference.

Women also need the support of knowledgeable and skilled carers to make sure that they are safe and healthy during childbearing. They need information so that they can make sensible choices about what happens to them. It is all too easy to look after a woman's physical needs and neglect other support. They need to have carers who are considerate and understand the importance of kindness and respect for their dignity. Women who do not feel respected may choose not to return for further care. They may also tell others who may then decide not to seek help either. So, unkind or inconsiderate words can kill.

■ Activity

Think of a custom or tradition in your area which may be responsible for women being less healthy than they could be for childbearing. Consider ways in which you could involve the community and bring about an improvement in women's health.

Who provides care?

There are many people who can help to provide care and support to childbearing women. The women's own mothers, grandmothers, friends and perhaps husbands can provide support and comfort. Traditional midwives, known by a variety of names but internationally as traditional birth attendants (TBAs), have a role that varies from one country to another.

In most countries, highly trained midwives are the people employed officially to provide care for childbearing women. They make a significant difference to women's well being when they themselves have good support and backup services. The World Health Organisation (WHO) emphasises the importance of having both skilled attendants, and good referral facilities. Together these are known as 'skilled attendants'.

Skilled attendance at birth

Having a properly trained attendant is the single most important factor in safe childbearing. Midwives, doctors and nurses who have the skills and knowledge to manage normal childbirth, prevent problems and provide basic emergency care are vital. These skills are known as 'midwifery skills'. Skilled attendants must be able to diagnose problems and act appropriately. They must be able to manage complications or refer women to a higher level of care. They may care for women either in hospital, clinics or in the home. Wherever they work, they need support, supervision and contact with colleagues. They must have well-planned referral systems so that they can get affordable help very quickly for women when emergency situations arise. This includes transport and communication.

Two levels of care are required in addition to normal care for pregnancy, labour, birth and the puerperium. These are Basic Emergency Obstetric Care and Comprehensive Emergency Obstetric Care. They are often called BEmOC and CEmOC.

Basic Emergency Obstetric Care consists of the provision of:

- Parenteral antibiotics, oxytocic drugs and anticonvulsants
- Manual removal of the placenta
- Manual vacuum aspiration of retained products
- Assisted vaginal delivery – ventouse extraction or forceps delivery.

Comprehensive Emergency Obstetric Care consists of the provision of the above plus:

- Blood transfusion
- Caesarean section and anaesthesia.

The role of the midwife

Midwives' roles extend beyond providing clinical care. They are well placed for gaining the confidence of women and their families. They are ideally placed to motivate and help parents and communities to bring about change (see Chapter 50). They also act as *advocates*, helping women and adolescents to improve their nutrition and well being. They have a responsibility to work with other care providers towards improving services for women and babies. Strong links make it easier to ensure that women have access to other services they need such as family planning, sexually transmitted infection clinics and voluntary counselling and testing for HIV. Family planning is especially important. Having children too close together is an important factor in the poor health or death of babies, older children and women themselves.

The role of the midwife and the scope of their practice vary between countries. Some work alongside medical colleagues, others may be very isolated. Some have a very wide clinical role; others will rarely have to carry out life-saving procedures themselves. The overall emphasis is on:

- supporting women through normal childbearing
- detecting when problems are arising
- dealing with emergencies while awaiting medical assistance.

It is important that national law supports midwives in their practice and the extent of what they are permitted to do is clear. This is often called 'enabling legislation' and means that midwives are legally covered. Giving oxytocin for active management of the third stage of labour is one example, performing manual vacuum aspiration or ventouse deliveries are others.

Most countries acknowledge the definition of the midwife accepted in 1992 by the International Confederation of Midwives, the Federation of International Gynaecologists and Obstetricians and the World Health Organisation. It is as follows:

'A midwife is a person who, having been regularly admitted to a midwifery educational programme, duly recognised in the country in which it is located, has successfully completed the prescribed course of studies in midwifery and has acquired the requisite qualifications to be registered and/or legally licensed to practise midwifery.

She must be able to give the necessary supervision, care and advice to women during pregnancy, labour and the postpartum period, to conduct deliveries on her own responsibility and to care for the newborn and the infant. This care includes preventative measures, the detection of abnormal conditions in the mother and child, the procurement of medical assistance and the execution of emergency measures in the absence of medical help. She has an important task in health counselling and education, not only for women, but also within the family and the community.

The work should involve antenatal education and preparation for parenthood and extends to certain areas of gynaecology, family planning and child care. She may practise in hospitals, clinics, health units, domiciliary conditions or in any other service.'

Making best use of available support for women

All women have the right to the best care in pregnancy, birth and the postnatal period. The ideal carer for childbearing women is considered to be a midwife or any person with midwifery skills; however the reality is that many countries do not yet have the resources to have enough persons to care for all women. It is important that health services make the best use of the people who are available to them. This may mean using a combination of fully qualified skilled attendants and others. The others may be nurses without midwifery skills, village health workers or TBAs. They may provide some parts of care working under the guidance and direction of skilled midwives.

Midwives have worked for many years with TBAs and their roles can overlap and complement each other. It is important to develop harmonious and respectful relationships and maintain good communication. In this way women can benefit from the best possible care available whatever the local situation may be. It is difficult to prove that TBAs, even trained ones, reduce the number of women dying through childbirth but they can make a real difference in other ways such as with the survival of the newborn. They can motivate and mobilise women and communities to make good choices, attend antenatal care and immunisations. Many women choose the care of TBAs for birth even if they have good access to hospitals because of the kindness they often receive. They also choose them for simple reasons like being given food to eat and hot water to bathe. TBA services may be cheaper to use. They may be prepared to accept payment in kind, or in instalments. They may be much nearer than a hospital or clinic and are often respected and selected by the community. The reality is that many women still have no access to skilled services and will use whatever support is available, whether the provider is trained and officially recognised or not.

In places where established TBAs continue to provide services that are officially recognised, midwives need to be involved with district health management teams to:
- maintain effective referral and communication systems for TBAs
- help them and the communities to plan reliable emergency transport systems
- stimulate, motivate and evaluate their work
- provide ongoing supervision and education.

Where authorities continue to select and train new TBAs, midwives need to assist to:
- select suitable people for training in conjunction with community leaders and women's groups
- design and organise training programmes that take into account the pre-existing knowledge and ideas of women working as TBAs.

Gradually the emphasis is changing to increasing women's access to skilled attendants in order to save more lives and this inevitably means changes for TBAs. Midwives will need to work with communities and their TBAs to develop their role in other fulfilling and appropriate ways. In this way they can then continue to feel they can use their strengths to help women and families.

34

Normal pregnancy and antenatal care

In this chapter there is information on what happens to the woman as she adapts to the needs of her fetus. It covers the normal physiological changes and some of the minor discomforts that affect women. Important aspects of providing pregnancy care are described, together with advice and help that might be given to pregnant women. The chapter includes short sections on nutrition in pregnancy and on providing information and preparing for birth.

Recognising pregnancy

Many women who have had previous pregnancies suspect they are pregnant before obvious signs and symptoms develop. Others may require guidance. The earliest symptoms may be nausea and tiredness, breast tingling, sudden dislike of particular foods or drink, and passing urine more frequently. The expected menstrual period does not occur (*amenorrhoea*) although some women have spotting of blood. This can confuse the diagnosis.

Skin colouration starts to darken after about 12 weeks. As well as breast pigmentation, most women have a dark line running from the umbilicus to the pubic hair called the linea nigra. Many women have darkening between the thighs, on the perineum and in underarm areas. Pigmentation often spreads across the nose and cheeks – the mask of pregnancy. This may be more obvious in lighter skinned women. Red stretch marks (striae gravidarum) appear later where the underneath skin layers stretch. These are commonest on the abdomen, breasts, thighs and buttocks. These eventually become silvery after the birth.

The fetal movements are first felt as internal fluttering sensations, known as quickening. This is felt at 18–20 weeks by *primigravid* women and 16-18 weeks by *multigravidae*. This is reliable so can confirm the probable birth date. However, some primigravidae believe it to be intestinal wind at first and even multigravidae can be deceived. The fetal heart can first be heard using a stethoscope around 20 weeks of pregnancy. Doppler ultrasound detects heart sounds at 12 weeks.

Other changes can be detected on vaginal examination by about 8 weeks. They can also be caused by anything that causes pelvic congestion so should not be used alone to diagnose pregnancy:

- The vagina and cervix are bluish in colour.
- The uterine artery pulsation can be detected in the vagina either side of the cervix (the lateral fornices) using gloved fingers.
- The isthmus of the cervix is soft and can be compressed between the internal fingers and external hand of the experienced examiner.

Pregnancy tests may be available if pregnancy needs to be confirmed early. Urine tests indicate pregnancy about 6 weeks after the beginning of the last menstrual period. Blood tests are positive at about 3 weeks.

A diagnosis of pregnancy can cause either great delight or distress so needs to be treated with great sensitivity.

Being healthy for pregnancy and birth

Healthy women are able to adapt to the needs of their babies but pregnancy can be a heavy burden for those who are not healthy. It is important that women have long enough gaps between pregnancies so that they can regain full strength. It is especially important that they prevent anaemia by rebuilding their body stores of iron and folic acid from food. Many young women are anaemic before even becoming pregnant. Girl children and women need to receive nourishing food so that they do not suffer problems in pregnancy and afterwards.

Women may need special advice about what is safe to do in pregnancy. Smoking tobacco and using other substances of addiction such as alcohol are very dangerous for the fetus. They may cause abnormalities and affect brain development. They also limit the efficiency of the placenta and may cause the fetus to be seriously underweight at birth. Women may be more vulnerable to sexually transmitted infections and HIV when pregnant so safe sex is vital. Malaria is also more of a problem for the woman and her fetus (see Chapter 36).

Physiology of pregnancy

The woman's body has to undergo great changes. Every system has to adjust to the pregnancy and the needs of the fetus. Emotional changes happen too. Many become more emotional than usual and cry or laugh more easily. Women may become forgetful and have difficulty in concentrating. Many want to sleep more than usual in early pregnancy then cannot sleep in later pregnancy. These are all due to combinations of *hormone* changes, their changing body shape, and tiredness.

Endocrine system

Hormone changes are considered first as they affect every system in the woman's body. They maintain the pregnancy and prepare for birth and lactation. Hormones are produced by the placenta and fetus as well as by the woman. They are interlinked in complex ways.

Hormones begin to alter immediately the fertilised ovum implants in the lining of the uterus (the endometrium). As the fertilised ovum begins to divide and develop, the outer cells produce hormones. These cells are known as the trophoblast and later become the placenta. They release a hormone known as human chorionic gonadatrophin (HCG). This enables the corpus luteum to keep producing oestrogen and progesterone. The corpus luteum is the scar left where the ovum was released from the ovary. The combined effect of these hormones is to allow the embryo to develop and not be rejected. HCG is probably one cause of early nausea and vomiting in pregnancy. Any condition where HCG levels are raised will result in excessive vomiting. Examples are multiple pregnancy and Hydatidiform mole, an abnormal development of the early cells of conception.

Placental hormones

The corpus luteum ceases to produce hormones by about 12 weeks gestation. The placenta then produces increasing quantities of oestrogen and progesterone. Progesterone is the hormone which causes relaxation of the smooth muscle in the woman and prevents the uterus from contracting before the fetus is mature. It is responsible for many of the other changes in pregnancy and the physiological effects experienced as discomforts by women. Oestrogen is mainly responsible for growth of uterine muscle and blood supply, and the preparation of the breasts for feeding. It also affects most other tissues. Oestrogen has an important role in the commencement of uterine contractions in labour. Hormones from the fetus play an important role in maintaining production in the placenta.

Human placental lactogen reduces the effects of insulin. This ensures that the fetus receives the carbohydrate and proteins it needs for survival and development. It causes varying blood sugar levels in the mother. She may feel nauseated if her blood sugar becomes low, especially on waking in the morning and in early pregnancy. This can be overcome by eating. The insulin needs of diabetic women may become very unstable in pregnancy.

Relaxin is produced by the placenta. Its main effect is to allow softening of the ligaments between the joints of the pelvis. This allows for their movement and widening in labour. This hormone is more efficient in second and subsequent pregnancies and is one reason why second labours are usually shorter than first labours.

Pituitary gland

The pituitary produces a variety of hormones. Oxytocin is important for uterine contractions and for the delivery of milk from the breasts during lactation. Oxytocin is produced by the posterior pituitary gland. The anterior pituitary produces prolactin in increasing amounts. Oestrogen and progesterone limit the effects of oxytocin and prolactin until they are needed for labour and lactation.

Thyroid gland

Changes in the thyroid encourage the woman's metabolism to change. Nutrient metabolism increases so the woman uses foods more efficiently. Some women show slight enlargement of the thyroid especially if their diet is low in iodine. These changes are normal but can cause confusion as they appear similar to thyroid problems. Thyroid function tests can help the diagnosis of true abnormality which can be serious.

Blood and the cardiovascular system

Blood

The blood volume increases greatly during pregnancy. It also becomes more dilute and less viscous; this is called haemodilution. This allows oxygen and nutrients to pass more easily across the placenta to the fetus. The dilution occurs because the fluid content, the *plasma*, increases more than the cells. Plasma increases by about 50 per cent. Red blood cells increase by 18 per cent. The woman will appear to be slightly anaemic when tested for haemoglobin and red cell count because of the lower proportion of red blood cells. This is sometimes known as physiological anaemia and is most obvious at about 32 weeks of *gestation*. The changes mean healthy women can cope with the extra demands of the pregnancy. They ensure that blood reaches the woman's own organs and the extra tissue such as the enlarged uterus. Healthy women can also bleed fairly heavily during the third stage of labour without suffering serious effects as quickly as they might when not pregnant. Remaining healthy depends on a supply of nourishing food to help to make the extra blood cells. Anaemia is very common when women cannot get good enough supplies of iron, folic acid and vitamin C from their food. Women who may become anaemic should receive daily iron supplements from about 16 weeks of pregnancy.

The metabolic rate rises in pregnancy by about 20 per cent. This generates heat. The extra blood reaching the skin helps to control this by allowing heat to be lost. This also causes women to feel hot and sweat more than when not pregnant.

The clotting of blood changes in pregnancy. This is important for controlling haemorrhage in the third stage of labour. It can, however, lead to *thrombo-embolism* in pregnancy and the puerperium. The level of blood coagulation factors increases and the break-down of clots is slowed.

The white cell count rises in pregnancy but the function of the immune system is reduced by hormonal changes. These changes prevent the fetus from being rejected by the mother's body. This means that women are more vulnerable to infections such as rubella, influenza, herpes, poliomyelitis and malaria. Malaria can also cause low birth weight and stillbirth because of parasites in the placenta. The reduced immune responses and HIV infection together can mean women suffer more from infections in pregnancy (see Chapter 32).

Cardiovascular system

Cardiovascular changes make many women feel very tired and they should be told that they may need extra rest. The heart works harder to supply the woman's body and the demands of the fetus. The uterus, placenta and enlarging breasts all make extra demands for blood supply. The heart enlarges to cope with the work of pumping the extra blood volume. The pulse rate increases and some women feel the rate change. This is normal. A woman with heart disease may have difficulty in coping with the extra demands of pregnancy (see Chapter 36).

Many women feel dizzy, nauseous and faint if they lie on their backs in the supine position. The enlarging uterus may reduce the blood flow back to the heart through the vena cava. This is called supine *hypotensive* syndrome. This can be prevented by avoiding laying the woman too flat when examining the abdomen. Her head and shoulders should be raised on pillows and examinations performed quickly. Feeling faint can be treated by sitting up or by lying on the left side.

Blood flow in the lower parts of the body and legs is slowed by the relaxation of the veins and by the pressure of the growing uterus. This may cause *oedema*, and *varicosities* in the legs and vulva and in the rectum, known as *haemorrhoids*. These are common in pregnancy and can cause severe discomfort.

Although the heart is working harder the blood pressure falls gradually in the first half of pregnancy. This lower blood pressure probably happens because blood vessels dilate. The resistance in their walls is reduced by rising pregnancy hormone levels. As the blood volume increases in the last *trimester* of the pregnancy the blood pressure returns to normal. It is normal for it to become very slightly higher than before pregnancy.

Slow venous return combined with *hypotension* may cause feelings of faintness when standing, known as postural hypotension. It is important to remember the advice to lay the woman on her left side, not flat on her back.

Respiratory system

The demand for oxygen increases as pregnancy develops and the fetus grows and the lungs have to work harder. The thoracic cavity changes in shape. The ribs and the diaphragm move more. This enables an increase in the air taken in and increased oxygenation of the blood, so meeting the demands of the growing fetus. As the fetus becomes larger, the rib cage and diaphragm are pushed up and the ribs move outward. Women become breathless more easily when pregnant and the changes can cause problems for women with lung disease as well as heart problems.

Renal system

The kidneys have to deal with more waste products in pregnancy and become larger under the effect of hormones. The extra demands come from the faster metabolism, from the fetus and the increased blood volume. The ureters lengthen and dilate. Some sections become lax and the heavy uterus may compress them. This causes slow passage of urine and a risk of infection.

The uterus presses on the bladder as it becomes larger. Women then need to pass urine more frequently, especially in early and late pregnancy. At the same time the inner urethral sphincter relaxes and many women suffer some stress incontinence. The bladder contracts less effectively and so women do not always empty it properly. Many women have bacteria in the urine without feeling symptoms so residual urine left in the bladder can easily become infected. The result of this is an increased incidence of urinary tract infection (UTI). The midwife should investigate fully if a woman has symptoms of UTI as this can cause premature labour and kidney infection and damage.

The *glomerular filtration rate* in the kidneys increases in pregnancy and reabsorption of glucose is reduced in the tubules. This results in glucose being lost in the urine which may show on urine tests. *Glycosuria* is usually just the result of these physiological changes. It can, however, be the first sign of diabetes so should be investigated.

Most pregnant women experience some fluid retention which may show in several ways but subsides after the birth:
- Swelling of their feet especially after standing
- Numbness and tingling in the fingers from increased pressure on the nerves in the wrist, known as Carpal tunnel syndrome
- Nasal congestion and reduced sense of smell and taste, even congestion of ears and eyes.

This oedema is normal and results from changes in electrolyte, serum protein and fluid balance. As oedema is associated also with pre-eclampsia the blood pressure should be checked and the urine examined for protein.

Gastro-intestinal system

Hormones such as progesterone affect the gastro-intestinal system too. Many women feel extra hungry and sometimes have strong desires for particular foods. This is called 'pica' and may include eating non-food items such as charcoal. They may also develop a dislike of particular foods. The extra appetite allows women to build up their fat stores to help provide energy for themselves and the fetus.

The gums may become swollen and may bleed. This is normal but inflammation can lead to bacterial infection. This is particularly important if the woman has heart disease as the infection can damage the *pericardium*. There is no evidence that pregnancy leads to loss of teeth through the fetus taking calcium as was once believed.

Excessive salivation, known as ptyalism, occurs sometimes and is said to be more common in African women than others. It can cause vomiting when women have to swallow the saliva repeatedly while feeing nauseated. It usually subsides as soon as the pregnancy has ended.

Hormones affect the activity of the whole tract and the enlarging uterus has a mechanical action. The cardiac *sphincter* of the stomach relaxes and the stomach is displaced upwards so reflux of gastric contents can occur into the oesophagus, known as heartburn. This is unpleasant and may cause inflammation, known as oesophagitis. Heartburn can be remedied using antacids. Antacid preparations inhibit the metabolism of iron and so should be used with caution.

It has long been believed that gastric emptying is delayed in pregnancy due to the influence of progesterone. Research now shows that this probably occurs only in labour. This must be considered when an anaesthetic is to be given. The stomach may not be empty even after several hours of fasting and there is a risk of aspiration of the undigested food and gastric acids.

Peristalsis is slowed and results in constipation and haemorrhoids. Eating food containing fibre, such as fruits, vegetables and grains, and drinking plenty of fluids, helps to deal with constipation.

Skeletal system – bones, muscles and ligaments

The joint capsules and the ligaments holding the bony skeleton together are affected by progesterone and relaxin. They become softer and more mobile during pregnancy and labour. This is most noticeable in the pelvis and makes the birth easier.

Pelvis

The pelvis is made up of several bones held tightly together by strong ligaments (see Figure 34.1). In men and non-pregnant women the bones become as one solid structure.

Looking at Figure 34.1 you can see:

- One central bone at the back – the curved sacrum. This is made of fused vertebrae.
- One large innominate bone each side – each made of the fused ileum, ischium and pubis.
- The two pubic bones meet at the front, the symphysis pubis joint.
- The two ilea meet the sacrum at the back, the sacroiliac joints.
- The coccyx is triangular and made of the last fused vertebrae. It meets the sacrum at the sacrococcygeal joint.

The pelvis can be divided into three areas: the inlet or brim, cavity, and outlet. The passage of the fetus is like passing head first through a tight rounded doorway (the brim), negotiating a small curved funnel-shaped room (the cavity) then squeezing through a diamond shaped doorway (the outlet).

The normal female pelvis is called gynaecoid. It is ideal for childbirth because:

- **The brim** is almost round. The sacral promontory protrudes slightly into it behind. When the fetus enters the pelvis, the widest diameter of the skull should fit into the widest, transverse, diameter of the brim. The fetus faces the woman's hips (see Figure 34.2a).

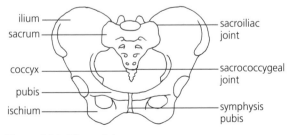

Figure 34.1 *The pelvis*

ilium
sacrum
coccyx
pubis
ischium

sacroiliac joint
sacrococcygeal joint
symphysis pubis

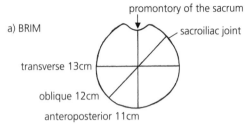

a) BRIM

promontory of the sacrum
sacroiliac joint
transverse 13cm
oblique 12cm
anteroposterior 11cm

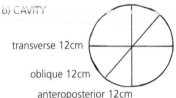

b) CAVITY

transverse 12cm
oblique 12cm
anteroposterior 12cm

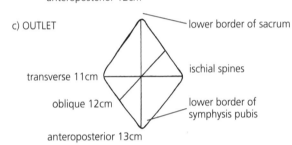

c) OUTLET

lower border of sacrum
ischial spines
lower border of symphysis pubis
transverse 11cm
oblique 12cm
anteroposterior 13cm

Figure 34.2 *Diameters of the pelvic brim, cavity and outlet*

- **The cavity** is a round and curved passageway. The back is deeper and formed from the sacrum; the front is shallow, the symphysis pubis. The circular shape helps the fetal head to rotate as it moves down to face the woman's back (see Figure 34.2b).
- **The outlet** is diamond shaped. The front point is the symphysis pubis, the rear is the coccyx. The side points are the ischial spines which should be shallow enough to permit the fetus to descend. As the fetus passes through the outlet, usually looking toward the coccyx, it must emerge under the sub-pubic arch. This needs to have an angle of at least 90 degrees to permit birth (see Figure 34.2c).

Other types of pelvis are described in Chapter 39.

The sacrococcygeal joint becomes more mobile in pregnancy. This enables the coccyx to move backwards as the baby descends through the pelvis in labour. This is restricted when women lie flat in labour so upright or lateral positions should be encouraged as they allow better expansion.

The sacroiliac joints also become more mobile so that they can expand. The sacrum can rock slightly as the fetal head passes through. This movement is also reduced by supine positions in labour see Chapter 37). The mobility can cause low backache or pain in pregnancy.

The symphysis pubis ligaments also soften to allow more room for the fetus in labour. Some women experience pain in pregnancy as the bones move against each other and the joint becomes less stable. This pain can be severe. Strapping or bandaging the pelvis from hip to hip with cloth may help a little. Physiotherapy is helpful following the birth if it is available.

Pelvic floor

The pelvic floor is made of muscles and ligaments that are attached to the bony pelvis on two layers (see Figure 34.3). It has several functions. It supports the internal organs and forms the sphincters that control the passage of urine and faeces. It also provides the outlet to the reproductive tract, the vagina and introitus. The muscles and ligaments are softened by hormones just as are all other connective tissues. This allows for the passage of the fetus.

The relaxation of these muscles can lead to stress incontinence and *prolapse* of the uterus, bladder and bowel after childbirth. It is important that inactive pregnant women are encouraged to keep these muscles well toned by deliberately exercising them (see below). Women who work hard should have stronger pelvic floor muscles.

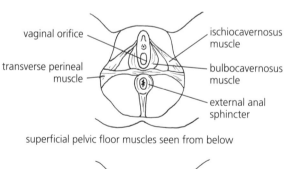

vaginal orifice

transverse perineal muscle

ischiocavernosus muscle

bulbocavernosus muscle

external anal sphincter

superficial pelvic floor muscles seen from below

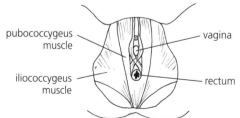

pubococcygeus muscle

iliococcygeus muscle

vagina

rectum

deep pelvic floor muscles (levator ani) seen from below

Figure 34.3 *The pelvic floor*

These muscles may be damaged by perineal lacerations occurring during birth. They are also cut when episiotomies are performed. It is vital that suturing is performed well if it is needed, and that good healing is promoted.

Spinal column

The spinal ligaments are also softened by hormones and the vertebrae become more mobile. The extra weight carried in front causes women to stand differently as their centre of gravity changes. Women tend to increase the lumbar curve, known as *lordosis* and lean back. This can cause backache and pain. Attempting to stand more upright can help. These problems are made worse if back and abdominal muscles are weak.

Reproductive tract

The changes in the reproductive tract are under constant hormone influence. This permits them to protect the growing fetus and allow for the supply of its needs. Then the softening effects allow for easier passage of the fetus through the birth canal. Tissues become more sensitive to particular hormones as the pregnancy develops. Figure 34.4 shows the female reproductive tract.

Uterus

The uterus is a round organ in its non-pregnant state. It is flattened from front to back, with an elongated end, the cervix (see Figures 34.4 and 34.5). It measures about 7.5 cm long, 5 cm wide and 2.5 cm deep. It is hollow, like a bag, but the cavity is flattened when there is no pregnancy. The uterus is tipped forward over the bladder and bent on itself (known as anteversion and anteflexion), see Figure 34.4. Growth in pregnancy is achieved by new muscle cells being made and existing

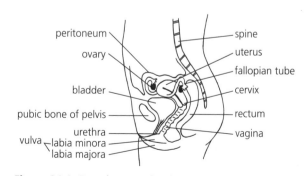

peritoneum

ovary

bladder

pubic bone of pelvis

urethra

vulva — labia minora
labia majora

spine

uterus

fallopian tube

cervix

rectum

vagina

Figure 34.4 *Female reproductive system*

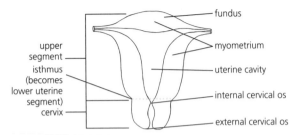

Figure 34.5 *Structure of the uterus*

ones becoming enlarged. By the end of pregnancy it is about 30 cm long, 25 cm wide and 20 cm deep, depending on the size of the fetus. A narrowed section, the isthmus, forms between the uterus and cervix.

The uterus has three layers of muscle forming the myometrium (see Figure 34.6). Each can stretch progressively to allow for fetal growth and also contract. These layers are the inner circular, middle oblique and outer longitudinal. They have different functions:

- Outer longitudinal fibres pass right over the uterus. They shorten and thicken progressively in labour. This pushes the fetus gradually down the birth canal.
- Inner circular fibres keep the cervix closed in pregnancy. They then allow it to dilate in labour to allow the fetus through.
- Oblique middle layer fibres are spiral and interlocking. They contract after the birth to control bleeding. They are often called 'living ligatures'.

The muscles have the ability to contract through pregnancy but this is held back by hormones. Contractions become more obvious as the fetus matures. These are known as Braxton Hicks contractions.

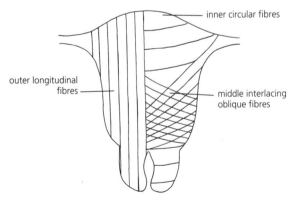

Figure 34.6 *Muscle layers of the uterus*

Braxton Hicks contractions are usually felt as painless, irregular tightenings and do not increase steadily in strength and frequency and become spasmodic as do labour contractions. However, some women may experience them as generally uncomfortable or even painful and they can last one minute or more. They may then give a false impression that labour has commenced.

In later weeks of pregnancy the contractions begin to reduce the size of the fundus and shorten and soften the lower segment. This begins the preparation and stretching of the cervix for labour (effacement).

The shape of the uterus changes from being flattened to become globular in early pregnancy. At about 28 weeks of pregnancy the isthmus elongates to become the lower uterine segment (see Figure 34.5). This thins progressively.

At first the growing uterus may cause a desire to pass urine frequently because it presses on the bladder. As it grows, it straightens and rises out of the pelvis. The rounded top (the fundus) can be felt as above the symphysis pubis at about 12 weeks of pregnancy (see below). Growth is then progressive.

During pregnancy, blood vessels and the blood supply to the uterus increase greatly to supply the placental site and the increased muscle and endometrium. The lining of the uterus, the decidua, becomes thicker and more vascular. This happens more in the upper part (the fundus) where the placenta is most likely to develop:

- The layer nearest the myometrium, the basal layer, develops new vessels to supply the placenta.
- The layer nearest the cavity becomes spongy.
- A 'compact' layer forms between the spongy layer and the uterus itself.

The compact layer is needed to allow separation of the placenta from the myometrium following the birth. The placental chorionic villi are prevented from penetrating the myometrium itself because this layer is dense. If this does occur it is called placenta acreta or percreta. Placenta acreta causes failure of the placenta to separate normally in the third stage of labour or pieces to remain behind. This leads to problems with haemorrhage and infection.

The cervix is tightly closed in pregnancy to contain the fetus and fluids, and prevent infection from entering from the vagina. A mucus plug, known as the operculum, forms in the cervical canal to act as a barrier. The cervix becomes softer and stretchy in later pregnancy in preparation for effacement and dilating in labour. The cervix opens from the inside (the internal os) before the external os begins to open. The mucus plug is often lost which shows the process is underway.

Vagina

The vagina becomes more elastic in pregnancy and stretches during the birth. Increased blood supply changes the colour to purple. Vaginal and cervical secretions increase but should remain white and non-irritant. These are known as leucorrhoea. Glycogen is produced by the cells of the vaginal lining. This allows the normal vaginal bacteria to produce more lactic acid to prevent infection. However, fungal Candida albicans organisms can still thrive and cause candidiasis (thrush). Thrush appears as severe irritation and soreness, white lumpy discharge and often, non-removable white patches on the *mucosa* of the vulva and vagina. The mucosa appears swollen and inflamed. Offensive discharge, yellow or greenish in colour, could be due to Trichomonal infection or gonorrhoea. Any of these symptoms should be investigated and treated (see Chapter 31).

Breasts

Breast changes start early in pregnancy. Tingling may be felt by women as early as the 6th week as the blood supply develops influenced by oestrogen and progesterone. This may be the first indication of pregnancy. The breasts can become tender and tight as the milk producing glands, the alveoli, develop. Veins become more obvious. By 12 weeks the nipples become more prominent and dark brown pigmentation appears around the nipple, called the primary areola. In this pigmented area are small sebaceous glands. These are called Montgomery's tubercles. Their secretions keep the area soft and supple and protect the skin when the baby starts to feed at the breast. A wider area of secondary pigmentation occurs around the primary areola. This is more obvious in darker skinned people. Around 16 weeks the breasts begin to secrete colostrum. This is the watery-looking fluid made in the breast before milk production commences 2 to 3 days after the birth. This can leak spontaneously in later pregnancy.

The nipples become larger in late pregnancy. If the nipples remain flat or turn inwards no treatment is needed. Inverted nipples will be 'brought out' by the infant during feeding.

We have taken a brief look at the systems of the body that change during pregnancy. It is clear from this that the midwife needs to care for the whole woman. It is important that the woman is in good health to enjoy a normal pregnancy and a healthy baby. Promoting good health in young women before they embark on a pregnancy is vital. Nutrition is very important.

Nutritional requirements in pregnancy

There is a relationship between poor nutrition and increased perinatal mortality, and also with the health and survival of women. Food is used more efficiently in pregnancy but women still need about 250 more calories per day to support the demands of the fetus without themselves suffering. During lactation this rises to about 500 extra calories. Some of this need can be met by decreasing activity but many women are not able to reduce their work load. A good mix of foods is important to obtain all the required nutrients.

Food availability is not the only factor that affects good nutrition. Levels of infection, work load and general health matter. So does local tradition which may restrict or encourage particular food for women, especially in pregnancy.

On average women gain about 20 per cent on their body weight if they have easy access to the foods they need. These foods are:

Protein: This is needed for the growth of new tissue and the repair of damaged tissue. Women often have insufficient protein in their diet because the men and boy children have the best portions of the protein available to the family. It is important for families to understand this, not just the women who may be powerless to make changes.

Carbohydrates: These provide energy. If women have insufficient carbohydrate then amino acids will be used to provide energy and this will deprive the fetus of necessary nutrients.

Fats: These are very important to provide energy and as sources of fat soluble vitamins. These are needed for the woman's own health as well as that of the fetus and for lactation, so women need to build good stores. Animal fats may have a role in preventing anaemia (see below).

Iron: This is essential for the health of the pregnant woman. Iron is discussed in the section on anaemia.

Folates and **Vitamin C:** These are both essential for the prevention of anaemia and for the health of the fetus. Both are contained in fruit and leafy vegetables. Folates are also found in beans and potatoes. Women whose diet is poor or who are anaemic may be given folic acid supplements in pregnancy.

Vitamin A: This is lacking from the diet in many areas but is needed to prevent anaemia. Vitamin A can be converted in the liver from fruit and vegetable sources, mainly yellow and orange foods and leafy vegetables. It is fat soluble so animal sources such as oily fish, liver and milk products are more effective.

Vitamins and minerals are known as micro-nutrients. A range of these is needed to prevent problems in women and babies. Other vitamins such as B vitamins, D and E vitamins all play a role in health and preventing infection. Midwives and nurses need to have local knowledge about what affordable foods are available in the area. For example, a diet of beans, groundnuts, spinach or pumpkin leaves, tomatoes, local fruit such as mangoes or bananas, a little dried fish, meat or eggs when possible, vegetable oil and a starchy food would provide adequate nutrients. Starchy carbohydrate sources such as maize or rice are better if ground or pounded with the husks as micro-nutrients and fibre are retained.

Antenatal care

The aims of antenatal care and contemporary approaches

The outcome of women's pregnancies is more likely to be good if they receive effective antenatal care. Complications are more likely to be recognised early and women can be referred to the most appropriate care. Measures can be taken to prevent many of the problems that cause women and their babies to become ill or die. Women can be helped to take responsibility for their own health. They can also be assisted to make plans for the birth.

Antenatal care has changed in recent years. An emphasis on detecting those at risk of birth complications did not produce very good results. Many women who were expected to experience problems did not actually do so. Those who were expected to have a normal birth might then encounter an emer-

gency without being prepared. Specific issues that can be addressed when you meet women in pregnancy are:

- Tetanus prevention is important to women and their babies. Give tetanus toxoid 0.5 ml IM at the first visit and repeat after 4 weeks and 6 months if she has not been immunised before. She should receive 2 more annual doses.
- Provide malaria prophylaxis where appropriate and discuss prevention such as the use of impregnated bed nets.
- Give iron, folic acid, vitamin C and A supplements where needed. Recommended doses are iron tablets 60 mg and folic acid 400 microgrammes, daily until 3 months postpartum. Give double the iron for anaemic women. Many women stop taking iron because of nausea and constipation. Advise them to take iron with food or at night and to drink plenty of water. Check that there are no fears about taking iron such as producing a big baby.
- Detection of pre-existing problems like anaemia or diabetes
- Detection of life-threatening problems such as pregnancy induced hypertension
- Fetal growth and condition can be assessed and abnormalities that will affect labour can be recognised. An appropriate place for the birth can then be organised.
- Education about health lifestyles, nutrition, rest and exercise, safe sex
- Provide information about available help so women can make sensible choices about issues such as place of birth and choice of carer.
- Encourage women and their families to plan ahead for emergencies such as deciding how to send messages and find transport during the day and night. This is often known as emergency preparedness and includes giving information about danger signs.
- Women may be willing to start thinking about family spacing (see Chapter 29).
- Some may wish to accept voluntary counselling and testing for HIV.

Providing antenatal care

Antenatal care needs to be accessible, affordable, acceptable and meet women's needs for safety, support, information and guidance.

It is essential that pregnant women feel that you are an expert and that you care about them. Greeting clients in a friendly, courteous and professional manner helps greatly. Women need to have privacy when talking to you and when being examined. They also need to have their dignity respected at all times and be confident that confidences will not be passed on to others. Poor attitudes of midwives and nurses are common complaints of childbearing women and can cause refusal to use services that have been provided.

You can make initial general assessments of women's health and well being while 'meeting and greeting'. Throughout the examination you should be alert for signs she may wish to talk to you about worries. You may be the only one she can approach about health concerns or problems at home such as violence.

Women need to receive an initial assessment as early as possible in pregnancy. Follow-up checks should occur at least three times, at about 6, 8 and 9 months. Many national policies recommend more antenatal checks. Advise women to return if they have not given birth within 2 weeks of their Expected Date of Delivery (EDD).

Record all findings for future reference. In many places women now carry their own record cards and produce them at each visit and in labour.

Initial assessment

Once a good relationship has been established then a thorough general history can be taken. You need to know about the woman's own health and, where possible, that of her family. The questions that can be used are shown in the information box.

Ask about her **menstrual history**. This permits an assessment to be made of the gestation, or stage of pregnancy. It enables progress to be watched over

---

Questions for antenal initial assessment

Question	Comment
Have you had any previous pregnancies? If so what happened? Have you experienced bleeding, operative delivery, convulsions, stillbirth or early death of the baby?	The woman who has had a previous full term, normal labour with a healthy baby will probably do so again. But some problems tend to repeat themselves. Also, babies are often born larger with successive pregnancies. An abnormal presentation or position and larger baby can cause problems this time.
Do you, or any of the people with whom you live, have a persistent cough?	Tuberculosis is a real risk to newborn babies. Treatment of women and family members before birth can protect the newborn.
Have you or your family been unwell recently, e.g. malaria, hepatitis, dysentery?	Hepatitis and malaria can be serious in pregnancy. Treatment can be provided and prevention discussed. This is a health promotion opportunity.
Do you smoke tobacco or drink alcohol?	The issues surrounding the woman's health and health of the fetus can be discussed.
Are your children healthy now? Have the children been immunised?	This provides information about whether help and guidance is needed by the family. A new baby to protect may encourage families to make changes.
Do you or your family suffer from any diseases, e.g. high blood pressure, diabetes, or heart disease?	These diseases tend to recur in families so the midwife needs to be particularly observant. It is especially important in relation to hypertensive disease of pregnancy.
Do you intend to breastfeed the baby? Did you breastfeed previous babies?	This question may not be considered to be relevant where breastfeeding is universal. Otherwise it provides opportunities to discuss the benefits and dispel misunderstandings. It may be local policy to discuss this with women living with HIV infection.

time. It also helps you to decide about the approximate date when the birth can be expected – the EDD. Many women will have a clear idea of their dates; others will have little knowledge. Midwives need to be patient if women take time to remember dates of menstruation. Many women do not have calendars and work it out in relation to an event. Here are some facts to assist calculation of the EDD:

- The EDD is said to be about 9 calendar months and 7 days from the first day of the last normal menstrual period. This is 280 days.
- Ovulation occurs on day 14 in a typical 28 day cycle.
- Fertilisation occurs within 48 hours of ovulation.
- This date is approximate as birth may happen 2 weeks earlier or later.
- Some people now believe that different races may have slightly longer or shorter pregnancies.
- This calculation does not take account of different length menstrual cycles so there is always potential for inaccuracy.
- If the woman's menstrual cycle is not regular then it is difficult to calculate her EDD.
- If a woman's cycle is normally 21 days, her EDD may be 7 days earlier than if she has a 28 day cycle.
- If her cycle is normally 35 days, then an extra 7 days should be added.
- Some women will know when conception must have taken place, perhaps if this was the only occasion when intercourse happened. EDD could then be calculated from this date.

This calculation is always approximate and women need to understand this. In fact many people now believe that an average pregnancy is about 3 days longer than was thought.

Many women calculate pregnancy as 10 lunar months. It is interesting to note that this is equivalent to the methods used above so ought not to be ridiculed.

In later visits: Ask the woman about her health and any worries. Ask her about:

- Whether the fetus is moving and growing
- Vaginal bleeding
- Offensive smelling vaginal discharge
- Headaches
- Burning or pain on urinating
- Constant low backache over the kidneys
- Regular or constant abdominal cramps

- How well she is eating and sleeping. Poor sleep can be helped by putting pillows or home-made pads behind the back, under the abdomen or under the upper leg.

Clinical examination

Blood tests

Laboratory examination of the blood should be done at the first visit. Test for anaemia, and if possible the blood group and Rhesus factor, for syphilis, hepatitis and rubella immune status. Some women will wish to have their HIV status assessed. Blood disorders such as sickle cell disease and thalassaemia can be detected on blood test (see Chapter 12).

Testing for anaemia: Do a full blood count at the first visit and repeat haemoglobin (Hb) estimation at 28 and 36 weeks, if possible. Four methods for Hb testing are:

- Laboratory testing – the most reliable
- Portable haemoglobin meters – reliable but expensive
- WHO Colour Scale – cheap and fairly useful
- Inspection of the conjunctiva of the eyes for pallor – for rapid assessment. This is the least reliable but is useful to find severe anaemia.

Ideally the Hb value should be above 11.0 g/dl falling to 10.5 g/dl in the second half of pregnancy. Low Hb only indicates the presence of anaemia. If the Mean Cell Volume is low, then it is desirable to check the woman's iron stores by measuring the serum ferritin. Anaemia is discussed in Chapter 36. If haemoglobin and iron stores are low, or there is a risk of anaemia, iron and folic acid supplements should be given to the woman.

ABO group: It saves time if the blood group is already known if a blood transfusion is needed.

Rhesus status: Rhesus immunisation may occur if there is incompatibility between a Rhesus negative woman and her Rhesus positive baby (see Chapter 42). This can be prevented if anti D gamma globulin is given to prevent the formation of Rhesus antibodies.

Syphilis: Syphilis is life-threatening for the fetus and can be detected on blood test. Treatment with penicillin before 20 weeks gestation may prevent fetal damage. The baby needs penicillin again after birth.

Urine tests

Test the urine at each visit for:

Protein: *Proteinuria* can indicate contamination from

vaginal secretions, the presence of bacteria, or pre-eclampsia. Many pregnant women have *bacteriuria* with no symptoms. If laboratory testing is possible, check the urine once more. If still positive order a test to detect infection. Urine infection can have consequences for the woman and fetus (see Chapter 35). Another sample will need to be tested and if still positive, look for other signs of pre-eclampsia. If other signs of pre-eclampsia exist then refer the woman for specialist help.

Glucose: *Glycosuria* occurs in some women after meals because of the lowered renal threshold for glucose. Pregnancy can also act as a trigger to cause diabetes. Investigate further if it persists.

Blood pressure

Monitor blood pressure as early as possible in pregnancy then at each antenatal visit. This helps to detect the onset of pre-eclampsia (see Chapter 35). Remember that a drop in blood pressure is normal between 10 and 22 weeks. If the diastolic blood pressure rises by more than 15 mm of mercury, the woman should be monitored closely. After 28 weeks gestation, check at least every 2 weeks. Check blood pressure weekly after 36 weeks. Nervousness can cause the blood pressure to rise. If you suspect this, take it again when the woman has had time to relax.

Look for:

- Oedema of the legs: this is normal unless accompanied by signs of pre-eclampsia (see Chapter 35).
- Face and finger oedema. This may indicate pre-eclampsia.
- Haemorrhoids and varicose veins of the legs and vulva. These are common but significant because they can be painful and leg thrombosis becomes more likely as blood clotting changes. Advise women not to stand around and to exercise, but to raise the legs when sitting. Avoiding constipation helps prevent haemorrhoids.

Abdominal examination

Some of the terms used in abdominal examination need to be defined before describing the methods, see information box on page 242.

How to examine the abdomen

Explain to the woman what you are going to do before starting. Encourage her to empty her bladder to make palpation easier and prevent discomfort. Ask her to make herself comfortable lying down with her head and shoulders raised on pillows, if possible, to prevent supine hypotension. Wash your hands and warm them to avoid a reaction to cold hands. Stand or kneel beside her. Talk to the woman as you examine her. She will be able to tell you where the baby is kicking her which can confirm what you are feeling. The abdominal examination should be carried out in three stages:

1. Inspection

Look for:

Size: Estimate the size of the abdomen in relation to the period of gestation. This is difficult in obese women.

Shape: A primigravida will have strong abdominal muscles. The abdomen will have an ovoid shape. Multigravid women will tend to have a rounder shape with less firm muscle tone. Some women with very poor tone have pendulous abdomens especially if they are overweight. It can then be difficult to decide on findings. Transverse lie is more likely with poor muscle tone. The abdomen may look wider than it is long. You may see a depression in the middle of the abdomen. This suggests that the fetal limbs are in front – a posterior position.

Scars: These indicate previous surgery that might affect the uterus such as caesarean section or fibroid removal. Ask about this.

2. Palpation of the uterus

Examine the uterus and fetus by touch. Try to imagine what you are feeling. Making a simple cloth doll helps with this. Look for:

Fundal height: The fundus of the uterus is palpated using flat hands. Find the top curve of the uterus using the hand that is nearest the woman's ribs. The height is decided in relation to average size for gestation. There are two ways of measuring:

- Measure from the upper edge of the pubic bone to the fundus. From 20 weeks gestation the fundal height should increase by about 1 cm per week so it is possible to use a tape measure to assess growth until the last month.
- Specific 'landmarks' on the woman's body are used (see Table 34.1 and Figure 34.10). These are the pubis, the umbilicus and lower edge of the sternum (xiphisternum). Measure using the number of fingers that fit between the fundus and the landmark

Definitions

Fundus: The upper rounded part of the uterus between the two fallopian tubes

Pole: The head or breech (pelvis and buttocks) of the fetus; may be used for the upper and lower parts of the uterus

Lie: The relationship of the fetal spine (often called the long axis) to the spine of the mother. Longitudinal lie is normal. The fetus has its spine parallel to the mother, head or breech in the lower part of the uterus and the other pole in the fundus. The lie is described as transverse if the head is out to the side and the spine at right angles to the mother's spine. The fetus cannot be born vaginally unless this changes to longitudinal lie (see Figure 34.7).

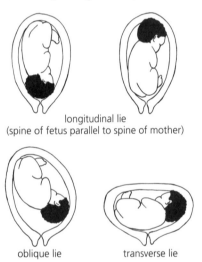

longitudinal lie
(spine of fetus parallel to spine of mother)

oblique lie   transverse lie

Figure 34.7 Lie of the fetus

Presentation: The part of the fetus that occupies the lowest part of the uterus. This may be cephalic (the head), vertex (flexed head), face or brow, breech, shoulder. Cephalic is normal, preferably head flexed into a vertex presentation. Persistent brow and shoulder presentations cannot be born vaginally (see Figure 34.8).

Denominator: The area on the presentation that is used to describe the position of the fetus in relation to the pelvis. In a cephalic presentation it is the occiput (back) of the skull. In a breech presentation it is the sacrum. In a face presentation it is the chin (mentum).

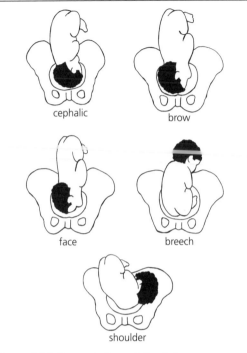

cephalic   brow

face   breech

shoulder

Figure 34.8 Presentation of the fetus

Position: This describes the relationship between the denominator of the fetal presentation to the maternal pelvis, for example left occipito-anterior (LOA) in cephalic presentation, or left sacro posterior (LSP) in breech presentation. LOA or ROA are the best positions for birth.

Attitude: The relationship of the fetal head and limbs to its body. A fetus may be partially flexed, partially extended or completely extended. The ideal attitude is full flexion, chin on the chest, with limbs curled up tightly (see Figure 34.9).

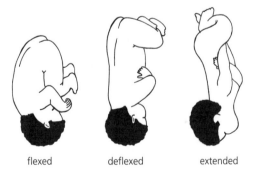

flexed   deflexed   extended

Figure 34.9 Attitude of the fetus

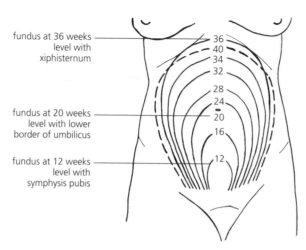

fundus at 36 weeks level with xiphisternum

fundus at 20 weeks level with lower border of umbilicus

fundus at 12 weeks level with symphysis pubis

Figure 34.10 *Assessment of uterine growth in weeks*

Table 34.1 Gestational landmarks

Gestation	Landmark
12 weeks	Just palpable above the symphysis pubis
16 weeks	Slightly more than midway between pubis and umbilicus
20 weeks	Just below the umbilicus
24 weeks	Just above the umbilicus
36 weeks	At the xiphisternum
40 weeks	2–3 finger breadths below the xiphisternum. The presentation has sunk into the softened lower uterine segment (lightening). It should be engaged in the pelvis in primigravidae.

(2–3 fingers for each four weeks). Alternatively, divide the space between the umbilicus and the sternum into five (2 weeks for each section). These are approximate guides as taller and shorter women, or different sized babies, can confuse the findings.

Note that the head or breech descends into the lower uterine segment around 38 weeks. This 'lightening' makes women feel more comfortable and able to breathe more easily.

If the fundus is too high in early pregnancy, the estimation of the gestation period is probably wrong, or there may be more than one fetus. More rarely there may be a hydatidiform mole. In later pregnancy, the increase in size could be due to polyhydramnios, an excessive amount of amniotic fluid.

A smaller than expected fundal height could suggest wrong dates or a fetus that is not growing well. The well being of the fetus should be assessed if possible. Growth delays are more likely to be recognised if the same person cares for the woman throughout her pregnancy.

Now you can proceed to lateral palpation – move to face the woman slightly.

Lie: Place hands either side of the abdomen and gradually move them downwards from the fundus. You can feel a longitudinal lie between the hands. You can feel the fetus lying across the abdomen in a transverse lie. The lie can be determined from about 28 weeks but can change frequently because the fetus still has room to move. It should be longitudinal by 32 weeks. Transverse lie has serious implications for labour (see Chapter 39) but is uncommon in primigravidae.

Presentation: Use both hands together to find the head and breech. The head feels hard and rounded. It can be moved from side to side unless fixed in the pelvic inlet. This is because the neck bends. The breech feels more irregular and does not bend. It can be difficult to tell the difference.

At 28 weeks, 25 per cent will be breech presentations. By 34 weeks most primigravidae will have cephalic presentations. By 38 weeks almost all are cephalic. Other presentations (face, brow or shoulder) have implications for labour (see Chapter 39).

Position: 'Walk' your hands across the abdomen. The fetal spine curves gently and feels harder than the front of the body which feels lumpy because of the limbs. The denominator will usually be in line with the spine.

- The spine nearer the midline indicates that the fetus is anterior position (the best position).
- The spine located near the woman's side indicates a lateral position.
- No spine felt suggests a posterior position.

The position of the fetus is relevant in late pregnancy because of its importance in labour. If the occiput is posterior, then progress in labour will be delayed.

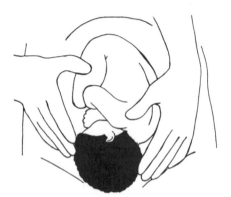

left occipito anterior position,
fetal head well flexed

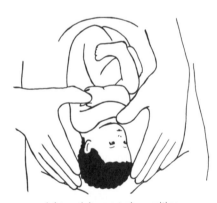

right occipito posterior position,
fetal head deflexed

Figure 34.11 *Abdominal palpation*

Attitude: Face toward the woman's feet. Feel the head between your flat fingers. Assess how well flexed the fetal head is. The back of the head (nearest the spine) should be lower than the front (flexed). A deflexed head feels very wide.

This becomes important as labour approaches as it needs to flex to enter the pelvis. If it does not flex, it may delay engagement (see Figure 34.11).

Engagement of the fetal head: This is the descent of the widest diameter of the fetal head into the pelvic inlet (brim). It usually happens in the last month in primigravidae and in labour with multigravidae.

Face the woman's feet. Place your hands both sides of the uterus. Feel down deeply, firmly and gently. It may help if the woman breathes in and holds her breath for a few seconds. Try to decide whether the widest part of the head can be felt. If the head is immovable and you are unable to feel the widest part, or can feel only the part of the head opposite the fetal spine, then it is engaged.

The usual way to describe what you feel is in the number of fifths of the head that are felt above the pelvis. 5/5 palpable is described as 'free', 3/5 means the head is not engaged, 2/5 means it is engaged (see Figure 34.12). Labour usually starts within 2 weeks of engagement of the fetal head. Engagement is likely to occur before term in primigravidae and not until labour begins in multigravidae. Once the head is engaged, labour is likely to progress without obstruction.

Head fitting test: If the head is not engaged in the last 2 weeks, then it is wise to check that there is room for it to do so. There are two methods. Both can be uncomfortable for the woman:

- Place the hand nearest the woman's feet on her lower abdomen, the little finger level with the symphysis pubis. Place two fingers on the fetal head. Ask the woman to raise herself up and lean back on her elbows (see Figure 34.13). If the head slips into the pelvis then the pelvis is probably large enough for vaginal birth providing the outlet

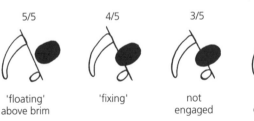

5/5	4/5	3/5	2/5	1/5	0/5
'floating' above brim	'fixing'	not engaged	just engaged	engaged	deeply engaged

Figure 34.12 *Engagement of the fetal head*

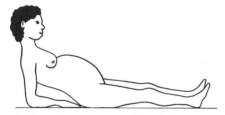

Figure 34.13 *Position as part of head fitting test*

of the pelvis is large enough. The outlet is assessed on vaginal examination.

- Ask the woman to stand up and lean forward over a table or chair. Palpate the head with one hand. If the head has slipped into the pelvis, then the pelvis is probably large enough for vaginal birth.

3. Auscultation

Listen to the fetal heart.

The heart beat can be heard best over the back of the fetus. A Pinard fetoscope is usually used. Alternatives are:

- hollowed out wood or bamboo, or strong cardboard tube
- listen with your ear on the woman's abdomen
- ordinary stethoscope
- electronic fetal heart monitor if available.

The heart beat can be heard from about 20 weeks gestation. It should be about twice the rate of the mother's heart beat.

Pelvic assessment

If you believe that the fetus may be too big for the woman you can examine the internal size of the pelvis and how well the head fits in late pregnancy. It is uncomfortable, especially in primigravidae, so must be done carefully. It is possible to assess the capacity of the inlet, cavity and outlet of the pelvis. Remember

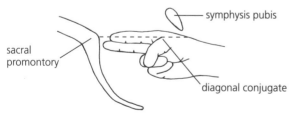

Figure 34.14 *How the diagonal conjugate can be measured*

that internal pelvic examination is not usually needed.

Inlet (brim): The sacral promontory projects slightly into the round brim of the pelvis. Midwives with long fingers may just reach the sacral promontory with two fingers in the vagina. The normal distance is 12–13 cm (known as the diagonal conjugate). Many female midwives cannot reach a normal sacral promontory. If it can be felt easily, the fetus may find it difficult to pass through the brim (see Figure 34.14).

Cavity: Sweep your fingers down from the sacral promontory to test the sacral curve. A rounded curve allows the fetal head to rotate properly. A flattened curve makes this difficult.

Try to feel the ischial spines each side of the cavity. If they are prominent they may 'catch' the fetal head. The spines make this one of the tightest parts of the pelvis the fetus has to pass through. Sometimes they cannot be felt at all when the pelvis is normal.

Outlet: Check the subpubic arch as you remove your fingers. You should be able to fit two fingers in the subpubic arch if it has a normal angle of 90 degrees between the pubic bones. This allows the fetal head to emerge under the bony arch.

Alternatively, a clenched fist held between the ischial tuberosities indicates a good size.

Remember that the relationship of the pelvis to the size of this particular fetus is the important issue. A big baby needs a big pelvis. A small baby does not. Also note that:

- The pelvis enlarges slightly in labour if the woman's position allows.
- The fetal head changes shape and the diameters become slightly smaller as the bones overlap (moulding).

■ Activities

1. You often have women arriving in labour at your maternity clinic who have not received antenatal care. Design a plan to find out why this is happening and discover ways of encouraging clinic attendance. Include a list of who could help you in the community.

2. You are given charge of an antenatal clinic in a small city health centre. You soon notice that many women are anaemic and very few can afford nutritious food in pregnancy. Work out a way of encouraging women to eat better, using cheap foods from the local market.

35

Abnormal pregnancy

This chapter covers important disorders of pregnancy. These disorders are hypertensive disease, bleeding, incarcerated uterus, hyperemesis gravidarum, hydatidiform mole, polyhydramnios and oligohydramnios.

Introduction

There are a number of disorders of pregnancy that can cause major problems for the woman and fetus and may be life-threatening. Disorders not specific to pregnancy, such as anaemia, are addressed in Chapter 36. Abnormal presentations such as breech are covered in Chapter 39. Where possible, obstetricians will lead in the care of these women, working in collaboration with midwives.

Pregnancy-induced hypertension (PIH)

Types of hypertensive disease

- Gestational hypertension. A woman with previously normal BP has a rise after 20 weeks of pregnancy to more than 140/90 mmHg, at rest, on two occasions and a few days apart. There is no *proteinuria* and normal *oedema*. The hypertension may disappear after the birth or persist.
- Chronic hypertension. BP more than 140/90 on two occasions before the 20th week of pregnancy.
- Pre-eclampsia. Proteinuria and hypertension develop in a woman whose BP was normal at the beginning of pregnancy. It may occur for the first time in labour or in the first postnatal days. Pre-eclampsia may still be diagnosed with only hypertension or proteinuria (see below).

- Pre-eclampsia may occur in a woman who has chronic hypertension. This is very dangerous with rapidly increasing BP and proteinuria.
- Eclampsia. Convulsions occur with pre-eclampsia. They may occur before pre-eclampsia is diagnosed.

Pre-eclampsia and eclampsia

About six per cent of women have some degree of pre-eclampsia but some are at greater risk than others, for example:

- Primigravidae, particularly those less than age 19
- Women having a new sexual partner since previous pregnancies
- Close family history of pre-eclampsia, especially own mother or sister
- Previous history of pre-eclampsia
- Pre-existing vascular disease, for example diabetes, chronic hypertension
- Multiple pregnancy or hydatidiform mole.

Causes

Although causes are uncertain, the placenta is probably involved because pre-eclampsia disappears following the birth. Current theories include genetic predisposition, dietary factors, vascular and auto-immune disorders. These all link to the predisposing factors listed above.

What happens in pre-eclampsia?

The process is probably initiated by an immune response that damages the epithelial linings of the woman's blood vessels. Changes are complex and inter-related. Widespread spasms of the blood vessels happen with hypertension leading to worsening of the hypertension. The hypertension leads to *ischaemia* and oedema from fluid leaking from the cells. There may be the formation of small blood clots. These changes cause damage in any or all organs and trigger each other off (sequelae):

- The placenta becomes inefficient (uteroplacental insufficiency). The fetus is deprived of oxygen and nutrients and does not grow well. It may become severely *hypoxic* and die or be born brain damaged.
- Pulmonary oedema. Giving too much intravenous fluid in pre-eclampsia is very dangerous.
- Renal damage may be permanent.
- Liver cell ischaemia results in oedema and haemorrhage. The woman complains of severe *epigastric* pain.
- The brain becomes oedematous. Signs and symptoms of this are exaggerated reflexes, severe headache, and visual disturbances (flashing lights, *photophobia*, blurring and double vision). Cerebral haemorrhage may result.
- Blood coagulation may be affected. Capillary damage causes widespread clotting, blockage of blood flow to the organs and placenta and using up of clotting factors. Disseminated intravascular coagulation (DIC) and haemorrhage can then follow. Fluid replacement may prevent this and fresh whole blood is needed to treat it.

'Fulminating pre-eclampsia' is often used to describe rapidly worsening pre-eclampsia.

'HELLP syndrome' is a label given to the interlinked events of **H**aemolysis of red cells, **E**levated **L**iver enzymes and **L**ow **P**latelets. This very serious condition causes many maternal and perinatal deaths.

The convulsions of eclampsia may follow without any warning.

Diagnosis of pre-eclampsia

The main signs of pre-eclampsia are hypertension and proteinuria. Oedema is often present but severe pre-eclampsia may exist without it. Similarly, proteinuria may not appear.

Hypertension: This is usually the first sign of pre-eclampsia. It is important to know the early pregnancy BP for comparison. A recording of 140/90 is classified as hypertension. However, a diastolic recording that has risen by 15 mmHg compared with the early reading, still indicates possible hypertension even if below 90. For example women may convulse with a BP of 130/80 having had an early pregnancy BP of 110/60.

Proteinuria: This is defined as:
- More than 300 mg of protein per litre in a 24 hour urine collection
- More than 100 mg of protein found in two urine samples taken at least 6 hours apart.

Remember that false results occur if the urine is contaminated by vaginal secretions, the receptacle is dirty or the woman had been standing for a long time.

Oedema: Abnormal oedema must be differentiated from physiological oedema seen in most pregnant women. Oedema of the face, hands or abdomen which does not subside with 12 hours of bed rest is abnormal. It may also show as excessive weight gain. Women do not have symptoms they can recognise as pre-eclampsia until the late stages. This means that regular BP measurement and urine testing is the only way of identifying it early. Antenatal care is vital to identify and treat this condition before the health and lives of women and babies are threatened.

Management

The only cure for pre-eclampsia is the birth of the baby. The aim of care is to prevent serious consequences while allowing the pregnancy to continue until it is mature enough to survive.

Mild pre-eclampsia: This is treated with rest and close observation so that birth can be hastened if the condition deteriorates. Women may need to be seen daily because pre-eclampsia can worsen rapidly. They can be monitored at home safely if facilities and emergency transport arrangements exist.

- Bed rest appears to improve pre-eclampsia and increase the blood flow to the placenta. However, rest should be encouraged only until the condition is stable in order to avoid thrombosis.
- Women and their families must know when to seek emergency help:
  - Significant swelling
  - Headaches, visual disturbances, abdominal pain.
- Fetal growth and well being is monitored. The birth should be hastened if this shows signs of deteriorating. Before 34 weeks gestation, corticosteroids should be given to the woman, if available, to make the fetal lungs mature faster.
- Labour should be induced before the pre-eclampsia becomes too serious. If progress is slow in the second stage, assisted delivery may be needed using forceps or vacuum extractor. Prolonged pushing can raise the BP to dangerous levels.

Note: Restricting food, fluid or salt intake is unhelpful and dangerous.

Severe pre-eclampsia: This is defined as BP 140/100 or more, or 20 mmHg or more above the normal reading, and/or rising proteinuria levels. The woman with severe pre-eclampsia needs:

- Admission to a unit with medical support
- Monitoring of her condition through BP, fluid balance and blood levels including clotting profiles
- Monitoring the fetal condition until mature enough for birth
- Readiness of resuscitation equipment
- Active management:
  - Antihypertensive therapy to protect against complications
  - Anti-convulsant therapy to prevent and control fits
  - Induction of labour or caesarean section.

Note: Drugs do not alter the course of the disorder. Table 35.1 lists the WHO recommended drug regime for severe pre-eclampsia and eclampsia.

For labour and postpartum period see Eclampsia.

Eclampsia: The state of convulsion. 'Eclampsia' means 'flashing lights'. This refers to the visual disturbances women may report prior to convulsions.

Caring for the woman with a rapidly worsening condition:

- Call for medical help.
- Assess for signs of impending eclampsia: epigastric pain, nausea, vomiting, severe headache, jaundice, confusion, restlessness, visual disturbances, rising BP, decreasing urinary output, heavy proteinuria, haematuria.
- Have oxygen and suction available.
- Provide a quiet, darkened room and limit visitors.
- Monitor blood status using bedside clotting test – more than 7 minutes to form a clot, or easy breakdown indicates abnormal clotting.
- Drug therapy as Table 35.1.

Convulsions: Like all epileptiform fits these have four stages:

1. Aura – flashing lights
2. Tonic phase – general rigidity
3. Clonic phase – spasmodic uncontrollable movements
4. Coma.

During a convulsion, remain with the woman and:

- Shout for help
- Protect her without restraining her

- Roll her onto her side (recovery position) when possible to reduce risk of aspiration of vomit, secretions and blood. This is a real risk.
- Ensure her airway is clear all the time
- Administer oxygen by face mask
- Observe and record the duration of the stages.

When the convulsion ceases:

- Aspirate her mouth and throat
- Intubate
- Check her blood pressure.

See Chapter 14 for more information on the care of the unconscious patient.

Labour and delivery with pre-eclampsia and eclampsia

- Deliver as soon as woman is stabilised, even if fetus is immature.
- Induce if vaginal delivery is likely within 12 hours (for eclampsia) or 24 (for severe pre-eclampsia) or fetus is dead.
- Caesarean section if the anticipated time to delivery is longer, or fetal heart rate is abnormal (provided no clotting problems exist).
- Do not leave the woman unattended.
- Monitor vital signs, fluid balance and blood clotting.
- Ergometrine and Syntometrine should not be used in the third stage of labour as they cause hypertension. Use Syntocinon 5-10 units IM.

Post partum care

- Monitor BP at least 4 hourly for 24 hours in pre-eclampsia.
- Continue anticonvulsive therapy for 24 hours after delivery or the last convulsion.
- Continue antihypertensive therapy until diastolic BP is lower than 110.
- Watch for convulsions for 24 hours.
- Speed of recovery depends on the severity of the disorder. The BP may remain high for some weeks.

Those who have pre-eclampsia in one pregnancy are slightly more likely to get it in subsequent pregnancies and so these women should be monitored carefully in the next pregnancy.

Haemorrhage in pregnancy

This section looks at bleeding in early and late pregnancy. These are major causes of maternal and neonatal *morbidity* and mortality.

Table 35.1 WHO recommended drug regime for severe pre-eclampsia and eclampsia

Drug	When used	Dose and route	Comments and warnings
Hydrallazine **Antihypertensive** to prevent cerebral haemorrhage	Diastolic 110 or more, aim to maintain diastolic 90–100	5 mg IV slowly every 5 minutes until BP lowered. Repeat hourly if BP rises. May give IM 12.5 mg every 2 hours.	Side effects: dizziness, faintness, headache, palpitations, tingling of extremities, disorientation. Breastfeeding should be delayed until 48 hours after discontinuation of drug.
or Labetalol	As above	10 mg IV, then 20 mg IV after 10 minutes if BP does not reduce below 110 diastolic. Can be increased to 40 mg after 10 minutes if response remains poor, then 80 mg	Side effects: nausea, vomiting, tingling, bronchospasm, heart failure, hypotension if combined with magnesium sulphate.
Magnesium sulphate **Anti-convulsive**	Convulsions, or to prevent them in severe pre-eclampsia	4 g IV of 20% solution, over 5 minutes and – immediately 10 g IM 50% solution (5 g deeply each buttock). Include 1 ml Lignocaine 2% in same syringe to minimise pain from the injection.	Feeling of warmth, nausea and weakness may be experienced. Before repeating ensure: respiratory rate at least 16/min., patellar reflexes present, urinary output at least 30 ml/hour for last 4 hours. Otherwise withhold or delay.
	If convulsions recur after 15 minutes	2 g IV of 50% solution magnesium sulphate over 5 minutes.	
	Maintenance	5 g IM of 50% solution and 1 ml Lignocaine 2% every 4 hours in alternate buttocks. Continue 24 hours after delivery or last convulsion.	Be prepared for respiratory arrest. Keep resuscitation equipment and antidote ready: calcium gluconate 1 g IV (10 ml 10% solution) slowly until respirations improve.
or Diazepam	If magnesium sulphate unavailable	10 mg IV slowly over 2 minutes loading dose	Neonatal respiratory depression is more likely.
	If convulsions recur	Repeat	Titrate to keep woman sedated but rousable. Giving more than 30 mg in 1 hour risks respiratory depression.
	Maintenance	40 mg IV in 500 ml normal saline or Ringer's lactate.	Do not give more than 100 mg in 24 hours.
	If IV not possible	Give rectally 20 mg in 10 ml syringe – can use rectal catheter.	
	If convulsions not controlled in 10 minutes	10 mg/hour or more depending on size and response	

Note: While receiving magnesium sulphate, the woman should be monitored constantly. Take the pulse, blood pressure and respiratory rate initially every 5 minutes and then every 15 minutes if satisfactory. Watch for signs of toxicity (respiratory depression, loss of reflexes, muscle weakness, nausea, warmth and flushing). Fluid intake and output must also be observed closely. Magnesium sulphate interacts with sedatives and many other drugs, or makes them work more powerfully, so care is needed for example with anaesthesia and with the infant following birth.

Early pregnancy bleeding

Threatened abortion (miscarriage)

Bleeding from the vagina in early pregnancy is usually an indication that the pregnancy is in danger. For what to do when women lose the pregnancy, see Chapter 30. Many women do not lose the fetus which continues to grow. They may have cramps and some bleeding but the cervical os stays closed and the bleeding stops. Usually the fetus grows normally but can be affected if the placenta is damaged. These women might need extra supervision of the fetal growth if facilities exist.

Missed abortion

When the fetus dies in the uterus but is not expelled the signs of pregnancy subside. There may be a stale brown vaginal blood loss. The woman often ceases to feel pregnant and pregnancy tests become negative. Evacuation of the uterus is needed. If the fetus is retained for a long time clotting factors may be affected and disseminated intravascular coagulation (DIC) may follow. The woman could then bleed heavily during the uterine evacuation. If the fetus dies very early in pregnancy the embryonic material is absorbed. A blood mole (sometimes called a carneous mole) may be all that remains. This can cause heavy vaginal bleeding and uterine evacuation may be necessary.

Ectopic (tubal) pregnancy

Implantation of the fertilised ovum occurs outside of the uterus. It may implant in the ovary, abdomen or cervix but the fallopian tube is the most common site, most often near the ovarian end (the ampulla) (see Figure 35.1). Ectopic pregnancy is a common cause of maternal death. Cervical pregnancy is rare but causes massive haemorrhage.

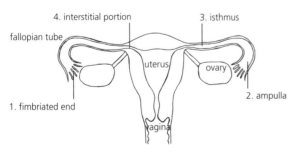

Figure 35.1 *Areas of implantation in ectopic pregnancy*

Predisposing factors: These are related to a narrowed tube:

- Congenital abnormality of the uterus and of the tube
- Scarring of the tubes from previous surgery or ectopic pregnancy. This slows or stops the passage of the fertilised ovum.
- Scarring of the tube from infection such as salpingitis and pelvic inflammatory disease, caused by gonorrhoea or chlamydia
- Use of intrauterine contraceptive device (see Chapter 29).

Diagnosis: Ectopic pregnancy may be confused with appendicitis, pelvic inflammatory disease and ovarian cysts. Normal changes of early pregnancy occur but many women do not yet realise they are pregnant. Symptoms usually arise by 8 weeks gestation:

- Amenorrhoea
- Slight vaginal bleeding or spotting
- Vomiting and diarrhoea sometimes occur
- Abdominal, pelvic or possibly shoulder tip or chest pain (from stimulation of the vagus nerve). Pain may be absent. Hiccups sometimes occur.
- The fertilised ovum may die. It may be expelled from the ovarian (fimbriated) end of the tube or be retained as a tubal mole. This results in a damaged tube and subsequent infertility.
- If the tube ruptures the woman may suddenly feel very unwell, have acute pain and become very shocked. She may collapse.
- Diagnosis can be confirmed with an ultrasound scan if available.

Ectopic pregnancy is very dangerous as massive haemorrhage can occur especially if accurate diagnosis and treatment are delayed.

Very occasionally a fetus will develop in the abdomen after the fertilised ovum has been expelled from the fallopian tube. It can grow to maturity with the placenta on an organ such as the intestines. The baby has to be delivered by *laparotomy*. The placenta may have to be left to disintegrate as removal may cause massive haemorrhage.

Management of tubal pregnancy: Surgery must be very prompt to save the woman's life:

- Blood should be cross-matched in case transfusion is needed. Sometimes the woman's own blood can be collected from the abdomen and re-infused.

- The products of conception may be removed with little damage to the tube. (This increases the risk of future tubal pregnancies.) More often the tube must be removed because of damage (salpingectomy).

Bleeding in late pregnancy

Antepartum haemorrhage is bleeding from or into the genital tract after the 24th week of pregnancy and before the birth of the baby. The term intrapartum haemorrhage may be used when bleeding occurs in the first and/or second stage of labour.

There are two main types of antepartum haemorrhage:

- Placenta praevia. Bleeding from the placenta which is partially or completely situated in the lower uterine segment. Normally, the placenta should be in the upper uterine segment.
- Placental abruption. Bleeding from a normally situated placenta which separates from the uterus before the third stage of labour. A small part may separate, such as an edge, or a large proportion of the placenta. Bleeding can be very severe. It is often known as 'accidental' antepartum haemorrhage.

Placenta praevia

The placenta is located low in the uterus near, or over, the cervix. There are four types of placenta praevia as shown in Figure 35.2.

Bleeding may commence in the last few weeks of pregnancy or earlier. As the lower segment of the uterus starts to grow the placenta begins to separate from it. The placenta does not always separate before labour begins. If it is very low, the birth of the fetus inevitably causes major bleeding and the fetus may die. The woman's life is at serious risk.

Predisposing factors: Scars on the uterus, for example from previous caesarean section or abortion, or many pregnancies, make a low placenta more likely; so may use of an intrauterine contraceptive device. Increasing age and smoking are also linked.

Diagnosis: There may have been occasional or slight blood loss on previous occasions gradually increasing in severity and in frequency. There may have been none.

- There is no pain. The uterus is not tender.
- Bleeding may be light and occasional, or sudden and very heavy.

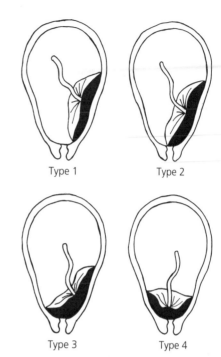

Type 1   Type 2

Type 3   Type 4

Figure 35.2 *Degrees of placenta praevia*

- The fetal presentation will not be engaged except with minor placenta praevia.
- The lie may be oblique or transverse, or unstable.
- The fetus may be moving normally, or less or more than usual (hypoxic responses).
- The diagnosis can be confirmed by ultrasound scan if it is available.

Management: A woman who has painless vaginal bleeding should be referred to a unit where caesarean section can be performed quickly if bleeding becomes severe.

Vaginal examination must not be performed unless caesarean section can be performed at once.

- If bleeding is not severe the woman should be admitted to hospital and her and her baby's condition should be monitored.
- Blood should be grouped, cross-matched and saved ready to give if needed.
- Normal resuscitation measures may be needed such as IV infusion of normal saline or Ringer's lactate.
- Vaginal delivery is permitted if the placenta is grade 1, possibly with grade 2 and bleeding is not heavy. Severe bleeding may occur in labour.
- Caesarean section is used once the fetus is mature for grades 3 and 4, or at once if bleeding becomes severe, or the fetus becomes hypoxic.

- Following the birth, severe bleeding may occur because the lower uterine segment does not contract effectively. There are no criss-cross muscle fibres to constrict or 'tie off' the blood vessels of the placental site very effectively. Syntocinon 20 units in 500 ml of IV fluid may be given to keep the uterus contracted.
- Family planning advice needs to be given because high parity raises the chances of placenta praevia (see Chapter 29).

Placental abruption

This is the separation of a normally located placenta, that is the placenta is implanted in the upper uterine segment. It happens in pregnancy or before the birth of the baby in labour. Bleeding then occurs in the uterine wall behind the placenta that further increases its separation. It may happen following the birth of a first twin.

Predisposing factors: These relate to damage caused somehow to the uterus and placenta:

- Severe pre-eclampsia
- High parity
- Folic acid deficiency
- Trauma to the abdomen
- Sudden reduction in size of the uterus, for example membrane rupture.

There are three **types** of bleeding that may occur:

- Revealed. The placenta separates. Blood flows behind the membranes and down through the vagina so is seen at the vulva. All the blood that is lost is revealed.
- Concealed. Blood lost from the placental site is retained behind the placenta and does not escape from the uterus. It may enter the uterine muscle and damage or saturate it (Couvelaire uterus). The woman complains of pain which can be very severe but no blood loss is seen.
- Mixed. Some of the blood escapes and can be seen, some remains concealed. The degree of shock may be more than expected from the visible blood loss.

Diagnosis: There is always some pain.

- There may be extreme abdominal tenderness with the pain.
- The woman may be shocked. This is difficult to assess properly if she has pre-existing hypertension but she may have a fast pulse rate.
- Abdominal girth measurements will increase and would be an indication of increasing retained loss.

- Blood examination reveals the presence of fibrin breakdown products from clotting.
- Ultrasound scan if available shows placental separation.
- There may be relevant history, for example a blow to the abdomen, membrane rupture, pre-eclampsia. (Women may be reluctant to reveal deliberate violence.)
- The fetus may show hypoxic activity.

Both woman and fetus are at risk:

- The fetus may become hypoxic as functioning placenta is reduced. This depends on the degree of separation.
- The uterus may function poorly, for example in the third stage if it is damaged or saturated with blood. It may then contract poorly. The woman will bleed excessively, labour cannot progress. Bleeding cannot be controlled during the third stage or after caesarean section.

Management: Immediate transfer to a place that can provide blood transfusion and caesarean section is essential.

- Resuscitation measures should be taken first such as commencing an IV infusion.
- Blood must be grouped and cross-matched. Adequate blood transfusion is very important.
- Pain relief may be needed. Pain increases shock.
- Sometimes the bleeding stops and it is possible to wait for the fetus to become mature enough before delivering it. Fetal condition needs to be monitored. The woman may need to remain in hospital.
- If the fetus is alive and bleeding is severe then caesarean section should be performed as soon as possible.
- If the fetus has died then labour should be induced using Syntocinon infusion and artificial rupture of membranes.
- Clotting factors are used up at the site of the bleed. Further bleeding may be more severe. DIC may occur and this has to be reversed by fresh whole blood transfusion to prevent the death of the woman.
- Oxytocin infusion may be needed for the third stage of labour because the damaged uterus cannot contract properly.

General care issues for women who have bled heavily

- Renal function may become impaired if blood volume decreases, so urinary output must be monitored.
- During the postnatal period the woman needs to have the haemoglobin checked and anaemia treated.
- Family planning advice needs to be given so that the woman has enough time to recover before starting another pregnancy.
- Very severe haemorrhage may result in hypoxia of the posterior lobe of the pituitary gland and permanent damage called Sheehan's syndrome. Lactation may fail to commence. Other effects may take at least 6 months to show because the body takes time to excrete all circulating pituitary hormones. Premature aging follows because the thyroid, ovaries and adrenal glands are affected.

Incarcerated uterus

The non-pregnant uterus is normally tipped forward (anteverted) and bent forward (anteflexed). In some women it is directed backwards (retroverted). This may make becoming pregnant difficult and cause bleeding and early pregnancy loss. If it does not straighten by about the 14th week, it may become trapped under the sacral promontory. This is called 'incarceration'. The bladder neck may be compressed. This can cause frequency of urination, abdominal and back pain, and bladder and kidney infection. In severe cases the uterus and bladder may rupture. The woman will need urgent help for urinary retention.

Management

It will be possible to palpate the bladder. It should be catheterised, using a suprapubic catheter if a urethral catheter cannot be passed. An indwelling catheter may be needed until the uterus has risen out of the pelvis. Adopting a knee-chest position may aid the correction of the problem.

Hyperemesis gravidarum

Nausea and some vomiting are normal in pregnancy. Hyperemesis gravidarum is a more serious condition that commences in the first 3 months of pregnancy and resolves itself by 5 months. Women are unable to eat or drink and vomiting can lead to dehydration, electrolyte imbalance, *ketosis*, jaundice and eventually, losing weight. Untreated, the condition may lead to *encephalopathy*, renal and liver damage.

The cause is unknown but there is usually an excess of placental hormones involved. It is more common in multiple pregnancies and hydatidiform mole. Both have extra placental tissue. Psychological factors may be involved. There is thought to be a higher incidence in women who have previously lost a baby or if this pregnancy is unwanted. It is a very depressing condition itself because of the nausea and vomiting and inability to eat.

Management

- Admit to a unit where intravenous fluids can be administered to treat the dehydration and electrolyte imbalance.
- Introduce oral fluids and food gradually.
- The woman needs rest and the opportunity to talk about anxieties.
- Consider other causes of nausea and vomiting and treat.

Hydatidiform mole

Hydatidiform mole is an abnormal growth of the fertilised ovum. It normally contains only an overgrowth of placental tissue although sometimes signs of a dead embryo may be found. The tissue grows rapidly and excessively, developing into water filled vesicles that look like grapes. There are non-invasive forms of the mole and invasive forms that erode the uterus and its blood vessels, and provoke growths elsewhere in the woman's body. In one form, these disappear once the tumour in the uterus is removed. Another form is highly malignant and known as choriocarcinoma.

Diagnosis

- Bleeding may follow *amenorrhoea* and vesicles may be seen in the blood loss.
- Signs of pre-eclampsia or even eclamptic fits occur as early as 16 weeks gestation. With pre-eclampsia before 24 weeks, hydatidiform mole should be considered.
- Anaemia is common.
- The uterus may be very large for dates with no fetal parts or heart beat.
- X-ray or ultrasound will confirm the absence of a fetal skeleton.
- Pregnancy or other hormonal tests are strongly positive.

Referral for careful evacuation of the uterus is essential. Manual vacuum aspiration is now recommended. Haemorrhage may occur. Choriocarcinoma may result if left untreated. Women should be followed up to ensure the pregnancy tests become, and remain, negative.

Polyhydramnios

Polyhydramnios is defined as more than 1500 ml of liquor amnii. The normal maximum is about 1000 ml, then reduces to about 800 ml at term. Liquor absorbs shocks and enables the fetus to move and develop normally. Excess fluid overstretches the uterus which causes problems, and the fetus is often abnormal. There is a risk of cord prolapse, placental abruption and maternal shock when the membranes rupture, and postpartum haemorrhage.

Predisposing factors

These are linked to conditions where excess fluid is produced or the fetus cannot swallow it:
- Diabetes with a large fetus and membranes
- Multiple pregnancy: excess production and an increased incidence of fetal abnormality
- Fetal abnormalities such as:
  - spina bifida: fetal cerebrospinal fluid leaks
  - exomphalos: fetal body fluids leave the fetus's open abdomen
  - oesophageal deformity: fluid is not swallowed by the fetus.

Diagnosis

- Diagnosis is difficult when liquor is below 2500 ml.
- The woman may be very uncomfortable and breathless.
- The uterus is large for dates, abdominal skin tight and shiny.
- Measuring the abdominal girth with a tape measure may indicate rapid increase over time.
- The fetus can be moved between the hands but identification of parts is difficult.
- Fetal heart sounds will be muffled.
- A fluid thrill may be felt if a hand is placed on one side of the abdomen, and the abdomen flicked on the other side. A ripple (thrill) can be felt under the hand.
- A large quantity of fluid will gush out when the membranes rupture.

Management

- Advise the woman with mild polyhydramnios to rest and seek help immediately the membranes rupture.
- Upright positions make breathing easier.
- She may be distressed by the discomfort. About 500 ml fluid can be withdrawn using a large needle (amniocentesis) to relieve the symptoms temporarily but it usually increases again. There is a risk of infection and provoking labour.
- It may be necessary to induce labour, attempting to release the fluid slowly when rupturing the membranes. Move the fetus into a longitudinal lie first. Note that rapid release of large quantities of fluid can cause placental abruption.
- Bed rest is needed once the membranes are ruptured until the fetal head or breech has engaged. This is to prevent cord prolapse. Observe the fetal heart to watch for signs of distress that might indicate cord prolapse.
- Syntocinon infusion may be required in labour if the uterus contracts poorly.
- Intravenous ergometrine or Syntocinon infusion should be ready in case postpartum haemorrhage occurs (see Chapter 39).
- Pass a nasogastric tube down the baby before permitting its first feed to check that the oesophagus and trachea are patent.
- The fetus may have severe abnormalities. The presence of these, if known, will be taken into account when deciding how to help the woman.

Oligo-hydramnios

A small reduction in liquor quantity is expected once the EDD is passed. This causes no problems. If there is significantly too little liquor in pregnancy, fetal movement is not possible. It may be confined in abnormal positions and be born with deformities such as twisted neck, squashed face, talipes of the feet or malformed lungs. Skin adhesions and severe dryness are common.

Common causes are inadequate placental function, non-functioning fetal kidneys, or early membrane rupture. There may be only 500 ml of liquor or less at term. The fetus may be growth retarded – underweight for its maturity.

Diagnosis

- Uterus feels small for dates on palpation.
- Fetal parts may be very easily palpated.
- Little liquor drains once the membranes rupture.

Management

Little can be done to improve the fetal safety except to induce labour if the fetus is becoming hypoxic or not growing. Labour may be unusually painful. Fetal distress may also occur in labour because of placental insufficiency and cord compression. The newborn infant must be examined to detect abnormalities caused by the lack of liquor amnii, and they should be treated if possible. Observe the baby to ensure he passes urine.

Fibroids

A fibroid is a benign tumour in the uterus composed of muscle and fibrous tissue. It is more common in African women than Caucasian and in women over 35.

Fibroids can enlarge slightly in early pregnancy and become soft with an increased blood supply. The effect that the fibroid has on pregnancy depends on the type of fibroid and where it is located:

- Early pregnancy loss
- Enlargement of the uterus
- Twisting of the fibroid causing abdominal pain
- Bleeding
- Infection
- Red degeneration – bleeding in the middle of the fibroid, acute and severe pain and slight high temperature
- Obstruction of the descent of the fetus
- Postpartum haemorrhage if the uterus cannot contract properly, or the placenta cannot separate.

Management

- Low fibroids may be felt on vaginal examination. Others can only be identified if ultrasound scanning is available.
- Women with signs of degeneration need only bed rest and analgesia.
- Fibroids may obstruct labour and caesarean section may be needed.
- Be prepared for postpartum haemorrhage, blood cross-matched and saved if possible, and oxytocin available.
- Removal of fibroids during caesarean section is not recommended because of the risk of bleeding.

Abdominal pain in pregnancy

Many women experience abdominal pain in pregnancy. Midwives need to be able to distinguish between low-risk abdominal pain and problems by examination and asking the right questions. Causes can be divided into two main types:

Those associated with pregnancy: Some causes are physiological but can be very painful. For example pain can be felt from stretching of the round ligaments that support the uterus. Most women experience heartburn, abdominal distension from gas, and constipation. Contractions in later pregnancy can be painful. The normal rotation of the uterus can go too far. This can be relieved by bed rest and change of position. Other conditions can be dangerous and women must be treated:

- Ectopic pregnancy
- Threatened and inevitable abortion
- Fibroids
- Urinary tract infection
- Severe pre-eclampsia
- Preterm labour
- Placental abruption
- Rupture of the uterus.

Incidental problems: Any problem that occurs in non-pregnant women can arise in pregnancy, or even in labour and the puerperium, for example:

- Urinary tract infection
- Ovarian cyst or twisted ovary
- Peptic ulcer
- Sickle cell crisis
- Malignant disease
- Acute inflammatory conditions of, for example, the appendix, gall bladder, bowel.

Women with these conditions need prompt medical care that takes their pregnancies into account.

Prolonged pregnancy

If a pregnancy continues beyond 42 weeks and the dates are accurate then it is considered to be prolonged. This is more common in primigravidae.

The problems associated are:

- Maternal frustration and discomfort
- Abnormal fetal heart rate patterns
- Reduced fetal movements
- Placental insufficiency
- Reduced amniotic fluid

- Meconium staining of the liquor
- Increased incidence of perinatal mortality
- Significant increase in the birth weight of the baby. Some advocate induction of labour at 41 weeks gestation. Others wait until 42 weeks, by which time most women will have given birth. Membrane sweep on vaginal examination may help to stimulate labour to begin.

Membrane sweep: The midwife places her fingers through the internal os of the cervix and gently separates the membranes from the endometrium in the area of the lower uterine segment that is immediately above the internal os.

Nipple stimulation may help to start labour and if the couple have sexual intercourse labour may begin. This may not be culturally acceptable.

It may be necessary to cause labour to begin artificially. This is called induction of labour.

Induction of labour

Indications

Labour may need to be started artificially using hormones or rupturing the membranes surgically. This may be needed for the well being of the mother or the fetus if there is:
- Pre-eclampsia
- Placental abruption
- Renal disease
- Diabetes that is difficult to control
- Hyperemesis gravidarum
- Post term pregnancy
- Reduced fetal movement
- Poor fetal growth
- Intrauterine death
- Haemolytic disease in rhesus isoimmunisation
- Large baby (macrosomia)
- Possibility of a breech presentation.

Contraindications

- Cephalopelvic disproportion
- Oblique lie or shoulder presentation
- Poor fetal condition: labour may endanger the fetus and the best management may be caesarean section.
- Cardiac disease in the mother because any infection may cause endocarditis
- Placenta praevia

The success of the induction depends on how ready the cervix is to respond to attempts to start labour. The Bishop's score is used to make this assessment during a vaginal examination. This is shown in Table 35.2.

Prostaglandins

If the cervix is not ready for induction then prostaglandins (hormones) can be given to 'ripen' the cervix (that is, to cause it to become more ready for labour with an increase in Bishop's score). Prostaglandins can be put into the vagina for this purpose. The pharmacist prepares the medication and the dose needs to be carefully assessed as hypertonic uterine action may result. During the administration the condition of the mother and fetus must be monitored carefully.

Rupture of the membranes (surgical induction or amniotomy)

Once the membranes are ruptured the birth should take place within 24 hours as ascending infection becomes a risk to the mother and the fetus. This means that a caesarean section may have to be performed with all the risks associated with this. Surgical induction should only be undertaken in a place where caesarean section can be performed if labour fails to commence.

Table 35.2 The Bishop's score

Assessment features score	0	1	2	3
Dilatation of the cervix in centimetres	0	1–2	3–4	5–6
Consistency of the cervix	firm	medium	soft	–
Length of cervical canal (cm)	>2	1–2	0.5–1	<0.5
Position of cervix	posterior	mid	anterior	–
Station of presenting part in relation to ischial spines – means above spines, + means below spines	–3	–2	–1	+1 +2

Note: The symbol < means 'less than', and > means 'more than'. Induction is likely to be successful with a Bishop's score of 6 or more.

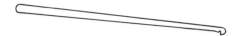

Figure 35.3 *An amnihook*

If the presenting head or breech is engaged in the pelvis then the membranes can be ruptured with an amniotomy hook (see Figure 35.3). If the head or breech is high then the rupturing of the amnion may result in cord prolapse. Another complication is rupture of a fetal blood vessel in membranes lying across the cervical os (vasa praevia).

- The procedure should be as sterile as possible to reduce the risk of infection.
- Note the time of rupturing the membranes.
- The colour and amount of the liquor should be noted.
- Record the fetal heart frequently.
- Wash the vulval area frequently with soap and water to keep it clean.
- Change soiled bed linen as soon as it is soiled.
- Observe the fetal heart before and after the procedure.

Contractions will often begin within a few hours of amniotomy.

Oxytocin

If labour does not begin once the cervix is 'ripe' and the membranes have been ruptured then an intravenous infusion (IVI) of dextrose saline or Hartman's solution is commenced with Syntocinon (synthetic oxytocin) 5 to 10 units in the fluid. The infusion should be started slowly and the rate increased gradually until contractions are established. Specific complications may occur:

- Some women react very quickly and tonic contractions (contractions which come too frequently or which last too long) can occur. Contractions should last no longer than 1 minute or commence more often than every 2 minutes. If this happens the midwife must adjust the rate or discontinue the IVI. Hypertonic contractions can cause the mother great distress and the fetus quickly becomes hypoxic because the oxygen supplied via the placenta is reduced.
- The uterus can rupture if strong contractions continue and the fetus is in an abnormal position.
- The blood pressure may rise.
- It is possible to overload the woman's circulation with the IV fluid.
- The uterus may become dependent on the Syntocinon: if administration stops, the contractions becoming weaker or ceasing. This can cause delay in progress of the labour or lead to postpartum haemorrhage in the third stage of labour.
- Women are more likely to need analgesia in labour with oxytocin.

Urine output should be monitored and the woman encouraged to empty her bladder. Close observation of mother and fetus must continue throughout. The partogram should be maintained to record observations made in labour (see Chapter 36).

■ Activities

1. Jessica tells you she has bled lightly from her vagina on a few occasions recently after having intercourse. She is 28 weeks gestation and tells you she felt no pain. She says her fetus is moving normally. Jessica has walked to your clinic with her mother from six miles away. Decide what you would do next and write a care plan for her.

2. An 18 year old primigravid woman comes to the antenatal clinic in the health centre at 37 weeks gestation. She has a blood pressure of 145/95 with +++ protein in her urine. What action should you take?

36

Medical disorders in pregnancy and childbirth

This chapter considers the effect of some of the medical disorders which may cause difficulties for women during pregnancy and birth. The disorders included are diabetes mellitus, cardiac disease, anaemia, haemolytic disorders, thyroid disease, tuberculosis and malaria.

Introduction

The care of women who have disorders in pregnancy and childbirth needs to be supervised by doctors, especially for diagnosis and medication. It may be necessary for obstetricians and physicians to collaborate in providing care. There may also be specialist nurses involved, for example diabetes specialists. However, midwives must be familiar with women's needs and the conditions. They have an important role in the ongoing support and supervision of women with chronic medical disorders, for example around dietary advice, blood sugar control in diabetes, and weight reduction.

Sexually transmitted infections and HIV are covered in Chapters 31 and 32.

Diabetes

Diabetes becomes more difficult to control during pregnancy because of the effect of the placental hormones, in particular human placental lactogen. The placental hormones enable the body to use glucose more efficiently by reducing its sensitivity to insulin. Some women have difficulty with carbohydrate metabolism but are normally symptom free; these women may present with diabetes during pregnancy. These women may have *glycosuria* and be identified during routine antenatal care.

Diabetes affects the course of pregnancy, at the same time pregnancy affects the diabetes (see Chapter 19).

Effects of diabetes on pregnancy and the fetus

- Infertility – increased difficulty in becoming pregnant
- Early miscarriage
- *Hypoglycaemia* is more common in early pregnancy. Women and their families should be warned of this.
- Pre-eclampsia is more common.
- Diabetic *retinopathy* progresses faster.
- Urinary tract infections: bacteria multiply easily when there is glycosuria.
- Vaginal infections
- Polyhydramnios is common.
- Chorioamnitis (infection of the placental membranes) is more common leading to preterm birth, stillbirth, uterine and neonatal infection, and postnatal sepsis.
- Congenital abnormalities of the fetus are more common.
- The fetus grows larger than normal because of the mother's *hyperglycaemia*.
- The size of the baby means that cephalopelvic disproportion and shoulder dystocia are more common.
- Babies are often born early and have all the problems of prematurity even though they may be normal size or even large for dates (see Chapter 42).
- Stillbirth is more common.
- Neonatal hypoglycaemia is common. The baby produces large amounts of insulin in utero because of the mother's hyperglycaemia. After birth it takes a few days to adjust to lower glucose levels (see Chapter 42).

Effect of pregnancy on diabetes

- Insulin requirements increase during pregnancy. Women who are normally controlled on oral preparations will need to have insulin.
- Kidney problems may occur.
- Eye problems (diabetic retinopathy) may become worse.

Management of the pregnancy

- Women who have diabetes should, if possible, be counselled before becoming pregnant about the importance of controlling blood glucose before and during pregnancy.
- Women should be taught to monitor their own blood glucose levels so that they can adjust their diet to keep the glucose levels stable and as near normal as possible.
- As insulin requirements are higher, they may need short acting insulin twice a day.
- Antenatal care should include frequent blood pressure monitoring and checks on the fetus as it may deteriorate suddenly.

Management of labour

- Labour may need to be induced at about 38 weeks if:
  - the fetus is very large
  - the fetal condition deteriorates
  - control of the diabetes is poor
  - the woman's condition deteriorates.
- Women with stable blood sugar levels may be permitted to labour spontaneously. Induction of labour does not improve neonatal survival in these women.
- Caesarean section is only necessary if the woman's condition deteriorates.
- Blood glucose levels should be monitored hourly during labour and insulin given as necessary. A blood glucose level of less than 7 mmol/l is desirable.

The postnatal period

- Insulin requirements return to normal immediately after delivery. The diet and insulin requirements may need adjustment in breastfeeding women.
- Family planning/spacing should be discussed and methods considered carefully (see Chapter 29). A barrier method is probably the best choice. The contraceptive pill increases insulin demand and intrauterine devices may cause infection. Women who do not want any more children may be offered tubal ligation as risks increase with the age of the mother.

Care of the baby

Babies of diabetic mothers behave like immature babies (see Chapter 42). The blood sugar needs to be monitored and feeding commenced immediately, as hypoglycaemia is common.

Cardiac disease in pregnancy

The most common form of heart disease seen during pregnancy is valve damage due to rheumatic heart disease. This may not be known about before pregnancy. The physiological changes of pregnancy in the cardiovascular system cause heart problems to become worse partly because cardiac output is increased (see Chapters 11 and 34). This is even more noticeable in multiple pregnancies. Extra cardiac load is experienced at three particular times and women may be at greater risk of heart failure then:

- 28–32 weeks of pregnancy when the blood volume is at its greatest
- During labour contractions
- During the third stage of labour and first few postnatal hours when blood is diverted from the uterus into the circulation. Digoxin and diuretics may be needed.

Recognising and treating cardiac failure

See Chapter 11 for signs and symptoms and general advice. **Note:** Heart failure can result from nutritional deficiency and anaemia.

Management of cardiac disease during pregnancy

- Iron and folic acid supplements should be given to prevent anaemia and reduced oxygen supplies.
- Infection (gums, teeth, chest or urinary) may cause heart valve infection so antibiotics should be given if infection is suspected.
- Blood pressure monitoring, and perhaps medication, are necessary as hypertension increases the risk.
- Obesity increases the risk so women who are overweight should be given advice about their diet.
- Tobacco smoking should be avoided.

- Women who have cardiac disease are more likely to develop *thrombosis*. If bed rest or surgery is required, heparin may be needed to prevent this. Warfarin can cause fetal abnormalities and death. Long support stockings should be worn if they are available.

Management during labour

- The woman should be admitted to a centre where there is a doctor available if possible.
- Labour should be allowed to commence spontaneously; medical induction is more stressful and surgical induction is more likely to cause infection, perhaps resulting in endocarditis.
- Vaginal birth is safer than caesarean section; heart failure is not a reason for surgery. However, women should be prepared for caesarean section if significant obstetric problems are anticipated, as emergency surgery always has a greater risk of serious consequences than planned surgery.
- Careful monitoring of the woman's condition is essential. She may need oxygen therapy.
- Keeping a careful fluid balance record is important as it is easy to cause overload with intravenous fluids.
- Antibiotics are given to prevent bacterial endocarditis.
- Women should labour in as comfortable position as possible.
  - The upright or left lateral positions are safer than lying flat as compression of the vena cava is a greater risk to a woman with a diseased heart.
  - The lithotomy position should be avoided if possible as this can lead to a sudden severe rise in the blood pressure and increases the risk of deep vein thrombosis and pulmonary embolus.
- Pain causes extra stress and anxiety so appropriate analgesia is important. Epidural analgesia can reduce the cardiac load and decrease pulmonary oedema so is useful if available. Extra care is needed when the epidural is discontinued as the blood pressure may rise at this point. Spinal anaesthesia is not advised.
- Sedation and regional anaesthesia may be used for caesarean section.
- Long pushing efforts can cause the cardiac output to fall. It is safer for the woman to make several short pushes during expulsive contractions as she feels the urge. Assisted delivery with ventouse extraction or forceps and episiotomy may be required if cardiac problems increase during pushing.
- Avoid active management of the third stage. Ergometrine must not be given as it causes rapid, strong contractions of the uterus. The sudden increase in the blood volume that results from compression of uterine vessels leads to increased cardiac problems. Intramuscular Syntocinon 10 units can be given to reduce haemorrhage.
- If oxytocin infusion is needed by a woman in heart failure, the WHO advises giving an intravenous infusion of Syntocinon at double dose but slow rate to avoid fluid overload. Frusemide 40 mg IV should be given at the same time to avoid pulmonary oedema.

Postnatal care

- Antibiotics are continued for 10 days until there is no risk of infection at the placental site.
- The woman's cardiac condition must be closely monitored as she is at risk of pulmonary oedema. Diuretics may be necessary.
- Anticoagulants are given to prevent thrombosis.
- Breastfeeding should be encouraged. If the woman is on cardiac drugs that are likely to affect the baby, she may need to be advised.
- Family planning advice will help the woman to avoid pregnancy until her condition has stabilised.
- Extra help at home will enable the woman to rest more after the birth.

Late cardiac failure occurs in some parts of Africa and may be related to traditional practices such as giving large amounts of food to increase the weight. 'Heating' or 'smoking' postnatal women over fires is common in several parts of the world and increases the risk of heart failure. Weather conditions such as high humidity and heat, and high sodium diets, appear also to be involved. This happens more often with older and *multiparous* women and in multiple pregnancy. Digoxin and diuretics may be given and bed rest and low salt diet advised. Women improve but the condition may recur in future pregnancies. Also many women develop hypertension, heart failure and embolism later.

Anaemia in pregnancy

For further information see Chapters 12 and 35.

Anaemia is common in pregnancy and causes

particular problems for malnourished women, those who have had frequent pregnancies, those who have malaria or are living with HIV or have AIDS. Anaemia can be implicated in many instances of maternal death. Women often compensate for anaemia in early pregnancy. Then in late pregnancy they may become breathless and easily tired, and may experience heart failure. In labour they are unable to compensate for bleeding and are more likely to die than non-anaemic women. Particular attention should be given to encourage adolescent girls to take a diet that helps to avoid anaemia as they approach childbearing years.

Anaemia also causes placental insufficiency, fetal hypoxia, intrauterine death and preterm labour. Fetal hypoxia in labour, growth retardation, prematurity and neonatal anaemia is common. Babies may need iron and folic acid supplementation after 3–4 weeks to make up for depleted iron stores. They build their iron stores naturally in pregnancy only.

The WHO defines pregnancy anaemia as haemoglobin of less than 11 g/dl, or 10.5 g/dl in late pregnancy. The physiological changes during pregnancy cause a drop in the Hb concentration, so a pregnant woman might not be considered to be anaemic until the Hb is less than 10 g/dl. Hb levels of 7 g/dl or less are common in women in developing countries.

Causes

- Deficiencies in the diet, especially micro-nutrients such as iron, folates, vitamins A, C and B12
- Excessive haemolysis of red blood cells due to haemoglobinopathies, such as sickle cell disease, thalassaemia, Glucose 6 phosphate dehydroginase (G6PD) deficiency, infections and, very commonly, malaria. Common infections causing anaemia are urinary, tuberculosis and HIV.
- Decreased bone marrow production of red blood cells, such as in the presence of infection
- Increased blood loss, for example hookworms and other parasites in endemic areas
- Frequent pregnancies which deplete the iron stores needed to make red blood cells.

Signs and symptoms

- Moderate anaemia 7–10 g/dl. Women usually compensate but may tire or become breathless more easily. Some pallor of mucosa, conjunctiva, nails and palms may be noticed.
- Severe anaemia 4–7 g/dl. There may be headaches,

dizziness, rapid heart beat, breathlessness, fatigue and inability to work. Pallor is noticeable. Common signs and symptoms are systolic heart murmurs, and neck pulses may be visible. The diastolic blood pressure may fall while the systolic BP rises slightly or remains the same. The woman may have leg, and eventually generalised, oedema. As proteinuria can also occur, severe anaemia may be mistaken for pre-eclampsia.
- Very severe anaemia less than 4 g/dl. Cardiac failure and low circulating blood volume occurs. In cardiac failure the heart muscle lacks oxygen. Half of untreated women are likely to die.

Note: Signs and symptoms will always include those of any underlying disease.

Investigations for anaemia

- Review the diet.
- Blood specimens should go to the laboratory for haemoglobin and/or haematocrit, and serum ferritin and serum folate levels if possible:
  - Haemoglobin estimation
  - Haematocrit (packed cell volume) provides an accurate estimation. Less than 20 per cent indicates severe anaemia.
  - Serum ferritin measures the woman's iron stores.
  - A blood picture will tell what size the cells are. Iron deficiency anaemia causes the cells to be small (microcytic), folic acid deficiency results in large, immature cells (macrocytic or megaloblastic anaemia).
- Blood smear for malaria where appropriate
- Stool specimen for parasitic infection in areas of high prevalence
- Urine for infection

Management

- Malaria prophylaxis or treatment should be given to pregnant women where appropriate. The physiological changes that take place during pregnancy reduce any immunity they may have built up. Non-immune women may be severely affected.
- Parasitic infections or urinary tract infections should be treated.
- Give advice on achieving a diet high in iron, folates, and vitamin A and C, and with some animal fat if possible (see Chapter 34).
- Anaemic women need oral iron, folic acid and

vitamin supplements but may find them difficult to take (see Chapter 34). **Note:** Women with haemolytic disorders should not be given iron unless blood examination indicates the need. The following regime may be followed for iron-deficiency anaemia:

- Ferrous sulphate 200 mg twice daily
- Folic acid 1 mg daily (5 mg or more may be advised)
- Vitamin A 5000 iu daily.

- Some women respond poorly to oral iron or cannot take it. Severe iron-deficiency anaemia may also be discovered late in pregnancy. These women may be given intramuscular iron. This must be given deep into the muscle as it stains the skin.
- It may be necessary to give the iron as an intravenous infusion, in the form of iron dextran. A test dose must be given first as it may cause anaphylactic shock (see Chapter 5).
- Blood transfusion of packed cells can be life-saving but should be given only to the most anaemic women because of the risks of HIV and hepatitis B infection:
  - Very severe anaemia less than 4 g/dl with heart failure
  - Severe anaemia less than 7 g/dl if major surgery is needed

  Frusemide 40 mg should be given IV with each unit.
- Intravenous infusions can cause pulmonary oedema and death so should only be used with great care in labour and early postnatal period.
- Minimise blood loss by:
  - avoiding episiotomy if possible and repairing damage immediately
  - active management of the third stage. Ergometrine may cause circulation overload in severe anaemia and should not be given in heart failure (see above).
- IV Frusemide, oxygen and sitting the women up helps if overload or pulmonary oedema occurs.

Haemolytic disorders

(See Chapter 12)

Sickle cell trait

Women who have the sickle cell trait do not usually have symptoms, even though there is an increased demand for oxygen during pregnancy. They are likely to have a high serum iron, so should not be given iron

supplements. They should be protected from severe stresses.

Sickle cell disease

This is an important cause of maternal death especially in women with less access to services. Some women appear well in pregnancy, others have severe haemolytic anaemia and skeletal changes such as contracted pelvis. Cardiac and renal failure may occur. Crises are more likely with advancing pregnancy through to a few days after delivery. *Haemolysis* is especially severe in women who have falciparum malaria as well as sickle cell. A condition similar to pre-eclampsia may occur but with systolic hypertension instead of diastolic, and proteinuria with no oedema. Sedatives must be avoided. Blood transfusion may be needed for severe anaemia or heart failure but iron overload is a risk.

- Screening for sickle cell disease is advisable if available.
- Regular antenatal checks are needed to detect complications and monitor haemoglobin levels.
- Iron supplements should be given only if there is a low serum iron.
- Folic acid 5 mg daily must be given as demand is increased.
- A blood transfusion may be necessary but only to correct severe anaemia.
- Malarial treatment and prevention is vital.
- Sickle cell crisis should be prevented by:
  - Avoiding exposure to cold, excessive physical exertion, dehydration, infection and acidosis
  - Careful infection prevention
  - Adequate oral fluid intake, which is important especially in labour and the early puerperium
  - Avoiding hypoxia during labour
  - Giving oxygen before, during and after anaesthesia
  - Ensuring blood is available for transfusion if needed in labour
  - Giving antibiotics in labour
  - Avoiding blood loss in labour (see severe anaemia)
  - Avoiding prolonged labour.
- Prophylactic antibiotics may be given in the postnatal period to prevent infection. Wound infection is more likely.
- Women should be encouraged to breastfeed and keep very well hydrated.

Thalassaemia

The general principles of care are the same as for sickle cell anaemia. The prevention of anaemia and infection are the priorities to prevent red blood cell breakdown. Folic acid supplementation is very important. Iron is avoided unless iron stores are low. Malaria prophylaxis and treatment are important. Women may have contracted pelves so prolonged and obstructed labour is important to avoid, or identify and treat. Placental insufficiency, low birth weight, fetal hypoxia and birth asphyxia may occur and the fetus may die in pregnancy. The seriousness of thalassaemia depends on the type and whether the faulty genes have been inherited from one or both parents. This varies in different populations, thalassaemia being more common in parts of the Middle East and Mediterranean and some parts of Asia.

Thyroid disease
(See Chapter 12)

Thyroid problems can be difficult to diagnose in pregnancy because they may be similar to the normal changes that occur (see Chapter 34).

Hypothryoidism

Development of the fetus will be affected if there is insufficient iodine for healthy growth. Women who take medicines for an under-active thyroid may need to have the drugs adjusted whilst breastfeeding. These women need a higher intake of iodine in their diets. This can be difficult to achieve when they have no access to sea fish. However, iodised salt is available in many countries now.

Hyperthyroidism or thyrotoxicosis

Pregnancy is uncommon as hyperthyroidism causes infertility. Some women experience a sudden increase of normal thyrotoxic symptoms. This is more likely in labour or because of caesarean section or infection. It can lead to collapse and severe breathing difficulties and needs to be treated with fluid replacement, cooling and medication to reduce the action of the thyroid.

During pregnancy, thyrotoxic women need:

- Extra calories in the diet
- Good fluid intake especially if diarrhoea occurs
- Propylthiouracil, which is better than Carbimazole in pregnancy and during breastfeeding as it has less effect on the baby
- Monitoring of the pulse rate.

- A partial thyroidectomy may be needed during the second trimester to avoid cardiac failure.

Treatment given to the mother may affect the fetal thyroid gland. Growth retardation, preterm labour and perinatal death can occur. Pre-eclampsia is more common which may have similar effects on the fetus.

Tuberculosis See Chapter 25

Diagnosis of tuberculosis (TB) may be delayed in pregnant women because symptoms such as tiredness and feeling unwell are similar. It is important to consider TB when women have *pyrexia* without explanation, or suffer abortion or preterm labour. Women with HIV need to be tested for TB in pregnancy. Chest X-rays may have to be done and the fetus must be protected using a lead apron. Treatment needs to be started as early as possible to reduce the effects of TB on mother and baby and the risk of death of either. Early treatment also protects the newborn infant from infection.

- Drug treatment can be the same as for non-pregnant TB patients (see Chapter 25). It is now thought that all drugs, including rifampicin, can be given in pregnancy, although streptomycin can cause deafness in the infant.
- Women with tuberculosis are likely to be anaemic. Each condition makes the other worse and both must be treated.
- Assisted or operative delivery may be needed for women who are breathless, preferably avoiding inhalational anaesthesia.
- Haemorrhage and sepsis can re-activate TB.
- Good nutrition after the birth and extra help at home are very important to prevent re-activation of TB.
- Women should be advised to delay the next pregnancy until TB has been controlled for 2 years. Oral contraceptives are less effective when using rifampicin.

Babies may be born prematurely and underweight (see Chapter 42). The newborn needs to be protected from TB as soon as possible as the bacillus is transmitted in breast milk as well as by droplet infection. Breastfeeding is, however, very important because of the risks of artificial feeding. The regime is as follows:

- Isoniazid syrup 5 mg per kg weight given daily for 6 weeks (This may be given for 6 months if the woman has positive sputum.)
- Tuberculin testing is carried out after 3–6 weeks.
- If negative then BCG vaccine is given.

- If positive the baby is assessed and treated.

Isoniazid may not protect the baby adequately, making the early treatment of the mother even more important.

Vitamin K should be given to the baby, if possible, to prevent haemorrhage as a side effect of the mother's medication.

Malaria

Malaria affects pregnant women in different ways depending on the level of *immunity* they have. Falciparum malaria is thought to cause more problems than other types (see Chapter 26). Midwives providing antenatal care have an essential role in preventing problems. Communities and traditional birth attendants are important in motivating women.

Immunity and transmission of malaria in pregnancy

All women have an increased susceptibility to malaria when pregnant because they have suppressed immune systems. Women living with HIV are also more vulnerable to malaria because of reduced immunity. For pregnant women on low incomes, these factors lead to a deadly combination of malaria, anaemia, poor nutrition and HIV.

The degree of immunity women have developed is the main factor that influences how malaria affects them and their babies (see Chapter 26). Because of the reduced time exposed to malaria, young primigravid women may be more seriously affected than multigravid women. Non-immune travellers to a malarial area are at most risk, or pregnant women who have stopped using preventive treatment, or have lost their immunity after a period away.

Pregnant women with some immunity: Anaemia and parasites in the placenta are the main causes of problems:

- Women may start the pregnancy anaemic.
- They may not have obvious fever and other symptoms.
- They may have enlarged spleens and an increasing number of parasites in the blood. Parasite levels can rise rapidly once pregnant but drop in later weeks. These changes are most marked in younger and primigravid women.
- The effect on the woman of having malaria repeatedly can still be severe. Parasites continue

to invade and destroy red blood cells so haemolytic anaemia increases. Later, women become short of folates. This happens because the bone marrow works harder to make new cells causing *megaloblastic* anaemia.

- *Antibodies* pass across the placenta to the fetus which then has *passive immunity*. This *passive immunity* protects the infant for a short time after the birth (see Chapter 46).

Pregnant women with low immunity or none: These women are more likely to have a malaria attack than those with some immunity and are more badly affected by the infection itself. The effect on these women is as follows:

- High fever, and extreme weakness during an attack
- High probability of spontaneous abortion or preterm labour because of fever
- Hypoglycaemia may occur especially with quinine therapy.
- Cerebral malaria may be confused with eclampsia.
- They may die of a malaria attack or because of severe anaemia.

Note: Women with low immunity are much more likely to have malaria when pregnant than when not pregnant.

Effects of malaria common to both:

- Any woman who has high fever may abort, suffer a late intrauterine death, or commence labour early.
- The fetus may suffer growth retardation, become *hypoxic* in labour and be born with low birth weight.
- Anaemia and placental parasites increase these risks to the fetus.
- Placental parasites are very common, particularly in first pregnancies and very young women. The damage is to placenta function. Parasites do not cross to the fetus.
- Women can have placental parasites without symptoms of malaria.

Prevention and treatment of malaria in pregnancy

- At least 2 doses of locally effective antimalarial drugs should be given in pregnancy (see Chapter 34). Regular preventive treatment is safer but expensive. If mefloquine is used, it should be commenced in the second trimester because it can harm the fetus.
- Oral iron and folic acid supplements must be given in pregnancy.

- Women should be advised to use insecticide treated bed nets.
- Women who have symptoms must be treated:
  - With oral antimalarials if symptoms are mild
  - Under close observation for those unlikely to be immune, or who have severe symptoms, or signs of abortion or labour.
- Labouring women may need IV antimalarial therapy. Blood loss must be minimised because of the anaemia.
- A malaria attack in the postnatal period may be confused with postnatal *sepsis*. Mild sepsis can be life-threatening when combined with malaria and anaemia.

■ Activities

1. Plan the care you would give to Mumtaz who comes to the antenatal clinic where you work at 18 weeks of pregnancy. She has diseased heart valves from having rheumatic fever as a child. Consider also what support she might need at home and how you could help her to get this.

2. Jasmin tells you she wants to have another baby soon but is feeling tired and unwell. She suffered a malaria attack at 34 weeks in her first pregnancy. Her baby was born prematurely and died. What would you advise her to do now to increase her chances of having a healthy baby, and what are the special points to be thought about when she does become pregnant?

37

Normal labour

This chapter provides information about what happens in normal labour and the influences on it. It describes the care that women need in normal labour to ensure that the normal process continues without being disturbed and becoming abnormal. Also included are the midwifery activities needed to monitor mother and baby and detect problems that may arise.

Introduction

You may need to refer to Chapter 34 where the changes that happen to women's bodies in pregnancy are described.

Note: Vaginal examinations and assisting at the birth involve the use of aseptic techniques and universal precautions (see Chapter 6). This is to protect the woman and her baby, and also the midwife.

Childbirth is a continuous process that commences gradually in the late stages of pregnancy and ends with a healthy baby and a healthy lactating woman. It is normally divided into three stages to make it easier to describe. It is important to remember that these stages are not necessarily well divided in real life:

First stage: From the onset of regular painful contractions until the cervix of the uterus is fully dilated

Second stage: From full cervical dilatation until the completed birth of the baby

Third stage: From the birth of the baby until the placenta and membranes have been completely expelled, including the control of haemorrhage

Progress in labour depends on three main factors. These are often known as the powers, the passage and the passenger. The powers are the contractions of the uterus and the effect they have on the cervix. Progress also depends on the reproductive tract through which the fetus must pass – the passage. Success also depends on the fetus – the passenger – and the way its shape and size influence the descent through the pelvis. (Bear in mind that the fetus is not entirely an inactive 'passenger' as it influences labour with the hormones it produces.)

Preparing for action

How labour starts is still unclear. Oestrogen increases and becomes more dominant than progesterone as the pregnancy reaches its last weeks. This results in the release of prostaglandins from the decidua (the thickened endometrial lining of the uterus). Prostaglandins allow the oxytocin that is circulating in the woman to become active and enable the myometrium (the uterine muscle) to contract. The fetus also produces oxytocin and a type of oestrogen. Contractions of the myometrium increase gradually and become rhythmic until women become aware of them during the last two months of pregnancy. These Braxton Hicks contractions can be uncomfortable and may be painful, so making women think they are in labour. This is sometimes known as 'false' labour.

The contractions of the outer longitudinal muscle layer become more coordinated gradually, spreading down from the fundus. During these weeks the lower uterine segment has formed and the part of the fetus that is presenting will have sunk down into it (known as lightening, see Chapter 34). It should have engaged in the pelvis in primigravid women. A ring forms between the upper and lower uterine segments called a retraction ring.

With each contraction the longitudinal muscle fibres become shorter (known as 'retraction'). As they contract and retract, they pull upwards on the cervix where the circular muscle fibres are becoming relaxed. The connective tissue in the cervix is being softened by relaxin and the canal begins to widen (known together as 'ripening'). The effect of these processes is to change the shape of the ripening cervix:

- First the internal cervical os disappears into the lower uterine segment (being 'taken up'). The cervix thins. In the primigravid the cervix is taken up before thinning and dilatation, in the multigravid woman this all happens together.
- A sticky mucus plug (the operculum) that is streaked with blood may be lost from the cervix. This is often called the 'show'.

This preparation process can be felt on vaginal examination. It does not mean that labour has commenced yet. These changes can be seen in Figure 37.1. This process begins in the last 2 weeks or so of pregnancy in primigravidae, and during early labour in multigravidae.

Many women become very energetic. Some say that the burst of energy and work, such as scrubbing floors, may even help the fetus to take up a good position. Others become increasingly tired with loss of sleep and problems with finding comfortable positions. Reassurance is needed and encouragement to keep active. Many women stop having sexual intercourse around this time for reasons of discomfort or because of local traditions and taboos. There is no physical reason to cease intercourse as long as the membranes are intact. It is possible that it may help to initiate

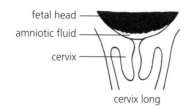

cervix long

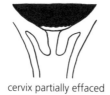

cervix partially effaced

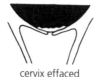

cervix effaced

Figure 37.1 *Effacement of the cervix*

labour when the woman is ready. Women need to know that they do not normally need to go to the planned place of birth until regular painful contractions come at decreasing intervals. This finally depends on the distance from the place of birth, and the transport facilities available. Some women may take advantage of opportunities to travel before the onset of labour and lodge with relatives or in a maternity hostel or 'waiting home'. Meanwhile they should keep active, eat and drink normally and rest when tired.

The first stage of labour
Contractions: the power behind labour

The first signs of labour are usually contractions that become more frequent, powerful and painful and the 'show'. Some women will begin to lose liquor amnii. This is usually considered as a reason for calling the midwife or preparing to go to the birth facility. There is risk of infection once the membranes have ruptured, and of cord prolapse if the head is not engaged (see Chapter 39).

The contractions of labour are considered painful by most women. This may be due to the *ischaemia* which occurs in the muscle when contractions last for 30 seconds or more. The contractions of the longitudinal myometrial fibres begin to pull back the stretchy cervical os so that it begins to open or dilate.

Contractions increase in intensity and frequency because of a feed-back mechanism. The contractions, and the pressure of the fetal presenting part on the cervix, bring about further release of prostaglandins and oxytocin. A fetus in a good position leads to labour being more efficient. This process continues until the birth of the baby.

Gradually the cervical os dilates and becomes part of the lower uterine segment. One continuous passage develops between the vagina and the uterus and no cervix can be felt on vaginal examination (see Figure 37.2). This is called 'full dilatation' and this is the end of the first stage of labour.

Contractions normally begin irregularly and then settle into a regular pattern of one contraction every 10 to 15 minutes, lasting a few seconds. They gradually get closer together until they start every 2 to 3 minutes and last 45 seconds or more. There are two distinct phases to the first stage of labour, the first is often called the latent phase when dilatation of the cervix is slow. This can take many hours. During this

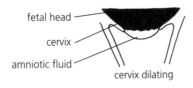

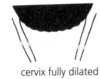

cervix fully dilated

Figure 37.2 *Dilatation of the cervix*

time the woman is better off in her home surroundings and does not normally need monitoring. Then the woman enters the active phase when contractions are stronger and closer together and dilatation speeds up. This is considered to be when the cervical os has dilated to about 3–4 cm diameter.

At some point during the first stage of labour, or during the second stage of labour, the membranes will rupture and the woman will lose liquor amnii from the vagina. This occurs when the bag of membranes comes under such tension from contractions that it bursts and the liquor is released. This causes a release of prostaglandins from the decidua and so contractions become more frequent. Membrane rupture should be allowed to happen spontaneously because:

- Rupturing membranes artificially, using toothed forceps or an amnihook, may introduce infection and so puts the mother and baby at risk.
- Cervical dilatation usually progresses more smoothly if there is a 'bag' of liquor formed in front of the fetal presenting part (the 'forewaters').
- Intact membranes help to protect the fetal umbilical cord from being compressed which would reduce the fetal oxygen supply.

If labour is not progressing well artificial rupture of membranes is sometimes considered (see Chapter 39).

Midwives need to observe and record this process as follows:

- Watch the behaviour of the woman. With experience this can provide some idea of progress and how she is reacting.
- Assess the strength, frequency and duration of contractions using one hand laid on the woman's abdomen. Make sure there are at least 60 seconds between contractions to allow the fetus to obtain enough oxygen.

- Observe for bleeding or the presence of liquor amnii and its colour. Brown or green colouring indicates that the fetus is passing meconium (faeces) and may be *hypoxic*.
- Assess the descent of the presenting part by abdominal examination (see Chapter 34).
- Record the rate of descent of the fetal presenting part through the vagina.
- Record the rate of cervical dilatation so that delay is recognised.

Vaginal examination (VE) is needed for the last two points: assessing cervical dilatation and descent of the presenting part. VE is uncomfortable, presents an infection risk and many women find it very upsetting. It should therefore be performed only when essential, not because of routines. If the woman is obviously progressing well, VE is probably not needed.

The passage

This is the bony canal of the pelvis and the soft tissues – the cervix, vagina and introitus. The normal gynaecoid pelvis permits a normal sized and positioned fetus to pass through without problems (see Chapter 34). Other types of pelvis can cause serious delays and obstruction (see Chapter 39). Women with abnormally shaped pelves need to give birth in facilities where caesarean section can be performed if necessary.

The passenger

The progress of labour is hindered or prevented if the fetus is too big or has an abnormal lie or presentation or position (see Chapter 34). The fetus needs to be in the best possible situation in order for labour to progress normally.

The fetal skull

The largest part of the fetus is its head. The fetal head fits well in the maternal pelvis and passes through it in labour without problems provided:

- It is not too big.
- It remains tucked down (flexed) onto its chest throughout.
- The diameters reduce slightly in size (see 'moulding' below).
- The fetus commences labour in a normal cephalic presentation and anterior position.
- The pelvis is normally shaped with no deformities and is not too small.

- The pelvic joints are not prevented from opening apart slightly.
- There are good labour contractions.

The head changes shape in labour. The main skull bones are soft and curved, and are not yet joined together by bone. There is only membrane between them. The places where two bones meet are the sutures. The larger gaps where three or four meet are the fontanelles. These sutures and fontanelles allow the brain to grow rapidly during pregnancy and babyhood while allowing for the presenting diameters to become a little smaller and the head to change shape.

The head changes shape in labour through a process known as moulding. It quickly returns to a rounded shape after the birth. Moulding happens in two ways:

- The flat bones overlap slightly (see Figure 37.3).
- The head is squeezed by the tight birth canal. It takes on a slightly elongated and compressed shape. The shape resulting from a normal labour is shown in Figure 37.3.

It is important to understand the features of the fetal skull as these are used to describe what happens in labour and make sure the normal process is happening. The drawings in Figures 37.4 and 37.5 show the main parts of the skull from the side and from the top. The most useful features to know are the areas of the skull that are used to describe the position of the head

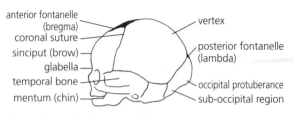

Figure 37.4 *The fetal skull (side view)*

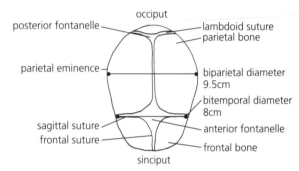

Figure 37.5 *The fetal skull (top view)*

during labour. These are the ones you will feel on abdominal examination and on vaginal examination.

Notice that the two fontanelles are different:

- The anterior fontanelle, just above the baby's forehead, is diamond-shaped. Four bones meet here, two frontal bones and two parietal bones. Between the frontal bones is the frontal suture. Between the parietal bones is the sagittal suture. Between the parietal and frontal bones is the coronal suture. This fontanelle will be felt as crossed-over bones in labour because of moulding.
- The posterior fontanelle, at the back of the head, is triangular and very small. It is the place where the occipital bone (back of the head) meets the two parietal bones. The suture between the parietals is again the sagittal. Between the parietal and the occipital bone is the lambdoidal suture. The bones overlap here in labour because of moulding.

Perhaps the easiest way to remember the difference between fontanelles is that three sutures = posterior fontanelle, and four sutures = anterior fontanelle. The posterior fontanelle should be easier to feel during a vaginal examination. Feeling a lot of the anterior fontanelle suggest the head is deflexed (see below). But it is easy to become confused as you will not be able to feel them all. Some will be higher up behind bone, and

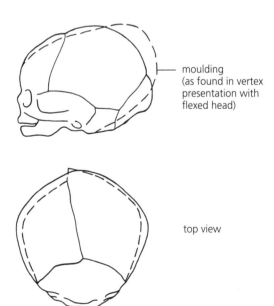

Figure 37.3 *Moulding of the fetal head*

269

there is often some swelling caused by pressure from the cervix on the scalp of the fetus (caput succedaneum).

The head needs to remain flexed because this puts the smallest and roundest shape through the pelvis and also dilates the cervix best. If the head is deflexed, or extended, then much wider parts try to pass through and may become stuck if they are too large. The term used to indicate how wide the different positions are is 'diameter'. You can see how different the diameters are and what they are called from Figure 37.6.

Small drawings called 'touch pictures' are often used to indicate what can be felt on vaginal examination. They can be used in women's care notes to record what you have felt. Figure 37.7 is an example showing a normal position near the end of labour.

This shows a posterior fontanelle to one side nearer the front (woman's symphysis pubis). This would be felt just as a slight dent, or as crossover between the bones if the head is moulded. There are two short lambdoidal sutures meeting the long sagittal suture in a Y shape. The sagittal suture is at an angle showing the head is rotating.

Abdominal examination in labour

The skills of detecting the lie, presentation and position on abdominal examination are vital ones for midwives (see Chapter 34).

The same observations need to be made as in pregnancy, with the addition of others:

- Fundal height and size of the uterus: Is the fetus small or large?
- Number of fetuses: Make sure that there are not undiagnosed twins.
- Lie of the fetus
- Presentation: Breech presentation can go undetected in pregnancy but must be identified at the onset of labour as it will influence management of the labour.
- Position: Knowing whether the occiput is anterior or posterior will influence the position you may encourage the woman to take in labour. You may be able to tell if it is rotating by the position of the fetal back.
- Descent and engagement of the fetal head: Flexing of the head and descent of the presentation part can be determined on palpation.
- Uterine activity: Frequency, duration, strength and length of contractions can be noted.

You may need to confirm abdominal findings by vaginal examination. At the same time you can decide on progress toward the birth:

- Confirming the onset of labour
- Assessing the state of the cervix and its dilatation
- Assessing the descent of the fetus.
- You will also decide whether there is umbilical cord in front of the presenting part.

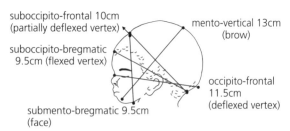

suboccipito-frontal 10cm
(partially deflexed vertex)

mento-vertical 13cm
(brow)

suboccipito-bregmatic
9.5cm (flexed vertex)

occipito-frontal
11.5cm
(deflexed vertex)

submento-bregmatic 9.5cm
(face)

Figure 37.6 *Diameters of the fetal head*

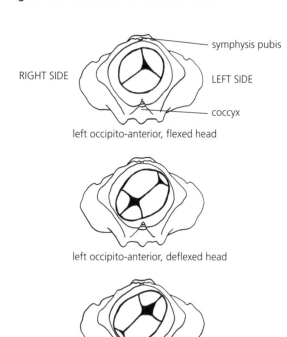

symphysis pubis

RIGHT SIDE

LEFT SIDE

coccyx

left occipito-anterior, flexed head

left occipito-anterior, deflexed head

right occipito-posterior, deflexed head

Figure 37.7 *Touch pictures of the fetal head in relation to the symphysis pubis*

Pp Ten steps of vaginal examination (VE) in labour

1. Check with the woman that there has been no bleeding in the last half of pregnancy. If there

time:										
09.00	10.00	11.00	12.00	13.00						
fetal heart (bpm):										
140	142	155	141	144						
maternal pulse (bpm):										
80	82	80	78	81						
maternal bp:										
110/ 70	112/ 70	110/ 68	110/ 70	112/ 68						
maternal temperature:										
36.5c				36.6c						
frequency, strength and length of contractions:										
2:10 Moderate 45 secs		3:10 strong 60 secs		4:10 strong 60 secs						
liquor:										
	clear	clear	pink	pink						
descent of presenting part and cervical dilatation:										
2/5 palp ceph, −2 3cm				1/5palp −1 7cm						
position of presenting part:										
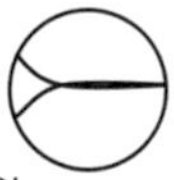 ROL				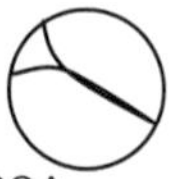 ROA						
food and fluid intake:										
tea and toast	water	water		water						
urinary output:										
100ml			200ml							
drugs/medication:										
other information:										
	SRM 09.50									

Figure 37.8 *A partogram*

has – stop! Examining her vaginally could cause a life-threatening haemorrhage.

2. Explain what you plan to do to the woman and ask for her agreement.

3. If this is given, help her into a comfortable position (lying semi-upright or on her side, standing, squatting, on her knees are all possible positions for VE).

4. Wash your hands and put on sterile gloves.

5. Using the hand you are not using for the actual VE, wash her vulva from front to back with clean water, using a new swab for each side.

6. Hold the labia apart with these same fingers. Lubricate two fingers of the other hand (usually the right) and introduce them carefully into the vagina. Pass them in the direction of the vagina, inwards and backwards.

7. Tell the woman what you are doing as you go and look at her to reassure her.

8. Picture what you are feeling to help you decide and note the points listed in the information box on page 273.

9. Remove your fingers, clean the woman and help her to get comfortable.

10. Discuss your findings with the woman and record them.

Recording the progress of labour

Using a chart called a partogram to record all the events of labour in one place can help to detect complications early and prevent the problems of prolonged labour (see Figure 37.8 and Appendix D). The partogram includes:

- The condition of the woman: maternal pulse, BP, temperature
- Membranes: intact or ruptured, colour of liquor
- Fetal heart rate, the presence or absence of meconium
- The progress of her labour:
  - contraction frequency
  - cervical dilatation
  - descent of the presenting part.
- Fluid intake and output
- Urine analysis
- Drugs given
- There may be space to draw 'touch pictures' of fetal position felt on VE.

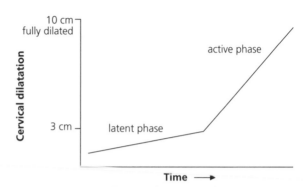

Figure 37.9 *A time line to show rate of dilatation*

Some versions of the partogram include space to record cervical dilatation and descent of the presenting part against time lines (see Figure 37.9). These lines indicate normal and abnormal progress. There is an alert line which gives warning of possible slow progress, and an action line which indicates when the woman and fetus may be in danger. It is, however, important to make individual decisions for women. Healthy women do not always follow standard patterns and the alert and action lines are guides rather than rules to be followed rigidly. If the alert and action lines are to be used to make decisions, the partogram should be commenced only when active labour is diagnosed. Remember active labour is more than 3 cm dilatation with regular painful contractions increasing in frequency.

Looking after the fetus

Placental function is affected by each contraction and this has an effect on the fetus rather like holding your breath. The fetus can cope with normal length contractions if the placenta is supplying him well with oxygen. If labour goes on for a prolonged period of time, or if the contractions are abnormally long, then harm can be done. The fetus receives too little oxygen for his vital organs to function and his brain can be damaged. Passing meconium into the liquor amnii is an indication of this, but this is seen only if the membranes have ruptured. The fetal heart (FH) rate should be between 110 and 150 beats per minute. There should be regularity of rhythm with some variation in speed. This is healthy and shows the fetus can react well to stresses.

It is important to monitor the FH at frequent intervals, and for a full minute to detect variability. It may slow during contractions but should recover immediately after the contraction finishes. It is difficult to

Points to look for on vaginal examination in labour

You are looking for	It should be	Comments
Swelling, varicosities, injury, scarring, redness of the vulva, offensive or coloured discharge	Unscarred, clear white discharge, or 'show'	Note scars e.g. from previous perineal laceration, episiotomy, genital cutting
Liquor amnii	Present or absent, clear with some blood specks from show	Green or brown indicates fetal meconium passed and possible hypoxia
Temperature of the vagina	Warm and moist	Heat and dryness can indicate infection or obstruction
The cervix – feel for position, length, effacement and dilatation	Easy to reach and effaced Fully effaced, thin, dilating up to 3 cm Dilated 4–9 cm Dilated 8–9 cm, thick lip of cervix Dilated 9 cm, thin lip of cervix at the front No cervix felt	Pre-labour Latent phase Active labour, first stage Wait and discourage pushing. Transition to second stage. Wait Fully dilated, second stage. **Note**: Dilatation should progress at about 1 cm/hour in primigravid women in active labour, faster in multigravid women.
Presentation	Hard rounded head with overlapping skull bones (moulding) Does the presenting part fit well down ('applied') onto the cervix?	For other presentations see Chapter 39. Poor application suggests a poor position or a tight fit of the fetal head.
Fetal membranes	Tight bulge indicates the forewaters (bag in front of the cervix) are not ruptured.	Can be confused with caput succedaneum.
Caput succedaneum (swelling on the head caused by pressure from the cervix	Some caput is normal.	Excess suggests slow progress and can confuse assessment of descent.
Moulding: Do the skull bones overlap a little or much more?	(Moulding and excessive moulding) Some moulding is normal as the head squeezes through the pelvis.	Excess moulding suggests the head is large and progress may be delayed.
Position: Identify the overlapping bones	They will be as Figure 37.7 for LOA and ROA positions.	For other positions see Chapter 39.
Attitude: Is the head flexed or deflexed?	Flexed (see Chapter 34)	Deflexed head, see Chapter 34 and 39.
Station of the presenting part: Is it above or below the ischial spines?	Above the spines, the presenting part is not engaged. Below the spines, it is engaged. See Chapter 34.	Descent should be noted on abdominal and vaginal examination. Measured as 1–5 above – or 1–5 below (+) the spines for VE.

Points to look for on vaginal examination in labour *continued*

You are looking for	It should be	Comments
Rotation of the presenting part as it descends through the pelvis	Where are the sutures and fontanelles of the fetal skull in relation to previous VEs?	The occiput should be felt rotating toward the woman's pubis.
If the presenting part is not engaged, assess the pelvis: cavity and prominence of the ischial spines	Cavity should be round, the sacral promontory hard to reach, the spines not prominent.	See Chapters 34 and 39.
Size of the outlet	Two fingers width under the angle of the sacral arch, or a fist width between the ischial tuberosities indicates good size.	

listen during contractions unless an electronic device is available. However, fetal stethoscopes, or using the ear direct, are adequate. Late slowing and return to normal of the FH are signs of fetal distress and hypoxia and this needs urgent action (see Chapter 39). If this happens, ask the woman to change her position, perhaps into the left lateral. This may be enough to cure the problem.

General care of the woman in the first stage of labour

Most women find the first stage of labour very difficult. They need midwives and other attendants who are kind and respect them, and whom they feel they can trust. Women labour more effectively when cared for in a way that makes them feel confident and positive. They are therefore more likely to have a good birth and a healthy baby. Those who have companions with them in labour, such as their mothers, sisters, friends or male partners, have been found to need less analgesia and progress better. In some places, women specialise in providing such non-professional companionship when women do not have others to fulfil this role.

Advocacy: Midwives have a vital role in acting as advocates for labouring women and ensuring they receive the care they need for their comfort and safety. They may also need to safeguard their rights to proper care and to making decisions for themselves. When frightened and in pain, women may find it very difficult to express their needs and what they want to happen.

Preventing infection: Protecting labouring women and their babies from infection is a key midwifery role.

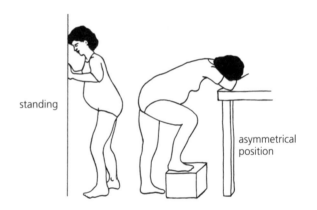

standing

asymmetrical position

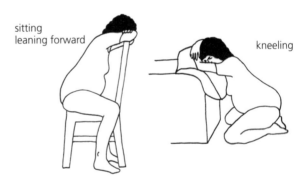

sitting leaning forward

kneeling

Figure 37.10 *Positions for labour*

They must ensure their own practice, and that of others, is safe. Hand washing before and after procedures is vital. Also very important is the cleanliness of equipment, for example beds, linen, instruments and gloves, and sterility where appropriate (see Chapter 6).

Positions for labour: Women often progress faster in labour when they move around and stay upright. The pressure on the cervix probably causes contractions to be more effective. Upright positions and movement may even encourage the fetus to rotate and descend. Women are also able to move around to relieve backache. Some women like to kneel forward resting on the hands (see Figure 37.10). They naturally rock back and forwards with contractions. In some cultures there is a tradition of rotating the hips to help labour. Women may need physical support and help to move. They may also appreciate massage during contractions, especially of the lower back or light abdominal massage.

Women can safely remain upright after membrane rupture provided that the presenting part has entered the pelvis, which prevents cord prolapse (see Chapter 39). If the head is not engaged, the cord can slip down (see Chapter 39), then the left lateral is probably the safest position for both woman and fetus. Left lateral avoids pressure on the main blood vessels behind the uterus, faintness and fetal hypoxia (see Chapter 34).

If the woman wishes to rest, she should likewise lie on her side, preferably the left, or be semi-upright with a slight left tilt. The most dangerous position is lying flat on the back. This may slow labour down and she may feel more pain and distress.

Food and drink: Women need energy in labour and should be encouraged to take light, easily digested food (including carbohydrates) and as much fluids as they wish, to prevent *ketosis* and dehydration. Ketosis can hinder effective contractions and so prolong labour. Food and fluid intake should be recorded in case emergency anaesthesia becomes necessary. Food should only be withheld if problems are anticipated that may lead to giving an anaesthetic. Stomach emptying slows and almost stops in labour. Fluid intake will be controlled but some water may be permitted even if anaesthesia is anticipated.

Monitoring the woman's condition: Women's temperature and blood pressure are normally taken every 4 hours, and pulse counted when the FH is listened to.

Emptying the bladder: It is important that this is done frequently for comfort and because a full bladder can prevent good progress. The urine should be tested for ketones and protein whilst membranes are intact. The presence of liquor amnii will give a false impression of *proteinuria* once the membranes have ruptured. A full bladder can be recognised on palpation as it becomes displaced into the abdomen.

Pain in labour and psychological support: Most women will cope with the powerful nature of contractions even if they see them as painful as well as powerful. Others find this harder. Knowing what to expect from experience, or just from being given information by the midwife, helps women to deal with labour with a positive attitude. It is important for women to know what labour contractions are doing and what is probably going to happen next. Seeing labour as a challenge rather than as a threat may help. An important task is to support the woman and help her find ways of dealing with what she is feeling. Women also need reassurance that they can give birth successfully, that they can cope with contractions and keep going, and that every contraction is achieving something.

Some facilities will have access to analgesia suitable for labour for women who need it. Commonly used preparations are:

- Nitrous oxide and oxygen by self-administered inhalation (such as Entonox). This is safe for the woman and fetus and can be used in most positions.
- Narcotics. These cause respiratory depression in both the woman and newborn. The woman cannot normally leave her bed after administration of the narcotics.
- Epidural analgesia. This is normally only given by an anaesthetist experienced in the technique. Usually effective, but there are risks attached for the woman and fetus. Many women need operative delivery as they have a reduced expulsive urge. It may slow fetal rotation. Women are confined to bed and need intravenous fluids in case of complications.

Women may have taken traditional herbal pain relief before seeking help from professional midwives. It is important to know what is used in your area and whether these have harmful effects.

The transition stage

As the second stage of labour approaches, many women pass through a period of wanting to give up. They may become difficult or abusive. They can become particularly distressed if they experience the urge to push when the midwife knows the cervix is not yet fully dilated. Resisting pushing can be assisted by lying on the side or kneeling forward onto the elbows. It can also help to breathe in ways that help to resist the urge. A common way is to chant 'hoo hoo haaa' and blow out on the 'haaa'. You can do this with the woman and look her in the eyes as you do so. If the woman cannot resist, then it is probably safe to push. It is important to treat women as individuals and let them do what feels right.

This period is often called the **transition stage**. Recognising it, and informing the woman why she is feeling this way, makes it easier. This difficult period may be less likely to happen if the woman is upright.

Wanting to push before the cervix is fully dilated can indicate an occipito-posterior position (or even breech presentation). Resisting the expulsive efforts until full dilatation occurs; allows time for the longer rotation process of the fetal head.

Some women start to push because they think they must. The expulsive urge is essential for the natural process to work properly. The internal tissues of the vaginal wall and pelvic floor may be over-stretched by forced early pushing. The bladder and rectum are displaced upwards out of the way if pushing is not hurried.

The second stage of labour

The second stage of labour is from full dilatation of the cervix until the complete birth of the baby. Contractions become longer, change their character and may last as long as 70 or 80 seconds. Around this time many women experience a quieter period when contractions slow temporarily. This has been called the 'rest and be thankful' stage. They may even stop completely for a few minutes. The contractions soon become very powerful and the urge to push the fetus out becomes irresistible.

External signs of full dilatation

The only way to be absolutely sure the cervix is fully dilated is to perform a vaginal examination. However, the external signs, and the woman's behaviour, are normally adequate indicators:
- Expulsive contractions. The woman wants to push and may not be able to resist it.
- The perineum bulges and begins to appear shiny.
- The anus 'pouts', that is it protrudes and looks like bulging lips.

If there is no obvious descent of the fetus with pushing, then a VE should be performed to detect any cervix still present below the head. This is usually found to the front (anterior lip).

Many women feel much more positive from now onwards because they feel they can do something. Many will grunt or groan loudly when pushing. This may be helpful and does not have to be discouraged. Natural pushing should follow the woman's urges. It usually involves several efforts per contraction rather than just two or three very long ones. The effort will vary depending on what the woman feels. Encouraging women to hold their breath as long as possible, while making long expulsive efforts, reduces the oxygen supply to the fetus dangerously. It may also raise the woman's blood pressure.

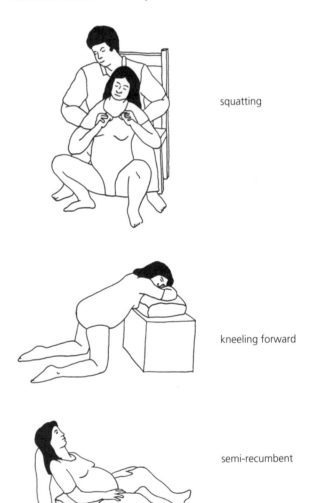

squatting

kneeling forward

semi-recumbent

Figure 37.11 *Positions for delivery*

Positions for birth

The same principles are as important for the second stage as the first:

- Comfort and mobility for the woman
- Good oxygen supply to the fetus
- No interference with the progress of labour.

Most labour positions are suitable for birth. If upright, women can be held under the arms by another person when pushing. They may squat, kneel, sit on a birthing stool or someone's knees or lie on the left side. Some use hammocks, or support themselves using furniture, suspended ropes or a roof beam. These positions allow the maximum expansion of the softened pelvic joints, rocking of the sacrum and movement backward of the coccyx. They also allow good oxygen supplies to the fetus. If using the semi-recumbent or lithotomy positions, the woman's head and shoulders must be raised. Figure 37.11 illustrates these positions.

Kneeling forward facing the head of the bed provides a good compromise in mobility and comfort for the woman and convenience for the midwife. Lying flat and the lithotomy position make pushing harder as well as reducing the blood supply to mother and fetus.

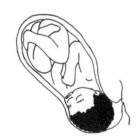

DESCENT of the fetus, FLEXION of
the fetal head

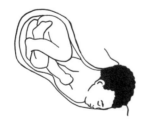

INTERNAL ROTATION of the fetal head,
so that the sagittal suture of the fetal head is
in the antero-posterior diameter of the pelvis

Figure 37.12 *Mechanism of labour*

Some positions require the midwife to be alert and prepared for delivery away from a bed. Floor delivery is acceptable if you are ready to provide a clean surface such as plastic sheet. You also have to rethink how the fetus will be born if you are used to women lying down. Understanding the mechanism of labour will help you to visualise what the fetus will do.

The mechanism of normal labour

This is the term given to the movements a fetus has to make as he descends through the birth canal (see Chapter 34 for terms used).

- The head flexes and descends through the pelvic inlet (the brim). The head will face the woman's side. The smallest diameter of the fetal skull will come through the pelvis, that is the sub occipito-bregmatic diameter.
- The head starts to rotate in the round pelvic cavity, the occiput moving forward.
- The occiput reaches the sloping gutter-shaped pelvic floor first. This makes it rotate and slide forward to come under the pubic bone. The fetus is now facing the woman's back, head still flexed. You can see fetal scalp.
- The occiput escapes under the pubic arch. The perineum is very thin and bulging now and the vaginal introitus stretching open. You can see more of the fetal scalp.
- Crowning takes place, that is the widest diameter of the fetal head crosses the perineum. The introitus is fully stretched with the head half through it.
- The head is born by extension. The face and chin emerge toward the woman's back.
- Restitution takes place, that is the head turns back to line up with the shoulders which are still rotating in the cavity.
- Internal rotation of the shoulders. The shoulders turn so that they are in the antero-posterior diameter of the outlet of the pelvis. The anterior shoulder usually meets the pelvic floor first and is born, followed by the posterior shoulder.
- External rotation of the head. The baby's head turns straight on the shoulders again. The baby is now looking at the mother's leg.
- The baby is born by lateral flexion. The trunk and legs follow the curve of the sacrum in order to be born.

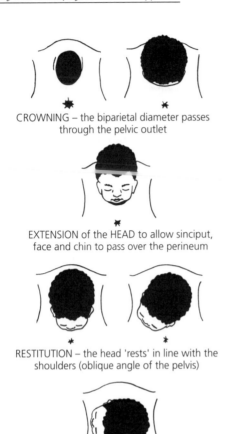

CROWNING – the biparietal diameter passes through the pelvic outlet

EXTENSION of the HEAD to allow sinciput, face and chin to pass over the perineum

RESTITUTION – the head 'rests' in line with the shoulders (oblique angle of the pelvis)

INTERNAL ROTATION of the SHOULDERS into the antero-posterior diameter of the pelvis, LATERAL FLEXION (downward flexion) of the head

Figure 37.13 *Mechanism of labour*

It is useful to practise these movements with a doll which can easily be made of old cloth. If a model pelvis is available, this is even better. A substitute can be made from a box, with stretchy cloth with a hole cut in it to act as a perineum.

As the fetus descends, the pelvic floor muscles are pulled up and sideways as the fetus passes through. They then return to their original position. The perineum is flattened as it stretches and becomes thinner. This pressure on the perineum causes a natural feedback mechanism which causes contractions to become even stronger (known as Ferguson's reflex). At some point the membranes will rupture and the liquor amnii be released. This usually happens with a contraction.

This whole process usually takes longer with primi-gravid women than those who have given birth previously. This is probably because the soft tissues are stretching for the first time. Many people expect the second stage to be complete in about 2 hours in primiparous women, and much shorter in women who have given birth previously. The condition of the woman and the fetus are probably more important than the time that has elapsed. If timing the second stage, you must be certain that the woman is fully dilated, otherwise operative delivery may be performed unnecessarily.

Assisting the woman in the second stage

The midwife should interfere as little as possible when assisting a woman to give birth. In most instances the woman's efforts and the uterine contractions are enough to push out the baby without any assistance except someone to reassure and encourage her.

- Simple actions such as giving sips of fluid and washing her face between contractions will refresh her.
- Many women pass faeces because of compression of the bowel. These should be removed without fuss and her buttocks and vulva should be washed. This improves her sense of well being and maintains clean surfaces for the birth.
- Encourage her to empty her bladder at intervals if she can.
- Listen to the fetal heart after each contraction. Expect some slowing (bradycardia) after each one but this should recover quickly. There should be a period of normal rate before the next contraction starts.
- Continue to monitor the woman's BP and pulse at frequent intervals, about every 15 minutes.
- Watch the perineum for signs of pressure from the head.
- Some women feel few expulsive contractions and may give birth very fast. This can cause stress and internal brain injury to the baby and perineal trauma to the woman. The left lateral and kneeling forward positions can help to slow such rapid progress by reducing the expulsive urges.

Controlling the birth

It is uncertain how important it is for midwives to control the stretching of the perineum and birth of the head. It is not known how much perineal damage this prevents or even causes.

- Keep the hands poised to prevent the head from escaping too quickly and causing tears. It may be necessary also to encourage flexion to ensure that the smallest diameter of the fetal head stretches the introitus.
- Once the head is out, feel gently around the neck to detect a tight cord. If it is tight, loosen it and slide it carefully over the head. It should still be pulsating and providing oxygen. Clamp and cut it, and unwind the coils, only if it is so tight as to cause asphyxia in the fetus or delay the birth.
- Clean the eyes and apply eye drops to prevent gonococcal infection if this is local policy.
- Clean the mouth and the nose to reduce the inhalation of fluids if there is time. Use cloth that is not fluffy to prevent the inspiration of fibres.
- The baby will be born with the next contraction. Hold the baby both sides of the head and then around the ribs when free (see Figure 37.14).

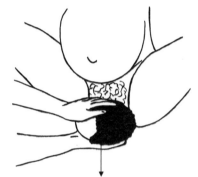

position of hands to aid lateral flexion of the head

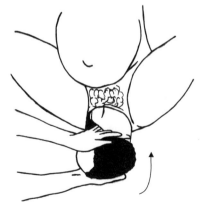

as the body delivers, the little finger on upper hand is placed under the axilla, in order to deliver baby onto mother's abdomen

Figure 37.14 *Delivery of the fetal head*

Follow its movements toward the woman's back and then forward as it:
- undergoes restitution of the head
- frees the anterior shoulder (usually), then the posterior shoulder
- frees the body by lateral flexion.
- If local custom allows, take the baby straight up and over to the woman to hold. Skin to skin contact helps to keep the baby warm and appears to be helpful emotionally. It may also encourage uterine contraction especially if the baby is placed near the nipples and begins to suckle. Some babies will seek the nipple eagerly.
- It is not necessary to hold the baby upside down. Most babies spit out the fluids from their mouth and upper airways.
- Dry the baby and wrap it in dry cloth, or wrap it together with the mother.
- Observe the condition of the baby using the Apgar score (see Chapter 41).

The perineum

The muscles of the pelvic floor and the perineum are designed to support the internal organs and to stretch to accommodate the birth of the baby (see Chapter 34). The structures often tear slightly during the birth of the head and shoulders. Once the birth is over, the perineum, vulva and lower vagina must be inspected for trauma. Most small tears heal well without suturing. There may, however, be tears which need sutures just to control bleeding. There are four levels of tear (known as lacerations) (see Figure 37.15):
- First degree: involves perineal skin only
- Second degree: also involves pelvic floor muscle layers
- Third degree: also involves the external mucosa of the rectum and the muscle ring of the anal sphincter
- Fourth degree: complete tear through the anal sphincter and internal mucosa.

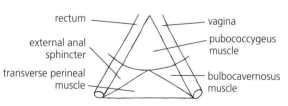

Figure 37.15 *Perineal body*

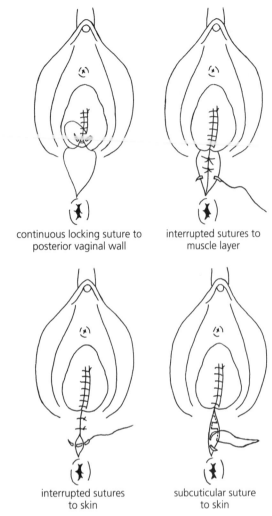

continuous locking suture to
posterior vaginal wall

interrupted sutures to
muscle layer

interrupted sutures
to skin

subcuticular suture
to skin

Figure 37.16 *Suturing the perineum*

Third and fourth degree tears need very good analgesia or even anaesthesia to repair properly so that
continence is preserved. Local policy may indicate
that repairs should be done by doctors if available.
Other tears can be repaired by midwives who have
learnt the technique (see perineal suturing in Figure
37.16).

Occasionally there is a need to make an incision
into the perineum in order to allow the birth of the
baby or speed up the delivery because there is a
problem. This incision is called episiotomy.

Episiotomy

Most women do not need an episiotomy and it should
never become a routine:

- Episiotomy should be done for serious fetal
  distress or risk of severe maternal trauma only.
- Episiotomy does not prevent second and third
  degree tears or alter the long-term consequences.
  Perineal pain, painful intercourse and continence
  difficulties are the same for lacerations and
  episiotomy.
- The woman who does not have an episiotomy may
  end up with no significant damage at all.
- Episiotomy can be considered an abuse if
  performed unnecessarily.
- Cutting without the woman's consent is an abuse
  of the right to self-determination (see Chapter 2).
- Episiotomy increases blood loss which is
  important to avoid in anaemic women.
- There is a serious risk of HIV transmission to the
  fetus and to the midwife in HIV positive women. It
  should be avoided.

Pp Performing an episiotomy

If an episiotomy must be made, the perineum should be
injected with local anaesthetic, 5 ml of 1% Lignocaine:
- Insert the needle at the fourchette and along the
  line where you plan to cut.
- Withdraw the plunger a little to check you are not
  in a blood vessel.
- Withdraw the needle slowly injecting one third.
  Keeping the tip under the skin, angle the needle
  again on both sides and repeat.
- Allow 5 minutes for it to take effect.

The cut must only be made when the perineum is well
stretched by the fetal head. This minimises bleeding
and allows time for the pelvic floor muscles to slide
away (see Figure 37.17).
- Insert two fingers into the vagina to protect the
  head.
- Insert the scissor blade between the fingers.
- Wait for a contraction to fully distend the
  perineum.
- Make a single cut of 4–5 cm in a medio-lateral
  direction, ensuring that the incision starts at the
  fourchette so that the Bartholin's glands are not
  damaged.

Episiotomy needs careful repair to restore the function of the pelvic floor and to stop bleeding. This may
be profuse as the vessels may have been cut before
they have fully stretched. Note that lacerations usually

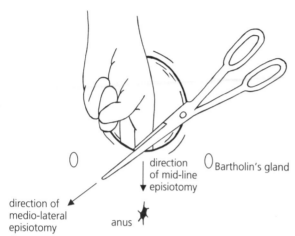

Figure 37.17 *Performing an episiotomy*

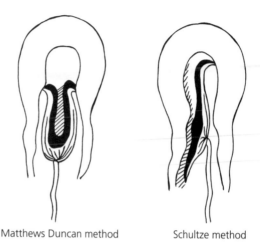

Matthews Duncan method   Schultze method

Figure 37.18 *Separation and expulsion of the placenta*

bleed less because of stretching and narrowing of blood vessels.

The third stage of labour

The third stage of labour lasts from the birth of the baby to the expulsion of the placenta and membranes. The natural length of this stage is from 5 minutes up to 1 hour. As with the second stage, the woman's condition is more important than actual time. Up to 500 ml of blood loss is common but this may be too much for anaemic women. Even small blood loss can lead to complications for them (see Chapter 36). The control of haemorrhage is very important. Blood loss should not be too rapid. Brisk loss may be a warning that a haemorrhage is occurring. However, women can easily lose large amounts unnoticed with a slow continuous trickle or if they are lying down. (See Chapter 39 for Postpartum haemorrhage.)

The physiology of the third stage of labour

The uterine contraction that expels the body of the baby is very strong. This begins to separate the placenta:

- The area the placenta is attached to becomes smaller.
- The placenta is compressed.
- Blood vessels burst behind it and start to force the placenta off.

There are two ways this happens:

Schultze separation: This is the most common type. The placenta separates from the centre and a clot forms behind it. This encourages more separation. Its own weight then separates the rest off and it falls into the lower segment. The shiny fetal surface of the placenta appears at the introitus of the vagina. The blood clot is inside it and the membranes trail behind.

Matthews Duncan separation: If the placenta separates from the edge first it will slide sideways into the lower segment. Blood is lost with it. The maternal surface of the placenta is seen at the vagina. The Matthews Duncan separation is associated with a low lying placenta and so bleeding may be heavier. There is less oblique muscle in the lower segment to form the 'living ligature' action around the blood vessels of the placenta site (see Chapter 34). Membranes may be ragged and bits may be left behind which can cause infection and later bleeding (see Figure 37.18).

With either separation type, the placenta will fall into the lower uterus. The woman will feel a contraction, and may want to push to expel the placenta and membranes. This happens more easily in upright positions when they often just fall out. Once the uterus is empty, the uterus contracts down hard. It will feel lower and firmer on abdominal palpation.

The spiral muscle fibres of the myometrium tighten around the blood vessels and so control the bleeding.

The contraction of the myometrium brings the muscular surfaces close together. This applies pressure to the blood vessels and further controls bleeding.

Management

There are two main ways of managing the third stage of labour: 'physiological' and 'active' management. Active management is the WHO recommended practice for three reasons:

- It is thought impossible to predict reliably who might bleed. All women are considered at risk.
- It leads to lower blood loss which may be vitally important to anaemic women.
- Fewer blood transfusions are needed.

Some women may have particular reasons for refusing this intervention. These have to be respected.

Physiological or expectant management: This needs confidence and patience, and no interference as this will divert the process from the normal.

- Palpate the fundus gently to ensure that the uterus is well contracted. It will be broad and felt below the umbilicus while the placenta is still in the upper segment. Do not manipulate it as this can cause relaxation and bleeding.
- Observe the vaginal blood loss constantly to ensure it is not too heavy.
- Leave the cord intact until it stops pulsating. The woman can meanwhile continue to hold the baby. Clamp the cord in two places once pulsation has stopped and cut between the clamps with sterile scissors or a clean new razor blade.
- Watch for signs of descent of the placenta into the lower segment:
  - The cord will lengthen a little
  - There is usually a small blood loss
  - The fundus of the uterus will rise and become narrow under the palpating hand, and more mobile.
- Encourage the woman to push. If lying down, it can be helpful to the woman to push against your hand lying flat over the lower abdomen.
- Catch the placenta and membranes, helping them out carefully to avoid tearing.
- Check again that the uterus is hard and well contracted. If it becomes soft or 'boggy' this suggests there is blood collecting.
- Record the time of expulsion of the placenta and the blood loss.
- Watch for bleeding and relaxation of the uterus.
- Putting the baby to the breast to feed may help the process.

Active management of the third stage: This starts as the baby is born. It combines:

- giving a uterotonic drug with
- clamping the umbilical cord and
- performing controlled cord traction to remove the placenta and membranes immediately the uterus contracts firmly.

There are a number of drugs that can be used:

- Ergometrine 0.5 mg with oxytocin 5 international units, given IM. The oxytocin causes rapid contraction (in 2½ minutes) and the ergometrine acts more slowly to sustain it for some hours. A commonly used band name is Syntometrine.
- Oxytocin can be given alone if ergometrine cannot be given (in cardiac disease and hypertension). Give oxytocin 5 international units IM. It can be given IV but only very slowly as it can cause severe hypotension and death.
- Ergometrine 0.25 mg IV. This acts in 45 seconds but can cause retained placenta. It is now recommended that it be used only for severe postnatal haemorrhage to make the uterus contract.
- Efforts are being made to develop an oral oxytocic that does not depend on cold storage as do injectable drugs.

Note: Uterotonic drugs must not be given after the birth of a first twin as the resulting contraction will kill the second twin.

Pp A standard management procedure of the third stage

- Give IM Syntometrine to the woman as the baby's anterior shoulder is born.
- After the birth, clamp the umbilical cord in two places and cut between this with sterile scissors or a clean, new razor blade. (Some people leave the maternal end to drain into a basin to reduce the size of the placenta. This may make separation quicker and removal easier.) Do not confuse it with maternal blood loss.
- Palpate the uterus gently to check it has contracted. Do not manipulate it as this can cause relaxation and bleeding.
- Wait for signs of separation (see physiological management). Some people do not wait for signs of separation but pulling immediately can lead to slightly more bleeding.
- When it is contracted, hold the uterus back with one hand. Never pull without this 'counter-traction'. To do this, place the hand above the pubic bone with the palm facing toward the umbilicus. Press down. Draw the placenta and membranes out firmly and steadily with the other hand. Winding the cord round the fingers helps.

Follow the curve of the birth canal downwards and backwards, then upward at the introitus. Stop traction if the uterus relaxes, as this can cause a uterine inversion (see Figure 37.19).
- Catch the placenta and membrane and help them out carefully to prevent tearing. Put aside in a basin.
- Record the time and approximate blood loss.
- Keep a check on the uterus and vaginal bleeding.

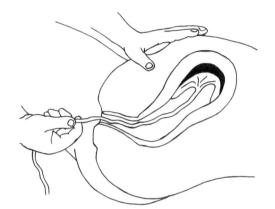

Figure 37.19 *Active management of the third stage*

Examination of the placenta

The placenta and membranes must be examined to make sure they are complete. If any part of the placenta has been retained then the uterus will need to be evacuated as bleeding and infection can follow. Examine:
- The maternal surface of the placenta for ragged areas or holes that may indicate missing cotyledons (see Figure 37.20).
- The edge of the placenta for blood vessels that run off the edge to a hole in the membrane. This could indicate that a piece has been retained. (This is a succenturiate lobe, a separate piece of placenta with its own blood vessels.)
- The cord, which may be inserted at the edge of the placenta (Battledore insertion) or which may terminate and the vessels run through the membrane before entering the placental mass (Velamentous insertion), see Figure 37.21 and Chapter 39 (vasa praevia).
- The cord to ensure that there are two arteries and one vein. One artery only can indicate congenital abnormality of the baby's heart or renal system.
Record your findings.

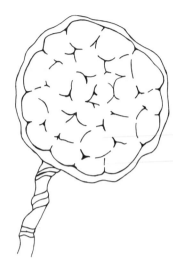

Figure 37.20 *Maternal side of the placenta*

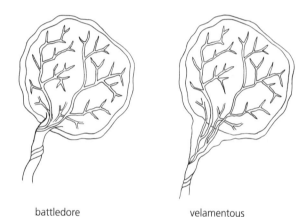

battledore   velamentous

Figure 37.21 *Battledore and Velamentous insertion of the cord*

General care following the birth

If needed, suturing of the perineum must be completed early to stop bleeding and promote good healing. The woman's temperature, pulse and blood pressure also need to be recorded. Once these essential tasks have been completed the woman needs to have a drink and light food if she wishes. Tea and porridge are popular choices. She also needs the opportunity to bathe and to have clean sheets and clothing. She will need rest and sleep. However, her vaginal blood loss and the contraction of her uterus must be checked at intervals.

The baby should stay with his mother so that she can put him to the breast whenever he wants to suckle. For further care, see Chapter 40.

38

Multiple pregnancy and preterm labour

This chapter will consider the issues related to multiple pregnancy which is a natural and normal occurrence except when treatment for infertility has been given. Some difficulties may be experienced by women with a multiple pregnancy and these situations will be explored. Because pre-term labour is often a feature of multiple pregnancy, pre-term labour will be explored here.

Multiple pregnancy

Why does multiple pregnancy happen?

Africa and Asia have higher incidences than elsewhere. Other factors which influence the number of babies conceived are:

- Older and multigravid women
- Genetic factors – family history of twinning is common
- Some infertility treatments
- Following the use of the contraceptive pill.

Types of twinning

- Monozygotic. One sperm and one ovum. The cell mass divides into two. These are identical twins and are the same sex. There will be one or two chorions, amnions and placentas, depending on when the division occurred.
- Dizygotic. Two ovum and two sperm. Each develops separately. These are non-identical twins and may be different sexes. There will always be two chorions, amnions and placentas. The placentas may fuse and look like one.
- In the case of triplets or even more multiples, the spilt will be either three ways, or may be a combination of identical and non-identical embryos.

Disadvantages of multiple pregnancy

Multiple pregnancy puts a greater strain on the woman. Minor disorders, and also most serious disorders present greater problems, for example pre-eclampsia, anaemia, diabetes, heart failure, polyhydramnios (see Chapters 35 and 36).

- The babies more often have low birth weight or are born prematurely.
- They may have unequal access to nutrients and oxygen so one grows better than the other. One may fail to develop and die.
- Identical twins may transfuse each other through the placenta. One becomes anaemic and underweight. The other has too many red cells and circulation overload. Heart failure can then happen in labour.
- Identical twins may be joined together.
- Cords may become tangled leading to hypoxia and death (one amnion).
- Lack of space often causes abnormal lie and presentation.
- Labour can become complicated and the risk of postpartum haemorrhage is greater. The heads may lock during labour making a caesarean section essential.
- Families may be under more stress which increases marriage breakdown, violence and child abuse.
- Twins may be welcome in some societies and unwelcome in others.
- Risks become greater with more than two babies.

Diagnosis

History

- Rapid increase in size and weight
- Minor disorders of pregnancy are more troublesome
- Extra fetal movements

Clinical examination

- Inspection. The abdomen appears large for dates. Fetal movements may be clearly visible.
- Palpation. The uterus is large for dates. It may be difficult to identify the presenting parts. You may find three poles (heads or breeches) instead of two. If there are even more fetuses it is more difficult to identify fetal parts on palpation.
- Listening. Two fetal hearts are difficult to distinguish from one heard in two places. Only a large difference in rates (at least 10 beats per minute), heard by separate listeners at the same time, might be significant.

Special investigations

- X-rays must only be used if essential because of risk to the fetuses.
- Ultrasound scan will confirm twinning and their positions (if available).

Management of multiple pregnancy

- Give iron and folic acid supplements as the demand on the woman's iron stores is huge.
- Monitor for anaemia and hypertensive disorders.
- Indigestion may be severe but antacids (if available) can make anaemia worse. Advise about meal size, food types, sleeping positions etc. and other remedies such as peppermint and ginger.
- *Advocacy* may be needed to help women organise the extra help and rest they need.
- Advise the woman to make emergency plans as premature labour is more common, and to reach the birth place before labour begins if she can. Advise her to use a facility providing Comprehensive Emergency Obstetric Care and care for sick or premature babies.

Multiple birth

Multiple birth should be a normal event without problems but it is included here because difficulties often arise. The difficulties which may affect labour are as follows:

- Preterm labour is common.
- The babies may have unequal access to oxygen and nutrients so one may be at more risk of hypoxia. They may also become tangled which threatens their oxygen supplies if cords are affected.

- All conditions arising in pregnancy or medical problems that existed before pregnancy are more common and increased in effect, for example anaemia, pre-eclampsia, heart problems, placenta praevia.
- Twins can lock together and become unable to pass into the pelvis.
- Undiagnosed twin birth makes extra problems. Giving oxytocin after the birth of twin 1 is likely to kill twin 2.

Management of multiple labour and birth

See Chapter 37 for normal labour as all the principles of care described there will apply to this labour. If there are three or more babies, caesarean section may be considered the safer option.

First stage

- Give care appropriate to the presentation and position of the first fetus, for example cephalic or breech.
- Group and cross-match the woman's blood.
- Ensure IV infusion equipment and oxytocic drugs are accessible.
- Ensure you have an amnihook (for rupturing the second amniotic sac), two razor blades or scissors for cutting the cords, and extra cord clamps or ties – for labelling the maternal end of the cord of twin 1, and the babies in birth order.

Second stage

- The process and management continue as appropriate for the first baby until it is born. Note the time.
- Clamp and cut the cord as usual including the maternal end. Label twin 1 and the maternal end of cord 1 with extra ties or clamps.
- Do not try to deliver the placenta. Do not give oxytocin now.
- Monitor and record the remaining fetal heart.
- Check for cord prolapse.
- Check the lie of the second twin. Correct it to longitudinal if necessary, using the principle described in the section on external cephalic version (page 298). If this fails, an experienced attendant may attempt internal version, bringing down one foot into the vagina so making the lie into a breech that can be manipulated.
- Wait for contractions to return and membranes to

rupture if intact. (Some people rupture the membranes at once if intact. An assistant holds the presenting part in the brim.) Check again for cord prolapse.

- Commence an oxytocin infusion if the contractions do not re-establish within 1 hour (some say 15 minutes). Use a low dose at first and increase rapidly. You could first try getting twin 1 to suckle to stimulate contractions. The cervix may need to dilate again.
- Monitor the condition of the second twin. Listen to the fetal heart every 5 minutes.
- The risk of hypoxia to twin 2 increases with time. Its condition determines how fast you need to act.
- Deliver the second twin according to its presentation.
- Give oxytocin for active management of the third stage (see Chapter 37) once you are certain there are no more babies.
- Be prepared for twin 2 to need resuscitation.
- Caesarean section will be needed if obstruction occurs.

Third stage

Note: The active management of the third stage must not commence until the last baby is born. Do not assume there are only two babies.

- Deliver the placenta(s) by pulling on both cords together once the uterus is contracted.
- Haemorrhage is common as delay in the second birth increases intrapartum bleeding, the uterus has been overstretched, and the placental site is large.
- One placenta, or the single placenta, may be expelled before twin 2 which may then die.

You may be expected to decide on whether twins are identical or not. The only combinations that can give a definite answer without expensive testing are:

- One placenta with one chorionic (outer/maternal side) membrane = identical twins
- Different sexes = non-identical twins.

Caring for twins

These may be healthy or small, premature, hypo-glycaemic and hypoxic (see Chapter 42).

Postnatal period

- Observe closely for haemorrhage or heavy lochia.
- Check the haemoglobin and provide iron and folic acid supplements.

- Give extra support with establishing feeding.
- Family spacing advice is important because of the extra workload and the need to increase depleted iron stores (see Chapter 30).
- Women and families who lose one twin are emotionally vulnerable. The enjoyment of the surviving baby is made difficult by grieving for the other.

Preterm onset of labour

Definition

Preterm onset of labour is labour that begins before the completion of the 37th week of pregnancy.

Causes

In many instances the labour begins spontaneously but sometimes it is necessary to induce labour prematurely to preserve the health of the mother, for example in pre-eclampsia, diabetes, renal disease or infection. Sometimes the fetus is at risk if the pregnancy continues, for example haemolytic disease, premature rupture of the membranes, placental abruption.

Preterm rupture of membranes

When the membranes rupture labour may begin soon after. The woman should be admitted to a unit which has facilities to meet the needs of a premature baby.

A cervical swab should be taken to detect any infection that may be present and an appropriate antibiotic then given.

Medication which can be given

Corticosteroids: To avoid the risk of respiratory distress syndrome (see Chapter 42) to which a preterm baby is prone, Dexamethasone 12 mg intramuscularly is given to the mother twice at 12 hourly intervals. This will stimulate the production of surfactant in the lungs of the baby and will aid in good lung expansion at birth.

It takes 24 hours for the drug to be effective and the effect lasts for about 7 days.

Antibiotics: Chorioamnionitis may be present and antibiotic therapy has been shown to reduce the risks of infection to both mother and baby.

Tocolytic drugs: Ritodrine hydrochloride or Salbutamol are both drugs which relax smooth muscle and may help to prevent the uterus from contracting. These drugs can cause a rapid fall in the blood pressure and so the mother's pulse and blood pressure should be monitored frequently during the administration of these drugs. Local policy will determine whether this medication should be given intravenously or orally and what dose should be given.

Management of labour and delivery

- Pain relieving drugs such as Pethidine should not be given, as this will depress the respiration of the baby. Epidural anaesthesia may be administered and Entonox is safe to use.
- If possible, a paediatrician should be present for the birth to resuscitate the baby.
- An obstetrician should be present to perform a forceps delivery if there is any delay.
- An episiotomy may be performed to reduce pressure on the head of this baby and so minimise trauma to the cerebral membranes.
- The cord should be cut, leaving at least 12 cm on the baby so that it can be used to give care to the baby in the special care baby unit.

- Vitamin K 0.5 mg should be given to the baby intramuscularly.
- The mother is likely to be very anxious about her baby's health and may need much encouragement to handle a baby which seems so fragile. Care must be taken to give her help and support.
- Every effort should be made to help this mother establish lactation, particularly as the baby may be unable to feed at the breast in the first days after birth.

■ Activities

1. Consider a birth plan that would be suitable for a 19 year old woman having her first pregnancy, which has been diagnosed as a twin pregnancy. Think about her physical and social and emotional needs.
2. How can a midwife help a woman to establish lactation when she has a preterm baby unable to feed at the breast?

39

Abnormal labour

This chapter provides information about difficulties that may occur in labour because of:
- The powers: the uterus not functioning normally
- The passenger: the fetus not being in a normal presentation or position
- The passage and the passenger: the fetal head is unable to pass easily through the woman's pelvis because it is too big for her, called 'cephalopelvic disproportion'
- Problems with the cord
- Postpartum haemorrhage or retained placenta.

There are also sections on other emergencies arising in labour, and on operative procedures for delivery.

Introduction

Some of the main causes of maternal and fetal death and disability occur during labour. These are prolonged and obstructed labour, uterine rupture, eclampsia and postpartum haemorrhage (see Chapter 35 for eclampsia). They all need prompt recognition and action to save lives. These conditions are debilitating and involve invasive treatments so contribute to postnatal infection, another major cause of maternal death.

Although it is impossible to predict difficult labour with accuracy, some women are more obviously at risk and need to be delivered where Comprehensive Emergency Obstetric Care is easily available. Risk factors are as follows:
- Very young women with immature pelves
- Short stature, for example less than 140 cm
- High parity
- Known pelvic deformity
- Very large fetus

- Previous difficult labour
- Previous caesarean section or scarred uterus, for example previous repair of a rupture
- Abnormal presentation or unstable lie
- First pregnancy
- Multiple pregnancy:
  - Lie may be unstable because of weak abdominal muscles, leading to abnormal presentations
  - Cephalopelvic disproportion may arise for the first time as babies each become larger.

Some women, with the following problems, should be advised not to attempt labour:
- Transverse lie
- Severely contracted pelvis
- If they had a previous caesarean section, particularly those who had a previous Caesarean section for cephalopelvic disproportion
- Repeated postpartum haemorrhage.

These lists do not include women with pre-existing medical disorders or pregnancy problems.

In most circumstances a doctor will be involved once the midwife realises that the woman is experiencing problems with her labour. Midwives must, however, know how to deal with emergencies.

Note: There are many procedures described in this chapter that need to be carried out with full aseptic techniques and using universal precautions (see Chapter 6). These situations include any that involve internal examinations and surgical procedures. This is to protect the woman and her baby, and also the midwife or doctor.

Prolonged and obstructed labour

The first four sections of this chapter consider the different problems that can lead to prolonged and obstructed labour. They are closely interlinked.

Labour may be called prolonged because it does not match specific expectations such as dilating 1cm/hour, but the woman and her fetus may be healthy. However, prolonged labour can mean the fetus is in a difficult position, the uterus is not working properly, or there is cephalopelvic disproportion.

Prolonged labour can have serious effects on the woman and the fetus:

- Maternal exhaustion and dehydration
- Internal damage from prolonged pressure of the fetal head. This leads eventually to a hole (fistula) between the vagina and the bladder (vesico-vaginal fistula) or rectum (recto-vaginal fistula).
- Postpartum haemorrhage because the uterus works less well after prolonged labour
- Eclampsia may arise without prior warning in prolonged labour.
- Postnatal infection is highly likely especially with internal manipulation, perhaps done by untrained people with poor *aseptic* techniques.
- Fetal *hypoxia*, stillbirth, *neonatal asphyxia* and death, and long-term brain damage.

Labour may become obstructed if the fetus cannot pass through the maternal pelvis. This may be because of cephalopelvic disproportion, or because of abnormal presentation or position of the fetus, but the effect will be the same. The uterus will continue to contract to try to push the fetus through. The uterus will eventually rupture (see Labour Emergencies), the fetus will die and the woman will die of haemorrhage and shock. These situations are avoidable if women have skilled attendants and good access to Comprehensive Emergency Obstetric Care.

Abnormal uterine action

The uterus may contract inadequately or in a disordered manner. It may also contract excessively strongly. Remember that abnormal contractions may occur because of abnormal pelvic shapes or malposition or malpresentation of the fetus. These problems may be why other emergencies occur such as cord prolapse, shoulder dystocia or postpartum haemorrhage.

General care of women with abnormal uterine action

Slow labour will make the woman exhausted and depressed whatever the cause.

- She will need extra support, and pain relief if available.

- Correct fluid and electrolyte balance.
- Monitor the condition of the woman and her fetus.
- Use a partogram to help to monitor the labour and act quickly if progress does not improve.

Hypotonic uterine action

Contractions may not increase in frequency, strength and length as they should once active labour has commenced. This leads to slow progress.

Diagnosis

- It has been confirmed that the woman is in active labour.
- Contractions are weak and short.
- The cervical os is dilating slowly or not at all.
- The fetus usually remains in a good condition.

If the contractions are like this from the onset of labour, this is primary hypotonic action. If the contractions become hypotonic after a period of normal activity, this is secondary hypotonic action.

Causes and predisposing factors

Primary hypotonic action may be associated with:

- the first birth
- occipito-posterior position of the fetus, or
- there may be no obvious cause.

Secondary hypotonic uterine action is associated with:

- cephalopelvic disproportion
- poor presentation or position of the fetus
- maternal exhaustion or dehydration
- epidural analgesia.

Management

Make sure there is no cephalopelvic disproportion.

Are you sure the woman is in the active phase of labour?

Are you sure the presenting part is engaged in the pelvis? If so then:

- Try asking her to walk around if she can. If still no improvement:
- Rupture the membranes with an amnihook or toothed forceps. Wait for good contractions, 3 every 10 minutes lasting about 40 seconds.
- If no good pattern is established after 1 hour, augment labour with an IV infusion of oxytocin. (To augment labour is to improve the strength and rhythm of contractions so they can work more effectively.) Follow your local protocol for

administration in gradually increasing concentrations of oxytocin. This can cause ruptured uterus and fetal and maternal distress so do not use:

- If the uterus is scarred from previous surgery
- There is any suspicion of cephalopelvic disproportion
- Caesarean section is not easily available.

Hypotonic action can be a sign of exhaustion of the uterus with cephalopelvic disproportion. Hypertonic contractions and uterine rupture may then follow if prompt caesarean section is not performed. This happens mostly with multigravid women.

Rupturing membranes: Try to avoid rupturing membranes for as long as possible in areas of high HIV prevalence. Explain what you want to do to the woman and seek her permission.

- Palpate the abdomen to check lie, presentation and position.
- Check the fetal heart.
- Perform a vaginal examination (see Chapter 37). Identify the membranes through the cervix. Insert an amnihook or toothed forceps along the fingers and catch the membranes carefully to make a hole.
- Let the liquor drain and note the colour.
- Check the fetal heart again.

Hypertonic uterine action

Diagnosis

- Contractions are frequent and very intense.
- The resting time between contractions is reduced.
- Pain is severe.
- The fetus becomes distressed. This is indicated by:
  - The heart rate drops below 110 beats/minute after contractions and is slow to return to normal.
  - The fetus may pass meconium which becomes visible if liquor is draining.

Causes

- Obstructed labour especially in a multigravid woman, perhaps following a period of hypotonic 'resting' of the uterus. The fetus must be delivered quickly by caesarean section.
- The over-use of oxytocin infusion. This is especially dangerous for multigravid women and those with uterine scars.
- Traditional herbal oxytocic medicines. These may have toxic effects as well as causing hypertonic

contractions. These may have been taken while still at home, or may have been brought secretly into hospital.

Bandl's ring: It is normal for a 'contraction' ring to form between the upper and lower segments of the uterus (see Chapter 37). Bandl's ring is an abnormal continuation of this process. It indicates that the lower segment is becoming dangerously thin and could rupture at any time. A caesarean section should be carried out as soon as possible.

- Contractions will have been very strong and/or excessively long.
- The woman will complain of supra-pubic pain.
- The ring may be palpable or visible on the abdomen as a ridge or a groove rising gradually higher up the abdomen.

Incoordinate uterine action

The upper and lower uterine segments do not work together despite strong contractions. Contractions work in random ways, or upwards, rather than down from the fundus. Pain is felt before contractions become palpable and continues after they die away. Cervical dilatation may be slow or absent. Placental blood flow will be reduced resulting in fetal distress. A common reason for this is poor position of the fetus or cephalopelvic disproportion.

Constriction ring, diagnosis and management: A ring of tight muscle can form around the body or neck of the fetus. This constriction ring forms if the uterus continues to contract without the fetus descending or the cervix dilating. It does not relax between contractions:

- The woman may have pain which does not go away.
- It may be palpable on the abdomen or visible in thin women.
- The abdomen may take on the shape of an hourglass or figure 8.
- It may be diagnosed on vaginal examination: the presenting part may rise up with contractions rather than descend.

A caesarean section is needed. A muscle relaxant such as IM Sparine 50 mg may be given to reduce the spasm and make delivery easier.

Precipitate labour

This is probably the result of hypertonic contractions and relaxed pelvic floor so is most common in multigravid women. The baby is born after a very short strong labour. The woman may notice very few contractions. Possible complications are:

- Perineal damage
- Postpartum haemorrhage
- Fetal hypoxia and birth asphyxia
- Intracranial damage caused by rapid compression then sudden expansion of the fetal head
- The baby may be cold or injured from the uncontrolled birth.
- The infection risk is higher because of inadequate cleanliness at the birth.

Women with histories of rapid labours should be advised to try to reach their chosen birthplace before the expected date.

Abnormal position of the fetus

See Chapter 37 for normal positions and terms used.

Occipito-posterior position

This is the most common malposition. It is the commonest reason for the head not to be engaged at term in primigravid women. The fetus commences labour head down but looking toward the woman's umbilicus. It has to rotate during labour to face her back. The outcome of this situation depends on the efficiency of the uterine contractions and whether the head flexes or extends as it descends. It may start as a normal anterior position but the fetus turns' abnormally during labour. It is common with android pelves (see Table 39.2).

Causes

- The placenta may be situated on the anterior wall of the uterus.
- A pelvis that has most space at the back of the brim (android): The back of the fetal head fits this more easily.
- A pelvis with a brim that is narrowed sideways and longer front to back (oval anthropoid) (see Table 39.2): the direct occipito-posterior position of the fetal head fits better into this long diameter.
- A flat sacrum interferes with available space for rotation.

Diagnosis

The lie is longitudinal, presentation cephalic, the occiput is in the posterior part of the brim of the pelvis,

the head is not properly flexed, the diameter of the head presenting is large (see Figure 39.1).

- History. The woman may complain of backache. She may feel most limb movement at the front.
- Inspection. You see a bulge looking like a full bladder and a dip around the umbilicus. Alternatively a flat area may be seen below the umbilicus.
- *Palpation*. The head is high above the brim. The limbs are felt centrally. The fetal spine is impossible to find if it is against the woman's spine.
- *Auscultation*. The fetal heart is heard most clearly in the midline or out in the flank.
- Vaginal examination. Identifying landmarks on the skull may be difficult because of swelling (caput succedaneum).

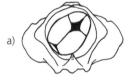

a) right occipito-posterior position, vertex deflexed

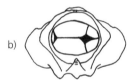

b) right occipito-lateral position, vertex beginning to flex

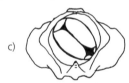

c) right occipito-anterior position, further flexion of vertex

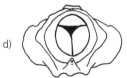

d) occipito-anterior position, vertex well flexed

Figure 39.1 *Progress from occipito-posterior to occipito-anterior position*

Features of the labour

- Persistent backache. The hard back of the fetal skull presses against the sacral nerves. Turning onto her knees, leaning forward or walking may be

Table 39.1 Outcomes of occipito-posterior position

Outcome	Mechanism	Management
Long rotation to anterior position (born facing the coccyx)	Head descends and flexes. The occiput meets the pelvic floor first and rotates forward 3/8 of a circle. The occiput slides under the sub-pubic arch and stretches the perineum.	See Figure 39.1 Progresses as normal birth (see Chapter 37).
Short rotation to persistent occipito-posterior position	Head descends without flexing. The sinciput (forehead) reaches the pelvic floor first and rotates 1/8 of a circle forward. The face is in the woman's sacral curve. On vaginal examination the anterior fontanelles can be felt behind the symphysis pubis. The sinciput slides under the sub-pubic arch. A wider part of the head stretches the perineum so it becomes highly distended. Tears are likely which may commence in the middle of the perineum (button-holing).	If undiagnosed, the lack of visible hair and feeling the anterior fontanelles may be the first indication of face to pubis birth. Keep two fingers flat between the eyebrows to help flex the head. Grasp the back of the head (parietal eminences) with the other hand and free the face (see Figure 39.2).
Deep transverse arrest (cannot be born unaided)	The fetus descends and begins to flex. The occiput reaches the pelvic floor first and starts to rotate forwards. Rotation is inadequate. The head becomes caught between the ischial spines, a narrow part of the outlet. The sagittal suture is transverse and both fontanelles can be felt (see Figure 39.1b). The causes may be weak contractions, a flat sacrum, abnormally prominent spines and narrow outlet (Android pelvis).	Help the woman to resist pushing by position change and breathing. During vaginal examination, push the sinciput up above the spines and allow the head to flex with contractions. It should rotate to occipito-anterior and a normal birth. Vacuum extraction: apply the cup as near to the occiput as possible so traction can encourage flexion and rotation. Rotation forceps may be used but can cause major pelvic organ and vaginal trauma to the mother, and brain damage to the fetus.
Face presentation	The occiput may feel large and fetal parts difficult to identify. A deep groove may be felt between the head and the back. On vaginal examination you may feel high up: soft mouth with hard gums, nose and eyebrow ridges (see Figure 39.3). Swelling may make this difficult. The head enters the brim fully extended so the face presents. The face descends and either: • The chin meets the pelvic floor first and rotates forward. The chin comes under the pubic arch. The face is born by extension, the rest of the head by flexion. • The sinciput (forehead) reaches the pelvic floor first, rotates forward, chin to the rear. Labour will obstruct. Caused by either an android pelvis with flat sacrum, weak abdominal muscles with the uterus tipped forward, sudden gush of fluid on membrane rupture with polyhydramnios, or fetal deformity.	Check for cord prolapse by vaginal examination when membranes rupture. Assess descent by palpation and vaginal examination. Decide which is lower – the chin or sinciput. Delivery of the face with chin anterior: hold back the sinciput with two fingers so the chin can emerge under the pubic arch. Then let the head flex round the symphysis pubis to be born.

Table 39.1 Outcomes of occipito-posterior position *continued*

Outcome	Mechanism	Management
Brow presentation (can only be born vaginally if head is small and pelvis is very large, or fetus is dead)	The head feels very large and high in early labour. It is partly extended with the sinciput lower than the occiput. The brow tries to enter the brim. It begins to extend instead of flexing. Extension is not complete. This is too large to pass through the pelvis (see Figure 39.4). On vaginal examination, the anterior fontanelle will be to one side, the eyebrow ridges to the other if they can be reached (see Figure 39.4). The head may become impacted if contractions continue. Labour becomes obstructed.	Caesarean section is needed unless: • The brow extends fully to a face presentation or flexes and become anterior. • The head is very small and the pelvis large. Manipulation to a flexed or fully extended position is sometimes possible using Ritodrine. Uterine rupture is a real risk. Craniotomy may be used if the fetus is dead.

more comfortable and help the fetus to turn forward. Deep back massage is helpful.

- Contraction pain. This may be severe and felt mainly in the back. Women become tired and frustrated and may need analgesia if available.
- Prolonged labour is common. There is a poor fit between the deflexed head and the cervix. This reduces the stimulus to stronger contractions.
- Early rupture of membranes. This occurs because the fetal head does not fit tightly against the cervix.
- Slow progress. The long rotation process takes time.
- Early pushing caused by pressure on the woman's bowel from the back of the fetal head. This leads to cervical oedema and further delay. Changing position may help her to resist the urge (see Chapter 37).
- Perineal damage may be severe.

Problems for the fetus

- Cord prolapse can occur when the head is still high.
- Severe facial bruising can make feeding difficult. Tube feeding may be needed. The bruising may cause jaundice.
- Abnormal moulding of the head may cause cerebral haemorrhage.
- Hypoxia and birth asphyxia.

Management

- Augment contractions with rupture of membranes and oxytocin infusion if progress is slow. Make sure there is no cephalopelvic disproportion first.
- Use a partograph to keep track of progress.

Possible outcomes of occipito-posterior position
– see Table 39.1.

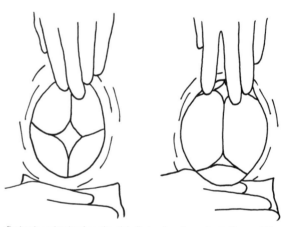

flexion is maintained on the glabella to allow the vertex to flex, and the occiput to deliver

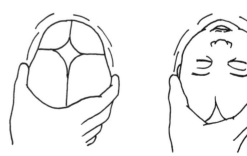

the two parietal eminences are grasped, and the head delivered by extension

Figure 39.2 *Delivering the head with a persistent posterior position of the occiput*

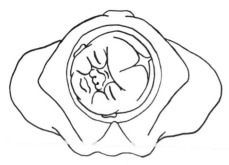

Figure 39.3 *Touch picture of face presentation*

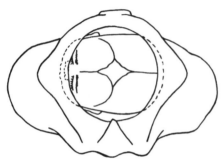

Figure 39.4 *Touch picture for brow presentation*

Abnormal pelvic shapes

These may be genetic or caused by malnutrition in childhood, or injury. They are a major cause of prolonged and obstructed labour. Some may be impossible barriers for the fetus.

See Chapter 34 for the normal gynaecoid pelvis. Small gynaecoid is the same shape but with overall reduction in size. Problems arise in labour and birth unless the fetal head is also small.

Abnormal presentations of the fetus

Presentations other than the vertex cause specific difficulties in labour. These presentations are face, brow, compound, shoulder and breech. The presenting parts fit poorly onto the cervix and may result in early rupture of membranes, poor uterine action and prolonged labour. Labour may become obstructed.

Face presentation

If the head is fully extended and the face is over the internal os then the fetus is said to be presenting by the face.

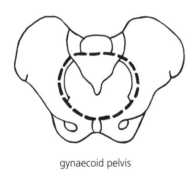

gynaecoid pelvis

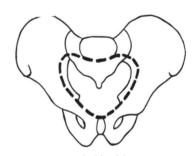

android pelvis

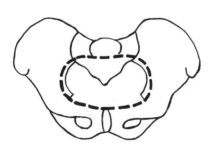

platypelloid pelvis

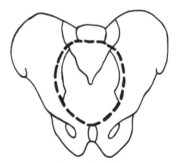

anthropoid pelvis

Figure 39.5 *Types of pelvis*

Table 39.2 Variations in pelvic shape.

	Funnel-shaped android	Long oval anthropoid	Flat platypelloid	Tilted high assimilation	Deformed pelvis e.g. from rickets or trauma
Inlet / brim	Heart-shaped with a narrow front. The widest diameter is at the back so the widest part of the fetal head fits better there. The fetus may engage in the occipito-posterior position.	Narrow transverse and long antero-posterior diameters. The head engages direct occipito-anterior or direct occipito-posterior.	Antero-posterior diameter is reduced so the brim is kidney shaped. The head may engage with difficulty. It may make a sideways rocking movement to put in one side at a time, known as asynclitism.	5th lumbar vertebra is fused with the sacrum so the antero-posterior diameter is smaller. The pelvis is tilted forward. Engagement of the head may be delayed.	In rickets the brim may be flat and badly deformed from the weight of the body on soft bones. The head cannot enter the pelvis except possibly by asynclitism.
Cavity	The sacrum is straight or flat. The fetal head may be unable to rotate to an anterior position. The ischial spines may be prominent. This reduces the transverse diameter. The head may arrest there.	The walls become wider. The fetus has room to rotate but may remain as occipito-posterior.	Flat sacrum but side walls widen so there is room for rotation.	Normal	The cavity may be deformed, with a straight sacrum.
Outlet	The sub-pubic arch is narrow. The fetus cannot pass close under. Causes perineal damage.	Wide	Wide	Normal	Flared and enlarged but the coccyx may bend inward.
	Similar to a male pelvis narrowing towards the outlet. Women are often short, wide and obese. They may be unusually hairy.	Women are often tall and slim.	Slow engagement then often rapid labour.	Associated with tall African women.	Cephalopelvic disproportion is a common feature of deformed pelves. The pelvis may be completely squashed. Obstructed labour is probable.

It is a primary face presentation if the head has extended fully before labour begins. This can be caused by fetal abnormality and other factors:

- Fetal goitre
- Anencephaly
- Flat pelvic sacrum
- Lax uterine muscle tone
- Prematurity
- Polyhydramnios
- Multiple pregnancy.

Diagnosis is difficult in pregnancy and is usually diagnosed in labour as described above in posterior position of the occiput. It is important to determine if the chin is anterior or posterior as the persistent mentoposterior cannot deliver vaginally.

It is said to be a secondary face presentation if the head extends in labour as it may do in a posterior position of the occiput.

If the chin remains posterior it will come into the hollow sacral curve and there will be no more progress in labour as the extended head and the fetal chest would all be trying to enter the pelvis together. Labour will be obstructed and, although it may be possible to rotate the head with forceps, it will usually be necessary to perform a caesarean section.

Brow presentation

Primary brow presentation is when the head is extended until the mento-vertical diameter is the presenting diameter. This may occur before the onset of labour, for example if the cord is round the neck several times or congenital goitre is present. Identification on abdominal palpation is difficult but it gives the overall impression of being a very large presenting part. This is unlikely to deliver vaginally unless it is fully extended to a face presentation or flexes.

Secondary brow presentation can be the outcome of an occipito-posterior position (see Table 39.1 on page 292).

Persistent brow presentation would need to born by caesarean section.

Compound presentation

A cephalic presentation may be complicated by a hand slipping down beside it. Before membrane rupture the hand may withdraw. Usually the hand slides out of the way as the fetal head descends. It is rarely necessary to attempt to move the arm. If the membranes have ruptured, it can sometimes be pushed away when the cervix is fully dilated. Vacuum extraction can then bring down the head. Caesarean section may be used.

Shoulder presentation and transverse or oblique lie

The fetus that lies across the abdomen in pregnancy may turn to a longitudinal presentation in time for labour, either cephalic or breech. It may instead drop into a shoulder presentation or an arm may pass into the pelvis. Sometimes the arm may prolapse through the vagina and may be seen at the vagina. The fetus cannot be born vaginally like this and obstructed labour will follow.

Causes

- Lax abdominal muscles as in grand multiparity
- Contracted pelvis or a placenta praevia which prevents the head entering the pelvis
- An abnormally shaped uterus may force the fetus into this presentation.
- Multiple pregnancy – lack of space may force one fetus into a shoulder presentation.

Diagnosis

On abdominal examination the head and buttocks will probably be felt at the sides of abdomen (transverse lie). They may be felt diagonally across the abdomen (oblique lie). There will be no presenting part over the brim.

On vaginal examination the soft shoulder and possibly the rib cage may be felt very high up.

Note: There is a high risk of provoking a haemorrhage if placenta praevia exists, causing the lie to be abnormal.

Management

- External version may be successful in late pregnancy or early labour (only if the membranes are intact). This involves turning the fetus from transverse to longitudinal lie, either cephalic or breech presentation.
- Caesarean section is needed if this is unsuccessful or if the arm has prolapsed. The uterus will rupture during labour without it.
- If transverse lie has been noted in pregnancy, the woman should be advised to go to a facility that can provide caesarean section (if needed) before labour commences.

- Check for cord prolapse and continue to observe for this.
- Attempts at manipulation are dangerous as uterine rupture can follow.

Breech

This is a longitudinal lie with the buttocks, feet or knees entering the pelvis first.

Types

There are four types of breech presentation:

- Flexed or complete. The knees are bent so the fetus squats in the pelvis.
- Extended or frank. The hips are bent with legs extended straight up the fetal body, feet at the shoulders. This is normally impossible to turn by external cephalic version (ECV). It is most common in primigravid women whose firm abdominal muscles prevent the fetus from bending the legs.
- Footling. One or both of the legs are extended so that a foot (or feet) enters the birth canal.
- Knee presentation. One or both hips are extended with the knee(s) below the buttocks (partly kneeling) (see Figure 39.6).

The position of the fetus is described relating its sacrum to the maternal pelvis.

Causes

- Pelvic brim abnormality
- Obstructions in the lower uterine segment so that the head cannot enter, for example placenta praevia, fibroids or pelvic tumours
- Fetal abnormality

- Premature labour. About 25 per cent of women have a breech presentation around 28 weeks gestation. Most turn to cephalic presentation by about 37 weeks. Prematurity is the commonest reason for breech presentation.

Diagnosis

- History of previous breech presentation
- The woman may report discomfort under the ribs and kicking below the umbilicus.
- On abdominal examination:
  - Inspection appears normal.
  - Palpation. A hard round mass in the fundus that can be 'bounced' between the hands (the head is 'ballotable')
  - The presenting part may feel less hard and is not ballotable.
  - **Note:** This can be confused with a deeply engaged head. It is important to palpate the fundus carefully to exclude the presence of a head there.
  - Expect thick meconium in the second stage of labour.
- Auscultation. The fetal heart may be heard above the umbilicus.
- On vaginal examination. It may be difficult to decide between a head and a buttock especially with a frank breech. The buttock can feel like caput succedaneum. It may be possible to feel the sacrum and the anal cleft.

Management of breech presentation

Some women try changing the position of the fetus by resting with their hips raised for about 15 minutes,

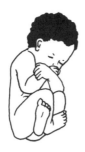 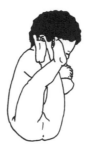 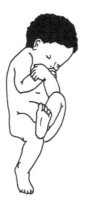 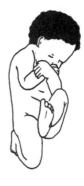

flexed or complete breech   extended or frank breech   footling presentation   knee presentation

Figure 39.6 *Types of breech presentation*

3 times a day. They then walk for 5 minutes. If they believe the fetus has turned head down, they should get this checked then stop the exercise.

External cephalic version (ECV): Breech birth has risks for both fetus and the woman. ECV may be successful in primigravid women at 35 weeks gestation and multigravid after 37 weeks gestation. Contraindications are:

- Known cephalopelvic disproportion
- Ruptured membranes
- Oligo-hydramnios (see Chapter 35)
- Rhesus negative mother
- Antepartum haemorrhage
- Pre-eclampsia or hypertension
- A scarred uterus
- Multiple pregnancy
- Fetal abnormality.

Method of ECV:

- Explain the process and seek the woman's permission. The procedure should not be uncomfortable and if it is then attempts to turn the fetus must be stopped.
- Ask her to empty her bladder and lay down.
- Listen to the fetal heart and record.
- Raise the foot end of the couch if possible. This helps to free the breech from the pelvis.
- Identify the fetal back and the direction of flexion of the fetus. The fetus must be turned so that this flexion is maintained.
- Grasp the head and breech and apply gentle pressure so that the fetus turns 'following his nose'.
- Check the fetal heart again once the fetus has turned (or you have abandoned the attempt). If it changes significantly – turn the fetus back as the cord may be under tension.
- The fetus may immediately return to its breech presentation.
- Observe for signs of membrane rupture, the onset of labour or indications of placental separation (see Chapter 37).

If this is an antenatal ECV, the woman may return home if no problems have arisen after 30 minutes.

The management of breech labour

The mechanism:

- The principles are the same as for cephalic presentation:
  - Lie: longitudinal

- Presentation: breech
- Denominator: sacrum
- Positions: right or left sacro-anterior or sacro-posterior
- Presenting diameter: across the hips of the fetus. This is smaller than the head.
- Leading part: anterior buttock.
- Descent takes place through the brim and cavity with good uterine contractions.
- The anterior buttock meets the pelvic floor. It rotates forward to come under the pubic arch. The anterior buttock is born by lateral flexion of the trunk.
- The anterior shoulder rotates forward and comes behind the symphysis pubis. The anterior shoulder and arm come under the pubic arch. The posterior shoulder comes across the perineum.
- The occiput rotates to come under the pubic arch; the face is in the hollow of the sacrum. The face is born by flexion.

Risks to the fetus:

- Placental separation may occur before the baby is completely born.
- The baby may inhale before the head is born. Cold air can stimulate breathing.
- Cord compression occurs when the body and cord are in the vagina together.
- Intracranial haemorrhage may occur due to rapid descent through the pelvis and from hypoxia.
- Skeletal and nerve damage may result from manipulation.
- Bruising of internal organs may occur if they are compressed by the hands during manipulation.
- Genitals may become bruised and oedematous. Maternal tissues may also be damaged.

Caesarean section: This should be performed when serious doubt exists about the success of vaginal breech birth and especially with:

- Abnormal pelvis
- Large fetus
- Both feet presenting (double footling)
- Deflexed or extended head
- Previous caesarean section because of cephalopelvic disproportion.

Note that:

- Caesarean section is more dangerous for the woman than uncomplicated vaginal breech birth. The main risk to the woman is of the after-coming head becoming stuck in the pelvis. Symphisiotomy is an option.

- Caesarean section should not be performed if the fetus is dead. A destructive delivery should be performed instead.
- Prematurity is not an indication for caesarean section alone as the fetal outcomes are no better than vaginal breech birth.

Vaginal breech delivery: This is safe when attended by staff skilled in breech birth, and with caesarean section easily available.

- Use of the partogram is advised to monitor progress. Dilatation may be slightly slower than for cephalic presentation. However, the alert and action lines are still relevant (see Chapter 37).
- Monitor the maternal and fetal condition.
- Meconium during the first stage of labour may indicate fetal hypoxia. During the second stage it usually indicates pressure on the fetal pelvic floor.
- Encourage the woman to walk around and change position as she wishes during labour unless there is risk of cord prolapse (ruptured membranes and poorly fitting presenting breech).
- Teach her 'no pushing' breathing and alternative positions if she feels the urge to push.
- The woman needs to maintain her fluid intake in labour. Whether or not she is allowed to eat easily digested food depends on local policy and the risk of caesarean section (see Emergency Procedures below).
- Encourage her to empty her bladder frequently.
- Perform a vaginal examination immediately the membranes rupture to exclude cord presentation (see below).
- Confirm full dilatation by vaginal examination as women experience the need to push prematurely. The body may pass through the cervix before it is dilated enough for the head to descend. This can lead to fetal hypoxia and death.
- She may adopt a supported upright (standing) position. The lithotomy position with raised shoulders may be used. Position the woman at the edge of the bed or on a stool so that the fetus can be allowed to 'hang' and use its body weight to bring the head down into the vagina and to aid rotation of the occiput to the front.

Assisting the birth: Note that the birth will often occur almost unaided, especially if the woman is upright.

- Limit handling of the fetus to the minimum needed to ensure his safety. Handling will stimulate the fetus to inhale before the airways are clear.
- Perform an episiotomy when the buttocks are distending the perineum if it is tight enough to cause serious difficulty.
- The buttocks will be born under the pubic arch with the sacrum toward the woman's thigh. It then turns the sacrum toward the woman's pubis.
- Free the feet if needed by flexing them. If the legs are caught deliver one first, then the other. Pushing behind the knee makes the leg bend, abduct the hip, then hold the foot by the ankle and pull it down. Do the same to the other leg. For extended legs see 'Delivery difficulties'.
- No further handling is needed until the umbilicus is born.
- Pull down a loop of cord if it is under tension.
- Allow the fetus to descend keeping your hands poised to support if needed.
- Wait for the shoulder blades to show. The body will face the woman's thigh again.
- If it is necessary to handle the fetus, handle gently around the pelvic girdle so that there is no risk of damaging the fragile organs of the abdomen.
- Arms will slip out if over the chest. The shoulders will be born spontaneously. Lift the buttocks up to free the posterior shoulder if needed.
  - If the first arm does not slip out, place a finger in the elbow to bend the arm, sweep the hand down over the face inside the vagina.
  - If the arms are extended upward, free them using Lovset's manoeuvre (see below) as they and the head will not fit in the pelvis together.
  - If the anterior arm cannot be delivered first, lift the baby upwards by the legs and toward the woman's thigh to free the posterior shoulder first. Then lower the baby to free the anterior shoulder.
- The head has entered the pelvis facing sideways. Let the baby hang down unsupported for 1–2 minutes. Its weight will help to bring the head through the pelvis and keep it flexed. The occiput turns forward as it meets the pelvic floor and emerges under the sub-pubic arch. The hair line appears.
- Deliver the baby's head slowly using either the

Burns-Marshall or Mauriceau-Smellie-Veit manoeuvres (see below). Obstetric forceps can be used following the same principles of maintaining flexion and slow delivery.

Lovset's manoeuvre: This is for freeing extended arms.

- Grasp the baby round the pelvis, thumbs on the sacrum and pull gently until one underarm is visible.
- Rotate the baby halfway round (180°) keeping the back uppermost to bring the posterior shoulder forward under the pubic arch. Pull gently at the same time.
- Free that arm forward over the baby's face as though it is washing its face.
- Repeat the rotation still keeping the back uppermost. The new anterior arm can be freed. This may have to be repeated.

Burns-Marshall manoeuvre: This is used for delivering the head.

- Let the baby hang from the vagina so that its own weight brings down the head. Do not touch the baby but watch for rapid descent.
- When the sub-occipito region is visible, grasp the ankles with one hand. Hold the head back with the other hand on the perineum to prevent its sudden delivery.

- Apply gentle traction (see Figure 39.7). Rotate the baby upward, or forward and outward, so that the sub-occipito region stays under the pubic arch and the face emerges slowly from the vagina. Avoid bending the baby's spine backward.
- The face will come free of the perineum. Deliver the head very slowly so no rapid change in head pressure occurs to cause internal haemorrhage.

Mauriceau-Smellie-Veit manoeuvre: Traction is applied to the shoulders to bring down the fetal head while using the jaw to keep it flexed.

- Put your arm under the baby's body, one leg and arm on each side. Lift the baby level with the woman's body. (Imagine a cat or leopard sleeping astride the branch of a tree.)
- Place three fingers of this hand in the vagina. Put the middle finger on the baby's chin or in its mouth, the other two fingers each side on the cheek bones.
- Place the middle finger of the other hand on the occiput and one finger each side hooked over the shoulders (see Figure 39.8).
- The baby is then gently and slowly brought down with the head being flexed as it descends. An assistant may need to apply supra-pubic pressure.

Note: Flexion should always come before traction.

This method is used particularly if the head is extended. You may need to rotate and flex the head, and rotate it back, if the sinciput (forehead) is held up in the pelvis. Supra-pubic pressure may help to flex the head.

Note: These manoeuvres are described for a woman lying in lithotomy. They can be adapted for women who are upright. Little manipulation may then be needed other than ensuring flexion of the head. You need to encourage breathing to slow the birth of the head.

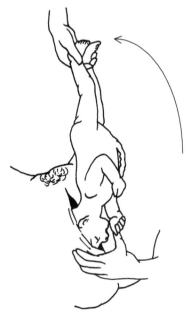

Figure 39.7 *Burns-Marshall manoeuvre*

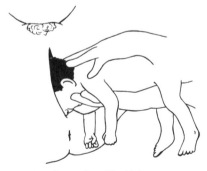

Figure 39.8 *Mauriceau-Smellie-Veit manoeuvre*

Delivery difficulties

Delay in descent of the buttocks: Either caesarean section or 'breech extraction' may be used. Anaesthesia is needed for breech extraction. The experienced attendant reaches for a foot along the sacral curve, brings it down and follows the full mechanism of labour using traction and manipulation. The risk of fetal damage is high.

Extended legs: The baby's body is splinted by its legs so that lateral flexion is difficult. Place two fingers along one thigh with the fingertips behind the knee to bend it and sweep it across the abdomen. That foot will be freed. Repeat with the other foot.

Extended arms: If the arms are extended over the head then the diameter of the head plus the arms is too big to descend through the pelvis. Lovset's manoeuvre is performed.

Impacted head: Caesarean section is essential if the head cannot be moved. Craniotomy might be performed if the fetus is dead. If a live baby is partly born, vaginal tissues could be held away from the face using fingers or a speculum to allow air in while waiting.

Labour emergencies

Intrapartum haemorrhage

Placenta praevia

Painless bleeding from placenta praevia may occur for the first time in labour. Descent of the fetus may be obstructed by the placenta. Caesarean section may be the only way to save the mother and fetus. This depends on their condition, the placement of the placenta and severity of the haemorrhage. Watch for postpartum haemorrhage.

Placental separation (abruption)

Abdominal pain and tenderness may be felt between contractions. It may be with or without blood loss (see Chapter 35).

- Severe haemorrhage with maternal or fetal condition threatened:
  - Complete the birth as quickly as possible, by vacuum extraction if fully dilated, or caesarean section if not.
- If the maternal condition is not immediately threatened:
  - Rupture the membranes and augment labour if contractions are poor.

- Use vacuum extraction to speed up delivery if the fetal heart is abnormal.
- Caesarean section if vaginal delivery is not possible.

Note: Fetal hypoxia may result in both types from a reduced functioning area of placenta.

Ruptured uterus

This acute emergency can kill the fetus immediately and the mother very quickly. Alternatively the mother may die of exhaustion, infection and secondary haemorrhage. It may be:

- Complete with a tear right through the uterus. The fetus may be in the abdominal cavity.
- Incomplete rupture not involving the outer surface. An old caesarean section scar may give way. Blood loss may be minimal or show up in the third stage.

Causes

- Obstructed labour, that is powerful contractions and a fetus that cannot descend further
- Previous caesarean section or perforated uterus, for example from unsafe abortion
- High parity
- Excessive or inappropriate use of oxytocin or prostaglandins (by professional staff) or the use of traditional herbal oxytocic by women and untrained attendants. **Note:** The tradition exists among professional staff in some regions to use IM oxytocin injections to speed labour. This is highly dangerous.
- Cervical lacerations (spontaneous or from instrumental delivery) may extend upwards.
- Injury to the abdomen

Diagnosis

Early signs are rapid maternal pulse, scar tenderness, abnormal fetal heart, bleeding and poor progress. Later:

- Maternal shock
- Severe abdominal pain
- Bleeding from the vagina (unless the fetal head is deeply engaged)
- Fetal heart sounds and movements will stop.
- Fetal parts are easy to palpate.
- The uterus may be palpated as a separate mass from the fetus.
- Abnormal abdominal shape. It may be distended.

Management

- Resuscitate with IV fluids, for example normal saline or Ringer's lactate.
- Urgent caesarean section and uterine repair or hysterectomy will be needed. The cervix and vagina may also need to be repaired.
- Give broad-spectrum antibiotics. Anaerobic organisms are a special risk.
- If possible, monitor later for long-term damage such as fistulae.

Women who have hysterectomy or long-term damage may suffer serious social consequences through loss of their childbearing capacity, or from problems such as incontinence.

Shoulder dystocia

Difficulty with the birth of the shoulders may arise unexpectedly but can often be anticipated. The shoulders are too large, or in the wrong position to get through the bony pelvis. The posterior shoulder should enter first, then the anterior. The anterior shoulder may become trapped behind the symphysis pubis. The other is in the cavity or caught by the sacral promontory. The fetus may die quickly.

Predisposing factors

- Small pelvis but normal fetus, or normal pelvis and large fetus, for example woman with much taller partner. **Note:** Women may have small pelves from childhood malnourishment, and then improve their nutrition so produce normal-sized babies.
- Maternal diabetes or obesity
- Older and multiparous women
- Previous history of shoulder dystocia
- Labour augmented with oxytocin

Warning signs and diagnosis

- Slow delivery of the head
- Difficulty with the birth of the chin, or it remains hard against the vulva once the head is born because the shoulder is still above the brim
- The shoulders cannot emerge under the symphysis pubis.

Management

- Do not press on the fundus or pull on the fetal head – this will worsen the situation.
- Call for help immediately.
- Ask the woman to change her position, for example kneel forward, stand or squat or roll on her side. Try lithotomy.
- If unsuccessful use the manoeuvres below, external ones first.
- Symphisiotomy may be performed to provide more space (see below).
- Episiotomy may provide more space to manipulate the fetus but does not alter the dystocia.
- Fracturing a clavicle may reduce the shoulder width although nerve damage to the baby may follow. Fracture may happen accidentally.
- Manipulation can cause maternal haemorrhage, injury to the reproductive tract and uterine rupture. The fetus may be asphyxiated and have nerve damage to the neck and arm.

Knees on chest (McRobert's manoeuvre): Lay woman flat with knees bent hard onto her chest. Assistants may push on her knees to increase flexion and abduct the hips. This puts pressure on the abdomen and tilts the pelvis (see Figure 39.9).

Supra-pubic pressure: Pull down firmly but carefully on the head to free the anterior shoulder while an assistant presses on the fetal back through the abdomen to move the shoulder from against the pubis and to rotate the shoulders from the antero-posterior diameter of the brim to the larger oblique or transverse diameter.

The following manoeuvres involve manipulating the fetus in the vagina. Use the knees on chest position, or lithotomy with buttocks free of the bed to permit greater pelvic expansion. The kneeling forward position may be helpful.

Consider performing a wide episiotomy to improve access and prevent internal damage.

Decrease the shoulder width (Rubin's manoeuvre): Find the posterior shoulder of the fetus in the vagina. Apply pressure from behind. Alternatively press the anterior shoulder toward the posterior one. This reduces the shoulder width and turns them.

Deliver the posterior arm: Find the posterior

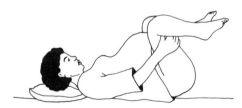

Figure 39.9 *The McRobert's position*

shoulder in the sacral curve. Move it to the antero-posterior diameter of the outlet if not already there. Hold the upper part of this arm and bend it at the elbow. Grasp the forearm and pull it forward across the chest and out. Rotate the shoulders round or decrease their width if the other shoulder does not come free.

Shoulders that are wedged across the outlet: May have to be pushed up to free them from the ischial spines.

Caesarean section may be needed if these actions are unsuccessful. The fetus will need to be manoeuvred and rotated backwards, reversing the mechanisms of birth to allow delivery through the abdomen (Zavenelli manoeuvre).

Uterine inversion

The uterus is turned partially or completely inside out. The main cause is poor management:
- Cord traction on an uncontracted uterus, and without counter-traction (see Chapter 37)
- Fundal pressure on a poorly-contracted uterus, or combining it with cord traction
- Withdrawing the hand after manual removal of placenta before the uterus is contracting
- Very short umbilical cord

Diagnosis

- Partial inversion: a depression can be felt in the fundus.
- Complete inversion: the inner surface of the uterus is visible in the vagina or may be reached. No fundus is palpable.
- Severe pain and maternal shock
- Massive haemorrhage

Management

- Do not remove the placenta until the uterus is back in position as it will bleed and be unable to contract.
- Replace immediately: grasp the uterus and push it through the cervix, fundus last, using a flat hand.
- Commence IV infusion after taking blood for cross-matching.
- If immediate replacement is not possible:
  - Compress the uterus with a sterile, warm, moist towel.
  - Give analgesia, for example morphine, or IV pethidine and IV diazepam separately.
  - Re-insert the uterus once it has taken effect.

- If still unsuccessful, use water (hydrostatic) pressure to relax any constriction and make the uterus return to its right place. Raise the foot of the bed high. Run 2–3 litres warmed sterile saline into the vagina using a douche nozzle and giving set. Hold the container very high to increase the hydrostatic pressure. Seal the introitus with the hand. The uterus should replace itself.
- Replacement under general anaesthesia may succeed.
- Once back, hold the fundus in place through the vagina until the uterus contracts.
- Give IV ergometrine 0.5 mg only when the uterus is replaced.
- Remove the placenta manually if necessary.
- Give antibiotics.
- Replacement can be done via an abdominal incision as a last resort.

Cord problems

Umbilical cord problems arise when the cord is malformed or gets into a position that threatens the oxygen supply to the fetus. The main problems arise in labour but twins can entangle themselves. Occasionally an active single fetus will make a knot that tightens during the birth.

Cord presentation

The cord slides down in front of the presenting part of the fetus. The membranes are intact.

Causes: The presenting part of the fetus does not fit well in the mother's pelvis and there is room for the cord to slip down, for example when:
- The fetus is premature or small for dates.
- There is malpresentation, particularly a flexed breech.
- The presenting part is high in the pelvis.

This is more likely with:
- Polyhydramnios, when the extra fluid in the uterus makes more space
- Twin birth, when the cord may present in front of the second twin.

Diagnosis: Cord presentation is often undiagnosed until a vaginal examination is performed. The cord can be felt pulsating through the liquor and membranes. You may suspect it when listening to the fetal heart, especially during contractions. You may hear an alteration in the rate or rhythm if the cord is compressed. A vaginal examination may then confirm cord presentation.

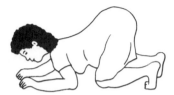

Figure 39.10 *Knee–chest position*

Management: Having felt the pulsating cord:

- Remove your examining fingers from the vagina.
- Put the mother into the knee–chest position (see Figure 39.10) or lying on the side opposite to the cord with the end of the bed raised. This reduces pressure on the cord.
- Arrange for caesarean section if the fetus is alive and mature enough to survive.
- If caesarean section is not quickly available, raise the foot of the bed as high as possible and push up the presenting part with your fingers to allow the cord to float upwards. Be aware the membranes may rupture as you do this, causing cord prolapse and fetal death unless birth takes place very quickly.

Cord prolapse

The cord is in front of the presenting part of the fetus and the membranes have ruptured. The cord escapes with the flow. The fetus can die quickly from hypoxia.

Diagnosis: Perform a vaginal examination as soon after membrane rupture as possible if the presenting part is not engaged. This detects cord prolapse. The cord may be in the vagina or visible at the vulva. If fetal distress is detected with no explanation for it, always check for cord prolapse.

Management: This depends on the stage of labour. It also depends partly on whether the woman is primigravid or multigravid and where she is when it happens.

- If the birth is expected in the next few minutes, encourage her to push.
- Perform an episiotomy if it might speed up the birth.
- Use vacuum extraction to achieve birth more quickly.
- Transfer the woman immediately for caesarean section if in the first stage.
- Use the knee–chest position while travelling to keep the pressure off the cord. Alternatively keep her on her side with buttocks raised. Listen to the

fetal heart frequently. Surgery should not be performed if the fetus dies.

- If you know others are around:
  - Keep your fingers in the vagina to push back the presenting part and reduce cord compression.
  - Turn the woman to the knee–chest position.
  - Shout for help.
  - Remain like this if possible until the baby is delivered, even when travelling.
- Handle the cord as little as possible. If it is outside, keep it warm and moist until the baby can be delivered or the fetus dies. Re-insert the cord into the vagina or apply warm towels.

Vasa praevia

This means 'blood vessels in front'. This may happen when the cord is inserted into the membranes (see Chapter 37) and the placenta is low-lying. The blood vessels are not protected as they are in the cord. If they run in front of the presenting part they may be compressed and the fetus will become hypoxic. They may tear when the membranes rupture and the fetus quickly bleeds enough for it to die.

Diagnosis: Pulsating blood vessels may be felt in front of the presenting part on vaginal examination. Sometimes there is sudden fetal distress on rupture of the membranes, accompanied by a small blood loss. Similar loss from placenta praevia would not cause such fetal distress.

Management: If the fetus is mature enough to survive and the woman is in the first stage of labour, caesarean section is used. If she is in the second stage, a forceps delivery may be attempted. Vacuum extraction must not be performed as it could cause severe haemorrhage from the fetus. The baby will probably need a blood transfusion.

Primary postpartum haemorrhage and retained placenta

Postpartum haemorrhage (PPH) is blood loss from the genital tract of 500 ml, or any amount which causes deterioration in the condition of the mother. It occurs after the birth of the baby and at any time up to 24 hours following the birth.

Note: Blood loss estimates are usually low.

Predisposing factors

PPH mainly occurs from poor contraction of the uterine muscle following birth. The blood vessels supplying the placental site are not properly compressed. The predisposing factors to this are:

- Uterine fibroids
- Over-stretched uterus from multiple pregnancy or polyhydramnios (see Chapters 38 and 35)
- More than four pregnancies
- Placenta praevia or
- Placenta abruption (see Chapter 35)
- Prolonged labour with poor uterine contractions
- Mismanagement of the third stage, for example manipulating the fundus so disturbing normal contraction
- Partially separated placenta or retained pieces
- Full bladder.

Other causes are:

- Trauma to cervix, vagina or perineum
- Uterine rupture
- Uterine inversion
- Clotting defects will also cause PPH:
  - Hypertensive disease and HELLP syndrome (see Chapters 36 and 35)
  - Amniotic fluid embolism
  - Retained dead fetus
  - Clotting factors being used up by previous haemorrhage.

Prevention

Previous PPH is a warning!

- Improving hypotonic uterine action (augmentation) provided there is no cephalopelvic disproportion or obstruction
- Active management of the third stage especially for those at risk
- Women's bladders should be empty in the third stage.
- As a precaution:
  - Cross-match blood for women at risk.
  - Prepare IV ergometrine 0.5mg for women having a fourth or more babies, in case it is needed.

Diagnosis

- Obvious bleeding from the vagina
- Shock
- There may be abdominal pain (uterine rupture).
- Soft uncontracted uterus
- Large, bulky and soft uterus may be filling with blood.
- Contracted uterus suggests cervical, vaginal or perineal trauma.
- Absent fundus suggests inversion.

Management

- Shout for help.

If the placenta is in the uterus and the woman is bleeding heavily:

- 'Rub up' a contraction.
- Administer intravenous ergometrine 0.5 mg.
- Catheterise the bladder.
- As soon as the uterus contracts, apply controlled cord traction.
- Manual removal of the placenta if needed (see Figure 39.11).

Note: A placenta that is completely attached to the uterus is less likely to cause immediate haemorrhage but the risk remains high.

If the placenta is out and the woman is bleeding heavily:

- Take the above actions.
- Carry out bimanual compression of the uterus to control the bleeding (see below).
- Examine the placenta to see if it is complete.
- Empty the uterus of retained products if necessary.

If the uterus is contracted, examine the cervix, vagina and perineum for trauma and bleeding. Apply pressure or clamps to bleeding points and suture.

- Monitor the blood clotting using the 7 minute bedside test (see Chapter 35).
- IV infusion should be commenced as soon as possible. If the woman must travel, this should be done first.
- Record all actions, observations and blood loss.
- Continue to monitor blood loss postpartum.
- Check haemoglobin after 24 hours.

Retained placenta

This is defined as a placenta that has not been expelled by 1 hour after completion of the second stage (time depends on local policy). If there is no bleeding and the woman's condition is good, you can wait this long before performing manual removal. The placenta will often separate in time. Do not leave the woman, and observe her uterus and blood loss closely.

- Use IM oxytocin 10 IU. Do not use ergometrine now as it will cause tonic contraction making removal difficult.
- If the cord has broken, try maternal effort, upright positions, emptying the bladder. These will work

well if the placenta is in the vagina and often when in the lower segment.

- Downward fundal pressure can be applied to expel the separated placenta if no other action has been successful. However, it can cause deep shock and inverted uterus. Make sure:
  - The uterus is well contracted.
  - The placenta has separated.
  - An oxytocic drug has been given.

If the placenta is attached fast to the uterine wall, it will not deliver on its own or with the aid of oxytocic drugs. It will be necessary to remove it manually (see below).

Bimanual compression of the uterus to stop bleeding

- External. An open hand is placed externally on the abdomen to one side. The other hand is clenched into a fist. The two hands are brought firmly together to compress the uterus.
- Internal. Insert the hand, shaped like a cone, high in the vagina. Make a fist against the abdominal wall. Press externally into the abdomen behind the uterus with the other hand until the uterus contracts and bleeding stops (see Figure 39.11).

Manual removal of retained placenta

Midwives should remove the placenta manually when no doctors are available. You need:

- An intravenous infusion in progress
- Blood available, preferably ready cross-matched
- The woman anaesthetised (general, spinal or epidural) or sedated with IV diazepam 10–20 mg
- Lithotomy position.

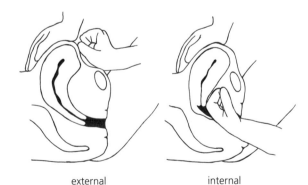

external   internal

Figure 39.11 *Bimanual compression*

Procedure

- Hold the cord with one hand. Work the other hand up the cord into the uterus and find the lower edge of the placenta.
- Release the cord and use that hand to support the uterus abdominally.
- Separate the placenta by sliding the hand carefully from side to side behind it. Keep the back of the hand against the uterine wall.
- Gradually move up the uterus until it is completely separated.
- Remove the complete placenta by cord traction. If removing it in pieces make sure no bits remain.
- Examine the cavity to ensure it is empty.
- Give IM or IV ergometrine 0.25 mg or 0.5 mg. Remove the hand only when the uterus begins to contract.
- Continuous infusion of oxytocin 10 to 20 units in 1 litre of fluid may be needed to keep the uterus contracted.
- Give broad spectrum antibiotics.

If the placenta cannot be removed because it has grown into the uterus, then it may be left to absorb. The risk of infection and secondary PPH is very high (see Chapter 40). PPH may follow if any part separates.

Retained products: These can be removed manually after spontaneous expulsion of the placenta.

Instrumental delivery and emergency procedures

Vacuum extraction

Vacuum extraction uses suction apparatus to enable you to assist the progress of the second stage and increase rotation of the head. A vacuum cup is attached to the scalp and sealed using a vacuum pump. It causes an area of oedema on the scalp. Vacuum pumps may be hand or electrically operated.

Women having vacuum extraction will need constant reassurance and explanation. Inhalational analgesia or local anaesthetic block should be used if available.

Vacuum extraction must be used on the skull, not the face or breech, and when:

- The head is engaged – at or below the ischial spines and no more than 1/5 palpable above the brim.

- The occiput can be located.
- The cervix is fully dilated or almost so.
- There is no cephalopelvic disproportion.

Advantages over forceps

- It uses no extra space in the pelvis.
- It increases flexion as the head descends when correctly applied.
- An episiotomy may not be needed.
- It can be used before full dilatation of the cervix.
- It causes less injury to the fetal skull.

Use it when there is:

- Delay in late first or the second stage
- Occipito-posterior position or transverse arrest
- Fetal distress
- Maternal exhaustion
- Need to reduce pushing, for example women with hypertension, heart disease, severe anaemia.

Contraindications

- Marked cephalopelvic disproportion
- Prematurity
- Abnormal presentation
- Dead fetus that has begun to deteriorate (macerated). The cup will not attach properly.

Pp Procedure for vacuum extraction

- Prepare the vacuum cup which must be sterile and check the suction apparatus and connections. If using a hand pump you need an assistant capable of working the pump. Check the vacuum against your hand.
- Lithotomy position is used.
- Insert an indwelling urinary catheter.
- Check the fetal heart and repeat between each contraction.
- Select the largest cup that will fit in the vagina without risk of damaging it. Usually a 5 cm cup is adequate.
- Check the position of the fetus.
- Insert the cup into the vagina sideways and place it on the head over the posterior fontanelle. Centre it 1 cm forward of the fontanelle. A small amount of sterile Vaseline may improve the seal (see Figure 39.12).
- Check that none of the cervix or vaginal wall has been included in the cup.
- Instruct the assistant to pump up the vacuum

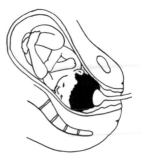

Figure 39.12 *Vacuum extraction delivery*

gradually until there is suction of 0.2 kg/cm^2. Check again for maternal tissue caught in the cup.
- Increase the vacuum to 0.8 kg/cm^2.
- Pull steadily but gently with contractions and maternal effort. (Do not pull without a contraction.) Keep a finger of the other hand on the cup and one on the head. This keeps the cup in place and detects slipping:
  - Three pulls with good contractions should be enough. Do not exceed 20 minutes traction.
  - Pulls should follow the curve of the birth canal. Angle them to correct obvious head tilt or deflexion.
  - If there is no descent – stop.
- If the cup comes off, check for serious cephalopelvic disproportion and review the direction of pull. It must follow the curve of the birth canal to achieve descent. Do not reapply more than twice.
- Perform an episiotomy only if essential once the head is stretching the perineum, or earlier if:
  - Access is too difficult to achieve accurate cup placement
  - You cannot get the right angle of pull.
- Remove the cup once the head has crowned.
- Active management of the third stage is strongly recommended.
- Record what you do, with results and times.

If vacuum extraction fails you may try it following symphisiotomy (see below). Otherwise caesarean section is needed. Some obstetricians will use forceps.

Care of the baby

Handle gently as there is a risk of intracranial damage. Give 1 mg of neonatal vitamin K. Keep grazes and cuts on the head clean and dry. The swelling will disappear in a day or so. A *haematoma* may form under the covering of the skull bones. This disappears in about one month.

Symphysiotomy

The cartilage of the symphysis pubis is cut to enlarge the pelvic inlet and outlet by 2–3 cm when obstructed labour occurs. Used with vacuum extraction, it can be life-saving for the fetus and woman when caesarean section is unavailable or undesirable. Future births should be easier as the separation is usually permanent.

The fetus must be alive and the cervix (normally) fully dilated. The head should be no more than 3/5 above the brim with no over-riding of the symphysis pubis. It is safer to keep to 2/5 palpable.

Indications

- Cephalopelvic disproportion
- Prolonged second stage despite augmentation
- Vacuum extraction alone is unsuccessful or expected to be so
- Shoulder dystocia – but maternal injury is more likely
- Trapped after-coming head in breech birth. (This needs more experience than cephalic presentations because of the urgency.)

Complications

- Long-term walking problems and pain
- Injury to the urethra and bladder
- Infection

Method

Note: Double gloving is advised to reduce the risk to the operator. Finger guards are available but reduce sensitivity.

- Explain the procedure and provide emotional support.
- Insert an indwelling urinary catheter.
- Clean the pubic skin with antiseptic solution.
- Infiltrate lignocaine 0.5% over the symphysis pubis and above and below. Ensure you are not in a blood vessel each time you reposition the needle. Check after 2 minutes that it is working. Allow longer if necessary.
- Position the woman lying down with legs bent up and no more than 90° apart. Assistants should help her to maintain this. They must be ready for

sudden separation which can cause serious tearing of the ligaments, urethra and bladder.

- Insert two fingers inside the vagina and find the catheter. Use the catheter to move the urethra sideways to protect it from being cut.
- Using a strong scalpel blade, cut down centrally into the cartilage, blade towards the woman's head. Cut down until you can feel pressure from the blade on the internal finger, without cutting into the vagina (or your finger). Cut to the top edge of the cartilage. Remove and reinsert the blade facing the other way. Cut the lower portion of the cartilage until the symphysis pubis separates.
- Remove the catheter to prevent urethral injury.
- The woman may now feel an urge to push; the fetus descends and is born. Vacuum extraction can be used but not forceps.
- Resuscitate the fetus if needed.
- Suture the pubic fat and skin.
- Re-insert an indwelling catheter.

Post-delivery care

- Applying elastic strapping across the hips can help to stabilise the pelvis and decrease pain.
- Bed rest for about 5 days. Encourage walking with help when she is ready. A walking frame may help. Encourage exercise to prevent deep vein thrombosis.
- Allow continuous drainage from the catheter for 5 days.
- Encourage the woman to drink to increase urinary output.
- Give analgesics as needed.
- Watch for infection. Broad-spectrum antibiotics may be needed.

Forceps delivery

This is less common now vacuum extraction is more widely accepted and routinely performed by midwives. There is a greater risk of fetal and maternal injury such as skull fracture, vaginal and cervical lacerations and uterine rupture. Indications may be:
- Fetal distress in the second stage of labour
- Maternal distress, when the woman is unable to push and cooperate
- To protect the fetal head in a preterm baby
- To deliver a face presentation or the after-coming head in a breech.

The procedure is as follows:
- Ensure the cervix is fully dilated.
- Empty the bladder.
- Confirm the position of the sutures and fontanelles on the fetal head so that the forceps can be placed correctly. Finding the fetal ear makes this easier.
- Provide a local anaesthetic block of the pudendal nerve to relax the pelvic floor and reduce pain.
- Episiotomy only needs to be used if access or the birth of the head is difficult.
- Forceps used:
  - Short handled (Wrigley's) if the head is at the perineum
  - Longer-handled forceps if the head is mid-cavity
  - For rotation, vacuum extraction should be used rather than Kiellands forceps as previously.
  - Pull should be the minimum force needed to achieve descent, and usually only with two contractions, (see Figure 39.13).
- Give IM vitamin K 1 mg to the baby if possible.
- Grazes and bruises to the baby's face heal quickly. Some have slight cerebral irritation. They should be treated gently but still be fed and cuddled as usual. Facial nerve damage usually recovers without treatment. Skull fractures or crushing may cause brain injury and death.

Destructive delivery

These procedures are used when labour is obstructed but the fetus is dead. A caesarean section should be avoided when the fetus is dead. All procedures are invasive for the woman although much less so than caesarean section. Caesarean section will be needed if the procedures fail to allow delivery of the baby.

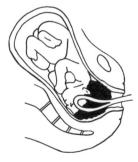

Figure 39.13 *Forceps delivery*

There must be no signs present of uterine rupture.
- Support of the woman is essential. She may need diazepam or local anaesthetic block.
- Intravenous infusion may be needed.
- Use the lithotomy position.
- Consider episiotomy to improve access.
- Catheterise and leave in until the absence of urethral or bladder injury is confirmed.
- Check for, and repair cervical and vaginal tears after the birth.
- Antibiotics may be given.
- Encourage good fluid intake and monitor urinary output.

Cleidotomy

This reduces the shoulder width by cutting the baby's clavicles with large scissors while protecting the maternal tissues. It may be difficult to gain access when the head is tight against the outlet.

Craniotomy

The skull is perforated so reducing its size. It can be used in cephalic and face presentations or when an after-coming head is trapped in the pelvis.

Cephalic presentations: The head must be fixed in the pelvis, or moulding must be enough to permit reaching it. The cervix is fully dilated.

Using a craniotome, strong pointed scissors or strong scalpel, make a cross-shaped incision of about 3 cm in the lowest point of the skull, cutting first one way, then the other. A hole can be made instead. Guide the instrument with your fingers to protect the woman's tissues. Use the instrument to enlarge the hole and break up the contents to allow them to escape.

Grip the skull bone edges with toothed forceps (several if possible). Pull and rotate the occiput under the pubic arch to bring the baby down. The skull will reduce in size as it descends. Make sure jagged bone does not tear the cervix or vagina.

Face presentation: Use the orbits of the eyes to enter the skull.

Breech: Insert the instrument through the skin at the base of the neck and tunnel upwards. Enter the skull through the occiput and widen the hole. It can also be inserted through the roof of the mouth.

Craniocentesis

This is used when the fetus has hydrocephalus (excess fluid in the skull) so has enlarged fontanelles and sutures. Using a wide-bored spinal needle, enter through the fontanelle or suture. Aspirate cerebrospinal fluid to allow the head to reduce in size. If the breech presents, enter through the roof of the mouth. Alternatively enter through the base of the skull.

Caesarean section

Caesarean section carries the risks of any abdominal surgery and anaesthesia but can be life-saving. The scarred uterus may tear in future pregnancies or labours. It should be used only as a last resort in those situations where women may not be able to get skilled care in future pregnancies. Caesarean section may be planned but is often done in an emergency. This means the normal preparations for anaesthesia may be difficult to achieve.

Preparation

The woman needs information and reassurance. She may fear for her baby's life and her own. She may also worry about reactions from her husband and relatives who may lose respect for her if she cannot give birth normally.

Special points about anaesthesia and surgery in pregnant women:

- Starving women in labour is distressing and results in inefficient uterine action so should not be done routinely. If surgery is not expected, they should drink freely and eat easily digested food. However, stomach emptying in labour is delayed. This is made worse by anxiety and narcotic analgesics such as pethidine. During anaesthesia, the weight of the uterus increases gastric reflux. Give an antacid and medication to reduce gastric acid production if available, especially if caesarean section is likely. When surgery is expected, food will be withheld but small quantities of water should be given. Local policy may exist.
- IV infusion, and having ready cross-matched blood from HIV negative donors, is essential.
- Shaving causes invisible cuts and grazes in which bacteria grow so should not be used on pregnant women. Hair may be clipped.

- Empty the bowels if possible, for example with glycerine suppositories. Insert an indwelling catheter to keep the bladder empty.
- The risk of deep vein thrombosis is high in pregnancy. Correctly sized graduated pressure stockings should be used if available.

Care during surgery should be as follows:

- Aspiration of stomach contents is a major cause of maternal death. *Cricoid pressure* should be applied during *intubation*.
- Administer oxygen to the woman by face mask for a few minutes before anaesthetising her to improve fetal oxygen levels.
- Tilt the operating table slightly to the left or place a wedge of foam under the woman's right hip to avoid supine hypotension (see page 232).
- Broad-spectrum antibiotics are routinely given.

Post-operative care

Examine the placenta and membranes for completeness while she is still anaesthetised. See Chapter 40 for postnatal care.

■ Activities

1. Consider what you would do if a woman came to your antenatal clinic complaining of pain in her abdomen and bleeding from her vagina. She is 39 weeks pregnant, this is her second pregnancy and she has just started to contract. Write a care plan for her, including getting her to a place that can provide all the care she may need. Discuss with your colleagues how you could overcome difficulties you might meet.
2. Devise a programme with your colleagues for encouraging local communities to be ready for emergencies. Include how you would teach them the danger signs and when they should get help for women.
3. Some midwives in your unit have never delivered a breech baby. Make a plan for getting together and practising breech birth using a doll. If you do not have a pelvis, think of something else to use instead.

40

The postnatal period

Postnatal care is described in this chapter. It also reviews the changes that happen to women once their babies are born and the problems that sometimes occur. It provides details about how to care for women and prevent such difficulties. Also included is what to do when abnormalities occur.

Introduction

The six weeks following the birth of the baby are known as the postnatal period or the puerperium. During this time the mother's body returns to the state it was in before pregnancy, apart from the cervix which never quite closes at the external os and the breasts which produce the baby's milk. Postnatal care includes ensuring these changes take place normally and detecting abnormalities. It includes supporting the mother, dealing with any problems and helping with feeding.

Another important part of postnatal care is helping the woman as she learns to care for her infant. She may lack confidence especially if she does not have female relatives or friends to help her. She will also need advice on contraception before she leaves the midwife's care.

Most women experience a healthy and happy change to motherhood. Others may have problems that can become life-threatening. Haemorrhage, infection and embolism are major causes of maternal death that occur in this period. It is also possible for eclamptic fits to take place.

It is important to assess the woman's condition and progress systematically. You also need to reassure her about what is normal and tell her about warning signs. To do this you need to understand what is normal. The particular points to assess are:

- Pulse rate, temperature and blood pressure should all be within the normal range.
- The calf muscles in the legs should not be tender, reddened or swollen which might suggest venous thrombosis or inflammation.
- The uterus should be reducing in size progressively.
- The vaginal discharge (called the lochia) should be changing from bright red, to brown then to white and reducing in quantity with no bad odour.
- Passing urine; the woman should be urinating regularly and without pain apart from soreness of the perineum.
- The perineum should be clean and healing if it has been damaged.
- Breasts which become enlarged and tender as lactation commences then settle down.
- The woman's ability to care for her own hygiene (she may need help).
- The woman's mental state and how she behaves with her baby.

Physiology and related problems

Changes in the uterus, cervix and vagina

Immediately after the birth of the baby the uterus can be felt just below the umbilicus. It should be central and feel hard from being well contracted. Gradually the uterus reduces in size until it can no longer be felt above the symphysis pubis after about 10 days. By 6 weeks the uterus weighs about 60 g again as it did before pregnancy. This happens because:

- Placental oestrogen levels have fallen.
- The blood vessels to the uterus are constricted. This reduces the blood supply and oxygen reaching the tissues causing *ischaemia*. This causes muscle fibres to become smaller or *atrophy*.

- The *myometrium*, connective tissue and fat cells are broken down and digested. This self digestion process is called *autolysis*. Autolysis is caused by *proteolytic* enzymes and cells called *macrophages*.

The raw placental site heals by having a protective layer of leucocytes laid down on it. The *decidua* is shed and is discharged from the body via the vagina. The discharge is called the *lochia*. Lochia changes throughout the postnatal period.

- Lochia rubra is red, lasts for about 2 days and consists mostly of blood.
- Lochia serosa is pinkish-brown because it has less blood and more decidual tissue. It continues for about 7 to 10 days.
- Lochia alba is yellowish white and lasts until about 4 to 8 weeks following birth.

The loss may become red again when women start to be more active. Blood loss is sometimes heavier during breastfeeding because hormones make the uterus contract. This can often be felt as 'afterpains' especially by multipara.

The cervix gradually becomes firmer and the canal closes. The external *os* never closes as tightly as it was before the first labour.

Lacerations and bruising in the vagina heal and the *rugae* return by 3 weeks after the birth.

Perineal tears take about 7 to 10 days to heal.

Changes in the circulation

A *diuresis* occurs in the first 24 hours to reduce the amount of fluid in the body. This means that women will pass urine frequently or in large quantities. The dilated pelvis of the kidney gradually returns to normal and takes about 3 months to do so.

Haemodilution in pregnancy will have resulted in a reduction in the concentration of haemoglobin circulating. As the diuresis occurs, the blood becomes more concentrated again so the haemoglobin level rises. This is known as *haemoconcentration*. These changes in the cardiovascular system put a strain on the heart. Healthy women can cope with this but those with cardiac problems may go into heart failure.

Blood clotting occurs more easily to prevent bleeding from the raw placental site in the uterus. This is caused by high *fibrinogen* and platelet levels in the blood and haemoconcentration. This increases the risk of clotting problems. It is important that postnatal women move about as soon as possible after the birth. If movement is restricted, they must at least move their legs. This is particularly important for women who have had surgery as the risk of clotting problems is increased. Emboli forming in the leg or pelvic veins can move to the lungs and cause rapid death.

Blood loss and infection

It is important that you should know what happened to women during labour and birth. You need to know whether the placenta and membranes were complete, as retained products of conception may lead to infection and haemorrhage.

Retained products or infection of the uterus exist if you detect the following:

- Uterus is soft, not contracted well or larger than you expect (known as sub-involution).
- The uterus is tender on palpation.
- The blood loss is excessive and the colour is reddish even if it has been pinker. The smell may be very offensive. Large clots may be passed.
- The woman may be feverish, have a rapid pulse and feel unwell.

Note: The danger of bleeding does not stop once the birth is safely completed and the placenta and membranes are delivered. Infection of the uterus can cause serious bleeding.

A secondary post partum haemorrhage: This is abnormal bleeding from the genital tract occurring from 24 hours following birth up to 6 weeks after delivery.

Excessive blood loss or signs of infection – what to do

- Assess the vaginal loss. If it is offensive, ensure that there is no infection.
- Examine the uterus for sub involution and tenderness.
- Take the temperature, and ask the woman how she feels, as a general feeling of being unwell is also an indication of infection.
- Assess the pulse rate.
- Send a high vaginal swab to the laboratory to detect any organisms which may be causing the infection. This test should also indicate the sensitivity of the organisms to antibiotics.

If there are signs of infection but blood loss is not excessive, the woman needs to be treated with antibiotics. You may need to consult a doctor. Failure to treat infection quickly may result in generalised infection (*septicaemia*), salpingitis and even peritonitis. These can kill the woman or result in subsequent infertility. Life-threatening haemorrhage could also result if treatment is delayed.

Severe life-threatening haemorrhage

- Summon medical help if it is available.
- Palpate the uterus and massage the fundus. Your aim is to make the uterus contract and expel any clots that are in the uterus. Clots will prevent it from contracting.
- Administer intravenous ergometrine 0.5mg. This should bring about uterine contraction in 45 seconds. **Note:** Ergometrine should not be given to women who have cardiac conditions unless the haemorrhage is a greater risk to life than the heart disease.
- Catheterise the bladder. A full bladder may prevent the uterus from contracting.
- Commence an intravenous infusion. A blood transfusion may be needed.
- The uterus will need to be evacuated, usually under general anaesthetic.
- Administer broad-spectrum antibiotics, preferably giving the first dose intramuscularly or intravenously.
- Observe the clotting of the blood. Delayed clotting will indicate *hypofibrinogenaemia*. This may result in disseminated intravascular clotting and later lead to massive bleeding. It may be fatal.

Note: Record keeping is vital and an accurate record of blood loss and the woman's condition should be kept.

Urinary problems

Urinary problems which may occur in the postnatal period are:

- Difficulty in passing urine and retention
- Urinary tract infection
- Stress incontinence
- Fistulae between the bladder and the vagina.

Difficulty in passing urine: This most commonly occurs after difficult labours, for example prolonged labour, instrumental delivery, epidural or spinal anaesthesia, and caesarean section. It is important that the bladder is not allowed to become excessively distended. This can cause long-term damage. The bladder should be emptied by catheter. Often this is all that is needed. Sometimes a pool of urine is left in the bladder after the woman has passed urine. There is an increased risk of infection if this keeps happening. This can be de-

tected by catheterising to measure the 'residual urine' after the woman has emptied her bladder. Sometimes an indwelling catheter is left in situ and released at 4 hourly intervals. This ensures that proper emptying takes place. The catheter can then be removed after 48 or 72 hours and the woman should be able to urinate normally.

Urinary tract infection: This is the presence of bacteria in the urine which may cause the following signs and symptoms:

- Urinary frequency
- Pain on passing urine
- Supra-pubic discomfort and pain in the side
- Nausea and vomiting
- Pyrexia.

Treatment consists of antibiotic therapy such as amoxicillin. The course should continue for at least a week. It is advisable to examine the urine in the laboratory to ensure the organisms have been removed. Organisms that remain can cause the infection to recur and this may damage the kidneys.

Stress incontinence: The bladder and urethra are relaxed during pregnancy by the naturally high progesterone levels. The same happens to the muscles that make up the pelvic floor. The bladder is pushed up from the pelvis into the abdominal cavity in labour. This results in the stretching of the urethra which also gets squashed by the descending head. All of these factors result in poor control over the urethral

---

Pelvic floor exercises

The pelvic floor is likely to have been traumatised during childbirth. Research indicates that activity and exercises may limit this damage. The following is an example of the kind of exercises which may be encouraged:

- Get into a comfortable position lying, standing or sitting.
- Pretend you are trying to stop yourself from passing urine by squeezing and lifting the muscles gently around the front and back passages.
- Do this about 10 times each day during the 6 weeks after the birth. You should aim at being able to hold the muscles for about 10 seconds once you are used to it.

sphincters. Women find themselves less able to control their urine flow and urine may leak out. This usually recovers spontaneously with activity and pelvic floor exercises may help (see information box on page 313). If incontinence persists the woman must be investigated and the presence of a vesico-vaginal fistula excluded as the cause.

Urinary fistula: A fistula is a hole between the vagina and urinary tract through which urine leaks uncontrollably. It is usually caused by injury from the pressure of the fetal head during prolonged labour. This causes *ischaemia* and a hole results when the tissues die. The woman needs to be referred to a doctor. These injuries do not often heal without treatment. The fistula should be repaired surgically within 3 months of the birth of the baby. This serious condition can destroy women's lives if it is not properly treated. They may become outcasts because of the leakage and smell which make them socially unacceptable.

Bowel problems

Constipation: This is difficulty in emptying the bowel and often occurs following childbirth. The best solution is to encourage the woman to drink plenty of fluids and eat foods containing fibre such as fruit and grains. Laxatives may be necessary. It is important to prevent prolonged constipation as this may result in an anal fissure. An anal fissure is a tear in the skin of the anal canal. It usually occurs in the posterior midline. Fissures cause pain and often bleeding on defaecation. Spasm of the anal sphincter may occur. The condition can become chronic and need surgical repair so simple preventative management of avoiding constipation is important.

Haemorrhoids: These occur when the veins around the anus become swollen. They may be known as 'piles' and can be very painful. There are four degrees of haemorrhoids:

- Visible but not prolapsed
- Prolapse with defeacation but return into the anal canal spontaneously
- Prolapse but need to be replaced manually
- Remain prolapsed outside of the anal canal.

As with difficulty in urinating, haemorrhoids occur as a result of the relaxing effect of the raised progesterone levels in pregnancy. They are made worse by pushing in the second stage of labour. Spontaneous recovery may result if constipation is avoided. Ligation with bands of rubber may be needed or even surgical

removal known as haemorrhoidectomy may be necessary.

Faecal incontinence: This is the involuntary passage of bowel contents which may occur after childbirth. It does not usually last long. If it does persist the woman needs to be examined for the presence of a recto-vaginal fistula. This fistula has the same cause as vesico-vaginal fistula and also needs to be repaired surgically.

Third degree tear: This is a tear of the perineum involving the anal sphincter. It may be called a fourth degree tear if the anal epithelium is involved. This condition may occur:

- If the fetus is very large
- In an instrumental delivery particularly using obstetric forceps
- When an episiotomy may extend into the anal sphincter
- When there is a long second stage of labour. The perineum may become over stretched, ischaemic and very easily damaged.

The laceration needs to be repaired very carefully and the midwife should refer the woman to a doctor. Following the operation the woman should be given laxatives to keep the faeces soft and antibiotics should be given to prevent infection. The midwife must follow the woman's progress and ensure there is no faecal incontinence.

Anaemia

See Chapters 34 and 36.

Iron stores are used during pregnancy to provide the iron necessary for the fetus, the extra blood cells in the mother and muscle growth. This continues while she is lactating. It is important to check that the woman is not anaemic in the postnatal period so that she is fit when she becomes pregnant again. Repeated pregnancies can seriously deplete iron stores and will result in raised maternal morbidity and mortality. Infections are also very important causes of anaemia so should be treated. Without this, no other treatment such as iron medication will be effective. HIV probably causes anaemia too.

Specific points to remember are:

- An anaemic woman should be given advice about delaying her next pregnancy until she has built up her iron stores (see Chapter 29).
- The anaemic woman may need to be given iron supplements for several weeks after the birth.

- A good varied diet is important so that all micro-nutrients such as vitamins A, B and C are included. These are essential to aid iron absorption.
- The best source of iron is red meat but this is usually very expensive and often impossible for women to obtain. However, even a little meat can help a woman to absorb iron from other foods such as vegetables.
- Supplements of vitamin A may be needed in areas where the diet is deficient in it.
- Good varied nutrition is also important for women who are breastfeeding.
- A woman who suffers from malaria should also be given antimalarial medication again after the birth.
- Parasites such as hookworms and schistosomiasis can cause anaemia.

Breastfeeding

Anatomy and physiology – how milk is made and reaches the baby

Milk is made in the woman's breast from her blood. An extensive network of blood vessels develops during pregnancy. This enables blood to be delivered throughout the lactation period to the milk producing units in the breasts (called alveoli).

Hormone changes in pregnancy, then at the birth, are responsible for the commencement of lactation. When the placenta is expelled the oestrogen level falls significantly. The pituitary gland responds to this by producing the hormone prolactin. This starts the production of milk. When the baby goes to the breast and stimulates the nipple, a neuro-hormonal reflex occurs. Milk is made and passes to the baby along the ducts. This is the process:

- There are sensory nerves in the nipple. When these are stimulated by suckling, messages pass to the posterior lobe of the pituitary gland.
- The posterior lobe of the pituitary gland produces the hormone oxytocin.
- Oxytocin makes the muscle cells surrounding the alveoli contract. The milk is squeezed into the ducts by the contracting muscle fibres.
- The ducts contract and the milk passes along them.
- The milk collects in widened areas of the ducts (ampullae) which lie just under the dark areola of the nipple and act as collecting chambers.

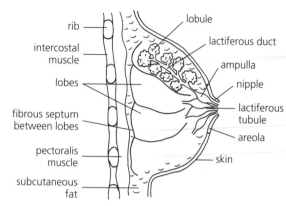

Figure 40.1 *Structure of breast and enlarged section of one duct*

- The baby's gum margins apply pressure to these ampullae and squirt the milk into its mouth. It is very important that the baby is positioned well at the breast to achieve this (see Figure 40.2).

Breastfeeding is vital for the health of infants (see Chapter 43). Most women can feed their babies on their own breast milk without any difficulty. Some problems can occur and may need special help from the midwife.

Painful nipples

These can be avoided by correct positioning of babies at the breast, see Figures 40.2 and 40.3 which show how babies should be positioned.

It is better not to use creams or other treatments for sore nipples as this stops the body's natural

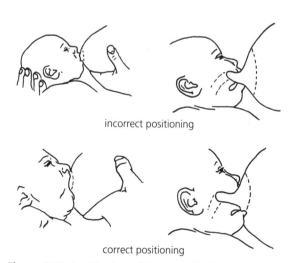

incorrect positioning

correct positioning

Figure 40.2 *Positioning of baby on the breast*

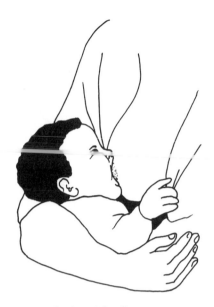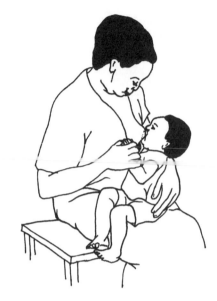

Figure 40.3 *Positions for breastfeeding*

healing processes from working. Bacteria can enter the breast and cause infection if inappropriate treatments are applied. Some traditional remedies can cause infections if bacteria are present in the remedies. Nipples should be kept clean and dry and the baby should continue to feed. It is important to pay particular attention to the way the baby has fixed to the breast to feed.

Inverted or 'non-protractile' nipples

Most women have nipples which stick out (protract). Some women have nipples that become turned inward (inverted) during pregnancy. It is very rare for this to prevent breastfeeding. Research has shown that it is not necessary to do anything special. Just encourage the baby to feed and this will bring the nipple out. Sometimes expressing the breast milk gently by hand will cause the nipple to stick out and so allow the baby to feed successfully.

Engorgement

Venous engorgement occurs in the breast as the blood supply increases very rapidly in the first 48 hours after birth. The breasts feel very full and often uncomfortable. This is normal. If the baby does not take enough milk, the alveoli in the breast will overfill and some milk will seep out into the surrounding tissues. This will cause inflammation. The woman may become feverish and her breasts will be hot and painful. The

best prevention and cure is to encourage the baby to feed frequently and until he has had enough.

In some cultures babies are not allowed to suckle until the milk comes in on the third day. This can increase the problem of engorgement so you should encourage early feeding. Both women and their female relatives may need information about the advantages of early feeding. Some people advise hand expressing of breast milk to relieve the symptoms. We now know from research that this is not necessary. It may also increase the amount of milk made and so make the problem worse. Stimulating the breast is part of the supply and demand of lactation.

Insufficient milk

Anaemia may be a cause of insufficient milk production so treating anaemia in the antenatal period is important. Lactation may be slow to start if a piece of placenta is retained in the uterus as the piece of placenta causes oestrogen levels to remain high. It is important to investigate this and treat it if necessary.

Mastitis

In mastitis the breast is inflamed and swollen with milk, known as milk engorgement. The flow of milk may be inhibited which results in too much pressure in the breast tissue. The breast may be infected or not. Mastitis is usually extremely painful and normally affects only one breast. Because there is poor milk flow, milk collects in the alveoli of the breast and this causes lumps to occur in the breast tissue. Even if it is not infected, women usually complain of feeling unwell. The symptoms are like those of influenza. Breast abscess is a common complication. Treatment should be started as soon as possible after the symptoms occur.

Treatment consists of:

- Encouraging the milk flow; this may need gentle massage and hand expression of the milk.
- Commence antibiotics if the condition does not improve within 6 hours.
- Observe closely for abscess formation. Should this happen then the woman must be treated with antibiotics. It is important to keep the milk flowing throughout. Once antibiotics have been started the baby should continue to breastfeed to keep the milk flowing. Research shows that aspiration of the abscess is better than incision.
- After completion of the treatment, the milk should be examined in the laboratory. This is to ensure that there is no residual infection as the breast will quickly become inflamed again. A recurrence of this very painful condition will damage the breast and make it difficult for the woman to ever successfully breastfeed a baby.

Mental health after the birth

Most women experience feelings of great emotion around the third or fourth day after the birth. It is sometimes called the 'third day blues'. Women may feel very miserable and tired, and may cry easily despite feeling happy about the baby. This is normal and passes quickly. However, some women become very ill. There are two conditions that can affect the mental health of women after the birth. These are depression and psychosis (see Chapter 49).

Care of women who have had a caesarean section

Women who have had a caesarean section will need extra care and support in the postnatal period. The immediate post-operative care will be the same as for anyone else who has had an anaesthetic and an operation (see Chapter 9). Some particular points are important:

- The woman may have become very dehydrated if labour was prolonged. Her IV infusion should be continued until bowel sounds have been heard and she is drinking well. It is important to watch

for *paralytic ileus* as the bowel is handled during the operation.
- Broad-spectrum antibiotics are normally given.
- Pain relief is important to help the woman to move around and to start to care for her baby.
- It is important for the woman to see her baby as soon as possible and to feed him as she would normally. She should not be left unattended with the baby until she is fully conscious. It is important to feed as soon as possible although most women need extra help at first.
- The abdominal wound and lochia must be monitored for blood loss and signs of infection. Some women will have perineal, vaginal or cervical lacerations or maybe an episiotomy, especially if they had a failed attempt at vaginal birth.
- Leg movements and early walking must be encouraged to prevent clotting in the leg veins which can lead to pulmonary embolism and death.
- There will be a urinary catheter. This needs to be removed when she can get to the toilet.
- Abdominal sutures and clips need to be removed.
- Haemoglobin estimation should be done on the third day and anaemia treated.
- Family planning advice should be given and the woman advised to wait two years before becoming pregnant again. This makes sure her wound is healed properly (see Chapter 29).
- The woman must be advised to give birth in hospital in future and to go there before labour begins. It is important to warn her that she has a scar on her uterus which might rupture next time. She may need a caesarean section again.
- The family of the woman needs to understand that she needs more help with domestic work than if she had given birth normally.

■ Activities

1. A woman in your care has heavy lochia 6 days after the birth. What could be the cause of this problem and what action would you take?
2. Aminatta is preparing to leave hospital with her first baby who is one day old. The baby was born normally but Aminatta has a second degree tear in her perineum which has been sutured with dissolvable stitches. She plans to walk home to her village accompanied by her mother. What advice would you give Aminatta and her mother before they leave?

41

Physiology and management of the newborn

This chapter covers the physiological changes that take place after babies are born that enable them to adapt to life outside the uterus. It covers the basic resuscitation procedures that may be required and the examination of the baby to ensure that any abnormalities are detected. It also outlines the care required by newborn babies.

Introduction

While they are in the uterus, fetuses are protected. They are fed, oxygenated by the mother's blood and kept warm. After birth every system of the baby has to adapt to life outside of the uterus. The most important changes take place in the cardio-respiratory systems.

Cardio-respiratory changes

In the fetus the pulmonary vascular resistance is high because the lungs have never expanded and the blood vessels are constricted. Only about 10 per cent of the fetal blood passes from the heart to the lungs. Therefore the pressure is higher in the right side of the heart than in the left.

In the fetus, blood returns to the right atrium in two ways:

- Oxygenated blood from the placenta passes into the right atrium, through the foramen ovale into the left side of the heart. From there it is pumped into the aorta. The oxygenated blood flows to all the organs.
- Most of the deoxygenated blood from the fetal tissues passes through the ductus arteriosus into the aorta and then returns to the placenta.

At birth changes take place:

- The stress of labour stimulates the fetus to produce *catecholamines*. (adrenaline, noradrenoline and steroids).
- This causes the lungs to stop producing fluid and to produce more *surfactant*. The surfactant reduces the surface tension in the alveoli and helps them to inflate more easily when the baby breathes in.
- The baby is bathed in amniotic fluid before birth. This is squeezed out of the lungs as the baby comes down through the birth canal. If there is infection in the fluid, the whole airway has been exposed to infection and causes serious intrapartum pneumonia.
- The baby is stimulated to breathe by handling and by the change in temperature from the inside of the uterus to outside.
- The pressure in the right side of the heart falls as the lungs expand. The cord is clamped and there is an increase in blood returning from the lungs to the left atrium. The pressure in the left side of the heart rises and is now greater than in the right side. This reduces the flow through the foramen ovale, which will soon fibrose.
- The rise in the *oxygen saturation* causes the ductus arteriosus to go into spasm. The blood in it clots and gradually the vessel fibroses and forms a ligament. If the baby becomes *hypoxic* for any reason, the ductus may reopen. This can cause problems as the blood will now flow from the left side of the heart, through the ductus, to the right side due to the change in pressures. Too much blood will now go to the lungs, causing heart failure. Drugs may be needed to close it again.
- The whole of the cardiac output will now go through the lungs.

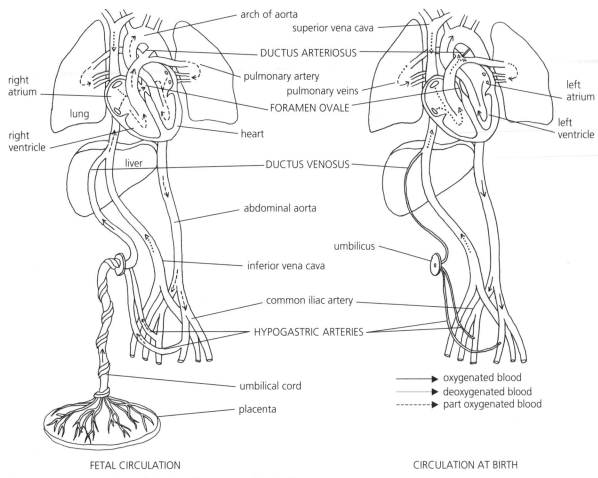

arch of aorta

superior vena cava

DUCTUS ARTERIOSUS

pulmonary artery

pulmonary veins

FORAMEN OVALE

right atrium

left atrium

lung

heart

left ventricle

right ventricle

liver

DUCTUS VENOSUS

abdominal aorta

umbilicus

inferior vena cava

common iliac artery

HYPOGASTRIC ARTERIES

umbilical cord

placenta

→ oxygenated blood
⋯▶ deoxygenated blood
--▶ part oxygenated blood

FETAL CIRCULATION

CIRCULATION AT BIRTH

Figure 41.1 *Comparison of fetal and newborn circulation*

Temperature control of the newborn

When babies are first born, they are very likely to lose heat. There are various reasons for this. Heat is lost from the body in four ways:

- Evaporation. Moisture evaporates from the skin to the air.
- Conduction. Heat is lost from the body to a cold surface.
- Radiation. Heat is lost from the body to cold objects in the area, such as a window.
- Convection. Loss of heat to the surrounding air. Draughts will increase this loss.

Babies are particularly at risk because:

- They are wet when they are born.

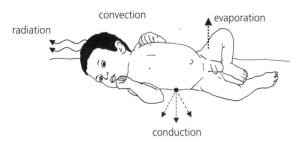

Figure 41.2 *Four ways a newborn baby may lose heat to the environment*

- They have a proportionately larger surface area than an adult and so can lose more heat through their skin.
- The head is large in comparison to the body, so heat loss through the head can be a particular

problem. During cold weather it is important to cover heads of babies.

- Babies are not able to shiver. Adults shiver and this produces heat.
- They need adults to care for them. They are not able to move to a warmer area or put on more clothes, as adults can.

Babies do have deposits of brown fat. This is a specialised fat which is laid down from 28 weeks gestation, mainly over the shoulders, the spine, around the chest, heart and kidneys. The purpose of this brown fat is to provide heat without using up glycogen. It can only do this if babies are breathing well and have a normal oxygen saturation. Babies who are cold will try to keep warm by increasing their metabolic rate. This uses up both energy and oxygen. The link between *hypothermia*, *hypoglycaemia* and hypoxia is sometimes known as the energy triangle, as each affects the other (see Figure 41.3).

To prevent hypothermia

- The delivery room must be warm, with no draughts. Babies should not be exposed to a cold environment during birth.
- Immediately after birth, dry the baby thoroughly with a warm towel to prevent heat loss through evaporation.
- Place babies next to their mothers' skin. Cover both mothers and babies to keep them warm.
- Breastfeeding should be started as soon as possible.
- If resuscitation is needed, babies should be dried carefully before treatment starts. They must not be placed on cold surfaces during treatment. Rooms must be kept warm and free of draughts.

Signs of hypothermia

- Babies may feel cold to touch, especially the hands and feet.

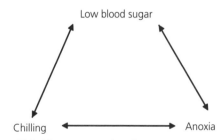

Figure 41.3 *The energy triangle*

- They may be reluctant or unable to feed.
- Weak cries and reduced activity.

Management of hypothermia

If there is reason to suspect that a baby is cold, an axillary temperature should be recorded immediately using a low reading thermometer. If the temperature is below 36.5°C, the baby is suffering from cold stress. If it is between 32° and 36°C, they are moderately hypothermic. If it is below 32°C, they are severely hypothermic.

They need to be rewarmed immediately. Check that they are thoroughly dry. Remove any wet cloths or napkins. Place next to the mother's skin and cover both mother and baby with warm cloths.

Assessing the baby's condition at birth

A scoring system called the APGAR score is used internationally. Five factors are assessed:

- Respiration
- Heart rate
- Colour
- Muscle tone
- Nervous system.

Each of these aspects of the baby's condition is given 0, 1 or 2 points and the sum of these points give a score out of 10.

To help remember this, you can use the following: **A**ppearance, **P**ulse, **G**rimace, **A**ctivity, **R**espiration (see Table 41.1).

The baby with a low Apgar score of 1 to 3 will need to be actively resuscitated.

The baby with an Apgar score of 4 to 7 will need suction and oxygen by face mask.

Table 41.1 Apgar chart

Sign	Score: 0	Score: 1	Score: 2
Heart rate	none	below 100	above 100
Breathing	none	slow, gasping, irregular	regular, crying
Muscle tone	limp	some bending of limbs	active movements
Response to stimulation	none	slight grimace	cry, cough, sneeze
Colour	white	blue	pink

The baby with an Apgar score of 8 or more can be dried, kept warm by wrapping and then given to the mother to be fed at the breast.

The Apgar score is first assessed at 1 minute after birth and then at 5 and again at 10 minutes. If it is low, it is repeated at 5 minute intervals until it is satisfactory. The score should be recorded as it gives an indication of the baby's condition at birth and possible future development. An Apgar score which is slow to recover may mean that the baby will have some developmental delay in the future.

Principles of neonatal resuscitation

- The baby must be dried and kept warm on a heated trolley or covered. A cold baby requires more oxygen. See above.
- Position the baby on his back, with the head tilted backwards. Extend the neck gently, do not over extend as this will prevent good air entry.
- Gently suction the oro-pharynx, using a mucus extractor or suction apparatus if available. Make sure all apparatus is clean and suction gently as it can cause laryngeal spasm.
- Stimulate the baby by rubbing with a towel. This may be enough to make the baby breathe.
- Give oxygen with a facemask. If the baby is not breathing well, oxygen should be given with a mask and bag. The jaw needs to be lifted slightly, taking care not to press on the soft tissue under the jaw as this will prevent good air entry.
- Ventilate the baby at about 50 breaths per minute. The baby's colour and pulse rate should show an immediate improvement.
- If the baby does not improve, tracheal intubation may be necessary. Midwives should be trained to carry out this procedure (see below).

Pp **Tracheal intubation**

- For a full term baby of normal weight 3.5 kg, use an endotracheal tube of 3.0 or 3.5 mm. A smaller tube will be needed for a baby who weighs less than 2.5 kg.
- Pass the laryngoscope over the tongue and depress it until the vocal cords are visible. This must be carried out gently.
- The endotracheal tube is passed into the trachea.

- Oxygen can then be given at a pressure of 20 to 25 cm of water, at a rate of 50 breaths per minute. If it is going well, the baby's chest will be seen to move. Listen with a stethoscope and you should be able to hear air entry.

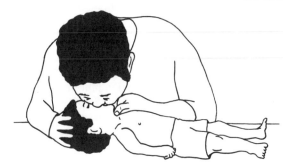

Figure 41.4 *Position of the newborn for ventilations*

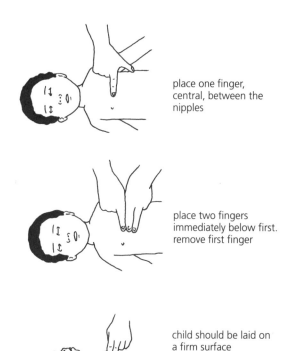

place one finger, central, between the nipples

place two fingers immediately below first. remove first finger

child should be laid on a firm surface

Figure 41.5 *Position of the newborn for cardiac massage*

If the baby does not recover quickly check that:
- The airway is not obstructed.
- The bag and mask are correctly applied.

- The endotracheal tube is in the correct position, not in the oesophagus or too far into the trachea. Both sides of the chest should be moving.
- The oxygen supply is connected.
- The inspiratory pressure being used is correct.

If all of these factors have been checked then other serious but rare possibilities must be considered.

- External cardiac massage may be needed if the heart remains at less than 60 beats per minute (see Figure 41.5).
- It may be necessary to give drugs. If the mother has had opiates administered in labour then a single intramuscular injection of naloxone 200 micrograms can be given. If the baby has been hypoxic for some time, it may be necessary to give calcium gluconate. This can be given via a naso-gastric tube
- After resuscitation, check the baby's temperature and blood sugar. He may have become hypothermic and hypoglycaemic. Rewarm and give intravenous glucose for any hypoglycaemia.
- It is important to avoid all unnecessary trauma or invasive procedures because of the risk of HIV infection (see Chapter 32).

Meconium aspiration syndrome

If there has been thick meconium staining of the liquor, meconium should be cleared from the baby's mouth and oro-pharynx as soon as the head is born. The meconium should then be aspirated from the vocal cords under direct vision with a laryngoscope using a wide-bore catheter before the baby takes his first breath. If the baby cries well at birth then no further action need be taken. If meconium is not cleared from the airways, pneumonia can develop.

The midwife must remember how anxious the mother will be during this time and give as much information and reassurance as she can.

Examination of newborn at birth

Parents need to know that their baby is well and healthy. The baby should be examined soon after birth in front of the parents. The room needs to be warm and well lit.

The head: The midwife feels the head and notes the size of the sutures and fontanelles. Wide sutures and large fontanelles may indicate that the baby is im-

mature or that there is increased intracranial pressure due to *hydrocephalus* or intracranial haemorrhage. The head circumference is measured around the occiput and the frontal bones and recorded. Any enlargement can be recognised.

The eyes: If *epicanthic* folds are seen, this could indicate the presence of Downs syndrome. The baby may be born without one or both eyes. Tetracycline eye ointment or 1% solution of silver nitrate drops to prevent gonococcal infection may be put into the eyes immediately after birth.

The nose: This is examined to ensure there are no abnormalities. Newborn babies are unable to breathe through their mouths. Listen to how the baby is breathing. A bloody discharge may indicate congenital syphilis.

The mouth: The palate is felt for a cleft. Any teeth that are present may need to be removed as they can be loose and could obstruct the baby's airway and are also uncomfortable for the mother when she breast-feeds.

The neck: A *sterno-mastoid* swelling may indicate that there is a tumour or that a haematoma has formed. This can happen if extra traction had been applied during the delivery if, for example, there had been a degree of shoulder dystocia.

The arms: The arms should be checked for any stiffness. Short arms may be a sign of *achondroplasia*. The fingers should be counted and any skin linking the fingers (webbing) should be noted. Extra digits can often be removed very simply by applying a ligature if there is no bone content to them.

The abdomen: Gentle palpation of the abdomen to determine enlargement of the liver or spleen is done as this could indicate a congenital infection such as toxoplasmosis or rubella.

External genitalia: In a boy the testes should be descended and the urethral opening should be at the end of the penis. The penis should be straight and the foreskin should not be too tight (see Chapter 28). In a girl the urethra and vagina should be checked for normality.

The hips: The hip joint should be examined for dislocation. The baby should be lying on his back on a firm surface. The knees and hips are flexed to 90° and the midwife holds each leg with the thumb on the inner aspect of the thigh and the middle finger on the greater trochanter. The leg is then gently *abducted* and a click is felt if the head of the femur slips back into the acetabulum of the pelvis from its dislocated position (see Figure 41.6). Sometimes no click is felt but the hip will not abduct, this too would indicate dislocation. Treatment is to keep the baby's hips abducted by placing him on his mother's back.

The feet: Talipes can be recognised when the feet are not in alignment with the baby's legs (see Chapter 42).

The toes: These are counted and checked for webbing.

The back: The midwife should look for any swelling and run her finger along the length of the spine to see if there is any evidence of spina bifida. If there is an open lesion, a myelomeningocele, it should be covered with a sterile dressing or plastic film. The baby should be seen by a neurosurgeon if possible.

The anus: This should be patent. Any abnormality should be referred immediately as it can cause an intestinal obstruction.

Neurological examination: Healthy newborn babies will have a startle reflex. This is shown by holding the infant in the supine position. One hand supports the sacrum, the other the upper back and head. The baby's head is then suddenly allowed to drop about 30°. The baby will then throw out his hands and legs and then bring his arms in, almost as if he is hugging himself. This is called the Moro Reflex. A healthy baby will also have a primitive walking reflex; if the baby is held up with the feet just touching a firm surface the baby takes steps just as if he is walking.

Muscle tone: Hold the baby in the *ventral* suspension. Normal babies will hold their heads in a straight line with the spinal column. Babies who have floppy legs and heads may be showing signs of cerebral irritation

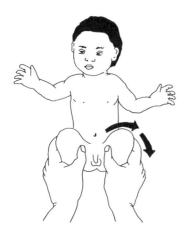

Figure 41.6 *Ortolani's test for congenital dislocation of the hips*

(hypoxic ischaemic brain damage).

Weight: The baby's weight should be recorded on a growth chart (see Appendix B). Tell the mother whether her baby is small or large.

Maturity: Assess the maturity of the baby. Post mature babies often have dry skins and long nails. Premature babies have thin skins, may be covered with *lanugo*, have some oedema. The ear may lack cartilage and folds forward easily, without springing back.

Remember to assess all babies including those who have been born at home and are then brought to hospital.

Note: If abnormalities are detected then the baby should be referred to the medical staff as soon as possible.

Many authorities recommend the administration of vitamin K 1 mg to every newborn baby to reduce the incidence of haemorrhagic disease in the newborn. This may be given orally or intramuscularly.

Daily care of the newborn

Hygiene

The midwife must wash her hands thoroughly before touching the newborn baby. A baby is at risk of picking up infection from those who care for him or from dirty equipment. Infection will be reduced by encouraging the mother to give the care as she will only be handling her own baby. Gloves should be worn when washing blood off the baby following delivery, in case the mother is HIV positive. He should be washed and dried carefully after passing urine or faeces.

Cord care

After birth the cord is no longer needed so, once it has been clamped and cut, it should be kept dry and clean and nothing should be applied to it. The blood vessels in the cord clot and then fibrose. The cord shrinks and it may be necessary to apply another ligature to prevent bleeding. The cord will then usually separate around the 5th to the 7th day. The cord separates by decaying and there is a danger that the umbilicus can become infected. The midwife must observe the area carefully and report any signs of infection, especially if the area around becomes inflamed. An infected cord can quickly lead to septicaemia (see Chapter 42). In some cultures, it is the tradition to apply a variety of substances to the cord area. This can be a dangerous practice as it can lead to tetanus. Studies have been carried out which make it clear that the cord area is more likely to heal quickly if it is just kept clean and dry. Mothers should be taught to care for the cord so that if they have their next baby at home, they are able to care for the cord safely.

Urinary tract

The midwife should record the first time that the baby passes urine, and record it. The mother can be asked to watch and report the stream of urine. A poor stream may indicate an abnormality.

Bowels

The first stool that a baby passes is called meconium. It is dark green in colour and of sticky consistency. It should be passed within 24 hours and is an indication that the lower bowel is normal. Any delay in passing meconium should be reported. Once the baby has been fed milk and the milk has passed through the alimentary tract, the stool will become pale green and will contain milk curds. The midwife should record this as it shows that the whole alimentary tract is working. This stool is referred to as a 'changing stool'.

Once breastfeeding has been established, the stool becomes deep yellow and is semi-fluid in consistency. Most babies will have a bowel movement each day. Any abnormality of the stools should be reported.

- Babies who are not getting enough milk will have a pale green stool.
- Babies with an intestinal infection will have an offensive green fluid. This should be treated quickly as the baby may become very ill.
- Blood in the stool may indicate haemorrhagic disease of the newborn. He will need vitamin K.

Temperature

A healthy newborn baby has a temperature of around 36.6°C. It is not necessary to take the baby's temperature with a thermometer but the baby's back should feel warm to touch although the hands and feet are often cool. It is important to prevent babies getting cold by keeping them close to their mothers. If they become infected, the temperature may be high or low (see Chapter 42).

Feeding

Breastfeeding should begin as soon as possible. Exclusive breastfeeding for the first 6 months is strongly recommended (see Chapters 40 and 43).

Love and contact

Babies thrive when they are handled with love and tenderness. Studies have shown that babies who are cuddled and handled gently by their mothers grow and thrive best.

Health promotion

The midwife must make sure that the mother is confident in caring for her baby before she takes him home. She should tell the mother to bring him back to the infant welfare clinic for his immunisations and for checking his weight.

■ Activity

A young girl of 13 years has just had her first baby. What advice would you give her to help her care for the baby?

42

Care of babies with neonatal problems

There are various problems that may affect newborn babies. They may be a normal weight but develop problems following delivery. They may be small, for example below 2500 g. This is either due to the fact they have been born before 37 weeks gestation or because they have not grown well in utero. They may be born with a congenital abnormality. This chapter covers the most common problems.

Hypoglycaemia

The blood sugar of some babies can fall too low, particularly if they have become cold. A low blood sugar causes the baby to become floppy and can cause fits. In severe cases they may suffer brain damage as a result. Newborn babies should be put to the breast to feed as soon as possible. If *hypoglycaemia* is proved and the baby will not suck, breast milk can be given with a cup and spoon, or if necessary via a nasogastric tube. Babies that are particularly at risk include:

Babies of diabetic mothers: They are particularly at risk as in utero they have been producing insulin in larger quantities than normal to deal with the hyperglycaemia of the mother. Once babies are born they may go on producing large quantities of insulin but are no longer getting the high glucose from the mother. These babies should have their blood glucose measured frequently over the first few days, as the blood glucose level can fall dramatically leading to brain damage or death. After a few days the baby will produce normal quantities of insulin so there will no longer be a problem.

Preterm and low birth weight babies: These babies have not built up the necessary glycogen stores before birth. They have either been born too early or have not received adequate nutrition in utero.

Any baby who convulses as a result of hypoglycaemia should be given intravenous glucose.

Jaundice of the newborn

Normal physiology: Red cells (erythrocytes) are formed mainly in the liver and spleen of the fetus. After birth they are formed in the red bone marrow of the body. Erythrocytes are continually being broken down (*haemolysis*). They live on average for 120 days in the adult, but only 90 days in the newborn baby. When broken down, the iron from the cells goes to the liver and can be re-used. The remainder is excreted as bilirubin.

Unconjugated bilirubin: This is fat soluble and is carried by the plasma proteins. It goes to the liver where it is acted on by a liver enzyme converting it to conjugated or water soluble bilirubin. When it rises above a certain level, it is laid down in fatty tissue, including the brain. High levels cause *kernicterus*, which can lead to fits, brain damage or death.

Conjugated bilirubin: This is water soluble and easily excreted as urobilinogen in the urine, giving urine its yellow colour, and stercobilinogen in the faeces, giving stools their brown colour (see Figure 42.1).

Causes of jaundice

Jaundice occurs when there has been rapid haemolysis or the liver is unable to clear the bilirubin. There are many possible causes:
- Physiological jaundice
- Breast milk jaundice
- Rhesus incompatibility
- ABO incompatibility
- G6PD deficiency
- Infection
- Neonatal hepatitis
- Biliary duct atresia.

Breakdown of red cells

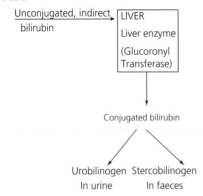

Figure 42.1 *Formation and excretion of bilirubin*

Physiological jaundice

This is the commonest form.

- At birth, babies have a very high red cell count. Before birth they receive their oxygen from their mothers. This is a less efficient way of receiving oxygen than by breathing. After babies are born, they do not need so many red cells, so the cells are broken down very quickly, leading to a high level of bilirubin.
- The liver of the newborn baby is relatively immature and cannot cope with this high level so the baby can become jaundiced.

Usually nothing needs to be done, as long as the baby feeds well. This will help to wash out the bilirubin. Sometimes the babies are sleepy and need a lot of encouragement to feed.

In physiological jaundice:

- The baby will be well.
- The jaundice appears at about the 2nd or 3rd day.
- It peaks at 5 days and has usually disappeared by 10 days, as the liver matures and the rate of breakdown of red cells is reduced.

Breast milk jaundice

Babies who are breastfed may remain jaundiced for longer, as breast milk contains a hormone which delays the breakdown of bilirubin. Breastfeeding must not be stopped.

Rhesus incompatibility (see Chapter 12)

This is when the mother of the baby is Rhesus negative, the father is Rhesus positive and the baby inherits the Rhesus factor from his father. The first Rhesus positive baby will not normally be affected, unless the mother has had a previous miscarriage, or a blood transfusion with Rhesus positive blood. However, she will develop *antibodies* to the Rhesus factor after the birth of this baby unless she is given the Anti D factor within 72 hours of giving birth. When she has her next baby, the antibodies in her blood react with the baby's blood in utero, causing excessive *haemolysis*. The baby is born anaemic and develops jaundice within 24 hours. The levels can be extremely high. As the bilirubin is conjugated, it can be laid down in the baby's brain causing kernicterus. Without treatment, each Rhesus positive baby that the mother has will be worse affected and she is likely to have stillborn babies. These may look very pale from the anaemia and oedematous from cardiac failure. This is known as Hydrops Foetalis. Babies who are born with Rhesus incompatibility may need an exchange blood transfusion using Rhesus negative blood, even though the baby is Rhesus positive. The mother's blood, which will still contain antibodies, will continue to break down the baby's blood if Rhesus positive blood is used.

ABO incompatibility

This is usually less severe than Rhesus incompatibility and occurs when the mother is blood group O and the baby either blood group A or B.

G6PD deficiency

This is an inherited condition, more common in boys, which results in the red cells breaking down very easily. This breakdown of the cells leads to anaemia and jaundice. The baby with this gene can be affected if the mother has been on certain drugs, for example anti malarials, sulphonamides, paracetamol or antibiotics and is breastfeeding. It can also be provoked by camphor or mentholatum used to keep clothes free of insects, or by substances applied to the cord by traditional birth attendants (TBAs). It is important to take a careful history in order to prevent a recurrence with future babies.

Infection

Babies who develop an infection will also break down more red cells than usual. The immature liver cannot deal with this and the baby may become jaundiced. All babies who develop jaundice for no other known reason should be suspected of having an infection.

Biliary duct atresia

This is where the bile ducts of the baby are blocked. Fortunately it is a rare condition as it is very difficult to treat and the majority of babies will die unless they can be referred to a paediatric surgeon quickly. Even then, the outlook is not good. In these babies the jaundice develops slowly and persists. The stools are pale and the urine dark as it is an obstructive jaundice and bile does not reach the gut. Neonatal hepatitis presents in a similar way. A liver biopsy is usually the only way in which an accurate diagnosis can be made.

Nursing care of the jaundiced baby

- Keep all babies well fed and hydrated as any jaundice is worse in a dehydrated baby. Mothers may need help to encourage a sleepy baby to feed.
- Expose jaundiced babies' skins to sunlight. If possible they should be nursed without clothes and placed in a sunny part of the nursery/room. They should be turned over every 2 hours. The sunlight acts on the bilirubin laid down in the subcutaneous fat and converts it to biliverdin which can be excreted. Make sure that babies do not get cold during this time.
- Phototherapy units may be available in major hospitals. This unit can be placed over the babies' cribs and the light from the unit will act in the same way as the sunlight. It is important to cover the eyes to avoid eye damage.
- Hydration. Both sunlight and phototherapy increase the fluid loss by evaporation, so the hydration of the baby must be monitored. Breastfed babies should be put to the breast at least every 3 hours. Babies receiving intravenous fluids or expressed breast milk should be given an extra 10% of fluid whilst under phototherapy or being treated with sunlight.
- Exchange transfusions may be necessary in cases

where the bilirubin rises to dangerous levels. This may only be possible in major units.

Table 42.1 shows when to consider phototherapy or exchange transfusion depending on serum bilirubin and age of the baby.

Risk factors include babies below 2.5 kg at birth, those born before 37 weeks, any baby with haemolysis or sepsis (WHO 2003).

Birth injuries

Sometimes the baby suffers some damage during birth.

Caput succedaneum

This is the name given to the swelling that sometimes occurs over the presenting part of the head. It is oedema caused by pressure on the tissues and is often obvious after vacuum extraction. It does not cause any problems and the oedema will be absorbed and the swelling disappear. Occasionally the caput can be seen over the face when there has been a face presentation. This can cause problems with feeding and it may be necessary to pass a nasogastric tube and feed with expressed breast milk.

Cephalhaematoma

This is where there has been some bleeding from the *periosteum* and the blood collects between the membrane and the bone. The swelling is localised by the edges of the skull bone so does not cross the midline. It may take some time to disappear and there may be a rise in the bilirubin as the blood is absorbed and broken down. This leads to jaundice.

Cerebral irritation (*Ischaemic* hypoxic brain damage)

A lack of oxygen before birth, during birth or after birth can cause swelling of the brain. Also if it has

Table 42.1 Indications for phototherapy and exchange transfusion

Age of baby	Phototherapy				Exchange transfusion			
	Healthy term baby		Any risk factor		Healthy term baby		Any risk factor	
	mg/dl	μmol/l	mg/dl	μmol/l	mg/dl	μmol/l	mg/dl	μmol/l
Day 1	Any visible jaundice				15	260	13	220
Day 2	15	260	13	220	25	425	15	260
Day 3	18	310	16	270	30	510	20	340
Day 4	20	340	17	290	30	510	20	340

been a prolonged labour, the pressure on the baby's head can also lead to swelling.

Signs and symptoms

- Slow to cry or an abnormal cry
- Slow to suck
- Floppy baby
- Irritability
- Convulsions

Some of these babies may suffer permanent brain damage, leading to cerebral palsy. Some will make a full recovery. Babies should be kept very quiet, handled as little as possible and kept warm. They may not feed well so mothers should be encouraged to express their milk. This can be given by cup and spoon or by nasogastric tube to avoid hypoglycaemia. It may be necessary to give anti-convulsants or sedation if the baby is having fits or is very irritable.

Facial palsy

Damage to the nerve supplying the face can cause a paralysis to one side of babies' faces. They will not be able to close the eye on the affected side, will have a droopy mouth and may have difficulty in sucking. There is no permanent damage and recovery is usually complete. During the first few days, mothers may need help to get them to suck from the breast. If necessary they can be fed via a nasogastric tube. The eye needs protection with eye drops to prevent the cornea from drying out (see Figure 42.2).

Erb's palsy

Damage to the *brachial plexus* during delivery can lead to paralysis of the arm. This usually recovers well, but it is important to keep the arm in a good position, and exercise it gently. The mother will need to be shown how to do this, so she can continue when she takes the baby home (see Figure 42.3).

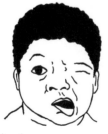

Figure 42.2 *Facial palsy*

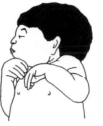
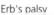

Erb's palsy   Erb's palsy undergoing correction by pinning baby's sleeve

Figure 42.3 *Erb's palsy*

Infection in the newborn

Newborn babies are very prone to infection for several reasons:

- They have a thin skin which is easily damaged.
- The gut has no normal *flora*. This means that they are more susceptible to gut infections.
- They have a poor inflammatory response, which means that infection is quickly spread around the body.
- Babies have also not had time to build up their own antibodies to infection. They do get some antibodies from their mothers, but their *immunoglobulin* levels will take a year to reach 50 per cent of an adult's immunoglobulin. Some pass across the placenta before they are born and they get some in breast milk. Babies develop antibodies to their mothers' bacteria quickly. Therefore the majority of the care should be given by the mother and other people should be involved as little as possible. The baby is then less likely to develop infection.

Some babies are infected before birth: This can happen if the membranes rupture and the baby is not born for some time. Or infection can pass from the mother's blood across the placenta to the baby's blood.

Some babies are infected during birth: If mothers have a vaginal infection, babies become infected as they pass down the birth canal. Eye infections caused by the gonococcus or chlamydia are examples of this (see Chapter 21). Infected amniotic fluid can cause intrapartum pneumonia (see Chapter 41). They can also be infected with HIV at this stage (see Chapter 32).

Some babies are infected after birth: The infection can enter through a break in the skin, or it can enter via the umbilicus. Before birth, three large blood vessels pass through the cord. When the umbilical cord is cut, these vessels will gradually wither away as they are no longer useful. However, this does take a few days and during this time it is easy for infection to enter via the umbilicus. When babies are born at home they may be admitted with an umbilical infection caused by local treatment of the umbilicus. The nurse needs to be aware of any local or traditional methods of treating the umbilicus of the newborn. Mothers and traditional birth attendants will need educating concerning safe practice. Neonatal tetanus is sometimes caused by local treatment of the umbilicus. This can be prevented by immunising the mother during the antenatal period. Babies can also develop respiratory infections or gastro-intestinal infections. Breastfeeding protects the baby from gut infections. Once babies become infected they can quickly develop a septicaemia. Figure 42.4 shows a baby with septicaemia resulting from an umbilical infection.

Signs and symptoms of infection in the newborn

The nurse needs to be very aware of the possibility of the newborn becoming infected as signs and symptoms are often non specific. Infection should be suspected when:

- Mothers tell you they are worried about their babies as they are not well.
- Babies who have been feeding well, become less interested in feeds.
- Babies fail to gain weight or even lose weight. It is normal for newborn babies to lose some weight

after birth but they should have regained this by the time they are 10 days old.
- Babies are dehydrated.
- Babies are hypothermic or have a raised temperature.
- Babies are jaundiced as haemolysis is increased during infection and there is a build up of bilirubin.
- The abdomen becomes distended. There may be signs of inflammation around the umbilicus.
- Pustules anywhere on the body.
- There is vomiting.
- The fontanelle becomes full. A sign of neonatal meningitis. Nurses should practise feeling normal fontanelles in babies, so that they know when the fontanelle is fuller than usual.
- Babies become drowsy and floppy.
- The respiratory rate is raised and respirations more laboured.
- There is tachycardia. The pulse may be of a poor volume.
- There is a discharge from the eyes, the ears or the umbilicus.
- Babies have albumin in the urine. This is a sign of a urinary tract infection.

Management

As babies have a poor resistance to infection, treatment should be started as soon as possible. Sometimes there is an obvious cause, the eyes may be swollen, red and discharging, or there is a discharge from the umbilicus. Often the cause of the infection is not obvious. If there are the facilities, the baby should have a full infection screen:

- Swabs from eyes, throat, umbilicus
- Full blood picture and blood culture
- Stool culture
- Lumbar puncture if meningitis is suspected
- Urine sent for culture. Ask the mother to help with collecting a sample. She can be given a clean container to place under the baby. If clean plastic bags are available, they can be taped over the penis of boys, or attached to the vulva of girls.
- Chest X-ray.

Sometimes it is not possible to do all these tests, in which case treatment should start with antibiotics which will cover both gram negative and gram positive organisms.

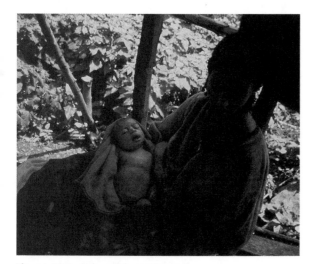

Figure 42.4 *Baby with septicaemia*

Antibiotic treatment

Most units will develop their own policy for deciding which antibiotics to use. These antibiotics may be changed once the results of the tests have been received. Penicillin and gentamycin are common combinations and are usually available.

Penicillin 150,000 units can be given 6 hourly for very sick infants, twice daily for the less sick. This is given with gentamycin 3 mg/kg every 12 hours. Gentamycin is a good drug but can cause kidney problems, so the dose must not be exceeded and the nurse needs to observe that the baby is passing urine well.

Ampicillin, cloxacillin and cefotaxime are other commonly used drugs. The doses will depend on the infection. Larger doses are given for neonatal meningitis.

Antibiotics should be given intravenously if possible. It is essential that the drugs are given at the right time, so that the blood level is kept constant. An intravenous infusion will need to be started. However, the nurse must be very careful to see that the infusion runs at the correct rate. This will depend on the maturity and age of the babies and whether they are to continue to breastfeed.

If the baby is still breastfeeding satisfactorily, the intravenous infusion should be run at 4 ml/hour (4 micro drops per minute).

It is very easy to give too much fluid and overload the baby's circulation, leading to cardiac failure. If it is not possible to give the drugs intravenously, they should be given intramuscularly, into the front or side of the thigh. It is advisable to avoid giving intramuscular injections into the buttock of the baby, as the buttock is small and it is easy to damage the *sciatic* nerve.

Nursing care

Babies with infection need constant observation as they can deteriorate quickly. They should be nursed as near to the nurses' station as possible and mothers should remain with them, as they are in a position to watch them all the time. The mothers will need to be told what they can do to help. They may be able to do some of the observations or they can be told what changes in the infants they should be looking for.

Prevention of cross-infection (See Chapter 6)

Nurses must wash their hands before and after handling sick infants. It is very easy to carry infection from one baby to another, either on the hands or on the clothes. Plastic aprons should be worn to protect the clothes. All equipment used for the baby must be very clean and not used for other babies. The ward area must be cleaned every day. If possible, they should be nursed in a different room to other newborn babies to reduce the chance of infection spreading.

Observations

- Take the temperature every 4 hours and record on the chart. If the baby is hypothermic, keep them close to the mother's body.
- Count the respiratory rate (normal is 30–60 per minute). Notice whether they have difficulty in breathing and the colour of the baby. It may be necessary to give them oxygen via nasal cannula. It may be possible to measure their *oxygen saturation*.
- Count the pulse rate (normal is 100–180 per minute). Sometimes it is hard to count the pulse rate of small babies. It may be easier to count the heart rate, using a stethoscope. If the rate suddenly rises, check that they are not getting too much fluid.

Feeding

If they are well enough, continue breastfeeding. They may need more frequent, smaller feeds. If they are unable to suck, help mothers to express their breast milk and give with a cup and spoon or via a naso gastric tube. See Table 42.2.

If intravenous fluids are not being given, a baby weighing 3 kg needs 450 ml on day 6. They can be given 40 ml every 2 hours. If they are having intravenous fluids as well, the amount given orally must be reduced. Assess their hydration level, check the elasticity of the skin, the fontanelle, the urine output and the mouth.

Care of intravenous infusion: Check the site frequently. Babies have fragile blood vessels and fluids can easily run into the tissues. Ensure the intravenous is running at the correct rate. Change the bag of fluid and giving set daily. They are a source of infection.

Table 42.2 Total daily feed and fluid volumes for mature babies from birth

Day of life	1	2	3	4	5	6	7
ml/kg body weight of feeds and/or fluid	60	80	100	120	140	150	160

(WHO 2003)

Hygiene

Sick infants do not tolerate being handled well. They should be left to rest as much as possible. Wipe their faces with warm water. Keep them clean from urine and faeces. As long as they are kept well hydrated, mouths should not need cleaning.

Drug treatment

Make sure that drugs are given at the right time.

Management of eye infections

Newborn babies are very likely to get eye infections as they do not produce tears until they are about 6 weeks old. Tears contain a natural antiseptic which helps prevent infection. In some centres, newborn babies are given one drop of 1% silver nitrate or tetracycline eye ointment to prevent infection. This is important if it is known that either parent has gonorrhoea or chlamydia. Sometimes babies' eyes become infected as they are being born. These babies are likely to present with red inflamed eyes, which may be discharging pus, 2 to 3 days after birth.

Gonococcal infection: This needs urgent attention as it can lead to *corneal* ulceration (see Chapter 21).

Chlamydia infection: These babies present with a less severe infection occurring a few days after birth. They can be treated with tetracycline or chloramphenicol eye ointment (see Chapter 21).

Neonatal tetanus

This is a very serious infection with a high mortality rate. It is also a failure in antenatal care, as mothers should have been immunised against tetanus. Babies will need very careful nursing if they are to survive. The tetanus bacterium is an *anaerobic* organism. The damage is caused by the toxins produced by the bacteria which affect the nervous system and cause the typical spasms. In the newborn, infection usually occurs at or after delivery, through the umbilicus. The cord may have been cut with a dirty instrument, or something may have been applied to the umbilicus according to local practice. Sometimes the infection occurs after *circumcision* (see Chapter 28).

Signs and symptoms

- Presents 3 to 10 days after delivery, when the toxins start affecting the nerve cells. The earlier the symptoms occur, the worse the prognosis.

- Mothers report that babies are having difficulty with feeding and do not open their mouths when they cry. They may have noticed them becoming rigid.
- Trismus (spasm of the muscles of the jaw, lockjaw)
- Jerks when touched or startled
- May have respiratory difficulty and *cyanosis*
- Temperature may be raised.
- The umbilicus may appear infected.

Nursing care of the baby with tetanus

The aim is to reduce the number of spasms the babies are having. They do not tolerate noise, handling or bright lights.

- They should be nursed in a room on their own but they must be clearly visible as they need constant observation.
- The light should be dimmed, but enough light available to be able to see them clearly.
- The room should be kept as quiet as possible. Nurses must avoid all unnecessary noise. Cover tables with cloths, to avoid noise when moving equipment.
- All nursing care should be given at the same time, to avoid constant disturbance. It should be given when the baby is well sedated.

Drugs

Sedation: This should be given immediately, and no further treatment given until it has had time to act. The treatment is aimed at preventing spasms without suppressing respirations.

- Diazepam I mg/kg body weight given intravenously, slowly over 3 minutes.

If diazepam is not available, give:

- Rectal paraldehyde 0.3 ml/kg body weight in arachis oil
- Repeat diazepam or paraldehyde if spasms do not stop in 30 minutes.
- If spasms still continue, repeat diazepam or paraldehyde after another 30 minutes. Do not give diazepam if respirations fall below 30 per minute.
- Diazepam or paraldehyde can be repeated every 6 hours if the spasms continue or recur.
- Phenobarbitone and chlorpromazine can be used instead of diazepam if necessary.

Give anti tetanus immunoglobulin (human) 500 units intramuscularly immediately, if available. If not, give tetanus antitoxin 5000 units IM. This will treat the circulating tetanus toxins.

Give intramuscular crystalline penicillin 125,000 units 2–4 times a day. The penicillin will treat the tetanus bacteria.

Care of the umbilicus

If this is thought to be the source of the infection, it should be cleaned carefully with methylated spirit or chlorhexidine.

Feeding

Once the baby is well sedated, a nasogastric tube should be passed and taped securely in place. Mothers will need to be helped to express their breast milk which can be given via the tube. Small, frequent feeds are usually needed. Initially babies will probably only be able to tolerate 75 ml/kg per day, but as they improve this should be increased to 150 ml/kg per day.

Prevention of *hypostatic pneumonia*

As babies are being kept well sedated, it is important to turn them from side to side, approximately every 3 hours. This gives each lung a chance to expand properly.

Temperature, pulse and respiration rates

These should be taken every 3 hours, when the baby is being turned. It is important to watch that they are not getting cold or developing respiratory problems.

Hygiene

These babies do not tolerate being handled, so they should just have their faces gently wiped and be kept clean from urine and faeces. This should be done at the same time as they are having their temperatures taken and are being turned.

Note: Remember to time the care to be given when the baby is well sedated, and give all care at the same time, to reduce handling.

Resuscitation equipment should be kept at the bedside and a chart to record the number of spasms. Babies may take several weeks to recover and even with careful nursing, many of them will die. Mothers will need a great deal of support as they will see that their babies are very ill and it will be several days before they see any improvement. The babies will not develop any immunity to tetanus, so will need the usual immunisations. Mothers should be given 0.5 ml of tetanus toxoid and be asked to return in 1 month for a second dose. This will protect both them and any future babies they may have.

Note: Neonatal tetanus can be prevented by giving pregnant women 2 injections of 0.5 ml of tetanus toxoid. TBAs should be taught about the causes of tetanus.

Care of the low birth weight baby

Babies may be small either because they have been born before 37 weeks gestation or because they have not been growing well in utero. Babies who are born before 30 weeks or are less than 1 kg are unlikely to survive unless they are being cared for in a unit which has the most up-to-date equipment and is very well staffed.

Low birth weight babies may have problems because they are small and also because some of their systems are immature.

Hypothermia (See Chapter 41)

Immature babies are more likely to get cold than a normal size baby, because they have been born before the brown fat has been laid down or they have not grown well. They are less well insulated with subcutaneous fat. They also have a relatively larger surface area compared to their body mass.

Hypoglycaemia

Low birth weight babies are more likely to get hypoglycaemic because they may not be able to suck well and also they can only take very small amounts at a time. If they did not grow well in utero, the stores of glycogen laid down before birth will be low. They also need more calories as they need to grow even faster than full term babies.

Respiratory distress syndrome

Babies with immature lungs may develop respiratory problems soon after being born. Surfactant, an enzyme which helps gas exchange in the lungs, may not be produced in sufficient quantities in the premature baby. The respiratory rate will rise, there may be periods of apnoea, increased movements of the chest wall and grunting respirations.

Apnoea attacks

These are common in immature babies because the respiratory centre is immature. Apnoea attacks are also a sign of hypoxia or infection. They need stimulation to start breathing again and treatment of any hypoxia or infection.

Infection

Low birth weight babies are even more prone to develop infection than normal babies because they have even lower levels of immunoglobulins. They are also likely to be handled by many different people and invasive procedures may be carried out.

Jaundice

The brains of immature babies are damaged at lower levels of bilirubin than full term babies because they have less fat to absorb the fat soluble bilirubin.

Anaemia

Immature babies may become anaemic as they may have been born before iron stores from their mothers have been laid down. These babies may also be having frequent blood sampling and iron is stored in the blood cells. They are also growing quickly so may grow out of these stores.

Vitamin deficiencies

Low birth weight babies are more likely to develop vitamin deficiencies as, once they are thriving, they are likely to grow more quickly than full term babies. Premature babies are more likely to develop rickets.

Nursing care of the low birth weight baby

Immediate care

Maintenance of body temperature and establishment of respirations: Immature babies must not be allowed to get cold. Ensure that the delivery room is warm and free of draughts. Dry them thoroughly as soon as they have been delivered. Check that they are breathing well, clear their airways if necessary and then place them between their mothers' breasts and cover them both. The mothers' body warmth is the best way of seeing that they do not lose heat. If resuscitation is needed, a heated trolley should be used, or a radiant heater placed above the surface on which they are being resuscitated.

Further care

If they are below 2000 gm, they are likely to need special care. Babies who weigh less than 1500 gm, are called Very Low Birth Weight Babies.

Prevention of infection

- Encourage the mothers to give most of the care. Discourage them from handling other babies.

- Keep them away from other babies with infections.
- Make sure there is a good supply of clean water for hand washing. Doctors and nurses must wash their hands thoroughly before touching them. Soap or an antiseptic wash should be used. Nails should be clean and short.
- All equipment used for their care must be kept clean and not used for other babies.
- Breast milk will give them the antibodies they require.

Nurses must watch them carefully for signs of infection, and if suspected, they should be given antibiotics as soon as possible.

Prevention of hypothermia

- They should be kept in a warm nursery, free from draughts.
- Their heads should be covered with a woollen hat. They must be kept clean and dry as heat loss from wet clothes is high.
- Keep them close to their mothers' body. Kangaroo nursing is an ideal method, especially if electricity supply is erratic (see Figure 42.5).
- Overhead heaters are used in some centres (see Figure 42.6).
- Hot water bottles must **not** be used. They should be forbidden as they are dangerous. They can cause burns and do not give a constant heat.
- Incubators are expensive and not always available. If they are used, they must be kept in good

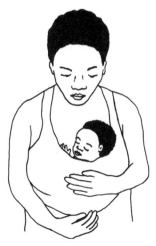

Figure 42.5 *Mother caring for her baby in the 'kangaroo' position*

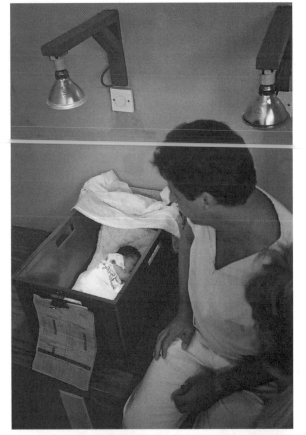

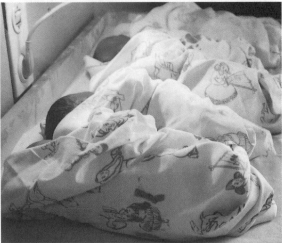

Figure 42.6 *Babies under overhead heaters*

working order and kept very clean. The warm wet atmosphere will cause any bacteria to multiply very quickly. The water in the incubator should be changed daily and the inside of the incubator

wiped clean. As it is difficult to clean an incubator thoroughly with a sick infant and all the equipment in it, it is better to change incubators once a week. However, this is only possible where there are sufficient incubators.

Nurses must be aware that if electricity (radiant heaters and incubators) is being used to maintain the temperature of these babies and there is a power cut, alternative methods must be used to keep them warm, for example kangaroo nursing.

Feeding

Immature babies may be able to suck and this should be encouraged.

- Put to the breast frequently so that they can take small amounts. If they are unable or unwilling to suck they can be given breast milk with a cup and spoon. Mothers will need help to express their milk.
- The very small baby may need feeding via a nasogastric tube. Nurses must check the position of the tube before each feed and also make sure that the stomach is emptying before feeding again.
- As they improve the feeds can become less frequent. They will be growing quickly so need more feeds per kg than full term babies of normal weight. They may need up to 250 ml/kg per day.

Care of respiratory problems

If they are having apnoea attacks:

- Watch carefully and teach their mothers how to stimulate them.
- Resuscitation equipment should be nearby.

Babies with respiratory distress syndrome will show signs within a few hours of birth. They will start to make a grunting noise as they breathe. There will be signs of recession. They will have *tachypnoea* and they may become cyanosed.

- They will need humidified oxygen given via nasal cannula. Do not give it at too high a concentration as this can cause a problem known as *retrolental fibroplasia* which causes blindness.
- Turn from side to side each time they are handled so that each lung is given a chance to expand.
- Count their respiratory rates and record on a chart. Note the amount of recession and cyanosis to monitor improvement or deterioration.

Planning for discharge

Mothers need to feel fully capable of looking after their small babies before they go home. They should be taught how to care for them throughout the hospital stay. Babies must be feeding well and gaining weight, although the weight may still be below an average birth weight. Check that the mothers have enough breast milk. Once the mothers start wanting to go home and are confident in the care, they should be discharged. This is better than insisting they stay and the mothers then run away.

- They will need to take iron supplements home with them to prevent anaemia. Ferrous sulphate 10 mg/kg/day is usually recommended. This should be continued until they start taking weaning food containing iron when they are 6 months old.
- Vitamin D supplements should be given to prevent rickets. Mothers can also be taught to expose their babies' skin to the sunlight each day as vitamin D is made by the skin in the sunlight.
- Mothers should be told to bring their babies back to the infant welfare clinic for weighing and immunisations.

Common congenital abnormalities

Mothers often feel very guilty when they have a baby who is born with an abnormality. They may be blamed and suffer *stigma*. They should be reassured that it is not their fault. There are many causes, some are genetic, some caused by infections such as rubella. However, the cause is often unknown.

Hydrocephalus

This is when the ventricles in the brain become too large, usually due to a blockage in the circulation of cerebrospinal fluid (CSF). The baby's head grows abnormally large and the increased pressure can cause brain damage. It can be treated in major centres by inserting some sort of shunt, which will help the drainage of CSF. It is often associated with myelo-meningocele. This is where part of the spinal cord of the baby is exposed. It may be possible for babies to have an operation to cover the defect. However, they will often be left with many abnormalities such as paralysis of the lower limbs and incontinence.

Cleft lip and palate

Sometimes these abnormalities occur together, sometimes separately. Because of the defect, babies

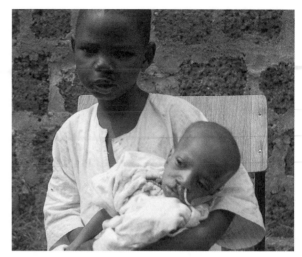

Figure 42.7 *Infant with a cleft lip*

may have difficulty in sucking so will need cup and spoon feeding. Their weight should be checked carefully as often these babies fail to grow well. It is possible for the defects to be repaired. See Figure 42.7.

Congenital heart disease

There are many different abnormalities that can affect the heart. Babies may go into cardiac failure, or they may be very cyanosed due to the abnormal circulation leading to poor oxygenation. Unless there is a major cardiac centre nearby most of these babies will not survive. They do not feed or grow well and are very prone to infection.

Gastro-intestinal problems

There may be an obstruction anywhere along the alimentary tract. Some are more easily treated than others. In imperforate anus, there is no opening from the rectum. This should be noticed at birth. It may be possible for the baby to have a colostomy to relieve the obstruction until more major corrective surgery can be carried out.

Talipes

Babies may be born with their feet in an abnormal position, (see Figure 42.8). It is important that this is corrected as soon as possible as, in the early days, the bones are easily moulded into a correct position. If left untreated, the child will be crippled without major corrective surgery. The feet should be manipulated by a doctor into an over corrected position and plaster of Paris applied. The type of plaster will depend on the

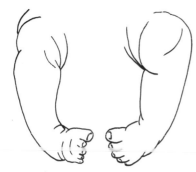

bilateral congenital talipes

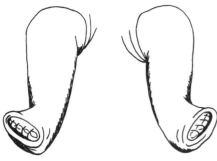

talipes undergoing correction
in plaster casts

Figure 42.8 *Talipes*

type of talipes. Following this, the nurse must ensure that the toes are pink, warm and are moving well. Plasters can cut off the circulation to the feet leading to gangrene.

Health promotion

Many of the problems that affect the newborn baby can be avoided by good antenatal care and good care during delivery (see Chapter 34).

- Identify women at risk of having problems during pregnancy and give extra advice and support.
- Prevention of malaria during pregnancy
- Giving anti tetanus toxoid to pregnant women
- Ensuring good nutrition for pregnant women
- Ensuring women are given safe care during labour and the postnatal period
- Preventing infection in the mother and newborn
- Preventing babies getting cold after delivery
- Helping mothers to breastfeed their babies

■ Activities

What are the three most important things to do to stop a newborn baby picking up an infection?

Part 5

Care of children

43

Nutrition and malnutrition in children

This chapter covers the important points about child nutrition and ways in which nurses can check on whether a child is getting enough of the right nutrients. It also covers *marasmus* and *kwashiorkor* and suggests ways to manage these conditions.

Introduction

Making sure that children are well fed is the basis of health during childhood. Many illnesses that affect children are more serious if the child is poorly nourished and may even kill them. Nurses and midwives have a very important role in assessing a child's nutritional status, advising the parents on which foods to give and when.

Children need relatively more food per kilogram than adults, as they burn up calories more quickly due to their higher metabolic rate, and also need extra calories to enable them to grow. Fat is the best way of increasing the calorie value of food and also makes it more appetising. Cooking oil is a readily available source of fat.

Table 43.1 Kilocalorie requirements per kilogram per 24 hours

Age	Kilocalories
0+	110
3+	100
5+	90
10+	70
Adults	35–45

Breastfeeding

Babies should be breast fed as breast milk has many advantages over artificial milks. The newborn baby should be put to the breast within the first hour after delivery, when he will get *colostrum*, a rich source of *antibodies*. Other nutritional advantages include:

Protein: The protein in breast milk is more easily digested than the protein in other milks.

Fats: The fats in breast milk provide most of the energy that the baby needs and are in the form of *polyunsaturated fats* which are important for the growth of the brain. Breast milk also contains the enzyme lipase which helps in the digestion of the fats.

Sugars: Lactose is the sugar found in breast milk and also provides energy for the baby. Lactose also encourages the growth of the lactobacillus which keeps the reaction in the gut acid and therefore helps prevent infection from harmful bacteria. The lactose also helps in the absorption of calcium which is important for healthy bone development.

Iron: Milk is not a good source of iron, but babies are born with iron stores which should last them until they are a few months old. The iron in breast milk is absorbed better than iron in artificial milks and breast fed babies do not become anaemic, unless they are born too early.

Minerals and vitamins: Breast milk contains the right amount of minerals and vitamins for babies. Cows milk contains too much of some minerals and can make a baby ill.

Other advantages in breastfeeding

Protection from infection: Breast milk contains antibodies and white blood cells which help prevent infection, as does the lactobacillus (see above). Breast milk is also clean and less likely to be contaminated than artificial milks. Breast milk also contains lactoferrin which inhibits the growth of the E Coli bacillus. The baby therefore gets protection from diarrhoeal diseases.

Bonding: Breastfeeding helps to develop a close relationship between the mother and the baby.

Availability: It is always available and the mother can feed the baby at any time, wherever she is.

Delaying the next pregnancy: If the mother breast-feeds regularly during the day and night, 10–12 times, with no long gaps between feeds, she is less likely to get pregnant again before the baby is 6 months old.

Saves money: Artificial milks are expensive. In Kenya, to feed a 6–10 month old baby with artificial milk can cost 60 per cent of a labourer's wages.

Less asthma and eczema: Babies who are breast fed are less likely to develop allergic diseases such as eczema and asthma.

WHO policy now encourages exclusive breastfeeding until the age of 6 months.

Problems with artificial milks

• They do not contain the best nutrients for the baby.
• They are expensive. If money is short, the mother may make the feeds too weak, so that the baby does not get enough calories to grow well.
• They are easily contaminated and can cause diarrhoea. In many areas the water is not clean and the baby may be given dirty feeds. Bottles and teats are difficult to keep clean and many parents are not able to clean and sterilise them properly.

Difficulties with breastfeeding

Most difficulties can be overcome with a good technique (see Chapter 40). If the baby has difficulty feeding because of a deformity, for instance cleft lip and palate, it may still be possible for the mother to breastfeed. If the baby cannot suck, the mother can be taught to express her milk and give it to her baby by cup and spoon. This is safer than using a bottle and teat, as the cup and spoon are more easily cleaned. In some countries, the use of bottles for feeding has been banned.

If the mother has died, see if there is another woman in the family who can breastfeed the child. There may be someone who is already feeding one baby, but has enough milk for two. Even if the woman has not had a baby herself, if the baby is put to the breast frequently, she may start producing milk (see Chapter 40).

Mothers who are HIV positive (see Chapter 32)

Unfortunately the virus is passed in the breast milk. Many studies are being carried out to find the best way of protecting the baby from becoming HIV positive. One study in Kenya found that 36.7 per cent of babies who were breast fed became HIV positive, as against 20.5 per cent of formula fed babies. However, one dose

of nevirapine to the mother during labour and another to her infant after delivery reduced transmission by 42 per cent in a study in Uganda. If the family has enough money to buy artificial milks and is able to see that the feeds are always clean, it is better to use artificial milks. In many circumstances, this is not possible. The baby is more likely to die from poorly prepared artificial milks, so it is better to continue with breastfeeding. Latest evidence suggests that if babies are given any food or fluid other than breast milk, the lining of the gut is damaged and when the mother breastfeeds, the virus is more likely to pass to the baby. These babies should therefore be **breast fed only**. Any oral infections in the baby should be treated quickly to reduce the chance of the virus being passed on.

Breastfeeding should continue for as long as is possible, for example up to two years. However, from the age of six months the child will need additional food as well as the breast milk. Continuing to breast-feed alongside the weaning diet, gives the child valuable extra calories.

Preparation of formula feeds

• Choose a milk powder that is specially adapted for infant feeding.
• Prepare a clean area for making up the feed.
• Use only boiled water.
• Clean all utensils thoroughly. It is safer to use cups and spoons than bottles and teats.
• Wash hands and make up the feed following the instructions on the tin. Never make feeds stronger or more dilute.
• Test the temperature of the feed before giving to the baby.
• Only make up one feed at a time, unless the feed can be stored in a refrigerator.
• Make sure the mother knows how to make up the feed safely before she goes home and that she has enough money to buy the milk.

Complementary feeding

When a baby is fed small amounts of food in addition to breast milk, this is known as complementary feeding. This is the most difficult period for the child as most diets are high in fibre and low in calories and the child has to eat great quantities to obtain the correct amount of energy. Foods are also easily contaminated and the child is at risk of getting diarrhoea.

Complementary feeding should start when the baby is around six months old. He then begins to need more calories than he can get from the breast milk alone. Most of the extra feeding starts by giving the baby a pap or porridge made from the staple cereal. This is usually soft and easily taken by the baby. However it may not contain enough nutrients and may be low in calories. It is essential that breastfeeding continues and is not reduced, to ensure the baby gets enough calories.

Improving food for the small child

Adding a little oil or fat (margarine or peanut paste) to the family food after cooking increases the energy and also makes the food easier for the baby to take. The volume of food that the child needs to take is much reduced when oil has been added. Most communities have a staple food that is commonly available, such as cassava, maize, potato, green bananas, rice or bread. These can provide some of the energy required but are usually a poor source of iron, zinc or calcium. The nurse needs to find out from the family the types of foods that are readily available and culturally acceptable before offering advice on the sort of foods to add to the diet. These may include some of the following:

- Mashed up egg or pulses to give protein
- Pounded groundnuts, which will give energy and other nutrients
- Mashed fish or meat
- Mashed dark green vegetables. These should not be overcooked as this will destroy the vitamins. These are good sources of vitamin A and C and also folate and iron, though the iron is not well absorbed.
- Mashed orange vegetables, such as pumpkin or carrots (vitamin A and C)
- Mashed tomatoes
- Mashed fruits, such as pawpaw and mango
- Iron rich foods which are well absorbed include liver, red meat and foods fortified with iron, such as fortified infant cereals.

There are also ways to make the porridge thinner and easier for the baby to take. This can be done by using a soured or fermented porridge, or germinated flour. Germinated or fermented cereals have been used traditionally in many countries for years. This practice should be encouraged. The advantage of using a fermented porridge is that bacteria are less likely to grow in it and it is therefore less likely to cause diarrhoea.

Germinated flour can either be used instead of a plain flour to make porridge, or it can be added to plain thick porridge, when the enzyme it contains will partly digest the cooked starch.

Small children need to eat more frequently than adults as their stomachs are smaller. They will need 5 to 6 feeds a day, as well as breast milk when they start on solid foods. Snacks between main meals should be encouraged. By the time they are nine months old, they need 4 to 5 feeds a day as well as breast milk. As the child grows, he will be able to take more food at each meal and the number of feeds will reduce. It is important to remember when feeding children that the calorie and micronutrient value of the food is as important as the protein content.

Iodine: This is necessary for the production of the thyroid hormones. Lack of these hormones damages the growth and development of the body and brain. If this happens before the child is born, it can cause mental retardation, or *cretinism*. After birth it can lead to poor development and the child is not able to learn easily (see Chapter19). It can be prevented by adding iodine to salt and in many countries this is now done routinely.

Iron: This is necessary to prevent anaemia.

Monitoring nutrition

One of the most important roles of the nurse is to see that children are getting enough of the right foods and are growing well.

Weight and growth charts

The child needs to be weighed each time he comes to the clinic and his weight plotted on a growth chart. It is then easy to see if he is growing at the right rate for his age. See Appendix B for growth chart and guidelines on how to fill it in.

However, growth charts are not always easily understood and mothers and guardians will need help in using them. Health personnel will need to be taught how to fill in the chart so that it becomes a useful measuring tool.

Arm circumference

Another way of seeing if the child is growing well, if there is no growth chart, is by measuring the arm circumference. Between the ages of one and five years, the muscles in a well fed, healthy child grow bigger, but the fat becomes less, so there is very little change in the arm circumference. Between these ages the arm circumference should be 16.5 cm. A child who has an arm circumference of less than 12.5 cm is very thin and badly nourished. The arm should be measured round the middle of the upper arm and can be done with an ordinary tape measure or a special insertion tape (see Figures 43.1 and 43.2). If no tapes are available, the nurse can learn to use her finger and thumb after practising.

The nurse then has to decide whether the child is well nourished, slightly malnourished or very malnourished. It is also necessary to find out whether any loss of weight is recent or whether the child has never

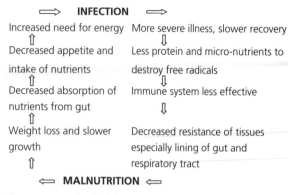

$$\Longrightarrow \quad \textbf{INFECTION} \quad \Longrightarrow$$

Increased need for energy	More severe illness, slower recovery
⇑	⇓
Decreased appetite and intake of nutrients	Less protein and micro-nutrients to destroy free radicals
⇑	⇓
Decreased absorption of nutrients from gut	Immune system less effective
⇑	⇓
Weight loss and slower growth	Decreased resistance of tissues especially lining of gut and respiratory tract
⇑	

$$\Longleftarrow \quad \textbf{MALNUTRITION} \quad \Longleftarrow$$

Figure 43.3 *The link between infection and malnutrition*

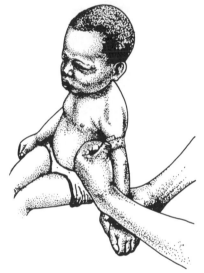

Figure 43.1 *Measuring arm circumference with a tape measure*

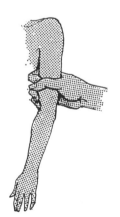

Figure 43.2 *Practise measuring a child's arm*

gained weight properly. In all cases, it is important to ask the mother or guardian whether he has been ill recently. Sick children do not eat well and if he has also had diarrhoea, this may be another reason for a loss in weight. Also when a child has an infection he needs more energy.

If the weight is not satisfactory, the nurse must give the mother advice on how to increase the calorie content of the meals. The child may need encouragement to eat and the mother should offer several small meals a day. Very malnourished children should be admitted to a nutrition unit if possible and their feeding supervised.

Protein-energy malnutrition

Marasmus

Marasmus is caused by children having a very low intake of energy and nutrients. It is most common during the period when solids are being introduced and often occurs when the child has been very ill or had several infections. It may also occur if the child is HIV positive.

Signs of marasmus

- Very low weight. The child will be below 60 per cent of normal and the third centile on the growth chart
- Extreme wasting. The child has lost fat and muscle, so he looks thin. The arms and legs are like sticks and the buttocks are wasted. The arm circumference is often below 10 or 11 cm.
- Looks old. The face is wasted and the child looks worried and anxious.

341

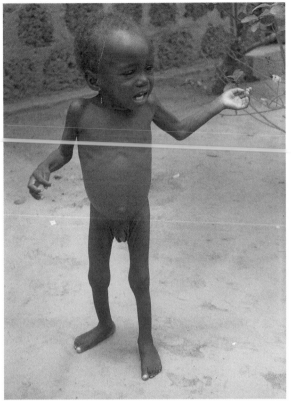
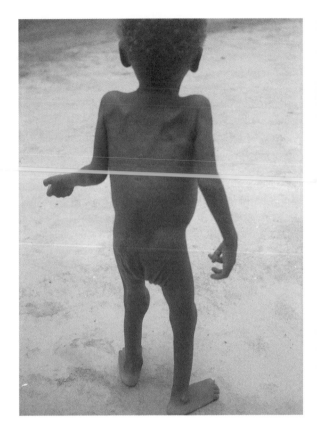
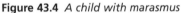

Figure 43.4 *A child with marasmus*

- Pot belly. The abdomen sticks out because the muscles of the abdominal wall are wasted and weak.
- Irritability. The child is fretful, he cries and complains.
- Hunger. He may be very hungry as long as he is not ill.

Kwashiorkor

Kwashiorkor is a more complicated form of malnutrition. It is mainly due to a very low intake of energy and nutrients as in marasmus but other factors are involved which are not completely understood. It is thought that it happens when malnourished children have an excess of *free radicals* which have not been destroyed by *antioxidants*. Free radicals are highly reactive molecules which are produced during infections and can damage body tissue. When children are healthy these are destroyed by antioxidants such as vitamin A and zinc. Protein also helps to remove them. The child may recently have had a severe infection such as measles. Large numbers of free radicals have

been produced, but as the child is already malnourished they cannot be removed. These free radicals then damage the tissues, causing the signs of kwashiorkor. Another reason why children may have too many free radicals is thought to be due to the presence of certain poisons, such as aflatoxin which is produced by a mould growing on groundnuts and maize.

Signs of kwashiorkor

- Oedema of the legs, arms and face
- Moon face
- Moderately underweight. He will not be as severely underweight as the child with marasmus, as he has oedema.
- Wasted and weak muscles. He may be unable to sit up or walk.
- Miserable and apathetic
- Poor appetite
- Pale, thin, peeling skin
- Pale, thin hair. The hair at the roots looks reddish in colour and can easily be pulled out.
- Enlarged liver which has become full of fat

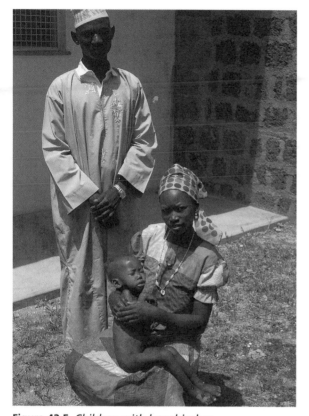

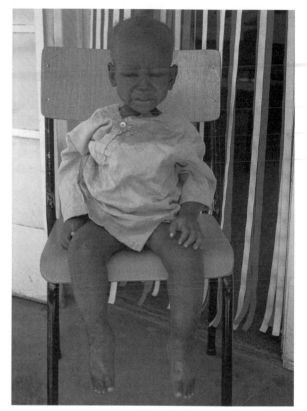

Figure 43.5 *Children with kwashiorkor*

Complications of malnutrition

- Diarrhoea. The child may have acute diarrhoea due to an infection (see Chapter 45). Sometimes the wall of the gut gets damaged and the child is not able to absorb nutrients so well. The diarrhoea can become chronic.
- Dehydration
- Infections. Often the child has an underlying infection but because he is malnourished may not have a fever. Common infections are otitis media, pneumonia, urinary tract infection and malaria. He may be HIV positive.
- *Hypoglycaemia*. The blood sugar may fall very low and if it is not treated can result in brain damage.
- *Hypothermia*. The child lacks the nutrients to burn to keep the body warm. This can lead to death.
- *Anorexia*
- Anaemia. Most very malnourished children are anaemic due to a deficiency of iron and sometimes folate as well.

- Other nutritional deficiencies. Other nutrients such as zinc and vitamin A may be lacking. This can be the reason for their low resistance to infection. Vitamin A deficiency can lead to severe and sudden eye damage (see Chapter 21).

Nursing care of the malnourished child – ten steps to recovery

If the child is severely malnourished, the first step should be to treat for hypothermia and hypoglycaemia.

1. Prevention of hypothermia

- Take his temperature regularly. It is preferable to have a special low reading thermometer available as normal ones do not go below 35° C. If no low reading thermometer is available, shake the normal one down to 35° C and if there is no reading assume hypothermia.
- Keep him close to his mother as her body warmth is the best way of keeping him warm. Use extra

343

clothes and blankets as necessary and keep the child away from any draughts. Cover his head. Change wet clothes quickly.

- Watch the child closely during the night as this is when the temperature is most likely to fall.
- Remember that the child will use up more calories to try to keep himself warm.

2. Prevention of hypoglycaemia

- Check for hypoglycaemia, using a dextrostix. If the blood sugar is below 3 mmol/litre, give glucose solution, orally or via a nasogastric tube.
- Immediate feeding, with starter feeds, should be commenced to prevent the blood sugar falling further. Feeds need to continue every 2 to 3 hours, and **this must continue during the night** (see Table 43.3).

Once the child has been checked for hypothermia and hypoglycaemia, a history can be taken.

History taking

It is most important to get a good history from the guardian. This must include the following questions:

- ■ Has the child lost weight recently or has he never gained weight? Check with any recent weights on the chart.
- ■ When did the guardian first notice there was a problem?
- ■ Has the child been ill recently? If so does the guardian know what was wrong, how it was treated and if so, is medicine still being given? Urinary tract infections are a common reason for children to fail to thrive. Tuberculosis and AIDS are also causes.
- ■ Is there a history of diarrhoea and if so how many episodes recently?
- ■ For how long was the child breast fed, when was complementary feeding started and what food was given?
- ■ What does the child normally eat?
- ■ How many other children are there in the family and is there a younger baby? Sometimes the weanling becomes malnourished when he is displaced at the breast by a new baby or the mother stops feeding when she becomes pregnant again.

---

3. Treat/prevent dehydration

The usual oral rehydration solution contains too much sodium and too little potassium for severely malnourished children. There is a special solution called ReSoMal. It has less sodium.

Table 43.2 ReSoMal formula

Water	2 litres
ORS	1 packet
Sugar	50 g
Electrolyte/mineral solution	40 ml

- Use a modified solution. This should taste no saltier than tears.
- If the child is dehydrated, give 5 ml/kg every 30 minutes for 2 hours, then 6-10 ml/kg for 4 to 10 hours.
- If the child has watery diarrhoea, replace the approximate volume of stool losses with the modified solution.

4. Correct electrolyte imbalance

Severely malnourished children have too much sodium in their bodies and may have too little magnesium and potassium. Oedema is partly due to these deficiencies. The children can be given an electrolyte/mineral solution which can be added to their feeds or to the rehydration fluid.

Table 43.3 Electrolyte/mineral solution

Potassium chloride	224 g
Tripotassium citrate	81 g
Magnesium chloride	76 g
Zinc acetate	8.2 g
Copper sulphate	1.4 g
Water – Make up to	2500 ml

This can be added to feeds.

5. Treat and prevent infection

- Treat any infection as soon as possible. He may not have a fever even if he has an infection. Observe for signs of pneumonia.
- Test for malaria and treat if necessary.
- Remember he may have tuberculosis or be HIV positive.
- Examine stools for worms and ova.
- Give a course of antibiotics as he is very susceptible to infection. Keep away from other children with infections.

- If he has not been immunised, measles vaccine should be given.
- He must be kept clean and all food and drink given to him must be clean.
- The nurse must wash her hands before giving him any care.

6. Correct *micronutrient* deficiencies

All severely malnourished children have vitamin and mineral deficiencies.

- He should be given a multivitamin supplement.
- Folic acid 1 mg per day (5 mg on the first day) should be given.
- Vitamin A should be given to all children who have not had a dose within the last month. Children whose eyes are affected should be given 2 further doses. Vitamin A protects the eyes and is also essential for the immune system (see Chapter 21).
- Iron can be started once he has started to gain weight.

7. Start cautious feeding

When a child is severely malnourished, the lining of the gut and other organs have often been damaged. Feeding has to be very carefully started as often the child will have diarrhoea or go into heart failure.

- The child needs small frequent feeds.
- The diet should be low in protein and sodium.
- Extra potassium and magnesium is needed.
- The child may be unwilling to feed. It may be necessary to pass a nasogastric tube.
- Feeds must continue during the night.

Table 43.4 Starter formula

Whole dried milk	35 g
Sugar	100 g
Vegetable oil	20 g
Electrolyte/mineral solution	20 ml
Or	
Dried skimmed milk	25 g
Sugar	100 g
Oil	30 g
Electrolyte/mineral solution	20 ml
Make up all mixtures to 1000 ml of water	

Starter feeds

- Give small frequent meals.
- Aim for 100 cal/kg/day.
- Continue breastfeeding.

8. Rebuild wasted tissues. Catch up growth

- Children now need plenty of food with high energy and nutrient content. They will usually start to feel hungry.
- Teach the guardian how to give the feeds and when to give them. The guardian is in a strange place and may not know what to do.
- Weigh children twice a week.

Catch up feeds

- Gradually change from starter formula to catch up formula.
- The child should have about 200 ml/kg per day of the formula.
- Continue breastfeeding.
- Gradually introduce family foods.

Table 43.5 Catch up formula

Whole dried milk	110 g
Sugar	50 g
Vegetable oil	30 g
Electrolyte/mineral solution	20 ml
Or	
Dried skimmed milk	80 g
Sugar	50 g
Oil	60 g
Electrolyte/mineral solution	20 ml
Make up with water to 1000 ml	

9. Stimulation and play

Severe malnutrition causes mental and physical delay, so children should be encouraged to play once their physical condition has improved. Smiling, happy children are a sign that they are getting better.

10. Preparation for discharge and follow up

- Teach the family about feeding the child in the future. There may be other families with the same problem, so it may be possible to give some group teaching sessions.

In many areas special nutrition units have been set up where mothers and children can stay together. The mothers learn about nutrition and the preparation of suitable food for the children. There is no point in getting the child well if he goes home to get sick again, because the family have not been given any help.

Health promotion

- Encourage exclusive breastfeeding until children are 6 months old, unless you suspect they may be HIV positive.
- Give advice about suitable complementary feeding diets.
- All children who are seen by a nurse, either in hospital or in a clinic, should be assessed to see if they are growing well and are well nourished. It is easier to treat malnutrition if it is identified in the earlier stages.
- Any child who is at risk of malnutrition should be followed up.
- Children who have frequent infections should be watched very closely.
- Children who are recovering from severe infections such as measles need extra care.

■ Activities

Hussein is 14 months old when he is brought to the clinic by his mother with moderate malnutrition. What observations will you make and what advice will you give his mother?

44

Children's nursing

Children who are admitted to hospital have special needs, they do not behave in the same way as adults and they have physiological differences. This chapter will outline some of these differences. It will also consider history taking and the assessment of a child.

The children's ward needs to be planned so that there is room for the guardians to sleep near the child. It may be easier to have adult sized beds, which can be shared by the sick child and the guardian. If cots are used, then there needs to be space beside the cot for the guardian to spread their mat. There will need to be a separate room where the guardians can keep their belongings and somewhere where they can do their cooking and washing.

Psychological differences

Young children rely on their guardians, usually their mothers, to look after them and care for them when they are ill. When they are ill and brought into hospital, they will be very frightened of all the strange people, the uniforms, the equipment and any treatment they may need to have. Their guardians should be included in every part of their care so that they can give the child the security they need. If children are separated from the people who usually look after them, they may behave in the following way:

Protest: First of all they get angry, they may shout, and try to get out of their cots.

Despair: Then they get very sad, they may cry quietly and refuse to eat. They think they have been abandoned.

Denial: Lastly they seem to settle down, but they may have lost their trust in their family to care for them.

Physiological differences

Children are very different and when they are sick their response to illness can be different. They get sick very quickly, but they also get better very quickly.

Many of the differences are because the child has a higher metabolic rate than the adult. The metabolic rate of the baby is twice that of the adult. The metabolic rate can be shown as:

Glucose + oxygen = Carbon dioxide + water + heat + energy.

As the oxygen needs are twice as high and the carbon dioxide is increased, the child needs to breathe more quickly and the heart needs to pump more quickly. The child also needs more calories per kilo than the adult, not just because of the increased metabolic rate, but also because he needs extra calories to grow.

Table 44.1 Physiological differences in children from newborn to 5 years

Age	Temperature	Pulse rate	Respiratory rate	Blood pressure
Newborn	37.5	100–180	30–60	$\frac{60-85}{20-60}$
6 months	37.5	80–150	30–45	$\frac{75-105}{40-70}$
2 years	37.2–37.7	80–120	25–35	$\frac{75-110}{45-80}$
5 years	37.0–37.2	70–110	20–30	$\frac{75-115}{45-80}$

The fluid requirements of a child are also different to the fluid requirements of an adult.

- Infants and children have different proportions of body fluids to adults. The total amount is proportionately greater. A newborn baby's body is 80 per cent water; an adult's body is 60 per cent water. Immediately after birth, a baby loses up to 10 per cent of his body weight, mainly water. The increase in body fluids in children is mainly outside the cells (extracellular).
- The baby has a larger surface area (skin) in proportion to his weight, than an adult. The preterm baby has a surface area (proportionately) 5 times that of an adult. The infant has a surface area 2–3 times that of an adult (proportionately). This larger surface area means that the amount of fluid the baby loses through his skin is greater than an adult. He also secretes proportionately more gastro-intestinal fluids than an adult.
- Kidney function is different. The baby's kidney is not as good at concentrating urine as the adult's. This means that when he is dehydrated, toxic wastes build up more quickly.
- The baby has a small circulating volume of fluid, only 100 ml per kilo. The adult has a circulating volume of blood of approximately $5\frac{1}{2}$ litres.

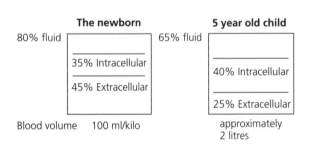

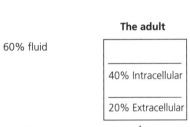

Figure 44.1 *Fluid compartments in children and adults compared*

Fluid requirements for 24 hours
- The full term baby needs 150 ml/kilo.
- The 5 year old child needs 100 ml/kilo.
- The adult needs 40–50 ml/kilo.

Defence against infection

Babies and children have fewer defences against infection than the adult. Their immune systems are less mature and they have not had time to build up defence against many of the common bacteria. In hospital there are many other sick children and it is important to see that the child does not pick up another infection while he is there.

The nurse must wash her hands well after caring for one child, before going to another. She must also wash her hands after handling any soiled linen or discharge from the child. Children with infectious diseases, such as whooping cough or measles, should be nursed in a separate room.

The ward should be kept very clean. The toilets and washing area are particularly important. Dirty toilets and washing areas can be a dangerous source of infection. Equipment should not be used on one child and then another, without washing or sterilising it.

Admitting the child to hospital

When children are being examined, they should always be sat on the lap of the mother or guardian. It is not necessary to put them on a bed or cot as they are likely to become more distressed and more difficult to examine.

It is important to get a good history from the guardian. Older children can also help with this.
- When was the child last well? The mother should be asked when he was last smiling and playing.
- How long has the child been ill?
- What are the symptoms?
- Is the child eating well, if not, how long since he ate well?
- Has the child been given any medicine recently, either from another clinic, or local medicine?
- Has he had his immunisations and is he on anti malarial drugs?

Specific questions

Convulsions: Has he had any convulsions? If so, when did they start, how long did they last, how many? Was the child unconscious at all? Did he have a fever at the time? Has he complained of a headache or stiff neck?

Fever: Has he had a fever? If so, for how long? Does it go up and down, or has it remained high? Has there been a rash at all? If so, what does it look like?

Cough: Has the child got a cough? Does it sound wet or is it a dry cough? Does he cough anything up? Remember, young children are likely to swallow any mucus they cough up.

Breathing difficulty: Has he been short of breath? Is he making a noise when he breathes, for example a stridor or wheeze.

Abdominal complaint: Has he any abdominal pain, any diarrhoea or vomiting? Has he passed any worms recently?

Diarrhoea and vomiting: It is normal for children to pass 2 stools per day, so the nurse needs to establish that he has got diarrhoea. How many times has he had diarrhoea? What does it look like: watery, bloody, any mucus? Does it smell? How many times has he vomited, is there any blood or bile in the vomit?

Genito-urinary: Has he complained of any pain on passing urine, any blood in the urine, any frequency?

Assessment of the child

General nutritional status

Weigh the child and plot his weight on a growth chart (see Appendix B). It is very helpful if the mother has a chart from the clinic, as it will then be possible to see if there has been a recent weight loss. Measure the child's arm circumference (see Chapter 43).

Does the child show signs of marasmus or kwashiorkor (see Chapter 43)?

Does he look underweight for his age? What does he normally eat?

Hydrational status

Has the child been drinking well? Is he showing any signs of dehydration, for example dry skin with a loss of elasticity, sunken fontanelles, sunken eyes, dry mouth, limp and apathetic, poor urinary output, rapid pulse (see Chapter 45)?

Respiratory

Count his respiratory rate. Notice any difficulty in breathing, for example using accessory muscles of respiration. Is there any *cyanosis* (see Chapter 47)?

Cardiovascular

Count his pulse rate, or in a baby the heart rate. Is the volume normal, or is the pulse rapid and thready? Are there any signs of anaemia? Check the colour of the *conjunctiva* and the mucous membranes of the mouth. Take and record his temperature.

Neurological

Note any convulsions, any stiff neck or reluctance to move, any paralysis. Check his level of consciousness.

Skin

Note if the skin looks healthy, or is it dry and flaky? Are there any blemishes or rashes, any birthmarks?

Eyes

Are the eyes bright, or dull and apathetic? Note any conjunctivitis, any swelling round the eyes, or any ulceration of the cornea.

Ears

See if there is any discharge or if the child is rubbing his ears.

Mobility

See if the child is moving normally, or does he appear to have pain. Look at his limbs to see if he moves them all. Note any weakness or paralysis.

Behaviour

Sick children are apathetic and not interested in playing. If he is very restless, it may mean he is in pain or is short of oxygen or he is frightened.

Growth and weight: Is he growing well? Is he gaining weight? Does he eat well?

Involvement of guardians in care

It is very important that the guardian is involved in every aspect of the care. Most children's wards are very busy and the nurses do not have time to give all the normal care that children require. The involvement of guardians also reduces the risk of cross-infection, as they are caring for one child only, and the nurse has many to care for. The guardians can almost always continue to wash the children, keep them company, give them drinks and food. However, if the child is very sick, the guardian needs to be taught how to give drinks and food. It is not enough to put the food or drink beside the child and expect the guardian to know what to do.

It is a good opportunity to give health education and if the child has become sick, because of poor care at home, this is a good opportunity to explain to the guardian how the sickness could have been avoided. The guardian will also be caring for the child on discharge, so if the child is going home on any treatment, or with any plasters or medicines, the guardian needs to be taught how to give the care.

The aim of medical and nursing care is to restore the child to health as soon as possible.

Always listen to what the mother or guardian is saying. She is the person who knows the child best and will be able to tell you whether he is improving or whether she has additional concerns.

Monitoring the child's condition is essential. The nurse should do any observations that are requested, and record them carefully on a chart. If the child appears to be getting worse, she must tell either a senior nurse or a doctor.

Make sure the child is eating and drinking enough and is passing urine. Note when he has his bowels open.

Give drugs and treatments at the correct time and watch for any side effects.

Discharge

When the child is ready to go home, check that the mother has any medicines that he is to continue with and that she knows how to give them.

Make sure that the mother knows if she needs to come back to the hospital for any further treatment or to see a doctor.

For children under 5 years old, encourage the mother to take the children to the clinic if she does not do so already. Explain the importance of watching the child's weight, growth and development and that he gets his immunisations at the right time.

■ Activities

1. Look at all the children on the ward. Are there any who need not have been admitted to hospital if their guardians had been able to get good advice at a clinic?
2. Think of ways in which you could prevent children coming in to hospital in the area in which you are working.

45

Nursing care of children with diarrhoea

This chapter explains why young children are more at risk of dying from diarrhoea than adults and covers the management of a dehydrated child.

Introduction

Children who are malnourished are at particular risk of dying from dehydration as their resistance to infection is often lowered. Children may suffer many episodes of diarrhoea over a short period of time. They are at risk of becoming dehydrated on each occasion and also lose important nutrients so that their malnutrition is likely to worsen with each attack. Children who are being weaned are particularly at risk, as they are being introduced to new foods and may be given fluids to drink that are contaminated. They are also mobile and put everything into their mouths. In a contaminated environment this is a risk.

Why children are more prone to dehydration than adults

- Young children require a proportionately higher fluid intake than adults and excrete more urine (see Figure 45.1 and Chapter 44).
- Adults who weigh about 50 kg will need to drink 1500 ml per day and will pass 1000 ml of urine. Adults need 30–50 ml of fluid per kg per day and have a blood volume of 5½ litres.
- Babies of 3 months who weigh 5 kg will need to drink 750 ml per day and will pass 500 ml of urine. These babies need 150 ml per kg per day and have a blood volume of approximately 100 ml per kg. For their size, infants need a much higher fluid intake and are more vulnerable to fluid deficits.

Note: Remember that these are average figures. In a hot dry climate the amount of fluid lost in sweat is great and the fluid intake will increase and the urine output fall. Children with a high fever or very rapid respirations will lose more fluid than healthy children.

- Children of 7 kg may lose 700 ml of fluid in diarrhoea; this is 10 per cent of their body weight and they are then obviously dehydrated.
- Children with diarrhoea do not only lose water, they also lose sodium, potassium, chloride and bicarbonate. At first the body can compensate, as the urine output will fall, but if more fluid is lost, children will start to show signs of dehydration.

Children become dehydrated more quickly than adults.

Enteral (gut) infections that cause diarrhoea

Table 45.1 Enteral infections that cause diarrhoea

Bacteria	Viruses	Protozoa
E. coli	Rotavirus	Amoebic dysentery
Salmonella	Adenoviruses	Giardia
Cholera		
Campylobacter		

Parenteral (non gut) infections that may cause diarrhoea

Most infections may be associated with diarrhoea in young children, but the most common are:

- Malaria
- Measles
- Pneumonia; .upper respiratory tract infections
- Urinary tract infections.

The child who is HIV positive may present with diarrhoea.

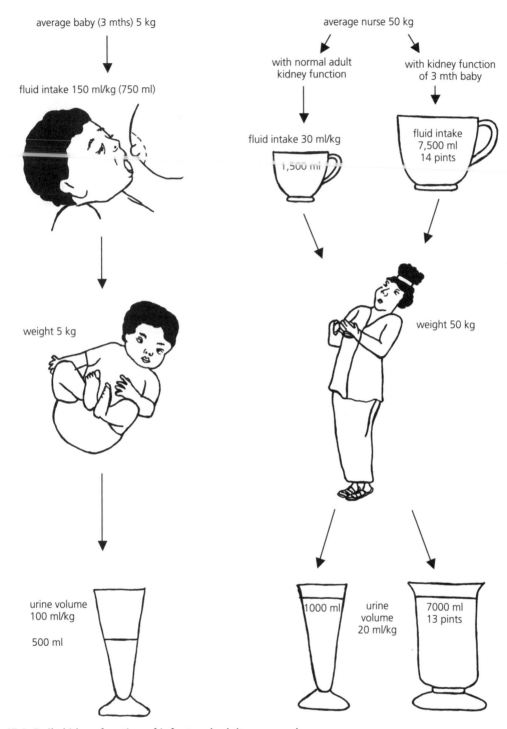

average baby (3 mths) 5 kg

fluid intake 150 ml/kg (750 ml)

weight 5 kg

urine volume
100 ml/kg

500 ml

average nurse 50 kg

with normal adult
kidney function

with kidney function
of 3 mth baby

fluid intake 30 ml/kg

1,500 ml

fluid intake
7,500 ml
14 pints

weight 50 kg

1000 ml

urine
volume
20 ml/kg

7000 ml
13 pints

Figure 45.1 *Daily kidney function of infant and adult compared*

Nursing care of the child with diarrhoea

Taking a nursing history

- How long has the child had diarrhoea? Diarrhoea that lasts for more than 2 weeks is called persistent diarrhoea and is dangerous.
- How many stools has the child had in the last 24 hours? What colour are they?
- Are they large or small stools?
- Are the stools watery? Nurses should ask guardians to save the next one passed for them to see.
- Is there any blood in the stools? This is evidence of dysentery.
- Are they vomiting? If so, how often and when did they last vomit?
- Do they appear thirsty, drinking eagerly?
- Are they able to drink or are they not drinking well?
- Are they still breastfeeding? If not, when did the mother stop?
- What food have they been having?
- Have they lost their appetite?
- Have they got a fever and if so when did it start?
- Are they coughing or are there any other symptoms?
- Have they had a rash at all recently?
- Have they been given any medicines, traditional or otherwise?

Nursing assessment

Weight: If they have been to a clinic before or if their mothers have weight charts with them, compare the present with the last known weight. Children who are moderately dehydrated will have lost 5–10 per cent of their weight. So a child who is normally 11 kg may only weigh 10 kg on admission. Children who are severely dehydrated will have lost more than 10 per cent of their weight. It is useful to reweigh them once they have been rehydrated to get more accurate weights. Even when children have been rehydrated, the diarrhoea is likely to continue for some time, so plotting weights on a growth chart gives some idea of how they are doing and can be reassuring to the mothers as they will be able to see that their weight is above their admission weight.

Hydration: Check to see whether the child is dehydrated or not.

Signs of dehydration

- Lethargic or unconscious
- Restless or irritable
- Sunken eyes
- Loss of elasticity of skin. Pinch the skin of the abdomen: if it takes 1–2 seconds to return to normal, dehydration is severe; 2 or more seconds, it is very severe. (If children are also very malnourished, this can be difficult to assess, particularly if they have recently lost weight.)
- Sunken fontanelles in babies
- Dry mouths. Children may be complaining of thirst, otherwise, having washed your hands, place a finger in their mouths to see if they are dry. Offer children drinks and observe the eagerness to drink.
- Poor urinary output. Mothers should be asked when they last passed urine. If the stools are very watery, try to see whether they have passed urine as well.
- Rapid pulse and respirations
- Cold extremities (severe dehydration)

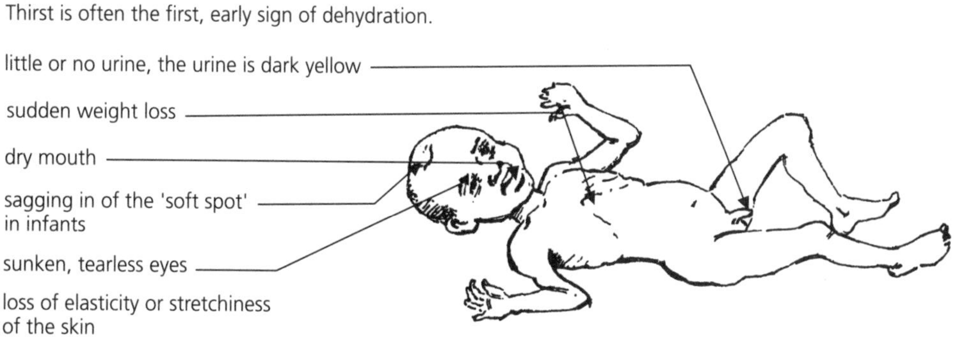

Thirst is often the first, early sign of dehydration.

little or no urine, the urine is dark yellow

sudden weight loss

dry mouth

sagging in of the 'soft spot' in infants

sunken, tearless eyes

loss of elasticity or stretchiness of the skin

Figure 45.2 *A child showing the signs of dehydration*

Nursing care of the dehydrated child

The most important aspect is to replace the water and salts as quickly as possible. Usually this can be done orally. Children need water, salt and glucose. The glucose increases the amount of salt and water that can be absorbed from the intestine.

ORS (oral rehydration solution)

The hospital or clinic may have packets of oral rehydration salts that can easily be made up into a solution.

If these are not available, it is very easy to make up a suitable solution:

- 1 litre of boiled or clean water
- $\frac{1}{2}$ a level teaspoon of salt (3 g)
- 4 level teaspoons of glucose or sugar (20 g).

Once the fluid has been made up, the mother or guardian should be shown how to give it to the child. Using a cup and spoon is the easiest way. The aim is to give the child at least 100 ml/kg over the first 4 hours + 100 ml for every loose stool passed. At first this may not be easy, as the child is sick and may be reluctant to drink, however with perseverance most children will be able to take the fluid. Most children with diarrhoea will also vomit and this can be a cause

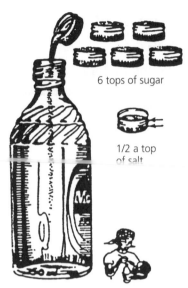

Figure 45.4 *Using a bottle and cap to make up ORS*

6 tops of sugar

1/2 a top of salt

Using the plastic spoon, add 1 large scoopful of sugar and 1 small scoopful of salt to 1 glass of water. Stir well.

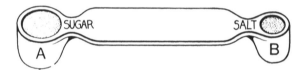

Figure 45.5 *Using a TALC spoon to make up ORS*

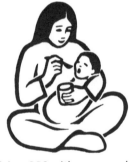

Figure 45.6 *Giving ORS with a cup and spoon*

of great concern to the mother. Vomit always appears to be of a larger quantity than it actually is. It may seem that the child is vomiting all the fluid that is taken. It may be worth giving the mother a small bowl to catch the vomit in. She will then be able to see that it is likely only to be $\frac{1}{4}$ of the amount taken in. So oral feeding should continue, in spite of vomiting.

UNICEF ORAL REHYDRATION SALTS

Sodium Chloride	3.5 g
Potassium Chloride	1.5 g
Sodium Bicarbonate	2.5 g
Glucose	20.0 g
Flavouring	0.5 g
Total weight	28.0 g

Directions

Dissolve in ONE LITRE of drinking water
To be taken orally —

Infants — over a 24 hour period
Children — over a 6 to 8 hour period
Or as otherwise directed
under medical supervision

**CAUTION
DO NOT BOIL SOLUTION**

Figure 45.3 *UNICEF formula for ORS*

Some children will not be able to drink this amount of fluid, and it may be necessary to pass a nasogastric tube and give the fluid in this way.

Children who are very severely dehydrated will need fluid given intravenously or into the bone.

Intravenous fluid

A scalp vein needle can be used and inserted into the scalp, the back of the hand, the wrist or the ankle. This takes practice but nurses can develop the skill after watching others and then doing it themselves. Sometimes a doctor will be available to insert the needle, but this is often not the case.

- The amount of fluid to be given should be worked out carefully, as it is easy to give too much fluid too quickly which can overload the circulation of a small child.
- Aim to give 50 ml/kg over the first hour.
- Then 50 ml/kg over the next 3 hours. This should be increased if the child is continuing to pass loose stools.
- Half strength Darrow's solution is the best solution to use, but if it is not available, use a glucose saline mixture, as this will give the water and salts that are necessary. The child may need extra potassium, but it is safer to give this orally.

Observing children while they are being rehydrated

Children must be carefully watched while they are being rehydrated to make sure that their condition is improving and they are becoming less dehydrated.

A fluid chart is essential for children on intravenous infusions

- Note the following:
  - The amount of fluid taken in
  - The number of vomits and approximate amount
  - The number and type of stools
  - The amount of urine passed
- It may be necessary to increase or decrease the amount of fluid given, depending on the number of stools and whether they continue to vomit.
- Observe the pulse rate and volume. As they improve, the pulse rate should slow down and the volume increase.
- Check the temperature. They may have been hypothermic when they first arrived, due to shock.

They should **not** be warmed up until they have been rehydrated, as this will take the blood supply away from the essential organs. As they improve, the circulation will improve and they will warm up. They may then develop a fever, if they have an infection.

- Check the respiration rate and the amount of effort being used to breathe. If intravenous fluids are being given, an increasing respiratory rate and effort can be a sign of overloading of the circulation. A puffy face and eyes are also signs of overloading. The amount of fluid being given must be reduced immediately.

Feeding the child with diarrhoea

It is important not to stop feeding, as many of these children are already malnourished. Breastfeeding should continue, along with the oral rehydration solution. Breastfeeding can also continue, even if the child has an intravenous infusion or has been given fluid into the bone. Mothers will need to be reassured over this, as every time the child feeds another stool may be passed due to the gastro colic reflex. However, they can be reassured that the food is not coming straight through as it has been estimated that 80–90 per cent of the food will be absorbed. The volume of the stool is also likely to be only half the volume of the stool of a child who is being starved.

Weaning diets can be reintroduced as the child improves. Food needs to be given often and in small amounts. Sometimes cow's milk will cause the child to have worse diarrhoea. This is because the diarrhoea can damage the villi of the intestine and there is a reduction in the amount of the enzyme lactase that is produced. The lactose in the milk is then not properly digested. This can lead to frothy, acid stools which can contain sugar. If this is a big problem, the milk should be stopped until the child improves.

Drug treatment in vomiting and diarrhoea

Unless there is a specific cause of the vomiting and diarrhoea, drugs should not be used. Few of them will do any good, and some will cause harm.

Drugs which reduce peristalsis should never be used (immodium, tinct opii). They can cause respiratory depression and also result in harmful toxins being retained in the body, instead of being expelled in the diarrhoea. They can also cause total paralysis of the gut.

Antibiotics should only be given if there is blood in the stool (dysentery) or a specific infection (otitis media, urinary tract infection). Many antibiotics cause diarrhoea as a side effect. However:

- Salmonella may be treated with chloramphenicol.
- Shigella may be treated with ampicillin or cotrimoxazole or chloramphenicol or nalidixic acid.
- Cholera may be treated with tetracycline.
- Amoebic dysentery may be treated with flagyl.
- Giardia may be treated with flagyl.
- Malaria should be treated with an appropriate anti malarial (see Chapter 46).

Conclusion

Diarrhoea still causes many young children to die every year. Most of these deaths are preventable with simple oral rehydration techniques. Many cases of diarrhoea could be prevented by teaching families public health measures.

■ Activities

1. Write out a care plan for a 2 year old child who is admitted with severe diarrhoea and is moderately dehydrated.
2. What observations will you make on this child while he is being rehydrated?

Health promotion

- Before children go home, it is most important to talk to mothers or guardians about preventing future attacks.
- Stress the importance of continuing with breastfeeding.
- If the mother is bottle feeding the child and there is no possibility of her breastfeeding again, suggest she uses a cup and spoon as it is easier to keep these clean. Discuss with her how she is making up the feeds and make sure she knows how important it is always to use clean, if possible boiled, water.
- Discuss the preparation and storage of food. The area where food is prepared should be clean and all the utensils used must be washed carefully before use. Once prepared, food should be covered to prevent contamination from flies. The food should not be kept too long and if possible kept in a cool place.
- Hands must be washed before any food preparation and before feeding children. Children should be taught to wash their hands after using the latrine and before eating.
- Make sure mothers/guardians know that flies can spread disease. Rubbish should be disposed of carefully and families should be encouraged to have proper latrines.
- Discuss the importance of good nutrition for all the family but in particular for the child who is being weaned (see Chapter 43).
- Make sure mothers or guardians know what to do if the child gets diarrhoea again. They should know how to make up a simple oral rehydration solution so that they can start treatment themselves. They also need to know what signs to look for so that they can bring children to a clinic or hospital if necessary.

46

Nursing care of children with malaria, meningitis and convulsions

This chapter will cover the main points to be considered when caring for a child with malaria or meningitis or who is suffering from convulsions.

Care of the child with malaria

Malaria is a common cause of illness and death in young children (see Chapter 26). Adults who live in an area where malaria is common usually build up a partial immunity. During pregnancy this immunity may break down, particularly with the first baby (see Chapter 36). Some immunity is passed on to the newborn baby, so that during the first 6 months of life attacks are usually mild. However, after this time attacks can become common and more severe. Most deaths occur during the first 2 years of life. By the time he goes to school, the child has usually built up some immunity so that attacks are less severe.

Between the ages of 6 months and 3 years, the child is at his most vulnerable. He is likely to have suffered several attacks of diarrhoea, he may be malnourished, he may have had measles. Frequent attacks of malaria are an added threat.

Signs and symptoms

Not all children with malaria will appear sick. Some who have malarial parasites will be running around. However, any sick child should be suspected of having malaria, as the symptoms can be so varied. He may present with:
- A high temperature; rapid pulse and respirations
- Diarrhoea and vomiting
- Cough
- Convulsions; drowsiness; coma
- Anaemia; jaundice as the parasite causes the red cells to break down.

- Children who have had several attacks may have very enlarged spleens.

Management

A positive blood smear will prove the child has malaria, but it is possible that he also has another infection such as meningitis. So the child must be carefully observed. A negative blood smear does not mean that the child has not got malaria. Even one dose of anti malarials can clear the parasites from the bloodstream, so the nurse needs to ask the guardian whether the child has already had any treatment.

All children with raised temperatures should be given anti malarials.

Most children can be treated in clinics and do not need to be admitted to hospital. However, the nurse should consider carefully before deciding which children need more intensive treatment.

The following need further consideration:
- Children who are convulsing. Should be admitted. May have cerebral malaria or meningitis.
- Children who are vomiting. May need anti-emetics or anti malarials by a route other than oral.
- Children who are very anaemic. May have sickle cell disease, may need a blood transfusion, may go into cardiac failure, or may need iron once malaria is under control.
- Children who have respiratory problems. May have pneumonia or bronchitis.
- Children who have diarrhoea. May be dehydrated.

Drug treatment for malaria

Chloroquine resistance is becoming an increasing problem. However, in many parts of Africa it is still the drug most commonly used as it is easily available and is cheap. Quinine is effective in managing severe malaria. A combination of drugs is often now used. The nurse should follow the local policy on which drug regime to follow as different areas will use different drugs.

Cerebral malaria

Cerebral malaria is a very serious condition and needs urgent treatment. 10–20 per cent of the children are likely to die and seven per cent are left with a permanent handicap. The parasites are found in the small blood vessels of the brain.

The child starts with a temperature, but quickly deteriorates. He may become drowsy, then starts convulsing before lapsing into coma and death if no treatment is given. Hypoglycaemia is common and dehydration may also occur. In some centres, children who are suspected of having cerebral malaria will have a lumbar puncture to ensure that they do not have a bacterial meningitis.

Children who are very drowsy should have their conscious levels monitored using a coma scale. The Blantyre coma scale has been adapted for use with children, including those who are too young to speak, from the Glasgow coma scale (see Chapter 14). The score goes from 0–5, a low score being the most serious. A state of coma has been reached when the score is less than 3. The conscious level should be monitored frequently as it will show deterioration or improvement (see Table 46.1).

Nursing care of the child with cerebral malaria

Care of the unconscious child

Children who are unconscious will need to be nursed in the recovery position to ensure that their airway is not obstructed. If they are likely to vomit, a nasogastric tube should be passed and their stomach aspirated to prevent vomiting.

Hydration

Children should be kept well hydrated. In severe malaria, this will mean that an intravenous infusion is necessary. Children who are fully conscious can be encouraged to drink.

Hypoglycaemia

This can occur, especially if children are unconscious. The blood sugar should be measured and children given intravenous dextrose.

Children who are conscious can be given small, frequent meals as soon as any vomiting has stopped.

Fever

The temperature should be monitored regularly. Tepid sponging and fanning can be used to reduce the temperature and antipyretics such as paracetamol given.

Management of convulsions

See below.

Unfortunately some of the children who do survive are left permanently damaged. It is necessary to assess each one carefully for mental retardation and for mobility problems. The parents may be very happy to begin with, because the child has survived. They will then need help to readjust to the problems in having a permanently handicapped child.

Care of the child with convulsions

There may be several reasons why children are having convulsions.
- They may be having a febrile convulsion.
- They may have cerebral malaria.
- They may have meningitis.
- They may have been given native medicine. Ask mothers if any other medicines have been given recently.

They may also have been treated for convulsions in an inappropriate way. The photograph in Figure 46.1 shows a child whose feet were put into a fire to stop a convulsion.

Nursing care for children during convulsions

- Turn them on their side to protect their airways. It is important that the tongue does not obstruct the airway and that they do not inhale vomit. Never

Table 46.1 Blantyre coma scale

Best motor response	Localises painful stimulus	2
	Withdraws limb from pain	1
	Non specific or absent response	0
Verbal response	Appropriate cry	2
	Moan or inappropriate cry	1
	None	0
Eye movements	Directed (e.g. follows mother's face)	1
	Not directed	0
	Total	**0–5**

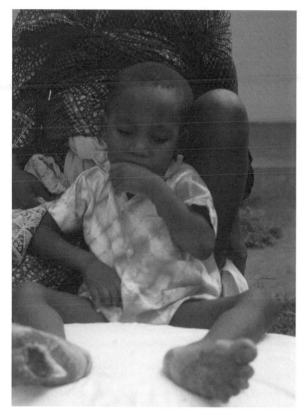

Figure 46.1 *Child whose feet were put in a fire*

force anything into their mouths as this can damage the teeth or cause other injury.

- Protect them from injuring themselves whilst they are convulsing. Remove any dangerous objects from the area.
- If they become *cyanosed*, first check that the airway is not obstructed, then give oxygen if it is available.
- Record how long the convulsion lasts.
- Notice whether it affects any particular part of the body, or whether it is generalised.
- Reassure the mothers/guardians, as it is a very frightening thing for anyone to see. They may think their children are dying, particularly if they appear not to be breathing.
- If they stop breathing for more than a few seconds, they need resuscitation.
- If convulsions last longer than 5 minutes, children need to be given anti-convulsants.

Diazepam: 2 mg for under 1 year
5 mg up to 3 years
10 mg in older children

This can be given rectally or intravenously. If given intravenously, it must be given slowly and stop as soon as the convulsion stops.

Or

Phenobarbitone: 10–15 mg/kg intramuscularly

Febrile convulsions

Many young children have convulsions when they have a high temperature. The reason is not fully understood but is thought to be due to the fact that in children, the rise in temperature is often more sudden and it goes higher. There is thought to be an increased electrical activity in the brain during this time. The children are usually between the ages of 6 months and 5 years and the convulsions are always generalised. Many children only have one febrile convulsion, others may have more than one and may go on to develop epilepsy.

It is important to reduce the temperature. This can be done in the following ways:

- Administer antipyretics:

Paracetamol: | | |
|---|---|
| 5–10 mg /kg | under 3 months |
| 60–120 mg | 3 months–1 year |
| 120–250 mg | 1–5 years |
| 250–500 mg | 6–12 years |

No more than 4 doses in every 24 hours.

Aspirin: 50 mg/kg per day

Note: Aspirin is the second choice for children, as it can cause *Reye's syndrome*, a life-threatening *encephalitis*. Use **only** if paracetamol is not available.

- Remove any thick clothes or blankets.
- Tepid sponge. Sponge the child down using warm water. The water should not be cold, as this causes *vasoconstriction* and prevents heat loss through the skin.
- If the child starts shivering, stop the sponging immediately, and cover with light clothes.
- Fans can be used, as long as they are not directed at the child. They increase heat loss through the skin by *convection*.
- Make sure the child drinks plenty of fluids.
- Young children are better placed on the mother's lap, rather than on her back, as this will help them to lose heat.

Meningitis (see Chapters 14 and 24)

This is a common infection and is a serious illness. Most cases are caused by the meningococcus and tend to occur in outbreaks particularly in the dry season. The meningococcus is carried in the nose and throat and most children who are infected will not develop meningitis. It is not known why some should.

Other organisms that may cause meningitis

- E.coli or Haemolytic Streptococcus B in young babies
- Haemophilus influenzae
- Pneumococcus
- Cryptococcus. This occurs in patients with AIDS.
- Trypanosomiasis
- Viral. No antibiotics given
- Tubercle bacillus. Drug treatment as for TB

Course of diseases

The infection spreads from a source of infection elsewhere, for instance the nasopharynx or mastoid sinuses. Sometimes the organism can enter via a wound. The meninges become inflamed, there is an *exudate* and a rise in intracranial pressure. The brain becomes oedematous and covered with pus. Infection can spread to the ventricles of the brain and there can be an obstruction to the flow of cerebrospinal fluid which may later result in *hydrocephalus*. Subdural effusions or cerebrovascular accidents can arise as late complications.

Signs and symptoms

- Sudden onset of fever, which may be high.
- Headache and stiff neck. Sometimes children arrive at the clinic/hospital with their heads bent right back (*opisthotonos*).
- *Kernig's* positive. Lie children on their backs. Take one of their legs and extend the leg with the hip flexed. This causes acute pain and distress in children with meningitis and they are unable to do it.
- Tripod sign. Sit children up. The back is so straight that they will put their arms out to steady themselves.
- Vomiting. Due to the raised intracranial pressure.
- Convulsions. These are not always present.

Children who have a meningococcal septicaemia, may present with widespread *petechial* haemorrhages. Look in the *sclera* of the eyes, as it is more easily seen there. This is a serious sign and the child may suddenly collapse with a very low blood pressure.

Children under 6 months often show no signs of a stiff neck and may not have a positive Kernig sign. They are also unable to say where the pain is so may not be able to show that they have a headache.

In babies the signs are even less obvious. Any baby who has a fever, is vomiting, has a convulsion, or is drowsy should be suspected of having meningitis. The anterior fontanelle may be full or bulging, but this is not always the case.

Diagnosis is by lumbar puncture, when the fluid is found to be under raised pressure and cloudy, except in viral or tubercular meningitis (see Chapter 25).

Nursing care

Antibiotics must be started immediately, preferably given intravenously until the child has started to improve. Broad spectrum antibiotics are given, as initially it may not be clear which organism is causing the disease. Paracetamol can be given for the pain and headache.

- Children with meningitis need very careful nursing. Initially they may not be able to drink so should be given intravenous fluids. However, it is necessary to be very careful. These children already have raised intracranial pressure, so it is safer to keep them slightly dehydrated, rather than over hydrated. If, after a few days, they are not eating, feeds can be given via a nasogastric tube.
- Their skin should be kept clean and dry. With a high temperature, they may be very sweaty and uncomfortable.
- Make sure that their mouth remains moist and clean. Apply Vaseline to the lips as necessary. Sometimes cold sores (Herpes simplex) occur. These can be treated with gentian violet.
- Monitor temperature, pulse and respirations carefully. Blood pressure should be taken at least every hour if children have a petechial rash. Report any sudden fall.

If there is no improvement and a late rise in temperature, there may be a subdural effusion. Any stiffness in arms and legs may be as a result of a cerebrovascular accident. Children should be checked thoroughly following an attack of meningitis to make sure there has not been permanent damage.

Health promotion

Prevention of malaria

- Avoid build up of stagnant water.
- Keep the bush cut back.
- Cover arms and legs when going out in the evening.
- Children should sleep under a cloth or mosquito net. The best nets are those treated with Permethrin.
- Young children can be protected by being given regular anti malarials. Check your national policy.

Prevention of fits

- Parents of children who have had fits due to a high temperature need to be taught how to sponge them down when the temperature goes up. They can also be advised to give them paracetamol to bring the temperature down.
- They should also give their children plenty of fluids to drink.
- Parents should be warned not to buy medicine from the market or from other patients. They may need advice if they are likely to use other methods to stop the fits, for example putting the child's feet in the fire.
- Teach the parents what to do if the child has another fit and give advice on when to seek further help.

■ Activity

What observations would you make on a child who is having a convulsion and why?

47

Nursing care of children with respiratory problems

This chapter covers the important anatomical and physiological differences between the respiratory tract of the child and the adult and outlines the assessment of respiratory function in the young child. It covers the management of the most common problems to affect babies and children: colds, otitis media, croup, whooping cough, pneumonia and asthma.

Anatomical and physiological differences

Young babies have to breathe through their noses. If they are blocked by mucus, they have difficulty in maintaining their oxygenation. The ribs of newborn babies lie in a horizontal position, whilst in adults, the ribs slope down. In adults the chest cavity is enlarged in inspiration by the contraction of the intercostal muscles which raises the ribs to a horizontal position. Because the ribs of babies are already in this position, they are not able to increase the size of the chest cavity in this way. Instead they rely on contracting their diaphragms and using their abdominal muscles. Watch newborn babies breathe and you will see that the abdomen moves with each breath. Young children also have smaller airways than adults. The adult's bronchus is about the size of a pencil, and the child's the size of a pencil lead. However, the lining of the bronchus is approximately the same thickness, therefore when the lining swells during infection, the airways become more easily blocked.

The respiratory tract is also shorter, which means that children are more susceptible to infections. The young baby also has a higher metabolic rate than the adult so needs relatively more oxygen and excretes more carbon dioxide than the adult. The respiratory rate is often irregular and may be in the range of 50–60 respirations per minute in the neonatal period, even when the baby is quite well.

Assessing the respiratory function

This is an important skill for the nurse to develop and should be carried out on all sick children. Wait until the child is resting quietly, as a crying child will have a raised respiratory rate for some time after the crying stops.

Respiratory rate: Count the number of respirations per minute and notice whether they are regular or irregular. (See Chapter 44 for normal rates.) In children from 0–2 months it should be less than 60 per minute, from 2–12 months it should be less than 50 per minute. Between the ages of 12 months and 5 years, it should be less than 40 per minute. Rates above these levels are an indication of pneumonia. (WHO)

Respiratory effort: Look to see how much effort the child is having to put into breathing. He may be using his accessory muscles of respiration which will be shown by flaring of the nostrils, *intercostal* recession and raising of the shoulders. *Subcostal* recession may indicate the child has pneumonia (see Figure 47.1).

Noise: Notice whether there is any noise as the child breathes. There may be a *stridor* on inspiration, (croup),

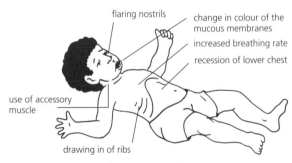

Figure 47.1 *Signs of respiratory distress*

or a wheeze on expiration (asthma). If there is a stridor, was the onset sudden? This could indicate an inhaled foreign body.

Cough: Ask the mother whether the child has a cough. If so, for how long has he had it? Observe any coughing. The cough may be dry and irritating, or it may be moist and productive. In whooping cough, there is a prolonged bout of coughing, followed by a characteristic whoop on inspiration. This may be followed by an *apnoeic* attack.

Sputum: See if the child is producing any sputum when he coughs. This is quite difficult as young children will swallow their sputum and not cough it out as adults will do. If any sputum is being produced notice the colour. If it is yellow/green it is a sign of a bacterial infection. Drooling from the mouth is a sign of epiglottitis.

Colour: Notice the child's colour. Is there any central *cyanosis*. Check inside the mouth, and the fingernails. Observe whether they are pale.

Behaviour: Children who are short of oxygen usually become very restless. Before deciding that the child is short of oxygen, make sure that he is not just frightened. If he becomes very *hypoxic*, he may suddenly become floppy. This is a dangerous sign and urgent action needs to be taken so that he does not have a respiratory arrest. He may need suction to remove a mucous plug and may require oxygen.

Hydration: Children who are having difficulty in breathing may also have difficulty in drinking. Also the increased respiratory rate means that there is an increased loss of fluid in respirations. Always ask the mother whether the child is drinking and encourage her to give frequent small sips of water. Dehydration leads to an increased stickiness of the sputum and makes it more difficult for the child to cough it out.

Vomiting: Children who are swallowing sputum may vomit. Look to see if there is any mucus in the vomit.

Temperature: Take the temperature to see whether there is a fever. A raised temperature indicates an infection.

Mouth: Check for signs of candida which is an indication of HIV.

Common respiratory problems

Colds

Young children may have frequent colds and although they are not serious, they can cause the child some problems. Colds are caused by viruses so children do not need antibiotics unless there is a secondary infection. They may have a fever whilst they have a cold, and also their noses may become blocked. Noses of young babies should be gently cleaned using cotton wool dipped in saline. The cotton wool can be twisted into a fine stick and gently pushed into the nose, then slowly withdrawn. Mucus will be drawn out. This is especially important before a feed, as babies may not be able to feed properly if their noses are blocked. Mothers can be taught how to clean the nose and they need to be informed that babies are more likely to take longer feeding whilst they have a cold and may need more frequent feeds.

Otitis media

Infection of the middle ear is very common in young children as the Eustachian tube (auditory tube) is short, wide and straight. It is easy for infection to pass from the throat to the middle ear and this can cause intense pain. Pus builds up within the middle ear and because there is no way for it to come out, it can result in a perforated eardrum. All sick children should have their ears examined for infection. The pinna of the ear is drawn back and the auriscope introduced gently. The drum normally looks silvery grey; with otitis media it will look red and opaque. Many of the infections will be caused by viruses, some will be caused by bacteria. Antibiotics may be given if it is thought that the infection is caused by bacteria. Frequent ear infections can lead to loss of hearing (see Chapter 20).

Croup – acute laryngo tracheo bronchitis

The child has usually had a cold during the last few days. Croup is also a common complication of measles. There is a loud inspiratory stridor and the child has difficulty in taking in enough air. Usually this is caused by a virus, but there may be other reasons for the stridor.

Inhaled foreign body: Young children have a habit of putting things in their mouths. It is then very easy for them to inhale something. Common objects include peanuts or small bits of plastic. Taking a careful history from the guardian may be helpful as the stridor is likely to have started very suddenly or there may have been an episode of coughing. The guardian may know that the child was eating peanuts or playing with a small object at the time that this happened. Sometimes these foreign bodies can be removed by turning the child upside down and squeezing the chest. If this does not work, the child may need to go to theatre so that the object can be removed under a general anaesthetic. If the inhaled foreign body is a peanut, it will need urgent removal as it can set up a severe inflammation. Sometimes the object has slipped into the lower respiratory tract and can then set up an infection. It is more difficult to remove in this case and the child will need to be encouraged to cough, after removal, to get rid of the sputum.

Epiglottitis: This is usually caused by the bacteria Haemophilus influenzae and is a serious threat to the child's life. The epiglottis becomes red and swollen and can obstruct the airway. The child needs urgent antibiotics and may need a tracheostomy or endotracheal intubation to relieve the obstruction. On no account should the nurse attempt to look in the throat of the child if epiglottitis is suspected as this can cause laryngeal spasm. Children with epiglottitis are likely to have a high temperature, and to have become ill quickly. They may also be flushed and drooling saliva.

Retropharyngeal abscess: Occasionally an abscess can form at the back of the pharynx and, if not incised, can obstruct the airway. The onset is usually slower, with fever and loss of appetite. Children then develop a stridor and, if the back of the throat is examined, the uvula is pushed to one side. These children need to go to theatre urgently to have the abscess incised.

Diphtheria: Diphtheria should be prevented by immunisation, but occasionally may occur in communities with low rates of immunisation. The child is usually very ill with a rapid pulse. A greyish membrane is seen to cover the back of the throat and the palate.

Nursing care of the child with croup

Children need continuous assessment of their respiratory function.

Hydration: They must be kept well hydrated to loosen the secretions. The mother should be taught to give frequent small sips of fluid. Breastfeeding should continue and, if necessary, the milk can be expressed and given by cup and spoon.

Humidity: Nursing the child in a humid environment also helps to loosen the secretions.

One way of increasing the humidity is to put wet sheets or towels near the child's bed. If the weather is hot, this will raise the humidity. Another way is to have the child in a small room with a cement floor.

Buckets of water can then be thrown on the floor and again the humidity will be raised.

Oxygen: If the child becomes increasingly distressed, it may be necessary to give oxygen. Small children do not like having oxygen masks put over their faces as this is frightening. A better way is to give the oxygen via nasal cannulae. However, it is very important to see that the oxygen is humidified first, as dry oxygen will make the condition worse.

Drug treatment: Sometimes IM hydrocortisone 100 mg can reduce the inflammation and in severe cases may be given. Alternatively the child may be given prednisolone 2 mg/kg per day. Check with local policies. Antibiotics may be used if bacterial infection is suspected.

Tracheostomy or intubation: In cases where the child continues to get worse and there is a danger of respiratory arrest, tracheostomy or intubation will be necessary, but can only be done in some hospitals. (See Chapter 20 for care of tracheostomy.)

Whooping cough (see Chapter 24)

This is an infectious disease caused by bacteria. Children should have been immunised against it. However, epidemics can occur and it is a serious illness in young babies who do not get any protection from the mother's antibodies. Most deaths occur in children who are under the age of 1 year.

It is passed easily from child to child, by droplet infection. There is an incubation period of 7–10 days and the child remains infectious for about 3 weeks. However, children may continue to whoop for the next year, whenever they get a respiratory illness. It is sometimes therefore called the 100 days cough.

The illness starts with a troublesome cough, which becomes spasmodic. The spasms of coughing all occur whilst children are breathing out, and there is then a characteristic 'whoop' as they struggle to breathe in. Some children will vomit at this stage. Babies may stop breathing and become cyanosed at the end of the attack and need immediate attention. Babies under 3 months may not whoop at all but have cyanotic attacks. If there is an epidemic of whooping cough at the time, then this should be suspected. Antibiotics are usually given as they shorten the illness.

Nursing care of a child with whooping cough

Barrier nursing: These children should be in a separate room, so that they do not spread the infection to other children.

Humidity: It may help the child to breathe if the environment is kept humid (as for croup).

Fluids: The mucus becomes very thick and stringy, so children should be given plenty of fluids to drink. Give the fluids after they have recovered from an attack of coughing, as they are then less likely to vomit.

Nutrition: In the early days children may not feel like eating. However, the illness can last some time and it is important to introduce food as soon as possible, especially in young children who may be malnourished. Food should be given once the coughing attack is over. Babies who vomit should be fed again. It may help to clean the nose before feeding. The weight should be recorded twice a week, so that extra feeding with energy dense foods can be introduced to children who are losing weight.

Temperature: Take the temperature every 4 hours in the first few days.

Respirations: The respiratory status of the child should be watched carefully as pneumonia is a common complication. Between attacks of coughing, the respirations should return to normal. If they are becoming laboured and faster, the child may need different antibiotics.

Management of apnoea attacks in young babies: These babies need very careful watching, each time they have a coughing attack. Suction equipment should be kept at the side of the cot. Often the apnoea is due to a plug of mucus which needs removing. Suction can be applied gently to the mouth, but care should be taken not to suction the back of the throat, as this can cause a further spasm of coughing. Slapping them on their backs may help. Once the mucus has been removed, if they are still not breathing, it may be necessary to use an ambu bag with a mask that fits securely over the babies' mouths and noses. A few assisted breaths may be all that is needed for them to recover.

Pneumonia

Pneumonia is a serious illness in young children and in severe cases has a high mortality rate. It is the commonest cause of death in some countries. It may occur as a complication of whooping cough or measles and can also occur in AIDS. It is thought that the high incidence can be related to the custom of burning grass, cow dung and wood for cooking purposes. These release toxic gases which cause damage to the immature lungs. Polythene shelters can also result in a high incidence due to the poor circulation of air.

Children present with a raised temperature, rapid pulse and distressed breathing. (See above for respiratory rates in pneumonia.) They are likely to be using their accessory muscles of respiration and may have painful sounding coughs. It is important to start treatment as soon as possible.

Nursing care of a child with pneumonia

Antibiotics: They will need antibiotic treatment as most cases are caused by bacteria, a few by viruses. The antibiotic to be used will depend on the ones available. Penicillin and gentamycin or chloramphenicol are usually the first choice. Check local policy.

Fluids: It is important that the fluid intake is maintained as this will help loosen the secretions. Breastfeeding should continue with extra fluids for the child who is being weaned. The guardian should be taught to give small amounts, frequently, by cup and spoon.

Nutrition: At first children will not want to eat. Once the temperature has reduced, food should be offered and small meals given frequently.

Positioning: Children should be nursed sitting up as this helps the expansion of the lungs. Small children may prefer to remain on their mother's back, but nurses must ensure that they can observe them closely. Sitting children on their mother's knee is another method, or propping them up with pillows.

Temperature: This may initially be high. Paracetamol can be given if it rises above 39° C. Tepid sponging will help bring the temperature down. Tepid water is better than cold water, as cold water causes *vasoconstriction*.

Fans can also be used, but should not be directed at the child.

Respiratory status: The children's respiratory status should be checked at least every 4 hours and any deterioration should be reported immediately.

Oxygen: Some children may require oxygen. This can be given by face mask for older children, by nasal cannula for babies and small children. Oxygen must always be humidified by running it through water to prevent drying of the mucous membranes. Oxygen may be available in cylinders or an oxygen concentrator.

Skin and mouth care: Children will be hot and sweaty, so need to have cool washes and change of sheets to keep them comfortable. Their mouths may become dry and the lips cracked. Giving extra fluids should help keep the mouth moist. Vaseline can be applied to the lips.

Asthma

Asthma is a chronic condition which occurs in children and adults. There are acute episodes but between the episodes, the airways return to normal. The airways become over sensitive and react in three ways. There is:

- Oedema of the mucous membranes of the airways
- Spasm affecting the smooth muscle of the bronchi and bronchioles. This makes the tubes smaller.
- Production of sticky mucus in the airways.

There are many causes. Often it is found that the child is allergic to a substance in their environment. It might be dust, pollen or animal *dander*. It can be caused by a sudden change in the weather, air pollution, strenuous exercise or by an emotional response. The effects can be mild or can become severe and life-threatening. The child presents with:

- A very obvious expiratory wheeze
- A paroxysmal dry cough.

If attacks are not treated, children become increasingly distressed. The lungs become over inflated as there is difficulty in breathing out. Due to the over inflation, there is increased breathlessness as it is difficult to take in sufficient oxygenated air. The shoulders are often raised in an effort to increase the size of the chest cavity and children will be using the accessory muscles of respiration. The pulse rate will increase and cyanosis can occur.

Treatment during an asthma attack

- Administration of bronchodilators such as salbutamol. This can be given by inhaler or nebuliser.
- Ensure the children remain well hydrated to loosen the sticky mucus.
- Steroids may be given, either by inhalation or orally. This helps reduce the oedema of the mucous membranes.
- Oxygen may be necessary.
- Encourage rest to reduce the body's need for oxygen.

- Give reassurance. Asthma is very distressing and fear makes the condition worse.

Once the acute attack is over, nurses should try to find out whether the parents know what caused the attack. It may be possible to reduce the number of future attacks by avoiding the cause. Some children may need to be discharged with inhalers containing a bronchodilator that they can use at home to prevent or reduce the severity of future attacks.

Conclusion

Respiratory illnesses are the cause of many deaths in young children. Early treatment and careful nursing can reduce this mortality. Good observation of the respiratory status of all sick children is essential.

Health promotion

- Children should be immunised against whooping cough. Keeping the level of immunisation high in the general population will reduce the number of epidemics and protect the young babies.
- Small children, under the age of 3, should not be allowed to play with small objects, which they can put in their mouths and then inhale.
- Advise mothers to protect their children from smoke from cooking fires.
- Where children are living in plastic shelters, encourage the circulation of air by raising one side when possible.

■ Activity

1. Why are children more prone to otitis media than adults?
2. How would you know whether a child with a respiratory problem was getting worse?

48

Nursing care of children with measles

Measles is a very dangerous illness in young children, causing many deaths and long-term problems. This chapter will cover the spread of measles and the care required by children with the infection (see Chapter 24).

Incidence, spread and long-term effects (see Chapter 24)

Measles is caused by a virus, which is easily spread by droplet infection. It can be prevented by immunisation, which is usually given from the age of 9 months onwards. Some countries with good immunisation records have seen the disappearance of the disease. It is not common to see measles in children under the ages of 7 months as before this time they are protected by *antibodies* from the mother. In a community where most children have been immunised, the young child gets protection from the fact that there is less likelihood of an epidemic as there are few children at risk. In unprotected communities, the risk is very high and epidemics can quickly spread. It is estimated that nine out of every ten unprotected children will develop the disease. It has long been thought that children who are already malnourished are likely to suffer more severe forms of the disease. However, more recent research shows that this theory is not totally correct. It is the amount of virus that the child is exposed to that determines the severity of the disease. Therefore the first child in a family to develop the illness is likely to have a milder course. He has probably been exposed to a child outside the home for a limited period of time, and so has a smaller virus load. Subsequent children in the family are more likely to get a severe form of the disease as they are in close contact with the child with measles for long periods and may share a bed or mat with them. The more crowded the home, the more severe the disease will be.

However, nutrition is an important factor, as malnourished children will likely suffer a deterioration in their nutritional status as a result of the infection. Malnourished children already have reduced immunity; an attack of measles will further reduce their ability to fight infection. As a result, following epidemics of measles, there is often an increase in the number of children with *marasmus* or *kwashiorkor* and more children may present with tuberculosis. Children under the age of 5 and those who have had a severe form of the disease have been shown to have a higher mortality rate for the next two years.

Care of the child with measles

Signs and symptoms

- The child presents with a high temperature and an upper respiratory tract infection.
- The eyes may become red and inflamed.
- *Koplik's* spots (white spots usually found inside the lips and cheeks of the mouth) may be seen. It is important to make sure these white spots are not milk curds or thrush. Milk curds can be wiped away, and thrush is likely to be widespread. Koplik's spots are usually discrete and localised.
- After 3–4 days, the typical red rash appears, spreading quickly all over the face and body. The rash is not only confined to the skin, but spreads into the mouth, the gastro-intestinal tract, the trachea and the rest of the respiratory tract.
- The temperature usually starts to fall a few days later, and the rash begins to fade. As the rash subsides there can be blackening of the skin from small haemorrhages. This is followed by dry peeling, *desquamation*.

Common complications of measles

- Laryngo tracheo bronchitis (croup)
- Pneumonia

- Otitis media
- Diarrhoea
- Stomatitis (sore mouth)
- Febrile convulsions
- Conjunctivitis, corneal ulcers, cloudy cornea, dry eye (*xeropthalmia*)
- Worsening nutritional status

Nursing care of the child with measles

Mild cases of measles can be managed at home with the child looked after by the family. However, it is important to tell the parents that they should return with the child to the clinic if the condition worsens. They should also be advised to give the child frequent small meals and to see that he is given plenty of fluids to drink. They will need to return with the child when he is recovered so that his weight can be checked to ensure that he regains the weight he will have lost while he is ill.

Children with the severe form of the disease and children who are malnourished should be admitted if at all possible. Children with complications need to be cared for under medical supervision.

Barrier nursing

As the illness is so infectious, the child should **not** be nursed in an open ward with other children who are sick. He can pass the infection on and also he is likely to pick up infections from other children whilst his immunity is low. Often during an outbreak, there are several cases in the community, so these children can be nursed in the same room. The problem is that often measles is not diagnosed until the rash appears, and if the child has been in the open ward, the virus will already have passed to other children. For this reason, it is practice in many countries to immunise all children on admission to a children's ward who have not already been immunised against measles.

Observations and management

Temperature: The temperature should be taken every 4 hours whilst it is raised. The child can be given paracetamol to help reduce the temperature. He can also be tepid sponged. A high temperature can result in febrile convulsions (see Chapter 46). Anti malarials should be given as the child may also have malaria.

Respiratory assessment (see Chapter 47): Observe the child's respiratory status carefully. If he develops an inspiratory stridor or a hoarse sounding cough, he may have croup. Increased humidity is necessary.

Increased difficulty in breathing may mean he has pneumonia and he will need antibiotics.

Nutritional status: The child should be weighed on admission and his weight plotted on a growth chart. The child who is already malnourished will need extra care and supervision. The metabolic rate (the rate at which he burns calories) is increased whilst he has an infection and if his mouth is sore, he is unlikely to want to eat. He may also have diarrhoea and be losing important nutrients in his stool. Breastfeeding should continue and frequent, small, high energy feeds be encouraged. If he has diarrhoea, his hydrational status also needs to be watched carefully, and oral rehydration fluids given (see Chapter 45).

Vitamin A capsules (50,000 iu) should be given once a day for 2 days to protect the eyes.

Under 6 months	1 capsule
6–12 months	2 capsules
1–5 years	4 capsules

Eye care: This is particularly important in the child who is already malnourished. In the early days there is often conjunctivitis. The eyes look red and watery and the child may complain that the light hurts his eyes (*photophobia*). If the eyes start discharging pus, there may be a secondary bacterial infection and this can be treated with chloramphenicol eye ointment. The child may be more comfortable if he is nursed in a room with subdued light.

Children who complain of very sore eyes, or where there is clouding of the cornea, may be developing *keratitis* or a corneal ulcer or xeropthalmia. If possible consult an eye worker for advice (see Chapter 21). The nurse should examine the child's eyes at least twice every day and ask the guardian to report at once if she is worried.

Follow-up care

Weigh the child before he goes home to see how much weight he has lost. Advise the guardian to bring him back to clinic for further weighing within 1 or 2 weeks.

Advise the guardian to give him frequent small meals with a high energy content, until he has regained his lost weight.

Explain that he will pick up infection very easily until he has regained weight. If possible she should keep him away from other sick children and overcrowded places. Avoid bringing him into contact with people who have troublesome coughs that may be tuberculosis.

If the child fails to thrive following an attack of measles, tuberculosis should be suspected. Unfortunately, in the child who has a lowered immunity, the tuberculin test may remain negative, in spite of the child having the disease.

■ Activity

1. Check the child's weight when measles is first diagnosed and weigh again in 2 weeks. See how much weight he has lost.
2. If the child had not been immunised against measles, ask the mother why not. It may be that she was too far from a clinic or was not aware of the importance.

Health promotion

- Advise parents to have their children immunised against infectious diseases, including measles.
- Prevent overcrowding if possible, especially in rooms where children are sleeping, to reduce the incidence of the severe form of the disease.
- Well nourished children will recover more quickly from measles than malnourished children. Encourage good nutrition for all children.
- Encourage parents to see that the child has a BCG vaccination after birth to protect against tuberculosis.

Part 6

Mental health

49

Care of people with
mental health problems

This chapter provides basic information on mental health nursing. It covers different types of illness, the effects they may have and important aspects of care provision. A life-span perspective is used because people experience difficulties and respond in different ways depending on their stage of development. Problems that are specific to a stage of development or to particular circumstances are described.

Introduction

Mental and physical health are closely connected as people try to adjust and adapt to experiences and difficulties in life. Physical signs and symptoms usually follow a physical stress such as infection. Sometimes mental problems can result. Likewise, emotional stress may cause mental health problems but also may cause physical problems like headache. Mental health is to do with thinking clearly, coping with difficulties and everyday activities, enjoying life and helping others to do so too. Mental illness affects people's emotions and their thoughts and behaviour. They may act in ways not expected by their families or society and cause difficulties for themselves and those close to them.

Several factors influence mental health. These include heredity, upbringing and life circumstances. Some illness is linked to damage or chemical changes in the brain. Illness may be mild or more severe, such as when people act in ways that others consider are unacceptable. Their behaviour may interfere with everyday activities, cause them to lose touch with reality and affect their judgement. Sometimes illness is easy to identify but obvious behaviour changes such as violence and extreme agitation are less common. HIV infection can cause mental health problems and they

are becoming more common because of it. The stress and social isolation of being HIV positive or having AIDS, losing relatives and friends, and the complicated nature of treatments can cause distress, anxiety and depression. Some drugs may cause side effects. The virus may affect the brain causing dementia, with loss of understanding and memory, behaviour and emotional changes, and poor coordination.

Attitudes to people who have mental health problems have changed over time and are different from one culture to another. Mentally ill people may be accepted as part of the family and their difficulties accepted. Some are left to wander around without proper care or treated brutally. In many countries they used to be put in big institutions to remove them from society. It is now understood that mentally ill people have the same rights as other ill people. They need to be assessed properly and receive appropriate treatment. Care can often be given at home or in community units and this has lessened the *stigma* associated with mental illness.

This chapter will help you understand mental illnesses and the care and support that are needed by ill people and their families in ideal situations. However, services may be very limited and specialist help may be difficult to obtain. Nurses and midwives can provide some support themselves and can act as *advocates* to encourage better services which do not have to be expensive. The chapter is not intended as a full guide to what to do. Details of resources that contain more information about treatments are listed in Sources and Further Reading.

Socio-cultural issues

Culture has great influence on mental illness and its treatment. What is labelled as mental illness in one culture may be seen as witchcraft in another, or just being odd or eccentric or mad. What is acceptable in one culture may be totally unacceptable in another.

For example we react differently to death. In one culture people may be expected to grieve quietly, in another people may cry and wail. Individuals react differently too. Nurses should treat everyone with respect and dignity and avoid imposing their own values on others. The way in which people see mental illness affects the services that are provided too. If it is not taken seriously, or considered to be untreatable, money is less likely to be dedicated to providing help. Prison may be the only place available for those who endanger others or themselves.

Another difference between people and cultures is the way in which they seek help. Some will try to hide mental illness. This is more common if it is seen as personal failure or shameful, or people fear being rejected by friends and family. Others will seek help from priests or pastors. They may see a traditional healer or diviner, or go straight to a doctor or psychiatrist. They may go from one to the other. Many people avoid seeking help because it means admitting that they are unwell. Some may not realise they are ill or may deny it.

What causes mental illness?

There have been many explanations for mental illness. Often these have been to do with the way people develop. It is now believed that causes are mostly genetic and biological or to do with the environment in which people live. An unhappy childhood, perhaps with violent or unkind treatment, can cause anxiety and depression and so can violence and abuse experienced as an adult. Difficult life circumstances such as lack of money or work, infertility, bereavement and being involved in disaster or conflict are common causes of illness. Some severe illnesses can be inherited from parents. Others can result from physical illness. Becoming disabled, for example after a car accident or a stroke, may cause severe depression. Being told that one has a chronic condition such as diabetes or terminal illness may cause depression too. Illnesses such as kidney failure, brain diseases, HIV and AIDS, epilepsy or injury may affect behaviour and thinking abilities. Medications may be responsible for bad effects, so too can drugs of addiction.

Types of mental health problems

Mental health problems can be divided into categories. Most of them can occur in some form at any age.

These categories are:

- Depression and anxiety that is severe enough to interfere with daily life
- Psychoses – severe disorders that cause abnormal ways of thinking and serious behavioural problems
- Dependency on drugs or alcohol
- Dementia
- Personality disorder.

Depression and anxiety

Depression is common and most people experience it at some time. However, it can make life difficult and then it should be seen as an illness. Depressive illness shows as sadness, loss of interest in activities, poor concentration and lack of energy. Depressed people may feel worthless, lose interest in sex and not want to spend time with others. They may experience feelings of guilt, be unable to sleep properly and have poor appetites. On the other hand, excessive sleep and over-eating can also be symptoms of depression. Depression often shows up just as aches and pains and tiredness.

People who are very depressed may feel there is no hope for them and suicide is a real possibility. Some who try to injure or kill themselves may succeed even if it was intended as a cry for help or to punish someone such as a family member or friend who has upset them. It may be a real attempt to die. Those who have made repeated attempts and who are seriously depressed are at serious risk. Some people provide verbal clues to their intention such as saying 'tomorrow this time I will be no more'. These need to be taken seriously and never ignored.

Sometimes it is possible to anticipate the risk of suicide and provide supervision to try to prevent it. This is very demanding of resources and a burden for a family. Hospital care, if it is available, may be helpful during the acute stage of an illness and following a suicide attempt. Anti-depressive medication may be used with careful supervision. Counselling can help people with depression. People need help to find support especially if this is not available from close family or friends.

Nurses may need to act as advocates for people who have attempted suicide. This is particularly important where suicide is against the law and the nurse may have important information about the reasons behind the attempt.

Anxiety is also something most people experience sometimes but it can interfere with their lives. They may become fearful and experience panic attacks. These can be felt as a sense that something dreadful is going to happen. Anxiety can cause fast heart beat, sweating, trembling, dizziness and feeling unable to breathe. In Africa and Asia people may say they feel insects crawling over their skin. It is common for those suffering from anxiety to avoid situations that they believe cause the problem, such as open spaces, small rooms, or travel. Fear like this is called phobia. Another form of anxiety is obsessive-compulsive disorder in which people repeat the same action over and over again. It can completely disrupt their lives. Hand-washing is a common obsession, or repeatedly checking that a door is locked.

Belonging to a group of others who have similar experiences may be enough to help people get over depression or anxiety. Nurses can provide a listening ear and help people to find their own solutions. They may need referral and treatment with anti-depressant medications and specialised counselling if symptoms are severe.

Psychosis

Psychosis is a group of disorders that cause unreal ideas known as delusions and can also cause hallucinations. Hallucinations are abnormal sensations that only the ill person experiences. These may be sights, sounds, smells or feelings which may be terrifying and very real to the person concerned. Two examples are of feeling ants crawling over the skin as with anxiety, or hearing voices. Delusions are strange beliefs such as thinking that one has special powers. Like hallucinations, they are not true but very real. These delusions and hallucinations cause severe difficulties in carrying out normal daily tasks.

Psychotic illnesses include schizophrenia and manic depression. Manic depression is often called 'bi-polar disorder' because people swing from extreme depression to extreme excitement, called mania. Psychosis can result from drug dependency, severe stress, and head injury as well as happening in the manic phase of manic depression. Infection of the brain such as in malaria or AIDS is another cause of psychotic behaviour (see Chapters 32 and 46). It is possible for short psychotic illnesses to happen and never be repeated. It may also arise shortly after childbirth. This is called postnatal or postpartum psychosis (see below).

People may lose contact with reality. They may be very confused and have little insight into their condition, lack judgment and act on impulse. They may neglect to care for themselves or try to harm themselves. They may make repetitive or ritualistic actions like head banging or hand rubbing and can be very frightened.

Seeking the help of a mental health worker is very important as people with psychotic illnesses need proper assessment and treatment. When psychosis happens suddenly it is important to make sure the person is not suffering from delirium. This can be brought on by a physical illness such as brain infection or injury, or a high temperature. It is a medical emergency and the cause needs to be identified and treated (see Chapter 14).

People in an acute psychotic state may need admission to hospital for their own safety or that of others. Management includes combining psychotherapy with medications. People with psychotic illnesses may need help with their basic physical needs including feeding, bathing and getting exercise. They may need help with developing skills for successful living. Individuals and their families will require ongoing support in the community. Recovery from psychotic illness can be good with proper care.

Schizophrenia

Schizophrenia usually begins in early adulthood. Women tend to become ill later than men and may respond better to treatment. The cause is unknown but it often occurs in more than one member of a family so it may be inherited. It often continues for years.

People suffering from schizophrenia may not believe that they are ill and may refuse help. They experience psychotic symptoms and may hear voices talking about them or believe others are telling them what to do. They may talk back to the voices. They may be unable to think clearly and feel they cannot resist the instructions of the voices. Schizophrenic people may even believe they have another being inside them. They may be depressed and lethargic and have no interest in eating or keeping themselves clean. They may withdraw into their own private world. Sometimes they become very restless or aggressive.

People with schizophrenia need to be referred for specialist help. They may need hospital admission for a period, then community care if available. It is important to teach family members how to cope at home and recognise the signs of increasing illness so they can seek help. Anti-psychotic medications are very important to relieve symptoms and prevent their recurrence. Nurses have an important role in helping schizophrenic people to take their medicines properly and to watch for side effects such as drowsiness, restlessness and agitation, weight gain and lowered white cell counts in the blood.

Manic depression

Manic depression can be difficult to identify except when the person becomes over-active. In the depressive phase they may seem no different from other depressed people. Extreme mood swings are common with periods when there are no symptoms. People may become deeply depressed, withdrawn and become suicidal. They may then become very happy and excited without any reason. They talk very fast and may act irresponsibly. Mania can cause people to take great risks, perhaps with money, or their own safety or that of others. They may engage in high-risk and promiscuous behaviour. Often they believe they have special abilities and can do anything. They may become very irritable and believe everyone is trying to harm them. Like schizophrenic people, they may not agree to treatment because they do not believe they are ill.

Specialist help is again important for these people if it can be arranged. They may need specific medication such as lithium carbonate or valproate for long periods. Careful monitoring of drug levels through blood testing is essential although this is less important with valproate. Therapy may include counselling and talking treatment.

Dependency on drugs and alcohol

Drug and alcohol dependency is often called substance abuse. Some substances are used just once or twice to try them out. They may be used on social occasions and in special rituals but lead to addiction in some people only. Other drugs such as cocaine are highly addictive and quickly lead to dependency. People become increasingly unable to control their intake and develop cravings if they cannot get hold of the substances to which they are addicted. The commonest drugs of addiction throughout the world are probably alcohol and tobacco. Other substances include sedatives, marijuana, cocaine, glues, opium and heroin. Part of the brain function begins to depend on the new chemical which takes the place of normal brain chemicals. This is called chemical dependency.

There are four stages in chemical dependency:
- Experimentation. Users feel happy and socially accepted.
- Seeking. Users actively seek out the substance in order to change their mood. Work or school and relationships begin to suffer.
- Preoccupation. Users believe they cannot cope without their chemicals and have lost control over their use. They develop tolerance to the drug and may begin to use higher doses or stronger substances. The chemical is now used to prevent withdrawal symptoms.
- Burnout. The pleasant 'high' feeling is no longer available. If the substance is stopped withdrawal symptoms will appear so users continue just to avoid these feelings. They may be unable to function normally now.

An addiction causes problems when people's health begins to suffer, or when those close to them are affected. Addiction often causes marriage problems, depression in family members, domestic violence, family break up, unemployment, poverty, homelessness, accidents and violence. People may steal or become prostitutes to buy drugs. Serious physical problems such as liver damage and convulsions may follow or depression, psychosis and suicide.

People who misuse drugs and alcohol may be depressed and feel guilty at their inability to control their cravings. They may be irritable and have problems sleeping. If they cannot get their drugs they can become agitated and suffer from tremors, anxiety, sweating and stomach cramp. These are called withdrawal symptoms and can include severe body pain, hallucinations and lead to death. Addicts who inject may have infected injection sites and skin rashes. Death is a constant risk through overdose. Injecting drug addicts are at high risk of blood-borne disease such as HIV and hepatitis especially if they share needles and syringes.

Counselling and support is important in helping substance abusers. People with severe symptoms may need hospital care. Help needs to be long-term to avoid returning to drug dependency.

Dementia and Alzheimer's disease

Dementia is a progressive condition of memory loss and abnormal behaviour that involves degeneration of the brain. It can start in early adulthood but is commonest in the elderly and occurs more often in women than in men. This may be due to the fact that women live longer than men in many societies. Dementia may not be recognised in countries where lives are short or where families usually cope alone. This is changing as people live longer and as family structures change but services may not be available to help.

Causes of dementia are unknown. However, some people with the commonest cause of dementia, Alzheimer's disease, may have inherited it. Familial Alzheimer's disease is very likely to occur again in close relatives. It can occur with other mental illnesses, following brain injury or from excess alcohol intake or infections like meningitis, syphilis or AIDS. It is more common in people with Down's syndrome.

Dementia is usually progressive. The person who suffers from it may change slowly over years or deteriorate very rapidly. Rapid change may occur in early onset Alzheimer's disease or be caused by several small strokes. People may have memory loss and be forgetful and unable to understand what they hear or see happening around them. Thinking and judgment deteriorates and capacity to learn new things is reduced. They may have no insight into their condition. Others know they have a problem in the early stages and this can be very distressing. People with dementia gradually become unable to work, look after themselves or relate to others. The main signs are:

- Loss of short and long-term memory, for example inability to recall names of people and places
- Not recognising people who they have known for years, for example spouse or children
- Getting lost, forgetting where they live, being confused about where they are
- Inability to concentrate or think logically
- Loss of skills learnt early in life
- Personality change: becoming withdrawn or aggressive and rude, suspicious or lazy
- Loss of inhibitions and behaving inappropriately
- Repetitive or inappropriate actions or speech.

The main goal of caring for people with dementia is to help them to lead lives that are as normal as possible. It is important to try to reduce the symptoms and provide support to families. Both the person with dementia and the family and care givers are affected and life can be very hard for care givers especially if there are not many others around to help. Meeting others who have relatives with dementia may be very helpful to the family. Care givers need to learn how to cope and

to encourage as much independence as possible. Involving people with dementia in making decisions about their care and retaining their dignity is important. Groups exist in some places for the person with dementia; this provides stimulus for them and gives carers a break. If such facilities do not exist despite there being a demand for them, nurses could help to get them started with minimal cost.

There is no known treatment or cure for dementia. However, medication may be provided to calm disturbed behaviour, encourage sleep and improve depression.

Personality disorders

Specialists in mental health and illness do not agree about whether personality disorders are illnesses. They are often described as ways of thinking, feeling and behaving that make it difficult to function normally and maintain stable relationships. People with personality disorders are often called psychopaths and their difficulties may start in adolescence. They are usually of normal ability but may never reach their full potential. They may be inflexible and antisocial and completely unaware of the feelings or needs of others. People with personality disorder may ignore moral standards and laws and cause harm to others. They may disregard other people's wishes and see no problem with engaging in sexual activity whenever and with whoever they wish. They do not believe they have any accountability for what they do. Some experts believe that such disorders are related to experiencing abuse in childhood.

There are other ways in which personality disorder may become obvious. Some people are very dependent on others and cannot make decisions. They may be dramatic and emotional, or completely indifferent to what happens around them. Other types of this disorder cause mistrust of others and the belief that harm is intended. This is called paranoia. People may be perfectionists or very unforgiving and manipulative, finding ways of making others do what they want. On the other hand they may worry constantly about what others think of them, or just appear odd and act in unusual but harmless ways.

Some people continue to show personality disorders throughout their lives. Others can change but it depends on whether they want to do so. They have to be prepared to accept help to change the way they think about themselves and those around them. Counselling and group therapy may be helpful.

Ways of helping those with mental health problems

The main treatments for mental illnesses can be divided into talking and drug therapy. People may also be taught how to relax, helped to learn to cope with their difficulties and will need support as they recover. It is important to involve family members and friends where appropriate. They may themselves need support. Mental health workers have experience of these therapies but some help can be provided by nurses and midwives when specialist help is not available.

Talking treatments

- Counselling is a way of helping people to help themselves. Counsellors encourage people to talk through their feelings and experiences, understand them, and make their own decisions. Counselling is often done without telling people what to do and must be done without being judgmental. People may be very reluctant to talk about themselves and need encouragement and plenty of time.
- The word 'counselling' may also be used to describe giving information about illnesses and advice about ways of overcoming specific difficulties. People need to feel confident about its accuracy.
- Group therapy may be used so that sufferers can meet together, listen to each other and help each other to solve problems and find ways of coping. The nursing role may be just to get people together, support them as they get to know each other and encourage them to talk.
- Problem solving is often a feature of talking treatments. Problems can be identified one by one, goals selected and ways found of solving them. It is important to identify what has worked and what has been less successful. In this way people learn the skills of problem solving and become more self-confident.
- Psychotherapy is a specialised form of talking treatment that may be used one-to-one or in a group. Proper training is essential. It is rarely available when health services are short of money because it is so specialised. One type is called cognitive behaviour therapy. This helps people to learn new ways of looking at themselves and at the

world, and new ways of behaving. It may be used over long periods with people with depression or personality disorders.

Drug therapy

Accurate diagnosis is vital for drug treatment to be effective. Monitoring must take place so that drugs can be changed or their dose altered depending on how successful they are in helping with the symptoms. Side effects may occur and this also needs to be monitored. The various drugs are divided into the following groups:

- Anti-depressants are used for depression and anxiety.
- Beta-blockers are used to help control the symptoms of anxiety.
- Anti-psychotics or tranquilisers can help stop extreme mood swings and control the symptoms of schizophrenia.
- Manic-depression drugs can prevent return of the illness.

You will find details of the most commonly available medicines, their dosage and side effects in Table 49.1.

Dealing with emergencies

Any nurse or midwife may find herself having to deal with emergency situations in hospital or community settings and support from professional mental health workers may not be available. These emergencies include aggression, confusion and agitation, and threatened or attempted suicide. Common causes you should ask about are drug treatments which may have these side effects, substance abuse and underlying medical conditions.

- Aggression. Make sure of your own safety by asking someone else to remain nearby and checking your way out of the room is unhindered. This is important even with children or the elderly. Find out what has triggered this aggression. There may be a known illness or the person may have been drinking or taking drugs. Try to find out what is troubling the person. Talk calmly and without threat. Refuse to remain with someone who has a weapon. If the person becomes increasingly agitated despite what you say, leave the room or at least call for help. If talking fails to prevent violence you may need to get help and restrain the person as a last resort.

Table 49.1 Basic medicines used for mental health problems

Note: All medicines should be given by mouth. If side effects occur, try reducing the dose or changing to another medicine of the same type if available. Medicines are often given in combination.

Condition	Medicine	Dose and administration	Side effects	Notes and cautions
Depression	Amitryptiline	Start 25 mg nightly, increase up to 75 mg, or 150 mg if needed. No more than 150 mg	Drowsiness, dry mouth, blurred vision, weight gain, constipation	Half dose for adolescents and elderly. Not under age 16 or for mania, avoid with heart disease, recent myocardial infarction, glaucoma. Usually needs 2 weeks to take effect, 4 weeks to full effect. Can bring on seizures. Overdose risk.
	Fluoxetine	20 mg in the morning (increase up to 60 mg if no significant improvement seen after 6 weeks).	Nervousness, fatigue, nausea, poor appetite, diarrhoea, sleep difficulties, sexual difficulties	Usually needs 2 weeks to take effect. Better tolerated than many other anti-depressants
Anxiety	Diazepam	5 mg nightly (increase up to 10 mg twice daily if no improvement seen)	Drowsiness, dizziness, dependence, overdose causes suppression of breathing.	Dependency possible when used for long periods. Avoid using more than 4 weeks. Can be given for alcohol withdrawal and sleeping problems. Half dose for elderly. Can cause memory and coordination problems. Can cause fetal malformations and later problems.
	Propanalol	Start with 20 mg twice daily, increase up to 40 mg twice daily.	Heart failure, asthma, fatigue, nausea	Beta-blocker, for physical symptoms of anxiety
Psychosis	Haloperidol	5 mg nightly, increase up to 10 mg. IM 5–10 mg twice daily	Stiffness, dry mouth, weight gain, restlessness, drowsiness, dizziness,	Tranquiliser for severe agitation/acute mania. Less sedative than chlorpromazine
	Chlorpromazine	25 mg nightly, increase up to 200 mg twice daily. IM 25–100 mg undiluted	sudden jerky movements	Tranquiliser for people with psychosis and sleep problems combined. Use for confusion, agitation and aggression. In mania, treat for 3 months after symptoms subside. Then commence long-term medicines for manic depression.
Side effects of anti-psychotic medicines are occurring	Procyclidine	2.5 mg twice daily, increase up to 5 mg three times daily	Dry mouth, constipation, blurred vision, urinary retention, confusion	Use for prevention or treatment of tremor and stiffness and other side effects of anti-psychotic drugs.
	Benzhexol	1mg once daily, increase up to 2.5 mg three times daily		

Table 49.1 Basic medicines used for mental health problems *continued*

Note: All medicines should be given by mouth. If side effects occur, try reducing the dose or changing to another medicine of the same type if available. Medicines are often given in combination.

Condition	Medicine	Dose and administration	Side effects	Notes and cautions
Manic depression	Sodium valproate	Start with 200 mg twice daily, increase in steps over 2 weeks to 600 mg twice daily.	Nausea, drowsiness, diarrhoea, weight gain, tremor, jaundice, liver failure, pancreatitis.	Mood stabiliser for long-term control of manic depression and epilepsy. Blood level monitoring is advised. Liver function tests advisable. Can cause fetal malformation when given in early pregnancy. Treatment for at least 2 years.
	Lithium carbonate	400–1200 mg single dose daily.	Nausea, diarrhoea, thirst, weight gain.	Mood stabiliser. Use for long-term control of manic depression. Treatment for at least 2 years. Takes 5–14 days to take effect so haloperidol may be given to control symptoms meantime. Very dangerous in excess. Use is not advised in rural settings and **never** give unless blood monitoring can be carried out. Blood level must be 0.6–1.2 mmol/l. May interact with non-steroidal anti-inflammatories and diuretics. Can cause fetal malformation when given in early pregnancy. Avoid dehydration and salt depletion.

Note: Intramuscular and intravenous routes may sometimes be used when patients refuse oral medicines. This does not apply to medicines used for anxiety or depression.

- Confusion and agitation. The person may be unaware of the surroundings and what is happening. They may become extremely agitated and violent. Enquire about possible causes as already described. Provide a quiet space for the person and a health worker or relative to supervise him. Sometimes restraint or medication may be needed to calm him. Sedative medications such as diazepam can be given by mouth. If the person refuses these they can be given intramuscularly or by slow intravenous injection. It is important to prepare medication before restraining the patient if this is needed.
- Threatened and attempted suicide. Emergency medical treatment may be needed if suicide has been attempted. Make sure the person is not in imminent danger. It is important that he is not left alone until he appears to have calmed down. Make sure access to dangerous items is prevented as much as possible. In the end it may be impossible to prevent suicide in someone who is determined to kill himself.

Once the immediate emergency is over, continuing support will be needed. During the crisis it is important to take care of normal needs for fluids, food and personal care.

Mental health problems through the life cycle
Childhood

Many of the mental or emotional problems diagnosed in adulthood are caused by experiences during childhood. They may experience physical and emotional insecurity, neglect, violence, being orphaned, and homelessness. It is every child's right to have a loving and supportive environment in which to grow and develop but many children do not have this security. Nurses need to be alert enough to identify problems and know what resources exist in the community to help those who need shelter, clothing, food, love and care.

The difficulties children experience may show up early as emotional and behavioural problems. Common signs of distress are:
- behavioural problems and poor concentration
- developmental and speech delays
- withdrawal, aggression, and inappropriate social interactions

- poor achievement at school
- anxiety, fear and general unhappiness
- difficulties in relating to people such as parents and those in authority
- eating and elimination disorders.

Conflict, abuse, neglect and violence

Conflict between parents and children happens everywhere. Some disagreement is normal but children need to know they are accepted and loved. They can experience anxiety and depression when they feel rejected or insecure. This can happen when parents become physically or mentally ill. Children may have received violent punishment or believe they have been punished unfairly. They may blame themselves for what happens. Nurses need to understand and support these children emotionally. A thorough assessment is important to determine their emotional state and what happens at home. Counselling both children and parents can be helpful.

Abused children are those experiencing some form of harm which may be physical, emotional or sexual. Neglect refers to children whose basic physical or emotional needs are not being met, but abuse and neglect really go together. Abuse may lead to later difficulties such as depression, post traumatic stress disorder and personality disorders. Children can experience abuse and violence as a result of conflict between adults too and this is worse if it happens repeatedly. They may feel intense helplessness, fear, or horror and experience nightmares and physical complaints such as stomach aches.

Child abuse is often hidden to protect the family from shame especially if it is sexual. A typical example is the child who is beaten or sexually abused by a father or uncle. The mother may know this and be abused too but says nothing for shame and fear that she will lose her home and support. Nurses again need to know where to get help for these children and their families. Sensitive counselling may be needed to help them to deal with their inner feelings as well as to stop the abuse. Health workers should aim at preventing abuse by educating children about it and the importance of reporting it to someone they trust. Children also need to understand that abuse is wrong even if their abusers are not strangers but close friends and relatives. Nurses may need to intervene to ensure they are protected from further harm. In some countries nurses have a legal duty to inform appropriate authorities and support services.

Protecting children sometimes involves removing them from their homes.

Child abuse is always a difficult subject as people have different ideas about what is abuse and what is discipline. Local customs can be difficult areas to address too. For example ritual sex with girls as young as nine may form a part of initiation and be condemned or encouraged by different sections of society. Common myths can lead to abuse too, such as believing that sex with a young girl will cure a person of AIDS.

Behavioural problems

Every child goes through periods of bad behaviour such as disobedience, lying and cheating or refusing to eat properly. This usually decreases as children become older but consistent guidance from parents is important. Children need to know the limits to what they can and cannot do. Parents who change their minds easily or punish and reward in inconsistent ways can confuse children. Violence in the family leads to more behavioural problems as children learn to deal with conflict by hitting out. Nurses can help parents and children to find out why they are behaving badly and develop plans to bring about change. Children need to know what to expect from day to day and have activities to keep them busy and interested. Their behaviour should be supervised, giving rewards and praise where possible.

Developmental problems

Common developmental problems include mental retardation, learning and communication disorders, autism and hyperactivity.

Mental retardation: Children with mental retardation problems should be thoroughly assessed. Nurses need to focus on meeting children's basic needs, providing safe environments and encouraging the development of life skills so that they can achieve their best.

Learning disorders: These are diagnosed when a child's achievement in reading and written tests routinely falls below the normal for children of the same age. These children may have low self-esteem. They may lack social skills, become discouraged and depressed and drop out of school early. Learning disorders are not the same as low potential ability. For example, dyslexic children can do very well with skilled help and encouragement. Early diagnosis, referral and assistance are very important.

Communication disorders: These show as difficulties with receiving messages from other people and sending them out to them. Stammering and problems with the pronunciation of words are examples of this. The cause is usually unknown but can be because of neurological or other medical conditions and problems with development. These disorders may interfere with children's everyday activities or their ability to achieve well academically. Children need love, patience and encouragement to help them to overcome these difficulties.

Pervasive development disorders: Children who have pervasive development disorders have difficulty interacting and communicating with other people, and learning new skills. The causes are unknown. These children may be slow to develop mentally or have congenital disorders as well. They may have suffered infections or have abnormal central nervous system functions. Autism is one disorder and begins in infancy or early childhood. Autistic children may speak and play in abnormal ways, and have a limited range of interest. It may be very difficult to communicate with them.

Attention deficit hyperactive disorder: Some children who seem badly behaved are suffering from attention deficit hyperactive disorder (ADHD). These children, especially boys, are always on the move, cannot concentrate and are easily distracted and angered. They can be very demanding and act without thinking. They do not achieve well at school and can be very difficult to handle at home. Their difficulties may continue as they grow older. They may be seen as badly behaved instead of having their illness recognised. Although there is no cure, parents can learn how to calm their children and avoid stimulating them too much. Children need to have routines and simple, clear directions about what to do and how to behave. Understanding that this is an illness helps parents, relatives and teachers to react calmly and to respect and encourage the children who may become very unhappy.

With all these conditions, children and their parents benefit from specialist help if it is available. Parents need to be flexible in what they expect of their children and may need help with this. It is important to work with parents, and involve children in decision making where possible as they get older. Programmes should be designed so that children's individual needs are met.

Adolescence

Adolescence is a period of great physical and emotional change and often, of turmoil and confusion.

Many young people experience some kind of emotional difficulty as they come to terms with physical changes and how they see themselves. From being pleasant, cooperative children they may change to being moody, unpredictable and emotional teenagers. Many adolescents become extremely private and refuse to talk to their families any more. They may feel awkward and inadequate and often worry about being different from friends (see also Chapter 27).

Social development is an important area for adolescents. Belonging to a group means they can identify with it as they break away from dependency on parents. They often feel they must conform to the group norms to avoid isolation. This can mean behaving in ways that they would not have done before and disregarding the values they have previously followed. They need understanding, patience, space and respect rather than judgemental attitudes, and parents who are there when they need them.

Many cultures mark the change from childhood to adolescence with special rituals and ceremonies. These may be helpful in establishing children's identity as adults but the physical and emotional changes still continue. Most societies experience change with modernisation and adolescents everywhere may find themselves in conflict with older people.

Most adolescents pass through these life changes successfully but some experience difficulty in adapting to being a young adult and become ill. These mental problems can arise from within or from external sources such as abuse and violence at home or desertion by a parent. They may have emotional problems or become involved with fighting, stealing, sexual activity or substance abuse. They may perform poorly or drop out of school and fail to live up to family expectations, become defiant of authority and aggressive.

As with children, abuse, harsh and inconsistent discipline and severe physical punishment can lead to these behaviours. A secure and stable environment is important with clear and sensible rules, boundaries and sanctions for bad behaviour.

Although this behaviour may be temporary, it can be the first sign of mental illness or disorder such as manic depression and schizophrenia.

Depression and schizophrenia

The anxiety and mood changes experienced by adolescents can be serious enough to lead to depression and withdrawal. They may feel worthless and hopeless; they may injure themselves or have suicidal ideas. Some will actually kill themselves. They may experience panic states, phobias, obsessive-compulsive disorders and, in some cultures, disordered eating patterns such as self-starving (anorexia) or excessive eating and deliberate vomiting (bulimia). These problems may not be recognised by family and friends especially if they believe the young person is just being moody and uncooperative.

Schizophrenia is less common than depression and substance abuse in adolescents but may appear for the first time. It mostly affects boys.

The role of nurses with emotionally distressed young people includes understanding the behaviour and making sure they have space and time to settle emotionally. Simply asking what is bothering them may help as some will feel they cannot talk to anyone. It can be useful to suggest sharing ideas, emotions, and feelings with others of the same age group. Nurses need also to help families to understand how important it is to support young people without pressure or criticism. Referral may be necessary to a mental health professional if depression is severe or schizophrenia is suspected.

Substance abuse

Many adolescents are tempted to try out new chemical substances either as an experiment or to conform to their peers. Some use chemical substances as a way of coping. Homeless children, for example, may sniff glue or drink alcohol to forget their difficulties for a short while. Accidents, violence, depression and engaging in risk behaviours happen as they do with adults. Adolescents under the influence of drugs or alcohol may be especially vulnerable to high-risk sexual behaviour. They may become sex workers at a young age or at least have casual sex for money when desperate for drugs or alcohol. Common early signs of substance abuse are failure to attend school, poor achievement, mood changes and conflict with families. Depression and suicide are real threats.

Nurses may need to work with other services such as those for homeless children and young people to identify those who need help. Safe environments are essential and prevention programmes and early recognition of drug abuse are more effective than dealing with addiction.

Mental health problems of adults

There is, of course, no firm division between adolescence and adulthood and the problems people encounter can be very similar. Young adults are faced with the challenge of developing individual identities, finding employment and becoming financially independent. They need to build stable relationships and make commitments. This is a time of finding marriage partners, creating families and parenting. People continue to take on new roles and challenges and leave others behind.

Most people respond to the stresses and changes of adulthood satisfactorily but many become mentally ill at some point. The main illnesses and disorders already described continue into adulthood or arise then for the first time. These illnesses can cause great strain on relationships and make the individual and family suffer severely.

Depression

The gap between the hopes and the reality of adults' lives may lead to disappointment and feelings of failure. Losing a job can be very traumatic as it damages self-esteem and causes increased financial worries. Providing for a family, poor living conditions, major life change and employment may be especially difficult. Adults may be caring for sick or older relatives and have no break from this. They may be bereaved or receive a diagnosis themselves of serious or chronic illness. They may have difficulties with sexual relationships. These are all experiences that can lead to depression in adults.

Suicide

Risk factors associated with suicide in adults include violence and conflict at home as with adolescents. Adults, however, are more likely to meet circumstances that make them feel suicidal such as alcoholism, breakdown of relationships, loneliness, chronic or terminal illness and experiencing major life change such as moving house. A key difference between adolescents and adults is that adults may have easier access to the means of killing themselves.

Psychotic illnesses

These disorders, described earlier, may arise for the first time when people are adults. They may continue to occur at intervals throughout life and can cause great difficulties to families. People with these illnesses may find it very hard to provide the reliable parenting that children need in order to develop properly themselves. They may also be unable to provide for them financially and knowing this may increase their own distress. Children may need substitute carers if neglect, violence or high-risk behaviour happens.

Substance abuse

Older adults have usually moved beyond trying substances for the sake of the experience. However, the social pressure to drink alcohol, smoke and take drugs can still be very high. It is the continuous use of a substance that has adverse effects on a person. Substances may have immediate and long-term physical and mental health effects but commonly lead to psychological dependency and chemical addiction over time.

Postnatal mental illness

Some women experience problems when they have just given birth and become very disturbed. They may suffer depression or psychosis, often called puerperal psychosis. It may happen in late pregnancy and unfortunately may happen again with future pregnancies. Depression may also occur after miscarriage or stillbirth and women need great understanding and reliable support at that time.

Postnatal depression: Most women experience feelings of great emotion around the third or fourth day following the birth. It is sometimes called the 'third day blues'. They may feel miserable and tired, and cry easily despite feeling happy about the baby. This is normal and passes quickly. Some women experience longer periods of 'the blues' but only need rest, support and understanding from families and health care workers until this mild depression improves. However, a more severe form of depression can cause great misery and may result in suicide.

Signs of postnatal depression are the same as for other depressed people but can also include:

- extreme tiredness
- oversensitivity
- guilt at feeling miserable when they think they should feel happy
- difficulty in relating to the baby
- irrational fears for the baby

- disturbed sleep patterns.

Tiredness, dizziness, 'thinking too much' and aches and pains may be the only symptoms a woman reports especially if the illness is not understood in the culture. Postnatal depression is often missed by health care workers and by families. The focus of attention is usually on the baby and the woman's mental state is not noticed. The first sign of depression may be that the baby is not thriving properly.

Treatment will depend on the severity of the condition. Support from other mothers and family may be all that is needed. Anti-depressants may be required but should be avoided if possible. Even mild depression must not be underestimated as it can cause great distress to the woman and her family. It may also affect her infant if she experiences difficulty in making a relationship with him and in giving him the contact and stimulation he needs.

Postnatal psychosis: This condition is less common than postnatal depression but is very serious. Some mental health specialists believe that it is actually schizophrenia. It is associated with disorders of thought processes and the woman may show the same symptoms described for psychosis and schizophrenia. Special characteristics are having strange ideas about the baby and his well being and extreme excitability. The mother may become hyperactive and violent. She needs close supervision to prevent her harming herself or her infant. She should be admitted to a psychiatric unit if one is available. The ideal place is a specialist unit for mothers and babies but these are uncommon in developing countries. If she stays at home, someone else must help to care for the baby. It is important not to take the baby away from the mother unless she is very disturbed. Tranquillisers and anti-psychotic medication may be needed for about 6 weeks but also only if the mother's behaviour is very psychotic. Anti-psychotic medication can pass through the breast milk. The family will need help and explanation as it is very frightening to see a woman become so disorientated and irrational. They need to know that the prognosis is good but that the illness may last several months. She will need to be followed up once she has left hospital.

Mental health problems of the elderly

People face many changes as they become older. These include physical illness, socio-cultural changes,

alterations in social roles and loss of income. The major factor in the lives of this group is 'loss'. They may lose a spouse. They may suddenly have no work, often no income and may lose self-esteem. If they have always grown their own food they may no longer be able to do so. Suddenly they may become dependent on others. On the other hand, they may find themselves with new responsibilities which may be stressful. Many elderly people now find themselves caring alone for the children of relatives who have died of AIDS. They may also find there is no-one to care for them as they become less able to cope alone because of these AIDS deaths. Traditionally, older people have remained within their families in developing countries and systems may not be in place for when they need help.

Dementia

Dementia is an important reason why some older people develop behavioural problems. Alzheimer's disease is the main form of dementia in the elderly. These problems may, of course, be added to difficulties they have faced all their lives. People do not necessarily become less psychotic, less anxious or drink less alcohol just because they are now elderly. At the same time, some alterations in memory and the ability to learn are normal as people become older.

Memory loss, confusion and inability to concentrate may be due to failing sight and hearing, or even boredom, poor sleep, alcohol, medications or pain. Any disorder that reduces the oxygen supply to the brain, such as under-active thyroid, Parkinson's disease and diabetes, can cause the same symptoms. Whatever the cause of problems may be, a proper diagnosis is essential. Older people are more sensitive to medication so doses must be adjusted, usually to half or two-thirds of the usual adult dose. They must be watched for side effects and may need extra help in giving themselves medications.

Depression

Depression is said to be the most common mental illness in the elderly. Predictors include poor physical health, poverty, lack of supportive social networks and stressful life events such as bereavement. Physical changes such as loss of hearing, vision or memory may bring about feelings of isolation and disorientation and lead to depression.

The usual symptoms of depression apply to the elderly too but it is easy to diagnose it wrongly as dementia. Someone showing several symptoms of depression should be considered to be depressed, not demented. Particularly important symptoms are poor appetite and being unable to sleep properly. They may not bother to prepare meals or want to go out.

Nurses can help by improving older people's environments and helping them to feel useful. A good way of helping mild depression is to involve older people in supporting others. Just putting older people in touch with each other can achieve a lot. Nurses can also encourage older people to restrict daytime sleep so they can sleep better at night. Talking about their feelings can help but many older people are unused to this and may resist. Just helping older people to make new friends and assisting them to meet them regularly may be all that is needed.

Mental health in special circumstances

Sexual difficulties

Concerns about sex are normal but few people discuss them with others. Many people complain of something physical such as tiredness rather than admit a problem with sex. They can cause personal distress and lead to difficulties with relationships or even depression. It may be the relationship problem that is causing the sexual difficulties. Problem sexual behaviour may be the early signs of manic depression, personality disorders or dementia. These people require proper help for the illness causing the behaviour.

Difficulties may be slightly different for adolescents and older people. Adolescents can experience problems establishing their sexual identity and developing confidence in themselves. Having strong sexual feelings and attractions is normal but can be confusing and cause shame and guilt. Knowing how to handle them without harming themselves and others is an important development task for adolescents. All young people have to learn to deal with pressure to conform to the sexual behaviour of others. This can cause conflict with parents and with the groups to which they belong. Some young people will deal with their anxiety by shutting themselves off from friends and can become lonely and depressed. It can also be very difficult for young people who feel attracted to their

own sex and feel confused by it, especially if shame and stigma are associated with homosexuality or it is illegal. They can become severely distressed and sometimes suicidal.

Adults who experience difficulties need to be checked for physical illness such as diabetes, high blood pressure and reproductive tract infections. Some medicines cause sexual problems and so may alcohol and tobacco smoking, anxiety, depression and tiredness.

Lack of interest in sex is common. Men may complain of failure to achieve an erection, known as impotence. Fear that this will happen makes sex even more difficult. Women may complain of pain on intercourse. Tension and fear are common causes and women may feel they have no control over when they have sex. Abuse in childhood makes sexual difficulties more likely.

Most problems disappear quickly. Providing information about normal sexual activities and preventing pregnancy and infections may be all that is needed. Advice about making sex more comfortable using lubricants such as vegetable oils or butter may also help. Couples may need encouragement to talk to each other about sex and perhaps sort out emotional difficulties and conflicts. Help for any underlying mental illness should be provided.

Post-traumatic stress disorder

Many traumatic situations can affect people's mental health. Common ones are gender-based violence and sexual abuse. Other events that may cause severe mental health problems as well as physical ones include:
- being involved in natural or man-made disasters
- getting caught up in war or civil conflict
- becoming homeless, perhaps witnessing the destruction of the home
- losing a child, parent or close relative or friend
- being raped or tortured
- witnessing others being hurt or dying
- becoming a refugee especially if separated from one's own people
- living in unsanitary and overcrowded places with an uncertain future
- loss of income and livelihood.

Young children may be very severely traumatised but may have no way of communicating their experiences. Older children and adults may be too frightened or ashamed. This shame reaction is particularly severe when women and girls have been raped. This can happen to men and boys too. They may say nothing but become deeply traumatised. People may be ashamed of being alive when others are not, or believe they could have done more to help others. Children may have been forced to fight and commit acts of violence. Men may be deeply affected by not being able to protect their families from harm.

Traumatised adults may respond by depression and withdrawal, by drinking, neglecting their families or themselves becoming abusive. Children may not eat, and eventually may fail to thrive. They may develop severe behavioural difficulties. Their development may be slowed or even reversed. People may have flashbacks to the events they experienced and may have very disturbed sleep and panic attacks. General symptoms of depression and anxiety may be experienced with feelings of hopelessness and suicidal thoughts. Physical symptoms such as headaches may take the place of mental symptoms.

Post-traumatic stress disorder (PTSD) is diagnosed when symptoms continue well after the first response. They may arise much later. These include:

- Preoccupation with the experience and reliving it repeatedly or inability to remember details
- Sleep disturbances
- Either numbness or being irritable, being always on guard and over-sensitive to events
- Avoidance of situations that act as reminders.

People with PTSD need counselling and opportunities to share what has happened with others, especially those who have had similar experiences. They need a secure place to stay and help with difficulties like anxiety and depression. Those in situations where violence continues, such as at home, need help to find ways to change this. Anti-depressants and beta-blockers (to calm hyper-arousal) may be needed for a short time. Early help may reduce the severity of PTSD symptoms.

HIV infection and AIDS

People who have been diagnosed with HIV or who have AIDS can experience mental health difficulties.

They may become fearful, anxious, depressed and withdrawn as with any life-threatening illness. This may be made worse by the stigma of HIV and AIDS and the discrimination they may suffer. They may feel guilty if there is a chance they have infected others or been sexually unfaithful. They may also feel bad because they may not be able to support their families in future and because treating HIV and AIDS is expensive. They may have to face blame from others and the loss of loving relationships. Misery and depression can happen because of feeling weak, ill and being in pain from AIDS related problems. Some people are helped by anti-depressants and, of course, relief of physical symptoms is important (see also Chapter 32).

The brain may be directly infected causing mental health problems including psychosis. Anti-psychotic medicines may be needed, such as chlorpromazine.

■ Activity

1. A group of people arrive at your clinic leading a man who looks untidy and dirty and is struggling to get away. They tell you Ahmed has become very agitated recently and is not bothering to look after himself. They have already taken him to the village healer but his treatment has not made any difference. Think about what you would do immediately and how you would plan his care for the future. You may find it helpful to discuss this with colleagues as you take into account the services available in your area.

2. Dalita comes to see you complaining about stomach pains. When you talk to her you find her husband has been beating her ever since her baby was stillborn three years ago. She is very miserable and starts crying. She tells you her husband has talked of marrying another wife and sending her away. He complains that Dalita no longer bothers to cook proper meals or clean the house and anyway she's no good without a son. Think of ways in which you might help Dalita.

Part 7

Promoting good health

50

Promoting health

This chapter outlines key ideas about promoting health. It emphasises the broad factors which influence healthy living and successful programmes, and considers who needs to be involved, and what needs to be done. The chapter builds upon Chapter 1 and health promotion activities throughout the book.

Health promotion and health education

Three phrases are commonly used to consider how to assist people to live healthier lives. These are health promotion, health education, and 'information, education and communication' (IEC). They are often used to mean the same although there are differences.

IEC suggests providing knowledge to people, and helping them to understand. Information is vital so people can make choices but people do not necessarily make appropriate choices just from having it given to them. Understanding matters, but something has to motivate them. They may have different views and priorities from others such as health care workers or policy-makers (see Chapter 1). For people to change the way they act, they must see some benefit and also believe the change is achievable.

Influences on change

There are many reasons why information and education alone may not lead to health changes (often known as 'health gains'). Some are shown in Figure 50.1.

Because education alone rarely leads to long-term improvements, health promotion also recognises other barriers to change that people experience. It focuses on communities, populations and individuals, and on why people find it difficult to stay healthy. It

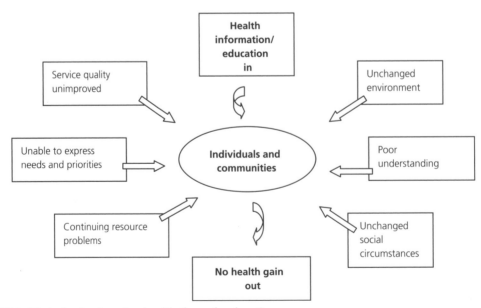

Figure 50.1 *Obstacles to changing health through education*

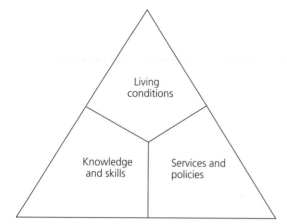

Figure 50.2 *Health promotion focuses on three areas*

considers the basic causes of poor health such as poverty, discrimination, poor quality services, bad roads, unsafe water supplies, and lack of power to make choices. These are often known as 'structural' difficulties. The areas that need to be addressed can be seen in Figure 50.2.

Health promotion also acknowledges that people may be unable to change even if they want to. They may be ignored by society, be unable to make their concerns known, or not have the skills they need. Promoting health also highlights the need to cooperate across other 'sectors' such as housing, social welfare, women's rights, and safety at work legislation. We often think 'health' only, or our own small area within it. Even then, unhelpful attitudes can act as a 'brick wall' and make successful health improvement difficult to achieve (see Figure 50.3).

Nursing and midwifery roles in health promotion

Understanding this helps us to promote health through everyday work and in special programmes but our roles may need to go further. Three particular areas for nurses and midwives are:

- Providing information and education
- Planning, supporting and implementing activities and programmes
- Advocacy for communities and empowering them to take responsibility for their own health and living circumstances.

These roles and activities need to address all three areas of health promotion shown in Figure 50.2 above.

Planning health promotion

It is easy to plan health promotion programmes but less easy to ensure they are welcomed, achieve their aims and are sustainable. Programmes have to be responsive to needs, and involve appropriate individuals and groups. Meeting community leaders is important as they are the gateway to others. Local people need to feel they own what is happening and that their concerns are addressed. Building trust, cooperation and respect is more successful than criticism and helps people to develop confidence in their own skills.

The process of planning can be broken down into the steps identified in Figure 50.4.

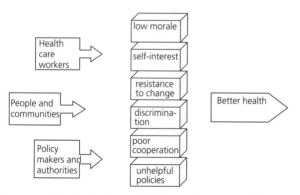

Figure 50.3 *The 'brick wall' of attitudes unhelpful to achieving health improvement*

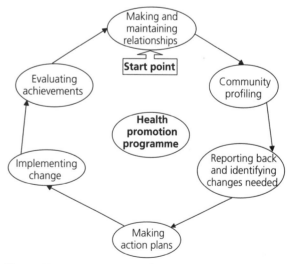

Figure 50.4 *A programme planning cycle*

389

You can see that the cycle can be continuous and that building relationships is the starting point but remains important throughout. The steps can be broken down further.

Community profiling

Identify needs and priorities, characteristics and problems, for example:

- Talents, skills and local resources
- Other health promotion initiatives and agencies
- Difficulties (for example contaminated water, impassable roads)
- Power structures and decision makers
- Communication networks
- Cultural and religious issues
- Health beliefs and practices
- Employment and income
- Women's and men's work-load
- Seasonal activities
- Seasonal disease patterns.

Community surveys are often carried out to identify such issues, using interviews and other data collection methods. Community members may help with this. Local authorities need to be involved and can provide access to existing records. (See resource list on page 397 for detailed help with profiling and surveys, and analysing them, and see Chapter 4 for research methods that can be adapted.)

Reporting back and identifying priorities

Giving feed-back to communities means that they continue to be involved and can give agreement or point out misunderstandings. It can help people to recognise problems they have not understood previously. They then become part of prioritising and identifying what needs to be done. Regular reporting to authorities is essential.

Making action plans

A clear aim and objectives are very important to help you to stay on track. An objective is a statement that shows exactly what you intend to achieve. It will help you plan, assess progress and avoid going astray. It should be SMART:

- **S**pecific (exactly what is to be done)
- **M**easurable (success can be determined)
- **A**chievable
- **R**elevant
- **T**ime-bound (a pre-planned time frame).

Once objectives are clear, you can begin to explore solutions and consider what activities to carry out, resources needed and who to involve, and an appropriate time for activities. This avoids failure because someone has been ignored, or people are too busy, for example with harvesting or during a religious fast.

It is easy to stray to less essential activities so it is useful to check them regularly against the SMART objective. Developing a clear framework that details all the steps needed makes keeping to target easier. One way of doing this is to focus on what you want to achieve, the structures (facilities) you need to have in place, and the processes that must take place for this to happen. This Structure, Process, Outcome model gives an example featuring immunisation, see page 391. It is also useful for implementing change and evaluating success (see below). You need to think about evaluation even when planning begins.

Implementing change

A good plan shows what needs to be done at each stage and should be checked to avoid wasting time and resources during its implementation. A coordinator such as a nurse or community health worker is usually selected. Coordinators need to:

- receive training
- have support and supervision from managers
- work with local health workers in the community, for example health care assistants and traditional birth attendants
- act as resources.

Supervision and support helps to ensure trust, for example that funds are being used wisely, and that workers do not become demoralised or overwhelmed by responsibilities.

Monitoring and evaluating achievements

Everyone involved will need to know that the health promotion activity is doing what it is intended to do. Evaluation will be expected by managers, policymakers and donors and helps to identify the strengths and weaknesses of what is happening and any unexpected effects (whether beneficial or not).

Achievements can be difficult to identify so a systematic way of doing so is helpful. The Structure, Process, Outcome model on page 391 can be used again for evaluation. Each point can be considered individually to help identify problems in achieving them. The activities on page 391 show how this can be done. It is important

Structure, Process, Outcome Model for planning and measuring achievements

Objective: To increase the number of infants receiving measles immunisation from 50% to 90% in two years. (Note this objective is SMART)

Structure	Process	Outcome
People and facilities needed	What needs to be done	Measurable achievements
Information materials	Collaborate with communities	Communities feel involved Communities understand need for immunisation Local beliefs do not hinder
Financial resources	Gain support of authorities	Authorities provide support e.g. funds
Staff (clinical and support e.g. drivers)	Staff training	Staff are confident in skills and knowledge
Work space		Space available for use
Vaccines, syringes, needles Storage facilities (including refrigeration) Means of transport Fuel	Ensure supplies keep flowing Keep supplies in good condition (clinical supplies, cold chain maintained, fuel, spares, vehicle maintenance etc.)	Vaccine, syringes and needles always available and in good condition Transport available and functioning
Record forms	Keep records current	Immunisation records are accurate and complete

to review progress at intervals (monitoring), not just at the end. This enables you to put things right quickly or change plans if necessary. Even at the end, it is usually appropriate to review what needs to happen next to maintain the benefit of the programme (see Figure 50.4).

At the end of the programme, a final review will be carried out. This is commonly done by people who have been uninvolved previously, such as external specialists.

■ Activity

Use the Structure, Process, Outcome model above to do questions 1 and 2:

1. Consider what methods could be used to decide whether objectives are being achieved. For example, community involvement could be tested by interviews or group discussions. Some items can be counted, for example journeys logged, vaccine supply, number of babies immunised.
2. Looking back, it was noticed that some clinics were cancelled on the actual morning. The following weeks, very few women turned up in these centres. How could you find out what went wrong? (Consider individual items in all three areas,

structures, processes and outcomes, to find possible problems.)
3. Having read about health promotion you could now try to apply this to a particular problem you are familiar with in the community or your workplace.

Work out a plan and decide who to involve and what help will be needed. Remember 'ownership' and 'sustainability', and involving appropriate groups, individuals and authorities.

Some ideas might be:

- A stop-smoking campaign amongst hospital and community care employees
- Increasing the use of impregnated bed-nets to prevent malaria among young children and pregnant women
- Working with health care assistants and hospital cleaners to prevent cross-infection
- Working with a community to improve their water supplies and food hygiene after noting how many children have been admitted with diarrhoea and dehydration
- A healthy eating campaign using local and affordable foods.

Fly trap

Making a Fly Trap with Plastic Bottles

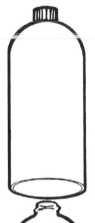

1. Start with two plastic bottles.
   Cut off the lower end of one.

   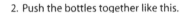

   Cut flaps at the bottom of the other one.

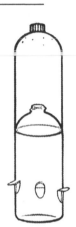

2. Push the bottles together like this.

   Make slits or small holes in the upper bottle for ventilation.

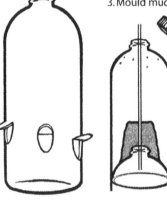

3. Mould mud around the neck of the lower bottle.

   Use a greased stick to make a hole in the mud.

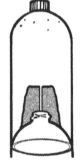

4. Once the mud has dried, you should have a small passage through the mud around the neck of the lower bottle.

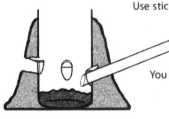

5. Now heap mud around the bottom of the trap. Use sticks to poke holes in the flaps.

   You can poke bait through the holes.

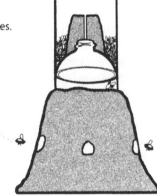

6. Flies enter the trap at the bottom, then they fly up into the top.

   They cannot get out and they die.

Bait with breast-fed baby's faeces - and wash hands carefully afterwards! Keep bait moist with urine.

Design and Illustration by David Gifford from an original design by David Morley.   Child-to-Child, Institute of Education UK.

Appendix B

Growth assessment chart

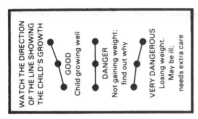

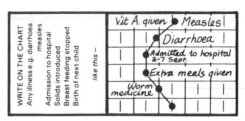

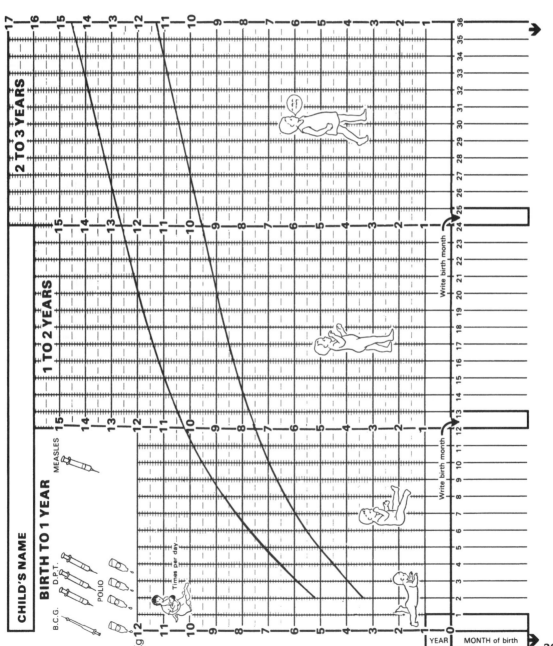

How to fill in the growth chart

1. Write the child's name at the top of the chart.
2. Write the month the child was born at the bottom of the chart and fill in the months following in the spaces.
3. Weigh the child.
4. If the child was born in January and it is now July, he is 6 months old. He may weigh about 6 kilogrammes.
5. You will see that the side of the chart shows the kilogrammes, and along the bottom of the chart you have the months of the year.
6. Follow up the side of the chart until you reach 6 kilogrammes and along the bottom until you reach July. Hold a piece of paper or ruler along the line running up from the month.
7. Make a dot where the line from July meets the line from 6 kilogrammes.
8. Look to see where dots were in earlier months. They should show a line going up from earlier dots. This will show that the child is growing and is healthy.
9. The child's weight should go up steadily, running between the lines on the chart.

Appendix C

Sympto-thermal chart

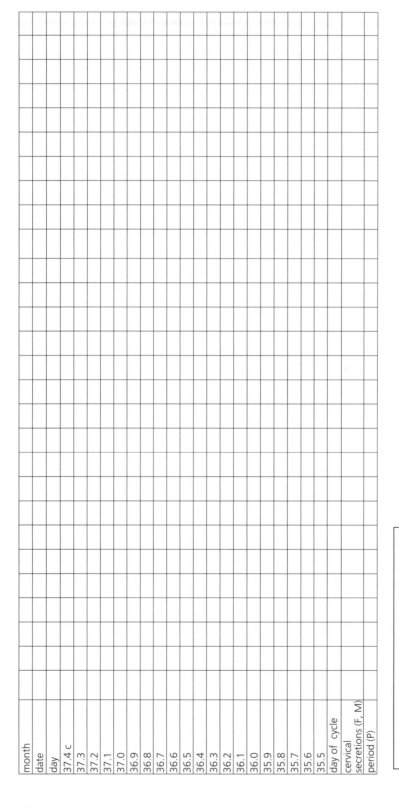

Key: cervical secretions

F = highly Fertile (wet, slippery, clear, stretchy)
M = Mucus (moist, thick, white, cloudy, sticky)

Simple observation chart
for a labouring woman

time:										

fetal heart (bpm):										

maternal pulse (bpm):										

maternal bp:										

maternal temperature:										

frequency, strength & length of contractions:										

liquor:										

descent of presenting part and cervical dilatation:										

position of presenting part:

○ ○ ○ ○ ○ ○ ○ ○ ○ ○

food & fluid intake:										

urinary output:										

drugs/medication:										

other information:										

Sources and further reading

Issues in nursing

Cormack D. (ed.) 2000. *The Research Process in Nursing*, 4th. edn. Oxford: Blackwell.

Couchman W., Dawson. J. 1995. *Nursing and Health-Care Research: a practical guide*, London: Scutari Press.

Digby A., Sweet H. 2002. Nurses as Culture Brokers in Twentieth Century South Africa, in Ernst W. (ed.) *Plural Medicine, Tradition and Modernity, 1800–2000*, London: Routledge.

International Confederation of Midwives. 2002. *International Code of Ethics for Midwives*. Available online at www.internationalmidwives.org

International Council of Nurses. 2002. *International Code of Ethics for Nurses*. Available online at www.icn.ch/

Sleep J., Grant A., Garcia J., Elbourne D., Spencer J., Chalmers I. 1984 West Berkshire perineal management trial. BMJ 289: 587–90.

United Nations Children's Fund 2001. *Poverty and Children: Lessons of the 90s for Least Developed Countries*, New York: UNICEF. Available online at www.unicef.org/publications/

Principles of care

Hubley J. 2004. *Communicating Health*, 2nd. edn. Oxford: Macmillan/TALC.

Lankester T. 2002. *Setting up Community Health Programmes*, 2nd. edn. Oxford: Macmillan/TALC.

Nicol M., Bavin C., Bedford-Turner S., Cronin P., Rawlings-Anderson K. 2004. *Essential Nursing Skills*, Edinburgh: Mosby. Available from TALC.

Pearson A., Vaughan B. and Fitzgerald M. 1996. *Nursing Models for Practice*, 2nd. edn. Oxford: Butterworth Heinemann.

Watson R. 2000. *Anatomy and Physiology for Nurses*, 11th. edn. Edinburgh: Bailliere Tindall/RCN. Available from TALC.

Patient care

Bastian G.F. 1993. *An Illustrated Review of the Skeletal and Muscular Systems*, New York: Harper Collins.

Berkow R., Fletcher M.B. 1990. *The Merck Manual*, Rahway, NJ, USA: Merck & Co Inc

Bickley L.S. 1999. *Bates Guide to Physical Examination and History Taking*, 7th. edn. Philadelphia PA: Lippincott.

Canizares O. 1993. *A Manual of Dermatology for Developing Countries*, 2nd. edn. Oxford: Oxford University Press.

Crofton J., Horne N. and Miller F. 1999. *Clinical Tuberculosis*, 2nd. edn. London: Macmillan/TALC.

De Haan M. 2001. *The Health of Southern Africa*, Cape Town: Juta and Co. Ltd.

Footner A. 1992. *Orthopaedic Nursing*, 2nd. edn. London: Balliere Tindall.

Jamieson E.M., McCall J.M., Blythe R., Whyte L.A. 2002. *Clinical Nursing Practices* 4th. edn. Edinburgh: Churchill Livingstone.

Kings College (University of London) Dept. of Palliative Care Policy, 2004. *Palliative Care in Sub Saharan Africa: an appraisal*, available online www.the workcontinues.org/

Leppard, B. 2002. *An Atlas of African Dermatology*, Abingdon: Radcliffe Medical Press.

Mallett J. and Dougherty L. 2000. *The Royal Marsden Hospital Manual of Clinical Nursing Procedures*, 5th. edn. Oxford: Blackwell Science.

Penzer, R. (ed.) 2002. *Nursing Care of the Skin*. Oxford: Butterworth Heinemann.

Powell M. 1986. *Orthopaedic Nursing and Rehabilitation*, 9th edn. Edinburgh: Churchill Livingstone.

Van den Berg R.H. and Viljoen M.J. 1999. *Communicable Diseases: a nursing perspective*, Cape Town: Maskew Miller Longman.

Vlok M.E. 1996. *Manual of Community Nursing: communicable diseases*. Cape Town: Juta and Co Ltd.

World Health Organization. 2003. *Tuberculosis Factsheets*, Available on line at http://www.who.int/gtb/

Reproductive and sexual health

CIRP. 2003. *Circumcision Information and Resources Pages*. Available online at http://www.cirp.org

Evian C. 2003. *Primary AIDS Care: A practical guide for primary health care personnel in the clinical and supportive care of people with HIV/AIDS*, 4th. edn. Jacana Education. Available from TALC.

Ministry of Health Uganda. 2000. *The National Policy Guidelines and Service Standards for Reproductive Health Services*.

Ministry of Health Uganda. 2001. *Essential Maternal and Neonatal Care Clinical Guidelines for Uganda*.

Post Abortion Care Consortium 2002. *Essential Elements of Post-abortion Care: an expanded and updated model*. Post Abortion Care Consortium. Available on line at http://www.ipas.org/

World Health Organization. 2000. *Managing Complications in Pregnancy and Childbirth: a guide for midwives and doctors*. Geneva: WHO Dept. of Reproductive Health and Research. Available online at www.who.int/

WHO/UNAIDS. *Guidance Modules on Anti-retroviral Treatments* (WHO/ASD/98.1 and UNAIDS/98.7) and documents available online at www.who.int/3by5/ publications/

World Health Organization. 2001. *Female Genital Mutilation: Information pack*. Available on line at www.who.int/docstore/frh-whd/FGM/infopack/

World Health Organization. 2001. *Female Genital Mutilation*: A *student's manual*. Geneva: WHO. Available online at www. who.int/mipfiles/

World Health Organization. 2003. *Guidelines for the Management of Sexually Transmitted Infections*. Geneva: WHO. Available online at www.who.int/

World Health Organization. 2003. *Scaling up Antiretroviral Therapy in Resource-limited Settings. Guidelines for a public health approach*. Geneva: WHO. Available online at www.who.int/

World Health Organization. 2002. *The use of Anti-retroviral Therapy: A simplified approach for resource constrained countries*. Geneva: WHO. Available online at www.who.int/

Maternal and child health

Ashworth A., Burgess A. 2003. *Caring for Severely Malnourished Children*. Oxford: Macmillan Education. Available from TALC.

Coad J. and Dunstall M. 2001. *Anatomy and Physiology for Midwives*, Edinburgh: Mosby. Available from TALC.

Crafter H. 1997. *Health Promotion in Midwifery*, London: Arnold.

Dean P., Ebrahim G.J. 1996. *Practical Care of Sick Children: a manual for use in small tropical hospitals*, London: Macmillan. Available from TALC.

Fraser D.M. and Cooper M.A. eds. 2003. *Myles Textbook for Midwives*, 14th. edn. Edinburgh: Churchill Livingstone. Available from TALC

ICM/FIGO/WHO. 1992. *International Definition of a Midwife*. Available online at www.internationalmidwives.org/ Statements/Definition

Johnston P., Floors K. and Spinks K. 2002. *The Newborn Child*. 9th. edn. Edinburgh: Churchill Livingstone. Available from TALC

Lawson J.B., Harrison K.A., Bergstrom S. eds. 2001. *Maternity Care in Developing Countries*, London: RCOG.

Morley D., Lovel H. 1986. *My Name is Today*. London: Macmillan. Available from TALC.

National Essential Drug List Committee. 1998. *Essential Drugs Programme South Africa: Primary Health Care*, Pretoria: National Department of Health.

National Essential Drug list Committee 1998. *Essential Drugs Programme South Africa*: Hospital Level, Pretoria: National Department of Health.

Savage-King F., Burgess A. 1993. *Nutrition for Developing Countries*. Oxford: Oxford University Press. Available from TALC.

Stables D. 1999. *Physiology in Childbearing with Anatomy and Related Sciences*, Edinburgh: Churchill Livingstone.

Stansfield P., Balldin B., Versluys Z. 1997. *Child Health*: A *manual for medical and health workers in health centres and rural hospitals*. 2nd. edn. Nairobi: African Medical Research Foundation. Available from TALC.

World Health Organization. 2000. *Complementary Feeding: Family foods for breast fed children*, WHO Department of Nutrition for Health and Development. Available online at www.who.int/child-adolescent-health/New_Publications/ NUTRITION/Complementary/_Feeding.pdf

World Health Organization. 2000. *Managing Complications in Pregnancy and Childbirth: a guide for midwives and doctors*. Geneva: WHO Dept. of Reproductive Health and Research. Available online at www.who.int/

World Health Organization. 2003. *Managing Newborn Problems: a guide for doctors, nurses and midwives*, Geneva: WHO Dept. of Reproductive Health and Research, available online www.who.int/reproductive-health/docs/mnp.pdf

Mental health

Patel V. 2003. *Where There is No Psychiatrist*. A *mental health care manual*, London: Gaskell. (Available from TALC)

Royal College of Psychiatrists, *Fact sheets on mental health*: www.rcpsych.ac.uk/info

World Health Organization. *Fact sheets on mental health*: Available online at www.who.org/int/inf-fs/

World Health Organization. 2003. *Essential Medicines*, WHO *Model List*. Available online at www.who.int/medicines/

Useful addresses

African Medical Research Foundation. www.amref.org

Cochrane Library of Evidence-based Medicine. www.cochrane.org

Healthlink Worldwide. Email publications@healthlink.org.uk
 Website. http://www.healthlink.org.uk
 International newsletters published include *Child Health Dialogue* and *Disability Dialogue*.

International Confederation of Midwives. www.international-midwives.org

International Council of Nurses. www.icn.ch

WHO Reproductive Health Library online at
 www.rhlibrary.com
 Free subscription for low income country healthcare workers,
 Email: rhl@who.int for CD

Linkages Program, www.linkagesproject.org
 Publishes FAQ Sheets, on frequently asked questions on breastfeeding, LAM, complementary feeding and maternal nutrition.

Teaching Aids at Low Cost. (TALC) PO Box 49, St Albans, Herts AL1 5TX. www.talcuk.org

UNICEF Division of Communication, 3 United Nations Plaza, H-9F, New York, NY 10017, USA. E-mail: pubdoc@unicef.org. Website: www.unicef.org

World Health Organization, CH-1211, Geneva 27, Switzerland. Website www.who.org

International Skin Care Nursing Group www.isng.soton.ac.uk

Glossary

Abductor – A muscle that draws a limb away from the midline of the body

Abortion – Expulsion of the products of conception from the uterus, before the 24th week of pregnancy

Achondroplasia – An inherited condition in which there is early union of the parts of the long bones which enable them to grow; growth is stopped and dwarfism results

Acidosis – Disturbance in the usual balance between the acidity and alkalinity of blood

Advocate – One who speaks in favour of

Advocacy – Giving active support to a person or a cause, interceding on their behalf

Alveolus – Air sac, the end part of the bronchioles or hollow structure in the breast

Amenorrhoea – Absence of menstruation

Amino acid – The end product of protein digestion; required for growth and replacement

Anaemia – Too few red blood cells, or too little haemoglobin in the cells

Anaerobic – An organism that only grows in conditions where there is no oxygen

Angina – Tight, strangling sensation of pain

Anorexia – Loss of appetite

Anticoagulant – A drug that delays clotting

Antibody – Protein produced in the body in response to an antigen

Antigen – A substance which can stimulate the production of an antibody

Antioxidants – Destroy free radicals; examples are zinc and vitamin A

Aplastic – Without the power to develop, e.g. aplastic anaemia when an individual cannot develop blood cells

Apnoea – Absence of breathing

Arrhythmias – Irregular heart rates

Arterioles – Small branches of the arteries

Ascites – Free fluid in the peritoneal cavity

Asepsis – Free from harmful bacteria

Asphyxia – Suffocation; e.g. neonatal asphyxia when a baby does not breathe at birth

Atherosclerosis – Fatty degenerative plaques of atheroma are accompanied by hardening and narrowing of the blood vessels.

Atopy – Over sensitivity to antigens (foreign proteins)

Atrio-ventricular node – Neurogenic tissue situated between the atrium and ventricle, transmits impulses

Atrophy – Wasting of any part of the body due to lack of use; degeneration of the cells; or lack of nourishment

Attenuation – A bacteriological process by which organisms are made less virulent by culture in artificial media

Autolysis – Breaking up of living tissue

Autonomy – The freedom to decide on one's own actions, behaviours

Beneficence – Doing good

Brachial plexus – Nerves supplying the arm

Bradycardia – Abnormally slow heart and pulse rate

Bronchioles – One of the smallest sub-divisions of the bronchi

Bronchospasm – Spasm caused by sudden constriction of the plain muscle in the walls of the bronchi

Capillaries – Minute vessel connecting arteriole and venule

Caput succedaneum – An oedematous swelling that forms on the presenting part of the fetus during delivery

Carcinogen – Substance or agent which can cause cancer

Carcinogenesis – The initiation of cancer

Catecholamines – A group of compounds that stimulate the sympathetic nervous system

Celibate – A person who decides not to have sexual intercourse

Cerebellum – Portion of the brain below the cerebrum and above the medulla oblongata

Cerebrum – Largest part of the brain, taking up most of the cranial space; divided into two hemispheres

Cilia – Small hair like structures arising from some epithelial cells such as in the bronchi

Circumcision – Removal of foreskin in male; incision in skin over clitoris in female

Coitus – Sexual intercourse between male and female

Colostrum – First yellowish milk produced by the breasts after delivery, rich in antibodies and white cells

Convection – Transmission of heat caused by movement of air

Commensal – Living on another organism without causing harm

Compliant – Obliging or agreeing

Conjunctiva – Delicate mucous membrane that covers the eyeball and lines the eyelid

Cornea – Transparent membrane covering the eyeball

Coryza – Acute infection of the upper respiratory tract

Cretinism – Condition arising from deficiency of thyroid hormone before birth resulting in dwarfism and mental retardation

Cyanosis – Bluish purple colour of skin and mucous membranes due to a lack of oxygen

Decidua – Name given to the endometrium of the uterus during pregnancy

Defaecation – Elimination of waste products and undigested food as faeces from the rectum

Defaulters – A person who fails to complete a programme

Degeneration – Loss of structure and function of cells or tissues

Deontology – The rightness of an action is dependent on the rules and codes which are followed.

Diastole – The phase of the cardiac cycle when the heart relaxes and blood flows into the ventricles

Diastolic pressure – The point at which the 'sounds' disappear when taking blood pressure

Dialysis – Process by which crystalline substances are passed through a semi permeable membrane

Diffusion – Spontaneous mixing of molecules of liquids or gas so that they become equally distributed

Diuresis – Increased production of urine

Dormant – Quiet and inactive

Dyspnoea – Difficulty in breathing

Dysfunction – Abnormality in the working of an organ or part

Dysuria – Difficulty in passing urine

Ectopic pregnancy – Pregnancy in which the fertilised ovum is implanted outside the uterus, often in the fallopian tube

Electrolyte – Salts that conduct electrical charges in the body; present in all cells

Electrolyte balance – The balance between electrolyte levels that is essential for health

Emphysema – Abnormal enlargement of terminal bronchioles, accompanied by destruction of alveolar walls

Encephalitis – Inflammation of the brain

Encephalopathy – Damage or disease to the brain leading to poor functioning

Endocardium – Membrane lining the heart

Endemic – A disease common in a particular region

Enterotoxins – Toxins produced by organisms that cause food poisoning

Enzymes – Protein which causes a biological reaction

Endocrine – Glands whose secretions flow directly into the bloodstream

Epicanthic folds – A fold of skin on either side of the nose

Epigastric – Region of the abdomen, situated above the stomach

Episiotomy – Incision made to enlarge the opening of the vagina during delivery of a baby

Erythrocytes – Red blood cells

Erythropoietin – Hormone produced by the kidney which stimulates the production of red blood cells in the marrow

Ethics – The science or study of morals; code of moral behaviour

Evert – Turn the eyelid outwards

Exacerbation – An increase in the severity of a disease

Exopthalmos – Protruding eyeballs

Expiration – To breathe out

Exudate – Serous fluid which has leaked from a blood vessel

Fetus – The developing baby, between the 8th week of pregnancy and delivery

Fibrinogen – Protein formed in the liver and present in the plasma, essential for clotting

Flaccid – Soft, flabby; usually refers to a type of paralysis

Flexures – Where two skin surfaces rub together

Flora (normal) – Organisms that normally grow on skin, gut or elsewhere without causing disease

Free radicals – Harmful chemicals produced during infections which can damage tissues

Fundus (of eye) – Posterior part of the inside of the eye, seen using an ophthalmoscope

Gangrene – Death of tissue due to interrupted blood supply, disease or injury

Gestation – Period of development of the baby from conception to birth

Glomerulus – The tuft of capillaries within the nephron

Glycosuria – Sugar in the urine

Haematuria – Blood in the urine

Haemoconcentration – Loss of fluid from the plasma; cells become more concentrated

Haemodialysis – The removal of wastes from the blood of a patient with renal failure by means of a dialyser or artificial kidney

Haemodilution – An increase in plasma in the blood in proportion to the cells

Haemolysis – Break down of red blood cells

Haemoptysis – Coughing up of blood

Haemorrhage – A loss of blood from the blood vessels

Haemothorax – Blood in the thoracic cavity

Haematoma – A swelling containing clotted blood

Hepatitis – Inflammation of the liver

Histamine – An enzyme which is released from body tissues and causes local vasodilation and increased permeability of the walls of blood vessels

Holistic – Characterised by the treatment of the whole person

Homeostasis – Biological systems maintain stability while adjusting to conditions which are best for survival

Hormones – Chemical messengers, secreted by endocrine glands, travel to another organ and cause activity

Hydrocephalus – Enlargement of the skull due to an abnormal collection of cerebrospinal fluid around the brain or in the ventricles

Hyperbilirubinaemia – High levels of bilirubin in the blood

Hyperglycaemia – High blood sugar

Hyperkalaemia – High potassium in the blood

Hypernatraemia – High sodium in the blood

Hypertension – High blood pressure

Hyperthermia – Very high body temperature

Hyperthyroidism – Overactive thyroid gland

Hyperventilation – Abnormally prolonged and deep breathing

Hyphaema – Blood in the anterior chamber of the eye

Hypocalcaemia – Low blood calcium

Hypofibrinogenaemia – Deficiency of fibrinogen in the blood; rare but serious cause of post partum haemorrhage

Hypoglycaemia – Low blood sugar, usually falling below 3.3 mmol/litre

Hyponatraemia – Low levels of sodium in the blood

Hypopyon – Pus in the anterior chamber of the eye

Hypostatic pneumonia – Pneumonia due to secretions in the lung being retained, because the patient is not moving well

Hypotension – Low blood pressure

Hypothermia – Low temperature, below 36° C

Hypothyroid – Under-active thyroid gland

Hypoxia – Low amount of oxygen in the tissues

Idiopathic – Applied to a condition, the cause of which is not known

Immunoglobulins – Protein molecules known as antibodies; five different types: IgG, IgM, IgA, IgE, IgD

Immunity – The resistance the body has to infectious diseases, foreign tissue, and other antigens

Impairment – Loss or abnormality of psychological, physiological or anatomical structure or function

Inspiration – To breathe in

Intercostal recession – Sucking in of the ribs by the muscles which connect them; a sign of difficulty in breathing

Interdigital spaces – Between the toes and fingers

Intravascular – Within the blood vessels

Ions – An atom or group of atoms having a positive or negative electrical charge

Ischaemia – Lack of blood supply to a part of the body

Justice – To act justly is to treat people equally and fairly

Keratitis – Inflammation of the cornea

Keratomalacia – Corneal ulcers

Keratolytic – Ointments which soften and remove scales of the skin

Kernicterus – Laying down of unconjugated (fat soluble) bilirubin in the brain cells leading to brain damage

Kernig's sign – Being unable or finding it painful to extend the leg with the hip flexed

Ketones – Waste product of fat metabolism

Ketonuria – Ketones in the urine

Kwashiorkor – Protein-energy malnutrition with wasting and oedema

Kyphosis – Backward curvature of the thoracic spine either congenital or due to disease

Lacrimation – An excessive secretion of tears

Lanugo – Fine hair that covers the body of the fetus and newborn baby; it is especially noticeable in the premature baby.

Laparoscopy – Viewing of the abdominal cavity by passing an endoscope (special instrument) through the abdominal wall

Laparotomy – Incision of abdominal wall for exploratory purposes

Lesions – A pathological or traumatic loss of tissue; broad term which covers wounds, sores, ulcers, tumours

Leucocytes – White blood cells: Neutrophils; Basophils; Lymphocytes and Monocytes

Lochia – The discharge from the uterus following childbirth or abortion

Lordosis – Abnormal forward curve of the lumbar spine

Lumen – The space inside a tube

Lymphoedema – Intercellular spaces contain abnormal amounts of lymph because of an obstruction in drainage

Macrophage – A large reticuloendothelial cell which can ingest cell debris and bacteria, present in inflammation

Malaise – A feeling of generalised illness

Marasmus – Protein-energy malnutrition with wasting

Melanin – Dark pigment found in hair, eye and skin

Meninges – Three membranes which cover the brain and spinal cord: dura mater, arachnoid mater and pia mater

Meningo-encephalitis – Inflammation of the brain and meninges

Menorrhagia – Excessive flow of menstrual fluid

Metabolism – All the chemical processes that take part in the body, which lead to production of energy and waste products and growth

Metastasis – Transfer of disease from one part of the body to another

Micro-nutrients – Vitamins and minerals that are needed in small amounts to keep a person healthy

Micturition – The act of passing urine

Miliary – In tuberculosis, a severe form which has spread throughout the body

Monogamy (ous) – Having one husband or wife over a period of time

Morals – Accepted standard of behaviour based on the sense of right and wrong

Mucosa – Mucous membrane

Mucolytic – A drug that softens the mucus and makes it less sticky

Multigravidae – Pregnant woman who has previously had more than one pregnancy

Multiparous – A woman who has had two or more children

Mutate – Change in the genetic make up of a cell causing it to show a new characteristic

Myocardium – Muscle tissue of the heart

Myometrium – Muscle of the uterus

Nausea – Feeling sick, wanting to vomit

Necrosis – Death of a portion of tissue

Neonatal – The four week period of life after birth

Nephritis – Inflammation of the kidney

Nephron – The functional unit of the kidney

Nephrotic syndrome – A syndrome where there is albumen in the urine, low plasma proteins and oedema.

Neurons – Nerve cell

Neuroglia – Special form of connective tissue supporting nerve cells

Neurotransmitters – Chemical substance produced by the neurons, e.g. noradrenaline, acetylcholine, dopamine

Nocturia – The production of large quantities of urine during the night

Non-maleficence – Doing no harm

Notifiable – Applied to such diseases which must by law be reported to health authorities

Nulliparous – A woman who has never given birth to a child

Oedema – Excessive amount of fluid in the body tissues

Oliguria – Very low secretion of urine

Oncotic/osmotic – Pressure exerted by the blood proteins which enables fluid to move from the tissues into the capillaries

Oophoritis – Inflammation of the ovaries

Opistothonos – Severe extension of the head, with pain on flexion; a sign of meningeal irritation

Optimal – Best possible

Orchitis – Inflammation of the testicles

Organic matter – Relating to or derived from living plants or animals

Osmosis – The passage of fluid from a low concentration solution to one of a higher concentration through a semi permeable membrane

Osteoblasts – Cells which help form bone and collagen tissue

Osteoclasts – Cells which break down bone

Osteomalacia – Painful, soft bones as a result of a deficiency of vitamin D

Osteomyelitis – Infection of the bone due to a pathogenic organism

Oxygen saturation – The amount of oxygen bound to haemoglobin in the blood

Paralytic ileus – Lack of peristalsis in the gut

Paraplegia – Paralysis of the legs and lower trunk

Parous – Having born one or more children

Pathogenesis – Ability of the organism to cause disease

Pericardium – Smooth membranous sac covering the heart, outer fibrous layer, inner serous coat

Periosteum – Thick fibrous two-layered membrane covering the surface of the bones

Peripheral – Relating to the periphery, near the surface

Peristalsis – Waves of involuntary muscular contractions that occur in various body tubes

Permeability – The degree to which a fluid can pass from one structure through a wall or membrane to another

Petechia – Small red spots on the skin due to leakage of blood from the capillaries

Phagocytosis – The engulfing and destruction of micro-organisms and foreign bodies by white blood cells

Phimosis – Tight foreskin (of penis)

Photophobia – Dislike of light

Plasma – Fluid part of the blood

Pleura – Membrane covering the lung

Pleural effusion – Collection of fluid between the two layers of the pleura

Pneumothorax – Air in the pleural cavity leading to collapse of the lung

Polypeptides – Chains of amino acids

Polyunsaturated fats – Fatty acid containing two or more double bonds (links between the carbon atoms); contains less hydrogen; found in oils

Polyuria – Large output of urine

Potency – Very powerful

Prepuce – Foreskin; loose fold of skin which covers the glans of the penis

Prevalent – Widespread or current

Primigravida – A woman who is pregnant for the first time

Prn – Where necessary

Prophylaxis – Measures taken to prevent a disease

Prosthesis – Artificial part e.g. eye, limb which replaces a missing one

Proteinuria – Protein in the urine

Proteolytic – Breaking down of proteins by enzymes

Pruritis – Extreme irritation of the skin

Pulmonary embolism – Clot of blood which has travelled to the lung

Pyoderm – Any purulent skin disease

Pyrexia – Fever

Quadriplegia – Paralysis of both legs and arms

Renal failure – Kidney failure

Renin – Enzyme which is released into the bloodstream when the kidneys are ischaemic, raises the blood pressure

Retrolental fibroplasias – Overgrowth of blood capillaries in the retina causing damage and leading to blindness; occurs in premature babies who have been given too much oxygen leading to a high oxygen saturation in the blood

Retinopathy – Any non inflammatory disease of the retina

Reye's syndrome – Rare syndrome which is linked to giving aspirin to young children; the liver becomes fatty and the brain oedematous.

Rickets – Deformity of the bones, occurs in young children who lack vitamin D

Rigors – An attack of intense shivering

Rugae – Ridges or creases of the mucosa of the stomach and squamous epithelium of the vagina

Sclera (of eye) – The white of the eye which covers the back of the eye and forms the cornea in the front. It is a fibrous coat.

Sciatic nerve – Nerve which runs down the back of the thigh and leg

Semi permeable – A membrane that allows some molecules to pass through, but not others

Sepsis – Infection from pus forming bacteria

Septicaemia – Blood poisoning. Micro-organisms in the bloodstream

Sequestrum – A piece of dead bone which gets separated from the original bone

Sino-atrial node – Pacemaker of the heart

Stigma – A mark of social disgrace, or being seen as an outcast

Stridor – A harsh, vibrating noise when breathing, heard in croup

Sub-costal recession – Sucking in of the sub-costal muscles, due to problems in breathing

Surfactant – A mixture of protein and fatty acid that reduces the surface tension of pulmonary fluids

Sympathetic nerve – Part of the autonomic nervous system; supplies involuntary muscles and glands

Synapse – The very small gap between two neurons

Syndrome – A group of signs or symptoms typical of a particular disease which often occur together and form a distinctive clinical picture

Systemic – Affecting the body as a whole

Systole – The period of contraction of the heart

Systolic pressure – The point at which the sounds are first heard when taking a blood pressure

Tachycardia – Fast pulse/heart rate

Tachypnoea – Fast respirations

Tetany – Increased excitability of nerves due to a lack of calcium, leads to painful muscle spasm of hands and feet

Thrombocytes – Platelets; essential for blood clotting

Thrombocytopaenia – Low levels of platelets

Thromboembolism – Obstruction of a blood vessel with a clot

Thrombosis – A stationary blood clot

Topical – Local or external application

Triad – Group of three

Triage – The assessment and classification of casualties according to the type and severity of their symptoms so that those most seriously ill are treated first

Trichiasis – In growing hairs around an opening, or in growing eyelashes

Trimester – A period of three months

Utilitarianism – Theory that the highest good is the greatest good for the greatest number of people

Vagal – Relating to the vagal nerve

Vascular – Relating to or largely consisting of blood vessels

Vasoconstriction – Narrowing of the blood vessels

Vasovagal – Vascular and vagal

Vectors – Organism, often an insect which carries a disease producing micro-organism from one person to another

Ventral – Relating to the front part of the body

Venules – Small branches of the veins

Viraemia – Presence of viruses in the blood

Xeropthalmia – A group of eye conditions which can lead to blindness. Usually due to a lack of vitamin A

Xiphisternum – A small cartilaginous process at the lower end of the sternum

Index

ENVIRONMENTAL TOXICANTS

ENVIRONMENTAL TOXICANTS

Human Exposures and Their Health Effects

SECOND EDITION

Edited by

Morton Lippmann
New York University School of Medicine

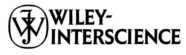

WILEY-INTERSCIENCE

A JOHN WILEY & SONS, INC., PUBLICATION

Published by John Wiley & Sons, Inc., Hoboken, New Jersey.
Published simultaneously in Canada.

For general information on our other products and services please contact our Customer Care Department within the U.S. at 877-762-2974, outside the U.S. at 317-572-3993 or fax 317-572-4002.

Wiley also publishes its books in a variety of electronic formats. Some content that appears in print, however, may not be available in electronic format.

Library of Congress Cataloging-in-Publication Data is available.

ISBN-13 978-0-471-78085-4
ISBN-10 0-471-78085-5

Printed in the United States of America.

10 9 8 7 6 5 4 3 2 1

CONTENTS

PREFACE

This second edition of *Environmental Toxicants: Human Exposures and Their Health Effects* updates and expands the range of current knowledge of environmental health challenges to people in our communities resulting from exposures to chemical and physical agents in the nonoccupational environments we inhabit. It remains a unique resource in terms of its depth of coverage on the limited number of environmental agents that have, or are highly likely to have, adverse health effects following exposures that are typical of current or recent ambient community levels. It contains 7 new chapters that complement the updated revisions of the original 23 chapters. These include 6 chapters on additional environmental agents or mixtures—namely particulate matter, chromium, mercury, noise, pesticides, and ultraviolet radiation—as well as a new chapter on the broad perspective of the application of environmental engineering perspectives to the management of environmental health risk.

I am grateful to all of the authors of the new and revised chapters, all recognized experts in their respective fields, for their thorough and insightful contributions. They are all exceptionally busy and productive people, and their willlingness and ability to find the time to produce such excellent reviews is greatly appreciated.

Although this second edition is more comprehensive than the first, it cannot be the last word. The existing chapters will need to be further updated in future editions as our generally still limited knowledge grows in the following areas: (1) exposures and their geographic and temporal distributions, (2) biological mechanisms responsible for the adverse effects produced by environmental agents, (3) susceptibility factors that account for the generally large interindividual variability in responses to exposure, and (4) exposure–response relationships for sensitive population segments. There may also be a need and justification for new chapters on additional environmental agents or mixtures. These might include aeroallergens, ethers such as MTBE, and / or wood smoke. As with the first edition, comments received from users of this book are welcome and may be used to determine the need for, and content of, future editions.

In addition to the chapter authors, there are several others who have made critically important contributions to the preparation of this edition. First and foremost are Toni Moore and Francine Lupino for their preparation of text materials and management of the editorial enterprise. Second is Gordon Cook for preparation of numerous illustrations used in the text. Finally, this undertaking would not have been possible without the cooperation and patience of my wife, Janet, during all of the extra hours of text preparation at home that were needed.

MORTON LIPPMANN
New York University School of Medicine

CONTRIBUTORS

RICHARD J. BULL, Ph.D. Battelle-PNL, Health Division, P.O. Box 999-P7-56, Richland, WA 99352, rj_bull@pnl.gov

JAMES S. BUS, Ph.D. Dow Chemical Company, Toxicology Research Laboratory, 1803 Building, Midland, MI 48674, usdowplx@ibmmail.com

LUZ CLAUDIO, Ph.D. Assistant Professor, Department of Community Medicine, Mount Sinai Medical Center, Box 1057, New York, NY 10029-6574, lclaudio@smtplink.mssm.edu

MITCHELL D. COHEN, Ph.D. New York University School of Medicine, Nelson Institute of Environmental Medicine, 57 Old Forge Road, Tuxedo, NY 10987, cohenm@env.med.nyu.edu

NORMAN COHEN, Ph.D. New York University School of Medicine, Nelson Institute of Environmental Medicine, 57 Old Forge Road, Tuxedo, NY 10987, norman@env.med.nyu.edu

FRANCIS COLVILLE, Ph.D. 5158 Blackhawk Road, Aberdeen Proving Ground, MD 21010-5403, Francis.Colville@APG.AMEDD.ARMY.MIL

MAX COSTA, Ph.D. New York University School of Medicine, Nelson Institute of Environmental Health, 57 Old Forge Road, Tuxedo, NY 10987, costam@env.med.nyu.edu

NIGEL A. CRIDLAND, D.Phil National Radiological Protection Board, Chilton, Didcot, Oxon, OX11 ORQ, England, nigel.cridland@nrpb.org.uk

MICHAEL J. DEVITO, Ph.D. NHEERL, Environmental Toxicology Division, Research Triangle Park, NC 27711, devito.mike@epamail.epa.gov

COLIN M. H. DRISCOLL, Ph.D., National Radiological Protection Board, Chilton, Didcot, Oxon, OX11 ORQ, England

MICHAEL A. GALLO, Ph.D. Environmental and Occupational Health Science Institute, 681 Frelinghuysen Road, Piscataway, NJ 08855-1179, magallo@eohsi.rutgers.edu

BERNARD D. GOLDSTEIN, M.D. Environmental and Occupational Health Science Institute, 681 Frelinghuysen Road, Piscataway, NJ 08855-1179, bgold@eohsi.rutgers.edu

PHILIPPE GRANDJEAN, Ph.D. Odense University, Department of Environmental Medicine, Winslowparken 17, Odense KD-5000, Denmark, p.grandjean@winsloew.ou.dk

NAOMI H. HARLEY, Ph.D. New York University, School of Medicine, Department of Environmental Medicine, 550 First Avenue, New York, NY 10016, harlen01@mcrcr6.med.nyu.edu

FRED D. HOERGER, Ph.D. Midland, MI 48674, (Retired)

DANIEL L. JOHNSON, Ph.D. 4719 Mile High Drive, Provo, UT 84604, danielljohnson@-compuserve.com

MICHAEL T. KLEINMAN, Ph.D. University of California at Irvine, Department of Community and Environmental Medicine, Irvine, CA 92717-1825, mtklein@uci.edu

PHILIP J. LANDRIGAN, M.D. M.SC. Mount Sinai Medical Center, Department of Community Medicine, Box 1057, New York, NY 10029-6574

MICHAEL D. LEBOWITZ, Ph.D. The University of Arizona, Health Science Center (Room 2332), College of Medicine, 1501 North Cambell Avenue, Tucson, AZ 85724-5030, lebowitz@resp-sci.arizona.edu

GEORGE D. LEIKAUF, Ph.D. University of Cincinnati Medical Center, Institute of Environmental Health, 231 Bethesda Avenue, Cincinnati, OH 45267

MORTON LIPPMANN, Ph.D. New York University School of Medicine, Nelson Institute of Environmental Medicine, 57 Old Forge Road, Tuxedo, NY 10987, lippmann@env.-med.nyu.edu

RAYMOND C. LOEHR, Ph.D. University of Texas at Austin, Department of Civil Engineering, 9102 ECJ Hall, Austin, TX 78712

KATHRYN R. MAHAFFEY, Ph.D. U.S. EPA, 401 M Street, SW, Washington, DC 20460, mahaffey.kate@epamail.epa.gov

JOE L. MAUDERLY, D.V.M., Inhalation Toxicology Research Institute, P.O. Box 5890, Albuquerque, NM 87185, jmauderl@lrri.org

JOHN J. MAURO, Ph.D. 209 Ueland Road, Red Bank, NJ 07701

ROB McCONNELL, M.D. Department of Preventive Medicine, University of Southern California, 1540 Alcazar St., Suite 236, Los Angeles, CA 90033, rmcconne@hsc.-usc.edu

JAMES McKINNEY, Ph.D. National Institute of Environmental Health Sciences, P.O. Box 12233, Research Triangle Park, NC 27709

LARS MØLHAVE, M.D. Institute of Environmental and Occupational Medicine. Aarhus Universitet, Universitet parken, bygning 180, DK-8000 Århus C, Denmark. lm@mil.aau.dk

JESPER BO NIELSEN, Ph.D. Odense University, Department of Environmental Medicine, Winslowparken 17, Odense KD-5000, Denmark

MARY KAY O'ROURKE, Ph.D. Environmental and Occupational Health, The University of Arizona, 1435 North Fremont Avenue, Tucson, AZ 85721-0468

LARRY W. RAMPY, Ph.D. Midland, MI 48674, (Retired)

DOUGLAS A. RAUSCH, Ph.D. Midland, MI 48674, (Retired)

J. ROUTT REIGART, M.D. Medical University of South Carolina, Department of Pediatrics, 171 Ashley Avenue, Charleston, SC 29425

JOSEPH V. RODRICKS, Ph.D. The Life Sciences Consultancy LLC, 750 17th Street, NW, Suite 1000, Washington, DC 20006, jrodricks@lstrust.com

JONATHAN M. SAMET, M.D., M.S. The Johns Hopkins University, Department of Epidemiology, 615 North Wolfe Street (Suite 6039), Baltimore, MD 21205-2179, jsamet@phnet.sph.jhu.edu

RICHARD B. SCHLESINGER, Ph.D.   New York University School of Medicine, Nelson Institute of Environmental Medicine, 57 Old Forge Road, Tuxedo, NY 10987, schlesinger@env.med.nyu.edu

DAVID H. SLINEY, Ph.D.   U.S. Army, USACH PPM (Building E-1950), Aberdeen Proving Ground, MD 21010-5422, dsliney@aeha1.apgea.army.mil

ARTHUR C. UPTON, M.D.   EOSHI-CRESP, 317 George Street, New Brunswick, NJ 08901, acupton@eoshi.rutgers.edu

MARK J. UTELL, M.D.   University of Rochester Medical Center, Pulmonary Unit, Box 692, Rochester, NY 14642-8692, mark_utell@urmc.rochester.edu

SOPHIA S. WANG, M.D.   The Johns Hopkins University, Department of Epidemiology, 615 North Wolfe Street (Suite 6039), Baltimore, MD 21205-2179

GISELA WITZ, Ph.D.   University of Medicine and Dentistry of New Jersey, Robert Wood Johnson Medical School, Experimental and Occupational Health Sciences Institute, 675 Hoes Lane, Piscataway, NJ 08854, witz@eohsi.rutgers.edu

ENVIRONMENTAL TOXICANTS

1 Introduction and Background

MORTON LIPPMANN, Ph.D.

This book identifies and critically reviews current knowledge on human exposure to selected chemical agents and physical factors in the ambient environment and the effects of such exposures on human health. It provides a state-of-the-art knowledge base essential for risk assessment for exposed individuals and populations to guide public health authorities, primary care physicians, and industrial managers having to deal with the consequences of environmental exposure.

Aside from professionals in public health, medicine, and industry who may use this book to guide their management functions, the volume can also be used in graduate and postdoctoral training programs in universities and by toxicologists, clinicians, and epidemiologists in research as a resource for the preparation of research proposals and scientific papers.

The subject is environmental toxicants, that is, agents released into the general environment that can produce adverse health effects among large numbers of people. Such effects are usually subclinical, except when cumulative changes lead to chronic effects after long exposure. Short-term responses following acute exposures are often manifest as transient alterations in physiological function that may, in some sensitive members of the population, be of sufficient magnitude to be considered adverse. Each of the specific topic chapters has a thorough discussion of the extent of human exposure as well as of toxic responses. The four closing chapters on the uses of the data for risk assessment, risk management, clinical applications, and industrial operations provide guidance for those performing individual and / or collective population hazard evaluations. The first provides individuals and public agency personnel with a basis for decisions on risk avoidance and relative risk assessment. The second outlines the operational philosophies and techniques used by environmental engineers in scoping and managing environmental risks. The third enables the primary care physician to recognize diseases and symptoms associated with exposures to environmental toxicants and to provide counsel to patients. The fourth assists decision makers in industry in evaluating the potential impacts of their plant operations and products on public health.

Although many books provide brief reviews of hundreds of chemicals encountered in the work environment at levels that can cause demonstrable health effects, both acute and chronic, they contain relatively little information on the effects of low-level exposures on large populations of primary interest in environmental health and risk assessment. This book has been designed to provide in-depth, critical reviews of the environmental toxicants of contemporary public health concern.

Environmental Toxicants: Human Exposures and Their Health Effects, 2/e. Edited by Morton Lippmann.
ISBN: 0-471-29298-2 © 2000 John Wiley & Sons, Inc.

CHARACTERIZATION OF CHEMICAL CONTAMINANTS

Concentration Units

In environmental science, confusion often arises from the use of the same or similar sounding terms having different meanings in different contexts. This is especially true in describing the concentrations of air and water contaminants. Solutes are frequently expressed in parts per million (ppm) or parts per billion (ppb). However, when used for air contaminants, the units are molar or volume fractions, whereas when used for water contaminants, they are weight fractions. This problem can be avoided by expressing all fluid contaminant concentrations as the weight of contaminant per unit volume (e.g., cubic meter, m^3, or liter, L) of fluid. In air, the units generally used are mg/m^3 or $\mu g/m^3$, whereas in water they are most often mg/L or $\mu g/L$.

Air Contaminants

Chemical contaminants can be dispersed in air at normal ambient temperatures and pressures in gaseous, liquid, and solid forms. The latter two represent suspensions of particles in air and were given the generic term "aerosols" by Gibbs (1924) on the basis of analogy to the term "hydrosol," used to describe disperse systems in water. On the other hand, gases and vapors, which are present as discrete molecules, form true solutions in air. Particles consisting of moderate- to high-vapor-pressure materials tend to evaporate rapidly, since those small enough to remain suspended in air for more than a few minutes (i.e., those smaller than about 10 μm) have large surface-to-volume ratios. Some materials with relatively low vapor pressures can have appreciable fractions in both the vapor and aerosol forms simultaneously.

Gases and Vapors

Once dispersed in air, contaminant gases and vapors generally form mixtures so dilute that their physical properties, such as density, viscosity, and enthalpy, are indistinguishable from those of clean air. Such mixtures may be considered to follow ideal gas law relationships. There is no practical difference between a gas and a vapor except that the latter is generally considered to be the gaseous phase of a substance that is normally a solid or liquid at room temperature. While dispersed in the air, all molecules of a given compound are essentially equivalent in their size and probabilities of contact with ambient surfaces, respiratory tract surfaces, and contaminant collectors or samplers.

Aerosols

Aerosols, being dispersions of solid or liquid particles in air, have the very significant additional variable of particle size. Size affects particle motion and, hence, the probabilities for physical phenomena such as coagulation, dispersion, sedimentation, impaction onto surfaces, interfacial phenomena, and light-scattering properties. It is not possible to fully characterize a given particle by a single size parameter. For example, a particle's aerodynamic properties depend on density and shape as well as linear dimensions, and the effective size for light scattering is dependent on refractive index and shape.

In some special cases all of the particles are essentially the same in size. Such aerosols are considered to be *monodisperse*. Examples are natural pollens and some laboratory-generated aerosols. More typically aerosols are composed of particles of many different sizes and hence are called *heterodisperse* or *polydisperse*. Different aerosols have different degrees of size dispersion. It is therefore necessary to specify at least two parameters in characterizing aerosol size: a measure of central tendency, such as a mean or median, and a measure of dispersion, such as an arithmetic or geometric standard deviation.

Particles generated by a single source or process generally have diameters following a log-normal distribution; that is, the logarithms of their individual diameters have a Gaussian distribution. In this case the measure of dispersion is the geometric standard deviation, which is the ratio of the 84.1 percentile size to the 50 percentile size (Fig. 1-1). When more than one source of particles is significant, the resulting mixed aerosol will usually not follow a single log-normal distribution, and it may be necessary to describe it by the sum of several distributions.

Particle Characteristics

There are many properties of particles, other than their linear size, that can greatly influence their airborne behavior and their effects on the environment and health. These include:

- *Surface.* For spherical particles, the surface varies as the square of the diameter. However, for an aerosol of given mass concentration, the total aerosol surface increases with decreasing particle size. Airborne particles have much greater ratios of external surface to volume than do bulk materials, and therefore the particles can dissolve or participate in surface reactions to a much greater extent than would massive samples of the same materials. Furthermore, for nonspherical solid particles or aggregate particles, the ratio of surface to volume is increased, and for particles with internal cracks or pores, the internal surface area can be much greater than the external area.
- *Volume.* Particle volume varies as the cube of diameter; therefore the few largest particles in an aerosol tend to dominate its volume concentration.
- *Shape.* A particle's shape affects its aerodynamic drag as well as its surface area and therefore its motion and deposition probabilities.

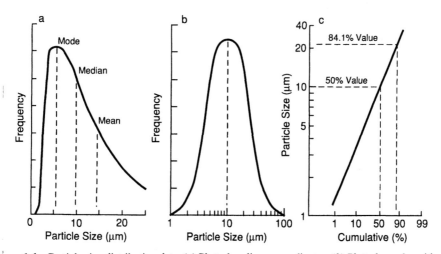

Figure 1-1   Particle size distribution data. (*a*) Plotted on linear coordinates. (*b*) Plotted on a logarithmic size scale. (*c*) In practice, logarithmic probability coordinates are used to display the percentage of particles less than a specific size versus that size. The geometric standard deviation (σ_g) of the distribution is equal to the 84.1% size / 50% size.

- *Density.* A particle's velocity in response to gravitational or inertial forces increases as the square root of its density.
- *Aerodynamic diameter.* The diameter of a unit-density sphere having the same terminal settling velocity as the particle under consideration is equal to its aerodynamic diameter. Terminal settling velocity is the equilibrium velocity of a particle that is falling under the influence of gravity and fluid resistance. Aerodynamic diameter is determined by the actual particle size, the particle density, and an aerodynamic shape factor.

Types of Aerosols

Aerosols are generally classified in terms of their processes of formation. Although the following classification is neither precise nor comprehensive, it is commonly used and accepted in the industrial hygiene and air pollution fields:

- *Dust.* An aerosol formed by mechanical subdivision of bulk material into airborne fines having the same chemical composition. A general term for the process of mechanical subdivision is *comminution*, and it occurs in operations such as abrasion, crushing, grinding, drilling, and blasting. Dust particles are generally solid and irregular in shape and have diameters greater than 1 μm.
- *Fume.* An aerosol of solid particles formed by condensation of vapors formed at elevated temperatures by combustion or sublimation. The primary particles are generally very small (less than 0.1 μm) and have spherical or characteristic crystalline shapes. They may be chemically identical to the parent material, or they may be composed of an oxidation product such as a metal oxide. Since they may be formed in high number concentration, they often rapidly coagulate, forming aggregate clusters of low overall density.
- *Smoke.* An aerosol formed by condensation of combustion products, generally of organic materials. The particles are generally liquid droplets with diameters of less than 0.5 μm.
- *Mist.* A droplet aerosol formed by mechanical shearing of a bulk liquid, for example, by atomization, nebulization, bubbling, or spraying. The droplet size can cover a very large range, usually from about 2 μm to greater than 50 μm.
- *Fog.* An aqueous aerosol formed by condensation of water vapor on atmospheric nuclei at high relative humidities. The droplet sizes are generally greater than 1 μm.
- *Smog.* A popular term for a pollution aerosol derived from a combination of smoke and fog. It is now commonly used for any atmospheric pollution mixture.
- *Haze.* A submicrometer-sized aerosol of hygroscopic particles that take up water vapor at relatively low relative humidities.
- *Aitken or condensation nuclei (CN).* Very small atmospheric particles (mostly smaller than 0.1 μm) formed by combustion processes and by chemical conversion from gaseous precursors.
- *Accumulation mode.* A term given to the particles in the ambient atmosphere ranging from 0.1 to about 2.5 μm. These particles generally are spherical, have liquid surfaces, and form by coagulation and condensation of smaller particles which derive from gaseous precursors. Being too large for rapid coagulation and too small for effective sedimentation, they tend to accumulate in the ambient air.
- *Coarse particle mode.* Ambient air particles larger than about 2.5 μm and generally formed by mechanical processes and surface dust resuspension.

Aerosol Characteristics

Aerosols have integral properties that depend on the concentration and size distribution of the particles. Mathematically these properties can be expressed in terms of certain constants or "moments" of the size distribution (Friedlander, 1977). Some integral properties such as light-scattering ability or electrical charge depend on other particle parameters as well. Some of the important integral properties are:

- *Number concentration.* The total number of airborne particles per unit volume of air, without distinction as to their sizes, is the zeroth moment of the size distribution. In current practice, instruments are available that count the numbers of particles of all sizes from about 0.005 to 50 μm. In many specific applications, such as fiber counting for airborne asbestos, a more restricted size range is specified.
- *Surface concentration.* The total external surface area of all the particles in the aerosol, which is the second moment of the size distribution, may be of interest when surface catalysis or gas adsorption processes are of concern. Aerosol surface is one factor affecting light scatter and atmospheric-visibility reductions.
- *Volume concentration.* The total volume of all the particles, which is the third moment of the size distribution, is of little intrinsic interest in itself. However, it is closely related to the mass concentration, which for many environmental effects is the primary parameter of interest.
- *Mass concentration.* The total mass of all the particles in the aerosol is frequently of interest. The mass of a particle is the product of its volume and density. If all of the particles have the same density, the total mass concentration is simply the volume concentration times the density. In some cases, such as "respirable," "thoracic," and "inhalable" dust sampling (Phalen et al., 1986), the parameter of interest is the mass concentration over a restricted range of particle size. In these applications, particles outside the size range of interest are excluded from the integral.
- *Dustfall.* The mass of particles depositing from an aerosol onto a unit surface per unit time is proportional to the fifth moment of the size distribution. Dustfall has long been of interest in air pollution control because it provides an indication of the soiling properties of the aerosol.
- *Light scatter.* The ability of airborne particles to scatter light and cause a visibility reduction is well known. Total light scatter can be determined by integrating the aerosol surface distribution with the appropriate scattering coefficients.

Water Contaminants

Chemical contaminants can be found in water in solution or as hydrosols; the latter are immiscible solid or liquid particles in suspension. An aqueous suspension in liquid particles is generally called an *emulsion*. Many materials with relatively low aqueous solubility will be found in both dissolved and suspended forms.

Dissolved Contaminants   Water is known as the universal solvent. Although there are many compounds that are not completely soluble in water, there are a few that do not have some measurable solubility. In fact the number of chemical contaminants in natural waters is primarily a function of the sensitivity of the analyses. For organic compounds in rivers and lakes, it has been observed that as the limits of detection decrease by an order of magnitude, the numbers of compounds detected increase by an order of magnitude, so that one might expect to find at least 10^{-12} g/L (approximately 10^{10} molecules per liter) of each of the million organic compounds reported in the literature (NIEHS, 1977). Similar considerations undoubtedly apply to inorganic chemicals.

Dissolved Solids   Water quality criteria generally include a nonspecific parameter called *dissolved solids*. However, it is customary to exclude natural mineral salts such as sodium chloride from this classification. Also water criteria for specific toxic chemicals dissolved in water are frequently exceeded without an excessive total dissolved-solids content.

Dissolved Gases   Compounds dissolved in water may also exist in the gaseous phase at normal temperatures and pressures. Some of these, such as hydrogen sulfide and ammonia, which are generated by decay processes, are toxicants.

Oxygen is the most critical of the dissolved gases with respect to water quality. It is essential to most higher aquatic life forms and is needed for the oxidation of most of the organic chemical contaminants to more innocuous forms. Thus a critical parameter of water quality is the concentration of dissolved oxygen (DO). Another important parameter is the extent of the oxygen "demand" associated with contaminants in the water. The most commonly used index of oxygen demand is the 5 day BOD (biochemical oxygen demand after 5 days of incubation). Another is the COD (chemical oxygen demand).

Suspended Particles   A nonspecific water quality parameter that is widely used is *suspended solids*. The stability of aqueous suspensions depends on particle size, density, and charge distributions. The fate of suspended particles depends on a number of factors, and particles can dissolve, grow, coagulate, or be ingested by various life forms in the water. They can become "floating solids" or part of an oil film, or they can fall to the bottom to become part of the sediments.

There are many kinds of suspended particles in natural waters, and not all of them are contaminants. Any moving water will have currents that cause bottom sediments to become resuspended. Also natural runoff will carry soil and organic debris into lakes and streams. In any industrialized area such sediment and surface debris will always contain some chemicals considered to be contaminants. However, a large proportion of the mass of such suspended solids would usually be "natural" and would not be considered as contaminants.

The suspended particles can have densities that are less than, equal to, or greater than that of the water, so the particles can rise as well as fall. Furthermore the effective density of particles can be reduced by the attachment of gas bubbles.

Gas bubbles form in water when the water becomes saturated and cannot hold any more of the gas in solution. The solubility of gases in water varies inversely with temperature. For example, oxygen saturation of fresh water is 14.2 mg/L at 0°C and 7.5 mg/L at 30°C, and in seawater the corresponding values are 11.2 and 6.1 mg/L.

Food Contaminants

Chemical contaminants of almost every conceivable kind can be found in most types of human food. Food can acquire these contaminants at any of several stages in its production, harvesting, processing, packaging, transportation, storage, cooking, and serving. In addition there are many naturally occurring toxicants in foods as well as compounds that can become toxicants upon conversion by chemical reactions with other constituents or additives or by thermal or microbiological conversion reactions during processing, storage, or handling.

Each food product has its own natural history. Most foods are formed by selective metabolic processes of plants and animals. In forming tissue, these processes can act either to enrich or to discriminate against specific toxicants in the environment. For animal products, where the flesh of interest in foods was derived from the consumption of other life forms, there are likely to be several stages of biological discrimination, and therefore

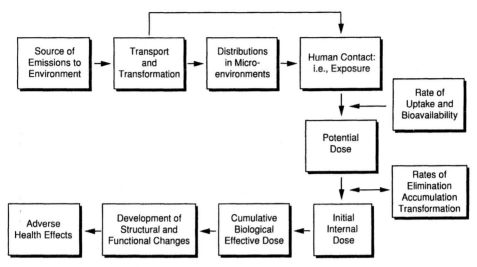

Figure 1-2 Environmental and biological modifiers of human exposure and health responses.

large differences between contaminant concentrations in the ambient air and / or water and the concentrations within the animals.

HUMAN EXPOSURES AND DOSIMETRY

People can be exposed to chemicals in the environment in numerous ways. The chemicals can be inhaled, ingested, or taken up by and through the skin. Effects of concern can take place at the initial epithelial barrier, namely the respiratory tract, the gastrointestinal (GI) tract, or the skin, or they can occur in other organ systems after penetration and translocation by diffusion or transport by blood, lymph, and so on. As illustrated in Figure 1-2, exposure and dose factors are intermediate steps in a larger continuum, ranging from release of chemicals into an environmental medium to an ultimate health effect.

Exposure is a key step in this continuum and a complex one. The concept of total human exposure has developed in recent years as essential to the appreciation of the nature and extent of environmental health hazards associated with ubiquitous chemicals at low levels. It provides a framework for considering and evaluating the contribution to the total insult from dermal uptake, ingestion of food and drinking water, and inhaled doses from potentially important microenvironments such as workplace, home, transportation, and recreational sites. More thorough discussions of this key concept have been prepared by Sexton and Ryan (1988), Lioy (1990), and the National Research Council (1991). Guidelines for Exposure Assessment have been formalized by the U.S. Environmental Protection Agency (U.S. EPA, 1992).

CHEMICAL EXPOSURES AND DOSE-TO-TARGET TISSUES

Toxic chemicals in the environment that reach sensitive tissues in the human body can cause discomfort, loss of function, and changes in structure leading to disease. This section addresses the pathways and transport rates of chemicals from environmental media to critical tissue sites as well as retention times at those sites. It is designed to provide a conceptual framework as well as brief discussions of (1) the mechanisms for, and some quantitative data on, uptake from the environment; (2) translocation within the body, retention at target sites, and the influence of the physicochemical properties of the chemicals on these factors; (3) the patterns and pathways for exposure of humans to chemicals in environmental media; and (4) the influence of age, sex, size, habits, health status, and so on.

An agreed on terminology is critically important when discussing the relationships between toxic chemicals in the environment and human health. The terms used in this book are defined as follows:

- *Exposure*. Contact with external environmental media containing the chemical of interest. For fluid media in contact with the skin or respiratory tract, both concentration and contact time are critical. For ingested material, concentration and amount consumed are important.
- *Deposition*. Capture of the chemical at a body surface site on skin, respiratory tract, or GI tract.
- *Clearance*. Translocation from a deposition site to a storage site or depot within the body, or elimination from the body.
- *Retention*. Presence of residual material at a deposition site or along a clearance pathway.
- *Dose*. Amount of chemical deposited on or translocated to a site on or within the body where toxic effects take place.
- *Target tissue*. A site within the body where toxic effects lead to damage or disease. Depending on the toxic effects of concern, a target tissue can extend from whole organs down to specific cells to subcellular constituents within cells.
- *Exposure surrogates or indexes*. Indirect measures of exposure, such as (1) concentrations in environmental media at times or places other than those directly encountered; (2) concentrations of the chemical of interest, a metabolite of the chemical, or an enzyme induced by the chemical in circulating or excreted body fluids; and (3) elevations in body burden as measured by external probes.

In summary, exposure represents contact between a concentration of an agent in air, water, food, or other material and the person or population of interest. The agent is the source of an internal dose to a critical organ or tissue. The magnitude of the dose depends on a number of factors: (1) the volumes inhaled or ingested; (2) the fractions of the inhaled or ingested material transferred across epithelial membranes of the skin, the respiratory tract, and the GI tract; (3) the fractions transported via circulating fluids to target tissues; and (4) the fractional uptake by the target tissues. Each of these factors can have considerable intersubject variability. Sources of variability include activity level, age, sex, and health status as well as such inherent variabilities as race and size.

With chronic or repetitive exposures, other factors affect the dose of interest. When the retention at, or effects on, the target tissues is cumulative and clearance or recovery is slow, the dose of interest can be represented by cumulative uptake. However, when the agent is rapidly eliminated, or when its effects are rapidly and completely reversible on removal from exposure, rate of delivery may be the dose parameter of primary interest.

CONCENTRATION OF TOXIC CHEMICALS
IN HUMAN MICROENVIRONMENTS

The technology for sampling air, water, and food is relatively well developed, as are the technologies for sample separation from copollutants, media, and interferences and for quantitative analyses of the components of interest. However, knowing when, where, how long, and at which rate and frequency to sample to collect data relevant to the exposures of interest is difficult and requires knowledge of temporal and spatial variability of exposure concentrations. Unfortunately, we seldom have enough information of these kinds to guide our sample collections. Many of these factors are discussed in detail in the chapters that follow as they apply to the specific environmental toxicants being discussed.

Water and Foods

Concentrations of environmental chemicals in food and drinking water are extremely variable, and there are further variations in the amounts consumed because of the extreme variability in dietary preferences and food sources. The number of foods for which up-to-date concentration data for specific chemicals are available is extremely limited. Relevant human dietary exposure data are sometimes available in terms of market basket survey analyses. In this approach, food for a mixed diet is purchased, cleaned, processed, and prepared as for consumption, and one set of specific chemical analyses is done for the composite mixture.

The concentrations of chemicals in potable piped water supplies depend greatly on the source of the water and its treatment history. Surface waters from protected watersheds generally have low concentrations of both dissolved minerals and environmental chemicals. Well waters usually have low concentrations of bacteria and environmental chemicals but often have high mineral concentrations. Poor waste disposal practices may contribute to ground water contamination, especially in areas of high population density. Treated surface waters from lakes and rivers in densely populated and/or industrialized areas usually contain a wide variety of dissolved organics and trace metals, whose concentrations vary greatly with season (because of variable surface runoff), with proximity to pollutant sources, with upstream usage, and with treatment efficacy.

Uptake of environmental chemicals in bathing waters across intact skin is usually minimal in comparison to uptake via inhalation or ingestion. It depends on both the concentration in the fluid surrounding the skin surface and the polarity of the chemical, with more polar chemicals having less ability to penetrate the intact skin. Uptake via skin can be significant for occupational exposures to concentrated liquids or solids.

Air

Although chemical uptake through ingestion and the skin surface is generally intermittent, inhalation provides a continuous means of exposure. The important variables affecting the uptake of inhaled chemicals are the depth and frequency of inhalation and the concentration and physicochemical properties of the chemicals in the air.

Exposures to airborne chemicals vary widely among inhalation microenvironments; the categories include workplace, residence, outdoor ambient air, transportation, recreation, and public spaces. There are also wide variations in exposure within each category, depending on the number and strength of the sources of the airborne chemicals, the volume and mixing characteristics of the air within the defined microenvironment, the rate of air exchange with the outdoor air, and the rate of loss to surfaces within the microenvironment.

Workplace Exposures to airborne chemicals at work are extremely variable in terms of composition and concentration, depending on the materials being handled, the process design and operation, the kinds and degree of engineering controls applied to minimize release to the air, work practices followed, and personal protection provided. Workplace air monitoring often involves breathing zone sampling, generally with passive samplers for gases and vapors or with personal battery-powered extraction samplers for both gases and particles; these operate over periods from 1 to 8 hours. Analyses of the samples collected can provide accurate measures of individual exposures to specific air contaminants.

Workplace air monitoring is also frequently done with fixed-site samplers or direct reading instruments. However, air concentrations at fixed sites may differ substantially from those in the breathing zones of individual workers. The fixed-site data may be relatable to the breathing zone when appropriate intercomparisons can be made, but otherwise, they represent crude surrogates of exposure. The characteristics of equipment used for air sampling in industry are described in detail in *Air Sampling Instruments* (ACGIH, 1995).

Residential   Airborne chemicals in residential microenvironments are attributable to their presence in the air infiltrating from out of doors and to their release from indoor sources. The latter include unvented cooking stoves and space heaters, cigarettes, consumer products, and volatile emissions from wallboard, textiles, carpets, and other materials. Personal exposures to choloroform, largely from indoor residential sources, are illustrated in Figure 1-3, and the influence of smoking in the home on indoor exposures to respirable particulate matter is illustrated in Figure 1-4. Indoor sources can release enough nitrogen dioxide (NO_2), fine particle mass (FPM), and formaldehyde (HCHO) that indoor concentrations for these chemicals can be much higher than those in ambient outdoor air. Furthermore their contributions to the total human exposure are usually even greater, since people usually spend much more time at home than in the outdoor ambient air.

Outdoor Ambient Air   For pollutants having national ambient air quality standards (particulate matter, SO_2, CO, NO_2, O_3, and Pb), there is an extensive network of fixed-site monitors, generally on rooftops. Although these devices generate large volumes of data,

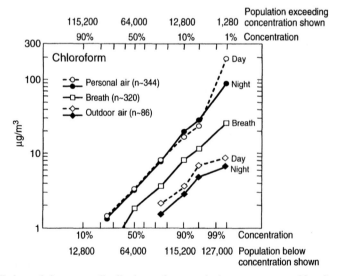

Figure 1-3 Estimated frequency distributions of personal air exposures to chloroform: outdoor air concentrations, and exhaled breath values in Elizabeth-Bayonne, New Jersey, area. Note that the air values are 12 hour integrated samples. Breath value was taken following the daytime air sample (6:00 a.m. to 6:00 p.m.). Outdoor air samples were taken near participants' homes. (Source: Wallace et al., 1985)

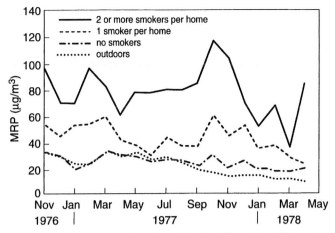

Figure 1-4   Respirable particle concentrations, six U.S. cities, November 1976 to April 1978. (Source: National Academy of Science, 1981)

the concentrations at these sites may differ substantially from the concentrations that people breathe, especially for tailpipe pollutants such as CO. Data for other toxic pollutants in the outdoor ambient air are not generally collected on a routine basis.

Transportation   Many people spend from one-half to three hours each day in autos or buses as they go to work, to school, or shopping. Inhalation exposures to carbon monoxide (CO) in vehicles and garages can represent a significant fraction of total CO exposures.

Recreation and Public Spaces   Recreational exposure while exercising may be important to total daily exposure because the increased respiratory ventilation associated with exercise can produce much more than proportional increases in delivered dose and functional responses. Spectators and athletes in closed arenas can be exposed to high concentration of pollutants. Spengler et al. (1978) documented high exposures to CO at ice rinks from exhaust discharges by the ice-scraping machinery.

INHALATION EXPOSURES AND RESPIRATORY TRACT EFFECTS

Deposition and Absorption

The surface and systemic uptake of chemicals from inhaled air depends on both their physical and chemical properties and on the anatomy and pattern of respiration within the respiratory airways. The basic structure of the respiratory tract is illustrated in Figure 1-5. The following discussion outlines some of the primary factors affecting the deposition and retention of inhaled chemicals. More comprehensive discussions are available in recent reviews (ICRP, 1994; NCRP, 1997; U.S. EPA, 1996). Figure 1-6, from the 1994 ICRP Report, summarizes the morphometry, cytology, histology, function, and structure of the human respiratory tract, while Figure 1-7 shows the compartmental model developed by ICRP (1994) to summarize particle transport from the deposition sites within the respiratory tract.

Gases and vapors rapidly contact airway surfaces by molecular diffusion. Surface uptake is limited for compounds that are relatively insoluble in water, such as ozone (O_3).

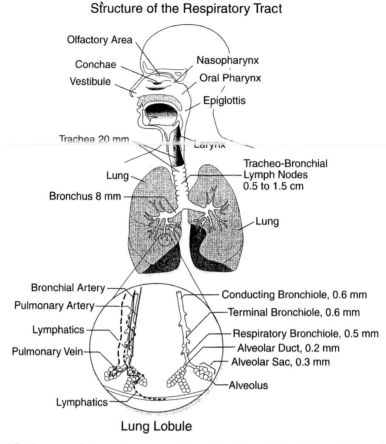

Figure 1-5 Structure of the respiratory tract. (Reproduced from National Research Council, 1979)

For such chemicals, the greatest uptake can be in the lung periphery, where the residence time and surface areas are the greatest. For more water-soluble gases, dissolution and/or reaction with surface fluids on the airways facilitates removal from the airstream. Highly water-soluble vapors, such as sulfur dioxide (SO_2), are almost completely removed in the airways of the head, and very little of them penetrates into lung airways.

For airborne particles, the most critical parameter affecting patterns and efficiencies of surface deposition is particle size. The mechanisms for particle deposition within respiratory airways are illustrated in Figure 1-8. Almost all of the mass of airborne particulate matter is found in particles with diameters greater than 0.1 μm. Such particles have diffusional displacements many orders of magnitude smaller than those of gas molecules, and they are small in relation to the sizes of the airways in which they are suspended. Thus the penetration of airborne particles into the lung airways is determined primarily by convective flow, namely by the motion of the air in which the particles are suspended.

Some deposition by diffusion does occur for particles <0.5 μm in small airways, where it is favored by the small size of the airways and the low flow velocities in such airways. For particles >0.5 μm, deposition by sedimentation occurs in small to midsized airways. For particles with aerodynamic diameters >2 μm, particle inertia is sufficient to cause particle motion to deviate from the flow streamlines, resulting in deposition by impaction

Figure 1-6 Morphometry, cytology, histology, function, and structure of the respiratory tract and regions used in the 1994 ICRP dosimetry model.

Functions	Cytology (Epithelium)	Histology (Walls)	Generation Number	Anatomy	New	Old*	Zones (Air)	Location	Airway Surface	Number of Airways
Air Conditioning; Temperature and Humidity, and Cleaning; Fast Particle Clearance; Air Conduction	Respiratory Epithelium with Goblet Cells; Cell Types: - Ciliated Cells - Nonciliated Cells: • Goblet Cells • Mucous (Secretory) Cells • Serous Cells • Brush Cells • Endocrine Cells • Basal Cells • Intermediate Cells	Mucous Membrane, Respiratory Epithelium (Pseudostratified, Ciliated, Mucous), Glands		Anterior Nasal Passages	ET_1	(N-P)	Conditioning — 0.175 x 10⁻³ (Anatomical Dead Space)	Extrathoracic / Extrapulmonary	2×10^{-3} m²	—
		Mucous Membrane, Respiratory or Stratified Epithelium, Glands		Nose / Mouth — Pharynx (Posterior) / Larynx / Esophagus	ET_2 LN_{ET}				4.5×10^{-2} m²	—
		Mucous Membrane, Respiratory Epithelium, Cartilage Rings, Glands	0	Trachea			Conduction	Thoracic		
			1	Main Bronchi						
		Mucous Membrane, Respiratory Epithelium, Cartilage Plates, Smooth Muscle Layer, Glands	2 – 8	Bronchi	BB	(T-B)			3×10^{-2} m²	511
	Respiratory Epithelium with Clara Cells (No Goblet Cells); Cell Types: - Ciliated Cells - Nonciliated Cells: • Clara (Secretory) Cells	Mucous Membrane, Respiratory Epithelium, No Cartilage, No Glands, Smooth Muscle Layer	9 – 14	Bronchioles	bb		0.2 x 10⁻³ m³		2.6×10^{-1} m²	6.5×10^4
		Mucous Membrane, Single-Layer Respiratory Epithelium, Less Ciliated, Smooth Muscle Layer	15	Terminal Bronchioles						
Air Conduction; Gas Exchange; Slow Particle Clearance	Respiratory Epithelium Consisting Mainly of Clara Cells (Secretory) and Few Ciliated Cells	Mucous Membrane, Single-Layer Respiratory Epithelium of Cuboidal Cells, Smooth Muscle Layers	16 – 18	Respiratory Bronchioles	LN_{TH}		Gas-Exchange Transitory	Pulmonary		
Gas Exchange; Very Slow Particle Clearance	Squamous Alveolar Epithelium Cells (Type I), Covering 93% of Alveolar Surface Areas	Wall Consists of Alveolar Entrance Rings, Squamous Epithelial Layer, Surfactant	**	Alveolar Ducts	AI	P	4.5×10^{-3} m³		7.5 m²	4.6×10^5
	Cuboidal Alveolar Epithelial Cells (Type II, Surfactant-Producing), Covering 7% of Alveolar Surface Area	Interalveolar Septa Covered by Squamous Epithelium, Containing Capillaries, Surfactant	**	Alveolar Sacs					140 m²	4.5×10^7
	Alveolar Macrophages			Lymphatics		L				

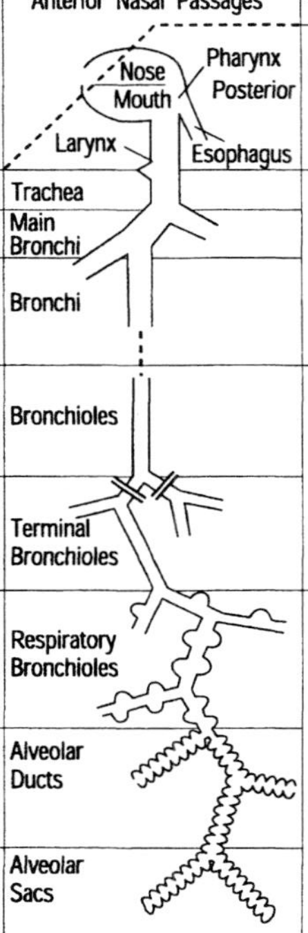

* Previous ICRP Model.

** Unnumbered because of imprecise information.

† Lymph nodes are located only in BB region but drain the bronchial and alveolar interstitial regions as well as the bronchial region.

13

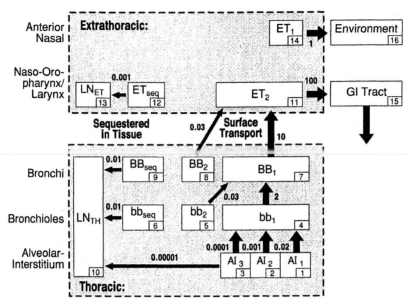

Figure 1-7 Compartment model to represent time-dependent particle transport from each region in 1994 ICRP model. Particle transport rate constants shown beside the arrows are reference values in d^{-1}. Compartment numbers (shown in the lower right-hand corner of each compartment box) are used to define clearance pathways. Thus the particle transport rate from bb_1 to BB_1 is denoted $m_{4,7}$ and has the value $2\ d^{-1}$.

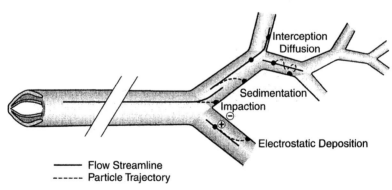

Figure 1-8 Schematic of mechanism for particle deposition in respiratory airways. (Source: Lippmann and Schlesinger, 1984)

on surfaces downstream of changes in flow direction, primarily in mid- to large-sized airways, which have the highest flow velocities. The concentration of deposition on limited surface areas within the large airways is of special interest with respect to dosimetry and the pathogenesis of chronic lung diseases such as bronchial cancer and bronchitis.

Although particle inertia accounts for much of the "hot-spot" deposition on the trachea below the laryngeal jet and at the bifurcations of large lung airways, some of the concentrated deposition is attributable to inertial airflow, which directs a disproportionately large fraction of the flow volume toward such surfaces and, at the same time, lessens the boundary layer thickness. Thus there is some preferential deposition of submicrometer-sized particles and gas molecules at airway bifurcations.

Quantitative aspects of particle deposition are summarized in Figures 1-9 through 1-12. It can be seen that deposition efficiencies in the major structural-functional regions of the human respiratory tract are both strongly particle-size dependent and highly variable among normal humans. Additional variability results from structural changes in the airways associated with disease processes. Generally, these involve airway narrowing or localized constrictions, which act to increase deposition and concentrate it on limited surface areas.

All of the preceding was based on the assumption that each particle has a specific size. For particles that are hygroscopic, there is considerable growth in size as they take up water vapor in the airways. Some hygroscopic growth curves for acidic and ambient aerosols are illustrated in Figure 1-13.

Materials that dissolve into the mucus of the conductive airways or the surfactant layer of the alveolar region can rapidly diffuse into the underlying epithelia and the circulating blood, thereby gaining access to tissues throughout the body. Chemical reactions and metabolic processes may occur within the lung fluids and cells, limiting access of the inhaled material to the bloodstream and creating reaction products with either greater or lesser solubility and biological activity. Few generalizations about absorption rates are possible.

Translocation and Retention

Particles that do not dissolve at deposition sites can be translocated to remote retention sites by passive and active clearance processes. Passive transport depends on movement on or in surface fluids lining the airways. There is a continual proximal flow of surfactant to

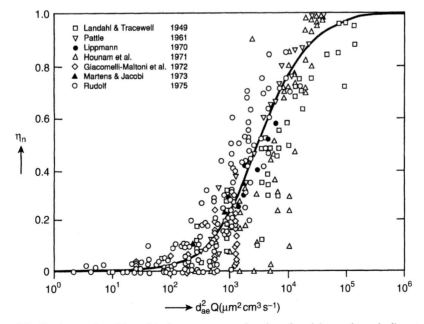

Figure 1-9   Inspiratory deposition of the human nose as a function of particle aerodynamic diameter and flow rate $(d_{ae}^2 Q)$. (From U.S. EPA, 1997)

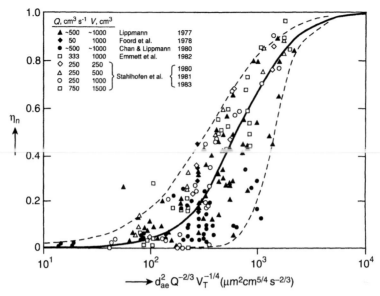

Figure 1-10 Inspiratory extrathoracic deposition data in humans during mouth breathing as a function of particle aerodynamic diameter, flow rate, and tidal volume ($d_{ae}^{2}Q^{2/3}V_{T}^{-1/4}$). (From U.S. EPA, 1997)

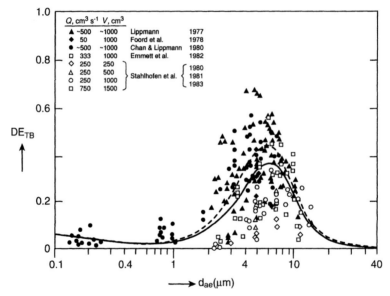

Figure 1-11 Tracheobronchial deposition data in humans at mouth breathing as a function of particle aerodynamic diameter (d_{ae}). The solid curve represents the approximate mean of all the experimental data; the broken curve represents the mean excluding the data of Stahlhofen et al. (From U.S. EPA, 1996)

and onto the mucociliary escalator, which begins at the terminal bronchioles, where it mixes with secretions from Clara and goblet cells. Within midsized and larger airways there are additional secretions from goblet cells and mucus glands, producing a thicker mucous layer having a serous subphase and an overlying more viscous gel layer. The

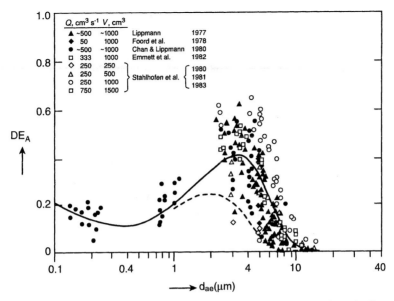

Figure 1-12 Alveolar deposition data in humans as a function of particle aerodynamic diameter (d_{ae}). The solid curve represents the mean of all the data; the broken curve is an estimate of deposition for nose breathing by Lippmann (1977). (From U.S. EPA, 1996)

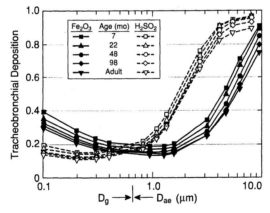

Figure 1-13 Tracheobronchial particle deposition as a function of particle size at various ages for both stable iron oxide particles and hygroscopic sulfuric acid droplets that grow in size in the warm moist respiratory airways. (Source: Martonen, 1990)

gel layer, lying above the tips of the synchronously beating cilia, is found in discrete plaques in smaller airways and becomes more of a continuous layer in the larger airways. The mucus reaching the larynx and the particles carried by it are swallowed and enter the GI tract.

The total transmit time for particles depositing on terminal bronchioles varies from about 2 to 24 hours in healthy humans, accounting for the relatively rapid bronchial clearance phase. Macrophage-mediated particle clearance via the bronchial tree takes place over a period of several weeks. The particles depositing in alveolar zone airways are ingested by alveolar macrophages within about 6 hours, but the movement of the particle-laden macrophages depends on the several weeks that it takes for the normal turnover of the resident macrophage population. At the end of several weeks, the particles not cleared to the bronchial tree via macrophages have been incorporated into epithelial and interstitial cells, from which they are slowly cleared by dissolution and / or as particles via lymphatic drainage pathways, passing through pleural and eventually hilar and tracheal lymph nodes. Clearance times for these later phases depend strongly on the chemical nature of the particles and their sizes, with half-times ranging from about 30 to 1000 days or more.

All of the characteristic clearance times cited refer to inert, nontoxic particles in healthy lungs. Toxicants can drastically alter clearance times. Inhaled materials affecting mucociliary clearance rates include cigarette smoke (Albert et al., 1974, 1975), sulfuric acid (Lippmann et al., 1982; Schlesinger et al., 1983), ozone (Phalen et al., 1980; Schlesinger and Driscoll, 1987), sulfur dioxide (Wolff et al., 1977), and formaldehyde (Morgan et al., 1984). Macrophage-mediated alveolar clearance is affected by sulfur dioxide (Ferin and Leach, 1973), nitrogen dioxide and sulfuric acid (Schlesinger et al., 1988), ozone (Phalen et al., 1980; Schlesinger et al., 1988), and silica dust (Jammet et al., 1970). Cigarette smoke is known to affect the later phases of alveolar zone clearance in a dose-dependent manner (Bohning et al., 1982). Clearance pathways as well as rates can be altered by these toxicants, affecting the distribution of retained particles and their dosimetry.

INGESTION EXPOSURES AND GI TRACT EFFECTS

Chemical contaminants in drinking water or food reach human tissues via the GI tract. Ingestion may also contribute to uptake of chemicals that were initially inhaled, since material deposited on or dissolved in the bronchial mucous blanket is eventually swallowed.

The GI tract may be considered a tube running through the body, the contents of which are actually external to the body. Unless the ingested material affects the tract itself, any systemic response depends on absorption through the mucosal cells lining the lumen. Although absorption may occur anywhere along the length of the GI tract, the main region for effective translocation is the small intestine. The enormous absorptive capacity of this organ results from the presence in the intestinal mucosa of projections, termed *villi*, each of which contains a network of capillaries; the villi result in a large effective total surface area for absorption.

Although passive diffusion is the main absorptive process, active transport systems also allow essential lipid-insoluble nutrients and inorganic ions to cross the intestinal epithelium and are responsible for uptake of some contaminants. For example, lead may be absorbed via the system that normally transports calcium ions (Sobel et al., 1938). Small quantities of particulate material and certain large macromolecules, such as intact proteins, may be absorbed directly by the intestinal epithelium.

Materials absorbed from the GI tract enter either the lymphatic system or the portal blood circulation; the latter carries material to the liver, from which it may be actively excreted into the bile or diffuse into the bile from the blood. The bile is subsequently secreted into the intestines. Thus a cycle of translocation of a chemical from the intestine to the liver to bile and back to the intestines, known as the *enterohepatic circulation*, may be established. Enterohepatic circulation usually involves contaminants that undergo metabolic degradation in the liver. For example, DDT undergoes enterhepatc circulation; a product of its metabolism in the liver is excreted into the bile, at least in experimental animals (Hayes, 1965).

Various factors serve to modify absorption from the GI tract, enhancing or depressing its barrier function. A decrease in gastrointestinal mobility generally favors increased absorption. Specific stomach contents and secretions may react with the contaminant, possibly changing it to a form with different physicochemical properties (e.g., solubility), or they may absorb it, altering the available chemical and changing translocation rates. The size of ingested particulates also affects absorption. Since the rate of dissolution is inversely proportional to particle size, large particles are absorbed to a lesser degree, especially if they are of a fairly insoluble material in the first place. For example, arsenic trioxide is more hazardous when ingested as a finely divided powder than as a coarse powder (Schwartz, 1923). Certain chemicals, for example, chelating agents such as EDTA, also cause a nonspecific increase in absorption of many materials.

As a defense, spastic contractions in the stomach and intestine may serve to eliminate noxious agents via vomiting or by acceleration of the transit of feces through the GI tract.

SKIN EXPOSURE AND DERMAL EFFECTS

The skin is generally an effective barrier against the entry of environmental chemicals. In order to be absorbed via this route (*percutaneous absorption*), an agent must traverse a number of cellular layers before gaining access to the general circulation (Fig. 1-14). The skin consists of two structural regions, the epidermis and the dermis, which rest on connective tissue. The epidermis consists of a number of layers of cells and has varying thickness depending on the region of the body; the outermost layer is composed of keratinized cells. The dermis contains blood vessels, hair follicles, sebaceous and sweat glands, and nerve endings. The epidermis represents the primary barrier to percutaneous absorption, the dermis being freely permeable to many materials. Passage through the epidermis occurs by passive diffusion.

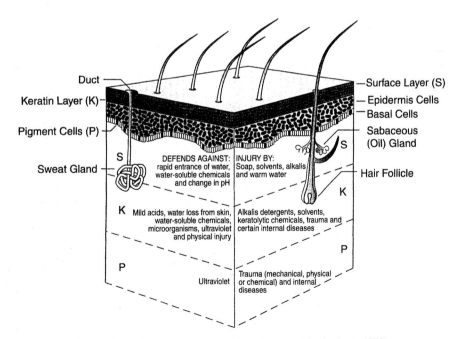

Figure 1-14 Idealized section of skin. (Source: Birmingham, 1973)

The main factors that affect percutaneous absorption are degree of lipid solubility of the chemicals, site on the body, local blood flow, and skin temperature. Some environmental chemicals that are readily absorbed through the skin are phenol, carbon tetrachloride, tetraethyl lead, and organophosphate pesticides. Certain chemicals, such as, dimethyl sulfoxide (DMSO) and formic acid, alter the integrity of skin and facilitate penetration of other materials by increasing the permeability of the stratum corneum. Moderate changes in permeability may also result following topical applications of acetone, methyl alcohol, and ethyl alcohol. In addition, cutaneous injury may enhance percutaneous absorption.

Interspecies differences in percutaneous absorption are responsible for the selective toxicity of many insecticides. For example, DDT is about equally hazardous to insects and mammals if ingested but is much less hazardous to mammals when applied to the skin. This is because of its poor absorption through mammalian skin compared to its ready passage through the insect exoskeleton. Although the main route of percutaneous absorption is through the epidermal cells, some chemicals may follow an *appendageal* route, namely entering through hair follicles, sweat glands, or sebaceous glands. Cuts and abrasions of the skin can provide additional pathways for penetration.

ABSORPTION THROUGH MEMBRANES AND SYSTEMIC CIRCULATION

Depending on its specific nature, a chemical contaminant may exert its toxic action at various sites in the body. At a portal of entry—the respiratory tract, GI tract, or skin—the chemical may have a topical effect. However, for actions at sites other than the portal, the agent must be absorbed through one or more body membranes and enter the general circulation, from which it may become available to affect internal tissues (including the blood itself). The ultimate distribution of any chemical contaminant in the body is therefore highly dependent on its ability to traverse biological membranes. There are two main types of processes by which this occurs: passive transport and active transport.

Passive transport is absorption according to purely physical processes, such as osmosis; the cell has no active role in transfer across the membrane. Since biological membranes contain lipids, they are highly permeable to lipid-soluble, nonpolar or nonionized agents and less so to lipid-insoluble, polar, or ionized materials. Many chemicals may exist in both lipid-soluble and lipid-insoluble forms; the former is the prime determinant of the passive permeability properties for the specific agent.

Active transport involves specialized mechanisms, with cells actively participating in transfer across membranes. These mechanisms include carrier systems within the membrane and active processes of cellular ingestion, namely phagocytosis and pinocytosis. Phagocytosis is the ingestion of solid particles, whereas pinocytosis refers to the ingestion of fluid containing no visible solid material. Lipid-insoluble materials are often taken up by active-transport processes. Although some of these mechanisms are highly specific, if the chemical structure of a contaminant is similar to that of an endogeneous substrate, the former may be transported as well.

In addition to its lipid-solubility characteristics, the distribution of a chemical contaminant is also dependent on its affinity for specific tissues or tissue components. Internal distribution may vary with time after exposure. For example, immediately following absorption into the blood, inorganic lead is found to localize in the liver, the kidney, and in red blood cells. Two hours later, about 50% is in the liver. A month later, approximately 90% of the remaining lead is localized in bone (Hammond, 1969).

Once in the general circulation, a containment may be translocated throughout the body. In this process it may (1) become bound to macromolecules, (2) undergo metabolic transformation (biotransformation), (3) be deposited for storage in depots that may or may not be the sites of its toxic action, or (4) be excreted. Toxic effects may occur at any of several sites.

The biological action of a contaminant may be terminated by storage, metabolic transformation, or excretion, the latter being the most permanent form of removal.

ACCUMULATION IN TARGET TISSUES AND DOSIMETRIC MODELS

Some chemicals tend to concentrate in specific tissues because of physicochemial properties such as selective solubility or selective absorption on or combination with macromolecules such as proteins. Storage of a chemical often occurs when the rate of exposure is greater than the rate of metabolism and / or excretion. Storage or binding sites may not be the sites of toxic action. For example, carbon monoxide produces its effects by binding with hemoglobin in red blood cells; on the other hand, inorganic lead is stored primarily in bone but exerts it toxic effects mainly on the soft tissues of the body.

If the storage site is not the site of toxic action, selective sequestration may be a protective mechanism, since only the freely circulating form of the contaminant produces harmful effects. Until the storage sites are saturated, a buildup of free chemical may be prevented. On the other hand, selective storage limits the amount of contaminant that is excreted. Since bound or stored toxicants are in equilibrium with their free form, as the contaminant is excreted or metabolized, it is released from the storage site. Contaminants that are stored (e.g., DDT) may remain in the body for years without effect. On the other hand, accumulation may produce illnesses that develop slowly, as occurs in chronic cadmium poisoning.

A number of descriptive and mathematical models have been developed to permit estimation from knowledge of exposure and one or more of the following factors: translocation, metabolism, and effects at the site of toxic action.

The use of these models for airborne particulate matter generally requires a knowledge of the concentration within specific particle size intervals or of the particle size distribution of the compounds of interest. Simple deposition models break the respiratory tract into regions (summarized by Phalen et al., 1986):

- *Head airways, nasopharynx, extrathoracic.* Nose, mouth, nasopharynx, oropharynx, laryngopharynx.
- *Tracheobronchial.* Larynx, trachea, bronchi, bronchioles (to terminal bronchioles).
- *Gas exchange, pulmonary, alveolar.* Respiratory bronchioles, alveolar ducts, alveolar sacs, alveoli.

Size-selective aerosol sampling can mimic the head airways and tracheobronchial airway regions so that airborne particle collection can be limited to the size fraction directly related to the potential for disease. More complex models requiring data on translocation and metabolism have been developed for inhaled and ingested radionuclides by the International Commission on Radiological Protection (ICRP, 1966, 1979, 1981, 1994).

INDIRECT MEASURES OF PAST EXPOSURES

Documented effects of environmental chemicals on humans seldom contain quantitative exposure data and only occasionally include more than crude exposure rankings based on known contact with or proximity to the materials believed to have caused the effects. Reasonable interpretation of the available human experience requires some appreciation of the uses and limitations of the data used to estimate the exposure side of the exposure-response relationship. The discussion that follows is an attempt to provide background for interpreting data, and for specifying the kinds of data needed for various analyses.

Both direct and indirect exposure data can be used to rank exposed individuals by exposure intensity. External exposure can be measured directly by collection and analysis of environmental media. Internal exposure can be estimated from analyses of biological fluids and in vivo retention. Indirect measures generally rely on work or residential histories with some knowledge of exposure intensity at each exposure site and/or some enumeration of the frequency of process upsets and/or effluent discharges that result in high-intensity short-term exposures.

Concentrations in Air, Water, and Food

Historic data may occasionally be available on the concentrations of materials of interest in environmental media. However, they may or may not relate to the exposures of interest. The more important questions to be addressed in attempts to use much data are as follows:

1. How accurate and reliable were the sampling and analytical techniques used in the collection of the data? Were they subjected to any quality assurance protocols? Were standardized and/or reliable techniques used?
2. When and where were the samples collected, and how did they relate to exposures at other sites? Air concentrations measured at fixed (area) sites in industry may be much lower than those occurring in the breathing zone of workers close to the contaminant sources. Air concentrations at fixed (generally elevated) community air-sampling sites can be either much higher or much lower than those at street level and indoors as a result of strong gradients in source and sink strengths in indoor and outdoor air.
3. What is known or assumed about the ingestion of food and/or water containing the measured concentrations of the contaminants of interest? Time at home and dietary patterns are highly variable among populations at risk.

Biological Sampling Data

Many of the same questions that apply to the interpretation of environmental media concentration data also apply to biological samples, especially quality assurance. The time of sampling is especially critical in relation to the times of the exposures and to the metabolic rates and pathways. In most cases it is quite difficult to separate the contributions to the concentrations in circulating fluids of levels from recent exposures and those from long-term reservoirs.

Exposure Histories

Exposure histories per se are generally unavailable, except in the sense that work histories or residential histories can be interpreted in terms of exposure histories. Job histories, as discussed below, are often available in company and/or union records and can be converted into relative rankings of exposure groups with the aid of long-term employees and managers familiar with the work processes, history of process changes, material handled, tasks performed, and the engineering controls of exposure.

Routine, steady-state exposures may be the most important and dominant exposures of interest in many cases. On the other hand, for some health effects, the occasional or intermittent peak exposures may be of primary importance. In assessing or accumulating exposure histories or estimates, it is important to collect evidence for the frequency and magnitude of the occasional or intermittent releases associated with process upsets.

CHARACTERIZATION OF HEALTH

Definitions of Health

There is no universally accepted definition of health. Perhaps the most widely accepted one today is that of the World Health Organization, which describes health as a state of complete physical, mental, and social well-being and not merely the absence of disease or infirmity. Unfortunately, by a strict interpretation of this rather idealistic definition, very few people could be considered healthy.

The discussion to follow is limited largely to physical well-being. The health effects discussed are those that can be recognized by clinical signs, symptoms, or decrements in functional performance. Thus, for all practical purposes, in this volume we consider health to be the absence of measurable disease, disability, or dysfunction.

Health Effects

Recognizable health effects in populations are generally divided into two categories: mortality and morbidity. The former refers to the number of deaths per unit of population per unit time, and to the ages at death. Morbidity refers to nonfatal cases of reportable disease.

Accidents, infectious diseases, and massive overexposures to toxic chemicals can cause excess deaths to occur within a short time after the exposure to the hazard. They can also result in residual disease and / or dysfunction. In many cases the causal relationships are well defined, and it may be possible to develop quantitative relationships between dose and subsequent response.

The number of people exposed to chemical contaminants at low levels is, of course, much greater than the number exposed at levels high enough to produce overt responses. Furthermore low-level exposures are often continuous or repetitive over periods of many years. The responses, if any, are likely to be nonspecific, such as an increase in the frequency of chronic diseases that are also present in nonexposed populations. For example, any small increase in the incidence of heart disease or lung cancer attributable to a specific chemical exposure would be difficult to detect, since these diseases are present at high levels in nonexposed populations. In smokers they are likely to be influenced more by cigarette exposure than by the chemical in question.

Increases in the incidence of diseases from low-level long-term exposure to environmental chemicals invariably occur among a very small percentage of the population and can only be determined by large-scale epidemiological studies (epidemiology is the study of the distribution and frequency of diseases in a specific population) involving thousands of person-years of exposure. The only exceptions are chemicals that produce very rare disease conditions, where the clustering of a relatively few cases may be sufficient to identify the causative agent. Notable examples of such special conditions are the industrial cases of chronic berylliosis caused by the inhalation of beryllium-containing dusts, liver cancers that resulted from the inhalation of vinyl chloride vapors, and pleural cancers that resulted from the inhalation of asbestos fibers. If these exposures had produced more commonly seen diseases, the specific materials might never have been implicated as causative agents.

Low-level chemical exposures may play contributory, rather than primary, roles in the causation of an increased disease incidence, or they may not express their effects without the coaction of other factors. For example, the excess incidence of lung cancer is very high in uranium miners and asbestos workers who smoke cigarettes but is only marginally elevated among nonsmoking workers with similar occupational exposures. For epidemiological studies to provide useful data, they must take appropriate account of smoking histories, age, and sex distributions, socioeconomic levels, and other factors that affect mortality rates and disease incidence.

Mortality   In industrialized societies there is generally good reporting of mortality and age at death but, with few exceptions, quite poor reporting of cause of death. In studies that are designed to determine associations between exposures and mortality rates, it is usually necessary to devote a major part of the effort to follow-up investigations of cause of death. The productivity of these follow-ups is often marginal, limiting the reliability of the overall study.

Morbidity   Difficult as it may be to conduct good mortality studies, it is far more difficult, in most cases, to conduct studies involving other health effects. Although there is generally little significant variability in the definition of death, there is a great deal of variation in the diagnosis and reporting of many chronic diseases. There are variations between and within countries and states, and these are exacerbated by the differences in background and outlooks of the physicians making the individual diagnoses. Furthermore there are some important chronic diseases that cannot be definitively diagnosed in vivo.

Many epidemiological studies rely on standardized health status questionnaires, and the success of these studies depends heavily on the design of the questionnaires. Of equal importance in many studies are the training and motivation of the persons administering the questionnaires.

Similar considerations apply to the measurement of functional impairment. The selection of the measurements to be used is very important; those functions measured should be capable of providing an index of the severity of the disease. Equally important here are the skills of the technicians administering these tests and their maintenance and periodic recalibration of the equipment.

Some studies try to avoid bias from the administrators of the questionnaires and functional tests by having the selected population enter the desired information themselves. They may be asked to make appropriate notations in notebook diaries or to call a central station whenever they develop the symptoms of interest. Other investigations use nonsubjective indexes such as hospital admissions, clinic visits, and industrial absenteeism as their indicators of the health effects to be associated with the environmental variables.

EXPOSURE – RESPONSE RELATIONSHIPS

Exposure–response relationships can be developed from human experience, but there are many chemicals that are known to be toxic in animals for which the extent of human toxicity, if any, is unknown. In order to use animal bioassay data for the prediction of human responses to environmental exposures, it is necessary to make two major kinds of extrapolation. One is to determine or estimate the relative responsiveness of humans and the animal species used in the bioassays. The second is to extrapolate from the observed effects resulting from relatively high administered doses to the much lower levels of effects still of concern at much lower levels of environmental exposure.

To deal with interspecies extrapolation, estimates are made on the basis of whatever is known about differences in uptake from environmental media, metabolic rates and pathways, retention times in target tissues, and so on, and tissue sensitivities. As uncertain as these extrapolations are, they are more straightforward than the low-dose extrapolation.

The goal of the dose–response assessment is to predict what response, if any, might occur, 10- to 1000-fold below the lowest dose tested in rodents (this is more representative of the range of doses to which humans are usually exposed). Because it would require the testing of thousands of animals to observe a response at low doses, mathematical models are used (Munro and Krewski, 1981). To appreciate the level of uncertainty in the dose extrapolation process and the typical regulatory use of low-dose models, it is useful to discuss the dose–response curve. However, reliance on the results of only one mathematical model is a potential pitfall in the dose–response assessment.

There are at least six different modeling approaches that may need to be considered when estimating the risks at low doses. These models include the probit, multihit, multistage, Weibull, one-hit, and the Moolgavkar-Knudson-Venzon (MKV) biologically based approaches (Moolgavkar et al., 1988). Nearly all of them can yield results that are plausible. No single statistical model can be expected to predict accurately the low-dose response with greater certainty than another. As discussed by Paustenbach (1990), one possible way to resolve this problem is to present the best estimate of the risk from the two or three models that are considered equally reasonable along with the upper- and lower-bound estimates. An alternate approach is to identify a single value based on the "weight of evidence," as the EPA did for dioxin (U.S. EPA, 1988).

Low-dose models usually fit the rodent data in the dose region used in the animal tests. However, they often predict quite different results in the unobserved low-dose region (Fig. 1-15). The results of the most commonly used low-dose models usually vary in a predictable manner because the models are based on different mathematical equations for describing the chemical's likely behavior in the low-dose region.

In general, the scientific underpinnings of the dose-response models are based on the present understanding of the cancer process caused by exposure to ionizing radiation and

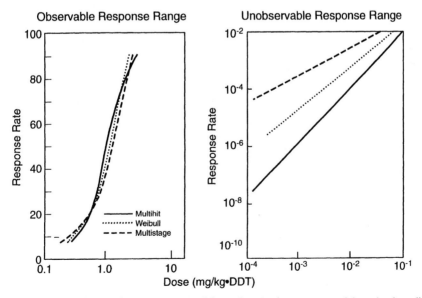

Figure 1-15 The fit of most dose–response models to data in the range tested in animal studies is generally similar. However, because of the differences in the assumptions on which the equations are based, the risk estimates at low doses can vary dramatically between different models. (Source: Paustenbach, 1990)

genotoxic chemicals (NRC, 1980). Both types of agents may well have a linear, or a nearly linear, response in the low-dose region. However, promoters and cytotoxicants (e.g., nongenotoxicants) would be expected to be very nonlinear at low doses and may have a genuine or practical threshold (a dose below which no response would be present) (Squire, 1987; Butterworth and Slaga, 1987). Thus the linearized multistage model may be inappropriate for dioxin, thyroid-type carcinogens, nitrolotriacetic acid, and, presumably, similar nongenotoxic chemicals (Paynter et al., 1988; Anderson and Alden, 1989). For these types of chemicals, the MKV model, or one of the other biologically based models, should be more appropriate (Moolgavkar, 1978; Ellwein and Cohen, 1988).

Summary of Exposure- and Dose-Related Responses

Studies of the specific responses of biological systems to varying levels of exposure can provide a great deal of information on the nature of the responses, their underlying causes, and the possible consequences of various levels of exposure. However, it must be remembered that the data are most reliable only for the conditions of the test and for the levels of exposure that produced clear-cut responses.

Generally, in applying experimental data to low-level environmental exposure conditions, it is necessary to extrapolate to delivered doses that are orders of magnitude smaller than those that produced the effects in the test system. Since the slope of the curve becomes increasingly uncertain, the further one extends it beyond the range of experimental data, the extrapolated effects estimate may be in error by a very large factor.

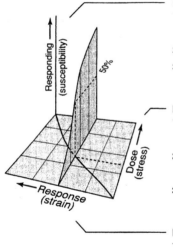

POPULATION RESPONSE SCALE

1. For test relationship
   Dose vs. % of test subjects responding, using sufficient numbers of appropriate subjects for valid statistical analysis.

2. Application of results from one population (or species) to another.

3. For practical dose - population - response relation
   Dose vs. probability of responding at different levels of effect for particular population at risk.

DOSE SCALE

1. For basic dose-response relation
   Quantitative scale of dose at critical site in body, expressed in terms of active form of stress agent at site.

2. Intervening events between portal of entry into body and critical site, which mediate between external level of exposure and effective dose at critical site.

3. For practical dose-response relation
   Magnitude of exposure to external conditions that give rise to stress, measured in appropriate terms for translation into effective dose.

RESPONSE SCALE

1. For basic dose-response relation
   Quanitative scale of response, expressed in terms of most basic event at critical site; response increments of equal value over entire scale.

2. Consequent events, leading to ill health.

3. For practical dose-response relation
   Magnitude of health risk (immediate or potential) to exposed individual.

Figure 1-16 Dose (population) response relationship with suggested distinction between basic (toxicological) and practical (health) scales on the three axes. The illustrative curve on the horizontal plane portrays the dose–response relationship for the middle (50%) of the exposed population; the curve on the vertical plane shows the percentages of population response of the indicated degree over the whole range of doses. The vertical line from the dose scale indicates the magnitude of dose needed to produce the indicated degree of response at the 50% population level. (Source: Hatch, 1968)

The basic dimensions of the dose-response relationship for populations were described by Hatch (1968), as illustrated in Figure 1-16. Many factors affect each of the basic dimensions.

Factors Affecting Dose

The effective dose is the amount of toxicant reaching a critical site in the body. It is proportional to the concentrations available in the environment: in the air breathed, the water and food ingested, and so on. However, the uptake also depends on the route of entry into the body and the physical and chemical forms of the contaminant. For airborne contaminants, for example, the dose to the respiratory tract depends on whether they are present in a gaseous form or as an aerosol. For contaminants that are ingested, uptake depends on transport through the membranes lining the gastrointestinal tract and, in turn, is dependent on both aqueous and lipid solubilities.

For contaminants that penetrate membranes, reach the blood, and are transported systemically, subsequent retention in the body depends on their metabolism and toxicity in the various tissues in which they are deposited.

In all of these factors, there are great variations within and between species, and therefore great variations in effective dose for a given environmental level of contamination.

Factors Affecting Response

The response of an organism to a given environmental exposure can also be quite variable. It can be influenced by age, sex, the level of activity at the time of exposure, metabolism, and the competence of the various defense mechanisms of the body. The competence of the body's defenses may, in turn, be influenced by the prior history of exposures to chemicals having similar effects, since those exposures may have reduced the reserve capacity of some important functions. The response may also depend on other environmental factors, such as heat stress and nutritional deficiencies. These must all be kept in mind in interpreting the outcomes of controlled exposures and epidemiological data and in extrapolating results to different species and across various age ranges, states of health, and the like.

REFERENCES

ACGIH. 1995. *Air Sampling Instruments*, 8th ed. Cincinnati, OH: American Conference of Governmental Industrial Hygienists.

Albert, R. E., J. Berger, K. Sanborn, and M. Lippmann. 1974. Effects of cigarette smoke components on bronchial clearance in the donkey. *Arch. Environ. Health* 29: 99–106.

Albert, R. E., H. T. Peterson Jr., D. E. Bohning, and M. Lippmann. 1975. Short-term effects of cigarette smoking on bronchial clearance in humans. *Arch. Environ. Health* 30: 361–367.

Andersen, R. L., and C. L. Alden. 1989. Risk assessment for nitrilotriacetic acid (NTA). In *The Risk Assessment of Environmental and Human Health Hazards: A Textbook of Case Studies*, ed. D. J. Paustenbach, pp. 390–426. New York: Wiley.

Birmingham, D. J. 1973. Occupational dermatoses: Their recognition and control. In *The Industrial Environment: Its Evaluation and Control*. Washington, DC: U.S. Department of Health, Education and Welfare.

Bohning, D. E., H. L. Atkins, and S. H. Cohn. 1982. Long-term particle clearance in man: Normal and impaired. *Ann. Occup. Hyg.* 26: 259–271.

Butterworth, B. E., and T. Slaga. 1987. *Nongenotoxic Mechanisms in Carcinogenesis* (Banbury Report 25), pp. 555–558. New York: Cold Spring Harbor Press.

Ellwein, L. B., and S. M. Cohen. 1988. A cellular dynamic model of experimental bladder cancer: Analysis of the effect of sodium saccharin. *Risk Anal.* 8: 215–221.

Ferin, J., and L. J. Leach. 1973. The effect of SO_2 on lung clearance of TiO_2 particles in rats. *Am. Ind. Hyg. Assoc. J.* 34: 260–263.

Friedlander, S. D. 1977. *Smoke, Dust and Haze.* New York: Wiley.

Gibbs, W. E. 1924. *Clouds and Smoke.* New York: Blakiston.

Hammond, P. B. 1969. Lead poisoning: An old problem with a new dimension. In *Essays in Toxicology*, ed. F. R. Blood. New York: Academic Press.

Hatch, T. F. 1968. Significant dimensions of the dose–response relationship. *Arch. Environ. Health* 16: 571–578.

Hayes, W. J., Jr. 1965. Review of metabolism of chlorinated hydrocarbon insecticides especially in mammals. *Ann. Rev. Pharmacol.* 5: 27–52.

International Commission on Radiological Protection. 1966. Task Group on Lung Dynamics. Deposition and retention models for internal dosimetry of the human respiratory tract. *Health Phys.* 12: 173.

International Commission on Radiological Protection. 1979. *Limits for Intakes of Radionuclides by Workers.* Part 1. New York: Pergamon.

International Commission on Radiological Protection. 1981. *Limits for Intakes of Radionuclides by Workers.* Part 3. New York: Pergamon.

ICRP. 1994. Human Respiratory Tract Model for Radiological Protection. ICRP Publ. 66. Annals ICRP; 24 (Nos. 1–3). Oxford: Elsevier.

Jammet, H., J. LaFuma, J. C. Nenot, M. Chameaud, M. Perreau, M. LeBouffant, M. Lefevre, and M. Martin. 1970. Lung clearance: Silicosis and anthracosis. In *Pneumoconiosis, Proc. International Conference, Johannesburg 1969*, ed. H. A. Shapiro. Capetown: Oxford University Press.

Lioy, P. J. 1990. Assessing total human exposure to contaminants. *Environ. Sci. Technol.* 24: 938–945.

Lippmann, M., and R. B. Schlesinger. 1984. Interspecies comparison of particle deposition and mucociliary clearance in tracheobronchial airways. *J. Toxicol. Environ. Health* 13: 441–469.

Lippmann, M., R. B. Schlesinger, G. Leikauf, D. Spektor, and R. E. Albert. 1982. Effects of sulphuric acid aerosols on the respiratory tract airways. *Ann. Occup. Hyg.* 26: 677–690.

Martonen, T. B. 1990. Acid aerosol deposition in the developing human lung. In *Aerosols—Science, Industry, Health and Environment*, Vol. 2, eds. S. Masuda and K. Takahashi, pp. 1287–1291. Oxford: Pergamon.

Moolgavkar, S. H. 1978. The Multistage theory of carcinogenesis and the age distribution of cancer in man. *J. Natl. Cancer Inst.* 61: 49–52.

Moolgavkar, S. H., A. Dewanji, and D. J. Venzon. 1988. A stochastic two-stage model for cancer risk assessment: The hazard function and the probability of tumor. *Risk Anal.* 8(3): 383–392.

Morgan, K. T., D. L. Patterson, and E. A. Gross. 1984. Frog palate mucociliary apparatus: Structure, function, and response to formaldehyde gas. *Fundam. Appl. Toxicol.* 4: 58–68.

Munro, I. C., and D. R. Krewski. 1981. Risk assessment and regulatory decision-making. *Food Cosmet. Toxicol.* 19: 549–560.

National Academy of Science. 1981. *Indoor Pollutants.* Washington, DC: National Academy Press.

NCRP. 1997. Deposition, Retention and Dosimetry of Inhaled Radioactive Substances. NCRP Report 125, National Council on Radiation Protection and Measurements, Bethesda, MD, 20814–3095.

National Research Council. 1979. *Airborne Particles.* Baltimore: University Park Press.

National Research Council. 1980. *The Effects on Populations of Exposure to Low Levels of Ionizing Radiation*, pp. 21–23. Washington, DC: National Academy Press.

National Research Council. 1991. *Human Exposure Assessment for Airborne Pollutants.* Washington, DC: National Academy Press.

NIEHS. 1977. Second Task Force for Research Planning in Environmental Health Science. *Health and the Environment-Some Research Needs.* DHEW Publ. NIH77-1277.

Paustenbach, D. J. 1990. Health risk assessment and the practice of industrial hygiene. *Am. Ind. Hyg. Assoc. J.* 51: 339–351.

Paynter, O. E., G. J. Burin, and C. A. Gregorio. 1988. Goitrogens and thyroid follicular cell neoplasia: Evidence for a threshold process. *Regul. Toxicol. Pharmacol.* 8: 102–119.

Phalen, R. F., J. L. Kenoyer, T. T. Crocker, and T. R. McClure. 1980. Effects of sulfate aerosols in combination with ozone on elimination of tracer particles inhaled by rats. *J. Toxicol. Environ. Health* 6: 797–810.

Phalen, R. F., W. C. Hinds, W. John, P. J. Lioy, M. Lippmann, M. A. McCawley, O. G. Raabe, S. C. Soderholm, and B. O. Stuart. 1986. Rationale and recommendations for particle size-selective sampling in the workplace. *Appl. Ind. Hyg.* 1: 3–14.

Schlesinger, R. B., and K. E. Driscoll. 1987. Mucociliary clearance from the lungs of rabbits following single and intermittent exposures to ozone. *J. Toxicol. Environ. Health* 20: 120–134.

Schlesinger, R. B., B. D. Naumann, and L. C. Chen. 1983. Physiological and histological alterations in the bronchial mucociliary clearance system of rabbits following intermittent oral or nasal inhalation of sulfuric acid mist. *J. Toxicol. Environ. Health* 12: 441–465.

Schlesinger, R. B., K. E. Driscoll, B. D. Naumann, and T. A. Vollmuth. 1988. Particle clearance from the lungs: Assessment of effects due to inhaled irritants. *Ann. Occup. Hyg.* 32(S1): 113–123.

Schwartz, E. W. 1923. The so-called habituation to "arsenic": Variation in the toxicity of arsenious oxide. *J. Pharmacol. Exp. Ther.* 20: 181–203.

Sexton, K., and P. B. Ryan. 1988. Assessment of human exposures to air pollution: Methods, measurements and models. In *The Automobile and Public Health*. Washington, DC: National Academy Press.

Sobel, A. E., O. Gawson, and B. Kramer. 1938. Influence of vitamin D in experimental lead poisoning. *Proc. Soc. Exp. Biol. Med.* 38: 433–437.

Spengler, J. D., K. R. Stone, and F. W. Lilley. 1978. High carbon monoxide levels measured in enclosed skating rinks. *J. Air Pollut. Control Assoc.* 28: 776–779.

Squire, R. A. 1987. Ranking animal carcinogens: A proposed regulatory approach. *Science* 214: 877–880.

U.S. EPA. 1996. *Air Quality Criteria for Particulate Matter.* EPA / 600 / P-95 / 001F. Washington, DC: U.S. Environmental Protection Agency.

U.S. EPA. 1988. *A Cancer Risk-Specific Dose Estimate for 2, 3, 7, 8 TCDD*, pp. 1–31. EPA / 600 / 6-88 / 007. U.S. Environmental Protection Agency, Washington, DC: Office of Health and Environmental Assessment.

U.S. EPA. 1992. *Guidelines for Exposure Assessment.* EPA / 600 / Z-92-001. Washington, DC: Risk Assessment Forum, U.S. Environmental Protection Agency.

Wallace, L. A., E. D. Pellizzari, and S. M. Gordon. 1985. Organic chemicals in indoor air: A review of human exposure studies and indoor air quality studies. In *Indoor Air and Human Health*, eds. R. B. Gammage, and S. V. Kaye. Chelsea, MI: Lewis Publishers.

Wolff, R. K., M. Dolovich, G. Obminski, and M. T. Newhouse. 1977. Effect of sulfur dioxide on tracheobronchial clearance at rest and during exercise. In *Inhaled Particles IV*, ed. W. H. Walton. Oxford: Pergamon.

2 Ambient Particulate Matter

MORTON LIPPMANN, Ph.D.

A broad variety of processes produce suspended particulate matter (PM) in the ambient air in which we live and breathe, and there is an extensive body of epidemiological literature that demonstrates that there are statistically significant associations between the concentrations of airborne PM and the rates of mortality and morbidity in human populations. The PM concentrations have almost always been expressed in terms of mass, although one recent study indicates that number concentration may correlate better with effects than does mass (Peters et al., 1997). Also, in studies that reported on associations between health effects and more than one mass concentration, the strength of the association generally improves as one goes from total suspended particulate matter (TSP) to thoracic particulate matter, a.k.a. PM less than $10 \, \mu m$ in aerodynamic diameter (PM_{10}), to fine particulate matter, a.k.a. PM less than $2.5 \, \mu m$ in aerodynamic diameter ($PM_{2.5}$). The influence of a sampling system inlet on the sample mass collected is illustrated in Figure 2-1.

The $PM_{2.5}$ distinction, while nominally based on particle size, is in reality a means of measuring the total gravimetric concentration of several specific chemically distinctive classes of particles that are emitted into or formed within the ambient air as very small particles. In the former category (emitted) are carbonaceous particles in wood smoke and diesel engine exhaust. In the latter category (formed) are carbonaceous particles formed during the photochemical reaction sequence that also leads to ozone formation, as well as the sulfur and nitrogen oxide particles resulting from the oxidation of sulfur dioxide and nitrogen oxide vapors released during fuel combustion.

The coarse particle fraction, namely those particles with aerodynamic diameters $> 2.5 \, \mu m$, are largely composed of soil and mineral ash that have been mechanically dispersed into the air. Both the fine and coarse fractions are complex mixtures in a chemical sense. To the extent that they are in equibrium in the ambient air, it is a dynamic equilibrium in which they enter the air at about the same rate as they are removed. In dry weather, the concentrations of coarse particles are balanced between dispersion into the air, mixing with air masses, and gravitational fallout, while the concentrations of fine particles are determined by rates of formation, rates of chemical transformation, and meteorological factors. PM concentrations of both fine and coarse PM are effectively depleted by rainout and washout associated with rain. Further elaboration of these distinctions is provided in Table 2-1.

In the absence of any detailed understanding of the specific chemical components responsible for the health effects associated with exposures to ambient PM, and in the presence of a large and consistent body of epidemiological evidence associating ambient air PM with mortality and morbidity that cannot be explained by potential confounders

Environmental Toxicants: Human Exposures and Their Health Effects, 2/e. Edited by Morton Lippmann.
ISBN: 0-471-29298-2 © 2000 John Wiley & Sons, Inc.

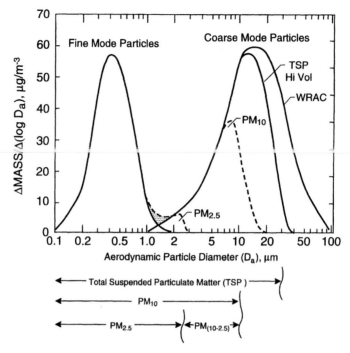

Figure 2-1 Representative bimodel mass distribution as a function of aerodynamic particle diameter for Phoenix, Arizona, showing effect of size-selective sampling inlet on mass collected for (*a*) wide-ranging aerosol classifier (WRAC), (*b*) standard total suspended particulate (TSP) high-volume sampler, (*c*) sampler following EPA's (PM$_{10}$) criteria for thoracic dust, and (*d*) sampler following EPA's criteria for fine particulate matter (PM$_{2.5}$). (Source: U.S. EPA, 1996a, b)

such as other pollutants, aeroallergens, or ambient temperature or humidity, public health authorities have established standards based on mass concentrations within certain prescribed size fractions.

This chapter summarizes the nature and extent of the health effects associated with gravimetric ambient air PM concentrations. Further discussions of the health effects of some of the specific constituents of the ambient air PM are discussed in the chapters on asbestos and other mineral fibers, Diesel exhaust, lead, nitrogen oxides, sulfur oxides, and trace metals.

SOURCES AND PATHWAYS FOR HUMAN EXPOSURE

As indicated in Table 2-1, fine and coarse particles generally have distinct sources and formation mechanisms, although there may be some overlap. Primary fine particles are formed from condensation of high-temperature vapors during combustion. Secondary fine particles are usually formed from gases in three ways: (1) nucleation (i.e., gas molecules coming together to form a new particle), (2) condensation of gases onto existing particles, and (3) by reaction of absorbed gases in liquid droplets. Particles formed from nucleation also coagulate to form relatively larger aggregate particles or droplets with diameters between 0.1 and 1.0 μm, and such particles normally do not grow into the coarse mode. Particles form as a result of chemical reaction of gases in the atmosphere that lead to products that either have a low enough vapor pressure to form a particle or react further to

TABLE 2-1 Comparison of Ambient Fine and Coarse Mode Particles

	Fine Mode	Coarse Mode
Formed from	Gases	Large solids / droplets
Formed by	Chemical reaction; nucleation; condensation; coagulation; evaporation of fog and cloud droplets in which gases have dissolved and reacted	Mechanical disruption (e.g., crushing, grinding, abrasion of surfaces); evaporation of sprays; suspension of dusts
Composed of	Sulfate, SO_4^-; nitrate, NO_3^-; ammonium, NH_4^+; hydrogen ion, H^+; elemental carbon; organic compounds (e.g., PAHs, PNAs); metals (e.g., Pb, Cd, V, Ni, Cu, Zn, Mn, Fe); particle-bound water	Resuspended dusts (e.g., soil dust, street dust); coal and oil fly ash; metal oxides of crustal elements (Si, Al, Ti, Fe); $CaCO_3$, NaCl, sea salt; pollen, mold spores; plant / animal fragments; tire wear debris
Solubility	Largely soluble, hygroscopic and deliquescent	Largely insoluble and non-hygroscopic
Sources	Combustion of coal, oil, gasoline,-Diesel, wood; atmospheric transformation products of NO_x, SO_2, and organic compounds including biogenic species (e.g., terpenes); high temperature processes, smelters, steel mills, etc	Resuspension of industrial dust and soil tracked onto roads; suspension from disturbed soil (e.g., farming, mining, unpaved roads); biological sources; construction and demolition; coal and oil combustion; ocean spray
Lifetimes	Days to weeks	Minutes to hours
Travel distance	100s to 1000s of kilometers	< 1 to 10 s of kilometers

Source: EPA Staff Paper (1996b),[3] which credited Wilson and Suh (1996).

form a low-vapor-pressure substance. Some examples include (1) the conversion of sulfur dioxide (SO_2) to sulfuric acid droplets (H_2SO_4); (2) reactions of H_2SO_4 with ammonia (NH_3) to form ammonium bisulfate (NH_4HSO_4) and ammonium sulfate ($NH_4)_2SO_4$; and (3) the conversion of nitrogen dioxide (NO_2) to nitric acid vapor (HNO_3), which reacts further with NH_3 to form particulate ammonium nitrate (NH_4NO_3). Although directly emitted particles are found in the fine fraction (the most common being particles less than 1.0 μm in diameter from combustion sources), particles formed secondarily from gases dominate the fine fraction mass.

By contrast, most of the coarse fraction particles are emitted directly as particles, and result from mechanical disruption such as crushing, grinding, evaporation of sprays, or suspensions of dust from construction and agricultural operations. Basically most coarse particles are formed by breaking up bigger masses into smaller ones. Energy considerations normally limit coarse particle sizes to greater than 1.0 μm in diameter. Some combustion-generated particles, such as fly ash, are also found in the coarse fraction.

Fine and coarse mode particles generally have distinct chemical composition, solubility, and acidity. Fine mode PM is mainly composed of varying proportions of several major components: inorganic ions (H^+, NH_4^+, NO_3^-, and $SO_4^=$), elemental carbon, organic carbon compounds, trace elements, and water. By contrast, coarse fraction constituents are primarily crustal, consisting of oxides of Si, Al, Fe, and K (note that small amounts of Fe and K are also found among the fine mode particles, but they stem from different sources). Biological material such as bacteria, pollen, and spores may also be found in the coarse mode. As a result of the fundamentally different chemical compositions and sources of fine and coarse fraction particles, the chemical composition of the sum of these two fractions, PM_{10}, is more heterogeneous than either mode alone.

Figure 2-2 presents a synthesis of the available published data on the chemical composition of $PM_{2.5}$ and coarse fraction particles in U.S. cities by region. Each fraction also has regional patterns resulting from the differences in sources and atmospheric conditions. In addition to the larger relative shares of crustal materials in the west, total concentrations of coarse fraction particles are generally higher in the arid areas of the western and southwestern United States.

In general, fine and coarse particles exhibit different degrees of solubility and acidity. With the exception of carbon and some organic compounds, fine particle mass is largely soluble in water and hygroscopic (i.e., fine particles readily take up and retain water). Except under fog conditions, the fine particle mode also contains almost all of the strong acid. By contrast, coarse mineral particles are mostly insoluble, nonhygroscopic, and generally basic.

Fine and coarse particles typically exhibit different behavior in the atmosphere. These differences affect several exposure considerations including the representativeness of central-site-monitored values and the behavior of particles that were formed outdoors after they penetrate into homes and buildings where people spend most of their time.

Fine accumulation mode particles typically have longer atmospheric lifetimes (i.e., days to weeks) than coarse particles, and they tend to be more uniformly dispersed across an urban area or large geographic region, especially in the eastern United States. Atmospheric transformations can take place locally, during atmospheric stagnation, or during transport over long distances. For example, the formation of sulfates from SO_2 emitted by power plants with tall stacks can occur over distances exceeding 300 km and 12 hours of transport time; therefore the resulting particles are well mixed in the air shed. Once formed, the very low dry deposition velocities of fine particles contribute to their persistence and uniformity throughout an air mass.

Larger particles generally deposit more rapidly than small particles; as a result total coarse particle mass will be less uniform in concentration across a region than are fine particles. Because coarse particles may vary in size from about 1 μm to over 100 μm, it is important to note their wide range of atmospheric behavior characteristics. For example, the larger coarse particles (>10 μm) tend to rapidly fall out of the air and have atmospheric lifetimes of only minutes to hours depending on their size, wind velocity, and other factors. Their spatial impact is typically limited by a tendency to fallout in the proximate area downwind of their emission point. The atmospheric behavior of the smaller particles within the "coarse fraction" ($PM_{10-2.5}$) is intermediate between that of the larger coarse particles and fine particles. Thus some of the smaller coarse fraction particles may have lifetimes on the order of days and travel distances of up to 100 km or more. In some locations, source distribution and meteorology affect the relative homogeneity of fine and coarse particles, and in some cases, the greater measurement error in estimating coarse fraction mass precludes clear conclusions about relative homogeneity.

Nevertheless, because fine particles remain suspended for longer times (typically on the order of days to weeks as opposed to days for coarse fraction particles) and travel much farther (hundreds to thousands of kilometers) than coarse fraction particles (tens to hundreds of kilometers), all else being equal, fine particles are theoretically likely to be more uniformly dispersed across urban and regional scales than coarse fraction particles. In contrast, coarse particles tend to be less evenly dispersed around urban areas and exhibit more localized elevated concentrations near sources, especially under windy conditions.

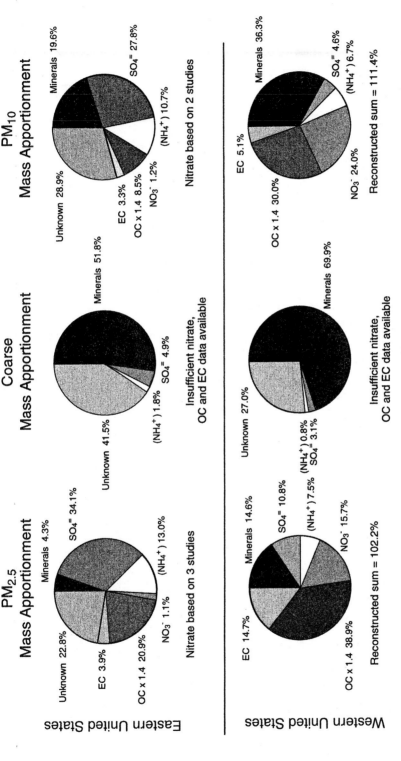

Figure 2-2 Major constituents of PM$_{2.5}$, coarse fraction, and PM$_{10}$. SO$_4^=$, NH$_4^+$, and organic carbon account for most of the PM$_{2.5}$ mass. Eastern PM$_{2.5}$ has more SO$_4^=$, whereas many western sites have a larger NO$_3^-$ contribution and twice the proportion of organic carbon compounds of eastern sites. By contrast, minerals dominate the coarse fraction, ranging from over 50% in the eastern United States to 70% in the western United States. Total concentrations of coarse fraction particles are generally higher in the arid areas of the western and southwestern United States than in the eastern United States. The unknown fraction of the fine mass is assumed to be mainly water. (Source: U.S. EPA, 1996a, b)

35

AMBIENT AIR PM CONCENTRATIONS

This discussion will focus primarily on the concentrations of thoracic PM (PM_{10}) and fine PM ($PM_{2.5}$), on the basis that health considerations are our primary concern. This has the unfortunate effect of limiting our more detailed examination of temporal trends to the period beginning in the 1980s when such size-selective concentrations measurements were first made. There are, however, times when historic measurements of less current relevance can be useful for gaining a holistic appreciation of the effects of ambient PM on human health, and this section begins with a brief review of that experience of most relevance to today's concerns about excess mortality and morbidity in relation to ambient PM.

Up until the mid-1980s available PM concentrations in the United States were generally measured as TSP. Because TSP includes, and can be dominated by, particles too large to penetrate into the thorax, it is a poor index of inhalation hazard. Since the dispersion of large particles is limited, proximity of the sampler to local sources of dust has a major influence on measured TSP concentrations. The artifacts also vary with season and climate, and can be especially severe in the arid portions of the western United States. With these limitations in mind, it is still useful, in terms of historical perspective, to examine the major downward trend in TSP in large U.S. cities, such as New York City, from the 1930s when coal was used for domestic and commercial building heating, to the 1970s, when coal had been almost completely replaced by light oil and gas as fuels for such purposes. The approximately fivefold reduction in TSP that occurred is illustrated in Figure 2-3, as well as the further reduction into the late 1970s.

Some PM monitoring systems have determined PM concentrations by measuring the optical properties of the particles collected on a filter in terms of light reflectance (as for black smoke, or "British smoke" [BS] or in terms of light transmission through the filter (coefficient of haze [CoH]). This can lead to underestimation of the mass concentration of light-colored ash particles, and/or to overestimation of sample masses containing diesel engine soot. This complicates the interpretation of epidemiological data based on exposures determined using these optically based measurements.

On the other hand, when a major change in pollution sources is taking place, there are generally parallel reductions in all of the pollutants affected by those sources. Figure 2-4 shows that as coal smoke came under control in London, England between 1960 and 1980, there were essentially proportionate reductions in BS, SO_2, and the sulfuric acid content of ambient air PM.

Furthermore, even when there are relatively precise gravimetric measurements of sampled particles, there can be significant measurement artifacts. Positive artifacts can

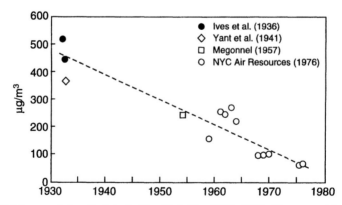

Figure 2-3 Total suspended particulates in New York City (1930–1976). (Data assembled by Eisenbud, 1980.)

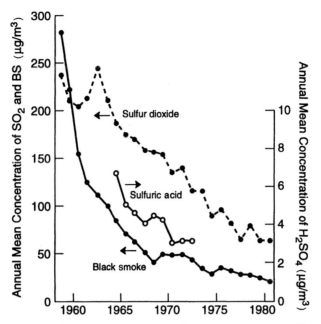

Figure 2-4 Long-term trends in annual mean atmospheric concentrations of BS and SO$_2$ at seven stations in Greater London, and annual mean concentration of H$_2$SO$_4$ at St. Bartholomew's Hospital in Central London.

occur when the filters, or the particles collected on the filters, extract gas phase pollutants from the sampling stream by chemical reaction or sorption. Negative artifacts can occur when the sampled particles are volatilized and carried away from the filter by the sampling stream. Volatile constituents of the ambient air PM include ammonium nitrate (NH$_4$NO$_3$) and some organics formed by photochemical reactions. In southern California, especially on hot summer days, particle volatilization can account for substantial underestimations of PM$_{10}$ concentrations, and even greater underestimations of PM$_{2.5}$ concentrations, since the volatile components are largely within the PM$_{2.5}$ fraction.

Despite the inherent limitations of (1) the assumption of equivalent toxicity of all sampled particles and (2) the sampling and analytical artifacts that limit the accuracy and precision of measured PM concentrations, there is a substantial body of epidemiological evidence for statistically significant associations between airborne PM concentrations and excess mortality and morbidity. Furthermore the mortality and morbidity effects appear to be coherent and not explicable on the basis of known potential confounding factors or coexisting gas phase pollutants (Bates, 1992; Pope et al., 1995a). The nature of this evidence will be discussed following a discussion of ambient air quality data and the relationships between ambient air PM concentrations and actual human exposures to PM.

PM Air Quality Patterns

This section outlines geographic distributions of PM as well as ambient concentration trends and background levels for PM$_{10}$ and fine particles.

PM Concentrations and Trends

PM$_{10}$ Concentrations and Trends   State and local air pollution control agencies have been collecting PM$_{10}$ mass concentration data using EPA-approved reference samplers

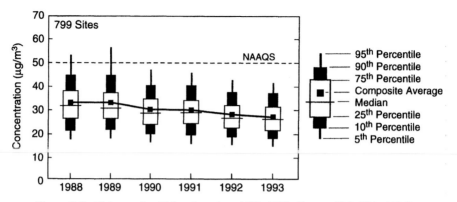

Figure 2-5   PM$_{10}$ trend at U.S. urban sites, 1988–1993. (Source: U.S. EPA, 1996b)

and reporting these data to EPA's publicly available Aerometric Information Retrieval System (AIRS) database since mid-1987. The national trend for the 6 year period from 1988 to 1993 is illustrated in Figure 2-5 for 779 trend sites, mostly from urban and suburban locations. There was a decline of about 20% over the 6 year period from 1988 to 1993, and annual average PM$_{10}$ concentrations ranged from 25 to 35 µg/m^3 for most U.S. regions by 1994.

Fine Particle Concentrations and Trends   The PM$_{2.5}$ concentration data are considerably more limited than for PM$_{10}$. From 1983 to 1993, fewer than 50 sites reported data to AIRS in any given year. These data generally do not include urban concentrations but represent the regional nonurban concentrations. The data show both the regional character of elevated fine particle levels in the eastern United States and California as well as a strong seasonality. In the eastern United States high fine particle levels, dominated by sulfates, occur in the summer, often in conjunction with elevated ozone levels.

National PM$_{2.5}$ trends are not available because of the limited number of sites measuring PM$_{2.5}$ and the sampling period at most sites is restricted to a few years. The development of national trends is further hindered because PM$_{2.5}$ is measured using a variety of sampling frequencies and a variety of nonstandard sampling equipment.

However, visibility data can be used as a reasonable surrogate to estimate fine particle trends because the extinction coefficient (B_{ext}) is directly related to fine particle mass. Sufficient visibility data are available to produce national trends from 137 U.S. sites (principally airports) since 1948. The location of these sites reflects suburban and urban locations with airports. Trends maps show significant regional and seasonal trends. In the northeastern states, winter haze shows a 25% decrease, while in the southeastern states, there is a 40% increase in winter haze. The summer haziness in the northeast shows an increase up to the mid-1970s followed by a decline. In the southeast there was an 80% increase in summer haziness, mainly occurring in the 1950s and 1960s. During the summer months, haziness in the east can be dominated by sulfate (with associated water and ammonium). In this situation, visibility trends may be a better surrogate for sulfate than for nonsulfate related fine particle components.

EXTENT OF POPULATION EXPOSURES TO AMBIENT AIR PM

The concentrations of constituents of PM in the ambient air are important determinants of human exposure to PM of outdoor origin, but other factors also greatly influence exposure.

For exposures occurring indoors, where most people spend most of their time, these include (1) limited penetrability, (2) removal to indoor surfaces, and (3) chemical transformations. Each of these factors tends to reduce exposures to particles of outdoor origin for people spending time indoors.

The penetrability of particles into the indoor environment varies with the air exchange between outdoors and indoors, which, in turn, varies with building size, type of construction, heating and cooling systems, and wind velocity. There will also be variations by season, with minimal air exchange in midwinter and, for air-conditioned homes, in midsummer. Particle size affects penetrability, especially when infiltration pathways are reduced in order to save energy. Under such conditions coarse particle penetration can be greatly reduced.

Once PM penetrates indoors, particle size and chemical composition become major determinants of its fate. Coarse particles deposit by sedimentation relatively rapidly under the generally quiescent conditions indoors. Ultrafine particles diffuse to and deposit on the walls and other indoor surfaces. Acidic particles will be neutralized by ammonia released into the indoor air by people, pets, and household products. Thus the indoor/outdoor concentration ratio can be close to unity for a component such as $SO_4^=$, which is (1) present in the ambient air almost entirely in the accumulation mode (0.1 to 1 μm), (2) chemically nonreactive, and (3) without indoor source in most circumstances. This is illustrated by the data from EPA's Particle Total Exposure Assessment Methodology (PTEAM) study in Riverside, California. As shown in Figure 2-6, the ratio of personal to outdoor $SO_4^=$ was $0.78 + 0.02$. For hydrogen ion (H^+) the ratio was much lower.

For many constituents of outdoor PM, there are significant indoor sources, and the ratio of personal exposure to outdoor concentration for many substances can be much greater than unity. Major PM sources indoors include smoking and cooking, as well as cleaning activities that release or resuspend PM such as dusting, sweeping, and conventional vacuum cleaning. Furthermore there is a major source associated with the personal cloud created by each of us as we engage in routine activities whereby our motions resuspend settled dust on floors, furniture, and other surfaces. In Figure 2-7 additional data from the PTEAM study show that elements enriched in settled dust can be enriched in the personal

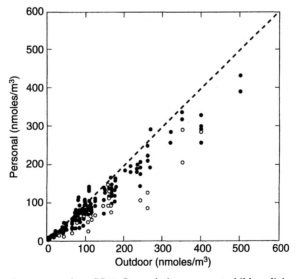

Figure 2-6   Personal versus outdoor $SO_4^=$. Open circles represent children living in air-conditioned homes; the solid line is the 1 : 1 line. (Source: U.S. EPA, 1996a)

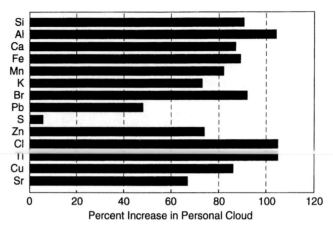

Figure 2-7 Increased concentrations of elements in the personal versus the indoor samples. (Source: U.S. EPA, 1996a)

cloud by a factor of about 2. Figure 2-8 provides an overall summary of PTEAM data on personal exposure, illustrating that, on average, personal activities were associated with 37% of overall personal PM exposure, as compared to 21% for identifiable indoor sources (cooking, environmental tobacco smoke, etc.), and 42% for PM of outdoor origin.

There are few such extensive data sets for locations other than Riverside, California, but less detailed data from other studies elsewhere indicate that the PTEAM results are not atypical (United States EPA, 1996a). Important lessons from such studies is that gravimetric PM concentrations indoors may bear little relation to ambient mass PM concentrations and that the compositions of indoor and outdoor PM can be very different. If the objective is to determine total exposure to PM of outdoor origin, then it may be best to use a conservative tracer of PM from outdoor sources, such as sulfate (by ion

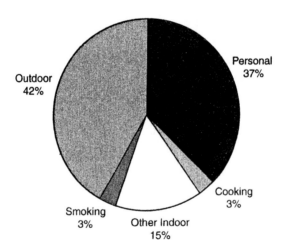

N = 166 Samples

Figure 2-8 Source apportionment of PTEAM PM_{10} personal monitoring data. "Other indoor" represents PM found by the indoor monitor for which the source is unknown. "Personal PM" represents the excess PM that cannot be attributed to either indoor or outdoor sources. (Source: Clayton et al., 1993)

chromatography) or sulfur (by X-ray fluorescence analysis), along with data on the ratio of $SO_4^=$ (or S) to ambient $PM_{2.5}$ or PM_{10}.

NATURE OF THE EVIDENCE FOR HUMAN HEALTH EFFECTS OF AMBIENT AIR PM

For ambient air PM, there is abundant evidence, to be discussed, for significant associations between elevated concentrations and excess human mortality, morbidity, and lost-time, as well as reduced lung function. However, except under the most extreme exposure conditions, such as in Donora, Pennsylvania, in 1948 (Schrenk et al., 1949), only a small percentage of the population has been observed to suffer these adverse effects. Furthermore the affected populations are generally limited to those who are very young or elderly, and within these groups, those with pre-existing disease or special sensitivity. In this context, the lack of confirming data and mechanistic understanding of the basis for the adverse effects from controlled human and animal inhalation studies should come as no great surprise. Short-term human exposure studies can seldom be ethically conducted on especially vulnerable subjects, and chronic long-term exposure studies on humans that may produce cumulative damage are both unethical and technically infeasible. Controlled inhalation studies on laboratory animals that have been pre-treated to produce enhanced sensitivity have recently been initiated, using concentrated ambient air PM, and the early results of some of these studies, to be discussed later in this chapter, have produced mortality and functional changes that may well be relevant to the epidemiological findings.

There is only one component of ambient air PM that has produced functional responses that can readily be related to some of the epidemiologic results following controlled inhalation exposures in healthy humans and laboratory animals, and that component is H^+. These studies are discussed in detail in Chapter 23 on the sulfur oxides. Other chapters that discuss the biological effects that can be produced by normal components of ambient air PM include Chapter 3 (mineral fibers), Chapter 7 (diesel exhaust), Chapter 13 (indoor bioaerosols), Chapter 14 (lead), and Chapter 18 (nitrogen oxides). However, the ambient air PM concentrations for each of these constituents are almost certainly much too low to account for the effects observed.

It is possible that the effects associated with ambient air PM are initiated by nonspecific responses or reactions to deposited particles by lung epithelial cells that can be triggered by most, if not all, deposited particles. In that case the appropriate index of challenge may be associated with the number of depositing particles, or the number having a surface area or volume greater than some threshold level. Much more research is needed before such speculations can be confirmed or refuted.

EPIDEMIOLOGICAL EVIDENCE FOR HUMAN HEALTH EFFECTS OF AMBIENT AIR PM

Quantitative information on adverse health effects associated with particulate matter dates back to the London episode of 1873. A summation of bronchitis mortality during and following the December 9–11, 1873, fog episode was tabulated in the Ministry of Health (1954) report of the December 5–9, 1952, episode. As shown in Table 2-2, various Nineteenth-century fog episodes produced excesses in bronchitis deaths that were comparable to that reported for the more famous 1952 episode. Also it is important to note the higher baseline bronchitis mortality for London in the late Nineteenth century, when

TABLE 2-2   Excess Bronchitis Deaths Associated with Historic London Fogs

Dates of Fog	Average weekly Bronchitis Martality in Previous 10 Years	Excess Bronchitis in Week of Fog and during Succeeding 3 Weeks				Total 4-Week Excess in Bronchitis Deaths
9–11 Dec. 1873		7–13 Dec.	14–20 Dec.	21–27 Dec.	28 Dec.–3 Jan.	
	228	133	424	129	102	788
26–29 Jan. 1880		25–31 Jan.	1–7 Feb.	8–14 Feb.	15–21 Feb.	
	294	258	939	453	167	1817
2–7 Feb. 1882		29 Jan.–4 Feb.	5–11 Feb.	12–18 Feb.	19–25 Feb.	
	357	14	324	186	31	555
21–24 Dec. 1891		20–26 Dec.	27 Dec.–2 Jan.	3–9 Jan.	10–16 Jan.	
	375	35	583	333	437	1388
28–30 Dec. 1892		25–31 Dec.	1–7 Jan.	8–14 Jan.	15–21 Jan.	
	451	− 55	208	154	2	309
26 Nov.–1 Dec. 1948		21–27 Nov.	28 Nov.–4 Dec.	5–11 Dec.	12–18 Dec.	
	65	14	84	33	20	151
5–9 Dec. 1952		1–6 Dec.	7–13 Dec.	14–20 Dec.	21–27 Dec.	
	86	− 3	621	308	92	1018

Source: Adapted from Ministry of Health (1954). Report 95 on Public Health and Medical Subjects. *Mortality and Morbidity during the London Fog of December 1952*. London: HMSO.

the population was below 3 million (compared to about 8 million in 1952), and at a time when that cigarette smoking could not have been a contributory cause.

As shown in Figure 2-9, the daily death rate rose rapidly with the onset of the fog on December 5, 1952, and peaked one day after the peak of pollution, as it was indexed by the measured pollutants, namely black smoke (BS) and sulfur dioxide (SO_2). There was also a rise in hospital emergency bed admissions, which peaked two days after the pollutant peaks. Both the deaths and hospital bed admissions remained elevated for several weeks after the fog lifted (see Table 2-2). Note also that hospital admissions exhibited declines on Sundays, a finding consistent with the known practices for hospital admissions.

The Ministry of Health (1954) report attributed an excess of 4000 deaths from all causes to the exposures during the 1952 episode. Deaths peaked in the first full week and were still above baseline levels two weeks after that. The specific cause with the greatest number of excess deaths over the four weeks was bronchitis (1156 excess deaths), and it had the greatest relative risk ($RR = 6.67$). The next greatest increase, for heart disease (737 excess deaths), had an RR of only 1.82. The all cause relative risk was somewhat higher (1.96). Most of the excess deaths occurred in individuals over 55 years of age (2616 excess deaths over the four weeks), but there was an excess for all age groups beyond four weeks of age. Overall, the excess mortality was concentrated among the elderly with pre-existing disease.

It is of particular interest to current concerns that while recent daily mortality studies show much lower absolute risk levels from the much lower peaks in PM pollution, the elevated relative risks among the very young and oldest cohorts and the risk rankings among causes of death are quite similar today to those of December 1952.

The Ministry of Health (1954) report also noted that there was a clear association between chronic air pollution and the incidence of bronchitis and other respiratory diseases. The death rate from bronchitis in England and Wales (where coal smoke pollution was very high) was much higher than in other northern European countries (with much lower levels of coal smoke pollution). The very high chronic coal smoke exposure in

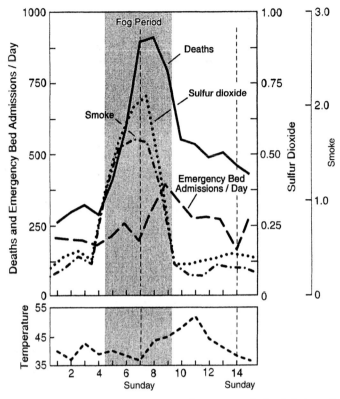

Figure 2-9 Metropolitan London total mortality and emergency bed admissions during the 1952 pollution episode in relation to black smoke, expressed as mg / m³, and sulfur dioxide, expressed as parts per million by volume.

the United Kingdom, associated with a high prevalence of chronic bronchitis, appears to have created a large pool of individuals susceptible to "harvesting" by an acute pollution episode.

The December 1962 London fog episode was the last to produce a clearly evident acute harvest of excess deaths, albeit a much smaller one than that of December 1952. Commins and Waller (1963) developed a technique to measure H_2SO_4 in urban air, and made daily measurements of H_2SO_4 at St. Bartholomew's Hospital in Central London during the 1962 episode. As shown in Figure 2-10, the airborne H_2SO_4 rose rapidly during the 1962 episode, with a greater relative increase than that for black smoke (BS).

The U.K. Clean Air Act of 1954 had led to the mandated use of smokeless fuels and, as shown in Figure 2-4, annual mean smoke levels had declined by 1962, to about one-half of the 1958 level. The annual average SO_2 concentrations had not declined by 1962, but dropped off markedly thereafter, along with a further marked decline in BS levels. For the period between 1964 and 1972, the measured levels of H_2SO_4 followed a similar pattern of decline.

During the later part of the coal smoke era in the United Kingdom, researchers begin to study the associations between long-term daily records of mortality and morbidity and ambient air pollution. In the first major time-series analysis of daily London mortality for the winter of 1958–1959, Martin and Bradley (1960) and Lawther (1963) used the readily available BS and SO_2 data. They estimated that both pollutants were associated with

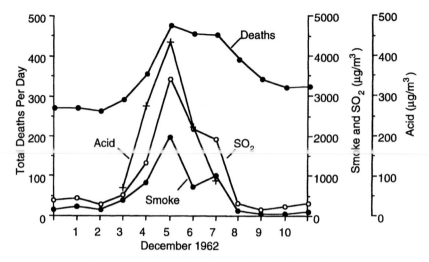

Figure 2-10   December 1962 London pollution episode.

excess daily mortality when their concentrations exceeded about $750 \, \mu g / m^3$. However, additional analyses of this data set led to different conclusions. For example, Ware et al. (1981) concluded that there was no demonstrable lower threshold for excess mortality down to the lowest range of observation (BS $\approx 150 \, \mu g / m^3$), as illustrated in Figure 2-11. Although $150 \, g / m^3$ is now near the upper end of observed concentrations rather than at the lower end, time-series analyses still indicate an increasing slope as concentrations decrease.

In terms of time-series analyses of morbidity, a study by Lawther (1970) reported the daily symptom scores of a panel of patients with chronic bronchitis in relation to the daily concentrations of BS and SO_2. There was a close correspondence between symptom scores and both pollutant indexes.

Chronic coal smoke exposure also affected baseline lung function. Holland and Reid (1965) analyzed spirometric data collected on British postal workers in 1965. By that time

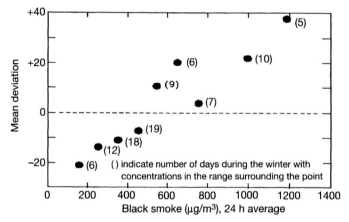

Figure 2-11   Martin and Bradley (1960) data for winter of 1958–1959 in London as summarized by Ware et al. (1981), showing average deviations of daily mortality from 15 day moving average by concentration of black smoke (BS).

pollution levels were well below their peaks, but the postal workers had been exposed out-of-doors for many years when pollution levels were higher. The London postal workers had lower forced expiratory volumes in one second (FEV_1) and peak expiratory flow rates (PEFR) than their country town counterparts. The deleterious effects of smoking were accounted for in these analyses. Within each smoking category, the differences between the London and country town means were attributed to pollution on the basis that pollution levels were, on average, twice as high in London as in the country towns.

The marked reduction in U.K. smoke pollution levels during the 1960s was shown to be associated with a marked reduction in annual mortality in County Boroughs by Chinn et al. (1981). As shown in Table 2-3, mortality rates in middle-aged and elderly men and women for the 1969–1973 period were no longer associated with an index of smoke pollution. By contrast, for both the 1948–1954 and 1958–1964 periods, the index of smoke exposure correlated strongly with annual mortality rates for both chronic bronchitis and respiratory tract cancers. On the basis of such evidence of improved health status, our U.K. colleagues considered air pollution to be a problem solved, and essentially halted further investigations for the next several decades.

Coal smoke pollution affected acute mortality and morbidity in the United States and in other countries as well as in the United Kingdom, but there was much less documentation and quantitative analyses prior to the mid-1960s. Among the notable non-U.K. reports are those of Firket (1936) on the December 1930 fog episode in the Meuse Valley in Belgium, and the reports on the October 1948 Donora, Pennsylvania, fog episode.

The December 1930 fog in the Meuse Valley was associated with 60 deaths from a population of about 6000, but the pollutant concentrations were not measured.

In Donora, a valley town of about 10,000 people at a bend in the Monongahela River south of Pittsburgh, there were steel mills, wire mills, zinc works, and a sulfuric acid plant along the river bank for the entire length of the town. As reported by Schrenk et al. (1949), a persistent valley fog was associated with 20 excess deaths as well as acute morbidity among 43% of the population. About 10% were reported to have severe effects requiring

TABLE 2-3   Standardized Annual Mortality Rate Regression Coefficients on Smoke for 64 U.K. County Boroughs

Sex	Age	Mortality in	Cancer of Trachea, Bronchus, Lung	Chronic Bronchitis
Males	45–64	1969–1973	0.07	0.02
		1958–1964	0.53[++]	0.32[+]
		1948–1954	0.71[+++]	0.48[+++]
	65–74	1969–1973	0.15	−0.06
		1958–1964	0.68[+++]	0.31
		1948–1954	0.87[+++]	0.37[+]
Females	45–64	1969–1973	−0.02	−0.02
		1958–1964	−0.64[++]	0.33[+]
		1948–1954	0.49[+]	0.49[++]
	65–74	1969–1973	0.07	0.03
		1958–1964	0.25	0.40[+]
		1948–1954	0.61[++]	0.31

Source: Adapted from Chinn et al. (1981).
Note: Based on index of black smoke pollution 20 years before death of Daly (*Br. J. Prev. Soc. Med.* 13: 14–27, 1959).
[+] $p < 0.05$.
[++] $p < 0.01$.
[+++] $p < 0.001$.

medical attention. In a ten-year follow-up of the affected population, Ciocco and Thompson (1961) reported greater mortality rates and incidences of heart disease and chronic bronchitis among the residents who had reported acute illness in 1948 in comparison to residents who did not report such illness.

As indicated in Figure 2-3, TSP levels in New York had declined markedly between the 1950s and 1970s, and similar declines had taken place in most other urban areas. Thus indexes of chronic effects of exposure to PM made in the early 1970s for U.S. populations could have been due to earlier and higher exposures as well as to contemporary levels of exposure. This is relevant background for a discussion of results obtained during the first National Health and Nutrition Examination Survey (NHANES I), which was conducted between 1971 and 1975. In one paper, Chestnut et al. (1991) studied the relationship between pulmonary function and quarterly average levels of TSP for adults who resided in 49 of the locations where the NHANES I was conducted. Statistically significant relationships were observed between TSP levels and FVC and $FEV_{1.0}$. Anthropometric measurements and socioeconomic characteristics of the subjects were included in the analysis, and the sample was restricted to "never" smokers. A one standard deviation increase (about $34 \, \mu g / m^3$) in TSP from the sample mean of $87 \, \mu g / m^3$ was associated with an average decrease in FVC of 2.25%. In another report of results from NHANES I, Schwartz (1993) examined reported rates of chronic respiratory illness by standardized questionnaire across 53 urban areas in the United States. Diagnosis of respiratory illness by an examining physician was also considered as an outcome. After controlling for age, race, sex, and cigarette smoking, annual average TSP was associated with increased risk of chronic bronchitis [odds ratio (OR) = 1.07, 95% confidence interval (CI) = 1.02–11.2] and of a respiratory diagnosis by the examining physician (OR = 1.06, 95% CI = 1.02–1.11). The odds ratios were for a $10 \, \mu g / m^3$ increase in TSP. When the analysis was restricted to never smokers, the associations remained, with a slight increase in the relative odds associated with airborne particles. Plots of relative odds by quartiles of TPS exposure, adjusting for covariates, showed dose-dependent increases in risk with increasing exposure.

In a study of the influence of chronic PM exposure on lung function of children and young adults (ages 6–24), Schwartz (1989) used TSP and NHANES II data for the period 1976–1980. TSP, NO_2, and O_3 were all significantly associated with reduced FVC, FEV_1, and PEFR, but SO_2 was not. For TSP and O_3, there appeared to be thresholds for response at about 40 ppb (daily average) O_3 and $90 \, \mu g / m^3$ TSP. The relationships held whether or not children with respiratory conditions or smokers were included. Demographic and geographic variables had little or no impact on the pollution relationships, which also held when only persons still residing in their state of birth were considered.

With the phasing out of bituminous coal as a fuel for domestic heating, the use of the optical density of smoke samples as an index of the health risk associated with ambient particulate matter became increasingly problematic. It has also become clear that total suspended particulate matter (TSP), the standard index of PM pollution in the United States prior to 1987 was also far from ideal. Under high-wind conditions, gravimetric TSP concentrations are dominated by PM too large to penetrate into the human thorax, even during oral inhalation. Some U.S. investigators chose the $SO_4^=$ content of TSP samples as an alternate index of PM associated health risk. Because of the nature of its sources, essentially all of the $SO_4^=$ in the ambient air is on fine particles below 2.5 µm in aerodynamic diameter ($PM_{2.5}$).

As discussed in Chapter 26, $SO_4^=$ is often a relatively large fraction of $PM_{2.5}$, it is nonvolatile, it is stable on filters used for air sampling, it can be easily extracted from the filters, and it can be accurately analyzed with relatively simple and inexpensive procedures. Furthermore it generally correlates with mortality and indexes of morbidity better than do other frequently measured PM indexes, such as TSP, BS, CoH, and PM_{10}.

During the 1990s there was a great increase in the number of peer-reviewed papers describing time-series studies of the associations between daily ambient air pollutant concentrations and daily rates of mortality and hospital admissions for respiratory diseases. Also results of two prospective cohort studies of annual mortality rates were published. In terms of morbidity there has been a rapid growth of the literature showing associations between airborne particle concentrations and exacerbation of asthma, increased symptom rates, decreased respiratory function, and restricted activities.

Much of the recent literature was summarized by Pope et al. (1995a). They converted historically measured values for CoH and TSP to estimated levels of PM_{10}, and remarked that very similar coefficients of response for the PM_{10}-daily mortality associations were determined in all locations. Table 2-4 shows Thurston's (1995) independent analysis of acute mortality studies in nine communities with measured PM_{10} concentrations, including four of the ten studies cited by Pope et al. (1995a). As indicated in this table, the coefficients of response tend to be higher when the PM_{10} is expressed as a multiple-day average concentration, and lower when other air pollutants are included in multiple-regression analyses. In any case, the results in each city (except for the very small city of Kingston, TN) indicate a statistically significant association.

It is also clear from recent research that the associations between PM_{10} and daily mortality are not seriously confounded by weather variables or the presence of other criteria pollutants. Figure 2-12 shows that the calculated relative acute mortality risks for PM_{10} are relatively insensitive to the concentrations of SO_2, NO_2, CO, and O_3. The results are also coherent as described by Bates (1992). Figure 2-13 shows that the relative risks (RRs) for respiratory mortality are greater than for total mortality, and the RRs for the less serious symptoms are higher than those for mortality and hospital admissions.

One aspect of the influence of PM on daily mortality that has recently come to light is its role in sudden infant death syndrome (SIDS). Woodruff et al. (1997) examined the

TABLE 2-4   Comparison of Time-series Study Estimates of Total Mortality Relative Risk (RR) for a $100\,\mu g/m^3$ PM_{10} Increase

Study Area (Reference)	Measured PM_{10} Concentrations		RR for $100\,\mu g/m^3$	95% CI for $100\,\mu g/m^3$
	Mean ($\mu g/m^3$)	Maximum ($\mu g/m^3$)		
Utah Valley, UT (Pope et al., 1992)	47	297	1.16[*][××]	(1.10–1.22)
St. Louis, MO (Dockery et al., 1992)	28	97	1.16[*][×]	(1.01–1.33)
Kingston, TN (Dockery et al., 1992)	30	67	1.17[*][×]	(0.88–1.57)
Birmingham, AL (Schwartz., 1993a)	48	163	1.11[*][××]	(1.02–1.20)
Athens, Greece (Touloumi et al., 1994)	78	306	1.07[*][×]	(1.05–1.09)
			1.03[**][×]	(1.00–1.06)
Toronto, Canada (Özkaynak et al., 1994)	40	96	1.07[*][×]	(1.05–1.09)
			1.05[**][×]	(1.03–1.07)
Los Angeles, CA (Kinney et al., 1995)	58	177	1.05[*][×]	(1.00–1.11)
			1.04[**][×]	(0.98–1.09)
Chicago, IL (Ito et al., 1995)	38	128	1.05[**][×]	(1.01–1.10)
Santiago, Chile (Ostro et al., 1995)	115	367	1.08[*][×]	(1.06–1.12)
			1.15[*][××]	(1.08–1.22)

[*] Single-pollutant model (PM_{10}).
[**] Multiple-pollutant model (PM_{10} and other pollutants simultaneously).
[×] One-day mean PM_{10} concentration employed.
[××] Multiple-day mean PM_{10} concentration employed.

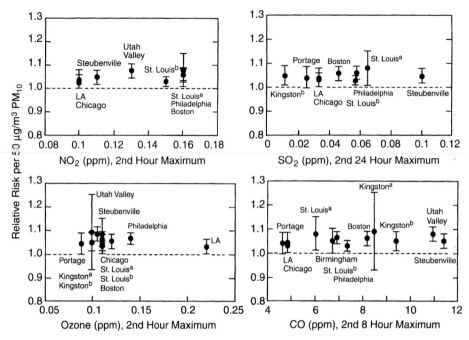

Figure 2-12   Relationship between *RR* for excess daily mortality associated with PM₁₀ and peak daily levels of other criteria pollutants. (Source: Adapted from Fig. V-3a of PM Staff Paper; U.S. EPA, 1996b)

relationship between postneonatal infant mortality and PM_{10} in the United States. The study involved analysis of cohorts consisting of approximately 4 million infants born between 1989 and 1991 in 86 metropolitan statistical areas (MSAs) in the United States. Data from the National Center for Health Statistics birth/infant death records were combined at the MSA level with measurements of PM_{10} from the EPA's Aerometric Database. Infants were categorized as having high, medium, or low exposures based on tertiles of PM_{10}. Overall postneonatal mortality rates were 3.1 among infants with low PM_{10} exposures, 3.5 among infants with medium PM_{10} exposures, and 3.7 among highly exposed infants. After adjustment for other covariates, the odds ratio (OR) and 95% confidence intervals (CI) for total postneonatal mortality for the high-exposure versus the low-exposure group was 1.10 (1.04, 1.16). In normal birth weight infants, high PM_{10} exposure was associated with respiratory causes [OR = 1.40 (1.05, 1.85)] and SIDS [OR = 1.26 (1.14, 1.99)]. For low birth weight babies, high PM_{10} exposure was associated, but not significantly, with mortality from respiratory causes [OR = 1.18 (0.86, 1.61)].

PM exposure, albeit at much high ambient levels, has been associated with pre-term delivery and low birth weight in Beijing, PRC. Xu et al. (1995) followed all registered pregnant women who lived in four residential areas of Beijing. The analysis included 25,370 women who gave first live births in 1988. Multiple linear regression and logistic regression were used to estimate the effects of air pollution on gestational age and preterm delivery (i.e., < 37 wk), with adjustment for outdoor temperature and humidity, day of the week, season, maternal age, gender of child, and residential area. Very high concentrations of ambient SO_2 (mean = 102 μg/m³, maximum = 630 μg/m³) and TSP (mean = 375 μg/m³, maximum = 1003 μg/m³) were observed. There was a significant dose-dependent association between gestational age and SO_2 and TSP concentrations. The estimated reduced duration of gestation was 0.075 wk (12.6 h) and 0.042 wk (7.1 h) for each

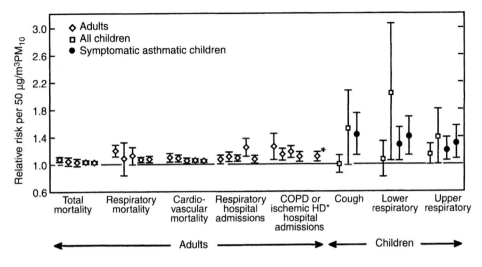

Total, Respiratory, Cardiovascular Mortality
1. Pope et al. (1992)   2. Schwartz (1993)   3. Styer et al. (1995)   4. Ostro et al. (1995a)
5. Ito and Thurston (1996)

Respiratory Hospital Admissions
1. Schwartz (1995) New Haven, CT   2. Schwartz (1995) Tacoma, WA   3. Schwartz (1996) Spokane, WA
4. Ito and Thurston (1994) Toronto, Canada

COPD or Ischemic HD* Hospital Admissions
1. Schwartz (1994f) Minneapolis, MN   2. Schwartz (1994c) Birmingham, AL
3. Schwartz (1996) Spokane, WA   4. Schwartz (1994d), Detroit, MI
*5. Schwartz & Morris (1995), Detroit, MI, Ischemic HD

Cough, Lower Respiratory, Upper Respiratory
1. Hoek and Brunekreef (1993)   2. Styer et al. (1994)   3. Pope & Dockery (1992), symptomatic children

Figure 2-13 Relationships between relative risks per $50 \mu g / m^3$ PM_{10} and health effects. (Source: Adapted from Fig. V-2 in PM Staff Paper; U.S. EPA, 1996b)

$100 \mu g / m^3$ increase in SO_2 and TSP 7-d lagged moving average, respectively. The adjusted odds ratio for preterm delivery was 1.21 (95% CI = 1.01–1.46) for each $\ln \mu g / m^3$ increase in SO_2, and was 1.10 (95% CI = 1.01–1.20) for each $100 \mu g / m^3$ increase in TSP. In addition the gestational age distribution of high-pollution days was more skewed toward the left tail (i.e., very preterm and preterm), compared with low-pollution days.

In a follow-on study, Wang et al. (1997) examined the relationship between maternal exposure to air pollution during periods of pregnancy (entire and specific periods) and birth weight in a well-defined cohort between 1988 and 1991. All pregnant women living in four residential areas of Beijing were registered and followed from early pregnancy until delivery. The sample for analysis included 74,671 first-parity live births with gestational age of 37 to 44 weeks. Multiple linear regression and logistic regression were used to estimate the effects of air pollution on birth weight and low birth weight (< 2500 g), adjusting for gestational age, residence, year of birth, maternal age, and infant gender. There was a significant exposure-response relationship between maternal exposures to SO_2 and TSP during the third trimester of pregnancy and infant birth weight. The adjusted odds ratio for low birth weight was 1.11 (95% CI, 1.06–1.16) for each $100 \mu g / m^3$ increase in SO_2 and 1.10 (95% CI, 1.05–1.14) for each $100 \mu g / m^3$ increase in TSP. The estimated reduction in birth weight was 7.3 g and 6.9 g for each $100 \mu g / m^3$ increase in SO_2 and in TSP, respectively. The birth weight distribution of the high-exposure group was more skewed toward the left tail (i.e., with higher proportion of births < 2500 g) than that of the low-exposure group.

While there is mounting evidence that excess daily mortality is associated with short-term peaks in PM_{10} pollution, the public health implications of this evidence are not yet fully clear. Key questions remain, including

- Which specific components of the fine particle fraction ($PM_{2.5}$) and coarse particle fraction of PM_{10} are most influential in producing the responses?
- Do the effects of the PM_{10} depend on co-exposure to irritant vapors, such as ozone, sulfur dioxide, or nitrogen oxides?
- What influences do multiple-day pollution episode exposures have on daily responses and response lags?
- Does long-term chronic exposure predispose sensitive individuals being "harvested" on peak pollution days?
- How much of the excess daily mortality is associated with life-shortening measured in days or weeks versus months, years, or decades?

The first four questions above are complex, and difficult to answer at this time on the basis of current knowledge. The discussion that follows will examine them in greater detail.

The last question above is a critical one in terms of the public health impact of excess daily mortality. If, in fact, the bulk of the excess daily mortality were due to "harvesting" of terminally ill people who would have died within a few days, then the public health impact would be much less than if it led to prompt mortality among acutely ill persons who, if they did not die then, would have recovered and lived productive lives for years or decades longer. An indirect answer to this question is provided by the results of two relatively recent prospective cohort studies of annual mortality rates in relation to long-term pollutant exposure.

Dockery et al. (1993) reported on a 14- to 16-year mortality follow-up of 8111 adults in six U.S. cities in relation to average ambient air concentrations of TSP, $PM_{2.5}$, fine particle $SO_4^=$, O_3, SO_2, and NO_2. Concentration data for most of these pollutant variables were available for 14 to 16 years. The mortality rates were adjusted for cigarette smoking, education, body mass index, and other influential factors not associated with pollution. The two pollutant variables that best correlated with total mortality (which was mostly attributable to cardiopulmonary mortality) were $PM_{2.5}$ and $SO_4^=$. The overall mortality rate ratios were expressed in terms of the range of air pollutant concentrations in the six cities. The rate-ratios (and 95% confidence intervals) for both $PM_{2.5}$ and $SO_4^=$ were 1.26 (1.08–1.47) overall, and 1.37 (1.11–1.68) for cardiopulmonary. The mean life-shortening was in the range of 2–3 years.

Pope et al. (1995b) linked $SO_4^=$ data from 151 U.S. metropolitan areas in 1980 with individual risk factor on 552,138 adults who resided in these areas when enrolled in a prospective study in 1982, as well as $PM_{2.5}$ data for 295,223 adults in 50 communities. Deaths were ascertained through December 1989. The relationships of air pollution to all-cause, lung cancer, and cardiopulmonary mortality was examined using multivariate analysis which controlled for smoking, education, and other risk factors. Particulate air pollution was associated with cardiopulmonary and lung cancer mortality but not with mortality due to other causes. Adjusted relative risk ratios (and 95% confidence intervals) of all-cause mortality for the most polluted areas compared with the least polluted equaled 1.15 (1.09–1.22) and 1.17 (1.09–1.26) when using $SO_4^=$ and $PM_{2.5}$, respectively. The mean life-shortening in this study was between 1.5 and 2 years. The results were similar to those found in the previous cross-sectional studies of Ozkaynak and Thurston (1987) and Lave and Seskin (1970). Thus the results of these earlier studies provide some confirmatory support for the findings of Pope et al. (1995b), whose results indicate that the concerns about the credibility of the earlier results, due to their inability to control for potentially confounding personal factors such as smoking and socioeconomic variables, can be eased.

The Dockery et al. (1993) study had the added strength of data on multiple PM metrics. As shown in Figure 2-14, the association becomes stronger as the PM metric shifts from TSP to PM_{10}. Within the thoracic fraction (PM_{10}) the association is much stronger to the fine particle component ($PM_{2.5}$) than for the coarse component. Within the $PM_{2.5}$ fraction, both the $SO_4^=$ and non-$SO_4^=$ fractions correlate very strongly with annual mortality, suggesting a nonspecific response to fine particles.

If, in fact, more people are dying of cardiopulmonary causes on a given day because of exposures to elevated concentrations of PM, it would be reasonable to expect higher daily rates of emergency hospital admissions and visits to emergency rooms and clinics for similar causes. This expectation is consistent with the results summarized in Table 2-5. These studies indicate that indexes of PM, such as daily concentrations of PM_{10}, $SO_4^=$, and BS are generally significantly associated with excess daily emergency admissions to hospitals for either respiratory diseases or cardiac diseases, or both. These studies have not shown associations with noncardiopulmonary· causes, and the influence of PM has generally been found to remain in multiple regression analyses that included other criteria pollutants. However, for respiratory diseases, the influence of summertime O_3 has generally been greater than that of PM. This is in contradistinction to excess daily mortality, where the influence of PM is generally much greater than that of O_3. For hospitalizations for cardiac diseases, the most influential criteria pollutants appear to be PM and CO. Further discussion on pollutant interactions and joint effects is provided in Chapters 21 and 24.

The importance of the fine particles as a risk factor for subnormal vital capacity in children is illustrated in Figure 2-15, which shows data collected in the Harvard-Health Canada cross-sectional study of 22 U.S. and Canadian communities (Raizenne et al., 1996). There was a significant association between the percentage of children with forced vital capacity (FVC) < 85% of predicted and fine particle mass concentration but no apparent association with the coarse component of PM_{10}. Actually the strongest association observed in this comparison was for the H^+ component of the fine particles. Most of the recent epidemiological studies have not had the advantage of available $PM_{2.5}$, $SO_4^=$ or H^+ data, and have had to rely on PM_{10} data. Summaries of such PM_{10} epidemiology are shown in Figure 2-13 and Table 2-6. There is coherence in the data, as defined by Bates (1992), in terms of the relative risk ratings, with mortality risks increasing from total to cardiovascular to respiratory, and with cough and respiratory conditions being more frequent than mortality.

The findings of Dockery et al. (1993) and Pope et al. (1995b), in carefully controlled prospective cohort studies, indicate that mean lifespan shortening is of the order of two years. This implies that many individuals in the population have lives shortened by many years, and that there is excess mortality associated with fine particle exposure greater than that implied by the cumulative results of the time-series studies of daily mortality.

In the absence of any generally accepted mechanistic basis to account for the epidemiological associations between ambient fine particles, on the one hand, and mortality, morbidity and functional effects, on the other, the causal role of PM remains questionable. However, essentially all attempts to discredit the associations on the basis of the effects being due to other environmental variables that may co-vary with PM have been unsuccessful. As shown in Figure 2-12, the relative risk for daily mortality in relation to PM_{10} is remarkably consistent across communities that vary considerably in their peak concentrations of other criteria air pollutants. The possible confounding influence of

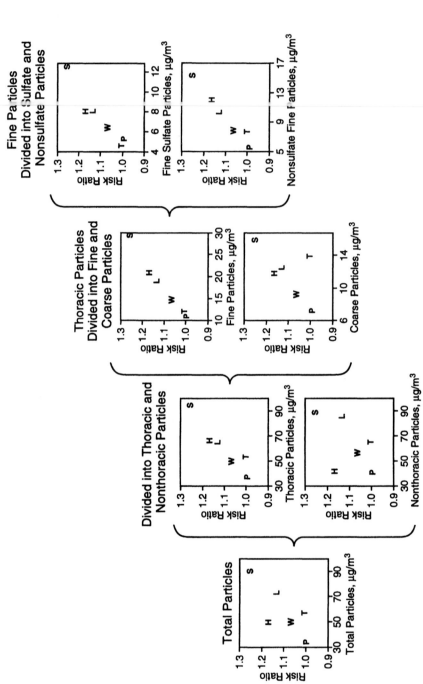

Figure 2-14 Adjusted relative risks for annual mortality are plotted against each of seven long-term average particle indexes in the six city study, from largest size range—total suspended particulate matter (*lower left*)—through sulfate and nonsulfate fine particle concentrations (*upper right*). Note that a relatively strong linear relationship is seen for fine particles, and for its sulfate and nonsulfate components. Topeka, which has a substantial coarse particle component of thoracic particle mass, stands apart from the linear relationship between relative risk and thoracic particle concentration. (Source: Adapted from Fig. V-5 of PM Staff Paper; U.S. EPA, 1996b)

TABLE 2-5 Summary of Recent Epidemiologic Study Findings: Associations of Ambient Air Particulate Matter with Hospital Admissions

Population	Pollutants Monitored	Effects Reported	Associated Pollutant(s)[a]	Reference
General Population				
Metropolitan Toronto Summers 1986–1988	TSP, PM_{10}, $PM_{2.5}$, $SO_4^=$, H^+, O_3	Increased hospital admissions for respiratory diseases	O_3, H^+, $SO_4^=$	Thurston et al. (1994a,b)
New York State: Buffalo, Albany, Bronx, Westchester Year-round 1988–1990	$SO_4^=$, H^+, O_3	Increased hospital admissions for respiratory diseases in Buffalo and Bronx	O_3, H^+, $SO_4^=$	Thurston et al. (1992a,b)
Ontario Summers 1983–1988	$SO_4^=$, O_3	Increased hospital admissions for respiratory diseases	O_3, $SO_4^=$	Burnett et al. (1994)
Montreal Summers 1984–1988	PM_{10}, $SO_4^=$, O_3	Increased hospital admissions for respiratory diseases	PM_{10}, $SO_4^=$	Delfino et al. (1994)
Ontario Year-round 1983–1988	$SO_4^=$, O_3	Increased hospital admissions for respiratory and cardiac diseases	$SO_4^=$	Burnett et al. (1995)
Denver, CO 1989–1992	PM_{10}, CO	Increased hospital admissions for cardiopulmonary diseases	PM_{10}	Fennelly and Bartelson (1996)
London, England 1987–1994	BS, CO, NO_2, SO_2, O_3	Increased hospital admissions for circulatory diseases, especially acute myocardial infarction	BS, CO, NO_2, SO_2	Poloniecki et al. (1997)
Population Older than 65				
Detroit Summers 1986–1989	PM_{10}, O_3	Increased hospital admissions for respiratory diseases	PM_{10}, O_3	Schwartz (1994c)
Minneapolis/St. Paul	PM_{10}, O_3	Increased hospital admissions for respiratory diseases	PM_{10}, O_3	Schwartz (1994b)
Birmingham, AL	PM_{10}, O_3	Increased hospital admissions for respiratory diseases	PM_{10}, O_3	Schwartz (1994c)
Spokane, WA	PM_{10}, O_3	Increased hospital admissions for respiratory diseases	PM_{10}, O_3	Schwartz (1996)

[a] Associations with $p \leq 0.05$.

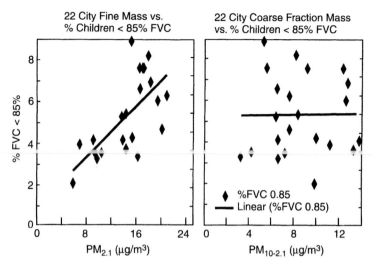

Figure 2-15 Plot appearing in PM Staff Paper (U.S. EPA, 1996). (Source: Based on data reported by Raizenne et al., 1996)

adjustments to models to account for weather variables has also been found to be minimal (Samet et al., 1997, Pope and Kalkstein, 1996).

While mechanistic understanding of processes by which ambient air PM causes human health effects remains quite limited, the credibility of ambient $PM_{2.5}$ as a cause of excess human mortality and morbidity has been enhanced by a series of animal inhalation studies in which rats were exposed to concentrated ambient accumulation mode PM. Godleski et al. (1996) exposed healthy and compromised rats to both filtered ambient air and Boston winter ambient accumulation mode PM that was concentrated up to 25X (yielding concentrations up to $250\,\mu g/m^3$) for six hours a day for three days. For two groups of compromised rats; one with SO_2-induced chronic bronchitis, and one with monocrotaline-induced pulmonary hypertension, there was excess mortality during and/or immediately following these exposures. None of the healthy rats died, and there was no lung inflammation and only minimal bronchoconstriction following exposure. The hypertensive rats has 19% mortality and evidence of acute inflammation in alveoli and lung interstitium. The bronchitic rats had 37% mortality and responses marked by airway inflammation, increased mucus, marked bronchoconstriction, interstitial edema, and pulmonary vascular congestion. Compromised rats exposed to filtered ambient air had no comparable responses. Since the animals exposed to filtered air were still exposed to the same pollutant gases (O_3, SO_2, NO_2, CO), the effects are linked to the $PM_{2.5}$. Coarse particles were removed at the inlet to the concentrator, and ultrafine particles ($< 0.15\,\mu m$) were not concentrated.

Godleski et al. (1977) also exposed tracheostomized dogs to concentrated Boston $PM_{2.5}$. The dogs had bronchoalveolar lavage (BAL) to establish baseline inflammation and implantation of subcutaneous electrocardiographic leads to monitor the electrocardiogram (ECG) several weeks prior to either sham or concentrated PM exposures. Twenty-four hours after the exposure protocol, BAL was repeated. The dogs were exposed two at a time by connecting their cuffed treacheostomy tubes to the output of the concentrator at $193.9\,\mu g/m^3$ ($26 \times$ ambient). The ECG had no changes during sham exposures in any dogs, but concentrated PM compared to sham exposures produced substantial PQ- and ST-segment changes in one dog. Increases in BAL neutrophils over preexposure levels (mean

TABLE 2-6   Summary of recent Epidemiologic Study Findings: Associations of Ambient Air Particulate Matter with Symptoms and Lung Function Indexes.

Children

Population	Pollutants Monitored	Effects Reported	Associated Pollutant(s)[a]	Reference
Asymptomatic and symptomatic children in Uniontown, PA Summer 1990	PM_{10}, $PM_{2.5}$, $SO_4^=$, H^+, O_3, SO_2	Reduced PEFR, symptoms	H^+, $SO_4^=$, O_3 H^+, $PM_{2.5}$, $SO_4^=$, SO_2, O_3	Neas et al. (1995)
Asymptomatic and symptomatic children in Austrian Alps Summer 1991	PM_{10}, $SO_4^=$, H^+, NH_4^+, O_3,	Reduced FVC and FEV_1, Pollen Increased medication usage	H^+, PM_{10} (not specified)	Studnicka et al. (1995a,b)
Asthmatic children in Conn. River Valley Summers 1991–1993	$SO_4^=$, H^+, O_3, pollen	Increased medication usage, symptoms, reduced PEFR	O_3, H^+, $SO_4^=$ O_3, H^+, $SO_4^=$ O_3, H^+, $SO_4^=$	Thurston et al. (1997)
Children in 7 U.S. cities Year-round 1985–1988	PM_{10}, $PM_{2.5}$, $SO_4^=$, H^+, O_3, SO_2, NO_2	Increased symptoms of bronchitis	H^+, $SO_4^=$, $PM_{2.5}$, PM_{10}	Damokosh (1993)
Children in 24 North American cities	PM_{10}, $PM_{2.1}$, $SO_4^=$, H^+, O_3, SO_2, NO_2	Increased symptoms of bronchitis	H^+, $SO_4^=$, $PM_{2.1}$, PM_{10}	Dockery et al. (1996)
Year-round 1988–1990		Decreased FVC and FEV_1	H^+, $SO_4^=$, $PM_{2.1}$, PM_{10}	Raizenne et al. (1996)
Children in 10 rural Canadian communities Year-round 1985–1986	PM_{10}, $SO_4^=$, O_3, NO_2, SO_2	Decreased FVC and FEV_1	$SO_4^=$, O_3	Stern et al. (1994)

[a] Associations with $p \leq 0.05$.

55

24.8%) were observed with exposure to concentrated PM. The findings suggest that ambient PM may adversely affect the lungs as well as the heart.

Rats have also been exposed to concentrated $PM_{2.5}$ in New York City. Gordon et al. (1997) exposed normal and monocrotaline-treated Fischer 344 rats to concentrated ambient urban PM for 3 hours and monitored for physiological, biochemical, and cellular changes up to 24 hours after exposure. At three hours postexposure, the percentage of neutrophils in peripheral blood of both normal and monocrotaline-treated rats was significantly elevated in PM-exposed animals ($p < 0.001$) while the percentage of lymphocytes was decreased ($p < 0.001$). No hematological changes were observed in animals exposed to HEPA-filtered air from the particle concentrator, suggesting that these changes were a result of exposure to the particulate and not the gaseous components of urban air. Moreover, in monocrotaline-treated but not normal rats, these systemic changes were accompanied by changes in lavage fluid parameters. Exposure of monocrotaline-treated rats to $360\,\mu g/m^3$ PM produced significant increases in lavage fluid protein and LDH at 24 hours after exposure. Heart rate and core temperature were monitored in unrestrained rats for 1 hour prior to, and 24 hours after, the 3-hour exposure to air or PM. In comparison to air-exposed monocrotaline rats, a significant increase in heart rate was observed in PM-exposed rats during the first hour postexposure. The observed pattern of hematological, biochemical, and cardiovascular changes suggests an activation of the sympathetic stress response.

The New York City concentrator has also been used by Zelikoff et al. (1997) to examine immunosuppression as a possible mechanism for PM-induced effects. In order to establish baseline information prior to studies with pneumonia-producing bacteria, six-months old rats were exposed either once for 3 hours or repeatedly (3 h/d for 4 d) to concentrated PM from NYC air at concentrations near the PM_{10} NAAQS ($150\,\mu g/m^3$). Rats were sacrificed 3 or 24 hours after exposure and effects on blood cell profiles, hematocrit/leukocrit, pulmonary histology, lavaged cell numbers/viability, macrophage (Mø) function, as well as on lung cell damage, were evaluated. In the absence of any histopathological changes, lung cell damage, or pulmonary inflammation, a single inhalation of concentrated $PM_{2.5}$ (about $200\,\mu g/m^3$) significantly depressed superoxide (O_2^-) production by macrophages, and altered the percentages of circulating neutrophils and lymphocytes in the blood 3 hours following exposure; after 24 hours, lavaged cell numbers were elevated, but production of O_2^- and blood cell values were similar to that of the filtered NYC air controls. Blood cell values were also significantly altered at the lower exposure concentration ($\sim 150\,\mu g/m^3$) after 3 hours. However, similar effects were not observed following repeated exposure.

Kleinman et al. (1996) examined the toxicology of PM10 components using laboratory-generated aerosols containing acidic ammonium bisulfate (ABS), and resuspended carbon black (C), a surrogate for combustion-generated carbonaceous aerosols using geriatric rats (about 24 months old) as a model. In vivo subchronic 4 week nose-only exposures (4 h/d, 3 d/wk) of rats ($n = 10$ per endpoint per atmosphere) were performed with atmospheres containing either C or ABS at concentrations of 60 and $70\,\mu g/m^3$, respectively, or to a mixture of C + ABS. Ozone (O_3) might be an important co-pollutant with PM10, therefore mixtures of C + O_3 and C + ABS + O_3 were also tested. Control groups were exposed to purified air or to O_3 alone. The particle size was $0.5\,\mu m$ mass median aerodynamic diameter for both C and ABS aerosols. Biological endpoints examined included permeability, inflammatory responses, macrophage functions, collagen synthesis, mucus production, and lung morphometry. Macrophages from rats exposed to either C + O_3 or C + ABS + O_3 showed functional changes that were significantly altered in comparison to those from rats exposed to O_3 alone. The O_3-containing mixtures induced significant changes in collagen concentrations in lung tissue and resulted in significant increases in lung cell turnover rates; both changes are suggestive of irritant effects on the lung.

Changes in both of these parameters were greatest following exposures to the mixture that contained ABS. Corresponding changes had not been seen in previous exposure studies using younger rats.

Collectively these animal inhalation studies indicate that diseased and elderly rats respond to PM inhalation with greater responses than healthy young animals, and they produce responses that appear relevant to excess mortality and morbidity in sensitive human populations. Future extensions of these studies using specific components of the ambient $PM_{2.5}$ could help to identify the most biologically active components of the ambient $PM_{2.5}$ mixtures, as well as the host factors that put an individual at greatest risk.

DISCUSSION AND CURRENT KNOWLEDGE ON THE HEALTH EFFECTS OF PM

The results of studies in recent years, summarized above, have made it possible to frame the remaining unresolved issues in a more coherent and focused manner.

One key issue is the role of $SO_4^=$, and why it consistently correlates with mortality and morbidity as well as, or better than, other metrics of PM pollution. It is extremely unlikely that $SO_4^=$, per se, is a causal factor. If it is not, then it must be acting as a surrogate index for one or more other components in the PM mixture. Evidence for and against an active role for some PM constituents is presented in Table 2-7.

One possibility is that the effects are really due to the $PM_{2.5}$ mass, irrespective of particle composition, and that $SO_4^=$ is a more stable measurement of airborne $PM_{2.5}$ than is the reported $PM_{2.5}$ itself. The ambient $PM_{2.5}$ includes nitrates (primarily ammonium nitrate) and organics formed by photochemical reactions in the atmosphere. There can be considerable volatilization of these species on sampling filters, resulting in negative mass artifacts whose magnitude varies with source strengths and ambient temperature.

Another possibility is that $SO_4^=$ is serving as a surrogate for H^+, a more likely active agent on the basis of the results of controlled exposure studies in humans and animals. The support for this hypothesis is summarized in Table 2-7 and discussed further in Chapter 23.

A third possibility is that the causal factor is the number concentration of irritating particles that would be dominated by the particles in the ultrafine mode (diameters below 50 nm) (Oberdörster et al., 1995). Epidemiologic support for this hypothesis has been provided by Peters et al. (1997), who reported closer associations between peak expiratory flow rates and symptoms in adult asthmatics with particle number concentration than with fine particle mass concentration in Erfurt, Germany.

A fourth possibility is that soluble transition metals in the ambient PM generate sufficient amounts of reactive oxygen species in the respiratory tract airways to cause inflammatory responses and chronic lung damage (Pritchard et al., 1996).

A fifth possibility has been proposed by Friedlander and Yeh (1996), that reactive chemical species, such as peroxides, are responsible for the health effects associated with fine particles and that $SO_4^=$, being a product of chemical reactions involving hydrogen peroxide, serves as a surrogate measure of the airborne peroxides.

It is also possible that effects are related to a hybrid of H^+ and ultrafines, namely acid-coated ultrafine particles. As discussed in Chapter 23, sulfuric acid coatings on ultrafine zinc oxide particles produce about the same responses as pure sulfuric acid for a given number of equivalently sized particles, yet the coated particles only had one-tenth of the acid content per unit volume of air. Thus the response may be related to the number of acidic particles that deposit on the lung surfaces rather than the amount of acid deposited. In other words, the total concentration of H^+ may be a better surrogate of the active agent

TABLE 2-7   Components of Ambient Air PM and Some or All Effects Associated with PM Exposures

Component	Evidence for role in Effects	Doubts
Strong acid (H^+)	• Statistical associations with health effects in most recent studies for which ambient H^+ concentrations were measured • Coherent responses for *some* health endpoints in human and animal inhalation and *in vitro* studies at environmentally relevant doses	• Similar PM-associated effects observed in locations with low ambient H^+ levels • Very limited data base on ambient concentrations
Ultrafine particles ($D \leq 0.2\,\mu m$)	• Much greater potency per unit mass in animal inhalation studies (H^+, Teflon, and TiO_2 aerosols) than for same materials in larger diameter fine particle aerosols • Concept of "irritation signaling" in terms of number of particles per unit airway surface	• Only one positive study on response in humans • Absence of relevant data base on ambient concentrations
Soluble transition metals	• Recent animal study evidence of capability to induce lung inflammation	• Absence of relevant data on responses in humans • Absence of relevant data on ambient concentrations
Peroxides	• Close association in ambient air with $SO_4^=$ • Strong oxidizing properties	• Absence of relevant data on responses in humans or animals • Very limited data base on ambient concentrations

than $SO_4^=$ or $PM_{2.5}$, but it still is a crude index for the number concentration of irritant particles. Amdur and Chen (1989) suggested that number concentration was important for sulfuric acid aerosol, and Hattis et al. (1987, 1990) gave the concept a name, "irritation signaling." Research of Chen et al. (1995) indicates that acid-coated particles much smaller than those discussed by Hattis et al. (1987, 1990) are capable of producing lung responses.

If the number concentration of acid-coated particles is the most relevant index of the active agent in ambient PM, then new sampling techniques will be needed to characterize ambient air concentrations and personal exposures.

Other components of the ambient ultrafine aerosol have not been well characterized either, and they may also be important health stressors. One class is the volatile trace metals (e.g., As, Cd, Cu, Pb, Zn) which condense as ultrafine particles in the effluent airstream of fossil fuel combusters (Amdur et al., 1986) and are inefficiently captured by air cleaners for fly ash collection. Another class is the ultrafine organics from atmospheric photochemical reaction sequences.

Any remaining inconsistency between the epidemiological findings and the results of the controlled exposure studies may be explicable on the basis that the relatively rare individuals who respond in the epidemiological populations are an especially responsive subset of the overall population, and that there is a low probability that such sensitive individuals would be included in the controlled exposure studies in the laboratory. An alternative hypothesis is that the controlled exposure atmospheres have not contained the highly toxic components or ultrafine particle sizes that may be present in ambient atmospheres.

In summary, in many communities in the United States and around the world, available pollutant concentration data are used to relate excess daily mortality and morbidity to ambient pollution at current levels. However, it is not at all clear whether any of the pollutant indexes used are causally related to the health effects, or if none of them are, which is the best index or surrogate measure of the causal factor(s). This gap can best be addressed by analyses of pollutant associations with mortality and morbidity in locations where a number of different pollutant metrics are available simultaneously, using analytic methods not dependent on arbitrary model assumptions.

STANDARDS AND EXPOSURE GUIDELINES

While more research is needed on causal factors for the excess mortality and morbidity associated with PM in ambient air, and on the characterization of susceptibility factors, responsible public health authorities cannot wait for the completion and peer review of this research. It is already clear that the evidence for adverse health effects attributable to PM challenges the conventional paradigm used for setting ambient air standards and guidelines, that is, that a threshold for adversity can be identified, and a margin of safety can be applied. Excess mortality is clearly an adverse effect, and the epidemiological evidence is consistent with a linear nonthreshold response for the population as a whole.

A revision of the Air Quality Guidelines of the World Health Organization-Europe (WHO-EURO) is currently nearing completion. The Working Group of WHO-EURO on PM, at meetings in October 1994 and October 1996 in Bilthoven, The Netherlands, determined that it could not recommend a PM Guideline. Instead, it prepared a tabular presentation of the estimated changes in daily average PM concentrations needed to produce specific percentage changes in (1) daily mortality, (2) hospital admissions for respiratory conditions, (3) bronchodilator use among asthmatics, (4) symptom exacerbation among asthmatics, and (5) peak expiratory flow. The concentrations needed to produce these changes were expressed in PM_{10} for all five response categories. For mortality and hospital admissions, they were also expressed in terms of $PM_{2.5}$ and $SO_4^=$. Using this guidance, each national or local authority setting air quality standards can decide how much adversity is acceptable for its population. Making such a choice is indeed a challenge.

In the United States the EPA administrator promulgated revised PM NAAQS in July 1997 (Federal Register 1997, 62:38762-38896) in recognition of the inadequate public health protection provided by enforcement of the 1987 NAAQS for PM_{10}. For PM_{10}, the $50\,\mu g/m^3$ annual average would be retained without change, and the 24-hour PM_{10} of $150\,\mu g/m^3$ would be *relaxed* by applying it only to the 98th percentile value (8th highest in each year) rather than to the 4th highest over 3 years. These PM_{10} standards would be supplemented by the creation of new $PM_{2.5}$ standards. The annual average $PM_{2.5}$ would be $15\,\mu g/m^3$, and the 24-hour $PM_{2.5}$ of $65\,\mu g/m^3$ would apply to the 98th percentile value. Implementation of the new $PM_{2.5}$ NAAQS will advance the degree of public health protection for ambient air PM, especially in the eastern United States and in some large cities in the west where fine particles are major percentages of PM_{10}.

In my view, the new PM NAAQS are not too strict. In terms of its introduction of a more relevant index of exposure and a modest degree of greater public health protection, it represents a prudent judgment call by the EPA administrator. These NAAQS may not be strict enough to fully protect public health, but there remain significant knowledge gaps on both exposures and the nature and extent of the effects that made the need for more restrictive NAAQS difficult to justify. It is essential that adequate research resources be applied to filling these gaps before the next round of NAAQS revisions during the first decade of the next century.

REFERENCES

Amdur, M. O., and L. C. Chen. 1989. Furnace-generated acid aerosols: Speciation and pulmonary effects. *Environ. Health Perspect.* 79: 147–150.

Bates, D. V. 1992. Health indices of the adverse effects of air pollution: The question of coherence. *Environ. Res.* 59: 336–349.

Burnett, R. T., R. E. Dales, M. E. Raizenne, D. Krewski, P. W. Summers, G. R. Roberts, M. Raad-Young, T. Dann, and J. Brook. 1994. Effects of low ambient levels of ozone and sulfates on the frequency of respiratory admissions to Ontario hospitals. *Environ. Res.* 65: 172–194.

Burnett. R. T., R. E. Dales, M. E. Raizenne, D. Krewski, R. Vincent, T. Dann, and J. Brook. 1995. Associations between ambient particulate sulfate and admissions to Ontario hospitals for cardiac and respiratory diseases. *Am. J. Epidemiol.* 142: 15–22.

Chen, L. C., C. Y. Wu, Q. S. Qu, and R. B. Schlesinger. 1995. Number concentration and mass concentration as determinants of biological response to inhaled irritant particles. *Inhal. Toxicol.* 7: 577–588.

Chestnut, L. G., J. Schwartz, D. A. Savitz, and C. M. Burchfiel. 1991. Pulmonary function and ambient particulate matter: Epidemiological evidence from NHANES I. *Arch. Environ. Health* 46: 135–144.

Chinn, S., C. Florey, V. du, I. G. Baldwin, and M. Gorgol. 1981. The relation of mortality in England and Wales 1969–73 to measurements of air pollution. *J. Epidemiol. Commun. Health* 35: 174–179.

Ciocco, A., and D. J. Thompson. 1961. A follow-up of Donora ten years after: Methodology and findings. *Am. J. Public Health* 51: 155–164.

Commins, B. T., and R. E. Waller. 1963. Determination of particulate acid in town air. *Analyst* 88: 364–367.

Damokosh, A. I., J. D. Spengler, D. W. Dockery, J. H. Ware, and F. E. Speizer. 1993. Effects of acidic particles on respiratory symptoms in 7 U.S. communities. *Am. Rev. Respir. Dis.* 147: A632.

Delfino, R. J., M. R. Becklake, and J. A. Hanley. 1994. The relationship of urgent hospital admissions for respiratory illnesses to photochemical air pollution levels in Montreal. *Environ. Res.* 67: 1–19.

Dockery, D. W., J. Schwartz, and J. D. Spengler. 1992. Air pollution and daily mortality: Associations with particulates and acid aerosols. *Environ. Res.* 59: 362–373.

Dockery, D. W., C. A. Pope III, X. Xu, J. D. Spengler, J. H. Ware, M. E. Fay, B. G. Ferris Jr., and F. E. Speizer. 1993. An association between air pollution and mortality in six U.S. cities. *N. Engl. J. Med.* 329: 1753–1759.

Dockery, D. W., J. Cunningham, A. I. Damokosh, L. M. Neas, J. D. Spengler, P. Koutrakis, J. H. Ware, M. Raizenne, and F. E. Speizer. 1996. Health effects of acid aerosols on North American children: Respiratory symptoms. *Environ. Health Perspect.* 104: 500–505.

Fennelly, K., and B. Bucher Bartelson. 1996. Cardiopulmonary morbidity associated with particulate air pollution in Denver, CO, 1989–1992. Abstract: *Proc. 2nd Colloquium on Particulate Air Pollution and Human Health*, eds. J. Lee and R. Phalen, pp. 3–41. Salt Lake City: University of Utah.

Firket, J. 1936. Fog along the Meuse Valley. *Trans. Faraday Soc.* 32: 1192–1197.

Friedlander, S. K., and E. K. Yeh. 1996. The submicron atmospheric aerosol as a carrier of reactive chemical species: Case of peroxides. In *Proceedings of 2nd Colloquium on Particulate Air Pollution and Human Health*, eds. J. Lee and R. Phalen, pp. 4–122 to 4–135. Irvine, University of California, Air pollution Health Effects Laboratory, December.

Godleski, J. J., C. Sioutas, M. Katler, and P. Koutrakis. 1996. Death from inhalation of concentrated ambient air particles in animal models of pulmonary disease. *Am. J. Respir. Crit. Care Med.* 153(4): A15.

Godleski, J. J., C. Sioutas, R. L. Verrier, C. R. Killingsworth, E. Lovett, G. G. Krishna Murthy, V. Hatch, J. M. Wolfson, S. T. Ferguson, and P. Koutrakis. 1997. Inhalation exposure of canines to concentrated ambient air particles. *Am. J. Respir. Crit. Care Med.* 155(4): A246.

Gordon, T., C. Nadziejko, L. C. Chen, C. P. Fang, and R. B. Schlesinger. 1997. Adverse health effects of ambient PM in compromised animal models. Abstract, 1977 Annual Conf. of Health Effects Inst., Annapolis, MD.

Hattis, D., J. M. Wasson, G. S. Page, B. Stern, and C. A. Franklin. 1987. Acid particles and the tracheobronchial region of the respiratory system — An "irritation-signaling" model for possible health effects. *J. Air Pollut. Control Assoc.* 37: 1060–1066.

Hattis, D. S., S. Abdollahzadeh, and C. A. Franklin. 1990. Strategies for testing the "irritation-signaling" model for chronic lung effects of fine acid particles. *J. Air Waste Manag. Assoc.* 40: 322–330.

Hoek, G., and B. Brunekreef. 1993. Acute effects of a winter air pollution episode on pulmonary function and respiratory symptoms of children. *Arch. Environ. Health* 48: 328–335.

Holland, W. W., and D. D. Reid. 1965. The urban factor in chronic bronchitis. *Lancet* 1: 445–448.

Ito, K., P. Kinney, and G. D. Thurston. 1995. Variations in PM10 concentrations within two metropolitan areas and their implications to health effects analyses. *Inhal. Toxicol.* 7: 735–745.

Ito, K., and G. D. Thurston. 1996. Daily PM_{10}/mortality associations: An investigation of at risk populations. *J. Expos. Anal. Environ. Epidemiol.* 6: 79–96.

Ives, J. E., R. H. Britten, D. W. Armstrong, et al. 1936. *Atmospheric Pollution of American Cities for the Years 1931 to 1933.* Public Health Bulletin 224, U.S. Public Health Service. Washington, DC: Government Printing Office.

Kinney, P. L., K. Ito, and G. D. Thurston. 1995. A sensitivity analysis of mortality/PM_{10} associations in Los Angeles. *Inhal. Toxicol.* 7: 59–69.

Kleinman, M. T., W. J. Mautz, R. F. Phalen, and D. K. Bhalla. 1996. Toxicity of constituents of PM_{10} inhaled by aged rats. In *Proceedings of 2nd Colloquium on Particulate Air Pollution and Human Health*, eds. J. Lee and R. Phalen, pp. 3–58. Irvine, University of California.

Lave, L. B., and E. P. Seskin. 1970. Air pollution and human health. The quantitative effect, with an estimate of the dollar benefit of pollution abatement, is considered. *Science* 169: 723–733.

Lawther, P. J. 1963. Compliance with the Clean Air Act: Medical aspects. *J. Inst. Fuel* 36: 341–344.

Lawther, P. J., R. E. Waller, and M. Henderson. 1970. Air pollution and exacerbations of bronchitis. *Thorax* 25: 525–539.

Martin, A. E., and W. H. Bradley. 1960. Mortality, fog and atmospheric pollution: An investigation during the winter of 1958–59. *Mon. Bull. Minist. Health Public Health Lab. Serv.* (BG) 19: 56–73.

Megonnel, W. H. 1957. *Historical Review.* Prepared for the Study of Air Pollution in the New York–Metropolitan Area conducted by Interstate Sanitation Commission. New York.

Ministry of Health. 1954. Mortality and Morbidity during the London Fog of December 1952. Her Majesty's Stationary Office, London.

Neas, L. M., D. W. Dockery, P. Koutrakis, D. J. Tollerud, and F. E. Speizer. 1995. The association of ambient air pollution with twice daily peak expiratory flow rate measurement in children. *Am. J. Epidemiol.* 141: 111–122.

NYC. 1976. *Department of Air Resources, Annual Report.* City of New York.

Oberdörster, G., R. M. Gelein, J. Ferin, and B. Weiss. 1995. Association of particulate air pollution and acute mortality: Involvement of ultrafine particles. *Inhal. Toxicol.* 7: 111–124.

Ostro, B., J. M. Sanchez, C. Aranda, and G. S. Eskeland. 1995. Air pollution and mortality: Results of a study of Santiago, Chile. *J. Expos. Anal. Environ. Epidemiol.* 6: 97–114.

Ozkaynak, H., and G. D. Thurston. 1987. Associations between 1980 U.S. mortality rates and alternative measures of airborne particle concentration. *Risk Anal.* 7: 449–461.

Ozkaynak, H., J. Xue, P. Severance, R. Burnett, and M. Raizenne. 1994. Associations between daily mortality, ozone, and particulate air pollution in Toronto, Canada. Presented at Colloquim on Particulate Air Pollution and Human Mortality and Morbidity, January, Irvine, CA. Air Pollution Health Effects Laboratory; Report 94–02. University of California at Irvine.

Peters, A., E. Wichmann, T. Tuch, J. Heinrich, and J. Heyder. 1997. Respiratory effects are associated with the number of ultrafine particles. *Am. J. Respir. Crit. Care Med.* 155: 1376–1383.

Poloniecki, J. D., R. W. Atkinson, A. Ponce de Leon, and H. R. Anderson. 1997. Daily time series for cardiovascular hospital admissions and pervious day's air pollution in London, UK. *Occup. Environ. Med.* 54: 535–540.

Pope, C. A. III, and D. W. Dockery. 1992a. Acute health effects of PM_{10} pollution on symptomatic and asymptomatic children. *Am. Rev. Respir. Dis.* 145: 1123–1128.

Pope, C. A. III, J. Schwartz, and M. R. Ransom. 1992b. Daily mortality and PM_{10} pollution in Utah Valley. *Arch. Environ. Health* 47: 211–217.

Pope, C. A. Jr., D. W. Dockery, and J. Schwartz. 1995a. Review of epidemiological evidence of health effects of particulate air pollution. *Inhal. Toxicol.* 7: 1–18.

Pope, C. A. III, M. J. Thun, M. Namboodiri, D. W. Dockery, J. S. Evans, F. E. Speizer, and C. W. Heath Jr. 1995b. Particulate air pollution is a predictor of mortality in a prospective study of U.S. adults. *Am. J. Resp. Crit. Care Med.* 151: 669–674.

Pope, C. A. III, and L. S. Kalkstein. 1996. Synoptic weather modelling and estimates of the exposure-response relationship between daily mortality and particulate air pollution. *Environ. Health Perspect.* 104: 414–420.

Pritchard, R. J., A. J. Ghio, J. R. Lehmann, D. W. Winsett, J. S. Tepper, P. Park, M. I. Gilmour, K. L. Dreher, and D. L. Costa. 1996. Oxidant generation and lung injury after particulate air pollution exposure increase with the concentrations of associated metals. *Inhal. Toxicol.* 8: 457–477.

Raizenne, M. E., R. T. Burnett, B. Stern, C. A. Franklin, and J. D. Spengler. 1989. Acute lung function responses to ambient acid aerosol exposures in children. *Environ. Health Perspect.* 79: 179–185.

Raizenne, M., L. M. Neas, A. I. Damokosh, D. W. Dockery, J. D. Spengler, P. Koutrakis, J. Ware, and F. E. Speizer. 1996. Health effects of acid aerosols on North American children: Pulmonary function. *Environ. Health Perspect.* 104: 506–514.

Samet, J. M., S. L. Zeger, J. E. Kelsall, J. Xu, and L. S. Kalkstein. 1997. Air pollution, weather, and mortality in Philadelphia 1973–1988. Report on Phase 1.B of the Particle Epidemiology Project. Health Effects Institute, Cambridge, MA 02139.

Schrenk, H. H., H. Heimann, G. D. Clayton, and W. M. Gafater. 1949. Air pollution in Donora, Pennsylvania, Public Health Bull. 306. Washington, DC: Government Printing Office.

Schwartz, J. 1989. Lung function and chronic exposure to air pollution: A cross-sectional analysis of NHANES II. *Environ. Res.* 50: 309–321.

Schwartz, J. 1993a. Air pollution and daily mortality in Birmingham, Alabama. *Am. J. Epidemiol.* 137: 1136–1147.

Schwartz, J. 1993b. Particulate air pollution and chronic respiratory disease. *Environ. Res.* 62: 7–13.

Schwartz, J. 1994a. PM$_{10}$, ozone, and hospital admissions for the elderly in Minneapolis, MN. *Arch. Environ. Health* 49: 366–374.

Schwartz, J. 1994b. What are people dying of on high air pollution days? *Environ. Res.* 64: 26–35.

Schwartz, J. 1994c. Air pollution and hospital admissions for the elderly in Detroit, Michigan. *Am. J. Respir. Crit. Care Med.* 150: 648–655.

Schwartz, J. 1995. Short term fluctuations in air pollution and hospital admissions of the elderly for respiratory disease. *Thorax* 50: 531–538.

Schwartz, J. 1996. Air pollution and hospital admissions for respiratory disease. *Epidemiol.* 7: 20–28.

Schwartz, J., and R. Morris. 1995. Air pollution and cardiovascular hospital admissions for cardiovascular disease in Detroit, MI. *Am. J. Epidemiol.* 142: 23–35.

Stern, B. R., M. E. Raizenne, R. T. Burnett, L. Jones, J. Kearney, and C. A. Franklin. 1994. Air pollution and childhood respiratory health: Exposure to sulfate and ozone in 10 Canadian rural communities. *Environ. Res.* 66: 125–142.

Studnicka, M. J., T. Frischer, R. Meinert, A. Studnicka-Benke, K. Hajek, J. D. Spengler, and M. G. Neumann. 1995a. Acidic particles and lung function in children. A summer camp study in the Austrian Alps. *Am. J. Respir. Crit. Care Med.* 151: 423–430.

Studnicka, M. J., T. Frischer, R. Meinert, A. Studnicka-Benke, K. Hajek, J. D. Spengler, and M. G. Neumann. 1995b. Acidic particles and lung function in children. A summer camp study in the Austrian Alps. *Am. J. Respir. Crit. Care Med.* 151: 423–430.

Styer, P., N. McMillan, F. Gao, J. Davis, and J. Sacks. 1995. The effect of airborne particulate matter on daily death counts. *Environ. Health Perspect.* 103: 490–497.

Thurston, G. D., J. E. Gorczynski, P. Jaques, J. Currie, and D. He. 1992a. An automated sequential sampling system for particulate aerosols: Description, characterization, and field sampling results. *J. Expos. Anal. Environ. Epidemiol.* 2: 415–428.

Thurston, G. D., K. Ito, P. L. Kinney, and M. Lippmann. 1992b. A multi-year study of air pollution and respiratory hospital admissions in three New York State metropolitan areas: Results for 1988 and 1989 summers. *J. Expos. Anal. Environ. Epidemiol.* 2: 429–450.

Thurston, G. D., J. E. Gorczynski, J. H. Currie, D. He, K. Ito, J. Hipfner, J. Waldman, P. J. Lioy, and M. Lippmann. 1994a. The nature and origins of acid summer haze air pollution in Metropolitan Toronto, Ontario. *Environ. Res.* 65: 254–270.

Thurston, G. D., K. Ito, C. G. Hayes, D. V. Bates, and M. Lippmann. 1994b. Respiratory hospital admissions and summertime haze air pollution in Toronto, Ontario: Consideration of the role of acid aerosols. *Environ. Res.* 65: 271–290.

Thurston, G. D. 1995. Personal communication of table prepared for draft EPA Criteria Document on Particulate Matter.

Thurston, G. D., M. Lippmann, M. Scott, and J. M. Fine. 1997. Summertime haze pollution and children with asthma. *Am. J. Respir. Crit. Care Med.* 155: 654–660.

Touloumi, G., S. J. Pocock, K. Katsouyanni, and D. Trichopoulos. 1994. Short-term effects of air pollution on daily mortality in Athens: A time-series analysis. *Int. J. Epidemiol.* 23: 1–11.

U.S. EPA. 1993. *Air Quality Criteria for Oxides of Nitrogen.* EPA/600/8-91/049F. Washington, DC: U.S. Environmental Protection Agency.

U.S. EPA. 1996a. *Air Quality Criteria for Particulate Matter.* EPA/600/P-95/001F. Washington, DC: U.S. Environmental Protection Agency.

U.S. EPA. 1996b. Review of the National Ambient Air Quality Standards for Particulate Matter: OAQPS Staff Paper. EPA-452/R-96-013. U.S. Environmental Protection Agency, Research Triangle Park, NC.

Wang, X., H. Ding, L. Ryan, and X. Xu. 1997. Association between air pollution and low birth weight: A community-based study. *Environ. Health Perspect.* 105: 514–520.

Ware, J. H., L. A. Thibodeau, F. E. Speizer, S. Colome, and B. G. Ferris Jr. 1981. Assessment of the health effects of atmospheric sulfur oxides and particulate matter: Evidence from observational studies. *Environ. Health Perspect.* 41: 255–276.

Woodruff, T. J., J. Grillo, and K. C. Schoendorf. 1997. The relationship between selected causes of postneonatal infant mortality and particulate air pollution in the United States. *Environ. Health Perspect.* 105: 608–612.

Xu, X, H. Ding, and X. Wang. 1995. Acute effects of total suspended particles and sulfur dioxide on preterm delivery: A community-based cohort study. *Arch. Environ. Health* 50: 407–415.

Yant, W. P., et al. 1941. Carbon Monoxide and Particulate Matter in Air of Holland Tunnel and Metropolitan New York. Report of Investigations, U.S. Department of Interior, Bureau of Mines, Washington, DC.

Zelikoff, J. T., C. P. Fang, C. Nadziejko, T. Gordon, R. B. Schlesinger, M. D. Cohen, and L. C. Chen. 1997. Immunosuppression as a possible mechanism for particulate matter (PM)-induced effects upon host mortality. *Am. J. Respir. Crit. Care Med.* 155(4): A245.

3 Asbestos and Other Mineral and Vitreous Fibers

MORTON LIPPMANN, Ph.D.

IMPORTANT SPECIAL PROPERTIES OF FIBERS

Asbestos

Asbestos is a geological term used to describe silicate minerals that display special qualities and properties (Langer and Nolan, 1986; Langer et al., 1990). The mineralogy and chemistry of asbestos fibers are summarized in Table 3-1. It is the fibrous habit or "asbestiform" nature of these minerals, as well as their occurrence as millimeter-long fibers, that separate them from other silicate minerals and gave them commercial importance. They are good thermal and acoustic insulators, those low in iron are good electrical insulators, and different varieties show good stability in alkaline and in acid environments. In particular, their high tensile strength and flexibility make them useful as reenforcing agents in building products. Over 200 commercial products have used asbestos (Zoltai, 1979). The minerals tremolite, actinolite, and anthophyllite have the same name for both their asbestos and their common rock-forming variety. Thus there has been some confusion in regard to the presence of the asbestos in some products and environments. The asbestos minerals may occur in greater than trace amounts as both asbestiform fibers and mineral cleavage fragments in other commercial minerals. When the asbestiform fiber content exceeds 1%, it becomes an asbestos-containing material (ACM) under the current EPA definition.

The asbestiform nature is brought about by crystallographic properties. The sheet silicate structure of the serpentine mineral known as chrysotile has a dimensional mismatch between its tetrahedral coordinate Si_2O_5 layer and the octahedral coordinated MgOH (Brucite) layer, resulting in a structural deformation that causes the sheets to roll up to form cylindrical or "tubular" fibrils (Whittaker and Zussman, 1956). Weak interatomic bonds can hold together many hundreds of these individual unit fibrils to form a fiber (Yada, 1966). The other asbestos minerals are all in a class known as amphiboles. They have a double-chain silicate structure. It is the crystal structure and defects (offset twin planes, cleavage planes, and chain-width errors) that facilitate the release of the ultimate amphibole asbestos fibers (Chisholm, 1983; Veblen, 1980).

The formation, geological origin, and crystal structure of chrysotile inhibit cation substitution, and apart from small percentages of iron, magnesium depletion from weathering is the main variation observed. In contrast, the amphiboles have a crystal structure more favorable to cation substitution. Most commercial amphibole deposits

Environmental Toxicants: Human Exposures and Their Health Effects, 2/e. Edited by Morton Lippmann.
ISBN: 0-471-29298-2   © 2000 John Wiley & Sons, Inc.

TABLE 3-1   Commercial Asbestos Fiber Types That May Be Found in Buildings

Commercial Name	Mineral Name	Mineral Group	Chemical Formula	Occurrence in Buildings [a]
Chrysotile	Chrysotile	Serpentine	$(Mg, Fe)_6(OH)_8Si_4O_{10}$	× × ×
Crocidolite	Riebeckite	Amphibole	$Na_2(Fe^{3+})_2(Fe^{2+})_3(OH)_2Si_8O_{22}(\pm Mg)$	×
Anthophyllite	Anthophyllite	Amphibole	$(Mg, Fe)_2(OH)_2Si_8O_{22}$	×
Amosite	Grunerite	Amphibole	$Fe_2(OH)_2Si_8O_{22}(\pm Mg, Mn)$	× ×
Actinolite	Actinolite	Amphibole	$Ca_2Fe_5(OH)_2Si_8O_{22}(\pm Mg)$	×
Tremolite	Tremolite	Amphibole	$Ca_2Mg_5(OH)_2Si_8O_{22}(Fe)$	×

Note: Chrysotile always occurs with the asbestos habit and is therefore always asbestiform. Actinolite *asbestos* is found as a contaminant of amosite from South Africa. It is not known to be exploited anywhere in the world. Tremolite *asbestos* is exploited commercially in Korea. Anthophyllite *asbestos* is no longer commercially worked anywhere in the world. Note that the amphibole minerals anthophyllite, actinolite, and tremolite do not have a separate mineral name for their asbestos varieties as do riebeckite (crocidolite) and grunerite (amosite).

[a] Occurrence in buildings, frequency of observation: × × ×, very commonly found if product is asbestos containing; × ×, commonly found; ×, uncommonly found.

show relatively little variation in their chemistry, and they can be reliably identified as individual fibers by modern analytical transmission electron microscopy (TEM). The chemistry, structure, and properties of asbestos have been reviewed in many texts (e.g., Walton, 1982; Chisholm, 1983; Langer and Nolan, 1986, 1988; Langer et al., 1990).

Each of the asbestos fiber types appears to possess its own size range in airborne and tissue evaluations (Pooley and Clark, 1980; Burdett, 1985). TEM airborne size distributions of asbestos were first reported by Lynch, Ayer, and Johnson (1970), and many measurements around mines and mills were reported by Gibbs and Hwang (1975, 1980) and Hwang and Gibbs (1981). These and other measurements were reviewed by Berman and Chatfield (1989). Their principal conclusion was that some 9% (range: 1–50%) of chrysotile, 4% (range: 1–18%) of crocidolite, and 25% (range: 8–43%) of amosite would meet the industrial hygiene definition of asbestos (i.e., fibers $> 5\,\mu m$ long, $> 0.25\,\mu m$ wide, and aspect (length / width) ratio $> 3 : 1$). Measurements in U.K. textile and friction product plants (Rood and Scott, 1989) showed that only about 4% of chrysotile fibers fell into this category. However, a NIOSH study (Dement and Wallingford, 1990) of the same industries reported some 20% of fibers that would be counted by the industrial hygiene definition. Evaluations by TEM reveal that (1) crocidolite may form very fine fibers that range between 0.04 and $0.15\,\mu m$ in diameter; (2) amosite fibers are found to be greater in diameter, between 0.06 and $0.35\,\mu m$; and (3) chrysotile's fibrils are smallest of all, some 0.02 to $0.05\,\mu m$ in diameter. Specific properties that affect the biological activity of asbestos fibers include fiber type, length, diameter, and their durability within the lungs and at other sites in the body.

Man-made Mineral (Vitreous) Fiber

Most of the man-made mineral fibers (MMMF) are also man-made vitreous fibers (MMVF). They are generally made by spraying or extruding molten glass, rock, or furnace slag. The production technology and its historical development have been summarized by Konzen (1984). Both fiber lengths and diameters are polydisperse, especially for sprayed fibers. Subsequent fabrication of fiber mats for commercial products such as insulation, filters and fiber-reinforced composites results in the breakage of fibers into shorter-length segments. Konzen (1984) reported that the average fiber diameters decreased from 10 to $12\,\mu m$ in the 1940s to about $7.5\,\mu m$ in present-day products, but that the percentage less than $1\,\mu m$ decreased from 2.8 to 1.7% over the same period. Smaller diameter fibers (microfibers) can be fabricated, but they require much more energy to produce and are much more expensive. The superior properties of microfibers for insulation and tensile strength lead to their use in special applications where the greater costs can be justified, such as space shuttle cabins and ear plugs. The chemical composition of MMMF varies with the source materials, and their mechanical properties and durability, both in the products and in the body after inhalation and deposition, can vary greatly with their composition.

Mineral, rock, and slag wools are terms used for vitreous products made from the precursor materials named by melting and then drawing, centrifugal spinning, and steam- or air-jet blowing. These processes produce discontinuous fiber; the resulting materials are short in length and generally not spinnable. Feldspar and kaolinite, now principally confined to use in ceramic manufacture, were once used to make mineral wool. Indiana limestone has been used for the production of rock wool. Slags, by-products from many sources including iron and steelmaking and base-metal and copper smelting, have been used as the precursor material in the production of slag wools. The bulk and trace metal chemistry of these products vary greatly depending on the slag source. The principal ceramic fiber in commerce in the United States is of alumina-silica composition. These fibers have great stability, which is thought to be imparted by the structural match of the aluminum and silicon tetrahedra units.

Durable man-made fibers can also be produced from pure chemicals. For example, DuPont developed Fybex (potassium octatitinate) and Kevlar, an aramid, as fibrous asbestos substitutes. They found that Fybex produced mesotheliomas in hamsters (Lee et al., 1981) and did not pursue commercial application. By contrast, Kevlar had biological effects similar to those associated with nuisance dusts (Lee et al., 1983). These "chemical" fibers will not be discussed in any detail here except insofar as toxicity data obtained using them sheds light on the properties of fibers affecting *in vivo* toxicity. The principal focus on MMMF in this section is on human exposures to widely used commerical fibrous glass and the health risks associated with such exposures. The principal basis for the assessment is (1) the epidemiological data on occupational exposures and their effects; (2) the biological responses to fiber suspensions inhaled by laboratory animals, or injected into their lungs or pleural or peritoneal spaces; and (3) the aerodynamics, deposition, and clearance of airborne fibers within the respiratory tract.

An underlying hypothesis is that the biological effects of MMMFs are essentially the same as those produced by asbestos fibers, varying in potency rather than in nature. This hypothesis is based on the morphological and toxicological similarities between MMMFs and asbestos fibers. The concern arises from the well-documented evidence that asbestos fibers can cause lung fibrosis (asbestosis), bronchial cancer, and mesothelioma in humans and that both asbestos and MMMFs can cause these diseases in animals. Glass fibers have been associated with dermatitis and eye irritation in industrial workers, but these nonrespiratory health effects will not be reviewed further in this chapter, since they are not likely to be relevant to the much lower levels of nonoccupational exposures.

Properties of Vitreous Fibers

Vitreous materials are unable to maintain periodic atomic order over long distances (hundreds of Angstrom units). However, short-range order *is* observed, with local structures formed in clusters (Hoare, 1976; Turnbull, 1976). High-silica glasses have been observed to contain short-range structures, ranging from open silica tetrahedra (cristobalite) to SiO_4O_{11} chains (an anhydrous amphibole), as reported by Galakhov and Varshall (1973).

If different cationic metals are present in silica melts, they may coordinate oxygen differently, as related to cation charge (Z) and ionic radius (r). Patches of orderliness will form following the general principles of crystal chemistry. However, if unlike polyhedra form during quenching, they may have a tendency to unmix. The immiscibility regions in glass melts is compositionally dependent, a function of Z/r^2 (the determining factor in influencing cation field strength).

Because of their different chemistries, MMVFs behave differently in biological hosts. The aluminum-silicon ceramic fibers are stable (similar Z/r^2 values) and are therefore long-lived in vivo (durable). Slag wools, rich in trace metals, are for the most part neither stable nor durable in biological hosts. High-soda glasses are most unstable in biological hosts. The issue of fiber durability may be of extreme biological importance. Because MMVFs are generally not stable in vivo, they appear to carry less risk of producing disease (Lippmann, 1990). It is crucial to stress that these vitreous fibers exhibit a range or properties (Dunnigan, 1990).

Most commercially available vitreous fibers, used in insulation, fire retardant, and acoustical applications have diameters that range from about 4 to 6 μm. These values are consistent with aerodynamic diameters in the range of 12 to 18 μm (Timbrell, 1972). Thus commercial MMVFs are too large for penetration into the thorax, providing one important basis for the conclusion that MMVFs are less biologically hazardous than asbestos fibers (Lippmann, 1990).

Insulating glasses may be coated with binders, such as, phenol formaldehyde resins, or with mineral oil lubricants in a range of concentrations. The biological significance of these coating materials for long-term, chronic, diseases is unknown.

Major Uses in Buildings

There are many asbestos-containing products found in buildings, including thermal system insulation, structural fireproofing, acoustical and decorative finishes, sheet products, floor and ceiling tiles, and asbestos-containing felts (Sawyer, 1989). A number of other construction products may contain asbestos fibers as well, such as spackling, patching, and plastering compounds used in dry-wall construction and interior repair. In addition to natural mineral fiber, many of these formulations contain man-made vitreous fibers in combination with asbestos. Over the last decade MMVFs have replaced asbestos in many applications. The major asbestos-containing items to be found in buildings have been outlined by Spengler et al. (1989).

EXPOSURES TO FIBERS

Exposure Indexes

There has never been a fully satisfactory method for measuring airborne fiber exposures relevant to health effects, and much confusion has arisen because the various methods used cannot be readily interconverted. Three different types of concentration indexes have been used for airborne asbestos. Initially the most widely used index was the number of particles per unit volume of air, expressed in millions of particles per cubic foot (MPPCF). It was determined from impinger samples analyzed by the now obsolete U.S. Public Health Service standard optical microscopic dust-counting technique. A 10 × objective lens was used to count the number of particles that settled to the bottom of a dust-counting cell that was initially filled with a liquid suspension of particles from the impinger flask.

Since there was no discrimination between fibrous and nonfibrous particles, and since fibers are a very variable fraction of the total dust in most cases, dust counting for occupational exposure evaluations was replaced by a technique that counts fibers only. At the time the fiber-counting technique was first adopted (in the United Kingdom), it was already clear that long fibers were of most concern. This, combined with the practical limitation that fibers shorter than 5 μm could not be reliabily identified by light microscopy, led to the adoption of a counting procedure that uses a 45 × phase-contrast objective to count the fibers collected on a membrane filter, provided that they have a length > 5 μm and an aspect ratio > 3 (ACGIH-AIHA Aerosol Hazards Evaluation Committee, 1975). The phase-contrast optical method (PCOM) is specified in the OSHA occupational health standard for asbestos. Table 3-2 summarizes recommended occupational exposure limits and standards used in the United States over the last 50 years. Detailed guidance on the use of the PCOM method has been provided by the World Health Organization (WHO, 1997).

The third type of concentration index that has been used is based on the mass concentration of asbestos or on the mass concentration passing a precollector meeting the British Medical Research Council (BMRC) or American Conference of Governmental Industrial Hygienists (ACGIH) sampler acceptance criteria for "respirable" dust. Some of the recent animal inhalation studies report the chamber concentrations in terms of the "respirable" mass based on samples collected using samplers that meet the BMRC criteria.

Environmental exposures have been measured either in terms of fiber count or fiber mass. Fiber counts have been made using both phase-contrast optical and electron microscopy. The reported concentrations have differed according to the size distributions of the fibers, the resolving power of the microscope, and whether there was any discrimination in the analyses according to fiber type. The fiber mass index was developed by Selikoff et al. (1972). The fibers and fiber bundles in the sample are mechanically reduced to individual fibers and fibrils, which are then identified and measured by electron microscopy. Mass concentrations in nanograms per cubic meter are calculated from the numbers of fibers and fibrils and their dimensions.

Use of these various exposure indexes has sometimes led to the development of a site- or industry-specific exposure-response relationship for one or more of the asbestos-related diseases, but it has not been possible to develop any generic relationships. This demonstrates the inadequacy of our current indexes of exposure.

Exposure Levels

Esmen and Erdal (1990) reviewed published data on human occupational and nonoccupational exposure to fibers. They concluded that for the traditionally defined

TABLE 3-2 Recommended Air Concentration Limits and Standards for Asbestos

Group	Year	Limit
ACGIH	1946	5×10^6 particles / ft^3
ACGIH	1968[a]	12 fibers[c] / mL or 2×10^6 particles / ft^3
ACGIH	1970,[a] 1974[b]	5 fibers / mL
OSHA	1972	5 fibers / mL
OSHA	1976	2 fibers / mL
NIOSH	1976	0.1 fiber / mL
ACGIH	1978,[a] 1980[b]	0.2 fiber / mL for crocidolite
		0.5 fiber / mL for amosite
		2.0 fiber / mL for chrysotile and other forms
ACGIH	1997[a], 1998[b]	0.1 fiber / mL for all forms
OSHA	1976	2.0 fiber / mL
OSHA	1986	0.2 fiber / mL
OSHA	1992	0.1 fiber / mL

[a] Notice of intent.
[b] Adopted as threshold limit value (TLV).
[c] All fiber limits based on phase-contrast optical determination at 400–450 × magnification.

asbestos fibers, namely $> 5\,\mu m$ long, large amounts of the available data suffer from the diversity of sample collection and analysis methods. Simple generalizations suggest that occupational exposures are several orders of magnitude higher than environmental exposures; currently extant data and the current routine measurement practices present significant difficulties in the consistent interpretation of the data with respect to health effects. The human exposure data to many nonasbestos minerals that do exist in fibrous habit are very scant, and in view of the biological activity of some of these fibers, this lack may be of significant concern.

With respect to asbestos exposures in buildings, the Literature Review Committee of the Health Effects Institute–Asbestos Research (HEI-AR, 1991) grouped building occupants into three main categories:

1. Bystanders or nonoccupationally exposed building occupants, such as office workers, visitors, students, and teachers.
2. Housekeeping or custodial employees who may disturb materials in the course of routine cleaning and service functions.
3. Maintenance or skilled workers who may disturb asbestos-containing material (ACM) in the course of making repairs, installing new equipment, or during minor renovation activity.

Two other categories not often dealt with in the context of building occupancy were identified as
4. Abatement workers or others involved in the removal or renovation of structures with ACM.
5. Firefighters and other emergency personnel who may be present during or after the fabric of the building has been extensively damaged by fire, wind, water, or earthquake.

Building employees and contractor employees may disturb asbestos-containing materials (ACM) during the course of their normal work assignments, especially during maintenance and custodial activities. They may or may not know that they are disturbing ACM, and if they do, they may or may not have the equipment and motivation to take the appropriate precautions to minimize their exposure to airborne asbestos. Exposures of such workers can be high and warrant special concern. By far the most numerous category are the C1 building occupants. Persons in categories C2–C5 fall under Occupational Safety and Health Administration (OSHA) regulations for personal monitoring if their exposures exceed the permissible exposure limit (PEL) of 0.1 fiber/mL $> 5\,\mu m$ in length as an 8-hour time-weighted average, or the OSHA excursion limit of 1 f/mL in a half-hour, respectively; both are determined by PCOM. Persons in category C1 are not covered by any federal exposure limits. Ambient standards have been enacted in some states, such as Colorado and North Carolina.

There are relatively few published data on the concentrations of airborne fibers in public buildings. The Health Effects Institute–Asbestos Research (HEI-AR) sponsored Literature Review Panel recently compiled the available data, both published and such unpublished data as it could assemble (HEI-AR, 1991). In their report, the panel concluded that

A large number of buildings in the U.S. and other countries have been examined for airborne asbestos fibers within the past 20 years, and have yielded many thousands of air measurements (most unpublished). However, few building environments have been characterized in sufficient detail or sampled with sufficient analytical sensitivity to describe adequately the exposures of general building (C1) occupants.... Specific details are especially lacking for episodic and point-source releases of fibers into the air of buildings from maintenance and engineering activities, from repair and renovation operations, and from normal custodial functions.

Such data as are now available on the airborne concentrations of asbestos fibers of the dimensions most relevant to human health (i.e., fibers $> 5\,\mu m$ long) generally show average concentrations on the order of 0.00001 f/mL for outdoor rural air (except near asbestos-containing rock outcroppings) and average concentrations up to about ten fold higher in the outdoor air of urban environments. However, outdoor urban average concentrations above 0.0001 f/mL have been reported in certain circumstances as a result of local sources; for example, downwind from, or close to, frequent vehicle braking or activities involving the demolition or spray application of asbestos products. Data on ambient indoor levels of asbestos from direct TEM measurements have been averaged for each of a number of individual buildings. The following data are based on some 1377 air samples obtained in 197 different buildings not involved in litigation. The overall means of the studies on these buildings range from 0.00004 to 0.00063 f/mL, with upper 90th percentiles ranging from 0.00002 to 0.0008 f/mL. Grouped by building category, the mean concentrations are 0.00051, 0.00019, and 0.00021 f/mL in schools, residences, and public and commercial buildings, respectively, with upper 90th percentiles of 0.0016, 0.0005, and 0.0004, respectively (see Fig. 3-1).

FIBER DEPOSITION IN THE RESPIRATORY TRACT

There are five mechanisms that are important with respect to the deposition of fibers in respiratory tract airways. These are impaction, sedimentation, interception, electrostatic precipitation, and diffusion (see Fig. 1-8).

Impaction and sedimentation probabilities are governed by the aerodynamic diameter of the fibers, which, for long mineral fibers, are close to three times their physical diameters (Stöber et al., 1970; Timbrell, 1972). Most impaction occurs downstream of air jets in the larger airways, where the flow velocities are high and the momentum of the fiber

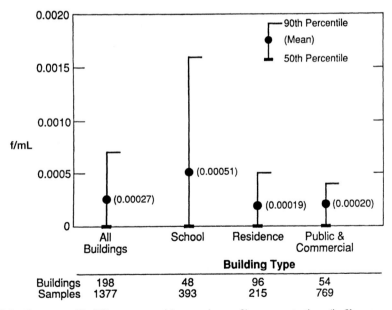

Figure 3-1 Summary of building average airborne asbestos fiber concentrations (in fibers per milliliter, with lengths $> 5\,\mu m$) in public and commercial buildings, (From data as reported by HEI-AR, 1991)

propels it out of the bending flow streamlines and onto relatively small portions of the epithelial surfaces. Sedimentation, on the other hand, is favored by low flow velocity, long residence times, and small airway size.

Electrostatic precipitation occurs primarily by image forces, in which charged particles induce opposite changes on airway surfaces. It is dependent on the ratio of electrical charge to aerodynamic drag. Little is known about the charge levels on MMMFs in the workplace. Jones, Johnston, and Vincent (1983) have shown that asbestos-fiber processing operations do generate fibrous aerosols with relatively high charge levels and that these charge levels are sufficient to cause an enhancement of fiber deposition in the lungs. Such an enhancement of fiber deposition for chrysotile asbestos in rats exposed by inhalation was demonstrated by Davis (1976).

Interception increases with fiber length. The greater the length, the more likely it is that the position of a fiber end will cause it to touch a surface that the center of mass would have missed.

Diffusional displacement results from collisions between air molecules and airborne fibers. For compact particles, diffusion becomes an important deposition mechanism for diameters smaller than about 0.5 µm. Fibers of similar diameter would be more massive and therefore be displaced less by a single molecular impact. Long fibers may have nearly simultaneous impacts from several gas molecules, and their random trajectories may tend to damp the net displacement. On the other hand, a single collision near a fiber end may rotate the fiber sufficiently to alter its interception probability. At the present time the role of diffusion in fiber deposition is poorly understood. Gentry et al. (1983) measured the diffusion coefficients of chrysotile and crocidolite asbestos fibers and found good agreement with theoretical predictions for chrysotile (0.4 µm mean diameter) but poor agreement with the more rodlike crocidolite (0.3 µm mean diameter).

The conductive airway region of the human lung consists of a series of bifurcating airways. The trachea is the only airway segment with a length-to-diameter ratio much greater than three. Single symmetrical fibers suspended in a laminar flow stream should tend to become aligned with the flow axis as they move through a lung airway. On the other hand, fiber agglomerates or nonfibrous particles would have more random orientations that would depend on their distributions of masses and drag forces. A fiber whose flow orientation differs from axial alignment would have an enhanced probability of deposition by interception.

A fiber's alignment is radically altered as it enters a daughter airway, and this loss of alignment with the flow at the entry of the daughter tube contributes to its deposition by interception at or near the carinal edge. To the extent that a fiber is entrained in the secondary flow streams that form at bifurcations, its deposition probability by interception should be further enhanced.

Sussman, Cohen, and Lippmann (1991a) performed an experimental study of fiber deposition within the larger tracheobronchial airways of the human lung using replicate hollow airway casts. For crocidolite fibers with diameters primarily in the 0.5 to 0.8 µm range, interception increased total deposition, with the effect increasing with fiber length, especially for fibers >10 µm in length. The effect was most pronounced at a high flow rate, such as 60 L/min. At a lower rate, such as 15 L/min, the effect was less pronounced, although still significant. This is consistant with greater axial alignment of the fibers during laminar flow within the airway.

Morgan and Holmes (1984) and Morgan et al. (1980) exposed rats for several hours by inhalation (nose only) to glass fibers 1.5 µm in diameter and 5, 10, 30 or 60 µm long. For fibers longer than 10 µm, essentially all of the fibers were deposited, mostly in the head. These results, together with the results of their earlier studies on asbestos fibers, indicate that penetrability of airborne fibers into the rat lung drops sharply with aerodynamic diameter above 2 µm. The results reported by Morgan and Holmes provide experimental verification that increasing fiber length increases lung deposition within the tracheobronchial airways.

Sussman, Cohen, and Lippmann (1990b) found that the deposition patterns of fibers in the larger lung airways are similar to those for particles of more compact shapes. In other words, the added deposition due to interception increased the deposition efficiencies without changing the pattern of deposition.

Most of the studies on particle deposition patterns and efficiencies in hollow bronchial airway casts of the larynx and the larger conductive airways of the human bronchial tree have been focused on deposition during constant flow inspirations. For studies of deposition during cyclic inspiratory flows, Gurman et al. (1984a, b) used a variable-orifice mechanical larynx model (Gurman et al., 1980) at the inlet in place of the fixed-orifice laryngeal models used in the prior constant-flow tests. In one series of tests, two replicate casts were connected in tandem. The corresponding terminal endings were connected with rubber tubing. Deposition in the downstream cast was analyzed to determine the deposition pattern and efficiencies during expiratory flow (Schlesinger et al., 1983).

Concern about sites of enhanced surface deposition density is stimulated by the observation that the larger bronchial airway bifurcations, which are favored sites for deposition, are also the sites most frequently reported as primary sites for bronchial cancer (Schlesinger and Lippmann, 1978).

Deposition patterns within the nonciliated airways distal to the terminal bronchioles may also be quite nonuniform. Brody et al. (1981) studied the deposition of chrysotile asbestos in lung peripheral airways of rats exposed for 1 hour to $4.3 \, \text{mg}/\text{m}^3$ of respirable chrysotile. The animals were killed in groups of 3 at 0, 5, and 24 hours and at 4 and 8 days after the end of the exposure. The pattern of retention on the epithelial surfaces was examined by scanning electron microscopy of lung sections cut to reveal terminal bronchiolar surfaces and adjacent airspaces. The rat does not have recognizable respiratory bronchioles, and the airways distal to the terminal bronchioles are the alveolar ducts. In rats killed immediately after exposure, asbestos fibers were rarely seen in alveolar spaces or on alveolar duct surfaces except at alveolar duct bifurcations. There were relatively high concentrations on bifurcations nearest the terminal bronchioles and lesser concentrations on more distal duct bifurcations. In rats killed at five hour, the patterns were similar, but the concentrations were reduced. Subsequent studies have shown that crocidolite asbestos (Roggli et al., 1987), Kevlar aramid synthetic fibers (Lee et al., 1983), and particles of more compact shape (Brody and Roe, 1983) also deposit in similar patterns and that the deposition patterns seen in the rat also occur in mice, hamsters, and guinea pigs (Warheit and Hartsky, 1990).

The sudden enlargement in air path cross section at the junction of the terminal bronchiole and alveolar duct may play a role in the relatively high deposition efficiency at the first alveolar duct bifurcation. Little has previously been known about the flow profiles in this region of the lung. However, Briant (1988) has shown that a net axial core flow in a distal direction and a corresponding net annular flow in a proximal direction take place during steady-state cyclic flow in tracheobronchial airways and that this could account for such concentrated deposition on the bifurcations of distal lung airways.

FIBER RETENTION, DISSOLUTION, AND TRANSLOCATION

The fate of fibers deposited on surfaces within the lungs depends on both the sites of deposition and the characteristics of the fibers. Within the first day, most fibers deposited on the tracheobronchial airways are carried proximally on the surface of the mucus to the larynx, to be swallowed and passed into the GI tract. The residence time for fibers on the surface of the tracheobronchial region is too short for any significant change in the size or composition of the fibers to take place.

Fibers deposited in the nonciliated airspaces beyond the terminal bronchioles are more slowly cleared from their deposition sites by a variety of mechanisms and pathways. These can be classified into two broad categories: translocation and disintegration.

Translocation refers to the movement of the intact fiber (1) along the epithelial surface to dust foci at the respiratory bronchioles, (2) onto the ciliated epithelium at the terminal bronchioles, or (3) into and through the epithelium, with subsequent migration to interstitial storage sites within the lung, along lymphatic drainage pathways, and for very thin short fibers, access via capillary blood to distant sites, as suggested by Monchaux et al. (1982). Boutin et al. (1996) suggested that thin fibers longer than 5 or 10 μm migrate toward the parietal pleura via the lymphatic pathway, where they accumulate preferentially in anthracotic "black spots" of the parietal pleura.

In a study by Dodson et al. (1990) comparing the fiber content of tissues from chronically exposed shipyard workers, they reported that while 10% of amphibole fibers in pleural plaque samples were longer than 5 μm and 8% were longer than 10 μm, the corresponding figures for chrysotile fibers were 3.1 and 0%. In lymph nodes, the corresponding figures for > 10 μm and > 5 μm lengths were 6.0 and 2.5% for amphiboles and 0 and 0% for chrysotile. In lung tissue, they were 41.0 and 20.0% for amphiboles and 14.0 and 4.0% for chrysotile. Boutin et al. (1996) noted that the black spots that concentrate longer fibers were in close contact with early pleural plaques. These studies indicate that fiber translocation is dependent on both fiber diameter and fiber length, and that length is an important determinant of biological responses. These issues will be discussed at greater length later in this chapter. Translocation may also occur after ingestion of the fibers by alveolar macrophages if the fibers are short enough to be fully ingested by the macrophages. Holt (1982) proposed that fibers phagocytosed by alveolar macrophages are carried by them toward the lung periphery by passing through alveolar walls and that some of these cells aggregate in alveoli near larger bronchioles and then penetrate the bronchiolar wall. Once in the bronchiolar lumen, they can be cleared by mucociliary transport.

Disintegration refers to a number of processes, including the subdivision of the fibers into shorter segments; partial dissolution of components of the matrix, creating a more porous fiber of relatively unchanged external size; or surface etching of the fibers, creating a change in the external dimensions of the fibers and/or complete dissolution. For MMMFs, fiber breakup is virtually all by length. The breakdown into smaller-diameter fibrils that is characteristic of asbestos fibers is seldom seen. For MMMFs, the relative importance of breakage into length segments, partial dissolution, and surface etching to the clearance of fibers depends on the size and composition of the fiber.

In the inhalation study of Brody et al. (1981) with chrysotile, their examination of tissues by TEM revealed that fibers deposited on the bifurcations of the alveolar ducts were taken up, at least partially, by type I epithelial cells during the 1 hour inhalation exposure. In the 5 hours period after exposure, significant amounts were cleared from the surfaces, and there was further uptake by both type I cells and alveolar macrophages. Within 24 hours after the exposure, there was an influx of macrophages to the alveolar duct bifurcations. The observations provide a basis for fiber penetration of the surface epithelium that does not hypothesize movement within macrophages.

Roggli and Brody (1984) exposed rats for one hour to a chrysotile aerosol and showed that fiber clearance was associated with sequential dimensional changes in the retained fibers and with a tendency for long, thin fibers to be retained within the interstitium of the lung parenchyma. Roggli, George, and Brody (1987) subsequently performed essentially the same study with a crocidolite aerosol. For the crocidolite there was a progressive increase in mean fiber length with increasing time post exposure, but the change was less pronounced than that for chrysotile. In addition there was no change in fiber diameter with time for the crocidolite. In contrast, the longitudinal splitting of the chrysotile into fibrils had caused a marked reduction of diameter with time.

Accumulation of fibers in distal lung airways may, by itself, slow the clearance of fibers and other particles from the lung. Ferin and Leach (1976) exposed rats by inhalation to 10, 5, or 1 mg/m^3 of UICC amosite or Canadian chrysotile for periods ranging from 1 hour to 22 days. Exposures at 10 mg/m^3 for 1–3 hours or for >11 days at 1 mg/m^3 suppressed the pulmonary clearance of TiO$_2$ particles.

Based on six-week inhalation studies of UICC amosite in rats, Bolton et al. (1983) at the Institute of Occupational Medicine (IOM) concluded that there is strong evidence for an overload of clearance at high lung burdens (exceeding about 1500 μg/rat), in which a breakdown occurs of the intermediate-rate clearance mechanisms (time constants of the order of 12 days). Their hypothesis is consistent with the results of other inhalation studies in rats with asbestos (Wagner and Skidmore, 1965), quartz (Ferin, 1972), and diesel soot (Chan et al., 1984). Vincent et al. (1985) modified the above hypothesis on the basis of additional rat inhalation studies at IOM for up to one year. They found the lung burden to scale directly in proportion to the exposure concentration in a way that seemed to contradict the overload hypothesis stated earlier. However, the general pattern exhibited by the results for asbestos is so similar to that for rats inhaling diesel fumes that they suggest that such accumulations are not specific to fibrous dust. They offered a modified hypothesis that whereas overload of clearance can take place at high lung burdens after exposure has ceased, it is cancelled by the sustained stimulus to clearance mechanisms provided by the continuous challenge of chronic exposure. The linearity of the increase in lung burden is explained in terms of a kinetic model involving sequestration of some inhaled material to parts of the lung where it is difficult to clear. The particular sequestration model favored by Vincent et al. (1985) is one in which the longer a particle remains in the lung without being cleared, the more likely it will be sequestrated (and therefore less likely be cleared).

Morrow (1988) developed a general hypothesis that dust overloading, which is typified by a progressive reduction of particle clearance from the deep lung, reflects a breakdown in alveolar macrophage (AM)-mediated dust removal as a result of the loss of AM mobility. The inabillity of the dust-laden AMs to translocate to the mucociliary escalator is correlated to an average composite particle volume per alveolar macrophage in the lung. When the volume of relatively nontoxic particles exceeds approximately 60 μm^3/AM, the overload effect appears to be initiated. When the distributed particulate volume exceeds 600 μm^3 per cell, the AM-mediated particle clearance virtually ceases, and agglomerated particle-laden macrophages remain in the alveolar region. For cytotoxic particles, these effects occur at lower loadings.

Oberdörster et al. (1990) performed additional lung instillation and inhalation studies to further explore the Morrow hypothesis and the respective roles of both AMs and polymorpho-nuclear leukocytes (PMNs), whose influx is indicative of a cellular inflammatory response. On the basis of their studies, they concluded that

- The delivered dose rate of particles to the lung is a determinant for the acute inflammatory PMN response: The same dose delivered over days by inhalation as opposed to sudden instillation leads to a very low response, conceivably reflecting the low release rate of phagocytosis-related inflammatory mediators (e.g., chemotactic factors) from AMs.
- The process of phagocytosis of "nuisance" particles by AMs rather than the interstitial access of the particles appears to initiate the influx of PMNs into the alveolar space.
- The surface area of the retained particles correlates best with inflammatory parameters rather than the phagocytized particle numbers, mass, or volume.

1. The surface area of the fraction of particles phagocytized by AMs correlates best with the influx of PMNs.
2. In contrast, another sign of inflammation, increase in alveolar epithelial permeability, correlates with the retained surface area of the particles in the total lung rather than with the surface area retained in the alveolar space.
3. Therefore, the two inflammatory parameters "alveolar PMN influx" and "alveolar epithelial permeability" are separate events likely to be triggered by different mechanisms.

- Interstitialization of particles appears to be important for inducing interstitial inflammatory responses including the induction of fibrotic reactions.
- If the interstitialized particle fraction exceeds the particle fraction remaining in the alveolar space, the influx of PMNs into the alveolar lumen decreases, conceivably reflecting a reversal of chemotactic gradients from alveolar space toward the interstitial space.

The IOM inhalation studies with UICC amosite were extended by Jones et al. (1988) to a lower concentration. In this study rats inhaled UICC amosite asbestos at an approximately constant concentration of $0.1 \, mg/m^3$ or, equivalently, $20 \, f/mL$ for 7 hours a day, 5 days a week, for up to 18 months. The lung burdens were compared with the previous results for higher-exposure concentrations of 1 and $10 \, mg/m^3$. Taken together, these results showed lung burdens rising pro rata with exposure concentration and exposure time. This accumulation of lung burden fit a kinetic model that takes account of the sequestration of material at locations in the lung from where it cannot be cleared.

Tran et al. (1997), at the IOM, showed that the overloading of the lung by fibers less than $15 \, \mu m$ long and particles follow the same kinetics, and are similarly affected by overloading. For long fibers ($> 25 \, \mu m$), the disappearance was independent of length and lung burden, implying that the clearance of such fibers occurs by dissolution and fragmentation into shorter lengths.

A differential lung clearance between fibers of chrysotile, a serpentine asbestos mineral, and the more rod-like amphibole asbestos fibers, such as amosite, anthophyllite, crocidolite, and tremolite was shown for rats that underwent chronic inhalation exposures (Wagner et al., 1974). The lung fiber burdens of the amphiboles rose continually throughout two years of exposure, and they declined slowly in the rats removed from exposure after 6 months. By contrast, the lung burdens in rats exposed to both Quebec and Zimbabwe chrysotile rose much more slowly during exposure, and seemed to decline after 12 months, even with further exposure.

Similar differential retention has been found in humans. Churg (1994) reported on analyses of lung tissue for 94 chrysotile asbestos miners and millers from the Thetford region of Quebec, Canada. The chrysotile deposit and exposure atmosphere contained a very small percentage of tremolite, yet the lungs contained more tremolite than chrysotile, and the tremolite content increased rapidly with the duration of exposure. Although most of the inhaled chrysotile was rapidly cleared from the lungs, a small fraction seemed to be retained indefinitely. After exposure ended, there was little or no clearance of either chrysotile or tremolite from the lungs of the Thetford miners and millers.

Albin et al. (1994) studied retention patterns in lung tissues from 69 Swedish asbestos-cement workers and 96 controls. They reported that chrysotile has a relatively rapid turnover in human lungs, whereas amphiboles (tremolite and crocidolite) have a slower turnover. They also noted that chrysotile retention may be dependent on dose rate, that chrysotile and crocidolite retention may be increased by smoking, and that chrysotile and tremolite retention may be increased by the presence of lung fibrosis.

The most direct evidence for the effect of altered dust clearance rates on the retention of inhaled fibers in humans comes from studies of the fiber content of the lungs of asbestos workers in various countries. Timbrell (1982) developed a model for fiber deposition and clearance in human lungs based on his analysis of the bivariate diameter and length distributions found in air and lung samples collected at an anthophyllite mine at Paakkila in Finland. At this particular mine the length and diameter distributions of the airborne dust were exceptionally broad, and historic exposures were very high. He observed that for workers with the highest exposure and most severe lung fibrosis (Ashcroft et al., 1988), the lung fiber distributions in some tissue segments approached those of the airborne fibers. Adjacent tissue, analyzed for extent of fibrosis, showed severe fibrotic lesions. He concluded that long-term retention was essentially equal to deposition in such segments. Figure 3-2 shows a series of retention curves for different degrees of lung fibrosis. These curves were determined by comparing the anthophyllite fiber size distributions in other tissue samples from the same lung with the distribution in the sample for which all fibers deposited were retained. Lung fibrosis is associated with increased fiber retention, and fiber retention is clearly associated with fiber length and diameter. More precise descriptions of the effect of fiber loading in the lung on fibrosis need to be based on the use of the most appropriate index of fiber loading.

Morgan, Holmes, and Davison (1982) and Morgan and Holmes (1984) studied the retention of 1.5 μm diameter glass fibers administered to rat lungs by intratracheal instillation. Retention at one year for 5 μm long fibers was 10%, whereas for 10 μm long fibers it was 20%. For the fibers which were 30 or 60 μm long, there was no measurable clearance during the first nine months. Further retention measurements were not made for these long fibers because of evidence that they were disintegrating and dissolving. This macrophage-mediated mechanical clearance is less effective for 10 μm fibers than for 5 μm fibers and is ineffective for fibers 30 μm long and longer. As confirmation, Morgan and Holmes (1984) cited work of Timbrell on the dimensions of anthophyllite fibers in the lungs of Finnish workers that suggest that the critical fiber length for mechanical clearance

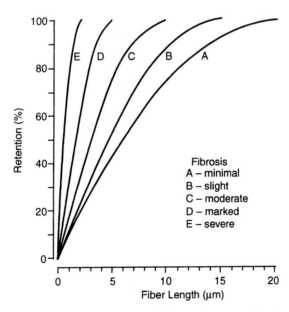

Figure 3-2   Effect of lung fibrosis on fiber retention in human lungs as a function of fiber length. The scores for fibrosis are *A*-minimal, *B*-slight, *C*-moderate, *D*-marked, and *E*-severe. (Source: Lippmann and Timbrell, 1990)

from the lungs is about 17 µm. They found that the solubility of MMMFs in rat lungs in vivo was dependent on both size and composition. The results were based on the sizes of fibers recovered from rats' lungs at various times following the inhalation exposures. For the glass fibers there was much less dissolution of the 5 and 10 µm fibers than of the 30 and 60 µm fibers. The dissolution of the long 1.5 µm diameter fibers was very nonuniform. Some were little changed in dimension, whereas others were reduced in diameter to 0.2 µm. On the other hand, for rockwool fibers >20 µm in length, there was no observable change in fiber dimensions after six months. Morgan and Holmes (1984) attributed the dependence of dissolution on fiber length to the differences and intra- and extracellular pH. The shorter fibers within macrophages are exposed to a pH of 7.2, whereas those outside were exposed to the extracellular pH of 7.4.

Bernstein et al. (1984) and Hammad (1984) also found evidence of substantial in vivo dissolution. LeBouffant et al. (1984) used X-ray analysis on individual fibers recovered from lung tissue to show the exchange of cations between the fibers and the tissues. For example, the fibers can lose calcium and gain potassium.

Insight on the solubility of fibers in vivo has also been obtained from in vitro solubility tests. Griffis, Henderson, and Pickrell (1981) found that glass fibers suspended in either buffered saline or serum simulant at 37°C for 60 days exhibited some solubility and that the sodium content of the residual fiber was reduced. Forster (1984) performed a comprehensive series of dissolution experiments. He used Gamble's solution for tests on samples of 18 different MMMFs at temperatures of 20°C and 37°C and for exposure times ranging from 1 hour to 180 days. There were static tests, tests with once-daily shaking, tests with continuous shaking, and tests with single fibers in an open bath. There was some solubility for all fibers. Klingholz and Steinkopf (1982, 1984) studied dissolution of mineral wool, glass wool, rock wool, and basalt wool at 37°C in water and in a Gamble's solution modified by omission of the organic constituents. Most of the tests used a continuous-flow system in which the pH was 7.5 to 8. There was relatively little dissolution in distilled water in comparison to that produced by the modified Gamble's solution. The alkali and alkali earth elements were leached out, and all glasslike compositions were homogeneously dissolved from the surface. Fibers with less alkaline reaction showed local pitting. Furthermore the surfaces developed a gel layer that, for the smaller diameters, extended throughout the fiber cross section. Thus the fibers can become both smaller in outline and more plastic to deformation.

Leineweber (1984) examined the stability of MMMFs in a lung fluid simulant that was passed slowly but continuously over the fibers at 65°C. He found among the glasses a wide range of solubility which was related to their composition.

Scholze and Conradt (1987) performed a comparative in vitro study of the chemical durability of industrial synthetic and natural mineral fibers in a simulated extracellular fluid under flow conditions. Seven viterous, three refractory, and three natural fibers were involved. Samples of the leachate were analyzed, and the silicon concentrations were used to roughly classify the fibers according to their chemical durability in terms of glass network dissolution. In order to establish a final classification, the effects of the fiber material and of the fiber geometry were separated by a mathematical procedure. A durability ranking of fiber materials was expressed in terms of a characteristic time required for the complete dissolution of single fibers of given diameter. MMMFs exhibited relatively poor durability (with network dissolution velocities ranging from 3.5 to 0.2 nm per day for a glass wool and an E glass fiber, respectively), whereas natural fibers were very persistent against the attack of the biological fluid (e.g. less than 0.01 nm per day for crocidolite).

Dissolution of glass fibers in rat lungs in vivo was also observed by Johnson, Griffiths, and Hill (1984), who exposed rats to MMMF aerosols at 10 mg/m^3 for 7 hours a day, 5 days a week for one year as compared to the single exposure of several hours duration used by Morgan and Holmes. The percentage of glass fibers with diameters less than 0.3 µm that were recovered from the lungs was consistently less than that in the original fiber suspension, and the reduction was more marked in the animals that were sacrificed following a period of recovery from the exposures than from those sacrificed at the end of the exposure. Furthermore morphological examination of the fiber surfaces revealed an etching of the surface, manifest as irregularities in outline, loss of electron density, and the appearance of pits along their edges. The degree of etching increased with residence times in the lungs. Glass wool with and without resin was also etched, but to a lesser extent, and the etching of the rock wool fibers was considerably less.

Bellmann et al. (1986) instilled reference suspensions of the International Union against Cancer (UICC) crocidolite and chrysotile A, as well as suspensions of glass fibers in rat lungs and examined the residual fibers after one day and 1, 6, 12, and 15 months. They reported that crocidolite fibers longer than $5\,\mu m$ did not decrease in number for over one year. The number of chrysotile fibers $> 5\,\mu m$ doubled, probably as a result of longitudinal splitting, while the number of glass fibers $> 5\,\mu m$ was reduced with a half-time of 55 days by dissolution. All fibers $< 5\,\mu m$ in length were cleared with half-times of 100 to 150 days. When the crocidolite fibers were pretreated in acid, there was no change in retention. On the other hand, acid-treated chrysotile and glass fibers had much more rapid clearance, with half-times of 2 and 14 days, respectively.

In a two-year follow-up study, Bellmann et al. (1987) reported the persistence of some MMMFs, crocidolite and chrysotile, in the rat lung after intratracheal instillation. Experiments were based on the assumption that thin, long, and durable fibers are of special importance for the carcinogenic potency of these types of substances. Parameters measured included number of fibers, diameter and length distribution of fibers retained in lung ash, and leaching of various elements from fibers longer than $5\,\mu m$. For a special type of glass microfiber and for ceramic wool, which both had a low alkaline earth content, the half-times of lung clearance were at a level similar to that of crocidolite. For another type of glass microfiber with a high alkaline earth content and a median diameter of about $0.1\,\mu m$, a very low half-time was reported. The glass and rock wools studied, which were thicker than the other fibers, had intermediate half-times.

In recent years there have been a series of much more detailed and focused studies on in vitro and in vivo rates of fiber dissolution in relation to fiber composition and size. Collier et al. (1994) studied the behavior of two experimental continuous filament glass fibers of $2\,\mu m$ diameter and cut to $50\,\mu m$ in length following intraperitoneal injections of 5 mg in rats. They had in vitro dissolution rates of 150 and $600\,ng\,/\,cm^2\,/\,h$. There were differences in dissolution when compared with durability in the lung. In the lung the diameters of the long fibers ($> 20\,\mu m$) were observed to decline at a rate consistent with their exposure to a neutral pH environment. The diameter of shorter fibers declined much more slowly, consistent with exposure to a more acidic environment such as is found in the phagolysosomes of alveolar macrophages. In the peritoneal cavity, all fibers, regardless of length, dissolved at the same rate as short fibers in the lung. The effect of dose on the distribution of fibers in the peritoneal cavity was investigated using similar experimental glass fibers and compared with that of a powder made from ground fibers. For both materials at doses up to 1.5 mg, material was taken up by the peritoneal organs roughly in proportion to their surface area. This uptake was complete one to two days after injection. At higher doses, the majority of the material in excess of this 1.5 mg formed clumps of fibers (nodules), which were either free in the peritoneal cavity or loosely bound to peritoneal organs. These nodules displayed classic foreign body reactions, with an associated granulomatous inflammatory response.

Collier et al. (1997) reported on the clearance of two stonewool fibers administered to rats by intratracheal instillation; one a conventional product (MMVF21) and the other an experimental, more soluble fiber (HTN). Unlike glasswool, stonewool is more soluble at the acid pH in macrophages than in the more neutral lung tissue. They found that

MMVF21 had relatively slow clearance, with somewhat faster clearance for short fibers. The clearance of HTN was much faster.

In an inhalation study by Eastes et al. (1995), suspensions of fibers were administered to rats by intratracheal instillation, and the numbers, lengths, and diameters of fibers recovered from the lungs at intervals up to one year after administration were measured by PCOM. Five different glass fibers were used that had dissolution rates ranging from 2 to 600 ng/cm^2/h measured in vitro in simulated lung fluid at pH 7.4. Examination of the diameter distributions of fibers longer than 20 μm showed that the peak diameter decreased steadily with time after instillation, at the same rate measured for each fiber in vitro, until it approached zero. Measurements of the total number of fibers remaining in the rats' lungs at times up to one year after instillation suggest that few of the administered fibers were being cleared by macrophage-mediated transport via the conducting airways. It was concluded that long glass fibers, at least those longer than 20 μm, are removed from the lung by dissolution at much the same rate measured in vitro.

In a study of dissolution of inhaled fibers by Eastes and Hadley (1995), rats were exposed for five days to four types of airborne, respirable-sized MMVF and to crocidolite asbestos fibers. The MMVF included two compositions of glass wool, and one each of rock and slag wool. After exposure, animals were sacrificed at intervals up to 18 months, and the number, length, and diameter of a representative sample of fibers in their lungs were measured. Long fibers (> 20 μm) were eliminated from the rats' lungs at a rate predicted from the dissolution rate measured in vitro for these fiber compositions. In particular, the long MMVF were nearly completely eliminated in several months, whereas the long crocidolite asbestos fibers remained in significant numbers at the end of the study. The number, length, and diameter distributions of fibers remaining in the rats' lungs agreed well with a computer simulation of fiber clearance that assumed that the long fibers dissolved at the rate measured for each fiber in vitro, and that the short fibers of every type were removed at the same rate as short crocidolite asbestos. The results provided evidence that long MMVF were cleared by complete dissolution at the rate measured in vitro, and that short fibers did not dissolve and were cleared by macrophage-mediated physical removal.

In another inhalation study, using nine fiber types, Bernstein et al. (1996) exposed rats to a respirable aerosol (mean diameter of about 1 μm) at a concentration of 30 mg/m^3, for 6 hours a day for 5 days, with postexposure sacrifices at 1 hour for 1 day, 5 days, 4 weeks, 13 weeks, and 26 weeks. At one hour following the last exposure, the nine fibers were found to have lung burdens ranging from 7.4 to 33×10^6 fibers per lung with geometric mean diameters (GMDs) of 0.40 to 0.54 μm, reflecting the different bivariate distributions in the exposure aerosol. The fibers were removed from the lung following exposure with weighted half-lives ranging from 11 to 54 days. The clearance was found to closely reflect the clearance of fibers in the 5 to 20-μm length range. An important difference in removal was seen between the long fiber ($L > 20$ μm) and shorter fiber (L between 5 and 20 μm and $L < 5$ μm) fractions depending on their composition. For all glass wools and the new stone wools, the longer fibers were removed notably faster than the shorter fibers. It was found that the time for complete fiber dissolution based on the acellular in vitro dissolution rate at pH 7.4 was highly correlated ($r = 0.97$, $p < 0.01$) with the clearance half-times of fibers > 20 μm in length. No such correlations were found with any of the length fractions using the acellular in vitro dissolution rate at pH 4.5. Examination of the fiber length distribution and particles in the lung from one hour through 5 days of exposure indicated that, especially for those fibers that form leached layers, a certain amount of fiber breakage may have occurred during this early period. These results demonstrate that for fibers with high acellular solubility at pH 7.4, the clearance of long fibers is very rapid.

Eastes and Hadley (1996) fitted much of the data cited above into a mathematical model of fiber carcinogenicity and fibrosis. Their model predicts the incidence of tumors and fibrosis in rats exposed to various types of rapidly dissolving fibers in an inhalation study or in an intraperitoneal (ip) injection experiment for which the response to durable fibers has been determined. It takes into account the fiber diameter and the dissolution rate of fibers longer than 20 μm in the lung, and it predicts the measured tumor and fibrosis incidence to within approximately the precision of the measurements. The underlying concept for the model is that a rapidly dissolving long fiber has the same response in an animal bioassay as a much smaller dose of a durable fiber. Long, durable fibers have special significance, since there is no effective mechanism by which these fibers may be removed. In particular, the hypothesis is that the effective dose of a dissolving long fiber scales as the residence time of that fiber in the extracellular fluid. The residence time of a fiber is estimated directly from the average fiber diameter, its density, and the fiber dissolution rate as measured in simulated lung fluid at neutral pH.

The incidence of fibrosis in recent chronic inhalation tests was well predicted by the model, and the observed lung tumor rates in these studies were consistent with the model. The model also predicts the incidence of mesothelioma in the ip model. The model allows one to predict, for an inhalation or ip experiment, what residence time and dissolution rate are required for an acceptably small tumorigenic or fibrotic response to a given fiber dose. For an inhalation test in rats at the maximum tolerated dose (MTD), the model suggests that less than 10% incidence of fibrosis would be obtained at the maximum tolerated dose of 1 μm diameter fibers if the dissolution rate were greater than 80 ng / cm^2 / h. The dissolution rate that would give no detectable lung tumors in such an inhalation test in rats is much smaller. Thus a fiber with a dissolution rate of 100 ng / cm^2 / h has an insignificant chance of producing either fibrosis or tumors by inhalation in rats, even at the maximum tolerated dose. This model provides manufacturers of MMMF with design criteria for fibrous products that minimize, if not eliminate, their potential for producing adverse health effects.

PROPERTIES OF MINERAL AND VITREOUS FIBERS RELEVANT TO DISEASE

Fiber dimensions, chemical composition, and surface properties are important factors in biological reactivity of mineral fibers. As discussed previously, fiber length influences the deposition, clearance, and translocation of fibers in the lungs. Fiber length also determines clearance from the pleural and peritoneal spaces — fibers longer than 8 μm are trapped at the mesothelial lining because the opening of lymphatic channels draining these spaces are 8 to 12 μm in diameter (Moalli et al., 1987). This provides an anatomic basis for the Stanton hypothesis that long fibers, regardless of their chemical composition, are more effective in producing mesotheliomas than shorter fibers, after direct intrapleural or intraperitoneal injection into rodents (Stanton et al., 1981).

Cations within the crystal lattice may affect the toxicity of asbestos fibers. Mg^{+2} ions on the surface of chrysotile asbestos are important in cytotoxicity and carcinogenicity; acid-leached fibers are less active than native fibers (Monchaux et al., 1981). The Fe^{+2} and Fe^{+3} content of amphibole fibers may be important because these cations can catalyze the Fenton or Haber-Weiss reactions, generating highly toxic and potentially mutagenic reactive oxygen species (Weitzman and Graceffa, 1984; Zalma et al., 1987).

ASBESTOS-RELATED DISEASES

Macrophages are the intial target cells of inhaled particles that are deposited in the terminal airways and alveolar spaces. Phagocytosis of mineral fibers by macrophages leads to generation of reactive oxygen species and release of lysosomal enzymes, arachidonic acid metabolites, neutral proteases, chemotactic factors, and growth factors (Adamson et al., 1991). The interactions among mediators released from macrophages and other inflammatory cells and the target cell populations can initiate a sequence of events culminating in fibrosis of the lungs and pleura, bronchogenic carcinoma, and malignant mesothelioma. However, for shorter exposures (two-weeks) to chrysotile, the early fibrotic lesions in rats were gradually resolved over the course of the following year (Pinkerton et al., 1997).

Diffuse, bilateral interstitial fibrosis of the lungs characterizes the disease asbestosis that usually develops in humans after prolonged exposure to high doses of asbestos fibers. Progressive scarring of the alveolar walls due to increased proliferation of fibroblasts and deposition of collagen produces radiographic evidence of disease, and interferes with gas exchange, leading to disability and premature death. The sequence of events that lead to the development of asbestosis includes

1. Asbestos fibers are phagocytized by alveolar and/or interstitial macrophages.
2. Release of reactive oxygen species from alveolar macrophages causes acute injury to the alveolar epithelial lining. (The importance of hydrogen peroxide in the pathogenesis of asbestosis was demonstrated by the protection against asbestos-induced pulmonary fibrosis provided by catalast conjugated to polyethylene glycol; Mossman et al., 1990).
3. Phagocytosis of asbestos fibers by alveolar or interstitial macrophages also triggers increased synthesis and release of growth factors for fibroblasts. Growth factors are released from macrophages exposed to asbestos fibers in vitro or in vivo: a homologue of platelet-derived growth factor (PDGF) (Bauman et al., 1990) and transforming growth factor-β (TGF-β) (Kane and McDonald, 1993).
4. Release of growth factors cause chemotaxis of inflammatory cells and fibroblasts, stimulation of collagen synthesis, and inhibition of collagen degradation.

Another reaction to asbestos exposure is the development of acellular fibrous scars, called pleural plaques, on the parietal pleural lining and diaphragm. Asbestos exposure may also lead to pleural effusions or diffuse fibrosis of the visceral pleura, but these reactions cause little disability. The most important reaction of the pleural and peritoneal linings to asbestos fibers is development of *diffuse malignant mesothelioma*, a rare neoplasm that is most closely associated with occupational or environmental exposure to amphibole forms of asbestos after a long latent period (up to 30–60 years). There is no increased incidence in cigarette smokers or in workers with asbestosis. This malignant neoplasm has a variable histology, ranging from epithelial to fibroblastic or mixed patterns. Malignant mesothelioma has usually spread diffusely when first diagnosed and responds poorly to radiation or chemotherapy (Craighead, 1987). The following sequence of events is hypothesized to lead to the development of diffuse malignant mesothelioma:

1. Fibers that reach the pleura or peritoneal lining are phagocytized by macrophages.
2. Release of reactive oxygen species causes acute injury to the mesothelial cell monolayer lining the pleural or peritoneal spaces. This injury can be prevented by coating the administered fibers with the iron chelator deferoxamine or exogenous superoxide dismutase or catalase (Goodglick and Kane, 1990; Kane and McDonald, 1993).
3. Acute injury to the mesothelial lining is repaired by proliferation of adjacent uninjured mesothelial cells. Growth factors released from macrophages following

phagocytosis of asbestos fibers may modulate mesothelial cell regeneration (Kane and McDonald, 1993).

4. Direct interaction of asbestos fibers with the regenerating mesothelial cell population may cause chromosomal aberrations and aneuploidy. Additional DNA damage may be produced by reactive oxygen species, especially the hydroxyl radical produced by the iron-catalyzed Haber-Weiss reaction (Barrett et al., 1989; Floyd, 1990).

5. Repeated episodes of mesothelial cell injury and regeneration may lead to the emergence of a subpopulation of autonomously proliferating cells.

6. Neoplastic mesothelial cells may produce growth factors that promote growth of an invasive tumor.

It is well established that workers exposed to asbestos fibers have an increased risk of developing bronchogenic carcinoma, and that workers who also smoke cigarettes have a much greater risk. Cancers can arise from the epithelial lining of the large airways or terminal bronchioles. Bronchogenic carcinomas have a variety of histologic appearances: adenocarcinoma, squamous cell carcinoma (presumably arising in areas of squamous metaplasia of the respiratory epithelium), large cell carcinoma, and small cell (oat cell) carcinoma. These are the same histologic types of cancer associated with cigarette smoking in the absence of asbestos exposure (Mossman and Craighead, 1987).

Lung cancer and mesothelioma are known to occur in people without radiographic evidence of lung fibrosis. DeKlerk et al. (1997) demonstrated that the level of radiographic fibrosis conferred additional risk for lung cancer beyond that associated with level of exposure but that asbestosis was not a prerequisite for asbestos-associated cancer.

Bronchogenic carcinomas that develop in cigarette smokers show multiple alterations in protooncogenes and tumor-suppressor genes. It is unknown whether similar molecular changes are present in those malignant tumors that result from cigarette smoking in combination with asbestos exposure. Most of the experimental evidence suggests that asbestos fibers act as a cocarcinogen or tumor promoter in the respiratory lining, in conjunction with multiple components of cigarette smoke that may act as initiators.

Some of these effects of asbestos fibers on the tracheobronchial epithelium may be mediated by reactive oxygen species, since they are decreased by addition of various scavenging enzymes (superoxide dismutase, catalase) to these in vitro model systems.

REVIEW OF BIOLOGICAL EFFECTS OF SIZE-CLASSIFIED FIBERS IN ANIMALS AND HUMANS

The pathological effects produced by fibers depend on both the characteristics of the fibers and their persistence at sensitive sites. A number of carefully designed studies have been performed in which the size distributions of fiber suspensions have been well characterized as well as their persistence and / or effects.

King, Clegg, and Rae (1946) instilled 100 mg of Rhodesian chrysotile into rabbit lungs at monthly intervals. One group received fibers microtomed to a length of 15 μm, and another group received fibers cut to 2.5 μm in length. At this huge dosage level, both groups showed foreign body reactions in the lungs. The long fiber produced a nodular reticulinosis, whereas the short fiber produced a diffuse interstitial reticulinosis.

Wright and Kuschner (1977) used short and long asbestos and synthetic mineral fibers in intratracheal instillation studies in guinea pigs. With suspensions containing an appreciable number of fibers longer than 10 μm, all of the materials produced lung fibrosis, although the yields varied with the materials used. However, with equal masses of short fibers of equivalent fiber diameters, none produced any fibrosis. The yields were lower for the long glass fibers than for the long asbestos, and this was attributed to their lesser durability within the lungs.

For fibers injected intraperitoneally (Davis, 1976; Pott et al., 1976; Wagner et al., 1976) or placed in a pledget against the lung pleura (Stanton and Wrench, 1972), a similar kind of fiber size and composition dependence was observed. The yield of mesotheliomas varied with fiber diameter and length and with dose, with very little response when long thin fibers were not included. Asbestos fibers were more effective than glass in these studies also. At a dose of 2 mg of chrysotile, crocidolite, or glass fiber, Pott, Friedrichs, and Huth (1976) found only slight degrees of fibrosis but tumor yields of from 16% to 38% in rats. When the chrysotile was milled to the extent that 99.8% of the fibers were shorter than 5 μm, the dose required to produce a comparable tumor yield (32%) was 50 times greater (100 mg).

Various hypotheses have been proposed to account for the pathological effects produced by asbestos. One was the contamination of the surface by trace metal and/or organic carcinogens. However, the studies of Stanton and Wrench (1972) found that surface contaminants played no role in mesothelioma yield, and they concluded that the carcinogenicity of asbestos and fibrous glass was primarily related to the structural shape of these fibrous materials rather than their surface properties.

The relative potencies of the various mineral forms of asbestos after inhalation exposure are still not firmly established. Crocidolite is generally considered the most hazardous because of its association with significant numbers of human mesotheliomas. The relative toxicity of various asbestos minerals have been compared in a variety of experimental inhalation studies on small animals, but the results are in apparent conflict. Wagner (1963) reported more asbestosis with amosite than with chrysotile in guinea pigs, rats, and monkeys. Wagner et al. (1974), in studies involving inhalation exposures of rats for 1 day to 2 years, found that amosite and crocidolite were the least fibrogenic of five types of UICC asbestos, the others being Canadian chrysotile, Rhodesian chrysotile, and anthophyllite (see Table 3-3). Holt, Mills, and Young (1965) found no differences in the fibrogenic potential of chrysotile, crocidolite, amosite, and anthophyllite. Davis et al. (1978) used UICC chrysotile A, amosite, and crocidolite in 12 month rat exposures at respirable mass concentrations comparable to those used by Wagner et al. (1974) and found a similar pattern; namely, chrysotile was the most fibrogenic, and amosite and crocidolite the least. Hiett (1978) exposed guinea pigs by inhalation for 9 and 18 days and also found that chrysotile was more fibrogenic than amosite. Davis et al. (1986b) subsequently repeated the protocol with amosite with fiber length both shorter and longer than UICC amosite. The short amosite produced virtually no fibrosis, whereas the long amosite was more fibrogenic than chrysotile. The most fibrogenic asbestos was tremolite (see Table 3-3).

It is generally believed that amphibole fibers account for much of the mesothelioma incidence among exposed workers, even when they are predominantly exposed to chrysotile, since amphibole fibers are more persistent in lung tissue. Pooley (1976) examined postmortem lung tissue from 20 workers with asbestosis in the Canadian chrysotile mining industry and found that amphibole and other fibers were present in 16 cases. In seven of these, they were more numerous than chrysotile. In a later study of lung asbestos in chrysotile workers with mesothelioma, Churg et al. (1984) reported that the concentration ratio between cases and controls was 9.3 for tremolite but only 2.8 for chrysotile. In a Norwegian plant using 91.7% chrysotile, 3.1% amosite, 4.1% crocidolite, and 1.1% anthophylite, Gylseth, Mowe, and Wannag (1983) reported that the percentage of chrysotile in lung tissue ranged between 0% and 9%, while the corresponding numbers for the amphiboles were 76% to 99%.

In their review of the assessment of mineral fibers from human lung tissue, Davis, Gylseth, and Morgan (1986) attributed the high amphibole/chrysotile ratios to the

TABLE 3-3 Summary of Results of Mineral Fiber Inhalation Studies in Rats

		Fiber Parameters					Number (%) of Rats with Tumors				Interstitial Fibrosis	
		Resp. Conc.	d_m	Length (% >)		Number of						
Reference	Fiber Type	(mg/m^3)	(μm)	5 μm	10 μm	Rats	Mesothelioma	Adenoma	Adeno-CA	Squam. CA	Score[a]	%[b]
Wagner et al. (1974)												
	UICC											
	Amosite	10	NR[c]	NR	NR	146	1(0.7)	19(13)	5(3.4)	6(4.1)	4.3	
	Anthophyllite	10	NR	NR	NR	145	2 (1.4)	22 (15)	8 (5.5)	8 (5.5)	6.2	
	Crocidolite	10	NR	NR	NR	141	4 (2.8)	26 (18)	7 (5.0)	9 (6.4)	4.8	
	Chrysotile											
	Canadian	10	NR	NR	NR	137	4 (2.9)	20 (15)	11 (8.0)	6 (4.4)	6.0	
	Rhodesian	10	NR	NR	NR	144	0	19 (13)	19 (13)	11 (7.6)	5.8	
Davis et al. (1978)												
	UICC											
	Amosite	10	0.38	16	2.7	43	0	2(4.7)	0	0		2.6
	Crocidolite	10	0.38	12	4	40	0	1(2.5)	0	0		1.4
	Crocidolite	5	0.38	12	4	43	0	2 (4.7)	0	0		0.8
	Chrysotile	10	0.42	30	16	40	0	7 (18)	6 (15)	2 (5.0)		9.2
	Chrysotile	2	0.42	30	16	42	1 (2.4)	6 (14)	1 (2.4)	1 (2.4)		3.5
Davis et al. (1985)	Tremolite	10	0.25	28	7	39	2 (5.1)	2 (5.1)	8 (21)	8 (21)		14.5
Davis et al. (1986)	Amostite-short	10	0.32	1.7	0.1	42	1 (2.4)	0	0	0		0.15
	Amosite-long	10	0.37	30	10	40	3 (7.5)	3 (7.5)	3 (7.5)	4 (10)		11.0
Wagner et al. (1985)	UICC crocidolite	10	0.30	53	12	28	0	0	0	1(3.6)		
	Erionite	10	0.22	44	7	28	27 (96)	0	0	0		
Davis (1987)	Chrysotile-short	10	0.17	5	0.7	40	1 (2.5)	1 (2.5)	6 (15)	0		2.4
	Chrysotile-long	10	0.18	12	2	40	3 (7.5)	8 (20)	6 (15)	5 (13)		12.6

[a] Relative scale where 1, nil; 2, minimal; 4, slight; 6, moderate; 8, severe at 24 months.
[b] Percentage of tissue with fibrosis at 27–29 months.
[c] Not reported.
Source: From Lippmann (1988).

dissolution of chrysotile within lung tissue. They suggested that the generally poor correlation between dust counts and mesothelioma is likely to be caused by the differences among the various asbestos types in the fraction that reaches the pleural surface and that this depends critically on the fiber dimensions. Amosite fibers need to be longer to produce pulmonary fibrosis and pulmonary tumors in experimental animals than to produce mesotheliomas after injection (Davis et al., 1986a). Davis (1987) notes that both chrysotile and amphibole asbestos fibers inhaled by rats are plentiful in the most peripheral alveoli bordering on the pleura, but penetration of the external elastic lamina of the lung appears to be a rare event. On the other hand, erionite causes a very high incidence of mesotheliomas in humans exposed to low environmental concentrations (Baris et al., 1987) and 100% incidence in rats exposed by inhalation (Wagner et al., 1985). Davis (1987) reported that the erionite used by Wagner et al. (1985) had a general appearance and fiber size distribution very close to that of UICC crocidolite which produces a much smaller mesothelioma yield in rats exposed by inhalation. He attributed the difference to the enhanced ability of erionite to cross the pleural membrane.

CRITICAL FIBER PARAMETERS AFFECTING DISEASE PATHOGENESIS

Critical Fiber Dimensions for Asbestosis

Asbestosis has been caused by respirable fibers of all of the commercially exploited kinds of asbestos. Within the respirable fraction, the fibers can differ in diameter and length distributions and in retention times.

The influence of these variables on fibrosis in the human lung has been systematically explored and described by Timbrell et al. (1987) through analyses of both retained fibers and fibrosis in lung samples from exposed workers. He analyzed the fiber distributions in 0.5-g lung samples from several hundred workers by a technique known as magnetic alignment and light scattering (MALS) that he had previously developed (Timbrell, 1982). Optical microscopy was applied to measure the degree of fibrosis in paraffin sections prepared from adjacent samples of the same specimens. Wide intra- and intersubject variations were observed in fiber concentration and fibrosis score. The quantitative relationships between fibrosis and amphibole fibers in mineworkers' postmortem lung specimens were determined for the main sources of amosite (Transvaal, South Africa), anthophyllite (Paakkila, Finland), and crocidolite (NW Cape and Transvaal, South Africa, and Wittenoom, Australia). As illustrated in Figure 3-3, the fibrosis-producing ability of the fibers was independent of amphibole type when normalized by the total surface area of long resident fibers per unit weight of lung tissue, presumably because the surface area determined the magnitude of the fiber-tissue interface. The wide range of the concentrations of retained fiber required to produce the same degree of fibrosis in the groups of mineworkers, when fiber quantity is expressed as number or total mass stemmed from the large differences between the distributions in diameter and length of the airborne fibers.

Although the main focus of the Timbrell et al. (1987) study was on amphibole asbestos, they also reported results for three Wittenoom workers whose dominant exposure was to chrysotile asbestos. For these workers, chrysotile produced a similar degree of fibrosis to Wittenoom crocidolite for equal fiber mass concentrations in the lungs. Long residence in the tissue had almost completely dispersed the chrysotile fibers into fibrils, to give them a ratio of total surface area to mass resembling that of the particularly fine Wittenoom fibers. The result indicates that the fibrogenicity of the retained chrysotile per unit of surface area within the lungs was similar to that of the amphiboles.

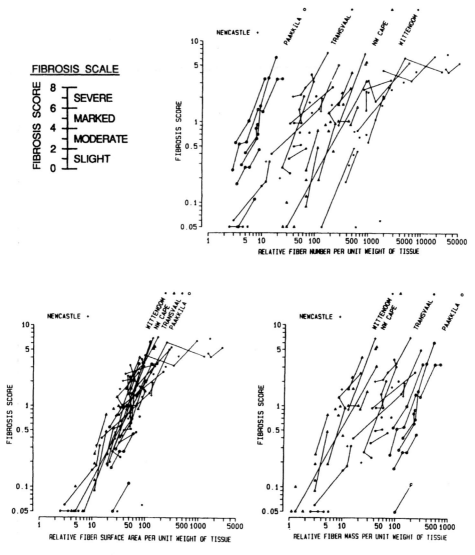

Figure 3-3 Relationships between lung fibrosis scale and relative concentrations of fibers per unit weight of dry lung tissue. The lines connect data points from the same subject. The relative fiber surface area normalizes the data better than either the relative fiber number concentration of the fiber mass concentration. (Source: Lippmann, 1988)

Timbrell et al. (1987) also reported that amphibole mineworkers with a given fiber mass concentration in their lungs showed much higher degrees of fibrosis than gold miners with roughly the same mass concentration of retained quartz grains. The amphibole and quartz produced about the same fibrogenicity per unit of surface area, but the smaller diameters and higher area/mass ratios of the amphibole fibers endowed them with the greater surface area and thereby the superior fibrosis-producing capability.

Knowledge of the interrelationships between retained fibers and fibrosis is critical in understanding the pathogenesis of the disease but is inadequate, by itself, in evaluating exposures to airborne fibers. This was recognized by Timbrell (1983, 1984), who developed a mathematical model relating fiber deposition and retention based on analysis of lung samples. Specifically, he used samples from a woman at Paakkila who worked at a job that gave her exposure to an amphibole (anthophyllite) at high concentrations of fibers with a range of diameters and lengths sufficiently wide to encompass the size limits of respirable fibers. Her lungs contained 1.3 mg fiber per gram of dry tissue, and she had asbestosis. One lung sample contained a fiber distribution matching the expected deposition. Timbrell speculated that severe fibrosis in the tissue in this sample had blocked the macrophage-mediated clearance. Another sample from the same lung yielded a retention pattern more closely matching those found in other Paakkila workers, with small fiber burdens and virtually no short fibers. He assumed that the latter represents long-term retention in the normal lung.

From the differences in retention, Timbrell developed a model for the retention of fibers as a function of length and diameter. Fiber retention rises rapidly with fiber lengths between 2 and 5 µm and peaks at about 10 µm. Fiber retention also rises rapidly with fiber diameters between 0.15 and 0.3 µm, peaks at about 0.5 µm, and drops rapidly between 0.8 and 2 µm. The utility of the model was demonstrated by applying it to predict the lung retention of Cape crocidolite and Transvaal amosite workers on the basis of the measured length and diameter distributions of airborne fibers. The predicted lung distributions did, in fact, closely match those measured in lung samples from a Cape worker (Timbrell, 1984) and, as shown in Figure 3-4, from a Transvaal worker (Timbrell, 1983). Thus fibrosis is most closely related to the surface area of fibers with diameters between 0.15 and 2 µm and lengths greater than 2 µm. The work of King, Clegg, and Rae (1946) showing that chrysotile with length of 2.5 µm produced interstitial fibrosis in rabbits following multiple intratracheal instillations is consistent with the retention shown in Figure 3-3 and a critical fiber length of about 2 µm.

Critical Fiber Dimensions for Mesothelioma

A National Research Council study (NRC, 1984) summarized mortality data for mesothelioma and lung cancer in asbestos-exposed occupational cohorts. In 20 studies in which there was an excess in respiratory cancer and / or mesothelioma, the percentage of the excess that was mesothelioma varied from 0% to 100%, with a mean ($\pm$ SD) of $38 \pm 29\%$. A study with 0% was that of Meurman, Kiviluoto, and Hakama (1974, 1979), who reported 44 observed lung cancers (vs. 22 expected) in a population of 1045 workers exposed to anthophyllite in Finland. Anthophyllite is an amphibole with larger fiber diameters than other forms of asbestos. By contrast, in several occupational cohorts the mesotheliomas accounted for more that 70% of the total. These included (1) the study of Newhouse, Berry, and Skidmore (1982) of 7474 British workers exposed to mixed asbestos, among whom there were 8 mesotheliomas and only three more than the 140 expected lung cancers; (2) the study of Rossiter and Coles (1980) of 6076 British shipyard workers exposed to mixed asbestos, among whom there were 31 mesotheliomas and 13 fewer lung cancers than the expected number of 101; (3) the study of Jones et al. (1980) of 578 British female workers exposed to crocidolite, among whom there were 17 mesotheliomas and 6 lung cancers more than the six expected; and (4) the study of Newhouse, Berry, and Skidmore (1982) of 3708 British female workers exposed to mixed asbestos, among whom there were 2 mesotheliomas and 5 fewer lung cancers that the 11 expected.

Timbrell (1983), Timbrell et al. (1987), and Harington (1981) have noted that animal inoculation experiments have been interpreted as suggesting a fairly high value of diameter, such as 1.5 µm (Stanton et al., 1977), 1 µm (Pott et al., 1976; WHO, 1986), and 0.25 µm (Wagner and Pooley, 1986); below this a fibrous material, so long as it is durable in lung fluids, can produce mesothelioma. In their view, these diameter limits are too high

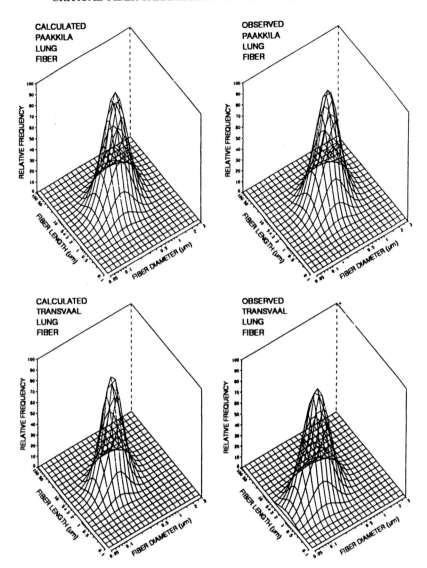

Figure 3-4 Distributions of fiber lengths and diameters of amosite asbestos in the lungs of a Transvaal worker. The predicted distribution at the left is based on the lengths and diameters of the airborne fibers and on the lung retention as a function of length and diameter. This corresponds closely to the distribution in the right panel, which was measured in samples from the worker's lung. (Source: Lippmann 1988)

for human fiber-induced mesothelioma. If fibers with diameters $>0.5\,\mu m$ produced mesothelioma, then the Paakkila mine, where the dust clouds contained on the order of $50\,f/mL$ (PCOM) and a high proportion of fibers in the 0.5 to $3\,\mu m$ diameter range, should have produced many mesotheliomas as well as excesses in fibrosis and lung cancer. As noted earlier, an average of 38% of the excess lung cancer plus mesothelioma in working populations exposed to asbestos was expressed as mesothelima. Despite the very high exposures of the Paakkila population, no mesotheliomas were observed.

Timbrell's (1983) examination of the size distributions and mesothelioma incidence at Paakkila and other asbestos mines worldwide led him to conclude that a good correlation

TABLE 3-4   Mesotheliomas Produced by Asbestos in Chronic Rat Inhalation Studies

Type of Asbestos	Source		Tumors / Animals
Zimbabwe Chrysotile			
Wagner et al. (1974)	$10\,mg/m^3$	UICC	0/44
Davis et al. (1978)	$10\,mg/m^3$	UICC	0/40
	$2\,mg/m^3$	UICC	1/42
Davis et al. (1980)	$10\,mg/m^3$(1 d/wk)	UICC	0/43
Overall			1/169 (0.6%)
Quebec Chrysotile			
Wagner et al. (1974)	$10\,mg/m^3$	UICC	4/44
Davis et al. (1988)	$10\,mg/m^3$	Short	1/40
	$10\,mg/m^3$	Long	3/40
Hesterberg et al. (1993)	$10\,mg/m^3$	NIEHS	1/69
Overall			9/193(4.7%)
Davis-Wagner subset			8/124 (6.5%)
Amphiboles			
Wagner et al. (1974)			
Crocidolite	$10\,mg/m^3$	UICC	2/44
Amosite	$10\,mg/m^3$	UICC	0/46
Anthophyllite	$10\,mg/m^3$	UICC	2/46
Davis et al. (1978)			
Crocidolite	$5\,mg/m^3$	UICC	1/43
Crocidolite	$10\,mg/m^3$	UICC	0/40
Amosite	$10\,mg/m^3$	UICC	0/43
Davis et al. (1980)			
Amosite	$50\,mg/m^3$(1 d/wk)	UICC	0/44
Wagner et al. (1985)			
Crocidolite	$10\,mg/m^3$	UICC	1/24
Davis et al. (1985)			
Tremolite	$10\,mg/m^3$	Korea	2/39
Davis et al. (1986)			
Amosite	$10\,mg/m^3$	Short	1/42
	$10\,mg/m^3$	Long	3/40
McConnell (1993)			
Crocidolite	$10\,mg/m^3$	UICC	1/69
Overall			13/520 (2.5%)
Davis-Wagner subset			12/451 (2.7%)

was obtained if the threshold diameter was reduced to 0.1 µm. The mesotheliomas that Paakkila fiber has produced in animals were, most likely, caused by the use of excessive doses, 10,000 times those observed in humans. Paakkila asbestos contains only 1% of fibers with diameters below 0.1 µm, but with such a large dose this represents an enormous absolute number. Harington (1981) noted that the data for the northwest Cape in South Africa, where numerous mesotheliomas have been reported, and for the northeastern Transvaal, where mesotheliomas are rare, are consistent with a low fiber-diameter limit. In the northwest Cape, about 60% of the fibers have diameters $< 0.1\,\mu m$, whereas for the Transvaal, only about 1% have diameters $< 0.1\,\mu m$, comparable to Paakkila.

Timbrell (1983) also noted that the length distributions at Paakkila and the northwest Cape point to a need to reduce the 10-μm threshold in Stanton's criteria. Paakkila had a high percentage of fibers longer than 10 μm, whereas the northwest Cape had virtually none. And yet the northwest Cape has been the major source of mesothelioma. Attributing potential carcinogenicity to shorter fibers by lowering the length threshold brings the estimated levels of significant fibers into closer line with the observed mesothelioma rates.

In reviewing the literature on mesothelioma induction in rats exposed by inhalation to fibrous aerosols, as summarized in Table 3-4, I concluded that, for mesothelioma, the relatively low tumor yields seemed to be highly dependent on fiber type. Combining the data from various studies by fiber type, the percentages of mesotheliomas were 0.6% for Zimbabwe (Rhodesian) chrysotile, 2.5% for the various amphiboles as a group, and 4.7% for Quebec (Canadian) chrysotile. This difference, together with the fact that Zimbabwe chrysotile has two to three orders of magnitude less tremolite than Quebec chrysotile, provides support for the hypothesis that the mesotheliomas that have occurred among chrysotile miners and millers could be largely due to their exposures to tremolite fibers. The chrysotile fibers may be insufficiently biopersistent because of dissolution during translocation from the sites of deposition to sites where more durable fibers can influence the transformation or progression to mesothelioma.

Combining the findings of Timbrell with the results of rat inhalation experiments reported by Davis et al. (1986) for studies with length-classified fibers leads to the conclusion that the critical fibers for mesothelioma induction have lengths between 5 and 10 μm. Davis et al. reported that intraperitoneal injections of short amosite (1.7%, $> 5\,\mu m$) produced only one mesothelioma among 24 rats (after 837 days), whereas UICC amosite (11% $> 5\,\mu m$; 2.5% $> 10\,\mu m$) produced 30 mesotheliomas among 32 rats and long amosite (30% $> 5\,\mu m$; 10% $> 10\,\mu m$) produced 20 mesotheliomas among 21 rats. Thus fibers shorter than 5 μm appear to be ineffective, and an appreciable fraction longer than 10 μm appears to be unnecessary.

Critical Fiber Dimension for Lung Cancer

Excess incidence of lung cancer has been reported for workers exposed to amphiboles (amosite, anthophyllite, and crocidolite), to chrysotile, and to mixtures of these fibers (NRC, 1984). But these studies have been uninformative with respect to the fiber parameters affecting the incidence. The series of rat inhalation studies performed by Davis et al. (1978), which have also produced lung cancers, have provided the most relevant evidence on the importance of fiber length on carcinogenicity in the lung.

The Wagner et al. (1974) study found that the yield of squamous cell carcinoma and adenocarcinoma was greatest with Rhodesian chrysotile, with decreasing yields for Canadian chrysotile, crocidolite, anthopyllite, and amosite, respectively. As shown in Table 3-3, Davis et al. (1978) reported two squamous cell carcinomas, six adenocarci-nomas, and seven adenomas in 40 rats exposed to $10\,mg/m^3$ of respirable chrysotile. In 42 rats exposed to $2\,mg/m^3$ of chrysotile, there were six adenomas, one adenocarcinoma, and one squamous cell carcinoma. There were also adenomas in the groups exposed to amosite at $10\,mg/m^3$ (two) and to crocidolite (one at $10\,mg/m^3$, two at $5\,mg/m^3$). Davis et al. (1978) attempted to examine the influence of fiber number concentration in relation to mass concentration in their inhalation studies. Their five exposure groups included three at the same respirable mass concentration of $10\,mg/m^3$, one each with chrysotile, crocidolite, and amosite. Of these, the amosite produced the lowest number concentration of fibers >5 μm in length. This fiber count was then matched with crocidolite ($5\,mg/m^3$ respirable mass) and chrysotile ($2\,mg/m^3$ respirable mass). In attempting to explain the greater fibrogenic and carcinogenic responses in the chrysotile-exposed animals than the crocidolite- or amosite exposed groups, they suggested it might have resulted, at least in part, from the greater number of $> 20\,\mu m$ long fibers in the chrysotile aerosol. The ratio of > 20 to $> 5\,\mu m$ long fibers in the chrysotile was 0.185 compared to 0.040 for crocidolite and 0.011 for amosite. The diameter distributions of all three types of asbestos were similar, with a median diameter of about $0.4\,\mu m$.

The importance of fiber length was further demonstrated by Davis et al. (1986) in inhalation studies with amosite aerosols both shorter and longer than the UICC amosite studied earlier with the same protocols. Both aerosols had median diameters between 0.3 and $0.4\,\mu m$. The short-fiber amosite (1.7% $> 5\,\mu m$) produced no malignant cancers in 42 rats, whereas the long-fiber amosite (30% $> 5\,\mu m$, 10% $> 10\,\mu m$) produced three adenocarcinomas, four squamous carcinomas and one undifferentiated carcinoma in 40 rats. In terms of adenomas, the frequencies were 3/40, 2/43, 0/42, and 1/81 for the long, UICC, short, and control groups, respectively. Davis et al. (1985) also studied tremolite asbestos using the same protocols. Its length distribution was similar to those of the chrysotile in the 1978 study and the long amosite in the 1986 study (i.e., 28% $> 5\,\mu m$, 7% $> 10\,\mu m$), but its median diameter was lower, $0.25\,\mu m$. It produced two adenomas, eight adenocarcinomas, and eight squamous carcinomas in 39 rats. Davis (1987) reported on a study comparing the carcinogenic effects of "long" and "short" chrysotile at $10\,mg/m^3$. Unfortunately, the discrimination between "long" and "short" fibers was less successful than that achieved for amosite. The fiber counts (PCOM) for the fibers $> 10\,\mu m$ in length for the "long" and "short" chrysotile were 1930 and $330\,f/mL$, whereas for the amosite they were 1110 and $12\,f/mL$, respectively. Despite the much more rapid clearance of the chrysotile from the lungs, the tumor yields were higher. For the "long" fiber, there were 22 tumors for the chrysotile compared with 13 for the amosite. For the "short" fiber, there were seven versus none. Davis (1987) concluded that fibers $< 5\,\mu m$ in length may be innocuous, since the tumors produced by the "short" chrysotile are explicable by the presence of $330\,f/mL$ longer than $10\,\mu m$.

In another study Wagner et al. (1985) exposed rats by inhalation to $10\,mg/m^3$ of respirable dust composed of either UICC crocidolite (52.7% $> 5\,\mu m$; 11.6% $> 10\,\mu m$; median diameter $0.30\,\mu m$) or Oregon erionite (44% $> 5\,\mu m$; 7.4% $> 10\,\mu m$; median diameter of $0.22\,\mu m$). The UICC crocidolite produced one squamous carcinoma in 28 rats (but no mesotheliomas), whereas the erionite produced no carcinomas in 28 rats but did produce 27 mesotheliomas.

In summary, Table 3-3 shows that $10\,mg/m^3$ of short amosite (about 0.1% $> 10\,\mu m$), UICC amosite (about 2.5% $> 10\,\mu m$), UICC crocidolite (about 3% $> 10\,\mu m$), and Oregon erionite (7.4%, $> 10\,\mu m$) failed to produce malignant lung cancers, whereas $10\,mg/m^3$ of UICC chrysotile, long amosite, and tremolite (all with $\geq 10\% > 10\,\mu m$) produced malignant lung tumors. Although there was no clear-cut influence of fiber diameter on tumor yield, the results suggest that carcinogenesis incidence increases with both fiber length and diameter. Since Timbrell (1983) has shown that fiber retention in the lungs peaks between 0.3 and $0.8\,\mu m$ diameter, it is likely that the thinner fibers, which are more readily translocated to the pleura and peritoneum, play relatively little role in lung carcinogenesis. Therefore it appears that the risk of lung cancer is associated with long fibers, especially those with diameters between 0.3 and $0.8\,\mu m$, and that substantial numbers of fibers $> 10\,\mu m$ in length are needed.

In my own review of the literature on the chronic rat inhalation studies with amosite, brucite, chrysotile, crocidolite, erionite, and tremolite (Lippmann, 1994), I found that for lung cancer, the percentage of lung tumors (y) could be described by a relation of the form $y = z + bf + cf^2$, where f is the number concentration of fibers, and a, b, and c are fitted constants. The correlation coefficients for the fitted curves were 0.76 for $> 5\,\mu m\,f/ml$, 0.84 for $> 10\,\mu m\,f/mL$, and 0.85 for $> 20\,\mu m\,f/mL$, and they seemed to be independent of fiber type. This supports the hypothesis that the critical length for lung cancer induction is in the 10 to 20 µm range. In terms of the critical sites within the lungs for lung cancer induction, it has been shown that brief inhalation exposures to chrysotile fiber produces highly concentrated fiber deposits on bifurcations of alveolar ducts, and that many of these fibers are phagocytosed by the underlying type II epithelial cells within a few hours. Churg (1994) has shown that both chrysotile and amphibole fibers retained in the lungs of former miners and millers do not clear much with the years since last exposure. Thus lung tumors may be caused by that small fraction of the inhaled long fibers that are retained in the interstitium below small airway bifurcations, where clearance processes are ineffective.

One reason that short fibers may be less damaging could be the fact that they can be fully ingested by macrophages (Beck et al., 1971) and can therefore be more rapidly cleared from the lung. The fibrogenic response to long fibers could result from the release of tissue-digesting enzymes from alveolar macrophages whose membranes are pierced by the fibers they are attempting to engulf (Allison, 1977). The fibers may also cause direct physical injury to the alveolar membrane. A positive association between asbestosis and lung tumors has been demonstrated by Wagner et al. (1974). The induction of fibrosis would impair clearance of deposited fibers, increasing the persistence of fibers in the lung.

The preceding implies that short fibers will have a low order of toxicity within the lung, comparable to that of nonfibrous silicate minerals. Within this concept, the critical fiber length would most likely be on the order of the diameter of an alveolar macrophage, namely about 10 to 15 µm. This line of reasoning leads to the same conclusion reached on the basis of the incidence of lung cancer in rats exposed to fibrous aerosols, that the hazard is related to the number of fibers longer than 10 µm deposited and retained in the lungs. The Timbrell (1983) model predicts alveolar retention of deposited fibers approaching 100% for 10 µm long fibers in the 0.3 to 0.8 µm diameter range. Airborne fibers longer than 100 µm may be much less harzardous than those in the 10 to 100 µm range because they do not penetrate deeply into the airways, since interception increases with fiber length.

Summary of Critical Fiber Parameters

The various hazards associated with the inhalation of mineral fibers, namely asbestosis, mesothelioma, and lung cancer, are all associated with fibers with lengths that exceed critical values. However, it now appears that the critical length is different for each disease, that is 2 µm for asbestosis, 5 µm for mesothelioma, and 10 µm for lung cancer. There are also different critical values of fiber diameter for the different diseases. For asbestosis and lung cancer, which are related to fibers retained in the lungs, only fibers with diameters > 0.15 µm need to be considered. On the other hand, for mesothelioma which is initiated by fibers that migrate from the lungs to the pleura and peritoneum, the hazard has been related fo fibers with diameters < 0.1 µm.

A recent study by Dufresne et al. (1996) of the fibers in lungs of Quebec miners and millers with and without asbestosis is supportive of the critical influence of long fibers on fibrosis and cancer incidence. They found that mean concentrations were higher in cases than in the controls for chrysotile fibers 5 to 10 µm long in patients with asbestosis with or without lung cancer; for tremolite fibers 5 to 10 µm long in all patients; for crocidolite, talc, or anthophyllite fibers 5 to 10 µm long in patients with mesothelioma; for chrysotile and tremolite fibers ≥ 10 µm long in patients with asbestosis; and crocidolite, talc, or anthophyllite fibers ≥ 10 µm long in patients with mesothelioma. Cumulative smoking index (pack-years) was higher in the group with asbestosis and lung cancer but was not statistically different from the two other disease groups.

Although all durable fibers of sufficient length can produce fibrosis and cancer, as documented in various animal studies, it appears that factors other than fiber size can - influence the extent of the response. For example, inhaled erionite appears to be much more potent for mesothelioma in both humans and animals because of its greater ability to penetrate the pleural surface. On the other hand, the animal and human data appear to differ on the ability of inhaled chrysotile to induce mesothelioma. Animal data indicate that chrysotile produces as much or more mesothelioma than the amphiboles, whereas human data more often implicate amphiboles, even when the predominant exposures are to chrysotile.

Examination of the fiber content of the lungs of asbestos workers and animals exposed by inhalation show that chrysotile is cleared much more rapidly than the amphiboles. It breaks down within the lungs both by disaggregation into fibrils and by dissolution. The differences between the responses in animals and humans may be in relative persistence (i.e., time of persistence of the long fibers in the lung relative to the time interval between exposure and the expression of the disease). In other words, the long fibers may be retained in the lung for a longer fraction of the lifespan in the rat.

Although all durable fibers in the right size range can cause the asbestos-related diseases, they may have different potencies and need different concentration limits. The remainder of this discussion addresses the indexes of exposure but not the concentration limits for the fibers that fall within the indexes. The concentration limits warrant separate and further discussion.

Implication of Critical Fiber Parameters to Exposure Indexes

Although the current occupational exposure index based on phase-contrast optical measurement of fibers with an aspect ratio > 3 and a length $> 5\,\mu m$ was a reasonable choice when it was made, it is now apparent that it cannot provide a fully adequate index for any of the several asbestos hazards.

A better index of the asbestosis hazard for the amphiboles is the total surface of fibers with diameters between 0.15 and $2\,\mu m$ and lengths greater than about $2\,\mu m$. This cannot be determined by optical microscopy, and electron microscopy is impractical for routine exposure assessments.

The applicability of this new index of asbestosis hazard for chrysotile is less well established than for the amphiboles. The long amphibole fibers clear very slowly from the lungs and do not dissolve, so the ratio of inhaled fiber surface area to lung-retained fiber surface area remains relatively constant. The chrysotile fibers dissolve and clear more rapidly, reducing the ratio of retained fiber surface to airborne fiber surface. On the other hand, the fibers split longitudinally within the lung, increasing the surface area of retained fibers. These issues need to be addressed in further experimental studies.

A better index of mesothelioma hazard is the number of fibers longer than $5\,\mu m$ and thinner than $0.1\,\mu m$. Since fibers with diameters less than $0.1\,\mu m$ cannot be resolved by optical microscopy, and only partially by scanning electron microscopy, analyses of relevant fiber counts must be done by transmission electron microscopy. The differences in fiber retention between chrysotile and the amphiboles may necessitate different concentration limits for the different fiber types.

A tentative proposal for a better index of lung cancer hazard is the number of fibers longer than $10\,\mu m$ that are retained within the lungs. Lung retention rises rapidly for diameters greater than about $0.15\,\mu m$. Thus the relevant fibers have diameters $> 0.15\,\mu m$ and lengths $> 10\,\mu m$. The current phase-contrast optical method of analysis of membrane filter samples is recommended for fibers with diameters between 0.25 and $3\,\mu m$ (WHO, 1986). Since lung retention of fibers with diameters between 0.15 and 0.25 m is relatively low (Fig. 3-5), PCOM analysis may provide a better index of hazard if the length limit is adjusted to $10\,\mu m$. Alternatively, analyses can be done by scanning electron microscope. Once again, the differences in fiber retention between chrysotile and the amphiboles may necessitate different concentration limits for the different fiber types.

Even if there were convenient and economical methods of sampling and analysis available for each of the three different asbestos hazards, it would undoubtedly be impractical to make three different kinds of exposure assessments at each potential exposure of concern. One option is to do a limited amount of detailed analyses of fiber size distribution initially by electron microscopy to determine if one or more of the potential hazards can be considered to be *de minimus*. For example, if there is negligable potential for exposure to fibers longer than 5 μm, there would be virtually no risk of either mesothelioma or lung cancer. For most nonoccupational exposures, there is virtually no risk of asbestosis, since prolonged exposure to high dust concentrations are needed to produce evidence of this disease.

If there were appreciable concentrations of fibers > 5 μm in length but with essentially all having fiber diameters larger than 0.15 μm, there would be virtually no risk for mesothelioma. In this case subsequent sampling could focus on the risk for lung cancer and asbestosis.

In essence, a rational preliminary examination would determine whether there was a controlling hazard at each potential asbestos exposure of concern, namely whether the fiber size distribution made it likely that the risk for asbestosis, mesothelioma, or lung cancer would dominate the others for that kind of exposure. If there was a dominant hazard, then only one kind of sampling and analysis protocol would be needed to demonstrate that the risk for all three hazards was under control. If two or more of the risks were approximately of equal concern, then monitoring for each would be needed.

It is not likely that regulatory authorities will adopt the dimensional criteria for hazardous fibers outlined above in the near future. One reason is that more research is needed to confirm their validity or to modify them in one aspect or another. Another reason is that essentially all current risk assessment models are based on exposure concentrations determined using other criteria, primarily the traditional industrial hygiene criterion of number concentration of fibers longer than 5 μm that are visible by phase-contrast optical microscopy, and such data cannot be reliably transformed to concentrations using different measurement criteria. Therefore, for the forseeable future, it would be desirable to use analytical protocols that permit the measurement of the lengths and diameters of all fibers longer than 2.5 μm so that the results can be tabulated according to the conventional criteria and any others adopted in future years. In the discussion of the human experience and risk assessments that follows, the exposure concentrations are based on the conventional 5 μm fiber-length criterion.

EXPOSURE–RESPONSE FOR ASBESTOS-RELATED LUNG CANCER AND MESOTHELIOMA: HUMAN EXPERIENCE

Epidemiologic Models

As noted by the HEI-AR Literature Review Committee (HEI-AR, 1991), the majority of published dose-specific estimates of the cancer risk caused by asbestos exposure have been based on models that assume the following:

1. The increase in relative risk for lung cancer is proportional to cumulative asbestos exposure, and the effects of asbestos and cigarette smoking multiply each other.
2. The increase in mesothelioma incidence caused by each brief period of exposure is propotional to the amount of that incremental exposure (exposure level × duration) and to a power of time since it occurred, independent of age or smoking. The power of time is approximately 2 or 3.

Similar risk assessment models were used in various government-sponsored reports, including those of the Environmental Protection Agency, the National Research Council, and the Consumer Product Safety Commission in the United States and comparable bodies in Britain and Canada. The validity of these models remains to be confirmed. Although dose-specific risk estimates differ substantially among cohorts, the results of analyses by different groups and authors for each cohort are similar.

For lung cancer the model implies that the effects of cigarette smoking and asbestos on lung cancer risk are multiplicative. This would mean that an exposure that doubles the rate among smokers (from a lifetime risk of about 0.1 to 0.2) will also double the rate among nonsmokers (from about 0.005 to 0.01). However, this may not be true. Lung cancer is so rare among nonsmokers, even after quite heavy asbestos exposure, that their risk cannot be estimated precisely. In fitting models, a major uncertainty is the choice of the lung cancer rate in unexposed workers. Local or national rates will not be appropriate if the workers' smoking habits are (or were, in the past) atypical.

Review of Epidemiological Data on Human Exposure – Cancer Response

The risk estimates (K_L) derived from different studies vary by two orders of magnitude. This in part reflects statistical variation, but Figure 3-5, in which 95% confidence limits are shown, indicates that there are highly significant differences between the different estimates. (Figure 3-5 is based on the risk estimates derived by the EPA, which are similar to those calculated in other reviews.) Possible reasons for this extreme heterogeneity include errors in the model, differences in hazard associated with different fiber types and dimensions, inaccuracies in exposure estimates, and the use of inappropriate lung cancer rates in calculating standardized mortality ratios (SMRs). The EPA review attempted a formal analysis of this variation between different studies (Nicholson, 1986). It presented explicit confidence limits for each estimate of K_L, taking account of statistical variation and assuming twofold (and in some cases greater) uncertainty in exposure estimates. For some cohorts, adjustments were made for suspected biases, particularly in the use of inappropriate lung cancer rates. Excluding the significantly lower risks per unit exposure observed for chrysotile mining and milling, this analysis gave a geometric mean for K_L of 0.01. The only study that gave a significantly higher-risk estimate than this central estimate was the Ontario asbestos cement products factor of Finkelstein (1983), but it had quite questionable exposure estimates and an inconsistant exposure-response relationship.

One of the studies with a higher than average risk coefficient was that of Dement et al. (1983a) in Figure 3-6. A follow-up study (Dement et al., 1994) confirmed the relatively high rate of lung cancer in this population, and attributed it to the high proportions of long fibers. Further modeling of the available data on this cohort was presented by Stayner et al. (1997), using a model designed to evaluate evidence of a threshold response. Lifetime risks of lung cancer and asbestosis were estimated with an actuarial approach that accounted for competing causes of death. They found a highly significant exposure–response relation for both lung cancer and asbestosis. The exposure–response relation for lung cancer seemed to be linear on a multiplicative scale, which is consistent with previous analyses of lung cancer and exposure to asbestos. By contrast, the exposure–response relation for asbestosis in this analysis seemed to be nonlinear on a multiplicative scale. There was no significant evidence for a threshold in models of either the lung cancer or asbestosis. The excess lifetime risk for white men exposed for 45 years at the current OSHA standard of 0.1 f / mL was predicted to be about 5 / 1000 for lung cancer, and 2 / 1000 for asbestosis.

One unsatisfactory aspect of the published literature on mesothelioma is the lack of adequately analyzed mortality data. The death rate rises sharply with time since exposure, yet only a few data sets have been analyzed by time since first exposure, and only four of

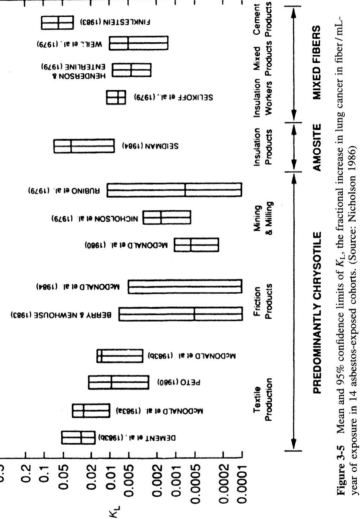

Figure 3-5 Mean and 95% confidence limits of K_L, the fractional increase in lung cancer in fiber/mL-year of exposure in 14 asbestos-exposed cohorts. (Source: Nicholson 1986)

these reports also provided estimates of average exposure level. Furthermore there are serious weaknesses in all four studies, particularly for assessing the effects of chrysotile. The exposure data and results for the cement factory workers' study reported by Finkelstein (1983) are of doubtful reliability for quantitative risk assessment, and there are no contemporary exposure data for the insulation workers (Selikoff et al., 1979) or the amosite textile workers (Seidman et al., 1979). Moreover none of these four cohorts was exposed only to chrysotile.

In the absence of any satisfactory basis for direct estimation of the dose-specific mesothelioma risk caused by any specific type of asbestos, particularly chrysotile, HEI-AR (1991) evaluated and modified previous predictions for mesothelioma by comparing observed and predicted ratios of mesothelioma to excess lung cancer in different cohorts. The predictive model for mesothelioma used by HEI-AR was proposed to explain the observation that mesothelioma incidence is independent of age and approximately proportional to the third power of time since first exposure. The model has been formally fitted in the only cohort for which individual exposure data were available (Peto et al., 1985). This limited analysis, based on only 10 cases, suggested that brief exposure causes less mesothelioma risk than that predicted.

The eventual lung cancer risk is assumed to be independent of age at exposure, but the predicted mesothelioma risk is much greater when exposure begins at an early age. These models therefore predict that the mesothelioma risk exceeds the lung cancer risk, even among smokers, for childhood exposure, whereas exposure in middle age causes a relatively trivial mesothelioma risk. Among nonsmokers, the lung cancer risk is much less than the mesothelioma risk irrespective of age at exposure.

Differences among Asbestos Types

Peritoneal Mesothelioma   The clearest difference in the effects of different fiber types is in the proportion of mesotheliomas that are present in the peritoneum. Almost all cases among chrysotile workers (usually with some exposure to crocidolite and / or tremolite) or among crocidilite miners are pleural, whereas workers with some amosite exposure have suffered similar and sometimes higher risks of peritoneal than pleural mesothelioma (Levin et al., 1998). The only exception appears to be female gas mask workers exposed mainly to crocidolite, among whom several mesotheliomas were peritoneal. The possibility of some amosite exposure in these workers was, however, not discussed by the authors of these reports. The inference that most peritoneal mesotheliomas are caused by amosite exposure is generally accepted (HEI-AR, 1991).

Pleural Mesothelioma   Direct comparison of workers employed for similar duration to different forms of asbestos (e.g., in mining or gas mask manufacture) indicates a much higher mesothelioma risk for amphiboles than for chrysotile. Chrysotile friction products workers in Britain suffered no detectable increase in lung cancer, and 11 of the 13 mesotheliomas in this cohort occurred in the subgroup of workers who were known to have been exposed to crocidolite (Berry and Newhouse, 1983; Newhouse and Sullivan, 1989). Chrysotile textile workers in Britain suffered a high risk of mesothelioma in contrast to those in South Carolina, although there was a substantial lung cancer risk in both cohorts. The only marked difference between these two textile plants was the use of some crocidolite (less than 5% of the fiber processed) in the British plant.

Mesothelioma and the "Amphibole Hypothesis"   As discussed previously, there have been marked differences between cohorts in the ratio of excess lung cancer to mesothelioma. Peritoneal mesotheliomas can usually be attributed to amosite exposure, but even when only pleural tumors are considered, the cancer ratio varies remarkably.

English shipyard workers with mixed exposure, including a substantial amount of crocidolite, suffered a high mesothelioma risk but no excess of lung cancer (Rossiter and Coles, 1980), whereas among workers at a South Carolina chrysotile textile plant there was a marked excess of lung cancer and a low incidence of pleural mesothelioma (McDonald et al., 1984; Dement et al., 1982, 1994). These data have been almost universally accepted as indicating that amphiboles, particularly crocidolite, cause a disproportionate mesothelioma risk.

Based on a pooling of various cohorts, Doll and Peto (1985) and Nicholson (1986) concluded that among men the ratio of excess lung cancer to pleural mesothelioma is about three times greater for chrysotile than crocidolite, varying from at least four for chrysotile to between one and two for crocidolite, with substantially lower ratios for women. However, such pooling of generally inconsistent data has dubious validity. In particular, it conceals the most extreme inconsistencies, most notably the marked excess of mesothelioma in the absence of any detectable excess of lung cancer observed among shipyard workers by Rossiter and Coles (1980) and in the subgroup of friction product workers with crocidolite exposure studied by Berry and Newhouse (1983).

Other investigators believe that virtually all mesotheliomas are due to amphibole exposure and that inhaled chrysotile fibers pose a negligible mesothelioma risk. The only strong evidence against the inference that mesothelioma is seldom, if ever, caused by chrysotile fibers alone is the observation of substantial numbers of cases among Quebec chrysotile miners and millers. It has, however, been suggested that these mesotheliomas are related to the presence of fibrous tremolite in this material (Mossman et al., 1990). Tremolite constituted less than 1% of the fiber extracted but more than half of the long ($> 5 \mu m$) fibers found in the lung tissue of the workers, apparently because chrysotile is cleared much more rapidly (Sebastien et al., 1989). Similarly, high levels of crocidolite were found in lung tissue from British textile workers who were exposed mainly to chrysotile but suffered a high incidence of mesothelioma (Wagner et al., 1982).

The early evidence that chrysotile fibers rarely causes pleural mesothelioma was consistent but not conclusive. There have been only two cohorts of heavily exposed asbestos workers who worked only with chrysotile (in both cases exposed to chrysotile from Quebec that is often contaminated with tremolite). There was an initial absence of pleural mesothelioma in the South Carolina plant despite the substantial risk of lung cancer (59 observed, 29.6 expected; Dement et al., 1982; McDonald et al., 1984). The Quebec chrysotile miners and millers suffered 230 lung cancers compared with 184.0 expected and 10 mesotheliomas, and lung burden studies show no marked differences between these cohorts in the type, size, or amount of either chrysotile or tremolite fibers (Sebastian et al., 1989).

In follow-up study of the South Carolina cohort by Dement et al. (1994) of 15 years of additional experience, there were two deaths attributable to mesothelioma, and the number of lung cancers had risen to 126. This was expressed as an increase in relative risk of 2.3% for each year of cumulative chrysotile exposure.

Begin et al. (1992) brought the experience in Quebec up to 1990. They concluded that the incidence of pleural mesothelioma in chrysotile miners and millers, while less than that for crocodolite workers, was well above the North American male rate.

A further examination of the Quebec asbestos cohort of some 11,000 chrysotile workers by McDonald and McDonald (1997), of whom 80% had already died, they addressed the amphibole hypothesis. They analyzed the deaths among almost 4000 miners employed by the largest company in the Thetford region. The number of cancer deaths by type were mesothelioma (21), lung (262), larynx (15), stomach (99), and colon and rectum (76). Risks, in relation to case referants, were analyzed by logistic regression separately for those working in the five chrysotile mines located centrally and for the ten mines located more peripherally, on the basis that tremolite concentrations were four times higher in the central region. Odds ratios were significantly and substantially elevated for workers at the centrally located chrysotile mines for mesothelioma and lung cancer but not for gastric, intestinal, or laryngeal cancers; while for the workers at the more peripherally located chrysotile mines, there was little or no elevation in odds ratio for any of the cancer groups. Dust exposures of the two groups were similar, and lung tissue analyses showed that the concentration of tremolite fibers was much higher in the lungs from the central area in comparison to those from workers at the peripheral mines (McDonald et al., 1997).

In an earlier study of Thetford mine workers by Gibbs (1979), pleural calcifications were also much more common among miners who had worked in the centrally located mines than those who worked in the peripherally located mines, suggesting that tremolite accounted for much of both pleural calcification and cancers of the lung and pleura. Furthermore the studies cited earlier by Dodson et al. (1990) and Boutin et al. (1996) suggest that some of this difference in potency was due to the greater retention of longer amphibole fibers in the lung and pleural lymph nodes than is the case for chrysotile. Additionally the experimental animal inhalation studies, summarized in Table 3-4 and discussed earlier, support the critical role of amphibole fibers in the causation of mesothelioma.

Thus, despite the continuing publication of contrary views (Frank et al., 1997; Smith and Wright, 1996; Stayner et al., 1996), the hypothesis that mesothelioma is largely, if not exclusively, caused by amphibole fibers remains consistent with the bulk of recently published evidence in humans and animals. No other epidemiological studies have addressed the mesothelioma-inducing potency of chrysotile directly. The substantial incidence of pleural mesothelioma in various cohorts exposed to both chrysotile contaminated by tremolite and by mixtures of chrysotile and other amphiboles is consistent with the hypothesis that these tumors were caused by amphibole exposure. However, it constitutes weak evidence that chrysotile per se does not cause mesothelioma. A prudent conclusion is that a very substantial proportion of the mesotheliomas in such cohorts are caused by amphibole exposure.

Measures of Asbestos Exposure Used in Past Epidemiologic Studies

The calculation of dose-specific risk depends as much on measurement of exposure as on estimation of excess risk, yet too little attention has been paid to the quality of these vital data. Only three cohorts in which substantial excess risks have been observed also have reasonably extensive historical dust measurements from which individual exposures can be estimated. In each case, however, there was little or no measurement of exposure in some of the dustiest areas, and conversion of particle to fiber counts was based on inconsistent measurements at relatively low levels. In one other study, of a United Kingdom friction products factory, extensive and probably reliable individual exposure estimates were calculated. The study does not provide a very useful dose-specific lung cancer risk estimate, however, since exposures were so low that the risk estimate (which was virtually zero) has very wide confidence limits.

RISK ASSESSMENT ISSUES: ASBESTOS

Assumption of Linear Dose – Response for Mesothelioma

The form of the mesothelioma dose response for chrysotile is not known. Some, although not all, carcinogens exhibit upward (possibly quadratic) curvature in dose response in cell transformation assays or in experimental tumor induction, and it has been suggested that the risk at low-dose levels may be negligible. There is, however, no good experimental evidence of such an effect for chrysotile. The prediction that risk is proportional to level of exposure at very low concentrations cannot be tested epidemiologically. Exposure levels have never been recorded accurately, and the predicted risks at low levels are far too low to be observable. The opposite belief, that the mesothelioma risk is anomalously high following very low exposure, is not supported by observation. In particular, the mesothelioma risk following short exposure to chrysotile may, if anything, be less than that predicted. Peto et al. (1985) studied approximately 18,000 men with no previous asbestos exposure employed in 1933 or later in a chrysotile textile plant. The incidence of mesothelioma was high among men with 20 or more years' exposure, but only two cases were observed among more than 16,000 men with under 10 years' exposure, and one of these seems certain not to have been caused by his employment, since the man was employed for only four months and died four years later. The current model for mesothelioma may thus overestimate the risk for brief (under 10 years) exposure, at least for chrysotile.

Assumption of Linear Dose – Response for Lung Cancer

The observation that excess lung cancer risk is roughly proportional to cumulative dose at high concentrations does not constitute very strong evidence of a linear relationship with fiber level, particularly at very low levels. This prediction is even more difficult to test directly for lung cancer than for mesothelioma, since lung cancer is so common in the general population, affecting more than 1 smoker in 10 and about 1 nonsmoker in 200, that even quite large increases in risk are difficult to estimate reliably. Prolonged low exposure to chrysotile in friction products, asbestos cement, and chrysotile mining has produced no detectable excess of lung cancer. Even in chrysotile textile production, the sector in which the highest dose- specific risks for chrysotile have been observed, over 10 years' exposure at low average levels (about 5 f/mL) produced little increase in risk in the U.K. study reported by Peto et al. (1985), although workers employed for fewer than 10 years in the South Carolina plant studied by Dement et al. (1983), who were more heavily exposed, suffered an increased risk (SMR = 1.9). Moreover there is evidence that the relative risk for lung cancer in chrysotile-exposed workers eventually falls after exposure to chrysotile has ceased (Walker, 1984; Peto et al., 1985). In the absence of evidence that the model used for lung cancer underestimates the long-term risk for brief or low exposure, and in view of the previously cited reassuring observations, the resulting predictions may, if anything, be too high for environmental exposure.

Dose – Response for Amphiboles

No extensive measurements of historical exposure levels are available for the cohorts exposed predominantly to crocidolite or amosite. Estimated levels have been published for the crocidolite miners of Western Australia (Armstrong et al., 1988) and varied from 20 to 100 f/mL. Most of this cohort were employed for less than a year, however, and more than half had estimated cumulative exposures of under 10 f/mL years, although only 5% exceeded 100 f/mL years. In a subsequent publication deKlerk et al. (1989) reported a case-control analysis indicating a significantly elevated lung cancer risk only in the minority of workers (about 3%) exposed for over five years, among whom the relative risk was 2.2, based on 11 deaths. No other study provides any useful exposure data for pure crocidolite, however, and this study alone is inadequate as a basis for a firm conclusion.

The situation for amosite is also unsatisfactory. The only study of amosite workers for which dose estimates have been provided (Seidman et al., 1979; see Nicholson, 1986, for updated lung cancer data) is a cohort of men manufacturing amosite insulation in Paterson, New Jersey, at the beginning of World War II. The dose estimates were based on very limited measurements taken more than 25 years later in two different factories using similar materials and equipment. There was a marked increase in lung cancer SMR, even in men employed for less than two months (SMR = 264, based on 15 deaths), and possible estimates of K_L vary from 0.01 (using the lung cancer rate in short-term workers as the baseline) to 0.04 (by regression on the SMR, based on local rates) (Nicholson, 1986). The SMR for men exposed for over two years was 650, and there were 14 mesotheliomas (7 pleural, 7 peritoneal). There are three major difficulties in interpreting this study: the lack of any direct exposure data, the anomalous pattern of SMR in relation to duration of exposure, and the uncertainties related to extrapolation from brief very high exposure to prolonged low exposure.

Both amosite and crocidolite have caused high risks of mesothelioma after brief exposure, which has not been observed for chrysotile. Brief amosite exposure can also cause a high lung cancer rate. Moreover there is consistent evidence that the ratio of mesothelioma to excess lung cancer is higher for amosite, and higher still for crocidolite, than for chrysotile alone.

One interesting inconsistency relates to the groups of workers exposed to some crocidolite who suffered a substantial risk of mesothelioma but no detectable excess of lung cancer, in contrast to the more heavily exposed crocidolite miners who appear to have suffered a larger excess of lung cancer than of mesothelioma. Perhaps the most plausible interpretation of these (and many other) differences is that different sizes have different effects, either in their ability to reach the bronchus or to reach the lung, and penetrate the pleura, or in their biological activity in different tissues. Unfortunately, however, our understanding of these processes is at present too limited to justify more specific conclusions.

Risks Associated with Nonoccupational Exposures

Mesothelioma among people not occupationally exposed to asbestos has been reported among people living near asbestos mining and processing areas, including members of households containing asbestos workers as well as those without. Presumably exposures to fibers were higher in homes with workers bringing home dust on their work clothing and shoes, but quantitative exposure data are lacking.

Wagner et al. (1960) reported that one-third of the mesothelioma cases reported in his South African population were not occupationally exposed to amphibole asbestos. Also three studies from Europe and one from the United States reported excess neighborhood cases around factories processing South African amphiboles (Newhouse and Thompson, 1965; Hain et al., 1974; Magnani et al., 1995; Hammond et al., 1979). In the United States, there was very heavy and visible community exposure to chrysotile asbestos in Manville, New Jersey (Borow and Livornese, 1973). Berry (1997) reported on the environmental, nonoccupational component of mesothelioma incidence among persons living in Manville. Prior to removal of occupational cases, residents of Manville had an average annual (1979–1990) mesothelioma rate of 636 male cases and 96 female cases per million population, about 25 times higher than average state rates. Cases were removed from the analysis when their "usual employment" was reported as being at the asbestos plant, as evidenced through union lists or occupational information from either the Cancer Registry or mortality records. Standardized incidence ratios (SIRs) were computed for residents of Manville and Somerset County (less the Manville population) by sex. New Jersey mesothelioma rates less than Somerset County contribution, 1979–1990, were used to generate the expected number of cases. The SIRs for Manville males and females were, respectively, 10.1 [95% confidence interval (CI): 5.8–16.4] and 22.4 (95% CI: 9.7–44.2). Male and female Somerset County mesothelioma incidence rates were 1.9 (95% CI: 1.4–2.5) and 2.0 (95% CI: 1.0–3.6). Some of these excesses were due to household exposures, but clearly the generally community exposures caused some of the excess.

Populations not occupationally exposed to mineral fiber may have very high incidences of mesothelioma. The most extreme case is the study of Baris et al. (1987) of people living in four villages in Central Cappadocia in Turkey. Three villages (Karain, Sarihidir, and Tuzkoy) were exposed to erionite, a fibrous zeolite, and a fourth (Karlik) lacked this exposure and served as a control. There were 141 deaths during the study period in the four villages, including 33 mesotheliomas, 17 lung cancers, 1 cancer of the larynx, 8 cancers of other sites, and 13 cancers not specified. Thus there were 72 cancers out of 141 deaths, with at least 33 of them due to mesothelioma. The age- and sex-specific mortality rates per 1000 person-years from mesothelioma and respiratory cancer for the four villages were 20.2, 13.5, 5.2, and 0 for males from Karain, Sarihidir, Tuzkoy, and Karlik, respectively. The corresponding rates for females were 10.9, 3.9, 4.9, and 0. Sebastien et al. (1984) examined ferruginous bodies in the sputum of residents of Karain, Tuzkoy, and Karlik. They found that the content of ferruginous bodies increased with age in Karain and Tuzkoy, but only one of 19 specimens from Karlik had any.

Mesotheliomas among nonoccupationally exposed people living near crocidolite-mining and -milling regions in South Africa and Western Australia have been known to occur for some time (Wagner and Pooley, 1986; Reid et al., 1990). For a population living near the Witenoom crocidolite mine in Western Australia, Hansen et al. (1997) were able to show a significant exposure-response relationship based on proximity and duration of exposure. Mesothelioma in nonoccupationally exposed residents of Cyprus has been attributed to tremolite by McConnochie et al. (1987).

For modeling purposes, however, risk extrapolations for community residents have had to rely on the quite considerable cancer risks associated with past occupational exposures. Within the range of observation, the models are consistent with the conservative assumption of a linear, nonthreshold response. Thus one can predict risks at the much lower exposure levels observed in schools and in commercial and public buildings. These predictions are unlikely to underestimate the risks and are more likely to overestimate them. Based on mean concentration data from Figure 3-1 and the lung cancer risk model of Doll and Peto (1985), the increase in cancer risk associated with 20 years of exposure to daily 8-hour exposures in commercial buildings, public buildings, and schools at average concentrations of fibers $> 5\,\mu m$ in length in such buildings of 0.0002 f / mL corresponds to a lifetime risk of about 2×10^{-6}. However, it should be noted that concentrations in buildings are seldom much higher than concentrations in the air outside the buildings, and therefore much of this small risk is related to the entry of outdoor fibers into the building with the ventilation air.

REVIEW OF EPIDEMIOLOGICAL EVIDENCE FOR HEALTH EFFECTS IN WORKERS EXPOSED TO MMMFs

Lung Cancer

The epidemiological literature on MMMFs has focused almost exclusively on lung cancer, and there have been no reports of mesothelioma in occupational groups without coexposures to asbestos. With respect to lung cancer, many of the studies of MMMF production workers have reported excess lung cancer among some cohorts, primarily those heavily exposed to slag wool and rock wool in earlier years, when exposure levels were largely uncontrolled (Enterline et al., 1983; Shannon et al., 1984; Saracci et al., 1984). Each of these studies was updated at the 1986 MMMF Symposium in Copenhagen (Enterline et al., 1987; Shannon et al., 1987; Simonato et al., 1986).

In the large multinational study in Europe involving approximately 22,000 MMMF production workers at 13 plants in seven countries, Saracci et al. (1984) reported a twofold excess in lung cancer mortality for the cohort having 30 years of follow-up since first employment but cautioned that the excess could not be clearly attributed to fiber exposure. In the follow-up study on this population reported by Simonato et al. (1986), the overall lung cancer SMR was 125, and the SMR for the subcohort with more than 30 years was 170. Adjustment for regional variations in mortality substantially reduced the excess lung cancer incidence for those workers exposed only to glass wool but not for those exposed to rock wool/slag wool. Within this group, most of the excess was accounted for by those with 20 to 29 years since first exposure (SMR of 270) and with 30 or more years (SMR of 244), who worked before dust controls were installed.

On the basis of measurements of airborne fiber concentrations made in the period 1977–1980 in the same European plants, Cherrie et al. (1986) reported that the average combined occupational group concentrations in the rock and glass wool plants were generally low (< 0.1 f/mL). In the glass continuous-filament factories the airborne fiber concentrations were very low (< 0.01 f/mL). The average plant median for fiber length ranged from 10 to 20 μm, and the corresponding median diameters ranged from 0.7 to 2 μm. In general, the glass wool fibers were thinner than the rock wool fibers. Higher levels (between 0.1 and 1.0 f/mL) were found in some insulation wool production, secondary production, and user industries. The highest levels (> 1.0 f/mL) occurred in very fine glass-fiber production and in other specialty insulation wool usage.

For the 17 U.S. plants producing and using ordinary fibrous glass insulation products that were studied by Enterline et al. (1983, 1987), Esmen (1984) reported that 35% of the airborne fibers were > 5 μm in length and that only 3.9% were < 1.0 μm in diameter. The average exposure concentrations, as determined by phase-contrast optical microscopy, were between 0.01 and 0.05 f/mL in 13 plants handling ordinary glass fibers. For a slag wool plant, the average was about 0.07 f/mL, while for a rock wool plant and a glass microfiber plant, the averages were about 0.25 f/mL.

Enterline et al. (1987) reported the 1946–1982 mortality experience of 16,661 MMMF workers employed six months or more during 1940–1963 at one or more of 17 U.S. manufacturing plants. Using local death rates to estimate expected deaths, there was a statistically significant excess in all malignant neoplasms and in lung cancer 20 or more years after first employment. For respiratory cancer the excess was greatest for mineral wool workers and workers ever exposed in the production of small diameter fibers. These two groups of workers are believed to have had mean exposures to respirable fibers of around 0.3 f/mL. For glass wool workers and glass filament workers, respiratory cancer SMRs were much lower. For these workers, exposures were estimated to be about 1/10 the level for mineral wool and small-diameter fiber workers. There were few positive relationships between respiratory cancer SMRs and duration of exposure, time since first exposure, or measures of fiber exposure. A smoking survey showed MMMF workers to have cigarette-smoking habits similar to all U.S. white males. In a case-referent study that controlled for smoking, there was a statistically significant relationship between fiber exposure and respiratory cancer for mineral wool workers but not for fibrous glass workers.

The historical prospective mortality study conducted by Shannon et al. (1987) at an insulating wool plant in Ontario, Canada, covered 2557 men who had worked for at least 90 days and were employed between 1955 and 1977, with follow-up to the end of 1984; 157 deaths were found in the 97% of men traced. Mortality was compared by the person-years method with that of the Ontario population. Overall mortality was below that expected (SMR = 84). Cancer deaths were slightly raised, owing entirely to an excess in lung cancer. The 21 deaths from this cause give a significantly high SMR of 176. All but two of these cases occurred among "plant-only" employees. However, the interpretation of these data remains difficult because the SMRs by length of exposure and time since first worked were not consistent with a causal relationship.

Another very large population studied by Engholm et al. (1987) for the incidence of respiratory cancer in relation to exposure to MMMFs was a large cohort of Swedish construction workers. The cohort comprised some 135,000 men, who were all examined at regular health checkups in 1971–1974. The cohort was followed for mortality through 1983 and for cancer incidence through 1982 by linkage to various national registries. A case-control study within the cohort was carried out on 518 cases diagnosed as having respiratory cancer. The subjects were classified into categories based on self-reported exposure and on estimates of average intensity of exposure in occupations concerned. Smoking habits and density of population were included as potential confounders. Overall, there was an excess of mortality from industrial accidents and an excess incidence of mesothelioma, but in other respects the mortality and the cancer incidence in this population compared favorably with those of the general Swedish population.

For lung cancer the overall incidence was below that expected, but there was a risk related to high asbestos exposure. The risk fell close to unity for MMMFs when both exposures were fitted simultaneously.

The human experience, based on long-term follow-up on 41,185 MMMF workers in the United States, Canada, and Europe, is encouraging. Many of these workers were exposed to very high concentrations of fibers in the 1940s and 1950s. As summarized by Doll (1987), the evidence of excess lung cancer among these workers appears confined to those subcohorts exposed to slag or rock wool or to small-diameter fibers as well as conventional fibrous glass. When he excluded short-term and office workers and compared the numbers of deaths with those that would have been expected had the workers experienced national mortality rates (or provincial rates in the Canadian series), he found that the mortality from lung cancer (SMR = 121) was raised but that the mortality from other cancers (SMR = 101), other respiratory disease (SMR = 103), and all other causes of death (SMR = 100) was close to that expected.

Division of the workers by type of product and time since first exposure showed that the mortality from lung cancer was highest in the rock or slag wool sector of the industry (SMR = 128), intermediate in the glass wool sector (SMR = 110), and lowest in the continuous-filament glass sector (SMR = 93) and that within the first two groups mortality rose with time since first exposure to a maximum after 30 or more years (rock or slag wool, SMR = 141; glass wool, SMR = 119). Within the U.S. glass wool industry, the mortality from lung cancer was higher in those men who had ever been exposed to small-diameter fibers (SMR = 124) than in others (SMR = 108). No relationship was observed with duration of employment or with cumulative fiber dose. In a case-control study, however, a weak relationship with cumulative fiber dose was observed in the rock and slag wool sectors of the industry after differences in smoking habits had been taken into account. No evidence was obtained of a risk of mesothelioma or any other type of cancer. Doll concluded that an occupational hazard of lung cancer has been demonstrated in the rock and slag wool section of the industry and possibly in the glass wool section. Uncertainty about fiber counts in the early years of the industry and about the extent to which other carcinogens were present in the atmosphere of the plants precludes an estimate of the quantitative effects of exposure to current fiber levels, except that it is unlikely to be measurable.

The results of the most recent epidemiologic study of MMMF workers in the United States were reported by Wong and Musselman (1994) for workers at nine plants that made or used slag wool. These included four plants previously studied and five additional plants. This was a nested case-control study based on 55 lung cancers. They analyzed lung cancer risk in relation to cumulative fiber exposure (concentration and duration) and smoking history, and controlled for other coexposures such as asbestos contamination. No increased lung cancer risk with exposure to slag wool fibers was found. This paper provided guidelines to estimate the magnitude of potential confounding effects of coexposures such as smoking.

Respiratory Morbidity

Quantitative data on exposure-response relationships in occupational groups exposed to MMMFs for effects other than lung cancer are sparse. The best-documented effects are for workers exposed to refractory ceramic fibers (RCFs). Lemasters et al. (1998) reported on an industrywide RCF cohort that was characterized as either production or nonproduction activities and duration of production employment. Both male and female production workers had significantly more respiratory symptoms. For male production workers there was a significant decline, over ten years, in FVC for both smokers and nonsmokers, while only the male smokers had a significantly greater decline in FEV_1. Female nonsmokers had a greater decline in FVC than their male counterparts. In an earlier report on this population, Lemasters and Lockery (1994) reported a correlation between pleural changes and RCF exposures.

By contrast, studies of a comparable industrywide cohort in Europe by Trethowan et al. (1995) found no excess in illness or chest X-ray abnormalities related to fiber exposures.

For symptoms, lung function changes related to exposures to other MMVFs, the epidemiologic evidence had been largely negative (Utidjian and deTreville, 1970; Hook et al., 1970; Nasr et al., 1971; Hill et al., 1973; Malmberg et al., 1984; Hughes et al., 1993). In terms of X-ray abnormalities, the only positive findings were reported by Hughes et al. (1993) on a population cohort exposed to very thin glass fibers.

RISK ASSESSMENT ISSUES: MAN-MADE MINERAL FIBERS

Although there has been a significant advance in our knowledge about the deposition and elimination of man-made mineral fibers (MMMFs) and other fibers in recent years, as well as some new knowledge about exposure-response in controlled animal inhalation studies, some further concern about lung cancer among heavily exposed workers in industry, and some new insight into the critical fiber dimensions affecting disease pathogenesis, there are also many important questions that remain to be addressed. In some cases the behavior and risks of airborne MMMFs can be inferred from those of either compact particles or asbestos fibers. On the other hand, the validity of such inferences depends on some critical assumptions about the aerodynamic properties of the various fibers and about the responses of lung and mesothelial cells to such fibers. The differences may be critical, and more in vivo studies with MMMFs should be performed in order to further clarify these issues. In the interim we already know a great deal about the nature and extent of fiber toxicity and the factors that modify its expression. This knowledge provides a good basis for a fairly definitive risk assessment for MMMFs.

MMMFs differ from asbestos fibers in several critical ways and tend to produce less lung deposition and more rapid elimination of those fibers that do deposit in the lungs. One difference is in diameter distribution. Except for glass microfiber, MMMFs tend to have relatively small mass fractions in diameters small enough to penetrate through the upper respiratory tract. Asbestos, on the other hand, usually contains more "respirable" fiber. Furthermore, once deposited, the asbestos fibers may split into a larger number of long thin fibers within the lungs. MMMFs rarely split but are more likely to break into shorter length segments.

There are also differences in solubility among the fibers that affect their toxic potential, among both the asbestos types and the MMMFs. Conventional glass fibers appear to dissolve much more rapidly than other MMMFs and asbestos. Dissolution of glass fibers takes place both by surface attack and by leaching within the structure. The diameters are reduced and the structure is weakened, favoring breakup into shorter segments. Since the smallest-diameter fibers have the greatest surface-to-volume ratio, they dissolve most rapidly. Thus the relatively small fraction of the airborne glass fibers with diameters small enough to penetrate into the lungs are the most rapidly dissolved within the lungs.

The more durable and less soluble MMMFs, namely slag and rock wool, some speciality glasses, and ceramic fibers, require a higher degree of concern because of their longer retention within the lungs. In vitro studies and studies of dissolution in simulated lung fluids can be very useful in preliminary evaluations of the toxic potential of the various MMMFs. On the other hand, the dissolution of MMMFs in vivo depends on many additional factors that cannot readily be simulated in model systems. For example, the differences in solubility in vivo of long and short fibers noted by Morgan and Holmes (1984) were attributed to small difference in intracellular and extracellular pH. The mechanical stress on fibers in vivo may also contribute to their disintegration, and this cannot readily be simulated in model systems. Thus hazard evaluations of specialty product MMMFs made for limited and specific applications should include detailed in vivo studies in which animals are exposed to appropriate sizes and concentrations of the fibers of interest.

In the case of conventional fibrous glasses, we have sufficient information to conclude that the occupational health risks associated with the inhalation of fibers dispersed during their manufacture, installation, use, maintenance, and disposal are unmeasurable (Doll, 1987) and hence of an extremely low order. The health risk from casual and infrequent indoor air exposure of building occupants to relatively low concentrations of fibrous glass is therefore essentially nil. These judgments are based on a series of interacting factors, each of which individually leads to a far lower order of risk for conventional glass fibers than asbestos. Specifically

1. Conventional glass fibers are less readily aerosolized than asbestos during comparable operations, as demonstrated by the much lower fiber counts measured at various industrial operations (Cherrie et al., 1986; Esmen, 1984).

2. A much smaller fraction of conventional glass fibers than asbestos fibers have small enough aerodynamic diameters to penetrate into lung airways (i.e., fibers with diameters below 3 µm) (Konzen, 1984).

3. The small fractions of glass fibers that can penetrate into the lungs are much less durable within the lung than asbestos. They tend to break up into shorter segments, so that fewer fibers longer than the critical length limits are retained at critical sites. They also tend to dissolve, further reducing their retention (Bernstein et al., 1984).

4. The inherent toxicity of conventional glass fibers is much lower than that of asbestos fibers of similar dimension, as shown by studies in which fiber suspensions are applied directly to target tissues by intratracheal instillation (Wright and Kuschner, 1977) or application of a fiber mat to the lung pleura (Stanton and Wrench, 1972).

In consideration of these factors, the risk for lung fibrosis is virtually nil unless there is continual exposure at concentrations high enough to maintain a high level of lung burden for this relatively rapidly cleared type of particulate. The risk of lung cancer is also virtually nil unless there is continual exposure to long fibers at high concentrations because of the relatively rapid breakup of long fibers into short fiber segments within the lungs. Finally the risk of mesothelioma from inhaled conventional glass fibers is virtually nil under almost any circumstances. There are hardly any glass fibers thin enough to cause mesothelioma in the aerosols, and the very few that may be present would dissolve rapidly within the lungs.

KEY FACTORS AFFECTING FIBER UPTAKE AND TOXICITY: RECAPITULATION AND SYNTHESIS

Critical Fiber Properties Affecting Toxicity

Review of the in vitro studies clearly indicates that fiber length, diameter, and composition are critical determinants of cytotoxicity and cell transformation. A review of the in vivo animal studies, both by inhalation and injection, shows that fiber dimensions and composition are important factors affecting pathological measures such as fibrosis and cancer yields. Review of human exposure shows that the proportions of the different diseases caused by asbestos, namely asbestosis, lung cancer, and mesothelioma, vary greatly among occupational cohorts and that the mesothelioma / lung cancer ratio tends to increase with decreasing fiber diameter for the durable amphibole forms of asbestos.

Influence of Fiber Diameter

Fiber diameter affects airborne fiber penetration into and along the lung airways and thereby the initial deposition patterns. The aerodynamic diameters of mineral fibers are about three times their physical diameters (Timbrell, 1972; Stöber et al., 1970). Thus fibers with diameters larger than 3 μm will not penetrate in the lungs (Lippmann, 1990). Fibers with diameters ≤ 0.1 μm are less well retained in the lungs than larger fibers (Lippmann and Timbrell, 1990). Their large surface-to-volume ratio favors dissolution (Lippmann, 1990). Those sufficiently durable not to dissolve can readily penetrate the epithelial surface and be translocated to the lung interstitium and pleural surfaces. The fibers that remain in the lungs can cause fibrosis and lung cancer, and those durable fibers that are translocated to pleural surfaces can cause mesothelioma. Thus, for asbestosis and lung cancer, the upper fiber diameter limit is on the order of 3 μm. For mesothelioma, the upper fiber diameter limit is likely to be much less for two reasons. First, the thinner fibers penetrate to the gas-exchange region to a greater extent. Second, fibers thinner than 0.5 μm are translocated from the deposition sites to postnodal lymphatic channels more than the thicker fibers and thus reach any organ of the body (Oberdörster et al., 1988).

Influence of Fiber Length

Fiber length can also affect fiber penetration into and along the airways. As the length increases beyond 10 μm, the interception mechanism begins to significantly enhance deposition (Sussman et al., 1991a, b). Thus longer fibers have proportionately more airway deposition and less deposition in the gas-exchange region. Lung retention also increases markedly with increasing fiber length above 10 μm, both on theoretical grounds (Yu et al., 1990) and on the basis of analysis of residual lung dust in humans (Pooley and Wagner, 1988; Churg and Wiggs, 1987; Timbrell et al., 1987) and animals (Morgan, 1979). Furthermore fibers shorter than 6 μm in length can readily penetrate through tracheobronchial lymph nodes and be translocated to more distant organs (Oberdörster et al., 1988).

Exact specification of the critical lengths for the different diseases remains difficult, since the experimental studies generally have had, of practical necessity, to use imperfectly classified fiber suspensions. Also the experimental studies have used very large concentrations, and apportioning attribution of the cytotoxicity and pathology produced to the effects of fiber size versus dust overload phenomena is difficult. In other words, the results described in the in vivo section of this review would be consistent either with short fibers having a much smaller effect than long fibers or with their contributing to the growth of fibrotic lesions caused by the relatively few long fibers in the tail of the fiber length distribution. In any case the fibers shorter than 5 μm have very much less toxicity, whereas fibers longer than 5 μm have the greatest impact on cytotoxicity and disease.

Influence of Fiber Composition

Comparative retention and toxicity studies with various kinds of asbestos and other fibrous minerals, ceramics and glasses indicate that properties other than fiber dimensions affect fiber retention and toxicity. Among these are solubility, specific surface area, and surface electrical charges that may contribute to redox reactions generating active oxygen species. Thus dimensional characteristics alone, although important, are insufficient indicators of fiber toxicity. It is now time to revise the Stanton hypothesis, which acknowledges the critical importance of fiber length and diameter in biological responses, and recognize the importance of the other physical-chemical properties that impart biological potential to fibers. A major research need is a systemic exploration of the surface properties and factors affecting solubility of fibers in lung fluids and cells so that due considerations can be given to fiber composition in hazard assessment.

ACKNOWLEDGMENTS

This research was performed as part of a Center Program supported by NIEHS (Grant ES 00260). It includes extensive review material from earlier review papers, specifically: Lippmann (1988, 1990, 1994) and Health Effects Institute–Asbestos Research (1991).

ACRONYMS

ACGIH	American Conference of Governmental Industrial Hygienists
ACM	Asbesto-containing material
AM	Alveolar macrophage
BMRC	British Medical Research Council
HEI-AR	Health Effects Institute–Asbestos Research
IOM	Institute of Occupational Medicine, Edinburgh
MALS	Magnetic alignment and light scattering
MMMF	Man-made mineral fibers
MMVF	Man-made vitreous fibers
MPPCF	Millions of particles per cubic foot
OSHA	Occupational Safety and Health Administration
PCOM	Phase-contrast optical method
PEL	Permissible exposure limit
PMN	Polymorphonuclear leukocytes
SMR	Standardized mortality ratio
TEM	Transmission electron microscopy
TLV	Threshold limit value

UICC   International Union against Cancer (English translation of name of organization in French

REFERENCES

ACGIH-AIHA Aerosol Hazards Evaluation Committee. 1975. Recommended procedures for sampling and counting asbestos fibers. *Am. Ind. Hyg. Assoc. J.* 36: 83–90.

Albin, M., F. D. Pooley, U. Strömberg, R. Atteweil, R. Mitha, L. Johansson, and H. Welinder. 1994. Retention patterns of asbestos fibres in lung tissue among asbestos cement workers. *Occup. Environ. Med.* 51: 205–211.

Allison, A. C. 1977. Mechanisms of macrophage damage in relation to the pathogenesis of some lung diseases. In *Respiratory Defense Mechanisms*, eds. J. D. Brain, D. F. Proctor, and L. M. Reid, part II, pp. 1075–1102. New York: Marcel Dekker.

Armstrong, B. K., N. H. DeKlerk, A. W. Musk, and M. S. T. Hobbs. 1988. Mortality in miners and millers of crocidolite in western Australia. *Br. J. Ind. Med.* 45: 5–13.

Ashcroft, T., J. M. Simpson, and V. Timbrell. 1988. Simple method of estimating severity of pulmonary fibrosis on a numerical scale. *J. Clin. Pathol.* 41: 467–470.

Baris, I., L. Simonato, M. Artvinli, F. Pooley, R. Saracci, J. Skidmore, and C. Wagner. 1987. Epidemiological and environmental evidence of the health effects of exposure to erionite fibers: A four-year study in the Cappadocian region of Turkey. *Int. J. Cancer.* 39: 10–17.

Barrett, J. C., P. W. Lamb, and R. W. Wiseman. 1989. Multiple mechanisms for the carcinogenic effects of asbestos and other mineral fibers. *Environ. Health Perspect.* 81: 81–89.

Bauman, M. D., A. M. Jetten, J. C. Bonner, R. K. Kumar, R. A. Bennett, and A. R. Brody. 1990. Secretion of a platelet-derived growth factor homologue by rat alveolar macrophages exposed to particulates *in vitro. Eur. J. Cell Biol.* 51: 327–334.

Bayliss, D. L., J. M. Dement, J. K. Wagoner, and H. P. Blejer. 1976. Mortality patterns among fibrous glass production workers. *Ann. NY Acad. Sci.* 271: 345–352.

Beck, E. G., J. Bruch, K. H. Friedricks, W. Hilscher, and F. Pott. 1971. Fibrous silicates in animal experiments and cell-culture in morphological cell and tissue reactions according to different physical chemical influences. In *Inhaled Particles III*, ed. W. H. Walton, pp. 477–486. Old Woking, U.K.: Unwin Bros.

Begin, R., J. J. Gauthier, M. Desmeules, and G. Ostiguy. 1992. Work-related mesothelioma in Quebec, 1967–1990. *Am. J. Ind. Med.* 22: 531–542.

Bellmann, B., H. Konig, H. Muhle, and F. Pott. 1986. Chemical durability of asbestos and of man-made mineral fibres *in vivo. J. Aerosol Sci.* 17: 341–345.

Bellmann, B., H. Muhle, F. Pott, H. Konig, H. Kloppel, and K. Spurny. 1987. Persistence of man-made mineral fibers (MMMF) and asbestos in rat lungs. *Ann. Occup. Hyg.* 31(4B): 693–709.

Berman, W., and E. J. Chatfield. 1989. Interim Superfund Method for the Determination of Asbestos in Ambient Air. Part II: *Technical Background Document.* Draft Report EPA Contract no. 68-61-7290, Task 117, USEPA, Region 9, San Francisco, CA 94105.

Bernstein, D. M., R. T. Drew, G. Schidlovsky, and H. Kuschner. 1984. Pathogenicity of MMMF and the contrasts to natural fibers. In *Biological Effects of Man-Made Mineral Fibers*, vol. 2, pp. 169–195, Copenhagen: WHO-EURO.

Bernstein, D. M., C. Morscheidt, H.-G. Grimm, P. Thévenaz, and U. Teichert. 1996. Evaluation of soluble fibers using the inhalation biopersistence model, a nine-fiber comparison. *Inhal. Toxicol.* 8: 345–385.

Berry, J., and M. Newhouse. 1983. Mortality of workers manufacturing friction materials using asbestos. *Br. J. Ind. Med.* 40: 1–7.

Berry, M. 1997. Mesothelioma incidence and community asbestos exposure. *Environ. Res.* 75: 34–40.

Bolton, R. E., J. H. Vincent, A. D. Jones, J. Addison, and S. T. Beckett. 1983. An overload hypothesis for pulmonary clearance of UICC amosite fibers inhaled by rats. *Br. J. Ind. Med.* 40: 264–272.

Bontin, C., P. Dumortier, F. Rey, J. R. Viallat, and P. DeVuyst. 1996. Black spots concentrate oncogenic asbestos fibers in the parietal pleura: Thorascopic and mineralogic study. *Am. J. Respir. Crit. Care Med.* 153: 444–449.

Borow, M., and L. L. Livornese. 1973. Mesothelioma following exposure to asbestos: A review of 72 cases. *Chest.* 201: 587–591.

Briant, J. K. 1988. *Distinction of reversible and irreversible convection by high-frequency ventilation of a respiratory airway cast.* Ph.D. disserfation. New York University.

Brody, A. R., and M. W. Roe. 1983. Deposition pattern of inorganic particles at the alveolar level in the lungs of rats and mice. *Am. Rev. Respir. Dis.* 128: 724–729.

Brody, A. R., L. H. Hill, B. Adkins Jr., and R. W. O'Connor. 1981. Chrysotile asbestos inhalation in rats: Deposition pattern and reaction of alveolar epithelium and pulmonary macrophages. *Am. Rev. Respir Dis.* 123: 670–679.

Burdett, G. 1985. Use of a membrane filter, direct-transfer technique for monitoring environmental asbestos releases. In *A Workshop on Asbestos Fiber Measurements in Building Atmospheres.* Mississauga, Ontario: Ontario Research Foundation.

Chan, T. L., P. S. Lee, and W. E. Hering. 1984. Pulmonary retention of inhaled diesel particles after prolonged exposures to diesel exhaust. *Fundam. Appl. Toxicol.* 4: 624–631.

Cherrie, J., J. Dodgson, S. Groat, and W. MacLaren. 1986. Environmental surveys in the European man-made mineral fiber production industry. *Scand. J. Work Environ. Health* 12 (suppl. 1): 18–25.

Chisholm, J. E. 1983. Transmission electron microscopy of asbestos. In *Asbestos*, eds. S. S. Chissick, and R. Derricott, pp. 86–167. New York: Wiley.

Churg, A. 1994. Deposition and clearance of chrysotile asbestos. *Ann. Occup. Hyg.* 38: 625–633.

Churg, A., and B. Wiggs. 1987. Accumulation of long asbestos fibers in the peripheral upper lobe in cases of malignant mesothelioma. *Am. J. Ind. Med.* 11: 563–569.

Churg, A., B. Wiggs, L. Depaoli, B. Kampe, and B. Stevens. 1984. Lung asbestos content in chrysotile workers with mesothelioma. *Am. Rev. Respir. Dis.* 130: 1042–1045.

Collier, C. G., O. Kamstrup, K. J. Morris, R. A. Applin, and I. A. Vatter. 1997. Lung clearance of experimental man-made mineral fibres, Preliminary data on the effect of fiber length. *Ann. Occup. Hyg.* 41 (suppl. 1): 320–326.

Collier, C. G., K. J. Morris, K. A. Launder, J. A. Humphreys, A. Morgan, W. Eastes, and S. Townsend. 1994. The behavior of glass fibers in the rat following intraperitoneal injection. *Regul. Toxicol. Pharmacol.* 20: S89–S103.

Craighead, J. E. 1987. Current pathogenetic concepts of diffuse malignant mesothelioma. *Human Pathol.* 18: 544–557.

Davis, J. M. G. 1976. Pathological aspects of the injection of fiber into the pleural and peritoneal cavities of rats and mice. In *Occupational Exposure to Fibrous Glass*, HEW Publ. (NIOSH) 76–151, pp. 141–199. Washington, DC: DHEW.

Davis, J. M. G. 1987. Experimental data relating to the importance of fibre type, size, deposition, dissolution and migration. In *Proceedings of 1987 Mineral Fiber Symposium*, Lyons, IARC.

Davis, J. M. G., B. Gylseth, and A. Morgan. 1986a. Assessment of mineral fibers from human lung tissue. *Thorax.* 41: 167–175.

Davis, J. M. G., J. Addison, R. E. Bolton, K. Donaldson, A. D. Jones, and B. G. Miller. 1985. Inhalation studies on the effects of tremolite and brucite dust in rats. *Carcinogenesis.* 6: 667–674.

Davis, J. M. G., J. Addison, R. E. Bolton, K. Donaldson, A. D. Jones, and T. Smith. 1986b. The pathogenicity of long versus short fiber samples of amosite asbestos administered to rats by inhalation and intraperitoneal injection. *Br. J. Exp. Pathol.* 67: 415–430.

Davis, J. M. G., S. T. Beckett, R. E. Bolton, P. Collings, and A. P. Middleton. 1978. Mass and number of fibers in the pathogenesis of asbestos-related lung disease in rats. *Br. J. Cancer.* 37: 673–688.

deKlerk, N. H., B. K. Armstrong, A. W. Musk, and M. S. T. Hobbs. 1989. Cancer mortality in relation to measures of occupational exposure to crocidolite at Wittenoom Gorge in western Australia. *Br. J. Ind. Med.* 46: 529–536.

deKlerk, N. H., A. W. Musk, J. J. Glancy, S. C. Pang, H. G. Lund, N. Olsen, and M. S. T. Hobbs. 1997. Crocidolite, radiographic asbestosis and subsequent lung cancer. *Ann. Occup. Hyg.* 41 (suppl. 1): 134–136.

Dement, J. M., and K. M. Wallingford. 1990. Comparison of phase contrast and electron microscopic methods for evaluation of occupational asbestos exposures. *Appl. Occup. Environ. Hyg.* 5: 242–247.

Dement, J. M., D. P. Brown, and A. Okun. 1994. Follow-up study of chrysotile asbestos textile workers: Cohort mortality and case-control analyses. *Am. J. Ind. Med.* 26: 431–447.

Dement, J. M., R. L. Harris, M. J. Symans, and C. Shy. 1982. Estimates of dose–response for respiratory cancer among chrysotile asbestosis workers. *Ann. Occup. Hyg.* 28: 869–887.

Dement, J. M., R. L. Harris Jr., M. J. Symans, and C. M. Shy. 1983. Exposures and mortality among chrysotile asbestos workers. Part II: Mortality. *Am. J. Ind. Med.* 4: 421–433.

Dodson, R. F., M. G. Williams Jr., C. J. Corn, A. Brollo, and C. Bianchi. 1990. Asbestos content of lung tissue, lymph nodes, and pleural plaques from former shipyard workers. *Am. Rev. Respir. Dis.* 142: 843–847.

Doll, R. 1987. Symposium on MMMF, Copenhagen, October 1986: Overview and conclusions. *Ann. Occup. Hyg.* 31(4B): 805–819.

Doll, R., and J. Peto. 1985. *Effects on Health of Exposure to Asbestos. A Report to the Health and Safety Commission.* London: Her Majesty's Stationery Office.

Dufresne, A., R. Bégin, S. Masse, C. M. Dufresne, P. Loosereewanich, and G. Perrault. 1996. Retention of asbestos fibres in lungs of workers with asbestosis, asbestosis and lung cancer, and mesothelioma in Asbestos township. *Occup. Environ. Med.* 53: 801–807.

Dunnigan, J. 1990. Author's reply. Comparing biological effects of mineral fibers. *Br. J. Ind. Med.* 47: 287.

Eastes, W., and J. G. Hadley. 1995. Dissolution of fibers inhaled by rats. *Inhal. Toxicol.* 7: 179–196.

Eastes, W., and J. G. Hadley. 1996. A mathematical model of fiber carcinogenicity and fibrosis in inhalation and intraperitoneal experiments in rats. *Inhal. Toxicol.* 8: 323–343.

Eastes, W., K. J. Morris, A. Morgan, K. A. Launder, C. G. Collier, J. A. Davis, S. M. Mattson, and J. G. Hadley. 1995. Dissolution of glass fibers in the rat lung following intratracheal instillation. *Inhal. Toxicol.* 7: 197–213.

Engholm, G., A. Englund, C. C. Fletcher, and N. Hallin. 1987. Respiratory cancer incidence in Swedish construction workers exposed to man-made mineral fibers and asbestos. *Ann. Occup. Hyg.* 31(4B): 663–675.

Enterline, P. E., and V. Henderson. 1975. The health of retired fibrous glass workers. *Arch. Environ. Health.* 30: 113–116.

Enterline, P. E., G. M. Marsh, and N. A. Esmen. 1983. Respiratory disease among workers exposed to man-made mineral fibers. *Am. Rev. Respir. Dis.* 128: 1–7.

Enterline, P. E., G. M. Marsh, V. Henderson, and C. Callahan. 1987. Mortality update of a cohort of U.S. man-made mineral fiber workers. *Ann. Occup. Hyg.* 31(4B): 625–656.

Esmen, N. A. 1984. Short-term survey of airborne fibres in U.S. manufacturing plants. In *Biological Effects of Man-made Mineral Fibers*, vol. 1, pp. 65–82. Copenhagen: WHO-EURO.

Esmen, N. A., and S. Erdal. 1990. Human occupational and nonoccupational exposure to fibers. *Environ. Health Perspect.* 88: 277–286.

Ferin, J. 1972. Observations concerning alveolar dust clearance. *Ann. NY Acad. Sci.* 200: 66–72.

Ferin, J., and L. J. Leach. 1976. The effect of amosite and chrysotile asbestos on the clearance of TiO_2 particles from the lung. *Environ. Res.* 12: 250–254.

Finkelstein, M. M. 1983. Mortality among long-term employees of an Ontario asbestos-cement factory. *Br. J. Ind. Med.* 40: 138–144.

Floyd, R. A. 1990. Role of oxygen free radicals in carcinogenesis and brain ischemia. *FASEB J.* 4: 2587–2597.

Forster, H. 1984. The behavior of mineral fibers in physiological solutions. In *Biological Effects of Man-Made Mineral Fibers*, vol. 2, pp. 27–59. Copenhagen: WHO-EURO.

Frank, A. L., R. F. Dodson, and M. G. Williams. 1997. Lack of tremolite in UICC reference chrysotile and the implications for carcinogenicity. *Ann. Occup. Hyg.* 41 (suppl. 1): 287–292.

Galakhov, F. Y., and B. G. Varshal. 1973. Causes of phase separation in glasses. In *The Structure of Glass, 8, Phase Separation Phenomenon in Glasses*, ed. E. A. Porai-Koshits, pp. 7–11. New York: Consultants Bureau.

Gentry, J. W., K. R. Spurny, J. Schormann, and H. Opiela. 1983. Measurement of the diffusion coefficient of asbostos fibers. In *Aerosols in the Mining and Industrial Work Environments*, eds. V. A. Marple and B. Y. H. Liu, vol. 2, pp. 593–612. Ann Arbor: Ann Arbor Science Publishers.

Gibbs, G. W. 1979. Etiology of pleural calcification: A study of Quebec asbestos miners and millers. *Arch. Environ. Health.* 34: 76–82.

Gibbs, G. W., and C. Y. Hwang. 1975. Physical parameters of airborne asbestos fibers in various work environments—Preliminary findings. *Am. Ind. Hyg. Assoc. J.* 36: 459–466.

Gibbs, G. W., and C. Y. Hwang. 1980. Dimensions of airborne asbestos fibres. In *Biological Effects of Mineral Fibres. Proceedings of a Symposium held at Lyons, September 25–27, 1979*, ed. J. C. Wagner, vol. 1, pp. 69–78. IARC Scientific Publications 30 Lyons: IARC.

Goodglick, L. A., and A. B. Kane. 1990. Cytotoxicity of long and short crocidolite asbestos fibers *in vitro* and *in vivo. Cancer Res.* 50: 5153–5163.

Griffis, L. C., T. R. Henderson, and J. A. Pickrell. 1981. A method for determining glass in rat lung after exposure to a glass fiber aerosol. *Am. Ind. Hyg. Assoc. J.* 42: 566–569.

Gurman, J. L., M. Lippmann, and R. B. Schlesinger. 1984a. Particle deposition in replicate casts of the human upper tracheobronchial tree under constant and cyclic inspiratory flow. I. Experimental. *Aerosol Sci. Technol.* 3: 245–252.

Gurman, J. L., P. J. Lioy, M. Lippmann, and R. B. Schlesinger. 1984b. Particle deposition in replicate casts of the human upper tracheobronchial tree under constant and cyclic inspiratory flow. II. Empirical model. *Aerosol Sci. Technol.* 3: 253–257.

Gurman, J. L., R. B. Schlesinger, and M. Lippmann. 1980. A variable-opening mechanical larynx for use in aerosol deposition studies. *Am. Ind. Hyg. Assoc. J.* 41: 678–680.

Gylseth, B., B. Mowe, and A. Wannag. 1983. Fiber type and concentration in the lungs of workers in an asbestos cement factory. *Br. J. Ind. Med.* 40: 375–379.

Hain, E., P. Dalquen, H. Bohlig, et al. 1974. Retrospective study of 150 cases of mesothelioma in Hamburg area. *Int. Arch. Argeitsmed.* 33: 15–37.

Hammad, Y. Y. 1984. Deposition and elimination of MMMF. In *Biological Effects of Man-Made Mineral Fibers*, vol. 2, pp. 126–142, Copenhagen: WHO-EURO.

Hammond, E. C., L. Garfinkle, I. T. Selikoff, et al. 1979. Mortality experience of residents in the neighborhood of an asbestos factory. *Ann. NY Acad. Sci.* 330: 417–422.

Hansen, J., N. H. deKlerk, A. W. Musk, J. L. Eccles, and M. S. T. Hobbs. 1997. Mesothelioma after environmental crocidolite exposure. *Ann. Occup. Hyg.* 41 (suppl. 1): 189–193.

Harington, J. S. 1981. Fiber carcinogenesis: Epidemiologic observations and the Stanton hypothesis. *J. Natl. Cancer Inst.* 67: 977–989.

HEI-AR. Health Effects Institute-Asbestos Research, 1991. Report of Literature Review Panel, Cambridge, MA.

Heitt, D. M. 1978. Experimental asbestosis: An investigation of functional and pathological disturbances. *Br. J. Ind. Med.* 35: 129–145.

Hoare, M. 1976. Stability and local order in simple amorphous packings. *Ann. NY Acad. Sci.* 279: 186–207.

Holt, P. F., J. Mills, and K. K. Young. 1965. Experimental asbestosis with four types of fibers. *Ann. NY Acad. Sci.* 132: 87–97.

Holt, P.R. 1982. Translocation of asbestos dust through the bornchiolar wall. *Environ. Res.* 27: 255–260.

Hook, H. L., G. Morrice Jr., and R. T. deTreville. 1970. Fiberglass manufacturing and health: Results of a comprehensive physiological study. October 13–14, 1970. Bulletin 44, pp. 103–111. Proc. 35th Annual Meeting of the Industrial Health Foundation, Pittsburgh, PA: IHF.

Hughes, J. M., R. N. Jones, H. W. Glindmeyer, Y. Y. Hammad, and H. Weill. 1993. Follow-up study of workers exposed to man-made mineral fibres. *Br. J. Ind. Med.* 50(7): 658–667.

Hwang, C. Y., and G. W. Gibbs. 1981. The dimensions of airborne asbestos fibres — I. Crocidolite from Kuruman area, Cape Province, South Africa. *Ann. Occup. Hyg.* 24: 23–41.

Johnson, N. F., D. M. Griffiths, and R. J. Hill. 1984. Size distributions following long-term inhalation of MMMF. In *Biological Effects of Man-Made Mineral Fibers*, vol. 2, pp. 102–125. Copenhagen: WHO-EURO.

Jones, A. D., A. M. Johnston, and J. H. Vincent. 1983. Static electrification of airborne asbestos dust. In *Aerosols in the Mining and Industrial Work Environments*, vol. 2, eds. V. A. Marple and B. Y. H. Liu, pp. 613–632. Ann Arbor: Ann Arbor Science Publishers.

Jones, A. D., C. H. McMillan, A. M. Johnston, C. McIntosh, H. Cowie, R. E. Bolton, G. Borzucki, and J. H. Vincent. 1988. Pulmonary clearance of UICC amosite fibers inhaled by rats during chronic exposure at low concentration. *Br. J. Ind. Med.* 45: 300–304.

Jones, J. S. P., F. D. Pooley, G. W. Sawle, R. J. Madeley, P. G. Smith, G. Berry, B. K. Wignall, and A. Aggarwal. 1980. The consequences of exposure to asbestos dust in a wartime gas-mask factory. In *Biological Effects of Mineral Fibres*, vol. 2, ed. J. C. Wagner, pp. 637–653. IARC Scientific Publications 30. Lyons: IARC.

Kane, A. B., and J. L. McDonald. 1993. Mechanisms of mesothelial cell injury, proliferation and neoplasia induced by asbestos fibers. In *Fiber Toxicology: Contemporary Issues*, ed. D. B. Warheit. pp. 323–347. San Diego: Academic Press.

King, E. J., J. W. Clegg, and V. M. Rae. 1946. The effect of asbestos, and of asbestos and aluminum, on the lung of rabbits. *Thorax* 1: 188–197.

Klingholz, R., and B. Steinkopf. 1982. Das Verhalten von Kunstlichen Mineralfasern in einer physiolo-gischen Modellflassigkeit und in Wasser. *StaubReinhalt. Luft.* 42: 69–76.

Klingholz, R., and B. Steinkopf. 1984. The reactions of MMMF in a physiological model fluid and in water. In *Biological Effects of Man-Made Mineral Fibers*, vol. 1, pp. 60–86, Copenhagen: WHO-EURO.

Konzen, J. L. 1984. Production trends in fibre sizes of MMMF insulation. In *Biological Effects of Man-Made Mineral Fibers*, vol. 1, pp. 44–63. Copenhagen: WHO-EURO.

Langer, A. M., and R. P. Nolan. 1986. The properties of chrysotile asbestos as determinants of biological activity. *Accom. Oncol.* 1(2): 30–51.

Langer, A. M., and R. P. Nolan. 1989. Fiber type and mesothelioma risk. In *Proceedings: Symposium on Health Effects of Exposure to Asbestos in Buildings*, Harvard University, December 14–16, 1988, pp. 91–140. Cambridge: Harvard University Energy and Environmental Policy Center.

Langer, A. M., R. P. and Nolan. 1988. Distinguishing between asbestiform tremolite and non-asbestiform tremolite. In *Proceedings Intl. Pneumoconioses Conference*, Pittsburgh, PA. DHHS (NIOSH) Publ. 90–108. Washington, DC: DHHS.

Langer, A. M., R. P. Nolan, and J. Addison. 1990. Physico-chemical properties of asbestos as determinants of biological potential. In *CRC Monograph Asbestos and Disease*, eds. K. Miller and D. Liddle. Boca Raton, FL: CRC Press.

LeBouffant, L., J. P. Henin, J. C. Martin, C. Normand, G. Tichoux, and F. Trolard. 1984. Distribution of inhaled MMMF in the rat lung — Long term effects. In *Biological Effects of Man-Made Mineral Fibers*, vol. 2, pp. 143–168. Copenhagen: WHO-EURO.

Lee, K. P., C. E. Barras, F. D. Griffith, R. S. Waritz, and C. A. Lapin. 1981. Comparative pulmonary responses to inhaled inorganic fibers with asbestos and fiberglass. *Environ. Res.* 24: 167–191.

Lee, K. P., D. P. Kelly, and G. L. Kennedy, Jr. 1983. Pulmonary response to inhaled Kevlar aramid synthetic fibers in rats. *Toxicol. Appl. Pharmacol.* 71: 242–253.

Leineweber, J. P. 1984. Solubility of fibers *in vitro* and *in vivo*. In *Biological Effects of Man-Made Mineral Fibers*, vol. 2, pp. 87–101. Copenhagen: WHO-EURO.

Lemasters, G., and J. Lockey. 1994. Radiographic changes among workers manufacturing refractory ceramic fibre and products. *Ann. Occup. Hyg.* 38 (suppl. 1): 745–751.

Lemasters, G. K., J. E. Lockey, L. S. Levin, R. T. Mckay, C. H. Rice, E. P. Horvath, D. M. Papes, J. W. Lu, and D. J. Feldman. 1998. An industry-wide pulmonary study of men and women manufacturing refractory ceramic fibers. *Am. J. Epidemiol.* 148: 910–919.

Levin, J. L., J. W. McLarty, G. A. Hurst, A. N. Smith, and A. L. Frank. 1998. Tyler asbestos workers: Mortality experience in a cohort exposed to amosite. *Occup. Environ. Med.* 55: 155–160.

Lippmann, M. 1990. Man-made mineral fibers (MMMF): Human exposures and health risk assessment. *Toxicol. Ind. Health.* 6: 225–246.

Lippmann, M. 1994. Deposition and retention of fibres: Effects on incidence of lung cancer and mesothelioma. *Occup. Environ. Med.* 51: 793–798.

Lippmann, M. and V. Timbrell. 1990. Particle loading in the human lung—Human experience and implications for exposure limits. *J. Aerosol Med.* 3: S155–S168.

Lynch, J. R., H. E. Ayer, and D. L. Johnson. 1970. The interrelationships of selected asbestos exposure indices. *Am. Ind. Hyg. Assoc. J.* 31: 598–604.

Magnani, C., B. Terracini, C. Ivaldi, M. Botta, A. Mancini, and A. Andrion. 1995. Pleural malignant mesothelioma and nonoccupational exposure to asbestos in Castale Monferrato, Italy. *Occup. Environ. Med.* 52: 362–367.

Malmberg, P., H. J. Hedenstein, B. Kolmodin-Hedran, and S. Krantz. 1984. Pulmonary function in workers of a mineral rock fibre plant. Biological effects of man-made mineral fibres. *Proceedings of a WHO / IARC Conference*, vol. 1, April 20–22, 1982. Copenhagen, Denmark. pp. 427–435.

McConnochie, K., L. Simonato, P. Mavrides, P. Christofides, F. D. Pooley, and J. C. Wagner. 1987. Mesothelioma in Cyprus: The role of tremolite. *Thorax* 42: 342–347.

McDonald, A. D., B. W. Case, A. Churg, A. Dufresne, G. W. Gibbs, P. Sebastien, and J. C. McDonald. 1997. Mesothelioma in Quebec chrysotile miners and millers: Epidemiology and Aetiology. *Ann. Occup. Hyg.* 41: 707–719.

McDonald, A. D., J. S. Fry, G. J. Woolley, and J. C. McDonald. 1984. Dust exposure and mortality in an American chrysotile asbestos friction products plant. *Br. J. Ind. Med.* 41: 151–157.

McDonald, J. C. and A. D. McDonald. 1997. Chrysotile, tremolite and carcinogenicity. *Ann. Occup. Hyg.* 41: 699–705.

Meurman, L. O., R. Kiviluoto, and M. Hakama. 1974. Mortality and morbidity among the working population of anthophyllite asbestos miners in Finland. *Br. J. Ind. Med.* 31: 105–112.

Meurman, L. O., R. Kiviluoto, and M. Hakama. 1979. Combined effects of asbestos exposure and tobacco smoking on Finnish anthophyllite miners and millers. *Ann. NY Acad. Sci.* 330: 491–495.

Moalli, P. A., J. L. Macdonald, L. A. Goodglick, and A. B. Kane 1987. Acute injury and regeneration of the mesothelium in response to asbestos fibers. *Am. J. Pathol.* 128: 425–445.

Monchaux, G., J. Bignon, A. Hirsch, and P. Sebastien. 1982. Translocation of mineral fibres through the respiratory system after injection into the pleural cavity of rats. *Ann. Occup. Hyg.* 26: 309–318.

Monchaux, G., J. Bignon, M. C. Jaurand, J. Lafuma, P. Sebastien, R. Masse, A. Hirsh, and T. Goni. 1981. Mesotheliomas in rats following inoculation with acid-leached chrysotile asbestos and other mineral fibers. *Carcinogenesis.* 2: 229–236.

Morgan, A. 1979. Fiber dimensions: Their significance in the deposition and clearance of inhaled fibrous dusts. In *Dusts and Disease*, eds. R. Lemen and J. M. Dement, pp. 87–96. Park Forest South, IL: Pathotox Publishers.

Morgan, A., A. Black, N. Evans, A. Holmes, and J. N. Pritchard. 1980. Deposition of sized glass fibers in the respiratory tract of the rat. *Ann. Occup. Hyg.* 23: 353–366.

Morgan, A., A. Holmes, and W. Davison. 1982. Clearance of sized glass fibers from the rat lung and their solubility *in vivo*. *Ann. Occup. Hyg.* 25: 317–331.

Morgan, A., and A. Holmes. 1984. The deposition of MMMF in the respiratory tract of the rat, their subsequent clearance, solubility *in vivo* and protein coating. In *Biological Effects of Man-Made Mineral Fibers*, vol. 2, pp. 1–17. Copenhagen: WHO-EURO.

Morrow, P. E. 1988. Possible mechanisms to explain dust overloading of the lungs. *Fundam. Appl. Toxicol.* 10: 369–384.

Mossman, B. T., and J. E. Craighead. 1987. Mechanisms of asbestos asssociated bronchogenic carcinoma. In *Asbestos-Related Malignancy*, eds. K. Antman, and J. Aisner, pp. 137–150. Orlando, FL: Grune and Stratton.

Mossman, B. T., J. P. Marsh, A. Sesko, S. Hill, M. A. Shatos, J. Doherty, J. Petruska, K. B. Adler, D. Hemenway, R. Mickey, P. Vacek, and E. Kagan. 1990. Inhibition of lung injury, inflammation, and interstitial pulmonary fibrosis by polyethylene glycol-conjugated catalase in a rapid inhalation model of asbestosis. *Am. Rev. Respir. Dis.* 41: 1266–1271.

Mossman, G. T., J. Bignon, M. Corn, A. Seaton, and J. B. L. Gee. 1990. Asbestos: Scientific developments and implications for public policy. *Science.* 247: 294–301.

Newhouse, M. L., and H. Thompson. 1965. Epidemiology of mesothelial tumors in the London area. *Ann. NY Acad. Sci.* 132: 579–588.

Newhouse, M. L., and K. R. Sullivan. 1989. A mortality study of workers manufacturing friction materials: 1941–86. *Br. J. Ind. Med.* 46: 176–179.

Newhouse, M. L., G. Berry, and J. W. Skidmore. 1982. A mortality study of workers manufacturing friction materials with chrysotile asbestos. *Ann. Occup. Hyg.* 26: 899–909.

Nicholson, W. J. 1986. *Airborne Asbestos Health Assessment Update, United States Environmental Protection Agency, Office of Health and Environmental Assessment.* EPA / 600 / 8-84 / 003F. Washington, DC: EPA.

NRC. 1984. *Asbestiform Fibers—Nonoccupational Health Risks.* Washington, DC: National Academy Press.

Oberdörster, G., J. Ferin, J. Finkelstein, S. Soderholm, and R. Gelein. 1990. Mechanistic studies on particle-induced acute and chronic lung injury. In Aerosols-Science, Industry, Health and Environment, vol. 2, eds. S. Masuda and K. Takahashi, pp. 1229–1233. Oxford: Pergamon Press.

Oberdörster, G., P. E. Morrow, and K. Spurny. 1988. Size dependent lymphatic short term clearance of amosite fibers in the lung. *Ann. Occup. Hyg.* 32(S1): 149–156.

Ontario Royal Commission. 1984. *Report of the Royal Commission on Matters of Health and Safety Arising from the Use of Asbestos in Ontario,* vols. 1–3. Toronto: Ontario Ministry of the Attorney General.

Peto, J., H. Seidman, and I. J. Selikoff. 1982. Mesothelioma mortality in asbestos workers: Implications for models of carcinogenesis and risk assessment. *Brit. J. Cancer.* 45: 124–135.

Peto, J., R. Doll, C. Hermon, W. Binns, R. Clayton, and T. Goffe. 1985. Relationship of mortality to measures of environmental asbestos pollution in an asbestos textile factory. *Ann. Occup. Hyg.* 29: 305–355.

Pinkerton, K. E., A. A. Elliot, S. R. Frame, and D. B. Warheit. 1997. Reversibility of fibrotic lesions in rats inhaling size-separated chrysotile asbestos fibres for 2 weeks. *Ann. Occup. Hyg.* 41 (suppl. 1): 178–183.

Pooley, F. D. 1976. An examination of the fibrous mineral content of asbestos lung tissue from the Canadian chrysotile mining industry. *Environ. Res.* 12: 281–298.

Pooley, F. D., and J. C. Wagner. 1988. The significance of the selective retention of mineral dusts. *Ann. Occup. Hyg.* 32 (suppl. 1): 187–194.

Pooley, F. D., and N. J. Clark. 1980. A comparison of fibre dimension in chrysotile, crocidolite, and amosite particles from samples of airborne dust and from post-mortem lung tissue specimens. In Biological Effects of Mineral Fibres, vol. 1, ed. J. C. Wagner, pp. 79–86. Lyons: International Agency for Research on Cancer

Pott, F., K. H. Friedrichs, and F. Huth. 1976. Results of animal experiments concerning the carcinogenic effect of fibrous dusts and their penetration with regard to the carcinogenesis in humans. *Zentralbl. Bakteriol. Hyg.* 162: 467–505.

Reid, G., D. Keilkowski, S. D. Steyn, and K. Botha. 1990. Mortality of an asbestos-exposed birth cohort: A pilot study. *S. Afr. Med. J.* 78: 584–586.

Robinson, C. F., J. M. Dement, G. O. Ness, and R. J. Waxweiler. 1982. Mortality patterns of rock and slag mineral wool production workers: An epidemiological and environmental study. *Br. J. Ind. Med.* 39: 45–53.

Roggli, V. L., and A. R. Brody. 1984. Changes in numbers and dimensions of chrysotile asbestos fibers in lungs of rats following short-term exposure. *Exp. Lung Res.* 7: 133–147.

Roggli, V. L., M. H. George, and A. R. Brody. 1987. Clearance and dimensional changes of crocidolite asbestos fibers isolated from lungs of rats following short-term exposure. *Environ. Res.* 42: 94–105.

Rood, A. P., and R. M. Scott. 1989. Size distributions of chrysotile asbestos in a friction products factory as determined by transmission electron microscopy. *Ann. Occup. Hyg.* 33: 583–590.

Rossiter, C. F., and R. M. Coles. 1980. H.M. Dockyard, Devonport: 1947 mortality study. In *Biological Effects of Mineral Fibres,* ed. J. C. Wagner, pp. 713–721. IARC Scientific Publ. 30. Lyons: International Agency for Research on Cancer.

Saracci, R., L. Simonato, E. D. Acheson, A. Anderson, P. A. Bertazzi, J. Claude, N. Charnay, J. Esteve, R. R. Frentzel-Beyme, M. J. Gardner, O. M. Jensen, R. Massing, J. H. Olsen, L. Teppo, P. Westerholm, and C. Zocchetti. 1984. Mortality and incidence of cancer of workers in the man-made vitreous fibres producing industry: An international investigation in 13 European plants. *Br. J. Ind. Med.* 41: 425–436.

Sawyer, R. N. 1989. Asbestos material inventory, control concepts and risk communications. In *Symposium on Health Aspects of Exposure to Asbestos in Buildings*, pp. 155–169. Cambridge: Harvard University Kennedy School of Government.

Schlesinger, R. B., and M. Lippmann. 1978. Selective particle deposition and bronchogenic carcinoma. *Environ. Res.* 15: 424–431

Schlesinger, R. B., J. Concato, and M. Lippmann. 1983. Particle deposition during exhalation: A study in replicate casts of the human upper tracheobronchial tree. In Aerosols in the Mining and Industrial Work Environments, vol. 1, eds. V. A. Marple and B. Y. H. Liu, pp. 165–176. Ann Arbor: Ann Arbor Science Publishers.

Scholze, H., and R. Conradt. 1987. An *in vitro* study of the chemical durability of siliceous fibers. *Ann. Occup. Hyg.* 31(4B): 683–692.

Sebastien, P., J. Bignon, Y. I. Baris, L. Awad, and G. Petit. 1984. Ferruginous bodies in sputum as an indication of exposure to airborne mineral fibers in the mesothelioma villages of Cappadocia. *Arch. Environ. Health.* 39: 18–23.

Sebastien, P., J. C. McDonald, A. D. McDonald, B. Case, and B. Harley. 1989. Respiratory cancer in chrysotile textile and mining industries: Exposure inferences from lung analysis. *Br. J. Ind. Med.* 46: 180–187.

Seidman, H., I. J. Selikoff, and E. C. Hammond. 1979. Short term asbestos work exposure and long term observation. *Ann. NY Acad. Sci.* 330: 61–90.

Selikoff, I. J., E. C. Hammond, and H. Seidman. 1979. Mortality experience of insulation workers in the United States and Canada: 1943–1976. *Ann. NY Acad. Sci.* 330: 91–116.

Selikoff, I. J., W. J. Nicholson, and A. M. Langer. 1972. Asbestos air pollution. *Arch. Environ. Health.* 25: 1–13.

Shannon, H. S., E. Jamieson, J. A. Julian, D. C. F. Muir, and C. Walsh. 1987. Mortality experience of Ontario glass fiber workers—Extended follow-up. *Ann. Occup. Hyg.* 31(4B): 657–662.

Shannon, H., M. Hayes, J. Julian, and D. Muir. 1984. Mortality experience of glass fibre workers. In *Biological Effects of Man-Made Mineral Fibers*, pp. 347–349. Copenhagen: WHO-EURO.

Simonato, L., A. C. Fletcher, J. Cherrie, A. Andersen, P. A. Bertazzi, N. Charney, J. Claude, J. Dodgson, J. Esteve, R. Frentzel-Beyme, M. J. Gardner, O. Jensen, J. Olsen, R. Saracci, L. Teppo, P. Westerholm, R. Winkelmann, P. D. Winter, and C. Zocchetti. 1986. Updating lung cancer mortality among a cohort of man-made mineral fibre production workers in seven European countries. *Cancer Lett.* 30: 189–200.

Smith, A. H., and C. C. Wright. 1996. Chrysotile asbestos is the main cause of pleural mesothelioma. *Am. J. Ind. Med.* 30: 252–266.

Spengler, J. D., H. Ozkaynak, J. F. McCarthy, and H. Lee. 1989. Summary of Symposium on Health Aspects of Exposure to Asbestos in Buildings. In *Symposium on Health Aspects of Exposure to Asbestos in Buildings*, pp. 1–26. Cambridge, MA: Harvard University Kennedy School of Government.

Stanton, M. F., and C. Wrench. 1972. Mechanisms of mesothelioma induction with asbestos and fibrous glass. *J. Natl. Cancer Inst.* 48: 797–821.

Stanton, M. F., M. Layard, A. Tegeris, E. Miller, M. May, and E. Kent. 1977. Carcinogenicity of fibrous glass: Pleural response in the rat in relation to fiber dimension. *J. Natl. Cancer Inst.* 58: 587–603.

Stayner, L. R. Smith, J. Bailer, S. Gilbert, K. Steenland, J. Dement, D. Brown, and R. Lemen. 1997. Exposure-response analysis of risk of respiratory disease associated with occupational exposure to chrysotile asbestos. *Occup. Environ. Med.* 54: 646–652.

Stayner, L. T., D. A. Dankovic, and R. A. Lemon. 1996. Occupational exposure to chrysotile asbestos and cancer risk: A review of the amphibole hypothesis. *Am. J. Public Health.* 86: 179–186.

Stöber, W., H. Flachsbart, and D. Hochrainer. 1970. Der aerodynamische Durchmesser von Latexaggregaten und Asbestfasern. *Staub-Reinhalt. Luft.* 30: 277–285.

Sussman, R. G., B. S. Cohen, and M. Lippmann. 1991a. Asbestos fiber deposition in a human tracheobronchial cast. I. Experimental. *Inhal. Toxicol.* 3: 145–160.

Sussman, R. G., B. S. Cohen, and M. Lippmann. 1991b. Asbestos fiber deposition in a human tracheobronchial cast. II. Empirical model. *Inhal. Toxicol.* 3: 161–179.

Timbrell, V. 1972. An aerosol spectrometer and its applications. In *Assessment of Airborne Particles*, eds. T. T. Mercer, P. E. Morrow, and W. Stöber, pp. 290–330. Springfield, IL: Charles C. Thomas.

Timbrell, V. 1982. Deposition and retention of fibers in the human lung. *Ann. Occup. Hyg.* 26: 347–369.

Timbrell, V. 1983. Fibers and carcinogenesis. *J. Occup. Health Soc.* 3: 3–12.

Timbrell, V. 1984. Pulmonary deposition and retention of South African amphibole fibers: Identification of asbestosis-related measure of fiber concentration. In *Proceedings of 6th International Pneumoconiosis Conference*, Bochum, Germany, 1983, vol. 2, pp. 998–1008. Geneva, ILO.

Timbrell, V., T. Ashcroft, B. Goldstein, F. Heyworth, L. O. Meurman, R. E. G. Rendall, J. A. Reynolds, K. B. Shilkin, and D. Whitaker. 1987. Relationships between retained amphibole fibers and fibrosis in human lung tissue specimens. In *Inhaled Particles VI*, ed. W. H. Walton. Oxford: Pergamon Press.

Tran, C. L., A. D. Jones, R. T. Cullen, and K. Donaldson. 1997. Overloading of clearance of particles and fibres. *Ann. Occup. Hyg.* 41 (suppl. 1): 237–243.

Trethowan, W. N., P. S. Burge, C. E. Rossiter, J. M. Harrington, and I. A. Calvert. 1995. Study of the respiratory health of employees in seven European plants that manufacture ceramic fibres. *Occup. Environ. Med.* 52(2): 97–104.

Turnbull, D. 1976. Relation of crystallization behavior to structure in amorphous systems. *Ann. NY Acad. Sci.* 279: 185 (Abstract).

Utidjian, H. M. D., and R. T. P. deTreville. 1970. Fibrous glass manufacturing and health: Report of an epidemiological study. Parts I and II. *Proc. 35th Annual Meeting of the Industrial Health Foundation.* October 13–14, 1970, pp. 98–102. Pittsburgh, PA. IHF Bulletin 44.

Veblen, D. R. 1980. Anthophyllite asbestos: Microstructures, intergrown sheet silicates and mechanisms of fiber formation. *Am. Mineral.* 65: 1075–1086.

Vincent, J. H., A. M. Johnston, A. D. Jones, R. E. Bolton, and J. Addison. 1985. Kinetics of deposition and clearance of inhaled mineral dusts during chronic exposure. *Br. J. Ind. Med.* 42: 707–715.

Wagner, J. C. 1963. Asbestosis in experimental animals. *Br. J. Ind. Med.* 20: 1–12.

Wagner, J. C., and F. D. Pooley. 1986. Mineral fibers and mesothelioma. *Thorax.* 41: 161–166.

Wagner, J. C., and J. W. Skidmore. 1965. Asbestos dust deposition and retention in rats. *Ann. NY Acad. Sci.* 132: 77–86.

Wagner, J. C., C. A. Steggs, and P. Marchand. 1960. Diffuse pleural mesothelioma and asbestos exposure in northwestern Cape Province. *Br. J. Ind. Med.* 17: 260–271.

Wagner, J. C., F. D. Pooley, G. Barry, R. M. E. Seal, D. E. Munday, J. Morgan, and N. J. Clark. 1982. A pathological and mineralogical study of asbestos-related deaths in the United Kingdom. *Ann. Occup. Hyg.* 26: 417–422.

Wagner, J. C., G. Berry, and J. W. Skidmore. 1976. Studies of the carcinogenic effects of fiber glass of different diameters following intrapleural innoculation in experimental animals. In *Occupational Exposure to Fibrous Glass*, pp. 193–197. HEW Publ. (NIOSH) 76–151. Cincinnati, Nat'l Inst. for Occup. Saftey and Health.

Wagner, J. C., G. Berry, J. W. Skidmore, and V. Timbrell. 1974. The effects of the inhalation of asbestos in rats. *Br. J. Cancer.* 29: 252–269.

Wagner, J. C., J. W. Skidmore, R. J. Hill, and D. M. Griffiths. 1985. Erionite exposure and mesotheliomas in rats. *Br. J. Cancer.* 51: 727–730.

Walker, A. M. 1984. Declining relative risks for lung cancer after cessation of asbestos exposure. *J. Occup. Med.* 26: 422–425.

Walton, W. H. 1982. The nature, hazards and assessment of occupational exposure to airborne asbestos dust: A review. *Ann. Occup. Hyg.* 25: 117–247.

Warheit, D. B., and M. A. Hartsky. 1990. Species comparisons of alveolar deposition patterns of inhaled particles. *Exp. Lung Res.* 16: 83–99.

Weitzman, S. A., P. Graceffa. 1984. Asbestos catalyzes hydroxyl and superoxide radical release from hydrogen peroxide. *Arch. Biochem. Biophys.* 288: 373–376.

Whittaker, E. J. W., and J. Zussman. 1956. The characterization of serpentine minerals by X-ray diffraction. *Min. Mag.* 32: 107–115.

WHO. 1986. Asbestos and other natural mineral fibers. *Environ. Health Criteria* 53, Geneva: World Health Organization.

WHO. 1997. *Determination of Airborne Fibre Number Concentrations.* Geneva. World Health Organization. 53 pp.

Wong, O., and R. P. Musselman. 1994. An epidemiological and toxicological evaluation of the carcinogenicity of man-made vitreous fiber, with a consideration of coexposures. *J. Environ. Pathol. Toxicol. Oncol.* 13: 169–180.

Wright, G. W., and M. Kuschner. 1977. The influence of varying lengths of glass and asbestos fibers on tissue response in guinea pigs. In *Inhaled Particles IV,* Part 2, ed. W. H. Walton, pp. 455–472. New York: Pergamon Press.

Yada, K. 1967. Study of chrysotile asbestos by a high resolution electron microscope. *Acta Crystallogr.* 23: 704–707.

Yu, C. P., B. Asgharian, and J. L. Abraham. 1990. Mathematical modeling of alveolar clearance of chrysotile asbestos fibers from the rat lungs. *J. Aerosol Sci.* 21: 587–594.

Zalma, R., L. Bonneau, J. Guignard, and H. Pezerat. 1987. Formation of oxy radicals by oxygen reduction arising from the surface activity of asbestos. *Can. J. Chem.* 65: 2338–2341.

Zoltai, T. 1979. Asbestiform and acicular mineral fragments. *Ann. NY Acad. Sci.* 330: 621–643.

4 Benzene

BERNARD D. GOLDSTEIN, M.D.
GISELA WITZ, Ph.D.

Understanding and preventing the threat of benzene to human health is one of the most important environmental issues facing national and international regulatory authorities. Benzene is a human leukemogen. Among the known human cancer-causing agents, benzene is the organic chemical of highest volume and broadest distribution. Further, as an integral component of our petrochemical era, benzene cannot simply be banned from use. Understanding the mechanisms by which benzene leads to adverse health effects is of crucial importance. Uncertainties about health effects must be balanced against the potential for substantial economic and societal costs in regulating benzene.

Current standards for benzene in the United States include a maximum permissible level in drinking water of 5 ppb. As with any carcinogen, EPA has set a drinking water goal of 0 ppb. The Occupational Safety and Health Administration (OSHA) has set a workplace standard for benzene of 1.0 ppm benzene as a time-weighted average for an eight-hour working day. The National Institute for Occupational Safety and Health (NIOSH) has recommended a workplace standard of 0.2 ppm. In addition the American Conference of Governmental Industrial Hygienists (ACGIH) threshold limit value (TLV), adopted in 1997, is 0.5 ppm as a time-weighted 8 hour average (TWA), 1.6 ppm as a short-term (15 min) exposure limit (STEL), and their revised Biological Exposure Index (BEI), namely S-phenylmercapturic acid in urine at end of a work shift is 25 μg / g creatinine. The control of benzene in ambient air by EPA is currently based on emission standards set for selected industrial sources. Under the 1990 Clean Air Act, maximum available control technology for all significant atmospheric benzene point sources will be required, followed by a risk-based approach that has yet to be clearly defined. Many states have developed their own drinking water or atmospheric standards for benzene.

Benzene (C_6H_6) is the smallest and most stable aromatic compound. It is a clear colorless liquid with a classic aromatic odor. It is minimally soluble in water (820 mg / L at 22°C; Chiou et al., 1977), has an octanol/water partition coefficient of 1.56 to 2.15 (Leo et al., 1971), a blood / air partition coefficient of 7.8 (Sato and Nakajima, 1979), and a vapor pressure of 0.125 atm at 25°C (Thibodeaux, 1981). It is thus a hydrophobic solvent that readily evaporates at room temperature and rapidly partitions into lipid. Benzene reacts with hydroxyl radicals and participates in the photochemical process leading to the formation of ozone and other components of oxidant smog.

Described below are a number of aspects of the toxicology and exposure pathways of benzene pertinent to understanding how the use of benzene in our modern society leads to the risk of adverse health effects. Pertinent review articles or documents include ATSDR

Environmental Toxicants: Human Exposures and Their Health Effects, 2/e. Edited by Morton Lippmann.
ISBN: 0-471-29298-2 © 2000 John Wiley & Sons, Inc.

(1989), Goldstein (1977, 1989a, b), U.S. HEW (1989), Mehlman (1989), Aksoy (1988), R. Snyder (1983), EPA (1997), Savitz and Andrews (1997), and Smith (1996).

BENZENE EXPOSURE

Benzene is a ubiquitous agent. As a component of petroleum it is widely distributed. Gasoline contains 1% to 2% benzene in the United States, and higher levels are reported elsewhere. Benzene is also an important starting agent for chemical synthesis. It is a valuable solvent, but its use in that regard has been decreasing, primarily because of health and safety concerns. Total global benzene production capacity in 1994 was 33.6 million tons (Mt) which is expected to increase to 38.2 Mt by 1998–99 (C&EN, 1997). Benzene exposure occurs in the workplace, in the general environment, and through the use of consumer products. Occupational exposures present the highest risks. Cigarette smoke contains relatively high levels of benzene. For nonsmokers, benzene sources in the home are usually the major component of exposure. Benzene is also present in a variety of foods but relatively little of the usual total daily body burden is likely to come from this source. The World Health Organization(WHO) estimates that total daily uptake from all sources ranges from 130 to 550 μg in nonsmokers (WHO, 1987).

   Much of what we know about the extent of individual benzene exposure in the general environment has come through a series of pioneering studies by EPA's Office of Research and Development. Through total exposure assessment methodology (TEAM) studies, researchers have developed a number of novel approaches to assess human exposures to volatile hydrocarbons, including miniaturized sampling and analytic techniques suitable for use as personal monitors, demographic sampling techniques to choose individuals representative of community exposure, and, most important, conceptual approaches allowing for integration of indoor and outdoor exposure data for individuals in conjunction with activity questionnaires (Wallace et al., 1985; Wallace, 1987). The sensitivity of the personal monitoring technique is in the low-ppb range, capable of picking up the difference in perchloroethylene exposure between those who visited a dry cleaner on a given day and those who did not. One of the large number of volatile air pollutants they have studied is benzene. Unfortunately, the absorbent that is used, Tenax[®], creates somewhat greater analytical problems for benzene than for other volatile organic compounds. Nevertheless, the data are of great value in understanding environmental benzene exposure.

   TEAM studies measuring individual exposures indoors and outdoors in conjunction with diaries recording individual activities have been done in different locations. Perhaps the most startling information concerning benzene has come from studies in northern New Jersey, near a major petrochemical refinery complex (Wallace et al., 1985; Wallace, 1987). Evaluation of 355 individuals, a representative sample of the 128,000 residents of Bayonne and Elizabeth, failed to reveal any statistically significant impact of proximity to the refinery on individual benzene exposure. It should be emphasized that this does not mean there was no impact; outdoor monitors confirmed the human olfactory perception of higher outdoor levels of petrochemical vapors, including benzene, in proximity to the refinery complex. However, the most notable finding was the large variability in indoor benzene levels, a variability so great that it swamped the relatively small differences caused by geographical proximity to the refinery. Not only were there large differences in indoor benzene exposure between neighbors, but for those with the higher individual levels of benzene exposure, namely those at greatest risk, the indoor sources clearly predominated. There is a similarity in indoor levels, and thus in total exposure, across a wide range of communities throughout the United States. In general, homes in northern communities have higher levels reflecting both the likelihood of attached garages and restricted outdoor ventilation in the winter. The TEAM methodology also was the basis for study of the risk of benzene exposure resulting from emissions from the Marine Oil Terminal in Valdez, Alaska. Despite exceptionally high emissions, personal monitoring coupled with extensive meteorological and tracer studies demonstrated that the Marine Oil Terminal circulated only minimally to the benzene cancer risk of the inhabitants of Valdez, located three miles away. (Goldstein, 1994)

The approaches pioneered by the TEAM study have continued to be adapted and improved, including use of breath analysis as a means of assessing body benzene burden (Brugnone et al., 1989; Yu and Weisel, 1996). These techniques should be considered as state of the art when exploring individual human exposures. In particular, regulatory decisions made about a pollutant source should no longer depend solely on simple modeling approaches to determine whether there is sufficient risk to warrant imposing control measures or closing the facility. With the availability of personal monitoring techniques for benzene, models should be relegated to use as scoping or priority-setting devices in assessing risk to individuals. The 1990 Clean Air Act Amendments provided, as part of its air toxics provisions, an emphasis on determining the risk to the maximally exposed individual, which should be a major spur to improved exposure assessment for benzene.

Benzene may also be measured in blood, and benzene metabolites can be measured in urine (ACGIH, 1997; Witz et al., 1993). A particularly valuable approach has been blood benzene analysis in 883 participants in the U.S. National Health and Nutrition Survey (Ashley et al., 1994). In addition to background levels of benzene from industrial sources in the community, the general public may be exposed to benzene in a number of ways. Some of the major ones are

1. *Cigarette smoking, including passive smoking.* Benzene levels in areas with significant levels of cigarette smoke have been reported to be elevated on the basis of breath measurements, and blood benzene levels have been shown to be higher in smokers than in nonsmokers (Wallace and Pellizari, 1986; Brugnone et al., 1989). One pack a day contributes about 600 µg benzene to the smoker (WHO, 1987).

2. *Home use of solvents or gasoline.* Many solvents contain benzene, in most cases at levels less than 0.1%. However, if allowed to evaporate freely, even at 0.1% (1000 ppm) solvents can be a major contributor to benzene levels in the home. Gasoline is often used as a solvent at home, particularly by those who have gasoline-fueled machinery such as automobiles or lawnmowers. Because gasoline may contain 1% to 2% benzene, this can be a significant source of exposure to the individual, involving dermal as well as inhalation exposure. In homes with attached garages, gasoline evaporation from storage cans, from the automobiles and from lawnmowers and other appliances can be a significant benzene source. Other consumer products that are sources of benzene include household cleaning agents, art and other hobby supplies, and glues.

3. *Leaky underground storage tanks.* Water supplies have become contaminated with benzene as a result of leaks from underground gasoline storage tanks. Many gasoline stations in the United States have underground storage tanks that were installed decades ago, and many of these have developed serious leaks. Contamination of groundwater has occurred, leading to human exposure through the three routes of ingestion, inhalation, and skin absorption. Inhalation and skin absorption can occur during such activities as showering with benzene-contaminated portable water (Weisel et al., 1996). Significant risk of benzene inhalation from groundwater contamination may occur even in situations in which a municipal water supply is unaffected. This can occur by off-gassing through

basement walls and floors. In one instance in Long Island, which has particularly porous sandy soils, a group of over 20 homes was sufficiently affected by a leaky underground storage tank from a nearby gasoline station that the gasoline levels in the basement reached potentially explosive concentrations and the families had to be evacuated. Eventually the decision about when it would be safe to return the families to their homes was based on arguments concerning the leukemia risk of residual air benzene concentrations. As is common in these unfortunate situations, after a period of living in a motel the families preferred to move elsewhere rather than return to their homes.

4. *Automotive sources.* Automobile emissions remain a substantial source of community exposure to benzene. Evaporation of ambient gasoline from carburetors and other parts of the fuel train have been largely, but still incompletely, controlled. However, release of benzene and other gasoline vapors during refueling remains a significant source of community benzene exposure, as well as exposure to the individual doing the refueling. Benzene is also emitted during the combustion of gasoline. The catalytic converter installed on automobile exhausts is an effective means of reducing benzene emissions, yet some benzene is still emitted.

A relatively neglected area of potential human benzene exposure is the interior of automobiles. We spend significant amounts of time in automobiles, often in heavy traffic. Inhalation of benzene while in an automobile can be a significant portion of total daily benzene burden.(Dor, 1995; Lawryk and Weisel, 1996)

UPTAKE

Absorption of benzene occurs through inhalation, ingestion, and across the skin. Except for unusual circumstances, inhalation of benzene is the major route. Benzene is readily absorbed in the lung, directly entering the bloodstream and being distributed to the tissues. Benzene within the blood is in direct equilibrium with the benzene in expired air. Thus measurement of end alveolar breath benzene concentration is a good indicator of body benzene concentration. Approximately 50% of benzene taken up into the body by any route is eventually exhaled, the extent being dependent on benzene dose and the rate of metabolism and respiratory mechanics (i.e., assisted ventilation following removal from the benzene source is an appropriate approach to removal of benzene from the body following acute central nervous system toxicity).

Ingested benzene is also assumed to be fully absorbed. The skin is more of a barrier. Studies of the absorption rate of liquid benzene across the skin have demonstrated significant uptake both in vitro and in vivo, with time in contact with the skin being a major factor (Franz, 1984; Loden, 1986). There is no evidence of transdermal absorption of benzene vapor. Much more needs to be done to understand the rate of skin absorption of benzene in liquid mixtures such as gasoline and commercial solvents. Furthermore it is at least theoretically possible that blends of gasoline with oxygenated fuels such as methyl-tertbutyl ether or ethanol will lead to a more rapid rate of benzene absorption across the skin.

METABOLISM AND DISPOSITION

Benzene is relatively inert to chemical additions, eliminations, oxidations, and reductions because it lacks substituents that can be altered and/or that confer chemical reactivity to the aromatic ring. Benzene is a nonpolar organic compound that partitions into fatty tissues. Numerous studies (Andrews et al., 1977; Sammett et al., 1979; Bolcsak and

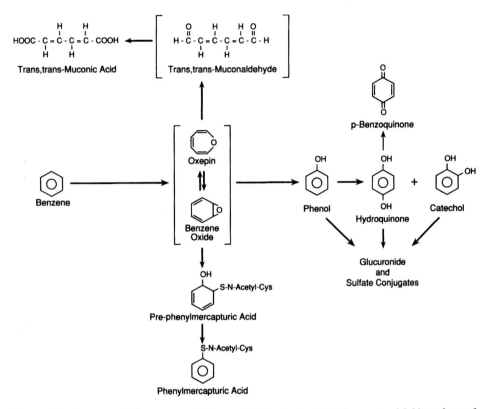

Figure 4-1 Structure of benzene metabolites and adducts investigated as potential biomarkers of benzene exposure. From Medeiros et al., 1997; Taylor and Francis, 1997, used with premission.

Nerland, 1983) suggest that benzene requires metabolism to reactive intermediates in order to be toxic. This discussion briefly reviews the essentials of benzene metabolism and disposition. For a detailed review, the reader is referred to Snyder and Kalf (1994).

In vivo Metabolism

The major pathways of benzene metabolism are shown in Figure 4-1. The earliest studies of benzene metabolism in vivo reported the formation of phenol (Schultzen and Naunyn, 1867), catechol, and hydroquinone (Nencki and Giacosa, 1880). Porteous and Williams (1949) found that phenol, catechol, p-benzoquinone, and hydroquinone are excreted as ethereal sulfates in the urine of rabbits dosed orally with benzene. Earlier, Jaffe (1909) and other investigators (Drummond and Finar, 1938) reported the urinary excretion of muconic acid, a ring-opened six-carbon diene dicarboxylic acid, in rabbits. In 1953, Parke and Williams, using [^{14}C]benzene, confirmed and extended the early studies on the metabolism of benzene to ring-hydroxylated metabolites and to trans,trans-muconic acid. In rabbits administered 0.3 to 0.5 ml/kg [^{14}C] benzene by gavage, the major metabolite formed was phenol. Catechol and hydroquinone were also detected. These, along with phenol, were eliminated in the urine, mainly as the ethereal sulfate or glucuronic acid conjugates. trans,trans-muconic acid (muconic acid) was also detected in the urine. Labeled carbon dioxide, indicating benzene ring opening, and phenylmercapturic acid were also detected. Metabolic fate studies indicated that 43% of the administered benzene dose was expired unmetabolized, 1.5% was exhaled as CO_2, 35% was recovered as urinary metabolites, and 5–10% was present in feces and body tissues. Urinary metabolites consisted of 23% phenol, 4.8% hydroquinone, 2.2% catechol, and 1–2% *trans,trans*-muconic acid. A second ring-opened metabolite, 6-hydroxy-*trans,trans*-2,4-hexadienoic acid (6-hydroxyhexadienoic acid, HHA), was recently identified by Kline et al. (1993) as a urinary metabolite of benzene in mice. In studies on benzene metabolism in the isolated perfused mouse liver, Hedli et al. (1997) found a significant difference between single-pass metabolism in the orthograde (normal) compared with the retrograde (reversed) direction. Although the amount of phenol plus its conjugates produced was the same regardless of the direction of perfusion, the amount of free phenol formed expressed as a percentage of total phenolic metabolites was twice as great following normal perfusion compared with reversed perfusion, indicating regional differences in the location of cytochrome P-450 and the conjugation enzymes. Phenol conjugates and small amounts of free and conjugated hydroquinone but no free phenol were detected after recirculation of products formed during single-pass orthograde perfusion. These results could in part explain why administration of phenol does not lead to bone marrow depression.

These major pathways of benzene metabolism, originally determined in rabbits, were subsequently established in rats and mice (Sabourin et al., 1988; for reviews see C. A. Snyder, 1987; Snyder et al., 1993). In general, in vivo metabolism of benzene results in the formation of ring-closed metabolites and the ring-opened metabolites muconic acid and 6-hydroxyhexadienoic acid. The latter two compounds can be formed by metabolism of *trans,trans*-muconaldehyde (Witz et al., 1990; Goon et al., 1992; Zhang et al., 1993), a reactive ring-opened microsomal metabolite of benzene (Latriano et al., 1986). The metabolism to phenol and subsequent formation of phenyl glucuronide or sulfate is a detoxication pathway, as is conjugation with glutathione and subsequent formation of the prephenylmercapturic acid [*S*-(1,2-dihydro-2-hydroxyphenyl)-*N*-acetyl cysteine]. Quinol thioethers were recently reported to be present in bone marrow of mice and rats administered 11.2 mmol / kg benzene twice daily for two days (Bratton et al., 1997). The quinol thioethers identified consisted of 2-(glutathione-*S*-yl) hydroquinone [2-(GSyl)HQ], 2-(cystein-*S*-yl-glycinyl)hydroquinone [2-(Cys-Gly) HQ],2-(cystein-*S*-yl)hydroquinone [2-(Cys)HQ], and 2-(*N*-acetyl-cysteine-*S*-yl) hydroquinone 2-(NAC)HQ. The metabolite 2-(GSyl)HQ is most likely derived by the reaction of glutathione with *p*-benzoquinone, a product formed by the oxidation of hydroquinone. Metabolism via the mercapturic acid pathway was demonstrated to lead to the quinol thioethers derived from 2-(GSyl)HQ

Metabolism of phenol to hydroquinone and of benzene to muconic acid are two pathways that are currently thought to lead to the formation of toxic benzene metabolites. Hydroquinone and *p*-benzoquinone, easily formed through the oxidation of hydroquinone, are reactive metabolites that also have been suggested to play a role in benzene toxicity (Schwartz et al., 1985; Irons, 1985; Sawahata et al., 1985). Muconaldehyde, a putative precursor of urinary muconic acid, is hematotoxic in mice (Witz et al., 1985) and may be responsible, in part, for benzene toxicity. A *p*-benzoquinone-glutathione adduct formation leading to quinol thioethers could potentially represent yet another pathway resulting in the formation of toxic benzene metabolites. Several quinol thioether metabolites of hydroquinone have been shown to inhibit erythropoiesis in rats (Bratton et al., 1997). Potential mechanisms for their bone-marrow toxicity could involve acylation of critical cellular molecules as well as oxidative damage by reactive oxygen species generated via redox cycling (Bratton et al., 1997; Rao, 1996).

Mechanism(s) of Metabolite Formation

The liver and, to a lesser extent, the bone marrow are the two organ systems examined for benzene metabolism. Studies by Sammett and others (1979) originally demonstrated that partial hepatectomy inhibits benzene hematotoxicity. It also decreases benzene metabolism by 70%. Coadministration of toluene, a competitive inhibitor of benzene metabolism, also reduces benzene hematotoxicity and decreases the amount of benzene metabolites excreted in the urine and found in the bone marrow, blood, liver, spleen, and fat tissue (Andrews et al., 1977). Based mainly on these studies, benzene toxicity is thought to be mediated by reactive metabolites that are formed via pathways including metabolism of benzene by the liver. This hypothesis does not preclude hepatic metabolism of benzene to intermediates that travel from the liver to the bone marrow, where they could be further metabolically activated to the ultimate myelotoxic species.

Many in vitro studies utilizing cellular fractions or reconstituted purified enzyme systems have been carried out in order to elucidate the mechanisms of benzene metabolite formation (for a review, see R. Snyder et al., 1981). Benzene is initially metabolized by a cytochrome P450-dependent monooxygenase to phenol. The formation of phenol is believed to involve the intermediate formation of benzene oxide followed by rearrangement to phenol (Jerina and Daly, 1974) or acid-catalyzed opening of the epoxide ring followed by aromatization via loss of a proton. A direct insertion of oxygen for aromatic hydroxylation may also account for the formation of appreciable amounts of phenol (Hanzlik et al., 1984). Urinary S-phenylmercapturic acid and N7-phenylguanine are adducts presumably derived from the reaction of benzene oxide with glutathione and DNA, respectively. Identification of these adducts (Parke and Williams, 1953; Norpoth et al., 1988) as well as of S-phenylcysteine (McDonald et al., 1994) in vivo after benzene exposure provides indirect evidence for the formation of benzene oxide as the initial benzene oxidation product. Using HPLC analysis, benzene oxide was tentatively identified as such by Lovern et al. (1997) in microsomal systems metabolizing benzene. Phenol can undergo further cytochrome P450-mediated oxidation to catechol and hydroquinone. Benzene oxide can also be metabolized by epoxide hydrolase to benzene-*trans*-dihydrodiol, a metabolite converted to catechol by the action of a dehydrogenase. The 1,2,4-benzenetriol observed in some in vitro metabolism systems is believed to be derived from the oxidation of dihydroxylated metabolites by cytochrome P450. The hydroxylated aromatic benzene metabolites can undergo further metabolic conversion to form sulfate or glucuronic acid conjugates. Benzene epoxide can also serve as substrate for glutathione-S-transferase, catalyzing the formation of the prephenylmer-capturic acid, which is aromatized by dehydration under acidic conditions to S-phenylmercapturic acid (Sabourin et al., 1988b). Tunek and others (1980) identified the glutathione conjugate of p-benzoquinone in an incubation of phenol and glutathione with microsomes. This product is thought to be formed mainly nonenzymatically (Lunte and Kissinger, 1983).

The cytochrome P450 isozyme primarily responsible for the initial oxidation of benzene is cytochrome P4502E1 (Johansson and Ingelman-Sundberg, 1988; Koop et al., 1989; Schrenk et al., 1992). This P450 isozyme is induced by many chemicals including ethanol, a chemical known to enhance benzene hematotoxicity in mice when administered in the drinking water (Baarson et al., 1982). In a study on benzene metabolism in relation to cytochrome P4502E1 activity, Seaton et al. (1994) reported that measured cytochrome P4502E1 activities varied 13-fold for microsomes prepared from human liver samples, and that the fraction of benzene metabolized in 16 minutes ranged from 10% to 59%. A model developed by the investigators predicted the dependence of benzene metabolism on the measured cytochrome P4502E1 activity in liver samples from humans, rats, and mice. The authors suggested that interindividual and interspecies variations in hepatic metabolism of benzene may be related to differences in liver cytochrome P4502E1 activity. Since benzene metabolism is required for toxicity, the findings suggest that interindividual differences in P4502E1 gene expression including differences in P4502E1 induction, as a result of alcohol consumption for example, could play a role in determining susceptibility to benzene toxicity. The relationship between cytochrome P450 expression and benzene metabolism and toxicity is further discussed below.

A reactive ring-opened metabolite of benzene, *trans,trans*-muconaldehyde (muconaldehyde), was identified by Latriano, Goldstein, and Witz (1986) as a microsomal metabolite of benzene but has not been identified in vivo. This metabolite, a six-carbon diene dialdehyde, is unique among individual benzene metabolites in its ability to cause bone-marrow depression in mice (Witz et al., 1985). Muconaldehyde was originally identified as a product formed via hydroxyl-radical-mediated ring opening in aqueous solutions of benzene irradiated with X-rays (Loeff and Stein, 1959). Studies by Latriano and others (1985) showed that muconaldehyde is formed from benzene in the presence of a hydroxyl-radical-generating Fenton system. In subsequent studies, both the *trans,trans*- and the *cis,trans*-isomer of muconaldehyde were identified in Fenton mixtures incubated with benzene (Zhang et al., 1995a). Identification of *cis,trans*-muconaldehyde, an isomer most likely derived by rearrangement of the less stable *cis,cis*-muconaldehyde, suggests that *cis,cis*-muconaldehyde is the initial product of benzene ring-opening in a Fenton system. Benzene dihydrodiol, a newly identified product derived from benzene incubated in the Fenton system, was shown to form phenol, catechol and ring-opened α,β-unsaturated aldehydes of unknown structure. These results indicate that although benzene dihydrodiol can be ring-opened to α,β-unsaturated aldehydic products, it is not the precursor of muconaldehyde formed from benzene in a Fenton system. Studies by Zhang et al. (1995b) suggest that Fenton chemistry plays a role in the formation of ring-opened as well as ring-hydroxylated compounds derived from benzene upon incubation with liver microsomes. Using microsomes prepared from the liver of mice treated with acetone for induction of cytochrome P4502E1, Zhang et al. showed that ring-opening and ring-hydroxylation were enhanced by micromolar concentrations of iron and inhibited by addition of oxy radical scavengers. Cytochrome P4502E1, the major isozyme responsible for the initial oxidation of benzene to benzene oxide, is known to produce large amounts of hydrogen peroxide (Wu and Cederbaum, 1994; Kukielka and Cederbaum, 1995). The possibility exists that the benzene ring-opening is mediated by reactive oxygen species generated during P4502E1 metabolism, and/or it involves a series of steps which include enzymatic and nonenzymatic transformations.

Oxidative and reductive metabolism of muconaldehyde leads to a variety of metabolites, some of which could be important in muconaldehyde toxicity, and consequently in benzene hematotoxicity (Witz et al., 1996). Of particular interest is 6-hydroxy-*trans,trans*-2,4-hexadienal, a reduced muconaldehyde metabolite shown to be hematotoxic in mice (Zhang et al., 1995c) and mutagenic in V79 cells (Chang et al., 1994). 6-Hydroxy-*trans,trans*-2,4-hexadienal is less reactive than muconaldehyde and, if formed in the liver (Grotz et al., 1994), is more likely than muconaldehyde to survive transport to the bone marrow, the target tissue of benzene. The mono-reduction of muconaldehyde is reversible (Zhang et al., 1995), a finding that could relate to the hematotoxicity observed for muconaldehyde as well as for 6-hydroxy-*trans,trans*-2,4-hexadienal.

The role of free radicals in benzene metabolism and benzene toxicity is relatively unexplored. Using a reconstituted system containing rabbit liver P450 isozyme LM2 as well as microsomes, Johansson and Ingelman-Sundberg (1983) demonstrated that phenol formation from benzene is inhibited by presumed hydroxyl radical scavengers including mannitol and DMSO and by catalase, horseradish peroxidase, and superoxide dismutase. The authors suggested that the cytochrome P450-dependent metabolism of benzene to phenol is mediated by hydroxyl radicals generated from hydrogen peroxide, thought to be formed by the spontaneous dismutation of superoxide anion radicals released by cytochrome P450. In this mechanism of phenol formation, the initial reactive intermediate is a hydroxy cyclohexadienyl radical formed by the addition of a hydroxyl radical to the benzene ring. This reaction takes place readily (Walling and Johnson, 1975), followed by phenol formation via loss of a hydrogen. In a subsequent study on the role of free hydroxyl radicals in the cytochrome P450-catalyzed oxidation of benzene and cyclohexanol, Gorsky and Coon (1985) concluded that in the presence of very low (micromolar) concentrations of benzene, the hydroxyl-radical-mediated formation of phenol is the dominant pathway, whereas at higher concentrations (millimolar), the direct oxidation by P450 is quantitatively of much greater importance. One implication of these studies is that a shift in metabolic pathways (free-radical-mediated compared with direct enzymatic conversion) may occur depending on the exposure dose or concentration of benzene.

The bone marrow, the target tissue of benzene, has been reported to contain small amounts of cytochrome P450 (Andrews et al., 1979) and to metabolize benzene to only a limited extent (Irons et al., 1980). Cytochrome P4502E1 was not detected in bone marrow of $B_6C_3F_1$ mice (Genter and Recio, 1994), but it is not known whether other strains of mice or other species also lack this major benzene-metabolizing P450 isozyme in the bone marrow. However, the hydroxylated metabolites of benzene are present in the bone marrow after benzene administration, and the levels of catechol and hydroquinone persist in this tissue (Rickert et al., 1979; Irons et al., 1982), suggesting a role for these metabolites in benzene toxicity. Peroxidases are present in appreciable levels in the bone marrow (Bainton et al., 1971), and recent studies suggest that they may play a role in the metabolism of hydroxylated benzene metabolites to reactive toxic intermediates. Using horseradish peroxidase (HRP) in the presence of hydrogen peroxide as a model for bone-marrow peroxidases, Sawahata and Neal (1982) demonstrated the formation of biphenols and of p-diphenoquinone from phenol. The formation of biphenols and covalent binding of ^{14}C to protein was also observed during the incubation of [^{14}C]phenol with a rat bone-marrow homogenate in the presence of hydrogen peroxide. The peroxidative oxidation of phenol and other hydroxylated benzene metabolites to reactive intermediates and the ability of hydroxylated benzene metabolites to serve as good reducing cosubstrates for peroxidases in the oxidation of benzene metabolites to reactive intermediates are well documented (Subrahmanyam and O'Brien, 1985; Smart and Zannoni, 1985; Eastmond et al., 1987; Sadler et al., 1988). The reactive toxic intermediates generated by metabolism of hydroxylated benzene metabolites by myeloperoxidase, the major peroxidase in the bone marrow, are quinones and free radical metabolite intermediates. The quinones can be detoxified by a 2-electron reduction by NAD (P) H:quinone acceptor oxidoreductase (NQO1), a process that regenerates the polyhydroxylated benzene metabolites. The balance of activation of hydroxylated benzene metabolites and detoxification by NQO1 has been suggested to be a determining factor in benzene bone-marrow toxicity (Ross, 1996). Results from a study by Rothman et al. (1997) support the hypothesis that high cytochrome P4502E1 activity along with low NQO1 activity are susceptibility factors for benzene-induced hematotoxicity.

Species and Strain Differences in the Metabolism of Benzene

Chronic toxicity studies by the National Toxicology Program (Huff, 1983) have shown that $B_6C_3F_1$ mice are more sensitive to the hematotoxic and carcinogenic effects of benzene than F344 / N rats. The greater sensitivity of mice compared with rats to benzene toxicity may be related to a greater metabolism of benzene to toxic intermediates, differences in detoxification of toxic metabolites, or greater inherent susceptibility of target tissues to the action of toxic metabolites. Differential toxicity as related to metabolic differences between $B_6C_3F_1$ mice and F344 / N rats was investigated when Sabourin et al. (1988a) quantitated water-soluble metabolites for four metabolic pathways. In animals exposed to 50 ppm benzene for 6 hours, phenylsulfate, a detoxification metabolite, was present in approximately equal concentrations in rats and mice. Hydroquinone glucuronide. hydroquinone, and muconic acid, which are thought to reflect pathways leading to potential toxic metabolites of benzene, were present in much greater concentration in the mouse than in the rat. These results suggest that greater metabolism to toxic intermediates may in part explain the higher susceptibility of $B_6C_3F_1$ mice to benzene-induced toxicity.

Significant differences in the metabolism of benzene to urinary muconic acid have also been demonstrated between DBA/2N and C57BL/6 mice (Witz et al., 1990), two strains previously reported to exhibit differences in benzene toxicity (Longacre et al., 1981). At hematotoxic benzene doses (220–880 mg/kg), benzene-sensitive DBA/2N mice excreted significantly more muconic acid than the less-benzene-sensitive C57BL/6 mice. No differences between the two strains were observed in urinary excretion of muconic acid after muconaldehyde administration or muconic acid administration. Assuming that urinary muconic acid is derived from muconaldehyde (Kirley et al., 1989), these findings suggest that strain sensitivity toward benzene may be related to differences in the metabolism of benzene to toxic intermediates, including toxic ring-opened compounds such as muconaldehyde. In contrast to the results at hematotoxic benzene doses, at lower benzene doses (0.5–2.5 mg/kg) C57BL/6 mice excreted significantly more muconic acid than DBA/2N mice. These findings may reflect a dose-dependent (and strain-specific) shift in the metabolic pathways of benzene analogous to that found by Gorsky and Coon (1985) for the in vitro metabolism of benzene.

The role of benzene metabolism in relation to toxicity was recently investigated by Valentine et al. (1996) in male mice lacking cytochrome P4502E1 expression (Lee et al., 1996). The CYP2E1 knockout mice and their wild-type counter parts were F_3 homozygous hybrids of SV/129 × C57BL/6N. After a 6 hour nose-only exposure to 200 ppm benzene along with a tracer dose of $[^{14}C]$-benzene, total urinary metabolites in the knockout mice were decreased to 13% compared with total urinary metabolites excreted by control wild-type mice. The amount of phenylsulfate excreted in the knockout mice constituted a significantly larger percentage of urinary total radioactivity than that in the wild-type mice, indicating a substantial role for cytochrome P4502E1 in the oxidation of phenol formed from benzene in normal mice. Toxicity studies in the knockout mice exposed by whole-body inhalation to 0 ppm or 200 ppm benzene 6 h/d for 5 days showed no effects on bone marrow cellularity and no benzene-induced genotoxicity using micronuclei formation in bone marrow and blood as an endpoint. In contrast, wild-type and $B_6C_3F_1$ mice exhibited severe bone-marrow cytotoxicity and genotoxic effects in bone marrow and blood. These studies indicate that cytochrome P4502E1 is the major benzene-metabolizing P450 isozyme in vivo and that benzene metabolism is required for toxicity. These conclusions are supported by other in vivo studies with male and female $B_6C_3F_1$ mice, which exhibited sex-dependent differences in the rate of benzene metabolism, these differences correlate with known differences in genotoxicity (Kreyon et al., 1996).

Disposition of Benzene

Benzene exposure in humans occurs by inhalation, ingestion, and dermal absorption, with inhalation most likely being the predominant exposure route. In humans the half-life of benzene is about 1 to 2 days, and essentially all absorbed benzene is gone from the body within a week following exposure. Thus long-term bioaccumulation of benzene or its metabolites is not of concern.

Ideally, in order to extrapolate results from animal experiments to humans, investigators should know the effects of dose, exposure rate, route of exposure, and species on the metabolism and disposition of benzene. These questions were recently addressed in a series of systematic studies in rats and mice. Sabourin et al. (1987) found virtually 100% absorption in F344/N and Sprague-Dawley rats and $B_6C_3F_1$ mice that had received oral administration of 0.5 to 150 mg / kg benzene. This differs from inhalation, where the percentage of benzene absorbed and retained during a 6-hour exposure decreases as the exposure concentration increases. For example, at 10 ppm benzene, mice and rats absorb and retain 33% and 50%, respectively, compared with 15% and 10% respectively, at 1000 ppm benzene. At oral doses below 15 mg / kg benzene, mice and rats excreted more than 90% of the administered dose as urinary metabolites. Above 15 mg / kg, increasing amounts of benzene were exhaled unmetabolized with increasing exposure concentration, suggesting saturation of metabolism of orally administered benzene in rats and mice. For inhalation exposures, saturation of metabolic routes occurred in mice but not in rats at higher exposure concentrations. The results indicate that a saturating dose, if given as a bolus by gavage, is not saturating when administered by inhalation over 6 hours.

The effects of exposure concentration, exposure rate, and route of administration on metabolism were studied by Sabourin et al. (1989) in F344 / N rats and $B_6C_3F_1$ mice. Animals were exposed orally to 1, 10, and 200 mg / kg benzene and, by inhalation for 6 hours to 5, 50, and 600 ppm benzene vapor. In addition, animals were exposed over different time intervals to the same total amount of benzene ($C \times T = 300$ ppm-h). As the exposure concentration or oral dose increased, there was a shift in metabolism from putative toxification pathways to detoxification pathways. In mice, hydroquinone glucuronide and muconic acid (markers of toxification pathways) represented a greater percentage of the administered dose at low benzene doses than was evidenced at high doses. The percentage dose excreted as the detoxification products phenylglucuronide and prephenylmercapturic acid increased with increasing dose. Similar results were obtained in the rat, except that hydroquinone glucuronide was a minor benzene metabolite at all concentrations. No simple relationship between oral dosing and inhalation was observed in terms of metabolite dose to tissues. These studies indicate that extrapolation from high-exposure toxicity studies to low-level exposures or from oral to inhalation exposures may not result in a true estimate for the parameter being extrapolated to humans. The authors concluded that if hydroquinone glucuronide and muconic acid are markers of toxic benzene metabolites and are formed in significant amounts in humans, then linear extrapolation of health effects from high exposures to low-level exposures could underestimate the toxicity of benzene.

MECHANISMS OF TOXICITY

Remaining as major uncertainties are the nature of the toxic metabolites responsible for benzene toxicity and the mechanisms of action of these toxic metabolites. Any hypothesis of benzene toxicity must account for the requirement of hepatic metabolism and the selective toxicity of benzene in the bone-marrow. As discussed above, benzene is metabolized in the liver mainly to phenol and minor amounts of hydroquinone and catechol. In contrast to muconaldehyde, the hydroxylated benzene metabolites administered singly do not cause bone marrow toxicity in experimental animals. Phenol and hydroquinone, which accumulate in bone marrow (Greenlee et al., 1981), have been shown to cause significant decreases in bone marrow cellularity when coadministered to mice (Eastmond et al., 1987). Since the bone marrow is rich in peroxidative enzymes including myeloperoxidase and potential oxidants such as hydrogen peroxide derived from leukocytes, it has been suggested (Eastmond et al., 1987; Smith et al., 1989) that a bone marrow-localized phenol-dependent stimulation of hydroquinone metabolism results in the formation of benzoquinone, the ultimate toxic benzene metabolite. Benzoquinone is a direct-acting alkylating agent. It readily reacts with sulfhydryls and has been shown to inhibit microtubule assembly by blocking the thiol-sensitive GTP binding site (Irons et al.,

1981). Benzoquinone also forms DNA adducts (Jowa et al., 1990), causes DNA strand breakage (Pellack-Walker and Blumer, 1986), and is genotoxic in V79 cells (Glatt et al., 1989). Thus binding of benzoquinone to critical cellular substituents may play a role in benzene myelotoxicity.

The bone marrow is a complex matrix harboring stem cells, progenitor cells of blood cells, and stromal cells, which provide growth factors necessary for the proliferation and differentiation of stem and progenitor cells (Tavassoli and Friedenstein, 1983). The stromal macrophage, a regulator of hematopoiesis (Bagby, 1987), has been proposed to be a specific target of benzene (Kalf et al., 1989). In DBA/2N and C57BL/6 mice, benzene caused a dose-dependent bone marrow depression and a significant increase in bone marrow prostaglandin E levels. Both effects were prevented by coadministration of indomethacin and other inhibitors of the cyclooxygenase component of prostaglandin H synthase (PHS). Benzene, or a reactive metabolite, is hypothesized to stimulate the release of arachidonic acid, which is further metabolized to the hydroperoxide PGG_2. In this mechanism of benzene toxicity, the decreased bone-marrow cellularity after benzene administration is attributed to the constitutive production of high levels of prostaglandins, known to be down-regulators of hematopoiesis, coupled with the genotoxic damage from reactive metabolites such as benzoquinone. Using hydroquinone or phenol as electron donors, the endoperoxidase would metabolize PGG_2 to PGH_2, the immediate precursor molecule for prostaglandins, with the concomitant formation of benzoquinone.

Phagocytic cells have the ability to produce a variety of toxic oxygen species including superoxide anion radical, hydrogen peroxide, and hydroxyl radical (Babior, 1984). Enhanced functional activity such as enhanced active oxygen production is indicative of cellular activation (Adams and Hamilton, 1984). Bone marrow macrophages and granulocytes from Balb/c mice treated with 880 mg/kg benzene were found to produce elevated levels of hydrogen peroxide on stimulation with phorbol myristate acetate compared with the same types of cells from control mice (Laskin et al., 1989). The authors suggested that toxic doses of benzene activate bone marrow macrophages and granulocytes, which, on the one hand, release toxic oxygen species responsible for bone-marrow cell killing. On the other hand, activated phagocytes can also produce elevated levels of immune mediators and cytokines including IL-1, which may contribute to benzene hematotoxicity by altering the proliferation of subpopulations of bone marrow cells. In addition to toxic oxygen species, Laskin et al. (1995) demonstrated that bone marrow leukocytes from mice administered hematotoxic doses of benzene or the metabolites hydroquinone, p-benzoquinone and 1,2,4-benzenetriol produced increased amounts of nitric oxide (NO) in response to the inflammatory mediators lipopolysaccharide (LPS) or interferon gamma (IFN-γ). The production of NO induced by the inflammatory mediators was further enhanced by granulocyte-macrophage- and macrophage colony-stimulating factor, which are the growth factors present in the bone marrow required for normal cell proliferation and differentiation. The authors suggested that elevated NO production in the bone marrow may be an important mediator of benzene-induced bone marrow suppression.

Despite many interesting hypotheses and fruitful lines of investigation, it is not now possible to identify a specific metabolic pathway leading to a specific toxic intermediate producing a specific pathogenetic mechanism resulting in either bone-marrow aplasia or leukemogenesis. In fact it has become more apparent that the effect of benzene is likely to be exerted through the action of multiple metabolites on multiple endpoints through multiple biological pathways (Goldstein, 1989b; Eastmond et al., 1987). An overall hypothesis for benzene-induced leukemia was recently proposed by Smith (1996). The key elements of this hypothesis consist of generally accepted knowledge on benzene metabolism and disposition of metabolites, cellular targets and effects leading to changes in chromosome structure that result in protooncogene activation and the inactivation of tumor suppressor genes. A stem cell thus affected would proliferate and develop a leukemic clone, which then develops into the disease state. Among the molecular targets of toxic metabolites suggested by Smith are tubulin, DNA, and topoisomerase II (topo II). The inhibitory effect of p-benzoquinone on tubulin formation has been known for some time (Irons et al., 1981).

In addition to DNA adduct formation which could lead to mutations and cancer discussed above, Kolachana et al. (1993) showed that mice administered benzene or its phenolic metabolites have increased levels of 8-hydroxydeoxyguanosine (8-OHdG) in bone marrow cell DNA. A study by Lagorio et al. (1994) in 65 filling station attendants in Rome, Italy, showed a dose-response relationship between personal exposure to benzene and urinary concentrations of 8-OHdG. Studies by Frantz et al. (1996) and Chen and Eastmond (1995) indicate that topoisomerase II is inhibited directly by p-benzoquinone and muconaldehyde, and by phenol and the polyhydroxylated metabolites after their peroxidase activation. Topo II is involved in breaking and resealing DNA strands during DNA replication and repair and inhibition of topo II could lead to chromosome breaks, and aneuploidy or cell death. It is of interest to note that the use of topo II inhibitors in chemotherapy is associated with a high risk of developing acute myeloid leukemia (1994). The inhibition of topo II by benzene metabolites could contribute to the clastogenic and carcinogenic effects of benzene. Synergistic clastogenic effects have been observed in bone-marrow erythrocytes of mice co-administered phenol and hydroquinone (Barale et al., 1990). The increase in micronuclei induction in the bone-marrow erythrocytes appears to originate mainly from breakage in the euchromatic region of mouse chromosomes (Chen and Eastmond, 1995).

Elevated levels of DNA–protein crosslinks have been demonstrated in bone-marrow cells of mice administered benzene and in HL-60 cells exposed to muconaldehyde (Schoenfeld et al., 1996). The induction of DNA–protein crosslinks by toxicants is often associated with DNA strand breaks (Cosma et al., 1988; Yamanaka et al., 1995), suggesting that DNA–protein crosslinks could contribute to the observed clastogenic effects observed after benzene exposure. Recent in vitro studies in bone-marrow cells and HL-60 cells indicate induction of apoptosis by exposure to phenolic metabolites and to muconaldehyde, suggesting that programmed cell death could be involved in benzene bone-marrow cytotoxicity (Moran et al., 1996; Hiraku and Kawanishi, 1996; Schoenfeld et al., 1997). Studies analyzing bone-marrow cell populations in mice administered benzene or hydroquinone (Hazel et al., 1996) and in vitro studies in model cell systems with reactive benzene metabolites (Irons and Stillman, 1996; Hedli et al., 1996; Hazel and Kalf, 1996; Kalf et al., 1996) indicate changes in cell differentiation and/or effects on signal transduction pathways which could play a role in the mechanism of benzene-induced leukemogenesis.

One particularly exciting area of benzene research can be loosely grouped under the heading of biological markers (NAS, 1989). As more is learned about the metabolism of benzene and the pathogenesis of its effects, it becomes possible to develop markers of exposure or effect suitable for assay in body fluids of laboratory animals or of humans. These should be of value in elucidating the mechanism of benzene hematotoxicity, in determining the extent of human exposure to benzene, and in establishing the appropriate dose–response curve for the effects of benzene. Substantial efforts have been made in the last 10 years toward the development of biological markers or biomarkers of benzene exposure and their application to exposed populations. Biomarkers have the advantage over external monitoring of integrating exposure from all routes and sources. Their measurement quantitates internal dose and reflects metabolism, where applicable, and disposition. Potential biomarkers of benzene exposure are the parent compound benzene, ring-hydroxylated- and ring-opened metabolites, glutathione-derived metabolite adducts

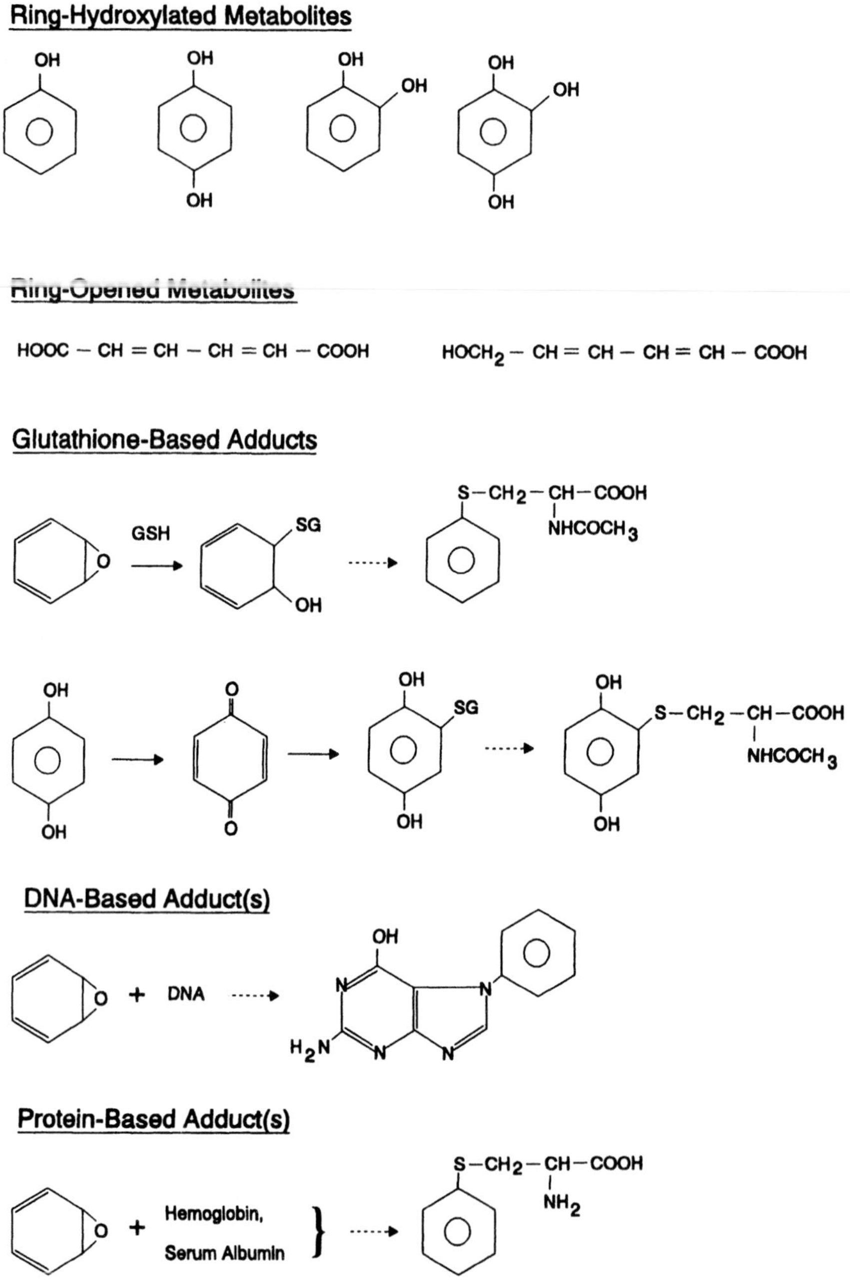

Ring-Hydroxylated Metabolites
OH
OH
OH
Ring-Opened Metabolites
HOOC – CH = CH – CH = CH – COOH
HOCH2 – CH = CH – CH = CH – COOH
Glutathione-Based Adducts
GSH
O
SG
OH
S–CH2–CH–COOH
NHCOCH3
O
SG
DNA-Based Adduct(s)
O
+ DNA
OH
N
H2N
Protein-Based Adduct(s)
Hemoglobin,
Serum Albumin
S–CH2–CH–COOH
NH2

Figure 4-2

and DNA- and protein-derived adducts (Fig. 4-2). Several reviews on biomarkers of benzene exposure have recently been published, and the reader is referred to them for a detailed description of individual biomarkers, their measurement in biological samples, and their usefulness in regard to serving as a biological index of benzene exposure (Bechtold and Henderson, 1993; Ong et al., 1995; Medeiros et al., 1997). A future goal is correlation of biomarkers with markers of susceptibility and effect for elucidation of the processes involved in benzene-induced hematotoxicity and leukemogenesis.

Hematological Effects

Pancytopenic Effects Benzene was first identified as a hematological toxicant in the nineteenth century. Experience since that time has amply confirmed the ability of benzene to destroy bone-marrow precursor cells responsible for the production of mature circulating blood cells in humans. Similar effects are noted in the many species of laboratory animals that have been experimentally exposed to benzene.

Human blood cells are generally considered to be of three types: red blood cells, whose primary function is to deliver oxygen to the tissues, white blood cells, which are involved in the body's defenses against infection; and platelets, which participate in normal blood coagulation. Exposure to benzene affects the formation of each of these cell types, and severe benzene toxicity produces aplastic anemia. This consists of a marked decrease in the cellularity of the bone marrow, which is often replaced by fat, and highly significant decrements in circulating red blood cells (anemia), white blood cells (leukopenia), and platelets (thrombocytopenia). Aplastic anemia is a frequently fatal disorder with death usually occurring from infection or hemorrhage.

The normal bone marrow has ample reserve. For example, under certain circumstances, six times as many red blood cells as normal can be made. Thus relatively low levels of a toxicant may decrease the bone-marrow reserve without causing any clinically recognizable decrease in blood counts. As toxicant levels get higher, initially one can see a decrease in blood counts within the normal range, a seemingly selective fall in one of the three blood cell types, then a mild decrease in each, known as pancytopenia, followed by full-blown aplastic anemia.

Benzene produces its pancytopenic and aplastic effects through damage to precursors within the marrow by its metabolites. The earliest bone marrow precursor is a pluripotential stem cell that can mature into precursors of red blood cells (erythoblastic cell line), platelets (megakaryocytic cell line), and granulocytic white blood cells (myelocytic cell line, resulting in polymorphonuclear leukocytes, basophils, and eosinophils). The pluripotential cell appears also to be a source of lymphocytic white blood cells. Circulating lymphocytes are relatively susceptible to benzene in laboratory animals (Wierda et al., 1981; C. A. Snyder et al., 1978; Rozen and Snyder, 1985) and in humans (Goldstein, 1988; Rothman et al., 1996).

A variety of potential mechanisms have been suggested to account for presumed differences in individual susceptibility to the pancytopenic effects of benzene including such factors as gender, increased bone-marrow turnover, and various metabolic factors (see above and Goldstein, 1988). Of particular interest is the recent observation by Rothman et al. (1997) that those individuals with both an elevation in the activity of cytochrome P4502E1, as measured by rapid fractional excretion of chlorzoxazone, and gene mutations reflecting a reduction in activity of NQO1, were associated with a 7.6-fold greater risk of benzene-induced pancytopenia. As discussed above, CYT P4502E1 is a major activator of benzene metabolism, and NQO1 is a presumed detoxifying enzyme of benzene metabolites. Either variation by itself showed a two- to three-fold increase in risk. This work needs to be confirmed and extended to the risk of benzene-induced neoplasia.

Neoplastic Effects Benzene is a known cause of acute myelogenous leukemia (AML), the adult form of acute leukemia that was almost uniformly fatal until recent advances in chemotherapy. Individual cases of AML in benzene-exposed individuals were first reported about six decades ago, but it was not until the 1970s that the causal relationship was fully accepted. Benzene exposure leads to cytogenetic abnormalities in bone-marrow cells and in circulating lymphocytes (Forni et al., 1971) consistent with alteration of the genome and in keeping with a somatic mutation leading to cancer.

More recent studies in benzene exposed Chinese workers have begun to apply molecular biological techniques to better understand the chromosomal effects of benzene. For example, Rothman et al. (1995) noted benzene-induced gene-duplicating but not gene-inactivating mutations at the glycophorin A locus in bone-marrow cells.

Of note is that hematologists have long recognized that anyone with an aplastic anemia from virtually any cause has an increased risk of developing AML. Thus radiation and alkylating agents used in chemotherapy produce both aplastic anemia and AML.

Unequivocal evidence of the causal relationship between benzene and AML has come through studies in a number of countries. An epidemic of aplastic anemia followed by AML was observed in Turkish leather workers due to introduction of a benzene-containing glue in their workshops (Aksoy, 1985a, b; Aksoy et al., 1971; Aksoy and Erdem, 1978). A cohort of workers in a pliofilm factory in Ohio has become among the most thoroughly studied in the history of occupational medicine, particularly in relation to reconstructing their past exposure history (Infante et al., 1977; Rinsky et al., 1981, 1987, Ward et al., 1996). In this cohort a total of 10 cases of myelogenous leukemia have been observed, with only two expected. Recent studies in China have again demonstrated the leukomogenic potential of benzene (Yin et al., 1987a,1996; Hayes et al., 1997).

Often individuals with aplastic anemia or some degree of pancytopenia are observed to go through a preleukemic stage of varying duration before developing frank AML. The manifestations observed, including morphological abnormalities of bone marrow precursors, have been classified together as the myelodysplastic syndrome (Layton and Mufti, 1987), a syndrome that is not unique to benzene hematotoxicity. Benzene also appears to share with radiation and with chemotherapeutic alkylating agents a predilection for a lag period between initial exposure and the development of frank myelogenous leukemia of 5 to15 years (Goldstein et al., 1991). This is relatively short for other types of cancers. Although the data for benzene are less clear-cut, a case can be made that it would be distinctly unusual for a benzene exposure to result in AML in less than 2 years, and there does appear to be a lessening of risk perhaps 10 to 15 years following cessation of exposure.

Benzene has also been associated with other neoplasms, both hematological and nonhematological (Young, 1989; Goldstein, 1977, 1990). In no case is the evidence as definitive as it is for AML (See Table 4-1). Evidence for other hematological neoplasms is reasonably good but not conclusive. An example is multiple myeloma. This is a bone-marrow tumor of plasma cells that are antibody-producing cells derived from β-lymphocytes. A few individual cases of multiple myeloma have been reported in association with benzene exposure, including four cases in the Turkish group (Aksoy, 1985a; Aksoy et al., 1984). Four deaths from multiple myeloma have been reported in the Ohio pliofilm cohort as compared to one expected, a statistically significant observation (Rinsky et al., 1987). A causal relationship is biomedically plausible in view of the fact that benzene unequivocally can cause a bone-marrow tumor, and β-lymphocytes, which are precursors of plasma cells, develop cytogenetic abnormalities following benzene exposure. Of note is that there is some evidence suggesting an international increase in the overall incidence of multiple myeloma, particularly in older age groups (Velez et al., 1982; Goldstein, 1990).

A related question is, if multiple myeloma is causally related to benzene exposure, why is the evidence less clear-cut than it is for AML? This important point is also pertinent when considering the relationship between benzene and other hematological and nonhematological neoplasms. There are three main considerations. The first is the relative risk per unit of benzene exposure for AML in comparison to multiple myeloma. It

TABLE 4-1   Causal Relation between Benzene Exposure and Various Hematological Disorders

- Causality proved
    - Pancytopenia aplastic anemia
    - Acute myelogenous leukemia and variants (including acute myelomoncytic leukemia, acute promyelocytic leukemia, erthroleukemia)
    - Myelodysplasia
- Causality probable
    - Non-Hodgkin's lymphoma
    - Chronic lymphocytic leukemia
    - Acute lymphoblastic leukemia
    - Paroxysmal nocturnal hemoglobinuria
    - Multiple myeloma
- Association suggested but unproved
    - Chronic myelogenous leukemia
    - Myelofibrosis and myeloid metaplasia
    - Hodgkin's disease
    - Thrombocythemia

Source: Modified from B.D. Goldstein (1983, 1989).

is conceivable, although speculative, that a given amount of benzene is more likely to produce the somatic mutation leading to AML than that it will produce the mutation responsible for multiple myeloma, or, similarly, benzene may be more likely to lead to AML cancer promotion or progression. The second consideration, which is not speculative, is that multiple myeloma is less common a cancer than is AML. Thus any multiplication of its original background risk caused by benzene exposure is less likely to be recognized given the usual size of cohorts (e.g., if the background incidence of death from tumor A is 10 in 1000 and of tumor B is 1 in 1000, then the doubling of risk by a carcinogen in a large cohort recording 1000 deaths would lead to 20 deaths as compared to 10 expected for tumor A, a statistically significant finding; however, for tumor B there would be a statistically unrecognizable two deaths as compared to one expected). The third point concerns the relatively short latency period for AML as compared to other tumors (Goldstein, 1989b, 1990). A greater delay between onset of exposure and eventual tumor complicates the likelihood of observing a causal relationship.

Similarly benzene is very likely to be a cause of non-Hodgkin's lymphoma (NHL). For NHL, the evidence is close to being conclusive. The recent findings in China of at least a borderline statistically significant increase in NHL (relative risk 3.0, 99% confidence interval 0.9–10.5) is particularly important in view of the low background incidence of lymphatic tumors in China. For those with 10 or more years of benzene exposure, the relative risk for NHL was 4.2 (95% CI. 1.1–15.9) (Hayes et al., 1997). A related study in the same cohort showed a statistically significant increase in risk for NHL (Yin et al., 1997).

The possibility that benzene might be the cause of nonhematological neoplasms, such as lung or liver cancer, has been raised by animal studies in which it has been difficult to demonstrate hematological neoplasms. Snyder et al. (1980) demonstrated an increased incidence of lymphoma in mice. A variety of solid tumors have been observed in two-year rodent studies performed by Maltoni, Conti, and Cotti (1983) in Italy and by the U.S. National Toxicology Program (Huff, 1983). However, there is at present no convincing evidence of nonhematological tumors occurring in humans as a result of benzene exposure. In predicting whether these would occur, it is of conceptual importance to determine whether the proximal carcinogen is uniquely formed within the bone marrow or whether the carcinogenic metabolites are made primarily in the liver and then travel throughout the circulation, the bone marrow being particularly susceptible because of its special dynamics, but as in radiation carcinogenesis, other organs also being at risk.

Nonhematological Effects

Central Nervous System   Benzene has an odor threshold in the range of 4 to 5 ppm (ATSDR, 1989). The acute central nervous system toxicity of benzene is similar to that of other alkyl benzenes and has much in common with the general anesthetic effects of lipophilic solvents. It appears to be a direct effect of benzene and not related to its metabolites. Symptoms following acute inhalation include drowsiness, lightheadedness, headache, delirium, vertigo, and narcosis leading to loss of consciousness. Benzene levels at which acute central nervous system effects become noticeable are at least above 100 ppm and are more likely to be in the few hundred or few thousand parts per million range. In view of the leukemogenicity of benzene, controlled human exposure studies of such effects are not appropriate. On structure-activity grounds, benzene might be expected to have acute central nervous system effects similar to toluene, albeit at a slightly lower dose for benzene. Chronic nervous system effects of benzene have not been unequivocally demonstrated. There is much debate about whether chronic nervous system effects may occur with alkyl benzenes, particularly in work groups such as commercial painters, and, if proved, such findings might conceivably be pertinent to chronic benzene exposure.

Reproductive and Developmental Effects   Davis and Pope (1986) have pointed out the need for thorough evaluation of the potential fetotoxicity of benzene. Keller and Snyder (1986, 1988) have shown hematological effects in the developing fetus at relatively low maternal exposure concentration. However, to date, animal studies have generally been negative, and there is no human evidence of reproductive or developmental toxicity from benzene despite substanital exposure of women of reproductive age.

Effects on the Immune System   There is no question that high levels of benzene produce effects on lymphocytes in laboratory animals exposed to benzene, and that these lymphocytopenic effects can result in deficits in immune function (Irons et al., 1983). Immune function decrements can occur in the absence of lymphocytopenic effects (Rosenthal and Snyder, 1985, 1987). However, there is currently no evidence whatsoever to suggest that immune function is affected following exposure of humans to allowable workplace levels of benzene or to the much lower levels present in the general environment.

RISK ASSESSMENT

Risk assessment for carcinogens as an organized process has developed rapidly in the last 15 years. The EPA's Carcinogen Assessment Group and similar groups at FDA have provided an impetus to what is now a broadly based approach to developing quantitative methods for assessing the extent to which cancer is likely to result from exposure to a chemical. In comparison to many other known or suspected carcinogens, benzene presents an intriguing paradox. There is comparatively good agreement about the risk-specific dose of benzene (Goldstein, 1985); yet the economic and societal stakes are so high as to make relatively small differences in interpretation highly controversial.

A major milestone in the use of risk assessment for regulatory purposes was a 1983 National Academy of Sciences report (NAS, 1983). This document provided an overview of the rationale for risk assessment for all endpoints, carcinogenic and noncarcinogenic, as well as a logical and consistent classification of the components of risk assessment. The four major components are hazard identification, dose–response estimation, exposure assessment, and risk characterization.

Hazard Identification

In terms of hazard identification, there is no question that benzene is a human carcinogen. This distinguishes benzene from many other compounds that are regulated on the basis of evidence in animal studies suggesting that they are probably human carcinogens, but without epidemiological confirmation. As discussed above, the unequivocal evidence for benzene carcinogenicity in humans is for acute myelogenous leukemia and its variants. Hazard identification of benzene as causal for other cancers remains equivocal. Benzene is also an identified hazard for producing pancytopenia and aplastic anemia, and it can produce acute central nervous system toxicity. Other effects, such as chronic CNS toxicity and fetal abnormalities, are of theoretical concern, but there is no direct evidence to support these hazards in humans.

Dose – Response Estimation

Dose–response estimation for benzene, as for other carcinogens, has generated controversy. Points of contention include the use of the standard EPA linearized multistage model, which in essence assumes that every single molecule of benzene has a finite chance of producing the somatic mutation responsible for acute myelogenous leukemia. Industry at times has argued that aplastic anemia is a necessary precursor of AML, based on observations of individuals with aplastic anemia who evolved through a preleukemic phase to AML, on the argument that many of the reported cases of benzene-associated AML have occurred in individuals with relatively high levels of exposure, and on the knowledge that aplastic anemia from seemingly any cause seems to predispose toward AML. There is clearly a threshold for aplastic anemia; that is there is a level of benzene exposure below which there is no apparent risk of aplastic anemia. Accordingly, if aplastic anemia is a necessary precursor of AML, then there must also be a threshold for benzene leukemogenesis, and this threshold must be well beyond any exposure level of environmental concern. However, the supporting evidence for such a threshold for AML is very weak. In terms of case reports, there have been numerous cases of benzene-associated AML in which there was no evidence of antecedent aplastic anemia, although some degree of pancytopenia cannot be ruled out because of lack of preceding blood counts. In addition a mechanism that depended solely on some leukemogenic process occurring in response to aplastic anemia would have difficulty explaining the cytogenic abnormalities that occur at levels of benzene that do not produce a frank pancytopenia (Yardley-Jones et al., 1988; Smith, 1996).

The slope of the dose–response curve for benzene leukemogenesis undoubtedly depends on the metabolism of benzene to proximal carcinogen(s). As described in detail above, the complex metabolic pathways leading to active species are in the process of being unraveled. Such information should be of great value in establishing the appropriate dose – response relationship for benzene leukemogenesis. This subject was recently considered in a conference that looked at the issue of whether there was sufficient information to establish a new dose response model for benzene (Smith, 1996). While a number of interesting proposals were considered, there was no scientific consensus to move away from the linearized multistage model.

Although it is difficult to overstate the importance of understanding benzene metabolism in relation to benzene leukemogenesis, it must also be emphasized that determining the kinetic relationship between benzene exposure and the formation of active species is not sufficient by itself to establish the dose–response relationship. One must also take into account the responsiveness of the target organ, which, through its own natural variation in sensitivity or in defense mechanisms, may play a role in determining the dose–response pattern. For example, Sabourin et al. (1990) and Witz et al. (1990) have shown that the percentage of benzene metabolized to the ring-opened form, as measured by muconic acid, is inversely proportional to the exposure level. This suggests that the dose pattern of concern might be chronic low-level exposure rather than the equivalent dose given as a short-term spike. However, Witz, Rao, and Goldstein (1985) have also shown that the bone marrow toxicity of *trans,trans*-muconaldehyde is greater with a single daily dose than it is with the same dose divided into three daily injections; that is the short-term spike of the toxic metabolite is more harmful to the target organ. Integrating physiologically based pharmacokinetics for benzene metabolites with the dose pattern responsiveness of the bone marrow will present an intriguing challenge to those interested in modeling dose–response patterns.

Because benzene is a known human carcinogen, it is appropriate and proper that the risk of benzene leukemogenesis be calculated by the seemingly conservative approach of the linear multistage model. Yet there seems to be no reasonable likelihood that aplastic anemia can be caused at the levels of exposure reported in the general environment. The threshold for aplastic anemia as a potentially crippling or fatal disease is likely to be significantly above the 10 ppm TWA (time–weighted–average) benzene standard that was the workplace norm for many years.

Attempts to use huge safety factors resulting in a sub-ppm benzene standard to protect against acute benzene effects or aplastic anemia are so much nonsense. Starting with animal data and then using a safety factor approach might be relevant for a new chemical but is simply inappropriate given the literally millions of person-years of data available for benzene. An example of the misapplication of this approach occurred recently in New Jersey where application of a 10 ppb indoor "acute action level" led to evacuation of homeowners and widespread community concern. The families were moved to a crossroads motel that likely contained higher indoor benzene levels than their homes. The level of 10 ppb is not uncommon in American basements. It was chosen as an acute action level by the state of Massachusetts based on an observation in one animal species, but not another, of cytogenetic abnormalities at 1 ppm benzene, plus a 100-fold safety factor. Risk assessment performed as a basis for regulatory decisions concerning benzene in the general environment should at present consider only cancer risk.

In view of the lack of positive data, no risk assessment for fetal abnormalities or chronic nervous system effects from benzene is currently indicated.

Exposure Assessment

Exposure assessment for benzene presents some current areas of intense controversy, both in terms of retrospective estimates of exposure of benzene-exposed cohorts with elevated leukemia incidence and in terms of the appropriate approach to exposure estimation from known benzene sources in a community.

Perhaps the most thorough retrospective evaluation of benzene exposure, or of any occupationally exposed cohort, has been that performed by Rinsky and his colleagues on the employees of a pliofilm plant whose benzene exposure resulted in a substantial risk of leukemia. The authors did a masterful job of reconstructing the location of each of the workers within the workplace and possible exposure levels. However, Rinsky et al. (1987) ended up with much lower exposure levels, particularly during the Second World War, when most of the leukemia cases were at work, than did Crump and Allen (1984), who built their exposure estimate on the base of the Rinsky study's efforts. The major distinction between the two approaches is the much higher levels posited by Crump and

Allen during World War II. The latter appears to be strongly supported by contemporary accounts of significant incidences of aplastic anemia and of central nervous system effects at pliofilm factories as a result of wartime conditions, which would also be expected to result in longer working hours and thus greater individual exposures. In addition Kipen et al. (1988, 1989a) have found that the historic blood counts of workers in this cohort had a statistically significant inverse correlation with the Crump and Allen exposure assessment but no relationship with the estimate of the Rinsky study (see also Hornung et al., 1989; Kipen et al., 1989b; Paxton et al., 1994a, b; Schnatter et al., 1996). Because almost all of the workers with AML had been in this cohort in the early 1940s, it appears that reliance on the Rinsky study's exposure estimation to perform a risk assessment may lead to an overestimate of the risk.

Similar to the pliofilm cohort, it can be anticipated that the extent to which the recent studies of benzene-exposed workers in China will affect the cancer risk potency for benzene will depend in large part on the scientific acceptability of the exposure assessment (Dosemici et al., 1994)

Risk Characterization

The EPA has characterized the risk of benzene-induced leukemia as being $8 \times 10^6 \, (\mu g / m^3$ benzene) per 70-year lifetime. This can be translated into a risk of 8 in 1 million of dying from benzene-induced leukemia from breathing $1 \, \mu g / m^3$ of benzene for 70 years. This risk is usually described as being the plausible upper boundary in that the conservative assumptions built into risk assessment are thought to make it unlikely that the risk is any higher, but it is conceivable that it is lower. The level of benzene responsible for a one in 1 million lifetime risk for drinking water has been similarly calculated by EPA to be 0.66 ppb.

REFERENCES

Adams, D. O., and T. A. Hamilton. 1984. The cell biology of macrophage activation. *Annu. Rev. Immunol.* 2: 283–318.

Aksoy, M. 1985a. Malignancies due to occupational exposure to benzene. *Am. J. Ind. Med.* 7: 395–402.

Aksoy, M. 1985b. Benzene as a leukemogenic and carcinogenic agent. *Am. J. Ind. Med.* 8: 9–20.

Aksoy, M., and S. Erdem. 1978. A follow-up study on the mortality and the development of leukemia in 44 pancytopenic patients associated with long-term exposure to benzene. *Blood.* 52: 285–292.

Aksoy, M., S. Erdem, G. Dincol. A. Kutlar, I. Bakioglu, and T. Hepyuksel. 1984. Clincial observations showing the role of some factors in the etiology of multiple myeloma. *Acta Haemat. I.* 71: 116–120.

Aksoy, M., K. Dincol, T. Akgun, S. Erdem, and G. Dincol. 1971. Haematological effects of chronic benzene poisoning in 217 workers. *Br. J. Ind. Med.* 28: 296–302.

American Conference of Governmental Industrial Hygienists (ACGIH). *1997 TLVs and BEIs.* Cincinnati, ACGIH, 1997.

Andrews, L. S., E. W. Lee, C. M. Witmer, J. J. Kocsis, and R. Snyder. 1977. Effects of toluene on the metabolism, disposition, and hemopoietic toxicity of ^{3}H-benzene. *Biochem. Pharmacol.* 26: 293–300.

Andrews, L. S., E. W. Lee, C. M. Witmer, and J. J. Kocsis. 1979. ^{3}H-Benzene metabolism in rabbit bone marrow. *Life Sci.* 25: 567–572.

Ashley, D. L., M. A. Bonin, F. L. Cardinali, J. M. McCraw, and J. V. Wooten. 1994. Blood concentrations of volatile organic compounds in a nonoccupationally exposed US population and in groups with suspected exposure. *Clin. Chem.* 40: 1401–1404.

Askoy, M., ed. 1988. *Benzene Carcinogenicity.* Boca Raton, FL: CRC Press.

ATSDR. 1989. *Toxicological Profile for Benzene.* U. S. Public Health Services. U. S. Environmental Protection Agency. Oak Ridge, TN: Oak Ridge National Laboratory.

Baarson, K. A., C. A. Snyder, J. D. Green, A. Sellakumar, B. D. Goldstein, and R. E. Albert. 1982. The hematotoxic effects of inhaled benzene on peripheral blood, bone marrow, and spleen cells are increased by ingested ethanol. *Toxicol. Appl. Pharmacol.* 64: 393–404.

Babior, B. M. 1984. Oxidants from phagocytes: Agents of defense and destruction. *Blood.* 64: 959–966.

Bagby, G. C. 1987. Production of multilineage growth factors by hematopoietic stromal cells: An intercellular regulatory network involving mononuclear phagocytes and interleukin-1. *Blood Cells.* 13: 147–159.

Bainton, D. F., J. L. Joan, and M. G. Farquar. 1971. The development of neutrophilic polymorphonuclear leukocytes in human bone marrow. *J. Exp. Med.* 134: 907–935.

Barale, R., A. Marrazzini, C. Betti, V. Vangelisti, N. Loprieno, and I. Barrai. 1990. Genotoxicity of two metabolites of benzene: phenol and hydroquinone show strong synergistic effects in vivo. *Mutat. Res.* 244: 15–20.

Bartczak, A.W., S. A. Kline, W. E. Bechtold, B. D. Goldstein, and G. Witz. 1993. An improved HPLC method for the determination of *trans,trans*-muconic acid in human urine. *Toxicologist.* 13: 441.

Bechtold, W. E., and R. F. Henderson. 1993. Biomarkers of human exposure to benzene. *J. Toxicol. Environ. Health.* 40: 377–386.

Bechtold, W. E., J. D. Sun, L. S. Birnbaum, S. Yin, G. L. Li, S. Kasicki, G. Lucier, and R. F. Henderson. 1992. *S*-phenylcysteine formation in hemoglobin as a biological exposure index to benzene. *Arch. Toxicol.* 66: 303–309.

Bolcsak, L. E., and D. E. Nerland. 1983. Inhibition of erythropoiesis by benzene and benzene metabolites. *Toxicol. Appl. Pharmacol.* 69: 363–368.

Bratton, S. B., S. S. Lau, and T. J. Monks. 1997. Identification of quinol thioethers in bone marrow of hydroquinone/phenol-treated rats and mice and their potential role in benzene-mediated hematotoxicity. *Chem. Res. Toxicol.* 10: 859–865.

Brugnone, F., L. Perbellini, G. B. Faccini, F. Pasini, B. Dansi, G. Maranelli, L. Romeo, M. Gobbi, and A. Zedde. 1989. Benzene in the blood and breath of normal people and occupationally exposed workers. *Am. J. Ind. Med.* 16: 385–399.

C&EN. 1997. Facts and Figures for the Chemical Industry. *Chemical and Engineering News.* (www. acsinfo. acs. org/cen/index. html).

Chang, R. L., C. Q. Wang, S. A. Kline, A. H. Conney, B. D. Goldstein, and G. Witz. 1994. Mutagenicity of *trans-trans*-muconaldehyde and its metabolites in V79 cells. *Environ. Mol. Mutagen.* 24: 112–115.

Chen, H., and D. A. Eastmond. 1995. Topoisomerase inhibition by phenolic metabolites: A potential mechanism for benzene's clastogenic effects. *Carcinogenesis.* 16: 2301–2307.

Chen, H., and D. A. Eastmond. 1995. Synergistic increase in chromosomal breakage within the euchromatin induced by an interaction of the benzene metabolites phenol and hydroquinone in mice. *Carcinogenesis.* 16: 1963–1969.

Cooper, L. R., and R. Snyder. 1988. Benzene metabolism. Toxicokentics and the molecular aspects of benzene toxicity. In *Benzene Carcinogenicity*, ed. M. Aksoy, pp. 33–58. Boca Raton, FL: CRC Press.

Cosma, G. N., R. Jamasbi, and A. C. Marchok. 1988. Growth inhibition and DNA damage induced by benzo(a)pyrene and formaldehyde in primary cultures of rat tracheal epithelial cells. *Mutation Res.* 201: 161–168.

Crump, K., and B. Allen. 1984. *Quantitative Estimates of risk of Leukemia from Occupational Exposure to Benzene.* OSHA Doket H-059B. Washington, DC: OSHA.

Davis, D. L., and A. M. Pope. 1986. Reproductive risks of benzene: Need for additional study. *Toxicol. Ind. Health.* 2: 445–451.

Dor, F., Y. LeMoullec, and B. Festy. 1995. Exposure of city residents to carbon monoxide and monocyclic aromatic hydrocarbons during commuting trips in the Paris metropolitan area. *J. Air Waste Manag. Assoc.*, 45(2): 103–110.

Dosemeci, M., G.-L. Li, R. B. Hayes, S.-N. Yin, M. Linet, W.-H. Chow, Y.-Z. wang, Z.-L. Jiang, T.-R. Dai, W.-U. Zhang, X.-J. Chao, P.-Z. Ye, Q.-R. Kou, Y.-H. Fam, X.-C. Zhang, X.-F. Lin, J.-F. Meng, J.-S. Zho,

S. Wacholder, R. Kneller, and W. J. Blot. 1994. Cohort Study Among Workers Exposed to Benzene in China: II. Exposure Assessment. *Am. J. Ind. Med.* 26: 401–411.

Drummond, J. C., and I. L. Finar. 1938. Muconic acid as a metabolic product of benzene. *Biochemistry.* 32: 79–84.

Eastmond, D. A., M. T. Smith, and R. D. Irons. 1987. An interaction of benzene metabolites repoduces the myelotoxicity observed with benzene exposure. *Toxicol. Appl. Pharmacol.* 91: 85–95.

Forni, A. M., A Cappellini, E. Pacifico, and E. C. Vigliani. 1971. Chromosome changes and their evolution in subjects with exposure to benzene. *Arch. Environ. Health.* 23: 385–391.

Frantz, C. E., H. Chen, and D. A. Eastmond. 1996. Inhibition of human topoisomerase II in vitro by bioactive benzene metabolites. *Environ. Health Perspect.* 104: 1319–1323.

Franz, T. J. 1984. Percutaneous absorption of benzene. In: *Advances in Modern Environmental Toxicology: Applied Toxicology of Petroleum Hydrocarbons,* vol. 6 eds. H. N. MacFarland et al. Princeton: Princeton Scientific Publishers.

Genter, M. B., and L. Recio. 1994. Absence of detectable P4502E1 in bone marrow of B6C3F1 mice: relevance to butadiene-induced bone marrow toxicity. *Fund. Appl. Toxicol.* 22: 469–473.

Glatt, H., R. Padykdula, G. A. Berchtold, G. Ludewig, K. L. Platt, J. Klein, and F. Oesch. 1989. Multiple activation pathways of benzene leading to products with varying genotixic characteristics. *Environ. Health Perspect.* 82: 81–89.

Goldstein, B. D. 1977. Hematotoxicity in humans. *J. Toxicol. environm. Health* (suppl.) 2: 69–105.

Goldstein, B. D. 1985. Risk assessment and risk management of benzene by the Environmental Protection Agency. In *Risk Quantitation and Regulatory Policy, Banbury Report,* vol 19, pp. 293–304. Cold Spring Harbor Laboratory, Cold Spring Harbor.

Goldstein, B. D. 1988. Benzene Toxicity. In *Occupational Medicine State of the Art Review:* The Petroleum Industry ed. N.K. Weaver, pp. 541–554. Philadelphia: Hanley and Beltus.

Goldstein, B. D. 1989a. Clinical hematotoxicity of benzene. In *Advances in Modern Environmental Toxicology,* Benzene: Occupational and Environmental Hazards — Scientific Update, vol. 16, pp. 55–65. Princeton: Princeton Scientific Publishing.

Goldstein, B. D. 1989b. Occam's razor is dull. *Environ. Health Perspect.* 82: 3–6.

Goldstein, B. D. 1990. Is exposure to benzene a cause of human multiple myeloma? *Ann. NY Acad. Sci.* 609: 225–334.

Goldstein, B. D., 1991. Lessons on the second cancers resulting from cancer chemotherapy. In *Biological Reactive Intermediates,* IV, Molecular and Cellular Effects and Their Impact on Human Health. Eds. C.M. Witmer et al., New York: Plenum Press.

Goldstein, B. D. 1994. Letter to the editor: Response to the Valdez Air Study Review Committee. *Risk Anal.* 14: 891–893.

Goon, D., X. Cheng, J. Ruth, D. R. Petersen, and D. Ross. 1992. Metabolism of *trans-trans*-muconaldehyde by aldehyde and alcohol dehydrogenase: Identification of a novel metabolite. *Toxicol. Appl. Pharmacol.* 114: 147–155.

Gorsky, L. D., and M. J. Coon. 1985. Evaluation of the role of free hydroxyl radicals in the cytochrome P-450 catalyzed oxidation of benzene and cyclohexanol. *Drug Metab. Disp.* 13: 169–174.

Greenlee, W. F., E. A. Gross, and R. D. irons. 1981. relationship between benzene toxicity and the disposition of ^{14}C-labeled benzene metabolites in rat. *Chem. -Biol. Interact.* 33: 285–299.

Grotz, V. L., S. Ji, B. D. Goldstein, and G. Witz. 1994. Metabolism of benzene and *trans-trans*-muconaldehyde in the isolated perfused liver to *trans-trans*-muconic acid. *Toxicol. Lett.* 70: 281–290.

Hanzlik, R. P., K. Hogberg, and C. M. Dugson. 1984. Microsomal hydroxylation of specifically deuterated monosubstituted benzenes. Evidence for direct aromatic hydroxylation. *Biochemistry.* 23: 3048–3055.

Hayes, R. B., S. -N. Yin, M. Dosemeci, G. -L. Li, S. Wacholder, L. B. Travis, C. -Y. Li, N. Rothman, R. N. Hoover, and M. S. Linet. 1997. Benzene and the dose-related incidence of hematologic neoplasms in China. *J. Nat. Cancer Inst.* 89: 1065–1071.

Hazel, B. A., A. O'Connor, R. Niculescu, and G. F. Kalf. 1996. Induction of granulocytic differentiation in a mouse model by benzene and hydroquinone. *Environ. Health Perspect.* 104: 1257–1264.

Hazel, B. A., and G. F. Kalf. 1996. Induction of granulocytic differentiation in myeloblasts by hydroquinone, a metabolite of benzene, involves the leukotriene D_4 receptor. *Receptors Signal Transduct.* 6: 1–12.

Hedli, C. C., N. R. Rao, K. R. Reuhl, C. M. Witmer, and R. Snyder. 1996. Effects of benzene metabolite treatment on granulocytic differentiation and DNA adduct formation in HL-60 cells. *Arch. Toxicol.* 70: 135–144.

Hedli, C. C., M. J. Hoffmann, S. Ji, P. E. Thomas, and R. Snyder. 1997. Benzene metabolism in the isolated perfused mouse liver. *Toxicol. Appl. Pharmacol.* 146: 60–68.

Hiraku, Y., and S. Kawanishi. 1996. Oxidative DNA damage and apoptosis induced by benzene metabolites. *Cancer Res.* 56: 5172–5178.

Hornung, R. W., E. Ward, J. A. Morris, and R. A. Rinsky. 1989. Letters to the editor. *Toxicol. Ind. Health.* 5: 1153–1155.

Huff, J. 1983. *National Toxicology Program. Technical Report on the Toxicology and Carcinogenesis Studies of Benzene (CAS No. 71-43-2) in F344/N Rats and B6C3F₁ Mice (Gavage Studies).* Research Triangle Park, NC: National Institutes of Environmental Health Sciences.

Infante, P. F., R. A. Rinsky, J. K. Waggoner, and R. J. Young. 1977. Leukemia in benzene workers. *Lancet.* 2: 76–78.

Irons, R. D., J. G. Dent, T. S. Baker, and D. E. Rickert. 1980. Benzene is metabolized and covalently bount in bone marrow in situ. *Chem. -Biol Interact.* 30: 241–245.

Irons, R. D., D. A. Neptun, and R. W. Pfeifer. 1981. Inhibition of lymphocyte transformation and microtubule assembly by quinone metabolites of benzene: Evidence for a common mechanism. *J. Reticuloendothel. Soc.* 30: 359–371.

Irons, R. D., W. F. Greenlee, D. Wierda, and J. S. Bus. 1982. Relationship between benzene metabolism and toxicity: A proposed mechanism for the formation of reactive intermediates from polyphenol metabolises. *Adv. Exp. Med. Biol.* 136: 229–243.

Irons, R. D. 1985. Quinones as toxic metabolites of benzene. *J. Toxicol. Environ. Health.* 16: 673–678.

Irons, R. D., and W. S. Stillman. 1996. Impact of benzene metabolites on differentiation of bone marrow progenitor cells. *Environ. Health Perspect.* 104: 1247–1250.

Jaffe, M. 1909. Uber die Aufspaltung des Benzolring im Organismus. I. Mitteilung. Das Auftreten von Muconsaure im Harn nach Darreichung von Benzol. *Hoppe-Seylers Z. Physiol. Chem.* 62: 58–67.

Jerina, D. M., and J. W. Daly. 1974. Arene oxides: A new aspect of drug metabolism. *Science.* 185: 573–582.

Johnasson, I., and M. Ingelman-Sundberg. 1983. Hydroxyl radical-mediated, cytochrome P450-dependent metabolic activation of benzene in microsomes and reconstituted enzyme systems from rabbit liver. *J. Biol. Chem.* 258: 7311–7316.

Johansson, I., and M. Ingelman-Sundberg. 1988. Benzene metabolism by ethanol-acetone-and benzene-inducible cytochrome P-450 (IIE1) on rat and rabbit liver microsomes. *Cancer Res.* 48: 5387–5390.

Jowa, L., G. Witz, R. Snyder, S. Winkle, and G. F. Kalf. 1990. Synthesis and characterization of deoxyguanosine-benzoquinone adducts. *J. Appl. Toxicol.* 10: 47–54.

Kalf, G. F. 1987. Recent advances in the metabolism and toxicity of benzene. *Crit. Rev. Toxicol.* 27: 399–427.

Kalf, G. S., M. J. Schlosser, J. F. Renz, and S. T. Pirozzi. 1989. Prevention of benzene-induced myeltoxicity by nonsteroidal anti-inflammatory drugs. *Environ. Health Perspect.* 82: 57–64.

Kalf, G. F., J. F. Renz, and R. Niculescu. 1996. *p*-Benzoquinone, a reactive metabolite of benzene, prevents the processing of pre-interleukins-1α and -1β to active cytokines by inhibition of the processing enzymes, calpain, and interleukin-1β converting enzyme. *Environ. Health Perspect.* 104: 1251–1256.

Keller, K. A., and C. A. Snyder. 1986. Mice exposed in utero to low concentrations of benzene exhibit enduring changes in their colony forming hematopoietic cells. *Toxicology.* 42: 171–181.

Keller, K. A., and C. A. Snyder. 1988. Mice exposed in utero to 20 ppm benzene exhibit altered numbers of recongizable hematopoietic cells up to seven weeks after exposure. *Fundam. Appl. Toxicol.* 10: 224–232.

Kipen, H. M., R. P. Cody, K. S. Crump, B. Allen, and B. D. Goldstein. 1988. Hematologic effects of benzene: A thirty-five year longitudinal study of rubber workers. *Toxicol. Ind. Health.* 4: 411–430.

Kipen, H. M., R. P. Cody, and B. D. Goldstein. 1989a. Use of longitudinal analysis of peripheral blood counts to validate historical reconstruction of benzene exposure. *Environ. Health Perspect.* 82: 199–206.

Kipen, H. M., R. P. Cody, and B. D. Goldstein. 1989b. Letters to the editor. *Toxicol. Ind. Health.* 5: 1156–1158.

Kirley, T. A., B. D. Goldstein, W. M. Maniara, and G. Witz. 1989. Metabolism of *trans, trans*-muconaldehyde, a microsomal hematotoxic metabolite of benzene by purified yeast aldehyde dehydrogenase and a mouse liver soluable fraction. *Toxicol. Appl. Pharmacol.* 100: 360–367.

Kolachana, P., V. V. Subrahmanyam, K. B. Meyer, L. Zhang, and M. T. Smith. 1993. Benzene and its phenolic metabolites produce oxidative DNA damage in HL-60 cells in vitro and in the bone marrow in vivo. *Cancer Res.* 53: 1023–1026.

Koop, D. R., C. L. Laethem, and G. G. Schnier. 1989. Identification of ethanol-inducible P450 isozyme 3a (P450IIE1) as a benzene and phenol hydroxylase. *Toxicol. Appl. Pharmacol.* 98: 278–288.

Kreyon, E. M., R. E. Kraichely, K. T. Hudson, and M. A. Medinsky. 1996. Differences in rates of benzene metabolism correlate with observed genotoxicity. *Toxicol. Appl. Pharmacol.* 136: 49–56.

Kukielka E., and A. I. Cederbaum. 1995. Increased oxidation of ethylene glycol to formaldehyde by microsomes after ethanol treatment: Role of oxygen radicals and cytochrome P450. *Tox. Lett.* 78: 9–15.

Lagorio, S., C. Tagesson, F. Forastiere, I. Iavarone, O. Axelson, and A. Carere. 1994. Exposure to benzene and urinary concentrations of 8-hydroxydeoxy-guanosine, a biological marker of oxidative damage to DNA. *Occup. Environ. Med.* 51: 739–743.

Laskin, D. L., L. MacEachern, and R. Synder. 1989. Activation of bone marrow phagocytes following benzene treatment of mice. *Environ. Health Perspect.* 82: 75–79.

Laskin, J. D., N. R. Rao, C. J. Punjabi, D. L. Laskin, and R. Snyder. 1995. Distinct actions of benzene and its metabolites on nitric oxide production by bone marrow leukocytes. *J. Leukocyte Biol.* 57: 422–426.

Latriano, A. Zaccaria, B. D. Goldstein, and G. Witz. 1985. Muconaldehyde formation from ^{14}C-benzene in a hydroxyl radical generating system. *J. Free Radical Med. Biol.* 1: 363–371.

Latriano, L., A. Zaccaria, B. D. Goldstein, and G. Witz. 1986. Formation of muconaldehyde, an open-ring metbolite of benzene in mouse liver microsomes: A novel pathway for toxic metabolites. *Proc. Natl. Acad. Sci.* 83: 8356–8360.

Lawyrk, N., and C. Weisel. 1996. Concentrations of volatile organic compounds in the passenger compartments of automobiles. *Environ. Sci. Tech.* 30: 810–816.

Layton, D. M., and G. J. Mufti. 1987. The myelodysplastic syndromes. *Br. Med. J.* 295: 227–228.

Lee, S.S.T., J. T. M. Buters, T. Pineau, P. Fernandez-Salquero, and F. J. Gonzalez. 1996. Role of CYP2E1 in the hepatotoxicity of acetaminophen. *J. Biol. Chem.* 15: 3012–3022.

Leo, A., C. Hansch, and D. Elkins. 1971. Partition coefficients and their uses. *Chem. Rev.* 71: 569.

Loden, M. 1986. The in vitro permeability of human skin to benzene, ethylene glycol, formaldehyde, and *n*-hexane. *Acta. Pharmacol. Toxicol.* 58: 382–389.

Loeff, I., and G. Stein. 1959. Aromatic ring opening in the presence of oxygen in irradiated solutions. *Nature* 184: 901.

Longacre, L. S., J. J. Kocsis, and R. Snyder. 1981. Influence of strain differences in mice on the metabolism and toxcity of benzene. *Toxicol. Appl. Pharmacol.* 60: 398–409.

Lovern, M. R., G. L. Kedderis, M. Turner, and P. M. Schlosser. 1997. Evidence for benzene oxide in vitro and in vivo. *Fund. Appl. Toxicol. Suppl. : The Toxicologist* 36: 164.

Lunte, S. M., and P. T. Kissinger. 1983. Detection and identification of sylfhydryl conjugates of *p*-benzoquinone in microsomal incubations of benzene and phenol. *Chem.-Biol. Interact.* 47: 195–212.

Maltoni, C., B. Conti, and G. Cotti. 1983. Benzene: A multipotential carcinogen. Results of long-term bioassays performed at the Bologna Institute of Oncology. *Am. J. Ind. Med.* 4: 589–630.

McDonald, T. A., K. Yeowell-O'Connell, and S. M. Rappaport. 1994. Comparison of protein adducts of benzene oxide and benzoquinone in the blood and bone marrow of rats and mice exposed to [^{14}C / ^{13}C$_6$] benzene. *Cancer Res.* 54: 4907–4914.

Medeiros, A. M., M. G. Bird, and G. Witz. 1997. Potential biomarkers of benzene exposure. *J. Toxicol. Environ. Health.* 51: 519–539.

Mehlman, M. A., ed. 1989. *Benzene: Occupational and Scientific Hazards — Scientific Update, Advances in Modern Environmental Toxicology*, vol. 16. Princeton: Princeton Scientific Publishing.

Moran, J. L., D. Siegel, X. -M. Sun, and D. Ross. 1996. Induction of apoptosis by benzene metabolites in HL-60 and CD34[+] human bone marrow progenitor cells. *Mol. Pharmacol.* 50: 610–615.

National Academy of Sciences. 1983. *Risk Assessment in the Federal Government: Managing the Process.* Washington, DC: National Academy Press.

National Academy of Sciences. 1989. *Biomarkers in Reproductive Toxicology.* Washington, DC: National Academy Press.

Nencki, M., and P. Giacosa. 1880. Uber die Oxydation der Aromatischen Wasserstoffe in Turkoyser. *Z. Physiol Chem.* 4: 325.

Norpoth, K., W. Stucker, E. Krewet, and G. Muller. 1988. Biomonitoring of benzene exposure by trace analysis of phenylguanine. *Int. Arch. Occup. Environ. Health.* 60: 163–168.

Ong, C. N., P. W. Kok, B. L. Lee, C. Y. Shi, H. Y. Ong, K. S. Chia, C. S. Lee, and X. W. Luo. 1995. Evaluation of biomarkers for occupational exposure to benzene. *Occup. Environ. Med.* 52: 528–533.

Parke, D. V., and R. T. Williams. 1953. Studies in detoxification. 44. The metabolism of benzene containing ^{14}C-benzene. *Biochem. J.* 54: 231–238.

Paxton, M. B., V. M. Chinchilli, S. M. Brett, and J. V. Rodricks. 1994. Leukemia risk associated with benzene exposure in the pliofilm cohort: I. Mortality update and exposure distribution. *Risk Anal.* 14: 147–154.

Paxton, M. B., V. M. Chinchilli, S. M. Brett, and J. V. Rodricks. 1994. Leukemia risk associated with benzene exposure in the pliofilm cohort: II. Risk estimates. *Risk Anal.* 14: 155–161.

Pellack-Walker, P., and J. L. Blumer. 1986. DNA damage in L5178YS cells following exposure to benzene metabolites. *Mol. Pharmacol.* 30: 42–47.

Porteous, J. W., and R. T. Williams. 1953. Studies in detoxication 49. The metabolism of phenol, catechol, quinol and hydroxyquinol from the ethereal sulfate fraction of the urine of rabbits receiving benzene orally. *Biochem. J.* 44: 56–61.

Rao, G. S. 1996. Glutathionyl hydroquinone: a potent prooxidant and a possible toxic metabolite of benzene. *Toxicol.* 106: 49–54.

Rickert, D. E., T. S. Baker, J. S. Bus, C. S. Barrow, and R. D. Irons. 1979. Benzene disposition in the rat after exposure by inhalation. *Toxicol. Appl. Pharmacol.* 49: 417–423.

Rinsky, R. A., R. J. Young, and A. B. Smith. 1981. Leukemia in benzene workers. *Am. J. Ind. Med.* 2: 217–245.

Rinsky, R. A., A. B. Smith, R. Hornung, T. G. Filloon, R. J. Young, A. K. Okun, and P. J. Landrigan. 1987. Benzene and leukemia: An epidemiological risk assessment. *N. Engl. J. Med.* 316: 1044–1050.

Rosenthal, G. J., and C. A. Snyder. 1985. Modulation of the immune response to *Listeria monocytogenes* by benzene inhalation. *Toxicol. Appl. Pharmacol.* 80: 502–510.

Rosenthal, G. J., and C. A. Snyder. 1987. Inhaled benzene reduces aspects of cell-mediated tumor surveillance in mice. *Toxicol. Appl. Pharmacol.* 88: 35–43.

Ross, D. 1996. Metabolic basis of benzene toxicity. *Eur. J. Haematol.* 57: 111–118.

Rothman, N., M. T. Smith, R. B. Hayes et al. 1997. Benzene poisoning, a risk factor for hematological malignancy, is associated with the NQO1 [609]$C \to T$ mutation and rapid fractional excretion of chlorzoxazone. *Cancer Res.* 57: 2839–2842.

Rothman, N., R. Haas, R. B. Hayes, G.-L. Li, J. Wiemels, S. Campleman, P. J. E. Quintana, L.-J. Xi, M. Dosemeci, N. Titenko-Holland, K. B. Meyer, W. Lu, L. P. Zhang, W. Bechtold, Y.-Z. Wang, P. Kolachana, S.-N. Yin, W. Blot, and M. T. Smith. 1995. Benzene induces gene-duplicating but not gene-inactivating mutations at the glycophorin A locus in exposed humans. *Proc. Natl. Acad. Sci.* 92: 4069–4073.

Rothman, N., G.-L. Li, M. Dosemeci, W. Bechtold, G. E. Marti, Y.-Z. Wang, M. Linet, L.-Q. Xi, W. Lu, M. T. Smith, N. Titenko-Holland, L.-P. Zhang, W. Blot, S.-N. Yin, and R. B. Hayes. 1996. Hematotoxicity among Chinese workers heavily exposed to benzene. *Amer. J. Indust. Med.* 29: 236–246.

Rozen, M. G., and C. A. Snyder. 1987. Inhaled benzene reduces aspects of cell-mediated tumor surveillance in mice. *Toxicol. Appl. Pharmacol.* 88: 35–43.

Sabourin, P. J., B. T. Chen, G. Lucier, L. S. Birnbaum, E. Fisher, and R. F. Henderson. 1987. Effect of dose on the absorption and excretion of [^{14}C] benzene administered orally or by inhalation in rats and mice. *Toxicol. Appl. Pharmacol.* 87: 325–336.

Sabourin, P. J., W. E. Bechtold, L. S. Birnbaum, G. Lucier, and R. F. Henderson. 1988a. Differences in the metabolism and disposition of inhaled [^{3}H] benzene by F344/N rats and B6C3F$_1$ mice. *Toxicol. Appl. Pharmacol.* 94: 128–140.

Sabourin, P. J., W. E. Bechtold, and R. F. Henderson. 1988b. A high pressure liquid chromatographic method for the separation and quantitation of water-soluable radiolabeled benzene metabolites. *Anal. Biochem.* 170: 316–327.

Sabourin, P. J., W. E. Bechtold, W. C. Griffith, L. S. Birnbaum, G. Lucier, and R. F. Henderson. 1989. effect of exposure concentration, exposure rate, and route of administration on metabolism of benzene by F344 rats and B6C3F$_1$ mice. *Toxicol. Appl. Pharmacol.* 99: 421–444.

Sabourin, P. J., J. D. Sun, J. T. MacGregor, C. M. Wehr, C. G. Birnbaum, G. Lucier, and R. F. Henderson. 1990. Effect of repeated benzene inhalation exposures on benzene metabolism, binding to hemoglobin, and induction of micronuclei. *Toxicol. Appl. Pharmacol.* 103: 452–462.

Sadler, A., V. V. Subrahmanyam, and D. Ross. 1988. Oxidation of catechol by horseradish peroxidase and human leukocyte peroxidase: Reactions of *o*-benzoquinone and *o*-benzosemiquinone. *Toxicol. Appl. Pharmacol.* 93: 62–71.

Sammett, D., E. W. Lee, J. J. Kocsis, and R. Sunder. 1979. Partial hepatectomy reduces both metabolism and toxicity of benzene. *J. Toxicol. Environ. Health.* 5: 785–792.

Sato, A., and T. Nakajima. 1979. Partition coefficents of some aromatic hydrocarbons and ketones in water, blood and oil. *Toxicol. Appl. Pharmacol.* 48: 49.

Savitz, D., and K. W. Andrews. 1997. Review of epidemiologic evidence on benzene and lymphatic and hematopoietic cancers. *Am. J. Ind. Med.* 31: 287–295.

Sawahata, T., and R. A. Neal. 1982. Horseradish peroxidate-mediated oxidation of phenol. *Biochem. Biophys. Res. Commun.* 109: 988–994.

Sawahata, T., D. E. Rickert, and W. F. Greenlee. 1985. Metabolism of benzene and its metabolites in bone marrow. In *Toxicology of the Blood and Bone Marrow,* ed. R. Irons, pp. 141–148. New York: Raven Press.

Schnatter, A. R., M. J. Nicolich, and M. G. Bird. 1996. Determination of Leukemogenic Benzene Exposure Concentrations: Refined Analyses for the Pliofilm Cohort. *Risk Anal.* 16: 833–840.

Schoenfeld, H. A., O. Mirochnitchenko, B. D. Goldstein, and G. Witz. 1997. Effects of *trans, trans*-muconaldehyde, a hematotoxic benzene metabolite, or DNA-protein crosslink levels and on apoptosis in mouse bone marrow cells. *Fundam. Appl. Toxicol., Suppl. The Toxicologist.* 31: 163.

Schoenfeld, H. A., R. Radbourne, B. D. Goldstein, and G. Witz. 1996. Mechanistic studies on benzene toxicity: formation of DNA-protein crosslinks induced by benzene in mice and muconaldehyde in HL-60 cells. *Fundam. Appl. Toxicol. Suppl. The Toxicologist.* 30: 232.

Schrenk, D. M. Ingelman-Sundberg, and K. W. Bock. 1992. Influence of P-4502E1 induction on benzene metabolism in rat hepatocytes and on biliary metabolite excretion. *Drug Metab. Disp.* 20: 137–141.

Schultzen, O., and B. Naunyn 1867. Uber das Verhalten des Kohlenwasserstoffes im Organisms. *Arc. Anat. Physiol.* 1: 349.

Schwartz, C. S., R. Snyder, and G. F. Kalf. 1985. The inhibition of mitochongrial DNA replication in vitro by the metabolites of benzene hydroquinone and *p*-benzoqinone. *Chem. -Biol. Interact.* 53: 327–350.

Seaton, M. J., P. M. Schlosser, J. A. Bond, and M. A. Medinsky. 1994. Benzene metabolism by human liver microsomes in relation to cytochrome P450 2E1 activity. *Carcinogenesis.* 15: 1799–1806.

Smart, R. C., and V. G. Zannoni. 1985. DT-diaphorase and peroxidase influence the covalent binding of metabolites of pehnol, the major metabolite of benzene. *Mol. Pharmacol.* 26: 105–111.

Smith, M. A., L. Rubinstein, and R. S. Ungerleider. 1994. Therapy-related acute myeloid leukemia following treatment with epipodophyllotoxins: estimating the risks. *Med. Pediat. Oncology.* 23: 86–98.

Smith, M. T., J. W. Yager, K. L. Steinmetz, and D. A. Eastmond. 1989. Peroxidase-dependent metabolism of benzene's phenolic metabolites and its potential role in benzene toxicity and carcinogenicity. *Environ. Health Perspect.* 82: 23–29.

Smith, M. T. 1996. The mechanism of benzene-induced leukemia: a hypothesis and speculations on the causes of leukemia. *Environ. Health Perspect.* 104: 1219–125.

Snyder, C. A. 1987. Benzene. In: *Ethel Browning's Toxicity and Metabolism of Industrial Solvents: Hydrocarbons,* 2nd ed., vol. 1, ed. R. Snyder, pp. 3–27. Amsterdam: Elsevier.

Snyder, C. A., B. D. Goldstein, and A. Sellakumar. 1978. Heamtotoxicity of inhaled benzene to Sprague-Dawley rats and AKR mice at 300 ppm. *J. Toxicol. Environ. Health.* 4: 605–618.

Snyder, C. A., B. D. Goldstein, A. R. Sellakumar, I. Bromberg, S. Laskin, and R. E. Alberts. 1980. The inhalation toxicology of benzene: Incidence of hematopoietic neoplasms and hematotoxicity in ARK/J and C57BL/6J mice. *Toxicol. Appl. Pharmacol.* 54: 323–331.

Snyder, R. and J. J. Kocsis. 1975. Current concepts of chronic benzene toxicity. *CRC Crit. Rev. Toxicol.* 3: 265–288.

Snyder, R., S. L. Longacre, C. M. Witmer, and J. J. Kocsis. 1981. Biochemical toxicity of benzene. In *Reviews in Biochemical Toxicology,* vol. 3, eds. E. Hodgson, J. R. Bend, and R. M. Philpot, pp. 123–153. New York: Elsevier.

Snyder, R., and G. Kalf. 1994. A perspective on benzene leukemogenesis. *Crit. Rev. Toxicol.* 24: 177–209.

Snyder, R., G. Witz, and B. D. Goldstein. 1993. The Toxicology of benzene. *Environ. Health Perspect.* 100: 293–306.

Snyder, R. 1983. The benzene problem in historical perspective. *Fundam. Appl. Toxicol.* 4: 692.

Subrahmanyam, V. V., and P. J. O'Brien. 1985. Pehol oxidation product(s) formed by a peroxidase reaction that bind to DNA. *Xenobiotica.* 15: 873–885.

Subrahmanyam, V. V., D. Ross, D. A. Eastmond, and M. T. Smith. 1991. Potential role of free radicals in benzene-induced myelotoxicity and leukemia. *Free Rad. Biol. Med.* 11: 495–515.

Tavassoli, M., and A. Friedenstein. 1983. Hemapoietic stromal microenvironment. *Am. J. Hematol.* 14: 195–203.

Thibodeaux, L. J. 1981. Estimating the air emissions of chemicals from hazardous waste landfills. *J. Hazard Mat.* 4: 235–244.

Tunek, A., K. L. Platt, M. Przybylski, and F. Oesch. 1980. Multistep metabolic activation of benzene. Effect of superoxide dismutase on covalent binding to mcirosomal macromolecules and identification of gluthathione conjugates using high pressure liquid chromatography and field desorption mass spectrometry. *Chem.-Biol. Interact.* 33: 1.

U. S. HEW. 1989. *Environmental Health Perspectives: Symposium on Benzene Metabolism, Toxicity and Carcinogenesis,* vol 82. Research Triangle Park, NC: National Institute of Environmental Health Sciences.

Valentine, J. L., S. S. -T. Lee, M. J. Seaton, B. Asgharian, G. Farris, J. C. Corton, F. J. Gonzalez, and M. A. Medinsky. 1996. Reduction of benzene metabolism and toxicity in mice that lack CYP2E1 expression. *Toxicol. Appl. Pharmacol.* 141: 205–213.

Velez, R., V. Beral, and J. Cuzick. 1982. Increasing the trends of multiple myeloma mortality in England and Wales; 1950–1979: Are the changes real? *J. Natl. Cancer Inst.* 69: 387–392.

Wallace, L. A., 1987. *The Total Exposure Assessment Methodology (TEAM) Study: Summary and Analysis: Vol. I.* EPA-600-6-87-002a. Washington, DC: U. S. EPA, Office of Acid Deposition, Environmental Monitoring and Quality Assurance.

Wallace, L. A. and E. D. Pellizzari. 1986. Personal air exposures and breath concentrations of benzene and other volatile hydrocarbons for smokers and nonsmokers. *Toxicol. Lett.* 35: 113–116.

Wallace, L. A., E. D. Pellizzari, T. D. Harwell, C. M. Sparacino, L. S. Sheldon, and H. Zelon. 1985. Personal exposures, indoor-outdoor relationships, and breath levels of toxic air pollutants measured for 355 persons in New Jersey. *Atoms. Environ.* 19: 1651–1661.

Walling, C., and R. A. Johnson. 1975. Fenton's reagent. V. Hydroxylation and side chain cleavage of aromatics. *J. Am. Chem. Soc.* 97: 363–367.

Ward, E., R. Hornung, J. Morris, R. Rinsky, D. Wild, W. Halperin, and W. Guthrie. 1996. Risk of low red or white blood cell count related to estimated benzene exposure in a rubberworker Cohort (1940–1975). *Am. J. Ind. Med.* 29: 247–257.

Weisel, C., R. Yu, A. Roy, and P. Georgopoulos. 1996. Biomarkers of environmental benzene exposure. *Environ. Health Perspect.* 104 (suppl. 5): 1141–1146.

WHO. 1987. *Air Quality Guideline for Europe.* Copenhagen: WHO Regional Publications.

Wiedra, D., R. D. Irons, and W. F. Greenlee. 1981. Immunotoxicity in C57BL/6 mice exposed to benzene and Aroclor 1254. *Toxicol. Appl. Pharmacol.* 60: 410–417.

Witz, G., G. S. Rao, and B. D. Goldstein. 1985. Short term toxicity of *trans, trans*-muconaldehyde. *Toxicol. Appl. Pharmacol.* 80: 511–516.

Witz, G., W. M. Maniara, V. J. Mylavarapu, and B. D. Goldstein. 1990. Comparative metabolism of benzene and *trans, trans*-muconaldehyde to *trans, trans*-muconic acid in DBA/2N and C57BL/6 mice. *Biochem. Pharmacol.* 40: 1275–1280.

Witz, G., Z. Zhang, and B. D. Goldstein. 1996. Reactive ring-opened aldehyde metabolites in benzene hematotoxicity. *Environ. Health Perspect.* 104: 1195–1199.

Wu, D., and A. I. Cederbaum. 1994. Characterization of pyrazole and 4-methylpyrazole induction of cytochrome P4502E1 in rat kidney. *J. Pharm. Exp. Ther.* 270: 407–413.

Yamanaka, K., H. Hayashi, K. Kato, A. Hasegawa, and S. Okada. 1995. Involvement of preferential formation of apurinic/apyrimidinic sites in dimethylarsenic-induced DNA strand breaks and DNA-protein crosslinks in cultured alveolar epithelial cells. *Biochem. Biophys. Res. Commun.* 207: 244–249.

Yin, S. N., G.-L. Li, F.-D. Tain, Z.-I. Fu, C. Jin, Y.-J. Chen, S.-J. Luo, P.-Z. Ye, J.-Z. Zhang, G.-C. Wang, X.-C. Zhang, H.-N. Wu, and Q.-C. Zhong. 1987a. Luekmia in benzene workers: A retrospective cohort study. *Br. J. Ind. Med.* 44: 124–128.

Yardley-Jones, A., D. Anderson, P. C. Jenkinson, D. P. Lovell, S. D. Blowers, and M. J. Davies. 1988. Genotoxic effects in peripheral blood and urine of workers exposed to low level benzene. *Br. J. Ind. Med.* 45: 694–700.

Yin, S.-N., R. B. Hayes, M. S. Linet, G.-L. Li, M. Dosemeci, L. B. Travis, C.-Y. Li, Z.-N. Zhang, D.-G. Li, W.-H. Chow, S. Wacholder, Y.-Z. Wang, Z.-L. Jiang, T.-R. Dai, W.-Y. Zhang, X.-J. Chao, P.-Z. Ye, Q.-R. Kou, X.-C. Zhang, X.-F. Lin, J.-F. Meng, C.-Y. Ding, J.-S. Zho, and W. J. Blot. 1996. A cohort study of cancer among benzene-exposed workers in China: Overall results. *Am. J. Ind. Med.* 29: 227–235.

Young, N. 1989. Benzene and lymphoma. *Am. J. Ind. Med.* 15: 495–498.

Yu, R., and C. Weisel. 1996. Measurement of Benzene in Human Breath Associated with an Environmental Exposure. *J. Expos. Anal. Environ. Epid.* 6: 261–277.

Zhang, Z., S. A. Kline, T. A. Kirley, B. D. Goldstein, and G. Witz. 1993. Pathways of *trans-trans*-muconaldehyde metabolism in mouse liver cytosol: Reversibility of monoreductive metabolism and formation of end products. *Arch. Toxicol.* 67: 461–467.

Zhang, Z., Q. Xiang, H. Glatt, K. I. Platt, B. D. Goldstein, and G. Witz. 1995a. Studies on pathways of ring opening of benzene in a Fenton system. *Free Rad. Biol. Med.* 18: 411–419.

Zhang, Z., B. D. Goldstein, and G. Witz. 1995b. Iron-stimulated ring-opening of benzene in a mouse liver microsomal system. Mechanistic studies and formation of a new metabolite. *Biochem. Pharmacol.* 50: 1607–1617.

Zhang, Z., F. Schafer, H. Schoenfeld, K. Cooper, R. Snyder, B. D. Goldstein, and G. Witz. 1995c. The hematotoxic effects of 6-hydroxy-*trans, trans*-2, 4-hexadienal, a reactive metabolite of *trans, trans*-muconaldehyde, in CD-1 mice. *Toxicol. Appl. Pharmacol.* 132: 213–219.

5 Carbon Monoxide

MICHAEL T. KLEINMAN, Ph.D.

Carbon monoxide (CO) is emitted from virtually all sources of incomplete combustion, including internal combustion engines (e.g., automobiles, trucks, and gasoline-fueled small engines); fires, both natural and man-made; improperly adjusted gas and oil appliances (e.g., space heaters, water heaters, stoves, and ovens); and tobacco smoking (Darbool et al., 1997; Clifford et al., 1997; Hampson and Norkool, 1992). Because of the large number and the ubiquity of CO sources with significant source strengths (e.g., tobacco smoke contains about 1% CO by volume, or 10,000 ppm CO), ambient CO concentrations show large temporal and spatial variations. The exposure of individuals to CO is therefore quite variable, depending on the types of activities in which a person is engaged and how long they are engaged in those activities (time-activity profiles), where the activity takes place (microenvironments: e.g., indoors, at a shopping mall; outdoors, in a vehicle; at work or school; in a parking garage; or even in a skating rink), (Viala, 1994; Levesque et al., 1990; Dor et al., 1995; Koushki et al., 1992) and the proximity to CO sources. Various methods have been used to document exposures, including the use of data from fixed site ambient monitors, the use of microenvironmental exposure assessment models, personal exposure monitoring methods, and biological monitoring methods. Controls on motor vehicle exhaust and the use of catalytic converters on vehicles sold in the United States have been very effective in reducing ambient CO emissions (Yu, 1996) and commuter exposures (Flachsbart, 1995).

CO EXPOSURE AND DOSIMETRY

CO competes with oxygen (O_2) for binding sites on the heme portion of the hemoglobin (Hb) molecules in red blood cells to form carboxyhemoglobin (COHb). The affinity of Hb for CO is about 240 to 250 times that for O_2 (Roughton, 1970). The formation of COHb by the binding of CO to circulating Hb reduces the oxygen-carrying capacity of blood. In addition, binding of CO to one of the four hemoglobin binding sites increases the O_2 affinity of the remaining binding sites, thus interfering with the release of O_2 at the tissue level. When O_2 content of blood (mL O_2 / mL blood) is plotted against O_2 partial pressure (mm Hg) in blood, the increased O_2 affinity is seen as the so-called leftward shift in the curve for blood partially loaded with CO (Longo, 1976). CO-induced tissue hypoxia is therefore a joint effect of the reduction in O_2 carrying capacity and the reduction of O_2 release at the tissue level. The brain and heart, under normal conditions, utilize larger fractions of the arterially delivered O_2 (about 75%) than do peripheral tissues and other organs (Ayers et al., 1970) and are therefore the most sensitive targets for hypoxic effects

Environmental Toxicants: Human Exposures and Their Health Effects, 2/e. Edited by Morton Lippmann.
ISBN: 0-471-29298-2 © 2000 John Wiley & Sons, Inc.

following CO exposures. The potential for adverse health effects is increased under conditions of stress, such as exercise, which increases O_2 demands at the tissue level to sustain metabolism.

The measure of biological dose that relates best to observed biological responses and deleterious health effects is the concentration of COHb expressed as a percentage of available, active Hb, thus representing the percent of potential saturation of Hb. COHb can be measured directly in blood or estimated from the CO content of expired breath (Lambert et al., 1988; Lee et al., 1994). It is currently accepted that the most accurate and reliable method for measuring COHb concentration is by gas chromatographic analysis (Dahms and Horvath, 1974; Vreman et al., 1984; Guillot, 1981). Spectrophotometric measures and instruments have been widely used in both clinical and occupational health settings. However, some instruments may have limited accuracy at COHb concentrations below 5% (Dahms and Horvath, 1974; and Allred et al., 1989). They can be very useful if calibrated properly, and if measurements are verified by a "gold standard," such as gas chromatography (Dahms and Horvath, 1974). When direct measurements cannot be made, it is possible to estimate COHb from ambient air CO concentrations (Ott et al., 1988), indoor air CO concentrations and personal CO monitoring data (Wallace and Ott, 1982) using pharmacokinetic and other models (Wallace and Ott, 1982; Forbes et al., 1945; Pace et al., 1946; Goldsmith et al., 1963; Coburn et al., 1965) that link the concentration of inhaled CO, breathing rate and volume, blood volume, metabolic production of endogenous CO, and rate of removal of CO. The Coburn-Forster-Kane (CFK) model (Coburn et al., 1965) has been widely used for this purpose. But perhaps more important, in the process of establishing ambient air quality guidelines, the CFK model has been the basis for associating ambient and workplace air CO concentrations with concentrations of COHb could be hazardous for sensitive exposed individuals. The CFK model has been experimentally verified for exposures at 25 to 5000 ppm, during rest and exercise (Peterson and Stewart, 1975; Tikuisis et al., 1987). Sensitivity analyses of CFK can be used to identify those model input parameters for which errors in the parameter values used will have the greatest errors in predicted COHb concentrations (McCartney, 1990). Validation of the CFK model under well-controlled conditions at environmental concentrations with larger numbers of subjects would be useful. However, Kleinman and associates (Kleinman et al., 1998) used the CFK model to successfully predict blood COHb concentrations in 17 human volunteers exposed to 100 ppm CO, suggesting that the CFK model is valid under such circumstances.

MECHANISMS OF CO TOXICITY

CO affects health indirectly by interfering with the transport of oxygen to tissues (especially the heart and other muscles and brain tissue). The resulting impairment of O_2 delivery cause tissue hypoxia and interferes with cellular respiration. Direct intracellular uptake of CO could permit interactions with hemoproteins such as myoglobin, cytochrome oxidase, and cytochrome P-450 and therefore interfere with electron transport processes and energy production at the cellular level. Thus, in addition to observed physiological effects and cardiovascular effects, CO can modify electron transport in nerve cells resulting in behavioral, neurological, and developmental toxicological consequences.

The possible role of CO as an etiologic factor in development of atherosclerosis and as a causative factor in cardiac arrhythmias, sudden cardiac arrest, and myocardial infarctions is an area of active research activity. The hemodynamic responses to CO have been reviewed by Penney (1988). Chronic CO exposures, usually at COHb concentrations greater than 10%, produce several changes. These may be adaptive responses to induced hypoxia, such as increases in numbers of red blood cells (polycythemia), increased blood volume, and increased heart size (cardiomegaly). In addition heart rate, stroke volume, and systolic blood pressure may be increased. Some of these effects have been seen in smokers. Other environmental factors, such as effects of other pollutants (both from conventional air pollution sources and from environmental tobacco smoke), interactions with drugs and medications, health and related factors (e.g., cardiovascular and respiratory diseases, anemia, or pregnancy), and exposures at high altitude are possible risk modifiers for the health effects of CO.

Exposures to high concentrations of CO due, for example, to fires and emissions from faulty appliances, result in nearly 4000 deaths per year and in illness sufficient to cause upward of 10,000 individuals to seek medical attention or to miss one or more days of work in the United States (U.S. Centers for Disease Control, 1982). The available data may substantially underestimate the total numbers of such cases, especially those related to unsuspected CO exposure in the home. Because some CO-related symptoms are similar to those of flu (headache and dizziness) and possibly to those of certain seizure disorders (Kirkpatrick, 1987; Heckerling et al., 1987, 1988), there is a potential that many cases may be misdiagnosed. Blood tests for COHb concentrations, or breath analyses for CO improve the accuracy of the diagnoses. This chapter will, however, deal for the most part with ambient environmental exposures and will focus on the recent health-based literature for examination of effects at COHb concentrations of 5% and below.

POPULATIONS AT RISK OF HEALTH EFFECTS DUE TO CO EXPOSURE

People with Cardiovascular Diseases

Ischemic heart disease, or coronary artery disease, which is a leading cause of disability and death in industrialized nations (Levy and Feinleib, 1984), is a clinical disorder of the heart resulting from an imbalance between oxygen demand of myocardial tissue and oxygen delivery via the bloodstream. The ability of the heart to adjust to increases in myocardial O_2 demands resulting from increased activity, or to reductions in O_2 delivery by arterial blood due, for example, to COHb or reduced partial pressure in O_2 in inspired air, by increasing O_2 extraction, is limited because the extraction rate in myocardial tissue is already high. Normally coronary circulation responds to such increased O_2 demands by increasing blood flow. Coronary artery disease, in which the coronary artery is occluded by lipid deposits, can impede augmentation of local coronary blood flow in response to increased O_2 demands, forcing the myocardium to extract more O_2 (resulting in reduced coronary venous and tissue O_2 tensions), which can lead to myocardial ischemia. Severe myocardial ischemia can lead to myocardial infarction (heart attack) and to abnormal cardiac rhythms, or arrhythmias. The association of acute CO exposure to heart attacks has been described (Mariusnunez, 1990).

Individuals with obstructed peripheral arteries (e.g., in their legs) may experience severe pain during relatively mild activities, such as walking (intermittent claudication). CO exposure could potentially exacerbate the imbalance between O_2 demand by exercising peripheral muscular tissue and O_2 delivery.

People with Anemia and Other Blood Disorders

Individuals with reduced blood hemoglobin concentrations, or with abnormal hemoglobin, will have reduced O_2 carrying capacity in blood. In addition disease processes that result in increased destruction of red blood cells (hemolysis) and accelerated breakdown of hemoproteins accelerate endogenous production of CO (Berk et al., 1974; Solanki et al.,

1988), resulting in higher COHb concentrations than in normal individuals. For example, patients with hemolytic anemia have COHb concentrations two to three times those seen in normal individuals (Coburn et al., 1966).

People with Chronic Lung Disease

Chronic lung diseases such as chronic bronchitis, emphysema, and chronic obstructive pulmonary disease (COPD) are characterized by impairment of the lung's ability to transfer O_2 to the bloodstream because diseased regions of the lung are poorly ventilated and blood circulating through these regions will therefore receive less O_2 (so-called ventilation-perfusion mismatch) (West, 1987). Exertional stress often produces a perception of difficulty in breathing, or breathlessness (dyspnea) in these individuals; although exercise increases ventilatory drive, they have a limited ventilatory capacity with which to respond (Sue et al., 1988). Reduction of blood O_2 delivery capacity due to formation of COHb could exacerbate symptoms and further reduce exercise tolerance in these individuals.

Potential Risks for Pregnant Women, Fetuses, and Newborn Children

A CO-induced leftward shift in the O_2Hb saturation curve may be significant for fetuses because the O_2 tension in their arterial blood is low (20 to 30 mm Hg) compared to adult values (100 mm Hg) and because fetal Hb has a higher O_2 affinity than does maternal Hb (Longo, 1976). Fortunately fetal blood has higher Hb concentrations than does maternal blood (Hellman and Pritchard, 1971). In pregnant women O_2 consumption is increased 15% to 25%, and hemoglobin concentration may be simultaneously reduced, lowering the O_2 carrying capacity of their blood (Pernoll et al., 1975).

REGULATORY BACKGROUND

The National Ambient Air Quality Standards (NAAQS) for CO were promulgated by the Environmental Protection Agency (EPA) in 1971 at levels of 9 ppm ($10 \, mg / m^3$) for an 8 h average and 35 ppm ($40 \, mg / m^3$) for a 1 h average, not to be exceeded more than once per year. (Primary and secondary standards were established at identical levels). The 1970 CO criteria document (National Air Pollution Control Administration, 1970) cited as the standard's scientific basis a study which indicated that subjects exposed to low levels of CO, resulting in COHb concentrations of 2% to 3% of saturation exhibited neurobehavioral effects (Beard and Wertheim, 1967). A reexamination of the scientific evidence, as reported in a revised CO criteria document (U.S. Environmental Protection Agency, 1979) issued in 1979, concluded that it was unlikely that significant, and repeatable, neurobehavioral effects occurred at COHb concentrations below 5%. Medical evidence, accumulated during the intervening years, however, indicated that aggravation of angina pectoris, and other symptoms of myocardial ischemia, occurred in men with chronic cardiovascular disease, exposed to low levels of CO resulting in COHb concentrations of about 2.7% (Aronow and Isbell, 1973; Aronow et al., 1972; Anderson et al., 1973). EPA proposed, in 1980, based in part on the above studies, to retain the 8 h 9 ppm primary standard level, to reduce the 1 h primary standard from 35 to 25 ppm, and to revoke the secondary CO standards (because no adverse welfare effects had been reported at near-ambient levels). Because of concerns regarding the validity of data on which the proposed reduction in the 1 h standard was based, EPA later decided to keep the 1 h standard at 35 ppm.

In 1984 EPA published an addendum to the 1979 CO criteria document that reevaluated the CO health effects data previously reviewed and took into account research that had been published in the interim (U.S. EPA, 1984). The document reviewed four effects associated with low-level CO exposure: cardiovascular, neurobehavioral, fibrinolytic, and perinatal. Dose–response data provided by controlled human studies allowed the following conclusions to be drawn:

1. *Cardiovascular effects.* Among those with chronic cardiovascular disease, a shortening of time to onset of angina was observed at COHb concentrations of 2.9% to 4.5%. A decrement in maximum aerobic capacity was observed in healthy adults at COHb concentrations at and above 5%. Patients with chronic lung disease demonstrated a decrease in walking distance when COHb concentrations were increased from 1.1–5.4% to 9.6–14/9%.

2. *Neurobehavioral effects.* Decrements in vigilance, visual perception, manual dexterity, and performance of complex sensorimotor tasks were observed at, and above, 5% COHb.

3. *Effects on fibrinolysis.* Although evidence existed linking CO exposure to fibrinolytic mechanisms, controlled human studies did not demonstrate consistent effects of carbon monoxide exposure on coagulation parameters.

4. *Perinatal effects.* While there were some epidemiological associations between CO exposure and perinatal effects, such as low birth weight, slowed postnatal development, and incidences of sudden infant death syndrome (SIDS), the available data were not sufficient to establish causal relationships.

In September 1985 the EPA issued a final notice that announced the retention of the existing 8 h 9 ppm and 1 h 35 ppm primary NAAQS for CO and the rescinding of the secondary NAAQS for CO.

The EPA completed the most recent CO criteria document in 1991, and this chapter reviews the health-based literature that has been published since the December 1991 criteria document Addendum (U.S. EPA, 1991) including controlled human clinical exposures and population based studies. There have also been inhalation studies using laboratory animal models. These studies have provided important insights into the possible mechanisms of toxic action of CO, in addition to those related to hypoxia, and illuminate effects not currently identified in human studies, or which might not be amenable to controlled human experimentation, such as perinatal and developmental effects. The existing NAAQS for CO were retained, and they form the current standards.

HEALTH EFFECTS OF CO

Population-Based Studies

Acute Exposures and Their Effects Most of the population-based studies in the literature relating to the health effects of CO in humans have been concerned with exposures to combustion and pyrolysis products from sources such as tobacco, fires, motor vehicle exhaust, home appliances fueled with wood (Pierson et al., 1989), gas, or kerosene, and small engines. The individuals in these studies are therefore exposed to variable, and usually unmeasured, concentrations of CO and also to high concentrations of other combustion products. Exposures to CO in occupational settings represent another substantial exposure classification, but such exposures are often accompanied by exposures to other contaminants as well.

Acute CO intoxication most commonly results in neurologic and / or myocardial injury, with approximately 10% of patients displaying delayed neurological sequelae (Thom and Keim, 1989). Parkinsonism, which can be viewed as an outcome of some neuropathological lesions, has been associated with exposures to certain neurotoxins, including CO (Bleeker, 1988). Necrosis of muscle tissue (myonecrosis) has been reported as an unusual sequelae to CO exposure (16–20 cases have been reported in the English-language literature) (Herman et al., 1988; Wolf, 1994). Some of the cases involve firefighters, and it is not clear that CO alone is a causal factor. Cyanide which is a frequent co-contaminant in fires has been suggested as a contributor to myonecrosis (Herman et al., 1989). Marius-Nunez (Marius-Nunez, 1990) reported a case of an individual who suffered an acute myocardial infarction (shown by ECG and serum enzyme findings) after an acute CO exposure. This case was of interest because the patient's medical profile was negative for coronary heart disease risk factors and because a coronary angiogram performed one week after admission failed to show coronary obstructive lesions. A similar case was reported by Ebisuno et al. (1986), and the circumstances of both cases suggest that contributing factors to the CO-induced reduction in oxygen supply to the myocardium might include induction of coronary artery spasm, inadequate myocardial perfusion, and a direct toxic effect on myocardial mitochondria. Leikin and Vogel (1986) reported that patients admitted to intensive care units with proven myocardial infarctions had higher COHb levels than a control group, but these differences could have been accounted for by smoking alone and a relationship to ambient urban CO could not be established.

Sokal and Kralkowska (1985) examined 39 cases of acute CO poisoning in Poland. The subjects were poisoned at home by emissions from household gas or coal stoves. The authors found that the duration of CO exposure and the degree of metabolic acidosis, indicated by lactate concentrations in the blood, were better predictors of the clinical severity of symptoms than the COHb concentration in blood at the time of admission to the hospital. The importance of exposure duration has been suggested in earlier evaluations of CO toxicity, and it is consistent with the possible involvement of myoglobin in CO toxicology.

The prognosis for patients who survive acute carbon monoxide (CO) poisoning is uncertain, particularly in those who develop delayed sequelae after their initial recovery. For example, Lee and Marsden (1994) followed 31 patients with CO poisoning sequelae for a year. Eight had a progressive course and four of the eight died. Twenty-three had a delayed relapse after an initial recovery period of approximately 20 days. Nine of these developed a Parkinsonian state with behavioral and cognitive impairment, but 14 of the cases progressed farther and were bed-bound; the deterioration to either condition occurred rapidly over a few days to a week and three died. The mean initial CO hemoglobin level was not different in the two groups. Brain computed tomography (CT) scans were obtained at the onset of sequelae in both groups. Ten patients had a normal CT scan; 13 had white matter, low-density lesions; and four had globus pallidus, low-density lesions. The mechanisms for these sequelae may involve ischemia / reperfusion injury (Mathieu et al., 1996) or cerebral biochemical and metabolic changes (Kristensen, 1989).

Chronic Exposures

Cardiovascular Effects   Kristensen (1989) examined the relationship between cardiovascular diseases and exposures in the work environment, and concluded that CO exposure increases the acute risk of cardiovascular disease, but that there was no lasting atherosclerotic effect. Stern et al. (1988) performed a retrospective study of heart disease mortality in 5529 bridge and tunnel officers. The socioeconomic and smoking characteristics of the two groups were well matched, and the populations were limited to individuals who were assigned their positions and did not transfer between groups. The bridge officers experienced significantly lower CO exposures than the tunnel officers. Significantly elevated risk of coronary artery disease was found in the tunnel officers relative to the bridge officers (61 deaths observed versus 45 deaths expected); however, the risk declined after cessation of exposure, dissipating substantially after 5 years. Although convincing evidence from animal studies is lacking (Penney et al., 1994), CO may elevate plasma cholesterol and does appear to enhance atherosclerosis when serum cholesterol is greatly elevated by diet (Penney and Howley, 1991).

Effects on Lung Function   In addition to cardiovascular effects, individuals exposed to relatively high concentrations of CO in both indoor and outdoor environments also may be at risk of lung function decreases. It should be noted, however, that in addition to CO, these individuals were also exposed to high concentrations of other products of combustion and pyrolysis as well, and it is difficult to separate the effects of CO from those of these other compounds, many of which are known to be respiratory system irritants. Firefighters exhibit losses of lung function associated with acute and chronic smoke and CO exposure (Sparrow et al., 1982), and decrements in function (days in which fires were fought compared to routine workshifts without fires) lasted for up to 18-h in some individuals (Sheppard et al., 1986). In a study of matched populations of tunnel and bridge officers whose primary job was to collect tolls, tunnel officers consistently had greater concentrations of COHb, compared to the population of bridge officers with a similar demographic profile that performed essentially similar work, but the differences were small. Lung function measures of forced vital capacity (FVC) and forced expiration volume in 1 s ($FEV_{1.0}$) were slightly reduced in tunnel vs. bridge officers (Evans et al., 1988). No changes in FVC or $FEV_{1.0}$ were observed in loggers who complained of dyspnea and eye, nose, and throat irritation after felling trees and cutting logs using chain saws (Hagberg et al., 1985). Exposures to typical ambient concentrations of CO, both outdoors and indoors, have not been significantly associated with pulmonary diseases (Lutz, 1983) or lung function decrements (Lebowitz et al., 1987; Alderman et al., 1987), although other components of ambient pollution do show some significant associations (ozone, particulate matter), as do the use of gas stoves and tobacco smoking.

Effects on Pregnancy Outcomes   Alderman et al. (1987) performed a case-control study of the association between low birthweight infants and maternal CO exposures in approximately 1000 cases in Denver. CO exposures were assigned to residential locations using fixed-site outdoor monitor data. After controlling for race and education (a surrogate for smoking behavior), no relationship was detected between the assigned CO exposure during the last 3 months of pregnancy and lower birth weights. The investigators suggested that failure to directly account for unmeasured sources of CO exposure, such as smoking, emissions from gas appliances and exposures to vehicular exhaust, were a limitation of the study design. They also noted that the use of personal monitors for CO would have permitted a more direct evaluation of the potential relationship (exposure evaluations could be made after cases were identified, the relationship of personal to fixed-site assignments could be established, and then applied to the retrospective fixed site data [author's note]). Fetotoxicity has been demonstrated in laboratory animal studies. Altered brain neurochemical development and growth retardation have been demonstrated in rats exposed to CO in utero (Storm and Fechter, 1985; Leichter, 1993).

Exposure and Relationship to COHb Concentrations   In a study of more than 1500 nonsmoking people sampled as part of the second National Health and Nutrition

Examination Survey (NHANES II), Wallace and Ziegenfus (1985) demonstrated that CO concentrations measured at fixed-site monitors only accounted for 3% of the variance in blood COHb concentrations, using Spearman rank order correlations between the fixed-site monitor readings and sampled blood COHb concentrations. They found that the correlations were not significant ($p < 0.05$) for 24 of the 36 sampling stations in 20 U.S. cities surveyed. The failure of 8-h average concentrations to correlate strongly with measured COHb concentrations indicates that outdoor monitoring data does not adequately reflect personal CO exposure.

Using data from personal monitors worn by a probability sample of more than 1500 residents of Denver and Washington, D.C., Akland et al. (1985) found that more than 10% of Denver residents and 4% of Washington residents were exposed during the winter to CO concentrations in excess of 9 ppm for 8 h, or longer.

Controlled Human Studies

Several clinically based studies have been published that have provided a relatively coherent picture of the effects of CO on the cardiopulmonary system. Some of the key studies cited in the 1991 CO criteria document (EPA, 1991), as well as those published since then, are described below.

Cardiovascular Effects

Individuals with ischemic heart disease have limited ability to compensate for increased myocardial oxygen demands during exercise, hence exercise testing is often used as a means for evaluating the severity of their cardiovascular impairment. Calvert et al. (1987) determined that four useful parameters of ischemia, measurable during exercise testing, were (1) ST segment depression (at least 1 mV of horizontal or downsloping depression of the ST segment of an electrocardiographic tracing persisting for 70 ms in 3 successive complexes); (2) exercise-induced angina (chest pain during exercise, which is increased with effort and then resolves with rest—some individuals may experience pain in the jaw, neck, or shoulder areas); (3) impaired work capacity (maximum work levels expressed as a percentage of nomographically predicted, normal values (Bruce et al., 1973); and (4) an inadequate blood pressure response to exercise (blood pressure that falls on exercise [test would be discontinued] or fails to rise more than 15 mm Hg at a work level of at least 40% of the predicted norm). There are some individuals who exhibit one or more of these responses during exercise who do not have angiographically abnormal coronary arteries, as determined by measuring luminal narrowing; however, these parameters, taken in combination, can identify 85–90% of people with coronary artery disease (Calvert et al., 1987). Since CO exposure impairs myocardial O_2 delivery, CO exposure would be expected to worsen symptoms of ischemia in individuals with coronary artery disease. Therefore, exercise tests of such individuals have been an important means of providing quantitative and dose-related estimates of the potential impact of CO on health.

Sheps et al. (1987) exposed 30 subjects with ischemic heart disease, aged 38–75 yr., to CO (100 ppm) or air, during a 3-day, randomized, double-blind protocol, to achieve an average post-exposure COHb concentration of 3.8% on the CO exposure day (COHb on the air exposure day averaged 1.5%). After exposure to either CO or air, subjects performed an exercise stress test. All exercise tests were performed with the subjects in a supine position using a cycle ergometer at the same time of day, with the subjects in a fasting state. The workload was set at 0 for the first min; was then increased to 200 kp-m for the next 4 min and was increased in 50 to 100 kp-m increments at 4 min intervals until a maximal level was achieved. Exercise was continued until anginal pain required cessation of exercise, fatigue precluded further exercise, or blood pressure plateaued or decreased, despite the increase in workload. All of the subjects were nonsmokers and had documented evidence of ischemic heart disease defined by either exercise-induced ST segment depression (1 mV or more) exercise-induced angina, or abnormal left ventricular ejection fraction response to exercise (failure to increase ≥ 5 units from rest). The study population included both men and women, and not all subjects reported exercise-induced angina. Sheps et al. (1987) reported small, but not significant, decreases in time to onset of angina (1.9%) and maximal exercise time (1.3%) following CO exposures. Times to significant ST decreases, double product (DP; heart rate $\times$ systolic blood pressure) at significant ST depression, and maximal DP were similar for both conditions. (Double products have been shown to correlate with measured myocardial O_2 consumption during dynamic exercise; Kitamura et al., 1972.) The change in ejection fraction (rest to maximal) was slightly lower for CO exposures (air = 3.5%, CO = 2%; $p = 0.049$). The authors concluded that there were no clinically significant effects of low-level CO exposures at COHb concentrations of 3.8%.

Adams et al. (1988) subsequently extended the above study to an average postexposure COHb concentration of 5.9%, during exercise, using an identical protocol and 30 subjects (22 men, 8 women; mean age 58 y). Not all of the subjects in this study experienced exercise-induced angina, and only 21 subjects reported angina on both exposure days. The time to onset of angina in these 21 subjects was slightly, but not significantly, decreased after CO exposure (10.3%) compared to air exposure. An actuarial analysis of the data from all subjects reporting angina indicated that subjects were likely to experience angina earlier during stress on the CO day ($p \leq 0.05$). The left ventricular ejection fractions at rest were the same after both air and CO exposures; however, the level of submaximal ejection fraction was significantly higher after air, when compared to the CO exposure (3.3%; $p \leq 0.05$) and the change in ejection fraction, from rest to submaximal exercise, was significantly lower after CO exposure, compared to air exposure (air = 1.6% and CO = -1.2%; $p \leq 0.05$). No statistically significant exposure-related differences were seen for either maximal ST-segment depression, time to onset of significant ST-segment depression, or maximal DP. The authors concluded that exposures to CO resulting in COHb concentrations of about 6% significantly impaired exercise performance in subjects with ischemic heart disease.

Kleinman et al. (1989) exposed 24 nonsmoking male subjects with stable angina and positive exercise tests to 100 ppm CO or air to achieve an average COHb concentration of 2.9%, during exercise, on the CO exposure day. Subjects ranged in age from 51 to 66 y, with a mean age of 59 y. All but one of the subjects had additional confirmation of ischemic heart disease, such as previous myocardial infarction, coronary artery bypass surgery, positive thallium isotope exercise test, or a positive angiogram or cardiac catheterization. Subjects were exposed to CO or to clean air in a randomized, double-blind protocol. Subjects performed an incremental exercise test on a cycle ergometer until the point at which they could detect the onset of their typical anginal pain, and then stopped exercising. Workload was set at 50 watts initially and was increased in 25 watt increments at 3 min intervals. Blood pressure was measured at the end of each 3 min of exercise, ECG tracings were taken at the end of each minute, and respiratory gas exchange was measured at 15 intervals and averaged for each minute. Data were analyzed statistically using a two-factor analysis of variance and one-tailed tests of significance. The time to onset of angina was decreased after CO exposure (5.9%; $p = 0.046$) relative to air exposure. The duration of angina was longer after CO exposure compared to air exposure (8.3%), but this change was not statistically significant. Oxygen uptake at the angina point was slightly reduced after CO exposure compared to air exposure (2.2%; $p \leq 0.04$), but the increase in oxygen uptake with increasing workload was similar on both exposure days. A subgroup of 11 subjects who, in addition to angina, exhibited arrhythmias or ST-segment depressions during exercise, showed a greater reduction in time to angina after CO exposure, compared to air exposure (10.6%; $p \leq 0.016$), than did the overall group. The time to significant ST-segment depression was significantly reduced for the eight subjects with this characteristic after CO exposure, compared to air exposure (19.1%; $p \leq 0.044$). The number of subjects exhibiting exercise-induced ST-segment depression identified in this study was small; however, those subjects in whom angina preceded detection of ST segment changes would not have been identified in the protocol used because exercise was stopped at the point of onset of angina.

The results of a multicenter CO exposure study, conducted in three different cities, have been reported by Allred et al. (1989) in which 63 men with documented coronary artery disease underwent exposure to air, 117 ppm CO or 253 ppm CO, on three separate days in a randomized, double-blind protocol, followed by an incremental treadmill exercise test. Average COHb concentrations of 2.2% and 4.3%, during exercise, were achieved on the two CO exposure days (2.0% and 3.9%, respectively, at the end of exercise). All of the subjects were males, aged 41 to 75 y (mean age of 62 y), with stable exertional angina and a positive exercise stress test with ST-segment changes indicative of ischemia. In addition all of the subjects had objective evidence of coronary artery disease indicated by at least one of the following: (1) angiographic evidence of at least 70% obstruction in one or more coronary arteries, (2) previous myocardial infarction, or (3) a positive thallium stress test. On each of the exposure days, the subject performed a symptom-limited treadmill exercise test, was exposed to one of the three test atmospheres (clean air, 117 ppm CO, or 253 ppm CO), and then performed a second exercise test. The subjects exercised until the subjects: (1) were too fatigued to continue, (2) experienced severe dyspnea, (3) experienced grade 3 angina (on a subjective scale where grade 1 indicated the first perception of angina and grade 4 represented the worst angina the subject had ever experienced), (4) exhibited ECG changes (ST depression ≥ 3 mV or important arrhythmias), (5) exhibited high systolic (≥ 240 mm Hg) or diastolic (≥ 130 mm Hg) blood pressure; (6) exhibited a 20 mm Hg drop in systolic blood pressure; or (7) made a request to stop. The time to onset of angina and the time to significant ST depression was determined for each test, and the percent changes (pre-vs. postexposure) for the two CO exposure days were compared to the same subject's response to the randomized clean air exposure. The time to onset of angina was significantly reduced by CO exposure, in a dose-dependent manner (4.2% at 2% COHb, $p = 0.054$; 7.1% at 4% COHb, $p = 0.004$). Linear regressions of time to angina versus COHb concentrations for each subject indicated that time to angina decreased $1.9 \pm 0.8\%$ for every 1% increase in COHb ($p \leq 0.01$). The time to onset of 1 mV ST-segment depression was also reduced by CO in a dose-dependent manner (5.1% at 2% COHb, $p = 0.02$; 12.1% at 4% COHb, $p \leq 0.0001$) compared to the clean air exposure. There was a decrease of approximately $3.9 \pm 0.6\%$ in time to ST depression for every 1% increase in COHb ($p \leq 0.0001$). There was a significant correlation between the percent change in the time to onset of angina and the time to onset of ST depression ≥ 1 mV ($p \leq 0.0001$).

There is some evidence that a level of hypoxia that can result in myocardial ischemia and reversible angina, can also lead to arrhythmias (Kerin et al., 1979; Carboni, 1987; Dahms et al., 1993). Hinderliter et al. (1989) exposed 10 subjects, with ischemic heart disease and no ventricular ectopy at baseline, to air, 100 ppm CO, and 200 ppm CO; COHb concentrations averaged 4% and 6% on the two respective CO exposure days. The exposures were randomized and double blinded. Following exposure, each subject performed a symptom-limited supine exercise test; ambulatory electrocardiograms were obtained prior to exposure, during exposure, during exercise, and over a 5 h postexercise period. The ECG's were analyzed for the frequency and severity of arrhythmias. Eight of the 10 subjects demonstrated evidence of ischemia on one or more of the exposure days (angina, 1 mV ST-segment depression, or abnormal ejection fraction response). There were no CO-related increases in the frequency of premature ventricular beats and no multiple arrhythmias were occurred. The authors concluded that low-level CO exposure (4% to 6% COHB) was not arrhythmogenic in patients with coronary artery disease and no ventricular ectopy at baseline.

However, researchers from this same team (Sheps et al., 1990), reported on a larger study population (41 subjects) with some evidence of ventricular ectopy, exposed to air, 100 ppm CO, and 200 ppm CO in a similar protocol to that described above. The frequency of single ventricular premature depolarizations (VPD's) per hour increased ($p \leq 0.03$) from 127 ± 28 (mean $\pm$ SD) after the air exposure to 168 ± 38 after exposure to achieve a COHb concentration of 6%. During exercise the frequency of multiple VPD's per hour increased approximately three fold at 6% COHb, compared to air exposure ($p \leq 0.02$). No significant differences in these parameters occurred after exposures that achieved COHb concentrations of 4%, compared to air exposures. The subjects who exhibited single VPD's with increased frequency after CO exposure were significantly older than the subjects who had no increased arrhythmias. The subjects who exhibited increased frequencies of multiple VPD's were older, exercised for longer durations, and had higher peak workloads during exercise, than those who did not have complex arrhythmias. Leaf and Kleinman have also reported evidence of effects of CO exposure on cardiac rhythm after relatively low CO exposures (3% COHb) in a small group of volunteers with coronary artery disease that exhibited abnormal rhythms on one or more exercise test (Leaf and Kleinman, 1996).

In all of the above clinical studies of CO-related effects, subjects with coronary artery disease were maintained on individualized regimens of medications, some of which might interact with CO-induced responses, increasing the apparent variations in observed responses. Specifically, blockade of beta-adrenergic receptors (Melinyshyn et al., 1988) and alpha-adrenergic receptors (Villeneuve et al., 1986) were shown to modify hemodynamic responses to CO in animal studies. Examination of the potential influence of medications on observed responses to CO could provide additional insights on the possible mechanisms of action of CO in individuals with coronary artery disease.

Cardiopulmonary Effects (Lung Function and Exercise Tolerance)

Normal Individuals   Reduction of O_2 delivery could reduce the ability to perform work in healthy individuals. Studies of the cardiopulmonary effects of CO have demonstrated that maximal oxygen uptake during exercise ($\dot{V}_{O_2}$ max) decreases linearly with increasing COHb concentrations, ranging from 2.3% to 35% COHb, in normals. The linear relationship can be expressed as percent decrease in $\dot{V}_{O_2}$ max $= 0.91$ [%COHb] $+ 2.2$. The specific studies on which these findings are based have been extensively reviewed in the 1979 CO criteria document (U.S., 1979), the 1984 Addendum to that document (U.S., 1984), Horvath (1981), and by Shephard (1984). Changes in $\dot{V}_{O_2}$ max are significant because they represent changes in an individual's maximal aerobic exercise (or work) capacity. Klausen et al. (1983) exposed 16 male smokers to CO (5.26% COHb) and compared the effects on maximal exercise performance to performance after 8 h without smoking and performance after smoking three cigarettes (4.51% COHb). Both exposures reduced $\dot{V}_{O_2}$ max by about 7%, but exercise time was decreased more after cigarette smoking than after CO exposure, suggesting that other components of smoke may contribute to the observed effects. Similar findings had been reported by Ekblom and Huot (1972).

Horvath et al. (1988) exposed 23 subjects (11 male, 12 female) to 0, 50, 100, and 150 ppm CO, at four different altitudes (55, 1524, 2134, and 3048 m); following each exposure performed an incremental exercise test. COHb concentrations ranged from 0.5 $\pm$ 0.2% to 5.6 $\pm$ 0.4% of saturation after sea-level exposures. The study showed a significant effect of increased altitude on decreased work performance and $\dot{V}_{O_2}$ max. CO exposure tended to slightly decrease these parameters at all altitudes; however, the statistical analyses did not demonstrate a CO × altitude interaction. The result suggests that these factors acted independently, and perhaps additively, but not synergistically. The female subjects appeared to be more resistant to the hypoxic effects of altitude than the male subjects. The rate of CO uptake (i.e., formation of COHb) decreased with increasing altitude, in part, due to the reduced driving pressure of CO at altitude. While this might be a mechanism by which CO could directly affect cardiac myoglobin, evidence for direct cardiotoxicity of CO is still lacking. Horvath and Bedi (1989) have demonstrated that longer-term, low-level (9 ppm for 8 h) exposures at 2134 m results in lower COHb concentrations than the same exposure at 55 m, again suggesting slower CO uptake during altitude exposure. McGrath (1989), however, has reported that endogenous CO production is increased in rats chronically maintained at high altitudes (1000 to 6000 m), suggesting that high altitude residents have higher initial COHb concentrations and might therefore achieve 2% or greater COHb levels (the COHb level associated with the CO NAAQS) more quickly than sea-level residents. It has been reported that unacclimated workers exposed to about 25 ppm CO at an altitude of 2.3 km above sea level exhibited significantly increased symptoms of headache, vertigo, fatigue, weakness, memory impairment, insomnia, and heart palpitations compared to local residents (Song, 1993). The subjects in these human clinical studies of exercise tolerance have been relatively young and all were in good health. There is not sufficient information available to determine if relationships between CO exposure, altitude, and COHb concentrations would be similar for individuals with coronary artery disease, chronic lung diseases, or anemias, or in pregnant women.

Kleinman and associates have demonstrated that hypoxia due to high altitude and CO exposure may cause additive effects on exercise tolerance, hemodynamic changes, and cardiologic parameters (Kleinman et al., 1998). The subjects in this study were older men with confirmed coronary artery disease.

Although Horvath et al. (1988) have reported that significant fractions of CO were moved to extravascular spaces during exercise, probably in temporary combination with myoglobin, when exercise levels exceeded 80% of $\dot{V}_{O_2}$ max. (COHb concentrations increased 5 min postexercise compared to concentrations measured at the point of maximum workload).

Individuals with Chronic Obstructive Pulmonary Disease (COPD)   Individuals with COPD usually have limited exercise tolerance because they have low ventilatory capacity, which can result in desaturation of arterial blood and hypoxemia (a relative deficiency of O_2 in the blood) and hypoxia (a relative deficiency of O_2 in some tissue) during exercise. Exercise performance in such individuals can be improved by providing supplemental O_2 (Lane et al., 1987). Reduced O_2 carrying capacity of blood due to formation of COHb could exacerbate this limitation; hence individuals with COPD could represent a potentially sensitive group. Aronow et al. (1977) exposed 10 men, aged 53 to 67 y, to 100 ppm CO for 1 h, achieving increases in COHb from baseline concentrations of 1.4% to postexposure concentrations of 4.1%. Mean exercise time was reduced by 33%. Calverley et al. (1981) exposed 6 smokers (who stopped smoking 12 h prior to testing) and 9 nonsmokers to 200 ppm CO for 20 to 30 min (increasing COHb concentrations to between 8% and 12% COHb above baseline COHb), and measured the distance each subject walked in a 12 min period. Significant decreases in walking distance were only seen in individuals with 12.3% COHb or greater. Some individuals with severe COPD, but without clinically apparent coronary artery disease, exhibit exercise-related cardiac arrhythmias. Cheong et al. (1990) reported that these arrhythmias were associated with arrhythmias at rest but were not related to the severity of pulmonary disease, O_2Hb desaturation, or ECG evidence of chronic lung disease. The Sheps et al. (1990) studies of exercise-related arrhythmias in CO-exposed subjects with coronary artery disease suggest that COPD subjects might be important to study as well. Overall, the information available on individuals with COPD are consistent with the hypothesis that they represent a population potentially at risk of CO-related health effects during submaximal exercise, as may occur during normal daily activities. The available data are, however, based on population group sizes that are too small and too diverse with respect to disease characteristics to draw firm conclusions.

Neurotoxicological and Behavioral Effects   The neurotoxic effects of relatively high level acute CO exposures have been well documented. Subtle neurotoxic effects associated with lower-level CO exposures may be underreported or not associated with CO exposure because the symptoms, which resemble those of a flu-like viral illness, may be misdiagnosed (Ilano and Raffin, 1990). Population-based studies on the potential neurotoxicological and behavioral effects of chronic CO exposure at ambient concentrations have not been reported. However, clinical studies of CO-related sensory effects have evaluated several different parameters, under controlled laboratory conditions. A study by Hudnell and Benignus (1989) demonstrated, in a double-blind study, that visual function in healthy, young adult males, as defined by measurements of contrast threshold, luminance threshold, and time of cone/rod break, was not affected by COHb concentrations maintained at 17% for over 2 h. Von Restorff and Hebisch (1988) reported no changes in time to dark adaptation and sensitivity after adaptation, at COHb concentrations ranging from 9% to 17%. The findings of these two recent studies are in general agreement with those of several earlier studies. Only one earlier study had demonstrated CO-induced visual threshold effects (McFarland et al., 1944). However, the number of subjects tested was small, and documentation of the study was scant. No recent studies of temporal resolution of the visual system have been reported. Two early studies by von Post-Lingen (1964) and Seppanen et al. (1977), in which large enough numbers of subjects ($n > 20$) were used to provide some confidence in the results but which were performed single blinded, had demonstrated changes in critical flicker fusion at COHb concentrations as low as 5%. However, a double-blinded study by Ramsey (1973) and a small ($n = 15$) double-blind repeat study by Seppanen et al. (1977) did not. Benignus et al. (1987) exposed 24 healthy nonsmoking males to 0 or 100 ppm CO for 4 h (mean COHb $= 8$%). They measured the subject's ability to perform fast and slow tracking tasks (maintaining the position of a moving point of light on a computer screen using a joystick) and monitoring tasks (judging the brightness of two red spots on a computer screen) once per hour during exposure. CO exposure increased tracking errors but did not interfere in the monitoring task. An earlier study by Putz et al. (1979) had shown significant decrements in both tracking and monitoring tasks at a COHb concentration of 4.6% but not at 3.5%. A large number of studies have investigated the effects of CO on several other behavioral parameters. However, effects in general are only seen at COHb concentrations above 5%, and there are inconsistencies between the study results. Of the studies, other than those discussed above, published in 1984 and later, Bunnell and Horvath (1988) showed interactive effects of exercise and CO exposure (>7% COHb) on cognitive tasks, Insogna and Warren (1984) demonstrated a significant decrement in video game performance (targets tracked and destroyed) at 2.1 to 4.2% COHb. (Both of these were single-blind studies with relatively small numbers of subjects—15 and 9, respectively). Although many earlier studies had demonstrated significant changes in brain electrical activity, Harbin et al. (1988) showed no changes in visually evoked response potentials in young (23 y) and older (69 y) subjects at 5.3% COHb. In general, neurotoxicity at COHb levels near 5% has not been convincingly demonstrated in normal healthy adults (Benignus et al., 1987).

Fetal Developmental and Perinatal Effects   Both theoretical reasons and supporting experimental data indicate that the fetus may be more susceptible to the effects of CO than the mother. Fetal Hb has greater affinities for CO and O_2 than does maternal Hb. The partial pressure of O_2 in fetal blood is about 20 to 30% of that in maternal blood because of the greater O_2 affinity of fetal Hb. In addition COHb shifts the O_2Hb dissociation curve to the left in maternal blood, reducing the transfer of O_2 across the placenta from maternal to fetal circulation. As in adults, the nervous and cardiovascular systems of the fetus are the most sensitive to the effects of CO. For humans, information is available for women who smoked during pregnancy or were acutely exposed to CO; however, most of the available reports do not characterize the relevant CO exposure levels and cannot, in general, rule out toxic effects of co-contaminants. Acute CO exposure plays a role in fetal death (Caravati et al., 1988), and environmental exposures, as well as maternal smoking, has been linked to sudden infant death syndrome (SIDS) (Hoppenbrouwers et al., 1981). Neonatal mortality and low birth weights are more prevalent in children born in high-altitude regions (Lichty et al., 1957; Grahn and Kratchman, 1963), suggesting a relation to high-altitude hypoxia, and further suggesting that these effects seen in children born to women who smoke are possibly a result of CO-induced hypoxia. High-level maternal CO exposures have significant neurotoxicological consequences for the fetus, but available data come from animal studies. Significant neurotoxic effects in prenatally exposed rats included disruption of neuronal proliferation and possible disruption of markers of neurochemical transmission (Fechter, 1987). Immune system changes have also been noted in rats exposed to CO prenatally (Giustino et al., 1993).

CO as a Risk Factor in Cardiovascular Disease Development   Evidence from population-based studies indicates that workers exposed to CO in combination with other combustion products from automobile exhaust (Stern et al., 1988) and other smoking co-workers (Kristensen, 1989) have increased risk of development of atherosclerotic heart disease. Also individuals hospitalized for myocardial infarction frequently exhibit higher COHb concentrations than individuals hospitalized for other reasons (Leikin and Vogel, 1986). Central to the development of atheromatous plaques is the deposition and retention of fibrinogen and lipids within the arterial wall. It is known that cigarette smoke increases the permeability of the arterial wall to fibrinogen. Allen et al. (1989) demonstrated in a canine model that both CO and nicotine in cigarette smoke might produce an atherogenic effect, but that they act via different mechanisms. CO increases arterial wall permeability and nicotine reduces clearance of deposited fibrinogen. Activation and dysfunction of blood platelets is also thought to be important in atherogenesis (Ross, 1986) and in cardiac-related sudden deaths due to the platelets role in the initiation of thrombosis. Nowak et al. (1987) reported biochemical evidence that cigarette smoking induced both platelet and vascular dysfunctions in apparently healthy individuals. Platelet dysfunction may also be a contributory cause of thrombosis during pregnancy and may increase fetal mortality and morbidity among women who smoke (Davis et al., 1987). Abnormalities in platelet aggregation after CO exposure have been seen in animal models (Kalmaz et al., 1980) and may be linked to guanylate cyclase activation (Brune and Ullrich, 1987). Davis et al. (1989) exposed 10 healthy nonsmokers passively to cigarette smoke (in hospital corridors) resulting in a small increase in COHb concentration, from 0.9% ± 0.3% to 1.3 ± 0.6%, before and after passive exposure, respectively. They showed evidence of changes in platelet aggregation and endothelial cell damage. The changes in endothelial cell counts (pre- to postexposure) were significantly correlated to changes in COHb concentrations from before to after exposure, but plasma nicotine levels were not. The contribution of carbon monoxide relative to other components of tobacco smoke in causing platelet dysfunction is not established.

SUMMARY AND CONCLUSIONS

The current CO ambient air standards are designed to protect susceptible individuals from exposures that would result in COHb concentrations of 2% and above. Occupational standards are designed to protect workers from concentrations of 5% COHb (U.S. Department of Health, Education and Welfare, 1972). Studies of individuals with coronary artery disease, and residents of New York, Denver, Washington, DC, and Los Angeles suggest that susceptible individuals frequently exceed 2% COHb in cities that frequently exceed NAAQS. Control of exposures is difficult because the sources of CO are widespread, the distribution of ambient CO is nonuniform, and emissions from unregulated sources, especially indoors, probably contribute substantially to individual CO doses. The distributions of COHb concentrations in workers are also very nonuniform but may often reach the 5% level.

The contribution of CO to the aggravation of symptoms of myocardial ischemia is reasonably well defined for a selected subset of people with existing coronary artery disease. The individuals comprising the populations tested in the various studies on which this conclusion was drawn were carefully selected to have sufficiently pronounced disease such that effects would be measurable, but they were also sufficiently healthy so that they could perform moderate levels of exercise with minimal risk. Thus more impaired individuals, who might presumably be at equal or greater risk of detrimental CO-induced health effects, and relatively asymptomatic individuals, so-called silent ischemics, have not been well characterized. Incorporation of broader, possibly more representative, subject populations into the clinical studies of Sheps et al. (1990) and Adams et al. (1988) significantly increased the variance in subject responses and increased the difficulty of attributing statistical significance to observed findings. As shown in Figure 5-1, there is a reasonable dose-response relationship over the range of 2% to 6% COHb for the decrease in time to onset of angina in data from five independent studies in which subjects with

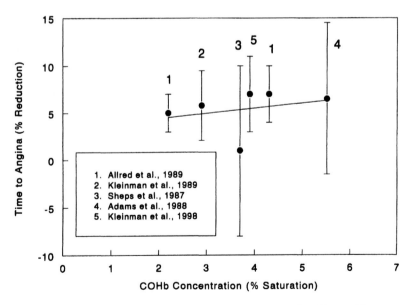

Figure 5-1   Reduction in time to angina (TTA) following CO exposure in subjects with coronary artery disease. Linear regression shows that TTA is reduced in a dose-dependent manner. Values shown are mean $\pm$ SE.

documented coronary artery disease were exposed to CO and then performed symptom-limited exercise tests.

Convincing documentation for effects of CO on other potentially susceptible individuals at ambient exposure levels is becoming available. The most extensive body of evidence of CO effects on pregnant women, fetuses, and neonates comes from the literature on smoking and from acute, high-level accidental CO exposures. In most cases actual CO exposures are poorly, if at all, documented and the contribution of co-pollutants to the observed effects cannot be assessed. However, animal studies demonstrating developmental changes and associations between environmental CO and SIDS indicates ~~that risks to pregnant women, fetuses, and neonates may be important.~~

The importance of occult CO exposures leading to clinically significant symptoms and effects is becoming well appreciated. The large number of such incidents suggests the potential that an equally large, or larger, number of events occur that lead to subclinical manifestations which are ignored if they are not serious enough to prevent relatively normal daily activities. The home indoor environment is very poorly characterized with respect to indoor pollutant levels and, given the apparently large potential for CO-related health effects in the home, should be the focus of significant study.

It would seem from this review that both occupational and ambient standards are placed at the limits at which significant effects are seen, albeit in sensitive individuals. The available information on the role of CO in the development of cardiovascular disease, and its possible role in infant mortality, is suggestive, but additional studies under well-controlled conditions with accurate estimates of CO exposure history are needed.

ACKNOWLEDGMENTS

This review was funded in part by the California Air Resources Board and by the UCI Center for Occupational and Environmental Health.

REFERENCES

Adams, K. F., G. Koch, B. Chatterjee, G. M. Goldstein, J. J. O'Neil, P. A. Bromberg, D. S. Sheps, S. McAllister, C. J. Price, and J. Bissette. 1988. Acute elevation of blood carboxyhemoglobin to 6% impairs exercise performance and aggravates symptoms in patients with ischemic heart disease. *J. Am. Coll. Cardiol.* 12: 900–909.

Akland, G. G., T. D. Hartwell, T. R. Johnson, and R. W. Whitmore. 1985. Measuring human exposure to carbon monoxide in Washington, D.C. and Denver, Colorado, during winter of 1982–1983. *Environ. Sci. Technol.* 19: 911–918.

Alderman, B. W., A. E. Baron, and D. A. Savitz. 1987. Maternal exposure to neighborhood carbon monoxide and risk of low infant birth weight, *Public Health Rep.* 102: 410–414.

Allen, D. R., N. L. Browse, and D. L. Rutt. 1989. Effects of cigarette smoke, carbon monoxide and nicotine on the uptake of fibrinogen by the canine arterial wall. *Atherosclerosis* 77: 83–88.

Allred, E. N., E. R. Bleeker, B. R. Chaitman, T. E. Dahms, S. O. Gottlieb, J. D. Hackney, M. Pagano, R. H. Selvester, S. M. Walden, and J. Warren. 1989. Short-term effects of carbon monoxide on the exercise performance of subjects with coronary artery disease *N. Engl. J. Med.* 321: 1426–1432.

Anderson, E. W., R. J. Andelman, J. M. Strauch, N. J. Fortuin, and J. H. Knelson. 1973. Effect of low-level carbon monoxide exposure on onset and duration of angina pectoris. *Ann. Internal Med.* 79: 46–50.

Aronow, W. S., and M. W. Isbell. 1973. Carbon monoxide effect on exercise-induced angina pectoris. *Ann. Internal Med.* 79: 392–395.

Aronow, W. S., C. N. Harris, M. W. Isbell, S. N. Rokaw, and B. Imparato. 1972. Effect of freeway travel on angina pectoris. *Ann. Internal Med.* 77: 669–676.

Aronow, W. S., J. Ferlinz, and F. Glauser. 1977. Effect of carbon monoxide on exercise performance in chronic obstructive pulmonary disease. *Am. J. Med.* 63: 904–908.

Ayers, S. M., S. Giannelli, Jr., and H. Mueller. 1970. Part IV. Effects of low concentrations of carbon monoxide. Myocardial and systemic responses to carboxyhemoglobin. *Ann. NY Acad. Sci.* 174: 268–293.

Beard, R. R., and G. A. Wertheim. 1967. Behavioral impairment associated with small doses of carbon monoxide. *Am. J. Public Health* 57: 2012–2022.

Benignus, V. A., K. E. Muller, C. N. Barton, and J. D. Prah. 1987. Effect of low level carbon monoxide on compensatory tracking and event monitoring. *Neurotoxicol. Teratol.* 9: 227–234.

Berk, P. D., F. L. Rodkey, T. F. Blaschke, H. A. Collison, and J. G. Waggoner. 1974. A new approach to quantitation of various sources of bilirubin in man. *J. Lab. Clin. Med.* 87: 767–780.

Bleeker, M. L. 1988. Parkinsonism, a clinical marker of exposure to neurotoxins. *Neurotoxicol. Teratol.* 10: 475–478.

Bruce, R. A., F. Kusumi, and D. Hosmer. 1973. Maximal oxygen uptake and nomographic assessment of functional aerobic impairment in cardiovascular disease, *Am. Heart J.* 85: 546–562.

Brune, B., and V. Ullrich. 1987. Inhibition of platelet aggregation by carbon monoxide is mediated by activation of guanylate cyclase. *Mol. Pharmacol.* 32: 497–504.

Bunnell, D. E., and S. M. Horvath. 1988. Interactive effects of physical work and carbon monoxide on cognitive task performance. *Aviat. Space Med.* 59: 1133–1138.

Calverley, P. M. A., R. J. E. Leggett, and D. C. Flenley. 1981. Carbon monoxide and exercise tolerance in chronic bronchitis and emphysema. *Br. Med. J.* 283: 878–880.

Calvert, A. F., G. Pater, D. Pye, J. Mann, D. Chalmers, and B. Ayres. 1987. A matched pairs comparison of cycle ergometry and treadmill exercise testing in the evaluation of coronary heart disease. *Aust. NZ J. Med.* 17: 472–478.

Caravati, E. M., C. J. Adams, S. M. Joyce, and N. C. Schafer. 1988. Fetal toxicity associated with maternal carbon monoxide poisoning. *Ann. Emergency Med.* 17: 714–717.

Carboni, G. P., A. Lahiri, P. M. M. Cashman, and E. B. Raftery. 1987. Mechanisms of arrhythmias accompanying ST-segment depression on ambulatory monitoring in stable angina pectoris. *Am. J. Cardiol.* 60: 1246–1253.

Cheong, T. H., S. Magder, S. Shapiro, J. G. Martin, and R. D. Levy. 1990. Cardiac arrhythmias during exercise in severe chronic obstructive pulmonary disease. *Chest* 97: 793–797.

Clifford, M. J; R. Clarke, and S. B. Riffat. 1997. Drivers' exposure to carbon monoxide in Nottingham, UK. *Atmos. Environ.* 31: 1003–1009.

Coburn, R. F., R. E. Forster, and P. B. Kane. 1965. Considerations of the physiological variables that determine the blood carboxyhemoglobin concentration in man, *J. Clin. Invest.* 44: 1899–1910.

Coburn, R. F., W. J. Williams, and S. B. Kahn. 1966. Endogenous carbon monoxide production in patients with hemolytic anemia. *J. Clin. Invest.* 45: 460–468.

Dahms, T. E., and S. M. Horvath. 1974. Rapid, accurate technique for determination of carbon monoxide in blood. *Clin. Chem.* 20: 553–557.

Dahms, T. E., L. T. Younis, R. D. Wiens, S. Zarnegar, et al. 1993. Effects of carbon monoxide exposure in patients with documented cardiac arrhythmias. *J. Am. Coll. Cardiol.* 21: 442–450.

Darbool, M. A., A. Bener, J. Gomes, and K. S. Jadaan. 1997. Carbon monoxide exposure from motor vehicles in United Arab Emirates. *J. Environ. Sci. Health, Part A—Environmental Science and Engineering and Toxic and Hazardous Substance Control* 32: 311–321.

Davidson, A. C., R. Leach, R. J. George, and D. M. Geddes. 1988. Supplemental oxygen and exercise ability in chronic obstructive airways disease. *Thorax* 43: 965–971.

Davis, J. W., L. Shelton, I. S. Watanabe, and J. Arnold. 1989. Passive smoking affects endothelium and platelets. *Arch. Int. Med.* 149: 386–389.

Davis, R. B., M. P. Leuschen, D. Boyd, and R. C. Goodlin. 1987. Evaluation of platelet function in pregnancy. Comparative studies in non-smokers and smokers. *Thrombosis Res.* 46: 175.

Dor, F., Y. Lemoullec, and B. Festy. 1995. Exposure of city residents to carbon monoxide and monocyclic aromatic hydrocarbons during commuting trips in the Paris metropolitan area. *J. Air Waste Manag. Assoc.* 45: 103–110.

Ebisuno, S., M. Yasuno, Y. Nishina, M. Hori, M. Imoue, and T. Kamada. 1986. Myocardial infarction after acute carbon monoxide poisoning: case report. *Angiology* 37: 621–624.

Ekblom, B., and R. Huot. 1972. Response to submaximal and maximal exercise at different levels of carboxyhemoglobin. *Acta Physiol. Scand.* 86: 474–482.

Evans, R. G., K. Webb, S. Homan, and S. M. Ayres. 1988. Cross-sectional and longitudinal changes in pulmonary function associated with automobile pollution among bridge and tunnel officers, *Am. J. Ind. Med.* 14: 25–36.

Fechter, L. D. 1987. *Neurotoxicity of prenatal carbon monoxide exposure.* Research Report, Health Effects Institute, Cambridge, MA.

Flachsbart, P. G. 1995. Long-term trends in United States highway emissions, ambient concentrations and in-vehicle exposure to carbon monoxide in traffic. *J. Expos. Anal. Environ. Epidem.* 5: 473–495.

Forbes, W. H., H. F. Sargent, and F. J. W. Roughton. 1945. The rate of carbon monoxide uptake by normal men, *Am. J. Physiol.* 143: 594–608.

Giustino A., R. Cagiano, M. R. Carratu, M. A. Desalvia, et al. 1993. Immunological changes produced in rats by prenatal exposure to carbon monoxide. *Pharmacol. Toxicol.* 73: 274–278.

Goldsmith, J. R., J. Terzaghi, and J. D. Hackney. 1963. Evaluation of fluctuating carbon monoxide exposures, *Arch. Environ. Health* 7: 647–663.

Grahn, D., and Kratchman, J. 1963. Variations in neonatal death rate and birth weight in the United States and possible relations to environmental radiation, geology and altitude. *Am. J. Hum. Genet.* 15: 329–352.

Guillot, J. G., J. P. Weber, and J. Y. Savoie. 1981. Quantitative determination of carbon monoxide in blood by head-space gas chromatography, *J. Anal. Toxicol.* 5: 264–266.

Hagberg, A. C., B. Kolmodin-Hedman, R. Lindahl, C. A. Nilsson, and A. Norstrom. 1985. Irritative complaints, carboxyhemoglobin increase and minor ventilatory function changes due to exposure to chain-saw exhaust. *Eur. J. Respir. Dis.* 66: 240–247.

Hampson N. B., and D. M. Norkool. 1992. Carbon monoxide poisoning in children riding in the back of pickup trucks. *JAMA* 267: 538–540.

Harbin, T. J., V. A. Benignus, K. E. Muller, and C. N. Barton. 1988. The effects of low-level carbon monoxide exposure upon evoked cortical potentials in young and elderly men. *Neurotoxicol. Teratol.* 10: 93–100.

Heckerling, P. S., J. B. Leikin, A. Maturen, and J. T. Perkins. 1987. Predictors of occult carbon monoxide poisoning in patients with headache and dizziness. *Ann. Intern. Med.* 107: 174–176.

Heckerling, P. S., J. B. Leikin, and A. Maturen. 1988. Occult carbon monoxide poisoning: validation of a prediction model. *Am. J. Med.* 84: 251–256.

Hellman, L. M., and J. A. Pritchard. 1971. *Obstetrics*, 14th ed. New York: Appleton-Century-Crofts.

Herman G. D., A. B. Shapiro, and J. Leikin. 1988. Myonecrosis in carbon monoxide poisoning. *Veterinary Hum. Toxicol.* 30: 28–30.

Hinderliter, A. L., K. F. Adams Jr., C. J. Price, M. C. Herbst, G. Koch, and D. S. Sheps. 1989. Effects of low-level carbon monoxide exposure on resting and exercise-induced ventricular arrhythmias in patients with coronary artery disease and no baseline ectopy. *Arch. Environ. Health* 44: 89–93.

Hoppenbrouwers, T., M. Calub, K. Arakawa, and J. Hodgeman. 1981. Seasonal relationship of sudden infant death syndrome and environmental pollutants. *Am. J. Epidemiol.* 113: 623–635.

Horvath, S. M. 1981. Impact of air quality on exercise performance. *Exercise Sport Sci. Rev.* 9: 265–296.

Horvath, S. M., and J. F. Bedi. 1989. Alteration in carboxyhemoglobin concentrations during exposure to 9 ppm carbon monoxide for 8 hours at sea level and 2134 m. *J. Air Poll. Contr. Assoc.* 39: 1323–1327.

Horvath, S. M., J. F. Bedi, J. A. Wagner, and J. W. Agnew. 1988. Maximal aerobic capacity at several ambient concentrations of CO at several altitudes. *J. Appl. Physiol.* 65: 2696–2708.

Hudnell, H. K., and V. A. Benignus. 1989. Carbon monoxide exposure and human visual function thresholds. *Neurotoxicol. Teratol.* 11: 363–371.

Ilano, A. L., and T. A. Raffin. 1990. Management of carbon monoxide poisoning. *Chest* 97: 165–169, 1990.

Insogna, S., and Warren, C. A. 1984. The effect of carbon monoxide on psychomotor function. In *Trends in Ergonomics/Human Factors I*, ed. A. Mital. Amsterdam: Elsevier/North Holland.

Kalmaz E. V., L. W. Canter, and J. W. Hampton. 1980. Effect of long-term low and moderate levels of carbon monoxide exposure on platelet counts of rabbits. *J. Environ. Pathol.* 4: 351–358.

Kamada, K., K. Houkin, T. Aoki, M. Koiwa, T. Kashiwaba, Y. Iwasaki, and H. Abe. 1994. Cerebral metabolic changes in delayed carbon monoxide sequelae studied by proton MR spectroscopy. *Neuroradiology* 36: 104–106.

Kerin, N. Z., M. Rubenfire, M. Naini, W. J. Wajszczuk, A. Pamatmat, and P. N. Cascade. 1979. Arrhythmias in variant angina pectoris: Relationship of arrhythmias to ST-segment elevation and R-wave changes. *Circulation* 60: 1343–1350.

Kirkpatrick, J. N. 1987. Occult carbon monoxide poisoning. *Western J. Med* 146: 52–56.

Kitamura, K., C. R. Jorgenson, G. L. Gebel, H. L. Taylor, and Y. Wang. 1972. Hemodynamic correlates of myocardial oxygen consumption during upright exercise, *J. Appl. Physiol.* 32: 516–522.

Klausen, K., C. Andersen, and S. Nandrup. 1983. Acute effects of cigarette smoking and inhalation of carbon monoxide during maximal exercise. *Eur. J. Appl. Physiol. Occup. Physiol.* 51: 371–379.

Kleinman M. T., D. M. Davidson, R. B. Vandagriff, V. J. Caiozzo, and J. L. Whittenberger. 1989. Effects of short-term exposure to carbon monoxide in subjects with coronary artery disease. *Arch. Environ. Health* 44: 361–369.

Kleinman, M. T., D. A. Leaf, E. Kelly, V. Caiozzo, K. Osann, and T. O'Niell . 1998. Urban angina in the mountains: Effects of carbon monoxide and mild hypoxemia on subjects with chronic stable angina. *Arch. Environ. Health*, 53: 388–397.

Koushki, P. A., K. H. Aldhowalia, and S. A. Niaizi. 1992. Vehicle occupant exposure to Carbon Monoxide. *J. Air Waste Manag. Assoc.* 42: 1603–1608.

Kristensen, T. S. 1989. Cardiovascular diseases and the work environment. A critical review of the epidemiologic literature on chemical factors. *Scand. J. Work Environ. Health* 15: 245–264.

Lambert, W. E., S. D. Colome, and S. L. Wojciechowski. 1988. Application of end-expired breath sampling to estimate carboxyhemoglobin levels in community air pollution exposure assessments, *Atmos. Environ.* 22: 2171–2181.

Lane, R., A. Cockcroft, L. Adams, and A. Guz. 1987. Arterial oxygen saturation and breathlessness in patients with chronic obstructive airways disease. *Clin. Sci.* 72: 693–698.

Leaf, D. A. and M. T. Kleinman. 1996. Urban ectopy in the mountains—Carbon monoxide exposure at high altitude. *Arch. Environ. Health* 51: 283–290.

Lebowitz, M. D., C. J. Holberg, B. Boyer, and C. Hayes. 1985. Respiratory symptoms and peak flow associated with indoor and outdoor pollution in the southwest, *J. Air Poll. Contr. Assoc.* 35: 1154–1158.

Lebowitz, M. D., L. Collins, and C. J. Holberg. 1987. Time series analysis of respiratory responses to indoor and outdoor environmental phenomena, *Environ. Res.* 43: 332–341.

Lee, M. S., and C. D. Marsden. 1994. Neurological sequelae following carbon monoxide poisoning clinical course and outcome according to the clinical types and brain computed tomography scan findings. *Movement Dis.* 9: 550–558.

Lee, P. S., R. M. Schreck, B. A. Hare, and J. J. McGrath. 1994. Biomedical applications of tunable diode laser spectrometry: Correlation between breath carbon monoxide and low level blood carboxyhemoglobin saturation. *Ann. Biomed. Eng.* 22: 120–125.

Leichter, J. 1993. Fetal growth retardation due to exposure of pregnant rats to carbon monoxide. *Biochem. Arch.* 9: 267–272.

Leikin, J. B., and S. Vogel. 1986. Carbon monoxide levels in cardiac patients in an urban emergency department. *Am. J. Emergency Med.* 4: 126–128.

Levesque B., E. Dewailly, R. Lavoie, D. Prud'Homme, and S. Allaire. 1990. Carbon monoxide in indoor ice skating rinks: Evaluation of absorption by adult hockey players. *Am. J. Pub. Health* 80: 594–598.

Levy, R. I., and M. Feinleib. 1984. Risk factors for coronary artery disease and their management. In *Heart Disease: A Textbook of Cardiovascular Medicine*, ed., E. Braunwald, Philadelphia: Saunders.

Lichty, J. A., R. Y. Ting, P. D. Bruns, and E. Dyar. 1957. Studies of babies born at high altitudes. I. Relation of altitude to birthweight. *AMA J. Dis. Child.* 93: 666–669.

Longo, L. D. 1976. Carbon monoxide: Effects on oxygenation of the fetus in utero. *Science* 194: 523–525.

Lutz, L. J. 1983. Health effects of air pollution measured by outpatient visits, *J. Fam. Pract.* 16: 307–313.

Mariusnunez, A. L. 1990. Myocardial infarction with normal coronary arteries after acute exposure to carbon monoxide. *Chest* 97: 491–494.

Marius-Nunez, A. L. 1990. Myocardial infarction with normal coronary arteries after acute exposure to carbon monoxide. *Chest* 97: 491–494.

Mathieu, D., M. Mathieu-Nolf, and F. Wattel. 1996. Carbon monoxide poisoning: Current aspects. *Bull. Acad. Nati. Med.* 180: 965–971.

McCartney, M. L. 1990. Sensitivity analysis applied to Coburn-Forster-Kane models of carboxyhemo-globin formation, *Am. Ind. Hyg. J.* 51: 169–177.

McFarland, R. A., F. J. W. Roughton, M. H. Halperin, and J. I. Niven. 1944. The effects of carbon monoxide and altitude on visual thresholds. *J. Aviat. Med.* 15: 381–394.

McGrath, J. J. 1989. Cardiovascular effects of chronic carbon monoxide and high altitude exposure. Research Report 27. Health Effects Institute, Cambridge, MA.

Melinyshyn, M. J., S. M. Cain, S. M. Villeneuve, and C. K. Chapler. 1988. Circulatory and metabolic responses to carbon monoxide hypoxia during beta-adrenergic blockade. *Am. J. Physiol.* 255: H77–84.

National Air Pollution Control Administration. 1970. *Air Quality Criteria for Carbon Monoxide*, Report No. NAPCA-PUB-AP-62, U.S. Dept. of Health, Education and Welfare, Washington, D.C., NTIS No. PB-190261.

Nowak, J., J. J. Murray, J. A. Oates, and G. A. FitzGerald. 1987. Biochemical evidence of a chronic abnormality in platelet and vascular function in healthy individuals who smoke cigarettes. *Circulation* 76: 6–14.

Ott, W., J. Thomas, D. Mage, and L. Wallace. 1988. Validation of the simulation of human activity and pollution exposure (SHAPE) model using paired days from the Denver, Colorado, carbon monoxide field study, *Atmos. Environ.* 22: 2101–13.

Pace, N., W. V. Consolazio, W. A. White Jr., and A. R. Behnke. 1946. Formulation of the principal factors affecting the rate of uptake of carbon monoxide by man, *Am. J. Physiol.* 145: 352–359.

Penney, D. G. 1988. A review: Hemodynamic response to carbon monoxide, *Environ. Health Perspect.* 77: 121–130.

Penney, D. G., and J. W. Howley. 1991. Is there a connection between carbon monoxide exposure and hypertension? *Environ. Health Perspect.* 95: 191–198.

Penney, D. G., A. A. Giraldo, and E. M. Vanegmond. 1994. Coronary vessel alterations following chronic carbon monoxide exposure in the adult rat. *J. Applied Toxicol.* 14: 47–54.

Pernoll, M. L., J. Metcalfe, T. L. Schenker, J. E. Welch, and J. A. Matsumato. 1975. Oxygen consumption at rest and during exercise in pregnancy. *Respir. Physiol.* 25: 285–293.

Peterson, J. E., and R. D. Stewart. 1975. Predicting the carboxyhemoglobin levels resulting from carbon monoxide exposures, *J. Appl. Physiol.* 39: 633–638.

Pierson, W. E., J. Q. Koenig, and E. J. Bardana Jr. 1989. Potential adverse health effects of wood smoke. *Western J. Med.* 151: 339–342.

Putz, V. R., B. L. Johnson, and J. V. Setzer. 1979. A comparative study of the effects of carbon monoxide and methylene chloride on human performance. *J. Environ. Pathol. Toxicol.* 2: 97–112.

Ramsey, J. M. 1973. Effects of single exposures of carbon monoxide on sensory and psychomotor response. *Am. Ind. Hyg. Assoc. J.* 34: 212–216.

Ross, R. 1986. The pathogenesis of atherosclerosis-an update. *New Engl. J. Med.* 314: 488–500.

Roughton, F. J. W. 1970. The equilibrium of carbon monoxide with human hemoglobin in whole blood. In: *Biological Effects of Carbon Monoxide*, Proceedings of a Conference, *Ann. NY Acad. Sci* 174 (Part 1): 177–188.

Seppanen, A., J. V. Hakkinen, and M. Tenkku. 1977. Effect of gradually increasing carboxyhemoglobin saturation on visual perception and psychomotor performance of smoking and nonsmoking subjects. *Ann. Clin. Res.* 9: 314–319.

Shephard, R. J. 1984. Athletic performance and urban air pollution. *Can. Med. Assoc. J.* 131: 105–109.

Sheppard, D., S. Distefano, L. Morse, and C. Becker. 1986. Acute effects of routine firefighting on lung function. *Am. J. Ind. Med.* 9: 333–340.

Sheps, D. S., K. F. Adams, P. A. Bromberg, G. M. Goldstein, J. J. O'Neil, D. Horstman, and G. Koch. 1987. Lack of effect of low levels of carboxyhemoglobin on cardiovascular function in patients with ischemic heart disease, *Arch. Environ. Health* 42: 108–116.

Sheps, D. S., M. C. Herbst, A. L. Hinderliter, K. F. Adams, L. G. Ekelund, J. J. O'Neil, G. M. Goldstein, P. A. Bromberg, J. L. Dalton, M. N. Ballenger, S. M. Davis, and G. Koch. 1990. Production of arrhythmias by elevated carboxyhemoglobin in patients with coronary artery disease. *Ann. of Internal Med.* 113: 343–351.

Sokal, J. A., and E. Kralkowska. 1985. The relationship between exposure duration, carboxyhemoglobin, blood glucose, pyruvate and lactate and the severity of intoxication in 39 cases of acute carbon monoxide poisoning in man. *Arch. Toxicol.* 57: 196–199.

Solanki, D. L., P. R. McCurdy, F. F. Cuttitta, and G. P. Schechter, 1988. Hemolysis in sickle cell disease as measured by endogenous carbon monoxide production: a preliminary report. *Am. J. Clin. Pathol.* 89: 221–225.

Song, C. P. 1993. Health effects on workers exposed to low concentration carbon monoxide at high altitude. *Chinese J. Preventive Med.* 27: 81–84.

Sparrow, D., R. Bosse, B. Rosner, and S. T. Weiss. 1982. The effect of occupational exposure on pulmonary function: a longitudinal evaluation of fire fighters and non fire fighters. *Am. Rev. Respir. Dis.* 125: 319–322.

Stern, F. B., W. E. Halperin, R. W. Hornung, V. L. Ringenburg, and C. S. McCammon. 1988. Heart disease mortality among bridge and tunnel officers exposed to carbon monoxide. *Am. J. Epidemiol.* 128: 1276–1288.

Storm, J. E., and L. D. Fechter. 1985. Alteration in the postnatal ontogeny of cerebellar norepinephrine content following chronic prenatal carbon monoxide. *J. Neurochem.* 45: 965–969.

Sue, D. Y., K. Wasserman, R. B. Moricca, and R. Casaburi. 1988. Metabolic acidosis during exercise in patients with chronic obstructive pulmonary disease. Use of the V-slope method for anaerobic threshold determination, *Chest* 94: 931–938.

Thom, S. R., and L. W. Keim. 1989. Carbon monoxide poisoning: A review of epidemiology, pathophysiology, clinical findings, and treatment options including hyperbaric oxygen therapy. *J. Toxicol. Clinical Toxicol.* 27: 141–156.

Tikuisis, P., H. D. Madhill, B. J. Gill, W. F. Lewis, K. M. Cox, and D. M. Kane. 1987. A critical analysis of the use of the CFK equation in prediciting COHb formation, *Am. Ind. Hyg. Assoc.* 48: 208–213.

U.S. Centers for Disease Control. 1982. Carbon monoxide intoxication—A preventable environmental health hazard, *Morb. Mortal. Weekly Report* 31: 529–531.

U.S. Department of Health, Education and Welfare, Health Services and Mental Health Administration, National Institute for Occupational Safety and Health, 1972. *Occupational Exposure to Carbon Monoxide*, Washington, DC.

U.S. EPA. 1979. *Air Quality Criteria for Carbon Monoxide*, EPA Report EPA-600/8-79-022. Environmental Criteria and Assessment Office. U.S. Environmental Protection Agency, Research Triangle Park, NC, NTIS No. PB81-244840.

U.S. EPA. 1984. *Revised Evaluation of Health Effects Associated with Carbon Monoxide Exposure: An Addendum to the 1979 EPA Air Quality Criteria Document for Carbon Monoxide*, EPA Report. EPA-600/9-83-033F. Environmental Criteria and Assessment Office, U.S. Environmental Protection Agency. Research Triangle Park, NC, NTIS No. PB85-103471.

U.S. EPA. 1991. *Air Quality Criteria for Carbon Monoxide*, EPA Report No. EPA-600/8-90-045F. Environmental Criteria and Assessment Office, U.S. Environmental Protection Agency. Research Triangle Park, NC, NTIS No. PB81-244840.

Viala A. 1994. Indoor Air Pollution and Health: Study of various problems. *Bull. Acad. Nati. Med.* 178: 57–66.

Villeneuve, S. M., C. K. Chapler, C. E. King, and S. M. Cain. 1986. The role of alpha-adrenergic receptors in carbon monoxide hypoxia. *Can. J. Physiol. Pharmacol.* 64: 1442–1446.

von Post-Lingen, M. L. 1964. The significance of exposure to small concentrations of carbon monoxide. *Proc. R. Soc. Med.* 57: 1021–1029.

von Restorff, W., and S. Hebisch. 1988. Dark adaptation of the eye during carbon monoxide exposure in smokers and nonsmokers. *Aviat. Space Environ. Med.* 59: 928–931.

Vreman, H. J., L. K. Kwong, and D. K. Stevenson. 1984. Carbon monoxide in blood: An improved microliter blood-sample collection system, with rapid analysis by gas chromatography, *Clin. Chem.* 30: 1382–1386.

Wallace, L. A., and R. C. Ziegenfus. 1985. Comparison of carboxyhemoglobin concentrations in adult nonsmokers with ambient carbon monoxide levels. *J. Air Poll. Contr. Assoc.* 33: 678–682.

Wallace, L. R., and W. R. Ott. 1982. Personal monitors: A state-of-the-art survey, *J. Air. Poll. Cont. Assoc.* 32: 601–610.

West, J. B. 1987. *Pulmonary Pathophysiology—The Essentials.* 3rd ed. Baltimore: Williams and Wilkens.

Yu, L. E., L. M. Hildemann, and W. R. Ott. 1996. A mathematical model for predicting trends in carbon monoxide emissions and exposures on urban arterial highways. *J. Air Waste Manag. Assoc.* 46: 430– 440.

6 Chromium

MITCHELL D. COHEN, Ph.D.
MAX COSTA, Ph.D.

Chromium (Cr) is abundant in the earth's crust, with both the hexavalent (Cr[VI]) and more predominant trivalent (Cr[III]) forms readily found in nature. Chromite ($FeCr_2O_4$) is the most important Cr-containing ore and is used for production of ferrochromium by direct reduction (Carson et al., 1986). Chemical treatment of chromite, followed by electrolysis, yields Cr metal. Commercially Cr compounds are commonly used directly in leather/pelt tanning and for electroplating, and as additives in production of pigments, catalysts, corrosion inhibitors, and wood preservatives. Chromium metal is widely used in the steel industry, as a superalloy for jet engines, and for the formation of other alloys. Exposure to Cr is primarily within the industrial setting or from contact with industrial effluents released into the general environment. Symptoms of acute toxicity include allergic contact dermatitis, skin ulcers, nasal membrane inflammation, and nasal ulceration, while chronic occupational exposure can result in nasal septum perforations, rhinitis, liver damage, pulmonary congestion, edema, and nephritis (Goyer, 1986). Increased incidences of lung and gastric cancers also occur among chronically exposed individuals, while elevations in other types of cancers are also evident (Costa, 1997). The toxicity and carcinogenicity of Cr are largely related to exposure to the metal in its hexavalent state.

ESSENTIALITY

A possible essential role of Cr(III) was demonstrated in 1955 when weanling rats that were fed a torula yeast-based diet developed small progressive impairments in their glucose tolerance (Mertz and Schwarz, 1955). Subsequent studies with other experimental animals showed that small Cr-deficiencies impaired their glucose tolerance, and that the rate of glucose removal was reduced to half its normal value (Schwarz and Mertz, 1959). In addition, severe Cr-deficiencies caused reductions in rodent growth, longevity, fertility, and sperm counts. Correspondingly there was an increase in glycosuria, aortic plaques, and a rise in the fasting blood glucose and cholesterol levels.

Evidence of the beneficial effects of Cr in human nutrition was obtained as a consequence of studies of patients who could no longer ingest food via the normal esophogeal-stomach-intestinal route due to disease or injury. In these patients, surgical implantation of a tube allows for parenteral delivery of fluids containing all essential nutrients. The beneficial effect of Cr was detected as a result of its omission from specially prepared total parental nutrition (TPN) regimens. Two case histories showed that the

Environmental Toxicants: Human Exposures and Their Health Effects, 2/e. Edited by Morton Lippmann.
ISBN: 0-471-29298-2 © 2000 John Wiley & Sons, Inc.

patients receiving chronic TPN developed considerable weight losses and hypoglycemia (Jeejeebhoy et al., 1977; Freund et al., 1979). These symptoms were reversed with Cr-supplementation (as Baker's yeast) of the parental fluids.

Since Cr-deficiency results in impaired glucose and lipid metabolism, the U.S. Department of Agriculture (USDA) recommended that a dietary intake of 50 to 200 μg Cr/d would be safe and adequate in adults (Food and Nutrition Board, NRC, 1980). This range was based on the absence of any symptoms associated with Cr-deficiency in a population known to consume an average of 60 μg Cr daily. However, metabolic studies estimated daily intake to be < 50 μg Cr/d (Andersen and Kozlovsky, 1985; Offenbaucer et al., 1986). Today Cr(III) picolinate is widely advertised as a supplement to enhance muscle mass. The picolinate form greatly enhances the absorption of Cr(III) into the body and into cells. The mechanism of an essential or pharmacological action of Cr(III) remains to be elucidated, although it seems to have a role in enhancing the effects of insulin on glucose transport. In diabetics that respond poorly to their insulin, Cr(III) picolinate helps control erratic blood glucose levels, but this effect could just as well be classified as pharmacological (i.e., Cr(III)) and not essential. The chemistry of Cr(III), with its ability to form tight kinetically inert bonds, makes it a most unusual essential element compared to others. If it has an essential function, it may be based upon a structural role.

ENVIRONMENTAL SOURCES AND STANDARDS

Occupational exposures to Cr occur during the various stages of its production. Because Cr can be used for many different purposes, there is the potential for exposure in a great variety of industries. The most likely risk of occupational exposure is through inhalation of Cr-bearing aerosols. These mixtures are thought to have a wide spectrum of biological activities and are frequently contaminated by other metals (Stern et al., 1984), as well as other known carcinogens such as benzo(α)pyrene. Additionally there are wide variations in the possible aerosol characteristics, such as the relative proportions of the major oxidation states of the Cr particles, as well as varying solubilities within these fractions (Hertel, 1986).

The Occupational Safety and Health Administration (OSHA) has established permissible exposure limits (PEL) for Cr and its compounds. The PEL for chromic acid and soluble chromates is 0.1 mg Cr/m^3, 0.5 mg Cr/m^3 for Cr(II) and Cr(III) compounds, and 1.0 mg Cr/m^3 for the Cr metal and its insoluble hexavalent salts. The threshold limit values (TLV) established by the American Conference of Government Industrial Hygienists (ACGIH) are 0.05 mg Cr/m^3 for chromate ore processing and water-soluble Cr(VI) compounds, 0.5 mg Cr/m^3 for Cr metal and Cr (III) agents, and 0.01 mg Cr/m^3 for insoluble Cr(VI) compounds (i.e., zinc chromate). These PEL and TLV values, while originally established to protect workers from irritation of the respiratory system as well as against renal and hepatic damage, are also intended to reduce the carcinogenic risk from exposure to Cr(VI) agents to acceptable levels (ACGIH, 1989; OSHA, 1989).

Chromium concentrations in soil can range from 0.1 to 250 ppm Cr, and in certain areas, soil content may be as high as 400 ppm Cr (Langard and Norseth, 1979). Overall, most soils have been shown to contain on average 50 ppm Cr (Hertel, 1986). However, industrial sources can contribute to significant elevations in the concentration of Cr found in soil. In cases of extensive Cr contamination, such as occurred in 42 Cr-contaminated sites in Hudson County, New Jersey, concentrations of Cr(VI) and Cr(III) up to 100 and 19,000 ppm, respectively, have been documented in the surrounding soils (Environmental Science and Engineering, 1989; Paustenbach et al., 1991; Sheehan et al., 1991). Other industrially contaminated sites which were deemed hazardous have included two sites in Odessa, Texas (total soil Cr levels ranging from 720 to 5000 ppm), and one site each in

Woburn, Massachusetts (total soil Cr of 1000 ppm), Dixiana, South Carolina (630 ppm Cr), and Vancouver, Washington (550 ppm Cr) (U.S. EPA, 1986, 1987a, b, 1988a, b).

Conversely, several agricultural regions throughout the world have been identified as being located upon Cr-deficient soils. This was demonstrated by the fact that both crop yield and quality were improved when Cr was added to the soil. However, it is not clear whether or not the beneficial aspects were due to an effect of the Cr upon the plants themselves or as a result of interactions of the introduced Cr with other elements or biological agents already present in the soil. While the presence of Cr in phosphate fertilizers is an important source of Cr for crop growth, the downside to the introduction of Cr into the normally Cr-deficient soils also provides a major means for introducing Cr into the environment as a pollutant.

Chromium in ambient air originates primarily from industrial sources (i.e., steel manufacturing and cement production) and the combustion of fossil fuels; the content in coal and crude oil varies from 1 to 100 μg Cr/L and from 0.005 to 0.7 μg Cr/L, respectively (Pacyna, 1986). Airborne particulate matter from coal-fired power plants have been shown to contain Cr in the range of 2.3–31 ppm Cr; however, these levels are reduced to 0.19/6.6 ppm Cr by fly ash collection processes (Goyer, 1986). In rural areas, Cr levels in the air are usually less than 10 ng Cr/m^3, whereas the concentrations were reported to vary from 10 to 100 ng Cr/m^3 in industrial cities (Fishbein, 1981; Nriagu and Nieboer, 1988). Overall, the distribution of Cr(III) to Cr(VI) is about 2:1 in atmospheric Cr emissions; this arises as a result of the fact that most Cr(VI) that enters the air is reduced by the action of many common environmental constituents and other ambient pollutants, including aerosolized acids and dissolved sulfides (ATSDR, 1989; Sheehan et al., 1991).

In general, removal of Cr from the atmosphere is the result of either precipitation events or dry deposition. In rural and urban areas, fallout rates for Cr average about 0.2–1.5 and 20–60 mg Cr/m^2/y, respectively (Nriagu et al., 1988); dry deposition rates in areas far away from the point source of emission average between 0.001 and 0.03 mg Cr/m^2/y.

The concentrations of Cr in water are variable and dependent on salinity. Average concentrations of Cr in American rivers and lakes range from 1 to 30 μg Cr/L; these values are considerably higher than those found in seawater (0.1–5 μg Cr/L) (NAS, 1974; U.S. EPA, 1984a). Drinking water has also been shown to contain higher Cr concentrations than that encountered in river water. For example, in a survey of 84 midwestern cities, the levels of Cr in tapwater were found to range from 5 to 17 μg Cr/L (U.S. EPA, 1975). A controllable source of Cr waste in water is from chromeplating and metal-finishing industries, as well as from textile and tanning plants. Industrial wastewater contains total Cr in the range of 0.005 to 525 mg Cr/L, with concentrations of Cr(VI) averaging from 0.004 to 335 mg Cr/L (U.S. EPA, 1980).

As noted previously, most of the Cr that can be encountered in both fresh water and seawater environs is the result of direct deposition of airborne Cr. Oddly, Cr that is associated with soil has been deemed not to pose a significant runoff hazard, nor does Cr present much of a threat to aquifers or groundwater supplies since it does not readily leach from soils (U.S. EPA, 1988a). This proposed low-risk scenario has been supported by the studies of groundwater Cr levels in the well-studied Hudson County sites; only about 1% of the total Cr found in the polluted soils was found to be leachable under stringent extraction procedures (ESE, 1989). The most likely explanation for this was that the majority of the Cr in the soils occured as water-insoluble Cr(III) (Rai et al., 1986, 1988; Sheehan et al., 1991).

However, there may not be a complete absence of a threat from Cr pollution of utilizable water supplies as a result of soil contamination. It might be concluded that under conditions wherein levels of natural reductants might be low in the soil, or the rate of deposition of Cr(VI) onto the soil exceeds that of normal reduction processes, increased amounts of soluble Cr(VI) may penetrate further into the soils and, possibly, reach water-bearing strata. Conditions have been documented in which residents in the vicinity of a Cr-contaminated site were potentially exposed to Cr(VI) in their drinking water at levels up to 10 ppm. For example, in Hinkley, CA, an electric power company pumping station utilizing water coolant laced with potassium chromate routinely discharged the solutions into unlined ponds in the desert. Over time, the Cr permeated into the local aquifer, as well as into wells used for drinking water (Costa, 1997).

EXPOSURE SCENARIOS

Significant nonoccupational Cr exposure of animals and humans is provided through the intake of Cr-containing foodstuffs. The largest sources of dietary Cr are found in meat, vegetables, and unrefined sugar, whereas fruit, fish, and vegetable oils contain fairly small quantities of the metal. Most food, with the exception of herbs and condiments, probably contain less than 100 ppb Cr; concentrations in meat range from 10 ppb to 60 ppb Cr wet weight (Guthrie, 1982; Kiovistoinen, 1982). Higher Cr concentrations have been measured in some beverages, with typical values in spirits, beer, and wine being 175, 300, and 450 µg Cr/ml, respectively (Jenning and Howard, 1980). The estimated daily intake by adults is between 100 and 200 µg Cr/d, although large interindividual variations of < 850 to 2620 µg Cr/d have been identified in several studies (Guthrie, 1982). The highest bioavailability of Cr is from the glucose tolerance factor (GTF) which is predominantly found in Baker's yeast, liver, and meat.

There are several factors regulating whether certain foodstuffs, primarily vegetables, can be a major source for Cr. Apart from the fact that the vegetables/fruits must be grown on a Cr-containing site, the levels of Cr in the soil must be in the range for which plant growth is not retarded, and the Cr taken up from the soil must localize to those portions that are edible. Plants growing on soil with a low Cr content have been estimated to contain 0.02 ppm Cr wet weight (Hertel, 1986). Even in soils with higher Cr concentrations, plants usually contain low levels of Cr, although a higher Cr content is often found in the roots. This may be related to the fact that only chelated Cr compounds, and not the soluble Cr molecules present in the soil, are absorbed by the plants (Kabata-Pendias and Pendias, 1984).

Because most sites containing the highest levels of soil Cr are located in urban areas, little commercial farming is expected, and the primary source for Cr-bearing vegetable/fruit consumption is via store-bought produce. However, a risk of consumption of Cr via ingestion of Cr-bearing soils in these environments still exists, primarily among children (those mostly 2 to 6 years of age; Calabrese et al., 1989) or those adults suffering from pica or geophagia. Among children, average consumption of soil/dirt has been found to range from 10 to 90 mg/d; an average rate of 10 mg/d has been calculated for those people above the age of 6 years (Paustenbach, 1987). Using these consumption rates for each age group, and factors including the amounts of time available for possible soil ingestion, average daily uptakes/intakes of Cr (primarily as Cr[III]) have been calculated to be 0.07 to 0.2 µg Cr/kg/d for children, and about 4 to 9 ng Cr/kg/d for adults, using the parameters of the most likely exposed individual (MLEI) or maximally exposed individual (MEI), respectively, during data analysis within each age group (Sheehan et al., 1991).

Ingestion of Cr from groundwater, especially from that around Cr-contaminated sites, is not considered a major risk factor. As noted earlier, the permeation of Cr from the contaminated soils is very limited, and so polluting of major water/deep aquifer supplies, including wells, is not likely. While contamination of shallow aquifers can occur over time, most often this water is not considered to be potable due to contamination by other pollutants or even sewage-associated microbes. The only possible source for consumption of significantly polluted water occurs after ponding; this is especially significant if soluble Cr(VI) agents are present in the contaminated soils.

In nonoccupational settings, the inhalation of suspended dust/soil particulates containing adsorbed Cr is one likely route of exposure that has been deemed to present a significant hazard to health. The amount of exposure to any Cr-bearing soil particles in residential environs is expected to be low, with outside soil particles representing no more than 10% (on average) of the total composition of home-associated dusts (Sheehan et al., 1991). In general, following inhalation, the Cr-bearing soil/dust particles are expected to undergo redistribution, with 25% being exhaled, 50% landing in the upper airways (and subsequently swallowed), and the remainder deposited in the lungs (Cowherd et al., 1985). Even within that small fraction that can reach the lungs, mucociliary clearance leads to the removal a significant amount of the Cr-bearing material. Using this redistribution profile, an assumption of a level of 1 ng Cr/m^3 air, and taking into account the differences in breathing rates as a function of age, deposition of Cr (as Cr[III]) at the MEI level can be estimated to be about 5 and 3.5 pg Cr/kg/d for an exposed child and adult, respectively. Correspondingly levels of Cr(VI) alone in the airborne particulates would be much lower in this model (i.e., 3 pg/m^3), so daily deposition levels would be on the levels of fg Cr(VI)/kg.

One other variable needs to be considered when discussing daily deposition of Cr within the lungs, namely cigarette smoking. Tobacco grown in the United States has been shown to contain 0.24 to 6.3 ppm Cr (IARC, 1980, 1990). However, no estimates on the amounts of Cr inhaled daily by smokers has yet been reported. The same equations used for determining the average daily dose of soil-associated Cr may no longer hold true in the case of smokers, due to smoking-induced changes in respiratory parameters/functions. In addition, cigarette usage among individuals is highly variable, even within defined age groups. As a result Cr deposition in the lungs arising from cigarette smoking is difficult to estimate.

The last major means for introduction of Cr into the body in nonoccupational situations is via dermal contact. Overall, Cr(III) is not dermally absorbed to any significant extent, since it binds readily to several constituents witihin the skin (Polak, 1983). Unless solubilized or suspended in solution, Cr in soil/dusts is very poorly absorbed through the skin. If soluble Cr(VI) is present in the contact sample, it can pass more readily through the epidermal barrier than its trivalent counterparts (Samitz and Katz, 1964). There are instances where contact surfaces may have elevated Cr levels (as observed on the cinderblocks used in many basement walls in Cr-contaminated sites in Hudson County, NJ), and the majority of the material is in the Cr(VI) form. This differs from a scenario involving skin contact with soil in that the cinderblocks are conducive to permeation by the solubilized Cr(VI) compounds while excluding Cr(III) agents (Sheehan et al., 1991). As a result of the differences in the potential risk posed between Cr(VI) and Cr(III) with respect to this route of exposure along with the apparent selective concentrating of Cr(VI) compounds on those surfaces most likely to pose a threat for human contact (i.e., basement walls), the MEI- and MLEI-associated values of average daily uptake via the dermal route, unlike those for intake via the diet or inhalation, are reported solely in terms of mg Cr(VI)/kg/d rather than Cr(III)/kg/d.

Not all nonoccupational dermal exposure to Cr is the result of contact with Cr-polluted waters, soils, or basement walls. Significant amounts of skin exposure can arise from daily contact with many household materials and clothing (reviewed in Paustenbach et al., 1992). In cleaning items such as bleaches and detergents, chromate has been included as both a stabilizing and a coloring agent; though this practice is not as common in the United States as it is in Europe, exposure to these Cr-containing cleaning agents has been associated with a condition known as "housewive's eczema." With clothing, particularly tanned leathers, sweat is the primary vehicle for both liberating Cr from the material and for providing a vehicle to concentrate Cr onto the skin during evaporation. Other less-frequently reported sources for dermal exposure to Cr include military uniforms, match heads, magnetic tapes, and green felt used on gaming tables. The oddest source of introducting a significant concentration of Cr directly onto the skin may be via tatooing, though Cr is probably not as widely in use today as it was in earlier decades when use of "chromium green" was common in tatoo application.

UPTAKE AND DISTRIBUTION

As noted above, exposure to Cr can occur through one of the three major routes: via absorption through the skin, by direct ingestion, or by inhalation of Cr-containing particles. The absorption of Cr is largely dependent on the oxidation state of the metal and the physical characteristics of the compound itself. Hexavalent Cr compounds can penetrate the skin more readily than trivalent forms, and uptake is enhanced with increases in the pH of the Cr-containing substances (Nriagu and Nieboer, 1988). While under normal conditions, absorption of Cr through the skin is limited due to ongoing chemical reduction, these processes can be circumvented; absorption of Cr(VI) may be increased by the presence of broken skin, as occurs frequently with workers bearing Cr-induced dermal ulcerations. There have been documented cases in which extensive absorption of Cr(VI) occurred following a chromic acid burn, and that the patient developed significant damage to tissues (i.e., kidney) at a distal site in the body (WHO, 1988).

Soluble Cr(VI) is readily absorbed from the respiratory system, whereas Cr(III) is absorbed to a much lesser degree. However, when present as insoluble particles, Cr in either valence state can by phagocytized by epithelial cells. Under normal exposure conditions (i.e., atmospheric Cr), absorption of Cr from the respiratory tract has been estimated to be $\ll 1\,\mu g\,Cr/d$ (Hertel, 1986); however, occupationally exposed individuals may inhale several micrograms per day. Absorption from the lung is dependent on the characteristics of the aerosol, including the size, shape, hygroscopicity, and overall electric charge of the Cr-containing particles (Stern et al., 1984; Hertel, 1986). Other factors that may influence the absorption of these particles include ambient temperature, solubility in body fluids, and reactions with other airborne agents. In the gastrointestinal tract, only 1% of an ingested dose of Cr(III) is absorbed, whereas absorption of Cr(VI) is 3% to 6% (Mertz, 1969; Offenbaucer et al., 1986). Recent studies suggest a wide variation in human absorption of Cr(VI) from drinking water, with some individuals absorbing >25% of an oral dose (Paustenbach, 1996). This variability may relate to reduction of Cr(VI) to the trivalent form by components of saliva and gastric juice.

The oxidation state of Cr is also the determining factor for its transportation via the bloodstream. Trivalent Cr is mainly transported via the serum, bound to the iron-binding transferrin and the μ-globulin fraction of serum proteins; however, at high concentrations Cr(III) binds to serum albumin or μ_1- or μ_2-globulin (Gray and Sterling, 1950; Harris, 1977). In contrast to Cr(III), Cr(VI) can readily cross the erythrocyte membrane and bind to the globulin portion of hemoglobin following oxidation of the heme group (Gray and Sterling, 1950; Saner, 1980; Nieboer and Jusy, 1986). Inside these cells, Cr(VI) is reduced to Cr(III) by glutathione and then becomes trapped intracellularly. Recent human studies where volunteers ingested Cr(VI) in drinking water showed that a substantial amount enters red blood cells; this indicated that not all Cr(VI) was reduced to Cr(III) in the GI tract (Paustenbach, 1996). Consequently the degradation products of erythrocytes may explain, in part, the high concentration of Cr found in the spleen and the slow excretion of Cr from the body.

The distribution of Cr from the bloodstream is dependent on its chemical state. Soluble chelated forms of Cr are rapidly cleared, whereas colloidal or protein-bound forms are cleared more slowly. The latter have a greater affinity for reticuloendothelial system components, such as the liver, spleen, and bone marrow (Hopkins, 1965; Langard, 1982). Accumulation of Cr also occurs in the kidney and testes, whereas retention is less in the heart, pancreas, lungs, and brain. The Cr retained in the liver and kidneys accounts for about 45% to 50% of total body Cr burdens (Saner, 1980).

Excretion of Cr also depends on the oxidation state and occurs primarily via urine and, to a lesser degree, the feces. Approximately 80% of a parental ^{51}Cr dose is excreted in the urine and 2% to 20% in the feces. The biological half-time of ^{51}Cr in humans has been estimated to be from 50 to 60 days (Nieboer and Jusy, 1986). Since urinary Cr is generally derived from the dialyzable fraction of serum, postglomerular reabsorption of Cr in renal tubuli results in an intrarenal circulation following exposure (Collin et al., 1961; Mutti et al., 1984). However, urinary excretion is generally $< 10\,\mu g$ Cr/d in the absence of excessive exposure (Underwood, 1977).

A minor route of excretion is through the skin and via sweat. Placental transfer of Cr has been indicated from animal studies; however, the transport across the placenta was time dependent (U.S. EPA, 1980). For example, insignificant amounts of Cr were transferred if the metal was administered at more than 10 days before birth, whereas larger amounts were transferred if the dose was given shortly before birth. This suggests that either inorganic Cr can cross the placenta or is converted to a form that can be readily transported (Danielsson et al., 1982). There were also considerable differences in distribution of Cr(III) and Cr(VI) in the fetal and embryonic tissues. On day 13 of gestation, the embryonic content of Cr(III) and Cr(VI) were 0.4% and 12%, respectively, and fetal concentrations increased with gestational age.

TOXICOLOGICAL EFFECTS

Chromium metal is biologically inert and has not been reported to produce toxic or other harmful effects in man or animal. The toxicity of Cr compounds has been largely associated with the Cr(VI) form, whereas Cr(III) is virtually inactive in vivo.

Following acute exposure of rats to Cr(VI) by various routes of administration, the main target organs affected included the liver and kidneys (U.S. EPA, 1980). The main toxic effects in the kidney were necrosis and desquamation of the epithelium of the convoluted tubules. Red blood cells were also found in the intertubular spaces. In rabbits, the effects of intraperitoneal administration of 2 mg Cr/kg (as $K_2Cr_2O_7$ or $Cr(NO_3)_3$) for a period of 3 or 6 weeks were largely relegated to alterations in the brain (Mathur et al., 1977). After a period of 3 weeks, these changes included occasional neuronal degeneration of the cerebral cortex, marked chromatolysis, and nuclear changes in the neurons. Six weeks of exposure resulted in marked degeneration of the cerebral cortex, accompanied by neuronophagic neuroglial proliferation and meningeal congestion. Hepatic changes have also been reported in a separate study using rabbits treated with these same compounds at similar doses (Tandon et al., 1978).

Soluble salts of chromates (CrO_4^{2-}) are highly toxic when administered parenterally, with an LD_{50} of 10–50 mg/kg as compared with LD_{50} values of 200–350 and 1500 mg/kg obtained with dermal and oral exposure, respectively (Carson et al., 1986). Large oral doses of chromate administered to rats primarily caused gastric corrosion (U.S. EPA, 1980). Hexavalent CrO_3 administered orally was found to be quite toxic in mice and rats with LD_{50} values of 137–177 and 80–114 mg/kg, respectively. Symptoms of acute toxicity included diarrhea, cyanosis, tail necrosis, and gastric ulcers; death occurred between 3 and 35 hours after dosing. Conversely, oral administration of Cr(III) compounds is relatively nontoxic. From this and other studies, oral LD_{50} values of 1.87, 11.26, and 3.25 g/kg were calculated for $CrCl_3$, $Cr(CH_3COO^-)_3$, and $Cr(NO_3)_3$, respectively (Smyth et al., 1969).

Cases of acute systemic poisoning are rare; however, they may follow deliberate or accidental ingestion. The oral LD_{50} of $Na_2Cr_2O_7$ in humans has been reported to be

50 mg / kg (NIOSH, 1979). Other effects of Cr(VI) poisoning include gastric distress, olfactory sense impairment, nosebleeds, liver damage, and yellowing of the tongue and teeth. Systemic toxicity may occur with both of the oxidation states (mainly due to increased absorption of Cr through the broken skin) resulting in renal chromate toxicosis, liver failure, and eventually, death.

In humans, the primary effects of Cr exposure occurs during and after its inhalation. Hexavalent Cr is highly corrosive and can cause chronic ulcerations and perforation of the nasal septum, although ulcerations of other skin surfaces occur (U.S. EPA 1980; Carson et al., 1986). These degenerative responses occur rapidly and are independent of the dose and any hypersensitivity reactions. As industrial hygiene practices (better worksite ventilation, increased usage of personal breathing masks, etc.) have improved, the reported incidence of nasomucosal ulceration/perforation by workers has decreased (Bidstrup, 1989). The possbility of similar ulcerative events occurring in nonoccupational environments is considered to be negligible; even in the heavily Cr-contaminated areas of northern New Jersey, there has yet to be any documentation of these pathologies.

Chromium compounds are also responsible for a wide range of respiratory effects. Prolonged inhalation of chromate dusts causes irritation of the respiratory tract, resulting in manifestation such as congestion and hyperemia, chronic rhinitis, congestion of the larynx, polyps of the upper respiratory tract, chronic inflammation of the lung, emphysema, chronic bronchitis, and bronchopneumonia. As with most metals, the solubility of the Cr(VI) agents impacts upon toxicity following inhalation. Insoluble Cr(VI) agents tend to have a greater retention in the lungs than do the soluble forms; however, with repeated inhalation over increasing periods of time, lung burdens eventually become roughly equivalent regardless of solubility (Cohen et al., 1997).

Contact dermatitis occurs as a result of exposure to both Cr(III) and Cr(VI), although as noted previously, ulcerative events are exclusively related to Cr(VI). Among the various Cr(VI) compounds, chromic acid is one of the more potent skin irritants (Adams, 1990); the majority of Cr(III) agents are not sensitizing under normal exposure conditions due to their poor solubility and low permeation of the dermis. However, if the concentration of the Cr(III) agent is high enough, and the exposure period prolonged enough, senzitization can be induced. Because of the disparity between the two valence states in inducing allergic contact dermatitis, only Cr(VI) compounds are utilized for patch testing for Cr sensitivity in exposed workers and residents of Cr-contaminated areas. Using standard patch test techniques, it has been shown that only about 10% of all occupationally Cr-exposed workers eventually developed allergic contact dermatitis (Peltonen and Fraki, 1983; Lee and Groh, 1988). Among the nonoccupationally exposed populace, the incidence of Cr sensitization is far lower; as of, 1996, it was estimated that the percentage of the American population senzitized to Cr (by contact with Cr in the environment and / or due to prolonged contact with leatherware) was about 0.08–1.00% (Sheehan et al., 1991; Proctor et al., 1998). To date, it is still unclear what is the threshold dose of Cr(VI) needed to induce sensitization in a previously non–Cr-exposed individual.

IMMUNOTOXICITY

Allergic contact dermatitis due to Cr is most commonly observed during occupational contact with low to moderate levels of chromates (Polak et al., 1973). This hypersensitivity usually occurs in the presence of other metal allergens (i.e., nickel or cobalt); however, the coexisting hypersensitivities are not due to immunologic cross-reactivities but rather to concomitant host sensitization (van Everdingen and van Joost, 1982; Polak, 1983). The elicited contact sensititivity is a four-stage hypersensitivity response that depends on T-lymphocyte activation rather than on formation of antibodies against any Cr-containing allergen (Arfsten et al., 1997). In the first phase (i.e., refractory period), following initial contact with the Cr compound, Cr(VI) ions penetrate cell membranes and undergo intracellular reduction; the resulting Cr(III) ions bind with cellular proteins to form Cr-protein complexes. If a level of damage sufficient enough to cause cell death occurs, the damaged / dead cell is engulfed and processed by resident antigen-presenting cells (APC). Similarly APC can engulf Cr-protein complexes if Cr-induced cell lysis occurs, and Cr-protein complexes are released into the tissue microenvironment. The APC then present the Cr-modified proteins to naive T-lymphocytes and initiate an expansion and proliferation of effector and memory lymphocytes specific for individual Cr-bearing protein/peptide complexes.

Any subsequent exposure of the individual to Cr will induce a hypersensitivity response characterized by both induction and elicitation (Haines and Nieboer, 1988). Induction occurs as a result of the APC presentation of Cr-protein/peptide complexes to memory T-lymphocytes. The elicitation arises from the subsequent release from activated T-lymphocytes of lymphokines which stimulate chemotaxis, inflammation, and edema. This cascade of cellular events also enhances further Cr-peptide / protein-specific effector T-lymphocyte proliferation. The final phase, persistence, is achieved through the continuous renewal of memory T-lymphocytes specific for each of the APC-expressed Cr-protein / peptide complexes.

That allergic contact dermatitis due to Cr exposure even occurs is peculiar in the sense that factors about Cr—including (1) a lack of universal contact sensitivity despite widespread Cr distribution in the environment, (2) a relatively weak allergenic potency for Cr itself, (3) variations in skin penetrability by different Cr compounds of equal or different valences, and (4) the long periods of exposure required for clinical manifestations to become evident—need to be overcome for the response to manifest. While the concentrations of Cr needed to induce sensitization are often only slightly greater than physiologic levels, Cr at very low or very high concentrations, or under conditions of repeated exposures, has been shown to induce states of immunological unresponsiveness (Polak et al., 1973; Vreeburg et al., 1984). The penetration of Cr(VI) through the epidermis is inversely concentration-dependent (Spruit and van Neer, 1966); however, once under the dermal layer(s), Cr(VI) reduction to Cr(III) and, ultimately, Cr(III)-protein conjugate hapten formation occur. Precisely which protein is conjugated is uncertain, but serum albumin, heparin, and glycosaminoglycans have been suggested as potential allergens (Rytter and Haustein, 1982).

Hosts that display Cr-dependent allergic contact dermatitis also display increased levels of serum IgM and IgA antibodies, increased Cr-induced lymphocyte transformation and proliferation, increased formation of immediate (E) rosettes, and decreased suppressor index values reflective of changes in the relative numbers of CD4$^+$ helper-T-lymphocytes (T$_H$) and CD8$^+$-supressor-T-lymphocytes (T$_S$) (Al-Tawil et al., 1985; Janeckova et al., 1989). An overall reduction in T$_S$ cell activity (either through a decrease in cell numbers or via Cr-mediated alterations in functionality) is thought to be responsible, at least in part, for the oberved increases in levels of circulating antibodies and immune complexes (Picardo et al., 1986). While the Cr-induced lymphocyte proliferation was found to be monocyte dependent (Al-Tawil et al., 1985), it is not clear whether monocytes (or mature macrophages) themselves, or even inflammation-associated polymorphonuclear leuko-cytes, are affected by Cr in ways that might contribute to the onset / development of the allergic response.

Because inhalation of Cr is the primary route of Cr exposure in industrial settings, studies have examined the impact of Cr compounds upon the cells critical to maintaining lung immuno-competence, namely lung macrophages. Morphologically, macrophages recovered from the lungs of animals following inhalation of either Cr(VI) or Cr(III) compounds display an increase in Cr-filled cytoplasmic inclusions, enlarged lysosomes, surface smoothing, and a decrease in membrane blebs utilized in mobility and for target contact (Johansson et al., 1986, 1987). Functionally these cells display reductions in phagocytic activity, rates of oxygen consumption following stimulation, and production of reactive oxygen intermediates used for target cell killing (Johansson et al., 1986; Galvin and Oberg, 1984; Glaser et al., 1985). The majority of the effects of Cr on macrophage structure and function have also been reproduced in vitro in alveolar macrophages from a variety of hosts. However, unlike in vivo, Cr(III) compounds are ineffective; this is most likely the result of valence-dependent differences in Cr ion entry into cells.

Immunotoxic effects arising from Cr exposure are also observed in lymphocytes. Lymphocytes exposed to Cr(VI) in vivo or in vitro display an increased incidence of chromosomal aberrations (Elias et al., 1989; Gao et al., 1992) (including DNA strand-breaks, gaps, interchanges) and increased levels of DNA-protein complex formation (Coogan et al., 1991; Toniolo et al., 1993). Although the implications from these defects are not certain, it has been suggested that changes in lymphocyte proliferation in vivo or under experimental conditions might arise as a result of the genetic alterations/damage to DNA integrity.

Functionally lymphocytes recovered from Cr-exposed hosts display altered mitogenic responsiveness (Kucharz and Sierakowski, 1987; Borella et al., 1990). At low concentrations, soluble Cr(VI) was slightly stimulatory, yet became inhibitory with increasing concentration; soluble Cr(III) was universally ineffective. An in vitro study using rat splenocytes in mixed lymphocyte cultures or in combination with B- / T-lymphocyte-specific mitogens also indicated a very narrow concentration-dependent biphasic (stimulatory / inhibitory) effect with Cr(VI) (Snyder, 1991). However, the mitogenic responsiveness of peripheral blood lymphocytes from Cr-exposed rats was enhanced overall, with even greater responsiveness when exogenous Cr was added. The basis for the discrepancies between the in vitro and in vivo studies may be (1) that Cr added to naive splenocyte cultures reacted with cell surface proteins (i.e., surface mitogen receptors) to block the proliferative effect, while (2) extended periods of in vivo exposure to Cr may have resulted in host sensitization and, ultimately, selection of lymphocyte populations that proliferate in the presence of Cr ions or Cr-conjugated protein haptens (as occurs during allergic contact dermatitis).

Other effects upon macrophages / lymphocytes induced by Cr include changes in the production/release of agents required for proper immune cell function and for induction of cellular activation critical to immunocompetency. These include decreased: levels of circulating antibody in response to viral antigens (Figoni and Treagan, 1975); formation of interferons in response to viruses/antigenic stimuli (Hahon and Booth, 1984; Christensen et al., 1992); and production of interleukin-2 (Treagan, 1975; Kucharz and Sierakowski, 1987) required for B-lymphocyte proliferation/differentiation during humoral immune responses. A disturbed immune cell intercommunication likely serves as the basis for Cr-induced reductions in cell-mediated and humoral immunity in vivo, and subsequently for the increased incidence/severity of infectious diseases and, possibly, cancers in hosts exposed to Cr compounds over extended periods of time.

CARCINOGENICITY AND TERATOGENIC EFFECTS

The carcinogenicity of Cr in experimental animals is well documented (reviewed in IARC, 1980, 1990; Cohen et al., 1993; Costa, 1997; Cohen and Costa, 1997). These studies also support the hypothesis that some of the most potent carcinogens are the slightly insoluble hexavalent compounds. An inhalation study with Wistar rats showed an increase in the incidences of lung cancers after long-term exposure to relatively low levels (i.e., $100 \, \mu g / m^3$) of $Na_2Cr_2O_7$ (Glaser et al., 1986). The three major forms of lung tumors that developed at this level of exposure included two adenomas and one adenocarcinoma, although a malignant tumor of the pharynx was also observed in one rat. No tumors were observed in the control group. In the group exposed to Cr(III), only one case of a primary adenoma of the lung was observed. Positive results were also obtained from a lifetime inhalation study employing mice (Nettesheim et al., 1971). The tumors obtained in this study were described as alveologenic adenomas and adenocarcinomas. From this and other studies, it was concluded that hexavalent Cr was a potent carcinogen. However, other variables such as exposure routes and choice of an animal model provided conflicting results regarding the absolute carcinogenicity of Cr compounds.

Studies using different routes of administration, such as the implantation of stainless steel wire mesh pellets containing chromate salts, demonstrated the inducibility of squamous cell carcinomas and adenocarcinomas in the lungs of rats exposed to $CaCrO_4$ (Laskin et al., 1970; Kuschner and Laskin, 1971). Similar studies using intrabronchial pellet implants showed positive carcinogenicities for $CaCrO_4$, $SrCrO_4$, and $ZnCrO_4$, whereas negative responses were obtained with chromite ore, Cr_2O_3 and CrO_3, Na_2CrO_4, and $Na_2Cr_2O_7$, as well as with $BaCrO_4$ and $PbCrO_4$ (Levy and Venitt, 1975a, b). The major drawback in the latter study with largely negative results was the use of only one dose (2 mg/kg) of each compound. In addition malignant tumors of the respiratory tract of rabbits, guinea pigs, rats, or mice were not produced by the administration of these various chromate salts either by inhalation and/or intratracheal injection (Steffee and Baetjer, 1965); studies with $Cr(CH_3COO^-)_3$ also failed to induce tumors in rats (Schroeder et al., 1965). Despite this conflicting evidence regarding the overall carcinogenicity of Cr, it can be concluded from these studies that some chromate and several Cr(VI) compounds are quite potent carcinogens.

Epidemiological studies of the incidence of cancer in occupationally exposed individuals have indicated that cancer mortality rates in the workers were 5 to 40 times higher than expected (Baetjer, 1950a, b; Mancuso and Hueper, 1951; Furst and Haro, 1969). An excess incidence of lung cancers has been reported in workers in the chromate producing industry and in pigment manufacturing plants (Davies, 1978; U.S. EPA, 1980). Cancer of the nasal cavities as well as of the larynx have been reported with a greater frequency in chromate workers. In addition gastric cancers have been associated with chromate exposure, although only five cases were reported in a small exposure population (U.S. EPA, 1980). A survey of three chromate pigment plants showed an increased risk of cancer in only one of the plants (Norseth, 1981). An increased risk of gastric cancer has been observed among electroplaters as well as in those employed in the ferrochromium plants (five incidences instead of three cases expected) (Langard et al., 1980). Other studies have shown that other types of cancer are elevated in Cr(VI)-exposed workers (Costa, 1997).

The teratogenicity of both Cr(III) and Cr(VI) has been demonstrated in animal studies. A study with Syrian golden hamster dams exposed to 5, 7.5, 10, or 15 mg CrO_3/kg on day 8 of gestation showed increased incidences of resorption and cleft palates in surviving pups in all treatment groups except for the lowest dosage (Gale, 1978). In addition to the craniofacial defects, the primary internal abnormalities were hydrocephaly as well as a wide range of skeletal defects. In a study employing $CrCl_3$, a dose of 19.5 mg Cr/kg administered intraperitoneally to mice on day 7, 8, or 9 of gestation resulted in increased anomalies in the litters of dams exposed on day 8 and 9 (Matsumato et al., 1976). Malformations included exencephaly and open eyelids as well as increased incidences of skeletal defects. To date, the teratogenicity of Cr has not been demonstrated in humans.

GENOTOXICITY AND MUTAGENICITY

The genotoxicity of Cr compounds have been well documented. The Cr(VI) ion is readily taken up into eukaryotic cells by anion-carrying proteins, after which it is reduced to

Cr(III) by a number of cytoplasmic reducing agents. During this reduction process, unstable intermediates of Cr(V) and Cr(IV) are formed by interacting with reduced glutathione. The final cellular form of Cr, Cr(III), becomes trapped intracellularly because it has low cell membrane permeability. This shift from Cr(VI) to Cr(III) allows a concentration gradient to be established such that a continual influx of Cr(VI) ions raises intracellular Cr levels until lethal burdens are achieved.

The reduction of Cr(VI) to Cr(III) causes the generation of oxygen radicals in cells which, in and of themselves, can produce DNA damage. Additionally the Cr(III) that is eventually formed can become adducted to the DNA. Recent studies have shown that Cr(VI) is very potent in forming DNA-protein crosslinks that involve the binding of Cr(III) to the phosphate backbone of DNA crosslinking a protein to the DNA. In addition to protein-DNA crosslinks, amino acids, such as cysteine, histidine, and glutamic acid are also crosslinked to DNA by Cr(III). These crosslinks are prevalent in cells exposed to Cr(VI) and are highly stable. They are likely to lead to mutagenic consequences and are probably more significant in determining the mutagenicity of Cr than the oxidative DNA damage produced by oxygen radicals generated during the reduction of Cr(VI) to Cr(III).

In many bacterial cells, almost all Cr(VI) compounds tested in either forward mutation or reversion assays demonstrated a mutagenic potential. In several *Salmonella typhimurium* his⁻ mutant strains, Cr(VI) caused basepair substitutions or frame-shift mutations that resulted in the recovery of histidine production (Lofroth and Ames, 1978; DeFlora, 1978; Levin et al., 1982; Nakamura et al., 1987; DeFlora et al., 1990). However, negative results were obtained with $K_2Cr_2O_7$ in a spot test using *S. typhimurium* strains TA1535, TA100, TA98, TA1537, and TA1538 (Kanematsu et al., 1980). In contrast, positive results were obtained with $K_2Cr_2O_7$ in some of these same tester strains using a plate test, while negative results were expectedly obtained with the trivalent $KCr(SO_4)_2$, $Cr(NO_3)_3$, and $CrCl_3$ agents (Petrelli and DeFlora, 1977, 1978a, b; Gava et al, 1989).

The positive mutagenic effects of Cr(VI) were demonstrated in the *Escherichia coli* strain WP2 (*try*⁻) reversion assay (Venitt and Levy, 1974). Similar results were observed with the *E. coli* WP2 *uvrA* (lacking error-prone excision repair mechanisms) strain (Nishioka, 1975) and in standard and fluctuation assays with K_2CrO_4 (Venitt and Bosworth, 1983). The *Bacillus subtillis* Rec-assay using both *rec*⁻ and *rec*⁺ strains yielded positive results with $K_2Cr_2O_7$ and K_2CrO_4 (Nishioka, 1975; Kanematsu et al., 1980; Gentile et al., 1981; Nakamura and Sayato, 1981) but not with $CrCl_3$ (Nishioka, 1975). The zone of inhibition that developed with Cr(VI) compounds was greater in the *rec*⁻ strain than in *rec*⁺ cells, indicating greater amounts of unrepaired DNA damage and cell death. Positive Rec-assay results with K_2CrO_4 were diminished by pretreatment of the host cells with the reducing agent Na_2SO_4; this suggests that the Cr(VI) oxidative state was necessary for DNA damage. While DNA damage was indicated by the Rec-assay, not all test agents displayed equal potencies; the overall order of mutagenic reactivity in this assay was $K_2Cr_2O_7 > K_2CrO_4 > CrO_3 > Cr(CH_3COO^-)_3 > Cr(NO_3)_3$ (Nakamura and Sayato, 1981).

In mammalian cells, while most Cr(VI) salts were mutagenic, Cr(III) compounds produced negative responses. Soluble salts of Cr such as $K_2Cr_2O_7$ and $ZnCrO_4$ have been shown to directly induce gene mutations in Chinese hamster V79 cells (Newbold et al., 1979). The loss of function of other target genes after Cr exposure, such as those for resistance to 6-thioguanine, ouabain, and 8-azaguanine, has also been documented (Newbold et al., 1979; Paschin and Kozachenko, 1982; Rainaldi et al., 1982). Overall, Cr(III) compounds are relatively nonmutagenic. However, one study indicated that $CrCl_3$ induced weak mutations in the human fibroblast 6-thioguanine resistance locus but that this effect was only observed with the insoluble (nonhydrated) form (Biedermann and Landolph, 1988).

A study on BHK cells exposed to $K_2Cr_2O_7$ indicated an inducible inhibition of DNA synthesis. This effect was more pronounced than the Cr-induced inhibition of either RNA or protein synthesis (Levis et al., 1978). In addition Cr compounds such as CrO_3 and $CrCl_3$ also affected the fidelity of DNA replication in vitro and in intact cells (Sirover and Loeb, 1976; DiPaolo and Casto, 1979; Tsapakos and Wetterhahn, 1983). Besides affecting DNA replication and repair mechanisms in vitro, DNA damage in the form of DNA intrastrand breaks and crosslinks, as well as DNA-protein crosslinks and Cr-DNA adducts, have been observed in rats and chick embryo tissues following in vivo exposure to Cr(VI) and not to Cr(III) (Tsapakos et al., 1983; Cupo and Wetterhahn, 1985; Hamilton and Wetterhahn, 1986; Standeven and Wetterhahn, 1989).

A number of studies have shown Cr to be capable of inducing chromosomal aberrations and enhancing cell transformation. The morphological transformation of BHK21 cells exposed to Cr(VI) was monitored by the loss of anchorage-independent growth (Hansen and Stern, 1985; Lanfranchi et al., 1988). Similar results were obtained in primary hamster embryo cells treated with $K_2Cr_2O_7$ (Hansen and Stern, 1985). In addition Cr(VI) salts increased the transformation of golden Syrian hamster embryo cells following exposure either in vivo or in vitro. Besides being the cause of direct transformation, Cr(VI) compounds (i.e., $CaCrO_4$, K_2CrO_4, and $ZnCrO_4$) altered the cell susceptibility to virally induced transformations (Casto et al., 1979).

A number of assays have shown that chromosomal aberrations can be induced by both valence states of Cr. Significant increases in the aberrations were observed in cultured BALB/c mouse and Chinese hamster V79 cells exposed to a number of Cr(III) or Cr(VI) salts (Tsuda and Kato, 1977; Newbold et al., 1979; Leonard and Deknudt, 1981; Loprieno et al., 1985). However, sister-chromatid exchange was produced in cultured lymphocytes with Cr(VI) salts exclusively (Ohno et al., 1982; Stella et al., 1982). An increase in the aberration frequency in cells obtained from occupationally-exposed individuals in Cr plating plants paralleled the observations from the in vitro studies (Bigaliev et al., 1977; Stella et al., 1982).

While both valence states of Cr are able to interact with DNA, Cr(III) ions are responsible for decreasing the fidelity of DNA replication. In addition, both Cr(III) and Cr(VI) exhibit a clastogenic potency; however, Cr(VI) possesses the greater activity and is also a powerful mutagen in many prokaryotic and eukaryotic cell systems. These properties of Cr(VI) support the claim that hexavalent compounds are likely to be active carcinogens, although it is more likely that the ultimate species responsible for the carcinogenic/mutagenic effects observed in vivo is the intracellularly derived trivalent form.

REFERENCES

ACGIH. 1989. *Documentation of the Threshold Limit Values and Biological Exposure Indices.*, 5th ed. Cincinnati: American Conference of Government Industrial Hygienists.

Adams, R. M. 1990. Allergic contact dermatitis. In *Occupational Skin Disease*, 2nd ed., e.d., R. M. Adams, pp. 26–31. Philadelphia: Saunders.

Al-Tawil, N. G., J. A. Marcusson, and E. Moller. 1985. HLA-class II restriction of the proliferative T-lymphocyte responses to nickel, cobalt, and chromium compounds. *Tissue Antigens* 25: 163–172.

Andersen, R. A., and A. S. Kozlovsky. 1985. Chromium intake, absorption and excretion of subjects consuming self-selected diets. *Am. J. Clin. Nutr.* 41: 1173–1183.

Arfsten, D. P., L. L. Aylward, and N. J. Karch. 1997. Immunotoxicity of chromium. In *Immunotoxicology of Environmental and Occupational Metals*, eds. J. T. Zelikoff and P. Thomas, pp. 63–92. London: Taylor and Francis Publishers.

ATSDR. 1989. *Toxicological Profile for Chromium.* Atlanta: Agency for Toxic Substances and Disease Registry.

Baetjer, A. M. 1950a. Pulmonary carcinoma in chromate workers: I. Reviews of literature and reports of cases. *Arch. Ind. Hyg. Occup. Med.* 2: 487–504.

Baetjer, A. M. 1950b. Pulmonary carcinomas in chromate workers: II. Incidence on basis of hospital records. *Arch. Ind. Hyg. Occup. Med.* 2: 505–516.

Bidstrup, P. L. 1989. Perspective on safety: Personal opinions. *Am. Ind. Hyg. Assoc. J.* 50: 505–509.

Biedermann, K. A., and J. R. Landolph. 1988. Influence of the valence state of chromium and solubility of chromium compounds on chromium uptake, cytotoxicity, mutagenesis, and induction of anchorage independence in diploid human fibroblasts (personal communication).

Bigaliev, A. B., M. N. Turebaev, R. K. Biganieva, and M. S. H. Elemesova. 1977. Cytogenetic examination of workers engaged in chrome production. *Genetika* 13: 545–547.

Borella, P., S. Manni, and A. Giardino. 1990. Cadmium, nickel, chromium, and lead accumulate in human lymphocytes and interfere with PHA-induced proliferation. *J. Trace Elem. Electrolytes Health Dis.* 4: 87–95.

Calabrese, E. J., R. Barnes, E. J. Stanek, H. Pastides, C. E. Gilbert, P. V. Veneman, X. Wang, A. Lasztity, and P. T. Kostechi. 1989. How much soil do young children ingest: An epidemiology study. *Regul. Toxicol. Pharmacol.* 10: 123–127.

Carson, B. L., H. V. Ellis, and J. L. McCann. 1986. *Toxicology and Biological Monitoring of Metals in Humans: Including Feasibilty and Need.* Chelsea, MI: Lewis Publishers.

Casto, B.C., J. Meyer, and J. A. Di Paolo. 1979. Enhancement of viral transformation for evualation of the carcinogenic or mutagenic potential of inorganic metal salts. *Cancer Res.* 39: 193–198.

Christensen, M. M., E. Ernst, and S. Ellerman-Eriksen. 1992. Cytotoxic effects of hexavalent chromium in cultured mouse macrophages. *Arch. Toxicol.* 66: 347–353.

Cohen, M. D., L. C. Chen, J. T. Zelikoff, and R. B. Schlesinger. 1997. Pulmonary retention and distribution of inhaled chromium: Effects of particle solubility and ozone co-exposure. *Inhal. Toxicol.* 9: 843–865.

Cohen, M. D., and M. Costa. 1997. Chromium compounds. In *Environmental and Occupational Medicine,* 2nd ed., ed. W. N. Rom, pp. 1045–1055. Boston: Little, Brown.

Cohen, M. D., B. Kargacin, C. B. Klein, and M. Costa. 1993. Mechanisms of chromium carcinogenicity and toxicity. *CRC Crit. Rev. Toxicol.* 23: 255–281.

Collin, R. J., P. O. Fromm, and W. D. Collings. 1961. Chromium excretion in the dog. *Am. J. Physiol.* 201: 795–798.

Coogan, T. P., J. Motz, C. A. Snyder, K. S. Squibb, and M. Costa. 1991. Differential DNA-protein crosslinking in lymphocytes and liver following chronic drinking water exposure of rats to potassium chromate. *Toxicol. Appl. Pharmacol.* 109: 60–72.

Costa, M. 1997. Toxicity and carcinogenicity of Cr(VI) in animal models and humans. *CRC Crit. Rev. Toxicol.* 27: 431–442.

Cowherd, D., G. E. Muleski, P. J. Englehart, and D. A. Gillette. 1985. *Rapid Assessment of Exposure to Particulate Emissions from Surface Contamination Sites.* U.S. EPA, Office of Health and Environmental Assessment, EPA/600-8-85/002.

Cupo, D. Y., and K. E. Wetterhahn. 1985. Binding of chromium to chromatin and DNA from liver and kidney of rats treated with sodium dichromate and chromium (III) chloride in vivo. *Cancer Res.* 45: 1146–1151.

Danielsson, B. R. G., E. Hassoun, and L. Dencker. 1982. Embryotoxicity of chromium: Distribution in pregnant mice and effects on embryonic cells in vitro. *Arch. Toxicol.* 51: 233–245.

Davies, J. M. 1978. Lung cancer mortality of workers making chrome pigments. *Lancet* 1: 384.

DeFlora, S. 1978. Metabolic deactivation of mutagens in the *Salmonella*-microsome test. *Nature* 271: 455–456.

DeFlora, S., M. Bagnasco, D. Serra, and P. Zanacchi. 1990. Genotoxicity of chromium compounds. A review. *Mutat. Res.* 238: 99–172.

DiPaolo, J. A., and B. C. Casto. 1979. Quantitative studies of in vitro morphological transformation of Syrian hamster cells by inorganic metal salts. *Cancer Res.* 39: 1008–1013.

Elias, Z., J. M. Mur, F. Pierre, S. Gilgenkrantz, P. Schneider, F. Baruthio, M. C. Daniere, and J. M. Fontana. 1989. Chromosome aberrations in peripheral blood lymphocytes of welders and characterization of their exposure by biological sample analysis. *J. Occup. Med.* 31: 477–483.

Environmental Science and Engineering., 1989. *Remedial Investigation for Chromium Sites in Hudson County, New Jersey*. New Jersey Department of Environmental Protection, Trenton, NJ.

Figoni, R. A., and L. Treagan. 1975. Inhibitory effect of nickel and chromium upon antibody response of rats to immunization with T-1 phage. *Res. Commun. Chem. Pathol. Pharmacol.* 11: 335–338.

Fishbein, L. 1981. Sources, transport, and alterations of metal compounds: An overview. I. Arsenic, beryllium, cadmium, chromium, and nickel. *Environ. Health Perspect.* 40: 43–64.

Food and Nutrition Board, National Research Council, 1980. *Recommended Dietary Allowances,* 9th ed., pp. 159–160. National Academy of Science. Washington, DC.

Freund, H., S. Atamian, and J. E. Fischer. 1979. Chromium deficiency during total parenteral nutrition. *J. Am. Med. Assoc.* 241: 496–498.

Furst, A., and R. T. Haro. 1969. A survey of metal carcinogenesis. *Prog. Exp. Tumor Res.* 12: 102.

Gale, T. F. 1978. Embryotoxic effects of chromium trioxide in hamster. *Environ. Res.* 16: 101–109.

Galvin, J. B., and S. G. Oberg. 1984. Toxicity of hexavalent chromium to the alveolar macrophage in vivo and in vitro. *Environ. Res.* 33: 7–16.

Gao, M., S. P. Binks, J. K. Chipman, L S.. Levy, R. A. Braithwaite, and S. S. Brown. 1992. Induction of DNA strand breaks in peripheral lymphocytes by soluble chromium compounds. *Human Exp. Toxicol.* 11: 77–82.

Gava, C. R., R. Costa, M. Zordan, P. Venier, V. Bianchi, and A. G. Levis. 1989. Induction of gene mutations in *Salmonella* and *Drosophila* by soluble Cr(VI) compounds: Synergistic effects of nitriloacetic acid (NTA). *Toxicol. Environ. Chem.* 22: 27–38.

Gentile, J. M., K. Hyde, and J. Schubett. 1981. Chromium genotoxicity as influenced by complexation and rate effects. *Toxicol. Lett.* 7: 439–448.

Glaser, U., D. Hochrainer, H. Kloppel, and H. Kuhnen. 1985. Low level chromium(VI) inhalation effects on alveolar macrophages and immune functions in Wistar rats. *Arch. Toxicol.* 57: 250–256.

Glaser, U., D. Hochrainer, H. Kloppel, and H. Oldiges. 1986. Carcinogenicity of sodium dichromate and chromium (VI/III) oxide aerosols inhaled by male Wistar rats. *Toxicology* 4: 219–232.

Goyer, R. A. 1986. Toxicity of metals. In *Toxicology*, eds. C. D. Klaassen, M. O. Amdur, and J. Doull, pp. 588–591. New York: Macmillan.

Gray, S. J., and K. Sterling. 1950. Tagging of red cells and plasma proteins with radioactive chromium. *J. Clin. Invest.* 29: 1604–1613.

Guthrie, B. E. 1982. The nutritional role of chromium. In *Biological and Environmental Aspects of Chromium*, ed. R. Vangard, pp. 117–148. Amsterdam: Elsevier Biomedical Press.

Hahon, N., and J. A. Booth. 1984. Effect of chromium and manganese particles on the interferon system. *J. Interferon Res.* 4: 17–27.

Haines, A. T., and E. Nieboer. 1988. Chromium hypersensitivity. In *Chromium in the Natural and Human Environments*, eds. J. O. Nriagu, and E. Nieboer, pp. 497–532. New York: Wiley-Interscience.

Hamilton, J. W., and K. E. Wetterhahn. 1986. Chromium (VI)-induced DNA damage in chick embryo liver and blood cells in vivo. *Carcinogensesis* 7: 2085–2088.

Hansen, K., and R. M. Stern. 1985. Welding fumes and chromium compounds in cell transformation assays. *J. Appl. Toxicol.* 5: 306–314.

Harris, D. C. 1977. Different metal-binding properties of the two sites of human transferrin. *Biochemistry* 16: 560–564.

Hertel, R. F. 1986. Sources of exposure and biological effects of chromium. *IARC Monographs* 71: 63–77.

Hopkins, L. L. 1965. Distribution in the rat of physiological amounts of ingested ^{51}Cr(III) with time. *Am. J. Physiol.* 209: 731–735.

IARC. 1980. Some Metals and Metallic Compounds. *IARC Monographs on the Evaluation of Carcinogenic Risks of Chemicals to Humans*, vol. 23, pp. 205–323. Lyon: International Agency for Research on Cancer, World Health Organization.

IARC. 1990. Chromium, Nickel, and Welding. *IARC Monographs on the Evaluation of Carcinogenic Risks of Chemicals to Humans*, vol. 49, pp. 49–256. Lyon: International Agency for Research on Cancer, World Health Organization.

Janeckova, V., S. Znojemska, L. Korcakova, M. Wagnerova, J. Kalensky, and J. Svobodova. 1989. The immune profile of contact allergy patients. *J. Hyg. Epidemiol. Microbiol. Immunol.* 33: 121–127.

Jeejeebhoy, K. N., R. C. Chu, E. B. Marliss, G. R. Greenberg, and A. Bruce-Robertson. 1977. Chromium deficiency glucose intolerance and neuropathy reversed by chromium supplementation in a patient receiving long-term total parenteral nutrition. *Am. J. Clin. Nutr.* 30: 531–538.

Jenning, M. E., and M. E. Howard. 1980. Chromium, wine and ischaemic heart disease. *Lancet* 2: 90–91.

Johansson, A., B. Robertson, C. Curstedt, and P. Camner. 1987. Alveolar macrophage abnormalities in rabbits exposed to low concentrations of trivalent chromium. *Environ. Res.* 4: 279–293.

Johansson, A., A. Wiernik, J. Jarstrand, and P. Camner. 1986. Rabbit alveolar macrophages after inhalation of hexa- and trivalent chromium. *Environ. Res.* 39: 372–385.

Kabata-Pendias, A., and H. Pendias. eds. 1984. *Trace Elements in Soils and Plants.* Boca Raton, FL: CRC Press.

Kanematsu, N., M. Hara, and T. Kada. 1980. Rec-assay and mutagenicity studies on metal compounds. *Mutat. Res.* 77: 109–116.

Kiovistoinen, P. 1982. Mineral element composition of Finnish food. *Acta Agric. Scand.* (suppl.) 22: 171.

Kucharz, E. J., and S. J. Sierakowski. 1987. Immunotoxicity of chromium compounds: Effect of sodium dichromate on the T-cell activation in vitro. *Arh. Hig. Rada Toksikol.* 38: 239–243.

Kuschner, M., and S. Laskin. 1971. Experimental models in environmental carcinogenesis. *Am. J. Pathol.* 64: 183–196.

Kuykendall, J. R., B. D. Kerger, E. J. Jarvi, G. E. Corbett, and D. J. Paustenbach. 1996. Measurement of DNA-protein crosslinks in human leukocytes following acute ingestion of chromium in drinking water. *Carcinogenesis* 17: 1971–1977.

Lanfranchi, G., S. Paglialunga, and A. G. Levis. 1988. Mammalian cell transformation induced by chromium (VI) compounds in the presence of nitrilotriacetic acid. *J. Toxicol. Environ. Health* 24: 251–260.

Langard, S. 1982. Absorption, transport and excretion of chromium in man and animals. In *Biological and Environmental Aspects of Chromium, Topics in Enviromental Health*, vol. 5, ed. S. Langard, pp. 149–169. Amsterdam: Elsevier Biomedical.

Langard, S., and T. Norseth. 1979. Chromium. In *Handbook on the Toxicology of Metals*, eds. L. Friberg, G. F. Nordberg, and V. B. Vouk, pp. 383–398. Amsterdam: Elsevier\North-Holland Biomedical.

Langard, S., A. Andersen, and B. Gylseth. 1980. Incidence of cancer among ferrochromium and ferrosilicon workers. *Br. J. Ind. Med.* 37: 114–119.

Laskin, S., M. Kuschner, and R. T. Drew. 1970. Studies in pulmonary carcinogenesis. In *Inhalation Carcinogenesis*, eds. M. G. Hanna, P. Nettesheim, and J. R. Gilbert, pp. 321–351. Oak Ridge, TN: U.S. Atomic Energy Commission.

Lee, H. E., and C. L. Goh. 1988. Occupational dermatitis among chrome platers. *Contact Dermatitis* 18: 89–93.

Leonard, A., and G. H. Deknudt. 1981. Mutagenicity test with chromium salts in mouse. *Mutat. Res.* 80: 287.

Levin, D. E., M. Hollstein, F. Christman, E. A. Schwiens, and B. N. Ames. 1982. A new *Salmonella* test strain (TA102) with A-T base pairs at the site of mutation detects oxidative mutagens. *Proc. Nat. Acad. Sci.* 79: 7445–7449.

Levis, A. G., M. Buttignol, V. Buchni, and G. Sponza. 1978. Effects of potassium dichromate on nucleic acid and protein syntheses and on precursor uptake in BHK fibroblasts. *Cancer Res.* 38: 110–116.

Levy, L. S., and S. Venitt. 1975a. Carcinogenic and mutagenic activity of chromium-containing materials. *Br. J. Cancer* 32: 254–255.

Levy, L. S., and S. Venitt. 1975b. Carcinogenicity and mutagenicity of chromium compounds: The association between bronchial metaplasia and neoplasia. *Carcinogenesis* 7: 831–835.

Lofroth, G., and B. N. Ames, 1978. Mutagenicity of inorganic compounds in *Salmonella typhimurium*: Arsenic, chromium, and selenium. *Mutat. Res.* 53: 65–66.

Loprieno, N., G. Boncristiani, P. Venier, A. Montaldi, F. Majone, V. Bianchi, S. Paglialunga, and A. G. Levis. 1985. Increased mutagenicity of chromium compounds by nitrilotriacetic acid. *Environ. Mutagen.* 8: 571–577.

Mancuso, T. F., and W. C. Hueper. 1951. A medical appraisal: I. Lung cancers in chromate workers. *Ind. Med.* 20: 358–363.

Mathur, A. K., K. K. Datta, S. K. Tandon, and T. S. Dikshith. 1977. Effect of nickel sulfate on male rats. *Bull. Environ. Contam. Toxicol.* 17: 241–248.

Matsumato, N., S. Iijima, and H. Katsunuma. 1976. Placental transfer of chromic chloride and its teratogenic potential in embryonic mice. *J. Toxicol. Sci.* 12: 1–13.

Mertz, W. 1969. Chromium occurrence and function in biological systems. *Physiol. Rev.* 49: 163–239.

Mertz, W., and K. Schwarz. 1955. Impaired intravenous glucose tolerance as an early sign of dietary necrotic liver degeneration. *Arch. Biochem. Biophys.* 58: 504–508.

Mutti, A., C. Pedroni, G. Arfinim, I. Franchini, C. Minoia, G. Micoli, and C. Baldi. 1984. Biological monitoring of occupational exposure to different chromium compounds at various valence states. *J. Environ. Anal. Chem.* 17: 35–41.

Nakamura, K., and Y. Sayato. 1981. Comparative studies of chromosomal aberration induced by trivalent and pentavalent arsenic. *Mutat. Res.* 88: 73–80.

Nakamura, S., Y. Oda, T. Shimada, I. Oki, and K. Sugimoto. 1987. SOS-inducing activity of chemical carcinogens and mutagens in *Salmonella typhimurium* TA1535/pSk1002: Examination with 151 chemicals. *Mutat. Res.*, 192: 239–246.

NAS. 1974. *Chromium*. Committee on Biological Effects of Atmosphere Pollutants. Washington, DC: National Academy of Science.

Nettesheim, P., M. G. Hanna, D. G. Doherty, R. I. Newell, and A. Hellman. 1971. Effect of calcium chromate dust, influenza virus and 100R whole body X-radiation on lung tumor incidence in mice. *J. Nat. Cancer Inst.* 47: 1129–1144.

Newbold, R. F., J. Ames, and J. R. Connell. 1979. The cytotoxic, mutagenic and clastogenic effects of chromium-containing compounds on mammalian cells in culture. *Mutat. Res.* 67: 55–63.

Nieboer, E., and A. A. Jusy. 1986. Biologic chemistry of chromium. In *Chromium in the Natural and Human Environment*, eds. J. O. Nriagu, and E. Nieboer, pp. 21–79. New York: Wiley Interscience.

NIOSH. 1979. *Registry of Toxic Effects of Chemical Substances* (RTECS). Washington, DC.

Nishioka, H. 1975. Mutagenic activities of metal compounds in bacteria. *Mutat. Res.* 31: 185–189.

Norseth, T. 1981. The carcinogenicity of chromium. *Environ. Health Perspect.* 40: 121–130.

Nriagu, J. O., and E. Nieboer, eds. 1988. *Chromium in the Natural and Human Environment*. New York: Wiley Interscience.

Nriagu, J. O., J. M. Pacyna, J. B. Milford, and C. I. Davison. 1988. Distribution and characteristic features of chromium in the atmosphere. In *Chromium in the Natural and Human Environment*, eds. J. O. Nriagu and E. Nieboer, pp. 125–172. New York: Wiley-Interscience.

Offenbaucer, E. G., H. Spencer, H. J. Dowling, and F. X. Pi-Sunyer. 1986. Metabolic chromium balance in men. *Am. J. Clin. Nutr.* 44: 77–82.

Ohno, H., F. Hanaok, and M. Yanada. 1982. Inducibility of sister-chromatid exchanges by heavy-metal ions. *Mutat. Res.* 104: 141–145.

OSHA. 1989. *Final Rule Air Contaminants—Permissible Exposure Limilts*. Title 29, Code of Federal Regulations, Part 1910.1000.

Pacyna, T. M. 1986. Emission factors of atmospheric elements. In *Toxic Metals in the Atmosphere*, eds. J. O. Nriagu, and C. Davidson, pp. 1–32. New York: Wiley.

Paschin, Y. V., and V. I. Kozachenko. 1982. The modifying effects of hexavalent chromate on the mutagenic activity of thio-TEPA. *Mutat. Res.* 103: 367–370.

Paustenbach, D. J. 1987. Assessing the potential environment and human health risks of contaminated soil. *Comments Toxicol.* 1: 185–220.

Paustenbach, D. J., P. J. Sheehan, J. M. Paull, L. M. Wisser, and B. L. Finley. 1992. Review of the allergic contact dermatitis hazard posed by chromium-contaminated soil: Identifying a "safe" concentration. *J. Toxicol. Environ. Health* 37: 177–207.

Peltonen, L., and J. Fraki. 1983. Prevalence of dichromate sensitivity. *Contact Dermatitis* 9: 190–194.

Petrelli, F. L., and S. DeFlora. 1977. Toxicity and mutagenicity of hexavalent chromium in *Salmonella typhimurium*. *Appl. Environ. Microbiol.* 33: 805–809.

Petrelli, F. L., and S. DeFlora. 1978a. Metabolic deactivation of hexavalent chromium mutagenicity. *Mutat. Res.* 54: 139–147.

Petrelli, F. L., and S. DeFlora. 1978b. Oxidation of inactive trivalent chromium to mutagenic hexavalent form. *Mutat. Res.* 58: 167–178.

Picardo, M., B. Santucci, R. Pastore, G. Valesini, D. Verducchi, and D. Bravi. 1986. Immune complexes in patients with contact dermatitis. *Dermatologica* 172: 52–53.

Polak, L. 1983. Immunology of chromium. In: *Chromium Metabolism and Toxicity*, ed. D. Burrows, pp. 51–136. Boca Raton, FL: CRC Press.

Polak, L., J. L. Turk, and J. R. Frey. 1973. Studies on contact hypersensitivity to chromium compounds. *Prog. Allergy* 17: 145–226.

Proctor, D. M., M. M. Frederick, P. K. Scott, D. J. Paustenbach, and B. L. Finley. 1998. The prevalence of chromium allergy in the United States and its implications for setting soil cleanup: A cost-effectiveness case study. *Regul. Texicol. Pharmacol.* 28: 27–37.

Rai, D., J. M. Zachara, L. E. Eary, D. C. Girvin, D. A. Moore, C. T. Resch, B. M. Sass, and R. L. Schmidt. 1986. *Geochemical Behavior of Chromium Species. Interim Report.* EPRI, EA-4544, pp. 3-1–3-16. Palo Alto: Electric Power Research Institute.

Rai, D., J. M. Zachara, L. E. Eary, C. C. Ainsworth, J. E. Amonette, C. E. Cowan, R. W. Szelmeczka, C. T. Resch, D. C. Girvin, and S. C. Smith. 1988. *Chromium Reactions in Geologic Materials. Interim Report.* EPRI, EA-5741. Palo Alto: Electric Power Research Institute.

Rainaldi, G., C. M. Colella, A. Piras, and T. Mariani. 1982. Thioguanine resistance and sister chromatid exchanges in V79/AP4 Chinese hamster cells treated with potassium dichromate. *Chem.-Biol. Interact.* 42: 45–51.

Rytter, M., and U. F. Haustein. 1982. Hapten conjugation in the leukocyte migration inhibition test in allergic contact eczema. *Br. J. Dermatol.* 106: 161–168.

Samitz, M. H., and S. Katz. 1964. A study of the chemical reactions between chromium and skin. *J. Invest. Dermatol.* 45: 35–43.

Saner, G., ed. 1980. *Chromium in Nutrition and Disease—Current Topics in Nutrition and Disease*, vol. 2, pp. 26–29. New York: Alan R. Liss.

Schroeder, H. A., J. J. Balassa, and W. H. Vinton. 1965. Chromium, cadmium, and lead in rats. Effects on life span, tumors, and tissue levels. *J. Nutr.* 86: 51–66.

Schwarz, K., and W. Mertz, 1959. Chromium(III) and glucose tolerance factor. *Arch. Biochem. Biophys.* 85: 292–295.

Sheehan, P. J., D. M. Meyer, M. M. Sauer, and D. J. Paustenbach. 1991. Assessment of the human health risks posed by exposure to chromium-contaminated soils. *J. Toxicol. Environ. Health* 32: 161–201.

Sirover, M. A., and L. A. Loeb, 1976. Infidelity of DNA synthesis in vitro: Screening for potential metal mutagens or carcinogens. *Science*, 194: 1434–1436.

Smyth, H. F., C. P. Carpenter, C. S. Weil, V. C. Pozzani, J. A. Striegel, and J. S. Nycum. 1969. Range finding toxicity data: List III. *Am. Ind. Hyg. Assoc. J.* 30: 470.

Snyder, C. A. 1991. Immune function assays as indicators of chromate exposure. *Environ. Health Perspect.* 92: 83–86.

Spruit, D., and F. C. van Neer. 1966. Penetration rate of Cr(III) and Cr(VI). *Dermatologica* 132: 179–182.

Standeven, A. W., and K. E. Wetterhahn. 1989. Chromium (VI) toxicity: Uptake, reduction, and DNA damage. *J. Am. Cell Toxicol.* 8: 1275–1283.

Steffee, C. H., and A. M. Baetjer. 1965. Histopathological effects of chromate chemicals. Report of studies in rabbits, guinea pigs, rats, and mice. *Arch. Environ. Health* 11: 66–75.

Stella, M., A. Mentaldi, R. Rossi, G. Rossi, and A. G. Levis. 1982. Clastogenic effects of chromium on human lymphocytes in vitro and in vivo. *Mutat. Res.* 101: 151–164.

Stern, R. M., E. Thomsen, and A. Furst. 1984. Cr(VI) and other metallic mutagens in fly ash and welding fumes. *Toxicol. Environ. Chem.* 8: 95–108.

Tandon, S. K., D. K. Saxena, J. S. Gaur, and S. V. Chandra. 1978. Comparative toxicology of trivalent and hexavalent chromium. Alterations in blood and liver. *Environ. Res.* 15: 90–99.

Toniolo, P., A. Zhitkovich, and M. Costa. 1993. Development and utilization of a new simple assay for DNA-protein crosslinks as a biomarker of exposure to welding fumes. *Int. Arch. Occup. Environ. Health* 65: S87–S89.

Treagan, L. 1975. Metals and the immune response, a review. *Res. Commun. Chem. Pathol. Pharmacol.* 12: 189–220.

Tsapakos, M. J., and K. E. Wetterhahn. 1983. The interaction of chromium with nucleic acids. *Chem.-Biol. Interact.* 46: 265–277.

Tsapakos, M. J., T. H. Hampton, and K. E. Wetterhahn. 1983. Chromium (VI)-induced DNA lesions and chromium distribution in rat kidney, liver, and lungs. *Cancer Res.* 43: 5662–5667.

Tsuda, H., and K. Kato. 1977. Chromosomal aberrations and morphological transformation in hamster embryonic cells treated with potassium dichromate in vitro. *Mutat. Res.* 46: 87–94.

U.S. EPA. 1975. Region V joint federal/state survey of organic and inorganics in selected drinking water supplies. Draft report, Chicago.

U.S. EPA. 1980. *Health Assessment Document for Chromium.* United States Environmental Protection Agency, Environmental Criteria and Assessment Office. Research Triangle Park, NC.

U.S. EPA. 1986. *Record of Decision for Industri-Plex. Woburn, MA.* U.S. Environmental Protection Agency, Research Triangle Park, NC.

U.S. EPA. 1987a. *Record of Decision for Frontier Hard Chrome. Vancouver, WA.* U.S. Environmental Protection Agency, Research Triangle Park, NC.

U.S. EPA. 1987b. *Record of Decision of Palmetto Wood Preserving. Dixiana, SC.* U.S. Environmental Protection Agency, Research Triangle Park, NC.

U.S. EPA. 1988a. *Record of Decision for Odessa Chromium I. Odessa, TX.* U.S. Environmental Protection Agency, Research Triangle Park, NC.

U.S. EPA. 1988b. *Record of Decision for Odessa Chromium II. Odessa, TX.* U.S. Environmental Protection Agency, Research Triangle Park, NC.

Underwood, E. J., ed. 1977. *Trace Elements in Human and Animal Nutrition.* New York: Academic Press.

van Everdingen, J. E., and T. van Joost. 1982. Hypersensitivity for nickel, chromium and cobalt; A continuous problem. *Ned. T. Geneesk* 126: 1088–1092.

Venitt, S., and D. Bosworth. 1983. The development of anaerobic methods for bacterial mutation assays: Aerobic and anaerobic fluctuation test of human fecal extracts and reference mutagens. *Carcinogenesis* 4: 339–345.

Venitt, S., and L. S. Levy. 1974. Mutagenicity of chromate in bacteria and its relevance to chromate carcinogenesis. *Nature* 250: 493–495.

Vreeburg, K. J., K. deGroot, B. M. von Blomberg, and R. J. Scheper. 1984. Induction of immunological tolerance by oral administration of nickel and chromium. *J. Dent. Res.* 63: 124–128.

WHO. 1988. *Chromium. Environmental Health Criteria No. 61.* Geneva: World Health Organization.

7 Diesel Exhaust

JOE L. MAUDERLY, D.V.M

HISTORICAL OVERVIEW

The compression ignition (diesel) engine was patented by Rudolf Diesel in 1892. The chief difference between diesel engines and spark-ignition gasoline engines is that the fuel–air mixture in diesel engines is ignited by the heat of compression alone. Diesel engines have several advantages over their gasoline counterparts. They are generally more efficient in converting fuel energy to work because they operate at higher compression ratios and temperatures, use no throttling of air at partial loads, and burn fuel that is higher in specific energy content. Diesel fuel is less highly refined than gasoline; indeed, Rudolph Diesel showed that compression ignition engines could burn a variety of low-grade fuels including coal dust. Diesel engines generally have greater durability than gasoline engines. It is not uncommon to find 30-year-old engines in regular operation in commercial fleets, and contemporary long-haul truck engines go multiple hundreds of thousands of miles between overhauls. Diesel fuel has a lower vapor pressure than gasoline, and thus contributes less to organic air pollution from evaporative emissions and presents a lower explosive hazard than gasoline.

On the other hand, diesel engines have historically been heavier and noisier than equivalent spark ignition engines, and were characterized by more vibration and less torque (slower acceleration) at low speeds. Diesel engines of the past were also characterized by much more visible and malodorous tailpipe emissions than equivalent gasoline engines. These characteristics, coupled with low gasoline prices, have limited their use in passenger cars and other light- and medium-duty vehicles in the United States. However, diesel engines are prevalent in applications in which fuel economy and durability offset the negative factors, such as heavy-duty trucks, buses, off-road heavy equipment, and railroad locomotives. Diesel-powered trucks were introduced into the western U.S. trucking fleet in the 1940s and into the rest of the country during the 1950s and 1960s. Diesel trucks constituted the majority of heavy-duty truck sales for the first time in 1961 (Motor Vehicles Manufacturers Association,1962), and they are now used in essentially all heavy-duty trucking, construction, and agricultural applications.

The dieselization of railroad locomotives occurred primarily after World War II. The approximate midpoint of dieselization was 1952, and by 1959, 95% of locomotives in the United States were diesel powered (U.S. Department of Labor,1972). Some railroads incorporated diesel locomotives earlier; the Baltimore and Ohio first used diesels in 1935 (Kaplan,1959). The penetration of diesel engines into above ground mining applications paralleled their penetration into the trucking and construction industries. The introduction of diesel engines into underground mines was more recent; approximately 1000 units were being used in coal mines in 1983 (Daniel,1984).

Environmental Toxicants: Human Exposures and Their Health Effects, 2/e. Edited by Morton Lippmann.
ISBN: 0-471-29298-2 © 2000 John Wiley & Sons, Inc.

Diesel engines are much more prevalent in light-duty applications in Europe than in the United States, largely because of the higher fuel prices. During recent years European concerns for emissions focused more on global warming than on particles, and diesels emit less carbon dioxide than equivalent gasoline engines. As a result the development of light-duty diesel engines with performance characteristics acceptable to individual consumers occurred primarily in Europe. This development demonstrated clearly that compression ignition engines can be made suitable for passenger car use.

There have been remarkable engineering advances in compression ignition engine technology in the United States during the past 10 years, driven both by market competition for fuel efficiency, durability, and performance and by the need to meet increasingly stringent emissions standards. Although still called "diesels," new technology compression ignition engines hardly resemble diesel engines of the past. Tailpipe emissions of soot particles and toxic gases are rapidly approaching the levels of those from gasoline engines, while fuel economy and durability continue to increase. The new diesel engines are finding increasing use in light-duty trucks (pickups) in the United States, and it appears likely that they will be used increasingly in the growing sport utility vehicle market. It now appears plausible that with continued technological development, compression-ignition, direct-injection engines might also find increasing use in passenger cars in the United States.

There are concerns for the potential adverse health effects of diesel exhaust because it contains trace amounts of toxic compounds and because occupational exposures are common and environmental exposures are widespread. Diesel exhaust is a ubiquitous component of air pollution. The contribution of soot from older engines to particulate pollution has received considerable attention recently, in parallel with heightened concerns for the health effects of fine particles in urban air. All people living in developed countries are exposed frequently to diesel exhaust at some concentration, although average exposures are low. While the potential for diesel exhaust to present a health hazard has been known for several decades, the current emphasis can be traced to the reporting in the late 1970s that extracts from diesel soot were mutagenic to bacteria. Research during the past 20 years focused almost exclusively on the potential contribution of diesel exhaust to human lung cancer risk.

Diesel exhaust is undoubtedly the most thoroughly studied complex environmental pollutant mixture in history. Nonetheless, it remains as remarkably true today as it was in 1982 (Williams,1982) that "the history of diesel emission studies is still being written." The history of diesel exhaust health concerns, research, and regulatory quandary is an excellent case study of the difficulties attendant to understanding and controlling environmental health risks. The purpose of this chapter is to provide an update on our understanding of the health effects of diesel exhaust from that contained in the first edition (Mauderly, 1992). Other excellent sources of information are the 1995 report by the Health Effects Institute (HEI,1995), the health assessment document developed by the California EPA (Cal EPA, 1998), and the draft health assessment document developed by U.S. EPA (1998). The California document has been recently finalized, but the EPA document is still a review draft, and does not yet represent the final Agency position.

EXPOSURES TO DIESEL EXHAUST

Composition of Diesel Exhaust and Potential Toxicity of Exhaust Components

Diesel exhaust is a complex and variable mixture of gases, vapors, and particles (soot), consisting of a very large number of elements and compounds. The complexity of diesel exhaust makes it difficult to associate adverse health effects with any single compound or class of compounds. For example, it is known that the organic fraction of diesel soot contains mutagenic activity, but over 450 organic compounds have been identified in diesel exhaust (Opresko et al., 1984). Few, if any, of the elements and compounds contained in the gas, vapor, and particulate phases of diesel exhaust are unique; most are also present in exhaust from other engines and in the effluents from other types of combustion of organic matter. This, along with the difficulty of determining exposure levels of occupational groups and the impossibility of identifying clearly unexposed populations, makes it difficult to determine with confidence whether or not environmental diesel exhaust exposures have caused adverse health effects in humans. This chapter does not describe the composition of diesel exhaust in detail. In addition to the references given, several compilations of exhaust composition and factors contributing to variations in composition have been published (Lewtas, 1982; Ishinishi, et al. 1986a; Johnson, 1988; International Agency for Research on Cancer [IARC], 1989; HEI, 1995). An abbreviated listing of the classes of compounds in diesel exhaust is presented in Table 7-1.

The complete combustion of petroleum fuel produces primarily carbon dioxide, water, and nitrogen; the other diesel exhaust emissions result largely from incomplete combustion and pyrosynthesis. Because the air entering diesel engines is not throttled, they can operate at air–fuel ratios other than that required for stoichiometric combustion. Fuel is injected under pressure into the combustion chamber in variable amounts to achieve different engine speeds and power outputs. Conditions promoting incomplete combustion are exacerbated before a new steady state is reached at each power setting, contributing to increases in emissions during load changes. The fuel is aerosolized under pressure by injection nozzles, and the air–fuel mixture is self-ignited by compression. Less than ideal injection timing, fuel aerosolization and distribution, and combustion chamber shape and temperature also contribute to incomplete combustion. The products of incomplete combustion include carbon monoxide and unburned fuel and lubricants, together with their additives. Nitrogen dioxide, although not a product of incomplete fuel combustion, is also an emission of concern.

Particulate Phase

Concern for the carcinogenicity of diesel exhaust centers on the organic hydrocarbons associated with soot particles. The soot consists of aggregates of spherical primary particles that form in the combustion chamber, grow by agglomeration, and are emitted as clusters having volume median diameters ranging from 0.1 to 0.5 m (Cheng et al., 1984). The elemental carbon core has a high specific surface area ($30-50\ m^2/g$: Frey and Corn, 1967) and serves as a nucleus for condensation of organic compounds formed and volatilized by combustion. As released to the environment, the portion of the mass of diesel soot consisting of adsorbed organic matter can range from 5% to 90% (Johnson, 1988), with values of 10% to15% representative of modern engines under most operating conditions. This adsorbed organic matter can be extracted from the elemental carbon core by solvents; however, heat and ultrasonic energy are required to separate all of the organic fraction from the inorganic carbon. Considerable effort has been expended in characterizing the types and biological activities of compounds contained in diesel soot extracts (Schuetzle et al., 1985; Schuetzle and Lewtas, 1986; Enya et al., 1997).

The size of diesel soot makes it readily respirable. Approximately 20% to 30% of the inhaled particles in diluted exhaust would be expected to deposit in the lungs and airways of humans (Snipes, 1989). The health risks lie in the small, poorly visible particles; the larger soot "flakes" visible in puffs of concentrated exhaust from older engines are too large to be readily respirable and few would be expected to enter the lung. Interestingly, as the mass emissions of soot are reduced by advances in combustion technology, the number of ultrafine (less than 0.1 μm) soot particles tends to increase (Bagley, 1996). Although it is speculated that ultrafine particles would have greater penetration into respiratory tissues,

TABLE 7-1   Abbreviated List of Classes of Compounds in Diesel Exhaust

Particulate Phase

Elemental carbon
Heterocyclics, hydrocarbons (C_{14}–C_{35}), and
   polycyclic aromatic hydrocarbons and derivatives:

Acids	Ketones
Alcohols	Nitriles
Aldehydes	Quinones
Anhydrides	Sulfonates
Esters	Halogenated and nitrated cpds.

Inorganic sulfates and nitrates
Metals

Gas and vapor phases

Acrolein
Ammonia
Carbon dioxide
Carbon monoxide
Benzene
1,3-Butadiene
Formaldehyde
Formic acid
Heterocyclics, hydrocarbons (C_1–C_{18}),
   and derivatives (as listed above)
Hydrogen cyanide
Hydrogen sulfide
Methane
Methanol
Nitric and nitrous acids
Nitrogen oxides
Sulfur dioxide
Toluene
Water

Source: Adapted from NRC 1983; Lies et al., 1986; Schuetzle and Frazier 1986; Carey 1987; Zaebst et al., 1988.

which coupled with their higher relative surface area per unit of mass may confer greater toxicity than larger soot particles, the health implications of reduced soot size are not known at this time.

Huisingh et al. (1978) reported that diesel soot extracts were mutagenic in the Ames *Salmonella typhimurium* assay and that the mutagenicity was "direct acting" and did not require metabolic activation. The extracts are also direct-acting mutagens in in vitro mammalian cell systems (Brooks et al., 1984; Morimoto et al., 1986; HEI, 1995; Enya et al., 1997). Considerable research has been done on the mutagenicity of diesel soot extracts, including variations in activity with engine and fuel type and operating conditions (Clark et al., 1981, 1984; Claxton, 1983; Brooks et al., 1984). Although the amount of solvent-extractable organic matter and its mutagenicity vary somewhat with these factors, the variation is typically less than an order of magnitude. All diesel soot extracts are mutagenic, and it appears reasonable to generalize among exhausts from a broad range of diesel applications when considering the toxicity of diesel exhaust.

The compounds responsible for the mutagenicity, and possibly carcinogenicity, of diesel soot extract and their potential bioavailability once the particles are deposited in the lung have been subjects of much research and debate. Summary lists of compounds found in soot extract and summaries of research efforts described briefly below can be found in Johnson (1988) and IARC (1989). Most concern has focused on the polycyclic aromatic hydrocarbons, a class that includes numerous known and suspected mutagens and carcinogens. Early attention focused largely on benzo(a)pyrene. More recently attention has turned to the more than 50 nitrated polycyclics, such as the nitropyrenes, that are present in lower concentrations but are considered to be responsible for a large part of the direct-acting mutagenic activity (Manabe et al., 1985; Howard, 1990). Enya et al. (1997) has identified 3-nitrobenzanthrone as a potent mutagen in soot extract. Although researchers will undoubtedly continue to identify the responsible chemical species, their identification does not change the long-recognized mutagenicity of the organic fraction of soot.

The extent of the availability of soot-borne organic compounds for interaction with DNA in cells in the lung, gastrointestinal tract, or elsewhere in the body remains uncertain. Early work suggested that little mutagenic activity would be released from soot in biological fluids and that inactivation or the reduction of mutagenesis would result from the binding of reactive compounds to proteins or other non-DNA molecules in the body (Brooks et al., 1981; King et al., 1981; Li, 1981). It was shown that cultured alveolar macrophages take up diesel soot in vitro and release metabolites back into the medium (Bond et al., 1984). It was also shown that substantial portions of the metabolites of inhaled soot-borne benzo(a)pyrene and nitropyrene are released from the soot, metabolized, and either bind to pulmonary tissues or are excreted (Sun et al.,1984; Bond et al.,1986). More recently Keane et al. (1991) demonstrated that diesel soot dispersed in simulated pulmonary surfactant has mutagenic activity.

Information on DNA adducts in lungs of rats exposed chronically to diesel exhaust does little to resolve the bioavailability of soot-borne organic mutagens. Early circumstantial evidence for bioavailability was provided by the finding that rats exposed repeatedly to diesel exhaust had increased levels of total DNA adducts in the respiratory tract (Wong et al., 1986; Bond et al., 1990a, b, c, d; Wolff et al., 1990). More recent results show that although total adduct levels may be increased during chronic exposure, the increases occur in adducts that are also present in controls and do not increase progressively with time (Randerath et al., 1995). Moreover increases in DNA adducts similar to those resulting from diesel exhaust exposure also occur in rats exposed similarly to mutagen-poor carbon black (Gallagher et al., 1994; Randerath et al., 1995) and titanium dioxide (Gallagher et al., 1994). The only suggestion of a diesel-specific adduct effect was the report by Gallagher et al. (1994) of one DNA adduct in diesel-exposed rats that was not found in rats exposed to carbon black or titanium dioxide. To date, there has been no report of a follow-up of this finding. Coupled with the finding that the organic fraction of diesel soot apparently plays little, if any, role in the carcinogenicity of soot in rats (described later), the present DNA adduct information from rats does not clarify the bioavailability of soot-borne organic mutagens.

While it remains plausible that at least a portion of the soot-borne organic material is released in the lung and is available to exert genotoxicity, the extent and rapidity of the bioavailability of the organic fraction and the relationship between these compounds and adduction of DNA and mutagenicity in vivo remain subjects of debate.

Gas and Vapor Phases

There has been less concern for the health effects of gases and vapors in diesel exhaust than for the soot. Diesel exhaust contains carbon monoxide, nitrogen oxides, and sulfur dioxide; irritants such as acrolein, ammonia, and acids; and a spectrum of low-molecular-weight vapor-phase organic compounds (Table 7-1). Emissions of carbon monoxide are typically lower than for gasoline engines and nitrogen oxide emissions are similar to those from comparable light-duty gasoline engines. Emissions of nitrogen dioxide from heavy-duty diesels are typically higher than those from comparable gasoline engines (Schuetzle and Frazier, 1986). Unfortunately, the engine design and operating factors that reduce emissions of nitrogen dioxide tend to increase emissions of particles, and vice versa. Considerable effort is being expended to optimize this engineering trade-off and achieve reductions of both pollutants.

The health effects of the inorganic gas phase of diesel emissions are not an issue unique to diesel exhaust and are not discussed here; much has been written about the effects of carbon, nitrogen, and sulfur oxides (see other chapters in this volume). The effect of diesel is simply to contribute to the environmental burdens of these ubiquitous pollutants.

The organic gases and vapors consist of C_1–C_{18} hydrocarbons, two- to four-ring polycyclic aromatic hydrocarbons, nitrated and oxygenated derivatives of C_1–C_{12} hydrocarbons, and two- to three-ring polycyclic aromatic hydrocarbons. Most of the C_1–C_{10} hydrocarbons result from the breakdown of larger hydrocarbons during combustion. The partitioning of compounds between the gas and particulate phases of exhaust depends on the vapor pressure, temperature, and concentration of each species (Hampton et al., 1983; Schuetzle, 1983). Few, if any, of the organic gases and vapors are uniquely emitted from diesel engines; most are also emitted from other petroleum fuel combustion sources. Although their potential effects are not well understood, little concern has been raised for the long-term health effects of these compounds. As described later, lung tumors are not induced in rats by chronic exposure to high concentrations of diesel exhaust if the exhaust is filtered and animals are exposed to only the gas and vapor phases. The volatile compounds, however, are not without adverse effects. People exposed to high concentrations of diesel exhaust complain about objectionable odor, headache, nausea, and eye irritation, symptoms thought to be primarily associated with the gas- and vapor-phase constituents. It is not known if there is any link between these transient symptoms and other health effects.

Emissions Standards and Current Exposure Levels

Tailpipe emissions standards for diesel engines have become progressively more stringent, and have been met largely by advances in engine technology. Particulate emission standards were first set at 0.6 g / mile for light-duty diesel cars and trucks in 1982; no standards were set at that time for heavy-duty vehicles. In 1987, the standards became 0.2 g / mile for light-duty cars and 0.26 g / mile for light-duty trucks. Standards for heavy-duty vehicles were first set at 0.6 g / brake horsepower-hour (bhp-h) in 1988. In 1991, the standard became 0.1 g / bhp-h for urban buses and 0.26 g / bhp-h for other heavy-duty vehicles. In 1994, the standard became 0.10 g / bhp-h for all heavy-duty vehicles, and sales-weighted averaging of emission rates among the engine families produced by each manufacturer was allowed. In 1996, the standard became 0.1 g / bhp-h.

Standards have also become progressively stringent for nitrogen oxides, the other pollutant class of major concern. The standard was 10.7 g / bhp-h in 1985, and it became 4.0 g / bhp-h in 1998.

The environmental concentrations of airborne pollutants derived from diesel emissions are not well characterized. There are only a few actual data for diesel soot concentrations in specific environmental locations and only rough estimates of average exposures. These data are based largely on elemental carbon on filter samples; few data are derived from more diesel-specific markers. Routine environmental air quality sampling does not distinguish among particles of different composition and only crudely distinguishes on the basis of particle size. Even in special studies aimed at source apportionment, it remains difficult to distinguish diesel soot from small carbonaceous particles emitted from other combustion sources. While diesel soot constitutes a minority of fine particulate matter in most urban settings, it constitutes a majority of particulate matter from on-road vehicles (HEI, 1995).

The U.S. EPA estimated that the U.S. annual average concentration of airborne diesel soot in 1990 was $1.80\,\mu g/m^3$, and that the urban and rural averages were 2.03 and $1.10\,\mu g/m^3$, respectively (U.S. EPA, 1993). The urban, rural, and nationwide average concentrations were predicted to fall to 0.44, 0.24, and $0.39\,\mu g/m^3$, respectively, by 2010. The California EPA recently estimated that annual average diesel soot concentrations in 1990 ranged from 0.2 to $3.6\,\mu g/m^3$ in different regions of that state, and that the current statewide population-weighted average exposure was $1.54\,\mu g/m^3$ (Cal EPA, 1998). Although these estimates involve a number of uncertainties, they suggest that the majority of the U.S. population is probably exposed to concentrations in the range of $1–3\,\mu g/m^3$.

There are few data for actual concentrations of diesel soot in occupational settings. Most estimates are based on filter samples of fine particles, or on analysis of elemental carbon concentrations adjusted to estimated soot concentrations on the basis of an assumed carbon–soot ratio. The best current review of our knowledge of occupational exposure levels is that reported by the Health Effects Institute (HEI, 1995). Workplace exposures of miners, truck drivers, vehicle operators, and other workers thought to have high exposures ranged from approximately 4 to $1700\,\mu g/m^3$. Workers in enclosed spaces, and particularly in mines, had the highest exposures, not uncommonly near or above $1000\,\mu g/m^3$.

Exposures of railroad workers and truck drivers are of particular interest because of the controversy about epidemiological data from those worker groups (described later). Woskie et al. (1988a) used personal air samplers to measure concentrations of total respirable particles in several work environments of four northern U.S. railroads. They measured the nicotine content of the collected particles and subtracted the estimated contribution of cigarette smoke. The smoke–adjusted geometric mean values for respirable particles were $17\,\mu g/m^3$ for office clerks, $39–73\,\mu g/m^3$ for engineers and firers, $52–191\,\mu g/m^3$ for brakemen and conductors, and $114–134\,\mu g/m^3$ for locomotive shop workers. If the authors' assumption that the smoke-adjusted particle concentration for office clerks represented nondiesel background was correct, the diesel soot concentrations for the most highly exposed groups were approximately $100\,\mu g/m^3$. These authors used a statistical model to estimate that the national average exposures for railroad workers was approximately $10\,\mu g/m3$ lower than the values for the northern railroads and that the exposure concentrations were probably constant from the 1950s to 1983 (Woskie et al., 1988b).

Perhaps the best data for exposures of truck drivers are those reported by Zaebst et al. (1991), who used personal samplers to measure exposures to elemental carbon. They reported geometric mean values of approximately $4\,\mu g/m^3$, which would imply soot exposures of approximately $7\,\mu g/m^3$ based on their assumption that soot was approximately 60% elemental carbon. Interestingly the soot exposures of the drivers were not much higher than roadside background levels, suggesting that their exposures resulted more from their presence in a roadway environment than from their position in truck cabs near exhaust stacks.

HEALTH EFFECTS

Concerns for adverse health effects of diesel exhaust have focused largely on lung cancer; thus, this issue is described in the most detail in the following sections. There has also been concern for other health effects of diesel exhaust, both because of its unique characteristics and because of its contribution to general air pollution. Because diesel soot is ubiquitous and comprises a variable portion of ambient particulate matter, it is included in current concerns for the effects of environmental particulate matter on mortality and morbidity. At this time there is little evidence that diesel soot plays any unique role other than its contribution to the fine particle mass generated from combustion sources. General particulate matter issues will not be described in this chapter; the reader is referred to Chapter 2 in this volume, a recent review (Vedal, 1997), and to the Criteria Document (1996a) and Staff Paper (1996b) developed by the U.S. EPA as part of the recent review of the national ambient air quality standard for particulate matter.

It is plausible that inhaled diesel exhaust might contribute to noncancer and extrapulmonary effects. Organic compounds in the vapor and soot phases of diesel exhaust, and their metabolites, might be transferred from the lung to other organs. Humans might also be affected by ingested diesel soot. Cuddihy et al. (1980), extrapolating from calculations derived from studies of airborne lead, estimated that much more diesel soot is ingested by humans than is deposited by inhalation.

Lung Cancer

Epidemiology   The most relevant information on the human health risks from exposures to potential toxicants is information obtained from studies of humans themselves, assuming that the information is adequate for establishing exposure-effects relationships with confidence. Numerous epidemiological studies of the relationship between diesel exhaust exposure and lung cancer have been reported, if one considers both the studies focusing specifically on diesel exhaust and those including occupations that may be presumed to have received substantial exposures to diesel exhaust. This body of information is large but weakened by the universal lack of direct measures of the exhaust exposures of the populations studied. The weight of the epidemiological evidence reviewed below suggests a positive effect of small magnitude, but confidence in conclusions drawn from this largely circumstantial evidence is eroded by uncertainties regarding exposure and potential confounding by cigarette smoking and other exposures. For additional perspectives, the reader is directed to other contemporary reviews of this same information (HEI, 1995; Cal EPA, 1998; U.S. EPA, 1998; HEI, 1999).

The level of confidence with which one can draw conclusions from the epidemiological studies of workers regarding cancer risks from lower environmental exposures is limited by the confidence one has in the accuracy of the estimates of worker exposures. The strongest evidence for an exposure-response relationship has been thought to be contained in the series of two studies of railroad workers (Garshick et al., 1987a, 1988) for which historical exposures were estimated from measurements in contemporary work environments. Four other studies used interviews or questionnaires, completed by the subjects or next of kin, that specifically addressed diesel exhaust exposure history (Lerchen et al., 1987; Boffetta et al., 1988; Siemiatycki et al., 1988; Swanson et al., 1993). In decreasing order of probable specificity for diesel exhaust, exposure classifications in other studies were derived from job history by interview of subject or family, job history from employment records, general occupational history from interview, general occupational history from death certificate or other individual record, and record of membership in a trade union.

Uncertainties in exposure assessment also result from the variable times that subjects in different studies were required to have spent in a particular job or occupation in order to have been considered "exposed." The classification of "ever" employed in an occupation and the requirement in some studies of employment in an occupation for only a short time (e.g., a little as six months) during a subject's working lifetime seriously compromise the usefulness of the results. Additional difficulties arise from the exposure of presumed "control" populations to diesel exhaust in the environment and the overlapping of the composition of diesel exhaust with those of other common pollutant mixtures. Finally information on tobacco smoking was only obtained in approximately one-half of the studies. Because the relative risk for lung cancer among smokers is 20–50 times greater than that suggested for diesel exhaust exposures, small imbalances in smoking among diesel exhaust "exposed" and "unexposed" groups, or small misclassifications of smoking histories, could have tremendous leverage on the apparent relationship between diesel exhaust exposure and lung cancer.

This chapter presents results from numerous studies, rather than only those from the few considered to be strongest. Readers can thus judge for themselves the weight of evidence for the association between diesel exhaust exposure and lung cancer. Forty-one epidemiological studies are grouped into 22 cohort studies, 18 case-control studies, and one combined analysis of the results of 9 studies. The studies are summarized in tabular form in order of publication date in Tables 7-2 and 7-3. Selected study characteristics and reported relative risks for lung cancer are presented for comparison. For reports listing multiple study groups or analyses, only the results considered most robust are presented. The 95% confidence intervals (CI) for the significantly elevated relative risks are given in the text if they were reported.

Cohort Studies   Reports of 20 retrospective and two prospective cohort studies of occupational groups thought to have substantial exposures to diesel exhaust are summarized in Table 7-2. These reports spanned 34 years, from 1957 to 1991, and examined truck and bus drivers, railroad workers, mechanics, miners, heavy equipment operators, dock workers, and vehicle examiners. The size of the total cohort populations ranged from fewer than 700 to over 476,000, and the numbers of deaths ranged from fewer than 100 to over 17,000. The time spans encompassing the data (study period) ranged from 3 months to 38 years.

Because of the importance of cigarette smoking as a confounding variable, the cohort studies listed in Table 7-2 are readily grouped for discussion into the 2 studies that considered smoking and the 20 studies that did not. Although the importance of tobacco smoking was acknowledged by virtually all investigators, only the study by Boffetta et al. (1988) incorporated adjustments for individual smoking. Garshick et al. (1988) did not adjust for smoking but collected information suggesting that the proportions of smokers were similar in their diesel exhaust-exposed and exhaust-unexposed cohorts. These two studies are further strengthened relative to the other 20 by the evaluation of large cohorts having large numbers of deaths and by using the strongest indexes of diesel exhaust exposure. In view of these strengths, it is particularly noteworthy that these two studies both demonstrated significantly elevated relative risks for lung cancer among subcohorts thought to have received substantial exposure to diesel exhaust.

Boffetta et al. (1988) examined the relationship between lung cancer and occupational exposure to diesel exhaust using data from a prospective mortality study begun in 1982 by the American Cancer Society. Living volunteer subjects from across the United States were enrolled in this study by completing a questionnaire that included, among many other items, information on smoking, occupation, job held for the longest period, and exposures to diesel exhaust. Cancer Society volunteers checked the status of enrollees every two years, and death certificates were obtained for decedents. The analysis by Boffetta et al. was limited to men 40 to 79 years old at enrollment, whose status was recorded at the end of the first two year follow-up (September 1984). Information was obtained for 11,044 decedents (1266 lung cancer cases) among 476,648 men, including 174 lung cancer cases among 378,622 men claiming to have been exposed to diesel exhaust. The reference population was men with no reported exposure or presumed occupational exposure to diesel exhaust.

Neither the relative risk for mortality from all causes nor the smoking-adjusted relative risk for lung cancer (1.18) was significantly increased among all men exposed to diesel

TABLE 7-2 Cohort Studies of the Relationship between Diesel Exhaust Exposure and Lung Cancer

Date	Author	Population	Population Size[a]	Number of Deaths	Study Period (years)[b]	Exposure Assessment	Control for Smoking	Relative Risk	Statistical Significance[c]
1957	Raffle	London transport employees	15,995 man-years	84	4	Job record	−	1.42, garage workers, 55–64 years	NR[d]
1959	Kaplan	Baltimore and Ohio railroad workers	6506	6506	5	Job record	−	0.88, most likely exposed	NR
1973	Waxweiler et al.	U.S. potash miners	3886	433	27	Diesel use in mine	−	(Reported lack of excess lung cancer)	
1978	Luepker and Smith	U.S. Teamsters' Union (central, southeast, and southwest)	179,756	245	0.25	Union membership	−	1.21, entire cohort	−
								1.37, age 50–59	+
1981	Ahlberg et al.	Swedish male truck drivers	34,027	NR	12	Job record	−	1.33, entire cohort	+
1981	Stern et al.	New Jersey vehicle examiners	1558	233	29	Years in job	−	1.02, entire cohort	NR
1981	Waller	London transport employees	20,000	NR	25	Job record	−	0.90, garage workers	−
1983	Howe et al.	Canadian railroad workers	43,826	16,812	12	Job at retirement	−	1.35, "probably exposed"	+
1983	Rushton et al.	London bus maintenance workers	8684	701	8	Job record	−	1.01, entire cohort	NR
1985	Wong et al.	U.S. heavy equipment operators	34,156	3243	14	Union membership	−	1.07, 20+ year members	+ (time trend)[e]
								1.30, retiring at age 65	+
1986	Gustafsson et al.	Swedish dock workers	6071	1062	20	Employment record	−	1.32, entire cohort	+
1986	Steenland	U.S. Teamsters	NR	7643	2	Job record	−	2.26, mechanics	NR
								1.54, truck drivers	NR
								1.32, dock workers	NR
								1.16, other	NR
1987	Edling et al.	Swedish bus company employees	689	195	32	Job record	−	All risk ratios < 1.0 for exposed cohorts	−
1988	Boffetta et al.	U.S. males	476,648	11,044	2	Job exposure by questionnaire	+	1.21, 16+ years of exposure	−
								2.67, miners	+
								2.60, heavy equipment	+
								1.59, railroad	−
								1.24, truck drivers	−
1988	Garshick et al.	U.S. railroad workers	55,407	17,127	21	Job contemporary measurements	±[f]	1.45, age 40–44 in 1959	+
								1.33, age 45–49 in 1959	+
								1.12, age 50–54 in 1959	−

1988	Netterstrom	Danish bus drivers	2465	15	6	Work record	−	0.87, entire cohort	−
1990	Gustavsson et al.	Swedish bus garage workers	695	17	26	Job and duration	−	1.22, entire cohort	−
1991	Rafnsson and Gunnardottir	Reykjavik taxi and truck drivers	868 truck	24	37	Union membership	−	2.14, all truck drivers	NR
			726 taxi	12	37			1.39, all taxi drivers	NR
1992	Guberan et al.	Swiss professional drivers	586	77	37	License records	−	1.50, entire cohort	+
1993	Hansen	Danish truck drivers	14,225	76	10	Occupation by census	−	1.60, all truck drivers	+
1994	Nokso-Koivisto and Pukkala	Finnish locomotive drivers	8391	236	38	Union membership	−	0.86, entire cohort	−
1994	Pfluger and Minder	Swiss professional drivers	218,848	284	4	License records	−	2.27, entire cohort	+

[a] Generally, the size of the total population studied, in some cases equal to the cohort size and in others larger than individual cohorts.

[b] In most cases the period over which data were collected (not necessarily time of exposure or since beginning of exposure).

[c] $p \leq 0.05$ for relative risk reported by author.

[d] NR = not reported.

[e] Relationship between relative risk and exposure length (time) significant at $p < 0.05$.

[f] Relative risks were not adjusted for smoking; however, ancillary data indicated no difference in smoking prevalence between exposed and unexposed.

TABLE 7-3 Case-Control Studies of the Relationship between Diesel Exhaust Exposure and Lung Cancer

Date	Author	Source of Cases and Controls	Number of Cases	Number of Controls	Sex	Exposure Assessment	Control for Smoking	Study Period (years)	Relative Risk	Statistical Significance[a]
1976	Menck and Henderson	204 hospitals and clinics in Los Angeles County	2716 (109)[b]	NR[c]	M	Last occupation by death certificate or admission record	−	5	1.65, truck drivers	+
1977	Decoufle et al.	Roswell Park Memorial Institute, Buffalo, NY	6434 (66)	NR (310)	M	Occupation by questionnaire	+	10	0.92, truck bus, and taxi drivers 0.94, train engineers and firemen	− −
1977	Williams et al.	U.S. Third National Cancer Survey	22 (22)	NR	M + F	Occupation by interview	+	3	1.52, male truck drivers	−
1983	Milne et al.	Alameda County, CA	747 (23)	3130 (53)	M	Occupation	−	4	1.6, truck drivers	+
1984	Coggon et al.	English-Welsh populations	598 (172)	1180 (281)	M	Occupation on death certificate	−	5	1.3, all diesel-exposed occupations 1.1, "high" exposure	+ −
1984	Hall and Wynder	18 U.S. hospitals (excluded "tobacco-related" disease)	502 (45)	502 (24)	M	Usual occupation by interview	+	2	1.4, total diesel exposed 1.9, heavy equipment repair and operators	− −
1985	Buiatti et al.	Florence, Italy hospitals	376 (20)	892 (25)	M + F	Occupation by interview	+	3	1.8, males ever driving taxis	NR
1987	Damber and Larsson	Northern Sweden population	589 (37)	1035 (25)	M	Occupation ≥ 1 year by mail questionnaire	+	6	1.2, professional drivers ≥ 20 years	−
1987a,b	Garshick et al.	U.S. railroad workers	1256 (251)	2512 (496)	M	Job, contemporary measurements	+	1	1.41, ≤ 64 years at retirement or death 1.64, ≥ 20 years of exposure	+ +
1987	Lerchen et al.	New Mexico population (excluded bronchioalveolar carcinoma)	506 (7)	721 (17)	M + F	Occupation and exposure by interview	+	3	0.6, all reporting exposure to diesel exhaust	NR
1988	Benhamou et al.	French population	1260 (285)	2084 (391)	M	Occupation by questionnaire	+	4	1.42, motor vechicle drivers 1.35, transport equipment operators	+ +
1988	Siemiatycki et al.	Montreal hospitals	857 (81)	1523 (NR)	M	Exposure by interview	+	NR	1.2, all diesel exposed versus squamous cell carcinoma	−
1989	Hayes et al.	FL, LA, NJ hospital and general populations	1444 (122)	1893 (113)	M	Occupation by interview	+	1–4	1.5, truck drivers >10 years 2.1, heavy equipment operator > 10 years	+ +

Year	Study	Population			Sex/Race	Exposure assessment	Direction[a]	No.[b]	Relative risk	[c]
1990	Boffetta et al.	18 U.S. hospitals	2584 (210)	5099 (324)	M	Occupation by interview of subject	+	10	0.92, all "probably exposed" occupations	–
									1.21, self-reported exposure	–
									2.39, self-reported exposure ≥ 31 years	NR
1990	Gustavsson et al.	Swedish bus garage workers	20	120	M	Job and duration	–	26	1.34, low exposure	NR
									1.84, medium exposure	NR
									2.43, high exposure	NR
1990	Steenland et al.	Central States Teamsters' Union	996 (219)	1085 (196)	M	Job by interview of next of kin	+	2	1.69, truck mechanic	–
									1.42, all diesel truck drivers	–
									1.89, diesel truck drivers ≥ 35 years	–
1993	Emmelin et al.	Nonsmoking Swedish dock workers	50	154	M	Job and duration	+	22	1.0, low-exposed time	NR
									1.6, medium-exposed time	NR
									2.9, high-exposed time	NR
1993	Swanson et al.	Detroit drivers of heavy trucks	3792 (325)	1966 (164)	M White	Job history and smoking by telephone interview	+	4	1.4, 1–9 years	–
									1.6, 10–19 years	–
									2.5, 20+ years	+
			(71)	(41)	Black				2.7, 1–9 years	–
									1.9, 10–19 years	–
									2.1, 20+ years	–

[a] $p < 0.05$ for relative risk as reported by author

[b] Number of cases or controls in parentheses are specific to populations for which relative risks are listed. Values not in parentheses represent total cases and controls in study.

[c] NR = not reported.

205

exhaust. When the data for all exposed men were stratified by length of exposure to diesel exhaust, the adjusted relative risk for lung cancer was not significantly increased (1.05) for men with 1 to 15 years of exposure; however, there was a slight increase in relative risk (1.21, $0.05 < p < 0.10$) among men with at least 16 years of exposure. These results suggest a positive trend of cancer risk with length of exposure.

Analysis by occupation demonstrated significantly elevated smoking-adjusted relative risks for lung cancer among miners (2.67, 95% CI $= 1.63 - 4.37$) and heavy equipment operators (2.60, 95% CI $= 1.12$–6.06), and slightly (insignificantly) elevated risks among railroad workers (1.59) and truck drivers (1.24). Analysis restricted to truck drivers demonstrated no significant difference between relative risks for lung cancer among men reporting diesel exhaust exposure (1.22) and those reporting no exposure (1.19). No information on exhaust exposure was available for some cases. Analysis by duration of diesel exhaust exposure among truck drivers yielded a positive time-response trend with relative risks of 0.87 for 1 to 15 years of exposure and 1.33 for 16 years or more of exposure. These results suggest a small positive association between lung cancer risk and occupations with high presumed exposure to diesel exhaust and a trend toward increasing lung cancer risk with time in those occupations.

Garshick et al. (1988) conducted a retrospective cohort study of lung cancer among 55,407 white male U.S. railroad workers, 40 to 64 years old in 1959, who had begun work 10 to 20 years earlier. The cohort was selected on the basis of job title in 1959 and followed through 1980 using records from the U.S. Railroad Retirement Board. Death certificates obtained for 17,127 decedents included 1694 lung cancer cases. Diesel exhaust exposure was a dichotomous (yes/no) variable based on job records. Exposures to diesel exhaust in various jobs were estimated from measurements in ancillary studies of contemporary railroads (Woskie et al., 1988a, b). Exposed workers included train crews and repairmen; unexposed workers included clerks, ticket and station agents, and signalmen. Jobs with the most likely exposure to asbestos were excluded. Although information on individual smoking was not used in the analysis, ancillary data (Garshick et al., 1987a, b) indicated that the prevalences of smoking in the diesel exhaust-exposed and exhaust-unexposed cohorts were similar. For analysis, the exposed cohort was subdivided by age in 1959, the time by which railroads had largely become dieselized. The youngest workers at that time therefore were thought to have the longest potential exposures to diesel exhaust.

Significantly elevated relative risks for lung cancer were found for exposed workers 40 – 44 years old in 1959 (1.45, 95% CI $= 1.11$–1.89) and 45–49 years old in 1959 (1.33, 95% CI $= 1.03$–1.73). The relative risks were smaller for workers older in 1959, with the oldest (60–64 years) having the lowest relative risk (0.95). These results suggest an association of a small lung cancer risk with occupational exposure to diesel exhaust and a positive trend toward increasing risk with length of exposure.

Although the other cohort studies did not address smoking, it is instructional to consider the results of the most robust studies, such as those examining cohorts among which 1000 or more deaths occurred (Table 7-2). Among these, only the study of railroad workers by Kaplan (1959) did not demonstrate an elevated risk for lung cancer. That study examined lung cancer among Baltimore and Ohio railroad workers dying between 1953 and 1958, and because diesel locomotives were introduced into that company between 1935 and 1958, the cohort might not have had sufficient exposure and latency time for effects to have been expressed.

Howe et al. (1983) conducted a retrospective cohort study of lung cancer among 43,826 male employees of the Canadian National Railway retired and alive in 1965 or retiring between 1965 and 1977. The total of 16,812 deaths included 933 deaths from cancer of the trachea, bronchi, and lung. The subjects were classified by job at the time of retirement into nonexposed, possibly exposed, and probably exposed. A highly significant relationship was found between relative lung cancer risk and the presumed level of exposure: nonexposed = 1.00; possibly exposed = 1.20 and probably exposed = 1.35. Although smoking was not considered in the Howe et al. study, it might be presumed that the prevalence of smoking was similar among diesel exhaust exposure groups if that was indeed the case for the similar job groups studied by Garshick et al. Similarities between the Howe et al. and Garshick et al. studies in the nature of the data bases, exposure classifications, and results bolster confidence that exposure to diesel exhaust in the railroad industry is likely to be associated with a small increased risk for lung cancer.

Wong et al. (1985) compared the incidence of lung cancer among male members of a heavy equipment operators' union in northern California, Utah, Nevada, Hawaii, and Guam to that among the entire U.S. white male population. The study cohort consisted of 34,156 men with at least one year of membership during 1964–1978 and included 3243 deaths, 309 of which were lung cancer cases. The authors reported a significant trend toward increasing lung cancer risk with duration of union membership; however, the relative risk for at least 20 years of membership was only 1.07. The positive trend was largely attributable to the very low relative risk among shorter-term members (< 5 years = 0.45; 5 – 9 years = 0.75). A significantly increased relative risk was found for all retirees (1.64), but this included men retiring early because of ill health. A lower but still significantly increased relative risk was found for members retiring at or after age 65 (1.30, 95% CI = 1.04 – 1.61).

Gustafsson et al. (1986) compared the incidence of lung cancer among male Swedish dock workers to that among the Swedish male population. Diesel trucks were introduced into Swedish ports in the late 1950s and became prevalent during the 1960s. The cohort consisted of 6071 men employed for a minimum of 6 months before 1974 and followed from 1961 to 1981. Twenty percent of the cohort had 30 or more years of service, and only 10% had less than 5 years of service. There were 70 cases of lung cancer among the 1062 cohort deaths. The relative risk for lung cancer among the dock workers was found to be significantly increased to 1.32 (95% CI = 1.05 – 1.66).

Steenland (1986) reported preliminary results from a proportionate mortality study comparing the incidence of lung cancer among decedent central U.S. members of the Teamsters' Union to that among the U.S. population. The subjects were 7643 long-term (length not specified) members who died during 1982 and 1983 and for whom job information was considered sufficient for classification into exposure groups. Although statistical significances were not reported, moderately to slightly elevated relative risks for lung cancer were reported for mechanics (2.26, 95% CI = 1.62–3.09), truck drivers (1.54, 95% CI = 1.44 – 1.66), dock workers (1.32, 95% CI = 0.99–1.75), and other Teamsters (1.16, 95% CI = 0.95–1.42). The authors noted that the apparent excess risks might be partially explained by a greater prevalence of smoking among teamsters than among the general population.

Most of the other studies listed in Table 7-2 which involved fewer numbers of deaths gave results similar to those described above. In addition to the study of railroad workers by Kaplan (1959), studies of bus garage workers by Waller (1981), bus drivers by Netterstrom (1988), and railroad locomotive drivers by Nokso-Koivisto and Pukkala (1994) yielded relative risks for lung cancer less than 1.0. The latter study is interesting because it involved a large, well-defined population (8391 drivers and 236 cancer deaths) observed over a 38-year period. Therefore, while most studies yielded positive results, there were certainly some that did not.

Case-Control Studies   Reports of 18 case-control studies including occupational groups thought to have substantial exposures to diesel exhaust are summarized in Table 7-3. Seven reports describe hospital-based studies, six describe population-based studies, and five describe studies focused on specific occupational groups. As in the cohort studies, the case-control studies largely used job or occupation as surrogates for exposure classification; two studies employed questions about diesel exhaust exposure, and one used contemporary measurements of diesel exhaust in workplaces. In contrast to the cohort studies, all but four of the case-control studies used smoking as a variable in the analysis of lung cancer risk. The strength of the 18 studies varies primarily in the number of cases within diesel exhaust-exposed subgroups. The cases among exposure groups for which relative risks are listed in Table 7-3 range in number from seven to 325. The following summary focuses primarily on the eight studies that included 100 or more cases in the relevant exposure groups; two based on single occupational groups and six including numerous occupations. Six of these studies included adjustments for smoking, and two did not.

The most robust study in terms of focus on exposed occupational groups, the number of relevant cases and controls, the establishment of exposure to diesel exhaust, the consideration of confounding factors, the length of exposures, and the depth of analysis is clearly that of Garshick et al. (1987a). These authors examined a population of 650,000 active and retired male U.S. railroad workers with 10 years or more of service, using records from the Railroad Retirement Board. Their study included a total of 1256 exposed cases and 2512 controls, assigned on the basis of job records and contemporary measurements of diesel exhaust concentrations in similar job environments (Woskie et al., 1988a, b). Cases and controls dying during a one year period (1981–1982) were matched by birth and death date. The cases and controls were classified by age, length of service, smoking (by interview of next of kin), and likely exposure to asbestos. The job categories within exposed and unexposed groups and other assumptions about exposures are described in the preceding section in relation to the cohort study by the same authors. The cases were divided at age 64 into younger and older groups, with the younger group presumed to have more years of diesel exposure because of the date of railroad dieselization, and years of exposure was used as a continuous variable.

A small positive association between exposure and lung cancer was found among the younger exposed group, similar to the association found in the related cohort study by the same investigators. After being adjusted for smoking (pack-years) and asbestos exposure (yes/no), the odds ratio for lung cancer among 251 cases and 496 controls was 1.41 ($p = 0.02$, 95% CI = 1.06–1.88). After similar adjustments, the odds ratio for workers with 20 or more years of diesel exposure was 1.64 (95% CI = 1.18–2.29). To exclude the effects of recent diesel exhaust exposure, the data were analyzed excluding exposures during the five years preceding death, and the relative risk for lung cancer remained similarly elevated (odds ratio = 1.43). The authors also tested the interaction between smoking and diesel exhaust exposure and found it to be insignificant ($p = 0.56$).

Steenland et al. (1990) reported a study of lung cancer among truck drivers in the Central States Teamsters' Union. The study population included a total of 996 cases and 1085 controls for whom death certificates were obtained, and information on work history, smoking, and asbestos exposure was obtained from next of kin. The subjects died in 1982 and 1983 after applying for pensions, which required a minimum of 20 years of union membership. Covariates included in the analysis were age, smoking, asbestos exposure, and jobs with diesel exposure. Among 219 cases including truck mechanics and diesel truck drivers, slightly elevated odds ratios were found for mechanics (1.69), drivers (1.42), and drivers for 35 years or longer (1.89). These increases in relative risk, although similar to or greater than those reported by Garshick et al. (see above), did not reach statistical significance by the analytical methods employed. A more recent analysis of the exposure–response relationship among the truck driver data yielded similar results but further demonstrated the sensitivity of the slope to assumptions about historic emissions factors (Steenland et al., 1998).

Benhamou et al. (1988) reported a case-control study of occupational risk factors among the French population. A total of 1260 male cases observed between 1976 and 1980 were matched by age, hospital of admission, and interviewer with 2084 controls, and information on occupation and smoking was obtained by interview. The smoking-adjusted relative risk for lung cancer among 285 cases and 391 controls was found to be significantly increased ($p = 0.01$) to 1.35 for transport equipment operators (95% CI = 1.05–1.75) and to 1.42 for motor vehicle drivers (95% CI = 1.07–1.89).

Hayes et al. (1989) reported a case-control study of lung cancer in motor-exhaust related occupations that used data from National Cancer Institute hospital- and population-based studies in Florida (1976–1979), Louisiana (1979–1983), and New Jersey (1980–1981). The study included a total of 1444 male cases and 1893 controls for which occupation and smoking information was obtained by interview. Among 122 cases and 113 controls, the smoking-adjusted odds ratios for lung cancer were significantly elevated for truck drivers for 10 years or longer (1.5, 95% CI = 1.1–2.0) and heavy equipment operators for 10 years or longer (2.1, 95% CI = 0.6–7.1). Although less specific for diesel exhaust, the odds ratio for cancer after 10 years or more of employment in all vehicle exhaust-related jobs was increased to 1.5. None of the job categories had elevated risks for lung cancer among those employed for less than 10 years.

The most recent report from a series of cancer studies conducted by the American Health Foundation using data from 18 U.S. hospitals (Boffetta et al., 1990) included a total of 2584 male cases of confirmed lung cancer and 5099 controls matched for age, date, and hospital of admission. Information on usual occupation and smoking was obtained by interview, and the more recent interviews included questions about diesel exhaust exposure. Data from 1977 to 1987 were divided into occupations with no, possible, and probable diesel exhaust exposure, and truck drivers were examined as a subgroup within the probably exposed group. The smoking-adjusted odds ratio for lung cancer among the group with probable exposure (210 cases) was 0.92 (95% CI = 0.75–1.12), and that among truck drivers (114 cases) was 0.83 (95% CI = 0.64–1.09). The odds ratios increased with duration of service in occupations with probable exposure, reaching 1.49 for 31 years or longer, but the trend did not reach significance ($p = 0.18$). There was no suggestion of an increasing odds ratio with length of service among truck drivers.

An analysis of data by years of self-reported diesel exhaust exposure was also conducted using a total of 477 cases and 946 controls accumulated since this question was incorporated into the interview. The adjusted odds ratio for lung cancer among those reporting exposure (35 cases) was 1.26. When these cases were further stratified by the years of self-reported exposure, the adjusted odds ratio for 31 years or more of exposure (12 cases) was increased to 2.39; however, the trend toward increasing risk with length of exposure did not reach significance ($p = 0.12$).

Swanson et al. (1993) reported lung cancer results from an occupational cancer incidence study of men in the Detroit area for the period of 1984 to 1987. Their study involved a total of 3792 cases and 1966 colon/rectum cancer controls, in which work and tobacco use histories were obtained by interviewing the subjects or close surrogates. This study is particularly interesting because it compared results from black and white men. Although numerous occupational groups were listed in the report, those likely to have had the greatest exposure to diesel exhaust were the drivers of heavy trucks. This category included 325 white and 71 black male cases, matched with 164 white and 41 black male controls. As shown in Table 7-3, the relative risk for lung cancer among white males was related to length of occupation as a truck driver, ranging from 1.4 (95% CI = 0.8–2.4) for 1 to 9 years to 2.5 (95% CI = 1.4–4.4) for 20 years or more. Although these results suggest an exposure-response relationship, the results from black men did not. Among black men, the relative risk ranged from 2.7 for 1 to 9 years to 2.1 for 20 or more years. The results for several other occupational groups also differed by race, suggesting both the need for caution in generalizing results to all groups and a possible source of variability of results in other studies.

The remaining two studies which included exposed groups of 100 or more cases did not include adjustments for smoking in their analyses. Menck and Henderson (1976) examined records from 204 hospitals and clinics in Los Angeles County for the periods 1968–1970 and 1972–1973 and reported a study involving a total of 2716 cases of lung cancer in white males. The subjects' last occupations were taken from death certificates and hospital admission records. The standard mortality ratio calculated for 109 cases among truck drivers indicated a significantly elevated relative risk among truck drivers (1.65, $p = 0.01$). Coggon et al. (1984) reported a study, including a total of 598 male cases and 1180 controls, derived from death certificates in England and Wales during 1975 to 1979. Occupations listed on the death certificates were classified into those with no exposure, some exposure, and high exposure to diesel exhaust. Among 172 cases and 281 controls, the relative risk for bronchial carcinoma was significantly increased to 1.3 (95% CI = 1.0–1.6, $p = 0.05$) for all exposed occupations, but the relative risk was not increased for occupations with high exposure (1.1).

Several of the studies that included target occupational groups with fewer than 100 cases demonstrated small increases in relative risks for lung cancer similar in magnitude to the increases demonstrated by most of the larger studies. In view of the small magnitude of the increases in risk, it is not surprising that most increases in risk did not reach statistical significance in the smaller studies. An exception was the study by Milne et al. (1983), in which the relative risk for lung cancer of 1.6 (95% CI not given) among 23 cases of male truck drivers was reported as significantly increased. Although Gustavsson et al. (1990) did not report statistical significance, their study of lung cancer cases among Swedish bus garage workers indicated a progression in risk with increasing exposure intensity length classification, ranging from 1.34 for the lowest to 2.43 for the highest exposure group. Similarly Emmelin et al. (1993) reported increasing relative risks for lung cancer with exposure time for 50 cases among nonsmoking Swedish dock workers ranging from 1.0 (no increase) for the lowest category to 2.9 for the highest.

Williams et al. (1977), using data from the Third U.S. National Cancer Survey, found the relative risk for lung cancer among truck drivers (22 cases) to be 1.52. In a study preceding that of Boffetta et al. (1990) described above, Hall and Wynder (1984) examined data from 18 U.S. hospitals and reported the relative risks for lung cancer to be 1.4 for all diesel-exposed occupations (45 cases) and 1.9 for heavy equipment repairmen and operators (10 cases). Buiatti et al. (1985) examined data from hospitals in Florence, Italy, and reported the relative risk for lung cancer among males having ever driven taxis to be 1.8 (20 cases).

Other small studies revealed even less, or no, increase in smoking-adjusted lung cancer risk. Decoufle et al. (1977) reported the relative risk among truck, bus, and taxi drivers and railroad engineers and firemen (total of 66 cases) to be approximately 0.9. Damber and Larsson (1987) reported the relative risk for lung cancer to be 1.2 among professional drivers in northern Sweden (37 cases). Lerchen et al. (1987) reported a relative risk of 0.6 for New Mexico cases of lung cancer other than bronchioalveolar carcinoma reporting exposure to diesel exhaust when interviewed, but only seven cases fell in this category. Siemiatycki et al. (1988) reported a relative risk of 1.2 for squamous cell carcinoma among 81 cases in Montreal hospitals reporting diesel exhaust exposure when interviewed.

Combined Analysis of Multiple Studies Dubrow and Wegman (1983) sought to identify occupations at high cancer risk by combining results from 12 occupational disease surveillance studies. The 12 studies had been described between 1961 and 1981, primarily in technical reports; only two (Decoufle et al., 1977; Williams et al., 1977) are reviewed individually in this chapter. Because the individual studies differed in their sources of data, adjustments for confounding factors, occupational groupings, analytical methods, and the availability of the raw data, this report does not represent a true meta-analysis of the data bases. Dubrow and Wegman based their synthesis of the results on the summary relative risks reported by the 12 studies rather than on the raw data.

To synthesize the results, the occupational cancer risk results from the 12 studies were first examined to select specific occupations for which the association was strongest. This was based on a significant association demonstrated in multiple studies—the number of studies reporting a relative risk for each association greater than 1.0 was significantly greater (binomial probability, $p < 0.05$) than the number reporting a relative risk less than 1.0 — and the authors' judgment that an association warranted further examination. Second, the occupational cancer risk associations thus chosen were combined from multiple studies into a single risk factor. This was done by arbitrarily allowing up to 20 "cases" from each contributing study. If a study reported more than 20 cases, it was assigned a value of 20, and the observed-to-expected ratio was adjusted for those 20 cases to match that reported for the larger number of cases in the original study. Unadjusted ratios were used for studies reporting 20 or fewer cases. The combined observed and expected values were then used to calculate an aggregate ratio.

This synthesis of the 12 studies indicated that the relative risks for cancer (aggregate observed-to-expected ratio) of the trachea, bronchus, and lung were slightly elevated for heavy equipment operators (1.27, seven studies), truck and tractor drivers (1.25, nine studies), bus drivers (1.24, eight studies), taxicab drivers and chauffeurs (1.21, eight studies), and motor vehicle drivers (1.20, six studies). Based on these results, Dubrow and Wegman recommended that the association of lung cancer with employment as a motor vehicle driver be one of the five priorities targeted for future evaluation.

More recently, Bhatia et al. (1998) reviewed the epidemiological data base and reported that 23 of 29 studies demonstrated elevated risks for lung cancer. A meta-analysis of the data by these authors resulted in a statistically significantly elevated risk of 1.33.

Summary of Epidemiological Evidence   The weight of the epidemiological evidence reviewed above suggests that long-term employment in jobs involving substantial exposures to diesel exhaust is statistically associated with a small increase in risk for lung cancer. However, the existing data do not allow confirmation of the increase, determination of its magnitude, or description of the exposure-response relationship with a high level of confidence. Many of the studies did not detect significant increases in risk because, although their central estimates of risk were positive, their 95% confidence limits included values indicating no increase or even reduced risk. The studies indicating statistically significant increases gave estimates of increases ranging from approximately 20% (relative risk of 1.2) to twofold (relative risk of 2.0). Increases in risk of less than twofold are difficult to assess with confidence from epidemiological data under any circumstances. Thus it may be unlikely that the issue will ever be resolved with a high degree of certainty by epidemiology, even if new prospective studies are conducted with much better assessments of exposure.

Animal Studies   In the absence of definitive data from humans, hazard characterization and risk assessment typically use data from animals exposed experimentally to the agent in question. Regarding the carcinogenicity of diesel exhaust, however, results from animals have not proved to be very helpful. The history of laboratory carcinogenicity studies of diesel exhaust is interesting because, despite the large amount of experimental data accumulated over the past 20 years and despite the dose-related lung tumor response of rats, our present knowledge indicates that this information should not be used for estimating human lung cancer risk, and that it is of questionable value in determining carcinogenic hazard. Regardless, the animal studies of the cancer risks from inhaled diesel exhaust are summarized in this chapter for historical perspective and as a foundation for understanding their lack of utility for estimating human cancer risk.

Unlike epidemiological studies, studies of the health effects of inhaled diesel exhaust in laboratory animals can be conducted under carefully controlled, well-documented experimental conditions that allow the effects to be quantitated precisely. Although the groups of animals are smaller (typically 50 to 200) than in most epidemiological studies, animal experiments gain statistical strength from their designs and the precision of the data. Nevertheless, studies of animals are bound by the same statistical rules as studies of humans, and even groups of 200 rodents do not have the statistical power to determine the significance of a 20% to 50% increase in lung tumor incidence against a variable background incidence of up to 3%. Statistics aside, the greatest difficulty with animal studies is the uncertainty of extrapolation across species. Confidence in extrapolating the results to humans is gained if similar responses are observed in more than one animal species. An increased tumor incidence in animals is generally accepted as signaling a potential carcinogenic hazard for humans. However, extrapolating the animal response to quantitative estimates of cancer risk requires confidence that (1) the mechanisms by which cancer occurred in animals are likely to also operate in humans and (2) the exposure–dose–response relationship observed in animals at high levels of exposure can be extended downward to the much lower levels of human exposure. The following information summarizes results from experimental exposures of rats, mice, and Syrian hamsters, the only species with which near-lifetime inhalation carcinogenesis bioassays of diesel exhaust have been conducted.

Studies of Rats   The published studies of pulmonary carcinogenicity in rats exposed chronically to diesel exhaust are summarized in Table 7-4. For studies described in multiple publications, the reference given is the most complete description. Early descriptions of several of the studies, in some cases presenting ancillary results not contained in the citations below, were published by Ishinishi et al. (1986). The experimental details are only briefly outlined, both because they were not reported in detail by all authors and because variables other than soot concentration and exposure time have not proved to strongly influence the outcome. Eight studies involved exposures of 24 months or longer and used groups of 50 or more rats, the minimum number generally considered adequate for testing carcinogenicity.

Heinrich et al. (1986) exposed 96 rats/group, 19 h/d, 5 d/w for 32 months to exhaust at 4.2 mg soot/m^3, resulting in a 15.8% incidence of lung tumors in contrast to none in controls. A key finding was that a parallel group (not listed in Table 7-4) exposed to the same concentration of exhaust with the soot removed by filtration had no increase in lung tumor incidence.

Mauderly et al. (1987) exposed 220 rats/group, 7 h/d, 5 d/w for 30 months at 0.35, 3.5, and 7.1 mg soot/m^3, resulting in lung tumor incidences of 1.3%, 3.6%, and 12.8%, respectively, in contrast to 0.9% among controls. The increases in tumor incidence were significant for the two higher concentrations. In another study conducted later using identical exposures, Mauderly et al. (1986, 1990b) exposed 80 rats/group, 7 h/d, 5 d/w for 30 months at 3.5 mg soot/m^3 and observed a 6.5% lung tumor incidence in contrast to none among controls.

Ishihara (1988) conducted concurrent studies of rats exposed 16 h/d, 6 d/w for 30 months to exhaust from light-duty and heavy-duty engines. The heavy-duty exhaust was administered at 0.5, 1.0, 1.8, and 3.7 mg soot/m^3, resulting in lung tumor incidences of 3.3% and 6.5% at the two highest levels, respectively. The highest tumor incidence was significantly elevated above the 0.8% incidence among controls.

TABLE 7-4 Studies of Lung Cancer in Rats Exposed Chronically to Whole Diesel Exhaust

	Animals						Exposure				Lung tumors	
Date	Author	Strain	Sex	Age at Start (weeks)	Number per Group[a]	Engine	Operating Mode	Hours/Day × Days/Week	Months	Soot Concentration (mg/m³)	Percentage with Tumors	$p < 0.05$
1981	Karagianes et al.	Wister	M	18	6	3-cyl, 43-hp electrical generator	Variable speed and load	6 × 5	20	0	0	
										8.3	16.7	−
1983	Kaplan et al.	F344	M	8	30	Odsmobile 5.7 L	Constant speed	20 × 7	15 (8)[b]	0	0	NR[c]
1983	White et al.									0.25	3.3	NR
										0.75	10.0	NR
										1.5	3.3	NR
1986	Heinrich et al.	Wister	F	8–10	96	Volkswagen 1.6 L	Variable, U.S. FTP[d]	19 × 5	32	0	0	
										4.2	15.8	+
1986	Iwai et al.	F344	F	7	24	2.4-L truck engine	Constant speed	8 × 7	24 (6)	0	4.5	
										4.9	42.1	+
1986	Takemoto et al.	F344	F	5	15	Yanmar 0.27 L	Constant idle	4 × 4	24	0	0	
										2–4	0	−
1987	Mauderly et al.	F344	M+F	17	220	Oldsmobile 5.7 L	Variable, U.S. FTP	7 × 5	30	0	0.9	−
										0.35	1.3	+
										3.5	3.6	+
										7.1	12.8	
1988	Ishihara	F344	M+F	5	123	1.8-L 4-cyl, light duty	Constant speed	16 × 6	30	0	3.3	−
										0.1	2.4	−
										0.4	0.8	−
										1.1	4.1	−
										2.3	2.4	
1988	Ishihara	F344	M+F	5	123	11-L, 6 cyl, heavy duty	Constant speed	16 × 6	30	0	0.8	−
										0.5	0.8	−
										1.0	0	−
										1.8	3.3	−
										3.7	6.5	+

TABLE 7-4 (*Continued*)

		Animals				Exposure					Lung tumor	
Date	Author	Strain	Sex	Age at Start (weeks)	Number per Group[a]	Engine	Operating Mode	Hours/Day × Days/Week	Months	Soot Concentration (µg/m³)	Percentage with Tumors	$p < 0.05$
1989	Brightwell et al.	F344	M+F	6-8	144	Volkswagen 1.5 L	Variable, U.S. FTP	16 × 5	24 (6)	0	1.2	
										0.7	0.7	−
										2.2	9.7	+
										6.6	38.5	+
1989	Lewis et al.	F344	M+F	(Weanling)	180	3304 Caterpillar 7.0 L with water scrubber	Variable, mine cycle	7 × 5	24	0	3.3	
										1.95	4.4	−
1990a	Mauderly et al.	F344	M	18	34	Oldsmobile 5.7 L	Variable, U.S. FTP	7 × 5	24	0	0	
										3.5	2.9	−
1990b	Mauderly et al.	F344	M+F	19	80	Oldsmobile 5.7 L	Variable, U.S. FTP	7 × 5	30	0	0	
										3.5	6.5	+
1995	Heinrich et al.	Wistar	F	7	100–200	Volkswagen 1.6 L	U.S. FTP	18 × 5	24 (6)	0	0.5	
										0.8	0	−
										2.5	2.0	−
										7.0	9.0	+
1995	Nikula et al.	F344	M+F	7–9	210–214	GM LH6 6.2 L	U.S. FTP	16 × 5	24	0	1.4	
										2.4	6.2	+
										6.3	17.9	+

[a] Number of rats examined for lung tumors.

[b] Value in parentheses is number of months rats were observed after cessation of exposure

[c] NR = not reported.

[d] FTP = Federal Test Procedure, EPA urban certification cycle (U.S.-72).

Brightwell et al. (1989) exposed 144 rats/group,16 h/d, 5 d/w for 24 months to exhaust at 0.7, 2.2, and 6.6 mg soot/m^3, and observed the rats for an additional 6 months. The lung tumor incidences at the two highest levels, 9.7% and 38.5%, were significantly increased above the 1.2% incidence among controls. In agreement with the Heinrich et al. (1986) study above, parallel groups of rats exposed to the two higher concentrations of exhaust with the particles removed by filtration (not listed in Table 7-4) had no increase in lung tumor incidence.

Lewis et al. (1989) exposed 180 rats/group, 7 h/d, 5 d/w for 24 months to water-scrubbed exhaust from a mine engine at 1.95 mg soot/m^3 and observed a slight but insignificant increase in lung tumor incidence.

Heinrich et al. (1995) exposed 100–220 rats/group 18 h/d, 5 d/w for 24 months to exhaust at 0.8, 2.5, and 7.0 mg soot/m^3 and observed the surviving rats for an additional 6 months. The lung tumor incidence was increased significantly at the highest-exposure level.

Nikula et al. (1995) exposed 210–214 rats/group 16 h/d, 5 d/w for 24 months to exhaust at 2.4 and 6.3 mg soot/m^3, and observed a dose-related increase in lung tumor incidence that was statistically significant at both exposure levels.

Only two of the above eight studies did not yield statistically significant increases in lung tumor incidence in rats, the light-duty engine study by Ishihara and the mine engine study by Lewis et al. Interestingly these two studies also yielded the highest incidences (3.3%) of lung tumors in control rats; control incidences in the other studies ranged from 0% to 1.2%. It is doubtful that a lower control incidence would have influenced the statistical outcome of the Ishihara et al. study, but a lower control incidence might have yielded significant increases in the Lewis et al. study. The highest-exposure level in both of these studies was approximately 2 mg soot/m^3 which proved to be just below the approximate threshold for a tumor response when data from all the studies were considered in aggregate.

Five of the studies listed in Table 7-4c used treatment groups of only 15 to 34 rats or exposure or observation periods that were too short for expression of carcinogenesis. Of those studies, however, only that of Takemoto et al. (1986) did not produce a greater incidence of lung tumors among exposed rats than among controls.

These results demonstrate clearly that the soot fraction of diesel exhaust is a pulmonary carcinogen in rats exposed in sufficient numbers at sufficiently high concentrations for sufficiently long times. The aggregate exposure–response relationship from the eight most robust studies is illustrated in Figure 7-1, in which the net (exposed minus control) tumor incidences are compared on the basis of the exposure rate, or weekly concentration-time product (mg·hr·m^{-3}). Two key points can be drawn from the graph. First, the data generally fall into three exposure-response groupings and strongly suggest a threshold. Exposure rates below approximately 100 mg·hr·m^{-3} produced no suggestion of a tumor response; that is., no suggestion of a response slope. Exposure rates between approximately 100 and 250 mg·hr·m^{-3} produced an intermediate zone of variable response, including some significant responses, some insignificantly elevated responses, and one group with no increase at all. All exposure rates above approximately 250 mg·hr·m^{-3} produced significant increases in tumor incidence. Second, diesel exhaust proved to be only a weak carcinogen in rats, even at the higher exposure rates. One group had a net tumor incidence of 37%, but none of the others exceeded 15%.

To explore the existence of a threshold in the rat lung tumor data more rigorously, Valberg and Crouch (1999) conducted a meta-analysis of the exposure–response data from eight long-term studies. Their analysis indicated a threshold in the range of 500–700 μg/m^3 and demonstrated that a positive slope did not exist when data below 600 μg/m^3 were analyzed separately.

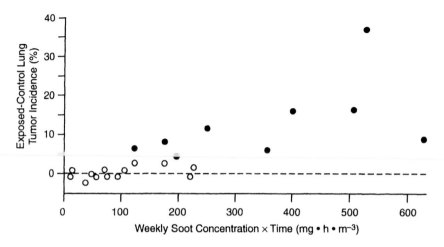

Figure 7-1 The relationship between diesel exhaust exposure and the rat lung tumor response is illustrated by aggregate data from the eight published studies including groups of 50 or more rats and exposures of 24 months or longer (Heinrich et al., 1986; Mauderly et al., 1987; Ishihara, 1988; Brightwell et al., 1989; Lewis et al., 1989; Mauderly et al., 1990b; Heinrich et al., 1995; Nikula et al., 1995). The lung tumor response is expressed as the net (exposed minus control) lung tumor incidence, and the dashed line represents the control incidence (no net increase) for each study. Because all studies used weekly repeating exposure patterns, exposures are normalized by expression as the weekly exposure rate (mg/m^3 times hours per week). Filled circles represent treatment groups with statistically significant increases above individual study control tumor incidences, and open circles represent exposed groups with no increase or statistically insignificant increases above the control incidences. The aggregate results indicate a response threshold. Exposure rates of 106 mg $\cdot$ hr $\cdot$ m^{-3} or below produced no suggestion of a tumor response among nine groups, including a total of 1359 rats exposed at five laboratories in four countries.

Studies of Mice There are six reports of carcinogenicity results from mice exposed chronically by inhalation to diesel exhaust (Table 7-5). Two studies used strains (Sencar and Strain A) which have high background incidences of lung tumors and were developed for their sensitivity to chemical carcinogens. Using exposures of only 7.5 to 15 months, these studies are a different type of carcinogenicity bioassay than the others conducted in mice, rats, and hamsters. The other four studies used longer-term exposures of strains commonly used in chronic inhalation cancer bioassays, and are more useful for inter-species comparisons.

Heinrich et al. (1986) exposed female NMRI mice 19 h/d, 5 d/w for 28 months to exhaust at 4.2 mg soot/m^3 and observed a significant increase in lung tumors. Interestingly parallel exposures of mice to the same dilution of exhaust with the soot removed by filtration (not shown) also increased the lung tumor incidence, in contrast to the finding of no increased carcinogenicity in rats exposed to filtered exhaust in the parallel study.

Takemoto et al. (1986) exposed male and female C57BL/6N and ICR/Jcl mice 4 h/d, 4 d/w for 28 months to exhaust at 2 to 4 mg soot/m^3 (mean concentration not reported) and observed modest increases in lung tumor incidence; the significance of the increases was not reported.

Heinrich et al. (1995) exposed female NMRI and C57BL/6N mice 18 h/d, 5 d/w for 23 (NMRI) or 24 months to exhaust at 4.5 mg soot/m^3. The lung tumor incidence of exposed NMRI mice was lower than that of controls, and that of exposed C57BL/6N mice was slightly, but not significantly, higher than that of controls. They also exposed female NMRI mice 18 h/d, 5 d/w to exhaust at 7.0 mg soot/m^3 for 13.5 months followed by a 9.5

TABLE 7-5 Stuides of Lung Cancer in Mice and Syrian Hamsters Exposed Chronically to Whole Diesel Exhaust

		Animals					Exposure				Lung tumors	
Date	Author	Strain	Sex	Age at Start (weeks)	Number per Group[a]	Engine	Operating Mode	Hours/Day × Days/Week	Months	Soot Concentration (mg/m³)	Percentage with Tumors	$p < 0.05$
							Mice					
1983	Pepelko and Peirano	Strong-A	F	6	56–58	Nissan 3.2 L	Variable, federal short cycle	8 × 7	7.5	0	6.9	
										6.0	25.0	+
		Strong-A	M	6	368–403	Nissan 3.2 L	Variable, federal short cycle	8 × 7	7.5	0	18.1	
										6.0	17.9	–
		Strong-A	M + F	6	80–87	Nissan 3.2 L	Variable, federal short cyele	8 × 7	7.5	0	24.1	
										12.0	12.5	+
		Strong-A	M + F	6	237–250	Nissan 3.2 L	Variable, federal short cycle	8 × 7 (dark)[b]	7.5	0	24.9	
										12.0	8.8	+
		Jackson-A	M	6	38–44	Nissan 3.2 L	Variable, federal short cycle	8 × 7	10.5	0	57.9	
										12.0	25.0	+
		Sencar	F	In utero[c]	104–111	Nissan 3.2 L	Variable, federal short cycle	8 × 7	15	0	7.2	
										6/12[d]	16.3	+
		Sencar	M	In utero[c]	101–105	Nissan 3.2 L	Variable, federal short cycle	8 × 7	15	0	3.8	
										6/12[d]	5.9	+
1983	Kaplan et al.	Jackson-A	M	8	388–399	Oldsmobile 5.7 L	Constant speed	20 × 7	8	0	33.5	
										0.25	33.8	–
										0.75	27.3	–
										1.50	25.0	+
1986	Heinrich et al.	NMRI	F	8–10	84–93	Volkswagen 1.6 L	Variable, U.S. FTP	19 × 5	28	0	13.0	
										4.2	32.0	+
1986	Tekemoto et al.	C57BL/6N	M + F	Birth	59–188	Yammar 0.27 L	Constant idle	4 × 4	28	0	1.7	
										2–4	9.0	NR[e]
		IRC/Jcl	M + F	Birth	96–105	Yammar 0.27 L	Constant idle	4 × 4	28	0	7.3	
										2–4	13.3	NR
1995	Heinrich et al.	C57BL/6N	F	7	120	Volkwagen 1.6 L	U.S. FTP	18 × 5	24	0	5.1	
										4.5	8.5	–
		NMRI	F	7	120				23	0	30.0	
										4.5	23.0	–
		NMRI	F	7	80				13.5(9.5)[h]	0	30.0	
										7.0	32.1	–

217

TABLE 7-5 *(Continued)*

Date	Author	Strain	Sex	Age at Start (weeks)	Number per Group[a]	Engine	Operating Mode	Hours/Day × Days/Week	Months	Soot Concentration (mg/m³)	Percentage with Tumors	$p < 0.05$
1996	Mauderly et al.	CD-1	M+F	16–18	155–186	Oldsmobile 5.7 L	U.S. FTP	7 × 5	24	0	13.4	
									0	0.35	14.6	—
										3.5	9.7	—
										7.1	7.5	—
						Syrian Hamsters						
1978	Cross et al.	Syrian golden	M	12	102	3 cyl, 43 hp electrical generator	Variable speed and load	6 × 5	20	0	0	
										7.3	0	
1982	Heinrich et al.	Syrian golden	F	8	48	Daimler-Benz 2.4 L	Constant speed and load	7–8 × 5	24	0	0	
										3.9	0	
1983	Kaplan et al.	Syrian golden	M	8	30	Oldsmobile 5.7 L	Constant speed	20 × 7	15	0	0	
										0.25	0	
										0.75	0	
										1.50	0	
1986	Heinrich et al.	Syrian golden	M+F	8–10	96	Volkswagen 1.6 L	Variable, U.S. FTP	19 × 5	Lifetime[f]	0	0	
										4.2	0	
1989	Brightwell et al.	Syrian golden	M+F	6–8	203–410	Volkswagen 1.5 L	Variable, U.S. FTP	16 × 5	24	0	0.2	
										6.6[g]	0	

[a] Number examined for lung tumors.
[b] Light cycle altered for exposure during dark period.
[c] Parents mated and offspring born in exposure atmospheres.
[d] Exposed to 6 mg/m³ to 12 weeks of age, then to 12 mg/m³.
[e] NR = not reported.
[f] Maximum possible exposure was 28 months, longest exposure of hamsters not reported.
[g] Exposures at 0.7 and 2.2 mg/m³ were also conducted, but detailed tumor results were not published.
[h] Value in parentheses is number of months mice were observed after cessation of exposure.

month observation period. The lung tumor incidences in exposed and control mice were nearly identical.

Mauderly et al. (1996) exposed male and female CD-1 mice 7 h/d, 5 d/w for 24 months to exhaust at 0.35, 3.5, and 7.1 mg soot/m^3, concurrent with the rat study reported earlier (Mauderly et al., 1987). The lung tumor incidence at the low level was slightly (insignificantly) higher than that of controls, and the incidences at the higher two levels were lower than that of the controls.

The studies of Pepelko and Peirano (1983) yielded mixed results using Strain A and Sencar mice. Exposures of Strong-A mice 8 h/d, 7 d/w for 7.5 months at a soot concentration of 6.0 mg/m^3 yielded a significantly positive response in a group of females but no increase in a parallel group of males. In contrast, two other combined male-female groups exposed at 12 mg soot/m^3 yielded significantly reduced lung tumor incidences. An exposure of male Jackson-A mice on the same weekly schedule for 10.5 months at a 12 mg soot/m^3 yielded a significantly reduced lung tumor incidence. Exposures of Sencar mice from birth on the same weekly schedule for 15 months at 6 mg soot/m^3 for the first 12 weeks and then 12 mg soot/m^3 for thereafter yielded a significantly positive response in females but not in males.

The above results indicate that mice have, at most, an equivocal lung tumor response to diesel exhaust. The positive results obtained in female NMRI mice by Heinrich et al. (1986) were not reproduced in their later study (Heinrich et al. 1995). All other results in common bioassay strains were negative. The results from genetically-susceptible strains were mixed. Overall, it is clear that the consistently positive response of rats produced by high-level exposures were not reproduced in mice. Although the life span of mice is typically shorter than that of rats, life-span shortening in exposed mice did not compromise the comparison to controls (Heinrich et al. 1995; Mauderly et al., 1996).

Studies of Syrian Hamsters   There are five reported studies of Syrian golden hamsters exposed chronically to diesel exhaust (Table 7-5). Groups of 30 to 410 male and female hamsters have been exposed for durations ranging from 15 months to their lifetime to exhaust at concentrations ranging from 0.25 to 7.3 mg soot/m^3. Not a single lung tumor has been observed in diesel exhaust-exposed hamsters; therefore diesel exhaust is clearly not a pulmonary carcinogen in Syrian hamsters exposed under conditions carcinogenic in rats.

Usefulness of Experimental Data for Assessing Lung Cancer Hazard and Risk   It is not broadly questioned that the organic fraction of diesel soot can be considered to present a carcinogenic hazard. The identification of hazard is fulfilled by the confirmed presence of mutagenic and carcinogenic chemical species, the mutagenicity of soot extract in bacteria and mammalian cells, and by its carcinogenicity in the mouse skin painting assay (Kotin et al., 1955). However, the identification of inhaled diesel soot as a lung cancer hazard is more controversial. As described above, lung tumor induction by inhaled soot has been consistently demonstrated only in rats, and it is not supported by results from other species. As described below, there is convincing evidence that the lung tumor response of rats to diesel soot should not be used for quantitative estimates of human lung cancer risk. For the same reasons it is doubtful that the rat lung tumor response is a useful indicator of lung cancer hazard for humans.

In the face of poor ability to confidently estimate quantitative lung cancer risks from environmental exposures to diesel exhaust from epidemiological data, it appeared logical to turn to the exposure-response relationships from the rat lung tumor data. A number of estimates of human lung cancer risk per unit of exposure have been derived by modeling the rat data (reviewed in Mauderly, 1992; HEI, 1995; Cal EPA, 1998; U.S. EPA, 1998), and at least one such estimate has been used by a regulatory agency to predict diesel exhaust-related cancer deaths (U.S. EPA, 1993). However, our current knowledge indicates that the rat lung tumor data should not be used for developing estimates of unit lung cancer risk for humans exposed to environmental levels of diesel exhaust (CASAC, 1995;1998; McClellan, 1996; Mauderly, 1998), and probably should not be used for estimating risks from even much higher occupational exposures. Although this conclusion is supported by a substantial base of information gained progressively over the last 15 years, it goes contrary to default risk assessment practices and is not well understood by all stakeholders in the issue. For these reasons the critical pieces of evidence for this conclusion are reviewed here.

1. The cellular responses of the rat lung to diesel soot are strikingly different from the responses of other rodents. During chronic exposure, soot accumulates in foci in the rat lung and causes a progressive inflammatory and fibrotic lesion accompanied by sustained increased proliferation of alveolar type II cells and bronchiolar Clara cells, the cell types thought to give rise to the lung tumors. Another characteristic response of the rat lung epithelium to heavy, chronic particle exposure is the development of squamous keratin cysts (Nikula et al., 1995; Mauderly 1996), which have sometimes been described as "benign keratinizing cystic squamous cell tumors" (Heinrich et al., 1995). Cuboidal and squamous epithelial metaplasias are typical of rat lungs after months of heavy exposure. Under identical conditions, soot tends to remain more widely dispersed in mouse lungs and has much less tendency to cause focal lesions (Mauderly, 1996). Although the size-adjusted lung burdens of soot are equivalent in rats and mice exposed identically, the inflammatory response is less in mice (Henderson et al., 1988). The magnitude and persistence of epithelial proliferation characteristic of rat lungs are not characteristic of mice (Mauderly, 1997). Although epithelial hyperplasia is sometimes observed in mice after long-term exposure, epithelial metaplasia is not common (Mauderly et al., 1996). Squamous keratin cysts are not a typical response of mouse lungs to particle exposure; only one lesion having similar characteristics has been reported in a diesel-exposed mouse (Mauderly et al. 1996). The same differences are found between rats and hamsters. This evidence indicates that the bronchiolar and alveolar epithelium of the rat is somehow predisposed to respond quite differently than the epithelia of mice and hamsters to chronic, heavy exposures to diesel soot and other particles. It seems likely that epithelial neoplasia (the formation of tumors) in exposed rat lungs is an extension of the hyperplastic and metaplastic epithelial changes typical of that species.

2. The epithelial response of rat lungs to diesel soot is not typical of nonhuman primates, and is not thought to be typical of humans. The key issue is not comparisons among animals but whether the lung epithelial proliferative changes in rats that appear to advance to neoplasia are characteristic of humans. Opinions of pathologists expert in human pulmonary responses to heavy dust exposure indicate that epithelial proliferative responses paralleling those of rats are not characteristic of human lungs (personal communications, Dr. F. H. Y. Green, University of Calgary, Alberta, Canada; Dr. N. V. Vallyathan, NIOSH, Morgantown, W.V.; and Dr. M. Schultz, Institut für Pathologie, Uchtspringe, Germany). Although direct comparisons between rats and humans known to be exposed identically are not possible, it is possible to directly compare responses of rats and nonhuman primates. Nikula et al. (1997) compared the pulmonary responses of rats and cynomolgus monkeys to identical chronic diesel exhaust exposures and observed clear differences between the species. They reported that although similar amounts of soot were retained in the lungs of the two species, the predominant site of retention was alveolar in rats and interstitial in monkeys. More important, the epithelial proliferative responses that occurred in rats were absent in the monkeys. Although the two year exposure was not sufficiently long to confirm a lack of tumor response in the monkeys, there were no

proliferative changes to suggest a progression that would lead to tumorigenesis. This information, along with knowledge of the typical responses of human lungs to particle loading, supports the conclusion that the proliferative response of the rat lung to diesel soot accumulation would not occur in humans.

3. Lung cancer risk from diesel soot cannot be extrapolated from rats to other rodents. The large base of information reviewed in the preceding section illustrates clearly that it is impossible to extrapolate lung cancer risk from rats to other rodents, even under extreme exposure conditions. This interspecies difference is not unique to diesel soot; it also occurs with chronic, heavy exposures to a number of other solid, respirable particles (reviewed in Mauderly, 1997). Twelve types of inhaled particles and fibers producing positive lung tumor responses in rats have been shown to be negative in mice. Few nonradioactive particles were positive in both species, and none were positive in mice and negative in rats. The positive carcinogenicity of the materials in rats is now attributed to a characteristic response of that species to exposures at rates that overwhelm the rate of clearance of particles from the lung, and "lung overload" has become a general term for the phenomenon. A symposium on the topic was summarized by Mauderly and McCunney (1996).

4. The threshold in the rat tumor response precludes extrapolation to low exposure levels. Even if the rat lung tumor response did mirror a likely human response, the threshold in the rat response would preclude linear projection of the exposure-response relationship down to environmental exposure levels. As described above, the data points in Figure 7-1 show a threshold for the rat lung tumor response at a weekly soot exposure rate of approximately 100 mg $\cdot$ hr $\cdot$ m^{-3}. The data are robust; confidence in the threshold is generated by the negative responses of nine exposed groups considered adequate for cancer bioassays. Further confidence in the threshold is generated by the absence of any slope among the data points within this range. Additional confidence is contributed by the negative results from detailed measurements of inflammatory, proliferative, fibrotic, and lung clearance effects at an exposure rate of 12.3 mg $\cdot$ hr $\cdot$ m^{-3}, despite the accumulation of small amounts of soot in the lungs (Mauderly et al., 1987; Henderson et al., 1988). These findings support the current view that not only tumors, but also significant nonneoplastic effects, occur in rats only if the exposure rate exceeds a functional threshold that allows substantial amounts of soot to accumulate progressively. The apparent exposure threshold for cancer of approximately 100 mg $\cdot$ hr $\cdot$ m^{-3}, if averaged over 24 h/d, 7 d/w, would represent a continuous exposure of approximately 600 µg/m^3, which is more than two orders of magnitude above estimated human environmental exposures. Even the nonneoplastic no-effects level of 12.3 mg $\cdot$ hr $\cdot$ m^{-3} would represent an average exposure of 73 µg/m^3, which is over an order of magnitude above environmental exposures.

The mathematical models that have been applied to the rat lung tumor data to estimate cancer risks from low-level exposures have generally been linearized models that assume no threshold. The assumption of a linear, no-threshold response is a common default practice in the absence of actual information on the nature of the exposure–response relationship. Because of the small numbers of exposure groups and small group sizes used in any single study, it is not surprising that even multistage linearized models applied to individual study data sets have not demonstrated a statistically significant threshold in the response. However, when the aggregate data in the low-exposure range are analyzed by meta-analysis, a threshold is demonstrated (Valberg and Crouch, 1999). Given the availability of a substantial data base from numerous treatment groups in adequately designed studies from several laboratories, the actual data provide a much better view of the exposure–response relationship than linearized models or default assumptions.

5. The lung tumors in rats are not caused by the organic fraction of soot. The concern for human lung cancer from inhaled diesel soot is founded on the soot-associated organic

mutagens, and these compounds are also key to the determination that diesel soot presents a carcinogenic hazard. Therefore the role of these compounds in the rat lung tumor response is key to the utility of that response for human risk assessment. Because of the large body of evidence that rat lungs respond similarly to a wide range of particles, many having no organic mutagens (Mauderly, 1997), independent studies were conducted in two laboratories to determine whether the organic fraction was necessary for the rat's response to diesel soot. Heinrich et al. (1995) exposed rats in parallel to diesel soot, mutagen-poor carbon black, and fine titanium dioxide particles. Nikula et al. (1995) exposed rats in parallel to diesel soot and a different mutagen-poor carbon black. Although the studies were designed differently, they yielded the same conclusion. Both studies demonstrated that the lung tumor exposure–response relationships to diesel soot and carbon black were identical, and the study by Heinrich et al. also produced an identical response to titanium dioxide. These findings indicate that the organic fraction of diesel soot played no significant role in its carcinogenicity in rats. This finding indicates that the rat lung tumor response to diesel soot is not relevant to carcinogenic hazard or lung cancer risk from the soot-associated organic mutagens.

Current Understanding of Human Lung Cancer Risk There have been numerous attempts over the past 20 years to develop quantitative estimates of the risks for human lung cancer per unit of diesel exhaust exposure, all based on exposure to the soot fraction. This effort continues, driven largely by the desire of regulatory agencies to make quantitative estimates of the effects of environmental exposures. The attempts have taken one of three approaches, which differ by the source of exposure–response data: (1) epidemiology, (2) rat lung carcinogenesis, and (3) comparative mutagenic potency. The first two are based on the information described in preceding sections. The third approach compared the mutagenic potency of the organic fraction of diesel soot to those of other materials for which human exposure-cancer response data exist, such as cigarette smoke or coke oven emissions. Previous risk estimates will not be reviewed in this chapter; several summaries are available (Mauderly, 1992; HEI, 1995; Cal EPA, 1998; U.S. EPA, 1998). To date, no approach using current data yields estimates with a high level of confidence. Epidemiological data should provide the soundest basis for estimating risk, but confidence in the result is limited by the confidence in our understanding of exposure–response relationships throughout the exposure range of interest. The current status of the three general approaches is summarized below.

Epidemiology The greatest barrier to deriving cancer risk estimates from epidemiological data is the lack of actual data on the exposures of the subjects. As described above, the weight of the epidemiological evidence suggests that high-level, long-term occupational exposures to diesel exhaust might be associated with a small increase in lung cancer risk. In the studies generally regarded to be the most robust, a positive effect can be obtained by comparing lung cancer rates of "exposed" and "unexposed" populations. The chief difficulty with mathematical extrapolation of risk from these data to environmental exposure levels lies in the uncertainty of the shape of the exposure–response relationship. The confidence with which an exposure–response slope can be derived and used to estimate risk at low environmental exposure levels from results of the occupational studies is pivotal to current risk estimating activities. Recent debates have centered largely on whether or not a significant exposure–response slope can be derived from the Garshick et al. railroad worker data (Garshick et al., 1987a, 1988). Under contract to the U.S. EPA, Crump et al. (1991) applied numerous modeling approaches to the Garshick et al. railroad worker data and determined that no exposure–response slope could be derived with confidence. In contrast, the California EPA (1998) contends that a suitable exposure–response slope can be derived from the Garshick et al. data.

The Health Effects Institute recently convened an independent panel to evaluate the usefulness of current epidemiological data sets for deriving an exposure–response relationship for lung cancer (HEI, 1999). The panel concluded that the existing railroad worker data reported by Garshick et al. (1987a, 1988) do not support the conclusion of a positive exposure–response relationship. The panel concluded that the truck driver data reviewed by Steenland et al. (1990, 1998) are potentially useful for exposure–response analysis, but required further evaluation to resolve critical issues, particularly regarding assumptions about exposures.

Rat Lung Tumor Data   Numerous estimates of human lung cancer risk have been derived from the rat lung tumor data since the first results became known in the mid-1980s. Since that time, the evidence against using the rat data, reviewed above, has accumulated progressively. At this time there appears to be no scientific basis for using the rat lung tumor data to either infer the existence of human lung cancer risk or to make estimates of its magnitude.

Comparative Mutagenic Potency   The comparative potency method was used in the earliest attempts to estimate human lung cancer risk from diesel exhaust (Albert et al., 1983; Harris, 1983; Cuddihy et al., 1984). This approach was intended to give a preliminary view of the general magnitude of risk, anticipating that more accurate estimates would later be derived from results of epidemiological and animal studies. The intake of mutagenic activity from the organic fraction of diesel soot was compared to the intakes of smokers and workers exposed to mutagenic material from other sources. The assumption was made that the relative cancer risks would parallel the relative doses of mutagenic material multiplied by the relative mutagenic potencies of the materials. A similar approach involves using the concentration of a single carcinogenic compound to predict the carcinogenicity of diesel exhaust from those of other exposures for which the cancer risk is known with greater confidence and assumed to be proportional to that compound. Heinrich et al. (1995) used this approach to estimate risk from the benzo[a]pyrene content of diesel soot, based on the comparative human cancer data reported by Pike and Henderson (1981). The comparative potency method has not been used recently to generate new risk estimates, although EPA included an earlier comparative potency estimate, along with other estimates, in its recent draft document (U.S. EPA, 1998).

In view of the current controversy surrounding the use of epidemiological and animal data for risk assessment, an updated comparative potency approach may yet provide a useful first approximation of human lung cancer risk from inhaled diesel exhaust. The key difficulties in using this approach lie in the need for assumptions regarding the bioavailability, and thus the absorbed dose, of the soot-borne mutagens, and the comparative relationships between mutagenicity and cancer risk among the materials being compared. Considerable uncertainty remains regarding the amount of soot-associated organic material that leaches from the particles in vivo, and the time course of that process. The extent to which carcinogenic risk parallels mutagenic potency also remains uncertain. Trosko (1997) recently reviewed the numerous difficulties in applying mutagenicity data and results from other in vitro assays in risk assessment, and highlighted the need to base such extrapolations on a knowledge of the carcinogenic mechanisms important for each type of agent. Despite these uncertainties a credible approximation of cancer risk might be derived using an updated comparative potency paradigm that integrates information from a range of cellular and molecular assays currently thought to be most relevant to the mechanisms by which soot-associated organic compounds might contribute to carcinogenesis.

Summary of Current Understanding of Lung Cancer Risk   At this time it is widely considered plausible that that diesel soot presents a carcinogenic hazard, but there is little consensus of opinion regarding the magnitude of lung cancer risk under current occupational exposure conditions and either the existence or magnitude of risk under current environmental exposure conditions. The aggregate epidemiological data suggest that past occupational exposures were associated with a small increase in lung cancer risk, but they do not provide a confident basis for quantitative estimates of risk. The validity of estimates from epidemiological data depend on the confidence with which an exposure–response slope can be derived, and that remains very uncertain. It now appears clear that ~~the rat lung tumor response should not be used to develop quantitative estimates of~~ human risk, regardless of the mathematical method applied. The comparative potency approach may yet yield useful approximations of risk, but this is also attended by considerable uncertainty.

Overall, it is reasonable to assume that if the inhalation of airborne mutagenic material is attended by cancer risk, then environmental diesel soot contributes in some measure to that pool of material and thus to the risk. It is also reasonable to assume that cancer risk might parallel the deposited dose of inhaled mutagenic material, depending on the bioavailability of the material and its mutagenic potency in humans. At present we face the yet-unresolved dilemma of acknowledging the plausibility of cancer risk but not being able to make quantitative estimates of that risk with good confidence. It appears doubtful that continuation of the present lines of debate over the existing epidemiological and animal data will resolve this dilemma. New approaches and new information will be required to move substantially from our present quandary.

During the past decade several health and regulatory agencies have reviewed the evidence for human carcinogenesis from inhaled diesel exhaust, with a primary emphasis on lung cancer. In 1988, the National Institute of Occupational Safety and Health (NIOSH) declared diesel exhaust a "potential occupational carcinogen" (NIOSH, 1988). In 1989, the International Agency for Research on Cancer (IARC) concluded that diesel exhaust was a "probable human carcinogen' (IARC, 1989). In 1995, the Health Effects Institute (HEI) noted that, although the weight of epidemiological evidence suggested an association between occupational exposure to diesel exhaust and lung cancer, several uncertainties precluded judging the level of risk with confidence (HEI, 1995). In 1996, the World Health Organization's International Programme on Chemical Safety (IPCS) classified diesel exhaust as "probably carcinogenic to humans" but noted that current epidemiological data were insufficient for estimating risk quantitatively (IPCS, 1996). California recently reviewed the carcinogenicity of diesel exhaust in view of its potential listing as a "toxic air contaminant" under state law. California considered the epidemiological data adequate to support a causal association between occupational exposures and lung cancer, and identified "diesel exhaust particulate matter," in contrast to diesel exhaust per se, as a toxic air contaminant (Cal EPA, 1998). In its most recent draft health assessment document, the U.S. EPA categorized diesel exhaust as "highly likely to be a human carcinogen" (U.S. EPA, 1998). In December 1998, the National Toxicology Program (NTP) reviewed "diesel exhaust particulates" for listing in its Report on Carcinogens (NTP, 1998). The Carcinogens Subcommittee of the NTP Board of Scientific Counselors voted to list diesel exhaust particulates as "reasonably anticipated to be a human carcinogen" but considered the evidence insufficient for the alternative listing as "known to be a human carcinogen." In aggregate, these designations portray a general consensus that diesel exhaust, most probably diesel soot, poses some level of human lung cancer risk at some exposure level but that present uncertainties prevent declaring diesel exhaust a known human carcinogen or estimating its carcinogenic potency with a high level of confidence.

Changes in Respiratory Function and Structure

The effects of inhaled diesel exhaust on respiratory function, lung structure, and noncancer respiratory disease have been reviewed in detail (HEI, 1995; Cal EPA, 1998;U.S. EPA, 1998) and will only be summarized in this chapter. The potential influence of diesel exhaust on allergic responses is reviewed separately in the next section. Experimental exposures of humans have induced pulmonary inflammatory responses. Workshift exposures to high concentrations of exhaust can cause transient decrements of respiratory function, and long-term occupational exposures have been associated with small increases in the incidence of respiratory symptoms and noncancer respiratory disease. Heavy, chronic exposures of animals cause changes in respiratory function that reflect progressive changes in lung structure.

Experimental Exposures of Humans   Battigelli et al. (1965) exposed subjects for 1 h to exhaust from a single-cylinder diesel engine and detected no decrements of airflow resistance. Although the soot concentrations were not given, the highest concentrations of 55 ppm carbon monoxide, 4.2 ppm nitrogen dioxide, and 1 ppm sulfur dioxide suggest that the highest soot concentration was in the range of a few mg/m^3.

Ulfvarson et al. (1987) exposed subjects for 3.7 h to exhaust from a 3.7 L engine at a soot concentration of 600 $\mu g/m^3$ and detected no decrement in forced expiratory parameters or the single-breath nitrogen washout.

Rudell et al. (1990) exposed subjects for 1 h to exhaust from an idling truck at a soot concentration of approximately 1 mg/m^3 and evaluated effects by bronchoalveolar lavage and the in vitro phagocytic ability of pulmonary macrophages removed by lavage. The exposure increased neutrophils and increased the T-helper to T-suppressor lymphocyte ratio in the lavage fluid, and decreased phagocytosis by macrophages.

These findings suggest that exposure of healthy subjects to diesel exhaust at a soot concentration in the mg/m^3 range for as little as 1 h causes a slight pulmonary inflammatory response and affects macrophage function but does not cause significant changes in ventilatory function.

Epidemiological Studies of Humans

Effects from a Single Workshift   There are six published evaluations of the effects of diesel exhaust exposure during a single workshift on respiratory function. These studies are complicated by the numerous other materials inhaled during the workshift by the miners, garage workers, stevedores, and ferryboat crewmen, and not all studies included control groups not exposed to diesel exhaust. In addition characterization of the personal exposures to diesel soot and other exhaust components varied considerably among the studies. All of these studies used forced expiratory performance as the respiratory function indicator. Ames et al. (1982) found that workshift changes in respiratory function did not differ between workers in mines where diesel engines were used or not used. The other five reports described workshift changes ascribed to diesel exhaust exposure.

Both Jörgensen and Swenson (1970) and Gamble et al. (1978) reported small workshift decrements in forced expiratory volumes and flow rates among miners. Gamble et al. (1987) measured small workshift decrements in function and found a stronger association with particle concentrations than with nitrogen dioxide. Ulfvarson et al. (1987) found small, but significant, workshift decrements in function among stevedores on roll-on, roll-off ships exposed to soot at 130 to 590 $\mu g/m^3$, but not in bus garage or car ferry workers exposed to soot at 100 to 460 $\mu g/m^3$. Ulfvarson and Alexandersson (1990) detected small workshift decrements of function among stevedores exposed to respirable particles at

$120 \,\mu g / m^3$. Overall, these findings support the premise that workshift exposures to high concentrations of diesel exhaust can cause small decrements in sensitive indicators of forced airflow performance.

Long-Term Effects The nine published evaluations of the effects of long-term occupational exposure to diesel exhaust on respiratory function and symptoms (listed in detail in HEI, 1995) yielded mixed results. Most studies found that long-term diesel exhaust exposure was associated with small increases in respiratory symptoms such as dyspnea, cough, and phlegm (Jörgensen and Svensson, 1970; Attfield et al., 1982; Reger et al., 1982; Gamble et al., 1983, 1987; Purdham et al., 1987), but some did not (Battagelli et al., 1964; Ames et al., 1984). As an example of the uncertainty regarding symptoms, Gamble et al. (1987) found that bus garage workers had higher age and smoking-adjusted incidences of cough, phlegm, and wheezing than controls, but they found no association between symptoms and length of employment. Similarly the studies produced mixed results concerning long-term decrements of respiratory function. Results to date do not show a consistent relationship between symptoms and respiratory function. Among the individual studies, some found decrements of function but no increase in symptoms, and others found the opposite. Jacobsen et al. (1988) found a relative risk of 1.7 for respiratory infections among British coal miners, a finding consistent with the impairment of alveolar macrophage function noted above (Rudell et al., 1990).

The relationship between long-term occupational exposure to diesel exhaust and mortality from noncancer respiratory disease is also uncertain. Among the nine studies evaluating this relationship (listed in detail in HEI, 1995), four showed a positive association and five did not. Just as for cancer, the epidemiological studies of noncancer disease contain uncertainties regarding exposure and smoking classification. Only two groups of investigators employed some form of adjustment for smoking, and both yielded positive results. In their case-control study of lung cancer among railroad workers, Garshick et al. (1987a) identified 575 cases of mortality from chronic respiratory disease and calculated a relative risk of 1.2 for workers exposed five years or longer. In their retrospective cohort study (Garshick et al., 1988), these investigators calculated a relative risk of 1.6 for chronic respiratory disease mortality among the group of railroad workers with the longest exposure to diesel exhaust. In their prospective mortality study of U.S. males, Boffetta et al. (1988) identified 1242 noncancer respiratory deaths during 1983 and 1984, and they calculated relative risks among diesel-exposed men of 1.2 for emphysema and other chronic obstructive pulmonary disease and 1.7 for respiratory infections. Overall, the risk for mortality from noncancer chronic respiratory disease associated with occupational exposure to diesel exhaust appears to be on the same order of magnitude as the risk for lung cancer, but the data are fewer and even more uncertain.

Animal Studies There is little additional information on the effects of inhaled diesel exhaust on respiratory function and lung structure of animals beyond that reviewed previously (Mauderly, 1994a,b, 1996; HEI, 1995). The largest body of information is derived from studies of rodents, and it reflects the species differences discussed briefly in the preceding section on lung cancer. Near lifetime repeated exposures of rats at concentrations of soot over approximately 1 mg/m^3 overwhelms the ability of normal particle clearance pathways and results in a progressive accumulation of soot in the lung. This accumulation is accompanied by persistent inflammation, focal epithelial proliferation and metaplasia, and fibrosis (Mauderly, 1996). The progressive structural changes are reflected by a progressive impairment of respiratory function which includes lung stiffening (loss of compliance), reduced lung volumes, uneven intrapulmonary gas distribution, and impaired alveolar-capillary gas exchange (Mauderly et al., 1988). This structure-function syndrome also occurs in rats exposed heavily to other solid, respirable particles (Mauderly, 1994b). Of importance from a human exposure viewpoint, no significant alterations of particle clearance (Wolff et al., 1987), inflammation, fibrosis (Henderson et al., 1988), or respiratory function or structure (Mauderly et al., 1988) resulted from chronic exposures of rats at 350 μg soot / m^3, even though small amounts of soot accumulated in the lungs. Under identical exposure conditions, mice accumulate similar amounts of soot in their lungs (Henderson et al., 1988), but the inflammatory, fibrotic (Henderson et al., 1988), and histopathological (Mauderly et al., 1996) responses are less than those in rats. Small reductions in lung volumes and compliance have also been observed in diesel-exposed Syrian (Heinrich et al., 1986) and Chinese (Vinegar et al., 1981) hamsters. Mice and hamsters have also been shown to have lesser functional and structural responses than rats to other solid respirable particles (Mauderly, 1994b).

A smaller, but perhaps more relevant, body of information comes from nonrodent species which have respiratory bronchioles (absent in rodents) and other lung features more similar to humans. Only two species have been chronically exposed to diesel exhaust. The U.S. EPA exposed male cats chronically to exhaust at 6 mg soot / m^3 for 61 weeks, and then at 12 mg/m^3 for the remainder of 27 months, followed by a 6 month recovery period (Pepelko and Peirano, 1983). A restrictive functional impairment with decreased lung volumes and uneven intrapulmonary gas distribution was observed at the end of the exposure (Moorman et al., 1985). Histopathology at the end of exposure included peribronchiolar fibrosis and epithelial metaplasia in terminal and respiratory bronchioles (Plopper et al., 1983). Interestingly, while the epithelial changes lessened during the 6 month recovery period, the fibrosis progressed. Lewis et al. (1989) exposed cynomolgus monkeys to diesel exhaust for 2 years at 2 mg soot / m^3 and reported that the forced expiratory flow rates were reduced at the end of exposure (Lewis et al., 1986). The lung histopathology of the monkeys differed from that of rats exposed concurrently (Nikula   et al., 1997). Soot was present in approximately the same tissue concentration in both species but was located predominantly in interstitial compartments in monkeys and in alveolar lumens in rats. The species had similar increases in pulmonary macrophages. The most striking difference was in the degree of epithelial proliferation, which was characteristically prevalent near accumulations of soot in rats, but essentially absent in monkeys. Although the data base is small, these results suggest that nonrodent species can develop fibrosis and epithelial responses under extreme exposure conditions, but they exhibit little structural response from chronic exposures at 2 mg soot / m^3.

Asthma and Allergic Rhinitis

There has been recent speculation about a possible association between inhaled diesel exhaust and allergic asthma and rhinitis. The evidence for a unique or specific effect of diesel is weak but worth noting as a current issue. Edwards et al. (1994) reported that children under the age of five years in Birmingham, U.K., were more likely to be hospitalized for asthma than for other reasons if they lived in an area of high traffic flow. Wade and Newman (1993) reported cases in which occupational exposure to diesel exhaust was thought to cause or contribute to the development of asthma, and coined the term, "diesel asthma." Keil et al. (1996) reported a positive correlation between the prevalences of wheezing and allergic rhinitis and traffic density among adolescents in German cities. Peters et al. (1997) reported that symptoms among adult asthmatics in Erfurt, Germany, was more closely related to the number of ultrafine particles than to fine particle mass. None of these reports demonstrate a relationship between diesel emissions and allergic disease, but diesel soot is frequently mentioned as a common constituent of fine and ultrafine particulate pollution, especially pollution related to vehicle emissions.

There is a growing body of experimental evidence suggesting that diesel soot might contribute to allergic symptoms by acting as an adjuvant in producing Th2-type immune responses. Much of our present information comes from laboratory studies in Japan. Takano et al. (1997) reported that intratracheally instilled diesel soot enhanced ovalbumin-induced lung inflammation, cytokine release, and ovalbumin-specific IgG and IgE antibodies in mice. Other Japanese investigators have demonstrated that inhalation (Fujimaki et al., 1997), intranasal instillation (Takafuji et al., 1987, 1989), and intratracheal instillation (Fujimaki et al., 1994) of diesel soot enhanced ovalbumin-specific IgE antibody production in mice. Diesel soot was also shown to enhance IgE antibody production in mice immunized intraperitoneally with ovalbumin or Japanese cedar pollen (Muranaka et al., 1986). Takenaka et al. (1995) reported that an extract of polycyclic aromatic hydrocarbons from diesel soot enhanced IGE antibody production by B lymphocytes in vitro. Finally Kobayashi et al. (1997) found that short-term exposure of guinea pigs to diesel exhaust increased the sneezing and nasal secretion responses to histamine, but they did not induce the responses in the absence of histamine.

A group in the United States reported that nasal challenge of humans with diesel soot increases local IgE antibody production (Diaz-Sanchez et al., 1994) and stimulates cytokine production (Diaz-Sanchez et al., 1996). They also found that combining diesel soot with ragweed allergen challenge markedly enhanced nasal ragweed-specific IgE and shifted cytokine production toward a Th2 pattern (Diaz-Sanchez et al., 1997).

Because diesel soot in sufficient quantity is known to have irritating effects on cells and to cause inflammation of the respiratory tract, it is plausible that at some dose, diesel soot might also act as an adjuvant in enhancing reactions to allergens. There are two issues critical to the assessment of the likely adjuvant effects of actual environmental exposures, and these issues remain to be resolved. First, it is not clear that environmentally or occupationally relevant exposures to diesel soot would have significant effects. Second, it is not clear if the adjuvant effects of diesel soot are a unique feature of its physical-chemical composition, or if other particles would act similarly. Unfortunately, the studies cited above did not compare responses to diesel soot and other particles. The only comparison published to date is that of Maejima et al. (1997), whose findings suggest that the adjuvant effects of diesel soot are not unique. Those investigators compared the effects of diesel soot, loam dust, fly ash, and carbon black instilled intranasally into mice exposed to aerosolized Japanese cedar pollen, and evaluated nasal irritation (rubbing) and antibody production. The particles all had similar effects, although the loam dust appeared to be most potent. Other comparisons will need to be made and exposure–response inhalation studies will have to be conducted to resolve the two issues.

Nonpulmonary Health Effects

Bladder Cancer   The bladder is the only organ other than the lung for which there has been significant concern for cancer associated with diesel exhaust exposure. There have been several studies of the incidence of bladder cancer among populations presumed to be heavily exposed to diesel exhaust. A few studies focused primarily on the relationship between bladder cancer and diesel exhaust exposure, but most included the bladder in the context of broader cancer surveys. Most of the difficulties described above for the studies of lung cancer are also inherent in the studies of bladder cancer. These include lack of quantitation of exposure, lack of uniqueness of the exposure materials to diesel exhaust, lack of clearly exposed and unexposed groups, the presence of several confounding factors, and potential misclassification. As for lung cancer, perhaps the most serious confounding factor for bladder cancer is cigarette smoking, but another is coffee drinking. Wynder et al. (1985) described potential confounding factors and reported that the odds ratio for bladder cancer from smoking alone was 3.5 in their hospital-based case-control study.

Information on the association between diesel exhaust exposure and bladder and other cancers was recently reviewed (HEI, 1995), and will not be presented in detail here. The weight of the present evidence suggests that as for lung cancer, there may be a small positive risk for bladder cancer among truck drivers and other long-term workers in occupations presumed to be highly exposed to diesel exhaust. Interestingly general population case-control studies tend to point toward a higher risk among truck drivers than the studies specifically addressing diesel-exposed cohorts. As for lung cancer, the apparent magnitude of relative risk for bladder cancer is at the approximate lower practical limit of detection by epidemiological studies, and the lower end of the 95% confidence interval for some of the positive studies includes a relative risk of 1.0. There are no clearly exposed and unexposed populations, and it is difficult to associate the small effect clearly with diesel exhaust. There is no evidence from animal studies for increased bladder cancer. Overall, the evidence for a diesel-related increase in bladder cancer risk is suggestive but even more uncertain than the lung cancer risk at this time.

Experimental Evidence for Other Nonpulmonary Effects   As predicted for humans, rodents exposed chronically to diesel exhaust would be expected to ingest more soot than is deposited and retained in the lung by inhalation. This route of exposure results largely from the grooming habits of rodents, which cause the ingestion of soot deposited on the fur. Wolff et al. (1982) examined the gastrointestinal tract intake of gallium oxide particles in rats exposed repeatedly by either nose-only or whole-body methods. They estimated that the intake was approximately 60% greater in rats exposed whole-body than in those exposed nose-only and attributed this difference to grooming. Because the size and morphological characteristics of the gallium oxide particles were similar to those of diesel soot, this result suggests that animals in the diesel exhaust studies listed in Tables 7-4 and 7-5 ingested substantial amounts of soot. These studies therefore constitute a reasonable examination of the hazard associated with ingestion and absorption of diesel exhaust vapors and soot-associated chemicals. Few of the reports of animal studies, however, gave detailed information on nonpulmonary health effects.

Nonpulmonary Cancer   Specific information on cancer in organs other than the respiratory tract was reported only for four studies of rats and one study of hamsters included in Tables 7-4 and 7-5. Karagianes et al. (1981) reported that no significant exposure-related lesions were found in the esophagus or stomach of rats. Kaplan et al. (1983) reported that no lesions were found in tissues other than the respiratory system of rats (and hamsters) that could be attributed to exposure. Ishihara (1988) reported that there were no differences between exposed and control rats in the incidences of leukemia, Leydig cell tumors, mammary gland tumors, or total nonpulmonary tumors. Lewis et al. (1989) examined 50 organs and gave detailed data for tumors in 11 nonpulmonary organs, including the bladder. They found no exposure-related difference in nonpulmonary carcinogenesis.

Although other reports did not detail nonlung findings, many studies (e.g., Heinrich et al., 1986; Mauderly et al., 1987; Nikula et al., 1995) included complete necropsies of all animals, which involved gross observations of all major organs. From published information and personal communications, it is evident that no increased incidence of nonlung cancers was observed in any of these studies.

Noncancer Effects   Three reports included information on noncancer, nonpulmonary health effects of chronic diesel exhaust exposures of animals. Among the variety of health endpoints that were evaluated, no consistent pattern of effects emerged; thus these reports are not reviewed in detail here. Only some of the results are mentioned below; the reader is referred to the original reports for details.

Pepelko and Peirano (1983) reported results of a series of studies that included exposures of fruit flies, mice, hamsters, rats, rabbits, and cats. These authors investigated a spectrum of nonpulmonary endpoints including spermatogenesis, heritable mutations, hematopoiesis, hematology, serum chemistry, xenobiotic-metabolizing enzymes, and neurophysiology, and the reader is referred to the report for details. Few significant exposure-related differences were observed. The learning ability of rats exposed soon after birth was reported to have been impaired. An increase in the fraction of banded neutrophils was found in the circulating blood of male cats exposed for 12 months to exhaust at $6 \, mg \, soot/m^3$.

Ishihara (1988) evaluated hematology, serum chemistry, and hematopoiesis in rats and mice exposed chronically. Hematopoiesis was unaffected in mice or rats. Elevations in circulating erythrocyte concentrations with reduced cell volume and hemoglobin concentration occurred in exposed rats. Several modest changes in serum chemistry were observed in rats, and these were resolved after cessation of exposure.

Lewis et al. (1989) exposed mice, rats, and monkeys chronically to diesel exhaust and evaluated hematopoiesis, hematology, serum chemistry, splenic lymphocyte blast transformation, spermatogenesis, and xenobiotic metabolic enzymes in liver. The fraction of banded circulating neutrophils was increased in rats, but few other exposure-related differences were observed.

The results of these studies indicate that other than modest alterations in hematology and serum chemistry, few nonpulmonary health effects are observed in animals exposed chronically to high concentrations of diesel exhaust. The experimental evidence therefore does not support concern for nonpulmonary effects.

CURRENT ISSUES AND RESEARCH NEEDS

Lung Cancer Risk from Environmental and Occupational Exposures

Clearly, the single most important and controversial issue continues to be the existence and magnitude of human lung cancer risk from both occupational and environmental exposures to diesel exhaust. Although regulatory agencies in other countries are involved, this issue is being largely driven at present by efforts of both the U.S. EPA and California EPA to estimate cancer risks from environmental exposures. As described above, there appears to be no method yielding answers at this time with a high level of confidence. Earlier issues concerning the use of the rat lung tumor response for this purpose have been resolved by the accumulation of information negating the value of these data for human risk assessment. Acceptance of the validity of results from mice and Syrian hamsters leads to the conclusion that contemporary exposures present negligible cancer risk. Progress in using animal data hinges on obtaining data from other species or other types of carcinogenesis assays having more relevance to human responses, and that pathway is not clear at this time. Progress in determining risk from epidemiological studies hinges on conducting new studies including the collection of more accurate exposure-response data from human populations. Progress in using the comparative potency method hinges on an improved understanding of the bioavailability and bioactivity of soot-associated organic mutagens, and the relationship between results of in vitro assays and cancer risk.

Measurement of Human Exposures to Diesel Exhaust

The accurate measurement of diesel exhaust concentrations in mixed pollutant atmospheres presents a technological challenge. The accuracy of estimates of health risks from diesel exhaust, whether derived by interpretation of epidemiological data or by extrapolation from animal studies, is dependent on the extent and accuracy of data for human exposures. As described in preceding sections, there are several estimates but few actual data for either environmental or occupational exposures to diesel exhaust. Historically few attempts have been made to distinguish concentrations of diesel exhaust among those of pollutants derived from other sources. The measurements that have been attempted were hampered by the overlapping compositions of diesel exhaust, other engine exhausts, and pollutants from other sources. Most attempts have focused on diesel soot because of its somewhat distinguishing physical and chemical characteristics. However, even the characteristics of diesel soot overlap those of other airborne particles in environmental and occupational settings. For both risk assessment and standards setting, it would be particularly useful to have good data on diesel exhaust concentrations in mine environments.

Methods used in attempts to determine the concentrations of diesel soot in the environment were described by HEI (1995). Cass et al. (1982) reported that the primary source of elemental carbon in urban particulate matter was diesel exhaust. Gray (1986) based estimates of environmental diesel exhaust concentrations on measurements of elemental and organic carbon. Estimates of the contribution of diesel soot to mine dust have relied primarily on particle size and to a lesser extent on composition (McCawley et al., 1989; Haney, 1990). Schenker et al. (1990) reported that phenanthrene might be a useful marker for diesel soot in respirable particulate matter collected in railroad environments. A combination of size-selective sampling and physical-chemical analysis will probably be required to distinguish diesel exhaust concentrations in both environmental and occupational settings.

A slightly different but similarly important and difficult technological challenge is the assessment of human exposure to diesel exhaust by sampling human subjects. The current drive to develop "biomarkers" of exposures to toxicants and resultant injury extends beyond diesel exhaust and beyond inhaled materials (National Research Council, 1989). The problem is similar to that of measuring airborne concentrations. The key is the identification of compounds unique to diesel exposures or effects that are accessible by noninvasive sampling, are present in measurable amounts, and persist for sufficient lengths of time after exposure. Although biomarkers are an active area of research, few researchers are pursuing markers of diesel exhaust exposure. Schenker et al. (1990) recently reported that the bacterial mutagenicity of urine was not a successful marker for diesel exhaust exposure among railroad workers. Urinary mutagenicity was correlated with cigarette smoking and dietary factors but was not independently correlated with diesel exhaust exposure. There are some efforts to link levels of DNA adducts in blood cells of workers to occupational exposures to diesel exhaust, but there is presently no known unique marker for diesel exhaust exposure.

Bioavailability and Bioactivity of Diesel Soot-Associated Organic Mutagens

The extent to which, and the time course with which, mutagenic activity is released from soot deposited in the lung and interacts with lung epithelium remain uncertain. This information would form the basis of improved knowledge on the dosimetry of mutagenic activity. We have an adequate knowledge of the relationship between exposure concentrations and the amount of mass deposited in different regions of the respiratory under different conditions of breathing and soot particle size. To complete the dosimetry picture, we need a better understanding of the relationship between the mass of deposited soot and the dose of mutagenic activity at critical cellular targets. Our lack of understanding is a barrier to placing the cancer risk of organic mutagens on diesel soot and other particles in its proper context. As described in preceding sections, this lack of understanding also limits our ability to estimate cancer risk by the comparative potency approach, or even to critically judge the usefulness of that approach.

Impact on Health Risk of Reduced Soot Particle Size

An emerging issue is presented by evidence suggesting that current engineering approaches to reducing the mass of soot in tailpipe emissions from diesel engines may tend to result in a larger fraction of the emitted soot falling into the ultrafine size range (less than $0.1\,\mu m$ diameter) (Bagley, 1996; personal communications with Drs. Robert Sawyer and John Johnson). At present, we have little understanding of whether the emission of larger numbers of ultrafine particles, albeit consisting of a small mass, has health implications. It is certainly plausible that ultrafine, poorly soluble particles could be more toxic than an equivalent mass of larger particles because of their greater penetration through tissue barriers and their higher surface to mass ratio. There is some experimental evidence for this (Oberdörster et al., 1995, 1996), although few studies have addressed the issue directly. There have been speculations about the potential role of ultrafine particles in the health effects associated with urban particulate matter (Oberdörster et al., 1995; Seaton et al., 1995; U.S. EPA, 1994), and there is some epidemiological evidence for their importance (Peters et al., 1997a, b). It is important to both engineering and regulatory decisions to develop a better understanding of the relative toxicities of fine and ultrafine soot particles. Two key issues are the irritant potential of ultrafine soot particles and their ability to deliver doses of surface mutagens and metals to cellular targets in the lung and elsewhere, relative to larger soot particles.

ACKNOWLEDGMENT

The years of research on diesel exhaust and the helpful reviews and suggestions by The Lovelace Respiratory Research Institute colleagues and the manuscript preparation support by the Institute's Technical Communications Unit are gratefully acknowledged. This chapter was prepared with support from the Office of Heavy Vehicle Technologies, the Office of Energy Efficiency and Renewable Energy, and the U.S. Department of Energy.

REFERENCES

Ahlberg, J., A. Ahlbom, H. Lipping, S. Norell, and L. Osterblom. 1981. Cancer among professional drivers—A problem-oriented register-based study (in Swedish.). *Lakartidningen* 78: 1545–1546.

Albert, R. E., J. Lewtas, S. Nesnow, T. W. Thorslund, and E. Anderson. 1983. Comparative potency method for cancer risk assessment: Application to diesel particulate emissions. *Risk Anal.* 3: 101–117.

Ames, R. G., M. D. Attfield, J. L. Hankinson, F. J. Hearl, and R. B. Reger. 1982. Acute respiratory effects of exposure to diesel emissions in coal miners. *Am. Rev. Respir. Dis.* 125: 39–42.

Ames, R. G., R. B. Reger, and D. S. Hall. 1984. Chronic respiratory effects of exposure to diesel emissions in coal miners. *J. Occup. Med.* 39: 389–394.

Attfield, M. D., G. D. Trabant, and R. W. Wheeler. 1982. Exposure to diesel fumes and dust at six potash miners. *Ann. Occup. Hyg.* 26: 817–831.

Bagley, S. T. 1996. *Characterization of Fuel and After-Treatment Device Effects on Diesel Emissions.* HEI Report 76.

Battigelli, M. C. 1965. Effects of diesel exhaust. *Arch. Environ. Health* 10: 165–167.

Battigelli, M. C., R. J. Mannella, and T. F. Hatch. 1964. Environmental and clinical investigation of workmen exposed to diesel exhaust in railroad engine houses. *Ind. Med. Surg.* 3: 121–124.

Benhamou, S., E. Benhamou, and R. Flamant. 1988. Occupational risk factors of lung cancer in a French case-control study. *Br. J. Ind. Med.* 45: 231–233.

Bhatia, R., P. Lopipero, and A. Smith. 1998. Diesel exhaust exposure and lung cancer. *Epidemiology* 9: 84–91.

Boffetta, P., S. D. Stellman, and L. Garfinkel. 1988. Diesel exhaust exposure and mortality among males in the American Cancer Society prospective study. *Am. J. Ind. Med.* 14: 403–415.

Boffetta, P., R. E. Harris, and E. L. Wynder. 1990. Case-control study on occupational exposure to diesel exhaust and lung cancer risk. *Am. J. Ind. Med.* 15: 577–591.

Bond, J. A., M. M. Butler, M. A. Medinsky, B. A. Muggenburg, and R. O. McClellan. 1984. Dog pulmonary macrophage metabolism of free and particle-associated [^{14}C]benzo[a]pyrene. *J. Toxicol. Environ. Health* 14: 181–189.

Bond, J. A., J. D. Sun, M. A. Medinsky, R. K. Jones, and H. C. Yeh. 1986. Deposition, metabolism, and excretion of 1-^{14}C nitropyrene and 1-^{14}C nitropyrene coated on diesel exhaust particles as influenced by exposure concentration. *Toxicol. Appl. Pharmacol.* 85: 102–117.

Bond, J. A., R. K. Wolff, J. R. Harkema, J. L. Mauderly, R. E. Henderson, W. C. Griffith, and R. O. McClellan. 1990a. DNA adduct distribution in the respiratory tract of rats exposed to diesel exhaust. In *Multilevel Health Effects Research: From Molecules to Man,* DOE Symposium Series, ed. R. A. Pelroy, pp. 349–355. Richland, WA: Battelle Pacific Northwest Laboratory.

Bond, J. A., J. R. Harkema, R. F. Henderson, J. L. Mauderly, R. O. McClellan, and R. K. Wolff. 1990b. The role of DNA adducts in diesel exhaust-induced pulmonary carcinogenesis. In *Mutation and the Environment, Part C: Somatic and Heritable Mutation, Adduction, and Epidemiology,* eds M. L. Mendelsohn and R. J. Albertini, pp. 259–269. New York: Wiley-Liss.

Bond, J. A., J. L. Mauderly, and R. K. Wolff. 1990c. Concentration- and time-dependent formation of DNA adduct in lungs of rats exposed to diesel exhaust. *Toxicology* 60: 127–135.

Bond, J. A., N. F. Johnson, M. B. Snipes, and J. L. Mauderly. 1990d. DNA adduct formation in rats alveolar type II cells—Cells potentially at risk for inhaled diesel exhaust. *Environ. Mol. Mutagen.* 16: 64–69.

Brightwell, I., X. Fouillet, A.-L. Cassano-Zoppi, D. Bernstein, E. Crawley, E. Duchosal, R. Gatz, S. Perczel, and H. Pfeifer. 1989. Tumours of the respiratory tract in rats and hamsters following chronic inhalation of engine exhaust emissions. *J. Appl. Toxicol.* 9: 23–31.

Brooks, A. L., R. K. Wolff, R. E. Royer, C. R. Clark, A. Sanchez, and R. O. McClellan. 1981. Deposition and biological availability of diesel particles and their associated mutagenic chemicals. *Environ. Int.* 5: 263–267.

Brooks, A. L., A. P. Li, J. S. Dutcher, C. R. Clark, S. J. Rothenberg, R. Kiyoura, W. E. Bechtold, and R. O. McClellan. 1984. A comparison of genotoxicity of automotive exhaust particles from laboratory and environmental sources. *Environ. Mutagen.* 6: 651–668.

Buiatti, E., D. Kriebel, M. Geddes, M. Santucci, and N. Pucci. 1985. A case control study of lung cancer in Florence, Italy. I. Occupational risk factors. *J. Epidemiol. Commun. Health* 39: 244–250.

California Environmental Protection Agency. 1998. *Part B: Health Risk Assessment for Diesel Exhaust, Proposed Identification of Diesel Exhaust as a Toxic Air Contaminant.* Office of Environmental Health Hazard Assessment, Air Resources Board, Sacramento.

CASAC (Clean Air Scientific Advisory Committee). 1995. *Review of Diesel Health Assessment Document.* EPA-SAB-CASAC-LTR-95-003. U.S. Environmental Protection Agency Research Triangle Park, NC.

CASAC (Clean Air Scientific Advisory Committee). 1998. *CASAC Review of the Draft Diesel Health Assessment Document.* EPA-SAB-CASAC-99-001. U.S. Environmental Protection Agency, Research Triangle Park, NC.

Cass, G. R., P. M. Boone, and E. S. Macias. 1982. Emissions and air quality relationships for atmospheric carbon particles in Los Angeles. In *Particulate Carbon: Atmospheric Life Cycle,* eds. G. T. Wolff and R. L. Klimisch. New York: Plenum Press.

Cheng, Y. S., H. C. Yeh, J. L. Mauderly, and B. V. Mokler. 1984. Characterization of diesel exhaust in a chronic inhalation study. *Am. Ind. Hyg. Assoc. J.* 45: 547–555.

Clark, C. R., R. E. Royer, A. L. Brooks, R. O. McClellan, W. E. Marshal, T. M. Naman, and D. E. Seizinger. 1981. Mutagenicity of diesel exhaust particle extracts: Influence of car type. *Fundam. Appl. Toxicol.* 1: 260–265.

Clark, C. R., J. S. Dutcher, T. R. Henderson, R. O. McClellan, W. E. Marshall, T. M. Naman, and D. E. Seizinger. 1984. Mutagenicity of automotive particulate exhaust: Influence of fuel extenders, additives and aromatic content. *Adv. Mod. Environ. Toxicol.* 6: 109–122.

Claxton, L. D. 1983. Characterization of automotive emissions by bacterial mutagenesis bioassay: A review. *Environ. Mutagen.* 5 : 609–631.

Coggon, D., B. Pannett, and E. D. Acheson. 1984. Use of job-exposure matrix in an occupational analysis of lung and bladder cancers on the basis of death certificates. *J. Natl. Cancer Inst.* 72: 61–65.

Cross, E T., R. E. Palmer, R. E. Filipy, R. H. Busch, and B. O. Stuart. 1978. *Study of the Combined Effects of Smoking and Inhalation of Uranium Ore Dust, Radon Daughters, and Diesel Exhaust Fumes in Hamsters and Dogs.* Report PNL-2744: UC-48. Richland, WA: Pacific Northwest Laboratory.

Crump, K. S., T. Lambert, and C. Chen. 1991. Assessment of risk from exposure to diesel engine emissions. USEPA Contract 68-02-4601; Appendix B in *USEPA, Health Assessment Document for Diesel Emissions.* vol. 2, EPA-600/8-90/057Bb.

Cuddihy, R. G., E. A. Seiler, W. C. Griffith, B. R. Scott, and R. O. McClellan. 1980. *Potential Health and Environmental Effects of Diesel Light Duty Vehicles.* DOE Research and Development Report, LMF-82. Springfield, VA: National Technical Information Service.

Cuddihy, R. G., W. C. Griffith, and R. O. McClellan. 1984. Health risks from light-duty diesel vehicles. *Environ. Sci. Technol.* 18: 14A–21A.

Damber, L. A., and L. G. Larsson. 1987. Occupation and male lung cancer: A case-control study in northern Sweden. *Br. J. Ind. Med.* 44: 446–453.

Daniel, J. H. 1984. The use of diesel-powered equipment in U.S. underground coal operations. Presented at the American Mining Congress International Coal Show, Chicago, May 3.

Decoufle, P., K. Stanislawczyk, L. Houten, J. D. J. Bross, and E. Viadana. 1977. *A Retrospective Survey of Cancer in Relation to Occupation.* DHEW(NIOSH) Publ. 77-178. Cincinnati, OH: U.S. Department of Health, Education, and Welfare.

Diaz-Sanchez, D., A. R. Dotson, H. Takenaka, and A. Saxon. 1994. Diesel exhaust particles induce local IgE production in vivo and alter the pattern of IgE messenger RNA isoforms. *J. Clin. Invest.* 94(4): 1417–1425.

Diaz-Sanchez, D., A. Tsien, A. Casillas, A. R. Dotson, and A. Saxon. 1996. Enhanced nasal cytokine production in human beings after in vivo challenge with diesel exhaust particles. *J. Allergy Clin. Immunol.* 98(1): 114–123.

Diaz-Sanchez, D., A. Tsien, J. Fleming, and A. Saxon. 1997. Combined diesel exhaust particulate and ragweed allergen challenge markedly enhances human in vivo nasal ragweed-specific IgE and skews cytokine production to a T helper cell 2-type pattern. *J. Immunol.* 158(5): 2406–2413.

Dubrow, R., and D. H. Wegman. 1983. Setting priorities for occupational cancer research and control: Synthesis of the results of occupational disease surveillance studies. *J. Natl. Cancer Inst.* 71: 1123–1142.

Edling, C., C.-G. Anjou, O. Axelson, and H. Kling. 1987. Mortality among personnel exposed to diesel exhaust. *Int. Arch. Occup. Environ. Health* 59: 559–565.

Edwards, J., S. Walters, and R. K. Griffiths. 1994. Hospital admissions for asthma in preschool children: Relationship to major roads in Birmingham, United Kingdom. *Arch. Environ. Health* 49(4): 223–227.

Emmelin, A., L. Nyström, and S. Wall. 1993. Diesel exhaust exposure and smoking: A case-referent study of lung cancer among Swedish dock workers. *Epidemiology* 4: 237–244.

Enya, T., H. Suzuki, T. Watanabe, T. Hirayama, and Y. Hisamatsu. 1997. 3-Nitrobenzanthrone, a powerful bacterial mutagen and suspected human carcinogen found in diesel exhaust and airborne particulates. *Environ. Sci. Technol.* 31(10): 2772–2776.

Frey, J. W., and M. Corn. 1967. Diesel exhaust particulates. *Nature* 216: 615–616.

Fujimaki, H., O. Nohara, T. Ichinose, N. Watanabe, and S. Saito. 1994. IL-4 production in mediastinal lymph node cells in mice intratracheally instilled with diesel exhaust particulates and antigen. *Toxicology* 92: 261–268.

Fujimaki, H., K. Saneyoshi, F. Shiraishi, T. Imai, and T. Endo. 1997. Inhalation of diesel exhaust enhances antigen-specific IgE antibody production in mice. *Toxicology* 116: 227–233.

Gallagher, J., U. Heinrich, M. George, L. Hendee, D. H. Phillips, and J. Lewtas. 1994. Formation of DNA adducts in rat lung following chronic inhalation of diesel emissions, carbon black and titanium dioxide particles. *Carcinogenesis* 15: 1291–1299.

Gamble, J., W. Jones, J. Hudak, and J. Merchant. 1978. Acute changes in pulmonary function in salt miners. In *Proceedings of an American Council of Governmental Industrial Hygiene Topical Symposium: Industrial Hygiene for Mining and Tunneling,* November 6–7, 1978. Cincinnati, OH: American Conference of Governmental Industrial Hygienists.

Gamble, J., W. Jones, and J. Hudak. 1983. An epidemiological study of salt miners in diesel and nondiesel mines. *Am. J. Ind. Med.* 4: 435–458.

Gamble, J., W. Jones, and S. Minshall. 1987. Epidemiological-environmental study of diesel bus garage workers: Chronic effects of diesel exhaust on the respiratory system. *Environ. Res.* 44: 6–17.

Garshick, E., M. B. Schenker, A. Munoz, M. Segal, T. J. Smith, S. R. Woskie, K. S. Hammond, and F. E. Speizer. 1987a. A case-control study of lung cancer and diesel exhaust exposure in railroad workers. *Am. Rev. Respir. Dis.* 135: 1242–1248.

Garshick, E., M. B. Schenker, S. Woskie, and E. E. Speizer. 1987b. Exposure to asbestos among active railroad workers. *Am. J. Ind. Med.* 12: 399–406.

Garshick, E., M. B. Schenker, A. Munoz, M. Segal, T. J. Smith, S. R. Woskie, K. S. Hammond, and E. E. Speizer. 1988. A retrospective cohort study of lung cancer and diesel exhaust exposure in railroad workers. *Am. Rev. Respir. Dis.* 137: 820–825.

Gray, H. A. 1986. Control of Atmospheric Fine Primary Carbon Particle Concentrations. In Final Report for the California Air Resources Board, Environmental Quality Laboratory Report 23, California Air Resources Board Project A1471-32. Pasadena: California Institute of Technology.

Gubéran, E., M. Usel, L. Raymond, J. Bolay, G. Fioretta, and J. Puissant. 1992. Increased risk for lung cancer and for cancer of the gastrointestinal tract among Geneva professional drivers. *Br. J. Ind. Med.* 49: 337–344.

Gustafsson, L., S. Wall, L.-G. Larsson, and B. Skog. 1986. Mortality and cancer incidence among Swedish dock workers—A retrospective cohort study. *Scand. J. Work Environ. Health* 12: 22–26.

Gustavsson, P., N. Plato, E.-B. Lidström, and C. Hogstedt. 1990. Lung cancer and exposure to diesel exhaust among bus garage workers. *Scand. J. Work Environ. Health* 16: 348–354.

Hall, N. E. L., and E. L. Wynder. 1984. Diesel exhaust exposure and lung cancer: A case-control study. *Environ. Res.* 34: 77–86.

Hampton, C. V., W. R. Pierson, D. Schuetzle, and T. M. Harvey. 1983. Hydrocarbon gases emitted from vehicles on the road. 2. Determination of emission rates from diesel and spark-ignition vehicles. *Environ. Sci. Technol.* 17: 699–708.

Haney, R. A. 1990. Diesel particulate exposures in underground mines. Presented at the Society for Mining, Metallurgy and Exploration, Inc. Annual Meeting, Salt Lake City, February 28–March 3.

Hansen, E. S. 1993. A follow-up study on the mortality of truck drivers. *Am. J. Ind. Med.* 23: 811–821.

Harris, J. E. 1983. Diesel emissions and lung cancer. *Risk Anal.* 3: 83–100.

Hayes, R. B., T. Thomas, D. T. Silverman, P. Vineis, W. J. Blot, T. J. Mason, L. W. Pickle, P. Correa, E. T. H. Fontham, and J. B. Schoenberg. 1989. Lung cancer in motor exhaust occupations. *Am. J. Ind. Med.* 16: 685–695.

HEI. 1995. *Diesel Exhaust: A Critical Analysis of Emissions, Exposure, and Health Effects.* A Special Report of the Institute's Diesel Working Group. Cambridge, MA: Health Effects Institute.

HEI. 1999. *Diesel Emissions and Lung Cancer: Epidemiology and Quantitative Risk Assessment.* A Special Report of the Institute's Diesel Working Group. Cambridge, MA: Health Effects Institute.

Heinrich, U., L. Peters, W. Funcke, E. Potts, U. Mohr, and W. Stöber. 1982. Investigations of toxic and carcinogenic effects of diesel exhaust in long-term inhalation exposure of rodents. In *Toxicological Effects of Emissions from Diesel Engines,* ed. J. Lewtas, pp. 225–242. Amsterdam: Elsevier.

Heinrich, U., H. Muhle, S. Takenaka, E. Ernst, R. Fuhst, U. Mohr, E Pott, and W. Stöber. 1986. Chronic effects on the respiratory tract of hamsters, mice and rats after long-term inhalation of high concentrations of filtered and unfiltered diesel engine emissions. *J. Appl. Toxicol.* 6: 383–395.

Heinrich, U., R. Fuhst, S. Rittinghausen, O. Creutzenberg, B. Bellmann, W. Koch, and K. Levsen. 1995. Chronic inhalation exposure of Wistar rats and two different strains of mice to diesel engine exhaust, carbon black, and titanium dioxide. *Inhal. Toxicol.* 7: 533–556.

Henderson, R. F., J. A. Pickrell, R. K. Jones, J. D. Sun, J. M. Benson, J. L. Mauderly, and R. O. McClellan. 1988. Response of rodents to inhaled diluted diesel exhaust: Biochemical and cytological changes in bronchoalveolar lavage fluid and in lung tissue. *Fundam. Appl. Toxicol.* 11: 546–567.

Howard, P. C., S. S. Hecht, and F. A. Beland. 1990. *Nitroarenes, Occurrence, Metabolism, and Biological Impact.* New York: Plenum Press.

Howe, G. R., D. Fraser, J. Lindsay, B. Presnal, and S. Z. Yu. 1983. Cancer mortality (1965–1977) in relation to diesel fume and coal exposure in a cohort of retired railway workers. *J. Natl. Cancer Inst.* 70: 1015–1019.

Huisingh, J. L., R. Bradow, R. Jungers, L. Claxton, R. Zweidinger, S. Tejada, J. Bumgarner, F. Duffield, M. Waters, F. V. F. Simmon, C. Hare, C. Rodriguez, and L. Snow. 1978. Application of bioassay to the characterization of diesel particle emissions. In: *Application of Short-Term Bioassays in the Fractionation and Analysis of Complex Environmental Mixtures,* eds. M. D. Waters, S. Nesnow, J. L. Huisingh, S. S. Sandhu, and L. Claxton, pp. 381–418. New York: Plenum Press.

IARC. 1989. *IARC Monographs on the Evaluation of Carcinogenic Risks to Humans,* vol. 46. Lyons: International Agency for Research on Cancer.

IPCS (International Programme on Chemical Safety). 1996. *Environmental Health Criteria 171: Diesel Fuel and Exhaust Emissions.* Geneva: World Health Organization.

Ishihara, T. 1988. *Diesel Exhaust and Health Risks.* Final Report of HERP Studies. Tsukuba, Japan: Health Effects Research Program.

Ishinishi, N., A. Koizumi, R. O. McClellan, and W. Stöber. 1986a. *Carcinogenic and Mutagenic Effects of Diesel Engine Exhaust.* Amsterdam: Elsevier.

Iwai, K., T. Udagawa, M. Yamagishi, and H. Yamada. 1986. Long-term inhalation studies of diesel exhaust on F344 SPF rats. Incidence of lung cancer and lymphoma. In *Carcinogenic and Mutagenic Effects of Diesel Engine Exhaust,* eds. N. Ishinishi, A. Koizumi, R. O. McClellan, and W. Stöber, pp. 349–360. Amsterdam: Elsevier.

Jacobson, M., T. A. Smith, J. F. Hurley, A. Robertson, and R. Roscrow. 1988. *Respiratory Infections in Coal Miners Exposed to Nitrogen Oxides.* Research Report 18. Cambridge, MA: Health Effects Institute.

Johnson, J. H. 1988. Automotive emissions. In *Air Pollution, the Automobile, and Public Health,* eds. A. Y. Watson, R. R. Bates, and D. Kennedy, pp. 39–75. Washington, DC: National Academy Press.

Jörgensen, H., and Å. Svensson. 1970. Studies on pulmonary function and respiratory tract symptoms of workers in an iron ore mine where diesel trucks are used underground. *J. Occup. Med.* 12: 348–354.

Kaplan, I. 1959. Relationship of noxious gases to carcinoma of the lung in railroad workers. JAMA 171: 97–101.

Kaplan, H. L., K. J. Springer, and W. F. MacKenzie. 1983. *Studies of Potential Health Effects of Long-Term Exposure to Diesel Exhaust Emissions.* Final Report 01-0750-103 (SWRI) and No. 1239 (SFRE). San Antonio, TX: Southwest Research Institute.

Karagianes, M. T., R. F. Palmer, and R. H. Busch. 1981. Effects of inhaled diesel emissions and coal dust in rats. *Am. Ind. Hyg. Assoc. J.* 42: 382–391.

Keane, M. J., S.-G. Xing, J. C. Harrison, T. Ong, and W. E. Wallace. 1991. Genotoxicity of diesel-exhaust particles dispersed in simulated pulmonary surfactant. *Mutat. Res.* 260: 233–238.

Keil, U., S. K. Weiland, H. Duhme, and L. Chambless. 1996. The international study of asthma and allergies in childhood (ISAAC): Objectives and methods; results from German ISAAC centres concerning traffic density and wheezing and allergic rhinitis. *Toxicol. Lett.* 86: 99–103.

King, L. C., M. J. Kohan, A. C. Austin, L. D. Claxton, J. Lewtas, and J. L. Huisingh. 1981. Evaluation of the release of mutagens from diesel particles in the presence of physiological fluids. *Environ. Mutagen.* 3: 109–121.

Kobayashi, T., T. Ikeue, T. Ito, A. Ikeda, M. Murakami, A. Kato, K. Maejima, T. Nakajima, and T. Suzuki. 1997. Short-term exposure to diesel exhaust induces nasal mucosal hyperresponsiveness to histamine in guinea pigs. *Fundam. Appl. Toxicol.* 38: 166–172.

Kotin, P., H. L. Falk, and M. Thomas. 1955. Aromatic hydrocarbons: III. Presence in the particulate phase of diesel-engine exhausts and the carcinogenicity of exhaust extracts. *Arch. Ind. Health* 11: 113–120.

Lerchen, M. L., C. L. Wiggins, and J. M. Samet. 1987. Lung cancer and occupation in New Mexico. *J. Natl. Cancer Inst.* 79: 639–645.

Leupker, R. V., and M. L. Smith. 1978. Mortality in unionized truck drivers. *J. Occup. Med.* 20: 677–682.

Lewis, T. R., F. H. Y. Green, W. J. Moorman, J. A. R. Burg, and D. W. Lynch. 1986. A chronic inhalation toxicity study of diesel engine emissions and coal dust, alone and combined. In *Carcinogenic and Mutagenic Effects of Diesel Engine Exhaust,* eds. N. Ishinishi, A. Koizumi, R. O. McClellan, and W. Stöber, pp. 361–380. Amsterdam: Elsevier.

Lewis, T. R., F. H. Y. Green, W. J. Moorman, J. R. Burg, and D. W. Lynch. 1989. A chronic inhalation toxicity study of diesel engine emissions and coal dust, alone and combined. *J. Am. Coll. Toxicol.* 8: 345–375.

Lewtas, J. 1982. *Toxicological Effects of Emissions from Diesel Engines.* New York: Elsevier.

Li, A. P. 1981. Antagonistic effects of animal sera, lung and liver cytosols, and sulfhydryl compounds on the cytotoxicity of diesel exhaust particle extracts. *Toxicol. Appl. Pharmacol.* 57: 55–62.

Maejima, K., K. Tamura, Y. Taniguchi, S. Nagase, and H. Tanaka. 1997. Comparison of the effects of various fine particles on IgE antibody production in mice inhaling Japanese cedar pollen allergens. *J. Toxicol. Environ. Health* 52: 231–248.

Manabe, Y., T. Kinouchi, and Y. Ohnishi. 1985. Identification and quantification of highly mutagenic nitroacetoxypyrenes and nitrohydroxypyrenes in diesel-exhaust particles. *Mutat. Res.* 158: 3–18.

Mauderly, J. L. 1992. Diesel exhaust. In Environmental Toxicants—Human Exposures and Their Health Effects, ed. M. Lippmann, pp. 119–162. New York: Van Nostrand Reinhold.

Mauderly, J. L. 1994a. Toxicological and epidemiological evidence for health risks from inhaled engine emissions. *Environ. Health Perspect.* 102(suppl. 4): 165–171.

Mauderly, J. L. 1994b. Non-cancer pulmonary effects of chronic inhalation exposure of animals to solid particles. In *Toxic and Carcinogenic Effects of Solid Particles in the Respiratory Tract,* eds. U. Mohr, D. L. Dungworth, J. L. Mauderly, and G. Oberdoerster, pp. 43–56. Washington, DC: ILSI Press.

Mauderly, J. L. 1996. Lung overload: The dilemma and opportunities for resolution. *Inhal. Toxicol.* 8 (Suppl.): 1–28.

Mauderly, J. L. 1997. Relevance of particle-induced rat lung tumors for assessing lung carcinogenic hazard and human lung cancer risk. *Environ. Health Perspect.* 105 (suppl. 5): 1337–1346.

Mauderly, J. L. 1998. Toxicology of diesel engine emissions. In *Health Effects of Particulate Matter in Ambient Air,* ed. J. Vostal, pp. 573–580. Air and Waste Management Association and Czech Medical Assopciation, Pittsburgh, PA.

Mauderly, J. L., and McCunney. 1996. *Particle Overload in the Rat Lung and Lung Cancer: Implications for Human Risk Assessment.* Washington, DC: Taylor and Francis.

Mauderly, J. L., E. B. Barr, D. E. Bice, A. F. Eidson, R. F. Henderson, R. K. Jones, J. A. Pickrell, and R. K. Wolff. 1986. Inhalation exposure of rats to oil shale dust and diesel exhaust. In: *Inhalation Toxicology Research Institute Annual Report,* DOE Research and Development Report LMF-115, pp. 273–278. Springfield, VA: National Technical Information Service.

Mauderly, J. L., R. K. Jones, W. C. Griffith, R. F. Henderson, and R. O. McClellan. 1987. Diesel exhaust is a pulmonary carcinogen in rats exposed chronically by inhalation. *Fundam. Appl. Toxicol.* 9: 208–221.

Mauderly, J. L., N. A. Gillett, R. F. Henderson, R. K. Jones, and R. O. McClellan. 1988. Relationships of lung structural and functional changes to accumulation of diesel exhaust particles. *Ann. Occup. Hyg.* 32(suppl. 1): 659–669.

Mauderly, J. L., D. E. Bice, Y. S. Cheng, N. A. Gillett, W. C. Griffith, R. F. Henderson, J. A. Pickrell, and R. K. Wolff. 1990a. Influence of pre-existing pulmonary emphysema on susceptibility to chronic inhalation exposure to diesel exhaust. *Am. Rev. Respir. Dis.* 141: 1333–1341.

Mauderly, J. L., Y. S. Cheng, and M. B. Snipes. 1990b. Particle overload in toxicological studies: Friend or foe? *J. Aerosol Med.* 3: S169–187.

Mauderly, J. L., D. A. Banas, W. C. Griffith, F. F. Hahn, R. F. Henderson, and R. O. McClellan. 1996. Diesel exhaust is not a pulmonary carcinogen in CD-1 mice exposed under conditions carcinogenic to F344 rats. *Fundam. Appl. Toxicol.* 30: 233–242.

McCawley, M., J. Cocalis, J. Burkhart, and G. Piacitelli. 1989. *Particle Size and Environmental Characterization of Underground Coal Mines: A Diesel/Non-diesel Comparison.* Final Report. Contract J0145006. Washington, DC: U.S. Department of the Interior, Bureau of Mines.

McClellan, R. O. 1996. Lung cancer in rats from prolonged exposure to high concentrations of carbonaceous particles: Implications for human risk assessment. *Inhal. Toxicol.* 8 (suppl.): 193–226.

Menck, H. R., and B. E. Henderson. 1976. Occupational differences in rates of lung cancer. *J. Occup. Med.* 18: 797–801.

Milne, K. L., D. P. Sandler, R. B. Everson, and S. M. Brown. 1983. Lung cancer and occupation in Alameda county: A death certificate case-control study. *Am. J. Ind. Med.* 4: 565–575.

Moorman, W. J., J. C. Clark, W. E. Pepelko, and J. Mattox. 1985. Pulmonary function responses in cats following long-term exposure to diesel exhaust. *J. Appl. Toxicol.* 5: 301–305.

Morimoto, K., M. Kitamura, H. Kondo, and A. Koizumie. 1986. Genotoxicity of diesel exhaust emissions in a battery of in-vitro short-term and in-vivo bioassays. In *Carcinogenic and Mutagenic Effects of Diesel Engine Exhaust,* eds. N. Ishinishi, A. Koizumi, R. O. McClellan, and W. Stöber, pp. 85–101. Amsterdam: Elsevier.

Motor Vehicle Manufacturers Association. 1962. *Facts and Figures.* Detroit: Motor Vehicle Manufacturers Association.

Muranaka, M., S. Suzuki, K. Koizumi, S. Takafuji, T. Miyamoto, R. Ikemori, and H. Tokiwa. 1986. Adjuvant activity of diesel-exhaust particulates for the production of IgE antibody in mice. *J. Allergy Clin. Immunol.* 77: 616–623.

National Research Council. 1989. *Biologic Markers in Pulmonary Toxicology.* Washington, DC: National Academy of Science.

Netterstrøm, B. 1988. Cancer incidence among urban bus drivers in Denmark. *Int. Arch. Occup. Environ. Health* 61: 217–221.

Nikula, K. J., M. B. Snipes, E. B. Barr, W. C. Griffith, R. F. Henderson, and J. L. Mauderly. 1995. Comparative pulmonary toxicities and carcinogenicities of chronically inhaled diesel exhaust and carbon black in F344 rats. *Fundam. Appl. Toxicol.* 25: 80–94.

Nikula, K. J., W. C. Griffith, K. J. Avila, and J. L. Mauderly. 1997. Lung tissue responses and site of particle retention differ between rats and Cynomolgus monkeys exposed chronically to diesel exhaust and coal dust. *Fundam. Appl. Toxicol.* 37: 37–53.

NIOSH (National Institute of Occupational Safety and Health). 1988. *Carcinogenic Effects of Exposure to Diesel Exhaust.* NIOSH Current Intelligence Bulletin 50, DHHS Publication 88–116. Atlanta: Centers for Disease Control.

Nokso-Koivisto, P., and E. Pukkala. 1994. Past exposure to asbestos and combustion products and incidence of cancer among Finnish locomotive drivers. *Occup. Environ. Med.* 51: 330–334.

NTP (National Toxicology Program). 1998. *Draft Report on Carcinogens: Background Document for Diesel Exhaust Particulates.* Research Triangle Park, NC: U.S. Department of Health and Human Services (NTP).

Oberdörster, G. 1996. Significance of particle parameters in the evaluation of exposure–dose-response relationships of inhaled particles. 1996. *Inhal. Toxicol.* 8(suppl.): 73–89.

Oberdörster, G., R. M. Gelein, J. Ferin, and B. Weiss. 1995. Association of particulate air pollution and acute mortality: Involvement of ultrafine particles? *Inhal. Toxicol.* 7: 111–124.

Opresko, D. M., J. W. Holleman, R. H. Ross, and J. W. Carroll. 1984. *Problem Definition Study on Emission By-product Hazards from Diesel Engines for Confined Space Army Workplaces.* ORNL Report 6017. Oak Ridge, TN: Oak Ridge National Laboratory.

Pepelko, W. E., and C. Chen. 1993. Quantitative assessment of cancer risk from exposure to diesel engine emissions. *Reg. Toxicol. Pharmacol.* 17: 52–65.

Pepelko, W. E., and W. B. Peirano. 1983. Health effects of exposure to diesel engine emissions. A summary of animal studies conducted by the US Environmental Protection Agency's Health Effects Research Laboratory at Cincinnati, OH. *J. Am. Coll. Toxicol.* 2: 253–306.

Peters, A., H. E. Wichmann, T. Tuch, J. Heinrich, and J. Heyder. 1997a. Respiratory effects are associated with the number of ultrafine particles. *Am. J. Respir. Crit. Care Med.* 155: 1376–1383.

Peters, A., A. Döring, H. E. Wichmann, and W. Koenig. 1997b. Increased plasma viscosity during an air pollution episode: A link to mortality? *Lancet* 349: 1582–1587.

Pfluger, D. H., and C. E. Minder. 1994. A mortality study of lung cancer among Swiss professional drivers: Accounting for the smoking related fraction by a multivariate approach. *Soz Präventivmed.* 39: 372–378.

Pike, M. E., and B. E. Henderson. 1981. Epidemiology of polycyclic aromatic hydrocarbons: Quantifying the cancer risk from cigarette smoking and air pollution. In: *Polycyclic Hydrocarbons and Cancer,* eds. H. V. Gellbond and P. O. P. Tso, pp. 317–334. New York: Academic Press.

Plopper, C. G., D. M. Hyde, and A. J. Weir. 1983. Centriacinar alterations in lungs of cats chronically exposed to diesel exhaust. *Lab. Invest.* 49: 391–399.

Purdam, J. T., D. L. Holness, and C. W. Pilger. 1987. Environmental and medical assessment of stevedores employed in ferry operations. *Appl. Ind. Hyg.* 2: 133–139.

Raffle, P. A. B. 1957. The health of the worker. *Br. J. Ind. Med.* 14: 73–80.

Rafnsson, V., and H. Gunnarsdóttir. 1991. Mortality among professional drivers. *Scand. J. Work Environ. Health* 17: 312–317.

Randerath, K., K. L. Putman, J. L. Mauderly, P. L. Williams, and E. Randerath. 1995. *Pulmonary Toxicity of Inhaled Diesel Exhaust and Carbon Black in Chronically Exposed Rats.* Research Report 68. Cambridge, MA: Health Effects Research Institute.

Reger, R., J. Hancock, J. Hankinson, F. Hearl, and J. Merchant. 1982. Coal miners exposed to diesel exhaust emissions. *Ann. Occup. Hyg.* 26: 799–815.

Rudell, B., T. Sandström, N. Stjernerg, and B. Kolmodin-Hedman. 1990. Controlled diesel exhaust exposure in an exposure chamber: Pulmonary effects investigated with bronchoalveolar lavage. *J. Aerosol Sci.* 21: S411–414.

Rushton, L., M. R. Alderson, and C. R. Nagarajah. 1983. Epidemiological survey of maintenance workers in London Transport executive bus garages and Chiswick works. *Br. J. Ind. Med.* 40: 34–45.

Schenker, M. B., S. J. Samuels, N. Y. Kado, S. K. Hammond, T. J. Smith, and S. R. Woskie. 1990. *Markers of Exposure to Diesel Exhaust in Railroad Workers.* In Health Effects Institute Report 33, Montpelier, VT: Capital City Press.

Schuetzle, D. 1983. Sampling of vehicle emissions for chemical analysis and biological testing. *Environ. Health Perspect.* 47: 65–80.

Schuetzle, D., and J. A. Frazier. 1986. Factors influencing the emission of vapor and particulate phase components from diesel engines. In *Carcinogenic and Mutagenic Effects of Diesel Engine Exhaust,* eds. N. Ishinishi, A. Koizumi, R. O. McClellan, and W. Stöber, pp. 41–63. Amsterdam: Elsevier.

Schuetzle, D., and J. Lewtas. 1986. Bioassay-directed chemical analysis in environmental research. *Anal. Chem.* 58: 1060A–1075A.

Schuetzle, D., T. E. Jensen, and J. C. Ball. 1985. Polar polynuclear aromatic hydrocarbon derivatives in extracts of particulates: Biological characterization and techniques for chemical analysis. *Environ. Int.* 11: 169.

Seaton, A., W. MacNee, K. Donaldson, and D. Godden. 1995. Particulate air pollution and acute health effects. *Lancet* 345: 176–178.

Siemiatycki, J., M. Gerin, P. Stewart, L. Nadon, R. Dewar, and L. Richardson. 1988. Associations between several sites of cancer and ten types of exhaust and combustion products: Results from a case-referent study in Montreal. *Scand. J. Work Environ. Health* 14: 79–90.

Snipes, M. B. 1989. Long-term retention and clearance of particles inhaled by mammalian species. *Crit. Rev. Toxicol.* 20: 175–211.

Steenland, K. 1986. Lung cancer and diesel exhaust: A review. *Am. J. Ind. Med.* 10: 177–189.

Steenland, N. K., D. T. Silverman, and R. W. Hornung. 1990. Case-control study of lung cancer and truck driving in the Teamsters' Union. *Am. J. Publ. Health* 80: 670–674.

Steenland, K., J. Deddens, and L. Stayner. 1998. Diesel exhaust and lung cancer in the trucking industry: Exposure-response analyses and risk assessment. *Am. J. Ind. Med.* 34: 220–228.

Stern, F. B., R. A. Curtis, and R. A. Lemen. 1981. Exposure of motor vehicle examiners to carbon monoxide: A historical perspective mortality study. *Arch. Environ. Health* 36: 59–66.

Sun, J. D., R. K. Wolff, G. M. Kanapilly, and R. O. McClellan. 1984. Lung retention and metabolic fate of inhaled benzo(a)pyrene associated with diesel exhaust particles. *Toxicol. Appl. Pharmacol.* 73: 48–59.

Swanson, G. M., C.-S. Lin, and P. B. Burns. 1993. Diversity in the association between occupation and lung cancer among black and white men. *Cancer Epidem. Bio. Prev.* 2: 313–320.

Takafuji, S., S. Suzuki, K. Koizumi, K. Tadokoro, T. Miyamoto, R. Ikemori, and M. Muranaka. 1987. Diesel-exhaust particulates inoculated by the intranasal route have an adjuvant activity for IgE production in mice. *J. Allergy Clin. Immunol.* 79(4): 639–645.

Takafuji, S., S. Suzuki, K. Koizumi, K. Tadokoro, H. Ohashi, M. Muranaka, and T. Miyamoto. 1989. Enhancing effect of suspended particulate matter on the IgE antibody production in mice. *Int. Arch. Allergy Appl. Immunol.* 90(1): 1–7.

Takano, H., Y. Toshikazu, T. Ichinose, Y. Miyabara, K. Imaoka, and M. Sagai. 1997. Diesel exhaust particles enhance antigen-induced airway inflammation and local cytokine expression in mice. *Am. J. Respir. Crit. Care Med.* 156: 36–42.

Takemoto, K., H. Yoshimura, and H. Katayama. 1986. Effects of chronic inhalation exposure to diesel exhaust on the development of lung tumors in di-isopropanol-nitrosamine-treated F344 rats and newborn C57BL and ICR mice. In *Carcinogenic and Mutagenic Effects of Diesel Engine Exhaust,* eds. N. Ishinishi, A. Koizumi, R. O. McClellan, and W. Stöber, pp. 311–327. Amsterdam: Elsevier.

Takenaka, H., K. Zhang, D. Diaz-Sanchez, A. Tsien, and A. Saxon. 1995. Enhanced human IgE production results from exposure to the aromatic hydrocarbons from diesel exhaust: Direct effects on B-cell IgE production. *J. Allergy Clin. Immunol.* 95(1 Pt 1): 103–115.

Trosko, J. E. 1997. Challenge to the simple paradigm that 'carcinogens' are 'mutagens' and to the in vitro and in vivo assays used to test the paradigm. *Mutat. Res.* 373: 245–249.

Ulfvarson, U., and R. Alexandersson. 1990. Reduction in adverse effect on pulmonary function after exposure to filtered diesel exhaust. *Am. J. Ind. Med.* 17: 341–347.

Ulfvarson, U., R. Alexandersson, L. Aringer, E. Svensson, G. Hedenstierna, C. Hogstedt, B. Holmberg, G. Rosen, and M. Sorsa. 1987. Effect of exposure to vehicle exhaust on health. *Scand. J. Work Environ. Health* 13: 505–512.

U.S. Department of Labor, Bureau of Labor Statistics. 1972. *Railroad Technology and Manpower in the 1970's.* Washington, DC: GPO.

U.S. EPA. 1993. *Motor Vehicle-Related Air Toxics Study.* EPA 420-R-93-005. Ann Arbor, MI: U.S. Environmental Protection Agency, Office of Mobile Sources, Emission Planning and Strategies Division.

U.S. EPA. 1998. *Health Assessment Document for Diesel Emissions.* EPA/600/8-90/057C. Washington, DC: U.S. Environmental Protection Agency, Office of Research and Development.

U.S. EPA. 1996a. *Air Quality Criteria for Particulate Matter,* vol 1–3 EPA/600/P-95/001aF. Washington, DC: U.S. Environmental Protection Agency, Office of Research and Development.

U.S. EPA. 1996b. *Review of the National Ambient Air Quality Standards for Particulate Matter: Policy Assessment of Scientific and Technical Information.* EPA-452/R-96-013. Research Triangle Park, NC: U.S. Environmental Protection Agency, Office of Air Quality Planning and Standards.

Valberg, P. A., and E. A. C. Crouch. 1999. Meta-analysis of rat lung tumors from lifetime inhalation of diesel exhaust. *Environ. Health Perspect.* 107: 693–699.

Vedal, S. 1997. Ambient particles and health: Lines that divide. *J. Air Waste Manag. Assoc.* 47: 551–581.

Vinegar, A., A. I. Carson, W. E. Pepelko, and J. G. Orthoefer. 1981. Effects of six months of exposure to two levels of diesel exhaust on pulmonary function of Chinese hamsters (abstract). *Fed. Proc.* 40: 593.

Wade III, J. F., and Newman, L. S. (1993). Diesel asthma: Reactive airways disease following overexposure to locomotive exhaust. *J. Occup. Med.* 35(2): 149–154.

Waller, R. E. 1981. Trends in lung cancer in London in relation to exposure to diesel fumes. *Environ. Int.* 5: 479–483.

Waxweiler, R. J., J. K. Wagoner, and V. E. Archer. 1973. Mortality of potash workers. *J. Occup. Med.* 15: 486–489.

White, H., J. J. Vostal, H. L. Kaplan, and W. F. MacKenzie. 1983. A long-term inhalation study evaluates the pulmonary effects of diesel emissions. *J. Appl. Toxicol.* 3: 332.

Williams, R. L. 1982. Diesel particulate emissions: Composition, concentration, and control. In *Toxicological Effects of Emissions from Diesel Engines,* ed. J. Lewtas, pp. 15–32. New York: Elsevier.

Williams, R. R., N. L. Stegens, and J. R. Goldsmith. 1977. Associations of cancer site and type with occupation and industry from the Third National Cancer Survey interview. *J. Natl. Cancer Inst.* 59: 1147–1185.

Wolff, R. K., L. C. Griffis, C. H. Hobbs, and R. O. McClellan. 1982. Deposition and Retention of 0.1 m 67Ga2O3 aggregate aerosols in rats following whole body exposures. *Fundam. Appl. Toxicol.* 126: 505–508.

Wolff, R. K., R. F. Henderson, M. B. Snipes, W. C. Griffith, J. L. Mauderly, R. G. Cuddihy, and R. O. McClellan. 1987. Alterations in particle accumulation and clearance in lungs of rats chronically exposed to diesel exhaust. *Fundam. Appl. Toxicol.* 9: 154–166.

Wolff, R. K., J. A. Bond, R. E. Henderson, J. R. Harkema, and J. L. Mauderly. 1990. Pulmonary inflammation and DNA adducts in rats inhaling diesel exhaust or carbon black. *Inhal. Toxicol.* 2: 241–254.

Wong, O., R. W. Morgan, L. Kheifets, S. R. Larson, and M. D. Whorton. 1985. Mortality among members of a heavy construction equipment operators union with potential exposure to diesel emissions. *Br. J. Ind. Med.* 42: 435–448.

Wong, D., C. E. Mitchell, R. K. Wolff, J. L. Mauderly, and A. M. Jeffrey. 1986. Identification of DNA damage as a result of exposure of rats to diesel engine exhaust. *Carcinogenesis* 7: 1595–1597.

Woskie, S. R., T. J. Smith, S. K. Hammond, M. B. Schenker, E. Garshick, and F. E. Speizer. 1988a. Estimation of the diesel exhaust exposures of railroad workers: I. Current exposures. *Am. J. Ind. Med.* 13: 381–394.

Woskie, S. R., T. J. Smith, S. K. Hammond, M. B. Schenker, E. Garshick, and F. E. Speizer. 1988b. Estimation of the diesel exhaust exposures of railroad workers: II. National and historical exposures. *Am. J. Ind. Med.* 13: 395–404.

Wynder, E. L., G. S. Dieck, N. E. L. Hall, and H. Lahti. 1985. A case-control study of diesel exhaust exposure and bladder cancer. *Environ. Res.* 37: 475–489.

Zaebst, D. D., D. E. Clapp, L. M. Blade, D. A. Marlow, K. Steenland, R. W. Hornung, D. Scheutzle, and J. Butler. 1991. Quantitative determination of trucking industry workers' exposures to diesel exhaust particles. *Am. Ind. Hyg. Assoc. J.* 52(12): 529–541.

8 Dioxins and Dioxin-like Chemicals

MICHAEL J. DE VITO, Ph.D.
MICHAEL A. GALLO, Ph.D.

Dioxins are a subset of the polyhalogenated aromatic hydrocarbons (PHAHs). The most well studied and most toxic of the class is 2,3,7,8-tetrachlorodibenzo-p-dioxin (TCDD). These chemicals are present in a variety of environmental media as well as in low-level contaminants of the food supply. The dioxin-like PHAHs consist in part of the polyhalogenated dibenzo-p-dioxin, dibenzofurans and biphenyls (PCBs and PBBs). These chemicals are sparingly soluble in water and are highly lipophilic. They are persistent in both environmental and biological samples with half-lives in humans ranging from 1 year to more than 20 years (Flesch-Janys et al., 1995). The dioxin-like chemicals induce similar toxicities in experimental animals. These toxicities are initiated in part by the binding and activation of these chemicals to an intracellular protein called the Ah receptor (AhR).

The health effects of dioxin and related chemicals in humans and wildlife are a hotly debated topic. The intensity of the debate is based as much on the uncertainty in risk assessments as it is on political, social, and economic causes. Despite being one of the most studied class of chemicals, risk assessments for dioxin by various governmental health and regulatory agencies throughout the world have resulted in tolerable daily intakes, or virtually safe doses, that range almost three orders of magnitude. This large discrepancy is because of the use of either threshold or linear models in risk estimates. The political and social issues revolve, in part, around the widespread background exposure to the "most toxic man-made chemical" as well as to the use of dioxin-contaminated herbicides during the Vietnam War. In addition, there have been a number of industrial accidents that resulted in human and wildlife exposure to these chemicals, and attempts to resolve these accidents have been widely criticized. It is unlikely that the debate on the health effects of dioxin and related chemicals will be resolved in the near future.

SOURCES

One of the problems in estimating potential health 'effects of dioxin is the coexposure to numerous dioxin-like chemicals originating from different sources. There are 75 different polychlorinated dibenzo-p-dioxin (CDDs), 135 dibenzofurans (CDFs), and 209 biphenyls (PCBs), depending on the number and position of the chlorine substitutions. Fortunately only a subset of these chemicals produce dioxin-like toxicities in experimental animals. The 2,3,7,8-substituted CDDs and CDFs are considered dioxin-like. Only 7 of 75 CDDs and 10 of the 135 CDFs are dioxin-like (Van den Berg et al., 1998). Of the 209 PCB congeners, only 12 have dioxin-like activity (Safe, 1994; Van den Berg et al., 1998). In

Environmental Toxicants: Human Exposures and Their Health Effects, 2/e. Edited by Morton Lippmann.
ISBN: 0-471-29298-2 © 2000 John Wiley & Sons, Inc.

addition brominated analogues have been found in the environment as well as in human tissues. The data available on the brominated analogues demonstrates that these compounds induce dioxin-like biochemical effects and toxicities, and they share a similar structure activity relationship with their chlorinated analogues (Safe, 1990).

Because dioxins consist of a broad class of chemicals with varying potencies, sources, and exposures, health risk assessments have used the toxic equivalency factor (TEF) methodology. This methodology is a relative potency scheme which compares the toxicity of all dioxins to the most potent, 2,3,7,8-tetrachlorodibenzo-p-dioxin (TCDD). Congeners are assigned relative potency values called toxic equivalency factors (TEFs) (Van den Berg et al., 1998). The concentration of a congener in a mixture is multiplied by its TEF, and this product is the TCDD or toxic equivalents (TEQ) for that congener. The TEQs for all chemicals in the mixture are summed to produce a TEQ for the entire mixture. It is assumed that the mixture will now behave as if it contained the TEQ concentration of TCDD alone. At present, only 29 chemicals are considered in the TEF scheme, and they consist of the 2,3,7,8-substituted CDDs/CDFs and 12 out of 209 PCBs (Van den Berg et al., 1998). TEF values for the brominated analogues have not been adopted by regulatory agencies. The development of this methodology is described in greater detail later in this chapter.

The CDDs and CDFs are unwanted products of several industrial processes. Combustion systems are a primary source for the production of CDDs and CDFs. Included in this category are waste incinerators, such as municipal solid waste, medical waste, sewage sludge, and hazardous waste incinerators. The burning of fuel such as coal, wood, and petroleum also produces CDDs and CDFs. Other high-temperature sources, such as cement kilns, produce significant amounts of dioxin. Iron ore sintering, steel production, and scrap metal recovery operations produce and release CDDs/CDFs into the air. In some parts of the United States, open burning of household trash is a common practice, and this results in the formation of CDDs/CDFs. The contribution of open burning of household trash to total emissions of dioxin into the environment cannot be quantified with any certainty at this time (U.S. EPA, 1997).

The formation of CDDs/CDFs is a by-product of several chemical manufacturing processes, the manufacture processes of herbicides such as Agent Orange or 2,4,5-trichlorophenoxy acetic acid and of chlorinated phenols such as pentachlorophenol have either been altered to eliminate dioxin production or the products have been discontinued. The manufacture of chlorine bleached wood pulp produces trace quantities of CDDs/CDFs, of which the octa- and heptachlorinated congeners predominate. It should be noted that many pulp and paper mills have re-engineered their processes and have decreased CDD/CDF production and emissions in these facilities by approximately 90% (Cleverly et al., 1998). The production of ethylene dichloride or vinyl chloride produces CDDs/CDFs; however, the date are insufficient to quantify emission estimates for these processes.

Several natural processes can result in the production of CDDs/CDFs. Hepta- and octa-chlorodibenzo-p-dioxin are the predominant congeners produced in forest fires. Under certain environmental conditions, such as composting, microorganisms can produce CDDs/CDFs from chlorinated phenolic compounds. Recently ball clay deposits in western Mississippi, Kentuckys and Tennessce were found to contain CDDs and CDFs. The CDDs/CDFs in these clay deposits are approximately 90% by weight 2,3,7,8-tetrachloro and 1,2,3,7,8-pentachlorodibenzo-p-dioxin. While this congener pattern is similar to that found in contaminated herbicides, the origin of these chemicals in the clay has not been determined, and natural occurrence is but one possibility.

Another source of CDDs/CDFs is redistribution and circulation of reservoirs of previously released CDDs/CDFs (U.S. EPA, 1994). Materials or places contaminated by previously released CDDs/CDFs can be considered reservoirs of these chemicals.

Contaminated sediments, soils and pentachlorophenol-treated wood are also considered reservoirs. Retrainment of these reservoirs may contribute significantly to overall exposure, but its exact contribution is uncertain.

While there are natural sources for CDDs/CDFs production, several lines of evidence indicate that current emissions and exposures are due to anthropogenic sources. Analysis of sediment cores in the United States and Europe show consistent patterns of CDD/CDF concentration changes over time. CDD/CDF concentrations in sediment started to increase in the 1920s and 1930s, peaked in the 1960s and 1970s and then began to decrease in the late 1970s through the 1980s (Czuczwa et al., 1985; Cleverly et al., 1996). These trends are consistent with the increase in general industrial activity in the 1930s and the promulgation of environmental regulations in the 1970s (Czuczwa et al., 1985). CDD/CDF concentrations are higher in human tissues from industrialized countries compared to those from underdeveloped nations (Schecter et al., 1994b, c). There are also data comparing present human tissue concentrations with those tissues taken from preserved 140 to 400 year-old human remains which show almost the complete absence of CDD/CDFs compared to tissues of the modern human (Schecter et al., 1994b, c). Finally no known large natural sources of CDD/CDFs have been identified. Current estimates of all emission sources suggest that forest fires are a minor source compared to anthropogenic sources (Cleverly et al., 1998).

The U.S. Environmental Protection Agency has developed an inventory of CDDs/CDFs sources for the years 1987 and 1995 (Cleverly et al., 1998). The year 1987 was chosen because prior to this year few potential sources in the United States had been characterized, and 1995 was chosen as the latest year for which significant data were available. This analysis indicates that the dominant source of dioxin releases to air in the United States is combustion. The estimate of releases from 1987 were 12 kg TEQ (range 5–30 kg) and from 1995 were 3 kg TEQ (range 1–8 kg). While there is uncertainty in these estimates, it is clear that emissions significantly decreased between 1987 and 1995. The reductions in emissions were due primarily to reductions in air emissions from municipal and medical waste incinerators (Cleverly et al., 1998).

Some dioxin-like chemicals were synthesized and sold commercially, such as the polychlorinated and polybrominated biphenyls, PCBs and PBBs, respectively. The PCBs were used as heat transfer fluids, flame retardants, paint additives, dielectric fluids for capacitors and transformers, and in several other industrial processes (DeVoogt and Brinkman, 1989). The PBBs were used predominantly as flame retardants in the early 1970s. Since 1929 approximately 1.5 million metric tons of PCBs were produced and sold. Numerous mixtures of PCBs were manufactured and sold worldwide, including Arochlor, Clophen, Fenclor, Kanechlor, Phenoclor and Pyralene among others. These mixtures were sold as blends based on their chlorine content. For example, Aroclor 1242, the most widely produced Aroclor, contained 42% chlorine, while Aroclor 1254 contained 54% chlorine. In the United States the sale of PCBs was banned in 1977. Since 1977 the disposal of PCBs have been strictly regulated under TSCA. If disposals of PCBs following TSCA guidelines are strictly followed, environmental release should be minimal. The majority of current PCB releases appear to be from re-release of these compounds from reservoir sources. Other current sources of PCBs are likely due to leaks and spills of still in-service PCBs from transformers, for example, or from illegal disposal of PCBs. Despite the ban on the production of PCBs in the United States and western Europe in the 1970s, PCBs were not banned in the former Soviet Union until the 1990s.

Environmental Fate and Transport

Much of the information on the fate and transport of CDDs/CDFs is based on the data for TCDD. Because CDDs/CDFs share many physical chemical properties, the fate and transport of these chemicals should be qualitatively similar. CDDs/CDFs enter the terrestrial food chain via atmospheric deposition (Fries and Paustenbach, 1990). Presently airborne sources of dioxin are dominated by the combustion of wastes and fuels. The CDDs/CDFs emitted from combustion sources are predominately bound to particulates, although there are some in the vapor phase. Once airborne, the CDDs/CDFs deposit on plants, soil, or water. Plant contamination by dioxins is mainly due to the deposition of contaminated particles on the leaves. While there is evidence that CDDs/CDFs in soil can be absorbed directly by the roots of plants, it is highly unlikely that this results in significant concentrations of the dioxins in the above ground plant (Insensee and Jones, 1971, Jensen et al., 1983). CDDs/CDFs also accumulate on soil through pesticide application and leakage from waste sites, although these pathways are more important for localized areas with specific problems.

Once deposited on the plants or soil, the dioxins either enter the food chain or degrade. The deposition of dioxins on plants and soil enter the food chain through direct ingestion of the plants or the incidental ingestion of soil by animals, resulting in the bioaccumulation of these chemicals in livestock (Fries and Paustenbach, 1990). Concentrations of CDDs/CDFs are higher in cows milk collected from the vicinity of a municipal waste incinerator than in commercial cows milk (Rappe et al., 1987). Dioxins can be degraded in the environment, but this appears to be a relatively slow process. Photolysis is the main degradation pathway for CDDs/CDFs in the environment and requires ultraviolet (UV) light and an organic hydrogen donor (Crosby, 1971). Because of the requirement for UV light, dioxins that are on the soil surface have shorter half-lives than those that are deeper in the soil. For example, the half-life of TCDD at the soil surface is estimated at 1 to 3 years while it is 10 to 12 years in the subsurface soil (diDomenico et al., 1982; Kimbrough et al., 1984).

Dioxins are sparingly soluble in water, and the concentrations of these chemicals in water are extremely low. Despite their low solubility, aquatic environments have significant amounts of dioxin as a result of their adsorption to sediments. Sediments of surface waters are thought to be the ultimate sink (or environmental reservoir) of CDDs/CDFs (Hutzinger et al., 1985), and the persistence of these compounds in water bodies results in bioaccumulation in aquatic organisms (Isensee and Jones, 1975). While deposition of particulates contaminated with dioxin appears to be the major source of water contamination, local events such as industrial effluents and herbicide runoff may also contribute to the dioxin burdens.

The PCBs and PBBs have similar physical chemical properties as the CDDs/CDFs, which result in qualitatively similar environmental fates and transports (Safe, 1994). Atmospheric concentrations of PCBs in urban centers $(1-10\,\text{ng}/\text{m}^3)$ have been approximately an order of magnitude higher than in nonurban areas $(0.1-0.5\,\text{ng}/\text{m}^3)$ (Atlas et al., 1986). Numerous factors including local sources, source emission strengths, and meteorological conditions influence ambient concentrations of PCBs. Surface waterways appear to be a major reservoir for PCBs (Tanabe and Tatsukawa, 1986) and the National Academy of Sciences (1979) estimated that 50% to 80% of the PCBs in the environment are contained within the waterways of the North Atlantic. Similar to the CDDs/CDFs, PCBs are predominantly found in the sediments of these waterways. PCBs are also found in soil to varying degrees from 0.01 to over 2000 ppm (Tatsukawa, 1976).

Photolysis and photoxidation appear to be major pathways for destruction of PCBs in the environment. All PCBs photodechlorinate, and the photolysis rate increases as the chlorine content increases (Tiedje et al., 1993). In addition to photolysis, PCBs are also sensitive to biological degradation. There are over two dozen strains of aerobic bacteria and fungi that are capable of degrading most PCB congeners with five or fewer chlorines (Tiedje et al., 1993). Many of these organisms are of the genus *Pseudomonas* or *Alcaligenes,* and they are widely distributed in the environment. The higher-chlorinated

PCBs are more resistant to biodegradation than are lower-chlorinated congeners. In addition PCBs substituted in two or more of the ortho positions are resistant to biodegradation.

Human Exposure

Exposure to dioxin can occur through occupational exposure, accidental exposures, or environmental exposures for the general population. The predominant hypothesis for environmental exposure focuses on the air to plant to animal hypothesis. This hypothesis focuses on the deposition of particulates onto plants and soil. The deposited dioxins then enter the food chain by ingestion of the contaminated substrates by either livestock or aquatic life where they bioaccumulate. Eventually the livestock or aquatic life are consumed by humans.

Estimates of daily human intake in the United States are approximately 3 to 6 pg TCDD equivalents/kg/d (Pinsky and Lorber, 1997; Schecter, 1994a), and these values are consistent with those reported from Western Europe (Schecter 1994b, c). Approximately half of the TCDD equivalents arise from PCBs, with only 10% attributable to TCDD itself (Schecter et al., 1994a–c). These daily intakes result in serum concentrations of approximately 40 to 60 parts per trillion TEQ, and body burdens of approximately 8 to 13 ng TEQ/kg (DeVito et al., 1995). In general, dioxin body burdens increase with age, and this is thought to be reflection of both higher exposure during the 1940s through the 1960s compared to present exposures (Pinsky and Lorber, 1997), as well as decreased metabolism of dioxin with age (Flesch-Janys, 1995).

A major route of elimination of dioxin in female humans, experimental animals, and mammalian wildlife is through breast milk. Breast milk has a high concentration of fat, and the dioxin distribute to fatty tissues. In women, nursing for at least seven months can decrease maternal serum concentrations of dioxin by up to 50% (Shecter et al., 1996). Exposure to nursing infants are much higher than maternal exposure and is estimated at 30 to 100 pg TEQ for the first year (Schecter et al., 1994a–c, 1996). These daily intakes are higher than all tolerable daily intakes defined by regulatory agencies throughout the world. In nursing infants, body burdens of dioxin at 12 months are two to four times higher than maternal burdens (Schecter et al., 1996). The potential health risks associated with these background exposures are uncertain; however, it should be noted that the benefits of breast feeding are well documented and far outweigh these potential risks from background dioxin exposures (Rogan and Gladen, 1993).

There are numerous incidents throughout the world where small populations have potentially been highly exposed to dioxin through industrial accidents, occupational exposures, wartime use of herbicides or environmental pollution. One of the most well characterized exposures occurred in Seveso, Italy in 1976. Approximately 1 kg of 2,3,7,8-tetrachlorodibenzo-p-dioxin was released following an explosion at a trichlorophenol manufacturing plant. In 1976 there were no validated methodologies available to determine serum concentrations of TCDD. Despite this fact a team of physicians, led by Dr. Paolo Mocarelli, collected and stored blood from over 30,000 patients in the area, both exposed and unexposed (Bertazzi and di Domenico, 1995). Initial chemical analysis of the serum from several children from the most highly exposed area found serum concentrations of dioxin up to 50,000 parts per trillion (Bertazzi and di Domenico, 1995). Based on the initial exposure estimates, the Seveso region was divided into three areas A, B, and R. Region A was thought to be more highly exposed than region B, and region R was the unexposed area. More recent characterization of the exposures in Seveso indicate that the average serum concentrations in regions A are lower than the initial studies indicated (Bertazzi and di Domenico, 1995).

Several industrial cohorts have been examined for dioxin exposure. Most of these workers are either farm workers spraying phenoxy herbicides or workers manufacturing herbicides or trichlorophenol (Fingerhut et al., 1991; Flesch-Janys et al., 1995). Workers in these studies have serum concentrations of dioxin ranging from 100 to 5000 ppt TEQ on a lipid-adjusted basis. TCDD is the predominant congener in the occupational exposures, in contrast to the low-level background exposure of the general population where TCDD contributes approximately 10% of the total TEQ.

Spraying of herbicides contaminated with TCDD during the Vietnam War exposed military personnel from both sides of the conflict as well as Vietnamese civilians. Exposures of members of the United States armed forces are the best characterized from these groups. Despite initial fears of high exposure during the war, it appears that with the exception of those directly involved in the formulation and spraying, most ground troops had limited exposure to these chemicals. The spraying occurred predominantly in the southern region of Vietnam. Civilians from South Vietnam have approximately 10 times the serum concentrations of TCDD compared to those in North Vietnam (Schecter et al., 1994b, c). Concentrations of dioxin are similar among residents of South Vietnam, United States, and Western Europe (Schecter et al., 1994b, c).

Accidental exposures to dioxin have occurred following consumption of contaminated rice oils. In 1968 a mass poisoning, called Yusho or oil disease, occurred in Fukuoka and Nagasaki prefectures in Japan due to ingestion of rice oil contaminated with Kanechlor-400, a commercial PCB mixture produced in Japan. It was subsequently discovered that the Kanechlor-400 mixture was contaminated with CDFs as well as s polychlorinated quarterphenyls (Masuda, 1995). A similar incident occurred in Yu-cheng, Taiwan, in 1979 (Hsu et al., 1995). These incidents are known as Yusho and Yu-cheng, respectively. The concentrations of dioxin in the Yusho population shortly after the accident were approximately 20 times higher than controls, while PCB concentrations are 20 to 50 times background (Masuda, 1995). Similar exposures were observed in the Yu-cheng incidence as well. While these populations have been intensively studied, it has been difficult to determine which of the effects seen were due to the dioxin, non-dioxin-like PCBs or to their coexposure.

Pharmacokinetics

The dioxin-like toxicity of these chemicals is due to the parent compound, and for the CDDs and CDFs, metabolism is a detoxification step. Dioxins have relatively long half-lives in biological systems. In rats the half-life of dioxin ranges from approximately one day for TCDF and 3,3',4,4'-tetrachlorobiphenyl to greater than six months for OCDD (Van den Berg et al., 1994). TCDD has a half-life ranging from nine days in mice (Birnbaum, 1986; Gasiewicz et al., 1983, 1984) to approximately one year in rhesus monkeys (Bowman et al., 1989). In humans the half-life of the CDDs and CDF range from months to over 20 years. Estimates of the half-life of TCDD ranges from 5.7 to 11.3 years, with an average of about 8 years (Flesch-Janys et al., 1998; Pirkle et al., 1984). The difference in the half-life for mice, rats, and humans is approximately 80- to 400-fold. Such large differences in half-life between species has significant impact on the dose metric used in comparing species sensitivity to these chemicals. Many of the earlier risk assessments were based on comparisons of daily dose or administered dose, and they did not accurately correct for the difference in the kinetics of these chemicals between species. More recent comparisons have used steady-state body burdens as the dose metric, which provides a more accurate comparison, although it has limitations depending on the endpoint of comparison (DeVito et al., 1995; Wang et al.,1997).

The term half-life must be used cautiously with dioxin for several reasons. First, in humans there is a relationship between percentage of body fat and half-life. The greater the percentage of body fat, the longer is the half-life (Flesch-Janys, 1995; 1998). In addition there are non-linear kinetics of these chemicals which preclude the use of a single half-life. The disposition of dioxin is dose-dependent due to hepatic sequestration (DeVito et al., 1997; Andersen et al., 1993). The liver contains CYP1A2, which is inducible by dioxin. CYP1A2 binds TCDD and sequesters dioxin in the liver. In CYP1A2 knockout mice, neither TCDD nor 4-PeCDF is sequestered in hepatic tissue (Diliberto et al., 1997). In the wild-type mice, the induction of CYP1A2 results in the sequestration of these chemicals in the liver. The dose-dependent hepatic sequestration has been demonstrated in rats, mice, hamster, guinea pigs, and humans (Van den Berg et al., 1994; Carrier et al., 1995). While TCDD is sequestered in the liver, other dioxins are sequestered to a greater degree (DeVito et al., 1998). Because of these nonlinearities in the kinetics of dioxin, using a single half-life value has limitations, is best used as an indication of the persistence of these chemicals, and may not be suitable for quantitative determination of exposures.

Intensive efforts have been made to develop physiologically based pharmacokinetics models for dioxin. Most of these models have focused on TCDD (Leung et al., 1990; Andersen et al., 1993; 1997; Kedderis et al., 1993); however, a few have examined other congeners such as 2,3,7,8-tetrabromodibenzo-p-dioxin, dibenzofurans and PCBs (DeJongh et al.,1993; Kedderis et al., 1993). These models not only describe the pharmacokinetics of dioxin, they are also the basis for response models examining gene transcription and hepatocarcinogensis (Kohn et al., 1996; Conolly and Andersen, 1997; Portier et al., 1996). These models have potential use in risk assessment, but at present they require further validation.

Congener-specific pharmacokinetics information for PCBs in humans is also available. Those chemicals that have been examined are persistent, with half-lives in humans ranging from months to years (GE data). However, there are significant differences between the metabolism and disposition of PCBs compared to CDDs and CDFs. While metabolism for the CDDs and CDFs is a detoxifying pathway, metabolism of some of the dioxin-like PCBs produces bioactive metabolites. For example, hydroxylation of PCBs 77, 105, and 118 results in metabolites that bind to transthyretin, one of the thyroxine-binding proteins in serum. It has been hypothesized that the binding to transthyretin displaces thyroxine and increases its elimination (Brouwer et al., 1998). Other hydroxylated PCBs bind to utero globulin and accumulate in tissues expressing this protein, particularly the lung. Similar to the CDDs and CDFs, PCBs 77, 126, and 169 are sequestered in hepatic tissue. In contrast, the mono-ortho dioxin-like PCBs do not accumulate in the liver (DeVito et al, 1998). There is also evidence of pharmacokinetics interactions among CDDs, CDFs, and PCBs (van der Plas et al., 1998; Van den Berg et al., 1994), so extrapolations of animal data on single congeners to human exposures must be viewed with caution.

TOXICOLOGICAL EFFECTS AND MECHANISM OF ACTION

In experimental animals, dioxins induce numerous toxicities including immunotoxicity, reproductive and developmental toxicities, and carcinogenicity (DeVito and Birnbaum, 1995; Safe, 1990; Pohjanvirta and Tuomisto, 1994). The lethal effects of dioxin are unique in that death occurs weeks after the initial exposure; it is preceded by a wasting syndrome. In acute exposure studies, the time to death appears independent of the dose, and increasing the dose does not decrease the time to death. More recent studies by Rozman and coworkers have determined that the lethal effects of dioxin are time dependent (Viluksela et al., 1997). Animals initially die from the wasting syndrome within weeks following the initial exposures. However, animals that survive the initial wasting syndrome may eventually die from other causes, such as anemia, months after the initial exposure. The time to death, while independent of dose, can be altered by hypophysectomy. Lethal effects of TCDD can be observed within the first 24 hours in hypophysectomized mice (DeVito et al., 1992a). While the dose-response and time course for TCDD-induced wasting syndrome and lethality have been well characterized, the exact cause of death is uncertain. The wasting syndrome is thought to be due to alterations in the body weight set point. While the wasting syndrome can be severe, it does not appear to be a direct cause of death. Pair-fed controls with the same weight loss as the TCDD-treated animals do not exhibit mortality (Seefield et al., 1984).

Carcinogenicity

The carcinogenicity of TCDD has been examined in rats, mice, hamsters, and Japanese medaka; it is positive in all four species (Huff et al., 1994). Several studies in rats and mice indicate that TCDD is carcinogenic when administered for the lifetime of an animal. Tumors are observed in both sexes at multiple sites including liver, thyroid, lung, and several other tissues (Huff et al., 1994). In hamsters, the species most resistant to the lethal effects of TCDD, epidermal tumors are observed after dosing once a month for six months by either oral gavage or subcutaneous injections (Rao et al., 1988). Few of the related dioxins have been examined for carcinogenicity in two-year bioassays. A mixture of HxCDDs induced liver tumors in female rats and thyroid tumors in the males. The Aroclors 1016, 1242, 1254, and 1260 mixtures have been tested for carcinogenicity, and all mixtures induce liver tumors, while 1242, 1254, and 1260 also increase the incidence of thyroid tumors (Mayes et al., 1998).

TCDD is negative in several short-term mutagenicity assays. In addition using methods that can detect one DNA adduct in 10^{11} nucleotides, no TCDD-derived adducts have been detected (Turtletaub, 1990). Carcinogenesis is a multistage process that requires discrete steps involving genetic alterations of cells that clonally expand and progress into tumors. In this multistage process, TCDD clearly acts as a tumor promotor, although it may act on multiple stages of this process. TCDD is one of the most potent tumor promoters (Pitot et al., 1980; Poland et al., 1982; Lucier et al., 1991). All of the dioxin-like chemicals tested in hepatic tumor promotion models have tested positive, including 1,2,3,7,8-pentaCDD, 2,3,4,7,8-pentaCDF, and PCBs 126, 169, 118, 105, and 156 (Hemming et al., 1993, 1995; Buchmann et al., 1994; Maronpot et al., 1993; Haag-Gronlund et al., 1997, 1998; Schrenk et al., 1994).

Much of the research on the carcinogenic effects of dioxin has examined the liver tumors in rats. In rats the development of hepatic tumors occurs only in the female (Kociba et al., 1978; NTP, 1982). Tumor promotion studies in ovariectomized rats indicate that TCDD does not promote liver tumors in rats without a functioning ovary (Lucier et al., 1991). However, in these studies, the ovariectomized rats developed lung tumors, while the intact rats only developed hepatic tumors (Lucier et al., 1991). It has been hypothesized that TCDD increases the metabolism of estrogens and results in the production of catechol estrogen metabolites (Lucier et al., 1991). These metabolites are thought to redox cycle, resulting in the production of oxygen free radicals, which then produce DNA damage (Tritscher et al., 1996). While the role of estrogen is critical in the TCDD-induced liver tumor in female rats, it should be noted that hepatic tumors were not observed in hamsters, and in mice, males were more responsive to the hepatic carcinogenic effects of TCDD than are females (NTP, 1982).

In rats and mice TCDD is an extremely potent carcinogen. The LOAEL for hepatic adenomas in rats is 10 ng/kg/d, while the NOEAL is 1 ng/kg/d (Kociba et al., 1978; NTP, 1982). These doses seem rather high compared to the human intake of 1 to 6 pg TEQ/kg/d. In order to make a appropriate comparison, the large difference in half-life between species must be taken into account. One method is to express dose as steady-state body burdens (ng/kg). Daily intake of a chemical will eventually result in a steady-state condition in which the amount ingested equals the amount eliminated. With persistent chemicals such as dioxin, small concentrations ingested daily can result in large accumulation of the chemical in the body. In rats 1 ng/kg/d results in a body burden of approximately 30 ng TCDD/kg body weight. In mice the LOAEL for hepatocarcinogenesis is 71 ng/kg/d (NTP, 1982), with a resulting steady-state body burden of 944 ng/kg (DeVito et al., 1995).

Developmental Toxicity

TCDD and several other congeners induce cleft palate and hydronephrosis in mice. Cleft palate can be induced in rats and hamsters, but only at doses that result in significant fetal mortality (Olson and McGarrigle, 1991). Studies in cultured developing palates indicate that mouse palates are approximately 100 to 1000 times more sensitive to the effects of TCDD than are human and rat palates (Abbott and Birnbaum, 1991; Abbott et al.,1994). In addition human and rat palate are equally sensitive to the effects of TCDD, suggesting that humans are unlikely to develop cleft palate from dioxin.

Other more subtle effects of dioxin have also been observed in developing animals. The developing reproductive system of rats and hamsters is extremely sensitive to the actions of TCDD and other AhR agonists. Prenatal exposure to TCDD decreases epididymal sperm counts in mice and epididymal and ejaculated sperm counts in rats and hamsters (Theobold and Peterson, 1997; Mabley et al., 1992a, b; Gray et al., 1995). Female rats and hamsters exposed to TCDD in utero and lactationally develop malformations of the phallus, clitoris, and incomplete opening of the vaginal orifice (Gray et al., 1995, 1997). These developmental alterations of the reproductive systems can occur at doses as low as 0.05 ug/kg when administered on gestational day 15 (Gray et al., 1995). In a multigenerational study, doses as low as 1 ng/kg/d decrease fertility in the F1 and F2 generation (Murray et al., 1979). The 1 ng/kg/d dose in the multigenerational study resulted in steady-state body burdens of approximately 30 ng/kg (DeVito et al., 1995).

Dioxin-like chemicals are also developmental neurotoxicants. Prenatal exposure to TCDD produces a permanent low frequency auditory deficiency in rats (Goldey et al., 1996). Similar effects were observed in animals prenatally treated with either Aroclor 1254 or PCB 126 (Goldey et al., 1995; Crofton and Rice, 1999). The development of the auditory system is dependent upon thyroid hormones (Goldey et al., 1996). TCDD and other dioxin decrease circulating thyroid hormones by inducing uridine diphosphate glucuronsyl transferase (UDPGT) (Henry and Gasiewicz, 1987). In rats, pre- and post-natal exposure to TCDD and other dioxins decrease circulating thyroid hormone concentrations during the period of cochlear development, particularly the regions of the cochlea responsible for low-frequency hearing (Goldey et al., 1995; 1996; Crofton and Rice, 1999). The auditory deficits in rats produced by TCDD is a relatively high-dose phenomena requiring at least 1 ug/kg on gestational day 18, which is approximately 20 times higher than the doses needed to alter the developing reproductive tract.

The developmental neurotoxicity of TCDD is also expressed as a permanent change in regulated body temperature in both rats and hamsters (Gordon et al., 1995, 1996). Several laboratories have demonstrated behavioral changes in animals exposed prenatally to dioxin-like chemicals. Schantz and Bowman (1989) have examined the neurological developmental effects of TCDD in rhesus monkeys. Rhesus monkeys were exposed prenatally and lactationally to TCDD with dams receiving as little as 5 to 25 ppt of TCDD in the diet. The offspring had alterations in object learning at the low dose, and at the high dose few of the dams were able to maintain pregnancy, with only one offspring from seven dams surviving (Schantz and Bowman, 1989). The rhesus monkeys fed a diet of 5 ppt TCDD averaged 151 pg/kg/d (Bowman et al., 1989), and this diet resulted in a body burden of approximately 42 ng/kg (DeVito et al., 1995).

Immunotoxicity

TCDD and related chemicals are immunotoxicants in several species (Harper et al., 1993). The immunotoxicity of dioxin is difficult to characterize, and there does not appear to be a unique dioxin-like immune response. The responses affected by TCDD depend on the species studied and the model used to examine the immune response. For example, the suppression of the plaque-forming cell response to sheep red blood cells in mice is one of the most consistent findings, with an ED50 of approximately 0.7 ug TCDD/kg (Smailowicz et al., 1994). Yet in rats, TCDD enhances the response to sheep red blood cells (Smailowicz et al., 1994). In contrast, exposure to the same doses of TCDD that enhance the response to sheep red blood cells, suppress host resistance to trichinella spiralis (Luebke et al., 1994, 1995). In influenza models, doses of TCDD as low as 10 ng/kg increase mortality in mice following exposure to influenza virus (Burelson et al., 1996). Other low-dose effects on the immune system by TCDD are altered lymphocyte subsets in marmoset monkeys exposed to 0.3 pg/kg/week for 24 weeks (Neubert et al., 1994). This dose results in body burdens of approximately 10 ng/kg (DeVito et al., 1995). The immunotoxicity is thought to be associated with changes in proliferation and differentiation in a variety of cell types in the immune system (Kerkvliet et al., 1995).

MECHANISM OF ACTION

Role of the Ah Receptor in the Biological Effects of Dioxin

Binding to and activating the aryl hydrocarbon receptor (AhR) is the initial step in the biological and toxicological effects of dioxin. Most if not all of the effects are mediated by this protein (Birnbaum, 1994; Scheuplein et al., 1991). The unliganded AhR is found in either the cytosol or nucleus as a multimeric complex that includes two molecules of a 90-kDa heat-shock protein and several other smaller molecular weight proteins (Whitlock et al., 1996). Upon ligand binding, the AhR dissociates from this complex and binds to the aryl hydrocarbon nuclear translocator (ARNT). The transformed AhR-ARNT complex then binds to specific dioxin-responsive enhacer (DRE) sequences located in the promotor region of the CYP1A gene and several other TCDD responsive genes. The binding of the activated AhR complex to the DREs alters chromatin structure and enhances the association of other components of the transcriptional machinery, resulting in the initiation of transcription. This transformation of the AhR into a nuclear-binding form can be attenuated by protein kinase C inhibitors, and phosphorylation events appear to be important in regulating the activity of these proteins (Whitlock et al., 1996).

   While the exact role of the AhR in normal biochemical and physiological processes is uncertain, there are several lines of evidence that suggest it plays an important function in developmental and homeostatic functions. AhR is a ligand activated transcription factor that is a member of the basic-helix-loop-helix-Per-Arnt-Sim (bHLH-PAS) superfamily. The AhR is a highly conserved protein that is present in all mammalian species examined, and it has been found in all vertebrate classes examined, including modern representatives of early vertebrates such as cartilaginous and jawless fish (Hahn, 1998). In addition a possible AhR homolog has been identified in *C. elegans* (Powell-Coffman, 1998). The bHLH-PAS superfamily consists of at least 32 proteins found in diverse organisms from *Drosophila*, *C. elegans*, to humans. These proteins are transcription factors, and they appear to require dimerization, either homo- or heterodimers, for functional effects. These proteins regulate circadian rhythms (*per* and *clock*), steroid receptor signaling (SRC-1,

TIF2, RAC3), or are involved in sensing oxygen tension (HIF-1, EPAS-1/HLF) (Hahn, 1998). It has been proposed that understanding the function of the bHLH-PAS family of proteins and the phylogenetic evolution of the AhR may lead to an understanding of the role of this protein in normal processes.

Other lines of evidence indicate that the AhR has important physiological functions based on its spatial and temporal expression in developing embryos. The AhR is expressed in a tissue- and cell-specific manner during development (Abbott et al., 1994, 1995, in press). It is highly expressed in the neural epithelium, which forms the neural crest during development (Abbott et al., 1995). AhR knockout mice have been produced using a targeted disruption of the *Ahr* locus (Fernandez-Salguero et al., 1997). While the results from the two laboratories are not identical, it is apparent that the AhR is not essential to life, since the knockout mice survive and reproduce. However, the AhR-/- mice develop numerous lesions with age (Fernandez-Salguero et al., 1997). Mortality begins to increase at about an age of 20 weeks, and by 13 months 46% of the mice either died or were ill. Cardiovascular alterations consisting of cardiomyopathy with hypertrophy and focal fibrosis, hepatic vascular hypertrophy and mild fibrosis, gastric hyperplasia, and T-cell deficiency in the spleen and dermal lesions were apparent in these mice, and the incidence and severity increased with age (Fernandez-Salguero et al., 1997). While male and female AhR-/-mice are fertile, the females have difficulty maintaining conceptuses during pregnancy, surviving pregnancy and lactation, and rearing pups to weaning. In one study only 46% of 39 pregnant AhR-/-females successfully raised pups to weaning (Abbott et al., in press).

Other groups have developed an ARNT knockout mouse. In contrast to the AhR-/-mice, the lack of its dimerization partner, ARNT, results in fetal mortality. Unlike the AhR, ARNT has several other dimerization partners including HIF1 alpha (Hahn, 1998). It has been suggested that some of the toxicity of AhR ligands such as TCDD may be due to sequestration of ARNT by the AhR, decreasing ARNTs availability for other members of the PAS family (Hahn, 1998).

The importance of the AhR in the toxicity of dioxin stems from several lines of evidence. First, structure activity relationships indicate a correlation between receptor binding affinity and in vivo toxicity in mice (Safe, 1990). Second there is genetic evidence in mice that is consistent with the AhR mediating the toxic effects of dioxin. The C57BL mice are the most sensitive to the toxic effects of dioxin, while the DBA/2J is the most resistant. The binding affinity of the AhR is approximately 10 to 20 lower in the C57BL compared to the DBA, and the C57BL mice are approximately 10 to 20 times more sensitive that are the DBA mice (Poland and Glover, 1980). In fact the sensitivity to dioxin in mice segregates nicely with several different alleles and the binding affinity of dioxin to these gene products (Poland and Glover, 1990). Finally the most powerful evidence is that the AhR-/- mice are resistant to the toxicities of TCDD (Mimura et al., 1997; Fernandez-Seguaro et al., 1996).

While the initial step in the toxicity of dioxin is binding to the bAhR, this binding is clearly not the sole determinant in the toxicity of these chemicals. In the mouse the different AhR alleles have different binding affinities to dioxin, and these differences can explain the differences in sensitivity to dioxin between these strains (Poland and Glover, 1980). The biochemical and biophysical properties of the AhR are similar between species with only slight differences in molecular mass and subunit stability (Gasiewicz and Rucci, 1984). Yet for some endpoints, such as lethality, there are significant differences in the ED50s between species (Pohjanvirta and Tuomisto, 1994). While the ED50s for some endpoints, such as fetal mortality and enzyme induction, are similar between the species (Olson and McGarrigle, 1991). Overall, these data indicate that the steps after AhR binding and activation are critical in understanding the species differences in response to dioxin.

Dioxin as Growth Dysregulators and Endocrine Disruptors

While dioxins appear to alter numerous systems, there are several underlying commonalities of the toxicity of these chemicals. Most of the toxicities are associated with alterations in proliferation and/or differentiation, such as cancer, immunotoxicity, and chloracne. Hyperplastic responses are observed in gastric mucosa and bile ducts in monkeys (McConnell and Moore, 1979), urinary bladder in guinea pigs, whereas hepatic and dermal hyperplasia occurs in several species. Hypoplasia occurs in lymphoid tissues in all mammalian species examined and in the gonads of mice, rats, rabbits, and mink. Squamous metaplasia is induced by TCDD in ceruminous and sebaceous glands in monkeys (Moore et al., 1979). Dysplastic responses of the nails and teeth have been observed in humans and nonhuman primates following prenatal exposure to dioxin (Moore et al., 1979; Masuda, 1995). Dioxins are potent growth dysregulators.

Dioxins alter the normal homeostatic processes by disrupting cell-signaling pathways through multiple mechanisms. Cells maintain homeostasis through a complex processes involving the release of paracrine or autocrine hormones or growth factors. These hormones and growth factors interact with specific receptors that can be localized to the cell membrane, cytosol, or nucleus. Activation of these receptors initiates a cascade of events that effect cell functioning. Dioxins alter cell signaling and homeostasis by altering hormones and growth factors, and their receptors, and by altering the signaling of the activated receptors. These effects of dioxin are often tissue and developmental stage specific (DeVito and Birnbaum, 1995).

TCDD alters many of the signaling pathways involved in the endocrine system as well, and it can be considered an endocrine disruptor. Dioxin alters serum concentrations of several pituitary hormones (Moore et al., 1989) and steroid hormones including androgens (Moore et al., 1985), glucocorticoids (Lin et al., 1991), and thyroid hormones (Henry and Gasiewicz, 1987; Kohn et al.,1996). In cell culture, TCDD increases estradiol metabolism by almost 100-fold (Spink et al., 1990). Estrogen receptors are decreased in several tissues including liver and uteri in mice and rats administered dioxin (DeVito et al., 1992a, b; Safe et al., 1991). Dioxins have frequently been described as antiestrogens because they decrease estrogen and estrogen receptor concentrations. However, this characterization should be viewed cautiously, since dioxins also increase the incidence and severity of endometriosis in monkeys (Reier et al., 1993) and increase endometriotic lesions in mice and rats (Cummings et al., 1996; Johnson et al., 1997). Endometriosis is dependent on estrogens for growth, so it is often treated with drugs that down-regulate ovarian function. Once again, this highlights the tissue-specific effects of these chemicals.

Human Health Effects Associated with Dioxin Exposure

The epidemiological data examining the potential carcinogenic effects of dioxin have focused mostly on several industrial cohorts of pesticide manufacturers (Kogevinas et al., 1997), American veterans of Vietnam, and the Seveso, Italy, cohorts. It has proved difficult to obtain a consensus on the interpretation of these studies. IARC recently evaluated the evidence for carcinogenicity for TCDD and other dioxins (McGregor et al., 1998). The IARC working group focused on the four cohorts with the highest exposure (Fingerhut et al., 1991; Hooiveld et al., 1998; Ott and Zober, 1996 and Flesch-Janys et al., 1995; Zober et al., 1994). In these studies the overall risk of developing cancer was significantly greater (approximately 1.4-fold) in the exposed populations (McGregor et al., 1998). Few site-specific cancer risks were consistent across the cohorts. However, evidence of increased risk of lung cancer was significant in all four studies (Fingerhut et al., 1991; Hooiveld et al., 1998; Ott and Zober, 1996; Flesch-Janys et al., 1995; Zober et al., 1994). One of the problems with interpretation of these studies is that an increase in risk for cancers at many sites was observed for only a few cases, as is the case for smoking exposure to ionizing radiation in atomic bomb survivors (McGregor et al., 1998). In contrast to TCDD, both smoking and ionizing radiation also increase site-specific tumors. The fact that TCDD is the only chemical that increased risk for all cancers without consistently increasing the risk for specific tumors suggests that the epidemiological data should be viewed with caution. The IARC workgroup considered the evidence for carcinogenicity as limited. However, the IARC workgroup also considered mechanistic information. Their overall evaluation was that TCDD is carcinogenic in humans (McGregor et al., 1998).

Immune effects of dioxin are observed in all species examined (Kerkvliet, 1995). However, human health has not been as consistently altered. Some of the best evidence comes from developmental studies in humans, which have suggested that there are developmental effects following exposure to CDDs, CDFs, and PCBs (Weisglas-Kuperus, 1995). In addition neurodevelopmental effects have been reported for a number of cohorts (Rogan and Gladen,1991; 1992; Jacobson et al., 1990; Jacobson and Jacobson, 1997). The Dutch studies of a cohort of infants has demonstrated relationships among high CDDs, CDFs, and PCBs exposure and decreases in thyroid hormones and delayed neurodevelopment (Koopman-Esseboom et al., 1994; Weisglas-Kuperus, 1995). While these studies indicate that exposure to this class of chemicals may be associated with alterations in the developing immune and neurological systems, these effects are subclinical, and extrapolation to the population at large is uncertain. However, it should be stressed that in the Dutch studies, this cohort is of women and infants with no known high exposures to PHAHs other than background exposures. The associations found in this cohort, while subclinical, warrants further research and concern.

Toxic Equivalency Factors

Estimating the risk associated with dioxin exposure can be problematic. These chemicals are present as trace contaminants of a complex mixture containing numerous dioxin-like chemicals. Initially risk assessments focused on TCDD alone, and all other dioxins were excluded. However, experimental evidence clearly indicates that these other dioxin-like chemicals cannot be ignored. If risk assessments are to include other dioxins, then either they must assume that all dioxin-like chemicals are as potent as TCDD or they must use some sort of relative potency scaling methodology. The experimental data clearly demonstrate that assuming all dioxin to be equally potent to TCDD would greatly overestimate the potential risk. Hence a relative potency scheme, described as toxic equivalency factors, was proposed to estimate the potential health risk following exposure to dioxin-like chemicals (Eadon et al., 1986).

The toxicological basis for the TEF methodology is the shared mechanism of action of these chemicals, namely activation of the AhR (Safe, 1990; Birnbaum and DeVito, 1995). The relative potency of a dioxin-like chemical is compared to TCDD, one of the most potent AhR ligands studied. The relative potency for a chemical from a particular study is described as a REP. A TEF is assigned by expert groups using all the available REP values for a particular chemical. The data available for assigning a TEF value for a chemical varies widely depending on the congener. For example, there are over 25 studies that examine the relative potency of PCB 126 compared to TCDD, with endpoints ranging from in vitro studies examining binding affinity and biochemical alterations to in vivo subchronic studies examining toxicological and biochemical effects (Van den Berg et al., 1998). For other chemicals, such as PCB 80, there are only in vitro studies suggesting a dioxin-like effect (Van den Berg et al., 1998). In determining the TEF value, the varying types of data are weighted according to relevancy. For example, data on binding affinity are weighted less than data from acute in vivo studies, which are weighted less than data from subchronic studies examining toxicological effects (Van den Berg et al., 1998). TEFs are considered *order of magnitude* estimates for several reasons, including the quality and quantity of the data available, the variability of the data, and the limited information on the species extrapolation of the relative potency of these chemicals (Van den Berg et al., 1998).

The relative potency of a chemical compared to TCDD is a function of its binding affinity to the AhR and its comparable pharmacokinetics properties, including absorption, disposition, metabolism, and elimination (DeVito et al., 1997; DeVito et al., in press). One example of the importance of pharmacokinetics in the relative potency of these chemicals is octachlorodibenzo-*p*-dioxin (OCDD). Originally OCDD was assigned a TEF value of 0 because it demonstrated no toxicological effects in acute studies in rodents, and binding data were unavailable due to the compound's insolubility in aqueous solutions. However, in subchronic studies in rats, OCDD demonstrated significant dioxin-like effects and was assigned a TEF value of 0.001. In short-term studies, very little OCDD is absorbed by the animal. However, because of its persistence, in longer-term studies OCDD will accumulate and eventually attain concentrations in the animal sufficient to produce toxicological effects (Birnbaum and Couture, 1988; Couture et al., 1988).

The TEF methodology assumes that the biochemical and toxicological effects of mixtures of dioxin can be predicted using a dose addition methodology. Several investigators have examined the TEF methodology, using simple mixtures containing 2, 3, or 4 congeners, or more complex mixtures from environmental samples, or laboratory prepared mixtures. The TEF methodology adequately predicted the immunotoxicity (Silkworth et al., 1989), lethality (Eadon et al., 1986), or biochemical changes (Van den berg et al., 1989) of complex environmental mixtures. Schrenck and coworkers used the TEF methodology to predict the tumor promotion potency of a laboratory prepared mixture of 49 different chlorinated dioxins. Rozman and coworkers examined the effects of a quarternary mixture of chlorinated dioxin and found the TEF methodology predicted both biochemical and toxicological responses of the mixture (Viluksela et al., 1998a, b).

While there are a number of papers demonstrating additivity and supporting the TEF methodology, there are still some unanswered questions. Recently the TEF methodology was expanded to include the coplanar PCBs and the mono-ortho-substituted PCBs. These chemicals, while demonstrating dioxin-like toxicities, have significant non-dioxin-like effects. For example, TCDD and other chlorinated dibenzo-p-dioxins decrease thyroxine concentrations by only 40% to 50% in rats. In contrast, PCBs 77 and 118 can produce a 90% decrease in thyroxine (Crofton et al., 1998). In a complex mixture consisting of two chlorinated dibenzo-p-dioxins, four chlorinated dibenzofurans, and six chlorinated biphenyls, the TEF methodology predicted the immunotoxicity and enzyme-inducing effects of the mixture, but it underpredicted the thyroxine decreases and porphyrin accumulation in rats administered the mixture compared to rats receiving TCDD.

One of the problems with the TEF methodology is the confusion as to what this method actually does. The TEF methodology only examines dioxin-like chemicals and assumes that there is no interactions between the dioxin and non-dioxin present in the mixture. In essence, the method allows one to estimate the potential health risk of a complex mixture by assuming that only TCDD is present. This method makes no attempt to predict interactions of dioxin and other classes of chemicals. Hence the method ignores potential nonadditive interactions, both antagonistic and greater than additive interactions.

While there is uncertainty in the use of the TEF methodology, one question to ask is whether using this method decreases or increases our uncertainty in the overall risk assessment. As described above, either excluding all other dioxin-like chemicals or considering other dioxin-like chemicals as potent as TCDD, increases uncertainty in risk assessments. At a recent workshop on the use of TEFs in ecological risk assessment sponsored by the U.S. EPA, the participants clearly agreed that the use of the TEF methodology decreases uncertainty. However, quantifying the uncertainty in the TEF methodology, and its effects on the uncertainty of the overall risk assessment, remain elusive (U.S. EPA, 1998). With no alternative methodology, one can argue that the TEF method decreases uncertainty in the overall risk assessment. Until alternative methodologies are developed, the TEF methodology is the most appropriate method to estimate the potential health risks of exposure to dioxin-like chemicals. Significant efforts should be made to clarify the uncertainty of this methodology to support risk assessors and managers until more accurate methods are developed.

Risk Characterization

Dioxins induce numerous toxicities in experimental animals. The toxicity of these chemicals is mediated through an interaction with the Ah receptor. The Ah receptor is a highly conserved protein throughout evolution. While the exact role of the Ah receptor is uncertain, inappropriate activation of this receptor by dioxins produces tissue-specific alterations in differentiation, proliferation- and apoptosis. These processes are critical in numerous biological systems including development, the immune system, and carcinogenesis, to name a few. While there may be outliers, either resistant or sensitive, to certain dioxin toxicities, most species respond at similar exposures (i.e., within an order of magnitude for dose). The available data suggest that for biochemical and some toxic responses, humans have similar sensitivities to experimental animals. For example, the steady-state body burdens in rodents that result in cancers are between 300 and 900 ng/kg (DeVito et al., 1995). In the epidemiological studies, the high end of exposures have body burdens ranging from 400 to 5000 ng/kg (DeVito et al., 1995). There is no evidence to suggest that humans are less sensitive to the potential effects of dioxin than are laboratory animals. Because of the consistency of effects observed in both humans and experimental animals and the evolutionary conservation of the structure and function of the Ah receptor, efforts should be made to limit exposure to this class of chemicals.

The available human data do not readily lend themselves to quantitative risk assessments for these chemicals. A reliance on the toxicity of dioxin in laboratory animals is required in order to understand and estimate the risks associated with exposure to these chemicals. In the past, regulators have relied on either linearized models for cancer risk assessments or safety factor methods. More recently a *margin of exposure* method was used to examine potential risks from these chemicals (DeVito et al., 1995). Present human background exposure is approximately 8 to 13 ng TEQ/kg. Responses in experimental animals have been observed at body burdens ranging from 5 to 900 ng/kg or more. In the low-dose range, immunotoxicity in rodents and monkeys, reproductive effects in multigeneration studies, and endometriosis in rhesus monkeys occur at body burdens between 5 and 64 ng/kg. If one divides the body burden in animals where effects are observed by the average human body burden, one obtains the margin of exposure. From the above data the margin of exposure ranges from less than one to approximately 10 (an order of magnitude). The margin of exposure does not imply that effects are occurring in the population. However, it compares the difference in present human exposure to that of animals exposed to toxic doses of a chemical. Typically the U.S. EPA, considers a margin of exposure of 100 reasonable for noncarcinogenic effects.

Recently the World Health Organization assessed the potential human health effects of dioxin. These experts suggested that the tolerable daily intake be set at 1 to 4 pg TEQ/kg/d. They also noted that present exposures throughout the world range from 2 to 6 pg TEQ/kg/d. These experts emphasized the results of the Dutch cohort studies and stressed that these data suggest that background exposures are associated with effects. In addition the working group noted that concentrations of dioxin have been decreasing in the environment over the last two decades.

The risk associated with exposure to dioxin remains uncertain. Recent studies suggest that present intakes are within the range where nonclinical responses are occurring in the population. While concentrations of dioxin are decreasing in the population, efforts should be made to continue monitoring this class of chemicals and identifying sources.

REFERENCES

Abbott, B. D., and L. S. Birnbaum. 1991. TCDD exposure of human embryonic palatal shelves in organ culture alters the differentiation of medial epithelial cells. *Teratology* 43: 119–132.

Abbott, B. D., L. S. Birnbaum, and G. H. Perdew. 1995. Developmental expression of two members of a new class of transcription factors: I. Expression of aryl hydrocarbon receptor in the C57BL/6N mouse embryo. *Dev. Dyn.* 204: 133–143.

Abbott, B. D., A. R. Buckalew, J. J. Diliberto, C. R. Wood, G. A. Held, J. A. Pitt, and J. E. Schmid. 1999. Adverse reproductive outcomes in the transgenic *ah* receptor-deficient mouse. *Toxicol. Appl. Pharmacol.* 155: 62–70.

Abbott, B. D., M. R. Probst, and G. H. Perdew. 1994. Immunohistochemical double-staining for Ah receptor and ARNT in human embryonic palatal shelves. *Teratology* 50: 361–366.

Andersen, M. E., J. J. Mills, M. L. Gargas, L. Kedderis, L. S. Birnbaum, D. Neubert, and W. F. Greenlee. 1993. Modeling receptor-mediated processes with dioxin: Implications for pharmacokinetics and risk assessment. *Risk Anal.* 13: 25–36.

Andersen, M. E., L. S. Birnbaum, H. A. Barton, and C. R. Eklund. 1997. Regional hepatic CYP1A1 and CYP1A2 induction with 2,3,7,8-tetrachlorodibenzo-p-dioxin evaluated with a multicompartment geometric model of hepatic zonation. *Toxicol. Appl. Pharmacol.* 144: 145–155.

Atlas, E., T. Bidleman, and C. S. Giam. 1986. Atmospheric transport of PCBs to the oceans. In *PCBs and the Environment.*, vol. 1, ed. J. S. Waid, pp. 79–100. Boca Raton, FL: CRC Press.

Bertazzi, P. A., and A. di Domenico. 1995. Chemical, environmental, and health aspects of the Seveso, Italy, Accident. In *Dioxins and Health,* ed. A. Schecter, pp. 587–632, New York: Plenum Press.

Birnbaum, L. S. 1986. Distribution and excretion of 2,3,7,8-tetrachlorodibenzo-p-dioxin in congenic strains of mice which differ at the Ah locus. *Drug Metab. Dispos.* 14: 34–40.

Birnbaum, L. S., and L. A. Couture. 1988. Disposition of octachlorodibenzo-p-dioxin (OCDD) in male rats. *Toxicol. Appl. Pharmacol.* 93: 22–30.

Birnbaum, L. S. 1994. Evidence for the role of the Ah receptor in response to dioxin. *Prog. Clin. Biol. Res.* 387: 139–154.

Birnbaum, L. S., and M. J. DeVito. 1995. Use of toxic equivalency factors for risk assessment for dioxins and related compounds. *Toxicology* 105: 391–401.

Birnbaum, L. S. 1995. Workshop on perinatal exposure to dioxin-like compounds. V. Immunologic effects. *Environ. Health Perspect.* 103 (suppl 2): 157–160.

Bowman, R. E., S. L. Schantz, N. C. A. Weerasinghe, M. L. Gross, and D. A. Barsotti. 1989. Chronic dietary intake of 2,3,7,8-tetrachlorodibenzo-p-dioxin (TCDD) at 5 or 25 parts per trillion in the monkey: TCDD kinetics and dose-effect estimate of the reproductive toxicity. *Chemosphere* 18: 243–252.

Brouwer, A., H. Hakansson, A. Kukler, K. J. Van den Berg, and U. G. Ahlborg. 1989. Marked alterations in retinoid homeostasis of Sprague-Dawley rats induced by a single i.p. dose of 10 micrograms/kg of 2,3,7,8-tetrachlorodibenzo-p-dioxin. *Toxicology* 58: 267–283.

Brouwer, A., D. C. Morse, M. C. Lans, A. G. Schuur, A. J. Murk, E. Klasson-Wehler, A. Bergman, and T. J. Visser. 1998. Interactions of persistent environmental organohalogens with the thyroid hormone system: mechanisms and possible consequences for animal and human health. *Toxicol. Ind. Health.* 14: 59–84.

Buchmann, A., S. Stinchcombe, W. Korner, H. Hagenmaier, and K. W. Bock. 1994. Effects of 2,3,7,8-tetrachloro- and 1,2,3,4,6,7,8-heptachlorodibenzo-p-dioxin on the proliferation of preneoplastic liver cells in the rat. *Carcinogenesis.* 15: 1143–1150.

Burleson, G. R., H. Lebrec, Y. G. Yang, J. D. Ibanes, K. N. Pennington, and L. S. Birnbaum. 1996. Effect of 2,3,7,8-tetrachlorodibenzo-p-dioxin (TCDD) on influenza virus host resistance in mice. *Fundam. Appl. Toxicol.* 29: 40–47.

Carrier, G., R. C. Brunet, and J. Brodeur. 1995. Modeling of the toxicokinetics of polychlorinated dibenzo-p-dioxins and dibenzofurans in mammalians, including humans. I. Nonlinear distribution of PCDD/PCDF body burden between liver and adipose tissues. *Toxicol. Appl. Pharmacol.* 131: 253–266.

Cleverly, D., M. Monetti, L. Phillips, P. Cramer, M. Heit, S. McCarthy, K. O'Rourke, J. Stanley, and D. Winters. 1996. A time-trends study of the occurrences and levels of CDDs, CDFs, and dioxin-like PCBs in sediment cores from 11 geographically distributed lakes in the United States. *Organohalogen Compounds* 28: 77–82.

Cleverly, D., J. Schaum, D. Winters, G. Schweer, and K. O'Rourke. 1998. The inventory of sources of dioxin in the United States. *Organohalogen Compounds* 36: 1–6.

Conolly, R. B., and M. E. Andersen. 1997. Hepatic foci in rats after diethylnitrosamine initiation and 2,3,7,8-tetrachlorodibenzo-p-dioxin promotion: evaluation of a quantitative two-cell model and of CYP 1A1/1A2 as a dosimeter. *Toxicol. Appl. Pharmacol.* 146: 281–293.

Couture, L. A., M. R. Elwell, and L. S. Birnbaum. 1988. Dioxin-like effects observed in male rats following exposure to octachlorodibenzo-p-dioxin (OCDD) during a 13-week study. *Toxicol. Appl. Pharmacol.* 93: 31–46.

Crofton, K. M., and Rice, D. C. 1999. Perinatal exposure to PCB126: Thyroid hormones and ototoxicity. *Neurotoxicol. Teratol.* 21: 299–301.

Crosby, D. G., A. S. Wong, J. R. Plimmer, and A. E. Woolson. 1971. Photodecomposition of chlorinated dibenzo-p-dioxins. *Science* 173: 748–749.

Cummings, A. M., J. L. Metcalf, and L. Birnbaum. 1996. Promotion of endometriosis by 2,3,7,8-tetrachlorodibenzo-p-dioxin in rats and mice: Time-dose dependence and species comparison. *Toxicol. Appl. Pharmacol.* 138: 131–139.

Czuczwa, J. M., F. Neissen, and R. A. Hites. 1985. Historical record of polychlorinated dibenzo-p-dioxins in Swiss lake sediments. *Chemosphere* 14: 1175–1179.

De Jongh, J., R. Nieboer, I. Schroders, W. Seinen, and M. Van den Berg. 1993. Toxicokinetic mixture interactions between chlorinated aromatic hydrocarbons in the liver of the C57BL/6J mouse: 2. Polychlorinated dibenzo-p-dioxins (PCDDs), dibenzofurans (PCDFs) and biphenyls (PCBs). *Arch. Toxicol.* 67: 598–604.

DeVito, M. J., T. Thomas, E. Martin, T. H. Umbreit, and M. A. Gallo. 1992a. Antiestrogenic action of 2,3,7,8-tetrachlorodibenzo-p-dioxin: tissue-specific regulation of estrogen receptor in CD1 mice. *Toxicol. Appl. Pharmacol.* 113: 284–292.

DeVito, M. J., T. Thomas, T. H. Umbreit, and M. A. Gallo. 1992b. Multi-site regulation of estrogen receptor by 2,3,7,8-tetrachlorodibenzo-p-dioxin. *Prog. Clin. Biol. Res.* 374: 321–336.

DeVito, M. J., L. S. Birnbaum, W. H. Farland, and T. A. Gasiewicz. 1995. Comparisons of estimated human body burdens of dioxinlike chemicals and TCDD body burdens in experimentally exposed animals. *Environ. Health. Perspect.* 103: 820–831.

DeVito, M. J., and L. S. Birnbaum. 1995. The importance of pharmacokinetics in determining the relative potency of 2,3,7,8-tetrachlorodibenzo-p-dioxin and 2,3,7,8-tetrachlorodibenzofuran. *Fundam. Appl. Toxicol.* 24: 145–148.

DeVito, M. J., J. J. Diliberto, D. G. Ross, M. G. Menache, and L. S. Birnbaum. 1997. Dose-response relationships for polyhalogenated dioxins and dibenzofurans following subchronic treatment in mice. I. CYP1A1 and CYP1A2 enzyme activity in liver, lung, and skin. *Toxicol. Appl. Pharmacol.* 147: 267–280.

DeVito, M. J., D. G. Ross, A. E. Dupuy Jr., J. Ferrario, D. McDaniel, and L. S. Birnbaum. 1998. Dose-response relationships for disposition and hepatic sequestration polyhalogenated dibenzo-p-dioxin, dibenzofurans, and biphenyls following subchronic treatment in mice. *Toxicol. Sci.* 46: 223–234.

Devoogt, P., and U. A. Brinkman. 1989. Production, properties and usage of polychlorinated biphenyls. In *Halogenated Biphenyls, Terphenyls, Naphthalenes, Dibenzodioxins and Related Products*, eds. R. D. Kimbrough and A. A. Jensen, pp. 3–45. Amsterdam: Elsevier.

di Domenico, A., G. Viviano, and G. Zapponi. 1982. Environmental persistence of 2,3,7,8-TCDD at Seveso. In *Chlorinated Dioxins and Related Compounds: Impact on the Environment*, eds. O. Hutzinger, R. W. Frei, E. Merian, and F. Pocchiari, pp. 105–114. Oxford: Pergamon Press.

Diliberto, J. J., D. Burgin, and L. S. Birnbaum. 1997. Role of CYP1A2 in hepatic sequestration of dioxin: studies using CYP1A2 knock-out mice. *Biochem. Biophys. Res. Commun.* 236: 431.

Eadon, G., L. Kaminsky, J. Silkworth, K. Aldous, D. Hilker, P. O'Keefe, R. Smith, J. Gierthy, J. Hawley, N. Kim, et al. 1986. Calculation of 2,3,7,8-TCDD equivalent concentrations of complex environmental contaminant mixtures. *Environ. Health Perspect.* 70: 221–227.

Fernandez-Salguero, P. M., J. M. Ward, J. P. Sundberg, and F. J. Gonzalez. 1997. Lesions of aryl-hydrocarbon receptor-deficient mice. *Vet. Pathol.* 34: 605–614.

Fingerhut, M. A., W. E. Halperin, D. A. Marlow, L. A. Piacitelli, P. A. Honchar, M. H. Sweeney, A. L. Greife, P. A. Dill, K. Steenland, and A. J. Suruda. 1991. Cancer mortality in workers exposed to 2,3,7,8-tetrachlorodibenzo-p-dioxin. *N. Engl. J. Med.* 324: 212–218.

Flesch-Janys, D., J. Berger, P. Gurn, A. Manz, S. Nagel, H. Waltsgott, and J. H. Dwyer. 1995. Exposure to polychlorinated dioxins and furans (PCDD/F) and mortality in a cohort of workers from a herbicide-producing plant in Hamburg, Federal Republic of Germany. *Am. J. Epidemiol.* 142: 1165–1175.

Flesch-Janys, D., K. Steindorf, P. Gurn, and H. Becher. 1998. Estimation of the cumulated exposure to polychlorinated dibenzo-p-dioxins/furans and standardized mortality ratio analysis of cancer mortality by dose in an occupationally exposed cohort. *Environ. Health Perspect.* 106 (suppl 2): 655–662.

Fries, G. F., and D. J. Paustenbach. 1990. Evaluation of potential transmission of 2,3,7,8-tetrachloro-dibenzo-p-dioxin-contaminated incinerator emissions to humans via foods. *J. Toxicol. Environ. Health* 29: 1–43.

Gasiewicz, T. A., L. E. Geiger, G. Rucci, and R. A. Neal. 1983. Distribution, excretion, and metabolism of 2,3,7,8-tetrachlorodibenzo-p-dioxin in C57BL/6J, DBA/2J, and B6D2F1/J mice. *Drug. Metab. Dispos.* 11: 397–403.

Gasiewicz, T. A., and G. Rucci. 1984. Cytosolic receptor for 2,3,7,8-tetrachlorodibenzo-p-dioxin. Evidence for a homologous nature among various mammalian species. *Mol. Pharmacol.* 26: 90–98.

Goldey, E. S., C. Lau, L. S. Kehn, and K. M. Crofton. 1996. Developmental dioxin exposure: Disruption of thyroid hormones and ototoxicity. 35th Annual Meeting of the Society of Toxicology, Anaheim, CA. *Toxicologist* 30: 225.

Gordon, C. J., L. E. Gray Jr., N. A. Monteiro-Riviere, and D. B. Miller. 1995. Temperature regulation and metabolism in rats exposed perinatally to dioxin: permanent change in regulated body temperature? *Toxicol. Appl. Pharmacol.* 133: 172–176.

Gordon, C. J., Y. Yang, and L. E. Gray Jr. 1996. Autonomic and behavioral thermoregulation in golden hamsters exposed perinatally to dioxin. *Toxicol. Appl. Pharmacol.* 137: 120–125.

Gray, L. E., Jr., W. R. Kelce, E. Monosson, J. S. Ostby, and L. S. Birnbaum. 1995. Exposure to TCDD during development permanently alters reproductive function in male Long Evans rats and hamsters: Reduced ejaculated and epididymal sperm numbers and sex accessory gland weights in offspring with normal androgenic status. *Toxicol. Appl. Pharmacol.* 131: 108–118.

Gray, L. E., C. Wolf, P. Mann, and J. S. Ostby. 1997. In utero exposure to low doses of 2,3,7,8-tetrachlorodibenzo-p-dioxin alters reproductive development of female Long Evans hooded rat offspring. *Toxicol. Appl. Pharmacol.* 146: 237–244.

Haag-Gronlund, M., Y. Kato, R. Fransson-Steen, G. Scheu, and L. Warngard. 1997. Promotion of enzyme altered foci in female rat 2,3,3',4,4',5-hexachlorobiphenyl. *Toxicol. Appl. Pharmacol.* 147: 46–55.

Haag-Gronlund, M., N. Johansson, R. Fransson-Steen, H. Hakansson, G. Scheu, and L. Warngard. 1998. Interactive effects of three structurally different polychlorinated biphenyls in a rat liver tumor promotion bioassay. *Toxicol. Appl. Pharmacol.* 152: 153–165.

Hahn, M. E. 1998. The aryl hydrocarbon receptor: A comparative perspective. *Comparative Biochemistry and Physiology Part C: Pharmacology, Toxicology and Endocrinology,* 121: 23–53.

Harper, N., K. Connor, and S. Safe. 1993. Immunotoxic potencies of polychlorinated biphenyl (PCB), dibenzofuran (PCDF) and dibenzo-p-dioxin (PCDD) congeners in C57BL/6 and DBA/2 mice. *Toxicology* 80: 217–227.

Hemming, H., S. Flodstrom, L. Warngard, A. Bergman, T. Kronevi, I. Nordgren, and U. G. Ahlborg. 1993. Relative tumour promoting activity of three polychlorinated biphenyls in rat liver. *Eur. J. Pharmacol.* 248: 163–174.

Hemming, H., Y. Bager, S. Flodstrom, I. Nordgren, T. Kronevi, U. G. Ahlborg, and L. Warngard. 1995. Liver tumour promoting activity of 3,4,5,3′,4′-pentachlorobiphenyl and its interaction with 2,3,7,8-tetrachlorodibenzo-p-dioxin. *Eur. J. Pharmacol.* 292: 241–249.

Henry, E. C., and T. A. Gasiewicz. 1987. Changes in thyroid hormones and thyroxine glucuronidation in hamsters compared with rats following treatment with 2,3,7,8-tetrachlorodibenzo-p-dioxin. *Toxicol. Appl. Pharmacol.* 89: 165–174.

Hooiveld, M., D. J. Heederik, M. Kogevinas, P. Boffetta, L. L. Needham, D. G. Patterson Jr., and H. B. Bueno-de-Mesquita. 1998. Second follow-up of a Dutch cohort occupationally exposed to phenoxy herbicides, chlorophenols, and contaminants. *Am. J. Epidemiol.* 147: 891–901.

Hsu, C.-C., M.-L. M. Yu, Y.-C. J. Chen, Y.-L. L. Gou, and W. L. Rogan. 1995. The Yu-cheng rice oil poisoning incident. In: *Dioxins and Health,* ed. A. Schecter. pp. 661–684. New York: Plenum Press.

Huff, J., G. Lucier, and A. Tritscher. 1994. Carcinogenicity of TCDD: Experimental, mechanistic, and epidemiologic evidence. *Ann. Rev. Pharmacol. Toxicol.* 34: 343–372.

Huisman, M., S. E. Eerenstein, C. Koopman-Esseboom, M. Brouwer, V. Fidler, F. A. Muskiet, P. J. Sauer, and E. R. Boersma. 1995. Perinatal exposure to polychlorinated biphenyls and dioxins through dietary intake. *Chemosphere.* 31: 4273–4287.

Hutzinger, O., M. J., Blumich, M. van den Berg, and K. Olie. 1985. *IARC Monographs on the Evaluation of Carcinogenic Risks to Humans. Overall Evaluations of Carcinogenicity: An Updating of IARC Monographs,* vols. 1–42 , Suppl. 7. Lyons: IARC.

Insensee, A. R., and G. E. Jones. 1971. Absorption and translocation of root and foliage applied 2,4-dichlorophenol, 2,7-dichlorodibenzo-p-dioxin and 2,3,7,8-tetrachlorodibenzo-p-dioxin. *J. Agr. Food. Chem.* 19: 1210–1214.

Insensee, A. R., and G. E. Jones. 1975. Distribution of 2,3,7,8-tetrachlorodibenzo-p-dioxin (TCDD) in an aquatic model ecosystem. *Environ. Sci. Technol.* 9: 668–672.

Jacobson, J. L., S. W. Jacobson, and H. E. Humphrey. 1990. Effects of in utero exposure to polychlorinated biphenyls and related contaminants on cognitive functioning in young children. *J. Pediatr.* 116: 38–45.

Jacobson, J. L., and S. W. Jacobson. 1997. Evidence for PCBs as neurodevelopmental toxicants in humans. *Neurotoxicology.* 18: 415–424.

Jensen, D. J., M. E. Getzendaner, R. A. Hummel, and J. Turley. 1983. Residues studies for (2,4,5-trichlorophenoxy) acetic acid and 2,3,7,8-tetrachlorodibenzo-p-dioxin in grass and rice. *J. Agr. Food. Chem.* 31: 118–122.

Johnson, K. L., A. M. Cummings, and L. S. Birnbaum. 1997. Promotion of endometriosis in mice by polychlorinated dibenzo-p-dioxins, dibenzofurans, and biphenyls. *Environ. Health Perspect.* 105: 750–755.

Kedderis, L. B., J. J. Mills, M. E. Andersen, and L. S. Birnbaum. 1993. A physiologically based pharmacokinetic model for 2,3,7,8-tetrabromodibenzo-p-dioxin (TBDD) in the rat: tissue distribution and CYP1A induction. *Toxicol. Appl. Pharmacol.* 121: 87–98.

Kerkvliet, N. I. 1995. Immunological effects of chlorinated dibenzo-p-dioxins. *Environ. Health Perspect.* 103 (suppl 9): 47–53.

Kimbrough, R. D., H. Falk, P. Stehr, and G. Fries. 1984. Health implications of 2,3,7,8-tetrachlorodibenzo-p-dioxin (TCDD) contamination of residential soil. *J. Toxicol. Environ. Health* 14: 47–93.

Kociba, R. J., D. G. Keyes, J. E. Beyer, R. M. Carreon, C. E. Wade, D. A. Dittenber, R. P. Kalnins, L. E. Frauson, C. N. Park, S. D. Barnard, R. A. Hummel, and C. G. Humiston. 1978. Results of a two-year chronic toxicity and oncogenicity study of 2,3,7,8-tetrachlorodibenzo-p-dioxin in rats. *Toxicol. Appl. Pharmacol.* 46: 279–303.

Kogevinas, M., H. Becher, T. Benn, P. A. Bertazzi, P. Boffetta, H. B. Bueno-de-Mesquita, D. Coggon, D. Colin, D. Flesch-Janys, M. Fingerhut, L. Green, T. Kauppinen, M. Littorin, E. Lynge, J. D. Mathews, M. Neuberger, N. Pearce, and R. Saracci. 1997. Cancer mortality in workers exposed to phenoxy herbicides, chlorophenols, and dioxins. An expanded and updated international cohort study. *Am. J. Epidemiol.* 145: 1061–1075.

Kohn, M. C., C. H. Sewall, G. W. Lucier, and C. J. Portier. 1996. A mechanistic model of effects of dioxin on thyroid hormones in the rat. *Toxicol. Appl. Pharmacol.* 136: 29–48.

Koopman-Esseboom, C., D. C. Morse, N. Weisglas-Kuperus, I. J. Lutkeschipholt, C. G. Van der Paauw, L. G. Tuinstra, A. Brouwer, and P. J. Sauer. 1994. Effects of dioxins and polychlorinated biphenyls on thyroid hormone status of pregnant women and their infants. *Pediatr. Res.* 36: 468–473.

Lin, F. H., S. J. Stohs, L. S. Birnbaum, G. Clark, G. W. Lucier, and J. A. Goldstein. 1991. The effects of 2,3,7,8-tetrachlorodibenzo-p-dioxin (TCDD) on the hepatic estrogen and glucocorticoid receptors in congenic strains of Ah responsive and Ah nonresponsive C57BL/6J mice. *Toxicol. Appl. Pharmacol.* 108: 129–139.

Lucier, G. W., A. Tritscher, T. Goldsworthy, J. Foley, G. Clark, J. Goldstein, and R. Maronpot. 1991. Ovarian hormones enhance 2,3,7,8-tetrachlorodibenzo-p-dioxin-mediated increases in cell proliferation and preneoplastic foci in a two-stage model for rat hepatocarcinogenesis. *Cancer Res.* 51: 1391–1397.

Luebke, R. W., C. B. Copeland, J. J. Diliberto, P. I. Akubue, D. L. Andrews, M. M. Riddle, W. C. Williams, and L. S. Birnbaum. 1994. Assessment of host resistance to Trichinella spiralis in mice following preinfection exposure to 2,3,7,8-TCDD. *Toxicol. Appl. Pharmacol.* 125: 7–16.

Luebke, R. W., C. B. Copeland, and D. L. Andrews. 1995. Host resistance to Trichinella spiralis infection in rats exposed to 2,3,7,8-tetrachlorodibenzo-p-dioxin (TCDD). *Fundam. Appl. Toxicol.* 24: 285–289.

Mably, T. A., D. L. Bjerke, R. W. Moore, A. Gendron-Fitzpatrick, and R. E. Peterson. 1992a. In utero and lactational exposure of male rats to 2,3,7,8-tetrachlorodibenzo-p-dioxin. 3. Effects on spermatogenesis and reproductive capability. *Toxicol. Appl. Pharmacol.* 114: 118–126.

Mably, T. A., R. W. Moore, R. W. Goy, and R. E. Peterson. 1992b. In utero and lactational exposure of male rats to 2,3,7,8-tetrachlorodibenzo-p-dioxin. 2. Effects on sexual behavior and the regulation of luteinizing hormone secretion in adulthood. *Toxicol. Appl. Pharmacol.* 114: 108–117.

Maronpot, R. R., J. F. Foley, K. Takahashi, T. Goldsworthy, G. Clark, A. Tritscher, C. Portier, and G. Lucier. 1993. Dose response for TCDD promotion of hepatocarcinogenesis in rats initiated with DEN: Histologic, biochemical, and cell proliferation endpoints. *Environ. Health Perspect.* 101: 634–642.

Masuda, Y. 1995. The Yusho rice oil poisoning incident. In *Dioxins and Health,* ed. A. Schecter, pp. 633–660. New York: Plenum Press.

Mayes, B. A., E. E. McConnell, B. H. Neal, M. J. Brunner, S. B. Hamilton, T. M. Sullivan, A. C. Peters, M. J. Ryan, J. D. Toft, A. W. Singer, J. F. Brown, Jr., R. G. Menton, and J. A. Moore. 1998. Comparative carcinogenicity in Sprague-Dawley rats of the polychlorinated biphenyl mixtures Aroclors 1016, 1242, 1254, and 1260. *Toxicol. Sci.* 41: 62–76.

Mimura, J., K. Yamashita, K. Nakamura, M. Morita, T. N. Takagi, K. Nakao, M. Ema, K. Sogawa, M. Yasuda, M. Katsuki, and Y. Fuji-Kuriyama. 1997. Loss of teratogenic response to 2,3,7,8-tetrachlorodibenzo-p-dioxin (TCDD) in mice lacking the Ah (dioxin) receptor. *Genes Cells* 2: 645–654.

McConnell, E. E., and J. A. Moore. 1979. Toxicopathology characteristics of the halogenated aromatic hydrocarbons. *Ann. NY Acad. Sci.* 320: 138–150.

McGregor, D. B., C. Partensky, J. Wilbourn, and J. M. Rice. 1998. An IARC evaluation of polychlorinated dibenzo-p-dioxin and polychlorinated dibenzofurans as risk factors in human carcinogenesis. *Environ. Health Perspect.* 106 (suppl 2): 755–760.

Michalek, J. E., J. L. Pirkle, S. P. Caudill, R. C. Tripathi, D. G. Patterson Jr., and L. L. Needham. 1997. Pharmacokinetics of TCDD in veterans of Operation Ranch Hand: 10-year follow-up. *J. Toxicol. Environ. Health* 47: 209–220.

Moore, J. A., E. E. McConnell, D. W. Dalgard, and M. W. Harris. 1979. Compartive toxicity of three halogenated dibenzofurans in guinea pigs, mice and monkeys. *Ann. NY Acad. Sci.* 320: 151–163.

Moore, R. W., C. L. Potter, H. M. Theobald, J. A. Robinson, and R. E. Peterson. 1985. Androgenic deficiency in male rats treated with 2,3,7,8-tetrachlorodibenzo-p-dioxin. *Toxicol. Appl. Pharmacol.* 79: 99–111.

Moore, R. W., J. A. Parsons, R. C. Bookstaff, and R. E. Peterson. 1989. Plasma concentrations of pituitary hormones in 2,3,7,8-tetrachlorodibenzo-p-dioxin-treated male rats. *J. Biochem. Toxicol.* 4: 165–172.

Murray, F. J., F. A. Smith, K. D. Nitschke, C. G. Humiston, R. J. Kociba, and B. A. Schwetz. 1979. Three-generation reproduction study of rats given 2,3,7,8-tetrachlorodibenzo-p-dioxin (TCDD) in the diet. *Toxicol. Appl. Pharmacol.* 50: 241–252.

National Academy of Sciences. 1979. PCB transport throughout the environment. In *Polychlorinated Biphenyls.* Washington: National Academy Press.

National Toxicology Program/National Cancer Institute. 1982. Carcinogenesis bioassay of 2,3,7,8-tetra-chlorodibenzo-p-dioxin (CAS No 1746-091-6) in Osborne-Mendel rats and B6C3F1 mice (gavage study). Technical Report 209, U.S. Department of Health, Education and Welfare, Public Health Service, National Institutes of Health, Bethesda Md.

Neubert, R., G. Golor, R. Stahlmann, H. Helge, D. Neubert. 1992. Polyhalogenated dibenzo-p-dioxin and dibenzofurans and the immune system. 4. Effects of multiple dose treatment with 2,3,7,8-tetrachlor-odibenzo-p-dioxin (TCDD) on peripheral lymphocyte subpopulations of a non-human primate (*Callithrix jacchus*). *Arch. Toxicol.* 66: 250–259.

Olson, J. R., and B. P. McGarrigle. 1991. Comparative developmental toxicity of 2,3,7,8-tetrachlorodi-benzo-p-dioxin. *Chemosphere.* 25: 71–74.

Ott, M. G., and A. Zober. 1996. Cause specific mortality and cancer incidence among employees exposed to 2,3,7,8-TCDD after a 1953 reactor accident. *Occup. Environ. Med.* 53: 606–612.

Pinsky P. F. and M. N. Lorber. 1998. A model to evaluate past exposure to 2,3,7,8-TCDD. *J. Expo. Anal. Environ. Epidemiol.* 8: 187–206

Pitot, H. C., T. Goldsworthy, H. A. Campbell, and A. Poland. 1980. Quantitative evaluation of the promotion by 2,3,7,8-tetrachlorodibenzo-p-dioxin of hepatocarcinogenesis from diethylnitrosamine. *Cancer Res.* 40: 3616–3620.

Pohjanvirta, R., and J. Tuomisto. 1994. Short-term toxicity of 2,3,7,8-tetrachlorodibenzo-p-dioxin in laboratory animals: Effects, mechanisms, and animal models. *Pharmacol. Rev.* 46: 483–549.

Poland, A., and E. Glover. 1980. 2,3,7,8-Tetrachlorodibenzo-p-dioxin: Segregation of toxicity with the Ah locus. *Mol. Pharmacol.* 17: 86–94.

Poland, A. and E. Glover. 1990. Characterization and strain distribution pattern of murine A receptor specificed by the Ah^d and Ah^b alleles. *Mol. Pharmacol.* 38: 306–312.

Poland, A., D. Phalen, and E. Glover. 1982. Tumour promotion by TCDD in skin of HRS/J hairless mice. *Nature.* 300: 271–273.

Portier, C. J., C. D. Sherman, M. Kohn, L. Edler, A. Kopp-Schneider, R. M. Maronpot, and G. Lucier. 1996. Modeling the number and size of hepatic focal lesions following exposure to 2,3,7,8-TCDD. *Toxicol. Appl. Pharmacol.* 138: 20–30.

Powell-Coffman, J. A., C. A. Bradfield, and W. B. Wood. 1998. Caenorhabditis elegans orthologs of the aryl hydrocarbon receptor and its heterodimerization partner the aryl hydrocarbon receptor nuclear translocator. *Proc. Natl. Acad. Sci. USA.* 95: 2844–2849.

Rao, M. S., V. Subbaro, J. D. Psada, and D. C. Scarpelli. 1988. Carcinogenicty of 2,3,7,8-tetrachlor-odibenzo-p-dioxin in the Syrian hamster. *Carcinogensesis* 9: 1677–1679.

Rappe, C., M. Nygren, G. Lindstrom, H. R. Buser, O. Blaser, and C. Wuthrich. 1987. Polychlorinated dibenzofurans and dibenzo-p-dioxins and other chlorinated contaminantes in cow milk from various locations in Switzerland. *Environ. Sci. Technol.* 21: 964–970.

Reier, S. E., D. C. Martin, R. E. Bowman, W. P. Dmowski, and J. L. Becker. 1993. Endometriosis in Rhesus monkeys (*Macca mulatta*) following chronic exposure to 2,3,7,8-tetrachlordibenzo-p-dioxin. *Fundam. Appl. Toxicol.* 21: 433–441.

Rogan, W. J., and B. C. Gladen. 1991. PCBs, DDE, and child development at 18 and 24 months. *Ann. Epidemiol.* 1: 407–413.

Rogan, W. J., and B. C. Gladen. 1992. Neurotoxicology of PCBs and related compounds. *Neurotoxicology.* 13: 27–35.

Rogan, W. J., and B. C. Gladen. 1993. Breast-feeding and cognitive development. *Early Hum. Dev.* 31: 181–193.

Safe, S. 1990. Polychlorinated biphenyls (PCBs), dibenzo-p-dioxins (PCDDs), dibenzofurans (PCDFs), and related compounds: Environmental and mechanistic considerations which support the development of toxic equivalency factors (TEFs). *Crit. Rev. Toxicol.* 21: 51–88.

Safe, S. H. 1994. Polychlorinated biphenyls (PCBs): Environmental impact, biochemical and toxic responses, and implications for risk assessment. *Crit. Rev. Toxicol.* 24: 87–149.

Safe, S., B. Astroff, M. Harris, T. Zacharewski, R. Dickerson, M. Romkes, and L. Biegel. 1991. 2,3,7,8-Tetrachlorodibenzo-p-dioxin (TCDD) and related compounds as antiestrogens: characterization and mechanism of action. *Pharmacol. Toxicol.* 69: 400–409.

Schantz, S. L., and R. E. Bowman. 1989. Learning in monkeys exposed perinatally to 2,3,7,8-tetra-chlorodibenzo-p-dioxin (TCDD). *Neurotoxicol Teratol.* 11: 13–19.

Schecter, A., J. Startin, C. Wright, M. Kelly, O. Papke, A. Lis, M. Ball, and J. R. Olson. 1994a. Congener-specific levels of dioxins and dibenzofurans in U. S. food and estimated daily dioxin toxic equivalent intake. *Environ. Health Perspect.* 102: 962–966.

Schecter, A., J. Stanley, K. Boggess, Y. Masuda, J. Mes, M. Wolff, P. Furst, C. Furst, K. Wilson-Yang, and B. Chisholm. 1994b. Polychlorinated biphenyl levels in the tissues of exposed and nonexposed humans. *Environ Health Perspect.* 102 (suppl 1): 149–158.

Schecter, A., P. Furst, C. Furst, O. Papke, M. Ball, J. J. Ryan, D. C. Hoang, C. D. Le, T. Q. Hoang, H. Q. Cuong, et al. 1994c. Chlorinated dioxins and dibenzofurans in human tissue from general populations: a selective review. *Environ Health Perspect.* 102 (suppl 1): 159–171.

Schecter, A., O. Papke, A. Lis, M. Ball, J. J. Ryan, J. R. Olson, L. Li, and H. Kessler. 1996. Decrease in milk and blood dioxin levels over two years in a mother nursing twins: Estimates of decreased maternal and increased infant dioxin body burden from nursing. *Chemosphere.* 32: 543–549.

Schrenk, D., A. Buchmann, K. Dietz, H. P. Lipp, H. Brunner, H. Sirma, P. Munzel, H. Hagenmaier, R. Gebhardt, and K. W. Bock. 1994. Promotion of preneoplastic foci in rat liver with 2,3,7,8-tetrachlor-odibenzo-p-dioxin, 1,2,3,4,6,7,8-heptachlorodibenzo-p-dioxin and a defined mixture of 49 polychlori-nated dibenzo-p-dioxins. *Carcinogenesis.* 15: 509–515.

Seefeld, M. D., S. W. Corbett, R. E. Keesey, and R. E. Peterson. 1984. Characterization of the wasting syndrome in rats treated with 2,3,7,8-tetrachlorodibenzo-p-dioxin. *Toxicol. Appl. Pharmacol.* 73: 311–322.

Silkworth, J. B., D. S. Cutler, and G. Sack. 1989. Immunotoxicity of 2,3,7,8-tetrachlorodibenzo-p-dioxin in a complex environmental mixture from the Love Canal. *Fundam. Appl. Toxicol.* 12: 303–312.

Smialowicz, R. J., M. M. Riddle, W. C. Williams, and J. J. Diliberto. 1994. Effects of 2,3,7,8-tetrachlorodibenzo-p-dioxin (TCDD) on humoral immunity and lymphocyte subpopulations: differ-ences between mice and rats. *Toxicol. Appl. Pharmacol.* 124: 248–256.

Spink, D. C., D. W. D. Lincoln, H. W. Dickerman, and J. F. Gierthy. 1990. 2,3,7,8-Tetrachlorodibenzo-p-dioxin causes an extensive alteration of 17 beta-estradiol metabolism in MCF-7 breast tumor cells. *Proc. Natl. Acad. Sci. USA.* 87: 6917–6921.

Tanabe, S., and R. Tatsukawa. 1986. Distribution, behavior, and load of PCBs in the oceans. In *PCBs and the Environment*, vol. 1 ed. J. S. Waid, pp. 143–161. Boca Raton, FL: CRC Press.

Tatsukawa, R. 1976. PCB pollution of the Japanese environment. In *PCB Poisoning and Pollution,* ed. K. Higuchi, pp. 147–179. Tokyo: Kodansha.

Theobald, H. M., and R. E. Peterson. 1997. In utero and lactational exposure to 2,3,7,8-tetrachlorodibenzo-p-dioxin: Effects on development of the male and female reproductive system of the mouse. *Toxicol. Appl. Pharmacol.* 145: 124–135.

Tiedje, J. M., J. F. Quensen, 3rd, J. Chee-Sanford, J. P. Schimel, and S. A. Boyd. 1993. Microbial reductive dechlorination of PCBs. *Biodegradation.* 4: 231–240.

Tritscher, A. M., A. M. Seacat, J. D. Yager, J. D. Groopman, B. D. Miller, D. Bell, T. R. Sutter, and G. W. Lucier. 1996. Increased oxidative DNA damage in livers of 2,3,7,8-tetrachlorodibenzo-p-dioxin treated intact but not ovariectomized rats. *Cancer Lett.* 98: 219–225.

Turtletaub, K. W., J. S. Felton, B. L. Gledhill, J. S. Vogel, J. R. Southon, M. W. Caffee, R. C. Finkel, D. E. Nelson, I. D. Proctor, and J. C. David. 1990. Accelerator mass spectrometry in biomedical dosimetry: Relationship between low-level exposure and covalent binding of heterocyclic amine carcinogens to DNA. *Proc. Natl. Acad. Sci. USA* 87: 5288–5292.

U.S. EPA. 1994. Estimating exposures to dioxin-like compounds. Vol. 2: Properties, sources, occurrence and background levels. External review draft. EPA/66/6-88/005Cb. Office of Research and Develop-ment, U.S. Environmental Protection Agency, Washington, DC.

U.S. EPA. 1997. Evaluation of emissions from the open burning of household waste in barrels. Vol. 1. Technical Report. EPA-600/r-97-134a. U.S. Environmental Protection Agency, Washington, DC.

Van den Berg, M., J. van Wijnen, H. Wever, and W. Seinen. 1989. Selective retention of toxic polychlorinated dibenzo-p-dioxins and dibenzofurans in the liver of the rat after intravenous admin-istration of a mixture. *Toxicology.* 55: 173–182.

Van den Berg, M., J. De Jongh, H. Poiger, and J. R. Olson. 1994. The toxicokinetics and metabolism of polychlorinated dibenzo-p-dioxins (PCDDs) and dibenzofurans (PCDFs) and their relevance for toxicity. *Crit. Rev. Toxicol.* 24: 1–74.

Van den Berg, M., L. Birnbaum, A. T. C. Bosveld, B. Brunstrom, P. Cook, M. Feeley, J. P. Giesy, A. Hanberg, R. Hasegawa, S. W. Kennedy, T. Kubiak, J. C. Larsen, F. X. R. van Leeuwen, A. K. D. Liem, C. Nolt, R. E. Peterson, L. Poellinger, S. Safe, D. Schrenk, D. Tillitt, M. Tysklind, M. Younes, W. R. F, and T. Zacharewski. 1998. Toxic Equivalency Factors (TEFs) for PCBs, PCDDs, PCDFs for Humans and Wildlife. *Environ. Health Perspect.* 106: 775–792.

van der Plas, S. A., J. de Jongh, M. Faassen-Peters, G. Scheu, M. van den Berg, and A. Brouwer. 1998. Toxicokinetics of an environmentally relevant mixture of dioxin-like PHAHs with or without a non-dioxin-like PCB in a semi-chronic exposure study in female Sprague Dawley rats. *Chemosphere* 37: 1941–1955.

Viluksela, M., B. U. Stahl, L. S. Birnbaum, K. W. Schramm, A. Kettrup, and K. K. Rozman. 1997. Subchronic/chronic toxicity of 1,2,3,4,6,7,8-heptachlorodibenzo-p-dioxin (HpCDD) in rats. Part I. Design, general observations, hematology, and liver concentrations. *Toxicol. Appl. Pharmacol.* 146: 207–216.

Viluksela, M., B. U. Stahl, L. S. Birnbaum, K. W. Schramm, A. Kettrup, and K. K. Rozman. 1998a. Subchronic/chronic toxicity of a mixture of four chlorinated dibenzo-p-dioxins in rats. I. Design, general observations, hematology, and liver concentrations. *Toxicol. Appl. Pharmacol.* 151: 57–69.

Viluksela, M., B. U. Stahl, L. S. Birnbaum, and K. K. Rozman. 1998b. Subchronic/chronic toxicity of a mixture of four chlorinated dibenzo-p-dioxins in rats. II. Biochemical effects. *Toxicol. Appl. Pharmacol.* 151: 70–78.

Wang, X., M. J. Santostefano, M. V. Evans, V. M. Richardson, J. J. Diliberto, and L. S. Birnbaum. 1997. Determination of parameters responsible for pharmacokinetic behavior of TCDD in female Sprague-Dawley rats. *Toxicol. Appl. Pharmacol.* 147: 151–168.

Weisglas-Kuperus, N., T. C. Sas, C. Koopman-Esseboom, C. W. van der Zwan, M. A. De Ridder, A. Beishuizen, H. Hooijkaas, and P. J. Sauer. 1995. Immunologic effects of background prenatal and postnatal exposure to dioxins and polychlorinated biphenyls in Dutch infants. *Pediatr. Res.* 38: 404–410.

Whitlock, J. P., Jr., S. T. Okino, L. Dong, H. P. Ko, R. Clarke-Katzenberg, Q. Ma, and H. Li. 1996. Cytochromes P450 5: Induction of cytochrome P4501A1: a model for analyzing mammalian gene transcription. *Faseb. J.* 10: 809–818.

Zober, A., M. G. Ott, and P. Messerer. 1994. Morbidity follow up study of BASF employees exposed to 2,3,7,8-tetrachlorodibenzo-p-dioxin (TCDD) after a 1953 chemical reactor incident. *Occup. Environ. Med.* 51: 479–486.

9 Drinking Water Disinfection

RICHARD J. BULL, Ph.D.

The disinfection of drinking water brings competing health concerns more sharply into focus than most other environmental problems. What is the contribution of drinking water disinfection to the control of infectious disease? What is the magnitude of carcinogenic risks associated with the by-products of disinfection reactions? Are there alternative methods that reduce one of these risks without exacerbating the other to unacceptable levels? The reciprocity implied by these questions does not imply that these risks really need to be "traded off." The questions do illustrate the need for systematic evaluation of each new approach to treatment to ensure that decisions are not made that put the public health at greater risk.

Waterborne infectious disease was common in the United States before the introduction of disinfection (Akin et al., 1982; Bull et al., 1990a). The introduction of chlorination and other improvements in drinking water treatment, particularly filtration, contributed to a very sharp decline in deaths from cholera, typhoid, and a variety of other infectious diseases (Akin et al., 1982). Waterborne infectious disease still does occur, and its occurrence is most frequently associated with inadequate disinfection or equipment failure (Craun, 1988; Bull et al., 1995). There is even some suggestion that endemic infectious diseases in large cities might well be attributed to well-designed and maintained urban water systems (Payment et al., 1990a, b). Although it is difficult to quantitatively estimate the impact of suspending the use of disinfectants in drinking water, recent history (ILSI, 1993) affords little doubt that the problem of waterborne infectious disease is a real, not an abstract, problem.

Thus the disinfection of drinking water is a well-established and effective means of preventing pathogenic organisms from being transmitted through public water supplies. Beginning in the 1970s, there has been an increasing amount of evidence that (1) by-products are generated in the use of disinfectants and (2) these compounds have toxicological properties that are of potential concern to human health. These data have been paralleled by epidemiological associations between the drinking of chlorinated water with an increased incidence of cancer.

Oxidants are added to drinking water for several reasons, but the most important is disinfection. There are usually two points where disinfectants are added. The first is made early in the treatment process, with the intent of inactivating all pathogenic microbes and viruses that might contaminate the source water. This is referred to as primary disinfection or preoxidation (Bull et al., 1990a). In most water supplies there is a second addition of disinfectant as the water leaves the treatment plant and occasionally at distal sites in the distribution system. These additions are referred to as postdisinfection or secondary disinfection. Their intent is to reduce colonization of the water distribution system and to

Environmental Toxicants: Human Exposures and Their Health Effects, 2/e. Edited by Morton Lippmann.
ISBN: 0-471-29298-2 © 2000 John Wiley & Sons, Inc.

minimize the impact of sources of contamination in the system (cross-connections, main breaks, etc.). Occasionally there will be other additions within the treatment plant. The overall process may involve successive additions of the same disinfectant or utilize different disinfectants in each of the locations to minimize operational as well as by-product formation issues.

CHEMICAL METHODS OF DISINFECTION

The chemical disinfectants most commonly utilized in public water supplies are chlorine, chloramine (chlorine + ammonia), ozone, and chlorine dioxide in approximate order of popularity. Iodine is also used, but it is limited to short-term emergency use (e.g. backpackers or the field situations by the military). While NASA plans to use iodine in its Space Station Freedom on which missions will last up to 180 days, iodine is to be removed before consumption. Recent studies have shown that relatively small intakes of iodine lead to elevations of thyroid-stimulating hormone (Robison et al., 1998). There are significant numbers of individuals in the population that may react adversely to levels of iodine needed to ensure disinfection (Carswell et al., 1970; Clark et al., 1990; Woeber, 1991). Thus iodine is not likely to be utilized in municipal systems.

The four commonly used disinfectants vary in their ability to achieve the goals of primary and secondary disinfection (Bull et al., 1990b). The high reactivity of ozone makes it an excellent primary disinfectant, but ozone has insufficient stability to be useful in secondary disinfection. Chloramine is weak as a primary disinfectant, requiring very long contact times for effective killing. However, its stability makes it an excellent choice for its bacteriostatic properties in the distribution system. Chlorine and chlorine dioxide are made effective for both situations if sufficient quantities are added to satisfy the disinfectant demand. Once the demand has been satisfied, reasonably stable residuals can be maintained in the distribution system. Therefore modification of a system's disinfectant treatment can introduce an additional risk of waterborne infectious disease if the switchover is not well managed.

When chlorine is used as the disinfectant, it is added either as chlorine gas that reacts to form hypochlorous acid in water or as a hypochlorite salt. Hypochlorous acid dissociates to hypochlorite and hydrogen ions with a pK_a of 7.5. At equivalent pH in the finished water, these processes yield the same reactive chemical species. The efficacy of OCl^- is considerably less than that of HOCl (Akin et al., 1982).

Chlorine dioxide is generally prepared in situ from chlorite or chlorate. In drinking water disinfection, generation from the acidification of chlorite is generally favored, whereas generation from chlorate is favored in bleaching of pulp and other industrial processes. The acidification of sodium chlorite is accomplished by the addition of mineral acid or with chlorine (Masschelein, 1989). As a consequence of its method of preparation and reactions of chlorine dioxide in solution, chlorine dioxide disinfected water will contain varying amounts of chlorite, chlorate, and free chlorine. Chlorine dioxide is as effective as chlorine as a disinfectant, but its effectiveness is less sensitive to modification by changes in pH (Akin et al., 1982).

Chloramine is prepared by addition of ammonia to chlorine. These additions can be made simultaneously or sequentially. The type of chloramine formed depends on the relative ratios of chlorine to ammonia and the pH. Generally speaking, every attempt is made to optimize for formation of monochloramine, since dichloramine and trichloramine create severe taste and odor problems. Since chloramine is less effective as a disinfectant than chlorine (Akin et al., 1982), the addition is most often made sequentially to take advantage of the disinfecting power of free chlorine. Once formed, however, chloramine is much more stable than chlorine, and for this reason it is preferred as a means of maintaining a disinfectant residual in the water distribution system (Olivieri et al., 1986).

Ozone is an extremely reactive chemical, and for this reason it is always generated on site (Faroog et al., 1977). Ozone is frequently used in combination with other disinfectants or oxidants (AWWA, 1982). Hydrogen peroxide used in conjunction with ozone facilitates formation of hydroxyl radical (Wolfe et al., 1989), increasing its effectiveness in breaking down various organic material in the source waters (Hoigne and Bader, 1975). A similar enhancement of hydroxyl radical can be accomplished by combining ozone use with ultraviolet radiation (Rice and Gomez-Taylor, 1986). As a primary disinfectant, ozone is the most effective chemical disinfectant currently in use. For example, it is quite effective in inactivating oocysts of *Giarida* and *Cryptosporidium*, two organisms that are known for their high resistance to chlorine. However, as noted earlier, its high reactivity with water makes ozone ineffective for postdisinfection. As ozone use increases in the United States, the use of a second disinfectant, such as chloramine, for postdisinfection is very likely to become popular.

Physical methods of disinfecting drinking water are not commonly used in the United States. Ultraviolet radiation is the most common process, and systems sufficiently large for application to municipal systems have been constructed and are known to be effective under the right conditions. A number of treatment systems based on electrolytic production of oxidants have also been developed. The reaction products from such systems have been very poorly described in the open scientific literature. Municipalities probably should not entertain electrolytic systems until both the oxidants produced and the potential for unusual by-product formation is better evaluated. Consequently they will not be further considered in this review.

Because the number of disinfectant by-products identified continues to expand, it is not possible to comprehensively review the field in the small space available. Consequently this chapter begins with a short general introduction to the chemical nature of disinfectant by-products and continues with an overview of epidemiological data. The bulk of the toxicological data on disinfectant by-products will focus on how the known toxicology of these compounds might contribute to an overall understanding of the problem that has been identified with chlorination. If the observations prove to be correct, then it is extremely important to make sure that problems that might be associated with the use of alternate disinfectants to chlorine have undergone a similar degree of scrutiny. Does it make sense to move away from chlorine as a disinfectant without a better appreciation of the hazards that could be associated with the alternatives?

CHEMICAL NATURE AND OCCURRENCE OF DISINFECTANT BY-PRODUCTS

Oxidation reactions as well as substitution reactions form disinfectant by-products. Table 9-1 is a partial list of compounds that are found as disinfectant by-products by general chemical class. There are three important points: (1) the most frequently identified by-products are halogenated, (2) there are nonhalogenated by-products associated with all disinfectants, and (3) by-products that are uniquely associated with a particular disinfectant are rare. The recognition that most by-products that are formed are halogenated is due in part to the ability of chlorine to chlorinate organic precursors. It is also related to the fact that halogen substitution is a telltale marker of by-products. Oxygen substituents that arise from oxidation reactions of disinfectants are not so unique. Naturally occurring humic and fulvic acids are the major precursors for disinfectant by-products in most water supplies (Thurman, 1986). These are very complex materials. The reaction of oxidants is actually quite extensive with these substrates. Therefore this simple

TABLE 9-1   By-products of Drinking Water Chlorination

Chemical Class	Concentration Range Found (ug/L)	References
	Trihalomethanes	
Chloroform	3–755	Bull and Kopfler (1991);[a] Baker and Bursill (1990)
Bromodichloromethane	1.6–228	Bull and Kopfler (1991);[a] Baker and Bursill (1990)
Dibromochloromethane	0.3–288	Bull and Kopfler (1991);[a] Baker and Bursill (1990)
Bromoform	<0.5–550	Bull and Kopfler (1991);[a] Baker and Bursill (1990)
	Haloacids	
Chloroacetate	<1.0–4	Jacangelo et al. (1989)
Dichloroacetate	8–79	Singer and Chang (1989)
Trichloroacetate	4–103	Singer and Chang (1989); Norwood et al. (1985)
Bromoacetate	<0.5–3.8	Jacangelo et al. (1989)
Bromodichloroacetate	Detected[b]	Stevens et al. (1990)
Dibromochloroacetate	Detected[b]	Stevens et al. (1990)
Dibromoacetate	0.7–19	Krasner et al. (1989a); Jacangelo et al. (1989)
Tribromoacetate	0.7–19	Krasner et al. (1989a); Jacangelo et al. (1989)
2-Chloropropanoate	0.7–19	Krasner et al. (1989a); Jacangelo et al. (1989)
2,2-Dichloropropanoate	0.7–19	Krasner et al. (1989a); Jacangelo et al. (1989)
3,3-Dichloropropanoate	0.7–19	Krasner et al. (1989a); Jacangelo et al. (1989)
Chlorobutanedioic acid	0.7–19	Krasner et al. (1989a); Jacangelo et al. (1989)
2,2-Dichlorobutanoate	0.7–19	Krasner et al. (1989a); Jacangelo et al. (1989)
	Haloacetonitriles	
Dichloroacetonitrile	<0.2–24	Reding et al. (1986)
Bomochloroacetonitrile	<0.2–10	Reding et al. (1986)
Dibromoacetonitrile	<0.2–2.5	Reding et al. (1986)
Trichloroacetonitrile	<0.029	Reding et al. (1986)
	Haloaldehydes	
Trichloroacetaldehyde	1.7–19	Jacangelo et al. (1989); Krasner et al. (1989a)
	Haloketones	
1,1-Dichloropropanone	0.38–1.4	Krasner et al. (1989a)
1,1,1-Trichloropropanone	<0.13–2.4	Coleman et al. (1984)
1,1,1,3-Tetrachloropropanone	Detected	Stevens et al. (1990)
1,1,3,3-Tetrachloropropanone	Detected	Stevens et al. (1990)
1,1-Dichloro-2-butanone	Detected	Stevens et al. (1990)
3,3-Dichloro-2-butanone	Detected	Stevens et al. (1990)
2,2-Dichloro-3-pentanone	Detected	Stevens et al. (1990)
3-chloro-4-(dichloromethyl)-5-hydroxy-2(5H)-furanone	0.002–0.067	Meier et al. (1987a)
	Halophenols	
2,4-Dichlorophenol	<0.01–1.4	Symons et al. (1975)
2,4,6-Trichlorophenol	Detected	Symons et al. (1975)
	Aldehydes (non-halogenated)	
Formaldehyde	8–13	Krasner et al. (1989a)
Acetaldehyde	4.6–11	Krasner et al. (1989a)
Benzaldehyde	Detected	Stevens et al. (1990)

TABLE 9-1   (*Continued*)

Chemical Class	Concentration Range Found (ug/L)	References
2-Methyl propanal	Detected	Hrudey et al. (1988)
2-Methyl butanal	Detected	Hrudey et al. (1988)
Phenylacetaldehyde	Detected	Hrudey et al. (1988)
Decanal	Detected	Daignault et al. (1987)
Methoxydimethyl octanal	Detected	Daignault et al. (1987)
C_2-Benzaldehydes	Detected	Daignault et al. (1987)
Carboxylic acids		
Benzoate	Detected	Stevens et al. (1990)
2,2-Dimethyl butanedioate		
Dodecanoate	Detected	Stevens et al. (1990)
Benzenedicarboxylate	Detected	Stevens et al. (1990)
Benzenetricarboxylate	Detected	Stevens et al. (1990)
Hexanedioate	Detected	Stevens et al. (1990)
Methylfurancarboxylate	Detected	Stevens et al. (1990)
Pentandioate	Detected	Stevens et al. (1990)
Hexanoate	Detected	Stevens et al. (1990)
Methylfurandicarboxylate	Detected	Stevens et al. (1990)
Nonanoate	Detected	Stevens et al. (1990)
Decanoate	Detected	Stevens et al. (1990)
Methylbenzenedicarboxylate	Detected	Stevens et al. (1990)
Octanedioate	Detected	Stevens et al. (1990)
Pentanoate	Detected	Stevens et al. (1990)
Propanedioate	Detected	Stevens et al. (1990)
Heptanoate	Detected	Stevens et al. (1990)
Miscellaneous		
Chloropicrin	< 0.2–5.6	Reding et al. (1986)
Cyanogen chloride	< 0.2–4.5	Krasner et al. (1989a)

[a] Review that includes results from a nubmber of studies.
[b] Detected as a chlorination by-product but not quantified.

listing represents a significant underrepresentation of the classes that are produced. Most of the uncharacterized by-products are not halogenated.

Exposure to disinfectant by-products, however, does not simply relate to the disinfectant that is used in a particular water supply. The total amount of by-product and its character depends on the characteristics of the water that is being treated. There are three major water variables that are important: total organic carbon (TOC) concentrations, bromide concentration, and pH. The relationship between total organic carbon and total disinfectant by-product formation is essentially linear, although the yield will vary depending on varying characteristics of the humic substances (Reckhow et al., 1990). However, the yield of individual by-products is modified more extensively by the other variables.

The pH affects the type of disinfectant by-product that is formed. Figure 9-1 provides some insight into how pH influences net disinfectant by-product formation. Compounds from different classes behave quite differently. Chloroform, provided as an example of the trihalomethane class, increases substantially in concentration as pH increases. Conversely, trichloroacetate concentrations decrease over the same pH range. The concentrations of

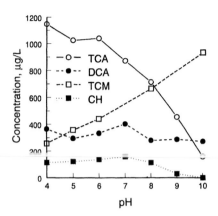

Figure 9-1   The effect of pH on the yield of several representative by-products of the chlorination of a concentrated solution of humic substances. TCA is trichloroacetate; DCA, dichloroacetate; TCM, chloroform; and CH, chloral hydrate. (Miller and Uden, 1983)

chloral hydrate also decrease with pH. On the other hand, dichloroacetate concentrations do not vary significantly with pH.

The influence of bromide on by-product formation is more complicated. First, bromide is oxidized in the presence of at least two disinfectants, chlorine and ozone. Therefore the form that gives rise to by-products is HOBr. HOBr and $^-$OBr are in an equilibrium that is controlled by pH. Acid pH favors the bromination of organic substrates (Stevens et al., 1989), while alkaline pH favors the formation of bromate when ozone is the disinfectant (Haag and Hoigne, 1983; Krasner et al., 1993).

In Table 9-2 the mean concentrations of various members of the trihalomethane (THM), halogenated acetate (HA), and haloacetonitrile (HAN) classes of by-products in the recent EPA/CDHS survey (McGuire et al., 1989) of 35 water supplies are compared to their concentrations in the water supply with the highest bromide concentrations (ca. 3 mg/L). Under such conditions, the brominated by-products predominate to the extent that bromoform is present at 66 times the concentration of chloroform, whereas the more general pattern is that chloroform is found in about 30-fold excess over bromoform. Very similar shifts in the distribution between chlorinated and brominated by-products are observed with the haloacetates and haloacetonitriles. Figure 9-2 illustrates the complexity of the situation by depicting the distribution of brominated and chlorinated haloacetic acids in different drinking waters that were sampled by Cowman and Singer (1996).

As a consequence of the above variables in source water quality, chlorinated drinking water cannot be considered to be the same entity at all locations. Therefore it is essential that the effects of different by-products be segregated from one another and from the effects that might be associated with the residual disinfectant.

In terms of the concentrations found in drinking water, the THMs and HAs are obviously the two most important groups of by-products. Mean or median concentrations for these by-product groups would fall into a range of 30 to 50 µg/L for the THMs (Krasner et al., 1989a) and 10 to 25 µg/L for the HAs (Singer and Chang, 1989; Cowman and Singer, 1996). Under appropriate circumstances these concentrations can be an order of magnitude higher as illustrated by experience in South Australia with THMs (Baker and Bursill, 1990).

Haloacetonitriles (HANs) and halogenated aldehydes and nonhalogenated aldehydes fall into a second tier of chlorination by-products. Within the HAN class, the dihaloacetonitriles are the most commonly found in finished drinking water. This is

TABLE 9-2 Impact of Bromide Concentration of Nature of Chlorination By-products

By-product	Mean Concentrations in 35 Utilities	Utility with highest Br$^-$ concentration (2.8–3.0 mg/L)
Trihalomethanes (THM)		
Chloroform	15 [a]	0.59
Bromodichloromethane	10	2.9
Dibromochloromethane	4.5	9.2
Bromoform	0.57	40
Total THM	44	53
Haloacetates (HA)		
Chloroacetate	1.2	< 1.0
Dichloroacetate	6.8	0.9
Trichloroacetate	5.8	< 0.6
Bromochloroacetate	NQ [b]	NQ
Dibromochloroacetate	NQ	NQ
Bromoacetate	< 0.5	1.2
Dibromoacetate	1.5	19
Total HA	20	21
Haloacetonitriles (HAN)		
Dichloroacetonitrile	1.1	0.34
Trichloroacetonitrile	< 0.012	< 0.012
Bromochloroacetonitrile	0.58	1.2
Dibromoacetonitrile	0.48	5.9
Total HAN	2.5	7.4

Note: Table adapted from Krasner et al. (1989a).
[a] Concentrations are all in μg/L
[b] NQ = not quantitated. These by-products were detected, but no standard was available to quantitate.

because the more heavily substituted compounds have limited stability in most drinking waters (Stevens et al., 1989a).

Trichloroacetaldehyde (existing as chloral hydrate in water) is clearly formed with chlorination of water (Miller and Uden, 1983; Krasner et al., 1989a). The formation of brominated analogs has apparently not been pursued in surveys. However, there can be little doubt that they occur. Formaldehyde and acetaldehyde are the most commonly measured nonhalogenated aldehydes in chlorinated water, but it is probable that other aldehydes are also present at appreciable concentrations because of analytical difficulties with this group of chemicals.

There has been repeated documentation that mutagenic activity is consistently increased in waters treated with chlorine (Meier et al., 1987a, b; Meier, 1988). A variety of halogenated aldehydes and ketones have been identified in studies of chlorinated humic and fulvic acids that probably contribute to this activity. Depending on the water supply, 8% to 60% of this activity can be accounted for by the potent bacterial mutagen, MX (Meier et al., 1987a; Kronberg and Vartiainen, 1988b; Romero et al., 1997). A few other chemicals are known to contribute to a lesser extent, including dichloroacetonitrile, 1,1-dichloropropanone, and 1,1,1-trichloropropanone (Krasner et al., 1989a). While most of the compounds identified are chlorinated, it is probable that their brominated analogues are also present in chlorinated drinking water (Romero et al., 1997). It is notable that many of these chemicals, as well as the mutagenic activity they

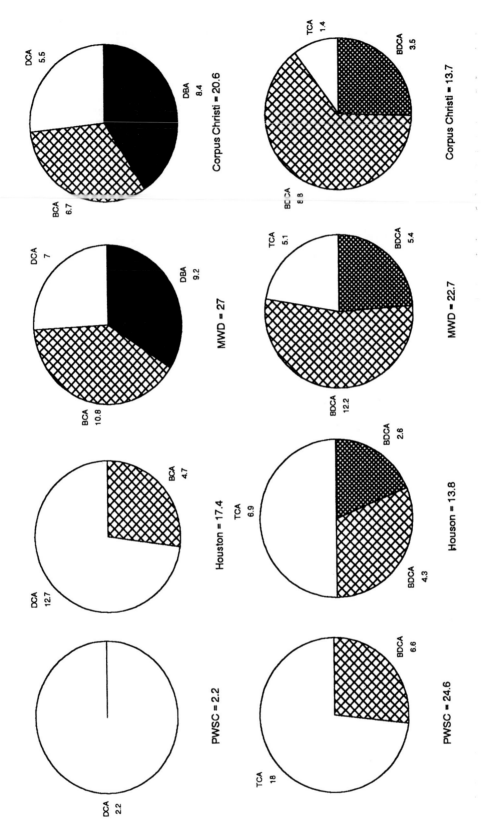

produce, are labile under the alkaline conditions easily found in many drinking waters (Meier et al., 1983).

In addition to the compounds identified above, there is a series of nonchlorinated acids whose concentrations in finished drinking water have not been documented. This group of compounds contains many normal constituents of the body, and at the low concentrations that can be anticipated (i.e., limited by the total organic carbon content of the water), these compounds are not of toxicological significance.

Chloramination by-products do not generally differ from those obtained from chlorination. The amounts of by-products formed depend on how the disinfectant is introduced into the system, namely whether free chlorine is allowed to exist for some minimum contact before the addition of ammonia, or chlorine and ammonia added simultaneously. Generally, water supplies that approach the current THM standard in their water when it has been treated with chlorine find that the least expensive alternative is to switch to one of these two methods of disinfection (Bull et al., 1990a). The total THM and HAN concentrations will be significantly decreased with a switch to chloramine (Jacangelo et al., 1989). Total concentrations of HAs are less readily predicted. Cyanogen chloride is actually formed at higher concentrations in chloraminated rather than chlorinated water (Krasner et al., 1989a). However, the median concentrations of cyanogen chloride observed was only 2.2 µg/L in plant effluents, and the compound appears to be relatively unstable in the distribution system.

The major by-products associated with the use of chlorine dioxide are chlorite and chlorate. Chlorite is the major by-product arising as the reduction product of chlorine dioxide when it oxidizes organic material in the water. Chlorate is produced by either disproportionation or by photodecomposition of chlorine dioxide (Masschelein, 1989). Somewhere between 40% and 80% of the applied dose of chlorine dioxide is ordinarily converted to chlorite (Lykins and Griese, 1986; Howe et al., 1989; Masschelein, 1989; Gordon et al., 1990). With doses of ClO_2 ranging as high as 4 to 6 mg/L (Gordon et al., 1990), several mg of chlorite can be expected in the water that is consumed. Chlorate yields are less predictable but are ordinarily lower in concentration than chlorite (Gordon et al., 1990; Masschelein, 1989).

A wide variety of aldehydes are formed by ozone (Glaze et al., 1989a, b), but of those identified, formaldehyde and acetaldehyde at levels of 5.8 to 31 and 2.1 to 15 µg/L, respectively, are reported at the highest concentrations in drinking water (Krasner et al., 1989a).

As with chlorine, ozonating waters containing significant amounts of bromide results in formation of brominated by-products. The by-products include bromoform, bromoacetates, bromoacetones, and bromoacetonitriles under simulated conditions in the laboratory (Haag and Hoigne, 1983; Krasner et al., 1989b).

An additional concern with ozonation is the formation of bromate (McGuire et al., 1989). Its formation appears to be facilitated by the addition of hydrogen peroxide (Krasner et al., 1993; von Gunten et al., 1996; Song et al., 1997). There is limited data on

◄——

Figure 9-2 Differing distribution of dihaloacetates (dichloroacetate, DCA; bromodichloroacetate, BCA; and dibromoacetate, DBA) and trihaloacetates (trichloroacetate, TCA; bromodichloroacetate, BDCA; and dibromochloroacetate, DBCA) in four different U.S. water supplies. The total haloacetate concentrations (including traces of the monohaloacetates) in the each system were PW SC, 27.1; Houston, 33.4; MWD, 52.6; and Corpus Christi, 34.3. These data illustrate that while total haloac etate levels are within a factor of two of one another, the differences in the distribution between dihaloacetates and trihaloacetates varies more widely between water supplies in different parts of the United States. The variation in the distribution of the individual haloacetates is even more dramatic. (Data taken form Cowman and Singer, 1996)

TABLE 9-3   **Distribution between Different THMs Dependent on Disinfectant**

	Mean Concentration		
Trihalomethane	Chlorine Only	Chlorine Followed by Ammonia	Chlorine plus Ammonia
Chloroform	26.4 ± 3.0^{a}	20.8 ± 3.1	3.3 ± 1.8
Bromodichloromethane	9.1 ± 1.5	15.2 ± 1.1	3.5 ± 0.8
Dibromochloromethane	5.7 ± 1.2	14.6 ± 2.0	4.8 ± 1.3
Bromoform	4.4 ± 1.3	8.5 ± 2.4	12.1 ± 4.8

Note: Data taken from Krasner from EPA/CDHS data base on 35 utilities (McGuire et al., 1989).
[a] Concentrations expressed as $g/L \pm SEM$

the concentrations of bromate that are produced in ozonated drinking water. A limited number of waters were examined by Krasner et al. (1993) where concentrations of < 5 (limit of detection) to 58 µg / L were observed under conditions that reasonably approximated actual disinfection conditions. Increasing ozone, however, can result in substantially higher levels of bromate.

The concept that more than one disinfectant can be used in water treatment to negate some of the disadvantages associated with the individual disinfectants has gained in popularity in recent years. In particular, water utilities are entertaining the utilization of ozone as a primary disinfectant followed by chloramine for maintaining microbiological water quality in the distribution system.

ASSOCIATIONS OF HUMAN DISEASE WITH DRINKING WATER DISINFECTION

Cancer

The relationships between human cancer and the chlorination of drinking water have received extensive epidemiological study. Many of the early studies were ecological, meant to be preliminary studies, and did not take into account many potentially confounding factors (Craun, 1988). An association between the use of chlorine and cancers of the rectum (Gottlieb et al., 1982), colon (de Rouen and Diem, 1977; Kuzma et al., 1977; Young et al., 1981), bladder (de Rouen and Diem, 1977; Kuzma et al., 1977; Cantor et al., 1978), and lung (Bean et al., 1982) were found with some consistency across geographical regions and study populations. Because of design difficulties, this group of studies have been frequently dismissed as being inconclusive (NAS, 1980).

Case-control and cohort studies have tended to support the relationship between the consumption of chlorinated drinking water and cancers at selected sites. These more recent studies are summarized in Table 9-4. An early case-control study (Alvanja et al., 1978) identified several tumor sites, the colon, bladder, liver and kidney, esophagus, pancreas, and stomach. Newer studies have focused on bladder and colon or colorectal cancers.

Seven, more or less independent, studies have found significant associations between bladder cancer and chlorinated drinking water consumption (Zierler et al., 1986, 1988; Cantor et al., 1987; McGeehin et al., 1993; Vena et al., 1993; King and Marrett, 1996; Cantor et al., 1998). Several of these studies have identified a dose-response relationships, primarily related to the duration of exposure to chlorinated water and / or the volume of water consumed (Cantor et al., 1987; Vena et al., 1993, McGeehin et al., 1993; King and Marrett, 1996). The lack of more specific measures of dose has been a major, and

TABLE 9-4 Case-control and Cohort Studies of Chlorinated Drinking Water

Author(s) Year	Population (Cases)	Exposure Variables	Analysis	Results
Alavanja et al., 1978	3446 GI and urinary tract cancer deaths	Chlorinated vs. unchlorinated water at residence	Stratified odds ratio with χ^2 test	Colon 1.99 men Bladder, 2.02 men Liver and kidney, 2.76 Esophagus, 2.39 Pancreas, 2.23 Stomach, 2.39, 2.23 Association of colon cancer with average daily chlorine dosage
Young et al., 1981	8029 cancer deaths	Chlorinated vs. unchlorinated water at residence	Logistic regression	Rectal, 1.35 women
Brenniman et al., 1980	3028 GI and urinary tract cancer deaths	Chlorinated vs. unchlorinated water	Odds ratios with Mantel Haenzel adjustment	Rectal, 1.68 Breast, 1.58
Gottlieb et al., 1982	10,205 kidney, bladder, stomach, liver and colorectal cancer deaths	Chlorinated vs. unchlorinated water at residence	Stratified odds ratio with χ^2 test	No statistically significant associations
Wilkins and Comstock, 1981	Diagnosis of cancer over 12 year period	Chlorinated water in Hagerstown vs. deep wells in County	Logistic regression	No statistically significant association with chloroform
Lawrence et al., 1982	395 colorectal cancer deaths	Modeled chloroform exposure in chlorinated surface vs. ground water	Logistic regression	Colorectal, 1.4 (1.1–1.7) to 3.4 (2.4–4.6) ages 6–89
Cragle et al., 1985	200 new cases of colon cancer	Years of exposure to chlorinated water	Logistic regression	Bladder, 1.7 (1.3–2.2)
Zierler, et al., 1986, 1988	51,645 kidney, bladder, stomach, pancreas, colon, lung, breast cancer deaths	Chlorinated vs. chloraminated drinking water from common source	Odds ratios with Mantel-Haenszel adjustment	Colon, 1.57 (1.04–2.37)
Young et al., 1987	347 new cases of colon cancer	Water consumption, chloroform	Logistic regression	Bladder, 1.43 (1.23–1.67)
Cantor et al., 1987	2982 new cases of bladder cancer	Residence, beverage consumption and water samples	Logistic regression	Pancreas, 2.23 (1.24–4.10)
Ijsselmuiden et al., 1992	101 pancreatic cancer cases	Chlorinated vs. unchlorinated water	Odds ratio	Bladder, 1.8 (1.1–2.9) for more than 30 years exposure
McGeehin et al., 1993	327 verified bladder cancer cases	Years of exposure to chlorinated drinking water	Odds ratio	Bladder, 2.62 (1.53–4.47) in individuals < 65 that drank 10–39 cups of water per day
Vena et al., 1993	351 bladder cancer cases	Tap water consumption—typically chlorinated	Odds ratio in quartiles of water intake	Bladder, 1.41 (1.09–1.81)
King and Marrett, 1996	696 bladder cancer cases	Chlorinated vs. unchlorinated water	Odds ratio	Brain cancer, 1.8, 20–39 years; 2.4, >40 years
Cantor et al., 1996	375 brain cancer patients	Duration of exposure to chlorinated water	Odds ratio	No association among non-smokers; significant interaction with smoking
Cantor et al., 1998	1,123 cases of bladder cancer	Duration of exposure to chlorinated drinking water	Odds ratio	Positive association with rectal cancer; none with colon cancer.
Hildesheim et al., 1998	560 colon cancer, 537 rectal cancer cases	Duration of exposure to chlorinated water and total trihalomethane exposure	Odds ratio	

acknowledged, shortcoming of these studies. The limited attempts to develop more specific measures of exposure have been limited to the THMs (Cantor et al., 1978; Lawrence et al., 1984; Young et al., 1987; Hildesheim et al., 1998). Tap water is not the only source of disinfectant by-products (Abdel-Rahman, 1982). The chemical composition of chlorinated water varies by location, and the THMs represent a limited fraction of the carcinogenic by-products that are present. A final concern is that no single disinfectant by-product or mixture of by-products has been shown capable of inducing bladder cancer.

Colon and colorectal cancer have also been frequently associated with chlorinated drinking water. An estimated odds ratio of 1.99 for chlorinated water relative to nonchlorinated water was reported by Alavanja et al. (1978) for male subjects. An association was also reported by Young et al (1981) for colon cancer. On the other hand, Brenniman et al. (1980) reported an odds ratio of 1.35 for rectal cancer in women. The inconsistencies between the colon and rectum continue through the studies of Gottlieb et al. (1982) identifying the rectum, the study of Cragle et al. (1985) implicating the colorectal area, and Young et al. (1987) again identifying the colon. Finally a recent study by Hildesheim et al. (1998) indicates little risk for colon cancer and significant risks for rectal cancer. The odds ratios of chlorinated to unchlorinated water in these studies ranged 1.35 to 1.68. In addition several studies failed to identify an association (Lawrence et al., 1982; Zierler et al., 1986, 1988) or found very inconsistent relationships (Bean et al., 1982). In contrast to the circumstance identified with bladder cancer, several chlorination by-products have been shown to induce cancer of the lower colon in rodents.

Additional target organs have been identified in case-control studies. Ijsselmuiden et al. (1992) found a significant association with pancreatic cancer (OR = 2.23). Brain cancer was found to be associated with the duration of exposure to chlorinated water (Cantor et al., 1996). Both of these sites were identified in the early study of Alavanja et al. (1978), but as yet additional studies have not been forthcoming to support these relationships. A weak response of pancreatic cancer has been observed in male rats treated with MX (Komulainen et al., 1997). There are some effects of the dihaloacetates on intermediary metabolism that may relate to effects on the pancreas that need to be kept in mind, and they will be discussed later. In addition there are familial links between pancreatic cancer and cancer of the colon that could be important. There has been no reports of the induction of brain cancer by disinfectant by-products in experimental animals.

Additional ecological studies have been conducted during the past decade. Koivusalo et al. (1994) found significant associations between mutagenicity in drinking water (produced by chlorination) with bladder (OR = 1.21), kidney (OR = 1.57), and colon cancer (OR = 1.39) in Finland. These findings confirm the general relationships found in other settings. However, considering the level of disinfectant by-products that have been reported in Finnish waters (Vartiainen and Liimatainen, 1986), the odds ratios seem modest. Perhaps there is a consistency in the quality and quantity of disinfectant by-products produced in Finnish drinking water that might be usefully contrasted with the more diverse sources of water used in other parts of the world, including the United States.

While epidemiological studies have yet to establish a clear association between the use of chemical disinfectants and the induction of cancer or other health effects, the case for associations with bladder, colon, or colorectal cancer continues to be strengthened by the further studies cited. The remaining weakness of these studies has been the lack of good measures of the exposure variables. The compounds produced in water treated with chemical disinfectants differ in potentially significant ways from place to place, depending on the nature of the water being treated. While it would be very expensive to attempt to relate cancer incidence to individual by-products and their exact concentrations in different places within the distribution system, there are approaches to exposure assessment that could be used in future studies. These studies should focus on those water and treatment variables that are likely to produce significant differences in the types and concentrations of by-products found in a particular drinking water. Investigating relationships with total organic carbon, pH, and bromide concentrations, as well as the type of disinfectant used, would seem more likely to produce more accurate estimates of exposure than a continuing pursuit of individual by-products, ad infinitum.

Reproductive and Developmental Effects

There have been a number of epidemiological investigations that have associated the chlorinated drinking water or particular disinfectant by-products with reproductive or developmental effects in humans. However, this literature is in a more primitive state of development than that focused on cancer incidence. Exposure assessment issues are essentially the same, but the firmer diagnostic criteria for cancer makes evaluation of the reality of the responses much more tractable. If compounds interfere with reproductive and developmental processes, they should produce concomitant and measurable effects on endocrine, paracrine, or autocrine factors in animals at very similar doses as found in the human population. Less specific mechanisms are not likely to occur without clear signs of toxicity in the mother. The resolution of the issue is, however, complicated by the relative high frequency of reproductive and developmental anomalies in human populations, in general.

Two studies have focused primarily on the relationship between chloroform in drinking water and measures of reproductive health. Kramer et al. (1992) conducted a case-control study of effects of drinking water containing high levels of THMs that were associated with low birth weights, premature birth, or intrauterine growth retardation (IUGR). The odds ratio for IUGR was 1.8 (1.1–2.9) in communities where chloroform exceeded $10\,\mu g/L$. The relationships between low birth weight and premature birth were not statistically significant. Bove et al. (1995) conducted an evaluation of chemicals in drinking water in areas near hazardous waste sites. In this case relationships with disinfectant by-products were essentially incidental to the original aims of the study. Nevertheless, odds ratios of > 1.5 were observed between total THM concentrations and small body size for gestational age, central nervous system defects, oral cleft defects, and major cardiac defects. Importantly the association with major cardiac defects did not relate to ventral septal defects.

A series of papers were published surrounding the observation of increased spontaneous abortion related to tap water consumption relative to bottled water consumption in California (Deane et al., 1989; Hertz-Picciotto et al., 1989; Fenster et al., 1991; Swan et al., 1992; Deane, et al., 1992; Wrensch et al., 1992; Hertz-Picciotto et al., 1992a; Windham et al., 1992; Fenster et al., 1992; Golub, 1992 Neutra et al., 1992). In part, these observations were accounted for by bias introduced by self-identification of cases and the fact that interviewers were not appropriately blinded (Hertz-Picciotto et al., 1992b). The authors felt that it was premature to abandon the possibility of a relationship entirely (Windham et al., 1992; Swan et al., 1992). The importance of considering by-products with differing modes of action than the THMs is discussed more fully in the review of the toxicological effects of disinfectant by-products.

TOXICOLOGY OF DISINFECTANTS

General Toxicological Properties of Chlorine (Chlorine / Hypochlorous Acid / Hypochlorite)

Until the 1980s little information existed concerning the toxicology of chlorine as it is consumed in water. In the past decade a series of studies have been published in which the general toxicology, carcinogenicity, and reproductive effects of chlorine have been studied by the oral route of exposure. There has been some variation in the protocols utilized, making comparison of results between studies difficult. In some cases chlorine gas has been bubbled into water until the desired concentration has been achieved. In others sodium hypochlorite has been utilized. At equivalent pH these methods of preparation yield identical chemical forms. Since the reactivity of chlorine for chlorination reactions varies with pH, studies conducted at different pHs cannot be considered equivalent. This is particularly true if the pHs at which studies have been conducted are on opposite sides of the pK_a of hypochlorous acid (7.5). Consequently the pH of the water utilized is provided, as available, in the present review. When this is not available in the original reference, the method of preparation is identified.

Animals tolerate concentrations of chlorine in their drinking water up to 625 mg/L. There is little indication of adverse effect beyond those that are secondary to reduced water consumption (Druckrey, 1968, using Cl_2 bubbled into water; Furukawa, 1980, Hasegawa et al., 1986, Kurokawa et al., 1986b, all using sodium hypochlorite). A recent study by Daniel et al. (1990) compared chlorine (pH 9.4) with chloramine and chlorine dioxide in rats. A series of clinical and hematological parameters were examined in addition to observations of gross pathology and effects on organ weights. Of these three disinfectants, chlorine was clearly the best tolerated, and the highest dose examined, 250 mg/L, produced no adverse effects. These data indicate that any adverse effects directly attributable to chlorine have to be quite subtle even at doses much above those utilized for water treatment.

Chlorine appears to have subtle effects on immune function. Administration of sodium hypochlorite in drinking water at levels of 25 to 30 mg/L was shown to reduce recovery of peritoneal exudate cells after one to four weeks of treatment (Fidler, 1977). The ability to stimulate the cytotoxic activity of macrophages in these cell populations toward B16 melanoma and UV-112 fibrosarcoma cells with the Conconavalin A macrophage-activating factor was decreased by approximately 50% relative to control animals receiving 0.5 to 1 ppm of chlorine in their drinking water. Subsequent experiments demonstrated that the in vivo phagocytic activity of macrophages recovered from the liver and spleen were also decreased (Fidler et al., 1982). The treatment led to an increase in the number of pulmonary metastases of injected B16-BL6 cells. Exon et al. (1987) attempted to correlate these effects with other parameters of macrophage function in Sprague-Dawley rats at doses of 0, 5, 15, and 30 mg chlorine/L as sodium hypochlorite. These authors did not observe a decrement in the in vitro phagocytic activity of peritoneal macrophages recovered by lavage. However, Exon et al. (1987) did observe impaired TPA-induced oxidative metabolism as measured by a chemiluminescence response. The most remarkable finding was that the production of prostaglandin E_2 was significantly increased in cells from animals receiving sodium hypochlorite. This latter effect was even greater in animals that were treated with an equivalent dose of monochloramine. Monochloramine appeared to suppress antibody production in response to keyhole limpet hemocyanin, raising the possibility that the effects of hypochlorite may depend on its conversion into monochloramine. These results are interesting primarily because of the relatively low doses at which some effect was observed. However, the extent to which these subtle effects reflect increasing disease burden in the population is difficult to determine.

Carcinogenic Properties of Chlorine and Chloramine

Administration of chlorine to rats or mice in drinking water at concentrations up to 250 mg/L has failed to produce any specific toxicological effects (Druckrey, 1968; Furukawa et al., 1980; Hasegawa et al., 1986; Kurokawa et al., 1986b). The National

Toxicology Program (NTP, 1990b) completed a carcinogenesis bioassay of sodium hypochlorite and chloramine in drinking water at concentrations up to 275 mg / L. There was little indication of pathology in either mice (B6C3F1) or rats (F344/N) with either disinfectant. There was a significant increase in mononuclear cell leukemia in female rats, which was discounted because the incidence in the concurrent control group was significantly lower than that of the historical controls (ca. 25%). Compared against historical controls, there was not significant increase in leukemia in either sex. Previous studies found no evidence that chlorine in drinking water was carcinogenic (Druckrey, 1968; Furukawa et al., 1980; Hasegawa et al., 1986; Kurokawa et al., 1986b). Consequently these data suggest that chlorine itself is not carcinogenic.

Hypochlorite does possess weak mutagenic activity in bacterial systems (Rosenkranz, 1973; Wlodkowski and Rosenkranz, 1975; Rosenkranz et al., 1976). Such responses are observed only at cytotoxic doses, however. The absence of other evidence of genotoxic activity, particularly in vivo, makes it difficult to assign much importance to these responses. Shih and Lederberg (1976) and Thomas et al. (1989) both reported that chloramine is also mutagenic in bacterial systems.

General Toxicological Properties of Disinfectant By-products

Inorganic By-products   Inorganic by-products of concern at this time appear to be limited to chlorite, chlorate, and bromate. Chlorate can occur as a result of the use of hypochlorite solutions in disinfecting drinking water (Bolyard et al., 1993) or potentially from the use of chlorine dioxide. Chlorite occurrence is specific to the use of chlorine dioxide, and bromate also appears unique to the use of ozone.

Early investigations of chlorite's toxic properties focused almost entirely on its potential ability to produce methemoglobin and hemolysis. Heffernan et al. (1979a, b) examined the ability of chlorite to induce methemoglobin in cats and Sprague-Dawley rats. When administered as an oral bolus, as little as 20 mg / kg resulted in formation of significant amounts of methemoglobin. Intraperitoneal doses of 20 mg / kg in rats also induced methemoglobin. However, when administered in drinking water, no significant elevation in methemoglobin was observed in cats (up to 1000 mg / L as sodium chlorite) or rats (up to 500 mg / L). Thus chlorite must enter into the systemic circulation at a rapid rate to induce methemoglobin. Harrington et al. (1995a) systematically assessed hematological parameters using single gavage doses ranging from 25 to 200 mg / kg subchronic doses by the same method for 13 weeks. Minor effects were observed at 25 and 50 mg / kg. At 100 mg/kg and above, signs of hemolytic anemia became apparent with decreases in red blood cell (RBC) count, hemoglobin concentration, and hematocrit accompanied by evidence of methemoglobinemia. These data clearly demonstrate that bolus doses of chlorite are effective in producing oxidative damage to RBCs.

Treatment of both cats and rats with chlorite in drinking water for extended periods (up to 90 days) did result in decreases in RBC counts, hemoglobin concentrations, and packed cell volume. These effects were observed with 500 mg sodium chlorite / L in cats and with as little as 100 mg / L in rats (Heffernan et al., 1979b). The changes in these blood parameters appeared to generally decrease in severity as the treatment was extended from 30 to 90 days, suggesting that adaptation to the treatment was occurring. However, in rats, decreases in the RBC content of glutathione and elevation of 2,3-diphosphoglycerate were maintained through 90 days of treatment. In the cat, increased turnover of erythrocytes was detectable at concentrations of 100 mg / L with no significant effect being observed at 10 mg / L. This latter concentration resulted in a daily dose of 0.6 mg / kg per day. RBCs drawn from rats treated with 100 mg chlorite / L had significantly less ability to detoxify hydrogen peroxide that was generated by the addition of chlorite, in vitro. These data show that while the anemia caused by hemolysis was largely compensated for in subchronic treatment of healthy rats, there was still evidence of oxidative stress being exerted by the chlorite treatment. Depletion of this reserve capacity could be of importance in individuals that are in a compromised state, or who might be exposed to other hemolytic agents. The lowest concentration at which glutathione was depleted significantly from control levels in rats was 50 mg / L, and no effect was observed at 10 mg / L.

The results of Heffernan et al. (1979b) have been generally confirmed by subsequent studies in a variety of species. Abdel-Rahman et al. (1980) and Couri and Abdel-Rahman (1980) obtained very similar effects in rats treated up to 11 months. Moore and Calabrese (1980, 1982) produced similar results in mice, and Bercz et al. (1982) demonstrated reduced RBC and decreased hemoglobin at similar doses in African green monkeys. More recently gavage doses of sodium chlorite were administered daily for 13 weeks to male and female Crl: CD (SD) BR rats (Harrington et al., 1995a). The doses of sodium chlorite were 0, 10, 25, or 80 mg / kg. This study is important because it included many of the standard parameters of subchronic toxicological studies, while previous studies had focused almost entirely on blood parameters. Gavage doses of 80 mg/kg produced death in a number animals. RBC counts were reduced slightly at doses of 10 mg / kg in male rats with further decreases being observed at 80 mg / kg. RBC counts were significantly depressed in female rats at doses of 25 mg / kg and above. Histopathological examination of necropsied tissues revealed squamous cell epithelial hyperplasia, hyperkeratosis, ulceration, chronic inflammation, and edema in the stomach of 7/15 males and 8/15 females given 80 mg / kg doses. This effect was observed in only 2/15 animals at the 25 mg / kg dose and was not observed at all at 10 mg / kg.

A clinical study of the effects of chlorite, chlorate, and chlorine dioxide was conducted in three parts a rising dose tolerance study in normal male volunteers (Lubbers and Bianchine, 1984), a 12 week subchronic study (Lubbers et al., 1981, 1982, 1984a) and a limited study in glucose-6-phosphate dehydrogenase-deficient male volunteers (Lubbers et al., 1984b). The 12 week study required subjects to drink 500 ml of water containing 5 mg / L chlorine dioxide, chlorite, or chlorate within a 15 minutes. period each day. Although there were significant, but small, trends in certain parameters, no physiological significance could be attributed to any of the results (Lubbers et al., 1984a). Three glucose-6-phosphate dehydrogenase-deficient individuals were studied under similar circumstances but were followed for an additional 8 weeks post-treatment. Again no significant trends could be identified in this small group of individuals (Lubbers et al., 1984b).

While chlorite appears most active in producing oxidative stress, chlorine dioxide appears to be most potent as an anti-thyroid agent. Bercz et al. (1982) found that administration of chlorine dioxide to primates at doses of 100 mg / L for six weeks produced a depression of serum thyroxine concentrations. This effect was not observed with up to eight weeks treatment with 400 mg / L sodium chlorite or sodium chlorate. A similar effect was observed when chlorine dioxide was administered to rats at levels of 100 mg / L or more (Orme et al., 1985; Harrington et al., 1986; Carlton et al., 1987).

Treatment of rats for 10 weeks with concentrations of $KBrO_3$ of 250, 500, 1000, 2000, and 4000 mg / L of drinking water established a maximally tolerated concentration of < 1000 mg / L. As treatments were extended to 13 weeks, there were elevated levels of serum enzymes associated with hepatic and renal damage. Perhaps most significant were elevations of blood urea nitrogen concentrations. Eosinophilic droplets were observed in the cytoplasm of the proximal renal tubule cells in male F344 rats at 600 mg / L (Onodera et al., 1985; cited in Kurokawa et al., 1990). These droplets were determined to be eosinophilic bodies rather than hyaline droplets. Lipofuscin pigments were also observed in the proximal tubular epithelium.

Organic By-products The long list of by-products and potential by-products of chlorination makes it difficult to discuss toxicities in a comprehensive way. Most effects of by-products are observed in the range of 1 to 100 mg / kg. The highest doses that could be anticipated for any one by-product in water is about 1 to 2 μg / kg. Thus it is difficult to determine whether the effects seen are of any relevance.

Attempts have been made to define the toxicity of chlorination by-products collectively by testing concentrated organic material from chlorinated water (Miller et al., 1986) or humic substances that have been chlorinated at high concentrations in the laboratory (Condie et al., 1985). The only clearly positive result that has been found is mutagenic activity measured in bacterial and / or in vitro systems (Bull et al., 1982; Meier et al., 1983, 1985b; Meier and Bull, 1985). While the negative data obtained in these studies are reassuring, there are methodological difficulties with such studies that are difficult to overcome. Experiments involving concentrates are plagued by questions of selective recovery, the potential for introduction of artifacts by the concentration technique, the possibility of increased reaction rates between components at the higher concentrations, the overwhelming concentrations of inorganic constituents of drinking water, and practical limits on the amount of organic material that can be recovered from drinking water. While chlorination of humic and fulvic acids at high concentrations obviates many of the difficulties with concentrates, such studies are frequently questioned on the basis of whether the products formed are truly representative of those seen in drinking water. A major problem has been that typically less than 10% of the organic material present in mixtures obtained from actual water or from chlorinated humic substances can be chemically characterized. This makes it difficult to overcome criticisms about the representative nature of either mixture. Additional objections are raised by the artificial limits on doses that can be administered. Cost is the principle limit on the amount of concentrate that can be prepared from drinking waters. Another problem, in the case of the model systems, is the production of hydrochloric acid as a by-product of chlorination reactions and the need to neutralize this material before providing it to experimental animals. The high salt concentrations result in an excessive osmolality that severely limits the concentrations of chlorinated humic or fulvic acid solutions that can be used as drinking water. Finally the large amount of biologically inert material limits the assessment of hazards associated with minor components that may be of toxicological significance when mixtures are prepared from actual drinking water or from model substrates.

As a consequence of the above, the assessment of toxicological hazards associated with chlorination still largely depends on what is known about the toxicology of individual by-products or what can be learned from the study of simple binary or tertiary mixtures of these chemicals. The five classes of chemicals that have received the most attention are the trihalomethanes, selected haloacids, haloacetonitriles, and some halogenated aldehydes and ketones. As discussed earlier, there are a variety of aldehydes, ketones, and organic acids that are associated with chlorine and other disinfectants. Few of these have received specific attention as disinfectant by-products, but they have in some cases received considerable study for other reasons. Some experimentation has been undertaken on by-products that have been thought to be more or less specific to disinfectants other than chlorine, including bromate, chlorite, and chlorate. Some large-scale experiments are underway as of this writing by the National Toxicology Program with chlorate, cyanogen chloride, and selected haloacetonitrile and haloacetates.

THMs Largely because of its long use as an anesthetic, chloroform has long been recognized for its ability to produce hepatic and renal damage in humans (Davidson et al., 1982). The cytotoxic effects of chloroform in the liver and kidney of rodents has received thorough study with short- and long-term treatments utilizing oral and inhalation exposure (Larson et al., 1994a, 1995a). In addition the nasal turbinates of the rat have been identified as a particularly sensitive target organ for chloroform (Larson et al., 1995b). The toxicity of other THMs also appears to largely involve cytotoxic effects to the liver and or kidneys (Chu et al., 1982a, b; Munson et al., 1982; Thornton-Manning et al., 1994; Lilly et al., 1997).

The toxicity of chloroform is dramatically affected by the vehicle in which it is administered, being significantly augmented when given in an oil vehicle (Bull et al., 1986; Larson et al., 1994a, 1995a, b, 1996). It has been suggested that these effects are primarily the result of altered kinetics of absorption and subsequent metabolism of chloroform, although this has not been rigorously demonstrated. Similar differences have been noted with short-term treatments with bromodichloromethane (Lilly et al., 1994), but in this case it was shown that separate treatments with corn oil and bromodichloromethane in an aqueous vehicle had no effect on its toxicity to the liver.

The toxicity of chloroform and the other THMs depends on their metabolism to reactive intermediates. This activation can occur by several mechanisms, oxidative metabolism to phosgene (Pohl and Krishna, 1978), reductive metabolism to free radical intermediates (Testai et al., 1990), or as a result of an reactive metabolite formed by the activity of glutathione-S-transferases of the theta class (Pegram et al., 1997).

HAs There are significant differences in the toxicities produced by various members of the HA class of disinfectant by-products. There are superficial parallels among dichloroacetate, bromochloroacetate, and dibromoacetate. All of the members of the dihaloacetate class are rapidly metabolized, but the brominated analogues are increasingly involved in processes, presumably metabolic, that induce lipid peroxidation and oxidative damage to nuclear DNA of the hepatocyte (Austin et al., 1997). A substantial fraction of the metabolism of dichloroacetate occurs in the cytosol (Lipscomb et al., 1995). Prior treatment of either humans (Curry et al., 1985) or rodents (Gonzalez-Leon et al., 1997) inhibits the metabolism that occurs in the cytosol. As bromine substitution increases, the metabolism of the HAs appears to shift from the cytosol to microsomal fractions. This shift perhaps accounts for the increasing evidence of formation of active oxygen species (Austin et al., 1996).

There has been considerable human experience with dichloroacetate because of early investigations of its potential as an orally active hypoglycemic agent (Crabb et al., 1976). The association of neurological deficits characterized by weakness of muscles in the lower extremities, face and fingers, diminished tendon reflexes and slowed nerve conduction velocity in individuals treated with does of dichloroacetate as low as 50 mg/kg per day for 16 weeks (Moore et al., 1979; Stacpoole et al., 1979) has limited its use in medicine. Subsequent to this work dichloroacetate was shown to cause hind limb weakness and/or paralysis in dogs and rats (Katz et al., 1981; Yount et al., 1982; Mather et al., 1990); Cicmanec et al., 1991).

In addition to peripheral neuropathy, dichloroacetate administered subchronically produces testicular abnormalities in rats and produce prostate glandular atrophy, cystic mucosal hyperplasia in the gall bladder, and ocular lesions in dogs (Katz et al., 1981; Yount et al., 1982; Mather et al., 1990). More recently dichloroacetate has been shown to produce a severe hepatomegaly and cytomegaly that is associated with large accumulations of glycogen in mice (Sanchez and Bull, 1990). Similar, but much less severe, hepatomegaly and glycogen accumulation were observed in rats (Bull et al., 1990b; Mather et al., 1990).

Accumulation of glycogen in heptatocytes is characteristic of the dihaloacetates, with dichloroacetate producing a more rapid accumulation, reaching a maximum level within one week of treatment. Significant increases of glycogen are observed with concentrations of dichloroacetate in drinking water as low as 0.2 g/L (Kato-Weinstein et al., 1998). The defect appears related to glycogen catabolism as the glycogen becomes progressively more resistant to mobilization by fasting. Substantial decreases in serum insulin are observed with treatments of 14 days longer in duration (Smith and Bull, 1995; Kato-Weinstein et al., 1998). Since this effect develops with a latency of about 14 days, it is suggested that it is a result of down-regulating some of the insulin-mimetic effects of dichloroacetate. The brominated dihaloacetates have the same properties, particularly in the liver, but there are qualitative differences. For example, dibromoacetate is less effective in producing accumulation of glycogen, but it produces a more pronounced hepatomegaly. Dibromoacetate is also more effective as a peroxisome proliferator than other dihaloacetates but is significantly less active than trichloroacetate.

The effects of high doses of dichloroacetate (e.g., > 15–200 mg / kg by an intraperitoneal or intravenous dosing regimen) on intermediary metabolism has been extensively studied. The principle interest has been in blood glucose, lactic acid, and lipid concentrations. These effects have been partially attributed to its ability to activate the pyruvate dehydrogenase complex through inhibition of the pyruvate dehydrogenase kinase (Blackshear et al., 1974; Whitehouse et al., 1974a, b; Crabb et al., 1976; Stacpoole, 1989). Although chloroacetate and trichloroacetate share this activity and are active at equivalent concentrations in pig heart mitochondria in vitro (Whitehouse et al., 1974a), their toxicological effects are distinct from that of dichloroacetate. Some of these differences may relate to the ability of dichloroacetate to be transported by the mitochondrial pyruvate carrier, while trichloroacetate apparently is not (Halestrap et al., 1978).

The lack of analytical information on systemic concentrations of dichloroacetate achieved by the administration of different doses by different routes renders strict comparison of effects of dichloroacetate across studies difficult. Some information is now becoming available about the concentrations of dichloroacetate that are observed in the blood of treated rodents in toxicological studies (Kato-Weinstein et al., 1998; Merdink et al., 1998c). These data suggest that the clinical studies in humans and animal studies that have been designed to mimic these responses have been conducted at doses much too high to be of interest for the long-term toxicological effects of dichloroacetate. For example, concentrations of 100 μM were required for 50% inhibition of the pyruvate dehydrogenase kinase in vitro (Whitehouse et al., 1974b). Peak concentrations observed with i.v. infusions of 30, 60, and 100 mg / kg in human subjects were 1 to 2.5 mM (Fox et al., 1996b). A further complication is that these high doses saturate the metabolism of dichloroacetate in rats. Saturation of dichloroacetate metabolism requires higher doses and tends to be more easily reversed in mice (the species in which effects on glycogen deposition and changes in insulin concentrations have been observed) in this dose range. Because of the high doses in humans, the apparent half-lives were extended for several hours, whereas lower doses in rodents (5–20 mg / kg, iv) are cleared with half-lives of 5 to 10 minutes. The blood concentrations that are associated with increased glycogen deposition in the liver of mice treated with dichloroacetate and modify serum insulin concentrations are in the range of < 1 to perhaps 10 μM (Kato-Weinstein et al., 1998). At the relatively high dose represented by 2 g / L in drinking water, blood concentrations in mice were as high as 300 μM during active consumption of the water, but the effects on glycogen accumulation were observed with concentrations in drinking water as low as 0.2 g / L. These data suggest that alterations induced in the insulin-signaling pathways may play a substantial role in the toxicology of the dihaloacetates at lower doses than those that have been studied for clinical applications.

The trihaloacetates produce a less marked hepatomegaly than the dihaloacetates (Sanchez and Bull, 1990; Kato-Weinstein et al., 1998; Stauber et al., 1998a.) Within the group, trichloroacetate is effective in the range of 0.5 to 2 g / L as a peroxisome proliferator, but it is not observed with bromodichloroacetate treatment in the same concentration range (Kato-Weinstein et al., 1998b). The ineffectiveness of bromine-substituted trihaloacetates as peroxisome proliferators may be related to their more rapid and complete metabolism (Austin et al., 1997). Dichloroacetate is the most potent of the dihaloacetates in terms of its effects on carbohydrate metabolism. Bromochloroacetate and dibromoacetate do increase glycogen deposition in liver with similar dose–response characteristics, but dichloroacetate produces the effect more rapidly. The dose–response for glycogen disposition relates closely to that observed for the hepatomegaly and induction of distortions of cell size for each of the dihaloacetates. In contrast to the centrilobular localization of glycogen seen with the dihaloacetates, glycogen deposition with trichloroacetate is much milder and appears to occur with a periportal distribution. Bromodichloroacetate, however, produces a distribution more similar to that of dichloroacetate, but it requires considerably more time to develop. It is likely that this is explained in part by the metabolism of bromodichloroacetate to dichloroacetate (Xu et al., 1995; Austin and Bull, 1995).

As with the dihaloacetates, the most prominent effects of the trihaloacetates are in the liver (Goldsworthy and Popp, 1987; Mather et al., 1990; Bull et al., 1990b; Sanchez and Bull, 1990). Trichloroacetate is without apparent cytotoxic effects in liver cells in vivo at dose rates of up to 300 mg / kg per day (Bull et al., 1990; Sanchez and Bull, 1990; Acharya et al., 1995) or in vitro at concentrations as high as 5 mM (Bruschi and Bull, 1993). Similar liver enlargement has been observed with bromodichloroacetate, but trihaloacetates with higher bromine substitution have not been studied.

HANs   The relationship between the metabolism of the HANs and their toxic effects are less well established. Pereira et al. (1984) found that from 2.3% to 14% of doses of chloroacetonitrile, dichloroacetonitrile, bromodichloroacetonitrile, dibromoacetonitrile, and trichloroacetonitrile were converted to thiocyanate in the urine. These data indicate that haloacetonitriles are cyanogens. Chronically, production of cyanide followed by conversion to thiocyanate is associated with adverse effects on the thyroid gland (Olusi et al., 1979). In addition to cyanide, Pereira et al. (1984) postulated that metabolism of the haloacetonitriles would yield the alkylating agents, formaldehyde with chloroacetonitrile, formyl chloride or formylhalide from the dihaloacetonitriles, and phosgene or cyanoformyl chloride from trichloroacetonitrile. These reactive metabolites may be associated with the mutagenic effects of these chemicals that will be discussed in the section on carcinogenicity of disinfectant by-products.

The HANs do not produce distinctive toxicological effects with treatments of 14 or 90 days in duration (Hayes et al., 1986). Dichloroacetonitrile is tolerated at daily doses as high as 8 mg / kg for 90 days in male and female CD rats. Dibromoacetonitrile was tolerated at doses of 23 mg / kg per day for 90 days.

3-Chloro-4-(dichloromethyl)-5-hydroxy-2[5H]-furanone (MX)   The general toxicology of MX, other than its carcinogenicity, has received very limited attention. Most research has focused on testing whether its potent mutagenic effects in bacterial systems and in vitro can be duplicated in vivo. It would appear from these studies that animals can tolerate dose rates of 32 mg / kg for up to 14 days (Meier et al., 1996). A dose rate of 64 mg / kg was overtly toxic. Little evidence of toxicity to specific organs was observed in the chronic bioassay of MX in Wistar rats (Komulainen et al., 1997).

Miscellaneous   Several groups of disinfectant by-products include mutagenic members. The more frequently identified compounds fall into the broad classes of haloaldehydes, haloketones, and halogenated hydroxy-furanones (Meier et al., 1988). With the exception of chloral hydrate, the metabolism of these compounds has received very little systematic study. Chloral hydrate is largely metabolized to trichloroethanol and trichloroacetate

(Merdink et al., 1998a; Merdink et al., 1998b). Lesser amounts may be converted to dichloroacetate, but the concentrations achieved in blood are quite low (Merdink et al., 1998c). Chloral hydrate has been used in high doses (500 to more than 2000 mg) as a sedative / hypnotic. This effect has been largely attributed to its conversion to trichloroethanol (Gessner and Cabana, 1970). These central nervous system depressant effects cannot occur at the very low doses of chloral hydrate derived from drinking chlorinated drinking water. Therefore most emphasis has been placed on the conversion of chloral hydrate to dichloroacetate and trichloroacetate, two established liver carcinogens in rodents.

Some work has been conducted examining the toxic properties of a limited number of the halogenated ketones that have been identified as chlorination by-products. Daniel et al. (1993) examined the effects of 1,1,1-trichloro-2-propanone. The only significant pathology was observed as hyperkeratosis in the stomach of rats treated by intubation at doses of 48 mg / kg and higher for up to 90 days. No effects were seen at 16 or 30 mg / kg per day. Other studies deal primarily with evaluations of the mutagenic effects of these chemicals and that will be discussed further below.

Carcinogenic By-products of Disinfectants

Inorganic By-products   The carcinogenicity of bromate poses some potentially serious problems for the use of ozone as a disinfectant in water supplies that contain significant quantities of bromide. Of all disinfectant by-products studied to date, bromate occurs at concentrations that are closer to those that produce overt effects in animals. It can be found at in concentrations of 10 to 50 μg / L. Bromate has been shown to induce renal tumors in two species, male and female F344 rats (Kurokawa et al., 1983, 1986a) and male Syrian Golden hamsters (Takamura et al., 1985). In addition, it induced mesothelioma and thyroid tumors in male rats (Kurokawa et al., 1983). Its minimally effective dose rate as a carcinogen is 2.7 mg / kg per day (Kurokawa et al., 1986a). Kasai et al. (1987) and Cho et al. (1993) have associated the development of renal tumors with the formation of excessive levels of 8-hydroxydeoxyguanosine adducts in DNA in a target organ specific manner. Sai et al. (1992) demonstrated that bromate generated free radicals that could be spin trapped in kidney cells or homogenate, but not by liver preparations. These data suggest that the carcinogenic effect in the kidney may be secondary to oxidative stress.

Chlorate and chlorite are the other inorganic by-products of concern that can occur at reasonably high concentrations in water disinfected by hypochlorite solutions (chlorate) or chlorine dioxide (both chlorate and chlorite). The carcinogenicity of chlorate has not been subjected to adequate testing. A study is currently underway sponsored by the National Toxicology Program. Some preliminary data are available on chlorite.

Sodium chlorite has been studied as a carcinogen at concentrations of 0, 300, and 600 mg / L of drinking water in F344 rats and 750 mg / L in B6C3F1 mice (Kurokawa et al., 1986b). The rats became infected with a Sendai virus in all groups which resulted in the termination of the study after only 85 weeks. There was a statistically significant increase in the incidence of hyperplastic nodules in male mice treated with 250 mg / L but not in females. The incidence of these lesions did not increase when the dose of chlorite was increased to 500 mg / L. Hepatocellular carcinomas were too few to add anything substantive to the evaluation. There were no other treatment-related changes in the incidence of other tumors in either male or female mice.

Yokose et al. (1987) examined the carcinogenicity of sodium chlorite in B6C3F1 mice in a chronic bioassay. The concentrations utilized in this study were 0.025% (250 mg / L) and 0.05% (500 mg / L) as sodium chlorite. A small, but statistically significant ($p < 0.05$)

increase in the incidence of lung adenomas was observed at 500 mg / L. The authors noted that this was not accompanied by the appearance of lung adenocarcinomas; thus it was not possible to conclude from these data that chlorite induced lung tumors.

Organic By-products Partly because of epidemiological evidence, a large portion of research directed at disinfectant by-products has focused on potential carcinogenic effects. A listing of the by-products that have been shown to induce cancer is provided in Table 9-5. Based on these data, it must be concluded that compounds produced in the chemical disinfection of drinking water do have carcinogenic properties. This qualitative conclusion, however, does not provide definitive support for the hypothesis that chlorinated water (or other disinfected water) induces tumors in humans. Definitive evidence must come from consideration of dose–response relationships, mechanisms by which the cancer is produced, intrinsic human susceptibility to the effects of these compounds relative to the amounts that are actually consumed in drinking water. A second consideration is whether the mixture of disinfectant by-products that is produced has some unique properties that result in effects at doses lower than could be anticipated from the sum of the carcinogenic activity of the individual compounds.

It is not feasible in this short review to do justice to the rich literature that has developed surrounding the carcinogenic effects of disinfectant by-products. With apologies to the authors of many excellent and important papers, it was necessary to focus on a few studies on the limited set of by-products for which a substantial database has developed.

THMs The THMs, particularly chloroform, have received the most study as carcinogens. Induction of liver tumors by chloroform is very dependent on the vehicle that is used. Jorgenson et al. (1985) were unable to demonstrate induction of liver tumors in female B6C3F1 mice when it was presented at higher doses and for a longer period of time than those required to produce an 80% incidence of tumors in the NCI (1976) study. Subsequent study demonstrated that the corn oil vehicle significantly enhanced the liver damage produced by chloroform (Bull et al., 1986; Larson et al., 1995a). This observation is consistent with the finding that high levels of polyunsaturated fat interact to increase the hepatocarcinogenic effects of N-nitrosodimethylamine in rats (Hietanen et al., 1990). Increasing levels of exhaled ethane with increasing levels of polyunsaturated fat in the diet indicated that there was an increase in the baseline level of lipid peroxidation in these animals. Evidence from initiation / promotion studies have shown that a corn oil vehicle can render chloroform as a hepatic tumor promoter in diethylnitrosamine-initiated rats (Deml and Osterle, 1985), but chloroform in drinking water was inactive in this regard (Herren-Freund and Pereira, 1986). It has been found that chloroform in drinking water was incapable of acting as a promoter of hepatic tumors in Swiss mice that were initiated with ethylnitrosourea (Herren-Freund and Pereira, 1986) or in B6C3F1 mice initiated with diethylnitrosamine (Klaunig et al., 1986). In point of fact, chloroform in drinking water inhibited diethylnitrosamine-induced liver tumors in B6C3F1 mice (Klaunig et al., 1986) and ethylnitrosourea-induced liver tumors Swiss mice (Pereira et al., 1985). This inhibitory activity of chloroform also results in reduced yields of dimethylhydrazine-induced gastrointestinal tract tumors (Daniel et al., 1989).

The apparent requirement for corn oil for induction of hepatic tumors raises serious questions about whether the induction of liver tumors in mice by chloroform should be utilized for estimating the magnitude of carcinogenic risks at all. A recent study by Pereira and Grothaus (1997) found that chloroform administered in drinking water could abolish the cell killing and cellular proliferation produced by chloroform administered by corn oil gavage in a dose–dependent manner. The lowest effective dose to inhibit the induction of hepatic necrosis by a high dose of chloroform in corn oil was 120 mg / L, or about 12 mg /

TABLE 9-5 By-Products of Disinfection That Have Been Shown to Produce Cancer in Animals

By-product	Species / Strain / Sex / Site	Vehicle / Route	Result
	Trihalomethanes		
$CHCl_3$	Mice / Strain A / F / Liver[a]	Olive oil / gavage	Positive
	Mice / B6C3F1 / M / Liver[b]	Corn oil / gavage	Positive
	Mice / B6C3F1 / F / Liver[b]	Corn oil / gavage	Positive
	Mice / B6C3F1 / F / Liver[c]	Drinking water	Negative
	Mice / ICI / M / Kidney[d]	Toothpaste / gavage	Positive
	Mice / ICI/M/Kidney[d]	Arachis oil / gavage	Positive
	Mice / C57BL / M[a]	Toothpaste / gavage	Negative
	Mice / CBA / M[a]	Toothpaste / gavage	Negative
	Mice / CF1 / M[a]	Toothpaste / gavage	Negative
	Rats / Osb.-M. / M / kidney[b]	Corn oil / gavage	Positive
	Rats / Osb.-M. / M / thyroid[b]	Corn oil / gavage	Positive
	Rats / Osb.-M. / M / kidney[c]	Drinking water	Positive
	Rats / Osb.-M. / M / thyroid[c]	Drinking water	Negative
$CHBrCl_2$	Mice / B6C3F1 / M / Kidney[e]	Corn oil / gavage	Positive
	Mice / B6C3F1 / F / Liver[e]	Corn oil / gavage	Positive
	Rats / F344 / M / Kidney[e]	Corn oil / gavage	Positive
	Rats / F344 / F / Kidney[e]	Corn oil / gavage	Positive
	Rats / F344 / M / Intestine[e]	Corn oil / gavage	Positive
	Rats / F344/F / Intestine[e]	Corn oil / gavage	Positive
$CHBr_2Cl$	Mice / B6C3F1 / M / Liver[f]	Corn oil / gavage	Positive
$CHBr_3$	Rats / F344 / M / Intestine[g]	Corn oil / gavage	Positive
	Rats / F344 / F/Intestine[g]	Corn oil / gavage	Positive
	Haloacetates		
$ClCH_2COOH$	Mice / B6C3F1 / M and F[h]	Water / gavage	Negative
	Rats / F344 / M and F[h]	Water / gavage	Negative
	Rats / F344 / M[i]	Drinking water	Negative
Cl_2COOH	Mice / B6C3F1 / M / Liver[j]	Drinking water	Positive
	Mice / B6C3F1 / M / Liver[k]	Drinking water	Positive
	Mice / B6C3F1 / M / Liver[l]	Drinking water	Positive
	Mice / B6C3F1 / F / Liver[m]	Drinking water	Positive
	Mice / B6C3F1 / M / Liver[n]	Drinking water	Positive
	Rats / F-344 / M / Liver[o]	Drinking water	Positive
Cl_3COOH	Mice / B6C3F1 / M / Liver[j]	Drinking water	Positive
	Mice / B6C3F1 / M / Liver[k]	Drinking water	Positive
	Mice / B6C3F1 / F / Liver[m]	Drinking water	Positive
	Mice / B6C3F1 / M / Liver[n]	Drinking Water	Positive
	Rats / F344 / M / Liver[l]	Drinking Water	Negative
	Bromate		
	Rats / F344 / M and F / Kidney[p]	Drinking water	Positive
	Rats / F344 / M / Kidney[q]	Drinking water	Positive
	Rats / F344 / M / thyroid[r]	Drinking water	Positive
	Rats / F344 / M / peritonium[p]	Drinking water	Positive
	Hamsters / Syr. / M / kidney[q]	Drinking water	Positive
	2,4,6-Trichlorophenol		
	Mice / B6C3F1 / M and F / Liver[s]	Diet	Positive
	Rats / F344/M and F / Leukemia[s]	Diet	Positive

TABLE 9-5   (*Continued*)

By-product	Species / Strain / Sex / Site	Vehicle / Route	Result
	Aldehydes		
Trichloroacetaldehyde	Mice / B6C3F1/Neo. / Liver[i]	Single oral	Positive
	Mice / B6C3F1 / M / Liver[i]	Drinking water	Positive
Formaldehyde	Rats / F344 / M and F / Nasal[u]	Inhalation	Positive
	Rats / Wistar / M / Nasal[v]	Inhalation	Positive
	Rats / S-D/M and F / Leukemia[w]	Drinking water	Positive
Acetaldehyde	Rats / Wistar / M and F / Nasal[x]	Inhalation	Positive
	Hydrogen peroxide		
	Mice / C57BL / M and F / Intestine[y]	Drinking water	Positive

[a] Eschenbrenner and Miller (1945)
[b] NCI (1976)
[c] Jorgenson et al. (1985)
[d] Roe et al. (1979)
[e] NTP (1986)
[f] Dunnick et al. (1985)
[g] NTP (1989)
[h] NTP (1990)
[i] DeAngelo et al. (1997)
[j] Herren-Freund et al. (1987)
[k] Bull et al. (1990)
[l] Daniel et al. (1992)
[m] Pereira et al. (1996)

[n] Stauber and Bull (1997)
[o] DeAngelo et al. (1996)
[p] Kurokawa et al. (1983)
[q] Kurokawa et al. (1986a)
[r] Takamura et al. (1985)
[s] NCI (1979)
[t] Rijhsinghani et al. (1986)
[u] Kerns et al. (1983)
[v] Johannsen et al. (1986)
[w] Soffriti et al. (1989)
[x] Woutersen et al. (1984)
[y] Ito et al. (1981)

kg per day. These doses are much below those required to produce liver cancer, even when administered in corn oil. Therefore these route- and vehicle-specific responses to chloroform are not simply related to differences in the pharmacokinetics and metabolism of chloroform. Similar caution should be exercised in accepting evidence of liver tumor induction with the other trihalomethane / corn oil combinations, bromodichloromethane (NTP, 1986) and dibromochloromethane (Dunnick et al., 1985), as being relevant to humans exposure through drinking water.

The weak mutagenic activity of chloroform calls into question its ability to initiate tumors. Evidence that chloroform is capable of inducing point mutations is largely negative (Bull et al., 1986). The few positive results found in bacterial or in vitro systems are counterbalanced by an inability to demonstrate covalent interactions with nucleic acids in vivo (Diaz-Gomez and Castro, 1980; Reitz et al., 1982). This includes lack of an ability of chloroform to induce unscheduled DNA synthesis in the liver of mice (Larson et al., 1994b).

While chloroform's carcinogenic properties appear to be limited primarily to the liver and kidney, bromodichloromethane and bromoform induce tumors of the colon (NTP, 1986, 1989). These responses required high doses, 50 and 200 mg / kg, respectively. Thus it seems unlikely that these chemicals have sufficient potency among themselves to account for the colorectal cancer observed in epidemiology studies. Colon cancer is rare in F344 rats. In the history of the National Toxicology Program, brominated compounds appear to commonly target the colon of the rat (Melnick et al., 1994). Therefore there may be reason to be concerned over the many brominated by-products found in chlorinated drinking water that have yet to be characterized toxicologically.

Bromodichloromethane, dibromochloromethane, and bromoform appear capable of inducing point mutation in *Salmonella* (Zeiger et al., 1990). All of the brominated THMs appear to be capable of inducing mutation in the mouse lymphoma assay. Moreover bromodichloromethane has been shown to produce stable adducts to DNA in the intestine (Bull et al., 1995) and one of its major target tissues in the rat (Lilly et al., 1997). It is probable that effects of these chemicals in the liver of mice and perhaps the kidney are similar to chloroform in that they all produce tissue damage and reparative hyperplasia at the doses they induce tumors. There are no specific data to demonstrate that a nongenotoxic mechanism could be responsible for the nonhepatic tumor sites resulting form treatment of animals with the brominated THMs.

HAs Dichloroacetate and trichloroacetate have been shown to be potent inducers of hepatic tumors in B6C3F1 mice (Herren-Freund et al., 1987; Bull et al., 1990b; DeAngelo et al., 1991, 1997; Daniel et al., 1992; Pereira, 1996; Stauber and Bull, 1997). A sharp upturn in the dose-response curve for dichloroacetate-induced liver tumors which has been associated with the doses that produce severe hepatic damage (Bull et al., 1990a) and the induction of reparative hyperplasia (Sanchez and Bull, 1990), suggests that these tumors may be partially caused by liver damage. The induction of acinar necrosis is seen irregularly at 2 g/L (Stauber and Bull, 1997) and in experiments lasting for a few months appears to be absent at lower doses that will ultimately induce a high incidence of hepatic tumors (Kato-Weinstein et al., 1998). Moreover Stauber et al. (1998a) has shown that dichloroacetate incorporated into the media will stimulate the growth of colonies obtained from suspensions of hepatocytes of male B6C3F1 mice in soft agar. The cells in these colonies had the same phenotype (c-Jun positive) that is found in tumors induced by dichloroacetate in vivo (Stauber and Bull, 1997). Anchorage-dependent growth is one characteristic of an initiated cell population. It is improbable that cytotoxicity could play a significant role in this response. Therefore these data strongly suggest that dichloroacetate is stimulating the growth of spontaneously initiated cells in the mouse liver. The number of cells isolated from mice that grew into colonies in the presence of dichloroacetate was significantly increased by 14 days of treatment prior to the isolation of hepatocytes (Stauber et al., 1998a). This pretreatment decreased the concentration of dichloroacetate required to produce significant growth from 500 to $20 \mu M$. It is probable that this increased sensitivity of hepatocytes obtained from pretreated mice is due to the less rapid metabolic clearance of dichloroacetate from pretreated animals (Gonzalez-Leon et al., 1997).

Considerable evidence is accumulating to suggest that the carcinogenic effects of dichloroacetate depend on its insulin-mimetic effects on the liver. Disturbances in glycogen metabolism are consistent with these effects (Kato-Weinstein et al., 1998a). Tumors induced by dichloroacetate express higher levels of the insulin receptor than surrounding normal tissue (Smith et al., 1998). Involvement of the insulin signaling pathway is of interest because of increasing evidence that individuals with diabetes mellitus are at greater risk for liver cancer than the general population (Wideroff et al., 1997). The glycogen storage abnormalities that are induced by dichloroacetate are also similar to pathology induced in individuals that suffer from glycogen storage diseases. Such individuals are at very high risk for liver cancer at young ages (Limmer et al., 1988; Narita et al., 1994).

Trichloroacetate-induced hepatocarcinogenesis in mice does not appear to depend on necrosis and reparative hyperplasia (Bull et al., 1990b; Sanchez and Bull, 1990; Stauber and Bull, 1997). Elcombe et al. (1985) suggested that the carcinogenic activity of trichloroacetate was dependent on its ability to induce peroxisome synthesis. Indeed a close correlation does exist between this response and hepatic carcinogenesis in mice (DeAngelo et al., 1989; Bull et al., 1990a; DeAngelo et al., 1991). Tumors induced by trichloroacetate carry a phenotype typical of peroxisome proliferators (Pereira, 1996; Stauber and Bull, 1997; Bannasch et al., 1997). It is perhaps related to a more frequent expression of the proto-oncogene, c-myc, in nodules within nodules induced by trichloroacetate than in those induced by dichloroacetate (Nelson et al., 1990). Tao et al. (1996) reported that trichloroacetate-induced tumors in female B6C3F1 mice lost heterozygosity in chromosome 6 much more frequently than those induced by dichloroacetate. A variety of other differences have been noted in the phenotypes of the tumors that are induced by the two compounds (Latendresse and Pereira, 1997). These seem to correlate to the more aggressive nature of trichloroacetate-induced liver tumors. Tumors induced by trichloroacetate do progress to carcinomas more readily than those of dichloroacetate when treatments were suspended after 37 weeks of treatment (Bull et al., 1990b) and actually appear to regress with intermittent exposure (Pereira, 1996). These observations held despite the fact that trichloroacetate-induced tumors were less frequent and smaller than dichloroacetate-induced tumors at dosing regimens utilizing 2 g/L of drinking water (Bull et al., 1990b).

Trichloroacetate also stimulates the growth of colonies of cells derived from liver suspensions from B6C3F1 mice on soft agar (Stauber et al., 1998a). Unlike dichloroacetate-induced colonies, those observed with trichloroacetate have a c-Jun negative phenotype. This is the same phenotype that is observed in trichloroacetate-induced tumors (Stauber and Bull, 1997). These data are consistent with the notion that the primary effect of trichloroacetate is to stimulate growth of spontaneously initiated cells present in the liver of B6C3F1 mice. It appears that the media concentrations required for this effect fall into the same range needed for the induction of peroxisome synthesis in vivo (DeAngelo et al., 1989).

Both dichloroacetate and trichloroacetate have been shown to be very effective tumor promoters in the liver of B6C3F1 mice. Pereira and Phelps (1996) found dose–response curves for the promotion of N-methyl-N-nitrosourea-initiated tumors to closely parallel the dose–response observed for whole carcinogenicity of these compounds. Dichloroacetate had a very shallow, if not flat, dose–response curve at concentrations below 1 g/L, but the slope was sharply increased to very large tumor yields at doses in excess of 2 g/L. This is very similar to the dose–response demonstrated by Bull et al. (1990b). In contrast, the dose–response for trichloroacetate was linear within the observable range. The phenotype of tumors in female mice whose growth was promoted by dichloroacetate was overwhelming eosinophilic, whereas those promoted by trichloroacetate were basophilic. These differences were observed in a second study by the same group (Pereira et al., 1997) where the effects of mixtures of dichloroacetate and trichloroacetate were used to promote tumors. These data provide strong evidence that much, if not all, of dichloroacetate and trichloroacetate's activities as carcinogens are as a tumor promoters. However, the available evidence indicates that the two chemicals select different phenotypes of initiated cells.

Monochloroacetate is apparently without carcinogenic properties. Recent studies by the National Toxicology Program (NTP, 1990a) and by DeAngelo et al. (1997) found no evidence that it could increase tumor incidence in either B6C3F1 mice or F344 rats.

There are several studies that suggest that the HAs are mutagenic. Some of the positive data available are difficult to interpret and at the same time there is a growing body of negative data. The most serious difficulty is the excessive concentrations administered in in vitro or bacterial assays, and those that are achieved in the systemic circulation by the consumption of high concentrations in drinking water. In general, concentrations achieved in vivo with 2 g/L in drinking water (near a maximally tolerated concentration) are approximately $300 \mu M$ at peak hours of drinking behavior (Kato-Weinstein et al., 1998), and this falls off to about $10 \mu M$ as drinking behavior decreases. In vitro studies frequently range into the high mM concentrations, and the use of intraperitoneal injections of 200 mg/kg increase the concentrations to an excess of 1 mM (Kato-Weinstein et al., 1998) in mice. Second, some of the test procedures have been conducted without ensuring that the media-buffering capacity was sufficient to prevent significant alterations in pH to occur when large amounts of these very strong acids are added to the system. Finally the design of in vivo studies that ostensibly provide evidence of in vivo mutagenic effects has been such as to make it very difficult to differentiate between mutagenesis and selection. Chloroacetate was found inactive in *Salmonella typhimurium* strain TA1535 (Rannug et al., 1976). Dichloroacetate produced a very weak mutagenic response in strain TA98 (i.e., less than the two fold increase over the spontaneous rate of reversion that is usually taken as minimum requirement for a positive result) and an equivocal response with TA1538 (Herbert et al., 1980). Trichloroacetate appears to be inactive in *Salmonella* (Nestmann et al., 1980). Recently, Bhunya and Behera (1987) tested trichloroacetic acid in vivo for induction of chromosome aberrations, micronuclei, and spermhead abnormalities. The authors reported induction of chromosome aberrations in bone marrow cells and micronuclei in lymphocytes. In an attempt to repeat these studies, MacKay et al. (1995) found that the induction of micronuclei in lymphocytes was probably related to the injection of trichloroacetic acid, since the response could not be repeated when the free acid was neutralized before testing.

Several attempts have been made to detect HA-induced damage to nuclear DNA or indications of mutagenic effects in the target organs. The most interesting of the studies is the increased recovery of mutant cells from the *lacI* transgenic mouse (Leavitt et al., 1997). Increases were observed when mice had been treated with 1 or 3.5 g/L for 60 weeks but not at shorter time intervals. While the authors took care to be sure that nodules and tumors were excluded from the sampling, Stauber and Bull (1997) demonstrated that there are numerous lesions that are smaller than nodules in B6C3F1 mice maintained on 2 g/L dichloroacetate for only 40 weeks. It was inevitable that these smaller lesions were included within the tissue samples described. Given the marked stimulation of cell replication that occurs within lesions in mice, it is not possible to determine if the effect reported by Leavitt et al. (1997) is due to mutagenic effects of dichloroacetate or if it demonstrated an ability to selectively stimulate the growth of tumor phenotype. It has also been argued that a change in mutation spectra in the H-ras codon 61 within dichloroacetate-induced tumors suggests that it is acting as a mutagen (Anna et al., 1994; Ferriera-Gonzalez et al., 1996). However, it has been pointed out that this effect can be explained by selection as easily as it can be by chemically induced mutation (Maronpot et al., 1995). It now appears that the increase in mutation in this codon is something that is highly dependent on when the animals are being sacrificed. In the case of dichloroacetate, tumors that are taken at one year and at lower doses (e.g., 0.5 g/L) do not display the spectra previously reported (Orner et al., 1998). Schroeder et al. (1997) have also shown that the mutation frequency and spectra seen in female mice were also more like that seen with other tumor promoters (Maronpot et al., 1995).

Austin et al. (1996) did find that dichloroacetate, when administered acutely in high doses, could increase the proportions of 8-hydroxy-2-deoxyguanosine to 2-deoxyguanosine in nuclear DNA of the mouse liver. However, significant elevations could not be detected in the liver of mice maintained on drinking water containing 2 g/L dichloroacetate (Parrish et al., 1996). Thus, while there are data that might suggest that dichloroacetate has some mutagenic properties, it is not clear that this weak activity plays any role in the induction of liver tumors. The data that suggest that dichloroacetate is mutagenic must be considered in the context of the fact that in vivo data strongly indicates that these compounds act primarily as tumor promoters.

Bromine substitution on the dihaloacetates appears to increase the probability that they possess mutagenic effects. In the *Salmonella* fluctuation assay and the SOS chromotest (Giller et al., 1997), dibromoacetate was 10 to 100 times as potent as dichloroacetate, and while monochloroacetate was negative, monobromoacetate was positive. Unlike previous studies, the inclusion of S9 as a means of increasing metabolism of the HAs decreased the potency of these chemicals in these tests. This is more consistent with the behavior of these chemicals in vivo. The much higher metabolic clearance of the brominated dihaloacetates (Schultz et al., personal communication) relative to dichloroacetate contrasts with the greater potency of dichloroacetate as a liver carcinogen. This suggests that dichloroacetate itself is responsible for the liver cancer. This is reinforced by the greater effectiveness of dichloroacetate in inducing colony formation from the liver of pretreated mice than naïve mice. As indicated above, such pretreatment sharply inhibits the metabolism of dichloroacetate, and it is assumed that is the reason for an increased sensitivity as exposure is extended out in time.

The carcinogenicity of the brominated HAs has not been studied extensively. Preliminary data from the author's laboratory clearly indicate that bromodichloroacetate, bromochloroacetate, and dibromoacetate produce dose-related increases in liver cancer in male B6C3F1 mice. The hepatocarcinogenic activity of the dihaloacetates all seem to be at least loosely associated with the disturbances in insulin signaling (Kato-Weinstein et al., 1998b). They are approximately equivalent in potency at low doses, but the short latency of induction of liver tumors concentrations of dichloroacetate in water of 2 g / L and above appears to be specific to dichloroacetate. As indicated earlier, these high doses of dichloroacetate also cause glycogen to be deposited in the liver much more rapidly as well (Stauber et al., 1998b; Kato-Weinstein et al., 1998b). Bromodichloroacetate also induces glycogen accumulation in the liver of mice, but this is delayed for three to four weeks. This and its apparent inability to induce peroxisome proliferation appear to distinguish bromodichloroacetate from trichloroacetate (Kato-Weinstein et al., 1998b). It is probable that the similarity with dichloroacetate is related to its metabolic conversion to that compound (Xu et al., 1995). Its more rapid metabolism is also likely responsible for bromodichloroacetate's ineffectiveness as a peroxisome proliferator.

There are trends in these preliminary data for the brominated HAs that suggest other target organs may be important as well. Lymphoma and lung tumor incidence are significantly elevated in B6C3F1 mice. In separate experiments, F344 rats developed aberrant crypt foci in the distal colon as a result of treatment with dibromoacetate (So and Bull, 1995). These preliminary data suggest that the brominated HAs may produce cancer in organs other than the liver.

The ability to induce oxidative damage to nuclear DNA of the liver of mice was also much higher with bromochloroacetate and dibromoacetate than with dichloroacetate, and bromodichloroacetate was much more effective than trichloroacetate (Austin et al., 1996). Increased levels of 8-hydroxy-2-deoxyguanosine were observed at concentrations in the drinking water that have been shown to be tumorigenic in vivo. Thus the production of oxidative damage to DNA may not play a big role in the induction of liver cancer, but this property could be important in other target organs of the haloacetates.

MX   The strong mutagen, 3-chloro-4-(dichloromethyl)-5-hydroxy-2(5H)-furanone (MX) has also been shown to be carcinogenic in male and female Wistar rats (Komulainen et al., 1997). MX was administered in drinking water at concentrations that resulted in average daily doses of 0.4, 1.3, and 5.0 mg / kg per day. The most prominent tumor site was follicular adenoma and carcinoma of the thyroid at all doses in both sexes. At the highest dose both males and females were also found to have cortical adenomas of the adrenal gland. In addition adenocarcinoma and fibroadenoma of the breast, cholangiomas and adenomas of the liver, and lymphoma and leukemia were found in female rats. Males were found to have an increased incidence of alveolar and bronchiolar adenomas and adenomas of the Langerhans cells of the pancreas only at the high dose. These data identify MX as the most potent carcinogen identified to date in drinking water. However, this higher potency does not offset the very low concentrations at which it occurs in drinking water.

Miscellaneous By-products   Members of other classes of chlorination by-product have only received cursory study as carcinogens. Several by-products of chlorination have been shown to be carcinogenic are produced in such small concentrations (e.g., 2,4,6-trichlorophenol) or are of questionable importance by the oral route of exposure (formaldehyde and acetaldehyde).

There is little question that inhalation of formaldehyde is a carcinogenic hazard at high dose levels (Kerns et al., 1983; Johannsen et al., 1986) In addition to being carcinogenic, however, formaldehyde is clearly genotoxic (Ma and Harris, 1988). Although one study which exposed rats to formaldehyde in drinking water indicated an increased incidence of leukemias (Soffriti et al., 1989), two more complete studies failed to produce such a response in other strains of rat (Til et al., 1989; Tobe et al., 1989). Even if the Soffriti studies are correct, the small concentrations of formaldehyde contribute very little to calculated risks of cancer attributed to identified chlorination by-products (Bull and Kopfler, 1991). There is no evidence that acetaldehyde is a carcinogen by the oral route of administration despite some evidence that it produces nasal tumors when inhaled (Woutersen et al., 1984; Woutersen and Feron, 1987).

Trichloroacetaldehyde presents a unique case. Rijhsinghani et al. (1986) found that a single oral dose of trichloroacetaldehyde administered to 15-day-old B6C3F1 mice resulted in hepatic tumors. The unconventional design and small numbers of animals used in this study makes it difficult to evaluate. Daniel et al. (1992a) have found increases in hepatic tumors with a more conventionally designed experiment. It is notable that trichloroacetaldehyde is metabolized to trichloroacetate (Cooper and Friedman, 1958; Gorecki et al., 1990; Ni et al., 1996) and to dichloroacetate (Abbas et al., 1991), and it appears to be weakly mutagenic in *Salmonella* (Waskell, 1978) and eukaryotic systems (Bronzetti et al., 1984; Crebelli et al., 1985). It also produced chromosomal aberrations and nondysjunction of chromosomes (Sora and Carone, 1987; Russo et al., 1984). Therefore its contribution to cancer might be mediated through several mechanisms. However, the metabolism of chloral hydrate is very rapid (Merdink et al., 1998a), and it seems improbable that the clastogenic effects reported at very high doses would be of any importance at the very low concentrations of chloral hyrate that are found in finished drinking water.

Several other chemicals that have been identified in drinking water have been shown to act as tumor initiators in the mouse skin when applied topically. Among these are chloroacetonitrile, bromochloroacetonitrile and dibromoacetonitrile (Bull et al., 1985), 2-chloropropenal, 2-bromopropenal, and 1,3-dichloropropanone (Robinson et al., 1989). Trichloroacetonitrile has been reported to induce micronuclei in gastrointestinal tract of mice (Lin et al., 1990). A number of these chemicals were generally direct acting mutagens in *Salmonella*, or they induced sister chromatid exchange in cultured mammalian cells (Bull et al., 1985; Meier et al., 1985b). Dichloroacetonitrile has been shown capable of binding to nucleic acids in vitro and the other HANs are capable of alkylating nucleophiles (Daniel et al., 1986). A number of other directly active mutagenic chemicals identified as by-products of chlorination were active as tumor initiators in the mouse skin (Robinson et al., 1989).

A general conclusion can be made that the addition of chemical disinfectants to drinking water results in the formation of chemicals that are capable of inducing cancer under controlled conditions in experimental animals. Thus, in a very nonspecific way, there is support for the epidemiological data that suggests that chlorination of drinking water may pose a carcinogenic hazard. However, as specifics of the toxicological findings are brought to bear, it is difficult to conclude that they provide strong support for the epidemiological findings. There are two problems. The first is that the target organs identified with most of the by-products that have been studied in animals are predominately the liver and kidney. This is especially true if each of the tested by-product's concentrations in drinking water are expressed as a ratio of the lowest dose in which they produce cancer in experimental animals. The prominent target organs in humans are the bladder, the colon, and the rectum. There is lesser support for other sites, such as the pancreas. A pattern that is emerging with the brominated by-products, however, suggests that the colon could be a significant target for these chemicals. On the other hand, it is difficult to suggest that the brominated by-products studied to date are sufficiently potent to account for the epidemiological findings.

Effects of Disinfectants and Their By-products on Reproduction

Inorganic By-products   Treatment with chlorine dioxide during the immediate postnatal period produced delayed exploratory behavior in 16 to 20-day-old rat pups (Orme et al., 1985) and decreased cell numbers in the cerebellum and forebrain in 11-day-old pups (Taylor and Pfohl, 1985). It was assumed that these effects were secondary to the depressed serum thyroxine levels produced at the same doses (14 mg/Kg per day). Subsequent work by Toth et al. (1990) failed to find effects on thyroid hormone levels or biologically significant effects on brain development in another strain of rat. Since the effects observed by Orme et al. (1985) and Taylor and Pfohl (1985) were modest, it is difficult to determine if the findings of Toth et al. (1990) are due to minor differences in strain sensitivity or if they are truly conflicting results.

Moore et al. (1980) reported that chlorite at a concentration of 100 mg/L reduced the conception rate and the number of pups alive at weaning in A/J mice. A significantly reduced pup weight at weaning was interpreted as indicating that chlorite retarded growth rate.

Carlton et al. (1987) examined the effects of 0, 1, 10, and 100 mg of sodium chlorite/L of drinking water administered for 14 days prior to mating and throughout the 10 days breeding period that was allowed to evaluate reproductive function in male Long-Evans rats. There was a significant increase in abnormal sperm morphology and a decrease in the progressive movement of sperm at 100 and 500 mg/L. Female rats were treated with concentrations of 0, 1, 10 and 100 mg/L throughout gestation and lactation. There was no sign of impaired reproductive function when males (treated as described above) were mated with these females. Decreases in the concentrations of tri-iodothyronine and thyroxine in blood were noted in both male and female rats treated with 100 mg/L. Apparently this group and the corresponding control group were the only ones examined for thyroid hormone levels, since no data were provided for the lower treatment concentrations.

Harrington et al. (1995b) examined the developmental toxicity of chlorite in New Zealand white rabbits. The rabbits were treated with 0, 200, 600, or 1200 mg sodium chlorite/L in their drinking water from day 7 to day 19 of pregnancy. The animals were necropsied on day 28. There were no dose-related increases in defects identified. Minor skeletal anomalies increased with increasing concentration of chlorite in water; food consumption was depressed.

Collectively the available data suggest that there are no significant reproductive or developmental hazards associated with chlorite as long as doses are kept well below concentrations that produce oxidative damage to erythrocytes. There may be some concern over changes in thyroid status identified in the Carlton et al. (1987) study. However, depressions of thyroid hormone levels have not been associated with chlorite treatment in other species (Bercz et al., 1982).

Organic By-products

HAs   Dichloroacetate does produce testicular toxicity when administered at high doses in drinking water. These effects were first noted in studies of the general toxicity of dichloroacetate (Katz et al., 1981) and were discussed above. Cicmanec et al. (1991)

followed up on these original observations in dogs a detected degeneration of testicular epithelium and syncytial giant cell formation at doses as low as 12.5 mg/kg.

Toth et al. (1992) conducted an examination of Dichloroacetate's ability to modify male reproductive function in Long-Evans rats. Reduced weights of accessory organ (epididymus, cauda epididymus, and preputial gland) weights were observed at doses as low as 31 mg/kg per day for 10 weeks. Epididymal sperm counts were found to be depressed, and sperm morphology increasingly abnormal at doses of 62 mg/kg and above. These latter effects were accompanied by changes in sperm motion analysis. Fertility was tested in overnight matings and was found to be depressed only at the highest dose evaluated 125 mg/kg per day.

Spermatotoxicity of dichloroacetate has been studied further by Linder et al. (1997b) who found effects at doses of 160 mg/kg per day. The authors found that the testicular toxicity of dichloroacetate in Sprague-Dawley rats increased significantly as the duration of exposure was extended in time. This progressive increase in testicular toxicity may be related to the reduced metabolic clearance of dichloroacetate that occurs as the result of pretreatment (Gonzalez-Leon et al., 1997).

A series of papers establish that dibromoacetate is significantly more potent than dichloroacetate as a testicular toxicant in Sprague-Dawley rats (Linder et al., 1994a, b; 1995). Dibromoacetate produced mild effects on spermiation at doses as low as 10 mg/kg with repeated doses (Linder et al., 1994b). Effects were progressively more severe as doses increased to 30, 90, and 270 mg/kg (Linder et al., 1997a). With prolonged exposure, the highest dose becomes severely toxic. At lower doses (50 mg/kg) there were no significant effects on male fertility, although mating behavior may have been altered (Linder et al., 1995).

Dichloroacetate was found to be more potent that trichloroacetate in inhibiting in vitro fertilization of B5D2F1 mouse gametes (Cosby and Dukelow, 1992). The percent of gametes fertilized dropped from 87% to 67.3% at the lowest concentration tested, 100 mg/L. At 1000 mg/L, 71.8% of the gametes were fertilized. Both responses were statistically different from their concurrent control groups.

HANs   The HANs appear to be the most specific reproductive toxins among chlorination by-products. Smith et al. (1987) found that dichloroacetonitrile and trichloroacetonitrile reduced fertility and early implantation loss in Long-Evans rats. Subsequent study demonstrated that trichloroacetonitrile, the most toxic member of this group, produced embryolethality and resorptions at doses of 7.5 mg/kg per day (Smith et al., 1988) A significant number of malformations were detected in the cardiovascular system in the same dose range and at doses considerably below those found to be maternally toxic. Dichloroacetonitrile did produce embryolethality at doses that were not maternally toxic but produced soft tissue malformations only at doses that were (Smith et al., 1989a). Thus trichloroacetonitrile may well be teratogenic in humans, but the doses expected from drinking water are still less than 1/1000 of those required to produce these effects in rats.

Effects on Development

THMs   Chloroform is the only THM that has been evaluated for teratogenic effects. Schwetz et al. (1974) noted some minor malformations in Sprague-Dawley rats exposed to high levels as chloroform vapor (30, 100, and 300 ppm) of the type that are associated with nonspecific delays in development. At the highest two doses there was clear evidence of embryolethality. In terms of systemic dose, these levels are orders of magnitude higher than exposures that are encountered in drinking water. Therefore reproductive and developmental effects by chloroform at doses that are not overtly toxic to the mother are unlikely.

HAs   Chlorinated acetates appear to be true developmental toxins. Trichloroacetate produced malformations in the cardiovascular system of Long-Evans rats at doses of 330 mg / kg and higher. Skeletal malformations were observed at doses of 1200 mg / kg, but these doses were maternally toxic (Smith et al., 1989b). Dichloroacetate also produced levocardia and malformations between the ascending aorta and right ventricle at doses of 140 mg / kg and above (Smith et al., 1992). Urogenital defects (bilateral hydronephrosis and renal papilla) and defects of the orbit were observed. While not grossly toxic, 140 mg / kg did produce the enlarged liver typical of dichloroacetate. Higher doses (400 mg / kg) resulted in weight loss and progressively more severe toxicity. Epstein et al. (1992) attempted to more finely define the period of susceptibility to dichloroacetate-induced aorta / ventricular septal defects. Very high single doses, 2400 and 3500 mg / kg, were required to produce effects. An increasing severity of developmental effects was observed when lower doses were administered for several days, suggesting that this progressive increase in toxicity is probably related to the inhibition of metabolism of dichloroacetate that occurs with prior treatment (Gonzalez-Leon et al., 1997). Evidence of teratogenic effects with dichloroacetate are clear, but the doses required to produce these effects were five orders of magnitude higher than those encountered in chlorinated drinking water.

Richard and Hunter (1996) explored the quantitative structure activity relationships involved in the developmental toxicology of the haloacetates in whole embryo culture. Strong associations were found with the lowest unoccupied molecular orbital and acid dissociation constants. While these relationships may not hold for in vivo potency of the class because of intervening mechanisms involved in their metabolism and disposition, they do suggest some commonality in the mechanisms involved in developmental toxicities. The in vitro data suggest greater activity of the monohaloacetates, with the trihaloacetates and dihaloacetates being approximately equal in their potency as developmental toxins.

SUMMARY AND CONCLUSIONS

The past decade has seen significant strengthening of the data that relate the use of chlorinated drinking water with cancer in epidemiological studies. Laboratory-based research has been successful in demonstrating that a number of disinfectant by-products are capable of inducing cancer in animals. Parallel to these findings is limited evidence of reproductive and developmental toxicities with chlorinated water. As with the cancer epidemiology, there are experimental data in animals to demonstrate that some by-products have the properties of reproductive and developmental toxicants.

Movement away from the use of chlorine as a disinfectant cannot be treated simply. First, the simplicity of chlorination as a process allows it to be employed in systems of all sizes with minimal training of plant operators. Second, it is not clear that alternate methods of disinfection are any less likely to increase cancer risk than chlorine. Finally, the fact that alternative methods do not leave stable residuals is not generally satisfactory for maintaining the microbial quality of water during distribution. This almost ensures that either chlorine or chloramination will continue play some role in the treatment of water in the foreseeable future. It is fortunate that the revival of concerns over the microbiological contaminants of drinking water has made it apparent why decisions should not be made in this area without assembling the data necessary to make full evaluation of all the risks that are associated with changes in treatment processes.

The critical role that disinfection plays in the delivery of safe water makes it necessary to understand the health risks involved with more clarity than is usually required for regulatory action. There must be a path that clearly reduces health risks, whether they are microbial or chemical, before the large investments that are involved in the continual process of expansion and upgrading municipal and other public water systems can move forward with confidence. Therefore it is important that research done today focus on the resolution of these larger issues as quickly as possible. The most critical question is whether the risks identified with chlorinated drinking water are significant in quantitative terms. In practical terms, resolution of this issue with some certainty determines whether it is *necessary* to move to different technologies or not. It must always be kept in mind that there are many valid and important reasons for changing the processes involved in treating water other than health effects. Experts in the field have suggested that there are a variety of new technologies that should be implemented in drinking water treatment over the next several decades irrespective of whether chlorination proves to be an unacceptable risk to health or not. Such changes will come regardless of the hazards that might be identified with chlorination or other disinfectant processes. The degree of hazard only tells us if the technology change should come sooner rather than later.

The problem associated with chlorination now appears to be more closely identified with the by-products it produces rather than with the disinfectant itself. Toxicological data developed in the past decade reduce concerns over chlorine and / or chloramine residuals as important contributors to carcinogenic and developmental toxicities. This statement cannot as easily be made for some alternatives to chlorine that have sufficiently stable residuals to maintain the microbiological integrity of the water in the distribution system.

Most of the early work done with disinfectant by-products focused on by-products produced with the use of chlorine as the disinfectant. Because of the availability of data (IARC, 1991), the problem has been viewed as one of a few chlorine-substituted organic by-products, primarily because these are the chemicals for which toxicological data exist. It is becoming increasingly clear that other disinfectants produce by-products that are of concern, and significant attention must now be directed at the many compounds that are bromine-substituted.

Research to resolve these issues must be properly focused. The problem with the organic by-products of disinfection is that efforts directed at measuring occurrence of by-products, and of identifying hazards associated with them, tend to result in interminable complexity. No by-products (except chlorite and chlorate) appear to present hazards as a result of disinfection reactions outside the categories of carcinogenesis and reproductive and developmental toxicities at concentrations likely to be found in drinking water. Consequently the problem reduces to a question of how likely it is that by-products with these properties pose significant hazards at the low concentrations found in drinking water. To simplify the ensuing discussion, carcinogenic effects are discussed. However, the reader should recognize that similar directions must be taken in the area of developmental toxicities.

The first important point is that the experiments demonstrating the carcinogenicity of chlorination by-products have all been conducted at dose rates that are very much higher than those that would be anticipated for humans drinking chlorinated drinking water. Therefore it is impossible to assert that these chemicals are carcinogenic in humans at the concentrations encountered in drinking water. It must also be admitted that the diversity of chlorination by-products makes it highly unlikely that epidemiological methods will be able to identify the individual or group of by-products that are responsible for carcinogenic activity in humans.

Second, the by-products whose carcinogenic properties have been established in animals clearly act by several different mechanisms. The prototypical disinfectant by-product, chloroform, appears to act entirely as a cytotoxic agent. Therefore it is improbable that it contributes to the induction of cancer at all. In contrast, the brominated

THMs, the haloacetonitriles, several halogenated aldehydes and ketones, and MX are clearly mutagenic. Because of the cumulative nature of mutagenic damage, it has been generally accepted that such compounds have some finite probability of producing an adverse outcome even at very low doses. Such effects may be vanishingly small. The haloacetates appear to act by differentially modifying cell-signaling processes involved in cell division and cell death in initiated and normal cells in the same tissue. There is little precedent for considering the risks from low doses of agents that act by such modes of action. However, it is difficult to accept that minor fluctuations induced by these compounds superimposed on much greater variations that are involved as a result of eating a meal, for example, could be a significant health hazard. Nevertheless, it is important to note that the three modes of action identified are likely to be highly synergistic with one another at doses ordinarily used in the safety testing of chemicals in animals. This brings up a serious question of whether interactions seen at the experimental range can extend to doses that are below those that modify cell-signaling pathways. That seems to be an improbable scenario as well.

There are other bases of sensitivity and interactions that must be considered. The first are the expression or lack of expression of enzymes that are involved in the activation or detoxification of by-products. For example, based on recent data, individuals that express glutathione-S-transferase theta at high levels are expected to be more sensitive to the carcinogenic effects of brominated trihalomethanes. Perhaps of greater importance are potential deficiencies in those enzymes that are responsible for the very rapid clearance of the dihaloacetates. These compounds are actually active in the low µM concentration range. If their rate of clearance from the body were to be as long as trichloroacetate, they would pose significant problems. In fact a much prolonged half-life for dichloroacetate is probably the reason that dogs are so much more sensitive to its testicular and neurotoxic effects than other species. An interesting and related question is whether mixtures of the disinfectant by-products can modify each other's metabolism. Again, the ability of the haloacetates to essentially eliminate one pathway for their own clearance is of interest (Gonzalez-Leon et al., 1997; Austin et al., 1997). However, the nature of this enzyme and its ability to participate in the metabolism of other disinfectant by-products has not been explored. Modifications of this magnitude have enormous implications for eliminating the efficient first-pass metabolism of low levels of disinfectant by-products. This could be one basis for the apparent differences in target organs that have been observed in epidemiological rather than laboratory experiments.

A second possibility that must be entertained is that the critical disinfectant by-products have yet to be identified or toxicologically characterized. The rate-limiting step is the toxicological evaluation because even members of major classes like the haloacetates and haloacetonitriles have yet to be studied in sufficient depth to deal with either their carcinogenic or developmental effects at low doses. If a sufficiently active by-product is not identified among these major by-products, there is a serious question of whether the larger issues associated with chlorinated drinking water can be resolved in reasonable time by utilizing the most advanced toxicological methods.

From this evidence emerges a purpose for further epidemiological study. While epidemiology does not have the ability to pinpoint the most important disinfectant by-products, it can focus on those conditions that give rise to differing by-products. As outlined in the section on the production of disinfectant by-products, pH and the presence of the bromide ion have major impacts on the types of by-products that are formed with chlorination or ozonation of water. If epidemiology establishes that one of these conditions results in significantly larger risks, it will

1. Add considerable support to the hypothesis that there is increased cancer risk from chlorinated water.

2. Provide a real and important insight into the type of by-products that should be pursued more aggressively with toxicological methods.

In conclusion, evidence that there may be some adverse health effects associated with the use of chemical disinfectants has continued to grow. There is little reason to suspect substantial differences in toxicological hazards or carcinogenic risks between disinfectants (Bull and Kopfler, 1991). Nevertheless, there are persistent relationships between chlorination of drinking water and the occurrence of bladder and colorectal cancer in human populations. The pursuit of this question by randomly testing by-products as they are identified is unlikely to yield definitive answers to the problem in the foreseeable future. Research in the area must take a more rigorous and formal approach to the testing of alternative hypothesis that could explain the epidemiological data. Such an approach needs to supplant much of the concentrated and rather narrow testing of individual by-products in a plethora of short-term assays that has characterized this field in the past. The testing data that have been developed form a valuable data base, but it is now time to work toward problem resolution. That dictates approaches that deal with risk in as quantitative terms as is possible.

GLOSSARY

Chloramine   A chemical or group of chemicals formed from mixing chlorine and ammonia in water. Depending on the relative amounts of chlorine and ammonia and pH, the actual chemical form can be monochloramine (most desired), dichloramine, or trichloramine. Chloramine is frequently used as a residual disinfectant because it is more stable than hypochlorous acid or hypochlorite. It is also referred to as combined chlorine.

Chloramination   Disinfection of water that utilizes chloramine.

Chlorination   Disinfection of water by adding chlorine gas or solutions of hypochlorite salts.

Chlorine   In water, the products of hydration following the introduction of chlorine into water. Depending on pH, the major forms are hypochlorite and hypochlorous acid which are in an equilibrium controlled by the pH of the water.

Chlorine dioxide   A disinfectant based on a dioxide of chlorine (i.e., ClO_2). It possesses and unpaired electron and is unstable as a gas, so it must be generated on site in water.

Cross-connections   Inadvertent connections of service pipes and mains intended to carry drinking water with counterparts intended for other purposes (i.e., conveyance of sewage)

Disinfection   A general description of a number of processes that can be employed to eliminate or control the growth of organisms in drinking water.

Primary disinfection includes processes employed early in the treatment of drinking water in order to inactivate all infectious agents hat might have contaminated a water being utilized as a source of drinking water. Disinfectants that are rapidly lethal (i.e., with the shortest contact time) are most desirable (ozone, chlorine, or chlorine dioxide). A secondary intent of these processes is to control microbial fowling of equipment in the treatment plant.

Secondary disinfection is intended to control the regrowth of organisms within the drinking water distribution system. Disinfectant is added as it leaves the treatment plant or in booster stations in the distribution system. The emphasis is to maintain effective concentrations of disinfectant throughout the distribution system. Within the distribution system there are inevitably areas of low flow or actual dead ends in where a residual disinfectant may need to be present for many days.

Postdisinfection is another term of secondary disinfection.

Distribution systems   For drinking water, includes the mains and pipes that deliver water from its source, with or without intervening treatment, to the consumers of the water.

Finished water   Water that has been treated to drinking water specifications.

Haloacetates   (Haloacetic acids, HAs) A group of important disinfectant by-products in which halogens (most frequently chlorine or bromine) are substituted on the alpha carbon of acetic acid. Dihalo-and trihalo-forms are the most common. Monochloro-and monobromo-acetates are generally found at significantly lower concentrations.

Haloacetonitriles   (HANs) The third most prevalent by-products of chlorination, with halogen substitution occurring on the alpha carbon of acetonitrile. Chlorine and bromine are the most common substituents.

Hypochlorous acid   The hydrated form of chlorine gas in water (HOCl).

Hypochlorite   The salt form of hypochlorous acid. The pKa of hypochlorous acid is approximately 7.5, so the predominate form of chlorine in water is a mixture of hypochlorous acid and hypochlorite.

MX   A commonly used abbreviation for a highly mutagenic chemical produced in the chlorination of drinking water. The proper chemical name is 3-chloro-4-(dichloromethyl)-5-hydroxy-2(5H)-furanone.

Preoxidation   The application of a oxidant chemical early in treatment to achieve a goal, one of which can be disinfection. Preoxidation is also used to control certain types of taste and odor or other aesthetic problems

Oxidants   Chemical used in disinfection, such as chlorine, ozone, or chlorine dioxide, as well as chemicals like potassium permanganate or hydrogen peroxide.

Raw water   Water as it is extracted from a source prior to treatment.

Residual disinfectant   The disinfectant that remains in the water after "demand" has been satisfied. Demand consists of natural organic matter, ammonia, and other reactants with a disinfectant. some of the demand, usually a small fraction, is accounted for by reactions with microorganisms that are present in the source water. See secondary disinfection.

Source water   A body of source (river, lake, or reservoir) or groundwater that serves as a source of drinking water.

Total organic carbon   (TOC) Determined by the oxidation of organic material present in a water sample and measuring the amount of CO_2. It is usually expressed as milligram equivalents per liter of water. The CO_2 present as carbonates is subtacted from the total analysis. This and related measures are simply ways of characterizing that amount of organic matter that might serve as precursors to disinfectant by-product formation.

Total organic halogen   (TOX) A measured amount of halogen present in a water that is substituted on carbon. In general, it is expressed in chlorine equivalents.

Trihalomethanes   (THMs) Methanes substituted in three of four possible positions on carbon. The halogens are primarily chlorine and bromine, although iodine can also be substituted if iodide and related salts are present in the treated water.

REFERENCES

Abbas, R. R., C. S. Seckel, J. K Kidney, and J. W Fisher. 1996. Pharmacokinetic analysis of chloral hydrate and its metabolism in B6C3F1 mice. *Drug Metabol. Dispos.* 24: 1340–1346.

Abdel-Rahman, M. S. 1982. The presence of trihalomethanes in soft drinks. *J. Appl. Toxicol.* 2: 165–166.

Abdel-Rahman, M. S., D. Couri, and R. J. Bull. 1980. Kinetics of ClO_2 and effect of ClO_2- and ClO_3- in drinking water on blood glutathione and hemolysis in rat and chicken. *J. Environ. Pathol. Toxicol.* 3: 431–449.

Acharya, S., K. Mehta, S. Rodrigues, J. Pereira, S. Krishnan, and C. V. Rao 1995. Administration of subtoxic doses of t-butyl alcohol and trichloroacetic acid to male Wistar rats to study the interactive toxicity. *Toxicol. Lett.* 80: 97–104.

Akin, E. W., J. C. Hoff, and E. C. Lippy. 1982. Waterborne outbreak control: Which disinfectant? *Environ. Health Perspect.* 46: 7–12.

Alavanja, M., I. Goldstein, and M. Susser. 1978. Case-control study of gastrointestinal and urinary tract cancer mortality and drinking water chlorination. In *Water Chlorination: Environment Impact and Health Effects*, vol. 2, eds. R. L. Jolley et al., pp. 395–409. Ann Arbor: Ann Arbor Science Publishers.

Anna, C. H., R. R. Maronpot, M. A. Pereira, J. F. Foley, D. E. Malarkey and M. W. Anderson. 1994. *Ras* proto-oncogene activation in dichloroacetic acid-, trichloroethylene- and tetrachloroethylene-induced liver tumors in B6C3F1 mice. *Carcinogenesis* 15: 2255–2261.

Austin, E. W., J. R. Okita, R. T. Okita, J. L. Larson, and R. J. Bull. 1995. Modification of lipoperoxidative effects of dichloroacetate and trichloroacetate is associated with peroxisome proliferation. *Toxicology* 97: 59–69.

Austin, E. W., J. M. Parrish, D. H. Kinder, and R. J. Bull. 1996. Lipid peroxidation and formation of 8-hydroxydeoxyguanosine from acute doses of halogenated acetic acids. *Fundam. Appl. Toxicol.* 31: 77–82.

Austin, E. W., and R. J. Bull. 1997. Effect of pretreatment with dichloroacetate or trichloroacetate on the metabolism of bromodichloroacetate. *J. Toxicol. Environ. Health* 52: 367–383.

AWWA (American Water Works Association). 1982. Disinfection Committee Report. *JWWA.* 74: 376–380.

Baker, C. C., and D. B. Bursill. 1990. South Australian water: A disinfection problem. In *Water Chlorination; Chemistry, Environmental Impact and Health Effects*, vol. 6, eds. R. L. Jolley et al., pp. 47–59. Chelsea, MI: Lewis Publishers.

Bannasch, P., F. Klimek, and D. Mayer. 1997. Early bioenergetic changes in hepatocarcinogenesis: Preneoplastic phenotypes mimic responses to insulin and thyroid hormones. *J. Bioenerget. Biomembranes* 29: 303–313.

Bean, J. A., P. Isacson, W. J. Hausler Jr., and J. Kohler. 1982. Drinking water and cancer incidence in Iowa. I. Trends and incidence by source of drinking water and size of municipality. *Am. J. Epidemiol.* 116: 912–923.

Bercz, J. P., L. Jones, L. Garner, D. Murray, D. A. Ludwig, and J. Boston. 1982. Subchronic toxicity of chlorine dioxide and related compounds in drinking water in the nonhuman primate. *Environ. Health Perspect.* 46: 47–55.

Bhunya, S. P. and B. C. Behera. 1987. Relative genotoxicity of trichloroacetic acid (TCA) as revealed by different cytogenetic assays: Bone marrow chromosome aberration, micronucleus and sperm-head abnormality in the mouse. *Mutation Res.* 188: 215–221.

Blackshear, P. J., P. A. Holloway, and K. G. Alberti. 1974. The metabolic effects of sodium dichloroacetate in the starved rat. *Biochem. J.* 142: 279–286.

Blazak, W. F., J. R. Meier, B. E. Stewart, D. C. Blachman, and J. T. Deahl. 1988. Activity of 1,1,1- and 1,1,3-trichloroacetones in a chromosomal aberration assay in CHO cells and the micronucleus and spermhead abnormality assays in mice. *Mutation Res.* 206: 431–438.

Bolyard, M., P. S. Fair, and D. P. Hautman. 1993. Sources of chlorate ion in U.S. drinking water. *JAWWA* 85: 81–88.

Bove, F. J., M. C. Fulcomer, J. B. Klotz, J. Esmart, E. M. Dufficy, and J. E. Savrin. 1995. Public drinking water contamination and birth outcomes. *Am. J. Epidemiol.* 141: 850–862.

Brenniman, G. R., J. Vasilomanolakis-Lagos, and J. Amsel. 1980. Case-control study of cancer deaths in Illinois communities served by chlorinated or nonchlorinated water. In *Water Chlorination: Environmental Impact and Health Effects*, vol. 3, eds. R. L. Jolley et al., pp. 1043–1057. Ann Arbor: Ann Arbor Science Publishers.

Bronzetti, G., A. Galli, C. Corsi, E. Cundari, R. D. Del Carratone, R. Nieri, and M. Paolini. 1984. Genetic and biochemical investigation on chloral hydrate *in vitro* and *in vivo*. *Mutation Res.* 141: 19–22.

Bruschi, S. A., and R. J. Bull. 1993. In vitro cytotoxicity of mono-, di- and trichloroacetate and its modulation by peroxisome proliferation. *Fundam. Appl. Toxicol.* 21: 366–375.

Bull, R. J., M. Robinson, J. R. Meier, and J. A. Stober. 1982. Use of biological assay systems to assess the relative carcinogenic hazards of disinfection by-products. *Environ. Health Perspect.* 46: 215–228.

Bull, R. J., J. R. Meier, M. Robinson, H. P. Ringhand, R. P. Laurie, and J. A. Stober. 1985. Evaluation of mutagenic and carcinogenic properties of brominated and chlorinated acetonitriles: By-products of chlorination. *Fundam. Appl. Toxicol.* 5: 1065–1074.

Bull, R. J., J. M. Brown, E. A. Meierhenry, T. A. Jorgenson, M. Robinson, and J. A. Stober. 1986. Enhancement of the hepatotoxicity of chloroform in B6C3F1 mice by corn oil: Implications for chloroform carcinogenesis. *Environ. Health Perspect.* 69: 49–58.

Bull, R. J., C. Gerba, and R. R. Trussell. 1990a. Evaluation of the health risks associated with disinfection. *Crit. Rev. Environ. Control* 20: 77–113.

Bull, R. J., I. M. Sanchez, M. A. Nelson, J. L. Larson, and A. J. Lansing. 1990b. Liver tumor induction in B6C3F1 mice by dichloroacetate and trichloroacetate. *Toxicology* 63: 341–359.

Bull, R. J., and F. C. Kopfler. 1991. *Health Effects of Disinfectants and Disinfectant By-products.* Denver, CO: AWWA Research Foundation and American Water Works Association.

Bull, R. J., L. S. Birnbaum, K. P. Cantor, J. B. Rose, B. E. Butterworth, R. Pegram, and J. Tuomisto. 1995. Water chlorination: Essential process or cancer hazard? *Fundam. Appl. Toxicol.* 155–166.

Cantor, K. P., R. Hoover, T. J. Mason, and L. J. McCabe. 1978. Associations of cancer mortality with trihalomethanes in drinking water. *J. Natl. Cancer Inst.* 61: 979–985.

Cantor, K. P., R. Hoover, P. Hartge, T. J. Mason, D. T. Silverman, R. Altman, D. F. Austin, M. A. Child, C. R. Key, L. D. Marrett, M. H. Myers, A. S. Narayana, L. I. Levin, J. W. Sullivan, G. M. Swanson, D. B. Thomas, and D. W. West. 1987. Bladder cancer, drinking water source, and tap water consumption: A case-control study. *J. Natl. Cancer Inst.* 79: 1269–1279.

Cantor, K. P., C. F. Lynch, and M. Hildeshiem. 1996. Chlorinated drinking water and risk of glioma: A case control study in Iowa, USA. *Epidemiology* 7: S83.

Cantor, K. P., C. F. Lynch, M. E. Hildesheim, M. Dosemeci, J. Lubin, M. Alavanja, and G. Craun. 1998. Drinking water source and chlorination byproducts. I. Risk of bladder cancer. *Epidemiology* 9: 211–228.

Carlton, B. D., D. L. Habash, A. H. Basaran, E. L. George, and M. K. Smith. 1987. Sodium chlorite administration in Long-Evans rats: Reproductive and endocrine effects. *Environ. Res.* 42: 238–245.

Carter, J. H., H. W. Carter, and A. B. DeAngelo. 1995. Biochemical, pathologic and morphometric alterations induced in male B6C3F1 mouse liver by short-term exposure to dichloroacetic acid. *Toxicol. Lett.* 81: 55–71.

Carswell, F., M. M. Kerr, and J. H. Hutchison. 1970. Congenital goitre and hypothyroidism produced by maternal ingestion of iodides. *Lancet* 1: 1241–1243.

CFR. 1989. Drinking water, national primary drinking water regulations; filtration, disinfection; turbidity, Giardia lamblia, viruses, Legionella and heterotrophic bacteria. *Fed. Reg.* 54(124): 27486–27541.

Chance, B., H. Sies, and A. Boveris. 1979. Hydroperoxide metabolism in mammalian organs. *Physiol. Rev.* 59: 527–605.

Chang, L. W., F. B. Daniel, and A.B. DeAngelo. 1992. Analysis of DNA strand breaks induced in rodent liver in vivo, hepatocytes in primary culture, and a human cell line by chlorinated acetic acids and chlorinated acetaldehydes. *Environ. Mol. Mutagen.* 20: 277–288.

Cho, D. H., J. T. Hong, K. Chin, T. S. Cho, and B. M. Lee. 1993. Organotropic formation and disappearance of 8-hydroxydeoxyguanosine in the kidney of Sprague-Dawley rats exposed to Adriamycin and $KBrO_3$. *Cancer Lett.* 74: 141–145.

Chu, I., D. C. Villeneuve, V. E. Secours, G. C. Becking, and V. E. Valli. 1982a. Toxicity of trihalomethanes: I. The acute and subacute toxicity of chloroform, bromodichloromethane, chlorodibromomethane and bromoform in rats. *J. Environ. Sci. Health* B17: 225–240.

Chu, I., D. C. Villeneuve, V. E. Secours, G. C. Becking, and V. E. Valli. 1982b. Trihalomethanes: II. Reversibility of toxicological changes produced by chloroform, bromodichloromethane, chlorodibromomethane and bromoform in rats. *J. Environ. Sci. Health* B17: 225–240.

Cicmanec, J. L., L. W. Condie, G. R. Olson, and S.-R. Wang. 1991. 90-day toxicity study of dichloroacetate in dogs. *Fundam. Appl. Toxicol.* 17: 376–389.

Clark, O. H., R. R. Cavalieri, C. Moser, and S. H. Ingbar. 1990. Iodide-induced hypothyroidism in patients after thyroid resection. *Eur. J. Clin. Invest.* 20: 573–580.

Coleman, W. E., J. W. Munch, W. H. Kaylor, R. P. Streicher, H. P. Ringhand, and J. R. Meier. 1984. Gas chromatography/mass spectroscopy analysis of mutagenic extracts of aqueous chlorinated humic acid. A comparison of the by-products to drinking water contaminants. *Environ. Sci. Technol.* 18: 674–681.

Condie, L. W., C. L. Smallwood, and R. D. Laurie. 1983. Comparative renal and hepatotoxicity of halomethanes: bromodichloromethane, bromoform, chloroform, dibromochloromethane and methylene chloride. *Drug Chem. Toxicol.* 6: 563–568.

Condie, L. W., R. D. Laurie, and J. P. Bercz. 1985. Subchronic toxicology of humic acid following chlorination in the rat. *J. Toxicol. Environ. Health* 15: 305–314.

Cooper, J. R., and P. J. Friedman. 1958. The enyzmic oxidation of chloral hydrate to trichloroacetic acid. *Biochem. Pharmacol.* 1: 76–82.

Cosby, N. C., and W. R. Dukelow. 1992. Toxicology of maternally ingested trichloroethylene (TCE) on embyonal and fetal development in mice and TCE metabolites on in vitro fertilization. *Fundam. Appl. Toxicol.* 19: 268–274.

Cotgreave, I. A., P. Moldeus, and S. Orrenius. 1988. Host biochemical defense mechanisms against prooxidants. *Ann. Rev. Pharmacol. Toxicol.* 28: 189–212.

Couri, D., and M. S. Abdel-Rahman. 1980. Effect of chlorine dioxide and metabolites on glutathione dependent systems in rat, mouse and chicken blood. *J. Environ. Pathol. Toxicol.* 3: 451–460.

Cowman, G. A., and P. C. Singer. 1996. Effect of bromide ion on haloacetic acid speciation resulting from chlorination and chloramination of aquatic humic substances. *Environ. Sci. Technol.* 30: 16–24.

Crabb, D. W., J. P. Mapes, R. W. Boersma, and R. A. Harris. 1976. Effect of dichloroacetate on carbohydrate and lipid metabolism of isolated hepatocytes. *Arch. Biochem. Biophys.* 173: 658–665.

Cragle, D. L., C. M. Shy, R. J. Strubaand, and E. J. Siff. 1985. Case-control study of colon cancer and water chlorination in North Carolina. In *Water Chlorination: Chemistry, Environmental Impact and Health Effects*, vol. 5, eds. R. L. Jolley, pp. 153–159. Chelsea, MI: Lewsi Publishers.

Craun, G. F. 1988. Surface water supplies and health. *JAWWA* 80: 40–52.

Crebelli, R., G. Conti, L. Conti, and A. Carere. 1985. Mutagenicity of trichloroethylene, trichloroethanol and chloral hydrate in *Aspergillus nidulans. Mutation Res.* 155: 105–111.

Curry, S. H., B. S. Pei-I Chu, T. G. Baumgartner, and P. W. Stacopoole. 1985. Plasma concentrations and metabolic effects of intravenous sodium dichloroacetate, *Clin. Pharmacol. Ther.* 37: 89–93.

Daignault, S. A., P. M. Huck, W. B. Anderson, R. C. von Borstel, E. Savage, G. A. Irvine, D. W. Rector, and D. T. Williams. 1987. Drinking water treatment alternatives as evaluated chemically and biologically at pilot scale. *1987 Annual Conference Proceedings, part 2. American Water Works Association*, Denver, CO, pp. 1031–1056.

Daniel, F. B., K. M. Schenck, J. K. Mattox, E. L. C. Lin, D. L. Haas, and M. A. Pereira. 1986. Genotoxic properties of haloacetonitriles: Drinking water by-products of chlorine disinfection. *Fundam. Appl. Toxicol.* 6: 447–453.

Daniel, F. B., A. B. DeAngelo, J. A. Stober, M. A. Pereira, and G. R. Olson. 1989. Chloroform inhibition of 1,2-dimethylhydrazine-induced gastrointestinal tract tumors in the Fisher 344 rat. *Fundam. Appl. Toxicol.* 13: 40–45.

Daniel, F. B., L. W. Condie, M. Robinson, J. A. Stober, R. G. York, G. R. Olson, and S.-R. Wang. 1990. Comparative 90-day subchronic toxicity studies on three drinking water disinfectants, chlorine, monochloramine and chlorine dioxide, in the Sprague-Dawley rats. *JAWWA* 82: 61–69.

Daniel, F. B., G. R. Olson, and J. A. Stober. 1991. The induction of G.I.-tract nuclear anomalies by 3-chloro-4-(dichloromethyl)-5-hydroxy-2(5H)-furanone, a chlorine disinfection by-product, in the male B6C3F1 mouse. *Environ. Mol. Mutagen.* 17: 32–39.

Daniel, F. B., A. B. DeAngelo, J. A. Stober, G. R. Olson, and N. P. Page. 1992a. Hepatocarcinogenicity of chloral hydrate, 2-chloroacetaldehyde, and dichloroacetic acid in male B6C3F1 mouse. *Fundam. Appl. Toxicol. 19*: 159–168.

Daniel, F. B., M., Robinson, J. A., Stober, N. P. Page, and G. R. Olson. 1992b. Ninety-day toxicity study of chloral hydrate in the Sprague-Dawley rat. *Drug Chem. Toxicol.* 15: 217–232.

Daniel, F. B., M. Robinson, J. A. Stober, G. R. Olson, and N. P. Page. 1993. Toxicity of 1,1,1-trihchloro-2-propanone in Sprague-Dawley rats. *J. Toxicol. Environ. Health* 39: 383–393.

Davidson, I. W. F., D. D. Sumner, and J. C. Parker. 1982. Chloroform: A review of its metabolism, teratogenic, mutagenic and carcinogenic potential. *Drug Chem. Toxicol.* 5: 1–87.

Deane, M., S. H. Swan, J. A. Harris, D. M. Epstein, and R. R. Neutra. 1989. Adverse pregnancy outcomes in relation to water contamination, Santa Clara County, California, 1980–1981. *Am. J. Epidemiol.* 129: 894–904.

Deane, M., S. H., Swan, J. A., Harris, D. M. Epstein, and R. R., Neutra. 1992. Adverse pregnancy outcomes in relation to water contamination, Santa Clara County, California, 1980–1981. *Epidemiology* 3: 94–97.

DeAngelo, A. B., F. B. Daniel, L. McMillan, P. Wernsing, and R. E. Savage, Jr. 1989. Species and strain sensitivity to the induction of peroxisome proliferation by chloroacetic acids. *Toxicol. Appl. Pharmacol.* 101: 285–298.

DeAngelo, A. B., F. B. Daniel, J. A., Stober, and G. R. Olson. 1991. The carcinogenicity of dichloroacetic acid in the male B6C3F1 mouse. *Fundam. Appl. Toxicol.* 16: 337–347.

DeAngelo, A. B., F. B. Daniel, B. M. Most, and G. R. Olson. 1996. The carcinogenicity of dichloroacetic acid in the male Fischer 344 rat. *Toxicology* 114: 207–221.

DeAngelo, A. B., F. B. Daniel, B. M. Most, and G. R. Olson. 1997. Two-year bioassay of monochloroacetic acid and trichloroacetic acid administered in the drinking water of male F344/N rats. *Toxicology* 114: 207–221.

DeMarini, D. M., E. Perry, and M. L. Shelton. 1994. Dichloroacetic acid and related compounds: induction of prophage in *E. coli* and mutagenicity and mutation spectra in Salmonella TA100. *Mutagenesis* 9: 429–437.

Deml, E., and D. Oesterle. 1985. Dose-dependent promoting activity of chloroform in rat liver foci assay. *Cancer Lett.* 29: 59–63.

De Rouen T. A., and J. E. Diem. 1977. Relationships between cancer mortality in Louisiana: Drinking water source and other possible causative agents. In *Origins of Human Cancer,* Book A, ed. H. H. Hiatt. Cold Spring Harbor Symposium, Cold Spring Harbor, ME.

Diaz-Gomez, M. I., and J. A. Castro. 1980. Covalent binding of chloroform metabolites to nuclear proteins-no evidence for binding to nuclear acids. *Cancer Lett.* 9: 213–218.

Druckrey, H. 1968. Chlorinated drinking water, toxicity tests, involving seven generations of rats. *Food Cosmetics Toxicol.* 6: 147–154.

Dunnick, J. K., J. K. Haseman, H. S. Lilja, and S. Wyand. 1985. Toxicity and carcinogenicity of chlorodibromomethane in Fischer 344/N rats and B6C3F1 mice. *Fundam. Appl. Toxicol.* 5: 1128–1136.

Elcombe, C. R. 1985. Species difference in carcinogenicity and peroxisome proliferation due to trichloroethylene: A biochemical human hazard assessment. *Arch. Toxicol.* Suppl. 8: 6–17.

Epstein, D. L., G. A. Nolen, J. L. Randall, S. A. Christ, E. J. Read, J. A. Stober, and M. K. Smith. 1992. Cardiopathic effects of dichloroacetate in the fetal Long-Evans rat. *Teratology* 46: 225–235.

Eschenbrenner, A. B., and E. Miller. 1945. Induction of hepatomas in mice by repeated administration of chloroform, with observations on sex differences. *J. Natl. Cancer Inst.* 5: 251–255.

Exon, J. H., K. D. Koller, C. A. O'Reilly, and J. P. Bercz. 1987. Immunologic evaluation of chlorine-based drinking water disinfectants, sodium hypochlorite and monochloramine. *Toxicology* 44: 257–269.

Fahroog, S., E. S. K. Chian and R. S. Engelbrecht. 1977. Basic concepts in disinfection with ozone. *J. Water Pollut. Control Fed.* 49: 1818–1831.

Fenster, L., S. H. Swan, G. C. Windham, and R. R. Neutra. 1991. Assessment of reporting consistency in a case-control study of spontaneous abortion. *Am. J. Epidemiol.* 133: 477–488.

Fenster, L., G. C. Windham, S. H. Swan, D. M. Epstein, and R. R. Neutra. 1992. Tap or bottled water consumption and spontaneous abortion in a case-control study of reporting consistency. *Epidemiology* 3: 120–124.

Ferreira-Gonzalez, A., A. B. DeAngelo, S. Nasim, and C. T. Garrett. 1995. Ras oncogene activation during hepatocarcinogenesis in B6C3F1 male mice by dichloroacetic and trichloroacetic acids. *Carcinogenesis* 16: 495–500.

Fidler, I. J. 1977. Depression of macrophages in mice drinking hyperchlorinated water. *Nature* 270: 735–736.

Fidler, I. J., R. Kirsh, P. Bugelski, and G. Poste. 1982. Involvement of macrophages in the eradication of established metastases following intravenous injection of liposomes containing macrophage activators. *Cancer Res.* 42: 496–501.

Fox, A. W., X. Yang, H. Murli, T. E. Lawlor, M. A. Cifone, and F. E. Reno. 1996a. Absence of mutagenic effects of sodium dichloroacetate. *Fundam. Appl. Toxicol.* 32: 87–95.

Fox, A. W., B. W. Sullivan, J. D. Buffini, M. L. Neichin, R. Nicora, F. K. Hochler, R. O'Rourke, and R. S. Randall. 1996b. Reduction of serum lactate by sodium dichloroacetate and human pharmacokinetic-pharmacodynamic relationships. *J. Pharmacol. Exp. Thera.* 279: 686–693.

Furukawa, F., Y. Kurata, T. Kokubo, M. Takahashi, and M. Nakadate. 1980. Oral acute and subchronic toxicity studies for sodium hypochlorite in F-344 rat. *Bull. Natl. Inst. Hyg. Sci.* 98: 62–69.

Fuscoe, J. C., A. J. Afshari, M. H. George, A. B. DeAngelo, R. R. Tice, R. Salman, and J. W. Allen. 1996. In vivo genotoxicity of dichloroacetic acid: Evaluation with the mouse peripheral blood micronucleus assay and the single cell gel assay. *Environ. Mol. Mutagen.* 27: 1–9.

Gessner, P. K., and B. E. Cabana. 1970. A study of the interaction of the hypnotic effects and of the toxic effects of chloral hydrate and ethanol. *J. Pharmacol. Exp. Thera.* 174: 247–259.

Giller, S., F. Le Curieux, F. Erb, and D. Marzin. 1997. Comparative genotoxicity of halogenated acetic acids found in drinking water. *Mutagenesis* 12: 321–328.

Glaze, W. H., M. Koga, D. Cancilla, K. Wang, M. J. McGuire, S. Liang, M. K. Davis, C. H. Tate, and E. M. Aieta. 1989a. Evaluation of ozonation by-products from two California surface waters. *JAWWA* 81: 66–73.

Glaze, W. H., M. Koga, and D. Cancilla. 1989b. Ozonation by-products. 2. Improvement of an aqueous-phase derivatization method for the detection of formaldehyde and other carbonyl compounds formed by the ozonation of drinking water. *Environ. Sci. Technol.* 23: 838–847.

Goldschmidt, B. M. 1984. Role of aldehydes in carcinogenesis. *J. Environ. Sci. Health* C2: 231–249.

Goldsworthy, T. L., and J. A. Popp. 1987. Chlorinated hydrocarbon-induced peroxisomal enzyme activity in relation to species and organ carcinogenicity. *Toxicol. Appl. Pharmacol.* 88: 225–233.

Golub, M. S. 1992. Reproductive toxicology of water contaminants detected by routine water quality testing. *Epidemiology* 3: 125–129.

Gonzalez-Leon, A., I. R. Schultz, and R. J. Bull. 1997. Pharmacokinetics and metabolism of dichloroacetate in the F344 rat after prolonged administration in drinking water. *Toxicol. Appl. Pharmacol.* 146: 189–195.

Gordon, G., B. Slootmaekers, S. Tachiyashiki, and D. W. Wood III. 1990. Minimizing chlorite ion and chlorate ion in water treated with chlorine dioxide. *JAWWA.* 82: 160–165.

Gorecki, D. K. J., K. W. Hindmarsh, C. A. Hall, D. J. Mayers, and K. Sankaran. 1990. Determination of chloral hydrate metabolism in adult and neonate biological fluids after single-dose adminstration. *J. Chromatography* 528: 333–341.

Gottlieb, M. S., J. K. Carr, and J. R. Clarkson. 1982. Drinking water and cancer in Louisiana: A retrospective mortality study. *Am. J. Epidemiol.* 116: 652–667.

Haag, H. B., and J. Hoigne. 1983. Ozonation of bromide-containing waters: Kinetics of formation of hypobromous acid and bromate. *Environ. Sci. Technol.* 17: 261–267.

Halestrap, A. P. 1978. Pyruvate and ketone-body transport across mitochondrial membrane: Exchange properties, pH, and mechanism of the carrier. *Biochem. J.* 172: 377–387.

Harrington, R. M., H. G. Shertzer, and J. P. Bercz. 1986. Effects of chlorine dioxide on thyroid function in the African green monkey and the rat. *J. Toxicol. Environ. Health* 19: 235–242.

Harrington, R. M., R. R. Romano, D. Gates, and P. Ridgway. 1995a. Subchronic toxicity of sodium chlorite in the rat. *J. Am. Coll. Toxicol.* 14: 21–33.

Harrington, R. M., R. R. Ramano, and L. Irvine. 1995b. Developmental toxicity of sodium chlorite in the rabbit. *J. Am. Coll. Toxicol.* 14: 108–118.

Hasegawa, R., M. Takahashi, T. Kokubo, F. Furukawa, K. Toyoda, H. Sato, Y. Kurokawa, and Y. Hayashi. 1986. Carcinogenicity study of sodium hypochlorite in F344 rats. *Food Chem. Toxicol.* 24: 1295–1302.

Hayes, J. R., J. W. Condie Jr., and J. F. Borzelleca. 1986. Toxicology of haloacetonitriles. *Environ. Health Perspect.* 69: 183–202.

Heffernan, W. P., C. Guion, and R. J. Bull. 1979a. Oxidative damage to the erythrocyte induced by sodium chlorite, in vitro. *J. Environ. Pathol. Toxicol.* 2: 1501–1510.

Heffernan, W. P., C. Guion, and R. J. Bull. 1979b. Oxidative damage to the erythrocyte induced by sodium chlorite, in vivo. *J. Environ. Pathol. Toxicol.* 2: 1487–1499.

Herbert, V., A. Gardner, and N. Coleman. 1980. Mutagenicity of dichloroacetate, an ingredient of some formulations of pangamic acid (trade name "vitamin B_{15}"), *Am. J. Clin. Nutr.* 33: 1179–1182.

Herren-Freund, S. L., and M. A. Pereira. 1986. Carcinogenicity of by-products of disinfection in mouse and rat liver. *Environ. Health Perspect.* 69: 59–65.

Herren-Freund, S. L., M. A. Pereira, M. D. Khoury, and G. Olson. 1987. The carcinogenicity of trichloroethylene and its metabolites, trichloroacetic acid and dichloroacetic acid, in mouse liver. *Toxicol. Appl. Pharmacol.* 90: 183–189.

Hertz-Picciotto, I., S. H. Swan, R. R. Neutra, and S. J. Samuels. 1989. Spontaneous abortions in relation to consumption of tap water: An application of methods from survival analysis to a pregnancy follow-up study. *Am. J. Epidemiol.* 130: 79–93.

Hertz-Picciotto, I., S. H. Swan, and R. R. Neutra. 1992. Reporting bias and mode of interview in a study of adverse pregnancy outcomes and water consumption. *Epidemiology* 3: 104–112.

Hietanen, E., H. Bartsch, J.-C. Bereziat, M. Ahotupa, A.-M. Camus, J. R. P. Cabral, and M. Laitinen. 1990. Quantity and saturation degree of dietary fats as modulators of oxidative stress and chemically-induced liver tumors in rats. *Int. J. Cancer* 46: 640–647.

Hildesheim, M. E., K. P. Cantor, C. F. Lynch, M. Dosemeci, J. Lubin, M. Alavanja, and G. Craun. 1998. Drinking water source and chlorination by-products. II. Risk of colon and rectal cancers. *Epidemiology* 9: 29–35.

Hoigne, J., and H. Bader. 1988. The formation of trichloronitromethane (chloropicrin) and chloroform in a combined ozonation/chlorination treatment of drinking water. *Water Res.* 22: 313–319.

Howe, E. W., E. M. Aieta, S. Liang, and M. J. McGuire. 1989. Removal of chlorite residuals with granular activated carbon; a case study. In *Chlorine Dioxide: Scientific, Regulatory and Application Issues* (A Workbook for the International Chlorine Dioxide Symposium), pp. 126–133, Washington, DC: Chemical Manufacturers Association.

Hrudey, S. E., A. Gac, and S. A. Daignault. 1988. Potent odour-causing chemicals arising from drinking water disinfection. *Water Sci. Technol.* 20: 55–61.

IARC. 1991. Monographs on the Evaluation of Carcinogenic Risks to Humans. *Chlorinated Drinking Water; Chlorination By-products; Some Other Halogenated Compounds; Cobalt and Cobalt Compounds*, pp. 45–296. Lyon, France: International Agency for Research on Cancer.

Ijesselmuiden, C. B., C. Gaydos, B. Feighner, W. L. Novakoski, D. Serwadda, L. H. Caris, D. Vlahov, and G. W. Comstock. 1992. Cancer of the pancreas and drinking water: A population-based case-control study in Washington County, Maryland. *Am. J. Epidemiol.* 136: 836–842.

ILSI. 1993. Part 1. Global perspectives on drinking water: Developed and developing countries. In *Safety of Water Disinfection: Balancing Chemical and Microbial Risks*, ed. G. Craun, pp. 1–30. Washington, DC: ILSI Press.

Jacangelo, J. G., N. L. Patania, K. M. Reagan, E. M. Aieta, S. W. Krasner, and M. J. McGuire. 1989. Ozonation: Assessing its role in the formation and control of disinfection by-products. *JAWWA* 81: 74–84.

Johannsen, F. R., G. J. Levinskas, and A. S. Tegeris. 1986. Effects of formaldehyde in the rat and dog following oral exposure. *Toxicol. Lett.* 30: 1–6.

Jorgenson, T. A., E. F. Meierhenry, C. J. Rushbrook, R. J. Bull, and M. Robinson. 1985. Carcinogenicity of chloroform in drinking water to male Osborne-Mendel rats and female B6C3F1 mice. *Fundam. Appl. Toxicol.* 5: 760–769.

Kasai, H., S. Nishimura, Y. Kurokawa, and Y. Hayashi. 1987. Oral administration of the renal carcinogen, potassium bromate, specifically produces 8-hydroxydeoxyguanosine in rat target organ DNA. *Carcinogenesis* 8: 1959–1961.

Kato-Weinstein, J., M. K. Lingohr, B. D. Thrall, and R. J. Bull. 1998. Effects of dichloroacetate-treatment on carbohydrate metabolism in B6C3F1 mice. *Toxicology* 130: 141–154.

Kato-Weinstein, J., A. J. Stauber, M. V. Templin, B. D. Thrall, and R. J. Bull. 1998b. Alterations in carbohydrate metabolism and peroxisome proliferation with haloacetate-treatment in B6C3-F1 mice. *Toxicology* (submitted).

Katz, R., C. N. Tai, R. M. Diener, R. F. McConnell, and D. E. Semonick. 1981. Dichloroacetate, sodium: 3-month oral toxicity studies in rats and dogs. *Toxicol. Appl. Pharmacol.* 57: 273–287.

Kerns, W. D., K. L. Pavkov, D. J. Donofrio, and E. J. Gralla. 1983. Carcinogenicity of formaldehyde in rats and mice after long-term inhalation exposure. *Cancer Res.* 43: 4382–4392.

King, W. D., and L. D., Marrett. 1996. Case-control study of water source and bladder cancer. *Cancer Causes Control* (November 1996).

Klaunig, J. E., R. S. Ruch, and M. A. Pereira. 1986. Carcinogenicity of chlorinated methane and ethane compounds administered in drinking water to mice. *Environ. Health Perspect.* 69: 89–95.

Komulainen, H., V.-M. Kosma, S.-L. Vaittinen, T. Vartiainen, E. Kaliste-Korhonen, S. Lotjonen, R. K. Tuominen, and J. Tuomisto. 1997. Carcinogenicity of the drinking water mutagen 3-chloro-4-(dichloromethyl)-5-hydroxy-2(5H)-furanone. *J. Natl. Cancer Inst.* 89: 848–856.

Koivusalo, M., J. J. K. Jaakkola, T. Vartianinen, T. Hakulinen, S.Karjalainen, E. Pukkala, and J. Tuomisto. 1994. Drinking water mutagenicity and gastrointestinal and urinary tract cancers: An ecological study in Finland. *Am J. Public Health* 84: 1223–1228.

Kramer, M. D., C. F. Lynch, P. Isacson, and J. W. Hanson. 1992. The association of waterborne chloroform with interuterine growth retardation. *Epidemiol.* 3: 407–413.

Krasner, S. W., M. J. McGuire, J. G. Jacangelo, N. L. Patania, K. M Reagen, and E. M. Aieta. 1989a. The occurrence of disinfection by-products in US drinking water. *JAWWA* 81: 41–53.

Krasner, S. W., W. H. Glaze, H. S. Weinburg, P. A. Daniel and I. N. Najm. (1993). Formation and control of bromate during ozonation of waters containing bromide. *JAWWA* 85: 73–81.

Kronberg, L., B. Holmbom, M. Reunanen, and L. Tikkanen. 1988a. Identification and quantitation of the Ames mutagenic compound 3-chloro-4-(dichloromethyl)-5-hydroxy-2(5H)-furanone and of its geometric isomer (E)-2-chloro-3-(dichloromethyl)-4-oxobutenoic acid in chlorine-treated humic water and drinking water extracts. *Environ. Sci. Technol.* 22: 1097–1103.

Kronberg, L. and T. Vartiainen. 1988b. Ames mutagenicity and concentration of the strong mutagen 3-chloro-4-(dichloromethyl)-5-hydroxy-2(5H)-furanone and of its geometric isomer (E)-2-chloro-3-(dichloromethyl)-4-oxobutenoic acid in chlorine-treated tap waters. *Mutation Res.* 206: 177–182.

Kurokawa, Y., Y. Hayashi, A. Maekawa, M. Takahashi, T. Kokubo, and S. Odashima. 1983. Carcinogenicity of potassium bromate administered orally to F344 rats. *J. Natl. Cancer Inst.* 71: 965–972.

Kurokawa, Y., S. Aoki, Y. Matsushima, N. Takamura, T. Imazawa, and Y. Hayashi. 1986a. Dose-response studies on the carcinogenicity of potassium bromate in F344 rats after long-term oral administration. *J. Natl. Cancer Inst.* 77: 977–982.

Kurokawa, Y., S. Takayama, Y. Konishi, Y. Hiasa, S. Asahina, M. Takahashi, A. Maekawa, and Y. Hayashi. 1986b. Long-term in vivo carcinogenicity tests of potassium bromate, sodium hypochlorite, and sodium chlorite conducted in Japan. *Environ. Health Perspect.* 69: 221–235.

Kurokawa, Y., Y. Matsushima, N. Takamura, T. Imazawa, and Y. Hayashi. 1987. Relationship between the duration of treatment and the incidence of renal cell tumors in male F344 rats administered potassium bromate. *Jap. J. Cancer Res.* 78: 358–364.

Kurokawa, Y. Y., A. Maekawa, M. Takahashi, and Y. Hayashi. 1990. Toxicity and carcinogenicity of potassium bromate—A new renal carcinogen. *Environ. Health Perspect.* 87: 309–335.

Kuzma, R. J., C. M. Kuzma, and C. R. Buncher. 1977. Ohio drinking water source and cancer rates. *A. J. Publ. Health* 67: 725–729.

Larson, J. L., and R. J. Bull. 1991. Metabolism and lipoperoxidative activity of trichloroacetate and dichloroacetate in rats and mice. *Toxicol. Appl. Pharmacol.* 115: 268–277.

Larson, J. L., D. C. Wolf, and B. E. Butterworth. 1994a. Induced cytotoxicity and cell proliferation in the hepatocarcinogenicity of chloroform in female B6C3F1 mice: Comparision of administration by gavage in corn oil vs. *ad libitum* in drinking water. *Fundam. Appl. Toxicol.* 22: 90–102.

Larson, J. L., C. S. Sprankle, and B. E. Butterworth. 1994b. Lack of chloroform-induced DNA repair in vitro and in vivo in hepatocytes of female B6C3F1 mice. *Environ. Mol. Mutagen.* 23: 132–136.

Larson, J. L., D. C. Wolf and B. E. Butterworth. 1995a. Induced regenerative cell proliferation in livers and kidneys of male F-344 rats given chloroform in corn oil by gavage or ad libitum in drinking water. *Toxicology* 95: 73–86.

Larson, J. L., D. C., Wolf, S. Mery, K. T. Morgan, and B. E. Butterworth. 1995b. Toxicity and cell proliferation in the liver, kidneys and nasal passages of female F-344 rats induced by chloroform administered by gavage. *Fed. Chem. Toxicol.* 33: 443–456.

Larson, J. L., M. V. Templin, D. C. Wolf, K. C. Jamison, J. R. Leininger, S. Mery, K. T. Morgan, B. A. Wong, R. B. Conolly and B. E. Butterworth. 1996. A 90-day chloroform inhalation study in female and male B6C3F1 mice: Implications for risk assessment. *Fundam. Appl. Toxicol.* 30: 118–137.

Latendresse, J. R., and M. A. Pereira. 1997. Dissimilar characteristics of N-methyl-N-nitrosourea-initiated foci and tumors promoted by dichloroacetic acid or trichloroacetic acid in the liver of female B6C3F1 mice. *Toxicologic Pathol.* 25: 433–440.

Lawrence, C. E., P. R. Taylor, B. J. Trock, and A. A. Reilly. 1984. Trihalomethanes in drinking water and human colorectal cancer. *J. Natl. Cancer Inst.* 72: 563–568.

Leavitt, S. A., A. B. DeAngelo, M. H. George, and J. A. Ross. 1997. Assessment of the mutagenicity of dichloroacetic acid in *lacI* transgenic B6C3F1 mouse liver. *Carcinogenesis* 18: 2101–2106.

Lilly, P. D., J. E. Simmons, and R. A. Pegram. 1994. Dose-dependent vehicle differences in the acute toxicity of bromodichloromethane. *Fundam. Appl. Toxicol.* 23: 132–140.

Lilly, P. D., T. M. Ross, and R. A. Pegram. 1997. Trihalomethane comparative toxicity: Acute renal and hepatic toxicity of chloroform and bromodichloromethane following aqueous gavage. *Fundam. Appl. Toxicol.* 40: 101–110.

Limmer, J., W. E. Fleig, D. Leupold, R. Bittner, H. Dischuneit, and H.-G. Berger. 1988. Hepatocellular carcinoma in type 1 glycogen storage disease. *Hepatology* 8: 531–537.

Lin, E. L. C., and C. W. Guion. 1989. Interaction of haloacetonitriles with glutathione and glutathione-S-transferase. *Biochem. J.* 38: 685–688.

Lin, E. L. C., T. V. Reddy, C. W. Guion, B. H. MacFarland, A. C. Roth, and F. B. Daniel. 1990. Macromolecular binding of trichloroacetonitrile in the rat. *Toxicologist* 10: 1005.

Linder, R. E., G. R. Klinefelter, L. F. Strader, J. D. Suarez, and C. J. Dyer. 1994a. Acute spermatogenic effects of bromoacetic acids. *Fundam. Appl. Toxicol.* 22: 422–430.

Linder, R. E., G. R. Klinefelter, L. F. Strader, J. D. Suarez, N. L. Roberts, and C. J. Dyer. 1994b. Spermatotoxicity of dibromoacetic acid in rats after 14 daily exposures. *Reprod. Toxicol.* 8: 251–259.

Linder, R. E., G. R. Klinefelter, L. F. Strader, M. G. Narotosky, J. D. Suarez, N. L. Roberts, and S. D. Perreault. 1995. Dibromoacetic acid affects reproductive competence and sperm quality in the male rat. *Fundam. Appl. Toxicol.* 28: 9–17.

Linder, R. E., G. R. Klinefelter, L. F. Strader, D. N. R. Veeramachaneni, N. L. Roberts, and J. D. Suarez. 1997a. Histopathologic changes in the testes of rats exposed to dibromoacetic acid. *Reprod. Toxicol.* 11: 47–56.

Linder, R. E., G. R. Klinefelter, L. F. Strader, J. D. Suarez, and N. L. Roberts. 1997b. Spermatotoxicity of dichloroacetic acid. *Reprod. Toxicol.* 11: 681–688.

Lingohr, M. K., B. D. Thrall, and R. J. Bull. 1998. Serum insulin levels and differential insulin receptor expression in livers and liver tumors of mice treated with dichloroacetate. *Toxical. Appl. Phamacol.* (in press).

Lipscomb, J. C., D. A. Mahle, W. T. Brashear, and H. A. Barton. 1995. Dichloroacetic acid: metabolism in cytosol. *Drug Metab. Dispos.* 23: 1202–1205.

Lubbers, J. R., and J. R. Bianchine. 1984. Effects of acute rising dose administration of chlorine dioxide, chlorate and chlorite to normal healthy male volunteers. *J. Environ. Pathol. Toxicol. Oncology* 5: 215–228.

Lubbers, J. R., S. Chauhan, and J. R. Bianchine. 1981. Controlled clinical evaluations of chlorine dioxide, chlorite and chlorate in man. *Fundam. Appl. Toxicol.* 1: 334–338.

Lubbers, J. R., S. Chauan, and J. R. Bianchine. 1982. Controlled clinical evaluations of chlorine dioxide, chlorite and chlorate in man. *Environ. Health Perspect.* 46: 57–62.

Lubbers, J. R., S. Chauhan, J. K. Miller, and J. R. Bianchine. 1984a. The effects of chronic administration of chlorine dioxide, chlorite and chlorate to normal healthy adult male volunteers. *J. Environ. Pathol. Toxicol. Oncology* 5: 229–238.

Lubbers, J. R., S. Chauhan, J. K. Miller, and J. R. Bianchine. 1984b. The effects of chronic administration of chlorite to glucose-6-phosphate dehydrogenase deficient healthy adult male volunteers. *J. Environ. Pathol. Toxicol. Oncology* 5: 239–242.

Lykins, B. W., and M. H. Griese. 1986. Using chlorine dioxide for trihalomethane control. *JAWWA* 78: 88–93.

Lynch, C. F., S. F. VanLier, and K. P. Cantor. 1990. A case-control study of multiple cancer sites and water chlorination in Iowa. In *Water Chlorination: Chemistry, Environmental Impact and Health Effects*, vol. 6, eds. R. L. Jolly et al., pp. 387–398. Chelsea, MI: Lewis Publishers.

Ma, T. H., and M. M. Harris. 1988. Review of genotoxicity of formaldehyde. *Mutation Res.* 196: 37–59.

Mackay, J. M., V. Fox, K. Griffiths, D. A. Fox, C. A. Howard, C. Coutts, I. Wyatt, and J. A. Styles. 1995. Trichloroacetic acid: Investigation into the mechanism of chromosomal damage in the in vitro human lymphocyte cytogenetic assay and the mouse bone marrow micronucleus test. *Carcinogenesis* 16: 1127–1133.

Maronpot, R. R., T. Fox, D. E. Malarkey, and T. L. Goldsworthy. 1995. Mutations in the *ras* proto-oncogene: Clues to etiology and molecular pathogenesis of mouse liver tumors. *Toxicology* 101: 125–156.

Masschelein, W. J. 1989. Historic and current overview of chlorine dioxide. In *Chlorine Dioxide: Scientific, Regulatory and Application Issues*, pp. 4–40, Washington, DC: Chemical Manufacturers Assoc.

Mather, G. G., J. H. Exon, J. J. Parnell, and L. D. Koller. 1990. Subchronic 90 day toxicity of dichloroacetic acid and trichloroacetic acid in rats. *Toxicology* 64: 71–80.

McGeehin, M. A., J. S. Reif, J. C. Becher, and E. J. Mangione. 1993. Case-control study of bladder cancer and water disinfection methods in Colorado. *Am. J. Epidemiol.* 138: 492–501.

McGuire, M. J., S. W. Krasner, K. M. Reagan, E. M. Aieta, J. G. Jacangelo, N. L. Patania, and K. M. Gramith. 1989. *Final Report for Disinfection By-products in United States Drinking Waters*, vol. 1. Washington, DC, U.S. EPA, California Department of Health Services.

Meier, J. R., R. D. Lingg, and R. J. Bull. 1983. Formation of mutagens following chlorination of humic acid, A model for mutagen formation during drinking water treatment. *Mutation Res.* 118: 25–41.

Meier, J. R., H. P. Ringhand, W. E. Coleman, J. W. Munch, R. P. Streicher, W. H. Kaylor, and K. M. Schenck. 1985a. Identification of mutagenic compounds formed during chlorination of humic acid. *Mutation Res.* 157: 111–122.

Meier, J. R., R. J. Bull, J. A. Stober, and M. C. Cimino. 1985b. Evaluation of chemicals used for drinking water disinfection for production of chromosomal damage and sperm-head abnormalities in mice. *Environ. Mutagen.* 7: 201–211.

Meier, J. R. and R. J. Bull. 1985. Mutagenic properties of drinking water disinfectants and by-products. In *Water Chlorination: Chemistry, Environmental Impact and Health Effects*, vol. 5, eds. R. L. Jolley et al., pp. 207–220. Chelsea, MI: Lewis Publishers.

Meier, J. R., R. B. Knohl, W. E. Coleman, H. P. Ringhand, J. W. Munch, W. H. Kaylor, R. P. Streicher, and F. C. Kopfler. 1987a. Studies on the potent bacterial mutagen, 3-chloro-4-(dichloro-methyl)-5-hydroxy-2(5H)-furanone: Aqueous stability, XAD recovery and analytical determination in drinking water and in chlorinated humic acid solution. *Mutation Res.* 189: 363–373.

Meier, J. R., W. F. Blazak, and R. B. Knohl. 1987b. Mutagenic and clastogenic properties of 3-chloro-4-(dichloromethyl)-5-hydroxy-2(5H)-furanone: A potent bacterial mutagen in drinking water. *Environ. Mol. Mutagen.* 10: 411–424.

Meier, J. R. 1988. Genotoxic activity of organic chemicals in drinking water. *Mutation Res.* 196: 211–245.

Meier, J. R., S. Monarca, K. S. Patterson, M. Villarini, F. B. Daniel, K. Moretti, and R. Pasquini. 1996. Urine mutagenicity and biochemical effects of the drinking water mutagen, 3-chlorp — 4-(Dichloromethyl)-5-hydroxy-2[5H]-furanone 9MX), following repeated oral administration to mice and rats. *Toxicology* 110: 59–70.

Melnick, R. L., J. K. Dunnick, D. P. Sandler, M. R. Elwell, and J. C. Barrett. 1994. Trihalomethanes and other environmental factors that contribute to colorectal cancer. *Environ. Health Perspect.* 102: 586–588.

Merdink, J. L., D. K. Stevens, R. D. Stenner, and R. J. Bull. 1999a. The effect of enterohepatic circulation on chloral hydrate and its metabolites in F344 rats. *J. Toxicol Environ. Health.* 57: 357–368.

Merdink, J. L., L. R. Robison, M. Hu, and R. J. Bull. 1999b. Metabolism and pharmacokinetics of chloral hydrate and its metabolites in male human volunteers. *Toxicology.* (in press).

Merdink, J. L., A. Gonzalez-Leon, R. J. Bull, and I. R. Schultz. 1998c. Dichloroacetic acid formation in B6C3F1 mice following administration of trichloroethylene or its metabolites. *Toxicol. Sci.* 45: 33–41.

Miller, R. G., F. C. Kopfler, L. W. Condie, M. A. Pereira, J. R. Meier, H. P. Ringhand, M. Robinson, and B. Casto. 1986. Results of toxicological testing of Jefferson Parish pilot plant samples. *Environ. Health Perspect.* 69: 129–140.

Miller, J. W., and P. C. Uden. (1983) Characterization of non-volatile aqueous chlorination products of humic substances. *Environ. Sci. Technol.* 17: 150–157.

Mink, F. L., W. E. Coleman, J. W. Munch, W. H. Kaylor, and H. P. Ringhand. 1983. In vivo formation of halogenated reaction products following peroral sodium hypochlorite. *Bull. Environ. Contam. Toxicol.* 30: 394–399.

Moore, G. S., and F. J. Calabrese. 1980. Effect of chlorine dioxide and sodium chlorite on erythrocytes of A/J and C57L/J mice. *J. Environ. Pathol. Toxicol.* 4: 513–524.

Moore, D. H., L. F. Chasseaud, S. K. Majeed, D. E. Prentice, and F. J. C. Roe. 1982. The effect of dose and vehicle on early tissue damage and regenerative activity after chloroform administration to mice. *Food Chem. Toxicol.* 20: 951–954.

Moore, G. W., L. L. Swift, D. R. Rabinowitz, O. B. Crofford, J. A. Oates, and P. W. Stacpoole. 1979. Reduction of serum cholesterol in patients with homozygous familial hypercholesterolemia by dichloroacetate. *Atherosclerosis* 33: 285–293.

Muller, G., M. Spassovski, and D. Henschler. 1974. Metabolism of trichloroethylene in man. II. Pharmacokinetics of metabolites. *Arch. Toxicol.* 32: 283–295.

Munson, A. E., L. E. Sain, V. M. Sanders, B. M. Kauffman, K. L. White Jr., D. G. Page, D. W. Barnes, and J. F. Borzelleca. 1982. Toxicology of organic drinking water contaminants: Trichloromethane, bromodichloromethane, dibromochlormethane and tribromomethane. *Environ. Health Perspect.* 46: 117–126.

Narita, T., H. Nakazawa, Y. Hizawa, and H. Kudo. 1994. Glycogen storage disease associated with Niemann-Pick disease: Histochemical, enzymatic and lipid analysis. *Modern Pathol.* 7: 416–421.

NAS. (National Academy of Sciences) 1980. *Drinking Water and Health*, vol. 3. Washington, DC: National Academy Press.

NAS. (National Academy of Sciences). 1987. *Drinking Water and Health: Disinfectants and disinfectant by-products*, vol. 7, pp. 50–60. Washington, DC: National Academy Press.

NCI. 1976. *Report on the Carcinogenesis Bioassay of Chloroform.* Bethesda, MD: National Cancer Institute, NTIS PB-264–018.

NCI. 1978a. *Bioassay of Chloropicrin for Possible Carcinogenicity.* Bethesda, MD: National Cancer Institute, U.S. Department of Health, Education and Welfare, Carcinogenesis Technical Report Series No. 65, DHEW Publ. (NIH) 78-1315, 82 pp.

NCI. 1978b. *Bioassay of Iodoform for Possible Carcinogenicity.* Bethesda, MD: National Cancer Institute, Technical Report Series NCI-CG-TR-110.

NCI. 1979. *Bioassay of 2,4,6-Trichlorophenol for Possible Carcinogenicity.* Bethesda, MD: National Cancer Institute, NCI-CG-TR-155.

NTP. 1986. *Toxicology and Carcinogenesis Studies of Bromodichloromethane in F344/N Rats and B6C3F1 Mice*, Research Triangle Park, NC: National Toxicology Program, Technical Report Series TRS No. 321, NIH No. 88–2537, CAS No. 75-27-4.

NTP. 1989. *Toxicology and Carcinogenesis Studies of Tribromomethane (Bromoform) in F344/N Rats and B6C3F1 Mice.* Research Triangle Park, NC: National Toxicology Program, Technical Report Series 350, NIH No. 89-2805, CAS No. 75-25-2.

NTP. 1990a. *National Toxicology Program Technical Report on the Toxicology and Carcinogenesis Studies of Monochloroacetic Acid in F344/N Rats and B6C3F1 Mice.* Research Triangle Park, NC: National Toxicology Program, Technical Report Series 396, NIH No. 90-2851.

NTP. 1990b. *Draft Technical Report on the Toxicology and Carcinogenesis Studies of Chlorinated and Chloraminated Water in F344/N Rats and B6C3F1 Mice.* Research Triangle Park, NC: National Toxicology Program. Technical Report Series 392, NIH No. 91-2847.

Nazar, M. A., and W. H. Rapson. 1982. pH stability of some mutagens produced by aqueous chlorination of organic compounds. *Environ. Mutagen.* 4: 435–444.

Nelson, M. A., and R. J. Bull. 1988. Induction of strand breaks in DNA by trichloroethylene and metabolites in rat and mouse liver in vivo. *Toxicol. Appl. Pharmacol.* 94: 45–54.

Nelson, M. A., I. M. Sanchez, R. J. Bull, and S. R. Sylvester. 1990. Increased expression of c-myc and c-H-ras in dichloroacetate and trichloroacetate-induced liver tumors in B6C3F1 mice. *Toxicology* 64: 47–57.

Nestmann, E. R., I. Chu, D. J. Kowbel, and T. I. Matula. 1980. Short-lived mutagen in Salmonella produced by reaction of trichloroacetic acid and dimethyl sulphoxide. *Can. J. Genet. Cytol.* 22: 35–40.

Neutra, R. R., S. H. Swan, I. Hertz-Picciotto, G. C. Windham, M. Wrensch, G. M. Shaw, L. Fenster, and M. Deane. 1992. Potential sources of bias and confounding in environmental epidemiologic studies of pregnancy outcomes. *Epidemiology* 3: 134–142.

Ni, Y.-C., T.-Y Wong, R. V. Lloyd, T. M. Heinze, S. Shelton, D. Casciano, F. F. Kadlubar, and P. P. Fu. 1996. Mouse liver microsomal metabolism of chloral hydrate, trichloroacetic acid, and trichloroethanol leading to induction of lipid peroxidation via a free radical mechanism. *Drug Metab. Dispos.* 24: 81–90.

Norwood, D. L., G. P. Thompson, J. D. Johnson, and R. F. Christman. 1985. Monitoring trichloroacetic acid in municipal drinking water. In *Water Chlorination: Chemistry, Environmental Impact and Health Effects*, vol. 5, eds. R. L. Jolley et al., pp. 1115–1122, Chelsea, MI: Lewis Publishers.

Olivieri, V. P., M. C. Snead, C. W. Kruse and K. Kuwata. 1986. Stability and effectiveness of chlorine disinfectants in water distribution systems. *Environ. Health Perspect.* 69: 15–29.

Olusi, S. O., O. L. Oke, and A. Odusote. 1979. Effects of cyanogenic agents on reproduction and neonatal development in rats. *Biol. Neonate.* 36: 233–243.

Orme, J., D. H. Taylor, R. D. Laurie, and R. J. Bull. 1985. Effects of chlorine dioxide on thyroid function in neonatal rats. *J. Toxicol. Environ. Health* 15: 315–322.

Orner, G. A., J. A. Malone, L. C. Stillwell, R. S. Chang, A. J. Stauber, L. B. Sasser, B. D. Thrall, and R. J. Bull. H-ras codon 61 mutation frequency and spectra in trichloroethylene, dichloroethylene and trichloroacetate-induced liver tumors in B6C3F1 mice. *Toxicol.* (submitted).

Parrish, J. M., E. W. Austin, D. K. Stevens, D. H. Kinder, and R. J. Bull. 1996. Haloacetate-induced oxidative damage to DNA in the liver of male B6C3F1 mice. *Toxicology* 110: 103–111.

Payment, P., L. Richardson, M. Edwardes, E. Franco, and J. Siemiatycki. 1990a. A prospective epidemiological study of drinking water related gastrointestinal illnesses. *International Association of Water Pollution Research and Contributory Symposium on Health Related Microbiology.* April 1–6, 1990, Eberhard-Kals-Universitat, Tubingen, Germany, p. 44.

Payment, P., L. Richardson, M. Edwardes, E. Franco, and J. Siemiatycki. 1990b. Drinking water-related gastrointestinal illness. *Abstracts of the 90th Annual Marketing of the American Society of Microbiology.* Abstract Q-ll, p. 290.

Pegram, R. A., M. E. Andersen, S. H. Warren, T. M. Ross, and L. D. Claxton. 1997. Glutathione-S-transferase-mediated mutagenicity of trihalomethanes in Salmonella tyhimurium: contrasting results with bromodichloromethane and chloroform. *Toxicol. Appl. Pharmacol.* 144: 183–188.

Pereira, M. A., L.-H. Lin, and J. K. Mattox. 1984. Haloacetonitrile excretion as thiocyanate and inhibition of dimethylnitrosamine demethylase: A proposed metabolic scheme. *J. Toxicol. Environ. Health* 13: 633–641.

Pereira, M. A., G. L. Knutsen, and S. L. Herren-Freund. 1985. Effect of subsequent treatment of chloroform or phenobarbital on the incidence of lung and liver tumors initiated by ethylnitrosourea in 15 day old mice. *Carcinogenesis* 6: 203–207.

Pereira, M. A. 1996. Carcinogenic activity of dichloroacetic acid and trichloroacetic acid in the liver of female B6C3F1 mice. *Fundam. Appl. Toxicol.* 31: 192–199.

Pereira, M. A., and J. B. Phelps. 1996. Promotion by dichloroacetic acid and trichloroacetic acid of N-methyl-N-nitrosourea-initiated cancer in the liver of female B6C3F1 mice. *Cancer Lett.* 102: 133–141.

Pereira, M. A., K. Li, and P. M. Kramer. (1997) Promotion by mixtures of dichloroacetic acid and trichloroacetic acid of N-methyl-N-nitrosourea-initiated cancer in the liver of female B6C3F1 mice. *Cancer Lett.* 115: 15–23.

Pereira, M. A., and M. A., Grothaus. 1997. Chloroform in drinking water prevents hepatic cell proliferation induced by chloroform administered by gavage in corn oil to mice. *Fundam. Appl. Toxicol.* 37: 82–87.

Piegorsch, W. W., and D. G. Hoel. 1988. Exploring relationships between mutagenic and carcinogenic potencies. *Mutation Res.* 196: 161–175.

Pohl, L. R., and G. Krishna. 1978. Deuterium isotope effect in bioactivation and hepatotoxicity of chloroform. *Life Sci.* 23: 1067–1072.

Rannug, U., R. Gothe, and C. A. Wachtmeister. 1976. The mutagenicity of chloroethylene oxide, chloroacetaldehyde, 2-chloroethanol and chloroacetic acid, conceivable metabolites of vinyl chloride. *Chem.-Biol. Interactions* 12: 251–263.

Reckhow, D. A., P. C. Singer, and R. L. Malcolm. 1990. Chlorination of humic materials: Byproduct formation and chemical interpretations. *Environ. Sci. Technol.* 24: 1655–1664.

Reding, R., P. S. Fair, C. J. Shipp, and H. J. Brass. 1986. Measurement of dihaloacetonitriles and chloropicrin in drinking water. Cincinnati, OH: U.S. EPA, Office of Drinking Water Technical Support Division.

Reitz, R. H., T. R. Fox, and J. F. Quast. 1982. Mechanistic considerations for carcinogenic risk assessment: Chloroform. *Environ. Health Perspect.* 46: 163–168.

Rice, R. G., and M. Gomez-Taylor. 1986. Occurrence of by-products of strong oxidants reacting with drinking water contaminants — Scope of problem. *Environ. Health Perspect.* 69: 31–44.

Richard, A. M., and E. S. Hunter III. 1996. Quantitative structure-activity relationships for the developmental toxicity of haloacetic acids in mammalian whole embryo culture. *Teratology* 53: 352–360.

Rijhsinghani, K. S., M. A. Swerdlow, T. Ghose, C. Abrahams, and K. V. N. Rao. 1986. Induction of neoplastic lesions in the livers of C57BLXC3HF1 mice by chloral hydrate. *Cancer Detection Prevention* 9: 279–288.

Robinson, M., R. J. Bull, G. R. Olson, and J. Stober. 1989. Carcinogenic activity associated with halogenated acetones and acroleins in the mouse skin assay. *Cancer Lett.* 48: 197–203.

Robison, L. M., P. W. Sylvester, J. P. Lang, and R. J. Bull. 1998. Comparison of the effects of iodine and iodide on thyroid function in humans. *J. Toxicol. Environ. Health.* 55: 93–106.

Romero, J., F. Ventura, J. Caizach, J. Rivera, and R. Guerrero. 1997. Identification and quantification of the mutagenic compound 3-chloro-4-(dichloromethyl)-5-hydroxy-2(5H)-furanone (MX) in chlorine-treated water. *Environ. Contam. Toxicol.* 59: 715–722.

Rosenkranz, H. S. 1973. Sodium hypochlorite and sodium perborate: Preferential inhibitors of DNA polymerase-deficient bacteria. *Mutation Res.* 21: 171–174.

Rosenkranz, H. S., B. Gutter, and W. T. Speck. 1976. Mutagenicity and DNA-modifying activity: A comparison of two microbial assays. *Mutation Res.* 41: 61–70.

Russo, A., F. Pacchierotti, and P. Metalli. 1984. Nondisjunction induced in mouse spermatogenesis by chloralhydrate, a metabolite of trichloroethylene. *Environ. Mutagen.* 6: 695–703.

Sai, K., S. Uchiyama, Y. Ohno, R. Hasegawa, and Y. Kurokawa. 1992. Generation of active oxygen species in vitro by the interaction of potassium bromate with rat kidney cell. *Carcinogenesis* 13: 333–339.

Sanchez, I. M., and R. J. Bull. 1990. Early induction of reparative hyperplasia in the liver of B6C3F1 mice treated with dichloroacetate and trichloroacetate. *Toxicology* 64: 33–46.

Sanders, V. M., B. M. Kauffman, K. L. White, Jr., K. A. Douglas, D. W. Barnes, L. E. Sain, T. J. Bradshaw, J. F. Borzelleca and A. E. Munson. 1982. Toxicology of chloral hydrate in the mouse. *Environ. Health Perspect.* 44: 137–146.

Schroeder, M., A. B. DeAngelo, and M. J. Mass. 1997. Dichloroacetic acid reduces Ha-ras codon 61 mutations in liver tumors from female B6C3F1 mice. *Carcinogenesis* 18: 1675–1678.

Schwetz, B. A., B. K. J. Leong, and P. J. Gehring. 1974. Embryo- and Fetotoxicity of inhaled chloroform in rats. *Toxicol. Appl. Pharmacol.* 28: 442–451.

Shih, K. L. and J. Lederberg. 1976. Chloramine mutagenesis in *Bacillus subtilis. Science* 192: 1141–1143.

Singer, P. C., and S. D. Chang. 1989. Correlations between trihalomethanes and total organic halides formed during water treatment. *JAWWA* 81: 61–65.

Smith, M. K., E. L. George, J. M. Manson, and J. A. Stober. 1987. Developmental toxicity of halogenated acetonitriles: Drinking water by-products of chlorine disinfection. *Toxicology* 46: 83–93.

Smith, M. K., J. L. Randall, D. R. Tocco, R. G. York, J. A. Stober, and E. J. Read. 1988. Teratogenic effects of trichloroacetonitrile in the Long-Evans rat. *Teratology* 38: 113–120.

Smith, M. K., J. L. Randall, J. A. Stober, and E. J. Read. 1989a. Developmental toxicity of dichloroacetonitrile, A by-product of drinking water disinfection. *Fundam. Appl. Toxicol.* 12: 765–772.

Smith, M. K., J. L. Randall, E. J. Read, and J. A. Stober. 1989b. Teratogenic activity of trichloroacetic acid in the rat. *Teratology* 40: 445–451.

Smith, M. K., J. L. Randall, E. J. Read, and J. A. Stober. 1992. Developmental toxicity of dichloroacetate in the rat. *Teratology* 46: 217–223.

Smith, M. K., B. D. Thrall, and R. J. Bull. 1997. Dichloroacetate (DCA) modulates insulin signaling. *Toxicologist* 36: 1133.

Snyder, R. D., J. Pullman, J. H. Carter, H. W. Carter, and A. B. DeAngelo. 1995. In vivo administration of dichloroacetic acid suppresses spontaneous apoptosis in murine hepatocytes. *Cancer Res.* 55: 3702–3705.

Soffriti, M., C. Maltoni, F. Maffei, and R. Biagi. 1989. Formaldehyde: An experimental mulitpotential carcinogen. *Toxicol. Ind. Health* 5: 699–730.

So, B.-J., and R. J. Bull. 1995. Dibromoacetate (DBA) acts as a promoter of abnormal crypt foci in the colon of F344 rats. *Toxicologist* 15: 1242.

Song, R., P. Westerhoff, R. Minear, and G. Amy. 1997. Bromate minimization during ozonation. *JAWWA* 89: 69–78.

Sora, S., and M. L. A. Carbone. 1987. Chloral hydrate methylmercury hydroxide and ethidium bromide affect chromosomal segregation during meiosis of *Saccharomyces Cerevisiae. Mutation Research* 190: 13–17.

Stacpoole, P. W., G. W. Moore, and D. M. Kornhauser. 1979. Toxicity of chronic dichloroacetate. *N. Engl. J. Med.* 300: 372.

Stacpoole, P. W. 1989. The Pharmacology of Dichloroacetate. *Metabolism* 38: 1124–1144.

Stauber, A. J., and R. J. Bull. 1997. Differences in phenotype and cell replicative behavior of hepatic tumors inducted by dichloroacetate (DCA) and trichloroacetate (TCA). *Toxicol. Appl. Pharmacol.* 144: 235–246.

Stauber, A. J., R. J. Bull, and B. D. Thrall. 1998a. Dichloroacetate and trichloroacetate promote clonal expansion of anchorage-independent hepatocytes in vivo and in vitro. *Toxicol. Appl. Pharmacol.* (in press).

Stauber, A. J., M. V. Templin, M. E. Bull, A. B. DeAngelo, D. H. Kinder, B. D. Thrall, and R. J. Bull 1998b. Effect of brominated haloacetates on hepatic tumor induction in male B6C3F1 mice. *Toxicology.* 150: 287–294.

Stenner, R. D., J. L. Merdink, M. V. Templin, D. K. Stevens, D. L. Springer, and R. J. Bull. 1997. Enterohepatic recirculation of trichloroethanol glucuronide as a significant source of trichloroacetic acid in the metabolism of trichloroethylene. *Drug Metab. Dispos.* 25: 529–535.

Stevens, A. A., L. A. Moore, and R. J. Miltner. 1989. Formation and control of non-trihalomethane disinfection by-products. *JAWWA* 81: 54–60.

Stevens, A. A., L. A. Moore, C. J. Slocum, B. L. Smith, D. R. Seeger, and J. C. Ireland. 1990. By-products of chlorination at ten operating utilities, In *Water Chlorination, Environmental Impact and Health Effects*, vol. 6, eds. R. L. Jolley et al., pp. 579–604, Chelsea, MI: Lewis Publishers.

Stevens, D. K., R. J. Eyre, and R. J. Bull. (1992) Adduction of hemoglobin and albumin in vivo by metabolites of trichloroethylene, trichloroacetate and dichloroacetate in rats and mice. *Fundam. Appl. Toxicol.* 19: 336–342.

Styles, J. A., I. Wyatt, and C. Coutts. 1991. Trichloroacetic acid: Studies on uptake and effects on hepatic DNA and liver growth in mice. *Carcinogenesis* 12: 1715–1719.

Swan, S. H., R. R. Neutra, M. Wrensch, I. Hertz-Picciotto, G. C. Windham, L. Fenster, D. M. Epstein, and M. Deane. 1992. Is drinking water related to spontaneous abortion? Reviewing the evidence from the California Department of Health Services studies. *Epidemiology* 3: 83–93.

Symons, J. M., T. A. Bellar, J. K. Carswell, J. DeMarco, K. L. Kropp, G. G. Robeck, D. R. Seeger, C. J. Slocum, B. L. Smith, and A. A. Stevens. 1975. National organics reconnaissance survey for halogenated organics. *JAWWA* 67: 634–647.

Takamura, N., Y. Kurokawa, Y. Matsushima, T. Imazawa, H. Onodera, and Y. Hayashi. 1985. Long-term oral administration of potassium bromate in male Syrian golden hamsters. *Report of the Research Institute for Tuberculosis and Cancer*, Tohoku University Series C (Medicine), 32: 43–46.

Tao, L., K. Li, P. M. Kramer, and M. A. Pereira. 1996. Loss of herterozygosity on chromosome 6 in dichloroacetic acid and trichloroacetic acid-induced liver tumors in female B6C3F1 mice. *Toxicol. Lett.* 108: 257–261.

Taylor, D. H., and R. J. Pfohl. 1985. Effects of chlorine dioxide on neurobehavioral development of rats. In: *Water Chlorination: Chemistry, Environmental Impact and Health Effects*, vol. 5, eds. R. L. Jolley et al., pp. 355–364. Chelsea, MI: Lewis Publishers.

Testai, E. and L. Vittozzi. 1986. Biochemical alterations elicited in rat liver microsomes by oxidation and reduction products of chloroform metabolism. *Chem. Biol. Interact.* 59: 157–171.

Thomas, E. L., M. M. Jefferson, J. J. Bennett, and D. B. Learn. 1987. Mutagenic activity of chloramines. *Mutation Res.* 188: 35–43.

Thorton-Manning, J. R., J. C. Seely, and R. A. Pegram. 1994. Toxicity of bromodichloromethane in female rats and mice after repeated oral dosing. *Toxicology* 94: 3–18.

Thurman, E. M. 1986. Dissolved organic compounds in natural waters. In: *Organic Carcinogens in Drinking Water*, eds. N. Ram et al. New York: Wiley.

Til, H. P., R. A. Woutersen, V. J. Feron, H. M. Hollanders, and H. E. Falke. 1989. Two-year drinking-water study of formaldehyde in rats. *Food Chem. Toxicol.* 27: 77–87.

Tobe, M., K. Naito, and Y. Kurokawa. 1989. Chronic toxicity study on formaldehyde administered orally to rats. *Toxicology* 56: 79–86.

Toth, G. P., R. E. Long, T. S. Mills and M. K. Smith. 1990. Effects of chlorine dioxide on the developing rat brain. *J. Toxicol. Environ. Health* 31: 29–44.

Toth, G. P., K. C. Kelty, E. L. George, E. J. Read, and M. K. Smith. 1992. Adverse male reproductive effects following subchronic exposure of rats to sodium dichloroacetate. *Fundam. Appl. Toxicol.* 19: 57–63.

Travis, C. C., S. A. Richter, E. A. C. Crouch, R. Wilson, and E. D. Klema. 1987. Cancer risk management: A review of 132 federal regulatory decisions. *Environ. Sci. Technol.* 21: 415–420.

Uden, P. C., and J. W. Miller. 1983. Chlorinated acids and chloral in drinking water. *JAWWA* 75: 524–527.

Vartiatainen, T., and A. Liimatainen. 1986. High levels of mutagenic activity in chlorinated drinking water in Finland. *Mutation Res.* 169: 29–34.

Vena, J. E., S. Graham, J. Freudenheim, J. Marshall, M. Zielezny, M. Swanson, and G. Sufrin. 1993. Drinking water, fluid intake, and bladder cancer in Western New York. *Arch. Environ. Health* 48: 191–198.

von Gunten, U., A. Bruchet, and E. Costentin. 1996. Bromate formation in advanced oxidation processes. *JAWWA* 88: 53–65

Waskell, L. 1978. A study of the mutagenicity of anesthetics and their metabolites. *Mutation Res.* 57: 141–143.

Whitehouse, S., R. H. Cooper, and P. J. Randle. 1974a. Mechanism of activation of pyruvate dehydrogenase by dichloroacetate and other halogenated carboxylic acids. *Biochem. J.* 141: 761–764.

Whitehouse, S., R. H. Cooper, and P. J. Randle. 1974b. The metabolic effects of sodium dichloroacetate in the starved rat. *Biochem. J.* 142: 279–286.

Wideroff, L., G. Gridley, L. Mellemkjaer, W.-H. Chow, M. Linet, S. Keehn, K. Borch-Johnsen, J. H. Olsen. 1997. Cancer incidence in a population-based cohort of patients hospitalized with diabetes mellitus in Denmark. *J. Natl. Cancer Inst.* 89: 1360–1365.

Wilkins, J. R. III, and G. W. Comstock. 1981. Source of drinking water at home and site-specific cancer incidence in Washington County, Maryland. *Am. J. Epidemiol.* 114: 178–190.

Windham, G. C., S. H. Swan, L. Fenster, and R. R. Neutra. 1992. Tap or bottled water consumption and spontaneous abortion: A 1986 case-control study in California. *Epidemiology* 3: 113–119.

Winterbourn, C. C. 1985. Comparative reactivities of various biological compounds with myeloperoxidase-hydrogen peroxide-chloride, and similarity of the oxidant to hypochlorite. *Biochem. Biophys. Acta* 840: 204–210.

Wlodkowski, T. J., and H. S. Rosenkranz. 1975. Mutagenicity of sodium hypochlorite for Salmonella typhumurium. *Mutation Res.* 31: 39–42.

Woeber, K. A. 1991. Iodine and thyroid disease. *Med Clin. North America* 75: 169–178.

Wolfe, R. L., M. H. Stewart, S. Liang, and M. J. McGuire. 1989. Disinfection of model indicator organisms in a drinking water pilot plant by using peroxone. *Appl. Environ. Micro.* 55: 2230–2241.

Woutersen, R. A., L. M. Appelman, V. J. Feron, and C. A. Vander Heijden. 1984. Inhalation toxicity of acetaldehyde in rats, II. Carcinogenicity study interim results after 15 months. *Toxicology* 31: 123–133.

Woutersen, R. A., and V. J. Feron. 1987. Inhalation toxicology of acetaldehyde in rats, IV. Progression and regression of nasal lesions after discontinuation of exposure. *Toxicology* 47: 295–305.

Wrensch, M., S. H. Swan, J. Lipscomb, D. M. Epstein, R. R. Neutra, and L. Fenster. 1992. Spontaneous abortions and birth defects related to tap water and bottled water use, San Jose, California, 1980–1985. *Epidemiology* 3: 98–103.

Xu, G., D. K. Stevens, and R. J. Bull. 1995. Metabolism of bromodichloroacetate in B6C3F1 mice. *Drug Metab. Dispos.* 23: 1412–1416.

Yokose, Y., K. Uchida, D. Nakae, K. Shiraiwa, K. Yamamoto, and Y. Konishi. 1987. Studies of the carcinogenicity of sodium chlorite in B6C3F1 mice. *Environ. Health Perspect.* 76: 205–210.

Young, T. B., M. S. Kanarek, and A. A. Tsiatis. 1981. Epidemiologic study of drinking water chlorination and Wisconsin female cancer mortality. *J. Natl. Cancer Inst.* 67: 1191–1198.

Young, T. B., D. A. Wolf, and M. S. Kanarek. 1987. Case control study of colon cancer and drinking water trihalomethanes in Wisconsin. *Int. J. Epidemiol.* 16: 90.

Yount, E. A., S. Y. Felten, B. L. O'Connor, R. G. Peterson, R. S. Powell, M. N. Yum, and R. A. Harris. 1982. Comparison of the metabolic and toxic effects of 2-chloropropionate and dichloroacetate. *J. Pharmacol. Exp. Thera.* 222: 501–508.

Zeighami, E. A., A. P. Watson, and G. F. Craun. 1990. Serum lipid levels in neighboring communities with chlorinated and nonchlorinated drinking water. *Fundam. Appl. Toxicol.* 6: 421–432.

Zeiger, E., J. K. Haseman, M. D. Shelby, B. H. Margolin, and R. W. Tennant. 1990. Evaluation of four in vitro genetic toxicity tests for predicting rodent carcinogenicity: Confirmation of earlier results with 41 additional chemicals. *Environ. Mol. Mutagen.* 16 (suppl 18): 1–14.

Zierler, S., R. A,. Danley, and L. Feingold. 1986. Type of disinfectant in drinking water and patterns of mortality in Massachusetts. *Environ. Health Perspect.* 69: 275–279.

Zierler, S., L. Feingold, R. A. Danley, and G., Craun. 1988. Bladder cancer in Massachusetts related to chlorinated and chloraminated drinking water: A case-control study. *Arch. Environ. Health* 43: 195–200.

10 Environmental Tobacco Smoke

JONATHAN M. SAMET, M.D., M. S.
SOPHIA S. WANG, Ph.D.

Extensive toxicological, experimental, and epidemiological data, largely collected since the 1950s, have established that active cigarette smoking is the major preventable cause of morbidity and mortality in the United States; see reports of the U.S. Department of Health Education and Welfare (DHEW), U.S. Environmental Protection Agency (EPA), National Center for Health Statistics (1979), and U.S. Department of Health and Human Services (DHHS, 1989). More recently, since the 1970s, involuntary exposure to tobacco smoke has been investigated as a risk factor for disease; it has also been found to be a cause of preventable morbidity and mortality in nonsmokers. The 1986 report of the Surgeon General on smoking and health and a report by the National Research Council, also published in 1986, comprehensively reviewed the data on involuntary exposure to tobacco smoke and reached comparable conclusions with significant public health implications (see (DHHS, 1986b; NRC, 1986a). Both reports concluded that involuntary smoking causes disease in nonsmokers. Subsequently the Environmental Protection Agency reached a similar conclusion in its 1992 risk assessment, which classified environmental tobacco smoke as a class A carcinogen (EPA, 1992). These conclusions have already had significant impact on public policy and public health.

This chapter summarizes the converging and now extensive evidence on the health effects of involuntary exposure to tobacco smoke. Although the initial research on involuntary smoking addressed respiratory effects, more recent investigations have examined associations with diverse health effects including nonrespiratory cancers, ischemic heart disease, age at menopause, sudden infant death syndrome, and birth weight. This chapter covers the findings on the respiratory effects of passive smoking and also the newer evidence on other effects published since the 1986 reports of the Surgeon General and the National Research Council. The evidence on involuntary exposure to tobacco smoke is now voluminous, and consequently this review is selective in its citations. The most recent compilation of the evidence can be found in the 1997 report of the California Environmental Protection Agency, "Health Effects of Exposure to Environmental Tobacco Smoke" (Cal EPA, 1997).

This review, which updates a 1991 publication, comprehensively covers the newer evidence, including cardiovascular disease, asthma and ear disease in children, and sudden infant death syndrome (SIDS). It does not attempt full coverage of the evidence on health effects of passive smoking for which causal conclusions had already been reached in 1991: lung cancer and respiratory symptoms and lung function in children. The California report provides in-depth reviews and citations to the literature. Respiratory effects of passive

Environmental Toxicants: Human Exposures and Their Health Effects, 2/e. Edited by Morton Lippmann.
ISBN: 0-471-29298-2 © 2000 John Wiley & Sons, Inc.

smoking have also been covered in a recent series of systematic reviews published in *Thorax* (Strachan and Cook, 1997, 1998a, b; Anderson and Cook, 1997, Cook and Strachan, 1997) and in the *British Medical Journal* (Hackshaw, Law, and Wald, 1997; Law and Hackshaw, 1997). These reviews provide the basis for conclusions on passive smoking in the 1998 Report of the Scientific Committee on Tobacco and Health from the United Kingdom (Scientific Committee on Tobacco and Health and HSMO, 1998).

EXPOSURE TO ENVIRONMENTAL TOBACCO SMOKE (ETS)

Characteristics of Environmental Tobacco Smoke

Nonsmokers inhale ETS, the combination of the sidestream smoke that is released from the cigarette's burning end and the mainstream smoke exhaled by the active smoker (First, 1985). The inhalation of ETS is generally referred to as passive smoking or involuntary smoking. The exposures of involuntary and active smoking differ quantitatively and, to some extent, qualitatively (NRC, 1981, 1986 a, b; DHHS, 1984, 1986a, b; EPA, 1992; Guerin, Jenkins, and Tomkins, 1992). Because of the lower temperature in the burning cone of the smoldering cigarette, most partial pyrolysis products are enriched in sidestream as compared to mainstream smoke. Consequently sidestream smoke has higher concentrations of some toxic and carcinogenic substances than mainstream smoke; however, dilution by room air markedly reduces the concentrations inhaled by the involuntary smoker in comparison to those inhaled by the active smoker. Nevertheless, involuntary smoking is accompanied by exposure to toxic agents generated by tobacco combustion (NRC, 1981, 1986a, b; DHHS, 1984,1986a, b; EPA, 1992).

Environmental Tobacco Smoke Concentrations

Tobacco smoke is a complex mixture of gases and particles that contains myriad chemical species (DHEW, 1979; DHHS, 1984; Guerin, Jenkins, and Tomkins, 1992). Not surprisingly, tobacco smoking in indoor environments increases levels of respirable particles, nicotine, polycyclic aromatic hydrocarbons, carbon monoxide (CO), acrolein, nitrogen dioxide (NO_2), and many other substances. Tables 10-1 and 10-2 provide summaries of data from some recent studies (Hammond, 1999), and Table 10-3 considers some earlier studies. The extent of the increase in concentrations of these markers varies with the number of smokers, the intensity of smoking, the rate of exchange between the indoor air and with the outdoor air, and the use of air-cleaning devices. Ott (1999) has used mass balance models to characterize factors influencing concentrations of tobacco smoke indoors. Using information on the source strength (i.e., the generation of emissions by cigarettes) and on the air exchange rate, researchers can apply mass balance models to predict tobacco smoke concentrations. Such models can be used to estimate exposures and to project the consequences of control measures.

Several components of cigarette smoke have been measured in indoor environments as markers of the contribution of tobacco combustion to indoor air pollution. Particles have been measured most often because both sidestream and mainstream smoke contain high concentrations of particles in the respirable size range (NRC, 1986; DHHS, 1986). Particles are a nonspecific marker of tobacco smoke contamination, however, because numerous sources other than tobacco combustion add particles to indoor air. Other, more specific markers have also been measured, including nicotine, solanesol, and ultraviolet light (UV) absorption of particulate matter (Guerin, Jenkins, and Tomkins, 1992). Nicotine can be measured with active sampling methods and also using passive diffusion badges (Leaderer and Hammond, 1991; Guerin, Jenkins, and Tomkins, 1992). Studies of levels of

TABLE 10-1 Occupational ETS Exposures in Non-office Settings (Nonsmokers Only)

Company Type	Year Sampled	Number of Samples	Mean	Standard Deviation	Geometric Mean	Concentration of Nicotine, $\mu g/m^3$		
						Minimum	Median	Maximum
			Smoking allowed					
Specialty chemicals	1991–92	8	0.60	0.91	0.24	<0.05	0.46	2.78
Railroad workers (personal)	1983–84	152	0.80	3.30	0.18	<0.1	0.10	38.10
Tool manufacturing	1991–92	13	1.59	1.05	1.16	0.15	1.85	3.40
Textile finishing b	1991–92	11	1.74	1.69	1.10	0.31	0.93	5.09
Labels and paper products	1991–92	1	2.31				2.31	
Die manufacturer	1991–92	12	2.70	1.27	2.46	1.23	2.41	5.42
Sintering metal	1991–92	12	2.88	2.59	2.11	0.62	2.24	9.72
Newspaper B	1991–92	5	2.96	1.37	2.68	1.23	2.78	4.63
Miscellaneous	<1990	282	4.30	11.80	1.70	<1.6	<1.6	126.00
Textile finishing, A	1991–92	11	4.33	8.82	1.77	0.46	1.39	30.71
Flight attendants (personal)	1988	16	4.70	4.00	2.32	0.10	4.20	10.50
Fire fighters A[a]	1991–92	16	5.39	3.81	4.08	1.20	4.84	13.42
Fire fighters B	1991–92	24	5.83	6.77	3.83	0.71	3.65	27.50
Barber shop (personal)	1986–87	2	8.80			4.00		13.70
Hospital (personal)	1986–87	5	24.80	22.80	16.80	6.30	10.00	53.20
			Smoking restricted					
Work clothing	1991–92	9	0.17	0.32	0.06	<0.05	<0.05	0.93
Filtration products	1991–92	10	0.32	0.87	0.08	<0.05	<0.05	2.78
Film and imaging	1991–92	6	0.82	0.83	0.39	<0.05	0.70	2.16
Fiber optics	1991–92	13	1.34	2.79	0.63	0.20	0.64	10.57
Newspaper A	1991–92	4	4.86	6.65	2.62	0.93	1.85	14.81
Valve manufacturer	1991–92	10	5.80	7.85	3.62	1.16	3.26	27.31
Rubber products	1991–92	2	5.85	5.36	4.18	2.06	5.85	9.64

321

TABLE 10-1 (*Continued*)

Company Type	Year Sampled	Number of Samples	Mean	Standard Deviation	Geometric Mean	Concentration of Nicotine, μg/m³		
						Minimum	Median	Maximum
			Smoking Prohibited					
Infrared and imaging systems	1991–92	1	<0.05				<0.05	
Hospital products	1991–92	5	0.08	0.17	<0.05	<0.05	<0.05	0.39
Weapons systems	1991–92	12	0.08	0.20	<0.05	<0.05	<0.05	0.63
Aircraft components	1991–92	12	0.20	0.18	0.13	<0.05	0.21	0.61
Radar communications components	1991–92	13	0.31	0.36	0.14	<0.05	0.26	1.08
Computer chip equipment	1991–92	10	0.51	0.33	0.41	0.15	0.39	1.08

Source: Hammond (1999).
[a] Omits one data point, 101 μg/m³.

TABLE 10-2 Nicotine Concentrations in Homes

	Year Sampled	Number of Samples	Mean	Concentration of Nicotine, $\mu g/m^3$			
				Standard Deviation	Minimum	Median	Maximum
North Carolina homes (weekly)	1988	13	1.50	1.10	1.00	1.40	4.40
Personal (each sampled 3 ×)	1988	15					
Males (personal: 16 hours)[a]	1993–94	86	2.13			1.29	>8.08
New York homes (weekly)	1986	47	2.20		0.10	1.00	9.40
Females (personal: 16 hours)[a]	1993–94	220	2.93			1.14	>7.81
North Carolina homes (14 hours: 5 p.m. to 7 a.m.)	1986	13	3.74			3.3[c]	6.5
Minnesota homes (weekly)	1989[c]	25	5.80		0.10	3.00	28.60

[a] 16 hour average; "away from work."
[b] Ninety-fifth percentile, as noted in the chapter.
[c] Assumed 16 hour exposure.

Source: Hammond (1999).

TABLE 10-3 Selected Studies of Tobacco Smoke Component Concentrations in Various Environments in the 1970s and 1980s

Reference	Location	Component	Mean Concentration
Badre et al. (1978)	Room, 18 smokers	Acrolein	$0.19\ \mu g/m^3$
Badre et al. (1978)	Room, 18 smokers	Benzene	$0.11\ \mu g/m^3$
Wallace (1987)	NJ homes, smokers	Benzene	$16\ \mu g/m^3$, overnight
	NJ homes, nonsmokers	Benzene	$8.4\ \mu g/m^3$, overnight
Chappell and Parker (1977)	Offices	Carbon monoxide	2.5 ppm, samples 2–3 min
Chappell and Parker (1977)	Nightclubs	Carbon monoxide	13.0 ppm, sampled 2–3 min
Hinds and First (1975)	Restaurant	Nicotine	$5.2\ \mu g/m^3$, sampled 2.5 h
Hinds and First (1975)	Train	Nicotine	$6.3\ \mu g/m^3$, sampled 2.5 h
Muramatsu et al. (1984)	Cafeterias	Nicotine	$26.4\ \mu g/m^3$
Weber and Fischer (1980)	Offices	Nitrogen dioxide	24 ppb
Repace and Lowrey (1980)	Cocktail party	Particles	$351\ \mu g/m^3$, 15 min sample
	Bowling alley	Particles	$202\ \mu g/m^3$, 20 min sample
	Bar	Particles	$334\ \mu g/m^3$, 26 min sample
Spengler et al. (1981)	Residences, ≥ 2 smokers	Particles	$70\ \mu g/m^3$, 24 h samples
	Residences, 1 smoker	Particles	$37\ \mu g/m^3$, 24 h samples
Henderson et al. (1989)	Residences, cigarette smoking	Nicotine	$3.4\ \mu g/m^3$, 14 h samples
	Residences, no cigarette smoking	Nicotine	$0.3\ \mu g/m^3$, 14 h samples

Source: Guerin, Jenkins, and Tomkins (1992).

ETS components have been conducted largely in public buildings; fewer studies have been conducted in homes and offices (NRC, 1986a; DHHS, 1986b).

The contribution of various environments to personal exposure to tobacco smoke varies with the time-activity pattern, namely the distribution of time spent in different locations. Time-activity patterns may heavily influence lung airway exposures in particular environments for certain groups of individuals. For example, exposure in the home predominates for infants who do not attend day care (Harlos et al., 1987). For adults residing with nonsmokers, the workplace may be the principal location where exposure takes place. A recent nationwide study assessed exposures of nonsmokers in 16 metropolitan areas of the United States (Jenkins et al., 1996). This study, involving 100 persons in each location, was directed at workplace exposure and included measurements of respirable particulate matter and other markers. The results showed that in 1993 and 1994, exposures to ETS in the home were generally much greater than those in the workplace.

The contribution of smoking in the home to indoor air pollution has been demonstrated by studies using personal monitoring and monitoring of homes for respirable particles. In one of the early studies, Spengler et al. (1981) monitored homes in six U.S. cities for respirable particle concentrations over several years and found that a smoker of one pack of cigarettes daily contributed about 20 $\mu g/m^3$ to 24 hour indoor particle concentrations. In homes with two or more heavy smokers, this study showed that the pre-1987 24 hour National Ambient Air Quality Standard (NAAQS) of 260 $\mu g/m^3$ for total suspended particulates could be exceeded. Because cigarettes are not smoked uniformly over the day, higher peak concentrations must occur when cigarettes are actually smoked. Spengler et al. (1985) measured the personal exposures to respirable particles sustained by nonsmoking adults in two rural Tennessee communities. The mean 24 hour exposures were substantially higher for those exposed to smoke at home: 64 $\mu g/m^3$ for those exposed versus 36 $\mu g/m^3$ for those not exposed.

In several studies, small numbers of homes have been monitored for nicotine, which is a vapor-phase constituent of ETS. In a study of ETS exposure of day-care children, average nicotine concentration during the time that the ETS-exposed children were at home was 3.7 $\mu g/m^3$; in homes without smoking, the average was 0.3 $\mu g/m^3$ (Henderson, et al., 1989). Coultas and colleagues (Coultas et al., 1990a measured 24 hour nicotine and respirable particle concentrations in 10 homes on alternate days for a week and then on five more days during alternate weeks. The mean levels of nicotine were comparable to those in the study of Henderson et al. (1989), but some 24 hour values were as high as 20 $\mu g/m^3$. Nicotine and respirable particle concentrations varied widely in the homes.

The total exposure assessment methodology (TEAM) study, conducted by the U.S. Environmental Protection Agency, provided extensive data on concentrations of 20 volatile organic compounds in a sample of homes in several communities (Wallace and Pellizzari, 1987). Indoor monitoring showed increased concentrations of benzene, xylenes, ethylbenzene, and styrene in homes with smokers compared to homes without smokers.

More extensive information is available on levels of ETS components in public buildings and workplaces of various types (Hammond, 1999; Guerin, Jenkins, and Tomkins, 1992) (Tables 10-1 and 10-3). Monitoring in locations where smoking may be intense, such as bars and restaurants, has generally shown elevations of particles and other markers of smoke pollution where smoking is taking place (DHHS, 1986b; NRC, 1986a). For example, Repace and Lowrey (1980) in an early study used a portable piezobalance to sample aerosols in restaurants, bars, and other locations. In the places sampled, respirable particulate levels ranged up to 700 $\mu g/m^3$, and the levels varied with the intensity of smoking. Similar data have been reported for the office environment (DHHS, 1986b; NRC, 1986a; Guerin, Jenkins, and Tomkins, 1992; Cal EPA, 1997). Recent studies indicate low concentrations in many workplace settings, reflecting declining smoking prevalence in recent years and changing practices of smoking in the workplace. Using passive nicotine samplers, Hammond (1999) showed that worksite smoking policies can sharply reduce ETS exposure.

Transportation environments may also be polluted by cigarette smoking. Contamination of air in trains, buses, automobiles, airplanes, and submarines has been documented (DHHS, 1986b; NRC, 1986a). A National Research Council Report (NRC, 1986b) on air quality in airliners summarized studies for tobacco smoke pollutants in commercial aircraft. In one study, during a single flight, the NO_2 concentration varied with the number of passengers with a lighted cigarette. In another study, respirable particles in the smoking section were measured at concentrations five or more times higher than in the nonsmoking section. Peaks as high as 1000 $\mu g/m^3$ were measured in the smoking section. Mattson and colleagues (1989) used personal exposure monitors to assess nicotine exposures of passengers and flight attendants. All persons were exposed to nicotine, even if seated in the nonsmoking portion of the cabin. Exposures were much greater in the smoking than in the nonsmoking section and were also greater in aircraft with recirculated air.

Biological Markers of Exposure

Biological markers can be used to describe the prevalence of exposure to environmental tobacco smoke, to investigate the dosimetry of involuntary smoking, and to validate questionnaire-based measures of exposure. In both active and involuntary smokers, the detection of tobacco smoke components or their metabolites in body fluids or alveolar air provides evidence of exposure to tobacco smoke, and levels of these markers can be used to gauge the intensity of exposure. The risk of involuntary smoking has also been estimated by comparing levels of biological markers in active and involuntary smokers.

At present, the most sensitive and specific markers for tobacco smoke exposure are nicotine and its metabolite, cotinine (NRC, 1986a; Jarvis and Russell, 1984; DHHS, 1988). Neither nicotine nor cotinine is usually present in body fluids in the absence of exposure to tobacco smoke, although unusually large intakes of some foods could produce measurable levels of nicotine and cotinine (Idle, 1990). Cotinine, formed by oxidation of nicotine by cytochrome P-450, is one of several primary metabolites of nicotine (DHHS, 1988). Cotinine itself is extensively metabolized, and only about 17% of cotinine is excreted unchanged in the urine.

Because the circulating half-life of nicotine is generally shorter than 2 hours (Rosenberg et al., 1980), nicotine concentrations in body fluids reflect more recent exposures. In contrast, cotinine has a half-life in the blood or plasma of active smokers of about 10 hours (DHHS, 1988; Kyerematen et al., 1982; Benowitz et al., 1983); hence cotinine levels provide information about more chronic exposure to tobacco smoke in both active and involuntary smokers. Whether cotinine has the same half-life in plasma, saliva, and urine has been uncertain, as is the choice of the optimal body fluid for measuring cotinine for research purposes (Jarvis et al., 1988; Wall et al., 1988; Haley et al., 1989). Concerns about nonspecificity of cotinine, arising from eating nicotine-containing foods, have been set aside (Benowitz, 1996). Thiocyanate concentration in body fluids, concentration of CO in expired air, and carboxyhemoglobin level distinguish active smokers from nonsmokers but are not as sensitive and specific as cotinine for assessing involuntary exposure to tobacco smoke (Hoffman et al., 1984; Jarvis and Russell, 1984).

Cotinine levels have been measured in adult nonsmokers and in children (Table 10-4) (Benowitz, 1996). In the studies of adult nonsmokers, exposures at home, in the workplace, and in other settings determined cotinine concentrations in urine and saliva. The cotinine levels in involuntary smokers ranged from less than 1% to about 8% of cotinine levels measured in active smokers. Smoking by parents was the predominant

TABLE 10-4 Cotinine Concentrations in Nonsmokers and Smokers (Selected Studies)

Study	Number of Subjects	Smoking Status	Exposure Level	Plasma or Serum Cotinine (ng/ml)	Urine Cotinine (ng/ml)	Salivary Cotinine (ng/ml)
Jarvis et al. (1984)	46	Nonsmokers	No exposure	0.8	1.5	0.7
	54	Nonsmokers	Exposed	2.0	7.7	2.5
Wald and Ritchie (1984)	101	Nonsmokers	Wife nonsmoker		8.5 (SE* ±1.3, median 5.0)	
	20	Nonsmokers	Wife smoker		25.2 (SE ±14.8, median 9.0)	
Wald et al. (1984)	43	Nonsmokers	0–1.5 hours ETS* exposure/week		1.8	
	47	Nonsmokers	1.5–4.5 hours ETS exposure/week		3.4	
	43	Nonsmokers	4.5–8.6 hours ETS exposure/week		5.3	
	43	Nonsmokers	8.6–29 hours ETS exposure/week		14.7	
	45	Nonsmokers	20–80 hours ETS exposure/week		29.6	
Jarvis et al. (1985)	269	Nonsmokers, children	Neither parent smoked			
	96	Nonsmokers, children	Father smoked			
	76	Nonsmokers, children	Mother smoked			
	128	Nonsmokers, children	Both parents smoked			
Coultas et al. (1986)	68	Nonsmokers aged < 5 years	No smoker in home			
	41	Nonsmokers aged < 5 years	1 smoker in home			
	21	Nonsmokers aged < 5 years	2 or more smokers in home			
	200	Nonsmokers aged 5–17 years	No smoker in home			
	96	Nonsmokers aged 5–17 years	1 smoker in home			
	25	Nonsmokers aged 5–17 years	2 or more smokers in home			
	316	Nonsmokers aged >17 years	No smoker in home			
	60	Nonsmokers aged >17 years	1 smoker in home			
	12	Nonsmokers aged >17 years	2 or more smokers in home			
Strachan et al. (1989)	405	Nonsmokers, age 7 years	No smokers in home			
	241	Nonsmokers, age 7 years	1 smoker in home			
	124	Nonsmokers, age 7 years	2 or more smokers in home			

TABLE 10-4 (Continued)

Study	Number of Subject	Smoking Status	Exposure Level	Plasma or Serum Cotinine (ng/ml)	Urine Cotinine (ng/ml)	Salivary Cotinine (ng/ml)
Thompson et al. (1990)	158	Nonsmokers	Lives alone or with nonsmoker		4.4 (geometric mean) (95% CI: 3.6–5.4)	
	26	Nonsmokers	Lives with smoker		11.4 (geometric mean) (95% CI: 8.9–18.9)	
Cummings et al. (1990)	162	Nonsmokers	No exposure past 4 days		6.2 (mean)	
	208	Nonsmokers	1–2 exposures past 4 days		7.8 (mean)	
	152	Nonsmokers	3–5 exposures past 4 days		9.8 (mean)	
	141	Nonsmokers	6 or more exposures		12.5 (mean)	
Tunstall-Pedoe et al. (1991)	1873	Nonsmokers, male		0.68 (median)		
	1940	Smokers, male		240 (median)		
	2270	Nonsmokers, female		0.10 (median)		
Cook et al. (1994)	1260	Nonsmokers, aged 5–7 years	No smokers in home			0.29 (geometric mean) (95% CI: 0.28–0.31)
	293	Nonsmokers, aged 5–7 years	Mother smoker			2.2 (geometric mean) (95% CI: 1.9–2.5)
	521	Nonsmokers, aged 5–7 years	Father smoker			1.2 (geometric mean) (95% CI: 1.1–1.3)
	553	Nonsmokers, aged 5–7 years	Mother and father smokers			4.0 (geometric mean) (95% CI: 3.7–4.4)
Riboli et al. (1990)	629	Nonsmokers, females from 10 countries	No home or work ETS exposure		2.7 ng/mg creatinine	
	210	Nonsmokers, females from 10 countries	Exposure at work but not at home		4.8 ng/mg creatinine	
	359	Nonsmokers, females from 10 countries	Exposure at home but not at work		9.0 ng/mg creatinine	
	124	Nonsmokers, females from 10 countries	Exposure at home and at work		10.0 ng/mg creatinine	
Pirkle et al. (1996)	1071	Nonsmokers, aged 4–11 years	No home ETS exposure	0.12 (geometric mean) (95% CI: 0.10–0.14)		

713	Nonsmokers, aged 4–11 years	Home ETS exposure only	1.13 (geometric mean) (95% CI: 0.98–1.34)
379	Nonsmokers, aged 12–16 years	No home ETS exposure	0.11 (geometric mean) (95% CI: 0.10–0.15)
268	Nonsmokers, aged 12–16 years	Home ETS exposure only	0.81 (geometric mean) (95% CI: 0.62–1.04)
3154	Nonsmokers, aged ≥17 years	No home or work ETS exposure	0.12 (geometric mean) (95% CI: 0.11–0.14)
1332	Nonsmokers, workers aged ≥17 years	No home or work ETS exposure	0.13 (geometric mean) (95% CI: 0.12–0.15)
779	Nonsmokers, workers aged ≥17 years	Work ETS exposure only	0.32 (geometric mean) (95% CI: 0.28–0.36)
315	Nonsmokers, workers aged ≥17 years	Home ETS exposure only	0.65 (geometric mean) (95% CI: 0.52–0.81)
246	Nonsmokers, workers aged ≥17 years	Home and work ETS exposure	0.93 (geometric mean) (95% CI: 0.76–1.13)

Source: Benowitz (1996).

determinant of the cotinine levels in their children. For example, Greenberg et al. (1984) found significantly higher concentrations of cotinine in the urine and saliva of infants exposed to cigarette smoke in their homes than in unexposed controls. Urinary cotinine levels in the infants increased with the number of cigarettes smoked during the previous 24 hours by the mother. In a study of school children in England, salivary cotinine levels rose with the number of smoking parents in the home (Jarvis et al., 1985). In a study of a national sample of participants in the Third National Health and Nutrition Examination Survey conducted in 1988 to 1991, 88% of nonsmokers had a detectable level of serum cotinine using liquid chromatography–mass spectrometry as the assay method (Pirkle et al., 1996). Cotinine levels in this national sample increased with the number of smokers in the household and the hours exposed in the workplace.

The results of studies on biological markers have important implications for research on involuntary smoking and add to the biological plausibility of associations between involuntary smoking and disease documented in epidemiological studies (Benowitz, 1996). The data on marker levels provide ample evidence that involuntary exposure leads to absorption, circulation, and excretion of tobacco smoke components. The studies of biological markers also confirm the high prevalence of involuntary smoking, as ascertained by questionnaire (Benowitz, 1996; Coultas et al., 1987; Pirkle et al., 1996). The observed correlations between reported exposures and levels of markers suggest that questionnaire methods for assessing recent exposure have some validity.

Comparisons of levels of biological markers in smokers and nonsmokers have been made in order to estimate the relative intensities of active and involuntary smoking. However, proportionality cannot be assumed between the ratio of the levels of markers in passive and active smokers and the relative doses of other tobacco smoke components. Nonetheless, several investigators have previously attempted to characterize involuntary smoking in terms of active smoking. For example, Foliart and colleagues (Foliart, Benowitz, and Becker, 1983) measured urinary excretion of nicotine in flight attendants during an 8 hour flight and estimated that the average exposure was 0.12 to 0.25 mg of nicotine. Russell, West, and Jarvis (1985) compared nicotine levels in nonsmokers exposed to tobacco smoke with levels achieved following infusion of known doses of nicotine. On the basis of this comparison, the investigators estimated that the average rate of nicotine absorption was 0.23 mg per hour in a smoky tavern, 0.36 mg per hour in an unventilated smoke-filled room, and 0.014 mg per hour from average daily exposure. In active smokers the first cigarette of the day resulted in absorption of 1.4 mg of nicotine.

Exposure Assessment

The information on the health effects of involuntary smoking has been largely derived from observational epidemiological studies. In these studies exposure to ETS has been estimated primarily by responses to questionnaires concerning the smoking habits of household members or of fellow employees; attempts have been made to quantitate exposure by determining the number of cigarettes smoked by family members and the duration of exposure. Biomarkers have also been used in some studies. Limitations of the questionnaire approach were discussed extensively in the 1986 report of the Surgeon General (DHHS, 1986b). The general topic is treated in a 1997 review by the Jaakkolas (Jaakkola and Jaakkola, 1997).

A number of studies have addressed questionnaires and biological markers for assessing exposure to ETS. In studies of lung cancer and passive smoking, questionnaires have been used to assess the smoking habits of spouses and, in a few studies, of parents. Two studies evaluated the reliability of questionnaires on lifetime exposure (Pron et al., 1988; Coultas, Peake, and Samet, 1989). Both showed a high degree of repeatability for questions concerning whether a spouse had smoked but lower reliability for responses concerning quantitative aspects of exposure. Because validity could not be assessed directly, reliability was used as a measure of information quality.

Several studies have assessed the validity of subjects' reports on smoking by parents and spouses. Sandler and Shore (1986) compared responses on parents' smoking given by cases and controls with responses given by the parents or siblings of the index subjects. Concordance was high for whether the parents had ever smoked. Responses concerning numbers of cigarettes smoked did not agree as highly. In a follow-up study of a nationwide sample, children's responses on smoking by their deceased parents closely agreed with the information given 10 years previously by the parents (McLaughlin et al., 1987). A number of studies have shown that people correctly report the smoking habits of their spouses (DHHS, 1990a). In a study of nonsmokers in Buffalo, index subjects' reports agreed well with reports from parents or siblings, spouse or children, and coworkers concerning exposure during childhood, at home, and at work, respectively (Cummings et al., 1989).

Nicotine is present primarily as a vapor-phase component in ETS and can thus be sampled using a diffusion-based monitor (Hammond and Leaderer, 1987). Coghlin, Hammond, Gann and colleagues (1989) described the use of a passive nicotine monitor as well as a questionnaire and diary approach for characterizing exposure to ETS. In a sample of 19 volunteers, they found a strong correlation between the monitored nicotine exposure and a questionnaire-based index. The sampling lasted only a week, however, and the diary method would be too cumbersome to implement among all participants in a large epidemiological study. Coultas et al. (1990b) measured personal exposure to ETS using a personal pump and a collection system for nicotine. In a small sample of volunteers, they established the feasibility of this approach.

Although biological markers have provided important evidence of population exposures, the utility of cotinine as an indicator of individual exposure has been questioned. Idle (1990) has reviewed the complex metabolism of nicotine and the many factors affecting the relationship between exposure to atmospheric nicotine and the concentration of cotinine in body fluids. He cautions against using any single determination of cotinine as a measure of exposure.

Several epidemiological studies support this concern about the limited validity of a single measurement of cotinine. Spot cotinine levels are not tightly predicted by questionnaire measures of exposures (Coultas, Peake, and Samet, 1989; Cummings et al., 1990), and cotinine levels are highly variable at any particular level of smoking in a household (Coultas et al., 1990a). Thus questionnaires remain the best method for characterizing usual exposure to ETS. However, biological markers and personal monitoring offer complementary approaches for developing more accurate exposure estimates for estimating dose and judging the extent of misclassification introduced by questionnaires.

HEALTH EFFECTS OF INVOLUNTARY SMOKING IN CHILDREN

Fetal Effects

Researchers have demonstrated that active smoking by mothers results in a variety of adverse health effects in children. Some of the health effects result predominantly from transplacental exposure of the fetus to tobacco smoke components. Recently studies have also investigated and demonstrated associations between adverse health effects in children and exposure to ETS. For example, paternal smoking in the presence of a pregnant mother may lead to perinatal health effects manifested upon birth of the baby, and either maternal or paternal smoking in the presence of a newborn child may lead to postnatal health effects in the developing child.

Potential health effects on the fetus resulting from ETS include fetal growth effects (decreased birth weight, growth retardation, or prematurity), fetal loss (spontaneous abortion and perinatal mortality), and congenital malformations. Health effects on the child postnatally, resulting from either ETS exposure to the fetus or to the newborn child, include sudden infant death syndrome (SIDS) and adverse effects on neuropsychological development and physical growth. Possible longer-term health effects of fetal ETS exposure include childhood cancers of the brain, leukemia, and lymphomas, among others.

Biological Plausibility

Fetal exposure to carbon monoxide and nicotine due to ETS may increase risk for perinatal health effects. Carbon monoxide in ETS may contribute to increased concentrations of carbon monoxide and carboxyhemoglobin in the fetus, and the fetus may not be able to physiologically compensate for the reduced oxygen delivery (DHHS, 1980), leading to fetal hypoxia. Chronic fetal hypoxia may lead to impaired development of the fetal central nervous system, with abnormal control of cardiorespiratory activity, and thus to SIDS (Harper and Frysinger, 1988). One study showed increased rates of central apnea in infants of smokers (Toubas et al., 1986).

Exposure to nicotine found in ETS can also alter an infant's catecholamine metabolism and response to hypoxia (Milerad and Sundell, 1993). Furthermore nicotine crossing the placenta may lead to decreased in utero placental perfusion, affecting the fetal cardiovascular system, gastrointestinal system, and central nervous system (Stillman, Rosenberg, and Sachs, 1986). Other constituents of cigarette smoke have also been demonstrated to adversely affect fetal growth (Cal EPA, 1996).

Association between ETS and childhood cancers is biologically plausible due to the presence of carcinogenic tobacco smoke components or metabolites, such as benzene, nitrosamines, urethane, and radioactive compounds, at organ sites of the cancers. In animal studies, neurogenic tumors as well as other tumors were induced after transplacental exposure to a number of compounds present in tobacco smoke, including several nitrosamines. Moreover Huel and colleagues (1989) measured aryl hydrocarbon hydroxylase activity in human placentas of passive smokers; levels were increased in placentas of women passively exposed to tobacco smoke.

Nonfatal Perinatal Health Effects

Fetal Growth   Most studies have used paternal smoking as the exposure measure to assess the association between ETS exposure and nonfatal perinatal health effects, such as reduced fetal growth. Low birth weight was first reported in 1957 to be associated with maternal smoking (DHHS, 1980). Extensive studies have since been conducted to assess ETS exposure and birth weight, accounting for gestational age at delivery, multiple births, maternal age, race, parity, maternal smoking, socioeconomic status, and pregnancy history (DHHS, 1994). Exposures have been measured with questionnaires that assess home and work exposure, and in some studies, with the use of biomarkers.

Recent studies continue to report lower birth weight for infants of nonsmoking women passively exposed to tobacco smoke during pregnancy (Martin and Bracken, 1986; Rubin et al., 1986). Haddow and colleagues (1988) used cotinine as a biomarker to measure exposure to ETS; they also adequately controlled for potential confounders. ETS exposure was defined as cotinine levels of 1.1 to 9.9 ng/mL in the fetus born to a nonsmoking mother. Their study demonstrated a decrease of 100 grams in birthweight for fetuses exposed to ETS. The most recent biomarker studies (Eskenazi and Bergmann, 1995; Eskenazi and Trupin, 1995; Martinez et al., 1994) support the findings of Haddow et al. (1988). Other epidemiologic studies assessed ETS exposure from multiple sources through questionnaire (Mainous and Hueston, 1994; Roquer et al., 1995; Rebagliato, Florey, and Bolumar, 1995). While not using a method as specific or sensitive as cotinine measurements, these studies still demonstrated decreases in mean birthweights after adjustment for confounders (20 to 40 g).

Other Effects Other nonfatal perinatal health effects possibly associated with ETS are growth retardation and congenital malformations. Martin and Bracken (1986) demonstrated a strong association with growth retardation in their 1986 study. More recent studies (Roquer et al., 1995; Mainous and Hueston, 1994) have supported this finding; however, these studies had small sample sizes and did not control for potential confounders.

The few studies (Zhang et al., 1992; Savitz, Schwingl, and Keels, 1991; Seidman, Ever-Hadani, and Gale, 1990) conducted to assess the association between paternal smoking and congenital malformations have demonstrated odds ratios ranging from 1.2 to 2.6. The most consistent associations have been found with the central nervous system or neural tube defects. However, due to possible effects of active smoke on the sperm, a causal association between ETS and congenital malformations cannot be concluded.

Fatal Perinatal Health Effects

ETS exposure to the fetus during its development may lead to fatal perinatal health effects such as spontaneous abortion and perinatal mortality. Very few studies have examined the association between ETS exposure and perinatal death. Eight studies have examined neonatal mortality in relation to paternal smoking; a few supported an increase in risk (Comstock and Lundin, 1967; Mau and Netter, 1974; Lindbohm, et al., 1991; Ahlborg, Jr. and Bodin, 1991).

Postnatal Health Effects

ETS exposure due to maternal or paternal smoking may lead to postnatal health effects related to SIDS, physical development, decrements in cognition and behavior, and cancers.

SIDS To date, 10 studies have been directed at the association between SIDS and postnatal maternal ETS exposure; 6 studies have addressed the association between paternal smoking and SIDS, and 4 studies have assessed household smoke exposure and SIDS (Table 10-5). While maternal smoking during pregnancy has been associated with SIDS, these studies measured maternal smoking after pregnancy, along with paternal smoking and household smoking generally. Effects of ETS exposure after birth and maternal smoking during pregnancy cannot be readily separated in many of these studies.

Mitchell and colleagues (Mitchell et al., 1993) demonstrated a significant association (odds ratio, OR = 1.7) between postnatal maternal smoking and SIDS; this association remained significant after adjustment for potential confounders. In their updated study Mitchell and colleagues (Mitchell, Scragg, and Clements, 1995) concluded that while SIDS was associated with postnatal maternal smoking, the elimination of postnatal maternal smoking did not reduce the risk of SIDS, and that prenatal exposure was still the more important risk factor. Similarly Schoendorf and Kiely (1992) demonstrated an adjusted odds ratio of 1.8 for SIDS associated with postnatal ETS exposure. In a larger study Klonoff-Cohen and colleagues (1995) found an adjusted odds ratio of 2.3 for postnatal ETS exposure. Three more studies assessing maternal smoking after pregnancy (Bergman and Wiesner, 1976; McGlashan, 1989; Mitchell et al., 1991) could not assess a possible independent relationship between postnatal smoking and SIDS due to extensive overlap between maternal smoking during and after pregnancy.

TABLE 10-5 Studies Investigating the Association between ETS and SIDS

Study Reference	Location	Outcome Assessed	Exposure	Exposure Ascertainment	Participants	OR	OR Adjusted for:
Bergman and Wiesner (1976)	United States (King County, Washington)	SIDS	Maternal smoking after pregnancy Paternal smoking	Mailed questionnaire	56 cases 86 controls	2.4 (1.2, 4.8) 1.5 (0.7, 3.2)	Matched on: date of birth, sex, and race Not adjusted for maternal smoking
McGlashan (1989)	Tasmania	SIDS	Maternal smoking during and after pregnancy Paternal smoking	Interviewed parents	167 cases 334 controls	1.9 (1.2, 2.9) "Significantly increased"	Matched on sex
Mitchell et al. (1991)	New Zealand	SIDS	Maternal smoking after pregnancy	Interview with parents or from medical records	128 cases 503 controls	1.8 (1.0, 3.3)	Demographic factors, social factors, breast-feeding, season, sleeping position
Nicholl and O'Cathain (1992)	United Kingdom	SIDS	Paternal smoking		242 cases 251 controls	1.4 (0.8, 2.4)	Spousal smoking matched for date and place of birth
Schoendorf and Kiely (1992)	United States (U.S. National Maternal and Infant Health Survey)	SIDS	Maternal smoking after pregnancy	Interview	435 cases 6000 controls	Whites: 1.8 (1.0, 3.0) Blacks: 2.3 (1.5, 3.7)	Maternal age, education, marital status
Mitchell et al. (1993)	New Zealand	SIDS	Maternal smoking after pregnancy Paternal smoking	Interview with parents of from medical records	485 cases 1800 controls	1.7 (1.2, 2.3) 1.4 (1.0, 1.8)	Region, season, breast-feeding, bed sharing, mother's marital status, SES, age, smoking during pregnancy, infant's age, sex, birth

Reference	Location	Outcome	Exposure	Sample size	Odds ratio (95% CI)	Confounders
Klonoff-Cohen et al. (1995)	United States (southern California)	SIDS	Maternal smoking after pregnancy	200 cases 200 controls	2.3 (1.0, 5.0)	weight, race, sleeping, position, smoking by mother, smoking by father, smoking by other household members
			Same-room, maternal smoking after pregnancy		4.6 (1.8, 11.8)	Birth weight, routine sleep position, medical conditions at birth, prenatal care, breast-feeding, maternal smoking during pregnancy
			Paternal smoking		3.5 (1.9, 6.8)	
			Same-room, paternal smoking		5.0 (2.4, 11.0)	
Blair et al. (1996)	United Kingdom	SIDS	Paternal smoking	195 cases 780 controls	2.5 (1.5, 4.2)	Maternal, age, marital status, SES, maternal smoking, drug and alcohol use, gestational age, sleeping position, breast-feeding, matched by age and region

Of the six studies conducted to assess the association between paternal smoking and SIDS, four (Nicholl and O'Cathain, 1992; Mitchell et al., 1993; Klonoff-Cohen et al., 1995; Blair et al., 1996) demonstrated elevated risks for SIDS while accounting for maternal smoking either by study design or through analyses, with odds ratios of 1.6, 1.4, 3.5, and 2.5, respectively. Two studies (Bergman and Wiesner, 1976; McGlashan, 1989) demonstrated elevated risks but did not adjust for maternal smoking.

Four studies assessed general household smoke exposure and SIDS. Dose–response relationships were observed by Blair and colleagues (1996), Mitchell and colleagues (1993), and Klonoff-Cohen and colleagues (1995). Klonoff-Cohen and colleagues reported adjusted odds ratios for 1 to 10, 11 to 20, and ≥ 21 cigarettes/day of 2.4, 3.6, and 22.7, respectively. Schoendorf and Kiely (1992) only demonstrated increased risk of SIDS in white infants.

Cognition and Behavior   While it is biologically plausible that ETS affects a child's neuropsychological development—perhaps through nicotine's effect on the central nervous system and through the effect of chronic exposure to carbon monoxide—few studies have provided the data needed to examine this relationship independent of prenatal exposure and maternal active smoking. Furthermore cognition and behavior are also measured through a variety of tests, making direct comparisons between studies difficult.

Makin, Fried, and Watkinson (1991) compared cognitive test scores of children of nonsmoking mothers exposed to ETS during pregnancy to children of unexposed mothers. Decrements in test scores were demonstrated for children whose mothers were exposed to ETS during their pregnancy. The much larger study conducted by Eskenazi and Trupin (1995), which used serum cotinine to ascertain ETS exposure, however, failed to detect such an association. Five more studies (Baghurst et al., 1992; Bauman, Koch, and Fisher, 1989; Bauman and Flewelling, 1991; Denson, Nanson, and McWatters, 1975; Weitzman, Gortmaker, and Sobul, 1992) assessing postnatal ETS exposure and cognitive endpoints in children also failed to produce consistent results. While four of the five studies demonstrated modest decrements in performance, the decrements demonstrated by Baghurst and colleagues (1992) were no longer found after adjustment for confounders; Bauman and colleagues (1991) did not demonstrate decrements for all ages, and results differed for two of the tests; Eskenazi and Trupin (1995) did not find a dose–response relationship. Results for the three studies (Denson, Nanson, and McWatters, 1975; Weitzman et al., 1992; Eskenazi and Trupin, 1995) examining postnatal ETS exposure and children's behavior are also conflicting. However, Weitzman and colleagues did demonstrate significant, dose-related associations between most categories of postnatal maternal smoking and a behavior problem index.

Cancers

Table 10-6 lists selected studies on ETS and childhood cancers. Due to the lack of distinction between true ETS exposure and maternal smoking during pregnancy, only studies associating paternal smoking and cancers are listed. The findings of these studies may be affected by confounding due to maternal smoking during pregnancy.

Brain Tumors   The association between ETS and brain tumors in children is biologically plausible due to the findings of endogenously formed N-nitroso precursors found in ETS; however, this association has yet to be demonstrated in adults. Associations between paternal smoking and risk of brain tumors were demonstrated in four studies (Preston-Martin et al., 1982; Howe et al., 1989; John, Savitz, and Sandler, 1991; McCredie, Maisonneuve, and Boyle, 1994), with odds ratios ranging from 1.4 to 2.2 and with

TABLE 10-6 Studies Investigating ETS and Childhood Cancers, Using Paternal Smoking as a Surrogate of ETS

Study Reference	Location	Outcome Assessed	Exposure	Exposure Ascertainment	Participants	OR
Preston-Martin et al. (1982)	United States (Los Angeles County)	Brain tumor	Paternal smoking during pregnancy	Interview	209 cases 209 controls	1.5 ($p < 0.05$)
Howe et al. (1989)	Canada (southern Ontario)	Brain tumor	Paternal smoking during pregnancy	Interview	74 cases 132 controls	1.1
Kuijten et al. (1990)	United States (Pennsylvania, New Jersey, Delaware)	Astrocytoma	Paternal smoking during pregnancy	Interview	163 cases 163 controls	0.8
John et al. (1991)		Brain tumor	Paternal smoking alone		48 cases 196 controls	1.9 (0.9, 4.2)
Gold et al. (1993)	United State (SEER)	Brain tumor	Paternal smoking alone	Interviews	361 cases 1083 controls	0.9
McCredie et al. (1994)	Australia (New South Wales)	Brain tumor	Paternal smoking during pregnancy	Interviews	82 cases 164 controls	2.2
Magnani et al. (1990)	Italy	Leukemia	Paternal smoking during pregnancy		73 cases 196 controls	1.7 (0.7, 3.8)
John et al. (1991)		Leukemia	Paternal smoking during pregnancy		187 cases 187 controls	No association
Severson et al. (1993)		Leukemia	Paternal smoking during pregnancy		22 cases 307 controls	0.9 (0.3, 2.1)
Magnani et al. (1990)		Non-Hodgkins lymphoma	Paternal smoking during pregnancy		19 cases	6.7 (1.0, 43.4)
John et al. (1991)		Lymphoma	Paternal smoking during pregnancy		26 cases	1.9 (0.7, 4.8)

statistically significant results in two of the studies (Preston-Martin et al., 1982; McCredie, Maisonneuve, and Boyle, 1994).

Leukemia   In animal studies, leukemia can be induced by transplacentally-acting carcinogens found in tobacco smoke and benzene, as a component of ETS is a leukemogen. The eight studies (Pershagen, Ericson, and Otterblad-Olausson, 1992; van Steensel-Moll et al., 1985; Stjernfeldt et al., 1986; McKinney et al., 1987; Buckley et al., 1986; Magnani et al., 1990; John, Savitz, and Sandler, 1991; Severson et al., 1993) on parental smoking and the risk of leukemia in children are conflicting. The only cohort study conducted did not demonstrate an association. Furthermore only two out of seven case-control studies demonstrated a positive association. These studies have been limited by not distinguishing between acute lymphocytic leukemia (ALL) and non-ALL and the lack of information on the patient's age of diagnosis. At the present time a positive association between ETS and leukemia cannot be supported.

Lymphomas   Six studies (Buckley et al., 1986; Stjernfeldt et al., 1986; Magnani et al., 1990; McKinney et al., 1987; John, Savitz, and Sandler, 1991; Pershagen, Ericson, and Otterblad-Olausson, 1992) have been conducted on ETS exposure and the risk of lymphomas and non-Hodgkin's lymphomas. While small increases in risk were observed, the data do not support a conclusion at this time.

Other Cancers   ETS exposure has also been assessed as a risk factor for neuroblastoma, germ cell tumors, bone and soft tissue sarcomas, and Wilm's tumor of the kidney. While it has been established that risk for neuroblastoma occurs through ETS exposure in utero, and a small increase in relative risk for neuroblastoma due to paternal smoking during pregnancy has been demonstrated (Kramer et al., 1987), more studies are needed. Several studies have also attempted to assess associations between ETS and germ cell tumors (McKinney et al., 1987), and also bone and soft-tissue sarcomas (Grufferman et al., 1982; McKinney et al., 1987; Hartley et al., 1988; Magnani et al., 1990). Lastly, active smoking is an established risk factor for cancers of the kidney and renal pelvis in adults, and animal studies have suggested that nitrosamines may have an etiologic role in these cancers. However, conclusive studies associating ETS with Wilm's tumor of the kidney in children have not yet been conducted.

Lower Respiratory Tract Illnesses in Childhood

Studies of involuntary smoking and lower respiratory illnesses in childhood, including bronchitis and pneumonia, provided some of the earliest evidence on adverse effects of ETS (Harlap and Davies, 1974; Colley, Holland, and Corkhill, 1974). Presumably this association represents an increase in frequency or severity of illnesses that are infectious in etiology and not a direct response of the lung to toxic components of ETS. Investigations conducted throughout the world have demonstrated an increased risk of lower respiratory tract illness in infants with smoking parents (Strachan and Cook, 1997). These studies indicate a significantly increased frequency of bronchitis and pneumonia during the first year of life of children with smoking parents. Strachan and Cook (1997) report a quantitative review of this information, combining data from 39 studies. Overall, there was an approximate 50% increase in illness risk if either parent smoked, with the odds ratio for maternal smoking being somewhat higher at 1.72 (95% confidence interval, CI: 1.55, 1.91). Although the health outcome measures have varied somewhat among the studies, the relative risks associated with involuntary smoking were similar, and dose–response relationships with extent of parental smoking were demonstrable. Although most of the studies have shown that maternal smoking rather than paternal smoking underlies the increased risk of parental smoking, studies from China show that paternal smoking alone can increase incidence of lower respiratory illness (Yue Chen, Wan-Xian, and Shunzhang, 1986; Strachan and Cook, 1997). In these studies an effect of passive smoking was not readily identified after the first year of life. During the first year of life, the strength of its effect may reflect higher exposures consequent to the time-activity patterns of young infants, which place them in close proximity to cigarettes smoked by their mothers.

Respiratory Symptoms and Illness in Children

Data from numerous surveys demonstrate a greater frequency of the most common respiratory symptoms: cough, phlegm, and wheeze in the children of smokers (DHHS, 1986; Cal EPA, 1997; Cook and Strachan, 1997). In these studies the subjects have generally been schoolchildren, and the effects of parental smoking have been examined. Thus the less prominent effects of passive smoking, in comparison with the studies of lower respiratory illness in infants, may reflect lower exposures to ETS by older children who spend less time with their parents.

By the mid-1980s results from several large studies provided convincing evidence that involuntary exposure to ETS increases the occurrence of cough and phlegm in the children of smokers, although earlier data from smaller studies had been ambiguous. In a study of 10,000 schoolchildren in six U.S. communities, smoking by parents increased the frequency of persistent cough in their children by about 30% (Ware, Dockery, and Spiro III, 1984). The effect of parental smoking was derived primarily from smoking by the mother. Charlton (1984) conducted a survey on cigarette smoking that included 15,709 English children aged 8 to 19 years. In the nonsmoking children, the prevalence of frequent cough was significantly higher if either the father or the mother smoked. For the symptom of chronic wheeze, the preponderance of the early evidence also indicated an excess associated with involuntary smoking. In a survey of 650 schoolchildren in Boston, one of the first studies on this association, persistent wheezing was the most frequent symptom (Weiss et al., 1980); the prevalence of persistent wheezing increased significantly as the number of smoking parents increased. In the large study of children in six U.S. communities, the prevalence of persistent wheezing during the previous year was significantly increased if the mother smoked (Ware, Dockery, and Spiros III, 1984).

Cook and Strachan (1997) conducted a quantitative summary of the relevant studies, including 41 of wheeze, 34 of chronic cough, 7 of chronic phlegm, and 6 of breathlessness. Overall, this synthesis indicates increased risk for respiratory symptoms for children whose parents smoke (Table 10-7) (Cook and Strachan, 1997). There was even increased risk for breathlessness (OR = 1.31; 95% CI = 1.08, 1.59). Having both parents smoke was associated with the highest levels of risk.

Childhood Asthma

Although involuntary exposure to tobacco smoke has been associated with the symptom of wheeze, evidence for association of involuntary smoking with childhood asthma was initially conflicting. Exposure to ETS might cause asthma as a long-term consequence of the increased occurrence of lower respiratory infection in early childhood or through other pathophysiological mechanisms including inflammation of the respiratory epithelium (Samet, Tager, and Speizer, 1983; Tager, 1988). The effect of ETS may also reflect, in part, the consequences of in utero exposure. Assessment of airways responsiveness shortly after birth has shown that infants whose mothers smoke during pregnancy have increased airways responsiveness compared with those whose mothers do not smoke (Young et al., 1991). Maternal smoking during pregnancy also reduced ventilatory function measured

TABLE 10-7 Asthma and Respiratory Symptoms: Summary of Pooled Random Effects Odds Ratios with 95% Confidence Intervals

	Either Parent Smokes			One Parent Smokes			Both Parents Smoke			Mother Only Smokes			Father Only Smokes		
	OR	95%CI	(n)	OR	95%CI	(n)	OR	95%CI	(n)	OR	95%CI	(n)	OR	95%CI	(n)
Asthma	1.21	1.10–1.34	(21)[c]	1.04	0.78–1.38	(6)	1.50	1.29–1.73	(8)	1.36	1.20–1.55	(11)	1.07	0.92–1.24	(9)
Wheeze[a]	1.24	1.17–1.31	(30)[c]	1.18	1.08–1.29	(21)	1.47	1.14–1.90	(11)	1.28	1.19–1.38	(18)[d]	1.14	1.06–1.23	(10)
Cough	1.40	1.27–1.53	(30)[c]	1.29	1.11–1.51	(15)	1.67	1.48–1.89	(16)	1.40	1.20–16.4	(14)[d]	1.21	1.09–1.34	(9)
Phlegm[b]	1.35	1.13–1.62	(6)	1.25	0.97–1.63	(5)	1.46	1.04–2.05	(5)						
Breathlessness[b]	1.31	1.08–1.59	(6)												

Source: Cook and Strachan (1997).

Note: Number of studies in parentheses.

[a] Excluding EC study, in which the pooled odds ratio was 1.20.

[b] Data for phlegm and breathlessness restricted as several comparisons are based on fewer than five studies.

[c] Two age groups for reference 80 included as separate studies.

[d] Reference 82 included as three separate studies.

shortly after birth (Hanrahan et al., 1992). These observations suggest that in utero exposures from maternal smoking may affect lung development, perhaps reducing relative airways size.

While the underlying mechanisms remain to be identified, the epidemiologic evidence linking ETS exposure and childhood asthma is mounting (Cal EPA, 1997; Cook and Strachan, 1997). The synthesis by Cook and Strachan (1997) shows a significant excess of childhood asthma if both parents or the mother smoke (Table 10-7).

Evidence also indicates that involuntary smoking worsens the status of those with asthma. The possibility that ETS adversely affects children with asthma was described as early as 1950 in a case report entitled "Bronchial Asthma due to Allergy to Tobacco Smoke in an Infant" (Rosen and Levy, 1950). More recently Murray and Morrison (1986; 1989) evaluated asthmatic children followed in a clinic. Level of lung function, symptom frequency, and responsiveness to inhaled histamines were adversely affected by maternal smoking. Population studies have also shown increased airways responsiveness for ETS-exposed children with asthma (O'Connor et al., 1987; Martinez et al., 1988). The increased level of airway responsiveness associated with ETS exposure would be expected to increase the clinical severity of asthma. In this regard exposure to smoking in the home has been shown to increase the number of emergency room visits made by asthmatic children (Evans et al., 1987). Asthmatic children with smoking mothers are more likely to use asthma medications (Weitzman et al., 1990), a finding that confirms the clinically significant effects of ETS on children with asthma. Guidelines for the management of asthma all urge reduction of ETS exposure at home (DHHS, 1997).

Lung Growth and Development

On the basis of the primarily cross-sectional data available at the time, the 1984 report of the Surgeon General (DHHS, 1984) concluded that the children of smoking parents in comparison with those of nonsmokers had small reductions of lung function, but the long-term consequences of these changes were regarded as unknown. In the two years between the 1984 and the 1986 reports, sufficient longitudinal evidence was accumulated to support the conclusion in the 1986 report (DHHS, 1986b) that involuntary smoking reduces the rate of lung function growth during childhood. Further cross-sectional studies have continued generally to confirm the evidence reviewed in the 1984 report of the Surgeon General (Burchfiel III, 1984; Tashkin et al., 1984; Tsimoyianis et al., 1987; Spengler and Ferris Jr., 1985), although not all studies have shown adverse effects of involuntary smoking on the lung function of children (Hosein and Corey, 1984; Lebowitz, 1984).

The effects of involuntary smoking on lung growth have been demonstrated in three separate major longitudinal studies with supporting findings from other less extensive studies (Samet and Lange, 1996). Based on cross-sectional data from children in East Boston, Massachusetts, Hosein, Mitchell, and Bouhuys (1977) reported that the level of FEF_{25-75}, a spirometric flow rate sensitive to subtle effects on airways and parenchymal function, declined with an increasing number of smoking parents in the household. In 1983 the investigative group of Tager and coworkers reported the results obtained on follow-up of these children over a 7 year period (see Tager et al., 1983). Using a multivariate technique, the investigators showed that both maternal smoking and active smoking by the child reduced the growth rate of the FEV_1. Lifelong exposure of a child to a smoking mother was estimated to reduce growth of the FEV_1 by 10.7%, 9.5%, and 7.0% after 1, 2, and 5 years of follow-up, respectively. Findings with additional follow-up were similar (Tager et al., 1985).

In 1983 the National Heart, Lung, and Blood Institute held a workshop on the respiratory effects of involuntary smoking. At that time adverse effects of parental smoking on children's lung function had been found in the East Boston study but not in another cohort study in Tucson, Arizona, that used similar methods for data collection. Subsequently two parallel analyses of data from these two cohort studies instigated as a result of that workshop have been reported (Tager et al., 1987; Lebowitz and Holberg, 1988). Both analyses showed that an adverse effect of parental smoking on lung growth could be demonstrated in East Boston but not in Tucson when the same analytical techniques were applied to the two data sets. The differing results could reflect higher exposures in East Boston related to the type of housing and the pattern of smoking or to other unmeasured differences in the populations.

Longitudinal data from the study of air pollution in six U.S. cities also showed reduced growth of the FEV_1 in children whose mothers smoked cigarettes (Berkey, Ware, and Dockery, 1986). The growth rate of the FEV_1 from ages 6 through 10 years was calculated for 7834 white children. The findings of a statistical analysis were that from ages 6 through 10 years, FEV_1 growth rate was reduced by 0.17% per pack of cigarettes smoked daily by the mother. This effect was somewhat smaller than that reported by Tager et al. (1983), although, if it is extrapolated to age 20 years, a cumulative effect of 2.8% is predicted. In the most recent analysis of these data, Wang and colleagues (1994) modeled exposures in a time-dependent fashion, classifying exposure during the first five years of life and cumulative exposure up to the year before follow-up. Current maternal smoking was found to affect lung growth.

Burchfiel and coworkers (Burchfiel III, 1984; Burchfiel et al., 1986) examined the effects of parental smoking on 15 year lung function change in subjects in the Tecumseh study, who had been enrolled at ages 10 through 19 years. In the female subjects who remained nonsmokers across the follow-up period, parental smoking did not affect lung function change. In nonsmoking males, parental smoking reduced the growth of the FEV_1, FVC, and v_{max50}, although the sample size was limited and the effects were not statistically significant. For the FEV_1 in males, the analysis estimated 7.4% and 9.4% reductions in 15 year growth associated with one or two smoking parents, respectively.

ETS and Middle Ear Disease in Children

Otitis media is one of the most frequent diseases diagnosed in children at outpatient facilities. Otitis media occurs as a result of dysfunction in the eustachian tube; serious, otitis media results when serous fluid effuses into the middle ear, and acute otitis media results when the serous fluid effused into the middle ear becomes infected. All stages lead to varying degrees of hearing loss.

We have identified 21 studies (Table 10-8) on the association between ETS and otitis media in children. ETS exposure in these studies is mostly assessed by questionnaire or interview of the parents. Two studies assessed ETS exposure objectively through the use of biomarkers (serum or salivary cotinine measurements in the children). Outcomes assessed in these 21 studies vary from acute, persistent, and recurrent otitis media or middle ear effusion, to consequences of otitis media such as hearing loss and ear surgery. In general, these studies support a positive association between ETS and middle ear disease.

There are four biologically plausible mechanisms by which ETS could lead to middle ear disease in children. First, ETS exposure could lead to decreased mucociliary clearance, increasing possible risk of dysfunction in the eustachian tube. Second, ETS may decrease eustachian tube patency due to adenoidal hyperplasia, a known risk factor for otitis media. Third, ETS may also decrease patency as a result of ETS-induced mucosal swelling. Fourth, ETS could decrease patency and mucociliary clearance by causing more frequent viral upper respiratory infections.

TABLE 10-8   Studies of Middle Ear Disease in Children

Source	Location	Outcome	Exposure Measurement	Age of Children	RR	95% CI
			Cohort			
Iversen (1985)	Denmark	MEE[a]	Questionnaire	0–7 years	Increase	$p < 0.05$
Tainio (1988)	Finland	>3 episodes of OM[b]	Questionnaire	0–2.5 years	1.7	1.1, 2.7
Teele (1989)	United States (Boston)	Acute OM	Questionnaire	0–1 year	Increase	
Etzel et al. (1992)		Incident OM with effusion	Serum cotinine	0–5.3 years	1.4 (idr)	1.2, 1.6
Ponka (1991)	Finland (Helsinki)	OM	Interview		No association	
Collet (1995)	Canada	Recurrent OM	Questionnaire	0–4 years	1.8	1.1, 3.0
Ey (1995)	United States	Recurrent OM	Questionnaire	0–1 year	1.8	1.0, 3.1
			Case control			
Kraemer (1983)		Persistent MEE	Interview		2.8	1.1, 7.0
Black (1985)		Ear surgery for secretory OM	Questionnaire		1.6	1.0, 2.6
Pukander (1985)	Finland	Acute OM		2–3 years	Trend	$p < 0.05$
Fleming (1987)	United States (Georgia)	OM	Interview	< 5 years	1.1	$p = 0.82$
Hinton (1989)		Ear surgery	Medical records	2–11 years	Trend	$p = 0.06$
Takasaka (1990)		OM			No association	
Kallail (1987)	United States (Kansas)	Hearing loss			No association	
Hinton (1988)		MEE	Questionnaire	1–11 years		
Zielhius (1989)		Incident OM with MEE	Interview	2–4 years	1.1	$p = 0.6$
Barr (1991)		Ear surgery		1.5–11.5 years	No association	
Green (1991)	West Germany	ENT clinic for ear pain and Hearing loss	Questionnaire	1.5–8 years	1.9	1.2, 2.9
Kitchens (1995)	United States	MEE, recurrent OM or adhesive OM	Questionnaire	≤ 3 years	1.7	$p = 0.05$
			Cross sectional			
Strachan (1989)	Scotland (Edinburgh)	MEE	Serum cotinine	6.5–7.5 years	1.3 trend	1.0, 1.3 $p < 0.05$
Ra (1992)		Hearing loss		10 months old		4.9 times

[a] MEE = middle ear effusion
[b] OM = otitis media

343

Epidemiologic Findings on Ear Disease

There have been 7 cohort studies, 2 cross-sectional, and 12 case-control studies (Table 10-8) conducted to determine the association between ETS and middle ear disease. Outcomes assessed vary from middle ear effusion in one study to different diagnostic categories of otitis media, such as recurrent episodes of otitis media, acute otitis media, and incident otitis media. Disease consequences such as ear surgery and hearing loss were also assessed. Exposure to ETS was usually assessed with a questionnaire or by interview and in some studies, ETS exposure was measured with serum cotinine assay (Etzel et al., 1992; Strachan, Jarvis, and Feyerabend, 1989).

Otitis Media   Six of the seven cohort studies demonstrated an increase in risk for otitis media or middle ear effusion; these studies were also cohorts that included children who were followed from birth to one or two years of age, therefore including the peak age of risk in which children are most likely to suffer from otitis media. Teele, Klein, and Rosner (1989) demonstrated an increase in risk for otitis media in children less than one year of age. Etzel and colleagues (1992) also demonstrated an increase in risk (RR:1.4; 95% CI: 1.2, 1.6) for incident otitis media with effusion for their cohort of children 0.5 to 3 years of age, using serum cotinine as a measure of ETS exposure. The study of Ponka (1991) was the only cohort study not showing an increase in risk for otitis media associated with ETS. However, this study has a potential limitation, since the otitis media outcome was not objectively measured but was assessed by parental reports. Collet et al. (1995), Ey et al. (1995), and Tainio et al. (1988) all measured recurrent episodes of otitis media and demonstrated increased risk for recurrent otitis media associated with ETS, reporting relative risks of 1.8 (95% CI: 1.1, 3.0), 1.8 (95% CI: 1.0, 3.1), and 1.7 (95% CI: 1.1, 2.7), respectively.

Results from case-control studies were inconsistent, with Pukander et al. (1985) demonstrating a significant positive trend but other studies not finding significant associations (Fleming et al., 1987; Takasaka, 1990; Zielhius et al., 1989).

Middle Ear Effusion   The only study assessing middle ear effusion as an outcome was that of Iversen et al. (1985); a significant increase in risk for middle ear effusion with ETS was demonstrated. The case-control studies consistently demonstrated an increased risk for middle ear effusion associated with ETS. Kraemer et al. (1983) and Kitchens (1995) both demonstrated increased risk for middle ear effusion with ETS, with odds ratios of 2.8 (95% CI: 1.1, 7.0) and 1.7 ($p < 0.05$), respectively. Hinton and Buckley (1988) demonstrated a positive increase and trend ($p = 0.06$) for middle ear effusion as a result of ETS exposure.

Consequences of Middle Ear Disease   Only one of three case-control studies demonstrated an increase in risk for ear surgery due to ETS-induced otitis media. Black (1985) demonstrated an odds ratio of 1.6 (95% CI: 1.0, 2.6) for ear surgery, Hinton and Buckley (1988) demonstrated a positive trend, and Barr and Coatesworth (1991) found no association.

Two case-control studies assessed the association between ETS and hearing loss due to middle ear disease. Green and Cooper (1991) demonstrated an increase in risk with an odds ratio of 1.9 (95% CI: 1.2, 2.9) for hearing loss. While Kallail, Rainbolt, and Bruntzel (1987) did not demonstrate an association, this study suffers from a major limitation; cases and controls were not subject to the same screening procedure. Ra's cross-sectional study (Ra, 1992) demonstrated that children exposed to ETS were 4.9 times more likely to suffer from hearing loss associated with middle ear diseases.

Conclusion

Issues of concern in these studies include possible misclassification of exposure or outcome. Exposure measured through questionnaire may not fully represent the extent of smoking behavior during pregnancy and after pregnancy. However, studies using objective measures of exposure such as salivary and serum cotinine measurements both demonstrated increase in risk for otitis media. Diagnosis of otitis media is also subject to misclassification, since it is subject to variation not only between different clinics but over time. However, while case-control studies are subject to screening differences and uses of different medical services in otitis media diagnosis, cohort studies reduce potential outcome misclassification and consistently demonstrated an increase in risk for otitis media.

Positive associations between ETS and otitis media have been consistently demonstrated in cohort studies but not as consistently in the case-control studies. This difference may have arisen because the cohort studies include children from birth to age 2 years, the peak age of risk for middle ear disease. The case-control studies, on the other hand, have been directed at older children who are not at peak risk for otitis media. Regardless of study type, however, increase in risk for middle ear disease is demonstrated when the outcome assessed is recurring episodes of middle ear effusion or otitis media, versus incident or single episodes of otitis media. In a 1997 meta-analysis Cook and Strachan (1997) found a pooled odds ratio of 1.48 (95% CI: 1.08, 2.04) for recurrent otitis media if either parent smoked, 1.38 (95% CI: 1.23, 1.55) for middle ear effusions, and 1.21 (95% CI: 0.95, 1.53) for outpatient or inpatient care for chronic otitis media or "glue ear."

The U.S. Surgeon General's Office (DHHS, 1986b), the National Research Council (NRC, 1986a), and the U.S. Environmental Protection Agency (EPA, 1992) have all reviewed the literature on ETS and otitis media, and they have concluded that there is an association between ETS exposure and otitis media in children. The evidence to date supports a causal relationship.

HEALTH EFFECTS OF INVOLUNTARY SMOKING IN ADULTS

Lung Cancer

In 1981 reports were published from Japan (Hirayama, 1981) and from Greece (Trichopoulos et al., 1981) that indicated increased lung cancer risk in nonsmoking women married to cigarette smokers. Subsequently this controversial association has been examined in investigations conducted in the United States and other countries. The association of involuntary smoking with lung cancer derives biological plausibility from the presence of carcinogens in sidestream smoke and the lack of a documented threshold dose for respiratory carcinogens in active smokers (DHHS, 1982; IARC, 1986). Moreover, genotoxic activity had been demonstrated for many components of ETS (Lofroth, 1989; Claxton et al., 1989; Weiss, 1989), although several small studies have not found cytogenetic effects in passive smokers (Sorsa et al., 1985; Husgafvel-Pursiainen et al., 1987; Sorsa et al., 1989). Experimental exposure of nonsmokers to ETS leads to their excreting NNAL, a tobacco-specific carcinogen, in their urine (Hecht et al., 1993). Non-smokers exposed to ETS also have increased concentrations of adducts of tobacco-related carcinogens (Maclure et al., 1989; Crawford et al., 1994).

Time trends of lung cancer mortality in nonsmokers have been examined with the rationale that temporally increasing exposure to ETS should be paralleled by increasing mortality rates (Enstrom, 1979; Garfinkel, 1981). These data provide only indirect evidence on the lung cancer risk associated with involuntary exposure to tobacco smoke. Epidemiologists have directly tested the association between lung cancer and involuntary smoking utilizing conventional designs: the case-control and cohort studies. In a case-control study, the exposures of nonsmoking persons with lung cancer to ETS are compared to those of an appropriate control group. In a cohort study, the occurrence of lung cancer over time in nonsmokers is assessed in relation to involuntary tobacco smoke exposure. The results of both study designs may be affected by inaccurate assessment of exposure to ETS, by inaccurate information on personal smoking habits that leads to classification of smokers as nonsmokers, by failure to assess and control for potential confounding factors, and by the misdiagnosis of a cancer at another site as a primary cancer of the lung.

Methodological investigations suggest that accurate information can be obtained by interview in an epidemiological study on the smoking habits of a spouse (i.e., never or ever smoker) (Pron et al., 1988; Coultas, Peake, and Samet, 1989; Cummings et al., 1989). However, information concerning quantitative aspects of the spouse's smoking is reported with less accuracy. Misclassification of current or former smokers as never-smokers may introduce a positive bias because of the concordance of spouse smoking habits (Lee, 1988). The extent to which this bias explains the numerous reports of association between spouse smoking and lung cancer has been controversial (Wald et al., 1986; Lee, 1988; EPA, 1992).

Use of spouse smoking alone to represent exposure to ETS does not cover exposures outside of the home (Friedman, Petitti, and Bawol, 1983), nor necessarily all exposure inside the home. The International Agency for Research on Cancer (IARC) has conducted a 13-center study to assess the contribution of the home and work environments to exposures of nonsmoking women to ETS (Saracci and Riboli, 1989). Overall, the data show that some women married to smokers receive little exposure at home and that the number of cigarettes smoked per day by the husband is only moderately correlated with "actual" exposure. The study shows a widely varying proportion of women exposed to ETS among the centers.

A U.S. study examined the contribution of spouse smoking to total exposure to ETS received at home (Sandler et al., 1989). Using 1963 data from the Washington County, Maryland, study, Sandler and colleagues found that for nonsmoking women, spouse smoking contributed 88% of the exposure, whereas for nonsmoking men, spouse smoking contributed 62% of the exposure.

In some countries, including the United States, smoking prevalence varies markedly with indicators of income and education, more recently tending to rise sharply with decreasing educational level and income (DHHS, 1989). In general, exposure to ETS follows a similar trend, and critics of the findings on ETS and lung cancer have argued that uncontrolled confounding by lifestyle, occupation, or other factors may explain the association. In fact, current data for the United States do indicate a generally less healthy lifestyle in those with greater ETS exposure (Matanoski et al., 1995). However, other than a few occupational exposures at high levels, as well as indoor radon, risk factors for lung cancer in never-smokers that might confound the ETS association cannot be proffered and the relevance to past studies of these current associations of potential confounders with ETS exposure is uncertain.

The first major studies on ETS and lung cancer were reported in 1981. Hirayama's (1981) early report was based on a prospective cohort study of 91,540 nonsmoking women in Japan. Standardized mortality ratios (SMRs) for lung cancer increased significantly with the amount smoked by the husbands. The findings could not be explained by confounding factors and were unchanged when follow-up of the study group was extended (Hirayama, 1984). Based on the same cohort, Hirayama also reported significantly increased risk for nonsmoking men married to wives smoking one to 19 cigarettes and 20 or more cigarettes daily (Hirayama, 1984). In 1981 Trichopoulos and colleagues also reported increased lung cancer risk in nonsmoking women married to cigarette smokers (see Trichopoulos et al., 1981). These investigators conducted a case-control study in Athens, Greece, which included cases with a diagnosis other than for orthopedic disorders. The positive findings reported in 1981 were unchanged with subsequent expansion of the study population (Trichopoulos, Kalandidi, and Sparros, 1983).

By 1986 the evidence had mounted, and three reports published in that year concluded that ETS was a cause of lung cancer. The International Agency for Research on Cancer of the World Health Organization (IARC, 1986) concluded that "passive smoking gives rise to some risk of cancer." In its monograph on tobacco smoking, the agency supported this conclusion on the basis of the characteristics of sidestream and mainstream smoke, the absorption of tobacco smoke materials during involuntary smoking, and the nature of dose–response relationships for carcinogenesis. In the same year the National Research Council (NRC, 1986a) and the U.S. Surgeon General (DHHS, 1986b) also concluded that involuntary smoking increases the incidence of lung cancer in nonsmokers. In reaching this conclusion, the National Research Council (NRC, 1986a) cited the biological plausibility of the association between exposure to ETS and lung cancer and the supporting epidemiological evidence. Based on a pooled analysis of the epidemiological data adjusted for bias, the report concluded that the best estimate for the excess risk of lung cancer in nonsmokers married to smokers was 25%. The 1986 report of the Surgeon General (DHHS, 1986b) characterized involuntary smoking as a cause of lung cancer in nonsmokers. This conclusion was based on the extensive information already available on the carcinogenicity of active smoking, on the qualitative similarities between ETS and mainstream smoke, and on the epidemiological data on involuntary smoking.

In 1992 the U.S. Environmental Protection Agency (EPA, 1992) published its risk assessment of ETS as a carcinogen. The agency's evaluation drew on the toxicologic evidence on ETS and the extensive literature on active smoking. A meta-analysis of the 31 studies published up to that time was central in the decision to classify ETS as a class A carcinogen — namely a known human carcinogen. The meta-analysis considered the data from the epidemiologic studies by tiers of study quality and location and used an adjustment method for misclassification of smokers as never-smokers. Overall, the analysis found a significantly increased risk of lung cancer in never-smoking women married to smoking men; for the studies conducted in the United States, the estimated relative risk was 1.19 (90% CI: 1.04, 1.35). Critics of the report have raised a number of concerns including the use of meta-analysis, reliance of 90% rather than 95% confidence intervals, uncontrolled confounding, and information bias. The report, however, was endorsed by the Agency's Science Advisory Board, and its conclusion is fully consistent with the 1986 reports.

Subsequent to the 1992 risk assessment, several additional studies in the United States have been reported (Brownson et al., 1992; Fontham et al., 1994; Kabat, Stellman, and Wynder, 1995; Cardenas et al., 1997). The multicenter study of Fontham and colleagues is the largest report to date, with 651 cases and 1253 controls. It shows a significant increase in overall relative risk (OR : 1.26; 95% CI : 1.04, 1.54). There was also a significant risk associated with occupational exposure to ETS.

Findings of an autopsy study conducted in Greece have further strengthened the plausibility of the lung cancer ETS connection. Trichopoulos and colleagues (1992) examined autopsy lung specimens from 400 persons, 35 years of age and older, in order to assess airways changes. Epithelial lesions were more common in nonsmokers married to smokers than in nonsmokers married to nonsmokers.

A more recent meta-analysis (Hackshaw, Law, and Wald, 1997) included 37 published studies. The excess risk of lung cancer for smokers married to nonsmokers was estimated at 24% (95% CI: 13%, 36%). The adjustment for potential bias and confounding by diet did not alter the estimate. This meta-analysis has supported the recent conclusion of the

U.K. Scientific Committee on Tobacco and Health (Scientific Committee on Tobacco and Health and HSMO, 1998) that ETS is a cause of lung cancer.

The extent of the lung cancer hazard associated with involuntary smoking in the United States and in other countries remains subject to some uncertainty, however (DHHS, 1986b; Weiss, 1986). The epidemiological studies provide varying and imprecise measures of risk, and exposures have not been characterized for large and representative population samples. Nevertheless, risk estimation procedures have been used to describe the lung cancer risk associated with involuntary smoking, but assumptions and simplifications must be made in order to use this method. The estimates of lung cancer deaths attributable to passive smoking have received widespread media attention and have figured prominently in the evolution of public policy on passive smoking.

Repace and Lowrey (1990) reviewed the risk assessments of lung cancer and passive smoking and estimated the numbers of lung cancer cases among U.S. nonsmokers that could be attributed to passive smoking. They provide nine estimates, covering both never-smokers and former smokers; the estimates ranged from 58 to 8124 lung cancer deaths for the year 1988, with a mean of 4500 or 5000 excluding the lowest estimate of 58. The bases for the individual estimates included the comparative dosimetry of tobacco smoke in smokers and nonsmokers using presumed inhaled dose or levels of nicotine or cotinine, the epidemiological evidence, and modeling approaches. A 1992 estimate by the Environmental Protection Agency, based on the epidemiologic data, was about 3000, including 1500 and 500 deaths in never-smoking women and men, respectively, and about 100 in long-term former smokers of both sexes.

More recently Repace and colleagues (1998) developed a model of risk to workers of lung cancer and heart disease arising from ETS exposure. The pharmacokinetic model incorporated nicotine as an indicator of exposure and cotinine as a measure of dose in order to estimate the risks. The model estimated that 400 lung cancer deaths occur annually from workplace exposure at a prevalence of 28% smoking in the workplace.

These calculations illustrate that passive smoking must be considered an important cause of lung cancer death from a public health perspective, since exposure is involuntary and not subject to control. The specific risk assessments require assumptions concerning the extent and degree of exposure to ETS, exposure-response relationships, and the lifetime expression of the excess risk associated with passive smoking at different ages. Moreover the calculations do not consider the potential contributions of other exposures, such as occupational agents and indoor radon. The current decline in the prevalence of active smoking and the implementation of strong clean indoor air policies will reduce the relevance of estimates based on past patterns of smoking behavior.

Other Cancers

In adults, involuntary smoking has been linked to a generally increased risk of malignancy and to excess risk at specific sites. Miller (1984) interviewed surviving relatives of 537 deceased nonsmoking women in western Pennsylvania concerning the smoking habits of their husbands. A significantly increased risk of cancer death (OR: 1.94; $p < 0.05$) was found in women who were married to smokers and also not employed outside the home. The large number of potential subjects who were not interviewed and the possibility of information bias detract from this report.

Sandler and colleagues (Sandler, Everson, and Wilcox, 1985; Sandler et al., 1985; Sandler, Wilcox, and Everson, 1985) conducted a case-control study on the effects of exposure to ETS during childhood and adulthood on the risk of cancer. The 518 cases included cancers of all types other than basal cell cancer of the skin; the cases and the matched controls were between the ages of 15 and 59 years. For all sites combined, significantly increased risk was found for parental smoking (crude OR : 1.6); and for marriage to a smoking spouse (crude OR : = 1.5); the effects of these two exposures were independent (Sandler, Wilcox, and Everson, 1985). Significant associations were also found for some individual sites: For childhood exposure (Sandler et al., 1985), maternal and paternal smoking increased the risk of hematopoietic malignancy, and for adulthood exposure (Sandler, Everson, and Wilcox, 1985), spouse's smoking increased the risk for cancers of the female breast, female genital system, and the endocrine system. The findings are primarily hypothesis-generating and require replication. In a case-control study, such as those reported by Sandler et al. (1985), information on exposure to ETS may be affected by information bias.

Other studies provide data on passive smoking and cancers of diverse sites. Hirayama (1984) has reported significantly increased mortality from nasal sinus cancers and from brain tumors in nonsmoking women married to smokers in the Japanese cohort. In a case-control study of bladder cancer, involuntary smoke exposure at home and at work did not increase risk (Kabat, Dieck, and Wynder, 1986). Cervical cancer, which has been linked to active smoking (DHHS, 1990a), was associated with duration of involuntary smoking in a case-control study in Utah (Slattery et al., 1989). In the Washington County (Maryland) study, colorectal cancer incidence rates were significantly increased for male passive smokers but not for female passive smokers; incidence rates were significantly reduced for female active smokers (Sandler et al., 1988). This pattern of findings cannot be readily explained.

These associations of involuntary smoking with cancer at diverse nonrespiratory sites cannot be readily supported with arguments for biological plausibility. Increased risks at some of the sites, such as cancer of the nasal sinus and female breast cancer, generally have not been observed in active smokers (DHHS, 1982, 1989, DHHS, 1990b). In fact the International Agency for Research on Cancer has concluded that effects would not be produced in passive smokers that would not be produced to a larger extent in active smokers (IARC, 1986). Thus investigation of cancer sites other than the lung should be guided by the data from active smokers and by appropriate toxicological evidence. For example, the plausibility of the passive smoking with cervical cancer would be supported by the demonstration of tobacco smoke components in the cervical mucus of exposed nonsmoking women. In investigations of cancer at sites not plausibly linked to passive smoking, associations may arise by chance or by the effect of bias, prompting further but possibly unnecessary investigations.

ETS and Coronary Heart Disease

Causal associations between active smoking and fatal and nonfatal coronary heart disease (CHD) outcomes have long been demonstrated (DHHS, 1989). This increased risk of CHD morbidity and mortality has been demonstrated for younger persons and the elderly, in men and women, and in ethnically and racially diverse populations. The risk of CHD in active smokers increases with amount and duration of cigarette smoking and decreases quickly with cessation. Active cigarette smoking is considered to increase the risk of cardiovascular disease by promoting atherosclerosis, increasing the tendency to thrombosis, causing spasm of the coronary arteries, increasing the likelihood of cardiac arrhythmias, and decreasing the oxygen-carrying capacity of the blood (DHHS, 1990a). It is biologically plausible that passive smoking could also be associated with increased risk for CHD through the same mechanisms considered relevant for active smoking, although the lower exposures to smoke components of the passive smoker have raised questions regarding the relevance of the mechanisms cited for active smoking.

Biological Plausibility   Glantz and Parmley (1991) have summarized the pathophysiological mechanisms by which passive smoking might increase the risk of heart disease. They suggest that passive smoking may promote atherogenesis, increase the tendency of platelets to aggregate and thereby promote thrombosis, reduce the oxygen-carrying capacity of the blood, and alter myocardial metabolism, much as for active smoking and CHD. The relevant data are presently limited in scope, but experimental models have been developed. Three separate experiments involving exposure of nonsmokers to ETS have shown that passive smoking affects measures of platelet function in the direction of increased tendency toward thrombosis (Glantz and Parmley, 1995). However, changes in these same types of assays of platelet function have not been consistently associated with active smoking (DHHS, 1990c). Glantz and Parmley also propose that carcinogenic agents such as polycyclic aromatic hydrocarbons found in tobacco smoke promote atherogenesis by effects on cell proliferation. Passive smoking may also worsen the outcome of an ischemic event in the heart; animal data have demonstrated that ETS exposure increases cardiac damage following an experimental myocardial infarction. Experiments on two species of animals (rabbits and cockerels) have demonstrated that not only does exposure to ETS at doses similar to exposure to humans accelerate the growth of atherosclerotic plaques through the increase of lipid deposits, but it also induces atherosclerosis.

In addition to its effects on platelets, passive smoke exposure affects the oxygen-carrying capacity of the blood. Even small increments, on the order of 1%, in the carboxyhemoglobin, may explain the finding that passive smoking decreases the duration of exercise of patients with angina pectoris (Allred et al., 1989). This is supported with evidence that cigarette smoking has been shown to increase levels of carbon monoxide in the spaces where ventilation is low or smoking is particularly intense (DHHS, 1986a).

Epidemiological Studies   Epidemiologic data first raised concern that passive smoking may increase risk for CHD with the report of Garland and colleagues (1985) based on a cohort study in southern California. We identified 22 studies on the association between environmental tobacco smoke and cardiovascular disease (Table 10-9), including 11 cohort and 10 case-control studies, and 1 cross-sectional study. These studies assessed both fatal and nonfatal cardiovascular heart disease outcomes, and most used self-administered questionnaires to assess ETS exposure. They cover a wide range of populations, both geographically and racially. While many of the studies were conducted within the United States; studies were also conducted in Europe (Scotland, Italy, and the United Kingdom), Asia (Japan and China), South America (Argentina), and the South Pacific (Australia and New Zealand). The majority of the studies measured the effect of ETS exposure due to spousal smoking; however, some studies also assessed exposures from smoking by other household members or occurring at work or in transit. Only one study included measurement of biomarkers.

As the evidence has subsequently mounted since the 1985 report, it has been systematically reviewed by the American Heart Association (Taylor, Johnson, and Kazemi, 1992) and the California Environmental Protection Agency(Cal EPA, 1997), and also in a recent meta-analysis done for the Scientific Committee on Tobacco and Health in the United Kingdom (Law, Morris, and Wald, 1997). The topic was not addressed in the 1986 Surgeon General's report nor in the 1992 EPA risk assessment of ETS because of the limited data available when these reports were prepared.

Cohort Studies

Fatal CHD Outcomes   Cohort studies assessing the association between ETS and fatal CHD outcomes have all demonstrated an increase in risk. In a cohort of nonsmoking Japanese women married to husbands who smoked, Hirayama (1984) demonstrated a modest increase in risk for death from ischemic heart disease. Hole and colleagues (1989)

TABLE 10-9 Studies Investigating ETS and CHD Outcomes

Study Reference	Location	Outcome(s) Assessed	Exposure	Participants	Combined RR	Men	Women	RR Adjusted for:
				Cohort				
Butler (1988 dissertation)	California (Loma Linda–Seventh Day Adventists)	Fatal CHD	Spousal (husband)	Spouse pairs: 87 female CHD deaths / 9785 nonsmoking women			1.4 (0.5, 3.8)	Age
			Household (years lived with smoker)	AHSMOG 76 male CHD deaths / 1489 never-smoking men		0: 1.0 1–10: 0.4 11+: 0.6	0: 1.0 1–10: 1.5 11+: 1.5	
			Work (years worked with smoker)	70 CHD female deaths / 3486 never-smoking women		0: 1.0 1–10: 1.3 11+: 0.8	0: 1.0 1–10: 1.8 11+: 1.9	
Garland et al. (1985)	California (San Diego)	Fatal CHD (ICDA-8: 410.0–414.9)	Spousal (husband)	19 female CHD deaths / 695 nonsmoking women			2.7	Age, systolic blood pressure, total plasma cholesterol, obesity, years of marriage
Helsing et al. (1988)	Maryland (Washington County)	Fatal CHD (ICD-7)	Household exposure	370 male CHD deaths / 3454 men; 988 female CHD deaths / 12,348 women	1.2	1.3 (1.1,1.6) Score: 0: 1.0 1–5: 1.4* 6–12: 1.3	1.2 (1.1, 1.4) Score: 0: 1.0 1–5: 1.2 6–12: 1.3*	Age, housing quality, schooling, marital status
Hirayama (1984, 1989, 1990)	Japan	Fatal CHD	Spousal (husband)	494 female deaths / 91,540 nonsmoking women			Cigarette/day: None: 1.0 1–19: 1.0 20+: 1.3*	Husband's age, occupation
Hole et al. (1989)	Western Scotland	Nonfatal angina Fatal ischemic heart disease	Cohabitees	525 IHD deaths / 3960 men 4037 women	1.1 (0.7, 1.7) 2.0 (1.2, 3.4)			Age, sex, social class, diastolic blood pressure, serum cholesterol, body mass index

351

TABLE 10-9 (*Continued*)

Study Reference	Location	Outcome(s) Assessed	Exposure	Participants	Combined RR	Men	Women	RR Adjusted for:
Humble et al. (1990)	Georgia (Evans County)	Fatal CVD (ICD8: 390–456)	Spousal (husband)	76 female CVD deaths / 185 never-smoking black women 328 never-smoking white women			1.6 (1.0, 2.6) Blacks 1.8 (0.9, 3.7) Whites Low SES: 1.8 High SES: 2.0 3.4	Age, blood pressure, cholesterol, body mass index
Hunt et al. (1986)	Utah	Incident fatal heart attack	Spousal (husband)	9172 spouse pairs				
Kawachi et al. (1997)	United States (Nurses' Health Study)	Incident CHD:	Home or work	152 CHD cases:			Home or work: None: 1.0 Any: 1.7* Occasional: 1.6 Regular: 1.8* Years with smoke: <1: 1.0 1–9: 1.2 10–19: 1.5 20–29: 1.1 30+: 1.5	Alcohol use, body mass index History of: hypertension, diabetes, hypercholesterolemia, menopausal status, hormone use, physical activity, vitamin E intake, fat intake, aspirin use, family history of CHD
		nonfatal MI		127 CHD cases			Home or work: None: 1.0 Any: 1.7 Occasional: 1.6 Regular: 1.9*	
		but fatal CHD		25 CHD cases			Home or work: None: 1.0 Any: 1.9 Occasional: 1.5 Regular: 2.6	

Reference	Location (study) / Cause of death	Exposure	No. of cases / population	Relative risk (95% CI)	Relative risk (95% CI)	Relative risk (95% CI)	Adjustment factors
LeVois and Layard (1995)	United States (CPS-I and CPS II) CPS-1 and II; Fatal CHD (ICD7: 420.0–420.2) ICD9: 410–414)	Spousal	7768 male CHD deaths/ 88,458 never-smoking men; 7133 female CHD deaths/247,412 never-smoking women; 1966 male CHD deaths/ 108,772 never-smoking men; 1099 CHD female deaths/ 226,067 never-smoking women	1.0 (0.97, 1.04) Cigarette/day: 1–19: 1.1 20–39: 1.1 40+: 1.0	1.0 (0.9, 1.1) Cigarette/day: 1–9: 1.0 20–39: 1.0 40+: 1.0; 1.0 (0.9, 1.1) Cigarette/day: 1–19: 1.4* 20–39: 1.3 40+: 1.1; 1.0 (0.9, 1.0) Cigarette/day: 1–19: 1.1 20–39: 1.1 40+: 0.9	1.1 (1.0, 1.1) Cigarette/day: 1–19: 1.0 20–39: 1.1 40+: 1.0; 1.0 (0.9, 1.1) Cigarette/day: 1–19: 1.1 20–39: 1.0 40+: 1.3; 1.0 (1.0, 1.1) Cigarette/day: 1–19: 1.1 20–39: 1.1 40+: 1.0	Age, race
Steenland et al. (1996)	United States (CPS-II); Fatal CHD (ICD-9:410–414)	Spousal	Analysis 1: 2494 male CHD deaths/ 101,227 men; 1325 female CHD deaths/ 208,372 women; Analysis 2: 1299 male CHD deaths/ 58,530 men; 572 CHD female deaths/ 99,821 women	1.2 (1.1, 1.4) Cigarette/day: < 20: 1.3* 20: 1.2 21–39: 1.1; 1.5 (1.2, 1.8) Cigarette/day: < 20: 1.1 20: 1.1 21–39:1.1 40+: 1.3*	1.1 (1.0, 1.3) Cigarette/day: < 20: 1.1 20: 1.1 21–39: 1.0 40+: 1.0; 1.2 (0.9, 1.5) Cigarette/day: < 20: 0.8 20: 1.0 21–39: 1.2 40+: 1.2		Age, history of heart disease, hypertension, diabetes, arthritis, body mass index, educational level, aspirin use, diuretic use, liquor consumption in men, wine intake in women, employment status, exercise, estrogen use in women

TABLE 10-9 *(Continued)*

Study Reference	Location	Outcome(s) Assessed	Exposure	Participants	Combined RR	Men	Women	RR Adjusted for:
				Analysis 3: 1180 male CHD deaths / 54,668 men; 426 female CHD deaths / 80,549 women		1.2 (1.0, 1.5) Cigarette/day: <20: 1.4* 20: 1.2 21–39: 1.1	1.2 (1.0, 1.5) Cigarette/day: <20: 1.2 20: 1.1 21–39: 1.0 40+: 1.3	
			Home			1.2 (1.0, 1.3)	1.1 (1.0, 1.2)	
			work			1.0 (0.9, 1.2)	1.1 (0.9, 1.3)	
			elsewhere	Analysis 4: 1751 deaths / 76,710 men; 768 deaths / 75,237 women		1.0 (0.9, 1.1)	0.9 (0.8, 1.0)	
Svendsen et al. (1987)	United States (MRFIT: 18 cities)	Fatal CHD	Spousal (wife)	13 male CHD deaths / 56 nonfatal CHD / 1245 never-smoking men		Fatal: 2.2 (0.7, 6.9) both: 1.6 (1.0, 2.7)		Age, baseline blood pressure, cholesterol, weight, drinks/week, education
		Fatal and nonfatal CHD	Coworkers			Fatal: 2.6 (0.5, 12.7) Both: 1.4 (0.8, 2.5)		Age, wives' smoking status
Case Control								
Ciruzzi et al. (1996)	Argentina (coronary care units)	Acute myocardial infarction	Household	336 AMI cases 446 hospital controls	1.7 (1.2, 2.3) 1.4 (0.9, 2.0)			Age, sex, education, body mass index, hyperlipidemia, family history of: diabetes, hypertension, history of CHD
			Spousal		Cigarette/day: 1–20: 1.3 > 20: 2.4			

Study	Country	Outcome	Exposure	Cases/controls	Men OR (95% CI)	Women OR (95% CI)	Adjusted for
Dobson et al. (1991)	Australia (New South Wales)	Fatal MI or fatal CHD (WHO MONICA)	Home	183 male cases / 293 nonsmoking male controls; 160 female cases / 532 nonsmoking female controls	0.97 (0.5, 1.9)	2.5 (1.5, 4.1)	Age, history of MI
			Work	75 male cases / 205 nonsmoking male controls; 17 female cases / 197 nonsmoking female controls	1.0 (0.5, 1.8)	0.7 (0.2, 2.6)	
He et al. (1989)	People's Republic of China	Nonfatal CHD (WHO)	Spousal (husband)	34 female CHD cases / 34 population / 34 hospital controls		3.0 (1.3, 7.2) Cigarette/day: < 20: 2.3 > 20: 6.8	Personal history of: hypertension, hyperlipidemia, Family history of: hypertension, CHD, drinking, physical exercise
He et al. (1994)	People's Republic of China (Xian)	Nonfatal CHD	Spousal (husband) and work	59 cases / 126 controls		1.2 (0.6, 2.7)	None
			Work only			1.9 (0.9, 4.0) Number of smokers: 0: 1.0 1–2: 1.2 3: 5.1 4 + : 4.1	Age, history of hypertension, personality type, total cholesterol, HDL cholesterol
Jackson (1989 dissertation)	New Zealand	Acute MI (WHO MONICA)		28 male AMI cases / 123 male controls; 11 female AMI cases / 112 female controls	1.0 (0.3, 4.3)	2.7 (0.6, 13)	Age, SES
		Fatal CHD		21 male CHD deaths / 61 male controls; 9 female CHD deaths / 62 female controls	1.1 (0.2, 4.5)	5.8 (1.3, 48)	

TABLE 10-9 *(Continued)*

Study Reference	Location	Outcome(s) Assessed	Exposure	Participants	Combined RR	Men	Women	RR Adjusted for:
La Vecchia et al. (1993)	Italy	Acute MI	Spousal	113 AMI cases 225 hospital controls	1.2 (0.6, 2.5) Cigarette/day: <15: 1.1 >15: 1.3	1.2 (0.6, 2.5)		Sex, age, education, coffee intake, body mass index, serum cholesterol, hypertension, diabetes, family history of MI
Layard (1995)	United States (National Mortality Follow-back Survey)	Fatal ischemic heart disease (ICD-9: 410–414)	Spousal	475 male IHD deaths/ 998 never smoking men; 914 female IHD deaths/ 1930 never smoking females		1.0 (0.7, 1.3) Cigarette/day: None: 1.0 1–14: 0.8 15–34: 1.1 35+: 0.9	1.0 (0.8, 1.2) Cigarette/day: None: 1.0 1–14: 0.9 15–34: 1.2 35+: 1.1	Age, race
Lee et al. (1986)	United Kingdom	Ischemic heart disease	Spousal Score: (home, work, travel, leisure)	66 IHD cases, 254 controls	1.0 (0.7, 1.6) Score: 0–1: 1.0 2–4: 0.5 5–12: 0.6	1.2 (0.6, 2.8) Score: 0–1: 0.1 2–4: 0.4 5–12: 0.4	0.9 (0.5, 1.7) Score: 0–1: 1.0 2–4: 0.6 5–12: 0.8	
Muscat and Wynder (1995)	United States (New York, Philadelphia, Chicago, Detroit)	Myocardial infarction (ICD-9: 410.0)	Adult	68 male cases/ 108 never smoking male controls; 46 female cases/ 50 never smoking female controls		Years exposed: None: 1.0 1–20: 1.7 21–30: 1.5 >30: 1.1	Years exposed: None: 1.0 1–20: 2.0 21–30: 0.9 >30: 1.7	Age, education, hypertension
Palmer et al. 1988 (abstract)	United States (MA–unknown)	Myocardial infarction	Spousal (husband)	336 cases 799 hospital controls			1.2	Age
Tunstall Pedoe et al. (1995)	Scotland	Nonfatal CHD	General	786 men 1492 never-smoking women	None: 1.0 Little: 1.2 Some: 1.5 A lot: 1.6			

Cross section

also reported significantly increased risk for ischemic heart disease mortality for passive smokers. Similarly Garland and colleagues' study (1985) on a San Diego cohort demonstrated an increase in risk for death from ischemic heart disease from spousal ETS exposure (RR : 3.6 for former smokers, 2.7 for current smokers). While study details are not described in detail, Hunt Martin, and Williams (1986) found a risk estimate of 3.4 for incident fatal heart attacks in a Utah cohort of nonsmoking women married to smoking husbands.

Helsing and colleagues (1988) reported on heart disease mortality of nonsmokers enrolled in a cohort study in Washington County, Maryland. In comparison with persons married to nonsmokers, both men and women married to smokers had significantly increased risk of dying from heart disease (RR: 1.3 for males, 1.2 for females). In another report based on a cohort study in the United States, passive smoking was found to increase the risk of cardiovascular death (RR: 1.59; 95% CI: 0.99, 2.57) in nonsmoking participants in the Evans County, Georgia, cohort study (Humble et al., 1990).

Fatal and Nonfatal CHD Outcomes   Several large cohort studies have been conducted that address both fatal and nonfatal CHD outcomes and ETS exposure. These studies include analyses of such large, national cohorts as the Nurses' Health Study, the American Cancer Society Cancer Prevention Study I and II (CPS-I and CPS-II), and the Multiple Risk Factor Intervention Trial (MRFIT). Except for the analyses of the CPS-I and CPS-II presented by LeVois and Layard (1995), all other studies demonstrated at least a modest increase in risk for fatal and nonfatal CHD due to ETS exposure.

Kawachi and colleagues' (1997) recent analysis of data from the Nurses' Health Study assessed both fatal CHD and nonfatal myocardial infarction due to exposure at home and work. Adjusting for a wide variety of CHD risk factors, any ETS exposure was associated with a risk of 1.71, occasional ETS exposure with a risk of 1.56 (95% CI: 0.9, 2.7), and regular ETS exposure with a risk of 1.97 (95% CI: 1.1, 3.3) for total CHD.

LeVois and Layard (1995), with support from the tobacco industry, analyzed data from the American Cancer Society's Cancer Prevention Study I and II (CPS-I and CPS-II). Males and females self-reported as never-smokers were not found to be more likely to die from CHD with increasing exposure to ETS. However, a significant increase in risk with passive exposure was reported for former smokers. Steenland and colleagues (1996) subsequently analyzed data from the same data set with the CPS-II cohort and conducted four different analyses on the data set. They found that nonsmoking men had a relative risk of 1.22 (95% CI: 1.07, 1.40) for ischemic heart disease (IHD) death when exposed to a current smoker. In fact, in all four analyses, significant positive associations were found for men currently exposed to ETS. Associations for women were nonsignificant.

The effect of involuntary smoking was also assessed among the nonsmoking male participants in the Multiple Risk Factor Intervention Trial (MRFIT); these men had been selected in 1973 to be in the upper 10% to 15% of risk for mortality for coronary artery disease, based on a score from the Framingham study (Svendsen et al., 1987). In comparison to men married to nonsmokers, never-smokers with smoking wives had increased risk for coronary heart disease (RR: 2.11; 95% CI: 0.69, 6.46); fatal or nonfatal coronary heart disease event (RR: 1.48; 95% CI: 0.89, 2.47), and death from any cause (RR: 1.96; 95% CI: 0.93, 4.11). These relative risks showed little change when former smokers were included in the analysis or when adjustments were made for other risk factors for coronary heart disease.

The unpublished dissertation of Butler (Grenier et al., 1992) on California Seventh Day Adventists also addressed nonfatal and fatal outcomes. This study assessed the risk of CHD due to spousal smoking, specifically on nonsmoking women married to husbands who smoked. Women exposed to husbands who were current smokers were found to have increased risk of CHD death (RR: 1.4; 95% CI: 0.5–3.8). Furthermore females working with smokers for 1 to 10 years and more than 11 years had relative risks of 1.85 and 1.86, respectively, compared with those working with nonsmokers.

Case-Control Studies

Fatal CHD Outcomes   While the data from the cohort studies consistently demonstrated an increased risk for fatal CHD, the findings of case-control studies have been inconsistent. Layard (1995) conducted a case-control study on fatal ischemic heart disease among decedents from the 1986 National Mortality Followback Survey. In this study no increase in risk or dose-response of risk with exposure was observed for either never-smoking men or women who were married to spouses who did smoke. In contrast, Dobson and colleagues (1991) conducted a study in Australia and found an elevated risk of fatal myocardial infarction for nonsmoking women exposed to ETS at home (OR: 2.46; 95% CI: 1.47, 4.13), after adjusting for age and history of myocardial infarction.

Nonfatal CHD Outcomes   A majority of the case-control studies investigated the association between ETS and nonfatal CHD outcomes. Ciruzzi and colleagues' recent (1996) case-control study in Argentina compared ETS exposure of acute myocardial infarction cases admitted into coronary care units to hospital controls. Persons exposed to one or more relatives who smoked had an odds ratio of 1.7 (95% CI: 1.2, 2.3) for acute myocardial infarction when compared to subjects exposed to relatives who did not smoke, after adjusting for a number of CHD risk factors. A similar hospital-based case-control study performed by La Vecchia and colleagues (1993) found an odds ratio of 1.2 for acute myocardial infarction in a cohort of men and women in Italy exposed to spouses who smoked, compared to never-smoking controls admitted to the same network of hospitals for acute diseases not related to cardiovascular risk factors. Risks were also demonstrated to be higher for persons with spouses smoking 15 or more cigarettes per day (RR: 1.3; 95% CI: 0.5, 3.4). Furthermore, in a hospital-based case-control study conducted in the United States, Muscat and Wynder (1995) observed an increased risk for myocardial infarction due to ETS exposure in both men and women. In this study, cases were defined as persons admitted to teaching hospitals in New York, Philadelphia, Chicago, and Detroit (OR: 1.5; 95% CI: 0.9, 2.6). However, a dose-response relationship was not observed. Palmer and colleagues (1989) also observed slightly higher risks for myocardial infarction in ETS-exposed women, although potential confounding risk factors were not accounted for.

Case-control studies have not shown an association between spousal smoking and either ischemic heart disease or stroke. For example, Lee, Chamberlain, and Alderson (1986) conducted a case-control study in England that failed to demonstrate an increased risk for ischemic heart disease or for stroke in nonsmokers married to smokers. However, the number of subjects in this study was small, and statistical power was accordingly limited.

The two studies conducted by He and colleagues in the People's Republic of China demonstrated elevated risks for nonfatal CHD. He and colleagues (1989) demonstrated an elevated risk for nonfatal CHD (OR: 3.0; 95% CI: 1.3, 7.2) for women married to husbands who were smokers, after adjusting for appropriate CHD risk factors. An increase in risk was also observed with the increasing number of cigarettes per day smoked by the husband. He and colleagues' second study in China (He et al., 1994) found that even though the risk for nonfatal CHD for women exposed to husbands and coworkers who smoked was not significantly increased, the risk did increase with the number of smokers to whom the women were exposed. The odds ratios for women whose husbands smoked was 1.24 (95% CI: 0.6, 2.7); however, like the initial 1989 study, this study had a modest sample size.

Fatal and Nonfatal CHD Outcomes   Jackson, Proulx, and Pelican (1991) also assessed risk for both nonfatal CHD and fatal CHD in men and women. Risks were only elevated in women and only significant for fatal CHD (OR: 5.8; 95% CI: 1.3, 48.0). However, no adjustments were made for any risk factors associated with CHD.

Conclusions

There are strengths and weaknesses to both the case-control and cohort study designs in investigating ETS and CHD outcomes. Many of the case-control studies have small sample sizes and lack the power to detect significant associations. Furthermore many studies also lack information on other risk factors for CHD, and therefore they may not adequately adjust for confounders. In contrast, many of the cohort studies have large sample sizes and do adjust for confounders. They also avoid information bias by assessing smoking status and exposure prior to the CHD outcome. However, cohort studies are more susceptible to exposure misclassification due to the cessation or resumption of smoking by the source of exposure; this risk of misclassification increases with the length of follow-up.

Although the risk estimates for ETS and CHD outcomes vary, they range mostly from null to modestly significant increases in risk, with the risk for fatal outcomes generally higher and more significant. In their meta-analysis Law, Morris, and Wald (1997) estimated the excess risk from ETS exposure as 30% (95% CI: 22, 38%) at age 65 years. The California Environmental Protection Agency (Cal EPA, 1997) recently concluded that there is "an overall risk of 30%" for CHD due to exposure from ETS. The American Heart Association's Council on Cardiopulmonary and Critical Care has also concluded that environmental tobacco smoke both increases the risk of heart disease and is "a major preventable cause of cardiovascular disease and death" (Taylor, Johnson, and Kazemi, 1992). This conclusion was echoed in 1998 by the Scientific Committee on Tobacco and Health (Scientific Committee on Tobacco and Health and HSMO, 1998).

RESPIRATORY SYMPTOMS AND ILLNESSES IN ADULTS

Only a few cross-sectional investigations provide information on the association between respiratory symptoms in nonsmokers and involuntary exposure to tobacco smoke. These studies have primarily considered exposure outside the home. Consistent evidence of an effect of passive smoking on chronic respiratory symptoms in adults has not been found (Spengler and Ferris Jr., 1985; Lebowitz and Burrows, 1976; Schilling et al., 1977; Comstock et al., 1981; Schenker, Samet, and Speizer, 1982; Euler et al., 1987; Hole et al., 1989).

Two studies suggest that passive smoking may cause acute respiratory morbidity. Analysis of National Health Interview Survey data showed that a pack-a-day smoker increases respiratory restricted days by about 20% for a nonsmoking spouse (Ostro, 1989). In a study of determinants of daily respiratory symptoms in Los Angeles, student nurses with a smoking roommate significantly increased the risk of an episode of phlegm, after controlling for personal smoking (Schwartz and Zeger, 1990). Leuenberger and colleagues (1994) describe associations between passive exposure to tobacco smoke at home and in the workplace and respiratory symptoms in 4197 randomly selected never-smoking adults in the Swiss Study on Air Pollution and Lung Diseases in Adults, a multicenter study in eight areas of the country. Exposed subjects were those who reported any exposure during the past 12 months; exposed persons were then asked about workplace exposure and also the number of smokers and the duration of exposure at home and work together. Involuntary smoke exposure was associated with asthma, dyspnea, bronchitis and chronic bronchitis symptoms, and allergic rhinitis. The increments in risk were substantial, ranging from approximately 40% to 80% for the different respiratory outcome measures. The increments were not reduced by control for educational level; dose response relationships were found with the quantitative indicators of exposure. For several of the outcome measures, the dose response relationships tended to be steeper for those also reporting workplace exposure.

Other recent studies have also shown adverse effects of involuntary smoking on adults. Robbins, Abbey, and Lebowitz (1993) examined predictors of new symptoms compatible with "airway obstructive disease" in a cohort study of 3914 nonsmoking participants in the Adventist Health Study. Significantly increased risk was identified in association with exposure during both childhood and adulthood. In a cross-sectional study Dayal and colleagues (1994) found that never-smoking Philadelphia residents with a reported diagnosis of asthma, chronic bronchitis, or emphysema had sustained significantly greater exposure to tobacco smoke than unaffected controls.

Neither epidemiological nor experimental studies have established the role of ETS in exacerbating asthma in adults. The acute responses of asthmatics to ETS have been assessed by exposing persons with asthma to tobacco smoke in a chamber. This experimental approach cannot be readily controlled because of the impossibility of blinding subjects to exposure to ETS. However, suggestibility does not appear to underlie physiological responses of asthmatics of ETS (Urch et al., 1988). Of three studies involving exposure of unselected asthmatics to ETS, only one showed a definite adverse effect (Shephard, Collins, and Silverman, 1979; Dahms, Bolin, and Slavin, 1981; Murray and Morrison, 1986). Stankus et al. (1988) recruited 21 asthmatics who reported exacerbation with exposure to ETS. With challenge in an exposure chamber at concentrations much greater than typically encountered in indoor environments, 7 subjects experienced a more than 20% decline in FEV_1.

Lung Function in Adults

With regard to involuntary smoking and lung function in adults, exposure to passive smoking has been associated in cross-sectional investigations with reduction of the FEF_{25-75}. White and Froeb (1980) compared spirometric test results in middle-aged nonsmokers with at least 20 years of involuntary smoking in the workplace to the results in an unexposed control group of nonsmokers. The mean FEF_{25-75} of the exposed group was significantly reduced, by 15% of predicted value in women and by 13% in men. This investigation has been intensely criticized with regard to the spirometric test procedures, the determination and classification of exposures, and the handling of former smokers in the analyses.

A subsequently reported investigation in France examined the effect of marriage to a smoker in over 7800 adults in seven cities (Kauffmann, Tessier, and Oriol, 1983). The study included 849 male and 826 female nonsmokers exposed to tobacco smoking by their spouses' smoking. At age above 40 years, the FEF_{25-75} was reduced in nonsmoking men and women with a smoking spouse. The investigators interpreted this finding as representing a cumulative adverse effect of marriage to a smoker. In a subsequent report the original findings in the French women were confirmed, but a parallel analysis in a large population of U.S. women did not show effects of involuntary smoking on lung function (Spengler and Ferris Jr., 1985).

The results of an investigation of 163 nonsmoking women in the Netherlands also suggested adverse effects of tobacco smoke exposure in the home on lung function (Brunekreef et al., 1985; Remijn et al., 1985). Cross-sectional analysis of spirometric data collected in 1982 demonstrated adverse effects of tobacco smoke exposure in the home, but in a sample of the women, domestic exposure to tobacco smoke was not associated with longitudinal decline of lung function during the period 1965 to 1982.

Svendsen and coworkers (1987) assessed the effects of spouse smoking on 1400 nonsmoking male participants in the Multiple Risk Factor Intervention Trial (MRFIT). The subjects were aged 35 to 57 years at enrollment and were at high risk for mortality from coronary artery disease. At the baseline visit the maximum FEV_1 was approximately 3% lower for the men married to a smoker.

Masi and colleagues (1988) evaluated lung function of 293 young adults, using spirometry and measurement of the diffusing capacity and lung volumes. The results varied with gender. In men, reduction of the maximal midexpiratory flow rate was associated with maternal smoking and exposure to ETS during childhood. In women, reduction of the diffusing capacity was associated with exposure to ETS at work.

In the study of a general population sample in western Scotland, nonsmokers living with another household member who was a smoker had significantly reduced lung function in comparison with unexposed nonsmokers (Hole et al., 1989); the reduction of FEV_1 associated with involuntary smoking was about 5%. Passive smokers with higher exposure had greater reduction of the FEV_1.

Masjedi, Kazemi, and Johnson (1990) investigated the effects of passive smoking on lung function of 288 nonsmoking volunteers living in Tehran. Ventilatory function was reduced significantly for men exposed at work, although an additional effect of exposure at home was not found. Passive smoking at home and at work did not reduce the lung function of the female subjects.

Other studies have not shown chronic effects of involuntary exposure to tobacco smoke in adult nonsmokers. In two cross-sectional studies marriage to a smoker was not significantly associated with reduction of ventilatory function (Schilling et al., 1977; Comstock et al., 1981) Jones and coworkers (1983) conducted a case-control study of 20- to 39-year-old nonsmoking women in the longitudinal study in Tecumseh. Subjects from the highest and lowest quartiles of the lung-function distribution had comparable exposure to smokers in the home. In a study conducted in Germany, the effects of involuntary and active smoking were examined in a population of 1351 white-collar workers (Kentner, Triebig, and Weltle, 1984). Self-reported exposure to ETS at home and at work was not associated with reduction of spirometric measures of lung function. In a study of young Canadian adults, Jaakkola et al. (1995) did not find effects of home and workplace exposures on a change in lung function during an 8-year follow-up. In persons less than 26 years of age at enrollment, workplace ETS exposure was associated with greater decline.

Several investigators have reported associations of involuntary smoking with chronic obstructive pulmonary disease in nonsmokers. In the Japanese cohort study, a nonsignificant trend of increasing mortality from chronic bronchitis and emphysema with increasing passive exposure of nonsmoking women has been reported (Hirayama, 1984). Kalandidi and co-workers (1987) conducted a case-control study of involuntary smoking and chronic obstructive pulmonary disease; the cases were nonsmoking women with obstruction and reduction of the FEV_1 by at least 20%. Smoking by the husband was associated with a doubling of risk. Dayal et al. (1994) conducted a case-control study of self-reported obstructive lung disease in 219 never-smoking residents of Philadelphia. Household ETS exposure from one or more packs per day was associated with a doubling of risk. In a prospective cohort study of 3914 nonsmoking Adventists, ETS exposure was associated with report of symptoms considered to reflective of "airway obstructive disease" (Robbins, Abbey, and Lebowitz, 1993). An association of passive smoking with chronic obstructive pulmonary disease seems biologically implausible, however, since only a minority of active smokers develop this disease, and adverse effects of involuntary smoking on lung function in adults have not been observed consistently (DHHS, 1984). The autopsy study of Trichopoulus et al. (1992) does show, however, that airways of nonsmokers can be affected by ETS.

A conclusion cannot yet be reached on the effects of ETS exposure on lung function in adults. However, further research is warranted because of widespread exposure in workplaces and homes.

Odor and Irritation

Tobacco smoke contains numerous irritants, including particulate material and gases (DHHS, 1986b). Both questionnaire surveys and laboratory studies involving exposure to ETS have shown annoyance and irritation of the eyes and upper and lower airways from involuntary smoking. In several surveys of nonsmokers, complaints about tobacco smoke at work and in public places were common (DHHS, 1986b): About 50% of respondents complained about tobacco smoke at work, and a majority were disturbed by tobacco smoke in restaurants. The experimental studies show that the rate of eye blinking is increased by ETS, as are complaints of nose and throat irritation (DHHS, 1986b). In the study of passive smoking on commercial airline flights reported by Mattson and colleagues (1989), changes in nose and eye symptoms were associated with nicotine exposure. The odor and irritation associated with ETS merit special consideration because a high proportion of nonsmokers are annoyed by exposure to ETS, and control of concentrations in indoor air poses difficult problems in the management of heating, ventilating, and air-conditioning systems.

Using a challenge protocol, Bascom and colleagues (1991) showed that persons characterizing themselves as ETS-sensitive have greater responses on exposure than persons considering themselves as nonsensitive.

Other Effects

Other associations of passive smoking with adverse effects have been reported, most in relation to the fetus and children. A study of children with cystic fibrosis suggested that exposure to ETS at home adversely affects growth (Rubin, 1990).

This finding was not confirmed in a study of 340 patients with cystic fibrosis (Kovesi, Corey, and Levison, 1993). The investigators found that cessation of smoking was more likely in households of patients having lower lung function, indicating the potential for bias from differential patterns of smoking cessation.

In a study of 261 women aged 35 and over, passive smoking was found to alter the age at natural menopause (Everson et al., 1986). Passive exposure was associated with an approximately twofold increased risk of being menopausal.

Total Mortality

Several cohort studies provide information on involuntary smoking and mortality from all causes. In the Scottish cohort study, total mortality was initially reported as increased for women living with a smoker but not for men (Gillis et al., 1984). On further follow-up, all-cause mortality was increased in all passive smokers (RR: 1.27; 95% CI: 0.95, 1.70). As described previously, total mortality was also increased among nonsmoking participants in MRFIT who lived with smokers (Svendsen et al., 1987). In contrast, mortality was not increased for nonsmoking female subjects in a study in Amsterdam (Vandenbroucke et al., 1984). Neither the study in Scotland nor the study in Amsterdam controlled for other factors that influence total mortality. In the cohort study in Washington County, all-cause mortality rates were significantly increased for men (RR: 1.17) and for women (RR: 1.15) after adjustment for housing quality, schooling, and marital status (Sandler et al., 1989). All-cause mortality was also increased for passive smokers in the Evans County cohort (RR: 1.39; 95% CI: 0.99, 1.94).

Wells (1988) has made an estimate of the number of adult deaths in the United States attributable to passive smoking. The total is about 46,000, including 3000 from lung cancer, 11,000 from other cancers, and 32,000 from heart disease.

The small excesses of all-cause mortality associated with passive smoking in the epidemiological studies parallel the findings for cardiovascular disease, the leading cause of death in these cohorts. The increased risk of death associated with passive smoking has public health significance as an indicator of the overall impact of this avoidable exposure.

SUMMARY

The effects of active smoking and the toxicology of cigarette smoking have been comprehensively examined. The periodic reports of the U.S. Surgeon General and other summary reports have considered the extensive evidence on active smoking; these reports have provided definitive conclusions concerning the adverse effects of active smoking, which have prompted public policies and scientific research directed at prevention and cessation and smoking.

Although the evidence on involuntary smoking is not so extensive as that on active smoking, health risks of involuntary smoking have been identified and causal conclusions reached, beginning in the mid 1980s. The 1986 Report of the U.S. Surgeon General (DHHS, 1986b) and the 1986 Report of the National Research Council (NRC, 1986a) both concluded that involuntary exposure to tobacco smoke causes respiratory infections in children, increases the prevalence of respiratory symptoms in children, reduces the rate of functional growth as the lung matures, and causes lung cancer in nonsmokers. These conclusions have been reaffirmed in subsequent reports (EPA, 1992; Cal EPA, 1997; Ott, 1999) and new conclusions added. Involuntary smoking is now considered a cause of asthma, and a factor in exacerbating asthma (EPA, 1992; Cal EPA, 1997; Ott, 1999), and a cause of heart disease (Cal EPA, 1997; Ott, 1999). At the present time the evidence on passive smoking and cancer at sites other than the lung does not support causal conclusions.

The adverse effects of involuntary exposure to tobacco smoke have provided a strong rationale for policies directed at reducing and eliminating exposure of nonsmokers to ETS (DHHS, 1986b). Complete protection of nonsmokers in public locations and the workplace may require the banning of smoking, since the 1986 Report of the Surgeon General (DHHS, 1986b) concluded that "the simple separation of smokers and nonsmokers within the same air space may reduce, but does not eliminate, the exposure of nonsmokers to environmental tobacco smoke."

REFERENCES

Ahlborg, G., Jr., and L. Bodin. 1991. Tobacco smoke exposure and pregnancy outcome among working women: A prospective study at prenatal care centers in Orebro County, Sweden. *Am. J. Epidemiol.* 133(4): 338–347.

Allred, E. N., E. R. Bleecker, B. R. Chaitman, T. E. Dahms, S. O. Gottlieb, J. D. Hackney, M. Pagano, R. H. Selvester, S. M. Walden, and J. Warren. 1989. Short-term effects of carbon monoxide exposure on the exercise performance of subjects with coronary artery disease. *N. Engl. J. Med.* 321: 1426–1432.

Anderson, H. R., and D. G. Cook. 1997. Passive smoking and sudden infant death syndrome: Review of the epidemiological evidence. *Thorax* 52: 1003–1009.

Baghurst, P. A., S. L. Tong, A. Woodward, and A. J. McMichael. 1992. Effects of maternal smoking upon neuropsychological development in early childhood: Importance of taking account of social and environmental factors. *Paediatr. Perinat. Epidemiol.* 6: 403–415.

Barr, G. S., and A. P. Coatesworth. 1991. Passive smoking and otitis media with effusion. *Br. Med. J.* 303(6809): 1032–1033.

Bascom, R., T. Kulle, A. Kagey-Sobotka, and D. Proud. 1991. Upper respiratory tract environmental tobacco smoke sensitivity. *Am. Rev. Respir. Dis.* 143(6): 1304–1311.

Bauman, K. E., and R. L. Flewelling. 1991. Parental cigarette smoking and cognitive performance of children. *Health Psychol.* 10: 282–288.

Bauman, K. E., G. G. Koch, and L. A. Fisher. 1989. Family cigarette smoking and test performance by adolescents. *Health Psychol.* 8(1): 97–105.

Benowitz, N. L. 1996. Cotinine as a biomarker of environmental tobacco smoke exposure. *Epidemiol. Rev.* 18(2): 188–204

Benowitz, N. L., F. Kuyt, P. Jacob, 3rd, R. T. Jones, and A. L. Osman. 1983. Cotinine disposition and effects. *Clin. Pharmacol. Ther.* 34: 604–611.

Bergman, A. B., and L. A. Wiesner. 1976. Relationship of passive cigarette-smoking to sudden infant death syndrome. *Pediatrics* 58(5): 665–668.

Berkey, C. S., J. H. Ware, and D. W. Dockery. 1986. Indoor air pollution and pulmonary function growth in preadolescent children. *Am. J. Epidemiol.* 123: 250–260.

Black, N. 1985. The aetiology of glue ear — A case-control study. *Int. J. Pediatr. Otorhinolaryngol.* 9: 121–133.

Blair, P. S., P. J. Fleming, D. Bensley, I. Smith, C. Bacon, E. Taylor, J. Berry, J. Golding, and J. Tripp. 1996. Smoking and the sudden infant death syndrome: Results from 1993–1995 case-control study for confidential inquiry into stillbirths and deaths in infancy. *Br. Med. J.* 313: 195–198.

Brownson, R. C., M. C. Alavanja, E. T. Hock, and T. S. Loy. 1992. Passive smoking and lung cancer in nonsmoking women. *Am. J. Public Health* 82(11): 1525–1530.

Brunekreef, B., P. Fischer, B. Remijn, R. Van Der Lende, J. Schouten, and P. Quanjer. 1985. Indoor air pollution and its effect on pulmonary function of adult nonsmoking women. III. Passive smoking and pulmonary function. *Int. J. Epidemiol.* 14: 227–230.

Buckley, J. D., W. L. Hobbie, K. Ruccione, H. N. Sather, W. G. Wood, and G. D. Hammond. 1986. Maternal smoking during pregnancy and the risk of childhood cancer. *Lancet* 1: 519–520.

Burchfiel, C. M., III. 1984. *Passive smoking, respiratory symptoms, lung function and initiation of smoking in Tecumseh, Michigan.* PhD dissertation. University of Michigan, Ann Arbor.

Burchfiel, C. M., M. W. Higgins, J. B. Keller, W. F. Howatt, W. J. Butler, and I. T. T. Higgins. 1986. Passive smoking in childhood: Respiratory conditions and pulmonary function in Tecumseh, Michigan. *Am. Rev. Respir. Dis.* 133: 966–973.

Cal EPA. 1996. *Evidence on Developmental and Reproductive Toxicity of Cadmium: Reproductive and Cancer Hazard Assessment Section.* Sacramento, California Environmental Protection Agency.

Cal EPA. 1997. *Health Effects of Exposure to Environmental Tobacco Smoke.* California Environmental Protection Agency.

Cardenas, V. M., M. J. Thun, H. Austin, C. A. Lally, W. S. Clark, R. S. Greenberg, and C. W. J. Heath. 1997. Environmental tobacco smoke and lung cancer mortality in the American Cancer Society's Cancer Prevention Study. II. *Cancer Causes Control* 8(1): 57–64.

Charlton, A. 1984. Children's coughs related to parental smoking. *Br. Med. J.* 288: 1647–1649.

Ciruzzi, M., O. Estaban, J. Roziosnik, H. Montagna, J. Caccavo, D. De La Cruz, D. Ojoda, J. Piskorz, J. De Ross, P. Pramparo, and H. Schargrodsky. 1996. Passive smoking and the risk of acute myocardial infarction. XVIIIth Congress of the European Society of Cardiology. *Eur. Heart J.* 309(suppl).

Claxton, L. D., R. S. Morin, T. J. Hughes, and J. Lewtas. 1989. A genotoxic assessment of environmental tobacco smoke using bacterial bioassays. *Mutat. Res.* 222(2): 81–99.

Coghlin, J., S. K. Hammond, and P. H. Gann. 1989. Development of epidemiologic tools for measuring environmental tobacco smoke exposure. *Am. J. Epidemiol.* 130(4): 696–704.

Collet, J. P., C. P. Larson, J. F. Boivin, S. Suissa, and B. Pless. 1995. Parental smoking and risk of otitis media in pre-school children. *Can. J. Public Health* 86: 269–273.

Colley, J. R. T., W. W. Holland, and R. T. Corkhill. 1974. Influence of passive smoking and parental phlegm on pneumonia and bronchitis in early childhood. *Lancet* 2: 1031–1034.

Comstock, G. W., and F. E. Lundin. 1967. Parental smoking and perinatal mortality. *Am. J. Obstet. Gynecol.* 98(5): 708–718.

Comstock, G. W., M. B. Meyer, K. J. Helsing, and M. S. Tockman. 1981. Respiratory effects of household exposures to tobacco smoke and gas cooking. *Am. Rev. Respir. Dis.* 124: 143–148.

Cook, D. G., and D. P. Strachan. 1997. Parental smoking and prevalence of respiratory symptoms and asthma in school age children. *Thorax* 52(12): 1081–1094.

Coultas, D. B., C. A. Howard, G. T. Peake, B. J. Skipper, and J. M. Samet. 1987. Salivary cotinine levels and involuntary tobacco smoke exposure in children and adults in New Mexico. *Am. Rev. Respir. Dis.* 136(2): 305–309.

Coultas, D. B., G. T. Peake, and J. M. Samet. 1989. Questionnaire assessment of lifetime and recent exposure to environmental tobacco smoke. *Am. J. Epidemiol.* 130: 338–347.

Coultas, D. B., J. M. Samet, J. F. McCarthy, and J. D. Spengler. 1990a. Variability of measures of exposure to environmental tobacco smoke in the home. *Am. Rev. Respir. Dis.* 142: 602–606.

Coultas, D. B., J. M. Samet, J. F. McCarthy, and J. D. Spengler. 1990b. A personal monitoring study to assess workplace exposure to environmental tobacco smoke. *Am. J. Public Health* 80(8): 988–990.

Crawford, F. G., J. Mayer, R. M. Santella, T. B. Cooper, R. Ottman, W. Y. Tsai, G. Simon-Cereijido, M. Wang, D. Tang, and F. P. Perera. 1994. Biomarkers of environmental tobacco smoke in preschool children and their mothers. *J. Natl. Cancer Inst.* 86(18): 1398–1402.

Cummings, K. M., S. J. Marbello, M. C. Mahoney, and J. R. Marshall. 1989. Measurement of lifetime exposure to passive smoke. *Am. J. Epidemiol.* 130: 122–132.

Cummings, K. M., S. J. Markello, M. Mahoney, A. K. Bhargava, P. D. McElroy, and J. R. Marshall. 1990. Measurement of current exposure to environmental tobacco smoke. *Arch. Environ. Health* 45(2): 74–79.

Dahms, T. E., J. F. Bolin, and R. G. Slavin. 1981. Passive smoking: Effect on bronchial asthma. *Chest* 80(5): 530–534.

Dayal, H. H., S. Khuder, R. Sharrar, and N. Trieff. 1994. Passive smoking in obstructive respiratory disease in an industrialized urban population. *Environ. Res.* 65(2): 161–171.

Denson, R., J. L. Nanson, and M. A. McWatters. 1975. Hyperkinesis and maternal smoking. *Can. Psychiatr. Assoc.* 20: 183–187.

DHEW. 1979. *Changes in Cigarette Smoking and Current Smoking Practices Among Adults: United States, 1978.* Washington, DC : U.S. Government Printing Office, Advance Data 52.

DHHS. 1980. *The Health Consequences of Smoking for Women: A Report of the Surgeon General.* U.S. Department of Health and Human Services, Public Health Service, Office of the Assistant Secretary for Health, Office of Smoking and Health.

DHHS. 1982. *The Health Consequences of Smoking: Cancer. A Report of the Surgeon General.* Washington, DC: U.S. Department of Health and Human Services, Public Health Service, Office on Smoking and Health, DHHS Publication (PHS) 82-50179.

DHHS. 1984. *The Health Consequences of Smoking — Chronic Obstructive Lung Disease. A report of the Surgeon General.* Washington, DC: U.S. Government Printing Office.

DHHS. 1986a. *Smoking and Health: A National Status Report to Congress.* Rockville, MD: U.S. Government Printing Office.

DHHS. 1986b. *The Health Consequences of Involuntary Smoking. A Report of the Surgeon General.* Washington, DC: U.S. Government Printing Office, DHHS Publication (CDC) 87-8398.

DHHS. 1988. *The Health Consequences of Smoking: Nicotine Addiction. A report of the Surgeon General.* Washington, DC: U.S. Government Printing Office.

DHHS. 1989. *Reducing the Health Consequences of Smoking: 25 years of progress. A report of the Surgeon General.* Washington, DC: U.S. Government Printing Office.

DHHS. 1990a. Current estimates from the National Health Interview Survey, 1990. Series 10: Data from the National Health Interview Survey. *Department of Health and Human Services* 181. DHHS Publication (PHS) 91-1509.

DHHS. 1990b. *Smoking, Tobacco, and Cancer Program, 1985–1989 Status Report.* Washington, DC: U.S. Government Printing Office, NIH Publication No. 90-3107.

DHHS. 1990c. *The Health Benefits of Smoking Cessation. A report of the Surgeon General*. Washington, DC: U.S. Government Printing Office.

DHHS, Public Health Service, Centers for Disease Control and Prevention (CDC), National Center for Chronic Disease Prevention and Health Promotion, and Office on Smoking and Health. 1994. *Preventing Tobacco Use among Young People: A Report of the Surgeon General*. Washington, DC: U.S. Government Printing Office.

DHHS. 1997. *Practical Guide for the Diagnosis and Management of Asthma*. NIH Report 97-4053.

Dobson, A. J., H. M. Alexander, R. F. Heller, and D. M. Lloyd. 1991. Passive smoking and the risk of heart attack or coronary death. *Med. J. Aust.* 154: 793–797.

Enstrom, J. E. 1979. Rising lung cancer mortality among nonsmokers. *J. Natl. Cancer Inst.* 62: 755–760.

EPA. 1992. *Respiratory Health Effects of Passive Smoking: Lung Cancer and Other Disorders*. Washington, DC: U.S. Government Printing Office, EPA/600/006F.

Eskenazi, B., and J. J. Bergmann. 1995. Passive and active maternal smoking during pregnancy as measured by serum cotinine, and postnatal smoke exposure. I. Effects on physical growth at age 5 years. *Am. J. Public Health* 142: S10–S18.

Eskenazi, B., and L. S. Trupin. 1995. Passive and active maternal smoking during pregnancy, as measured by serum cotinine, and postnatal smoke exposure. II. Effects on neurodevelopment at age 5 years. *Am. J. Public Health* 142: S19–S29.

Etzel, R. A., E. N. Pattishall, N. Haley, R. H. Fletcher, and F. W. Henderson. 1992. Passive smoking and middle ear effusion among children in day care. *Pediatrics* 90: 228–232.

Euler, G. L., D. E. Abbey, A. R. Magie, and J. E. Hodgkin. 1987. Chronic obstructive pulmonary disease symptom effects of long-term cumulative exposure to ambient levels of total suspended particulates and sulfur dioxide in California Seventh-Day Adventist residents. *Arch. Environ. Health.* 42(4): 213–222.

Evans, D., M. J. Levison, C. H. Feldman, N. M. Clark, Y. Wasilewski, B. Levin, and R. B. Mellins. 1987. The impact of passive smoking on emergency room visits of urban children with asthma. *Am. Rev. Respir. Dis.* 135: 567–572.

Everson, R. B., D. P. Sandler, A. J. Wilcox, D. Schreinemachers, D. L. Shore, and C. Weinberg. 1986. Effect of passive exposure to smoking on age at natural menopause. *Br. Med. J. (Clin. Res. Ed.)* 293: 792.

Ey, J. L., C. J. Holberg, M. B. Aldous, A. L. Wright, F. D. Martinez, and L. M. Taussig. 1995. Passive smoke exposure and otitis media in the first year of life. Group Health Medical Associates. *Pediatrics* 95(5): 670–677.

First, M. W. 1985. Constituents of sidestream and mainstream tobacco and markers to quantify exposure to them. In *Indoor air and human health*, ed. R. B. Gammage. Chelsea. MI: Lewis Publishers.

Fleming, D. W., S. L. Cochi, A. W. Hightower, and C. V. Broome. 1987. Childhood upper respiratory tract infections: To what degree is incidence affected by day-care attendance? *Pediatrics* 79(1): 55–60.

Foliart, D., N. L. Benowitz, and C. E. Becker. 1983. Passive absorption of nicotine in flight attendants. *N. Engl. J. Med.* 308: 1105.

Fontham, E. T. H., P. Correa, P. Reynolds, A. Wu-Williams, P. A. Buffler, R. S. Greenberg, V. W. Chen, T. Alterman, P. Boyd, D. F. Austin, and J. Liff. 1994. Environmental tobacco smoke and lung cancer in nonsmoking women: A multicenter study. *JAMA* 271(22): 1752–1759.

Friedman, G. D., D. B. Petitti, and R. D. Bawol. 1983. Prevalence and correlates of passive smoking. *Am. J. Public Health* 73: 401–405.

Garfinkel, L. 1981. Time trends in lung cancer mortality among nonsmokers and a note on passive smokers. *J. Natl. Cancer Inst.* 66(6): 1061–1066.

Garland, C., E. Barret-Connor, L. Suarez, M. H. Criqui, and D. L. Wingard. 1985. Effects of passive smoking on ischemic heart disease mortality of nonsmokers: A prospective study. *Am. J. Epidemiol.* 121(5): 645–650.

Gillis, C. R., D. J. Hole, V. M. Hawthorne, and P. Boyle. 1984. The effect of environmental tobacco smoke in two urban communities in the west of Scotland. *Eur. J. Respir. Dis.* 65: 121–126.

Glantz, S. A., and W. W. Parmley. 1991. Passive smoking and heart disease: Epidemiology, physiology, and biochemistry. *Circulation* 83: 1–12.

Glantz, S. A., and W. W. Parmley. 1995. Passive smoking and heart disease: Mechanisms and risk. *JAMA* 273(13): 1047–1053.

Green, R. E., and N. K. Cooper. 1991. Passive smoking and middle ear effusions in children in British servicemen in West Germany—A point prevalence survey by clinics of outpatient attendance. *J. Army Med. Corps* 137(1): 31–33.

Greenberg, R. A., N. J. Haley, R. A. Etzel, and F. A. Loda. 1984. Measuring the exposure of infants to tobacco smoke: Nicotine and cotinine in urine and saliva. *N. Engl. J. Med.* 310: 1075–1078.

Grenier, M. G., S. G. Hardcastle, G. Kunchur, and K. Butler. 1992. The use of tracer gases to determine dust dispersion patterns and ventilation parameters in a mineral processing plant. *Am. Ind. Hyg. Assoc. J.* 53: 387–394.

Grufferman, S., H. H. Wang, E. R. DeLong, S. Y. Kimm, E. S. Delzell, and J. M. Falletta. 1982. Environmental factors in the etiology of rhabdomyosarcoma in childhood. *J. Natl. Cancer Inst.* 68(1): 107–113.

Guerin, M. R., R. A. Jenkins, and B. A. Tomkins. 1992. *The Chemistry of Environmental Tobacco Smoke: Composition and Measurement*. Chelsea, MI: Lewis Publishers.

Hackshaw, A. K., M. R. Law, and N. J. Wald. 1997. The accumulated evidence on lung cancer and environmental tobacco smoke. *Br. Med. J.* 315(7114): 980–988.

Haddow, J. E., G. J. Knight, G. E. Palomaki, and J. E. McCarthy. 1988. Second-trimester serum cotinine levels in nonsmokers in relation to birth weight. *Am. J. Obstet. Gynecol.* 159(2): 481–484.

Haley, N. J., S. G. Colosimo, C. M. Axelrod, R. Hanis, and D. W. Sepkovic. 1989. Biochemical validation of self-reported exposure to environmental tobacco smoke. *Environ. Res.* 49: 127–135.

Hammond, S. K. 1999. Exposure of U.S. Workers to Environmental Tobacco Smoke. *Environ. Health. Perspect.* 107(suppl 2): 329–340.

Hammond, S. K., and B. P. Leaderer. 1987. A diffusion monitor to measure exposure to passive smoking. *Environ. Sci. Technol.* 21: 494–497.

Hanrahan, J. P., I. B. Tager, M. R. Segal, T. D. Tosteson, R. G. Castile, H. Van Vunakis, S. T. Weiss, and F. E. Speizer. 1992. The effect of maternal smoking during pregnancy on early infant lung function. *Am. Rev. Respir. Dis.* 145:1129–1135.

Harlap, S., and A. M. Davies. 1974. Infant admissions to hospital and maternal smoking. *Lancet* 1: 529–532.

Harlos, D. P., M. Marbury, J. M. Samet, and J. D. Spengler. 1987. Relating indoor NO_2 levels to infant personal exposures. *Atmos. Environ.* 21: 369–378.

Harper, R. M., and R. C. Frysinger. 1988. Supropontine mechanisms underlying cardiorespiratory regulation: Implications for the sudden infant syndrome. In *Sudden Infant Death Syndrome: Risk Factors and Basic Mechanism*, eds. R. M. Harper and J. H. Hoffman. New York: SP Medical and Scientific Books, pp. 399–412.

Hartley, A. L., J. M. Birch, P. A. McKinney, M. D. Teare, V. Blair, J. Carrette, J. R. Mann, G. J. Draper, C. A. Stiller, and H. E. Johnston. 1988. The Inter-Regional Epidemiological Study of Childhood Cancer (IRESCC): Case control study of children with bone and soft tissue sarcomas. *Br. J. Cancer* 58(6): 838–842.

He, Y., L. S. Li, Z. H. Wan, X. L. Zheng, and G. L. Jia. 1989. Women's passive smoking and coronary heart disease. *Chin. J. Prev. Med.* 23(1): 19–22.

He, Y., T. H. Lam, L. S. Li, R. Y. Du, G. L. Jia, J. Y. Huang, and J. S. Zheng. 1994. Passive smoking at work as a risk factor for coronary heart disease in Chinese women who have never smoked. *Br. Med. J.* 308: 380–384.

Hecht, S. S., S. G. Carmella, S. E. Murphy, S. Akerkar, K. D. Brunnemann, and D. Hoffmann. 1993. A tobacco-specific lung carcinogen in the urine of men exposed to cigarette smoke. *N. Engl. J. Med.* 93(21): 1543–1546.

Helsing, K. J., D. P. Sandler, G. W. Comstock, and E. Chee. 1988. Heart disease mortality in nonsmokers living with smokers. *Am. J. Epidemiol.* 127(5): 915–922.

Henderson, F. W., H. F. Reid, R. Morris, O. L. Wang, P. C. Hu, R. W. Helms, L. Forehand, J. Mumford, J. Lewtas, N. J. Haley, and S. K. Hammond. 1989. Home air nicotine levels and urinary cotinine excretion in preschool children. *Am. Rev. Respir. Dis.* 140: 197–201.

Hinton, A. E., and G. Buckley. 1988. Parental smoking and middle ear effusions in children. *J. Laryngol. Otol.* 102(11): 992–996

Hirayama, T. 1981. Non-smoking wives of heavy smokers have a higher risk of lung cancer: A study from Japan. *Br. Med. J. (Clin. Res. Ed.)* 282(6259): 183–185.

Hirayama, T. 1984. Cancer mortality in nonsmoking women with smoking husbands based on a large-scale cohort study in Japan. *Prev. Med.* 13: 680–690.

Hoffman, D., N. J. Haley, J. D. Adams, and K. D. Brunnemann. 1984. Tobacco sidestream smoke: Uptake by nonsmokers. *Prev. Med.* 13: 608–617.

Hole, D. J., C. R. Gillis, C. Chopra, and V. M. Hawthorne. 1989. Passive smoking and cardiorespiratory health in a general population in the west of Scotland. *Br. Med. J.* 299(6696): 423–427.

Hosein, H. R., C. A. Mitchell, and A. Bouhuys. 1977. Evaluation of outdoor air quality in rural and urban communities. *Arch. Environ. Health* 32(1): 4–13.

Hosein, R., and P. Corey. 1984. Multivariate analyses of nine indoor factors on FEV_1 of Caucasian children. *Am. Rev. Respir. Dis.* 129: A140

Howe, G. R., J. D. Burch, A. M. Chiarelli, H. A. Risch, and B. C. Choi. 1989. An exploratory case-control study of brain tumors in children. *Cancer Res.* 49: 4349–4352.

Huel, G., J. Godin, T. Moreau, F. Girard, J. Sahuquillo, G. Hellier, and P. Blot. 1989. Aryl hydrocarbon hydroxylase activity in human placenta of passive smokers. *Environ. Res.* 50(1): 173–183.

Humble, C., J. Croft, A. Gerber, M. Casper, C. G. Hames, and H. A. Tyroler. 1990. Passive smoking and 20-year cardiovascular disease mortality among nonsmoking wives, Evans County, Georgia. *Am. J. Public Health* 80(5): 599–601.

Hunt, S. C., M. J. Martin, and R. R. Williams. 1986. Passive smoking by nonsmoking wives is associated with an increased incidence of heart disease in Utah, 86 A.D., at Las Vegas, NV: Am Public Hlth Assoc Mtg.

Husgafvel-Pursiainen, K., M. Sorsa, K. Engstrom, and P. Einisto. 1987. Passive smoking at work: Biochemical and biological measures of exposure to environmental tobacco smoke. *Int. Arch. Occup. Environ. Health.* 59(4):337–345.

IARC. 1986. *IARC Monographs on the Evaluation of the Carcinogenic Risk of Chemicals to Humans: Tobacco Smoking.* Lyon, France: International Agency for Research on Cancer, World Health Organization, IARC.

Idle, J. R. 1990. Titrating exposure to tobacco smoke using cotinine — A minefield of misunderstandings. *J. Clin. Epidemiol* 43(4): 313–317.

Iversen, M., L. Birch, G. R. Lundqvist, and O. Elbrond. 1985. Middle ear effusion in children and the indoor environment: An epidemiological study. *Arch. Environ. Health* 40: 74–79.

Jaakkola, M. S., and J. J. K. Jaakkola. 1997. Assessment of exposure to environmental tobacco smoke. *Eur. Respir. J.* 10: 2384–2397.

Jaakkola, M. S., J. J. K. Jaakkola, M. R. Becklake, and P. Ernst. 1995. Passive smoking and evolution of lung function in young adults: An eight-year longitudinal study. *J. Clin. Epidemiol.* 48: 317–327.

Jackson, M. Y., J. M. Proulx, and S. Pelican. 1991. Obesity prevention. *Am. J. Clin. Nutr.* 91(6 suppl): 1625S–1630S.

Jarvis, M. J., and M. A. Russell. 1984. Measurement and estimation of smoke dosage to non-smokers from environmental tobacco smoke. *Eur. J. Respir. Dis.* 133 (suppl): 68–75.

Jarvis, M. J., M. A. H. Russell, N. L. Benowitz, and C. Feyerabend. 1988. Elimination of cotinine from body fluids: Implications for noninvasive measurement of tobacco smoke exposure. *Am. J. Public Health* 78: 696–698.

Jarvis, M. J., M. A. Russell, C. Feyerabend, J. R. Eiser, M. Morgan, P. Gammage, and E. M. Gray. 1985. Passive exposure to tobacco smoke: saliva cotinine concentrations in a representative population sample of nonsmoking school children. *Br. Med. J.* 291: 927–929.

Jenkins, M. A., J. R. Clarke, J. B. Carlin, C. F. Robertson, J. L. Hopper, M. F. Dalton, D. P. Holst, K. Choi, and G. G. Giles. 1996. Validation of questionnaire and bronchial hyperresponsiveness against respiratory physician assessment in the diagnosis of asthma. *Int. J. Epidemiol.* 25(3): 609–616.

John, E. M., D. A. Savitz, and D. P. Sandler. 1991. Prenatal exposure to parents' smoking and childhood cancer. *Am. J. Epidemiol.* 133(2): 123–132.

Jones, J. R., I. T. T. Higgins, M. W. Higgins, and J. B. Keller. 1983. Effects of cooking fuels on lung function in nonsmoking women. *Arch. Environ. Health.* 38: 219–222.

Kabat, G. C., G. S. Dieck, and E. L. Wynder. 1986. Bladder cancer in nonsmokers. *Cancer* 2: 362–367.

Kabat, G. C., S. D. Stellman, and E. L. Wynder. 1995. Relation between exposure to environmental tobacco smoke and lung cancer in lifetime nonsmokers. *Am. J. Epidemiol.* 142(2): 141–148.

Kalandidi, A., D. Trichopoulos, A. Hatzakis, S. Tzannes, and R. Saracci. 1987. Passive smoking and chronic obstructive lung disease. *Lancet* 2(8571): 1325–1326.

Kallail, K. J., H. R. Rainbolt, and M. D. Bruntzel. 1987. Passive smoking and middle ear problems in Kansas public school children. *J. Commun. Disord.* 20(3): 187–196.

Kauffmann, F., J. S. Tessier, and P. Oriol. 1983. Adult passive smoking in the home environment: A risk factor for chronic airflow limitation. *Am. J. Epidemiol.* 117: 269–280.

Kawachi, I., G. A. Colditz, F. E. Speizer, J. E. Manson, M. J. Stampfer, W. C. Willett, and C. H. Hennekens. 1997. A prospective study of passive smoking and coronary heart disease. *Circulation* 95(10): 2374–2379.

Kentner, M., G. Triebig, and D. Weltle. 1984. The influence of passive smoking on pulmonary function — A study of 1,351 office workers. *Prev. Med.* 13: 656–669.

Kitchens, G. G. 1995. Relationship of environmental tobacco smoke to otitis media in young children. *Laryngoscope* 105: 1–12.

Klonoff-Cohen, H. S., S. L. Edelstein, E. S. Lefkowitz, I. P. Srinivasan, D. Kaegi, J. C. Chang, and K. J. Wiley. 1995. The effect of passive smoking and tobacco exposure through breast milk on sudden infant death syndrome. *JAMA* 273(10): 795–798.

Kovesi, T., M. Corey, and H. Levison. 1993. Passive smoking and lung function in cystic fibrosis. *Am. Rev. Respir. Dis.* 148(5): 1266–1271.

Kraemer, M. J., M. A. Richardson, N. S. Weiss, C. T. Furukawa, G. G. Shapiro, W. E. Pierson, and C. W. Bierman. 1983. Risk factors for persistent middle-ear effusions: Otitis media, catarrh, cigarette smoke exposure, and atopy. *JAMA* 83(8): 1022–1025.

Kramer, S., E. Ward, A. T. Meadows, and K. E. Malojne. 1987. Medical and drug risk factors associated with neuroblastom: A case control study. *J. Natl. Cancer Inst.* 78(5): 797–804.

Kyerematen, G. A., M. D. Damiano, B. H. Dvorchik, and E. S. Vesell. 1982. Smoking-induced changes in nicotine disposition: Application of a new HPLC assay for nicotine and its metabolites. *Clin. Pharmacol. Ther.* 32: 769–780.

La Vecchia, C., B. D'Avanzo, M. G. Franzosi, and G. Tognoni. 1993. Passive smoking and the risk of acute myocardial infarction. *Lancet* 341: 505–506.

Law, M. R., and A. K. Hackshaw. 1997. A meta-analysis of cigarette smoking, bone mineral density and risk of hip fracture: Recognition of a major effect. *Br. Med. J.* 315(7112): 841–846.

Law, M. R., J. K. Morris, and N. J. Wald. 1997. Environmental tobacco smoke exposure and ischaemic heart disease: An evaluation of the evidence. *Br. Med. J.* 315(7114): 973–980.

Layard, M. W. 1995. Ischemic heart disease and spousal smoking in the National Mortality Followback Survey. *Regul. Toxicol. Pharmacol.* 21: 180–183.

Leaderer, B. P., and S. K. Hammond. 1991. Evaluation of vapor-phase nicotine and respirable suspended particle mass as markers for environmental tobacco smoke. *Environ. Sci. Technol.* 25: 770–777.

Lebowitz, M. D. 1984. The effects of environmental tobacco smoke exposure and gas stoves on daily peak flow rates in asthmatic and non-asthmatic families. *Eur. J. Respir. Dis.* 133: 90–97.

Lebowitz, M. D., and B. Burrows. 1976. Respiratory symptoms related to smoking habits of family adults. *Chest* 69: 48–50.

Lebowitz, M. D., and C. J. Holberg. 1988. Effects of parental smoking and other risk factors on the development of pulmonary function in children and adolescents. *Am. J. Epidemiol.* 128: 589–597.

Lee, P. N. 1988. *Misclassification of Smoking Habits and Passive Smoking.* Berlin: Springer Verlag.

Lee, P. N., J. Chamberlain, and M. R. Alderson. 1986. Relationship of passive smoking to risk of lung cancer and other smoking-associated diseases. *Br. J. Cancer* 54(1): 97–105.

Leuenberger, P., J. Schwartz, U. Ackermann-Liebrich, K. Blaser, G. Bolognini, J. P. Bongard, O. Brandli, P. Braun, C. Bron, M. Brutsche, et al. 1994. Passive smoking exposure in adults with chronic respiratory symptoms (SAPALDIA Study). Swiss Study on Air Pollution and Lung Diseases in Adults, SAPALDIA Team. *Am. J. Resp. Crit. Care. Med.* 150(5 Pt 1): 1222–1228.

LeVois, M. E., and M. W. Layard. 1995. Publication bias in the environmental tobacco smoke/coronary heart disease epidemiologic literature. *Regul. Toxicol. Pharmacol.* 21: 184–191.

Lindbohm, M. L., M. Sallmen, K. Hemminki, and H. Taskinen. 1991. Paternal occupational lead exposure and spontaneous abortion. *Scand. J. Work. Environ. Health* 17: 95–103.

Lofroth, G. 1989. Environmental tobacco smoke: Overview of chemical composition and genotoxic components. *Mutat. Res.* 222(2): 73–80.

Maclure, M., R. B. Katz, M. S. Bryant, P. L. Skipper, and S. R. Tannenbaum. 1989. Elevated blood levels of carcinogens in passive smokers. *Am. J. Public Health* 89(10): 1381–1384.

Magnani, C., G. Pastore, L. Luzzatto, and B. Terracini. 1990. Parent at occupation and other environmental factors in the etiology of leukemia's and non-Hodgkins lymphomas in childhood: A case-control study. *Stumori* 76: 413–419.

Mainous, A. G., and W. J. Hueston. 1994. Passive smoke and low birth weight: Evidence of a threshold effect. *Arch. Fam. Med.* 3: 875–878.

Makin, J., P. A. Fried, and B. Watkinson. 1991. A comparison of active and passive smoking during pregnancy: Long-term effects. *Neurotoxicol. Teratol.* 13(1): 5–12.

Martin, T. R., and M. B. Bracken. 1986. Association of low birth weight with passive smoke exposure in pregnancy. *Am. J. Epidemiol.* 124(4): 633–642.

Martinez, F. D., A. L. Wright, L. M. Taussig, and Group Health Medical Associates. 1994. The effect of paternal smoking on the birthweight newborns whose mothers did not smoke. *Am. J. Public Health* 84(9): 1489–1491.

Martinez, F. D., G. Antognoni, F. Macri, E. Bonci, F. Midulla, G. DeCastro, and R. Ronchetti. 1988. Parental smoking enhances bronchial responsiveness in nine-year-old children. *Am. Rev. Respir. Dis.* 138: 518–523.

Masi, M. A., J. A. Hanley, P. Ernst, and M. R. Becklake. 1988. Environmental exposure to tobacco smoke and lung function in young adults. *Am. Rev. Respir. Dis.* 138: 296–299.

Masjedi, M. R., H. Kazemi, and D. C. Johnson. 1990. Effects of passive smoking on the pulmonary function of adults. *Thorax* 45(1): 27–31.

Matanoski, G., S. Kanchanaraksa, D. Lantry, and Y. Chang. 1995. Characteristics of nonsmoking women in NHANES I and NHANES I epidemiologic follow-up study with exposure to spouses who smoke. *Am. J. Epidemiol.* 142(2): 149–157.

Mattson, M. E., G. Boyd, D. Byor, C. Brown, J. F. Callahan, D. Corle, J. W. Cullen, J. Greenblatt, N. J. Haley, K. Hammond, J. Lewtas, and W. Reeves. 1989. Passive smoking on commercial airline flights. *JAMA* 261: 867–872.

Mau, G., and P. Netter. 1974. The effects of paternal cigarette smoking on perinatal mortality and the incidence of malformations. *Dtsch. Med. Wochenschr.* 99(21): 1113–1118.

McCredie, M., P. Maisonneuve, and P. Boyle. 1994. Antenatal risk factors for malignant brain tumors in New South Wales children. *Int. J. Cancer* 56: 6–10.

McGlashan, N. D. 1989. Sudden infant deaths in Tasmania, 1980-1986: A seven-year prospective study. *Soc. Sci. Med.* 29: 1015–1026.

McKinney, P. A., R. A. Cartwright, J. M. Saiu, J. R. Mann, C. A. Stiller, G. J. Draper, A. L. Hartley, P. A. Hopton, J. M. Birch, and J. A. Waterhouse. 1987. The inter-regional epidemiological study of childhood cancer (IRESCC): A case control study of aetiological factors in leukaemia and lymphoma. Arch. Dis. Child. 62(3): 279–287. (Published erratum appears in *Arch. Dis. Child* 1987 Jun; 62(6): 644).

McLaughlin, J. K., M. S. Dietz, E. S. Mehl, and W. J. Blot. 1987. Reliability of surrogate information on cigarette smoking by type of informant. *Am. J. Epidemiol.* 126(1): 144–146.

Milerad, J., and H. Sundell. 1993. Nicotine exposure and the risk of SIDS. *Acta Paediatr. Scand.* 389(suppl): 70–72.

Miller, G. H. 1984. Cancer, passive smoking and nonemployed and employed wives. *West. J. Med.* 140: 632–635.

Mitchell, E. A., L. Scragg, and M. Clements. 1995. Location of smoking and the sudden infant death syndrome (SIDS). *Aust. N. Z. J. Med.* 25: 155–156.

Mitchell, E. A., R. P. K. Ford, A. W. Stewart, B. J. Taylor, D. M. O. Becroft, J. M. D. Thompson, R. Scragg, I. B. Hassall, D. M. J. Barry, E. M. Allen, and A. P. Roberts. 1993. Smoking and the sudden infant death syndrome. *Pediatrics* 91: 893–896.

Mitchell, E. A., R. Scragg, A. W. Stewart, D. M. O. Becroft, B. J. Taylor, R. P. K. Ford, I. B. Hassal, D. M. J. Barry, E. M. Allen, and A. P. Roberts. 1991. Results from the first year of the New Zealand cot death study. *NZ Med. J.* 104: 71–76.

Murray, A. B., and B. J. Morrison. 1986. The effect of cigarette smoke from the mother on bronchial responsiveness and severity of symptoms in children with asthma. *J. Allergy Clin. Immunol.* 77(4): 575–581.

Murray, A. B., and B. J. Morrison. 1986. The effect of cigarette smoke from the mother on bronchial responsiveness and severity of symptoms in children with asthma. *J. Allergy Clin. Immunol.* 77(4): 575–581.

Murray, A. B., and B. J. Morrison. 1989. Passive smoking by asthmatics: its greater effect on boys than on girls and on older than on younger children. *Pediatrics* 84(3): 451–459.

Muscat, J. E., and E. L. Wynder. 1995. Exposure to environmental tobacco smoke and the risk of heart attack. *Int. J. Epidemiol.* 24(4): 715–719.

Nicholl, J., and A. O'Cathain. 1992. Antenatal smoking, postnatal passive smoking, and the Sudden Infant Death Syndrome. In *Effects of Smoking on the Fetus, Neonate, and Child*, eds. D. Poswillo and E. Alberman. New York: Oxford University Press, p. 230.

NRC. 1981. *Indoor Pollutants*. Washington, DC: National Academy Press.

NRC. 1986a. *Environmental Tobacco Smoke: Measuring Exposures and Assessing Health Effects*. Washington, DC: National Academy Press.

NRC. 1986b. *The Airliner Cabin Environment: Air Quality and Safety*. Washington, DC: National Academy Press.

O'Connor, G. T., S. T. Weiss, I. B. Tager, and F. E. Speizer. 1987. The effect of passive smoking on pulmonary function and nonspecific bronchial responsiveness in a population-based sample of children and young adults. *Am. Rev. Respir. Dis.* 135: 800–804.

Ostro, B. D. 1989. Estimating the risks of smoking, air pollution, and passive smoke on acute respiratory conditions. *Risk Anal.* 9(2): 189–196.

Ott, W. R. 1999. Mathematical models for predicting indoor air quality from smoking activity. *Environ. Health Perspect.* 107(suppl 2): 375–381.

Palmer, J. R., L. Rosenberg, and S. Shapiro. 1989. "Low yield" cigarettes and the risk of nonfatal myocardial infarction in women. *N. Engl. J. Med.* 320(24): 1569–1573.

Pershagen, G., A. Ericson, and P. Otterblad-Olausson. 1992. Maternal smoking in pregnancy: Does it increase the risk of childhood cancer? *Int. J. Epidemiol.* 21(1): 1–5.

Pirkle, J. L., K. M. Flegal, J. T. Bernert, D. J. Brody, R. A. Etzel, and K. R. Maurer. 1996. Exposure of the US Population to Environmental Tobacco Smoke. The Third National Health and Nutrition Examination Survey, 1988 to 1991. *JAMA* 275(16): 1233–1240.

Ponka, A. 1991. Asthma and low level air pollution in Helsinki. *Arch. Environ. Health* 46: 262–270.

Preston-Martin, S., M. C. Yu, B. Benton, and B. E. Henderson. 1982. N-Nitroso compounds and childhood brain tumors: A case-control study. *Cancer Res.* 42(12): 5240–5245.

Pron, G. E., J. D. Burch, G. R. Howe, and A. B. Miller. 1988. The reliability of passive smoking histories reported in a case-control study of lung cancer. *Am. J. Epidemiol.* 127(2): 267–273.

Pukander, J., J. Luotonen, M. Timonen, and P. Karmer. 1985. Risk factors affecting the occurrence of acute otitis media among 2–3-year-old urban children. *Acta Otolaryngol.* 100: 260–265.

Ra, L. 1992. Passive smoking and hearing loss in infants. *Irish Med. J.* 85: 111–112.

Rebagliato, M., C. d. Florey, and F. Bolumar. 1995. Exposure to environmental tobacco smoke in nonsmoking pregnant women in relation to birth weight. *Am. J. Epidemiol.* 142(5): 531–537.

Remijn, B., P. Fischer, B. Brunekreef, E. Lebret, J. S. Boleij, and D. Noij. 1985. Indoor air pollution and its effect on pulmonary function of adult nonsmoking women: I. Exposure estimates for nitrogen dioxide and passive smoking. *Int. J. Epidemiol.* 14: 215–220.

Repace, J. L., and A. H. Lowrey. 1980. Indoor air pollution, tobacco smoke, and public health. *Science* 208: 464–472.

Repace, J. L., and A. H. Lowrey. 1990. Risk assessment methodologies for passive smoking-induced lung cancer. *Risk Analysis* 10: 27–37.

Repace, J. L., J. Jinot, S. Bayard, K. Emmons, and S. K. Hammond. 1998. Air nicotine and saliva cotinine as indicators of workplace passive smoking exposure and risk. *Risk Analysis* 18(1): 71–83.

Robbins, A. S., D. E. Abbey, and M. D. Lebowitz. 1993. Passive smoking and chronic respiratory disease symptoms in non-smoking adults. *Int. J. Epidemiol.* 22(5): 809–817.

Roquer, J. M., J. Figueras, F. Botet, and R. Jimenez. 1995. Influence on fetal growth of exposure to tobacco smoke during pregnancy. *Acta Paediatr.* 84: 118–121.

Rosen, F. L., and A. Levy. 1950. Bronchial asthma due to allergy to tobacco smoke in an infant: A case report. *JAMA* 144(8): 620–621.

Rosenberg, J., N. L. Benowitz, P. Jacob, and K. M. Wilson. 1980. Disposition kinetics and effects of intravenous nicotine. *Clin. Pharmacol. Ther.* 28: 517–522.

Rubin, B. K. 1990. Exposure of children with cystic fibrosis to environmental tobacco smoke. *N. Engl. J. Med.* 323(12): 782–788.

Rubin, D. H., P. A. Krasilnikoff, J. M. Leventhal, B. Weile, and A. Berget. 1986. Effect of passive smoking on birth-weight. *Lancet* 2(8504):415–417.

Russell, M. A., R. J. West, and M. J. Jarvis. 1985. Intravenous nicotine simulation of passive smoking to estimate dosage to exposed nonsmokers. *Br. J. Addict* 80: 201–206.

Samet, J. M., and P. Lange. 1996. Longitudinal studies of active and passive smoking. *Am. J. Resp. Crit. Care. Med.* 154(6 pt 2): S257–S265.

Samet, J. M., I. B. Tager, and F. E. Speizer. 1983. The relationship between respiratory illness in childhood and chronic airflow obstruction in adulthood. *Am. Rev. Respir. Dis.* 127: 508–523.

Sandler, D. P., A. J. Wilcox, and R. B. Everson. 1985. Cumulative effects of lifetime passive smoking on cancer risk. *Lancet* 1: 312–315.

Sandler, D. P., and D. L. Shore. 1986. Quality of data on parents' smoking and drinking provided by adult offspring. *Am. J. Epidemiol.* 124(5): 768–778.

Sandler, D. P., G. W. Comstock, R. J. Helsing, and D. L. Shore. 1989a. Deaths from all causes in non-smokers who lived with smokers. *Am. J. Public Health* 79: 163–167.

Sandler, D. P., K. J. Helsing, G. W. Comstock, and D. L. Shore. 1989b. Factors associated with past household exposure to tobacco smoke. *Am. J. Epidemiol.* 129(2): 380–387.

Sandler, D. P., R. B. Everson, and A. J. Wilcox. 1985. Passive smoking in adulthood and cancer risk. *Am. J. Epidemiol.* 121: 37–48.

Sandler, D. P., R. B. Everson, A. J. Wilcox, and J. P. Browder. 1985. Cancer risk in adulthood from early life exposure to parents' smoking. *Am. J. Public Health* 74: 487–492.

Sandler, R. S., D. P. Sandler, G. W. Comstock, K. J. Helsing, and D. L. Shore. 1988. Cigarette smoking and the risk of colorectal cancer in women. *J. Natl. Cancer Inst.* 80(16): 1329–1333.

Saracci, R., and E. Riboli. 1989. Passive smoking and lung cancer: current evidence and ongoing studies at the International Agency for Research on Cancer. *Mutat. Res.* 89(2): 117–127.

Savitz, D. A., P. J. Schwingl, and M. A. Keels. 1991. Influence of paternal age, smoking, and alcohol consumption on congenital anomalies. *Teratology* 44(4): 429–440.

Schenker, M. B., J. M. Samet, and F. E. Speizer. 1982. Effect of cigarette tar content and smoking habits on respiratory symptoms in women. *Am. Rev. Respir. Dis.* 125: 684–690.

Schilling, R. S., A. D. Letai, S. L. Hui, G. J. Beck, J. B. Schoenberg, and A. H. Bouhuys. 1977. Lung function, respiratory disease, and smoking in families. *Am. J. Epidemiol.* 106(4): 274–283.

Schoendorf, K. C., and J. L. Kiely. 1992. Relationship of sudden infant death syndrome to maternal smoking during and after pregnancy. *Pediatrics* 90: 905–908.

Schwartz, J., and S. Zeger. 1990. Passive smoking, air pollution, and acute respiratory symptoms in a diary study of student nurses. *Am. Rev. Respir. Dis.* 141: 62–67.

Scientific Committee on Tobacco and Health, and HSMO. 1998. *Report of the Scientific Committee on Tobacco and Health.* The Stationary Office, Report 011322124x.

Seidman, D. S., P. Ever-Hadani, and R. Gale. 1990. Effect of maternal smoking and age on congenital anomalies. *Obstetrics Gynecol.* 76(6): 1046–1050.

Severson, R. K., J. D. Buckley, W. G. Woods, D. Benjamin, and L. L. Robison. 1993. Cigarette smoking and alcohol consumption by parents of children with acute myeloid leukemia. An analysis within morphological subgroups—A report from the Childrens Cancer Group. *Cancer Epidemiol. Biomarkers Prev.* 2: 433-439.

Shephard, R. J., R. Collins, and F. Silverman. 1979. "Passive" exposure of asthmatic subjects to cigarette smoke. *Environ. Res.* 20(2): 392–402.

Slattery, M. L., L. M. Robison, K. L. Schuman, T. K. French, T. M. Abbott, J. C. Overall, and J. W. Gardner. 1989. Cigarette smoking and exposure to passive smoke are risk factors for cervical cancer. *JAMA* 261: 1593–1598.

Sorsa, M., K. Husgafvel-Pursiainen, H. Jarventaus, K. Koskimies, H. Salo, and H. Vainio. 1989. Cytogenetic effects of tobacco smoke exposure among involuntary smokers. *Mutat. Res.* 222(2): 111–116.

Sorsa, M., P. Einisto, K. Husgafvel-Pursiainen, H. Jarventaus, H. Kivisto, Y. Peltonen, T. Tuomi, S. Valkonen, and O. Pelkonen. 1985. Passive and active exposure to cigarette smoke in a smoking experiment. *J. Toxicol. Environ. Health* 16(3–4): 523–524.

Spengler, J. D., and B. G. Ferris Jr. 1985. Harvard air pollution health study in six cities in the U.S.A. *Tokai J. Exp. Clin. Med.* 10(4): 263–286.

Spengler, J. D., D. W. Dockery, W. A. Turner, J. M. Wolfson, and B. G. Ferris Jr. 1981. Long-term measurements of respirable sulfates and particles inside and outside homes. *Atmos. Environ.* 15: 23–30.

Spengler, J. D., R. D. Treitman, T. Tosteson, D. T. Mage, and M. L. Soczek. 1985. Personal exposures to respirable particulates and implications for air pollution epidemiology. *Environ. Sci. Technol.* 19: 700–707.

Stankus, R. P., P. K. Menan, R. J. Rando, H. Glindmeyer, J. E. Salvaggio, and S. B. Lehrer. 1988. Cigarette smoke-sensitive asthma: challenge studies. *J. Allergy Clin. Immunol.* 82: 331–338.

Steenland, K., M. Thun, C. Lally, and C. Heath Jr. 1996. Environmental tobacco smoke and coronary heart disease in the American Cancer Society CPS-II Cohort. *Circulation* 94(4): 622–628.

Stillman, R. J., M. J. Rosenberg, and B. P. Sachs. 1986. Smoking and reproduction. *Fertil Steril* 46(4): 545–566.

Stjernfeldt, M., K. Berglund, J. Lindsten, and J. Ludvigsson. 1986. Maternal smoking during pregnancy and risk of childhood cancer. *Lancet* 1: 1350–1352.

Strachan, D. P., and D. G. Cook. 1997. Health effects of passive smoking: 1. Parental smoking and lower respiratory illness in infancy and early childhood. *Thorax* 52(10): 905–914.

Strachan, D. P., and D. G. Cook. 1998a. Parental smoking and allergic sensitization in children. *Thorax* 53(2): 117–123.

Strachan, D. P., and D. G. Cook. 1998b. Parental smoking, middle ear disease and adenotonsillectomy in children. *Thorax* 53(1): 50–56.

Strachan, D. P., M. J. Jarvis, and C. Feyerabend. 1989. Passive smoking, salivary cotinine concentrations, and middle ear effusion in 7 year old children. *Br. Med. J.* 298(6687): 1549–1552.

Svendsen, K. H., L. H. Kuller, M. J. Martin, and J. K. Ockene. 1987. Effects of passive smoking in the multiple risk factor intervention trial. *Am. J. Epidemiol.* 126(5): 783–795.

Tager, I. B. 1988. Passive smoking-bronchial responsiveness and atopy. *Am. Rev. Respir. Dis.* 138: 507–509.

Tager, I. B., A. Muñoz, B. Rosner, S. Weiss, V. Carey, and F. E. Speizer. 1985. Effect of cigarette smoking on the pulmonary function of children and adolescents. *Am. Rev. Respir. Dis.* 131: 752–759.

Tager, I. B., M. R. Segal, A. Muñoz, S. T. Weiss, and F. E. Speizer. 1987. The effect of maternal cigarette smoking on the pulmonary function of children and adolescents: Analyses of data from two populations. *Am. Rev. Respir. Dis.* 136: 1366–1370.

Tager, I. B., S. T. Weiss, A. Muñoz, B. Rosner, and F. E. Speizer. 1983. Longitudinal study of the effects of maternal smoking on pulmonary function in children. *N. Engl. J. Med.* 309: 699–703.

Tainio, V. M., E. Savilahti, L. Salmenpera, P. Arjomaa, M. A. Siimes, and J. Perheentupa. 1988. Risk factors for infantile recurrent otitis media: Atopy but not type of feeding. *Pediatr. Res.* 23(5): 509–512.

Takasaka, T. 1990. Incidence, prevalence, and natural history of otitis media in different geographic areas and populations. *Ann. Otol. Rhinol. Laryngol.* 99: 13–14.

Tashkin, D. P., V. A. Clark, M. Simmons, C. Reems, A. H. Coulson, L. B. Bourque, J. W. Sayre, R. Detels, and S. Rokaw. 1984. The UCLA population studies of chronic obstructive respiratory disease: VII. Relationship between parental smoking and children's lung function. *Am. Rev. Respir. Dis.* 129: 891–897.

Taylor, A. E., D. C. Johnson, and H. Kazemi. 1992. Environmental tobacco smoke and cardiovascular disease: A position paper from the council on cardiopulmonary and critical care, American Heart Association. *Circulation* 86(2): 1–4.

Teele, D. W., J. O. Klein, and B. Rosner. 1989. Epidemiology of otitis media during the first seven years of life in children in greater Boston: A prospective cohort study. *J. Infect. Dis.* 160: 83–94.

Toubas, P. L., J. C. Duke, M. A. McCaffree, C. D. Mattice, D. Bendell, and W. C. Orr. 1986. Effects of maternal smoking and caffeine habits on infantile apnea: A retrospective study. *Pediatrics* 86(1): 159–163.

Trichopoulos, D., A. Kalandidi, and L. Sparros. 1983. Lung cancer and passive smoking: Conclusion of Greek study. *Lancet* 2: 677–678.

Trichopoulos, D., A. Kalandidi, L. Sparros, and B. MacMahon. 1981. Lung cancer and passive smoking. *Int. J. Cancer* 27(1): 1–4.

Trichopoulos, D., F. Mollo, L. Tomatis, E. Agapitos, L. Delsedime, X. Zavitsanos, A. Kalandidi, K. Katsouyanni, E. Riboli, and R. Saracci. 1992. Active and passive smoking and pathological indicators of lung cancer risk in an autopsy study. *JAMA* 268(13): 1697–1701.

Tsimoyianis, G. V., M. S. Jacobson, J. G. Feldman, M. T. Antonio-Santiago, B. C. Clutario, M. Nussbaum, and I. R. Shenker. 1987. Reduction in pulmonary function and increased frequency of cough associated with passive smoking in teenage athletes. *Pediatrics* 80(1): 32–36.

Urch, R. B., F. Silverman, P. Corey, R. J. Shephard, P. Cole, and L. J. Goldsmith. 1988. Does suggestibility modify acute reactions to passive cigarette smoke exposure? *Environ. Res.* 47: 34–47.

van Steensel-Moll, H. A., H. A. Valkenburg, J. P. Vandenbroucke, and G. E. van Zanen. 1985. Are maternal fertility problems related to childhood leukaemia? *Int. J. Epidemiol.* 14(4): 555–559.

Vandenbroucke, J. P., J. H. Verheesen, A. De Bruin, B. J. Mauritz, C. van der Heide-Wessel, and R. M. van der Heide. 1984. Active and passive smoking in married couples: Results of 25 year follow up. *Br. Med. J. (Clin. Res. Ed.)* 84: 1801–1802.

Wald, N. J., K. Nanchakal, S. G. Thompson, and H. S. Cuckle. 1986. Does breathing other people's tobacco smoke cause lung cancer? *Br. Med. J.* 293: 1217–1222.

Wall, M. A., J. Johnson, P. Jacob, and N. L. Benowitz. 1988. Cotinine in the serum, saliva and urine of nonsmokers, passive smokers, and active smokers. *Am. J. Public Health* 78: 699–701.

Wallace, L. A., and E. D. Pellizzari. 1987. Personal air exposures and breath concentrations of benzene and other volatile hydrocarbons for smokers and nonsmokers. *Toxicol. Lett.* 35(1): 113–116.

Wang, X., D. Wypij, D. Gold, F. E. Speizer, J. H. Ware, B. G. Ferris Jr., and D. W. Dockery. 1994. A longitudinal study of the effects of parental smoking on pulmonary function in children 6–18 years. *Am. J. Resp. Crit. Care Med.* 149(6): 1420–1425.

Ware, J. H., D. W. Dockery, and A. Spiro, III. 1984. Passive smoking, gas cooking, and respiratory health of children living in six cities. *Am. Rev. Respir. Dis.* 129: 366–374.

Weiss, S. T. 1986. Passive smoking and lung cancer: What is the risk? *Am. Rev. Respir. Dis.* 133: 1–3.

Weiss, B. 1989. Behavior as an endpoint for inhaled toxicants. In *Concepts in Inhalation Toxicology*, eds. R. O. McClellan and R. F. Henderson. New York: Hemisphere Publishing, pp. 475–493.

Weiss, S. T., I. B. Tager, F. E. Speizer, and B. Rosner. 1980. Persistent wheeze: Its relation to respiratory illness, cigarette smoking, and level of pulmonary function in a population sample of children. *Am. Rev. Respir. Dis.* 122: 697–707.

Weitzman, M., S. Gortmaker, and A. Sobul. 1992. Maternal smoking and behavior problems of children. *Pediatrics* 90(3): 342–349.

Weitzman, M., S. Gortmaker, D. K. Walker, and A. Sobol. 1990. Maternal smoking and childhood asthma. *Pediatrics* 85(4): 505–511.

Weitzman, M., S. L. Gortmaker, A. M. Sobol, and J. M. Perrin. 1992. Recent trends in the prevalence and severity of childhood asthma. *JAMA* 268(19): 2673–2677.

Wells, A. J. 1988. An estimate of adult mortality in the United States from passive smoking. *Environ. Int.* 14: 249–265.

White, J. R., and H. F. Froeb. 1980. Small airways dysfunction in nonsmokers chronically exposed to tobacco smoke. *N. Engl. J. Med.* 302: 720–723.

Young, S., P. N. Le Souef, G. C. Geelhoed, S. M. Stick, K. J. Turner, and L. I. Landau. 1991. The influence of a family history of asthma and parental smoking on airway responsiveness in early infancy. *N. Engl. J. Med.* 324(17): 1168–1173.

Yue Chen, B. M., L. I. Wan-Xian, and Y. Shunzhang. 1986. Influence of passive smoking on admissions for respiratory illness in early childhood. *Br. Med. J.* 293: 303–306.

Zhang, J., D. A. Savitz, P. J. Schwingl, and W. W. Cai. 1992. A case-control study of paternal smoking and birth defects *Int. J. Epidemiol.* 21(2): 273–278.

Zielhius, G. A., E. W. Heuvelmans-Heinen, G. H. Rach, and P. van den Broek. 1989. Environmental risk factors for otitis media with effusion in preschool children. *Scand. J. Prim. Health Care* 7(1): 33–38.

11 Food Constituents, Additives, and Contaminants

JOSEPH V. RODRICKS, Ph. D.

FOOD-RELATED HEALTH RISKS

Composition of Food

Food is by far the most chemically complex part of the environment to which humans are directly exposed. We have no reliable estimate of the number of distinct chemical compounds in the different items of food and drink we select for nourishment and pleasure, but it is surely in the hundreds of thousands. The chemical structures of most of these are unknown, but the known constituents display immense variety. To make matters more complex, the chemical composition of the human diet varies from culture to culture and over time within cultures. Food chemists will probably never know more than a small fraction of the chemicals we deliberately put into our mouths every day of our lives (NRC, 1996).

The major share of dietary chemicals is represented by the natural constituents of foods and beverages. In addition to the hundreds of distinct compounds that supply nutritional requirements, there are thousands more that impart flavor and color. Food plants contain large numbers of natural constituents that contribute neither nutritional nor aesthetic properties but are present because they play some role in the lives of these plants. It has been estimated, for one small example, that a freshly brewed cup of coffee contains more than 600 distinct (and mostly unidentified) compounds (Smith, 1991). We also need to note the additional burden of natural products from the hundreds of herbs and spices used in food preparation.

Also among the constituents of the human diet are substances that arise during food and beverage preparation. Fermentation, for example, produces numerous chemical alterations of organic compounds, yielding products bearing little chemical similarity to the starting materials. Little scientific skill, and not much gastronomic skill, is needed to recognize that each variety of wine and cheese possesses a unique chemical composition, and that none of these bears much resemblance to grape juice and milk. Roasting, broiling, baking, microwaving, smoking, and other means of preparing and processing foods each sets off dozens of chemical reactions. Because most methods of food preparation have been in use for centuries, people by now think of the products of preparation as "natural". This is perhaps appropriate, but strictly speaking, they actually result from human manipulation of raw food products.

Human beings have of course never been satisfied to leave nature as it is and have added substances to food to achieve any number of desirable technical effects. Food preservation

Environmental Toxicants: Human Exposures and Their Health Effects, 2/e. Edited by Morton Lippmann.
ISBN: 0-471-29298-2 © 2000 John Wiley & Sons, Inc.

using various inorganic salts was probably one of the earliest example of this practice, but adding substances to color, to sweeten, to emulsify, to flavor, and to alter taste perception is also a fairly ancient practice that continues to this day.

Many chemicals not directly added to food but that are intentionally used in food production, processing, and storage actually end up in the diet, although usually in very small concentrations. Among these indirectly added substances are residues of drugs and feed additives used in animal production, crop-use pesticides and their metabolites and degradation products, and migrants from materials used in food processing and packaging. Several thousand direct and indirect additives that may be present in foods add a significant increment to the uncounted numbers of natural substances resulting from food preparation.

Some foods may also contain contaminants—unwanted by-products of nature or human industry that somehow come to be present in food. Included are bacterial and fungal metabolites resulting from the growth on food of species of these organisms, organic chemicals of industrial origin, and various metals and other inorganic species that arise either because of their natural presence in soils and water used for food production or because they have locally accumulated to unusually high environmental levels as a result of mining, industrial, or other human activities. For completeness we need to include bacterial metabolites that are not produced directly in food but rather in the intestines following ingestion of foods contaminated with the offending organisms. Some contaminants are fairly regularly occurring constituents of certain foods, whereas others arise only occasionally (and unpredictably) because of a human or natural mishap. As with the other dietary constituents, the total number of possible dietary contaminants is unknown, although the most important ones are fairly well documented. The major categories of the constituents of food are summarized in Table 11-1.

Problem of Understanding Food-Related Health Risks

Given the complexity of food, it is no surprise that we find little uniformity in the study of the health risks associated with its constituents. One approach is that of epidemiologists interested in diet and health. Their studies of health trends in populations with different intakes of certain food constituents have revealed such significant associations as those between high intakes of calories and of animal fats and low intakes of fiber, on the one hand, and cardiovascular disease and certain forms of cancer on the other (NRC, 1991, 1996). Epidemiologists have also uncovered associations between excessive intakes of specific dietary constituents, such as salt, nitrates, oxalates, and aflatoxins, and specific human diseases, although epidemiological science is usually working close to its detection limits in such situations. Nutritionists rely on the tools of epidemiology but also turn to clinical studies and studies in experimental animals to learn about the risks and benefits of nutrients. Most of their efforts have focused on the major constituents and nutrients (Reddy and Cohen, 1986; NRC, 1996).

TABLE 11-1   Categories of Food Constituents

Natural components	Substances intentionally introduced (directly and indirectly)	Contaminants
Nutrients	Food and color additives	Naturally occurring substances
	Substances Generally Recognized as Safe (GRAS)	Industrial products and by-products
Nonnutrients	Veterinary drug residues and feed additives	
	Pesticide residues	

The contributions of toxicologists, whose main tool is experimental investigations, have generally been limited to the study of individual constituents. The efforts of toxicologists are primarily driven by regulatory requirements to establish limits on human exposure to additives and certain well-recognized contaminants. Up to the present, relatively little systematic study of the thousands of natural constituents of food, except for those that have made themselves known by high and easily detectable (usually acute) toxicity, has been carried out by epidemiologists, nutritionists, and toxicologists (Doull, 1981; NRC, 1996).

The tools available to study dietary risks are seriously limited. Certainly epidemiologists have been able to provide some highly important clues about health benefits and risks associated with certain obvious features of the diet, but so far they have been able to say little about the possible risks of the many thousands of individual constituents and contaminants. The clinician primarily studies health benefits. Clinical studies may detect unexpected side effects, but such studies are not carried out until preclinical toxicology data have been collected showing that, at the most, only minor and readily reversible adverse effects are to be expected under the proposed conditions of human dosing. Toxicology studies suffer from the obvious limitation that experimental animals are not the species of interest. They are also limited because they typically involve study of individual constituents (although there have been some efforts at wider application of this tool). It is almost certain that the collection of toxicology data on each of the individual constituents and contaminants of food (a clearly impossible task) would still not provide a thorough picture of dietary risks. The total health risk associated with food is surely not simply the sum of the risks associated with each of its individual constituents and contaminants. Moreover the picture is becoming increasingly complicated by the fact that many constituents of food, in addition to the nutrients, may confer substantial health benefits (NRC, 1996).

There is no single investigative tool that provides an evaluation of the total role of the diet in human health, nor are there adequate methods to acquire a thorough understanding of the interaction of diet and other environmental agents. Closer integration of the work of epidemiologists, clinicians, and toxicologists would seem an essential step toward the objective of understanding the total picture.

Scope and Limitations of This Chapter

Rather than attempting to provide a complete evaluation of the role of food in human health, we focus on individual constituents, additives, and contaminants and on the methods by which they are evaluated. Unlike most of the chapters in this volume, which deal with one or a few chemicals, we are forced somehow to consider thousands of individual substances. It seemed to make little sense to provide detailed exposure and toxicology reviews for a few important food substances, since little of general value can be learned by such an approach. Instead the choice has been made to emphasize the principles and methods for evaluating individual constituents, for assessing their health risks, and for establishing limits on human exposure to them. Broad surveys of the major categories of food constituents and contaminants are presented, and examples are drawn from several of these categories to illustrate certain principles and methods. Because it is the subject of Chapter 23, the problem of pesticides in food is omitted here.

Since much of what has been learned about food constituents and contaminants resulted from the scientific investigations that have been conducted because of legal requirements, we begin with a discussion of the regulatory framework under which these substances are treated. Following this, we proceed to surveys and examples of substances directly and indirectly added to food, contaminants of industrial origin, and constituents and contaminants of natural origin. The closing section deals with gaps in understanding and some suggestions regarding possible avenues toward improvements in knowledge.

LEGAL AND REGULATORY FRAMEWORK

Although this chapter emphasizes the scientific evaluation of risks from dietary constituents and contaminants, it is necessary to include some background on the legal and regulatory contexts. We do not propose to discuss the intricacies of the Federal Food, Drug and Cosmetic Act, the law governing food safety in the United States, but only to summarize certain broad features of it. Legal experts will recognize this summary as inadequate (but, we hope, not misleading). It is intended to provide scientists with some understanding of why certain categories of food constituents have received more extensive study than others, and about the role of risk information in decision making.

In connection with the risks of food constituents and contaminants, the Federal Food, Drug and Cosmetic Act recognizes and distinguishes among at least three categories (Roberts, 1981): (1) substances that are intentionally added to food, both directly and indirectly; (2) substances that are unavoidable contaminants of food; and (3) substances that are natural components of food (see Table 11-1).

The major federal agency responsible for enforcing the Act is the Food and Drug Administration (FDA). The Department of Agriculture has enforcement responsibility for the Federal Meat and Poultry Inspection Act, and most of its provisions dealing with potential food risks match those of the Food, Drug and Cosmetic Act. Although the law provides FDA with broad authority to act to ensure the safety of the food supply, it places different burdens on the agency and on the regulated industries for the different categories of food constituents and contaminants. For the first group listed above—substances intentionally added to food[1]—the FDA has been given power to prevent their addition unless certain safety criteria are met. The agency has responded to this legal mandate by specifying the types of toxicity studies that must be undertaken prior to the introduction of the added substance and the criteria by which safety is to be judged. In essence, such substances can be introduced only if they are "shown to be safe"; the sections of food law governing intentionally introduced substances do not permit other considerations (e.g., benefits conferred) to influence the decision about the acceptability of these substances—they are risk-only criteria. "Safe" is defined as the "practical certainty of no harm" under proposed conditions of use. The Delaney Amendment, introduced in 1958, further specifies that no additive found to induce cancer can be judged safe at any level of addition (clarification of the limits of applicability of the Delaney clause is reviewed later in this chapter). The burden of demonstrating safety falls primarily on those who would seek to add substances to food (the "petitioner"); FDA can prevent such actions simply by showing that the burden has not been met. Except for substances generally recognized as safe (GRAS), substances can be intentionally introduced into food only in conformance with written regulations, whose content in large part depends on the toxicology and human intake data supplied to FDA by the petitioner (Merrill, 1996).

Somewhat different burdens and criteria apply to contaminants. Clearly, if food is deliberately or accidentally contaminated, or if the contamination can readily be avoided by good manufacturing practice (e.g., botulism), the FDA has substantial authority to ban or otherwise limit human exposure to the contaminated food; it can take powerful emergency actions if the risks are judged substantial or imminent. The more difficult problem concerns contaminants the agency considers unavoidable that may be present at levels that

---

[1] This group consists of several subgroups, and distinctions are made among these; they are discussed later in this chapter.

possess significant (though perhaps not imminent) health risks. There are, for example, certain substances that may enter the food chain because of their widespread presence in the environment. Chemical pollutants such as mercury, lead, PCBs, and several chlorinated hydrocarbon pesticides can be found in certain foods on a fairly regular basis, mostly at low (but not always insignificant) levels. These substances are not present because of any deliberate act of food adulteration. They are present because of factors that are now beyond human control and, with the metals at least, because there is a certain level of natural occurrence. Obviously, with enough foresight, significant PCB and pesticide contamination of the environment might have been prevented by the institution of strict controls from the first days of their commercial production. But this was not done in a way that would be considered appropriate by today's standards, and the FDA is now faced with contamination that can be controlled only by banning or limiting consumption of the affected food itself. This situation is clearly different from that of the deliberately added substances, and under the law the FDA has authority to balance health risks from the contaminant against certain costs—notably the loss of portions of the food supply—in setting limits on human exposure. The FDA has also applied these criteria to certain contaminants of natural origin, such as the aflatoxins (Merrill, 1996).

Contaminants differ from intentionally added substances in another significant respect: No specific responsibility for developing the data necessary to characterize health effects, human exposures, and risks is assigned under the law. Generally, FDA, relying on its own or other governmental testing programs, or on data appearing in the scientific literature, has the burden of demonstrating the risks of contaminants prior to devising programs to control them. Thus, although some contaminants, such as lead and mercury, have received considerable scrutiny from toxicologists and epidemiologists because of their widespread environmental occurrence, many have been only poorly characterized as to the risks they pose, certainly far less than intentional additives.

Naturally occurring constituents (not contaminants) of food have received relatively little attention, in part because the law prefers not to tamper with food itself unless the risks are clearly substantial. Thus, for example, certain plants that might be considered suitable for food have been excluded, not by the FDA, but because they contain levels of toxicants sufficiently high to cause immediate adverse or even deadly effects. However, we readily accept many natural substances that produce subclinical effects under normal rates of intake or that produce serious, chronic toxicity at high doses in animal tests when it is clear their intentional addition to the diet would be prohibited because they fail to meet the safety criteria applied to additives. And, as with contaminants, no special responsibility is assigned under the law for the development of risk-related data on these substances. Not surprisingly, most investigations into the toxicity and risks of natural constituents of the diet (and they are very few in number relative to the size of this class of substances) tend to be of limited scope (Rodricks, 1981).

These various legal criteria (and others not mentioned here) help to explain why the extent of our knowledge of the classes of substances to be discussed later varies so greatly among them. They also reveal why different approaches to risk management have been taken for different constituents of the diet.

TOXICITY TEST REQUIREMENTS AND SAFETY CRITERIA

Acceptable Daily Intake

Except for carcinogens, one risk criterion for judging the acceptability of substances intentionally added to food is the acceptable daily intake (ADI). The ADI is a level of daily intake that is not expected to cause adverse health effects when maintained over a full lifetime (Joint Codex Alimentarius Commission, 1979; Food Protection Committee, 1970).

The ADI approach was introduced in the early 1950s by Arnold Lehman and O. Garth Fitzhugh of the FDA to assist regulation of food additives and pesticides. The ADI has been widely used in all areas of regulation; the FAO/WHO Joint Expert Committee on Food Additives has published ADIs for many food additives (some conditionally because of data gaps or uncertainties), and they are generally recognized as authoritative in member countries.

The theoretical basis for the ADI is that, for all toxic effects with the possible exception of carcinogenicity (see below), a threshold dose must be exceeded before the toxic response is produced. Experimentally measured thresholds, or "no-observed-adverse-effect levels" (NOAELs), are divided by various "safety factors" to estimate the corresponding threshold dose for the general human population. Safety factors are introduced to account for the possibility that humans may be more sensitive to the toxic effects of an agent than are test animals and because some members of the general population may be more sensitive than others (Dourson and Stara, 1983). The Environmental Protection Agency now uses the term toxicity Reference Dose (R_fD) for what is the practical equivalent of the ADI. The EPA also notes that the "safety factors" are in fact used to account for uncertainties regarding variabilities in suceptibility between animals and humans, and among members of the human population. For these and other scientific uncertainties associated with estimating a chemical's R_fD, the EPA has adopted the use of the term "uncertainty factor" (Table 11-2) (Dourson et al., 1995).

Typically a 100-fold safety factor is applied to NOAELs from chronic studies to derive a chronically applicable ADI. Exceptions to the use of a 100-fold factor are made when data are available to reduce uncertainties regarding inter- or intraspecies extrapolation or when certain data are lacking or are inadequate in some way, in which case larger factors are used (Table 11-2.) A substance can be added to foods as long as the total daily intake from all sources does not exceed its ADI.

The ADI is not a sharp dividing line between "safe and" "unsafe" intakes. It is by no means certain that intakes at or below the ADI are "risk-free" or that intakes above it pose significant risks. The ADI provides no insight into the question of risk because the generic safety factors used, and even those that are in part based on chemical-specific data, provide no information on the fraction of the population whose thresholds are below or above the ADI. Risk might be expressed in terms of those fractions (on the theory that thresholds are distributed in some regular fashion among members of the population), and policy decisions could then be made to ensure that no more than the tiniest fraction would, in theory, be exposed at intakes exceeding their thresholds; this is similar conceptually to the approach taken for carcinogens. No standardized methodology is available to estimate risks for threshold agents in this fashion; indeed, toxicology data are typically reported in

TABLE 11-2   Typical Safety Factors Used to Derive ADIs from Animal Toxicity Data

Source of Uncertainty or Variability[a]	Factors Typically Applied
Extrapolation from animal NOAEL to estimate NOAEL for "average" human[b]	10
Variability within human population; "average" to "most susceptible"	10
Chronic NOAEL from subchronic NOAEL	10
Chronic LOAEL to chronic NOAEL	2–10
Limited data base (e.g., data available from a single species only)	2–10

Note: Data available on specific compounds may allow departures from these standard ("default") factors.
[a] NOAEL = no-observed-adverse-effect level; LOAEL = lowest-observed-adverse-effect-level.
[b] Most sensitive species.

insufficiently quantitative terms to permit risk assessors to move toward more quantitative evaluations of risk for these classes of agents.

Toxicity Testing for Additives

The types and numbers of toxicity tests specified by the FDA were first described in detail in a publication entitled *Toxicological Principles for the Safety Assessment of Direct Food Additives and Color Additives Used in Food*. This document is commonly known as the "Red Book" because of the color of its cover when it was originally published in 1982 (FDA, 1982a).

The Red Book sets forth practices that have evolved over the years based on knowledge of toxicological properties associated with certain types of chemical compounds. It reflects an awareness of the need for toxicological information commensurate with the potential of an additive to cause safety concerns. Thus the extent of toxicological testing required for a food additive or a color additive used in food is determined on a chemical-specific basis, and this relates to its chemical structure (insofar as chemical structure reflects toxicological potential) and the extent of expected human exposure. The Red Book also provides guidance regarding the criteria used for food and color additive safety evaluations.

The Red Book invokes the term "Level of Concern" to establish a cost-effective system for gathering necessary safety information. This approach is based on the premise that the level of scientific testing and research needed for a safety evaluation should be related to the likelihood that the substance poses a potential public health risk.

Table 11-3 presents the Levels of Concern for various anticipated exposure levels for direct additives classified according to their structural similarity to compounds of known biological activity. Compounds in category C represent additives whose toxicological potency is likely to be high. For example, organic halides, compounds with highly reactive heterocyclic ring systems such as epoxides, or a, α, β-unsaturated lactones are structure C compounds. At the other extreme, substances such as sample aliphatic and noncyclic hydrocarbons, saturated, noncyclic straight-chain alcohols and carboxylic acids, and normal human metabolites, are placed in structure category A. Based on anticipated human exposure level, it is possible to derive a level of concern for a particular additive once it is classified according to chemical structure.

TABLE 11-3 Levels of Concern for Direct Food Additives of Specified Chemical Structure Category at Different Concentrations in the Diet

Expected Toxicity Based on Structure	Anticipated Human Exposure (ppm in Diet)	Concern Level[a] I (Least)	II	III (Most)
A. Low	1.0			+
	0.05		+	
	<0.05	+		
B. Moderate	0.5			+
	0.25		+	
	<0.025	+		
C. High	0.25			+
	0.0125		+	
	<.0125	+		

Note: Adapted from the Red Book (FDA, 1982a). See proposed revisions in the 1993 Red Book (FDA, 1993).
[a] Extent of toxicity testing needed increases with increasing Concern level.

TABLE 11-4   Minimum Required Studies for Direct Food Additive of Level III (Highest Level of Concern)

Two-generation reproduction study with a teratology phase
Rodent chronic feeding study of at least one year
Carcinogenicity bioassay in two rodent species (in utero exposure in rat)
Nonrodent long-term feeding study
Short-term tests for carcinogenic potential

Note: From FDA (1982a). Revisions proposed in the 1993 Red Book include requirements for additional neurotoxicity and immunotoxicity studies, and even clinical investigations.

Once a level of concern is determined, it then becomes possible to identify the studies required to support safety. Table 11-4 lists the studies required for a direct food additive with the highest level of concern. The list of studies does not include acute or subacute toxicity tests, but it is hard to imagine appropriate design and conduct of the studies listed here without this information. The example is, of course, illustrative, and the FDA should be consulted at early stages of planning to identify the specific information needed for a particular additive. Moreover, the need for additional information may arise as the results of testing become known (FDA, 1982b, 1993).

Information from Clinical Studies in Humans

Under the Food, Drug and Cosmetic Act, substantial clinical data are necessary to gain approval for a human drug. No such requirement exists for food additives; the basis for introducing such materials into the human diet can be founded on the results of animal studies only. This may seem odd, in that human exposure to some additives will ordinarily be much more widespread than drug exposure, and moreover additives are not introduced with the expectation that they directly confer health benefits. Neither is there a general requirement for postapproval monitoring of health effects, as there is for some drugs. Some manufacturers conduct some form of clinical investigation for additives when human exposure is expected to be relatively high, but this is not a legal requirement.

Because of major advances in food science and technology, the past decade has witnessed an enormous surge of interest in additives, such as noncaloric fat substitutes, that may be added to food in very large amounts. It seems clear that evaluation of the safety of such "macroingredients" cannot be resolved entirely through the use of animal studies, and it is now recognized that clinical data are necessary to assess adequately human risks. A fuller discussion of the problem of macroingredients is presented below.

The FDA has recognized that preapproval testing does not uncover all potentially adverse effects associated with the use of an approved food additive and that postmarketing surveillance techniques sometimes may be necessary. The Adverse Reaction Monitoring System (ARMS) was established by the FDA's Center for Food Safety and Applied Nutrition to handle reports of adverse health effects associated with specific foods, food and color additives, and vitamin and mineral supplements (Tollefson, 1988). Such a system is now in effect for the fat substitute Olestra.

Carcinogens and the Use of Risk Assessment

A demonstration of carcinogenicity by "appropriate" tests (interpreted by the FDA to mean tests by the oral route) invokes the Delaney Amendment; no "safe" intake level (no ADI) can be legally assigned to a substance having this property (Merrill, 1979). The FDA apparently has little scientific discretion to discount any positive finding because of possible irrelevance to humans or because the carcinogenic effect is likely secondary to toxic phenomena for which a threshold of action might be applicable, although there are cases (selenium, melamine, BHA) in which the FDA has found reasons to discount such data.

In 1973 the FDA proposed the use of risk assessment coupled with the notion of insignificant risk to deal with a certain class of intentionally added substances. The Delaney Amendment, as we have noted, applies to intentionally introduced substances, but in 1968, Congress modified the law to deal with carcinogenic animal drugs that were used in food-producing animals. Such drugs, Congress allowed, could be used as long as "no residue" of the drug could be found in food (meat, milk, eggs) from treated animals. One supposes that in the Congressional mind, "no residue" was not different from "no addition," as applied to directly introduced additives, but Congress modified "no residue" by adding "by a method of analysis approved by the Secretary" (read FDA). The FDA was then charged with the decision of whether any given "method of analysis" was adequate to show the absence of residues (Rodricks, 1988).

The critical question facing the FDA, of course, was the detection limit such methods should possess. In scientific terms, "no residue" meant only that the carcinogenic drug was not present above the detection limit of the analytical method used. In fact it was likely to be present in food at some nonzero level once an animal was treated and could be present at any level up to the detection limit.

The FDA introduced risk assessment as a regulatory tool to deal with this class of agents in the following way (FDA, 1979a):

1. The risks (or upper bounds thereon) of the particular animal drug would be quantified based on rodent bioassay data and the application of a linear, no-threshold model of the dose–response curve.

2. The level of daily intake of drug residue corresponding to an (upper-bound) lifetime cancer risk of 10^{-6} would be estimated.

3. An estimate would be made of the concentration of the drug in food (meat, milk, or eggs) that would yield, when the food is consumed, the level of daily intake estimated in step 2.

4. The petitioner would be required to demonstrate that a reliable analytical method is available that has a detection limit at least as low as the concentration estimated in step 3.

5. The petitioner would be required to show that under the proposed conditions of drug use, "no residue" remains in food when the analytical method of step 4 is applied.

This "sensitivity of the method" approach, as the FDA has dubbed it, constituted the first regulatory use of quantitative risk assessment for carcinogens and the first time regulations defined safety explicitly in terms of risk. The FDA noted that if the 10^{-6} level of lifetime (70 year) risk were accurate, and if every member of the U.S. population were exposed to it, the annual number of extra cancer cases associated with it would be $(240 \times 10^{6}$ persons $\times 10^{-6}$ lifetime risk per person$) = 240$ affected persons per 70 years, or three to four extra cases per year.

The agency then went on to qualify this estimate as follows:

1. The risk estimate is most likely an upper bound because of the conservative biological and statistical assumptions underlying it.

2. It is extremely unlikely that all food from treated animals would always contain the residue of carcinogen at a concentration just at (or slightly below) the detection limit of the analytical method.

3. It is extremely unlikely that every member of the population will consume meat (or milk or eggs) only from animals treated with the drug, and that they would do so on every day of their lives.

For these and several other similar reasons, the FDA concluded that the actual number of extra cancer cases associated with the 10^{-6} lifetime risk criterion, applied in this way, was likely to be far fewer than three to four per year, but that the actual number could not be quantified. The risk, the FDA concluded, was an insignificant burden on the public health (FDA, 1979a).

The presence in food of carcinogenic animal drugs can be detected only by the application of an analytical method. In this respect they are different from directly added substances but similar to migrants from packaging and other food contact materials (typically monomeric forms of polymers). Migrants become "additives" only if they can be detected in food. How far should we search? What analytical method, with what detection limit, should be used? The FDA seems satisfied if the methods that are used are shown capable of detecting residues at concentrations sufficient to create daily intakes corresponding to lifetime risks no greater than 10^{-6}. In the absence of a finding that a carcinogen has migrated from food contact materials, using an analytical method of sufficient detection power, there is no need to apply the Delaney restriction because no "additive" is introduced (Rodricks and Taylor, 1989).

Logic would have it that if a lifetime risk level of 10^{-6} is of insignificant public health concern for indirectly introduced food additives, it ought to hold that directly introduced substances that are carcinogenic but pose similarly small risks would be of no concern. Indeed, FDA attempted to apply this logic to some color additives (some of which showed lifetime risks of the order of 10^{-8} or less), but its efforts were thwarted by the U.S. Court of Appeals on the ground that the Delaney Amendment does not exempt substances because they cause negligible health risks: It is clearly a zero-risk (no addition) law (Merrill, 1979, 1996). So, although risk assessment has utility in helping to define the required characteristics of analytical methods used to search for indirectly introduced substances, the "no-risk" requirement of Delaney holds for directly introduced food and color additives, the presence of which in food does not depend on a search with analytical methods. As we will see later, FDA has also used risk assessment as a tool in the regulation of certain carcinogenic food contaminants.

Human Exposure Assessment — The EDI

The evaluation of carcinogenic and noncarcinogenic risks for food constituents depends not only on toxicity criteria (ADIs or carcinogenicity potencies) but also on estimates of human exposures to those constituents. The typical term used in food constituent risk assessment is the estimated daily intake (EDI). Generally, for intentionally introduced food constituents that are not carcinogenic, FDA's safety criteria (risk management goals) are satisfied if the constituent's EDI is less than its ADI. Carcinogenic risks are estimated by multiplying potencies (upper bounds on estimated lifetime risks per unit of daily intake) by EDIs.

EDIs are estimated for directly introduced constituents by multiplying the concentration of the constituent in the food by the weight of that item of food consumed per day (Pao et al., 1982). High-end consumers, at the 90th or 95th percentile of food consumption rates, are the usual targets for the risk assessment; if such users are protected, then it can be concluded that the safety standards set forth in law are satisfied (FDA, 1988). Estimating intakes for indirect additives (e.g., substances migrating from food contact surfaces and packaging) is more complex because it depends on analytical data regarding the amount of migration into food and the chemical identities of migrants. The FDA's *Recommendations for Chemistry Data for Indirect Food Additive Petitions* (FDA, 1988) sets forth procedures to be followed to collect relevant data. Various food-simulating solvents are used and extraction studies performed to estimate food concentrations; these data are combined with information on expected food contact surface areas and the daily intake of food to obtain the EDIs. The vinyl chloride example, presented below, illustrates the evaluation procedure.

By no means does the above summary of regulatory approaches do justice to the FDA's implementation of the federal food laws. Many subtle and not so subtle points have been omitted. But it does set the stage for our discussion of various categories of food constituents and contaminants. As noted earlier, in addition to describing these categories, we also provide examples to illustrate the general principles and methods discussed in the preceding sections.

SUBSTANCES INTENTIONALLY ADDED TO FOOD

Under the law, the term "food additive" has a specific meaning (Federal Food, Drug and Cosmetic Act, 21 United States Code):

> Any substance the *intended* use of which results or may reasonably be expected to result, *directly* or *indirectly*, in its becoming a component of or otherwise affecting the characteristics of any food (including any substance intended for use in producing, manufacturing, packing, processing, preparing, treating, packaging, transporting, or holding food; and including any source of radiation intended for any such use) (emphasis added).

The statute goes on to exclude:

- Substances generally recognized as safe (GRAS)
- Pesticide chemicals in or on *raw* agricultural commodities
- Color additives
- New animal drugs

These four categories of excluded substances (and some others as well) are certainly "intentionally introduced additives" in the popular and even technical use of the term, but legally they are not "food additives." For our purposes, many of the legal distinctions among these groups of additives are not important: Safety must be demonstrated for all of these various groups of additives, although data requirements and criteria for acceptability vary among them (Merrill, 1996).

GRAS Substances

When the food additive amendments to the Federal Food, Drug and Cosmetic Act were enacted in 1958, certain food ingredients that had long been in use were exempted from the premarket testing and approval process required for food additives. Ingredients in use prior to January 1, 1958, could be considered GRAS based on a common use in food or through scientific evaluation procedures. Any food ingredient can be classified as GRAS if it is "generally recognized, among scientific experts qualified by scientific training and experience to evaluate its safety ... to be safe under the conditions of its intended use." These criteria are quite general and basically leave the decision about GRAS status to scientific experts. Current notions that decisions regarding the acceptability of various chemical exposures should involve the scientific evaluation of risk and policy-based risk management choices do not seem to apply in a well-defined way to GRAS substances.

After public review of its proposals, FDA published a GRAS list with the following commentary (Roberts, 1981): "It is impracticable to list all substances that are generally recognized as safe for their intended use. However, by way of illustration, the Commissioner regards such common food ingredients as salt, pepper, sugar, vinegar, baking powder, and monosodium glutamate as safe for their intended use"

The FDA's published GRAS list includes more than 600 substances, but this list by no means includes every substance that is or could be considered GRAS. Indeed, classification of substances as GRAS could be made by any group of qualified experts. The Flavor and Extract Manufacturers Association (FEMA), for example, convened such a group in 1960, and the group listed more than 1000 flavoring ingredients and their levels of addition to food that could be considered GRAS; FDA has generally considered the FEMA process and lists as meeting the criteria set forth in the Act (Oser and Hall, 1977).

A selected list of GRAS substances is presented in Table 11-5. The levels of addition of these substances to food are specified for some, but for most, usage levels are simply defined according to the amounts consistent with "good manufacturing practice." For those substances having specified limits, new uses that would result in increased exposures have to be justified based on "scientific procedures" recognized by experts. The FDA may also "affirm" the GRAS status of substances by regulation (Merrill, 1979).

A presidential directive was issued in 1969 requiring FDA to undertake a review of GRAS substances. Two major groups were engaged by FDA to compile and evaluate the relevant data. Information on usage rates and daily intakes was collected by the National Research Council. An expert committee (Select Committee on GRAS Substances, SCOGS) was assembled by the Federation of American Societies of Experimental Biology to evaluate the scientific literature pertaining to the safety of GRAS substances. Most reviewed substances were reaffirmed as GRAS by SCOGS, including some (6%) with a recommendation for additional research (including BHT, BHA, carrageenan, oil of nutmeg, glutamates, caffeine). Insufficient data were available to affirm or judge safety on

TABLE 11-5   Some GRAS Substances Listed by FDA

Spices and other natural flavors		
Anise	Geranium	Parsley
Basil	Ginger	Spearmint
Capsicum	Glycyrrhiza	Vanilla
Elder flowers	Licorice	

Multipurpose substances	
Acetic acid	Hydrogen peroxide
Aluminum sulfate	Lecithin
Caffeine	Methylcellulose
Calcium carbonate	Papain
Caramel	Propane
Carbon dioxide	Rennet

Affirmed as GRAS by FDA regulations (incomplete list)	
Benzoic acid	Potassium iodide
Clove	Propyl gallate
Ethyl alcohol	Sorbitol
Garlic	Dextrans (indirect additive)
Guar gum	Gum tragacanth

another 8%. For substances in the last category, FDA sought additional data from industry and, if it did not appear, rescinded the GRAS status of the listed substance (SCOGS, 1981).

Most chemicals directly added to food are GRAS. Scrutiny of the highly abbreviated list presented in Table 11-5 reveals the presence of agents of diverse toxicological characteristics. Most are present because they have had a long history of use in food with no significant reports of adverse health effects. (The FDA cannot remove a substance from GRAS status unless evidence appears showing that it can no longer be considered safe for its intended use.) The quantity and quality of available toxicology data vary greatly among these substances, and decisions about the adequacy of these data bases to judge risk and safety have been in the hands of experts, both within and outside of the FDA.

It is difficult to generalize about the criteria used to affirm or judge GRAS status, since expert judgment is such an important part of the process. A comprehensive review of the scientific bases of the GRAS reviews that have been undertaken by SCOGS, FEMA, FDA, and others, would be needed before generalizations could be developed regarding the specific risk and safety criteria employed; no such review has been conducted.

Direct and Indirect Food Additives

As noted, there are hundreds of direct and indirect food ingredients listed as GRAS. There are also more than 100 direct and indirect food additives regulated as "food additives" in the legal sense of the term; that is, they have been the subject of a petition submitted to the FDA since 1958, containing toxicity and human intake data adequate to meet the FDA's safety criteria for food additives (as discussed above). Some major use categories for direct and indirect additives, along with specific examples, are given in Table 11-6 (Hall, 1979).

Toxicity Evaluation of a Direct Food Additive: Aspartame   The FDA's ban on cylamate and its proposed ban on saccharin (overridden by a special act of Congress) were highly controversial actions, for the most part because the demand for nonnutritive sweeteners is very high among consumers. The value of such agents for diabetics is fairly clear, but whether they play a significant role in weight control is debatable. Whatever the actual benefits of such agents, they certainly fill some need in many individuals.

In 1981 the FDA approved certain food uses of 1-methyl-N-L-aspartyl-L-phenylalanine, the sweetener otherwise known as aspartame, and has since permitted additional uses. The compound is a simple monomethylester of a dipeptide; per unit weight it yields about the same number of calories as sucrose (so it is not a nonnutritive agent, like saccharin or cyclamate), but it is 150 to 200 times sweeter than sucrose (FDA, 1983).

In aqueous solution, especially at elevated temperatures or at low pH, aspartame releases methanol when it hydrolyzes to the dipeptide. Because the dipeptide is bitter to the taste, aspartame cannot be used in baked goods or in highly acidic products that require prolonged storage. The dipeptide may also cyclize to a diketopiperazine (FDA, 1983).

The toxicity of the degradation products, most especially the diketopiperazine but also the methanol, was of substantial concern in the FDA review process.

Beginning in the 1960s, the petitioner, G.D. Searle Co., sponsored or conducted extensive toxicological studies on aspartame. All of the types of studies called for in the Red Book for a major-use food additive were conducted, and many more as well. The diketopiperazine degradation product was also subjected to extensive study. Metabolism studies in several species, including humans, were conducted to understand, among other things, the blood levels of phenylanlanine and methanol resulting from single and repeated exposures (the former compound because of concern about infant phenylketonurics). Although there is little reason to suspect that aspartame is carcinogenic, the diketopiperazine degradation product might undergo mono- or dinitrososation in the GI

TABLE 11-6 Functional Effects with Selected Examples of Direct and Indirect Food Additives Regulated by FDA

Major Categories of Direct Additives	Example	Notes
	Primary direct additives	
Food preservatives	BHA, BHT	GRAS for some uses
	Nitrites, nitrates	Antimicrobial actions, color fixation in meat, poultry, smoked fish; up to 2% in various foods
		Amount not to exceed 2% by weight of food
Anticaking agents	Silicon dioxide	Alcoholic beverages, 25 ppm limit on HCN
Flavoring agents	Elder tree leaves	Citrus fruits
Coating agents, films	Coumarone-indene resin	Used in minimum quantity required to produce intended effect
Gums, chewing gum bases	Arabinogalactan	as an emulsifier, stabilizer, binder, or bodying agent
Special dietary, nutritional agents	Nicotinamide-ascorbic acid complex	Source of ascorbic acid and nicotinamide in multivitamin preparations
	Multipurpose agents	
Emulsifiers	Sodium laurel sulfate	Egg white solids, etc.
Dough conditions	Azodicarbonamide	Also used for aging, bleaching of flour
Dispersing agent	Polysorbate 60	Also used as emulsifier, dough conditioner
Stabilizing agents	Propylene glycol alginate	Emulsifier, baked goods, cheeses, etc.
Nonnutritive sweeteners	Aspartame	See text
Secondary direct additives: processing aids		*Examples of use*
Polymers, resins	Acrylate-acrylamide resins	Clarification of juices
Enzyme preparations	Catalase derived from micrococcus lysodeikticus	Cheese production
Microbial agents	*Candida lipolytica*	Foods resulting from fermentation
Solvents, related agents	1,3-Butylene glycol	Extraction of flavors from spices, etc.
	Indirect food additives	
Adhesives and components of coatings	Acrylate ester copolymer coating	Approved for food contact
Paper and paperboard components	Acrylamide-acrylic acid resins	Specifications for monomer
Polymers	*n*-Butyl methacrylate	Approved for food contact
Adjuvants, production aids, and sanitizers	Hydrogen peroxide	For sterilizing food-contact surfaces

Note: Title 21, Code of Federal Regulations, Parts 170–199.

390

tract, yielding carcinogenic N-nitrosamines (both mono- and dinitrosopiperazine are carcinogenic in rats). Excess nonmalignant, uterine polyps result from long-term feeding of diketopiperazine to rats. (Note that these last references to diketopiperazine concern that specific compound, not the diketopiperazine derivative associated with aspartame.)

Two-year feeding studies of aspartame in mice, rats, and dogs yielded no evidence of carcinogenicity. The possibility of transplacental carcinogenicity has also been investigated in rats; animals were exposed beginning in utero and throughout their lifetimes to aspartame doses of 2 or 4 g/kg. No significant tumor excesses were observed. Bladder implantation studies involving both aspartame and the diketopiperazine degradation product also produced no evidence of carcinogenicity. Chronic administration of an aspartame/diketopiperazine mixture to rats revealed no evidence of carcinogenicity (FDA, 1983).

The potential neurotoxicity of aspartic acid also came under special scrutiny. Hypothalamic lesions, similar to but less severe than those produced by monosodium glutamate, were observed in neonatal mice orally administered aspartame at doses of 1 or 2 g/kg. Infant macaques administered 2 g/kg aspartame by gavage showed no evidence of brain damage. Feeding of aspartame at doses of 100 or 200 mg/kg to normal adults, one-year-old infants, and individuals heterozygous for phenylketonuria revealed rapid metabolism and only small increases in blood level of aspartate. The rapid rise necessary to induce brain lesions was not observed. Methanol levels in human subjects receiving these doses were also evaluated (Stegink et al., 1979).

Although several sources indicate an ADI for aspartame as 50 mg/kg per day, the source of this number is difficult to establish. Instead of an ADI, the commissioner's final decision on aspartame refers to a toxic threshold of 100 μmol/dL for plasma phenylalanine or for glutamic acid plus aspartic acid (FDA, 1981). The Decision of the Public Board of Inquiry (FDA Docket 75F-0355) also focuses on a figure of 100μmol/dL as the limit for the plasma level in order to protect against impaired brain development. In pregnant women the maternal plasma phenylalanine concentration need rise no higher than 50 μmol/dL for the fetal plasma concentration to reach 100 μmol/dL. To achieve a blood concentration of 50 μmol/dL would require a loading dose of 200 mg/kg or a daily intake of about 12 g in an adult. Usage of aspartame by the 99th percentile consumer yields an EDI of only about one-fifth this level (FDA, 1983).

Food Contact Material as a Food Additive: Vinyl Chloride   In 1975 the FDA proposed to prohibit some uses of vinyl chloride polymers (homo- and copolymers), including their use in semirigid and rigid food-contact articles such as bottles and sheet. The FDA withdrew this proposal in 1986 and in its place proposed to amend its regulations to provide for the use of vinyl chloride polymers. This change of position resulted from (1) improved production technology that reduced the level of residual vinyl chloride monomer by a factor of nearly one million and (2) new agency policy, as described earlier, concerning the regulation of food and color additives that may contain carcinogenic impurities (FDA, 1986).

The FDA concluded that vinyl chloride polymer will become a component of food, and the extent to which this occurs depends, at least in part, on the amount of monomer in the polymer. The FDA decided to regulate the use of vinyl chloride polymers to ensure that the polymer that is marketed does not contain unsafe levels of the monomer. The agency proposed that the Delaney clause is not triggered unless the additive as a whole (polymer) is found to induce cancer. An additive that has not been shown to induce cancer but that contains a carcinogenic impurity (vinyl chloride) is properly evaluated under the general safety clause of the statute, using risk assessment procedures to determine whether there is a reasonable certainty that no harm will result from the proposed use of the additive. The FDA has evaluated the safety of this additive under the general safety clause, using risk assessment procedures to estimate the upper-bound limit of risk presented by the carcinogenic chemical present as an impurity in the additive (as a by-product of polymer synthesis).

The FDA conservatively estimated that the lifetime average individual exposure to vinyl chloride monomer from the probable food-contact uses of vinyl chloride polymers (e.g., liquor bottles, wine bottles, oil bottles, vinyl chloride homopolymer film, vinyl chloride-vinylidene chloride copolymers including films and fresh citrus fruit coatings, and miscellaneous uses) will not exceed 25 ng per day. The agency used a quantitative risk assessment procedure (linear proportional model) to extrapolate from the doses in the animal carcinogenicity study on vinyl chloride to the very low doses of possible human exposure. The FDA calculated that the individual lifetime risk of cancer from exposure to vinyl chloride monomer at 25 ng per day is less than one in 10 million. The agency concluded that there is a reasonable certainty of no harm from these exposures. The monomer, though carcinogenic, need not be treated as an additive subject to the Delaney clause (FDA, 1986).

Color Additives

Color additives have wide use in foods, drugs, cosmetics, other consumer products, and medical devices. Specific colors are listed or approved for food uses under the FDA's color additive regulations. Synthetic colors have to be certified by the FDA on a batch-by-batch basis to assure that each new batch of the color additive meets certain standards of purity representative of the material tested for safety. Colors exempt from certification mainly include those of natural origin, such as beet powder, grape skin extract, titanium dioxide, and various fruit and vegetable juices. Of particular concern among the certified colors are trace constituents, typically starting materials used in color synthesis that are carcinogenic — certain azo compounds and aromatic amines.

Although there are some legal distinctions that result in different scientific requirements, safety criteria for color additives to be added to food are generally similar to those applicable to food additives. The Delaney Amendment applies. An issue of some importance, similar to the vinyl chloride polymer matter, concerns the presence of trace amounts of known carcinogens in some colors that, when tested in cancer bioassays, do not themselves provoke a detectable carcinogenic response. The color additive, including its trace constituents, is thus not carcinogenic, but it is known from other data that the trace constituent(s) is carcinogenic. Such outcomes are not surprising, given the limited detection power of cancer tests and the typically low level of the contaminant in the color additive. The FDA's "constituents" policy allows the use of such colors as long as application of risk assessment to the trace constituent reveals that carcinogenic risks associated with it are negligible. Thus, for example, the FDA found that the excess risks from p-toluidine, a trace contaminant of D&C Green No. 6, a well-tested and noncarcinogenic color, did not exceed 10^{-8} and permitted use of the color to continue (FDA, 1982b).

A particularly interesting example of the scientific dilemma created when emerging science encounters inflexible regulation (the Delaney Amendment) is presented by the recent events concerning the color additive, FD&C Red No. 3. This color is carcinogenic, producing excess thyroid tumors in rats. A substantial scientific basis exists for supposing that the increased incidence of rats with thyroid tumors resulting from chronic administration of FD&C Red No. 3 results from excessive stimulation of thyroid cells by thyroid-stimulating hormone (TSH), a hormone released from the hypothalamus–pituitary axis. It appears that the normal feedback mechanism by which TSH release is controlled, the elevation of blood levels of the hormone T_3 secreted from the TSH-stimulated thyroid, is interfered with by FD&C Red No. 3, perhaps because its structure mimics that of T_4 and allows it to compete for enzyme sites necessary to convert T_4 to T_3 Blockage of the $T_4 \rightarrow T_3$ pathway results in decreased control over TSH release, which in turn places thyroid cells at increased risk of neoplastic transformation. This phenomenon has been recognized for other agents that reduce controls on TSH release, such as the herbicide amitrole, several enthylene thiourea derivatives, and bridged-ring aromatic amines (Paynter et al., 1988; Hill et al., 1989). The important consequence of this hormonally mediated mechanism is the strong likelihood that no carcinogenic risk would exist unless levels of the color sufficient to interfere significantly with $T_4 \rightarrow T_3$ conversion were reached; this indirect mechanism of carcinogenesis seems to require a threshold dose to be exceeded. Although manufacturers of the color conducted studies that appeared to support this hypothesis, the crucial experiment of modulating the endpoint, follicular cell neoplasia, in a long-term bioassay was not undertaken.

The regulatory situation became complex because this color additive had been permanently listed for many years for use in food. The provisional uses were for cosmetics and externally applied drugs. Termination of the provisional listing and denial of a petition for these uses (FDA, 1990) are tantamount to banning the color additive for all uses, but this must be accomplished separately. Although the Delaney Amendment may have been invoked to support these actions, it is not clear what would have occurred had the secondary mechanism been established.

Animal Drug Residues

The issue of carcinogenic animal drugs, as we have already seen, gave rise to the incorporation of the risk assessment concept and the notion of negligible, or insignificant, risk into the FDA's regulatory process. Noncarcinogenic drugs are evaluated, like food and color additives, under the ADI approach; human intakes of drug residues in meat, milk, and eggs must be shown not to exceed the ADI for all uses of the drug combined.

A particularly difficult issue that arises in connection with the administration of drugs to food-producing animals concerns the fact that drug metabolism or degradation may lead to residues in edible food products of compounds other than the parent drug. A question arises whether toxicity studies on the parent drug alone are sufficient to characterize the toxicity of the total food residue. Although there are uncertainties, it may be argued that if the same profile of metabolites and degradation products is produced in the animal species used in the toxicity testing, then the resulting test data are reasonably representative of the toxicity of the total drug residue; indeed, this approach has been taken for some drugs. Alternatively, separate toxicity testing of metabolites or degradation products can be contemplated, but this may become impractical when many products are involved.

The issue of so-called bound residues has also caused difficulties. Not infrequently some drug metabolites covalently bind to tissues in treated animals and might be released when those tissues are consumed by people. How is the potential toxicity of such "bound residues" (which many times are found actually to represent incorporation of drug moieties into natural macromolecules) to be measured? Both this problem and the broader problem of "total residue" are still subjects of considerable debate, and completely satisfactory solutions have not been found (FDA, 1979a; Guest and Fitzpatrick, 1990).

Macroingredients: The New Class of Food Additives

Over the past decade intense interest in a variety of nontraditional additives has arisen. Among these are noncaloric substances designed to replace normal fats, novel sources and types of fiber, and other products designed to confer health benefits (so-called nutriceuticals). Advances in chemical technology, including the use of the tools of

TABLE 11-7   Comparison of "Traditional" and "New-Generation" Food Additives

Characteristics of many "traditional" food additives

1. No natural occurrence in diet
2. Low molecular weight; typically metabolized as foreign compound
3. Information on significant adverse effects obtainable only through animal studies
4. Little potential for identifying the "most relevant" animal model
5. Little potential for obtaining significant data concerning biological behavior in humans
6. Little potential to determine whether there are significant subpopulations of humans at especially high risk
7. Many likely to produce at least moderately serious toxicity at high doses
8. Useful animal testing possible without the confounding effects of dietary imbalances
9. Human intakes very low
10. Trace constituents unlikely to present risk

Characteristics of many "new-generation"food additives

1. Occur naturally in diet or closely related to compounds that do
2. Human intakes high
3. Metabolized to normal body constituents
4. Very low potential for toxicity
5. Traditional animal testing not possible without confounding effects of dietary imbalances
6. Substantial data can be obtained on humans (ADME, tolerance, allergic potential, effect on nutritional status)
7. Intakes of trace contaminants may not be negligible, especially problematic when ingredient derived from a novel source

modern biotechnology, have made practical the industrial synthesis of substances that may occur naturally in food only at very low levels. If such substances confer some benefits to consumers, then there exists the impetus and the wherewithal to add them to foods in greatly increased amounts. The term "macroingredients" has come into use to describe substances intended for addition to food at or near levels formerly associated only with macronutrients (fats, carbohydrates, proteins). In Table 11-7 are compared some of the characteristics of "traditional" and "new-generation" food additives.

The traditional methods for understanding the toxicity, intakes, and risks of food additives would appear to offer limited opportunities to understand these aspects of the "new-generation" additives. The traditional model of ensuring at least a 100-fold safety factor for chronic toxicity, which involves conducting toxicity studies at doses at least 100 times the human EDI, would not serve well, for example, to evaluate macroingredients intended for use at dietary levels of 0.1 % to 1%. Exaggerating doses to test animals to 100 times these levels makes animal diets completely unsuitable for understanding the toxicity of the additive, because of the substantial confounding effects on the animals of dietary imbalances created by administering such diets (the practical limit of dietary concentration for a test substance in animal experiments is usually put at 5%). Thus, while some information of value may be gleaned from animal studies, they may be most useful for guiding clinical investigations. The latter seem necessary to gauge the potential effects of macroingredients in regard to possible consequences not expected of most "traditional" additives: allergenicity, gastrointestinal tolerance, alterations of intestinal microflora, modification of nutritional status (Munro, 1990; FDA, 1993). The FDA has awarded a contract to the Federation of American Societies for Experimental Biology to evaluate the new and difficult problem of judging the health risks and safety of macroingredients.

FOOD CONTAMINANTS OF INDUSTRIAL ORIGIN

Classes and Sources

Two broad classes of food contaminants have been identified. The first are certain metals and some of their organic derivatives. It is misleading, however, to place all occurrences of metals and organometallics in the class of contaminants, in that a certain level of most of these substances can be found in food because of natural occurrence. Moreover, since background levels of substances such as lead, arsenic, mercury, and cadmium vary widely in soils and water from different geographic regions, it is not surprising that background levels in the diet depend heavily on the geographic sources of the various components of the diet. See Chapters 6, 14, and 16 for discussions of three important heavy metals, chromium, lead, and mercury and Chapter 16 for more abbreviated discussions of aluminum, arsenic, cadmium, and nickel.

Dietary levels of these same metals can, of course, be affected by industrial contamination. The nature and extent of this contamination depend on regional sources of the metals. A major element of the EPA's characterization of risks arising from Superfund and other hazardous waste sites concerns the migration of metals from such sites through air, soils, groundwater, and surface water into crops and livestock, with subsequent accumulation in food (Goyer, 1986; EPA, 1988).

Some organic chemicals of strictly industrial origin have been found on a fairly regular basis in foods. Of particular concern are various chlorinated hydrocarbons that exhibit moderate to high environmental stability and that bioaccumulate in fatty tissue. Table 11-8 contains a list of industrial compounds that have been of most concern as food contaminants.

Limiting Contaminant Exposure: PCBs in Fish

Food contaminants of the sort listed in Table 11-8 are unavoidable in the sense discussed in the earlier section on Legal and Regulatory Framework. Decisions about limits on exposures to these materials are somewhat different in character from those we have

TABLE 11-8   Some Food Contaminants of Industrial Origin

Chemical	Major Sources	Foods Subject to Contamination
Arsenic	Smelting, mining	Many, including fish[a]
Cadmium	Smelting, sewage sludge	Grains, vegetables, meat
Lead	Smelting, mining, solder in can seams, lead-glazed pottery and ceramic ware, automobile exhaust	Several, including acidic foods coming into contact with lead ceramic ware and pottery
Mercury, alkyl mercurials	Chlorine, soda lye manufacturing	Fish
Aldrin, dieldrin, DDT, mirex	Pesticide usage[b]	Fish, milk, eggs
Polychlorinated biphenyls	Electrical industry	Fish, human milk
Polychlorinated benzodioxins	Impurities in certain chemicals; incineration; bleached paper manufacturing	Fish, milk, beef fat

Source: From Munro and Charbonneau (1981). Note: The metals listed are also present in foods because of natural occurrence.

[a] Most of the arsenic in food appears to be organically bound. These forms are substantially less toxic than inorganic arsenic. EPA considers the latter form to be carcinogenic by ingestion.

[b] Pesticide residues in foods for which no official tolerance was ever granted, or was rescinded, are considered contaminants.

described for the various classes of intentional additives. In some instances imposition of an ADI or negligible cancer risk standard, derived using conventional methods, would require banning of certain foods altogether or very severe restrictions on the fraction of the available supply that could be marketed. Using the carcinogenic potency derived by the EPA for PCBs, for example, and a 10^{-6} upper limit on lifetime risk as the health protection standard would require maximum fish residue levels of approximately 1 to 5 ppb (the limit depends heavily on data and assumptions concerning fish consumption rates). At the present time PCB residues in commercial fish in several areas of the United States contain PCBs in the range of 1 to 5 ppm (FDA, 1979b; Maxim, 1989). Clearly, imposition of a 5 ppb limit would mean the end of much commercial fishing until environmental levels of PCBs declined to sufficiently low levels. The regulatory approach at the FDA has been to specify limits on PCBs in fish (commercial products moving in interstate commerce) at 2 ppm in edible portions. This tolerance level was chosen both to minimize health risk and to avoid an intolerable level of economic disruption in the affected industry. The risk level found tolerable by the FDA exceeded by more than 100 times the 10^{-6} lifetime risk level used as a guide in the various "insignificant risk" decisions discussed earlier (FDA, 1979b).

The PCBs represent a particularly difficult problem for the risk assessor. Most pertinent toxicology data have been collected on the commercial products: Aroclors in the United States, Clophens in West Germany, and Kaneclors in Japan. The difficulty for the risk assessor increases when it is realized that PCB mixtures are modified as they move through the environment. The mixtures of chlorinated biphenyl found in fish, for example, vary widely in composition according to source of PCB, length of time the chemicals have been in the environment, and the species and age of the fish that has accumulated the compounds. And none of these matches in composition the commercial products for which cancer bioassay are available. The risk assessor can do no better than to use dose–response data from the commercial product that most closely matches in composition the mixture found in fish. Of increasing interest is the potential for certain PCBs to display estrogenic-like properties, and to affect reproductive functions in animals. Certain isomers of PCBs bear structural similarities to certain chlorinated dibenzodioxins, and they may act through common, and apparently receptor-mediated, mechanisms. The EPA has suggested, in its current and continuing review of chlorinated dioxins, that normal human background levels of the combination of structurally related, chlorinated biphenyls, dibenzo-p-dioxins, and dibenzofurans, are within an order of magnitude of the level at which they may cause adverse effects on endocrine systems (EPA, 1997). Fatty foods are thought to constitute the major media through which human exposures are created. This issue remains one of intense debate (see Chapter 8).

In response to the EPA's suggestion that intake of fatty foods constitutes the major pathway by which humans become exposed to chlorinated dioxins and related compounds, the U.S. Department of Agriculture recently undertook a survey of beef; the Department has reported that no chlorinated dioxins or related compounds could be found. The Department did report detectable chlorinated dioxin levels in a small fraction of the poultry sampled, but only in birds from specific sources, and not on a countrywide basis. In this instance a "traceback" was conducted, and surprisingly, certain clays used as binders in the poultry feed were found to be the source of dioxins (Food Chemical News, 1997). Investigations of this unsuspected source are now underway, with the possibility that the dioxins may be of natural origin. It remains somewhat curious that some of the major postulated pathways of dioxin transfer to humans, beef and poultry (except for the isolated, clay-related samples), seem not to contain detectable levels. Inadequate sampling may offer one explanation; that the EPA's assessment is incorrect may be another.

TABLE 11-9   Toxic Food Constituents and Contaminants of Natural Origin

Categories	Sources	Examples
Intrinsic food components	Natural constituents of plants and animals	Natural pesticides in plants, puffer fish (fugu) toxin
Soil and water constituents	Natural mineral sources	Nitrate; metals such as mercury, arsenic
Microbial metabolites	Toxins from bacteria and fungi growing on food	Aflatoxin B_1, botulinum toxins
Contaminants of natural origin	Toxins accumulating in marine organisms and forage plants	Ciguatera, paralytic shellfish poison
Products of storage or preparation	Toxins arising in aged foods or in food preparation	Oxidized fats, polycyclic aromatic hydrocarbons

Source: From Rodricks and Pohland (1981).

CONSTITUENTS AND CONTAMINANTS OF NATURAL ORIGIN

Categories of Natural Constituents and Contaminants

It is convenient to group food constituents and contaminants of natural origin into five broad categories as shown in Table 11-9 (Rodricks and Pohland, 1981). These categories include the substances that are natural components of the food itself or that have become incorporated from the plant's environment or from the animal's food supply. Other substances become a part of the food after the food is collected and stored or during preparation.

Investigations into the possible risks to health of the enormous number of chemical compounds in these groups are limited to a relatively few members of each, particularly of the first. A brief survey of some selected examples of each group reveals that the range of health risks associated with these natural substances is wide and as potentially serious as that associated with additives and industrial contaminants.

Intrinsic Components of Foods: Oxalate   In this category are organic compounds that are natural constituents of the plants and animals we have chosen for our diets. Nutrients are included, but most of the many thousands of compounds in this group have no known nutritive value. Relatively few members of the group have been toxicologically investigated, although it seems clear that because of the enormous chemical diversity exhibited by these compounds, thorough toxicological study would reveal that they would display the full spectrum of toxic effects observed with synthetic chemicals. Some of those that have been studied are listed in Table 11-10 (Committee on Food Protection, 1973; Rodricks and Pohland, 1981; Ames, 1983a, b). A fuller discussion of one of these, oxalate, is presented below to illustrate both typical and unique problems associated with this huge and largely unstudied class.

Oxalic acid (HOOC – COOH) is the simplest of the dicarboxylic acids. Salts of oxalic acid are found in most plant and animal species, but certain common plants such as spinach, rhubarb, beet leaves, red beets, tea, cocoa, and cereal grains have especially high concentrations. Both soluble and insoluble oxalates occur in plants and animals, but free oxalic acid generally is not present in plants. Early interest in the toxicity of dietary oxalates centered about reported poisoning in humans and animals ingesting high-oxalate-containing plants. The occurrence in kidney stones of calcium oxalate also raised concern about the role of dietary oxalate in their formation (Committee on Food Protection, 1973).

TABLE 11-10   Some Intrinsic Components of Food of Known Toxicity

Compounds	Food Sources	Suspected or Known Toxic Endpoints
Salts of oxalic acid	See text	See text
Solanine, chaconine	White potato [a]	Nervous system
HCN	Many plants, as adducts, released when plant tissue is damaged	Hemoglobin, cyanosis
Vasoactive amines	Pineapple, banana, plum	Cardiovascular system
Xanthines (caffeine, theophylline, theobromine)	Coffee [b], tea, cocoa, kola nut	CNS stimulation, other biochemical changes, cardiac effects
Myristicin	Nutmeg, mace	Nervous system
Carotatoxin	Carrots, celery	Nervous system
Lathyrus toxins	Legumes of genus *Lathyrus*	Lathyrism (neurological disease)
Tannins	Tea, coffee, cocoa	Carcinogenic
Safrole and other methylenedioxy benzenes	Oil of sassafras, cinnamon, nutmeg anise, parsley, celery, black pepper	Carcinogenic (not all members of the class)
5- and 8-Methoxypsoralen (light activated)	Parsley, parsnip, celery	Carcinogenic, with UV light
Ethyl acrylate	Pineapple	Carcinogenic in animals
Estragole	Basil, fennel	Carcinogenic in animals

[a] Solanaceous glycoalkaloids are present in other solanaceae, including eggplant and tomato.

[b] Coffee contains more than 600 compounds in addition to caffeine. This is typical of natural foods. Included are many different classes of organic compounds.

By applying commonly used safety factors, ADIs for oxalates can be calculated based on three animal studies. These studies are listed in Table 11-11. For chronic, reproductive, and developmental toxicity studies, a 100-fold safety factor is usually applied. This safety factor can be further modified to reflect the seriousness of the effect, the duration of the study (e.g., subchronic rather than chronic data), and the quality of the data (e.g., small number of animals) (Kokoski and Flamm, 1984). Examples of possible safety and modifying factors are also shown in Table 11-11, along with the resulting ADIs.

The ADIs shown in Table 11-11 range from 0.2 to 3 mg/kg per day compared to an average oxalate consumption of 3.2 mg/kg per day from oxalate-containing food[2]. More specifically, the average U.S. intake of naturally occurring dietary oxalate is 4 to 17 times higher than the ADI for developmental effects and 1.6 times higher than the ADI for

TABLE 11-11   Animal Studies for Oxalate Suitable for Establishing an ADI

Study Type (species)	NOEL (LOEL) (mg/kg per day)	Safety Factor	Modifying Factor [a]	ADI (mg/kg per day)	Reference
Chronic (2-y) rat	600	100	2	3	Fitzhugh and Nelson (1947)
Reproduction (rat)	1975	100	10	2	Goldman et al. (1977)
Developmental toxicity	175	100	2–10	0.2–0.9	Sheikh-Omar and Schiefer (1980)

[a] Introduced to compensate for data limitations and severity of toxicity

[2] ENVIRON 1990, unpublished calculations of average daily oxalate consumption.

reproductive effects. Thus the background levels of oxalate exceed the acceptable daily intake levels that are suggested from the animal toxicity data available on this substance.

It is not unusual for intakes of naturally occurring components of food, such as oxalate, to exceed the ADI that could be derived for them using methods applicable to food additives. Such outcomes can be interpreted in at least two ways. Under one interpretation, oxalate and other such intrinsic food components actually create a risk of chronic toxicity. Although there are no data to suggest that this is the case for oxalate, this possibility appears not to have been thoroughly examined, either clinically or epidemiologically. Some evidence suggests, however, that oxalate is only poorly bioavailable, although it is not clear that it is greatly less bioavailable in people than it is in the animal species from which the toxicity data were derived.

A second interpretation is that the methods for deriving ADIs are excessively conservative and lead to acceptable intakes that are lower than they need to be. There seems to be no way to determine definitively which of these interpretations is correct; indeed, perhaps both are to a degree. But consideration of the toxicity data on many intrinsic components of food creates dilemmas not unlike that exhibited in the case of oxalate. (Committee on Food Protection, 1973; Rodricks and Pohland, 1981).

Naturally Occurring Pesticides   Substances with pesticidal properties that are found in plants are a particularly interesting subgroup of the toxic intrinsic constituents of food. For about a decade now, several biologists, most especially Bruce Ames, have been acquiring, organizing, and evaluating information on food plant metabolites displaying pesticidal activity. Ames and colleagues estimate daily intake of natural pesticides to be about 1.5 g, which they note is about 10,000 times the level of daily intake of human-made pesticides (Ames 1983a, b; Ames and Gold 1989). Thousands and probably tens of thousands of compounds having insecticidal and fungicidal activity and other types of toxicity toward predators are present in plants we use as food, frequently at concentrations in the parts-per-million to parts-per-thousand range. Moreover plant stress resulting from predator attack often induces biosynthesis of greater than normal concentrations. Most of these substances have not been evaluated toxicologically. Some of those that have been evaluated display the same range of toxic properties associated with synthetic chemicals. Ames and Gold (1989) list natural carcinogenic pesticides present in anise, apples, bananas, basil, broccoli, and about 40 other plant foods, herbs, and spices.

For reasons already stated, none of these findings has yet had a significant impact on regulation, either direct or indirect. Certainly there has been no attempt to regulate any of these natural carcinogens, and, until recently (see below), little effort has been devoted to evaluating the risks they may pose. Although regulation in any traditional sense would seem improbable, it may be possible to control the levels of these natural toxicants by breeding them out of plants. There seems to be little sign of interest in such an activity. Contrariwise, there are at least two instances in which plant breeders have inadvertently increased the level of natural toxicants—psoralens in celery and solanine in white potatoes—to levels sufficient to cause acute toxicity (rashes in the former case and cholinesterase inhibition in the latter). The dangerous variety of celery actually made it to market and had to be withdrawn; the problem in the new variety of white potato was discovered before marketing occurred (Ames and Gold, 1989). Surely one of the major concerns of regulators and public health officials with newer "bioengineered" foods is the potential for inadvertent introduction of dangerous levels of natural toxicants (many of which now are present at levels uncomfortably near the minimum toxic level).

Although the work of Ames and his associates, and others as well, has not yet had a major impact on the way health risks associated with environmental chemicals are viewed, the issue cannot forever be ignored. On the one hand, it may point to a significant role for natural food toxicants in chronic human diseases, including cancer. At the other extreme, it may suggest that our concerns over synthetic chemicals are wrongheaded, since it is clear that our risk assessment methodologies are inappropriate and greatly overstate low-dose risks (on the assumption that even the natural toxicants are not a significant health risk). It will require considerable research to untangle this issue, involving close collaboration between toxicologists and epidemiologists.

To confuse matters further, it is clear, as Ames himself has pointed out, that there are many naturally occurring dietary constituents that, probably by several mechanisms, protect against or reduce the risk of cancer. These dietary "anticarcinogens" are probably as prevalent as the carcinogens (Davis, 1989). In any event, risk evaluation requires consideration of both sets of naturally occurring food constituents.

A committee of the National Research Council recently reviewed the state of knowledge regarding dietary carcinogens and anticarcinogens (NRC, 1996). The committee concluded that, though our understanding is relatively poor, current evidence suggests that carcinogens naturally present in food far exceed those present because of human actions. Understanding the risks associated with such agents, and the benefits associated with naturally occurring anticarcinogens, is a formidable task; the committee nevertheless stressed the need to acquire that understanding, and set forth a program toward that end. Although the evidence for a significant role for natural dietary constituents in other chronic diseases was not reviewed, it seems likely that carcinogenesis is not the only disease process in which these substances play a significant role.

Accumulation of Chemicals from Water and Soils: Nitrate   The major members of this group are the metals and other elements that were discussed earlier in the section on industrial contaminants. A large number of metals and other elements beyond those discussed earlier are also naturally present in foods. Some are essential nutrients (copper, chromium, calcium, magnesium, iron, zinc), but many more that are present have no established nutritional value. Like lead, cadmium, arsenic, and mercury, some of these substances can, in limited geographic areas, accumulate to excessive levels because of industrial pollution, but for most of these, natural occurrence appears to be the dominant source (Munro and Charbonneau, 1981). The health risks from nitrates pose an interesting case, not only because the natural occurrence of nitrate is by far the greatest source but because nitrate itself is not the material of toxicological interest. Rather, derivatives of nitrate—nitrite and N-nitroso compounds—are formed as a result of chemical reactions and are responsible for harmful effects.

Several kinds of food plants accumulate naturally occurring nitrates from water and soil. The location of the plant and its variety, state of health, and moisture content determine how much nitrate a plant accumulates. The water and soil in the environment are the source of nitrate, and they in turn accumulate nitrate from nitrogen-based fertilizers as well as from nitrogenous wastes from humans and livestock. Certain food vegetables such as spinach, beets, cauliflower, lettuce, celery, radishes, kale, and mustard often contain high concentrations of nitrates (Committee on Food Protection, 1973).

Poisonings of human infants have been reported from high nitrate levels in well water used to prepare infant formulas, mostly in rural areas, and from high concentrations of nitrate in baby foods. The total daily intake of nitrate from all sources has been estimated as 75 mg/person, but in areas of high nitrate in water this can be doubled. Although these sound like large amounts, the real concern is with the conversion products of nitrates.

Nitrates are converted into nitrites by microorganisms in the mouth and gut through reactions with ammonia and other organic nitrogen-containing compounds. Nitrites in turn react with hemoglobin, the iron-containing respiratory protein in red blood cells, and convert it to methemoglobin. Methemoglobin is unable to combine with oxygen. Thus the blood of persons with too much methemoglobin, a condition known as methemoglobinemia, has a reduced oxygen-carrying capacity as well as a decreased capacity of residual oxyhemoglobin to dissociate and release oxygen to the tissues where it is needed. Infants are at a special risk from methemoglobinemia because their hemoglobin occurs in a form that is more easily oxidized. Furthermore, they are developmentally deficient in methemoglobin reductase, and the lower gastric acidity of infants permits nitrate-reducing microorganisms to thrive. Most episodes of methemoglobinemia in infants have been the result of high concentrations in well water (Menzer and Nelson, 1986).

Long-term carcinogenic effects of compounds formed from nitrate with other nitrogen-containing compounds are also of great concern. The reaction of nitrite with secondary amines to form nitrosamines in foods has been modeled in animal studies that show that feeding nitrate together with certain amines, for example, produces tumors in rats or mice. The nitrosamines are among the most potent animal carcinogens; single doses of certain nitrosamines are sufficient to cause cancer in experimental animals. The nitrosamines are discussed further in a later section of this chapter.

Microbial Metabolites: Aflatoxins   Mycotoxicoses—poisonings resulting from ingestion through foods and feeds of toxic fungal metabolites—have been and continue to be widely reported in the veterinary and medical literature. The best-known case is that of ergotism, which has been reported throughout the world periodically since the Middle Ages. Less widespread but equally serious human mycotoxicoses that have been associated with consumption of moldy foods include alimentary toxic aleukia, a hemorrhagic disease that occurred in the Soviet Union several times in the first half of this century; the related hemorrhagic disease, stachybotryotoxicosis; and yellow-rice disease, a neurotoxic disease reported from Japan. Veterinary outbreaks have been more numerous than human outbreaks because animals are more likely to receive moldy feeds. Fungi are enormously productive manufacturers of organic chemicals of immense and bewilderingly complex structural variety, and it is not surprising that many can produce serious forms of toxicity. Examples of some mycotoxins of potential concern as contaminants of food and feed are shown in Table 11-12 (Hayes and Campbell, 1986).

The discovery of the now well-known group of mycotoxins called aflatoxins (metabolites of *Aspergillus flavus* and *A. parasiticus*) in the early 1960s focused attention on several concerns that previously had not been considered. Notably scientists discovered that these mycotoxins could be found in foods not obviously moldy, indeed in foods showing no living mold on microscopic examination. Although partial destruction and elimination occur, the toxins can survive food-processing conditions that eliminate mold growth. The aflatoxins are detected in foods by chemical, not microbiological, analysis (Stoloff, 1977).

Aflatoxins are potent hepatic toxicants, but production of frank liver toxicity in either livestock or people is usually associated with the relatively high levels associated with heavily molded foods. The discovery during the 1963 to 1975 period that aflatoxins could

TABLE 11-12   Some Mycotoxins of Potential Concern as Food and Feed Contaminants

Mycotoxin	Health Concern	Source
Aflatoxins [a]	Carcinogenicity	Peanuts, corn, milk
Ergot alkaloids	Neurotoxicity	Grains
Ochratoxins	Nephrotoxicity	Grains
Trichlothecenes	GI, blood, and neurotoxicity	Grains
Zearalenone	Interference with reproduction	Grains, corn

Source: From Hayes and Campbell (1986).
[a] See text for discussion.

induce liver and other types of malignancies in rats, mice, monkeys, ferrets, guinea pigs, trout, and possibly humans provided the first suggestion that fungal toxins might present health risks on more than an intermittent basis—the aflatoxins turn out to be present in certain foods, albeit at very low levels, on a fairly regular basis (Stoloff, 1977).

In the Fisher strain of male rat, aflatoxin B_1 is a very potent carcinogen, exceeded only by 2,3,7,8-tetrachlorodibenzo-p-dioxin. Unlike dioxin, aflatoxin also displays genotoxicity. Application of a linear extrapolation model to the male rat data yields a low-dose potency of 2.5×10^3 per mg / kg per day (lifetime average daily dose). Potency does, however, vary greatly among species (Rodricks and Park, 1983). Based on epidemiological investigations reported recently from Southern Guangxi, China, Bechtel and Wilcock (1990) estimated the potency in humans to be 16.90 to 20 per mg / kg per day, significantly less than that observed for the male rat. These investigators were also able to estimate quantitatively the influence on hepatic cancer risk of hepatitis B infection and found it to have a potentiating effect on aflatoxin of about 33-fold. The studies from China and other locales point convincingly to a significant role for hepatitis B infection in aflatoxin-induced liver cancer in humans (Bechtel and Wilcock, 1990).

Given the relatively low level of aflatoxin intake in the United States, and the low rate of occurrence of hepatitis B infection, the compound is probably not a major contributor to liver cancer rates (Park and Stoloff, 1989). In some years, however, especially in corn grown in the southern states, aflatoxin levels increase dramatically, and contamination becomes widespread. This phenomenon is dependent on weather conditions and is, fortunately, intermittent. Livestock appear to experience the greatest threat, but some above-average increase in human health risk probably results as well. In areas of the world where aflatoxin contamination of food and human intake is substantial, and where hepatitis B virus infection rates are high, the contribution of these mycotoxins to human liver cancer is probably far from negligible (Van Rensburg et al., 1985).

Regulatory and manufacturing controls in the United States have greatly reduced aflatoxin intake over the past 25 years, but no way has been found to eliminate the problem.

Compounds Contaminating Edible Animal Products: Some Naturally Occurring Marine Toxicants   Fish and shellfish can accumulate some highly toxic substances from the natural marine environment. Paralytic shellfish poisoning, ciguatera intoxication, tetrodotoxin poisoning, and scombroid poisoning have been known for many years and continue to be significant problems in many areas of this world. Less well recognized than the marine toxins are those toxins that can be found in the edible tissues of animals grazing on plants containing them.

The oceans would be an inexhaustible source of human food but for the fact that thousands of species of marine organisms are too poisonous to consume. Only a small fraction of the compounds responsible for the toxicity of fish, molluscs, and other forms of ocean life have been identified, yet it is apparent that toxicants of marine origin display some of the most chemically and biologically complex properties of all known toxic chemicals. Many of these toxicants are endogenous constituents of seafood, but some of the important ones are actually metabolic products of marine organisms that are used as food by fish and shellfish. Ingestion of the organisms results in accumulation of their toxic metabolites in edible tissues, rendering them potentially hazardous. The paralytic shellfish toxins (PSTs) are the toxic contaminants of seafood of this group that have received the greatest public health attention and the greatest scientific investigation (Hayes and Campbell, 1986).

The PSTs are metabolites of several varieties of plankton or dinoflagellates. The principal organisms producing these toxins are *Gonyaulax catenella*, *G. tamarensis*, *G. acatenella*, and several species of *Gymnodinium*. Under certain conditions these organisms undergo rapid growth and color the ocean where this is occurring in various shades of red or yellow, creating the so-called red tide. The concentrations of PSTs in shellfish growing under these conditions may rise to levels that are seriously hazardous for those who might consume the shellfish. Many species of mussels, clams, cockles, oysters, and scallops are susceptible in dozens of regions of the earth (Halsted, 1978).

The PSTs are low-molecular-weight compounds (around 300) having extraordinarily potent neurotoxic properties. Seven such toxins have been identified and are simple chemical derivatives of saxitoxin, the principal member of the group. Saxitoxin is a tricyclic compound with a molecular weight of 283 containing two guanide functional groups. The estimated human LD_{50} for saxitoxin is 10 to 20 µg / kg. Although this value is not as low as some protein or polypeptide toxins, such as botulinum or cobra venom toxins, few compounds with molecular weights this low display such an extreme lethality. Unlike so many of the protein or polypeptide neurotoxicants, PSTs are chemically stable to a wide variety of conditions (Concon, 1988).

Respiration may be turned off almost immediately following ingestion of PSTs, depending on the dose received, or may be only partially depressed. Victims who recover from the initial CNS effects within 12 to 24 hr generally do not suffer any further manifestation of poisoning. The PSTs, or at least saxitoxin, act as sodium channel blockers and appear to prevent entry of Na^+ ions into the nervous system. The initial increase in sodium permeability associated with excitation is impaired, and nerve impulse transmission is blocked without depolarization. Paralysis of diaphragmatic muscles ensues. Hypotension is also frequently associated with PST poisoning (Concon, 1988).

In the United States, and in most areas of the world, PST poisoning is now quite uncommon, but this is only because the Public Health Service and similar agencies worldwide have maintained programs of shellfish monitoring and quarantine of affected beds. The cost of PST is thus not so much in human lives but rather an economic loss of potential sources of food (Halsted, 1978).

Ciguatera is a group of marine toxicants that are probably of algal origin and move up the marine food chain from smaller to larger fish. Their neurotoxicity appears to be based on anticholinesterase effects, although there are surely more complex pharmacological activities involved. Indeed, ciguatera poisoning is manifested in several ways, with gastrointestinal distress, leg cramps, burning sensations on the tongue and skin, metallic taste, dental pain, myalgia, headache, vertigo, and chills among the most common symptoms. Recovery from severe poisoning can be very prolonged (Concon, 1988). Dozens of common fish species, particularly those of tropical origin, are reported as ciguatoxic every year (Halsted, 1978; Lee, 1980). As in the case of PSTs, close monitoring is essential in preventing human poisonings. The chemistry of ciguatera poisons remains obscure, and analytic methods are accordingly less than ideal (Concon, 1988).

Many other examples of toxic contaminants of animal foods could be cited, including substances present in range plants that may remain as residues in tissues of grazing cattle or sheep. This is a little-explored area, in part because natural chemicals of marine or plant origin tend to be highly complex substances, and this creates difficulties for the analytical chemists. The importance of studies in animals, such as those recently reported by Tryphonas et al. (1990), cannot be overemphasized. These investigators found that the clinical picture in monkeys reflected that observed in patients who have recovered from toxic-mussel-induced brain damage from domoic acid. The establishment of this model makes it possible to clarify the role of certain complicating factors in fatal human cases.

Compounds Produced during Food Storage or Preparation: N-Nitrosamines   Substances such as oxidized fats, the polycyclic aromatic hydrocarbons, several types of heterocyclic compounds resulting from reactions taking place during cooking, the N-nitrosamines, and a variety of vasoactive amines are produced during food storage or preparation. The compounds that arise in processes that have been in use by humans for a long time are considered here to be of natural origin, although in theory some might legally be considered food additives or contaminants of industrial origin (Roberts, 1981).

Oxidized fats, which include a variety of epoxides and peroxides, pyrolysis products of L-tryptophan and other amino acids, and polycyclic aromatic hydrocarbons resulting from heating of foods, are all well-known and well-studied examples of potential food risks created during food storage or preparation (Concon, 1988). The N-nitrosamines, along with the related nitrosamines and nitrosoguanidines, are of particular interest because so many members of this class are animal carcinogens, some of considerable potency, and because some can form both in foods and in the alimentary tract when the appropriate precursors and conditions are present (Tannenbaum, 1988). The N-nitrosamine precursors along with nitrite, are either endogenous to or formed in many foods. Included are creatine, sarcosine, proline, pyrrolidine, and piperidine (meat and meat products), methyl guiaidine, diethylamine, and trimethylamine (fish), diethylamine and dipropylamine (cheese), and choline and lecithin (eggs and meat). There are also reports of N-nitrosamine formation from certain pesticides containing secondary amine or carbamate functions (Concon, 1988; Grasso, 1984).

The nitrosamines most commonly reported in foods are dimethylnitrosamine (DMN), diethylnitrosamine (DEN), nitrosoproline (N Pro), and nitrosopyrrolidine (N Pyr). The levels of these tend to fall below 10 µg/kg or 10 ppb, although levels up to several hundred micrograms per kilogram have been detected in certain smoked and nitrate-or nitrite-treated foods. In vivo formation of N-nitroso compounds from precursors associated with foods apparently creates a greater exposure than that created by preformed products (Grasso, 1984).

Dietary nitrosamine formation in food can be inhibited in several ways, particularly by limiting the acidity. But in many situations this is not practically achievable. Ascorbic acid is an effective inhibitor because it reacts quickly with nitrite to form nitric oxide and dehydroascorbic acid. There is some evidence that ascorbic acid also reduces in vivo formation of nitrosamines, although not all attempts to achieve such an effect experimentally have been successful. It is not clear whether the use of this vitamin results in a significant reduction in the human exposures to nitrosamines.

The principal reason for concern over nitrosamine formation in foods and beverages, and in other consumer and industrial products as well, is the marked carcinogenic activity exhibited by so many of these compounds in animals. Indeed, it is difficult to identify species of experimental animals that do not develop excess rates of tumors in response to exposures to nitrosamines and their chemical relatives. Typical targets following ingestion include the oral cavity, larynx, trachea, esophagus, liver, kidney, and skin. The multipotent properties of these substances are exemplified by DEN, which produces excess tumors at several sites in rats, mice, hamsters, guinea pigs, rabbits, dogs, monkeys, and several nonmammalian species. Although epidemiological evidence of nitrosamine involvement in human cancers is limited, it is difficult to imagine, given the nature of the animal evidence, that humans are somehow not among the susceptible species (Grasso, 1984; NRC, 1996).

No comprehensive evaluation of the risks of environmental nitrosamines and related substances or of the contribution of dietary sources of these compounds to the total burden of risk has been undertaken in recent years. A 1981 report from the National Research Council provided risk estimates based on data available before 1980. Total risks from these substances were estimated to fall in the range of 5.6×10^{-3} to 7.8×10^{-5} for the general population. The NRC committee included diet, drinking water, and various consumer and industrial products known to contain these substances. Diet, according to the committee, contributed approximately 16% to the total risk (NRC, 1981).

SUMMARY AND CONCLUSION

Because foods and beverages are so complex and variable in composition, health risks associated with them can be understood fully only through the continued pursuit of long-term epidemiological investigations. There seems to be little doubt that the composition of the human diet strongly influences health status, in both positive and negative ways. Current evidence suggessts that the major influences on long-term health status are those associated with total caloric intake and with the natural constituents of food, both nutritive and nonnutritive. A large impact from additives and contaminants seems unlikely, though the relative importance of these constituents, especially contaminants of both industrial and natural origin, varies considerably among the geographical regions of the earth. Recent evidence of large-scale pollution in rapidly developing countries suggests an increasing likelihood that food contamination could become a serious public health problem. As global trade in basic food commodities continues to increase, so will adverse public health impacts spread (Rodricks, 1993). Contamination by human pathogens—a not insignificant problem even in developed countries—is, on a global scale, almost certainly the most significant acute health problem associated with food.

A review of what is known and unknown about the risks associated with the chemical constituents and contaminants of food, as has been attempted in this chapter, demonstrates that on a chemical-specific basis, far more study has been devoted to substances intentionally added to food than to substances naturally present or contaminating food. This observation is confirmed by a recent NRC review of carcinogens and anticarcinogens in the diet (NRC, 1996). This state of affairs is perhaps largely explained by the fact that the laws under which foods are regulated, not only in the United States but around the world, require much closer examination of added substances, as we have earlier explained. The goal of understanding the effects on health of the diet as a whole, and of its myriad natural constituents and of its contaminants, is largely dictated by choices made in the research community and its funding agencies. If trends of the past decade are suggestive of the future, we can expect in the next decade or two a vastly increased understanding of the type of diet needed to maximize health benefits and to minimize the risks of chronic diseases. Of course, such an understanding will not, of itself, change individual behavior or that of the food production and distribution system, but without that understanding there is little hope for beneficial change.

ACRONYMS

ADI	Acceptable daily intake
ARMS	Adverse reaction monitoring system
CFSAN	Center for Food Safety and Applied Nutrition
CNS	Central nervous system
DEN	Diethylnitrosamine
DMN	Dimethylnitrosamine
EPA	Environmental Protection Agency
FAO / WHO	Food and Agriculture Organization/World Health Organization
FDA	Food and Drug Administration
FEMA	Flavor and Extract Manufacturers Association
GRAS	Generally recognized as safe
IFBC	International Food Biotechnology Council
NCI	National Cancer Institute

NOAELs	No-observed-adverse-effect levels
N Pro	Nitrosoproline
N Pyr	Nitrosopyrrolidine
NRC	National Research Council
PCB	Polychlorinated biphenyls
PST	Paralytic shellfish toxins
SCOGS	Select Committee on GRAS Substances
TSH	Thyroid-stimulating hormone
T_3	Triiodothyronine
T_4	Thyroxine

REFERENCES

Ames, B. N. 1983a. Dietary carcinogens and anti-carcinogens. *Science* 221: 1256–1264.

Ames, B. N. 1983b. Dietary carcinogens and anti-carcinogens, and changing patterns in cancer: Some speculation. *Environ. Res.* 50: 322–340.

Ames, B. N., and L. S. Gold. 1989. Pesticides, risk and apple sauce. *Science* 244: 757.

Bechtel, D. H., and K. E. Wilcock. 1990. Hepatitis B-independent hepatic cancer risk in aflatoxin exposed humans with estimation of a no-significant risk level. Paper presented at meeting of the Society Independent Epidemiologic Research. Snowbird, Utah.

Committee on Food Protection. 1973. *Toxicants Occurring Naturally in Foods.* Washington, DC: National Academy of Sciences.

Concon, J. 1988. *Food Toxicology*, pp. 511–603. New York: Marcel Dekker.

Davis, D. L. 1989. Natural anticarcinogens, carcinogens, and changing patterns in cancer: Some speculations. *Environ. Res.* 50: 322–340.

Doull, J. 1981. Food safety and toxicology. In *Food Safety*, pp. 289–293, ed. H. R. Roberts. New York: Wiley.

Dourson, M. L., and J. F. Stara. 1983. Regulatory history and experimental support of uncertainty (safety) factors. *Regul. Toxicol. Pharmacol.* 3: 224–238.

Dourson, M. L., Felter, S. P., and Robinson, D. 1996. Evolution of science-based uncertainty factors in noncancer risk assessment. *Reg. Toxicol. Pharmacol.* 24: 108–120.

Fitzhugh, O. G., and A. A. Nelson. 1947. The comparative toxicities of fumaric, tartaric, oxalic and maleic acids. *J. Am. Pharm. Assoc.* 36: 217–219.

Food Chemical News. 1997. EPA still wondering about dioxins in Mississippi clay. Washington, DC: CRC Press. Sept. 8: p. 4.

Food Protection Committee. 1970. *Evaluating the Safety of Food Chemicals.* Washington, DC: National Academy of Sciences/National Research Council.

Gartrell, M. J., J. C. Craun, D. S. Podrebarac, and E. L. Gunderson. 1986a. Pesticides, selected elements, and other chemicals in adult total diet samples, October 1980–March 1982. *J. Assoc. Off. Anal. Chem.* 69: 146–161.

Gartrell, M. J., J. C. Craun, D. S. Podrebarac, and E. L. Gunderson. 1986b. Pesticides, selected elements and other chemicals in infant and toddler total diet samples, October 1980–March 1982. *J. Assoc. Off. Anal. Chem.* 69:123–145.

Goldman, M., J. Doering, and R. G. Nelson. 1977. Effect of dietary ingestion of oxalic acid on growth and reproduction in male and female Long-Evans rats. *Res. Commun. Chem. Pathol. Pharmacol.* 18: 369–372.

Goyer, R. 1986. Toxic effects of metals. In *Casarett and Doull's Toxicology*, pp. 691–735, eds. C. D. Klaassen, M. O. Amdur, and J. Doull. New York: Macmillan.

Grasso, P. 1984. Carcinogens in food. In *Chemical Carcinogens*, 2nd edition, ed. C. E. Searle. ACS Monograph 182. Washington, DC: American Chemical Society.

Guest, G. B., and S. C. Fitzpatrick. 1990. Overview on bound residue issue – regulatory aspects. *Drug Metabol. Rev.* 22: 595–599.

Hall, R. L. 1979. Food additives and ingredients. In *Food Science and Nutrition: Current Issues and Answers*, pp. 6–12, ed. F. M. Clydesdale. Englewood Cliffs, NJ: Prentice-Hall.

Halsted, B. 1978. *Poisonous and Venomous Marine Animals of the World*, rev. edition. Princeton, NJ: Darwin Press.

Hayes, J. R., and T. C. Campbell. 1986. Food additives and contaminants. In *Casarett and Doull's Toxicology*, eds. C. D. Klaassen, M. O. Amdur, and J. Doull. New York: Macmillan.

Hill, R. N., L. S. Erdreich, O. E. Paynter, P. A. Roberts, S. L. Rosenthal, and C. F. Wilkinson. 1989. Thyroid follicular cell carcinogenesis. *Fundam. Appl. Toxicol.* 12: 629–697.

International Food Biotechnology Council. 1990. Biotechnologies and food: Assuring the safety of foods produced by genetic modification. *Regul. Toxicol. Pharmacol.* 12: part 2, pp. 202–410.

Joint Codex Alimentarius Commission. 1979. *Guide to the Safe Use of Food Additives*. Rome: Food and Agricultural Organization of the United Nations.

Kokoski, C. J., and W. G. Flamm. 1984. Establishment of acceptable limits of intake. In *Proceedings of the Second National Conference for Food Protection*. Washington, DC: DHHS.

Lee, C. 1980. Fish poisoning with particular reference to ciguatera. *J. Trop. Med. Hyg.* 83: 93–77.

Maxim, L. D. 1989. Problems associated with the use of conservative assumptions in exposure and risk analysis. In *The Risk Assessment of Environmental Hazards*, pp. 197–222, ed. D. J. Paustenbach. New York: Wiley.

Menzer, R. E., and J. O. Nelson. 1986. Water and soil pollutants. In *Casarett and Doull's Toxicology*, eds. C. D. Klaassen, M. O. Amdur, and J. Doull. New York: Macmillan.

Merrill, R. 1979. Regulating carcinogens in food: A legislator's guide to the food safety provisions of the Federal Food, Drug, and Cosmetic Act. *Mich. Law Rev.* 77: 179–184.

Merrill, R. 1996. Regulatory toxicology. In *Casarett and Doull's Toxicology*, 5th Edition, pp. 1011–1023, eds. C. D. Klaassen, M. O. Amdur, and J. Doull. New York: Macmillan.

Munro, I. C. 1990. Issues to be considered in the safety evaluation of fat substitutes. *Food Chem. Toxicol.* 28: 751–753.

Munro, I., and S. M. Charbonneau. 1981. Environmental contaminants. In *Food Safety*, pp. 189–211, ed. H. R. Roberts. New York: Wiley.

NRC/NAS. 1981. *The Health Effects of Nitrate, Nitrite, and N-Nitroso Compounds*. Washington, DC: National Academy Press.

NRC. 1991. *Improving America's Diet and Health*. Washington, DC: National Academy Press.

Oser, B., and R. L. Hall. 1977. Criteria employed by the expert panel of FEMA for the GRAS evaluation of flavouring substances. *Food Cosmet Toxicol.*, 15: 457–466.

Pao, E. M., K. H., Fleming, P. M., Guenther, and S. J. Mickle, 1982. Foods commonly eaten by individuals: Amount per day and per eating occasion. Washington, DC: U.S. Department of Agriculture.

Park, D. L., and L. Stoloff. 1989. Aflatoxin control — How a regulatory agency managed risk from an unavoidable natural toxicant in food and feed. *Regul. Toxicol. Pharmacol.* 9: 109–130.

Paynter, O. E., G. J. Burin, R. B. Jaeger, and C. A. Gregorio. 1988. Goitrogens and thyroid follicular cell neoplasia: Evidence for a threshold process. *Regul. Toxicol. Pharmacol.* 8: 102–119.

Reddy, B. S., and L. A. Cohen, eds. 1986. *Diet, Nutrition and Cancer: A Critical Evaluation*. Boca Raton, FL: CRC Press.

Roberts, H. R. 1981. Food safety in perspective. In *Food Safety*, pp. 4–21, ed. H. R. Roberts. New York: Wiley.

Rodricks, J. V. 1981. Regulation of carcinogens in food. In *Management of Assessed Risks from Carcinogens*, ed. W. S. Nicholson. New York: New York Academy of Sciences.

Rodricks, J. V., and A. E. Pohland. 1981. Food hazards of natural origin. In *Food Safety*, ed. H. R. Roberts. New York: Wiley.

Rodricks, J. V., and D. L. Park, 1983. General aspects of food safety and an illustration using aflatoxin. In *Proceedings of the International Symposium on Mycotoxins*, Cairo, National Information and Documentation centre (NIDOC) eds. K. Naguib, D. L. Park, and A. E. Pohland, pp. 1–22.

Rodricks, J. V. 1988. Origins of risk assessment in food safety decision-making. *J. Am. Coll. Toxicol.* 7: 539–542.

Rodricks, J. V. 1994. Health and nutrition. In *The Encyclopedia of the Environment*, eds. R. A. Eblen and W. R. Eblen, pp. 321–324. Boston: Houghton Mifflin.

Rodricks, J. V., and M. Taylor. 1989. Comparison of risk management in U.S. regulatory agencies. *J. Hazard. Mater.* 21: 239–253.

Select Committee on GRAS Substances. 1981. Evaluation of health aspects of GRAS food ingredients: Lessons learned and questions unanswered. *Fed. Proc.* 36: 2519–2562.

Sheikh-Omar, A. R., and H. B. Schiefer. 1980. Effect of feeding oxalic acid to pregnant rats. *Pertanika* 3: 25–31.

Smith, R. L. 1991. Does one man's meat become another man's poison?. *Trans. Med. Soc. London*, Nov. 11: 6–17.

Stagink, L. D. 1979. Aspartame metabolism in human subjects. In *Health and Sugar Substitutes*, pp. 97–102, ed. B. Guggenheim. Basel: S. Karger.

Stoloff, L. 1977. Aflatoxins — An overview. In *Mycotoxins in Human and Animal Health*, eds. J. V. Rodricks, C. W. Hesseltine, and M. Mehlman. Park Forest South, IL: Pathotox Publishing.

Stoloff, L. 1989. Aflatoxin is not a probable human carcinogen: The published evidence is sufficient. *Regul. Toxicol. Pharmacol.* 10: 272–283.

Tollefson, L. 1988. Monitoring adverse reactions to food additives in the U.S. Food and Drug Administration. *Regul. Toxicol. Pharmacol.* 8: 438–446.

Tryphonas, L., J. Truelove, and F. Iverson. 1990. Acute parental neurotoxicity of domoic acid in cynomolgus monkeys (M. *fascicularis*). *Toxicol. Pathol.* 18: 297–303.

U.S. EPA. 1988. *Superfund Exposure Assessment Manual. EPA 540/1-88/001.* Washington, DC: Office of Emergency and Remedial Response.

U.S. EPA. 1997. *Draft Health Assessment Document for 2,3,7,8-Tetrachlorodibenzo-p-dioxin (TCDD) and Related Compounds*, Ch. 8. Washington, DC: Office of Research and Development.

U.S. FDA. 1979a. Chemical compounds in food producing animals. *Federal Register* 44: 17070–17112.

U.S. FDA. 1979b. Polychlorinated biphenyls (PCBs): Reduction of tolerances, final rule. *Federal Register* 44: 37336-37403.

U.S. FDA. 1981. Aspartame: Commissioner's final decision. *Federal Register* 46: 38283–38308.

U.S. FDA (Bureau of Foods). 1982a. *Toxicological Principles for the Safety Assessment of Direct Food Additives and Color Additives Used in Food.* Washington, DC: U.S. Food and Drug Administration. Proposed revisions published by FDA in 1993.

U.S. FDA. 1982b. Policy for regulating carcinogenic chemicals in food and color additives: Advance notice of proposed rulemaking. *Federal Register* 47: 14464–14470.

U.S. FDA. 1983. *Food Additives Permitted for Direct Addition to Food for Human Consumption. Section 172.804. Aspartame. Title 21.* Washington, DC: Code of Federal Regulations.

U.S. FDA. 1986. Vinyl chloride polymers. *Federal Register* 51: 4173–4185.

U.S. FDA. 1988. Recommendations for chemistry data for indirect food additives. Washington, DC: Center for Food Safety and Applied Nutrition.

U.S. FDA. 1990a. Color additives: Denial of petition for listing of FD&C Red No. 3 for use in cosmetics and externally applied drugs; withdrawal of petition for use in cosmetics intended for use in the area of the eye. *Federal Register* 55: 3520–3543.

U.S. FDA. 1990b. Termination of provisional listings of FD&C Red No. 3 for use in cosmetics and externally applied drugs and of lakes of FD&C Red No. 3 for all uses. *Federal Register* 55: 3516–3519.

Van Rensburg, S. J., P. Cook-Mozafarri, D. J. Schalwyk, J. J. Van DerWatt, T. J. Vincent, and I. F. Purchase. 1985. Hepatocellular carcinoma and dietary aflatoxin in Mozambique and Transkei. *Br. J. Cancer* 57: 713–726.

12 Formaldehyde and Other Aldehydes

GEORGE D. LEIKAUF, Ph.D.

BACKGROUND

Human Environmental Exposure

Characterized by a reactive, polarized carbonyl group, low-molecular-weight aldehydes constitute a number of organic compounds useful in a large number of industrial processes. The simplest aldehyde, formaldehyde (HCHO), is one of the top-ten organic chemical feedstocks in the United States. Other commonly encountered aldehydes include acetaldehyde (CH_3CHO) and acrolein ($CH_2{=}CHCHO$); they differ from formaldehyde in carbon chain length and saturation.

Human aldehyde exposures result from exogenous sources and endogenous formation (i.e., biogenesis through metabolism) (Benedetti et al., 1980, 1984; Nilsson and Tottmar, 1987; Marnett, 1988). Environmental aldehydes can be formed naturally through tropospheric reactions of terpenes and isoprene released from foliage with hydroxyl radicals. In addition aldehydes are formed anthropogenically during incomplete combustion of alcohols, or they are released from polymeric substances and solutions. Formaldehyde may become a source of increasing significance with the addition of methanol to automotive fuels (Othmer, 1987). This chapter reviews both the environmental sources and potential health effects. Other valuable reviews on aldehyde toxicity include reports by the National Research Council (NRC, 1981), Beauchamp et al. (1985), Feinman (1988), Marnett (1988), Council on Scientific Affairs (1989), World Health Organization (WHO, 1989, 1992, 1995), Heck et al. (1990), McLaughlin (1994), and International Agency for Research on Cancer (IARC, 1982, 1985, 1995).

Indoor Air   Considering the average time-activity pattern, poor indoor air quality is the most common mode of aldehyde exposure. We typically spend less than 1 hour a day (18–42 min) outside (Fig. 12-1), so outdoor exposures constitute only 3% of our average daily exposure (Chapin, 1974; Samet et al., 1987, Samet and Spengler, 1991). Excluding the other activities such as time in transit (1.0–1.6 h/d) and occupational exposure for those working outside the home 5.2 to 6.7 hours per day, the remaining and primary exposure for most individuals occurs at home. Indoor exposure therefore equals 55% to 65% for those working outside the home and 85% for those working inside the home (Songco and Fahey, 1987). Aldehyde-generating activities in the home include tobacco smoking, wood burning, and cooking. Other common sources include release from

Environmental Toxicants: Human Exposures and Their Health Effects, 2/e. Edited by Morton Lippmann.
ISBN: 0-471-29298-2   © 2000 John Wiley & Sons, Inc.

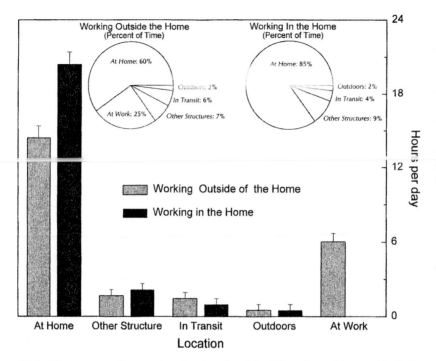

Figure 12-1 Time spent per day at various locations for adults. Values for working outside the home are for men and women and for working in the home are for women. Adapted from Chapin (1974); Samet et al. (1987).

structural materials, furnishings, clothing, cosmetics, and insulation (Pickrell et al., 1983; Feinman, 1988). Estimated contributions from three indoor sources of formaldehyde are listed in Table 12-1.

Another common source is urea-formaldehyde foam insulation, which can produce exposure averaging 120 ppb, with occasional concentrations as high as 4000 ppb (Gupta et al., 1982). Concentrations in older homes without foam insulation typically range from 30 to 90 ppb, whereas high-level exposures of up to 4200 ppb have been recorded in mobile homes (IARC, 1985, 1995). These concentrations are influenced by elevation of temperature or humidity. Formaldehyde is also released from polymeric resins such urea formaldehyde (used in particleboard, plywood, paper and textile treatments, and surface coatings), melamine formaldehyde (used in laminates, surface coatings, wood adhesives, and molding compounds), or phenolic resins (used in plywood adhesives and insulation) (WHO, 1989; Gerberich and Seaman, 1994).

In addition to formaldehyde, several other aldehydes are constituents of mainstream (that portion inhaled by the smoker), side stream (that portion emitted from a burning cigarette), and environmental tobacco smoke (the aged combination of side stream and exhaled mainstream smoke) (Table 12-2). Aldehydes are principally associated with the vapor phase of mainstream smoke, but they have been measured in the particulate phase (Ayer and Yeager, 1976; Godish, 1989). Of the various aldehydes present in mainstream smoke, acetaldehyde is the predominant compound by weight, accompanied by formaldehyde, acrolein, and propionaldehyde. Importantly, the aldehyde concentrations released in smoke from cigarettes between puffs at a lower temperature (600°C) are greater than those produced during smoking (900°C). Thus side stream aldehyde emissions are 8 to 17 times greater than mainstream levels. Because smokers inhale only

TABLE 12-1   Indoor Sources of Formaldehyde Exposure

Sources	Concentration
Cigarette smoke	
Dose per pack for smoke	0.38 mg / pack
Environmental tobacco smoke	0.25 ppm
Mainstream tobacco smoke (40 ml puff)	40 ppm
Clothing made with synthetic fibers	
Men's polyester cotton blend	2.7 µg / g per day
Women's dress	3.7 µg / g per day
Furnishings	
Particleboard [a]	0.4–8.1 µg / g per day
Plywood	1.5–5.3 µg / g per day
Paneling	0.9–21.0 µg / g per day
Draperies	0.8–3.0 µg / g per day
Carpet / upholstery fabric	≤ 0.1 ppm

Source: Pickrell et al. (1983); Feinman (1988).
[a] Made with urea-formaldehyde resin.

about 45% of each cigarette, side stream smoke can add significantly to the indoor aldehyde burden. For example, the contribution of cigarette smoke alone to indoor aldehyde concentrations can be as great as 250 ppb formaldehyde (Gammage and Gupta, 1984) and 75 ppb acrolein (Badre et al., 1978) in rooms where several individuals are smoking.

Occupational Exposures   Occupational exposure to low-molecular-weight aldehydes is extensive, primarily because of the usefulness of their reactive carbonyl in chemical synthesis. Of the several aliphatic aldehydes available, formaldehyde has the greatest production and usage. Over 5 billion pounds of formaldehyde are used in the United States each year, with about 90% being used as a chemical feedstock or an intermediate in the synthesis of a wide number of chemicals including urea-formaldehyde and phenol-formaldehyde resins, ethylene glycol, fertilizers, dyes, disinfectants, germicides, hardening agents, and as a preservative in water-based paints, cosmetics, and hair shampoos.

TABLE 12-2   Aldehydes in Cigarette Smoke

| Aldehyde [a] | Amount Released (mg / pack) | | |
	Mainstream	Side Stream	Environmental Tobacco Smoke [b]
Formaldehyde	3.4	14.5	1.3
Acetaldehyde	12.5	84.7	3.2
Acrolein	1.5	25.2	0.6
Propionaldehyde	1.3	18.8	0.9

Source: R.J. Reynolds Tobacco Company (1988).
[a] Other aldehydes in cigarette smoke include isobutylaldehyde, methacrolein, butylaldehyde, isovaleraldehyde, crotonaldehyde, and 2-methylvaleraldehyde.
[b] Environmental tobacco smoke = 2 hour integrated amount per pack.

Occupational exposure has been estimated to be over one million people to formaldehyde alone. This includes persons working in medical and health services (approximately one-third), funeral homes, textiles, furniture, paper, and agriculture industries (Consensus Workshop on Formaldehyde, 1984; IARC, 1995). Of these, over 20,000 individuals have routine exposure to concentrations greater than 1.0 ppm, with over 500,000 exposed to concentrations of 0.5 to 1.0 ppm (Occupational Safety and Health Administration, 1985). Along with inhalation, occupational exposures to low-molecular-weight aldehydes can also be topical, since these compounds are used as aqueous solutions (e.g., formalin, which is typically 37% formaldehyde in water and methanol) or as a polymerized solid (e.g. paraformaldehyde) Absorption through the skin is limited (typically <10%) because of the high reactivity and volatility of aldehydes.

Additional aldehydes with the greatest industrial production include acetaldehyde, acrolein, crotonaldehyde, chloroacetaldehyde, and furfural. The current recommended occupational threshold limit values (TLV) for these compounds are presented in Table 12-3. Of the compounds listed, acetaldehyde and acrolein have the greatest usage. Acrolein is used in the production of glycerine, synthetic methionine, glutaraldehyde, and other chemicals.

Ambient Air and Alternative Fuels Low-molecular-weight aldehydes are low-level contaminants of the urban environment. Concentrations in ambient air, however, are typically much lower than those encountered in occupational or indoor settings. Along with the direct release of aldehyde from stationary sources (home wood fires and incinerators), these compounds are either released directly from mobile sources (car, truck, or jet engines) or formed by secondary photochemical reactions from emitted hydrocarbons. Nonetheless, aldehydes are important components of atmospheric

TABLE 12.3 Occupational Threshold Limit Values (TLVs)

Low-Molecular-Weight Aldehyde	Time-Weighted Average[a] ppm (mg/m^3)	Ceiling[b] ppm (mg/m^3)	Carcinogenicity[c]	Skin[d]
Acetaldehyde	—	25 (45)	A3	—
Acrolein	—	0.1 (0.23)	A4	Skin
Chloroacetaldehyde	—	1.0 (3.2)	—	—
Crontonaldehyde	—	0.3 (0.86)	A3	Skin
Formaldehyde	—	0.3 (0.37)	A2	—
Furfural	2.0 (7.9)	—	A3	—
Glutaraldehyde	—	0.05 (0.2)	A4	—

Source: American Conference of Governmental Industrial Hygienists (1998).
[a] Mean concentration obtained normalized to an 8 hour work day and a 40 hour work week. At this concentration nearly all workers may be repeatedly exposed, day after day, without adverse effect.
[b] A concentration that should not be exceeded during any part of a working exposure. When continuous monitoring is not feasible, the sampling period should not exceed 15 minutes.
[c] Compounds that may cause or contribute to increased risk of cancer in workers. *A1 = confirmed human carcinogen. A2 = suspected human carcinogen.* This agent is carcinogenic in experimental animals at dose levels, by routes of administration, at sites, histological type, or by a mechanism considered relevant to worker exposure. Available epidemiologic studies are conflicting or insufficient to confirm the risk of cancer in exposed humans. *A3 = animal carcinogen.* This agent is carcinogenic in experimental animals at relatively high dose levels, by route of administration, at site, histological type, or by a mechanism not considered relevant to worker exposure. Available epidemiologic studies do not confirm an increased risk of cancer in exposed humans. Available evidence suggests that the agent is not likely to cause cancer in humans except under uncommon or unlikely routes or levels of exposure. *A4 = not classifiable as a human carcinogen.* Inadequate data exist on which to classify the agent as a carcinogen in either humans or animals.
[d] Agents with potential significant contribution of the overall exposure by the cutaneous route, including mucous membranes and the eyes, either by direct contact with vapors or, of probable greater significance, by direct skin contact with the substance.

chemistry because, as products of oxidation of almost all hydrocarbons, they are precursors of free radicals, ozone, and peroxyacyl nitrates (Grosjean, 1991, Grosjean et al., 1996, Tuazon et al., 1997). As such, aldehydes are an excellent species to evaluate predictions of ozone formation in kinetic models of urban air quality (Carter, 1990; Grosjean et al., 1992, Harley and Cass, 1995).

In urban areas, aldehyde levels, like those of other hydrocarbons, exhibit diurnal variations that precede ozone peaks. In the past, total aldehyde levels have occasionally reached maximums of 300 ppb but more typically were less than 40 ppb. Approximately 20% to 50% of the total aldehyde is in the form of formaldehyde, with typical values ranging from 5 to 30 ppb (with maximal values as high 50–86 ppb in urban air masses contained by atmospheric inversions). Historical episodic values recorded in Los Angeles for formaldehyde have reached 90 to 150 ppb; in contrast, ambient values in rustic environments can be as low as 0.8 ppb.

Other aldehydes are not routinely measured in urban air; thus few data exist on the ambient concentrations of most aldehydes. Acetaldehyde levels are often 2 to 39 ppb and thus are about 75% of formaldehyde levels (range 32–155%) (Grosjean et al., 1996). These levels are sufficient to make acetaldehyde the major aldehyde in the removal of hydroxyl radicals from the atmosphere. Other aldehydes important in this process include formaldehyde and nonanal. Estimates for acrolein are between 5% and 10% of the total aldehyde burden (or 5–30 ppb for peaks), and those for other aliphatic aldehydes between 35% and 40% of total aldehyde concentrations. Of these, higher molecular weight carbonyls (nine species: $C_8 – C_{14}$) typically account for 10% to 15% of the total aldehydes (Grosjean et al., 1996).

Between 55% and 75% of ambient aldehydes are from mobile sources, and proximity to such sources may produce greater localized exposures. For example, exposures near garages, tunnels, or in city street canyons may be much greater, since exhaust from passenger cars equipped with either spark-ignition or diesel engines can produce aldehydes. Estimated concentrations in emissions from warm gasoline-fueled automobiles (running at 40 mph cruising speeds) are about 1000, 200, and 100 ppb for formaldehyde, acrolein, and acetaldehyde, respectively (Swarin and Lipari, 1983). By contrast, starts of cold engines yield levels in which formaldehyde can exceed 5000 ppb. Diesel engines also produce significant amounts of formaldehyde, acrolein, and acetaldehyde, with levels produced by warm engines equaling about 4000, 500, and 1000 ppb, respectively.

Aldehydes are enriched in automotive emissions when fuels containing oxygenated additives (especially alcohols) are combusted (Grosjean, 1990; Carter, 1990: Shah and Singh, 1998). The formulation of these alternative fuels may vary and contain either methanol (from methane) or ethanol (from agricultural sources); these are likely to be mixtures of alcohol and gasoline (e.g., M-85, an 85% methanol–15% gasoline mixture). The addition of methanol to gasoline may markedly increase formaldehyde emissions, whereas ethanol is likely to increase acetaldehyde concentrations. Acetaldehyde concentrations, for example, for internal combustion engines using ethanol rather than gasoline can increase from <100 ppb to over 190,000 ppb following cold starts and from <100 ppb to 8400 ppb acetaldehyde from warm engines (Marnett, 1988). Formaldehyde concentration can also increase from 480 to 3600 ppb.

Cellular Exposure and Dosimetry

Nasal Deposition and Penetration   Regional deposition of an inhaled gas is controlled by water solubility, concentration, and physiological and pathological features of the respiratory tract. Measurements of formaldehyde deposition in rats (Dallas et al., 1985; Patterson, 1986) and in dogs (Egle, 1972) found essentially 100% total respiratory tract deposition. One interesting observation made in these studies was the secretion of low levels from control animals/individuals, presumably from biogenic formation. Aldehydes are highly soluble in water compared to other common air pollutants (Table 12-4) and the principal site of deposition of these compounds is the upper respiratory tract (Aharonson et al., 1974). When inhaled in low concentrations, almost all (>98%) of formaldehyde is deposited in the moist layers covering the nasal mucosa. This deposition occurs during the inspiration, with little (<2%) or no formaldehyde being exhaled (Egle, 1972; Heck et al., 1983; Dallas et al., 1985). In rats, Heck and coworkers reported that radiolabeled formaldehyde deposition was proportional to the concentration and length of exposure. Deposition rate decreased over a 6 hours exposure period, resulting, in part, from a decrease in ventilatory rate during exposure.

Aqueous solubility of aliphatic low-molecular-weight aldehydes decreases with increasing carbon chain length. For this reason greater nasal penetration has been noted for proprionaldehyde (CH_3CH_2CHO) and for acetaldehyde (CH_3CHO) than for formaldehyde (HCHO). Egle (1972), for example, reported approximately 60% retention (40% penetration) for proprionaldehyde and acetaldehyde as compared to >90% retention for formaldehyde in the canine upper respiratory tract during inspiration. Aliphatic aldehydes with carbon chain lengths greater than four carbon atoms are much less miscible in water, and penetration is therefore more likely to be greater than that for proprionaldehyde. Values vary for other gases of low solubility (e.g., 20–60% of ozone is retained in the upper respiratory tract of dogs), and few measures are currently available for aldehydes.

Additional physiological factors, such as altered clearance mechanisms (epithelial metabolism, mucociliary clearance, and possibly regional air and blood flow), also affect aldehyde dosimetry. This has been suggested for formaldehyde, since the magnitude of the decrease in the rate of deposition is not solely related to the decrease in ventilation. Studies with other inhalation hazards (sulfur dioxide and ozone) have suggested that other factors influencing nasal penetration include vascular congestion, respiratory flow rate, concentration, duration of exposure, and airway caliber.

Morris (1997) has proposed that aldehyde penetration, at least for the rat nasal passages, is strongly influenced by the metabolic capacity of the epithelium. Aldehydes are handled by a number of specific and nonspecific enzymes, including aldehyde dehydrogenases, aldehyde oxidases, or xanthine oxidase (Bohren et al., 1989). The predominant elimination pathway for aldehydes by dehydrogenation yields a carboxylic acid (e.g., formic acid from formaldehyde) through an irreversible step that requires glutathione (Lam et al., 1985; Bhatt et al., 1988) and a hydrogen carrier (e.g., nicotinamide adenine dinucleotide or its phosphate, NAD(P)). Formaldehyde deposits mainly (93%) within the respiratory epithelium with little in the olfactory epithelium of the rat nose (Kimbell et al., 1993; Cohen Hubel et al., 1997; Kimbell et al., 1997). Therefore the dose rate of low concentrations (< 5 ppm at a breathing rate of 200 ml/min) produces a tissue dose rate approximately equaling the maximal metabolic rate (Vmax) of formaldehyde dehydrogenase (estimated capacity 40 nmol/min) reported by CassanovaSchmitz et al. (1984) for the rat nasal epithelium. Likewise Morris (1997) proposed that 800 ppm acetaldehyde could produce a dose rate at the Vmax of aldehyde dehydrogenase of the rat respiratory epithelium. Accordingly doses greater than 800 ppm would have greater penetration. This proposition is in general agreement with the nasal depositions of 76%, 48%, 41%, and 26% for inspired acetaldehyde concentrations of 1, 10, 100, and 1000 ppm, respectively.

In addition differences in airflow patterns within the nasal passages produce different doses to various types of epithelium with the nose. For example, due to the difference of metabolic capacity and airflow over the olfactory epithelium, the acetaldehyde concentration necessary to overwhelm metabolism is lower, 300 ppm, than of the

TABLE 12-4   Physical and Chemical Properties of Aldehyde and Other Environmental Agents

Compound	Structure	Molecular Weight	Aqueous solution (g/L)	Organic solultion (most-least)[a]
I. Aldehydes				
A. SATURATED ALIPHATIC ALDEHYDES				
Formaldehyde		30.03	560.0	eth, ace, bz, al, chl
Acetaldehyde		44.05	200.0	eth, al, bz
Propionaldehyde		58.08	160.0	eth, al
Glutaraldehyde		100.12	–	al, bz
B. UNSATURATED ALIPHATIC ALDEHYDES				
Acrolein		56.06	210.0	eth, ace, al
Crotonaldehyde		70.09	181.0	bz, eth, ace,
C. AROMATIC OR CYCLIC ALDEHYDES				
Benzaldehyde		106.11	3.0	eth, al, ace, bz
Cinnamaldehyde		132.16	10.5	eth, al, chl
II. Other environmental agents and common inorganic molecules				
Sulfur dioxide	SO_2	64.07	106.4	chl, ether meth, al
Carbon dioxide	CO_2	44.01	1.74	–
Carbon monoxide	CO	28.01	0.03	eth, meth, eth ace, ace acid
Oxygen	O_2	32.00	0.04	–
Ozone	O_3	48.00	0.02	meth cl

Source: Comey and Hahn (1921); Seidell (1940, 1941), and Windholz (1983).

[a] Abbreviations: Eth, ethanol; ace, acetone; bz, benzene; al, alcohol; chl, chloroform; meth, methanol; eth ace, ethyl acetate; ace acid, acetic acid; meth cl, methylene chloride.

respiratory epithelium, 800 ppm (Morris, 1997). Because formaldehyde deposits more in the anterior respiratory epithelium, this difference has less of an effect for this compound (Monticello et al., 1996)

Relative reactivity of the inhaled aldehyde also influences retention in the upper respiratory tract (Aharonson et al., 1974). In the dog, nasal retention of acrolein (80%) is intermediate between those of formaldehyde (> 95%) and proprionaldehyde (60%). The difference between acrolein and proprionaldehyde, both three-carbon molecules, can only be partially explained by acrolein's higher solubility (acrolein = 210 g/L: propionaldehyde = 160 g/L; Table 12-4). The higher chemical reactivity of acrolein may also contribute significantly. Acrolein possesses both a reactive carbonyl group and an electrophilic β-carbon produced by the αβ-unsaturated carbon bond positioned next to the carbonyl group ($^+CH–C=CH–OH^-$). Presumably covalent binding with surface macromolecules, like mucin, is greater for acrolein than proprionaldehyde, and it should prevent acrolein reentry to a greater extent than that of proprionaldehyde (Bogdanffy et al., 1987).

Aldehydes that penetrate the nasal cavity or enter through oral breathing are almost completely deposited in the lower respiratory tract. Heck and associates (1983) examined deposition of [^{14}C]HCHO in nasal breathing rats and mice. In 6 hours tests with formaldehyde concentrations up to 24 ppm, approximately 250 nmol [^{14}C]HCHO/g tissue was deposited in the trachea as compared to 2200 nmol/g tissue in the nasal mucosa (the amount of deposition was nonlinear in relation to dose, with saturation at doses exceeding 6 ppm). Autoradiography of mouse and rat airways by Swenberg and associates (Chang et al., 1983; Swenberg et al., 1983) demonstrated the presence of radioactivity in the trachea and main bronchi following [^{14}C]HCHO exposure. Deposition of formaldehyde in the trachea and bronchi of monkey was greater than that of rats; this is presumably because rodents breathe principally through their nose. Humans typically breathe between 30% and 60% through their mouth at rest and more during exercise.

DNA-Protein Crosslinks and Molecular Dosimetry   Initial covalent interactions at the sites of exposure could serve as a sensitive indicator of the dose to the critical biological target site. If such interactions are irreversible and stable, these methods could enable a measure of regional molecular dosimetry. Aldehydes can form crosslinks, bridging macromolecules through attack of the electrophilic carbonyl carbon with various reactive groups on proteins, RNA, or DNA (French and Edsall, 1945; Naylor et al., 1988). One reactive group contained in proteins is the amino group, which is also contained in each of these types of macromolecules. Thus this reaction site can lead to mixed crosslinks (e.g., DNA–protein crosslinks) via a two-step process initiated by the formation of an unstable hydroxymethyl intermediate (through loss of water from a methylene Schiff base), followed by a nucleophilic attack on the carbon donated by formaldehyde by a second amino group contained on either DNA or a protein. Obviously bifunctional aldehydes, namely malondialdehyde or glutaraldehyde, are more effective at forming crosslinks. The resulting methylene bridge can either be repaired rapidly or become temporally stable, and an integrated measurement would thus reflect these competitive processes of formation and degradation (Graftstrom et al., 1984).

Although DNA–DNA crosslinks are possible, attempts at detection in intact cells have been met with limited success (Feldman, 1973; Chaw et al., 1980; Hemminki, 1981). On the other hand, DNA–protein crosslinks have been more readily measured (Wilkins and Macleod, 1976; Magana-Schwenke et al., 1978; Magana-Schwenke and Ekert, 1978; Graftstrom et al., 1984). The relationship between formaldehyde dose and DNA–protein crosslinks, however, has been found to be nonlinear over the range of 0.3 to 1 ppm

(Swenberg et al., 1983). This nonlinearity makes evaluation of cellular dose by measurements of DNA–protein alone difficult. Lastly, protein–protein crosslinks have been detected and are linear with dose; however, evidence suggests that this covalent binding is primarily between extracellular proteins, and therefore it does not reflect intracellular dose. This limitation may be important in the evaluation of dose in certain toxicological processes leading to cancer.

In addition to the instability of crosslinks formed by formaldehyde exposure (Grafstrom et al., 1984), a principal reason for the nonlinearity in the formation of DNA–protein crosslinks is likely to be simply the rapid enzymatic removal of aldehyde before crosslinks are formed. Depletion of glutathione alone increases the amount of detectable DNA–protein crosslinks and nearly restores the linearity of the dose–response relationship (Lam et al.,1985; Casanova and Heck, 1987), suggesting that this is an important defense mechanism at lower doses. Ultimately the carboxylic acid formed from each aldehyde is converted to CO_2 and H_2O, either through a multiple-step process involving tetrahydrofolate (initiated by formyl-THF synthetase) or a reaction catalyzed by catalase.

Conceivably other methods also prove useful in assessing regional aldehyde dosimetry. Such an indicator could be DNA-adduct levels, and two adducts, N^6-hydroxymethyl-deoxyadenosine (HOMedA) and N^2-hydroxymethyldeoxy guanosine (HOMedG), are possible. However, these hydroxymethyl adducts, like DNA–protein crosslinks, are not stable. Fennell (1990) has presented methods that stabilize these adducts so that they are suitable for ^{32}P or electrophore postlabeling. Such a technique could reduce the need for the use of radiolabeled formaldehyde.

Populations of Concern   At present, no specific population has been clearly identified to have an increased risk for adverse effects from aldehyde exposures. Previously persons with asthma were identified as being of special concern when the National Ambient Air Quality Standard was established for sulfur dioxide. By analogy, formaldehyde or other aldehydes with bronchoconstrictive properties, may also represent an added risk to this population (see below for more details). An aspect of this concern includes persons who have developed an immunologic hypersensitivity, but this is a complex issue (see below for details).

Aldehydes other than formaldehyde that can penetrate the upper respiratory tract, much like ozone, may produce adverse responses similar to ozone. Currently children have been suggested as a population of concern for ozone and environmental tobacco smoke exposure, and thus aldehyde effects among this population deserve attention.

Genetic differences in drug metabolism may also be predisposing risk factors for adverse responses to aldehyde exposure. Elimination of aldehydes is rapid and dependent on other aldehyde dehydrogenases, glutathione, tetrahydrofolate, and NAD(P). Alteration of the metabolism responsible for normal function of these defense mechanisms could therefore place individuals at risk. Currently 12 aldehyde dehydrogenase genes have been identified in humans (Yoshida et al., 1998). Studies of ethanol metabolism have identified NAD^+-dependent aldehyde dehydrogenase isoform (restriction length polymorphism) with reduced activity among Asians and Native Americans (Hsu et al., 1987; Card et al., 1989; Farres et al., 1989; Goedde and Agarwal, 1989; Kurys et al., 1989; Shibuya et al., 1989). Ingestion of ethanol by these individuals leads to the normal, but rapid, formation of acetaldehyde via an additional allelic variant in alcohol dehydrogenase (an NAD-dependent cytosolic enzyme contained principally in the liver) that increases aldehyde formation. Ethanol also is converted to acetaldehyde by microsomal ethanol-oxidizing system, or catalase (Crabb, 1990). Normally this acetaldehyde is rapidly converted to acetic acid; however, because of an alteration in aldehyde dehydrogenase (ALDH2), concentrations of this intermediate are elevated. This alteration is often due to a point mutation in ALDH2 (G → A transition in exon 12) that produces a Glu → Lys substitution at position 487. This allelic variant has been found in high frequency (40–60%) in Asians (Yoshida et al., 1998).

The accumulation of circulating acetaldehyde is responsible for a dysphoric response among these individuals following ethanol ingestion. It leads to sympathomimetic responses of facial flushing, tachycardia, and muscle weakness and a rise in circulating catecholamines. Aldehyde dehydrogenase can also be inhibited by disulfiram (tetraethylthiuram disulfide) (DeMaster and Stevens, 1988; Helander et al., 1988) and used clinically for the treatment of alcohol abuse, or its metabolites. The potential pathophysiological significance of depressed aldehyde dehydrogenase activity and its relationship to adverse reaction to aldehydes in the lung may be important in understanding individual susceptibility.

SINGLE-EXPOSURE HEALTH EFFECTS

Formaldehyde

Symptomatic Response in Controlled Human Exposures   Moderate concentrations of formaldehyde produce rapid responses including eye (50–2000 ppb) and upper respiratory tract (100–25,000 ppb) irritation which can become intolerable (Table 12-5). Eye irritation progresses to a greater extent with continuous exposure than with discontinuous exposure, whereas nose and throat irritation were significantly greater in discontinuous exposures (Weber-Tschopp et al.,1977). Tolerance to nose and throat irritation can develop in the same individual who continues to become increasingly sensitive to eye irritation during exposure (Anderson and Molhave, 1983).

TABLE 12-5   Symptomatic Responses in Humans to Formaldehyde

Formaldehyde Concentration (ppm)	Response	Reference
Eye irritation (blinking rate, lacrimation, conjunctivitis)		
0.01	Detectable by some	Schuck et al. (1966)
0.30	Slight but tolerable response	Rader (1977)
0.50	Intermediate response	Bourne and Seferian (1959)
0.80	Severe response	Wayne et al. (1977)
1.7–2.0	Marked eye blinking	Bender et al. (1983)
Upper respiratory tract irritation (nasal secretion or dryness, throat irritation)		
0.03	Minimal or no effect	Weber-Tschopp et al. (1977)
0.25–1.39	Moderate irritation	Kerfoot and Mooney (1975)
		Schoenberg and Mitchell (1975)
		Anderson and Molhave (1983)
1.7–2.1	Significant throat irritation	Weber-Tschopp et al. (1977)
3.1	Severe to intolerable irritation	Kane and Alaire (1977)
Odor threshold		
0.05	Odor threshold	Pettersson and Rehn (1977)
0.17	Detected by 50% exposed	Pettersson and Rehn (1977)
1.5	Detected by all subjects	Pettersson and Rehn (1977)

The characteristic odor of formaldehyde is detectable at concentrations below those that produce irritation. However, as with many compounds, the odor threshold (20–500 ppb) can vary widely among individuals, and acclimatization can occur during exposure (Berglund and Nordin, 1992). For these reasons the detection of odor or lack thereof cannot be used as an indicator of safety.

A sequel to massive acute exposure can include an aversion to the odor (Shusterman et al., 1988). This can be viewed as a psychoprotective response resulting from behavioral conditioning in which the initial single acute exposure accompanied by observable pathophysiological effects serves as the unconditional stimulus. The odor (at subirritant concentrations), re-exposure after the acute exposure, then serves as the conditioned stimulus. Following such a regimen, conditioned subjects can develop subjective (including those outlined above as well as a perception of poor air quality, discomfort, or a "desire to leave the room") or objective (changes in heart rate and breathing pattern) responses. Although the enhanced response is psychogenic in origin, generation is often involuntary and may involve minimal personality components.

In general, formaldehyde exposures of 50–150 ppb produce mild, transient, concentration-dependent responses in 10% to 50% of the persons exposed (Bernstein et al., 1984). These types of responses are common and often are the primary or solitary finding associated with low-level environmental exposure (see below). In one study 410 ppb formaldehyde exposure of 2 hours, increased mucosal inflammation (leukocytes and albumin recovered in nasal lavage recovered 4 and 18 hours after exposure) in healthy and asthma subjects (Pazdrak et al., 1993). Eye irritation develops frequently in the range of 1000 to 3000 ppb in most subjects, and upper respiratory irritation is frequent at concentrations of 1000 to 11,000 ppb (NRC, 1981; IARC, 1995). At concentrations of 4000–5000 ppb, many subjects cannot tolerate prolonged exposure (IARC, 1982; WHO, 1989; IARC, 1995).

Respiratory Mechanics in Laboratory Animals   Inhalation of formaldehyde decreases minute volume in laboratory animals, primarily as a result of a decrease in respiratory breathing frequency (more than through a decrease in tidal volume, which may even increase) (Table 12-6). Concomitantly, pulmonary resistance increases with or without a slight decrease in pulmonary compliance. These responses are rapid in onset, can remain constant during exposure (response plateau), and are readily reversible with exposure cessation.

The magnitude of the response plateau developed during exposure is dose dependent. The persistence of the response, however, varies somewhat with species. In studies with rats (F-344) and mice (Swiss-Webster but not B6C3F$_1$), decreases in minute volume are

TABLE 12-6   Acute Pulmonary Responses in Animals to Formaldehyde

Species	Concentration (ppm)			Reference
	Threshold	ED$_{25\%}$	ED$_{25\%}$	
Decreased minute volume/ respiratory rate				
Mice (Swiss-Webster)	0.50	0.8	3.1	Kane and Alaire (1977)
(B6C3F$_1$)[a]	0.50	1.8	4.4	Barrow et al. (1983)
Rats (F-344)[a]	0.95	3.1	13.1	Chang et al. (1981)
Guinea pig	0.30	11.0	>49.0	Amdur (1960)
Increased airway resistance				
Guinea pig	0.30	2.0	11–49	Amdur (1960)

[a] Tidal volume was noted to increase with exposure in animals during exposures ≥ 6.4 ppm.

not maintained during exposure, suggesting tolerance. In B6C3F$_1$ mice, the induced decrease in minute volume remained more consistent during exposure. These differences in minute volume, as noted by Barrow, Steinhagen, and Chang (1983), could alter the dose from exposure to 15 ppm (a dose found sufficient to induce nasal carcinoma in rats but not mice). In B6C3F$_1$mice, minute volume is decreased 75% as compared to 45% in F-344 rats. This would result in an estimated dose to the nasal epithelium of 0.076 in mice as compared to 0.156 g/min per cm^2. Changes in breathing pattern therefore may be viewed as protective.

The formaldehyde dose producing decreases in respiratory rate in mice is comparable to that producing increases in symptomatic responses in humans (see above). This led Alarie and associates to propose that evaluation of sensory irritation in mice might serve as a useful test system to evaluate relative irritation potential of various compounds (Kane and Alarie, 1977). From these findings the authors suggested that the threshold limit value should be set in the range of 0.03 to 0.3 ppm to prevent irritant responses.

Respiratory Mechanics in Humans after Single Exposure   When inhaled alone in controlled exposure chambers, few changes in respiratory mechanics have been reported among healthy subjects either during or shortly after single formaldehyde exposure at environmentally relevant levels (Table 12-7). After exposures ranging from 0.3 to 7.5 ppm, essentially no change has been noted in this group. For example, Day et al. (1984) exposed 18 volunteers to 1.0 ppm formaldehyde, with 9 subjects having complained of various nonrespiratory adverse effects from the urea-formaldehyde foam insulation in their homes. No effects were noted in subjects who exposed to 1.0 ppm formaldehyde for 90 minutes or 1.1 ppm formaldehyde (produced from urea-formaldehyde foam insulation) for 30 minutes. Exposure to 3.0 ppm for 60 minutes did produce a small change in forced expiratory volumes and flows (Green et al. 1987), but this response was transient and reversed when exposures were extended to 120 to 180 minutes (Sauder et al., 1986).

Formaldehyde's ability to alter pulmonary function has also been tested among two additional, possibly more susceptible, populations. The first population, persons with asthma, was selected based on the observation that another soluble irritant, like SO$_2$, had lower dose thresholds to initiate bronchoconstriction in this group compared to control subjects (Sheppard et al., 1980). One study involved oral breathing (mouthpiece) for 10 minutes of 1 to 3 ppm (Sheppard et al., 1984); another involved chamber exposures for 40 minutes to 2.0 ppm (Witek et al., 1987). In both studies, subjects failed to develop an increase in pulmonary resistance or a decrease in flow rate when tested at rest or with exercise. In the latter study, however, airway reactivity may have been altered (see below).

The second clinical population tested are persons with previous occupational exposure. The major objective of these studies is to determine across-shift changes in pulmonary function. This effect is often evident and discussed below under Effects of Multiple Exposure. Another objective of these studies is to uncover an immunologically based response in subjects referred to the clinic for a direct bronchial provocation. Such investigations have documented immediate and delayed responses, much like those found in antigen-induced immediate hypersensitivity reactions, but these responses appear to be rare (occurring in 12 of 230 persons tested, or 5% in one study). Given the widespread exposure to formaldehyde and documented formaldehyde skin sensitization (see below), these results suggest that there are remarkably few cases of pulmonary hypersensitivity. This implies that sensitization by aldehyde inhalation is not a primary mechanism for respiratory effect, but rather, observed effects are associated with a direct (nonimmuno-specific) irritant effect. This limited role for immunologic sensitization is particularly evident if hypersensitivity is narrowly defined as a response to extremely low doses of a compound, well below the dose necessary to induce irritation.

TABLE 12-7 Respiratory Function of Humans Exposed to Formaldehyde

Formaldehyde Concentration (ppm)	Length of Exposure (min)	Route of Exposure	Findings[a] (number of Subjects)	References
*Healthy individual (nonsmoking) in clinical studies*
0.3–1.6	300	Oronasal (chamber)	No change in FVC, $FEV_{1.0}$, $FEF_{25-75\%}$ or R_{aw} $(n=16)$	Anderson and Molhave (1983)
0.5–3.0	180	Oronasal (chamber, with or without exercise)	No change in FVC, $FEV_{1.0}$, $FEF_{25-75\%}$ sG_{aw} $(n=9-10)$	Kulle et al. (1987)
2.0	40	Oronasal (chamber)	No change in FVC, $FEV_{1.0}$, MMEF $(n=15)$	Schachter et al. (1986)
3.0	60	Oronasal (chamber, with exercise)	2.5–3.8% change in FVC and $FEV_{1.0}$ $(n=22)$	Green et al. (1987)
3.0	180	Oronasal (chamber, with exercise)	2–7% change in FVC, and $FEV_{1.0}$ in 60 min; no change in FVC and $FEV_{1.0}$ at 180 min	Sauder (1986)
7.5	2	Oral (mouthpiece)	No change in $FEV_{1.0}$ or R_{aw}	Radar (1977)
*Individual with asthma in clinical studies*
2.0	40	Oronasal (chamber, with exercise)	No change in FVC, $FEV_{1.0}$, MMEF (1987) $(n=12)$	Witek et al. (1987)
3.0	10	Oral (mouthpiece, with exercise)	No change in sR_{aw}	Sheppard et al. (1984)
3.0	60	Oronasal (chamber)	No change in FVC, $FEV_{1.0}$, $FEF_{25-75\%}$ SG_{aw}	Green et al. (1987)
*Individual with occupational exposure*
0.3–0.6	8 hour work	Oronasal (at work)	Small (≥ 200 ml) change in FVC and $FEV_{1.0}$ $(n=38)$	Alexandersson and Hedenstierna (1988)
2.0	40	Oronasal (chamber, with exercise)	No change in FVC, $FEV_{1.0}$, MMEF $(n=15)$	Schachter et al. (1987)
0.1–3.0	20	Oronasal (face mask)	$12 \pm 2\%$ decrease in $FEV_{1.0}$ as compared to $8 \pm 3\%$ in control; little or no change in MMEF and other measures	Frigas et al. (1984)
1.8	30	Oronasal (chamber)	13% decrease in $FEV_{1.0}$ $(n=4)$	Burge et al. (1985)
2.0	20	Oronasal (chamber)	Decreases in R_{aw} in 12 of 230 (5%) persons	Nordman (1985)
3.2	30	Oronasal (chamber)	12% decrease in $FEV_{1.0}$ $(n=8)$; three with decrease $>25\%$ in $FEV_{1.0}$	Burge et al. (1985)

[a] Abbreviations: FVC, forced vital capacity; $FEV_{1.0}$, forced expiratory flow at 1.0 second; $FEF_{25-75\%}$, mean of forced expiratory flow at 25% and 75% vital capacity; $(s)R_{aw}$, (specific) airway resistance; MMEF, midmaximal expiratory flow; $(s)G_{aw}$, (specific) airway conductance.

Few data exist comparing possible formaldehyde effects on minute volumes in humans with this well-documented effect noted in laboratory animals. This is unfortunate because this information would be useful if directly compared to the symptomatic responses noted within the same species.

Airway Reactivity Following an initial, transient bronchoconstriction (typically produced only at high, i.e., ≥ 10 ppm, concentrations), aldehydes can influence the underlying bronchial reactivity of the airways. Several other irritants (sulfur dioxide, ozone, and toluene diisocyanate) that induce an immediate bronchoconstriction also can induce bronchial hyperreactivity. Hyperreactivity is experimentally defined as heightened responsiveness to inhaled methacholine (a stable form of acetylcholine) or histamine and is a diagnostic feature of asthma (Boushey et al., 1980; Barnes et al., 1989). Following a single initial exposure of healthy individuals, this condition is typically reversible; it lasts for 12 to 48 hours. In persons with asthma, however, this condition can persist for several years. Hyperreactivity frequently lacks an immunologic component and is thus termed nonspecific. In these cases no identifiable causative antigen can be found, and a general heightened response is noted after a wide range of irritant stimuli. The relationship between each phase of the dual responses (e.g., an immediate and/or a delayed decrease in $FEV_{1.0}$) after antigen presentation/challenge and hyperreactivity is currently unclear.

Previously this laboratory reported that formaldehyde exposure of guinea pigs for 2 hours produced a small change in pulmonary resistance with an estimated half-maximal change in bronchial reactivity of 8.0 ppm (Swiecichowski et al., 1993). When the duration of exposure was extended to 8.0 hours, 1.1 ppm formaldehyde produced a significant increase in reactivity. This study suggests that low-level exposures of several hours may have effects not detectable with shorter (≤ 2 h) exposures.

Bronchial reactivity has been examined in humans, and no changes have been recorded in healthy persons after exposures up to 3.0 ppm formaldehyde for three hours (Sauder et al., 1986; Kulle et al.,1987; Green et al.,1987). In studies with persons with asthma, however, Witek et al. (1987) reported a decrease in the dose of methacholine necessary to produce a 20% decrease in forced expiratory volume in 1 second in 8 of 12 individuals following a 40 minute exposure to 2 ppm formaldehyde. The mean response for all 12 subjects was not statistically different from control; thus further study is required before any conclusions on the effect of formaldehyde on airway reactivity can be drawn. Burge et al. (1985) also has suggested that a relationship exists between bronchial responses of subjects with previous occupational exposure to formaldehyde and their underlying bronchial reactivity.

Mucociliary Clearance Formaldehyde markedly inhibits mucociliary clearance in animals and humans (Table 12-8). This effect was noted as early as 1942 by Cralley (1942), who observed an inhibition and complete stasis of ciliary beating after formaldehyde exposure. As concerns arose about the health effects of cigarette smoke, several investigators (Guillerm et al., 1961; Wynder and Hoffman, 1963; Falk, 1963; Kensler and Battista, 1963; Carson et al., 1966; Dalhamn and Rosengren, 1971) confirmed that aldehydes in smoke can alter ciliary function and extended this observation, finding that formaldehyde exposure as short as 12 seconds could reversibly inhibit ciliary activity.

The onset and duration of the effects of formaldehyde on mucociliary clearances are dose dependent. Formaldehyde exposures initially diminish the movement of the surface mucus layer before decreasing ciliary beat frequency (Morgan et al., 1984). Morgan et al. (1984) have proposed that this results from covalent reactions of formaldehyde with macromolecules in the mucus that impair the physical (rheologic) properties essential for effective energy coupling with the underlying cilia. In addition Hastie et al. (1990) have

TABLE 12-8 Formaldehyde Inhibition of Mucociliary Clearance in Laboratory Animals

Cotncentration	Duration of Exposure	Response	Species	Reference
20 ppm	10 min	Depression of ciliary activity without recovery	Rabbit	Cralley (1942)
10 ppm	—	Cilia stasis in 20%	Rabbit	Dalhamn and Rosengren (1971)
52 ppm	—	Cilia stasis in 90%	Rabbit	Dalhamn and Rosengren (1971)
32 ppm	11.5 min	Cilia stasis	Guinea pig	Oomichi and Kita (1974)
20 ppm	4 hours	Decrease early clearance of particles; no effect on delayed clearance (alveolar)	Rat (Sprague Dawley)	Mannix et al. (1983)
9.6 ppm	30 min	Increase mucus flow rate at 2 min; muco- and cilia stasis at 2 and 3 min	Frog palate	Morgan et al. (1984)
4.4 ppm	30 min	Mucostasis in 8 min	Frog palate	Morgan et al. (1984)
1.4 ppm	30 min	Increase in clearance	Frog palate	Morgan et al. (1984)
0.2 ppm	30 min	No effect	Frog palate	Morgan et al. (1984)
66 $\mu g/cm^2$	60 min	Reduced ciliary activity within 10 min	Rabbit and pig	Hastie et al. (1990)
33 $\mu g/cm^2$	60 min	Reduced ciliary activity within 10–20 min	Rabbit and pig	Hastie et al. (1990)
16 $\mu g/cm^2$	60 min	Reduced ciliary activity within 30–40 min	Rabbit and pig	Hastie et al. (1990)

demonstrated that doses of formaldehyde sufficient to inhibit ciliary activity can also reduce the number of cilia extractable from exposed tissue preparations. In cilia recovered from exposed epithelia, the specific activity of ATPase and dyneins and tubulin protein content are decreased. These responses were reversible in less than two hours after exposure, suggesting that recovery is not dependent on de novo protein synthesis and that ciliary loss and recovery are a dynamic process. In isolated tissue preparations, responses to formaldehyde are dose dependent, and a single exposure to a concentration of 1 to 5 ppm produces no effect or increases mucus transport rates, whereas concentrations between 5 and 10 ppm depress transport (Table 12-8). In animals, depression of overall particle clearance has been noted at a concentration of 20 ppm (4 hour exposure) in rats (Mannix et al., 1983; Adams et al., 1987). In humans, however, nasal particle clearance was depressed at concentrations as low as 0.24 ppm (4–5 h), with maximal effects observed at concentrations of 0.4 ppm (Anderson and Molhave, 1983). These effects on clearance are most prominent in the anterior portion of the nose.

Clearance is dependent on mucus composition, mucus quantity, and ciliary function. Clearance can be compromised in humans at concentrations below those necessary to produce single effects in preparations in vitro (i.e., decreased ciliary beat frequency). This suggests that this compound acts through interference with more than a single cellular or extracellular process. For example, it is probable that ciliary proteins are sensitive to formaldehyde (Hastie et al., 1990) and that protein–protein methylene crosslinks in mucus can alter the tertiary structure of this glycoprotein (Morgan et al., 1984). Acting together, these effects could diminish clearance at lower doses.

Effects of Aerosol-Formaldehyde Coexposures   Amdur (1960), the creator of many innovative insights in inhalation toxicology, reported that formaldehyde-induced increases in the respiratory resistance of guinea pigs were potentiated by the simultaneous administration of submicrometer sodium chloride aerosol (sodium chloride alone produced no effect). A response induced by a formaldehyde concentration delivered as a formaldehyde-aerosol mixture when breathed through the nose was greater than the response to the same formaldehyde dose (gas alone) when administered directly to the lung through a tracheal cannula. This interesting observation suggests that the increment added by the aerosol is not solely a result of the transfer of more formaldehyde to the lungs but that it may reflect additional factors. Similarly Kilburn and McKenzie (1978) reported that coexposure of formaldehyde with carbon particles produces greater recruitment of leukocytes into the airway epithelium and epithelial cytotoxicity (cytoplasmic vacuolization and nuclear aberrations) in trachea and bronchi of Syrian golden hamsters. This effect peaked 24 to 48 hours after exposure. Because many environmental exposures involve coexposure to ambient and occupational aerosols, future investigations clarifying these issues would add greatly to our understanding of how complex mixtures act in concert to exert aldehyde toxicity.

Other Aldehydes

Symptomatic Responses and Respiratory Mechanics   The decrease in respiratory rate induced by a wide array of aldehydes has been tested in mice by Steinhagen and Barrow (1984). In this experimental system, α,β-unsaturated aliphatic aldehydes, acrolein, and crotonaldehyde decreased respiratory rate at half-maximal concentration (ED_{50}) of 1.0 and 3.5 ppm as compared to 3.1 ppm for formaldehyde. In contrast, the half-maximal dose for acetaldehyde was much greater (> 2845 ppm). Saturated aliphatic aldehydes with two or more carbons (e.g., butyraldehyde or propionaldehyde) had half-maximal concentrations of 750 to 4200 ppm, whereas cyclic aldehydes (e.g., 3-cylcohexane-1-carboxyldehyde or benzaldehyde) exerts its effects in intermediate doses ranging from 60 to 400 ppm. Thus the relative potency was acrolein > crotonaldehyde ≥ formaldehyde > benzaldehyde > acetaldehyde.

This apparent relationship holds for most other toxic endpoints, including measures of pulmonary function in humans (Pattle and Cullumbine, 1956), half-maximal lethal dose in mice, guinea pigs, and rabbits (Salem and Cullumbine, 1960), and nasal pathology in rats (Lam et al., 1985, Roemer et al., 1993, Cassee et al., 1996b).

Acrolein at doses less than 1.0 ppm can produce a number of pulmonary effects. Murphy, Klingshirn, and Ulrich (1963) reported increases in pulmonary resistance and decreases in respiratory rate in guinea pigs exposed to 0.4–1.0 ppm acrolein. As with exposure to formaldehyde, these changes were rapid in onset, remained somewhat constant (response plateau) during exposure, and reversed within 60 minutes after exposure. Atropine inhibited the acrolein-induced change in resistance, suggesting that involvement of a vagally mediated cholinergic pathway. That this response is so readily reversible with cessation of exposure also suggests that continuous occupancy of an irritant receptor by acrolein during inhalation is necessary for the initiation of this reflex. Microelectrode recordings of trigeminal nerve fibers during inhalation of aldehydes (Kulle and Cooper, 1975) are consistent with involvement of this neural pathway in the decrease in respiratory rate (Kane and Alaire, 1977). The role of specific sensory afferent pathways was further examined by Lee et al. (1992), who reported that acrolein inhalation evoked an inhibitory effect on breathing with a prolongation of expiration and bradycardia. Through a number of interventions, these authors found that acrolein stimulated both vagal C-fiber active afferents and rapidly adapting irritant receptors, and that the elongation of expiration was due to stimulation of the former afferent pathway.

Airway Reactivity   In addition to the transient increase in baseline pulmonary resistance, acrolein exposure of 0.8 ppm (2 h) can produce in bronchial reactivity in guinea pigs (Leikauf et al., 1989a). Hyperreactivity occurred as early as 1 hour after exposure to 1.3 ppm, became maximal at 2 to 6 hours, and lasted for longer than 24 hours. This response was accompanied by an increase in three bronchoactive eicosanoids (prostaglandin $F_{2\alpha}$, thromboxane B_2, and leukotriene C_4) in bronchoalveolar lavage fluid. Inhibition of 5-lipoxygenase diminished the response (Leikauf et al., 1989b), indicating lower respiratory tract epithelial injury. An increase in leukocyte infiltration was also noted, occurring 6 to 24 hours after exposure. These findings suggest that acrolein-induced hyperreactivity occurred by a pathway dependent on acute injury to the airway epithelium and mediator release. In addition migration of leukocytes into the airway does not precede hyperreactivity, suggesting that injury to cells normally present in the lung during exposure produces the mediators responsible for hyperreactivity. Ben-Jebria et al. (1995) found that lumenal exposure of isolated ferret trachea to 0.3 ppm acrolein for 1 hour decreased the contractile dose of cholinergeric agonists (carbachol or acetylcholine) and increased the maximal contraction (indicative of increased smooth muscle reactivity).

Subsequently Turner et al. (1993a) examined airway responses to intravenous substance P following acrolein exposure. Guinea pigs were exposed twice to 1.6 ppm acrolein (7.5 h/d on 2 consecutive days) and followed for up to 28 days. Again, pulmonary inflammation and epithelial damage were prominent one day after acrolein exposure. Neutral endopeptidase (NEP) activity was decreased in the lungs, trachea, and liver 1 and 7 days after acrolein exposure. Twenty-eight days after exposure, NEP activity in the lungs and liver was not significantly different in vehicle- and acrolein-exposed guinea pigs, but it was still reduced in tracheal tissue. Acrolein increased airway reactivity to substance P that lasted for up to 28 days following exposure. Thiorphan, a NEP inhibitor, potentiated this response. To further investigate the role of neuropeptides in acrolein-induced airway responses, a subsequent study with capsaicin-treated guinea pigs exposed to acrolein was performed (Turner et al., 1993b). Capsaicin depletes neuropeptides from C-sensory fibers, and this resulted in 100% mortality (12 of 12 guinea pigs) within 24 hours of two 7.5 h × 1.6 ppm exposures. This result compared with only 14% mortality in guinea pigs exposed to acrolein alone. Pretreatment with capsaicin also exacerbated pulmonary inflammation and epithelial necrosis and denudation. Thus acrolein activates airway C-fibers, which release neuropeptides and alter breathing. The resulting shallow breathing patterns may be protective by reducing deposition in the distal airways.

Human studies have been performed with acetaldehyde. Myou et al. (1993) found that nine subjects with asthma had a dose-dependent decrease in $FEV_{1.0}$ following 2 minute inhalations of an aerosol of saline and acetaldehyde (0, 5, 10, 20, and 40 mg/ml) solution. In control subjects without alcohol sensitivity acetaldehyde had no effect on lung function. Five of the subjects with asthma also had alcohol-induced bronchoconstriction, a common feature among Japanese. As stated above, alcohol sensitivity is due to a dual inheritance of a rapid isoform of alcohol dehydrogenase with a slow isoform of aldehyde dehydrogenase-2. This allelic combination increases the formation of acetaldehyde and decreases it with subsequent clearance; it is carried by 20% of persons of Asian lineage. It is further enriched among Japanese asthma patients, among whom over 50% were found to have alcohol intolerance (Gong et al. 1981; Watanabe, 1991). However, this factor did not explain the effect of inhaled acetaldehyde observed by Myou et al. (1993), since 4 of the 9 asthma patients were not alcohol intolerant, yet they responded like the patients that were alcohol intolerant. Although the sample size of these populations is small, it is possible that persons with asthma may be at greater risk to the bronchoconstrictive effects of acetaldehyde. These results are much like the immediate bronchoconstriction that has been noted after sulfur dioxide exposure (Sheppard et al., 1984).

Mucociliary Clearance and Defense Mechanisms   Along with studies with formaldehyde, mucociliary function have been studied with other aldehydes. Unlike reported bronchoconstriction, Dalhamn and Rosengren (1971) found that the effects and dosimetry of formaldehyde were comparable to acrolein and crotonaldehyde in potency in the inhibition of cilia beating. Acetaldehyde was much less potent. Changes in ciliary beat can also be accompanied by alteration in mucus load. Borchers et al. (1998) found that acrolein exposure increases mucin (predominately MUC5ac) transcript and protein levels in rats.

Because acrolein has greater penetration of the upper respiratory tract than formaldehyde, effects of acrolein on other lung defense mechanisms have been examined. Exposure to 1 to 2 ppm acrolein significantly suppresses intrapulmonary killing in mice challenged with bacteria (Jakab, 1977; Astry and Jakab, 1983; Aranyi et al., 1986; Jakab, 1993), suggesting that host defense mechanisms of distal airway and alveolus are impaired. Macrophage activation and dysfunction induced by acrolein have also been observed in vitro (Leffingwell and Low, 1979; Grundfest et al.,1982; Sherwood et al., 1986; Jakab, 1993; Li, 1997). Thus damage to the lower respiratory tract is more likely after exposures to aldehydes other than formaldehyde, and some of these compounds (i.e., unsaturated aliphatic aldehydes) have equal or greater potency than formaldehyde.

Even though acrolein can penetrate to the distal lung more than formaldehyde, the effects of acrolein (2.5 ppm) can be enhanced by coexposure with carbon black particulate matter (10 mg/m³). Following exposure to each agent or coexposures of 4 h/d for four days, Jakab (1993) challenged Swiss mice with different infectious agents: *Staphylococcus aureus* to evaluate alveolar macrophage (AM) surveillance, *Proteus mirabilis* to evaluate AMs and polymorphonuclear leukocytes (PMNs) surveillance, *Listeria monocytogenes* to evaluate lymphokine-mediated cellular immunity, and influenza A virus for the cytotoxic T-cell-mediated cellular immunity. Only coexposure-produced effects suppressed the intrapulmonary killing of *S. aureus* a day after exposure, with a return to control levels by day 7. In contrast, the coexposure enhanced the intrapulmonary killing of *P. mirabilis* possibly resulting from a significant increase in PMNs recovered in lung lavage fluid (also only noted following coexposure with infection). Combined exposure to carbon black and acrolein also impaired elimination of *L. monocytogenes* and influenza A virus from the lungs. Exposure of alveolar macrophage to these concentrations directly, suppressed Fc-receptor-mediated phagocytosis for up to 11 days (Jakab and Hemenway, 1993), which agrees with diminished *S. aureus* surveillance. However, the effect was short-lived in vivo.These studies suggest that the carbon black particle acts as a carrier for acrolein to enhance penetration to the distal airway and alveolar regions of the lung.

EFFECTS OF MULTIPLE EXPOSURES

Formaldehyde

Carcinogenesis Formaldehyde is a probable human carcinogen based on (1) in vitro and in vivo genotoxic studies, (2) sufficient evidence in experimental animals (inhalation studies), and (3) limited evidence in humans (epidemiological studies) (IARC, 1995). Of these three types of studies, the findings from long-term animal exposures are the most convincing.

Formaldehyde has genotoxic effects in a wide number of in vitro systems (Auerbach et al., 1977; Ma and Harris, 1988; WHO, 1989; Feron et al., 1991; IARC, 1995). The level of activity in many experimental systems is often either weak or moderate compared to other known mutagens and can depend on what are sometimes unique experimental conditions. Regardless of these caveats, formaldehyde is clearly capable of reacting with cellular macromolecules (see above), and DNA damage induced by formaldehyde includes DNA–protein crosslinks and single-strand breaks (Fornance, 1982; Fornance et al., 1982; Graftstrom et al.,1984, IARC, 1995). DNA–protein crosslinks have been found in vivo in the nasal passages of Fisher 344 rats and rhesus monkeys (Heck et al., 1989, Casanova et al., 1991). Graftstrom et al. (1984) also found that DNA single-strand breaks could accumulate in the presence of DNA excision repair inhibitors and that formaldehyde can inhibit repair.

Studies examining genotoxic effects in bacteria, yeast, fungi, and *Drosophila* produce varied responses. For example, mutations in *Drosophila* are only noted in male larvae under culture conditions requiring adenosine, adenylic acid, or RNA medium supplementations. In mammalian systems the results are also subtle, complex, and varied. As noted by Boreiko and Ragan (1983), formaldehyde has been found to induce sister-chromatid exchange in Chinese hamster ovary cells by one investigator (Obe and Beck, 1979), but not by another (Brusick 1983). In addition formaldehyde is not mutagenic in either of these cells (Hsie et al., 1979). Another illustration of the complexity associated with the evaluation of formaldehyde's genotoxic effects is that it can induce unscheduled DNA synthesis, which has been recorded in HeLa cells (Martin et al., 1978) but not in monkey kidney cells (Nocentini et al., 1980). In vivo dominant lethal assays in mice have been found to be negative or transiently positive (Epstein, 1972; Fontignie-Houbrechts, 1981). In any case, formaldehyde has been found to facilitate malignant transformation of mouse embryo C3H10T1/2 C18 fibroblasts, acting through either an "initiating" or a "promoting" mechanism (Ragan and Boreiko, 1981; Boreiko and Ragan, 1983; Frazelle et al., 1983), and to directly cause DNA single-strand breaks and DNA–protein crosslinks (Graftstrom et al., 1984).

Mutational spectrum induced by formaldehyde was studied in human lymphoblasts in vitro, in *Escherichia coli* and in naked pSV2gpt plasmid DNA (Crosby et al., 1988). In lymphoblasts large visible deletions of some or all the X -linked hprt bands were detect by Southern blot analysis (Liber et al., 1989). In *E. coli*, mutations in the xanthine guanine phosphoribosyl transferase (gprt) gene included large insertions (41%), large deletions (18%), and point mutations (41%). Many of the point mutations were GC transversions. Higher doses of formaldehyde yielded 92% point mutations, 62% of which were single AT transitions. Therefore formaldehyde-induced genetic alterations in *E. coli* are concentration dependent. Exposure of a SV2gpt plasmid DNA (with transformation into *E coli)* resulted in frame shifts mutations.

Chronic inhalation of formaldehyde induces squamous cell carcinoma in the nasal cavity of rats (Swenberg et al., 1980; Albert et al., 1982; Kerns et al., 1983, Sellakumar et al., 1985, Feron et al., 1988; Woutersen et al., 1989). Exposure to 14.3 ppm formaldehyde (6 h/d × 5 d/wk × 24 wk) produced carcinomas in 103 of 240 (43%) Fischer 344 rats and in two of 240 C57BL/6 × C3H F1 mice (Kerns et al., 1983; Morgan et al., 1986). Subsequently Recico et al. (1992) examined 11 rat nasal squamous cell carcinomas and found point C or G mutations in regions II–V of the tumor suppressor gene, p53, in five tumors. These mutations particularly a CpG dinucleotide at rat codon 271, i.e., (codon 273 in humans) were mutational hot spots occurring in many human cancers. Sprague-Dawley rats also respond to 14.2 ppm formaldehyde, but the time to onset was delayed and the total carcinoma incidence was less (38 squamous cell carcinoma, or 38% and 10 polyps or papillomas in 100 rats) (Albert et al., 1982). Wistar rats yielded 6 tumors in 132 animals exposed to 20 ppm formaldehyde for 4 to 13 weeks, and followed by observation to 126 weeks (Feron et al., 1988). Although the exposure period and concentration varied, these results suggest that strain differences exist in rats (Fisher 344 ≥ Sprague-Dawley > Wistar strain) and that rats are more sensitive than mice.

The formaldehyde concentration — carcinoma response relationship is nonlinear in rats. In Fisher 344 rats, exposure to 5.6 ppm formaldehyde resulted in two rats (of 240 exposed) with squamous carcinomas, and 2.0 ppm produced no carcinomas (Kerns et al., 1983). Similarly Woutersen et al. (1989) found squamous-cell carcinoma in 1 of 26 Wistar rats exposed to 10 ppm for 28 months. (However, 15 of 58 rats developed carcinomas when the nasal epithelium was injured before exposure.) Swenberg and associates (1983) ascribed this nonlinearity in response to be due to nonlinearity in the formaldehyde dosimetry to its macromolecular target site. This nonlinear dosimetry results in part from variability of the breathing pattern during exposure, which influences the inhaled dose. (As noted above, formaldehyde deposition in mice exposed to 14 ppm were equivalent to those in rats exposed to 5.6 ppm. Consistent with this dosimetry estimate was the incidence of carcinomas: 2/240 in mice after 14 ppm and in rats after 5.6 ppm.) In addition to altered breathing pattern, these investigators have ascribed the nonlinearity in the dose–response relationship to the nonlinearity of cytotoxicity and overloading of protective mechanisms (including metabolic biotransformation, mucociliary clearance, and DNA repair) induced at higher formaldehyde concentrations.

In Syrian golden hamsters, 10 ppm formaldehyde alone (5 h/d × 5 d/wk for life) did not produce nasal carcinomas (Dalbey, 1982). In the exposed group, however, the mortality was marked, with only 20 of 88 animals surviving 10 weeks of treatment. In these animals, nasal epithelial cell hyperplasia or metaplasia was observed. When hamsters were exposed to formaldehyde before exposure to another carcinogen, diethylnitrosamine, the incidence of respiratory carcinomas increased. Formaldehyde (30 ppm) exposures were for 48 hours before subcutaneous injections with 0.5 mg diethylnitrosamine (each once a week for 10 weeks). About twice as many tracheal adenomas (per tumor-bearing hamster) were observed when compared to hamsters exposed to diethylnitrosamine alone. When formaldehyde was given after diethylnitrosamine, no increase in adenomas was observed. Formaldehyde clearly produces nasal carcinomas in rats, and although mice and hamsters are less sensitive than rats, nasal tumors have been observed in mice, and nasal hyper- and metaplasia have been observed in hamsters.

The nasal epithelial disruption has been investigated in several species including mice, rats, hamsters, and monkeys (Chang et al., 1983; Rusch et al., 1983; Maronpot et al., 1986; Morgan et al., 1986; Al-Abbas et al., 1986; Zwart et al., 1988; Monticello et al.,1989; Monticello et al., 1991; Bhalla et al., 1991; Cassee et al., 1996b; Cohen Hubal et al., 1997). In each species tested, the anterior nasal epithelium portion is most affected, although there are some species differences in the regional distribution of epithelial lesions. Repeated exposures to nearly comparable concentrations (about 5–6 ppm) produced loss of cilia and various stages of hyperplasia and squamous metaplasia of pseudostratified columnar respiratory epithelium and leukocyte infiltration. In Fischer 344 rats these changes were most severe in the maxilloturbinate, the lateral aspect of the nasoturbinate, and the wall of the lateral meatus (Morgan et al.,1986), whereas in the rhesus monkey changes were most severe in the middle turbinate. In both species many of the effects found after a single exposure become more persistent, and the percentage of nasal surface area affected progressed when exposures are extended.

Formaldehyde also increases nasal epithelial proliferation rate. In monkeys, the effects were more persistent than those observed in rats. In rats the proliferation rate returned to control values after 3 to 9 days at 1 to 6 ppm (Morgan et al., 1986; Cassee et al., 1996a, 1989). In contrast, in monkeys the proliferation rates remained elevated longer and areas of effected epithelium were more widespread. Increases in cell proliferation were observed in the nasopharynx, trachea, and carina of the lungs of monkeys as compared to only in the anterior nasal cavity of rats (Monticello et al.,1989). Since monkeys, like humans, breathe through both the nose and the mouth, the involvement of the lower respiratory tract may also be possible in humans.

Epidemiological studies have examined the cancer mortality among persons with occupational and residential exposure to formaldehyde. This topic remains controversial, and it has been reviewed extensively elsewhere (Blair et al., 1990; Feron et al., 1991; Partanen, 1993; McLaughin, 1995; IARC, 1995, Collins et al., 1997). Considering animal toxicological data, most concern has been directed at carcinomas of the nasal cavity. Remarkably, conclusive evidence supporting an association between formaldehyde and nasal cancer in humans is lacking. Increased relative risk for nasal cancer has been associated with formaldehyde exposure in several case-control studies (Olsen et al., 1986; Hayes et al., 1986; Roush et al.,1987; Vaughan et al., 1989; Luce et al., 1993) but not in two others (Hernberg et al., 1983; Brinton et al., 1985). This association has not always been supported by comparable increases in the standard mortality ratio in several cohort studies for nasal cancer (Marsh, 1982; Acheson et al., 1984a,b; Levine et al., 1984; Stroup et al., 1986; Blair et al., 1986; Hayes et al., 1990;Gardner et al., 1993; Marsh et al., 1994).

In contrast to nasal cancer, positive associations of formaldehyde exposure have been noted more frequently with nasopharyngeal cancer. This association has been noted in 3 of 4 case-control (Olsen et al., 1984, 1986; Vaughan et al., 1986; Roush et al., 1987; West et al., 1993) and 2 of 5 cohort (Blair et al., 1986; Hayes et al., 1990; Gardner et al., 1993; Marsh et al., 1994; Andjelkovich et al., 1995) epidemiological studies. Three meta-analyses (Blair et al., 1990; Partanen, 1993; Collins et al., 1997) of the later data suggest a small to moderate increase in relative risk (1.2–2.1). This relationship was further reconsidered by Collins et al. (1997) who proposed that underreporting (when no nasopharyngeal cancer is observed in a number of studies of small sample size) influenced the outcome. They found that when studies of small sample size are added to the meta-analysis, the meta-relative risk for cohort studies decreases to 1.0 (with 95% confidence interval of 0.5–1.8). It is also important to consider the small number of observed cases (less than 10 nasopharyngeal cancer in total) used in these analyses.

However, none to slight increases in risks for other cancers have been noted, these include respiratory (buccal cavity, oropharynx, pharynx, and lung) (Walrath and Fraumeri,

1983; Acheson et al., 1984b; Liebling et al.,1984; Sterling and Arundel, 1985; Stayner et al.,1986; Vaughan et al.,1986a; Bertazzi et al., 1986; Blair et al., 1987) and nonrespiratory sites (brain, lymphatic and hematopoietic, prostate, and skin) (Harrington and Shannon, 1975; Walrath and Fraumeri, 1984; Blair et al., 1986; Hagmar et al., 1986; Stayner et al., 1988). Most of the increases in cancer risk at other sites lack correlation with duration or intensity of exposure. This lapse has been explained in part as a strong self-selection effect because of irritant responses (healthy worker effect in occupational populations), difficulties in retrospective assessments of exposure, and potential confounding factors (e.g., wood dust exposure) (Acheson et al.,1967; Olsen et al.,1984; Sterling and Weinkam, 1988; Blair and Stewart, 1990; IARC, 1995; Collins, 1997). For example, an increased risk of nonrespiratory cancer mortality has often been associated with formaldehyde exposure in embalmers, and these individuals have exposures to complex mixtures of materials. Formaldehyde alone is also unlikely to be responsible for these systemic carcinomas, given its rapid metabolism at sites of entry.

Cytology of the nasal mucosa has also been examined in formaldehyde-exposed workers (Berke, 1987; Edling et al., 1988; Holmstrom, 1989; Boysen et al., 1990). Abnormalities observed include loss of cilia, goblet cell hyperplasia, squamous metaplasia, and mild dysplasia, but as with cancer mortality, these changes do not exhibit dose–response relationships and are confounded by coexposure to particulate matter, including wood dust. Increases in squamous metaplasia in individuals living in homes with urea-formaldehyde insulation have also been inconsistent with exposure (Broder et al., 1988; Broder et al., 1991). In contrast, Ballarin et al. (1992) found significant levels of epithelial abnormalities in 15 subjects exposed to urea-formaldehyde glue in a plywood factory. Exposed workers had higher frequencies of micronuclei and dysplasia of nasal epithelial cells and nasal inflammation (leukocyte infiltrates) when compared to age-and sex-matched control subjects.

In summary, formaldehyde produces a complex array of genotoxic effects in in vitro systems and consistently has been found to induce squamous carcinoma in the nasal cavity of laboratory animals (at concentrations exceeding 5.0 ppm) with correlated histopathological changes (at concentrations exceeding 1.0 ppm). Available epidemiological studies are conflicting or insufficient to confirm an increased risk of cancer in exposed humans. Evidence of an increased risk of nasopharyngeal cancer in humans from epidemiological studies is suggestive but controversial, and evidence for nasal cancer is limited. Evidence for cancer at other sites (including lung) is equivocal and hard to reconcile with exposure. Together these findings indicate that formaldehyde should remain a Group 2A Suspected (or Probable) human carcinogen (IARC, 1995; ACGIH, 1998), and exposures should be restricted accordingly.

Other Responses to Multiple Exposure   Repeated formaldehyde exposure can result in eye and upper respiratory tract irritation, declines in pulmonary function, and can initiate skin sensitization. Except for skin sensitization, these effects are often readily reversible with cessation of exposure and depend more on the exposure concentration (threshold dose) than on the exposure duration (cumulative dose). Such effects may be viewed as repeated immediate responses to acute exposure rather than persistent, irreversible dysfunction produced by cumulative degradation of defense mechanisms and initiation of compensatory processes.

Eye, nose, and throat irritation are often the most common compliant of individuals with occupational or residential formaldehyde exposures. In occupational studies, Alexandersson and Hedenstierna (1988), for example, found that exposures of 0.3 to 0.5 ppm during a work shift led to symptoms. Likewise Horvath et al. (1988) found that across-shift responses of sore throat and burning nose increased at concentrations ≤ 0.4 ppm. Control responses were 3% to 4%, and after exposure 8% to 15% responded. These responses followed a dose–response relationship with 22% to 36% and 33% to 55%, responding at < 1.0 and < 3.0 ppm, respectively. Although these exposures occurred in a population with repetitive exposure, the threshold dose or frequency of reported symptoms does not differ remarkably from that observed after a single exposure (Anderson and Molhave, 1983; Bender et al., 1983).

Residential exposures demonstrate similar results with one difference: effects, particularly eye irritation, are noted with greater frequency at low concentrations. For example, whereas Horvath et al. (1988) found about 8% to 15% positive respondents after occupational exposure, Hanrahan et al. (1984) and Ritchie and Lehnen (1987) found 22% to 32% positive respondents for eye irritation after residential exposure to nearly equivalent concentrations (0.3 ppm). Ritchie and Lehnen (1987) also found nearly 90% of persons exposed to ≥ 0.3 ppm reporting eye irritation. One reason for this difference may be that residential exposures are of longer duration (Fig.12-1). As mentioned previously, Anderson and Molhave (1983) also found that reports of eye irritation increase, whereas nose and throat irritation complaints decreased during extended exposure. Because these responses are subjective, this difference may also be explained by a greater willingness to tolerate symptoms at work than at home. Lastly, these study populations differ in sex and age distributions. Together these studies suggest that irritant-related responses will occur in humans at concentrations of ≥ 0.3 ppm.

Pulmonary function after repeated formaldehyde exposure in occupational settings has also been examined. One type of study involves comparison of forced expiratory flows and volumes (e.g., $FEV_{1.0}$) before and after an 8 hours work shift. Exposures in these studies ranged from 0.1 to 3.0 ppm (typically averaging 0.5 ppm) and yielded slight declines that are associated with single exposures (Schoenberg and Mitchell, 1975: Gamble et al., 1976; Alexandersson et al., 1982; Kilburn et al., 1985; Horvath et al., 1988; Uba et al., 1989; Khamgaonkar and Fulare, 1991).

Baseline values obtained Monday morning (after no exposures for two days) in each of these studies, however, typically showed no difference from control values, indicating that the cross-shift declines are reversible and are unlikely to lead to a persistent pulmonary dysfunction. In one study by Alexandersson and Hedenstierna (1988), however, such a Monday-morning decrement in $FEV_{1.0}$ and FVC was noted, suggestive of a persistent change. However, these changes correlate neither with peak exposure nor with duration of employment and thus offer only limited support for the contention that persistent changes are a consequence of repetitive exposure.

In each of the six above cross-shift studies, small but measurable decreases in $FEV_{1.0}$ were observed. In most cases these changes resulted from exposure to concentrations ≤ 0.5 ppm. This dose threshold is in good agreement with that of the acute respiratory effect reported in guinea pigs by Amdur (1960), which equaled 0.3 ppm. However, numerous studies of healthy subjects or persons with asthma (exposed in inhalation chambers) failed to observe effects on respiratory function, even at concentrations of 3.0 ppm. Possible explanations include the following: (1) occupational exposures involve a complex atmosphere that may or may not include particulate matter or other contaminants (Amdur, 1960; Kilburn and McKenzie, 1978; Jakab, 1993), (2) the extended occupational exposures (8 h) produce greater effects than 10 to 120 minute tests even at equivalent doses (concentration × time) (Leikauf and Doupnik, 1989, Swiecichowski, 1993), or (3) repeated exposure lowers the threshold of responsiveness without producing chronic effects.

Because symptomatic responses (e.g., eye irritation) occur at a greater frequency following residential exposures of 0.1 to 0.3 ppm formaldehyde when compared to occupational exposures to equivalent concentrations, residential exposure of 0.1 to 0.3 ppm may also produce pulmonary effects. Inasmuch as the current occupational threshold limit value has been set at 0.3 ppm (ACGIH, 1998), a prudent environmental/indoor air level might be between 0.05 and 0.1 ppm, a value recommended by Ritchie and Lehnen (1987). This value may be difficult to achieve, however, unless indoor cigarette smoking is curtailed (see Indoor Air). Epidemiological evidence supportive of this proposal has been obtained by Krzyzanowski et al. (1990), who found an increased pulmonary morbidity (prevalence of asthma and bronchitis) among children living in homes with 0.060 to 0.12 ppm formaldehyde when compared to children living in homes with ≤ 0.04 ppm. Decrements in peak expiratory flow rates were also correlated with formaldehyde exposure. Confirmation of this possible effect has also been reported in an abstract by Czap et al. (1993). These investigators found that the prevalence of physician-diagnosed asthma and asthma-related symptoms were about double for individuals living in home with formaldehyde levels averaging about 0.050 ppm as compared to controls that averaged about 0.005 ppm. Similarly Norback et al. (1995) and Wieslander et al. (1997) reported formaldehyde exposure (mixed with other volatile organic compounds) is associated with an increase in prevalence of asthma, asthma-related symptoms, and blood eosinophil counts. Thus these studies suggest that persistent respiratory effects can result from low-level indoor formaldehyde exposures, and that environmental exposures produce effects at concentration below those that produce observable effects in short-term clinical studies.

Along with direct irritation, topical application of formalin (37% formaldehyde in methanol : water) can initiate allergic reactions including contact dermatitis or systemic responses (anaphylactic shock). Such reactions may result from formaldehyde usage in industrial processes, histological laboratories, dental procedures, or kidney dialysis (reviewed in Chapters 3–13 in Feinman, 1988, and by Bardana and Montanaro, 1991). The mechanisms of these immunologic reactions are still somewhat unclear, but it appears that formaldehyde reactions involve both immediate (antibody-antigen-mediated) and delayed (cell-mediated) hypersensitivity. In immediate hypersensitivity, formaldehyde acts as an incomplete antigen (hapten) through its covalent binding to constituent proteins in the skin or blood, forming new antigenic determinants (Horsfall, 1934). Antibodies to formaldehyde-hemolytic red blood cell membrane protein or formaldehyde-human serum albumin conjugates have been identified and include immunoglobin (Ig)E, IgG, and IgM subtypes (Sandler et al., 1979; Lynen et al., 1983; Maurice et al., 1986; Wilhelmsson and Holmstrom, 1987; Thrasher et al., 1987, 1988; Broughton and Thrasher, 1988; Patterson et al., 1989). Gorski et al. (1992) reported that neutrophils isolated from persons with formaldehyde contact sensitivity who had been exposed to 400 ppb formaldehyde for two hours had higher responses (activation measured by chemiluminescence) than neutrophils isolated from control subjects. Concentrations of formalin causing immediate or delayed skin hypersensitivity (30–55 ppm) in human volunteers are typically lower than those causing irritation (2000 ppm) (Feinman, 1988).

Modulation of cell-mediated immunity, on the other hand, is not as well documented (Pross et al., 1987; Thrasher et al., 1988; Patterson et al., 1989). It also remains unclear whether allergic reaction involving the lung can be initiated solely by inhalation exposure (Hendrick and Lane, 1975, 1977; Hendrick et al., 1982; Lee et al., 1984; Patterson et al., 1989, Bardana and Montanaro, 1991), but it does appear that, although rare, documented dual (immediate and delayed) pulmonary reactions can be evoked in persons with previous occupational exposure (Nordman, 1985; Burge et al., 1985). Although formaldehyde is a weak sensitizing agent in allergic reactions, it may modulate immunity to other more common allergens. Enhancement of sensitization has been demonstrated in mice by Tarkowski and Gorski (1995) who found higher IgE ovalbumin antibody titers following exposure to 1.6 ppm formaldehyde for 10 days after presentation of antigen. Similarly guinea pigs exposed to 0.13 or 0.25 ppm formaldehyde for 5 days before presentation of antigen developed higher IgG ovalbumin antibody levels (ELISA units) when compared to guinea pigs exposed to filtered air (Reidel et al., 1996). These changes were associated with greater epithelial pathology and eosinophilic infiltrates. This suggests that immunologically based bronchial hypersensitivity can occur following formaldehyde exposure alone but that this response is rare. More frequently formaldehyde may enhance sensitization to other, more common respiratory antigens (based on recent animal experimental evidence).

Repeated Exposure to Other Aldehydes

Mutagenicity and Carcinogenicity of Other Aldehydes   Like formaldehyde, several other aldehydes have been found to be genotoxic in microbial, insect, and mammalian systems (Grafstrom, 1990: Feron et al., 1991, Grafstrom et al., 1994, WHO, 1995). Of the more common environmental aldehydes, acetaldehyde, acrolein, benzaldehyde, crotonaldehyde, furfural, and glutaraldehyde can be mutagenic in in vitro assay systems (Vegheli and Osztovics, 1978; Izard and Libermann, 1978; Obe and Beck, 1979; Hemminki et al., 1980; Marnett and Tuttle, 1980; Neudecker et al., 1981; Bird et al., 1982; Marnett et al., 1985; Cooper et al., 1987, Galloway et al., 1987; Reynolds et al., 1987; Hadi et al., 1989, He and Lambert, 1990; Grafstrom et al., 1994, Vaca et al., 1998). Acrolein, for example, can induce DNA single-strand breaks and DNA–protein crosslinks in human bronchial cells (Grafstrom et al., 1988) and guanosine adducts (Chung et al., 1984). Acrolein also was found to affect growth, membrane integrity, and differentiation in human bronchial epithelial cells. These responses may be mediated in part through acrolein's action on cell thiol status (Graftstrom et al., 1988; Grafstrom, 1990), cytoplasmic free Ca^{2+} (Trump et al., 1988), or eicosanoid metabolism (Doupnik and Leikauf, 1990).

When various aldehydes are compared in various geno- and cytotoxic assays, acrolein is often at least as potent as formaldehyde, and both compounds are markedly more potent than acetaldehyde. Interestingly inhalation studies with acetaldehyde, but not acrolein, produce tumors in vivo. Like formaldehyde, acetaldehyde is a suspected human carcinogen because acetaldehyde can induce nasal adeoncarcinoma and squamous cell carcinoma in rats (Woutersen et al., 1986; Woustersen and Feron, 1987) and laryngeal carcinoma in hamsters (Feron and Kruyse, 1977, Feron et al., 1982). The sites of tumors are somewhat different with acetaldehyde than with formaldehyde inasmuch as acetaldehyde (750 ppm) has produced adenocarcinomas of the olfactory epithelium in rats (Woutersen et al., 1986). Histopathological correlates at lower acetaldehyde concentrations (400–1000 ppm) include hyper- and metaplasia, principally in the nasal olfactory epithelium rather than the anterior respiratory epithelium (Appelman et al., 1982; Woustersen et al., 1984, 1986; Cassee et al., 1996b; Morris, 1997). In addition acetaldehyde shares an ability to enhance the tumorigenicity of benzo(a)pyrene in hamsters with formaldehyde (Feron, 1979). In contrast to the animal evidence for acetaldehyde, the animal inhalation studies with acrolein lack evidence for carcinogenesis (Feron et al., 1991; WHO, 1995).

The histological findings following repeated acrolein exposure are similar and dissimilar to those developed after repeated formaldehyde inhalation. Like formaldehyde, but unlike acetaldehyde, the effects of 3.0 ppm acrolein (6 h/d × 5 d/wk × 3 wk) in the nasal cavity are primarily limited to the respiratory epithelium and include degenerative change, squamous metaplasia, and neutrophilic inflammation (Feron et al., 1978; Leach et al., 1987; Monticello et al., 1991; Cassee et al., 1996a). In contrast to formaldehyde, acrolein can also produce effects in the mid- to distal rather than solely anterior portions of the rat nasal cavity (Leach et al., 1987) and can alter the epithelium of the lower respiratory tract (conductive airways and alveolar regions) (Lyon et al., 1970; Kutzman et al., 1985; Costa et al., 1986; Astry and Jakab, 1983; Borchers et al., 1998).

Besides acetaldehyde, malondialdehyde has also been found to be mutagenic in in vitro assays (Mukai and Goldstein, 1976; Shamberger et al., 1979; Yau 1979; Bird et al., 1982; Basu and Marnett, 1983; Marnett et al.,1985) and carcinogenic to mice (Shamberger et al., 1974). This naturally occurring compound, a three-carbon dialdehyde ($O=CH-CH_2-CH=O$), is produced from auto-oxidation (peroxidation) of unsaturated fatty acids (Bernheim et al., 1948; Esterbauer et al., 1982) or during synthesis of prostaglandins (Hamberg and Samuelsson, 1967; Marnett and Tuttle, 1980). Other related compounds, β-ethoxyacrolein and β-methoxyacrolein, are 25 to 40 times more mutagenic than malondialdehyde. Inasmuch as these compounds are the result of common biogenic pathways, they carry potential importance as mediators of spontaneous carcinogenesis, particularly with respect to background-level age-related tumor incidence .

Other Responses to Repeated Exposure   The noncarcinogenic effects of repeated exposure to low-molecular-weight aldehydes other than formaldehyde are less studied. Extended exposure to certain aldehydes may lead to similar symptomatic (upper respiratory tract irritation) effects as formaldehyde (NRC, 1981; Feinman, 1988). These compounds may also produce respiratory effects (WHO, 1992, 1995).

The chronic effects of acrolein and acetaldehyde are the most studied of the various aldehydes. Persistent decrements in pulmonary function in rats have been noted by Costa et al. (1986) after 4.0 ppm acrolein (62 d × 6 h/d × 5 d/wk). Airflow dysfunction was accompanied by focal peribronchial lesions and alterations of structural proteins (elastin). In tests with rats, guinea pigs, dog, and monkey, 0.7 ppm acrolein produced squamous metaplasia of the lungs in monkey (Lyon et al., 1970). This study, like those of Monticello et al. (1989) with formaldehyde and Morris (1997), suggests that obligatory nasal breathers (mouse, rats, and guinea pigs) are somewhat less responsive to chronic lower respiratory effects than oronasal breathers (dogs and monkeys). For example, Lyon et al. (1970) report histopathological effects of 0.22 ppm acrolein (24 h × 90 d) in the lungs of dogs and monkey that were only apparent after 1.0 to 1.8 ppm exposure in rats and guinea pigs. Rats, hamsters, and rabbits were compared after exposures to 0.4, 1.4, and 4.9 ppm acrolein (6 h/d × 5 d/wk × 13 wk) by Feron et al. (1978), who found rats to be more susceptible, responding at 0.4 ppm, whereas hamsters and rabbits were non-responsive at this level.

Low acrolein concentrations (≥ 0.2 ppm) may produce persistent changes in lung function observed at higher doses of formaldehyde (≥ 2 ppm). Unsaturated aliphatic aldehydes (e.g., acrolein) are more chemically reactive and irritating than formaldehyde. Animal studies clearly demonstrate that exposure to 0.3 ppm acrolein can initiate bronchial hyperreactivity, mediator release, and changes in pulmonary histology (Leikauf et al., 1989a, b), and two exposures to 1.6 ppm produced a persistent airway hyperreactivity that lasted up to 28 days in guinea pigs (Turner et al., 1993a). These observations parallel a human account of persistent respiratory effects following a single accidental exposure (Champeix et al., 1966). Acrolein and other compounds are less water soluble than formaldehyde and thus affect the lower, in addition to the upper, respiratory tract.

High (250 ppm) acetaldehyde concentrations will diminish lung function about as much as > 2 ppm formaldehyde. Acetaldehyde produces nasal lesions in the rat at concentrations of 400 ppm (6h/d × 5 d/wk × 4 wk) (Appelman et al., 1982), and in the hamster at concentration of 4000 ppm (6 hr/d × 5 d/wk × 13 wk) (Kruysse et al., 1975). The nasal area most damaged was the olfactory epithelium. In hamsters, tracheal epithelial metaplasia was also noted following the 4000 ppm and a lower 1340 ppm exposure, suggesting that the nasal passages of the hamster are less sensitive than those of the rat. Acetaldehyde may alter lung function in that in Wistar rats exposed to 243 ppm acetaldehyde (8 h/d × 5 d/wk × 5 wk) had altered functional residual capacity, residual volume, total lung capacity, and respiratory frequency (Saldiva et al., 1985).

The potential pulmonary effects of repeated exposures to other aldehydes are unknown. Longer-chain saturated aliphatic aldehydes (e.g., propionaldehyde) are less-toxic, but cyclic aldehydes (e.g., benzaldehyde) have intermediate toxic potency when compared to formaldehyde. Inasmuch as a number of environmental exposures involve the cogeneration of these aldehydes with formaldehyde, the need exists for more details on the extent of environmental exposure (through routine environmental sampling) and toxicological structure–activity relationships of these compounds. Lastly, a number of aldehydes, for example, malondialdehyde or hexanal, are naturally occurring or produced metabolically during oxidative metabolism. A better understanding of the molecular and cellular toxicology of these and other aldehydes is warranted and may be useful to establish a relationship between human exposure and spontaneous carcinogenesis and perhaps even chronic pulmonary disease.

REFERENCES

ACGIH. American Conference of Governmental Industrial Hygienist. 1998. *1998 TLVs and BEIs: Threshold Limit Values for Chemical Substances and Physical Agents Biological Exposure Indices.* Cincinnati. ACGIH.

Acheson, E. D., E. H. Hadfield, and R. G. Macbeth. 1967. Carcinoma of the nasal cavity and accessory sinuses in woodworkers. *Lancet* 1: 311–312.

Acheson, E. D., H. R. Barnes, M. J. Gardner, C. Osmond, B. Pannett, and C. P. Taylor. 1984a. Formaldehyde in the British chemical industry. *Lancet* 1: 611–616.

Acheson, E. D., H. R. Barnes, M. J. Gardner, B. Pannett, C. P. Taylor, and C. Osmond. 1984b. Formaldehyde in process workers and lung cancer. *Lancet* 1: 1066–1067.

Adams, D. O., T. A. Hamilton, L. D. Lauer. and J. H. Dean. 1987. The effect of formaldehyde exposure upon the mononuclear phagocyte system of mice. *Toxicol. Appl. Pharmacol.* 88: 165–174.

Aharonson, E. F., H. Menkes, G. Gatner, D. L. Swift, and D. F. Procter. 1974. Effect of respiratory airflow on the removal of soluble vapors by the nose. *J. Appl. Physiol.* 27: 654–657.

Al-Abbas, A. H., D. Krajci, and K. B. Ibrahim. 1986. The effect of formaldehyde vapour on the tracheal epithelium of albino rat. *Acta Univ. Palacki Olomuc Fac. Med.* 113: 35–52.

Albert, R. E., A. R. Sellakumar, S. Laskin, M. Kuschner, N. Nelson, and C. A. Snyder. 1982. Gaseous formaldehyde and hydrogen chloride induction of nasal cancer in the rat. *J. Natl. Cancer Inst.* 68: 597–603.

Alexandersson, R., and G. Hedenstierna. 1988. Respiratory hazards associated with exposure to formaldehyde and solvents in acid-curing paints. *Arch. Environ. Health* 43: 222–227.

Alexandersson, R., B. Kolmodin-Hedman, and G. Hedenstierna.1982. Exposure to formaldehyde: Effects on pulmonary function. *Arch. Environ. Health* 37: 279–284.

Amdur, M. O. 1960. The response of guinea pigs to inhalation of formaldehyde and formic acid alone and with a sodium chloride areosol. *Int. J. Air Poll.* 3: 201–220.

Anderson, I., and L. Molhave.1983. Controlled human studies in formaldehyde. In *Formaldehyde Toxicity,* ed. J. E. Gibson. Washington, DC: Hemisphere.

Andjelkovich, D. A., D. B. Janzen, M. H. Brown, R. B. Richardson, and F. J. Miller. 1995. Mortality of iron foundry workers. IV. Analysis of a subcohort exposed to formaldehyde. *J. Occup. Med.* 37: 826–837.

Appelman, L. M., R. A. Woutersen, and V. J. Feron. 1982. Inhalation toxicity of acetaldehyde in rats. I. Acute and sub-acute studies. *Toxicology* 23: 293–307.

Aranyi, C., W. J. O'Shea, J. A. Graham, and F. J. Miller. 1986. The effects of inhalation of organic chemical air contaminants on murine lung host defenses. *Fund. Appl. Toxicol.* 6: 713–720.

Astry, C. L., and G. J. Jakab. 1983. The effects of acrolein exposure on pulmonary antibacterial defenses. *Toxicol. Appl. Pharmacol.* 67: 49–54.

Auerbach, C., M. Moutschen-Dahman, and J. Moutschen. 1977. Genetic and cytogenetic effects of formaldehyde and related compounds. *Mutat. Res.* 39: 317–362.

Ayer, H. E., and D. W. Yeager. 1976. Irritants in cigarette smoke plumes. *Am. J. Public Health* 72: 1283–1285.

Badre, R., R. Guillerme, N. Abram, M. Bourdin, and C. Dumas. 1978. Pollution atmospherique par la fume'e de tabac. *Ann. Pharm. Fr.* 36: 443–452.

Ballarin, C., F. Sarto, L. Giacomelli, G. Bartolucci Battista, and E. Clonfero. 1992. Micronucleated cells in nasal mucosa of formaldehyde-exposed workers. *Mutat. Res.* 280: 1–7.

Bardana, E. J. Jr., and A. Montanaro. 1991. Formaldehyde: An analysis of its respiratory, cutaneous, and immunologic effects. *Ann. Allergy* 66: 441–452.

Barnes, P. J., I. W. Rodger, and N. C. Thomson. 1989. *Asthma: Basic Mechanisms and Clinical Management.* London: Academic Press.

Barrow, C. S., W. H. Steinhagen, and J. C. F. Chang. 1983. Formaldehyde sensory irritation. In *Formaldehyde Toxicity.* ed. J. E. Gibson. Washington, DC: Hemisphere.

Basu, A. K., and L. J. Marnett. 1983. Unequivocal demonstration that malondialdehyde is a mutagen. *Carcinogenesis* 4: 331–333.

Beauchamp, R. Q., Jr., K. T. Morgan. A. D. Kligerman, D. A. Anjelkovich, and H. A. Heck. 1985. A critical review of the literature on acrolein toxicity. *CRC Crit. Rev. Toxicol.* 14: 309–380.

Bender, J. R., L. S. Mullin, G. J. Graepel, and W. E. Wilson. 1983. Eye irritation response of humans to formaldehyde. *Am. Ind. Hyg. Assoc. J* 44: 463–465.

Benedetti, A., M. Comport I, and H. Esterbauer. 1980. Identification of 4-hydroxynonenal as a cytotoxic product originating from the peroxidation of liver microsomal lipids. *Biochim. Biophys. Acta* 620: 281–296.

Benedetti, A., M. Comport I, R. Fulceri, and H. Esterbauer. 1984. Cytotoxic aldehydes originating from the peroxidation of liver microsomal lipids. *Biochim. Biophys. Acta* 792: 172–181.

Ben-Jebria, A., Y. Crozet, M. L. Eskew, B. L. Rudeen, and J. S. Ultman. 1995. Acrolein-induced smooth muscle hyperresponsiveness and eicosanoid release in excised ferret trachea. *Toxicol Appl. Pharmacol.* 135: 35–44.

Berglund, B., and S. Nordin. 1992. Detectability and preceived intensity for formaldehyde for smokers and non-smokers. *Chem. Senses.* 17: 291–306.

Berke, J. H. 1987. Cytologic examination of the nasal mucosa in formaldehyde-exposed workers. *J. Occup. Med.* 29: 681–684.

Bernheim, F., M. L. C. Bernheim, and K. C. Wilbur. 1948. The reaction between thiobarbituric acid and the oxidation products of certain lipids. *J. Biol. Chem.* 174: 257–264.

Bernstein, R. S., L. T. Stayner, L. J. Elliott, R. Kimbrough, H. Falk, and L. Blade. 1984. Inhalation exposure to formaldehyde: An overview of its toxicology, epidemiology, monitoring, and control. *Am. Ind. Hvg. Assoc. J.* 45: 778–785.

Bertazzi, B. A., A. C. Pesatori, L. Radice, C. Zocchetti, and T. Vai. 1986. Exposure to formaldehyde and cancer mortality in a cohort of workers producing resins. *Scand. J. Work Environ. Health* 12: 461–468.

Bhalla D. K., V. Mahavni, T. Nguyen, and T. McClure 1991. Effects of acute exposure to formaldehyde on surface morphology of nasal epithelia in rats. *J. Toxicol. Environ. Health.* 33: 171–188.

Bhatt, H. S., S. B. Lober, and B. Combes. 1988. Effect of glutathione depletion on aminopyrine and formaldehyde metabolism. *Biochem. Pharmacol.* 37: 1581–1589.

Bird. R. P, H. H. Draper, and P. K. Basrur. 1982. Effect of malonaldehyde and acetaldehyde on cultured mammalian cells. Production of micronuclei and chromosomal aberrations. *Mutat. Res.* 101: 237–246.

Blair, A., and B. A. Stewart.1990. Correlation between different measures of occupational exposure to formaldehyde. *Am. J. Epidemiol.* 131 : 510–516.

Blair, A., P. Stewart, M. O'Berg, W. Gaffey, J. Walrath, J. Ward, R. Bales, S. Kaplan, and D. Cubit. 1986. Mortality among industrial workers exposed to formaldehyde exposure. *J. Natl. Cancer Inst.* 76: 1071–1084.

Blair, A., P. Stewart, M. O'Berg, W. Gaffey, J. Walrath, J. Ward, R. Bales, S. Kaplan, and D. Cubit. 1987. Cancers of the nasopharynx and oropharynx and formaldehyde. *J. Natl. Cancer Inst.* 78: 191–192.

Blair, A., P. A. Stewart, and R. N. Hoover. 1990. Mortality form lung cancer among workers employed in formaldehyde industries. *Am J. Ind. Med.* 17: 683–699.

Bogdanffy, M. S., P. H. Morgan, T. B. Starr, and K. T. Morgan. 1987. Binding of formaldehyde to human and rat nasal mucus and bovine serum albumin. *Toxicol. Lett.* 38: 145–154.

Bohren, K. M., B. Bullock, B. Wermuth, and K. H. Gabbay.1989. The aldo-keto reductase superfamily. *J. Biol. Chem.* 264: 9547–9551.

Borchers, M. T., S. E. Wert, and G. D. Leikauf. 1998. Acrolein-induced MUC5ac expression in rat airways. 1998. *Am J. Physiol.* 274: L573–L581.

Boreiko, C. J., and D. L. Ragan. 1983. Formaldehyde effects in the C3H/10T-1/2 cells transformation assay. In *Formaldehyde Toxicity*, ed. J. E. Gibson. Washington, DC: Hemisphere.

Bourne, H. G., and S. Seferian. 1959. Formaldehyde in wrinkle-proof apparel produces tears for milady. *Ind. Med. Surg.* 28: 232–233.

Boushey, H. A., M. J. Holtzman, J. R. Sheller, and J. A. Nadel. 1980. Bronchial hyperreactivity. *Am. Rev. Respir. Dis.* 121: 389–413.

Boysen, M., E. Zadig, V. Digernes, V. Abeler, and A. Reith. 1990. Nasal mucosa in workers exposed to formaldehyde: A pilot study. *Br. J. Ind. Med.* 47: 116–121.

Brinton, L. A., W. J.Blot, and J. F. Fraumeri. 1985. Nasal cancer in the textile and clothing industries. *Br. J. Ind. Med.* 42: 469–474.

Broder, I., P. Corey, P. Cole, M. Lipa, S. Mintz, and J. R. Nethercott. 1988. Comparison of health of occupants and characteristics of houses among homes and homes insulated with urea formaldehyde foam. II. Initial health and house variable and exposure-response relationships. *Environ. Res.* 45: 156–178.

Broder, I., P. Corey, P. Brasher\, M. Lipa, and P. Cole,. 1991. Formaldehyde exposure and health status in households. *Environ. Health Perspect.* 95:101–104.

Broughton, A., and J. D. Thrasher. 1988. Antibodies and altered cell mediated immunity in formaldehyde exposed humans. *Comments Toxicol.* 2: 155–174.

Brusick, D. J. 1983. Genetic and transforming activity of formaldehyde. In *Formaldehyde Toxicity*, ed. J. E. Gibson. Washington DC: Hemisphere.

Burge, P. S., M. G. Harries, W. K. Lam, I. M. O'Brien, and P. A. Patchett. 1985. Occupational asthma due to formaldehyde. *Thorax* 40: 255–260.

Card, S. E., S. F. Tompkins, and J. F. Brien. 1989. Ontogeny of the activity of alcohol dehydrogenase and aldehyde dehydrogenases in the liver and placenta of the guinea pig. *Biochem. Pharmacol.* 38: 2535–2541.

Carson, S., R. Goldhamer, and R. Carpenter. 1966. Mucus transport in the respiratory tract. *Am. Rev Respir. Dis.* 93: 86–92.

Carter, W. P. L. 1990. A detailed mechanism for the gas-phase atmospheric reactions of organic compounds. *Atmos. Environ.* 24A: 481–518.

Cassanova-Schmitz, M., R. M. David, and H. d'A. Heck. 1984. Oxidation of formaldehyde and acetaldehyde by NAD^+-dependent dehydrogenases in rat mucosal homogenates. *Toxicol. Appl. Pharmacol.* 33: 1137–1142.

Cassanova, M., and H. d'A. Heck.1987. Further studies of the metabolic incorporation and covalent binding of inhaled [^{3}H]- and [^{14}C]-formaldehyde in F-344 rats: Effects of glutathione depletion. *Toxicol. Appl. Pharmacol.* 89: 105–121.

Cassanova, M., K. T. Morgan, W. H. Steinhagen, J. I. Everitt, J. A. Popp,and H. d'A. Heck. 1991. Covalent binding of inhaled formaldehyde to DNA in the respiratory tract of rhesus monkeys: pharmacokinetics, rat-to-monkey interspecies scaling, and extrapolation to man. *Fund. Appl. Toxicol.* 17: 409–428.

Cassee, F. R., J. H. E. Arts, J. P. Groten, and V. J. Feron. 1996a. Sensory irritation to mixtures of formaldehyde, acrolein, and acetaldehyde in rats. *Arch. Toxicol.* 70: 329–337.

Cassee, F. R., J. P. Groten, and V. J. Feron. 1996b. Changes in the nasal epithelium of rats exposed by inhalation to mixtures of formaldehyde, acetaldehyde, and acrolein. *Fundam. Appl. Toxicol.* 29: 208–218.

Champeix J., L. Courtial L., E. Perche, and P. Catilina. 1966. Broncho-pneumopathie aigue par vapeurs d'acroline. *Arch. Mal. Prof.* 27: 794–796.

Chang, J. C. F., W. H. Steinhagen, and C. S. Barrow. 1981. Effect of single or repeated formaldehyde exposure on minute volume of B6C3F$_1$ mice and F-344 rats. *Toxicol. Appl. Pharmacol.* 61 :451–459.

Chang, J. C. F., E. A. Gross, J. A. Swenberg, and C. S. Barrow. 1983. Nasal cavity deposition, histopathology, and cell proliferation after single and repeated formaldehyde exposures in B6C3F$_1$ mice and F-344 rats. *Toxiol. Appl. Pharmacol.* 68: 161–176.

Chapin, F. S., Jr. 1974. *Human Activity Patterns in the City.* New York: Wiley-Interscience.

Chaw, U. F. M., L. E. Crane, P. Lange, and R. Shapiro. 1980. Isolation and identification of crosslinks from formaldehyde treated nuclei acids. *Biochemistry* 19: 5525–5531.

Chung, F. L., R. Young, and S. S. Hecht. 1984. Formation of cyclic l, N^2-propanodeoxyguanosine adducts in DNA upon reaction with acrolein or crotonaldehyde. *Cancer Res.* 44: 990–995.

Cohen Hubal, E. A., P. M. Schlosser, R. B. Conolly, and J. S. Kimbell. 1997. Comparison of inhaled formaldehyde dosimetry predictions with DNA-protein cross-link in the rat nasal passages. *Toxicol. Appl. Pharmacol.* 143: 47–55.

Collins, J. J., J. F. Acquivella, and N. A. Esmen. 1997. An updated meta-analysis of formaldehyde exposure and upper respiratory tract cancers. *J. Occup. Med.* 39: 639–651.

Comey, A. M., and D. A. Hahn. 1921. *Dictionary of Chemical Solubilities: Inorganic.* New York: Macmillan, pp. 158, 635, 900.

Consensus Workshop on Formaldehyde. 1984. Deliberations. *Environ. Health Perspect.* 58: 323–328.

Cooper, K. O., G. Witz, and C. M. Witmer. 1987. Mutagenicity and toxicity studies of several α,β-unsaturated aldehydes in *Salmonella typhimurium* mutagenicity assay. *Environ. Mol. Mutagen.* 9: 289–295.

Costa, D. L., R. S. Kutzman, J. R. Lehmann, and R. T. Drew. 1986. Altered lung function and structure in the rat after sub chronic exposure to acrolein. *Am. Rev. Respir. Dis.* 133: 286–291.

Council on Scientific Affairs. 1989. Formaldehyde. *JAMA.* 261: 1183–1187.

Crabb, D. W. 1990. Biological markers for increased risk of alcoholism and for quantitation of alcohol consumption. *J. Clin. Invest.* 85: 311–315.

Cralley, L. V. 1942. The effect of irritant gases upon the rate of ciliary activity. *J. Ind. Hyg. Toxicol.* 24: 193–198.

Crosby, R. M., K. K. Richardson, T. R. Kraft, K. B. Benforado, H. L. Liber, and T. R. Skopek. 1988. Molecular analysis of formaldehyde-induced mutations in human lymphoblasts and *E. coli. Environ. Mol. Mutagen.* 12: 155–166.

Czap, C., T. Nicolai, R. Wolf, and E. von Mutius. 1993. Asthma, bronchial hyperreactivity and formaldehyde exposure in children living near a chip-board factory. *Eur. Respir. J.* 6: 235s.

Dalbey, W. E. 1982. Formaldehyde and tumors in hamster respiratory tract. *Toxicology* 24: 9–15.

Dalhamn, T., and A. Rosengren. 1971. Effect of different aldehydes on tracheal mucosa. *Arch. Otolanngol. Head Neck Surg.* 93: 496–500.

Dallas, C. E., J. C. Thetas, R. B. Harrist, and E. J. Fairchild.1985. Effect of subchronic formaldehyde inhalation on minute volume and nasal deposition in Sprague-Dawley rats. *J. Toxicol. Environ. Health* 16: 553–564.

Day, J. H., R. E. M. Lees, R. H. Clark, and P. L. Pattee. 1984. Respiratory response to formaldehyde and off-gas of urea formaldehyde foam insulation. *Can. Med. Assoc. J.* 131: 1061–1065.

DeMaster, E. G., and J. M. Stevens. 1988. Acute effects of the aldehyde dehydrogenase inhibitors, disulfiram, pargyline and cyanamide, on circulating ketone body levels in the rat. *Biochem. Pharmacol.* 37: 229–234.

Doupnik, C. A., and G. D. Leikauf. 1990. Acrolein stimulates eicosanoid release from bovine airway epithelial cells. *Am J. Physiol.* 259: L222–229.

Edling, C., H. Hellquist, and L. Odkvist. 1988. Occupational exposure to formaldehyde and histopathological changes in the nasal mucosa. *Br. J. Ind. Med.* 45: 761–765.

Egle, L., Jr. 1972. Retention of inhaled formaldehyde, propionaldehyde, and acrolein in the dog. *Arch. Environ. Health* 25: 119–124.

Epstein, S. S. 1972. Detection of chemical mutagens by dominant lethal assay in the mouse. *Toxicol. Appl. Pharmacol.* 23: 288–298.

Esterbauer, H., K. H. Cheesman, M. U. Dianzani, G. Poli, and T. F. Slater. 1982. Separation and characterization of aldehydic products of lipid per oxidation stimulated by ADP-Fe^{+2} in rat liver microsomes. *Biochem. J.* 208: 129–140.

Falk, H. L. 1963. The response of mucus-secreting epithelium and mucus to irritants. *Ann. NY Acad. Sci.* 106: 583–608.

Farres, J., K.-L. Guan, and H. Weiner. 1989. Primary structures of rat and bovine liver mitochondrial aldehyde dehydrogenases deduced from cDNA sequences. *Eur. J. Biochem.* 180: 67–74.

Feinman, S. E. 1988. *Formaldehyde Sensitivity and Toxicity.* Boca Raton, FL CRC Press.

Feldman, M. Y. 1973. Reactions of nuclei acids and nucleoproteins with formaldehyde. *Prog. Nucleic Acid Res. Mol. Biol.* 13: 1–19.

Fennel, T. R. 1990. Development of methods for measuring formaldehyde exposure. In *Proceedings Seventh Annual Health Effects Institute Conference.* Cambridge, MA: Health Effects Institute.

Feron, V. J. 1979. Effects of exposure to acetaldehyde in Syrian hamsters simultaneously treated with benzo(a)pyrene or diethylnitrosamine. *Prog. Exp. Tumor Res.* 24: 162–173.

Feron, V. J., and A. Kruysse. 1977. Effects of exposure to acrolein vapor in hamsters simultaneously treated with benzo(a)pyrene or diethylnitrosamine. *J. Toxicol. Environ. Health* 3: 379–394.

Feron, V. J., A. Kruysse. H. P. Til. and H. R. Immel. 1978. Repeated exposure to acrolein vapor: Subacute studies in hamsters, rats, and rabbits. *Toxicology* 9: 47–57.

Feron, V. J., A. Kruysse, and R. A. Woutersen.1982. Respiratory tract tumours in hamsters exposed to acetaldehyde vapour alone or simultaneously to benzo(a)pyrene or diethylnitrosamine. *Eur. J. Cancer Clin. Oncol.* 18: 13–22.

Feron, V. J., J. P. Brruyntjes, R. A. Woustersen, H. R. Immel, L. M. Appelman. 1988. Nasal tumours in rats after short-term exposure to cytotoxic concentrations of formaldehyde. *Cancer Lett.* 39: 101–111.

Feron, V. J., H. P. Til, F. deVrijer, R. A. Wostersen, F. R. Cassee, and P. J. van Bladeren. 1991. Aldehydes: occurrence, carcinogenic potential, mechanism of action and risk assessment. *Mutat. Res.* 259: 363–385.

Fontignie-Houbrechts, N. 1981. Genetic effects of formaldehyde in the mouse. *Mutat. Res.*88: 109–119.

Fornace, A. J., Jr. 1982. Detection of DNA single-strand breaks produced during the repair of damage by DNA-protein cross-linking agents. *Cancer Res.* 42: 145–140.

Fornace, A. J., Jr., J. F. Lechner, R. C. Graftstrom, and C. C. Harris. 1982. DNA-repair in human bronchial epithelial cells. *Carcinogenesis* 3: 1373–1377.

Frazelle, J. H., D. J. Abernethy, and C. J. Boreiko. 1983. Weak promotion of C3H/l0T-1/2 cell transformation by repeated treatments with formaldehyde. *Cancer Res.* 43: 3236–3239.

French, D., and J. T. Edsall. 1945. The reactions of formaldehyde with amino acids and proteins. *Adv. Protein Chem.* 2: 277–335.

Frigas, E., W. V. Filley, and C. E. Reed. 1984. Bronchial challenge with formaldehyde gas: Lack of bronchoconstriction in 13 patients suspected of having formaldehyde-induced asthma. *Mayo. Clin. Proc.* 59: 295–299.

Galloway, S. M., M. J. Armstrong, C. Reubin, S. Coleman, B. Brown, C. Cannon, A. D. Bloom, F. Nakamura, M. Ahmed, S. Duk, J. Rimpo, B. H. Margolin, M. A. Resnick, B. Anderson, and E. Zeiger. 1987. Chromosome abberations and sister chromatid exchanges in Chinese hamster ovary cells: Evaluations of 108 chemicals. *Environ. Mol. Mutagen.* 10 (suppl): 1–175.

Gamble, J. F., A. J. McMichael, T. Williams, and M. Battigelli. 1976. Respiratory function and symptoms: An environmental / epidemiologic study of rubber workers exposed to phenoformaldehyde resin. *Am. Ind. Hyg. Assoc. J.* 37: 499–512.

Gammage, R. B., and K. C. Gupta. 1984. Formaldehyde. In *Indoor Air Quality*, eds. P. J. Walsh, C. S. Dabney, and E. D. Copenhaver. Boca Raton, FL: CRC Press.

Gardner, M. J., B. Pannett, P. D. Winter, and A. M. Cruddas. 1993. A cohort study of workers exposed to formaldehyde in the British chemical industry: An update. *Br. J. Ind. Med.* 50: 872–834.

Gerin, M., J. Siemiatycki, L. Nadon, R. Dewar, and D. Krewski. 1989. Cancer risk due to occupational exposure to formaldehyde: Results of a multi-site case-control study in Montreal. *Int. J. Cancer* 44: 53–58.

Gerberich, H. R., and G. C. Seaman. 1994. In *Kirk-Othmer Encyclopedia of Chemical Technology*. eds. J. I. Kroschwitz and M. Howe-Grant. New York: Wiley .

Godish, T. 1989. Formaldehyde exposures from tobacco smoke: A review. *Am. J. Public Health* 79: 1044–1045.

Goedde, H. W., and D. P Agarwal. 1989. Pharmacogenetics of aldehyde dehydrogenase (ALDH). *Pharmacol. Ther.* 45: 345–371.

Gong, H., Jr, D. P. Tashkin, and B. M. Calvarsee. 1981. Alcohol-induced bronchospasm in an asthmatic patient. Pharmacologic evaluation of the mechanism. *Chest.* 80: 167–173.

Gorski, P., M. Tarkowski, A. Krokowiak, and M. Kiec-Swierczynska. 1992. Neutrophil chemiluminescence following exposure to formaldehyde in healthy subjects and in patients with contact dermatitis. *Allergol. Immunopath.* 20: 20–23.

Graftstrom, R. C., A. Fornace Jr., and C. C. Harris. 1984. Repair of DNA damage caused by formaldehyde in human cells. *Cancer Res.* 44: 4323–4327.

Graftstrom, R. C., J. M. Dypbukt, J. C. Willey, K. Sundqvist, C. Edman, L. Atzori, and C. C. Harris.1988. Pathobiological effects of acrolein in cultured human bronchial epithelial cells. *Cancer Res.* 48: 1717–1721.

Graftstrom, R. C. 1990. *In vitro* studies of aldehyde effects related to human respiratory carcinogenesis. *Mutat. Res.* 238: 175–184.

Graftstrom, R. C., J. M. Dypbukt, K. Sundqvist, L. Atzori, I. Nielsen, R. D. Curren, and C. C. Harris.1994 Pathobiological effects of acetaldehyde in cultured human bronchial epithelial cells and fibroblasts. *Cancinogenesis* 15: 985–990.

Green, D. J., L. R. Sauder, T. J. Kulle, and R. Bascom.1987. Acute responsed to 3.0 ppm formaldehyde in exercising healthy nonsmokers and asthmatics. *Am. Rev. Respir. Dis.* 135: 1261–1266.

Grosjean, D. 1990. Atmospheric chemistry of toxic contaminants 2. Saturated aliphatics acetaldehyde dioxane ethylene glycol ethers propylene oxide. *J. Air Waste Manage. Assoc.* 40: 1522–1531.

Grosjean D. 1991. Ambient levels of formaldehyde, acetylaldehyde, and formic acid in Southern California: Results of a one-year base-line study. *Environ. Sci. Technol.* 25: 710–715.

Grosjean, D., E. L. Williams, and J. H. Seinfeld 1992. Atmospheric oxidation of selected terpenes and related carbonyls gas-phase carbonyl products. *Environ. Sci. Tech.* 26: 1526–1533.

Grosjean, E., D. Grosjean, M. P. Fraser, and G. R. Cass. 1996. Air quality model evaluation data for organics. 2. C_1–C_{14} carbonyls in Los Angeles air. *Environ. Sci. Technol.* 30: 2687–2703.

Grundfest, C. C., J. Chang, and D. Newcombe. 1982. Acrolein: A potent modulator of lung macrophage arachidonic acid metabolism. *Biochim. Biophys. Acta* 713: 149–159.

Guillerm R., R. Badre, and B. Vignon. 1961. Effects inhibiteurs de la fumé e de tabac sur l'activie ciliaire de l'epithélium respiratoire et nature tea compsants responsables. *Bull. Acad. Natl. Med.* 145: 416–423.

Gupta, K. C., A. G. Ulsamer, and P. W. Preuso. 1982. Formaldehyde in indoor air: Sources and toxicity. *Environ. Int.* 8: 349–354.

Hadi, S. M., H. Shahabuddin, and A. Rehman. 1989. Specificity of the interaction of furfural with DNA. *Mutat. Res.* 225: 101–106.

Hagmar, L., T. Bellander, V. Englander, J. Ranstam, R. Attewell, and S. Skerfring. 1986. Mortality and cancer among workers in a chemical factory. *Scand. J. Work Environ. Health* 12: 545–551.

Hamberg, M., and B. Samuelsson. 1967. Oxygenation of unsaturated fatty acids by the vesicular gland of sleep. *J. Biol. Chem.* 242: 5341–5354.

Hanrahan, L. P., K. A. Dally, H. A. Anderson, M. S. Kanarek, and J. Ralkin. 1984. Formaldehyde vapor in mobile homes: A cross sectional survey of concentrations and irritant effects. *Am. J. Public Health* 74: 1026–1027.

Harley, R. A., and G. R. Cass. 1995. Modeling the atmospheric concentrations of individual volatile organic compounds. *Atmos. Environ.* 29:905–922.

Harrington, J. M., and H. S. Shannon. 1975. Mortality study of pathologists and medical laboratory technicians. *Br. Med. J.* 4: 329–332.

Hastie, A. T., H. Patrick, and J. E. Fish. 1990. Inhibition and recovery of mammalian respiratory ciliary function after formaldehyde exposure. *Toxicol. Appl. Pharmacol.* 102: 282–291.

Hayes, R. B., J. W. Raatgever, A. De Bruyn, and M. Gerin. 1986. Cancer of the nasal cavity and paranasal sinuses, and formaldehyde exposure. *Int. J. Cancer* 37: 487–492.

Hayes, R. B., A. Blair, P. A. Stewart, R. F. Herrick, and H. Mahar. 1990. Mortality of U. S. embalmers and funeral directors. *Am J. Ind. Med.* 18: 641–652.

He, S.-M., and B. Lambert. 1990. Acetaldehyde-induced mutation at the *hprt* locus in human lymphocytes *in vitro*. *Environ. Mol. Mutagene.* 16: 57–63.

Heck, H. d'A., T. Y. Chin, and M. C. Schmitz. 1983. Distribution of ^{14}C formaldehyde in rats after inhalation exposure. In *Formaldehyde Toxicity*, ed. J. E. Gibson. Washington, DC: Hemisphere.

Heck, H. d'A., M. Cassanova, W. H. Steinhagen, J. L. Everitt, K. T. Morgan. and J. A. S. Popp. 1989. Formaldehyde toxicity: DNA–protein cross-linking studies in rats and nonhuman primates. In: *Nasal Carcinogenesis in Rodents: Relevance to Human Risk*, eds. V. J. Feron and M. C. Bosland. Wageningen: Pudoc.

Heck, H. d'A., M. Cassanova, and T.B. Starr. 1990. Formaldehyde toxicity—new understanding. *CRC Crit. Rev. Toxicol.* 20: 397–426.

Helander, A., S. Carlsson, and O. Tottmar.1988. Effects of disulfiram therapy on aldehyde dehydrogenase activity in human leukocytes and erythrocytes. *Biochem. Pharmacol.* 37: 3360–3363.

Hemminki, K. 1981. Reactions of formaldehyde with guanosine. *Toxicol. Lett.* 9: 161–164.

Hemminki, K., K. Falck, and H. Vainio. 1980. Comparison of alkylation rates and mutagenicity of directly acting industrial and laboratory chemicals. *Arch. Toxicol.* 46: 277–283.

Hendrick, D. J., and D. J. Lane. 1975. Formal in asthma in hospital staff. *Br. Med. J.* 1 : 607–608.

Hendrick, D. J., and D. J. Lane. 1977. Occupational formal in asthma. *Br J. Ind. Med.* 34:11–18.

Hendrick, D. J., R. J. Rando, D. J. Lane, and M. J. Morris.1982. Formaldehyde asthma: Challenge exposure levels and fate after five years. *J. Occup. Med.* 24:893–897.

Hernberg, S., P. Westerholm, K. Schults-Larsen, R. Degerth, E. Kuosma, A. Englund, U. Engzell, H. S. Hansen, and P. Mutanen. Nasal and sinonasal cancer. *Scand. J. Work Environ. Health* 9: 315–326.

Holmstrom, M., B. Wilhelmsson, and H. Hellquist. 1989. Histological changes in the nasal mucosa in rats long-term exposure to formaldehyde and wood dust. *Acta Otolaryngol.* 108: 274–283.

Horsfall, F. L. 1934. Formaldehyde hypersensitiveness: An experimental study. *J. Immunol.* 27: 569–581.

Horvath, E. P., Jr., H. Anderson Jr., W. E. Pierce, L. Hanrahan, and J. D. Wendick. 1988. Effects of formaldehyde on the mucous membranes and lungs: A study of an industrial population. *JAMA* 259(5): 701–707.

Hsie, A. W., J. O'Neill, J. R. San Sabastian, O. B. Couch, P. A. Brimen W. N. C. Sun, J. C. Fucoe, N. L. Forbes, R. Machanoff, J. C. Riddle, and M. H. Hsie. 1979. Quantitative mammalian cell toxicology: Study of the cytotoxicity and mutagenicity of seventy individual environmental agents related to energy technologies and three subfractions of a crude synthetic oil in the CHO/HGPRT system. EPA. Report 600/9-78-027, pp. 293–315.

Hsu, L. C., R. E. Bendel, and A. Yoshida. 1987. Direct detection of usual and atypical alleles on the human aldehyde dehydrogenase-2 (ALDH2) locus. *Am. J. Hum. Genet.* 41: 966–1001.

IARC. International Agency for Research on Cancer. 1982. *Some Industrial Chemicals and Dyestuffs.* IARC Monographs on the Evaluation of the Carcinogeneic Risk of Chemicals to Humans, vol. 29. Lyon: International Agency for Research in Cancer.

IARC. International Agency for Research on Cancer 1985. *Allyl Compounds, Aldehydes, Epoxides, and Peroxides.* IARC Monographs on the Evaluation of the Carcinogeneic Risk of Chemicals to Humans. vol. 36. Lyon: International Agency for Research in Cancer.

IARC. International Agency for Research on Cancer 1995.*Wood dust and Formaldehyde.* IARC Monographs on the Evaluation of the Carcinogeneic Risk of Chemicals to Humans. vol. 62. Lyon: International Agency for Research in Cancer.

Izard, C., and C. Liberman. 1978. Acrolein. *Mutat. Res.* 47: 115–138.

Jakab, G. J. 1977. Adverse effect of a cigarette smoke component, acrolein, on pulmonary antibacterial defenses and on viral-bacterial interactions in the lung. *Am. Rev. Respir. Dis.* 115: 33–38.

Jakab, G. J. 1993. The toxicologic interactions resulting from inhalation of carbon black and acrolein on pulmonary antibacterial and antiviral defenses. *Toxiclol. Appl. Pharmaacol.*121: 167–175.

Jakab, G. J., and D. R. Hemenway. 1993. Inhalation coexposure to carbon black and acrolein suppresses alveolar macrophage phagocytosis and TNF-α release and modulates peritoneal macrophage phagocytes. *Inhalation. Toxicol.* 5: 265–279.

Kane, L. E., and Y. Alarie.1977. Sensory irritation to formaldehyde and acrolein during single and repeated exposures in mice. *Am. Ind. Hyg. Assoc. J.* 38: 509–522.

Kensler, C. J., and S. P. Battista. 1963. Components of cigarette smoke with ciliary-depressant activity. *N. Engl. J. Med.* 269: 1161–1166.

Kerfoot, E. J., and T. F Mooney. 1975. Formaldehyde and paraformaldehyde study in funeral homes. *Am. Ind. Hyg. Assoc. J.* 36: 533–537.

Kerns, W. D., K. L. Pavkov, D. J. Donofrio, E. J. Gralla, and J. A. Swenberg. 1983. Carcinogenicity of formaldehyde in rats and mice after long-term inhalation exposure. *Cancer Res.* 43: 4382–4392.

Khamgaonkar, M. B., and M. B. Fulare. 1991. Pulmonary effects of formaldehyde exposure. An environmental-epidemiological study. *Indian J. Chest Dis. Allied Sci.* 33: 9–13.

Kilburn, K. H., and W. N. McKenzie. 1978. Leukocyte recruitment to airways by aldehyde-carbon combinations that mimic cigarette smoke. *Lab. Invest.* 38: 134–142.

Kilburn, K. H., B. C. Seidman, and R. Warshaw.1985. Neurobehavioral and respiratory symptoms of formaldehyde and xylene exposure in histology technicians. *Arch. Environ. Health* 40: 229–233.

Kimbell, J. S., E. A. Gross, D. R. Joyner, M. N. Godo, and K. T. Morgan. 1993. Application of computational fluid dynamics to regional dosimetry to inhaled chemicals in the upper respiratory tract of the rat. *Toxicol. Appl. Pharmacol.* 121: 253–263.

Kimbell, J. S., E. A. Gross, R. B. Richardson, R. B. Conolly, and K. T. Morgan. 1997. Correlation of regional formaldehyde flux predictions with the distribution of formaldehyde-induced squamous metaplasia in F344 rat nasal passages. *Mutat. Res.* 380: 143–154.

Kruysse, A., V. J. Feron, and H. P. Til. 1975. Repeated exposure to acetaldehyde vapor. Studies in Syrian golden hamsters. *Arch. Environ. Health.* 30:449–452.

Krzyzanowski, M., J. J. Quackenboss, and M. D. Lebowitz. 1990. Chronic respiratory effects of indoor formaldehyde exposure. *Environ. Res.* 52: 117–125.

Kulle, T., and G. Cooper. 1975. Effects of formaldehyde and ozone on the trigeminal sensory system. *Arch. Environ. Health* 30: 327–333.

Kulle, T. J., L. R. Sauder, J. R. Hebel, D. J. Green, and M. D. Chatham. 1987. Formaldehyde dose–response in healthy nonsmokers. *J. Air Pollut. Control Assoc.* 37: 919–924.

Kurys, G., W. Ambroziak, and R. Pietruszko. 1989. Human aldehyde dehydrogenase. *J. Biol. Chem.* 264: 4715–4721.

Kutzman, R. S., E. A. Popenoe, M. Schmaeler, and R. T. Drew. 1985. Changes in rat lung structure and composition as a result of subchronic exposure to acrolein. *Toxicology* 34: 139–151.

Lam, C.-W., M. Cassanova, and H. d'A. Heck. 1985. Depletion of nasal mucosal glutathione by acrolein and enhancement of formaldehyde-induced DNA–protein cross-linking by simultaneous exposure to acrolein. *Arch. Toxicol.* 58: 67–71.

Leach, C. L., N. S. Hatoum, H. V. Ratajczak, and J. M. Gerhart. 1987. The pathologic and immunologic effects of inhaled acrolein in rats. *Toxicol. Lett.* 39: 189–198.

Lee, B. P., R. F. Morton, and L.-Y. Lee. 1992. Acute effects of acrolein on breathing: Role of vagal bronchopulmonary afferents. *J. Appl. Physiol.* 72: 1050–1056.

Lee, H.-K., Y. Alarie, and M. H. Karol. 1984. Induction of formaldehyde sensitivity in guinea pigs. *Toxicol. Appl. Pharmacol.* 75: 147–155.

Leffingwell, C. M., and R. B. Low. 1979. Cigarette smoke components and alveolar macrophage protein synthesis. *Arch. Environ. Health* 34: 97–102.

Leikauf, G. D., and C. A. Doupnik. 1989. Formaldehyde induced bronchial hyperresponsiveness in guinea pig. *Am. Rev. Respir. Dis.* 139:A392.

Leikauf, G. D., L. M. Leming, J. R. O'Donnell, and C. A. Doupnik.1989a. Bronchial responsiveness and inflammation in guinea pigs exposed to acrolein. *J Appl. Physiol.* 66: 171–178.

Leikauf, G. D., C. A. Doupnik, L. M. Leming, and H. E. Wey. 1989b. Sulfidopeptide leukotrienes mediate acrolein-induced bronchial hyperresponsiveness. *J. Appl. Physiol.* 66: 1838–1845.

Levine, J. R., D. Anjelkovich, and L. K . Shaw. 1984. The mortality of Ontario undertakers and a review of formaldehyde related mortality studies. *J. Occup. Med.* 26: 740–746.

Li, L., R. F. Hamilton Jr., D. E. Taylor, and A. Holian. 1997. Acrolein-induced cell death in human alveolar macrophages. *Toxicol. Appl. Pharmacol.* 145: 331–339.

Liber, H. L., K. Benforado, R. M. Crosby, D. Simpson, and T. R. Skopek. 1989. Formaldehyde-induced and spontaneous alterations in human *hprt* DNA sequence and mRNA expression. *Mutat. Res.* 226: 31–37.

Liebling, T., K. D. Rosenman, H. Pastides, R. G. Griffith, and S. Lemeshow. 1984. Cancer mortality among workers exposed to formaldehyde. *Am. J. Ind. Med.* 5: 423–428.

Luce, D., M. Gerin, A. Leclerc, J. F. Morcet, J. Brugere, and M. Goldberg. 1993. Sinonasal cancer and occupational exposure to formaldehyde and other substances. *Int. J. Cancer* 53: 224–231.

Lynen, R., M. Rothe, and E. Gallasch. 1983. Characterization of formaldehyde-related antibodies in hemodialysis patients at different stages of immunization. *Vox Sang.* 44: 81–89.

Lyon, J. P., L. J. Jenkins, R. A. Jones, R. A. Coon, and J. Siegel. 1970. Repeated and continuous exposure of laboratory animals to acrolein. *Toxicol. Appl. Pharmacol.* 17: 726–732.

Ma, T. H., and M. M. Harris. 1988. Review of the genotoxicity of formaldehyde. *Mutat. Res.* 196: 37–59.

Magana-Schwenke, N., and B. Ekert. 1978. Biochemical analysis of damage induced in yeast by formaldehyde. II. Induction of crosslinks between DNA and protein. *Mutat. Res.* 51: 11–19.

Magana-Schwenke, N., B. Ekert, and E. Moustacchi. 1978. Biochemical analysis of damage induced in yeast by formaldehyde. 1. Induction of single-strand breaks in DNA and their repair. *Mutat. Res.* 50: 181–193.

Mannix, R. C., R. F. Phalen, R. B. Walters, and T. T. Kurosaki. 1983. Effects of sulfur dioxide and formaldehyde on particle clearance in the rat. *J. Toxicol. Environ. Health* 12: 429–440.

Marnett, L. J. 1988. Health effects of aldehydes and alcohols in Mobil source emissions. In *Air Pollution, the Automobile, and Public Health.* Washington DC: National Academy Press.

Marnett, L. J., and M. A. Tuttle. 1980. Comparison of the mutagenicities of malondialdehyde and side products formed during its chemical synthesis. *Cancer Res.* 40: 276–282.

Marnett, L. J., H. K. Holly, M. C. Hollstein, D. E. Levin, H. Esterbauer, and B. N. Ames. 1985. Naturally occurring carbonyl compounds are mutagens in *Salmonella* tester strain TA104. *Mutat. Res.* 148: 25–34.

Maronpot, R. R., R. A. Miller, W. J. Clarke, R. B. Westerberg, J. R. Decker, and O. R. Moss. 1986. Toxicity of formaldehyde vapor in B6C3F, mice exposed for 13 weeks. *Toxicology* 1: 253–266.

Marsh, G. M. 1982. Proportional mortality patterns among chemical plant workers exposed to formaldehyde. *Br. J. Ind. Med.* 39: 313–322.

Marsh, G. M., R. A. Stone, N. A. Esmen, and V. L. Henderson. 1994. Mortality patterns among chemical plant workers exposed to formaldehyde and other substances. *J. Natl. Cancer Inst..* 86: 384–386.

Martin, C. N., A. C. McDermid, and R. C. Garner. 1978. Testing of known carcinogens and non-carcinogens for their ability to induce unscheduled DNA synthesis in HeLa cells. *Cancer Res.* 38: 2621–2627.

Maurice, F, J.-H. Rivory, P. H. Larsson, S. G. O. Johansson, and J. Bouquest. 1986. Anaphylactic shock caused by formaldehyde in a patient undergoing long-term hemodialysis. *J. Allergy Clin. Immunol.* 77: 594–597.

McLaughlin, J. K. 1994. Formaldehyde and cancer: A critical review. *Int. Arch. Occup. Environ. Health* 66: 295–301.

Monticello, T. M., K. T. Morgan, J. I. Everitt, and J. A. Popp. 1989. Effects of formaldehyde gas on the respiratory track of rhesus monkeys. *Am. J. Pathol.* 134: 515–527.

Monticello, T. M., F. J. Miller, and K. T. Morgan. 1991. Regional increases in rat nasal epithelial cell proliferation following acute and subchronic inhalation of formaldehyde. *Toxicol. Appl. Pharmacol.* 134: 515–527.

Monticello, T. M., J. A. Swenberg, E. A. Gross, J. R. Leininger, J. S. Kimbell, S. Selikop, T. B. Starr, J. E. Gibson, and K. T. Morgan.1996. Correlation of regional and nonlinear formaldehyde-induced cancer with proliferating populations of cells. *Cancer Res.*56: 1012–1022.

Morgan, K. T., D. L. Patterson, and E. A. Gross. 1984. Frog palate mucociliary apparatus: Structure, function, and response to formaldehyde gas. *Fundam. Appl. Toxicol.* 4: 58–68.

Morgan, K. T., D. L. Patterson, and E. A. Gross. 1986. Responses of the nasal mucociliary apparatus of F-344 rats to formaldehyde gas. *Toxicol. Appl. Pharmacol.* 82: 1–13.

Morris, J. B. 1997. Uptake of acetaldehyde vapor and aldehyde dehydrogenase levels in the upper respiratory tracts of the mouse, rat, hamster, and guinea pig. *Fundam. Appl. Toxicol.* 35: 91–100.

Mukai, F. H., and B. D. Goldstein. 1976. Mutagenicity of malondialdehyde, a decomposition product of peroxidized polyunsaturated fatty acids. *Science* 191: 868–869.

Murphy, S. D., D. A. Klingshirn, and C. E. Ulrich. 1963. Respiratory response of guinea pigs during acrolein inhalation and its modification by drugs. *J. Pharmacol. Exp. Ther.* 141 : 79–83.

Myou, S., M. Fujimura, K. Nishi, T. Ohka, and T. Matsuda. 1993. Aerosolized acetaldehyde induces histamine-mediated bronchoconstriction in asthmatics. *Am. Rev. Respir. Dis.* 148: 940–943.

National Research Council. 1981. *Formaldehyde and Other Aldehydes*. Washington, DC: National Academy Press.

Naylor, S., R. P. Mason, J. K. M. Sanders, D. H. Williams, and G. Moneti. 1988. Formaldehyde adducts of glutathione. *Biochem. J.* 249: 573–579.

Neudecker, T., D. Lutz, E. Eder, and D. Henselher. 1981. Crotonaldehyde is mutagenie in a modified *Salmonella typhimurium* mutagenieity testing system. *Mutat. Res.* 91: 27–39.

Nilsson, G. E., and O. Tottmar. 1987. Effects of biogenic aldehydes and aldehyde dehydrogenase inhibitors on rat brain tryptophan hydroxylase activity *in vitro*. *Brain Res.* 409: 374–379.

Nocentini, S., S. Moreno, and J. Coppey. 1980. Survival, DNA synthesis and ribosomal RNA transeription in monkey kidney cells treated by formaldehyde. *Mutat. Res.* 70: 231–240.

Norback, D., E. Bjornsson, C. Jansen, J. Widstrom, and G. Borman. 1995. Asthmatic symptoms and volatile organic compounds, formaldehyde, and carbon dioxide in dwellings. *Occup. Environ. Med.* 52: 388–395.

Nordman, H. 1985. Formaldehyde asthma—rare or overlooked? *J. Allergy Clin. Immunol.* 75: 91–99.

Obe, G., and B. Beck. 1979. Mutagenic activity of aldehydes. *Drug Alcohol Depend.* 4: 91–94.

Occupational Safety and Health Administration. 1985. Occupational exposure to formaldehyde: Proposed rule and notice of hearing, 29 CFR Part 1920. *Federal Register* 50:50412.

Olsen, J. H., S. Plough-Jensen, M. Hink, K. Faurbo, N. O. Breum, and O. Moller Jensen. 1984. Occupational formaldehyde exposure and increased nasal cancer risk in man. *Int. J. Cancer* 34: 639–644.

Olsen, J. H., and S. Asneas. 1986. Formaldehyde and the risk of squamous cell carcinoma of the sinonasal cavities. *Br. J. Ind. Med. 43*: 769–774.

Oomichi, S., and H. Kita. 1974. Effect of air pollutants on ciliary activity of respiratory tract. *Bull. Tokyo Med. Dent. Uniu* 21 : 327–343.

Othmer, D. F. 1987. Methanol to gasoline? *Chem. Eng. News* 30: 2–3.

Partanen, T. 1993. Formaldehyde exposure and respiratory cancer — A meta-analysis of the epidemiologic evidence. *Scand. J. Work Environ.* Health. 11: 409–415.

Patteson, D. L., E. A. Gross, M. S. Bogdanffy, and K. T. Morgan. 1986. Retention of formaldehyde gas in the nasal passages of Fisher-344 rats. *Toxicologist* 6:55.

Patterson, R., M. S. Dykewicz, R. Evans III, L. C. Grammer, P. A. Greenberger, K. E. Harris, I. D. Lawrenee, J. J. Pruzansky, M. Roberts, M. A. Shaughnessy, and C. R. Zeiss. 1989. IgG antibody against formaldehyde human serum proteins: A comparison with other IgG antibodies against inhalant proteins and reactive chemicals. *J. Allergy Clin. Immunol.* 9: 359–366.

Pattle, R. E., and H. Cullumbine. 1956. Toxicity of some atmospheric pollutants. *Br. Med. J.* 2: 913–916.

Pazdrak, K., P. Gorski, A. Krakowiak, and U. Ruta. 1993. Changes in nasal lavage fluid due to formaldehyde inhalation. *Int. Arch. Occup. Environ. Health* 64: 515–519.

Pettersson, S., and T. Rehn. 1977. Determination of the odor threshold for formaldehyde. *Hygien. Miljo.* 10: 53–59.

Pickrell, J. A., L. C. Griffs, B. V. Mokler, G. M. Vanapilly, and C. H. Hobbs. 1983. Release of formaldehyde from various consumer products. *Environ. Sci. Technol.* 17: 753–764.

Pross, H. F., J. H. Day, R. H. Clark, and R. E. M. Lees. 1987. Immunologic studies of subjects with asthma exposed to formaldehyde and urea-formaldehyde foam insulation (UFFI) off products. *J. Allergy Clin. Immunol.* 79: 797–810.

Rader, J. 1977. *Irritative Effects of Formaldehyde in Laboratory Halls.* J. D. dissertation, University of Wurzberg.

Ragan, D. L., and C. J. Boreiko.1981. Initiation of C3H/10T-1/2 cells transformation by formaldehyde. *Cancer Lett.* 13: 325–331.

Recio, L. S. Sisk, L. Phutts, E. Bermudez, E.A. Gross, Z. Chen, K. Morgan, and C. Walker. 1992. *p53* mutations in formaldehyde-induced nasal squamous cell carcinomas in rats. *Cancer Res.* 52: 6113–6116.

Reidel, F., E. Hasenauer, P. J. Barth, A. Koziorowski, and C. H. L. Reiger. 1996. Formaldehyde exposure enhances inhalative allergic sensitization in the guinea pig. *Allergy* 51: 94–99, 1996.

Reynolds, S. H., S. J. Stowers, R. M. Patterson, R. R. Maronpot, S. A. Aaronson, and M. W. Anderson. 1987. Activated oncogenes in B6C3HF1 mouse liver tumors: implications for risk assessment. *Science* 237: 1309–1316.

Ritchie, L. M., and R. G. Lehnen. 1987. Formaldehyde-related health complaints of residents living in mobile and conventional homes. *Am. J. Public Health* 77: 323–328.

R. J. Reynolds Tobacco Company. 1988. Chemical composition of new cigarette smoke. In *Chemical and Biological Studies on New Cigarette Prototypes That Heat Instead of Burn Tobacco.* Winston-Salem, NC: R. J. Reynolds Tobacco Company.

Roemer, E., H. J. Anton, and R. Kindt. 1993. Cell proliferation in the respiratory tract of the rat after acute inhalation of formaldehyde or acrolein. *J. Appl. Toxicol.*13: 103–107.

Roush, G. C., J. Walrath, L. T. Stayner, S. A. Kalplan, J. T. Flannery, and A. Blair. 1987. Nasopharyngeal cancer, sinonasal cancer, and occupations related to formaldehyde: A case-control study. *J. Natl. Cancer Inst.* 79: 1221–1224.

Rusch, G. M., H. F. Bolte, and W. E. Rinehart. 1983. A 26-week inhalation toxicity study with formaldehyde in the monkey, rat, and hamster. In *Formaldehyde Toxicity,* ed. J. E. Gibson. Washington, DC: Hemisphere.

Saldiva, P. H., M. P. do Rio Caldeira, E. Massad, D. F. Calheiros, L. M. Cardoso, G. M. Bohm, and C. D. Saldiva. 1985. Effects of formaldehyde and acetaldehyde inhalation on rat pulmonary mechanics. *J. Appl. Toxicol.* 5: 288–292.

Salem, H., and H. Cullumbine. 1960. Inhalation toxicities of some aldehydes. *Toxicol. Appl. Pharmacol.* 2: 183–187.

Samet, J. M., M. C. Marbury, and J. D. Spengler. 1987. Health effects and sources of indoor air pollution. Part 1. *Am. Rev. Respir. Dis.* 136: 1486–1508.

Samet, J. H., and J. D. Spengler. 1991. *Indoor Air Pollution.* Baltimore. Johns Hopkins University Press.

Sandler, S. G., R. Sharon, M. Stroup, and B. Sabo. 1979. Formaldehyde-related antibodies in hemodialysis patients. *Transfusion* 19: 682–687.

Sauder, L. R., M. D. Chatham, D. J. Green, and T. J. Kulle. 1986. Acute pulmonary response to formaldehyde exposure in healthy nonsmokers. *J. Occup. Med.* 28: 420–424.

Schachter, E. N., T. J. Witek Jr., T. Tosun, B. Leaderer, and G. J. Beck. 1986. A study of respiratory effects from exposure to 2 ppm formaldehyde in health subjects. *Arch. Environ. Health* 41: 229–239.

Schachter, E. N., T. J. Witek Jr., D. J. Brody, T. Tosun, G. J. Beck, and B. P. Leaderer. 1987. A study of respiratory effects from exposure to 2.0 ppm formaldehyde in occupationally exposed workers. *Environ. Res.* 44: 188–205.

Schoenberg, J. B., and C. A. Mitchell. 1975. Airway disease cause by phenolic (phenolformaldehyde) resin exposure. *Arch. Environ. Health* 30: 574–577.

Schuck, E. A., E. R. Stephens, and J. T. Middleton. 1966. Eye irritation responses at low concentrations of irritants. *Arch. Environ. Health* 13: 570–575.

Seidell, A. 1940. *Solubilities of Inorganic and Metal Organic Compounds.* New York: D. Van Nostrand.

Seidell, A. 1941. *Solubilities of Organic Compounds.* New York: D. Van Nostrand.

Seinfeld, J. H. 1983. *J. Air Waste Manage. Assoc.* 28: 616–645.

Sellakumar, A. R., C. A. Synder, J. J. Solomon, and R. E. Albert. 1985. Carcinogenicity of formaldehyde and hydrogen chloride in rats. *Toxicol. Appl. Pharmacol.* 81: 401–406.

Shamberger, R. J., T. L. Andreone, and C. E. Willis. 1974. Antioxidants and cancer IV. Initiating activity of malonaldehyde as a carcinogen. *J. Natl. Cancer Inst.* 53: 1171–1773.

Shamberger, R. J., C. L. Corlett, K. D. Beaman, and B. L. Kasten. 1979. Antioxidant reduce the mutagenic effect of malondialdehyde and 13-propiolactone. Part IX. Antioxidants and cancer. *Mutat. Res.* 66: 349–355.

Shah J. J., and H. B. Singh 1998. Distribution of volatile organic chemicals in outdoor and indoor air. *Environ. Sci. Techol.* 22: 1381–1388.

Sheppard, D., W. S. Wong, C. F. Uehara, J. A. Nadel, and H. A. Boushey. 1980. Lower threshold and greater bronchomotor responsiveness of asthmatic subjects to sulfur dioxide. *Am. Rev. Respir. Dis.* 122: 873–878.

Sheppard, D., W. L. Eschenbacher, and J. Epstein. 1984. Lack of bronchomotor response to up to 3 ppm formaldehyde in subjects with asthma. *Environ. Res.* 35: 133–139.

Sherwood, R. L., C. L. Leach, N. S. Hatoum, and C. Aranyi.1986. Effects of acrolein on macrophage functions in rats. *Toxicol. Lett.* 32: 41–49.

Shibuya, A., M. Yasunami, and A. Yoshida. 1989. Genotypes of alcohol dehydrogenase and aldehyde dehydrogenase loot in Japanese alcohol flushers and nonflushers. *Hum. Genet.* 82: 14–16.

Shusterman, D., J. Salines, and J. Cone. 1988. Behavioral sensitization to irritants/odorants after acute overexposures. *J. Occup. Med* 30: 565–567.

Songco, G., and P. J. Fahey. 1987. Indoor and outdoor air pollutants and health. *Compr. Ther.* 13: 41–48.

Stayner, L., A. B. Smith, G. Reeve, L. Blade, L. Elliott, R. Keenlyside, and W. Halperin. 1985. Proportionate mortality study of workers in the garment industry exposed to formaldehyde. *Am. J. Ind. Med* 7: 229–240.

Stayner, L. T., L. Elliott, L. Blade, R. Keenlyside, and W. Halperin. 1988. A restrospective cohort mortality study of workers exposed to formaldehyde in the garment industry. *Am. J. Ind. Med.* 13: 667–681.

Steinhagen, W. H., and C. S. Barrow. 1984. Sensory irritation structure-activity study of inhaled aldehydes in B6C3F, and Swiss-Webster mice. *Toxicol. Appl. Pharmacol.* 72: 495–503.

Sterling, T., and A. Arundel. 1985. Formaldehyde and lung cancer. *Lancet* 2: 1366–1367.

Sterling, T. D., and J. J. Weinkam. 1988. Reanalysis of lung cancer mortality in a National Cancer Institute study on mortality among industrial workers exposed to formaldehyde. *J. Occup. Med.* 30: 895–901.

Stoup, N. E., A. Blair, and G. E. Erikson. 1986. Brain cancer and other causes of death in anatomists. *J. Natl. Cancer. Inst.* 77: 1217–1224.

Swarin, S. J., and F. Lipari. 1983. Determination of formaldehyde and other aldehydes by high performance liquid chromatography with fluorescence detection. *J. Liq. Chromatogr.* 6: 425–444.

Swenberg, J. A., W. D. Kerns, R. I. Mitchell, E. J. Gralla, and K. L. Pavkov. 1980. Induction of squamous cell carcinomas of the rat nasal cavity by inhalation exposure to formaldehyde vapor. *Cancer Res.* 40: 3398–3402.

Swenberg, J. A., E. A. Gross, J. Martin, and J. A. Popp.1983. Mechanisms of formaldehyde toxicity. In *Formaldehyde Toxicity*, ed. J. A. Gibson. Washington DC: Hemisphere.

Swiecichowski, A., K. J. Long, M. L. Milller, and G. D. Leikauf. 1993. Formaldehyde-induced airway hyperreactivity *in vivo* an ex vivo in guinea pigs. *Environ. Res.* 61: 185–199.

Tarkowski, M., and P. Gorski. 1995. Increased IgE antiovalbumin level in mice exposed to formaldehyde. *Int. Arch. Allergy Immunol.* 106: 422–424.

Thrasher, J. D., A. Wojdani, G. Cheung, and G. Heuser. 1987. Evidence for formaldehyde antibodies and altered cellular immunity in subjects exposed to formaldehyde in mobile homes. *Arch. Environ. Health* 42: 347–350.

Thrasher, J. D., A. Broughton, and P. Micevich. 1988. Antibodies and immune profiles of individuals occupationally exposed to formaldehyde: Six case reports. *Am. J. Ind. Med.* 14: 479–488.

Trump, B. F., M. W. Smith, M. Miyashita, P. C. Phelps, R. T. Jones, and C. C. Harriss. 1988. The effects of aldehydes on cytosolic Ca^2 of normal and transformed human bronchial cells. *J. Cell. Biol.* 107:72a.

Tuazon, E. C., S. M. Aschmann, J. Arey, and R. Atkinson 1997. Products of the gas-phase reactions of O_3 with a series of methyl-substituted ethenes. *Env. Sci. Tech.* 31: 3004–3009.

Turner, C. R., R. B. Stow, S. J. Hubbs, B. C. Gomes, and J. C. Williams. 1993a. Acrolein increases airway sensitivity to substance P and decreases NEP activity in guinea pigs. *J. Appl. Physiol.* 74: 1830–1839.

Turner, C. R., R. B. Stow, S. J. Hubbs, S. D. Talerico, E. P. Christian, and J. C. Williams. 1993b Protective role for neuropeptides in acute pulmonary response to acrolein in guinea pigs. *J. Appl. Physiol.* 75: 2456–2465.

Uba, G., D. Pachorek, J. Bernstein, D. H. Garabrant, J. R. Salines, W. E. Wright, and R. B. Amar. 1989. Prospective study of respiratory effects of formaldehyde among healthy and asthmatic medical students. *Am. J. Ind. Med.* 15: 91–101.

Vaca, C. E., J. A. Nilsson, J. L. Fang, and R. C. Grafstrom. 1998. Formation of DNA adduct in human buccal epithelial cells exposed to acetaldehyde and methylglyoxal *in vitro*. *Chemico-Biol. Interact.* 108: 197–208.

Vaughan, T. L., C. Strader, S. Davis, and S. Daling. 1986a. Formaldehyde and cancers of the pharynx, sinus, and nasal cavity. 1. Occupational exposures. *Int. J. Cancer* 38: 677–683.

Vaughan, T. L., C. Strader, S. Davis, and J. R. Daling. 1986b. Formaldehyde and cancers of the pharynx, sinus and nasal cavity. II. Residential exposures. *Int. J. Cancer* 38: 685–688.

Vegheli, P. V., and M. Osztovics. 1978. The alcohol syndromes: The intrarecombigenic effects of acetaldehyde. *Experientia* 34: 195–201.

Walrath, J., and J. F. Fraumeri Jr. 1983. Mortality patterns among embalmers. *Int. J. Cancer* 31: 407–411.

Walrath, J., and J. F. Fraumeri Jr. 1984. Cancer and other causes of death among embalmers. *Cancer Res.* 44: 4638–4641.

Watanabe, T. 1991. Mechanism of ethanol-induced bronchoconstriction in Japanese asthmatic patients. *Japan. J. Allergy* 40: 1210–1217.

Wayne, L. G., R. J. Bryan, and K. J. Ziedman. 1977. *Irritant Effects of Industrial Chemicals: Formaldehyde.* US DHEW, PHS, NIOSH Publication 77:117.

Weber-Tschopp, A., T. Fisher, and E. Grahdjean. 1977. Reizwirkugen tea Formaldehyds (HCHO) auf den Menschen. *Int. Arch. Occup. Environ. Health* 39: 207–218.

West, S., A. Hildesheim, and M. Dosemeci. 1993. Non-viral risk factors for nasopharyngeal carcinoma in the Phillipines: Results from a case-control study. *Int. J. Cancer* 55: 722–727.

WHO. World Health Organization. International Programme on Chemical Safety. 1989. *Environmental Health Criteria 89. Formaldehyde.* Geneva: World Health Organization.

WHO. World Health Organization. International Programme on Chemical Safety. 1992. *Environmental Health Criteria 127. Acrolein.* Geneva:. World Health Organization.

WHO. World Health Organization. International Programme on Chemical Safety. 1995. *Environmental Health Criteria 167. Acetaldehyde.* Geneva: World Health Organization.

Wieslander, G., D. Norback, E. Bjornsson, C. Janson, and G. Borman. 1997. Asthma and the indoor environment: The significance of emission of formaldehyde and volatile organic compounds from newly painted indoor surfaces. *Int. Arch. Occup. Environ. Health* 69: 115–124.

Wilhelmsson, B., and M. Holmstrom. 1987. Positive formaldehyde-rast after prolonged formaldehyde exposure by inhalation. *Lancet* 2:164.

Wilkins, R. J., and H. D. Macleod. 1976. Formaldehyde induced DNA-protein cross links in *E. coli. Mutat. Res.* 36: 11–16.

Windholz, M. 1983. *Merck Index.* Rahway, NJ: Merck and Co.

Witek, T. J., Jr., E. N. Schachter, T. Tosun, G. J. Beck, and B. P. Leaderer. 1987. An evaluation of respiratory effects following exposure to 2.0 ppm formaldehyde in asthmatics: Lung function, symptoms, and airway reactivity. *Arch. Environ. Health* 42: 230–237.

Woutersen, R. A., L. M. Appelman, V. J. Feron, and A. van Garderen-Hoetmer. 1986. Inhalation toxicity of acetaldehyde in rats. II. Carcinogenicity study: Interim results after 15 months. *Toxicology* 31: 123–133.

Woutersen, R. A., L. M. Appelman, A. van Garderen-Hoetmer, and V. J. Feron. 1986. Inhalation toxicity of acetaldehyde in rats. III. Carcinogenicity study. *Toxicology* 41: 213–231.

Woutersen, R. A., and V. J. Feron. 1987. Inhalation toxicity of acetaldehye in rats. IV. Progression and regression of nasal lesions after discontinuation of exposure. *Toxicology* 47: 295–305.

Woutersen, R. A., A. van Garderen-Hoetmer, J. P. Bruitntjes, A. Zwart, and V. J. Feron. 1989. Nasal tumours in rats after severe injury to the nasal mucosa and prolonged exposure to 10 ppm formaldehyde. *J. Appl. Toxicol.* 9: 39–46.

Wynder, E. L., and D. Hoffman. 1963. Ein experimenteller Beitrag zur Tabakrauchkanzerogenese. *Dtsch. Med. Wochenschr* 88: 623–628.

Yau, T. M. 1979. Mutagenicity and cytotoxicity of malonaldehyde in mammalian cells. *Mech. Aging Dev.* 11: 137–144.

Yoshida, A., A. Rzhetsky, L. C. Hsu, and C. Chang. 1998. Human aldehyde dehydrogenase gene family *Eur. J. Biochem.* 251: 549–557.

Zwart, A. R., A. Woutersen, J. W. G. M. Wilmer, B. J. Spit, and V. J. Fe Ron. 1988. Cytotoxic and adaptive effects in rat nasal epithelium after 3-day and 13-week exposure to low concentrations of formaldehyde vapour. *Toxicology* 51: 87–99.

13 Indoor Bioaerosol Contaminants

MARY KAY O'ROURKE, Ph.D.,
MICHAEL D. LEBOWITZ, Ph.D.

SOURCES

Bioaerosols fall into two classes: (1) airborne viable particles like fungi, bacteria, and viruses capable of multiplying under the right conditions and (2) biogenic particles like pollen, airborne antigen, and particles shed by animals and arthropods; these particles are subject to fragmentation but not independent reproduction. Bioaerosols have complex and varied organic structures; thus they differ from air pollutants (NRC, 1981). When they are present, even in small quantities, they can have very large health effects. These effects are due to infection, irritation, hypersensitivity, and inflammatory responses. Effects are characterized by human biological reactions ranging from uncomfortable to disabling (Pope et al., 1993; WHO, 1990; WHO/EURO, 1982; Lebowitz et al., 1972). Bioaerosols are both produced and concentrated in indoor environments; indoor exposure accounts for most of the attributable risk. In response, indoor bioaerosols were the focus of much research during the past decade.

A portion of indoor bioaerosols reflect natural seasonal increases, especially when growing conditions are favorable (O'Rourke et al., 1996, 1993, 1989; O'Rourke and Lebowitz, 1995; Meldrum et al., 1993). Pathogenic organisms, especially bacteria and fungi, can multiply in indoor microclimates, including ventilation systems (Pope et al., 1993; Burge, 1990; Bernstein et al., 1983). Viruses are host dependent; they do not multiply indoors but may spread among humans and from a few animal sources to humans and other animals. The airborne spread of viral disease can be facilitated by crowding of people, or through the spread of airborne virus by the ventilation system. Airborne contagion produces acute respiratory infections, which are often considered the largest single cause of morbidity (NCHS, 1988; Fox et al., 1970).

Arthropods and animals can introduce by-product aerosols that may precipitate airway hyperresponsiveness (van der Heide et al., 1997) including asthma attacks (Rosenstreich et al., 1997), and initiate a variety of allergic and irritant reactions among building occupants (RIVM, 1989; Andersen and Korsgaard, 1986). In most settings it is difficult to separate the confounding effects of multiple indoor exposures. Sporik et al. (1995) attempted this by working with school children in Los Alamos, New Maxico, where air pollution and household mite levels were low. Cat antigen loads were high in a number of homes, and asthma remained a major cause of morbidity among children (6.3%). Presence of dog in a home is associated with allergy in some, but it is rarely associated with asthma.

Environmental Toxicants: Human Exposures and Their Health Effects, 2/e. Edited by Morton Lippmann.
ISBN: 0-471-29298-2 © 2000 John Wiley & Sons, Inc.

Infiltration from outdoors is responsible for most indoor pollen (O'Rourke and Lebowitz, 1995, 1984; O'Rourke et al., 1989) with a negligible contribution by indoor plants. However, moist potting soil can produce abundant fungal spores. In many homes, particularly in regions with equable climates, indoor concentrations of fungi closely resemble those found outside the home with infiltration as the major spore source (Li and Kuo, 1994; Meldrum et al., 1993). Fungal concentrations become elevated in buildings where water damage has occurred and dampness is sustained (Morey, 1996; Johanning et al., 1996; Flannigan and Miller, 1994; Pope et al., 1993; Burge, 1990; Solomon and Burge, 1975). Some investigators (Ahern et al., 1995; Ezeonu et al., 1994; Rao, unpubl.) are evaluating fungal growth on various building materials. Many of these bioaerosols end up in house dust, to be resuspended with activity (Yli-Panula and Rantio-Lehtimaki, 1996; Verhoeff et al., 1994; Pope et al., 1993; Nevalainen et al., 1987).

A sizable proportion of the population has been or is capable of being sensitized (i.e., can develop a hypersensitivity) to bioaerosol contaminants over their lifetime. Allergy is thought to affect over 35 million people in the United State at some point in their lives (Pope et al., 1993). Asthma is a more dramatic disease. Death rates have risen for 0.8 per 100,000 in 1977 to 2.1 per 100,000 in 1994 (Sly and O'Donnell, 1997). The annual cost of asthma in the United States is estimated at $6.2 billion (Weiss et al., 1992). The combined effect of all bioaerosol contaminants indoors is thought to account for a substantial proportion of absenteeism in schools and workplaces, and days of restricted activity or performance. (In the general population 5 to 15 days of restricted activity per year may result; WHO, 1990; NCHS, 1988).

To understand health responses derived from bioaerosol exposures, WHO (1990) suggests evaluating (1) the species/type and nature of the suspended viable organisms or biologically derived particles; (2) the exposure to bioaerosols, including their sources, sites of multiplication, reservoirs, and means of dispersion; (3) the nature and mechanisms of the morbidity effects associated with bioaerosol exposure, including the range and distribution of sensitivity in the population; and (4) the methods of evaluation and control.

BIOLOGICAL FACTORS

In the environment, viable bioaerosols occupy three, sometimes overlapping, modalities: habitation in a reservoir, amplification, and dissemination (Burge and Freeley, 1991). Bacteria and viruses are usually brought indoors in human hosts (the major reservoir) and spread person to person (WHO, 1983a; CDC, 1987). Sometimes microorganisms become incorporated in house dust or attached to surfaces. Under the right conditions viable microorganisms reproduce, and their numbers, if not their virulence, increase. Such amplification minimizes the effects of dilution when dissemination occurs and results in the greater probability of infecting a new host. Some bacteria (e.g., *Pseudomonas*, TB) and some viruses (e.g., measles, chicken pox) can be disseminated through coughing, sneezing, and shedding of skin scales; the virus may remain as viable particles on surfaces and fabric. These particles may enter the ventilation systems (Riley, 1982; LaForce, 1986; Zeterberg, 1973), disperse, and infect other humans (Couch, 1981). Air transfer models explain most infection patterns fairly well. Recent studies also implicate direct contact among humans by hand or through fomites, or direct contact with contaminated surfaces to spread viruses like respiratory syncytial virus (RSV) (Madge et al., 1992) and influenza (Morens and Rash, 1995). Washing hands and surfaces and wearing protective gowns and gloves significantly reduced transmission of RSV, suggesting other routes of dispersal in addition to air (Madge et al., 1992).

Growth Indoors

Spores and viable bacteria are ubiquitous; they will grow virtually anywhere given the right balance of nutrient, moisture, and temperature. Specific growth requirements vary among organisms. In the indoor environment, spores and bacteria are found in house dust, which is often resuspended as bioaerosols by human or animal activity. When growth occurs, additional contaminants are produced. Bacterial endotoxins (Rix, 1997; Teeuw et al., 1994), fungal mycotoxins (Smoragiewicz et al., 1993; Hendry and Cole, 1993), and mycological volatile organic compounds (mVOCs) (Bjurman et al., 1997; Pasanen et al., 1996) may be released to further contaminate the indoor environment.

Ventilation will affect the introduction and removal, growth and control (moisture and temperature), of organisms and their resulting detritus (particles) (LaForce, 1986; Yoshizawa et al., 1987; Schata et al., 1989). Soil from indoor plants, food, and vegetal remains can support fungal growth (Raza et al., 1989). Fungal spore sizes range from 2 to 200 μm in diameter, with most spores being about 10 μm (Andersen and Korsgaard, 1986).

Moisture

Most construction materials, especially wood products, their sealants and finishes, can support microbial growth (NRC, 1981). Moisture is the major factor that promotes or limits microbial growth indoors (WHO, 1990). When the relative humidity (rh) of surfaces reaches 25%, fungal growth can occur; spore concentrations will elevate as humidity increases up to 70%. Beyond 70%, spore output does not increase (Burge, 1985) although hyphal growth may expand. Morey (1996) reports that mold will be found where rh exceeds 65% to 70% on finished surfaces. Moisture or water may penetrate into the structures, air ducts, and furnishings through diffusion, leakage, or condensation. With excess moisture the microbial growth starts immediately (Jantunen et al., 1987). This growth will lead to deterioration of building materials, which can produce more bioaerosols (NRC, 1981). Humid winter climates promote continuous problems (RIVM, 1989; Andersen and Korsgaard, 1986).

Elevated humidity indoors promotes the reproduction and expansion of mite populations inside homes. They can be found in carpets, furnishings, and fabrics where suitable nutrient (detritus) is available (Bischoff et al., 1986; Bishoff, 1989; Arlian, 1992). Mites require specific temperature and humidity regimes to thrive (Arlian, 1989, 1992; Arlian et al., 1990). Mite populations expand when indoor rh is 60% to 75% or above at temperatures of 60° to 75 °F (Arlian et al., 1982; Platts-Mills et al., 1987). Based on laboratory results, the critical equilibrium humidity for fasting *Dermatophagoides pteronyssinus* is 73% rh at 25 °C, 10 and 55% to 75% rh proportional to temperatures of 15° to 35 °C for *D. farinae* (Arlian, 1975a). Most mites die in 1 to 3 days at 40% or 50% rh, but some mites survive for 4 to 8 days (Arlian, 1975b, Arlian and Veselica, 1981, Brandt and Arlian, 1976). Since mites require relatively high humidity for survival, most surveys find the greatest mite prevalence in humid, temperate regions and the least in arid regions.

Water reservoirs associated with heating, ventilating, air conditioning, and humidification are favorable habitats for microbial growth (Burge and Freeley, 1991; Burge, 1985; Woods et al., 1989; Volk and Wheeler, 1980; WHO/EURO, 1982). Sediment collections are habitats for the bacteria, fungi, actinomycetes, algae, and amoebae. *Acinetobacter* and *Pseudomonas* have been found in cool-mist vaporizers (Volk and Wheeler, 1980; Smith, 1977). Depending on the temperature, the flora may contain thermophilic (heat-related) organisms. *Legionella* bacteria are frequently found in potable waters (WHO/EURO, 1982; WHO/EURO, 1986). Mechanical disturbance of contaminated water may produce bioaerosols; evaporation alone does not appear to do so. Very low moisture levels in air can enhance spore-release of fungi (Jantunen et al., 1987).

Ventilation

Ventilation systems serve two main functions: (1) to replace "old" dirty air with clean, "fresh" air and (2) to limit the spread of unwanted contaminants among rooms by removing pollutants from air being recycled (Seppanen, 1996). Dilution of indoor air with "fresh" outdoor air reduces the concentrations of bioaerosol contaminants circulating inside a building. Ventilation rates are generally calculated based on the floor area of a building (home) or based on the number of people expected to occupy an area (office). Seppanen reports (1996) the potential pollution load of an area plays little or no role in determining the ventilation provided to an area at the present time. Seppanen (1996) discusses air exchange rates reported by studies in several countries. In general, most studies examining air exchange in homes report mean rates of 0.3 to 0.5 air changes per hour. Mendell (1993) reviewed the ventilation literature related to sick building syndrome (SBS) in offices buildings. He reported when ventilation rates are $< 10 \, L/s$ per person, there are greater complaints of SBS. Seppanen reports that in the average Finnish school, ventilation rates are $3.5 \, L/s$ and well below the $6.0 \, L/s$ values set by the building code. Both figures are lower than the threshold value for SBS complaints reported by Mendell (1993), and dissatisfaction abounds among headmasters at the schools (Seppanen, 1996).

Addition of outdoor air to indoor environments affects indoor humidity levels and thermal loads, and thus growth of viable outdoor contaminants. When not properly maintained, mechanical ventilation systems can become sources of bioaerosols. For example, air filters that are not routinely replaced can provide nutrients and strata for microbial growth, and handling the system increases dispersal (Yoshizawa et al., 1987; Elixmann et al., 1989; Pope et al., 1993). Air exchange in winter reduces indoor moisture and promotes the use of humidifying equipment. In summer, air exchange can increase indoor moisture, and promote the use of dehumidifiers. In sealed buildings, energy conservation measures may reduced ventilation rates, so there is an excess of human-sourced biological air contaminants (Tobin et al., 1987a,b). When there are adequate rates of airflow throughout the space, ventilation assists in drying any wet building material.

Biologically Derived Particles

Biologically derived bioaerosols consist of antigen from arthropods and their feces, especially house dust mites and cockroaches (Colten et al., 1977; Tovey et al., 1981a,b; Pope et al., 1993). Also included are fecal matter and urine from rodents, dander from humans and animals (dogs and cats), secretions, fragments or other products derived from animals and plants (i.e., horse hair, kapok), and some potential parasites from animals. Cat antigen is derived primarily from saliva deposited on fur; as it dries the saliva flakes off as particles 1 to 10 µm in diameter; other body fluids may contribute some antigen. Dog antigen may be liberated in a similar fashion. Wood et al. (1988) found cat and dog antigen in 106 Baltimore homes regardless of whether a pet actually lived at or in the residence. Later work (Bollinger et al., 1996) compared *Fel d 1* antigen levels in 37 homes with resident cats and 40 homes lacking cats. As expected, all homes lived in by cats had detectable antigen in the air and dust sampled. Interestingly 25% of the cat-free homes had elevated levels of cat antigen in the air, and 100% of the cat-free homes had cat antigen present in the house dust, albeit in generally lower levels. Yet antigen loading in the cat-free homes was sufficient to evoke symptoms in susceptible individuals.

The composition of biologically derived particles can vary according to the production site (regional, local, microenvironmental). Biogenic particles are found in house dust, surfaces, fabrics, building materials, food, and pet enclosures. Dander and secretions from animals may be brought in from outside. Domestic mites (*Dermatophagoides spp, Blomia tropicalis, Euroglyphus maynei*, and storage mites) are widespread allergens found indoors

(Arlian et al., 1992; Kneist, 1989; Spieksma et al., 1969; Sinha and van Bronswijk, 1971). Their food source includes fungi, as well as human and other animal epidermal scales, and they are well adapted to indoor environments. Their excrement is a major proportion of the allergen in house dust (Bischoff, 1989). Mite excreta are sticky pellets about 20 μm in diameter (Tovey et al., 1981a), and the antigen contained in the pellets is water soluble (Tovey et al., 1981b) and can be found on particles less than 5 μm in diameter (Swanson et al., 1985). The humidity in the particular indoor environment is the determining feature of the species. *D. farinae* tolerates slightly lower humidity. Allergic diseases from house dust mites are most frequent in damp temperate climates. Mattresses and bedding (because of moisture from the sleeper), upholstery, and carpets (because the floor is cooler and humidity higher) are their main habitats. House dust mite antigen may be undetectable in undisturbed areas, but increase with activity (Tovey et al., 1981b). The homes of patients who have asthma associated with house dust allergy are more humid and have more mites than control homes in the same community (Tovey et al., 1981a; Korsgaard, 1983a,b).

Pollen

Both whole pollen grains and biogenic antigen particles of identical composition (airborne antigen) can be found in indoor environments (O'Rourke and Lebowitz, 1984, 1995; O'Rourke et al., 1989; Schumacher et al., 1988; Rantio-Lehtimaki et al., 1994; Yli-Panula and Rantio-Lehtimaki, 1996). The airborne antigen can be amorphous and be submicrometer in size. The submicrometer size facilitates particle penetration into the lower airways (Schumacher et al., 1988). To date over 700 homes have been sampled in the Tucson area for indoor pollen. None contain pollen attributable to house plants; a few fern spores were identified.

Most pollen found inside homes originates from outside sources. It enters the indoor environment through passive or active ventilation, on shoes, clothing, or pets. Pollen are generally spherical, oblate spheroids, or prolate. They range in size from 5 to 200 μm, though they generally are 15 to 50 μm. Most pollen settles on the floor fairly rapidly, but it can be resuspended through occupant activity. Pollen production outside is seasonal, and the quantity also varies greatly. The dominant species in any region depends on the composition of the local flora. Airborne pollen spectra vary among regions, and among years, in response to climatic variability (WHO, 1990; Holberg et al., 1987; Levetin, 1998; Rogers, 1997).

EXPOSURE

Environmental Measurement and Sampling

Sampling for bioaerosols is expensive and time-consuming. Prior to sampling, a visual inspection of the site should always be made, and obvious problems should be remediated. Only if complaints persist, should bioaerosol sampling be undertaken. Burge (1989) provided a useful approach to evaluating the workplace setting: Visually inspect the building, particularly the ventilation system, its filters, air intake, and ducts. Understanding the design and operation of the ventilation system is important. Make sure that there is an adequate supply of fresh air. Look for dampness along walls, ceilings, roofs, and in basements. Survey building users to identify special problem areas and chronic complainers. Preassessment of a building is a necessary initial phase for any investigation of SBS. Develop a sampling strategy for each room and for the ventilation system in response to symptom patterns. Choose appropriate samplers and sample consistently. Duplicate samples should be taken whenever possible, and a control, noncomplaint, building of similar design should be simultaneously sampled along with outdoor control samples. Consider the boundary layer effects of walls and all furniture, including room dividers, when placing samplers Recommendations for remedial action must be based on clear differences among areas sampled.

The building inspection should help define the problem under investigation. Woods et al. (1989) point out some of the critical issues that must be examined prior to investigation a building. They include four essential issues: (1) determining what to measure (through consultation, qualitative, and quantitative diagnostics), (2) determining appropriate instrumentation, (3) determining how results of measurements will be interpreted, and (4) predicting appropriate building performance.

Once the problem is defined, the investigator selects the sampling equipment that best implements the study design. Bioaerosol sampling in air, in water, and from surfaces should be performed when the presence of such agents is suggested, especially when confirmation of the presence of an agent is needed or to rule out the presence of one or more specific agents (Nevalainen, 1993; WHO, 1990; Jantunen et al., 1987; Burge, 1989; NRC, 1981). In general, there are no standard methods for sampling and analysis of microbiological agents in indoor air, so it is difficult to interpret the acquired data. For collection of regional outdoor pollen and spores, the American Academy of Allergy, Asthma and Immunology has a standard protocol, but none for indoor environments. The American Conference of Governmental Industrial Hygienists (ACGIH) has developed a generic protocol for workplaces (ACGIH, 1990). Together standard protocols help establish quantitative data bases.

Sampling protocols must address the potential spatial and temporal distribution of the biological agents (NRC, 1981; Wood et al., 1989; WHO, 1990). Standard environmental questionnaires help identify factors and locations favoring growth and dispersion (Lebowitz et al., 1989a,b). Sampling has to be accompanied by detailed information concerning the site and the circumstances of collection. Spore release and pollen production are highly dependent on environmental factors, especially temperature and humidity (NRC, 1981) but also light, location, and so on. Outdoor sampling for comparisons is deemed essential. In outdoor air, seasonal variations may produce differences of several orders of magnitude. Similar problems probably exist for bacteria and their endotoxins. Therefore indoor and outdoor collections should be paired, and the building should be sampled in different seasons. Ideally air sampling should be conducted utilizing active monitors (Burge, 1989; O'Rourke and Lebowitz, 1995; O'Rourke, 1996).

Collected samples take several forms: (1) Pollen and spores can be directly deposited on slides or tapes, and impacted bioaerosols are mounted and identified morphologically using compound light microscopy. (2) Fungi and bacteria can be directly deposited on a growth media, cultured and examined dissecting and compound microscopy. (3) Biological particles can be directly deposited on filters. The bioaerosols can be eluted, plated, and cultured, or they may be eluted and assayed using an immunological technique like ELISA. (4) Liquid impingers are used to capture bioaerosols, and the liquid is sampled and plated or examined immunochemically. (5) Samples can be collected from reservoirs of bioaerosols. This may involve collection of water from cooling towers, collection of surface wipes, or collection of dust samples. These samples may be plated directly, eluted and plated, or extracted and assayed immunochemically. Most of these collection methods rely on suction devices; some are described below. Other articles describing these samples include Ogden et al. (1974), Solomon (1988), Ausdenmoore (1988), Burge (1990), Macher et al., 1995; O'Rourke and Lebowitz (1995), and O'Rourke (1996).

In addition to the workings of air samplers, there are many important areas that bear further investigation by the novice. Many issues, ranging from the field to the lab, have entire volumes dedicated to them, and they include (1) sampler placement, (2) growth media, (3) the physics of air and samplers, (4) adhesives for particle collection, (5) mounting media and particle stains, (6) filter characteristics, (7) elution techniques and duration, (8) choice of assay (plates, antibodies, antisera, conjugates, labels, standards, etc.), and other potential issues that may have been overlooked. Justifiable, valid choices related to these areas will make developing standardized methods for bioaerosol sampling difficult, if not impossible. At this time the equipment is fairly standard, but operational choices vary widely.

Collected air samples must adequately address the study's objectives. For instance, some collection devices rely on enumeration of intact particles. Breakage of the particles would result in inflated measurement. By contrast, immunochemical techniques quantify specific proteins incidental to the number of particles collected. One method may be better than another at addressing a specific study aim. Macher et al. (1995) provide an excellent summary of commercially available equipment, factors related to equipment operation, and equipment limitations. Sample collection is commonly achieved through impaction, impingement, filtration, and gravitational settling.

Prior to selecting a sampler, the investigator should know the aerodynamic size of the particle of interest. Then the investigator can select the sampler with the correct cutpoint and measurable particle sampling efficiency. The investigator should be careful to select a sampler best representing airborne particle concentrations (not over- or undersampling particles). Further the investigator should adhere to "good field practice" (GFP) standards for bioaerosol collection: (1) Calibration checks should be made with every use of a sampler. (2) All sampler openings should be unobstructed. (3) Sterile collection protocols with field spikes and field blanks should be employed. (4) Duplicate samples should be collected. (5) Appropriate handling and shipping conditions should be observed (e.g., cold shipment). (6) Samples should be collected under isokinetic conditions by adjusting sample suction to match air velocity.

The sample collections described by Macher et al. (1995) are used to measure the biological exposure through air. Surfaces can also be assayed. Clinical handbooks describe wipe techniques for hard surfaces. Bacteria and viruses are frequently sampled from surfaces. As an outgrowth of research related to house dust mites, researchers began evaluating dust using enzyme-linked immunosorbent assay (ELISA). Dust collection techniques are varied. Arlian et al. (1992) and O'Rourke et al. (1996) employed consistent and internally standard techniques to sample dust that complied with the recommendations of the WHO (World Health Organization) working group on house dust mites and asthma (WHO, 1986b; Platts-Mills et al., 1989). These reports recommend vacuuming a fixed area, for a fixed time, using the same vacuum in all locations used for comparison. (O'Rourke et al., 1996, vacuumed 1 m^2, for 2 minutes with a 2.2 hp Hoover Port-a-Power vacuum cleaner; dust was deposited on a filter held in special wand attachment). Dust from carpets, floors, and furniture is evaluated for a many allergens (i.e., domestic mites, cockroaches, cat, dog, and a variety of pollen and mold types) using immunochemical techniques. The approach may present a good picture of biological contaminant in the carpet reservoir, but does it accurately represent bioaerosol exposure?

O'Rourke and Lebowitz (1984) evaluated house dust for pollen content, which was abundant and strongly correlated with the regional airborne pollen of the season. Chew et al. (1996) have performed preliminary analysis of house dust for culturable fungi. Preliminary indications suggest a limited relationship between the cultured fungi and the airborne fungi by type. The most dominant carpet type, yeast, either fails to become airborne or is not readily plated from air samples. The study is ongoing and results are preliminary. Today numerous investigators are currently using immunochemical evaluation of the reservoir of biological contaminant found in house dust, and they are relating these assays to observed health effects. The extent to which a single dust measure represents a cumulative exposure requires careful consideration for each potential bioaerosol considered.

Exposure Assessment

Investigations of populations require techniques differing substantially from those appropriate for evaluating individuals. Population studies depend on reliable epidemiologic techniques, particularly the comparison of representative unbiased population samples exposed to different indoor air environments (WHO, 1983a,b; Finnegan et al., 1984).

Questionnaires are the basis for investigations (Lebowitz et al., 1989a,b). They should be validated in the community to be studied in terms of comprehensibility, reproducibility, and their power to identify the conditions under study. They should also be used to help define exposure, and to measure the major confounding factors (other factors that modify the outcome being assessed). Questionnaire responses may be altered by the method of administration and the biases of the population being studied (WHO, 1983b).

Exposure to antigenic material, either infectious agents or allergens, can be estimated by specific antibody determinations in populations. This is particularly appropriate for the study of exposure to *Legionella*, other bacteria, and viruses (WHO/EURO, 1986). It is also appropriate for the study of sensitization to aeroallergens causing rhinitis, conjunctivitis, and asthma (specific IgE and IgG estimations) and alveolitis or humidifier fever (specific IgG estimations) (Riley, 1982; Rom, 1983; Turner-Warwick, 1978; WHO/EURO, 1982; NRC, 1981; Thorn et al., 1996; Rosenstreich et al., 1997). The measurement of infectious agents can be done in the living reservoirs, human or animal (Benenson, 1985; Wilks et al., 1995). These measurements are necessary for the presence of specific agents and also for identifying sources. The quantitative assessment of exposure for individuals is probably not necessary for most agents. Isolation of *Legionella* or *Stachybotrys chartarum* from the air is a definite health hazard, regardless of how many colony forming units are detected (WHO/EURO, 1982, Johanning et al., 1996).

Exposure to allergens can be assessed by measuring airborne antigens (described above). Airborne antigen levels can be a very good measure of exposure, especially when related to time activity information (WHO, 1983a). Sufficiently good methods exists to make airborne monitoring appropriate for some important indoor allergens such as the antigens from the house dust mite *(Dermatophagoides)* (Pope et al., 1993). One should determine the presence of pets or pests and antigens they release, since they can be responsible for important contamination of indoor air with nonviable allergenic bioaerosols. The determination of sources of allergens and of exposure can be made by questionnaire or by examination of the indoor and measurements. Dampness (moisture sources and/or humidity) can be determined in all three ways. A comparison of occupants' subjective impressions of dampness with home characteristics (visible mold growth, damp stains, bugs, bad smells, wet/humid crawl spaces) and with measurements of fungi and bacteria indicate that the subjective impressions were not related to counts (van Wageningen et al., 1987).

Case studies of exposure assessment without health assessment have been provided by several groups, starting with a well-known study by Solomon and Burge (1975). Other recent studies include those on fungi (Samson, 1985; Flannigan, 1987; Strieifel et al., 1989; Ohkge et al., 1987; Jantunen et al., 1987). Humidity effects were obvious. There have been studies of fungi and bacteria (Reponen et al., 1989; Binnie, 1987; Nevalainen et al., 1987), and of other bioaerosols (RIVM, 1989; Hawthorne et al., 1989, Custovic et al., 1996). RIVM (1989) found that 15% of Dutch homes had problems with fungi and mites due to dampness. Bischoff (1989) and Colloff (1991) reviewed studies of mites (WHO, 1986b).

Most recently, Verhoeff and Burge (1997) examined results from nine residential, population based studies of fungi associated with symptom responses. Their goal was to determine risk assessment based guidelines for permissible fungi concentrations in homes.

They concluded that based on the best of the current literature, there is insufficient data to determine guidelines for permissible fungal levels. More work needs to be done with sensitized populations, using health outcomes specific for allergic disease. Appropriate aerobiological measures need to be collected in duplicate and repeated over time, and other "confounder" allergens and air pollutants should be evaluated.

The most intense health effects caused by exposure are usually found in workplaces that specialize in producing a specific product or service. Bioaerosols are a risk in certain occupations and many of the exposures occur indoors. Unlike other workplace environments, responses to bioaerosols occur after a short period of exposure, not after years. As a result workers with host susceptibility are more likely to leave the job (healthy worker syndrome) and subsequent studies of occupational health only identify subtle effects. Some occupations have known health outcomes. Farmers have long been subject respiratory diseases like "farmers lung" in response to mold (*Micropolyspora faeni*) exposures (Miadonna et al., 1994; Kokkarinen et al., 1994), and more recently "farmer's fever" (Cormier et al., 1993). Dairy farmers are more prone to chronic bronchitis than control populations when controlling for smoking (Dalphin et al., 1993; Jorna et al., 1994). Pig farmers have frequent exposure to endotoxins (Preller et al., 1995a, b, c; Dornham et al., 1995), as do solid waste handlers and processors of recycled waste (Poulsen et al., 1995a, b). Other industrial workers, such as, metalworkers exposed to bacteria (Robins et al., 1997) and fiber glass manufacturers exposed to endotoxin (Milton et al., 1995, 1996), have also contracted respiratory disease in response to bioaerosol exposure.

MORBIDITY EFFECTS

Description of Morbidity

The wide variety of biological agents and derived materials in the indoor environment are associated with a range of illnesses (NRC, 1981). The frequency and severity of these illnesses also varies by environmental and host conditions. Their contribution to total illness is quite large. However, attributable risk is not known. Of the many diseases that have been associated with contaminants indoors (NRC/NAS, 1987; Lebowitz, 1983), some are specifically associated with or caused by bioaerosols. Some of these illnesses may have other causes unrelated to the indoor environment. The size of the bioaerosol is important to potential reactions. Large bioaerosols (10–50 μm MMAD) deposit in the nose, whereas intrathoracic airway deposition occurs with smaller bioaerosols (1 to 10 μm), and terminal airway-alveoli deposition occurs most frequently for those under 1 μm (Martonen and O'Rourke, 1991, 1992).

Infectious processes (due to bacteria and viruses) include Legionnaires' disease (a pneumonia caused by the bacterium *Legionella pneumophila*), and other lower, or upper, respiratory tract illnesses. Drinking water contaminated with *Legionella* fails to cause legionellosis. Inhalation of aerosolized water containing *Legionella* is required (WHO/EURO, 1982). Currently dose-specific information for allowable levels of *Legionella* bacteria in potable water is unknown. Hospital respiratory equipment (humidifiers and nebulizers) are routinely cleaned with tap water that may be contaminated. The "cleaned" respiratory equipment may serve as a secondary source for hospital-acquired legionellosis (Woo et al., 1992). *Legionella* pneumonia accounts for less than 5% of community-acquired pneumonia but may be particular to buildings in about 30% of cases, namely hotels and hospitals (WHO/EURO, 1982). Bates et al. (1992) attempted to identify the agent(s) responsible for hospital-acquired pneumonia. They examined 198 patients with 204 cases; a direct agent was found in only half the cases. Extensive diagnostic procedures were performed on all cases. *Legionella* was the most common pathogen identified.

Four common acute or chronic local inflammatory reactions often occur together and may be produced by bioaerosols (Rom, 1983; Wasserman, 1988; Middleton et al., 1988; NRC/NAS, 1987; WHO, 1983a). These conditions may be due to infection, allergy, or nonallergic mechanisms. Rhinitis (itching, sneezing, runny, or stuffy nose) is commonly related to the indoor environment (NRC/NAS, 1987); it may be due also to dryness or coldness of the air or air pollutants. The others are conjunctivitis, (eye itching, soreness, watering, or discharge), sinusitis (pain or fullness in the face, possibly headache), and otitis (in the external or internal ear, which may cause pain and impair hearing). Allergy will be defined as a physiological event mediated via a variety of immunological mechanisms induced by specific allergens (WHO, 1990; Weill and Turner Warwick, 1981; Rom, 1983; Wasserman, 1988; Middleton et al., 1988; Ring and Burg, 1986). Pseudoallergic reactions may be similar physiological reactions but without immunological specificity. They may be caused by direct release of mediators, complement activation, enzyme defects, or psychoneurogenic effects (Ring, 1993).

Asthma (variable airways obstruction) may be precipitated by bioaerosols. Most affected patients have multiple trigger factors (e.g., exercise and cold air, air pollutant irritants, allergens and infections). Indoor-related asthma symptoms may deteriorate within minutes or hours of exposure and improve after leaving the site of exposure. It may occur or reoccur 6 to 12 hours after exposure to an allergic stimulus (the late phase of dual phase asthma), which can occur due to indoor-related (or occupational) allergens; house dust is a good example of such a stimulus (Weinberger, 1992; Wasserman, 1988; Booij-Noord et al., 1971). Bronchopulmonary aspergillosis is a rare, complicated, specific form of asthma due to allergy to the fungus *Aspergillus* (Mrouch and Spock, 1994, Amitani et al., 1995). The same fungus may cause rhinitis and alveolitis (pneumonitis) (Malmburg et al., 1993), may produce mycetomas, fungal balls (Aspergilloma; also see Yoshida et al., 1992, for *Penicillium decumbens* fungal balls), and may be invasive in immunocompromised patients (Crissley et al., 1995; Kauffman, 1996).

Alveolitis (inflammation of the air sacs) results in breathlessness. It may be caused by nonspecific mechanisms, but indoor bioaerosols only are associated with allergic alveolitis (or hypersensitivity pneumonitis-HP)(de Hoyas et al., 1993). Most HP is caused by contaminated humidifiers (Reed et al., 1983), containing many fungi and bacteria, possibly amoebae, mostly soluble products rather than single whole organisms. The most well-known agents are thermophilic bacilli (e.g., actinomycetes) (WHO, 1990). HP is the most common illness from exposure to bird antigens, in their fecal matter (Weinberger, 1992). Pigeon fanciers can have a other immune system responses to the bird antigens (Rodriguez de Castro et al., 1993; Hasani et al., 1992). The problem is more serious since pulmonary fibrosis can occur before diagnosis. Humidifier fever is an influenzalike illness developing shortly after exposure to aerosols from microbiologically contaminated humidifiers. Recovery can occur within days, even with continuing exposure. It often occurs on the first day of re-exposure after a break from exposure. Although antibodies have been found to certain organisms, endotoxins are suspected to be the dominant cause (WHO, 1990). Experimental exposure of symptomatic workers to humidifier antigens can induce headache, rhinitis, and lethargy, as well as asthma and alveolitis; similar exposures do not cause symptoms in previously unexposed individuals. Organic dust toxic syndrome (ODTS) occurs in response to exposure to inhalation of dusts derived from products like cotton, grain, mulch, and wood chips. Wintermeyer et al. (1997) report some of the immune system changes that may be in response to endotoxin exposure.

Mycotoxicosos is an acute toxic response to products from certain molds. It is marked mostly by fatigue and irritability, and subtle alterations in immune function. There are many mycotoxin producing species that need to be considered (Jarvis, 1986; Samson, 1985; Croft et al., 1986; Flannigan, 1987; Tobin et al., 1987b; Sorenson et al., 1987; WHO, 1990). Perhaps the mycotoxin of greatest concern today is Satratoxin derived from

Stachybotrys chartarum (atra). This fungus grows under very wet conditions. It is mostly found in water-damaged buildings and prefers growing on high cellulose material. Spores rarely become airborne, so it is not routinely detected in air samples. Johanning et al. (1996) evaluated office workers who had been exposed to the fungi and toxin. They reported impairment to the respiratory and central nervous systems of some workers who experienced prolonged exposure. Mycotoxin exposure is very difficult to diagnose.

There are also skin conditions also associated with bioaerosols: Contact dermatitis (an acute or chronic inflammation) is caused by allergic, toxic, or irritant effects, from both physical contact (including constituents from flowers) and aerosols (Benezra et al., 1985; Lovell, 1993). Atopic eczema (chronic relapsing itching skin rash) commonly occurs first in infancy or early childhood, and it is sometimes aggravated by bioaerosols. Perspiration with high ambient temperatures may increase eczema as well. Contact urticaria (acute or chronic skin rash with itching) has allergic and nonallergic causes (Middleton et al., 1988).

Finally there is the sick building syndrome. It consists of a number of symptoms that are common in the general population but may, in a temporal sense, be related to a particular building. A substantial increase in the prevalence of the symptoms above background levels provides the link between the building and its occupants (WHO, 1983b; Woods et al., 1989; Redlich et al., 1997). The main symptoms are eye, nose, and throat irritation (WHO, 1986); sensation of dry mucous membranes; skin erythema; mental fatigue, headaches, nausea, and dizziness; high frequency of airway infection and cough; and hoarseness, wheezing, and unspecified hypersensitivity. There appear to be multiple causes of sick building syndrome. It has been related epidemiologically to sealed buildings, increased temperature and dust levels, environmental tobacco smoke, and psychogenic or social factors. There is also a likely role for bioaerosols, though mostly for true building-related illness (WHO, 1986; Woods et al., 1989; Wessen and Schoeps, 1996; Jarvis et al., 1996). There is epidemiological evidence that buildings with humidifiers and chillers have more symptomatic workers than buildings without, and that very dry air (< 30% RH), which is common during the heating season in very cold climates, increases many sick building symptoms (Reinikainen et al., 1988).

Health Hazards Related to Infection

The risk associated with exposure to infectious agents is determined by a number of factors to the pathogenic agents, to their exposure in the indoor environment, and to host-specific factors (Benezra et al., 1985; Fox et al., 1970). Dose–response relationships do exist. However, threshold infectious doses are not known for most viable agents. Thus the presence of pathogenic bacterial or viral species in the indoor air constitutes a health hazard per se. Emission of viruses depends on human behavior (sneezing, emission of droplets during talking, etc.) (Riley, 1982; Benenson, 1985). Droplet nuclei are 0.5 to 5.0 μm in diameter (Knight et al., 1980).

Transmission efficiency depends on the location of sources with respect to receptors. Transmission is further affected by mechanical reservoirs, air-cleaning systems, and air circulation. Other suspended aerosols can be efficient carriers of microbes. Temperature and humidity influence transmission by altering particle size, thus affecting their settling time (Benenson, 1985; Fox et al., 1970). At humidity levels higher than 65%, the incidence of upper respiratory illness can increase, and have adverse effects in asthmatics and allergics (WHO, 1990).

Some microbiological agents enter the indoor environment as diseases of pets (e.g., toxoplasmosis in cats or rabbits, psittacosis in birds), which may be transmitted (by handling) to humans. There are some animal viruses (e.g., cat leukemia virus) that may be transmittable as well, but there is insufficient information about such viruses (Benenson, 1985).

Individual susceptibility to infections is most important in determining the actual risk of developing (Rom, 1983; Turner-Warwick, 1978; Wasserman, 1988; Tobin et al., 1987a,b). Infancy, early childhood, and old age are associated with increased susceptibility. It may be increased due to various conditions — including existing disease, such as chronic lung disease; immunosuppression, as occurring under drug therapy, or during certain diseases (e.g., cancer, AIDS, other chronic affections); smoking habits and alcohol consumption, diet (i.e., low in necessary nutrients, vitamins, and minerals); occupational or ambient exposure to airway irritants which may damage the pulmonary defensive system (mucociliary cells, macrophages, etc.) — and with warm temperatures. Human susceptibility to infections decreases as a result of immunization (CDC, 1987).

Health Hazards Related to Allergens

Separate dose–response relationships exist for different populations. In a previously unsensitized population, the risk of sensitization is likely to depend on the potency of the allergen, the level of exposure, and the length of exposure (Rom, 1983; Turner-Warwick, 1978; Wasserman, 1988). Indoor air antigens vary in their potency. For example, house dust mite antigens are often considered potent, pollen relatively potent, and mold antigens less potent. Cockroach antigen may be very potent and can cause asthma, especially in inner city lower socioeconomic residents (Homberger et al., 1979; Colten et al., 1977; Rosenstreich et al., 1997; Sarpong et al., 1997).

Current evidence suggests that a considerable percentage of the population is capable of developing IgE-mediated sensitization (also referred to as *atopy*). The figure reaches around 60% of the population exposed to environmental allergens in Tucson, Arizona (Barbee et al., 1987; Sears et al., 1989). In occupational settings, this figure may be higher, reaching, for example, around 75% in biological detergent workers exposed to antigens for *Bacillus subtilis* (Turner-Warwick, 1978). Thus most of the population should be considered at potential risk for allergy. Once sensitization has developed, only a proportion will develop clinical disease related to it. Expression of disease depends on the dose, on the level of antibodies in the individual, and on nonspecific amplification mechanisms (bronchial responsiveness for asthma, releasability of mediators, skin reactivity, etc.) (Sorenson et al., 1987; NRC, 1981). Sears et al. (1989) have shown a very significant relationship between house dust and cat sensitivities with bronchial reactivity in nonasthmatics and with asthma; outdoor grass pollen had no such relationship. Di Pede et al. (personal communication) have shown similar relationships of house dust and dog to bronchial responsiveness in nonasthmatics in Tucson. In both cases IgE was implicated as the mediator.

High levels of exposure to allergens for a short period of time is likely to result in more sensitization than a similar total dose over a longer period of time. Therefore cumulative exposure is less relevant than exposure to recurrent peak levels (Turner-Warwick, 1978). Much lower doses are required to elicit disease in the sensitized individuals than to induce sensitization. Sensitized individuals that have become symptomatic often will respond similarly to other biological agents and to chemical agents, such as formaldehyde and particles, due to heightened tissue reactivity (Rom, 1983; Turner-Warwick, 1978).

Health Hazards Related to Irritants

Gram negative bacteria growing indoors can liberate endotoxins. These phospholipid-polysaccharide macromolecules are a integral part of bacterial cell walls and are water soluble. They may be distributed through the indoor environment via the ventilation system, particularly if water has seeped into the system and bacteria are growing there. Endotoxin inhalation may cause an acute illness with fever, sweating, muscle aches, headache, and sometimes rhinitis, asthma, and breathlessness. Symptoms usually start within hours after exposure and resolve within a day. Repeated continuous exposures lead to tolerance. However, an interruption may stop symptoms, but then symptoms will start again with repeat exposure. Endotoxin exposure is a possible cause of humidifier fever and may be relevant to some of the symptoms of sick building syndrome or building-related illness (Woods et al., 1989). A substantial growth of fungi may produce mycotoxins, which in sufficient doses have potentially serious health effects. House dust may produce its effects by nonspecific irritant effects, as well as by allergy to individual components (similar to formaldehyde).

Little is known in real environments (i.e., outside of animal exposure chambers) about possible interactions between bioaerosol irritants with temperature, humidity, and other air contaminants (e.g., inorganic particulates). Lower moisture levels (below 20%) and irritants may aggravate skin diseases and produce mucosal symptoms. Some individuals may be more sensitive to these other irritants, or odors; up to 20% have eye hypersensitivity (Weber, 1984). Those individuals who are allergic often also react more strongly to irritants as well especially where their allergy manifests itself. Individuals with existing airway disease, up to 10% of the population, may have an aggravated reaction to irritants and may show bronchospastic responses.

Exposure to abnormal concentrations of spores or mycelial fragments of certain species of filamentous/toxigenic fungi or substrate particles should be considered hazardous (Jarvis, 1986; Samson, 1985; Croft et al., 1986; Flannigan, 1987; Tobin et al., 1987b; Sorenson et al., 1987). For example, inhalation of the spores of the aflatoxin-producing *Aspergillus* species from harvesting corn (grain) or groundnuts or working in processing facilities where these commodities are handled has been shown to induce the associated mycotoxicosis (liver cancer). The mycotoxins may be ingested as well, such as with *Aspergillus flavus* contaminated peanuts, indicating multimedia exposure.

HAZARD ASSESSMENT

The assessment of the effect of bioaerosols has to be made for individuals (for diagnoses and medical management) and for populations. Hazard assessment is made for populations. It is complicated by the varied biological processes that may result from exposure, separately or jointly, by antigen and irritant challenges (NRS, 1981). Some questionnaire responses are capable of validation under field conditions, such as lung function tests (with and without challenges) to validate asthma (Lebowitz, 1982). Some responses are not easily capable of validation, such as lethargy and headache. Daily diaries of symptoms can be used as well to document longitudinal and time-specific responses in relation to exposures (WHO, 1983b) The health hazard assessments differ sufficiently with the different mechanisms (allergic, infective, or irritant/toxic), and they will be discussed separately.

Hazard Assessment for Infectious Responses

Immunity toward some infectious agents can be measured by serum immunological tests, which determine the specific antibody titer, or skin tests assessing the cell-mediated immune response. Accuracy of the methods is very important, especially if such testing leads to probability distributions of immunity in populations (Fox et al., 1970). (The detection of serum antibodies against *Legionella pneumophila* is of value in the diagnosis of legionellosis in patients, but its significance as an indicator of immunity in healthy individuals is unknown (WHO/EURO, 1982).

Significant exposure to indoor infectious agents should be suspected when (1) there are several important sources, (2) there are amplifiers or conditions favoring the micro-organism survival, (3) there are highly susceptible individuals or known carriers, (4) there are complaints or epidemics of diseases, or (5) a microbiological laboratory reports many positive cultures or high rates of seropositivity. Also buildings with high occupant densities have an increased risk of airborne transmission of infectious diseases, especially during endemic seasons.

A classic study was performed by Riley and colleagues (1959, 1962) on tuberculosis. They evaluated air vented from a TB ward into exposure chambers. The guinea pigs exposed were previously tuberculin negative but became positive after exposure, indicating infection. This was confirmed by a study on a submarine (Houk et al., 1968) in which one seaman with active TB exposed other seamen for six months. The submarine, of course, used recirculated air. Of 308 seamen, 140 became infected. Since few had direct contact with the index case, it demonstrated the infectivity of circulated droplet nuclei. Many other studies since have documented such infectious routes (Riley, 1982).

Fungal infections can lead to serious disease, as demonstrated by Staib and colleagues (1987). In HIV positive cases, they found a 3.6% prevalence rate of crytococcosis. All had been exposed to the fecal matter of caged birds or feral pigeons. In two of the cases, the isolates from sputum and cerebrospinal fluid were identical biochemically with isolates from the fecal matter of the birds to which they were known to be exposed. These investigators also isolated the same species of *Aspergillus* and Mucoraceae from hospitalized cases and from both the soil of potted plants and surrounding air.

Epidemic mathematical models help describe the spread of viruses through susceptible populations. The accuracy of such models is a function of the characteristics and size of the target population, the place and time models have been developed for tuberculosis, measles, varicella, rubella, pseudomonas, and staphylococcus. They take into account their viability in and out of the human reservoir, their passage (e.g., atmospherically, as fomites, through ventilation systems), their incubation period, pathogenicity, and virulence. Epidemic models of tuberculosis risk (spread within populations) have been better defined in general and have been discussed for indoor environments (Lebowitz et al., 1972). TB occurs about 10 times more frequently than legionellosis. Epidemic models have been discussed for certain outbreaks of legionellosis, but it does not occur frequently enough for general health hazard assessment. The other models have not been specified for different types of buildings, although attack rates and spread are more population oriented than they are building oriented (Lebowitz et al., 1972). The models are in the form of compound epidemic curves, which continue to be compounded by the influx of new susceptibles. Thus each model has parameters determined by the exposure, time, and the proportion of susceptibles. These compound distributions can represent the risk assessment exposure–response relationships; they can be defined for different populations. The risk assessment models for different indoor settings in different populations should be defined for risk management.

Hazard Assessment for Allergic Responses

Sensitization to allergens can be measured by finding specific IgE antibodies in the population, by finding positive allergy skin tests to the allergens, by finding IgG precipitins or immunoflourescent antigen-antibody reactions to the allergens, and especially by challenging the nose and airways with the allergen and measuring the response (Rom, 1983; Turner-Warwick, 1978; Middleton et al., 1988; Weill and Turner-Warwick, 1981). For example, precipitins to avian protein, especially as it waxes and wanes with symptomatology, are indicative of sensitization. As shown for HP, bronchoalveolar lavages may be useful; higher proportions of Tiells, low helper to suppresser Tiell ratios, and increased mast cells (2 + %) are indicative of allergic response (Turner-Warwick, 1978).

Responses to aeroallergens can be determined by symptoms, increased bronchial responsiveness using peak flows, increased medication use, visits to physicians or emergency rooms, and / or hospitalization. The techniques are highlighted in the studies discussed.

Fungal Reactions

Nevalainen and colleagues (1987) have reported more allergic symptomatology in occupants with elevated fungal levels, but challenge tests and other causes were not evaluated. In contrast, Licorish et al. (1985) challenged mildly asthmatic subjects and provoked asthma attacks using spores of *Alternaria* and *Penicillium* at concentrations found in doses that subjects could encounter in natural settings.

Schata and colleagues (1989) performed an experimental study with fungal antigens. They studied 150 patients, aged 32 to 47, with allergic diseases whose symptoms were reported to occur after exposure in air-conditioned rooms. (A previous report stated that 38% of allergic patients were sensitive to fungi.) The antigen extracts included 14 fungal species; they removed the mycotoxins. The extracts were used for skin tests and challenges. Four percent reacted to the control skin test, and between 11% and 73% had skin test positive results for fungi. The three most reactive antigens were all to *Penicillium* (62–73%), 13% to 51% reacted to seven *Aspergillus* species (of which *A. niger* was the highest), 47% reacted to *Cladosporium*, and 32% to *Alternaria*. However, the ultimate test, the challenge, yielded a maximum of 36% reactivity, confirming that skin test responses are not equivalent to allergic disease (but only predisposition). (The rank orders were the same for the two types of tests.) Thus, with both sets of results, one sees that sensitivity and specificity of allergic complaints are not optimum. However, desensitization for up to three years reportedly removed symptoms in 76% of patients who underwent the treatment. Others estimate that the incidence of asthma and rhinitis produced by fungi among allergics is 5% to 29% (Prince and Meyer, 1976).

Woods et al. (1989) reported a study of allergic respiratory disease, with episodes of fever, cough, and chest tightness in a workplace. The index case had a positive serology to *Aureobasidium pullulans*, a common fungus. As others complained during summer, they hypothesized that this fungus produced disease, amplified by humid conditions. Airborne fungi air sampling indicated the presence of several fungi, in descending rank order: *Aureobasidium, Cladosporium, Alternaria, Aspergillus niger*; outdoors, the order was: *Cladosporium, Alternaria, Penicillium, Aspergillus*. They concluded that *Aureobasidium* was amplified indoors, and analysis of stagnant water in fan coil drain pans showed heavy contamination of the unit by *Aureobasidium*. Thus they concluded that this was the allergic cause. However, challenge tests were not performed on occupants.

Mite, Cockroach, Cat, and Dog Reactions

Voorhorst (1967) had shown that allergic and atopic asthmatics, with specific hypersensitization to house dust mite, had clinic visits that correlated very well with mite growth curves in homes. This has been confirmed by others (Andersen and Korsgaard, 1986; Tovey et al., 1981a,b). Korsgaard (1983a) compared the occurrence of house dust mites in homes of 25 mite-specific asthmatics and 75 controls (same sex, age, and family size). The homes with asthmatics had much higher mean levels of mites (490 vs. 1 per gram mattress dust) with a clear dose–response curve. Clark and colleagues (1976) found a reduction in peak flows of children with asthma associated with house dust when house-cleaning increased particle concentration in the air; specifically, the relation was with particles less than 2 μm. Clinical improvement in patients was seen when they were removed from their homes, either to high altitude (Verveloet et al., 1979) or kept in the hospital (Platts-Mills et al., 1982). In the latter study, 7 adult patients in the hospital for

2 months showed a 47% increase in peak flow and a tenfold decrease in histamine reactivity. However, trying to change mites in houses through moisture control in one study (Korsgaard, 1983b) has not been beneficial.

Chan-Yeung et al. (1995) recruited 120 asthmatic subjects and evaluated them for the severity of their reactions to 13 common allergens. They collected seasonal dust samples from each of the homes. There was no relationship between skin test reactivity and the levels of the cat and mite allergens. However, among mite positive children daily symptom scores were elevated and peak flow scores declined. The relationship did not hold true for adults.

Rosenstreich et al. (1997) examined the role of cockroach allergy with exposure and morbidity among children with asthma who lived in 8 innercity areas in the northeast quarter of the United States; 476 asthmatic children were recruited. Skin test reactivity was recorded for specific indoor allergens (cockroach: 36.8%; mite: 34.9%; cat: 22.7%), and house dust was collected and evaluated for allergen content. High dust allergen levels were found in 50.2% for cockroach, 9.7% for house dust, and 12.6% for cat. Children with cockroach-specific skin tests who lived in highly contaminated environments experienced three times the rate of hospitalization when compared with other children. Similar results were not found among children with cat and mite skin test response.

By contrast, Sporik et al. (1995) and Platts-Mills et al. (1995) recruited 57 asthmatic children from the "perfect" high-altitude (about 7200 ft) town of Los Alamos, New Mexico. The area was considered a perfect study site because outdoor air was generally free of pollution/particulate, and there was a low probability of elevated mite and roach infestation in homes, thus limiting causal agents for asthma attacks. Pets were the dominant indoor contaminant, and allergen was found in homes in sufficient amounts to cause sensitization and the associated risk of asthma. Asthma remained a major cause of morbidity. They conclude that the specific antigen to which a person becomes sensitized is incidental. Rather it is the sensitization in conjunction with other factors that lead to the disease. They hypothesize that changes in housing conditions are driving the disease increase. Other lifestyle changes may also play a role (Platts-Mills and Pollart Squillace, 1997).

Pneumonitis / Alveolitis and Humidifier Fever

Hypersensitivity pneumonitis (HP), or allergic alveolitis, can be appraised also by other immunological tests, mostly IgG related, and inhalation challenge tests. HP has been found in occupational settings where workers are exposed to isocynates (Baur, 1995), wood dust (Halpin et al., 1994), and shell dust (Mitani et al., 1995). HP has further been shown in studies to be due to contaminated air conditioners, heating systems (Banaszek et al., 1970; Fink et al., 1971; Reed et al., 1983), and humidifiers (Burke et al., 1977). Reed and colleagues (1983) studied and outbreak of HP. They used antiserum from affected workers to test slime from a spray wash air-conditioning system. It contained antigens that reacted with the IgG antibodies from the workers. These antigens also produced positive inhalation challenge tests. They also found the antigens in the air through immunochemical procedures.

Humidifier fever (HF) has been studied in a similar fashion. Malmon et al. (1993) studied 28 workers from a small print shop. A contaminated humidifier contained fungi, amoebae, and endotoxin producing gram negative bacteria. Serological tests showed positive responses to extracts from the humidifier, but the specific agent was never identified although the endotoxins were suspected. Finnegan and colleagues (1987) studied 25 workers with HF and 90 workmates. They found positive immunofluorescent antibodies and precipitin reactions to the antigens of amoebae found in four different contaminated humidifiers; the two techniques correlated well. However, positive results did not correlate with the HF⁻ or work-related symptoms. Extracts from contaminated water can produce HF by inhalation challenge, but the exact cause is unknown still; the agent could be a bacillus, an endotoxin, or an amoebae. Prevalence studies of SBS / building-related illnesses have found fungal-related illnesses of various kinds (Finnegan et al., 1984; Morey, 1989; Andersen and Korsgaard, 1986); only some of them were specific enough to indicate allergic disease (as defined).

Hazard Assessment for Irritants, Toxic Responses, and Combined Effects

Such assessment follows the protocols for other irritants, specifically indoor air pollutants (WHO, 1989, 1990). These methods are well developed; they are discussed elsewhere (Lebowitz, 1981). Physiological effects from irritants have to be distinguished from effects of temperature and humidity (NRC, 1981) and other irritants.

Experimental and epidemiological studies have been used to evaluate toxicological effects. For example, trichothecene toxicosis has been explored (Croft et al., 1986). Bacterial endotoxin from organic dust has been experimentally studied by Rylander and colleagues (1989). Their last study exposed 77 naive subjects to endotoxin (isolated or attached to bacterial cells) from *Enterobacter agglomerans* (a major bacteria found in many organic dusts). The major physiological effect was a dose-related decrease in diffusing capacity. It was accompanied by a smaller decrease in spirometry, fever, and subjective feelings of chest tightness. Some bronchial reactivity occurred after four hours of exposure. The results support epidemiological studies showing endotoxin-produced acute reactions seen after exposure to many organic dusts.

Mixed Effects from Combined Exposures

A study in Edinburgh (Strachan, 1988) reported over 3.7 times more wheeze in children where molds in the bedroom were reported, but there was no relationship to actual bronchial lability. This indicates probable overreporting bias, which is strengthened by the extremely high rate of wheeze reported in positive homes (over 38%).

An epidemiological study of the respiratory effects of dampness and mold was conducted in the Netherlands in 210 houses (202 children and 328 parents) using A WHO CNSLD questionnaire, an environmental questionnaire, and monitoring in 36 houses (van Wageningen et al., 1987). The health questionnaire yielded prevalence rates of symptoms and potential confounders. The environmental questionnaire had questions about dampness (see above) and potential confounders. Fungal spores were measured in 25 "damp" and 11 "dry" houses using modified Andersen samplers, and bacterial concentrations (using agar plates with the same samplers). Comparisons were made with symptom responses in homes with sampling but without questions about dampness. The latter substudy indicated serious reporting bias (overreporting) when dampness questions are asked: Odds ratios for symptoms, comparing prevalence rates in damp vs. dry subjects, with such questions were over 3 (3.4 – 19.1) for many symptoms, while without such questions being asked (i.e., in children) they were only 1.7 to 2.9 and significant only for cough and total CNSLD (a combination of symptoms). Further the odds ratios were often greater using the subjective "dampness" compared to the moisture index. The odds ratios were higher for those exposed to environmental tobacco smoke. An attempt to avoid such biases must be made by utilizing more objective health and exposure data without subjective data. This was confirmed by the lack of significant correlation between the moisture index and both fungal and bacterial data, especially the latter. No relation of symptoms to bacteria were found, and direct fungal-symptom relations were not presented. The authors thought that unmeasured house dust mites might be related to the symptoms; if so, they were not as related as shown in patient studies, nor to the allergic-asthma symptoms expected by mite exposures in children (Sears et al., 1989).

A major study of home dampness and symptoms in children was performed in six U.S. cities (Brunekreef et al., 1989). Similar questions were asked to detect dampness; questions were also asked about water in the basement. Nine symptom rates were adjusted for age, sex, parental education, and smoking by city. The dampness index ranged from 45.7% to 58.2%. Adjusted odds ratios were almost always significantly greater than 1.0 for molds and for "dampness" and were usually greater than the unadjusted odds ratios. (Symptoms were highly intercorrelated.) However, only cough was significantly greater in asthmatics, and all symptoms except chest illnesses were significantly greater in nonasthmatic nonwheezers. Spirometric differences were not impressive. Unfortunately, no bioaerosols were actually measured, no relation to indoor humidity was presented, and no joint analyses with other indoor air pollutants were reported (although previous analyses in this population showed effects of passive smoking and possibly nitrogen dioxide). A later abstract (Su et al., 1989) reported that total colony-forming units, derived from Andersen samplers and cultures in 250 of these homes in three of the cities, did not relate to indoor humidity or temperature; they were higher in gas-cooking homes. Preliminary results did not show correlations between CFUs and symptoms, though case-by-case analysis showed trends.

A study in England of 200 children reported relations between respiratory illnesses and bedroom humidity, nitrogen dioxide, and some effects of passive smoking (Melia et al., 1982). Attributable and combined risks were not presented, and bioaerosols were not measured. Other confounding factors were controlled in analyses.

A study of 117 asthmatic and nonasthmatic families (229 subjects) from a representative community population sample in Tucson was monitored over a three-year period using daily diaries and peak flows (Lebowitz et al., 1982, 1985). Simultaneous microindoor and outdoor monitoring was conducted in a representative sample of houses for air pollutants, pollen, fungi, algae, and climate. Macromonitoring of air pollutants and pollen was conducted simultaneously. The relationship of indoor to outdoor and micro to macro factors can be demonstrated from this study. Suspended particulate matter and pollen independently were related to symptoms in asthmatics and nonasthmatics. The use of gas stoves was qualitatively related to symptoms. Fungi were not related to symptoms or peak flow after accounting for the other environmental factors. Algae, and other contaminants of evaporative coolers, did not appear to be important in producing symptoms. *Bacillus* species found in cooler water were not related to immunological tests in occupants.

Factor-based scales, which are climate and season specific, are developed for the environmental variables (Holberg et al., 1987). Three pollutant/meteorological scales represent summer, winter, and humidity. Four pollen scales represent early and late spring, summer, and fall pollen types. Relationships among the environmental variables, respiratory symptoms, and peak expiratory flow are analyzed with path diagrams, after accounting for age, sex, smoking habits, and stove type. The different effects of the environment on asthmatics, allergics, and airways obstructive disease (AOD) subjects were demonstrated. The pollutant and meteorological variables are related to respiratory symptoms and peak flow directly, as well as through interactions with pollen types, specifically rhinitis and attacks of wheezing in asthmatics, and the attack and decreased peak flow in subjects with AOD. Some of the largest positive coefficients are seen in association with seasonal pollen types, specifically rhinitis in allergics. Micropollen was significantly related to peak flow decrements in asthmatics.

A time-series analysis was utilized to evaluate the respiratory responses to outdoor and indoor air pollutant and aeroallergen exposures in the sensitive adults (Lebowitz et al., 1987). The time-series analysis helped determine appropriate lags between environmental stimuli and health responses. Asthmatics showed that most respiratory responses, while asymptomatics showed no significant responses. Outdoor ozone, nitrogen dioxide, aeroallergens, meteorological factors, and indoor gas stoves were significantly related, independently and interactively, with symptoms and peak flow. Pollen did not show any time lag.

O'Rourke et al. (1989) have monitored the regional/macro pollen rain in 4 representative vegetational clusters, using a Burkard 7 day pollen and spore sampler, whose tape can be analyzed by 2 hour segments. Indoor and outdoor pollen concentrations were determined in 93 households located within those clusters, using mini-Burkard samplers. Results for one spring indicate an order of magnitude difference among regional (rooftop), micro-outdoor (1.5 m above ground level), and indoor (1.5 m above floors) pollen concentrations. Based on questionnaire responses, immediate hypersensitivity skin tests, and bronchial responsiveness, 121 individuals were classified into four categories: asymptomatic, allergic, asthmatic, and symptomatic for other chronic obstructive lung disease (COLD). Individual responses were monitored with daily symptom diaries and peak flow measurements of lung function; their houses were monitored for air contaminants. (Peak flow values have been standardized based on the 2–4 daily values using the mini-Wright meter.) Analytically, multifactorial analysis of covariance is used to control for covariables and confounders in the evaluation of the effects of daily pollen and mold concentrations on daily symptom incidence and prevalence rates, and on peak flow variability. This approach evaluates the interactions of pollen and mold, meteorological and air pollutant variables, in regard to these health effects. It adjusts for other effects, whether interactions are completely additive, synergistic, or inhibitive. The regional daily mean pollen values were compared with the daily diary scores. Regional daily mean pollen concentrations reflected pollen encountered by subjects throughout the day, and the result was a compromise for exposures between pollen encountered indoors and outdoors. In contrast to "normals," "atopics" and "peak flow responsive" subjects showed increased nasal symptom responses with increased pollen concentrations.

The analysis showed a direct relationship between rhinitis and ragweed and mulberry pollen in sensitive subjects. Unfortunately, the pollen season for these two taxa was so similar that effects were undifferentiated. One may be able to differentiate these effects by assessing individuals who are allergic to specific antigens (i.e., mulberry- and ragweed-specific individuals).

The careful characterization of subjects was essential to this study. None of the "normals" showed an increase in symptom response with increased pollen prevalence. Decline in lung function, as measured by the evening peak expiratory flow, was associated with high concentrations of Morus (mulberry) pollen, but only for individuals defined as "peak flow responsive." More results will be forthcoming from this study. One can expect results in the near future from other studies with both bioaerosol and air pollution monitoring (Hawthorne et al., 1989; RIVM, 1989).

Recent work evaluates the relationship between pollen exposure and changes in peak expiratory flow. We hypothesized that persistent and elevated grass or cheno-am pollen exposures will be associated with a decline in lung function as measured by peak expiratory flow rate (PEFR). We tested this hypothesis in a previously recruited and characterized population of Pima County (Arizona) employees and their families. We visited 559 households and evaluated changes in daily respiratory symptoms, including PEFR, in over 1000 residents. Residents completed standard respiratory health questionnaires and were prick tested with *Cynodon dactylon*, *Amaranthus palmeri*, *Chenopodium alba*, and 21 other antigens and positive and negative controls. Regional daily pollen concentrations were evaluated using the Burkard 7 day regional pollen and spore sampler. Indoor and outdoor household pollen assemblages were evaluated using Burkard Personal Monitors. Daily time/activity logs were completed by subjects. From these measures, daily grass and cheno-am pollen exposures were calculated for each subject. Since daily pollen concentrations and daily lung function are both highly autocorrelated, random effect models were used to control for autoregressive factors. The

REM models can deal with irregularity in collection periods, missing data and lagged responses. We generated two types of models to examine relationships. The first model relied exclusively on local measurements of pollen inside and outside subject homes. The values collected by short-term grab samples were assumed to be stable over a 1 to 2 week period. The second model assumed that indoor / outdoor pollen ratios were stable. Variable daily pollen concentrations were reported from regional sites, and the pollen was apportioned as a function of the grab sample ratios. We controlled for gender, height, age, skin test response, and smoking behavior. Although smoking outweighs all other factors, we found a significant decline in PEFR associated with elevated grass and cheno-am pollen exposure on the preceding day during years with typical patterns of pollen production / dispersal. During nontypical years, other factors, possibly air toxics or weather conditions, confound the relationship.

CONTROLS

Strategies for the control of bioaerosols fall into two categories, those relating to the host and those relating to the physical environment. Prevention in the host can occur through immunization (for infectious agents), avoidance of sensitization (see above), allergic desensitization, and avoidance of exposures that exacerbate symptoms in the sensitized. Behavior and socioeconomic factors are very important in control. Avoidance of irritant exposures (as recommended clinically to asthmatics), including physical measures in indoor air, is predominantly based on avoiding conditions that favor bioaerosol growth. If bioaerosols succeed in growing , then the contaminants must be contained and removed. (Pope et al., 1993; NRC, 1981; WHO, 1990).

Socioeconomic Influences and Behavior

The socioeconomic conditions related to bioaerosol exposure cut both ways. Tighter buildings, recirculated air with humidifiers, deep pile carpets, overstuffed furniture, wall hangings, and heavy draperies are societal indicators of wealth. These amenities are commonly found in the homes of the middle class and wealthy. They can promote humid interiors with enhanced habitat. Once educated, the middle and upper class have the funds to remediate their environment. Generally, they will take some steps (usually modification of the ventilation system), but unless the illness is extreme, people rarely forgo comfort. Eliminating carpeting is unlikely, and removal of pets rarely happens.

By contrast those living in public housing complexes, dormitories, and rental units have control of only a small portion of their housing environment. Given appropriate education, people may effect changes in their immediate environment, but they have little or no control over their building. They have neither the means nor the power to alter the ventilation system. Residents may effectively eradicate rodents and arthropods from their units for a short period of time. Soon the vermin will return from adjacent units.

Call et al. (1993) state that "Inner city children have the highest prevalence and the highest mortality rates for asthma in the United States." They investigated homes of 122 asthmatic children (plus 22 control) in Atlanta, Georgia, for exposure to mite, cat, and cockroach allergens in dust. They demonstrated that black children in innercity Atlanta were exposed to high levels of allergen and that the combined sensitization was a major risk factor for asthma in this population. A survey in New York City (Carr et al., 1992) found that hospitalization and death rates from asthma were 3 to 5.5 time greater for African-Americans and Hispanics than for Caucasians. They concluded that there was disproportionate morbidity and mortality borne by poor and minority populations.

Behavioral controls a major determinant on the impact of indoor contamination (Pope et al., 1993; WHO, 1983a, 1986a). Modification of the behaviors that influence indoor air quality and resultant exposure often is the simplest, least expensive, and most effective means of reducing adverse health effects. For bioaerosols, these factors include a range of activities such as education, personal behavior, and social practices (WHO, 1990).

Education includes the dissemination of information to occupants on actions they could take to reduce/eliminate indoor bioaerosols and the ability to recognize situations (e.g., source and source use) that can contribute to bioaerosol concentrations. Use of the information will depend on the motivation of the individual and available resources. Individuals could use available information to reduce their exposures or remove themselves from contaminated environments in which they experience adverse health effects.

Platts-Mills and Pollart Squillace (1997) have observed a marked change in the play patterns of children over the last 30 years. Children's play used to be very active. Like adults, today's children spend leisure time watching television or playing with the computer. Lack of play with exercise eliminates the direct beneficial effect on the lung, and sitting without exercise may induce a breathing pattern that is harmful. They cite evidence suggesting that allergen exposure yields greater rates of bronchospasm with sedentary inhalation rates. They hypothesize that this change in behavior (active to passive play) allows the development of asthma in children who have become allergic to indoor allergens. Can the trend toward asthma increases be resolved by changing the play behavior of children? Will a society that is encouraging computer use by children both at home and in school now encourage a new behavior? Proposed changes in play behavior present an innovative, well-balanced, and integrated approach to resolving a disease trend.

Society can exert considerable pressure, or provide/promote incentives to control sources of contamination (NRC/NAS, 1987). In addition societal pressure can result in establishing adequate ventilation standards (ASHRAE, 1988) and ensure the institution of building maintenance practices that will minimize the potential for bioaerosol contamination. To protect the public, some governmental guidelines for reduction of biological contamination have been established in Canada (Department of National Health and Welfare, 1987). In the case of contagious diseases caused by bacteria and viruses, public health laws provide specific standards. For example, if a case of smallpox or tuberculosis is found, then standards require quarantine, source investigation, and preventive measures against further spread (CDC, 1987).

Although difficult, the financial burden associated with bioaerosols and their control should be adequately estimated. For asthma alone (regardless of attributable causal agent), costs were $6.2 billion in 1990 and are expected to exceed $14.5 billion in the year 2000 (Weiss et al., 1992; CDC, 1997). The relationship between the annual cost of heating, ventilation, and air conditioning in a given building and the annual payroll cost of the employees served is such that the annual salary costs are 100 to 200 times the total HVAC costs, when both are measured in terms of unit of floor area. This suggests that even if the HVAC costs were to be doubled in order to reduce biological (and other) indoor air contaminants, only a very minor increase in employee productivity would be required to offset such increased costs (WHO, 1990).

Physical methods

These methods of source control have been categorized into four groups by a WHO working group (WHO, 1990). Because several of these controls can have the opposite effect for other contaminants, it was stated that they should be used with caution.

Proper design and construction of buildings is the most desirable control means to avoid bioaerosol contamination from buildings and their system-related sources (NRC, 1987). The structure should consist of nondeteriorating materials so as not to offer a substrate for microbial growth. Construction materials should be chosen to effectively control moisture, which is the most important factor governing microbial growth in a building. Design should avoid the conflicts between energy conservation and effective moisture control, and where the control of one source of moisture (e.g., sealing out of rain water by a tight building envelope) will aggravate another source (e.g., moisture generated by cooking or by dense building occupancy rates). The design of the structure should allow for the removal of any condensed moisture through adequate ventilation. The construction site should be well drained.

Source modification offers several possibilities for control of biological pollution. Changes of temperature or relative humidity (two interrelated parameters) can be used to control some sources, but this will often have an opposite effect on other sources.

Maintenance, repair, and cleaning are common control strategies. They are important for moisture control, especially for *Legionella* and *Stachybotrys chartarum* (WHO/ EURO, 1986; Johanning et al., 1996). In this group chemical treatment with biocides and UV irradiation have also been included, but the use of these methods should be limited because of the health risks for occupants (WHO, 1990). Keeping filters clean has been shown to be advantageous (Streifel et al., 1989).

Removal of pollutants from air can be accomplished by increasing effective ventilation and / or by air cleaning (NRC, 1987). These methods, although in principle applicable to reduce emission deriving from all sources, are in practice only of importance in few cases (Streifel et al., 1989; WHO, 1990).

These recommendations were also espoused by the Committee on the Health Effects of Indoor Allergens constituted by the Institute of Medicine (Pope et al., 1993). Other recommendations were also made by this group. They addressed issues of health care, engineering, educational programs, and the research agenda. Three important recommendations not covered above include (1) the development of an exposure assessment infrastructure that can be used by medical professional to evaluate bioaerosol contamination and causation in homes, (2) an emphasis on the role of carpets as sources and reservoirs of bioaerosols, and (3) the development of focused, appropriate, and sensitive educational materials for populations of disparate socioeconomic and educational characteristics.

SUMMARY AND CONCLUSIONS

In the past two decades there has been a major shift in the study of bioaerosols. From the 1920s through the 1970s skin test extracts focused primarily on exposures outside the home (pollen and mold). Because the outdoor environment contains such massive seasonal doses of specific allergens, physicians recommended that allergy and asthma patients avoid exposures by spending as much time indoors as possible. A few patients had problems with indoor allergens from kapok, feathers, and pets. They were encouraged to eliminate these sources. With the discovery of the house dust mite in the 1960s and the development and characterization of the allergy extract, clinicians initiated the evaluation of indoor bioaerosols in earnest during the 1980s. Immunologists and clinicians were also beginning to understand the relationships between bioaerosol exposure and asthma in the genetically susceptible, sensitized host, both in terms of development and exacerbation.

While the science of immunology was expanding its investigation of allergy and asthma, players in the world's political area found a new weapon in oil. Energy was being used to shape political policy. Energy became more costly in the late 1970s, and engineers and contractors responded with changes in building materials (better insulation, tighter buildings) and altered designs in ventilation (lower air exchange rates). Indoor relative humidity began to climb. With greater energy costs and lower profitability, public institutions and corporate entities espoused the mantra "do more with less." Building maintenance and support of infrastructure were among the first areas cut. Unmaintained ventilation systems became sources of bioaerosols. Clinicians began seeing an elevation in asthma rate and outbreaks of respiratory diseases like Legionnaire's disease.

Concurrently a paradigm shift occurred in the field of exposure assessment. Data collected using time-activity diaries demonstrated what was known, but not thought about. People spend the majority, over 90%, of their time *indoors* (Samet and Spengler, 1991), and with energy and cost-cutting policies, contaminants in indoor air were becoming as great a health risk as contaminants in the outdoor air.

The indoor environment contains low-level persistent doses of bioaerosols posing a year-round, cumulative health hazard. In some settings (i.e., homes with cats, public housing with cockroaches) the airborne and dust loads of antigen can be extremely high and pose a real health threat to residents and their buildings. Research to define problems associated with bioaerosols and factors that promote their growth and spread has been ongoing. Today researchers, clinicians, and engineers, are identifying mitigation strategies to clean and maintain the quality of air inside our buildings.

A substantial portion of disease and disability are due to respiratory infections, allergic episodes, irritation, and inflammation from indoor bioaerosol exposure. Since these exposures are often due to building-related factors, such morbidity could be reduced significantly. Concentrations of bioaerosols indoors vary greatly in time and space. Methods for environmental sampling of bioaerosols need to be standardized to the extent possible. Only methods for pollen, specific bacteria, and viral sampling approach being "standard." Further studies on exposure and response are needed to provide useful information for risk assessment and management. These include specific programs aimed at young children.

Bioaerosols indoors are often caused by persistent moisture and/or inadequate ventilation, for which proper design, construction, and maintenance are essential in exposure prevention. Other useful controls include removal of pests and pets, plants, furnishings that provide homes for mites and other arthropoda, behavior changes, and vaccination.

REFERENCES

ACGIH. 1990. *Guidelines for the Assessment of Bioaerosols in the Indoor Environment.* Cincinnatti, OH: American Conference of Governmental Industrial Hygienists.

Ahern, D. G., R. B. Simmons, D. L. Price, L. Ajello, S. A. Crow, S. K. Mishra, and D. L. Pierson. 1995. Fungal colonization of synthetic substrates for use in space craft. *J. Indust. Microbiol.* 14: 26–30.

Amitani, R., T. Murayama, R. Nawada, W. J. Lee, A. Niimi, K. Suzuki, E. Tanaka, and F. Kuze. 1995. *Aspergillus* culture filtrates and sputum sols from patients with pulmonary aspergillosis cause damage to human respiratory ciliated epithelium in vitro. *Eur. Respir. J.* 8: 1681–1687.

Andersen, I., and J. Korsgaard. 1986. Asthma and the indoor environment: Assessment of the health implications of high indoor air humidity. *Environ. Int.* 12: 121–127.

Arlian, L. G. 1975a. Water exchange and effect of water vapour activity on metabolic rate in the house dust mite, *Dermatophagoides. J. Insect. Physiol.* 21: 1439.

Arlian, L. G. 1975b. Dehydration and survival of the European house dust mite *Dermatophagoides pteronyssinus. J. Med. Entomol.* 12: 437.

Arlian, L. G. 1989. Biology and ecology of house dust mites, *Dermatophagoides* spp. and *Euroglyphus* spp. *Immunol. Allergy Clin. N. Am.* 9: 339.

Arlian, L. G. 1992. Water balance and humidity requirements of house dust mites. *J. Exper. Appl. Acarology.* 16: 15–35.

Arlian, L. G., and M. M. Veselica. 1981. Effects of temperature on the equilibrium body water mass in the mite *Dermatophagoides farinae. Physiol. Zool.* 54: 393.

Arlian, L. G., I. L. Bernstein and J. S. Gallagher. 1982. The prevalence of house dust mites, *Dermatophagoides* spp. and associated environmental conditions in homes in Ohio. *J. Allergy Clin. Immunol.* 69: 527.

Arlian, L. G., C. M. Rapp, and S. G. Ahmed. 1990. Development of the house dust mite *Dermatophagoides pteronyssinus. J. Med. Entomol.* 27: 1035.

Arlian, L. G., D. Bernstein, I. L. Bernstein, S. Friedman, A. Grant, P. Lieberman, M. Lopez, J. Metzger, T. A. E. Platts-Mills, M. Schatz, S. Spetor, S. I. Wasserman, and R. S. Zeiger. 1992. Prevalence of dust mites in the homes of people with asthma living in eight different geographic areas of the U.S. *J. Allergy Clin. Immunol.* 90: 292.

ASHRAE Standard 62-1981R. 1988. *Ventilation for Acceptable Air Quality.* Draft for Public Review. American Society of Heating, Refrigerating and Air Conditioning Engineers, Inc., Atlanta GA.

Ausdenmoore, R. W. 1990. Aeroallergens and Environmental Factors. In *Manual of Allergy and Immunology*, eds. G. J. Lawler and T. S. Fischer, Boston: Little, Brown, pp. 3–45.

Banaszak, E. F., W. H. Thiede, and J. N. Fink. 1970. Hypersensitivity pneumonitis due to contamination of an air conditioner. *N. Engl. J. Med.* 283: 271.

Barbee, R. A., W. Kaltenborn, M. D. Lebowitz, and B. Burrows. 1987. Longitudinal changes in allergen skin test reactivity in a community population sample. *J. Allergy Clin. Immunol.* 79: 16–24.

Bates, J. H., G. D. Campbell, A. L. Barron, G. A. McCracken, P. N. Morgan, E. B. Moses, and C. D. Davis. 1992. Microbial etiology of acute pneumonia in hospitalized patients. *Chest* 101: 1005–1012.

Baur, X. 1995. Hypersensitivity Pneumonitis (extrinsic allergic alveolitis) induced by isocyanates. *J. Allergy Clin. Immunol.* 95 (part 1): 1004–1010.

Benenson, A. S. 1985. *Control of Communicable Disease in Man*, 14th edition Washington, DC: American Public Health Association.

Benezra, C., G. Ducombs, Y. Sell, and J. Fousserau. 1985. *Plant Contact Dermatitis.* St. Louis: Mosby.

Bernstein, R. S., W. G. Sorenson, D. Garabrant, C. Reux, and R. D. Treitman. 1983. Exposures to respirable, airborne *Penicillium* from a contaminated ventilation system: Clinical, environmental and epidemiological aspects. *Am. Ind. Hyg. Assoc.* 44: 161–169.

Binnie, P. W. H. 1987. Airborne microbial flora in Florida homes (preliminary study). In *Indoor Air '87*, eds. B. Seifert, H. Esdorn, M. Fischer, H. Ruden, and J. Wegner, pp. 660–664. Berlin: Institute for Water, Soil and Air Hygiene.

Bischoff, E. 1989. Sources of pollution of indoor air by mite allergen-containing house dust. *Environ. Int.* 15: 181–192.

Bischoff, E., B. Krause-Michel, and D. Nolte. 1986. Zur Bekaempfungdes Hausstaubmilbens in Haushalten von Patienten mit Milbenasthma. *Allergologie* 9: 448–457.

Bjurman, J., E. Nordstrand, and J. Kristensson. 1997. Growth-phase-related production of potential-volatile organic tracer compounds by moulds on wood. *Indoor Air* 7: 2–7.

Bollinger, M. E., P. A. Eggleston, E. Flanagan, and J. A. Wood. 1996. Cat antigen in homes with and without cats may induce allergic symptoms. *J. Allergy Clin. Immunol.* 97: 907–914.

Booij-Noord, H., N. G. M. Orie, and K. DeVries. 1971. Immediate and late bronchial obstructive reactions to inhalation of house dust and protective effects of disodium cromoglycate and prednisolone. *J. Allergy Clin. Immunol.* 48: 344–354.

Brandt, R. L., and L. G. Arlian. 1976. Mortality of House dust mites, *Dermatophagoides farinae* and *D. pteronyssinus*, exposed to dehydrating conditions or selected pesticides. *J. Med. Entomol.* 13: 327.

Brunekreef B., D. W. Dockery, F. E. Speizer, J. H. Ware, J. D. Spengler, and B. G. Gerris. 1989. Home dampness and respiratory morbidity in children. *Am. Rev. Respir. Dis.* 140: 1363–1367.

Burge, H. A. 1985. Indoor sources for airborne microbes. In *Indoor Air and Human Health*, eds. R. B. Gammage and S. V. Kaye, pp. 139–148. Chelsea, MI: Lewis Publishers.

Burge, H. A. 1989. Bioaerosols: Data collection. In *Design and Protocol for Monitoring Indoor Air Quality*, ASTM STP 1002, eds. N. Nagda, and J. P. Harper, pp. 119–120. Philadelphia: American Society for Testing and Materials.

Burge, H. A. 1990. Bioaerosols: Prevalence and health effects in the indoor environment. *J. Allergy Clin. Immunol.* 86: 687–705.

Burge, H. A., and J. C. Freeley. 1991. The Indoor air pollution and infectious disease. In: *Indoor Air Pollution*, eds. J. M. Samet, and J. D. Spengler pp. 273–284. Baltimore: Johns Hopkins University Press.

Burke, G. W., C. B. Carrington, J. N. Fink, E. A. Gaensler, and R. Strauss. 1977. Allergic alveolitis caused by home humidifiers: Unusual clinical features and electron microscopic findings. *J. Am. Med. Soc.* 238: 2705–2708.

Call, R. S., T. F. Smith, E. Morris, M. D. Chapman, and T. A. Platts-Mills. 1992. Risk factors for asthma in inner city children. *J. Peds.* 121: 862–866.

Carr, W., L. Zeitel and K. Weiss. 1992. Variations in asthma hospitalizations and deaths in New York City. *Am. J. Pub. Health* 82: 59–65.

CDC (Centers for Disease Control). 1987. *Communicable Disease 15th edition* Atlanta, GA: Office of Communication.

CDC (Centers for Disease Control). 1997. *Facts about Asthma*. Atlanta, GA: Office of Communication.

Chan-Yeung, M., J. Manfreda, H. Dimich-Ward, J. Lam, A. Ferguson, P. Warren, E. Simons, I. Broder, M. Chapman, T. Platts-Mills, and A. Becker. 1995. Mite and cat allergen levels in homes and severity of asthma. *Am. J. Respir. Crit. Care Med.* 1995 152: 1805–1811.

Chew, G., M. Mulienberg, D. Gold, and H. Burge. 1996. Is dust sampling a good surrogate for dust exposure to airborne fungi? *J. Allergy Clin. Immunol.* 97(1 part 2): 419.

Clark, R. P., D. C. Cordon-Nesbitt, S. Malka, T. D. Preston, and L. Sinclair. 1976. The size of airborne dust particles precipitating bronchospasm in house dust sensitive children. *J. Hygiene* (Camb.) 77: 321–325.

Colloff, M. 1991. Practical and theoretical aspects of the ecology of house dust mites (Acari: Pyroglyphidae) in relation to the study of mite-mediated allergy. *Rev. Med. Vet. Entomol.* 79: 612–630.

Colten, H. R., F. J. Picone, J. So, R. S. Strunk, and F. J. Twarog. 1977. Immediate hypersensitivity to cockroach: Isolation and purification of the major antigens. *J. Allergy Clin. Immunol.* 59: 154–160.

Cormier, Y., M. Fournier, and M. Laviolette. 1993. Farmer's Fever Systemic manifestations of farmer's lung without lung involvement. *Chest* 103: 632–634.

Couch, R. B. 1981. Viruses and indoor air pollution. *Bull. NY* Acad. *Med.* 57: 907–921.

Crissey, J. T., H. Lang, and L. C. Parish. 1995. *Manual of Medical Mycology.* Cambridge, MA: Blackwell Science.

Croft, W. A., B. B. Jarvis, and C. S. Yatawara. 1986. Airborne outbreak of trichothecene toxicosis. *Atmos. Environ.* 20: 549–552.

Custovic, A., R. Green, S. C. Taggart, A. Smith, C. A. Pickering, M. D. Chapman, and A. Woodcock. 1996. Domestic allergens in public places: Dog (Can f1) and cockroach (Bla g2)allergens in dust and mite, cat dog and cockroach allergens in the air in public buildings. *Clin. Exper. Allergy* 26: 1246–1252.

Dalphin, J. C. H., D. Pernet, A. Dubiez, D. Debreuviere, H. Allemand, and A. Depierre. 1993. Etiologic factors of chronic bronchitis in dairy farmers. *Chest* 103: 417–421.

Department of National Health and Welfare. 1987. *Exposure Guidelines for Residential Indoor Air Quality.* Ottawa, Ont. Canada.

Donham, K. J., S. J. Reynolds, P. Whitten, J. A. Merchant, L. Burmeister, and W. J. Popendorf. 1995. Respiratory dysfunction in swine facility production workers: Dose–response relationships of environmental exposures and pulmonary function. *Am. J. Indust. Med.* 27: 405–418.

Elixmann, J. H., H. F. Linskens, M. Schata, and W. Jorde. 1989. Can airborne fungal allergens pass through an air-conditioning system? *Environ. Int.* 15: 193–196.

Ezeonu, I. M., J. A. Nobel, R. B. Simmons, D. L. Price, S. A. Crow, and D. G. Ahearn. 1994. Effect of relative humidity on fungal colinization of fiberglass insulation. *Appl. Environ. Microbiol.* 60: 2149–2151.

Fink, J. N., E. F. Banaszak, W. H. Thiede, and J. J. Barboriak. 1971b. Interstitial pneumonitis due to hypersensitivity to an organism contaminating a heating system. *Ann. Intern. Med.* 74: 80.

Finnegan, M. J., C. A. C. Pickering, and P. S. Burge. 1984. The sick building syndrome — Prevalent studies. *BMJ* 289: 1573–1575.

Finnegan, M. J., A. C. Pickering, P. S. Davies, P. K. C. Austwick, and D. C. Warhurst. 1987. Amoeba: The cause of humidifier fever? In *Indoor Air '87*, eds. B. Seifert, H. Esdorn, M. Fischer, H. Ruden, and J. Wegner, pp. 648–652. Berlin: Institute for Water, Soil and Air Hygiene.

Flannigan, B. 1987. Mycotoxins in air. *Int. Biodeteriora*tion 23: 73–78.

Flannigan, B., and J. D. Miller. 1994. Health Implications of fungi in indoor environments—An overview. In *Health Implications of Fungi in Indoor Environments*, eds. R. Samson, B. Flannigan, and M. Flannigan, et al. pp. 3–28. Amsterdam: Elsevier.

Fox, J. P., C. E. Hall, and L. R. Elveback. 1970. *Epidemiology. New York: Macmillan.*

Halpin, D. M., B. J. Graneek, M. Turner-Warwick, and A. J. Newman Taylor. 1994. Extrinsic allergic alveolitis and asthma in a sawmill worker: Case report and review of the literature. *Occup. Environ. Med.* 51: 160–164.

Hasani, A., M. Johnson, D. Pavia, J. Agnew, and S. Clarke. 1992. Impairment of lung mucociliary clearance in pigeon fanciers. *Chest* 102: 887–891.

Hawthorne, A. R., C. S. Dundee, R. L. Tyndall, T. Vo-Dinh, M. A. Cohen, J. D. Spengler, and J. P. Harper. 1989. Case study: Multipollutant indoor air quality study of 300 homes. In *Design and Protocol for Monitoring Indoor Air Quality*, ASTM STP 1002, eds. N.L. Nagda and J. P. Harper, pp. 129–147. Philadelphia: American Society for Testing and Materials.

Hendry, K. M., and E. C. Cole. 1993. A review of mycotoxins in indoor air. *J. Toxicol. Environ. Health* 38: 183–198.

Holberg C. J., M. K. O'Rourke, and M. D. Lebowitz. 1987. Multivariate analysis of ambient environmental factors and respiratory effects. *Int. J. Epidemiol.* 16(3): 399–410.

Homburger, H., B. Kang, D. Vellody, and J. W. Yunginger. 1979. Cockroach cause of allergic asthma: Its specificity and immunologic profile. *J. Allergy Clin. Immunol.* 63: 80–86.

Houk, V. N., D. C. Kent, J. H. Baker, and K. Sorensen. 1968. The epidemiology of tuberculosis infection in a closed environment. *Arch. Environ. Health* 16: 26–35.

de Hoyos, A., D. L. Holness, and S. M. Tarlo. 1993. Hypersensitivity pneumonitis and airway hyper-reactivity induced by occupational exposure to *Penicillium. Chest* 103: 330–304.

Jantunen, M. J., A. Nevalainen, A. L. Rytkonen, M. Pellikka, and P. Kalliokosi. 1987. The effect of humidification on indoor air fungal spores counts in apartment buildings. In *Indoor Air '87*, eds. B. Seifert, H. Esdorn, M. Fischer, H. Ruden, and J. Wegner, pp. 643–647. Berlin: Institute for Water, Soil and Air Hygiene.

Jarvis, B. 1986. Potential air pollution problems associated with macrocyclic trichothene by producing fungi. Working Paper provided to the Health and Welfare Canada Working Group on Fungi and Indoor Air. Environmental Health Directorate, Health and Welfare Canada, Ottawa Ont. K1A 0L2.

Jarvis, B. B., Y. Zhou, J. Jiang, S. Wang, W. G. Sorenson, E. L. Hintikka, M. Nikulin, P. Parikka, R. A. Etzel, and D. G. Dearborn. 1996. Toxigenic molds in water damaged buildings: Dechlorogrisofulvins from *Memnoniella echinata. J. Natl. Proud* 59: 553–554.

Johanning, E., R. Biagini, D. Hull, P. Morey, B. Jarvis, and P. Landsbergis. 1996. Health and immunology study following exposure to toxigenic fungi (*Stachybotris chartarum*) in a water-damaged office environment. *Int. Arch. Occup. Environ. Health* 68: 207–218.

Jorna, T. H., P. J. Born, J. Valks, R. Houba, and E. F. Wouters. 1994. Respiratory symptoms and lung function in animal feed workers. *Chest* 106: 1050–1055.

Kaplya, M., and A. Penttinen. 1981. An evaluation of the microscopical counting methods of the tape in Hirst-Burkard pollen and spore trap. *Grana* 20: 131–141.

Kauffman, C. A. 1996. Opportunistic infections: The filamentous fungi. *J. Respir. Dis.* 17: 17–27.

Kokkarinen J., H. Tukianinen, and E. Terho. 1994. Mortality due to farmer's lung in Finland. *Chest* 106: 509–512.

Kneist, F. M. 1989. Reduction and joined colorimetric quantification of allergen sources: A case study. *Environ. Int.* 15: 197–201.

Knight, V. 1980. Viruses as agents of airborne infection. In *Airborne Contagion*, ed. R. B. Kundsin, pp. 147–156. *Ann. NY Acad. Sci.* no. 353. New York : New York Academy of Sciences.

Korsgaard, J. 1983a. Mite asthma and residency. A case-control study on the impact of exposure to house-dust mites in dwellings. *Am. Rev. Respir. Dis.* 128: 231–235.

Korsgaard, J. 1983b. Preventive measures in mite asthma. A controlled trial. *Allergy* 38: 93–102.

LaForce, F. M. 1986. Airborne infections and modern building technology. *Environ. Int.* 12: 137–146.

Lebowitz, M. D. 1981. Respiratory Indicators. *Environ. Res.* 25: 225–235.

Lebowitz, M. D., E. J. Cassell, and J. R. McCarroll. 1972. Health in the Urban Environment: The incidence and burden of minor illness in a healthy population. *Am. Rev. Respir. Dis.* 106: 824–841.

Lebowitz, M. D., M. K. O'Rourke, R. Dodge, C. J. Holberg, G. Corman, R. W. Hoshaw, J. L. Pinnas, R. A. Barbee, and M. R. Sneller. 1982. The adverse health effects of biological aerosols, other aerosols, and indoor microclimate on asthmatics and nonasthmatics. *Environ. Int.* 8: 375–380.

Lebowitz, M. D. 1983. Health effects of indoor pollution. *Ann. Rev. Public Health* 4: 203–221. (Republished in *Indoor Air Pollution: The Architects' Response*, ed. K. Collins. San Francisco: AIA, 1984).

Lebowitz, M. D., C. J. Holberg, B. Boyer, and C. Hayes. 1985. Respiratory symptoms and peak flow associated with indoor and outdoor air pollutants in the Southwest. *Air Pollution Control Assoc.* 35(11): 1154–1158.

Lebowitz, M. D., L. Collins, and C. J. Holberg 1987. Time series analysis of respiratory responses to indoor and outdoor environmental phenomena. *Environ. Res.* 43: 332–341.

Lebowitz, M. D., J. J. Quackenboss, M. L. Soczek, M. Kollander, and S. Colome. 1989a. The new standard environmental inventory questionnaire for estimation of indoor concentrations. *J. Air Pollution Control Assoc.* 39(11): 1411–1419.

Lebowitz, M. D., J. J. Quackenboss, M. L. Soczek, S. D. Colome, and P. J. Lioy. 1989b. Workshop: Development of questionnaires and survey instruments. In *Design and Protocol for Monitoring Indoor Air Quality*, ASTM STP 1002, eds. N. L. Nagda and J. P. Harper, pp. 203–216. Philadelphia: American Society for Testing and Materials.

Levetin, E. 1998. Oklahoma Tree Pollen: A longterm study of winter and early spring tree pollen, in the Tulsa, oklahoma, atmosphere. *Aerobiologia*, 14: 21–28.

Li, C. S., and Y. M. Kuo. 1994. Characteristics of airborne microfungi in subtropical homes. *Sci. Total Environ.* 155: 267–271.

Licorish, K., H. S. Novey, P. Kozak, R. D. Fairshter, and A. F. Wilson. 1985. Role of *Alternaria* and *Penicillium* spores in the pathogenesis of asthma. *J. Allergy Clin. Immunol.* 76: 819–825.

Lind, P. 1985. Purification and partial characterization of two major allergens from the house dust mite *Dermatophagoides pteronyssinus*. *J. Allergy Clin. Immunol.* 76: 753–761.

Lovell, C. R. 1993. *Plants and the Skin*. Oxford: Blackwell Scientific Publications.

Macher, J. M., M. A. Chatigny, and H. A. Burge. 1995. Sampling airborne microorganisms and aeroallergens. In: *Air Sampling Instruments*, 8th edition, eds. B. S. Cohen and S.V. Hering, Cincinnati: ACGIH.

Madge, P., J. Y. Paton, J. H. McColl, and P. L. Mackie. 1992. Prospective controlled study of four infection-control procedures to prevent nosocomial infection with respiratory syncytial virus. *Lancet* 340: 1079–1083.

Malmberg, P., A. Rask-Andersen, and L. Rosenhall. 1993. Exposure to microorganisms associated with allergic alveolitis and febrile reactions to mold dust in farmers. *Chest* 103: 1202–1209.

Mamolen, M., D. M. Lewis, M. A. Blanchet, F. J. Satunk, and R. L. Vogt. 1993. Investigation of an outbreak of "humidifier fever" in a print shop. *Am. J. Indust. Med.* 23: 483–490.

Martonen, T. B., and M. K. O'Rourke, 1991. Deposition patterns of ragweed pollen in the human respiratory tract. *Grana* 30: 82–86.

Martonen, T. B. and M. K. O'Rourke, 1992. Deposition of mulberry pollen in the human respiratory system: A mathematical model. *Grana* 32: 290–301.

Meldrum, J., M. K. O'Rourke, P. Boyer-Pfersdorf, and L. Stetzenbach. 1993. The relationship between mold spores and colony counts as representatives of airborne fungi. In *Proc. 6th International Conference on Indoor Air Quality,* Helsinki, vol. 4, eds. P. Kalliokoski, M. Jantunen and O. Seppanen, pp. 189–194.

Melia, R. J. W., C. du V. Florey, R. W. Morris, B. Goldstein, H. Joh, C. Clark, I. Craighead, and J. Mackinlay. 1982. Childhood respiratory illness and the home environment II. Association between respiratory illness and nitrogen dioxide, temperature and relative humidity. *Int. J. Epidemiol.* 11: 164–169.

Mendell, M. J. 1993. Non specific symptoms in office workers: a review and summary of the epidemiologic literature. In: *Proc. 6th International Conference on Indoor Air Quality,* Helsinki, vol. 3, eds. P. Kalliokoski, M. Jantunen and O. Seppanen, pp. 227–236.

Miadonna, A. A. Fesci, A. Tedeschi, G. Bertorelli, M. Arquati, and D. Olivieri. 1994. Mast cell and histamine involvement in farmer's lung disease. *Chest* 105: 1184–1189.

Middleton, E., C. E. Reed, and E. F. Ellis. 1988. *Allergy, Principles and Practice,* 3rd St. Louis: Mosby.

Milton, D. K., J. Amsel, C. E. Reed, P. L. Enright, L. R. Brown, G. L. Aughenbaugh, and P. R. Morey. 1995. Cross-sectional follow-up of a flu-like respiratory illness among fiberglass manufacturing employees: Endotoxin exposure associated with two distinct sequelae. *Am. J. Indust. Med.* 28: 469–488.

Milton, D. K., M. D. Walters, K. Hammond, and J. S. Evans. 1996. Worker exposure to endotoxin phenolic compounds, and formaldehyde in a fiberglass insulation manufacturing plant. *Am. Indust. Hyg. Assn. J.* 57: 889–896.

Mitani, M., K. Satoh, T. Kobayashi, Y. Kawase, N. Hosokawa, H. Takashima, S. Kobayashi, and M. Tanabe. 1995. Hypersensitivity Pneumonitis in a pearl nucleus worker. *J. Thor. Imaging* 10: 134–137.

Morens, D. M., and V. M. Rash. 1995. Lessons form a nursing home outbreak of influenza A. *Infection Control Hospital Epidemiol.* 16: 275–280.

Morey, P. R. 1989. Role of ventilation in the causation of building associated illness. *Occup. Med.* 4: 625–642.

Morey, P. 1996. Mold growth in buildings: Removal and prevention. In *Indoor Air '96. Proc. 7th International Conference on Indoor Air Quality and Climate* vol. 2, eds. K. Ikeda and T. Iwata, pp. 27–36.

Morey, P., H. Burge, M. Chatigny, J. Feeley, K. Kreiss, J. Otten, and K. Peterson. 1987. Assessment of non-pathogenic bioaerosols in indoor environments. In *Indoor Air '87,* eds. B. Seifert, H. Esdorn, M. Fischer, H. Ruden, and J. Wegner, pp. 622–625. Berlin: Institute for Water, Soil and Air Hygiene.

Mroueh, S., and A. Spock. 1994. Allergic Bronchopulmonary Aspergillosis in patients with cystic fibrosis. *Chest* 105: 32–36.

NCHS (National Center for Health Statistics) 1988. Current estimates from the National Health Interview Survey, United States, 1987, pp 66-159-DHHS Publication (PHS), Washington, DC.

Nevalainen, A. 1993. Microbial contamination of buildings. In: Proc. *6th International Conference on Indoor Air Quality,* Helsinki, vol. 4 eds. P. Kalliokoski, M. Jantunen, and O. Seppanen, pp. 3–13.

Nevalainen, A., M. Jantunen, M. Pellikka, E. Pitkanen, and P. Kalliokoski. 1987. Airborne bacteria, fungal spores and ventilation in Finnish day-care centers. In *Indoor Air '87,* eds. B. Seifert, H. Esdorn, M. Fischer, H. Ruden, and J. Wegner, pp. 678–680. Berlin: Institute for Water, Soil and Air Hygiene.

NRC/NAS. 1981. *Indoor Pollutants.* Washington DC: National Academy Press.

NRC/NAS. 1987. *Policies and Procedures for Control of Indoor Air Quality.* Committee on Indoor Air Quality, Washington DC: National Academy Press.

Ogden E. C., G. S. Raynor, J. V. Hayes, D. M. Lewis, and J. H. Haines. 1974. *Manual for Sampling Airborne Pollen.* New York: Hafner Press.

Ohgke, H., A. Geers, and J. Bercket. 1987. Fungal load of indoor air in historical and newly constructed buildings used by public services. In *Indoor Air '87,* eds. B. Seifert, H. Esdorn, M. Fischer, H. Ruden, and J. Wegner, pp. 681–684. Berlin: Institute for Water, Soil and Air Hygiene.

O'Rourke, M. K. 1996. Medical Palynology. In: *Palynology: Principles and Applications,* vol. 3, eds. J. Jansonius, and D. C. McGregor, pp. 935–955.

O'Rourke, M. K., and M. D. Lebowitz. 1984. A comparison of regional atmospheric pollen with pollen collected at and near houses. *Grana* 22: 1–10.

O'Rourke, M. K., and M. D. Lebowitz. 1995. The importance of environmental allergens in the development of chronic and obstructive lung diseases. In: *Environmental Respiratory Disease*, eds. S. L. Demeter, E. Cordasco, and C. Zenz, pp. 295–336. New York: Van Nostrand Reinhold.

O'Rourke, M. K., J. J. Quackenboss, and M. D. Lebowitz. 1989. An epidemiological approach investigating respiratory disease response in sensitive individuals to indoor and outdoor pollen exposure in Tucson, AZ. *Aerobiologia* 5: 104–110.

O'Rourke, M. K., L. Fiorentino, D. Clark, M. Ladd, S. Rogan, J. Carpenter, D. Gray, L. McKinley, and E. Sorensen. 1993. Building materials and importance of house dust mite exposure in the Sonoran Desert. In: *Proc. 6th International Conference on Indoor Air Quality,* Helsinki, vol. 4, eds. P. Kalliokoski, M. Jantunen, and O. Seppanen, pp. 155–160.

O'Rourke, M. K., C. L. Moore, and L. G. Arlian. 1996. Prevalence of house dust mites from homes in the Sonoran Desert, Tucson, Arizona. In: *Aerobiology*, eds. M. Mulienberg, and H. Burge, pp. 67–80. Chelsea: Lewis Publishers.

Passanen, A. L., S. Lappalaninen, A. Korpi, P. Pasanen, and P. Kalliokoski. 1996. Volatile metabolic products of moulds as indicators of mould problems in buildings. In *Indoor Air '96 Proc. 7th International Conference on Indoor Air Quality and Climate*, vol. 2 eds. K. Ikeda, and T. Iwata, pp. 669–674.

Platts-Mills, T. A. E., and M. D. Chapman. 1987. Dust mites: Immunology, allergic disease, and environmental control. *J. Allergy Clin. Immunol.* 80: 755.

Platts-Mills, T. A. E., and S. Pollart Squillace. 1997. Allergen sensitization and perennial asthma. *Int. Arch. Allergy Immunol.* 113: 83–86.

Platts-Mills, T. A. E., E. R. Tovey, E. B. Mitchell, H. Moszoro, P. Nock, and S. R. Wilkins. 1982. Reduction of bronchial hyper-reactivity during prolonged allergen avoidance. *Lancet* 2: 675 – 678.

Platts-Mills, T. A. E., de Werk, A. L. et al., 1989. Dust mite allergens and asthma—A worldwide problem. *J. Allergy Clin. Immunol.* 83: 416.

Platts-Mills, T. A. E., R. Sporik, J. M. Ingram, and R. Honsinger. 1995. Dog and cat allergens and asthma among school children in Los Alamos, New Mexico, USA: Altitude 7,200 feet. *Int. Arch. Allergy Immunol.* 107: 301–330.

Pope, A. M., R. Patterson, and H. Burge. 1993. *Indoor Allergens: Assessing and Controlling Indoor Health Effects*. Institute of Medicine. Washington, DC: National Academy Press.

Poulsen, O. M., N. O. Breum, N. Ebbehoj, A. M. Hansen, U. I. Ivens, D. van Lelieveld, P. Malmros, L. Matthiasen, B. H. Nielsen, and E. M. Neilsen. 1995a. Collection of domestic waste. Review of occupational health problems and their causes. *Sci. Total Environ.* 170: 1–19.

Poulsen, O. M., N. O. Breum, N. Ebbehoj, A. M. Hansen, U. I. Ivens, D. van Lelieveld, P. Malmros, L. Matthiasen, B. H. Nielsen, and E. M. Neilsen. 1995b. Sorting and recycling of domestic waste. Review of occupational health problems and their possible causes. *Sci. Total Environ.* 168: 33–56.

Preller, L., H. Kromhout, D. Heederik, and M. J. Tielen. 1995a. Modeling long-term average exposure in occupational exposure–response analysis. *Scand. J. Work Environ. Health* 21: 504–512.

Preller, L., D. Heederik, H. Kromhout, J. S. Boleij, and M. J. Tielen. 1995b. Determinants of dust and endotoxin, exposure of pig farmers: Development of a control strategy using empirical modeling. *Ann. Occ. Hygiene* 39: 545–557.

Preller, L., D. Heederik, J. S. Boleij, P. F. Vogelzang, and M. J. Tielen. 1995c. Lung function and chronic respiratory symptoms of pig farmers: focus on exposure to endotoxins and ammonia and use of disinfectants. *Occ. Environ. Med.* 52: 654–660.

Prince, H. E., and G. H. Meyer. 1976. An up-to-date look at mould allergy. *Ann. Allergy* 37: 18–25.

Rantio-Lehtimaki, A., M. Viander, and A. Koivikko. 1994. Airborne birch pollen antigens in different particle sizes. *Clin. Exper. Allergy* 24: 23–28.

Raza, S. H., R. Kausar, and M. S. R. Murthy. 1989. Indoor aerobiological pollution in certain indian domestic environments. *Environ. Int.* 15: 209–215.

Redlich, C. A., J. Sparer, and M. R. Cullen. 1997. Sick-building syndrome. *Lancet* 349: 1013–1016.

Reed, C. E., M. C. Swanson, M. Lopez, A. M. Ford, J. Major, W. B. Witmer, and T. B. Valdes. 1983. Measurement of IgG antibody and airborne antigen to control in industrial outbreak of hypersensitivity pneumonitis. *J. Occup. Med.* 25: 207–210.

Reinikainen, L. M., J. J. K. Jaakkola, and O. P. Heinanen. 1988. The effect of air humidification on different symptoms in an office building: An epidemiological study. *Proc. Healthy Buildings Conference*, Stockholm: Almquist and Wiksel. vol. 3, pp. 207–215.

Reponen, T., A. Nevalainen, and T. Raunemaa. 1989. Bioaerosol and particle mass levels and ventilation in Finnish homes. *Environ. Int.* 15: 203–208.

Riley, R. L. 1982. Indoor airborne infection. *Environ. Int.* 8: 317–320.

Riley, R. L., C. C. Mills, W. Nyka, N. Weinstock, P. B. Storey, L. U. Sultan, M. C. Riley, and W. C. Wells. 1959. Aerial dissemination of pulmonary tuberculosis: A two-year study of contagion in a tuberculosis ward. *Am. J. Hyg.* 70: 185–196.

Riley, R. L., C. C. Mills, F. O'Grady, L. U. Sultan, F. Wittestadt, and D. N. Shivpuri. 1962. Infectiousness of air from a tuberculosis ward: Ultraviolet irradiation of infected air; comparative infectiousness of different patients. *Am. Rev. Respir. Dis.* 85: 511–525.

Ring, J., and G. Burg. 1986. *New Trends in Allergy II*. Berlin: Springer.

Ring, J. 1993. Pseudo-allergic reactions. In *Allergy, Theory and Practice*, 2nd edition, eds. P. E. Korenblat and H. J. Wedner. Orlando: Grune and Stratton.

RIVM. 1989. Indoor environment. In *A National Environmental Survey 1985–2010, Concern for Tomorrow*, ed. Ir. F. Langeweg, pp. 243–254. Bilthoven, The Netherlands: National Institute of Public Health and Environmental Protection.

Rix, B. A. 1997. Exposure to endotoxins in the environment: Occurrence and health hazards. *Ugeskrift for Laeger* 159: 2529–2533.

Robins, T., N. Seixas, A. Franzblau, L. Abrams, S. Minick, H. A. Burge, and M. A. Schork. 1997. Acute respiratory effects on workers exposed to metalworking fluid aerosols in an automotive transmission plant. *Am. J. Indust. Med.* 31: 510–524.

Rodriguez de Castro, F., T. Carrillo, R. Castillo, C. Blanco, F. Diaz, and M. Cuevas. 1993. Relationships between characteristics of exposure to pigeon antigens. *Chest* 103: 1059–1053.

Rogers, C. A. 1997. An aeropalynological study of metropolitan Toronto. *Aerobiologia*, 13: 243–257.

Rom, W. N., ed. 1983. *Environmental and Occupational Medicine*. Boston. Little, Brown.

Rosenstreich, D. L., P. Eggleston, M. Kattan, D. Basker, R. G. Slavin, P. Gergen, H. Mitchell, K. McNiff-Mortimer, H. Lynn, D. Owenby, and F. Malveaux. 1997. The role of cockroach allergy and exposure to cockroach allergen in causing morbidity among inner-city children with asthma. *N. Engl. J. Med.* 336: 1356–1363.

Rylander, R., B. Bake, J. J. Fischer, and I. M. Helander. 1989. Pulmonary function and symptoms after inhalation of endotoxin. *Am. Rev. Respir. Dis.* 140: 981–986.

Samet, J. M., and J. D. Spengler, eds. 1991. *Indoor Air Pollution*. Baltimore: Johns Hopkins University Press.

Samson, R. A. 1985. Occurrence of moulds in modern living and working environments. *Eur. J. Epidemiol.* 1: 54–61.

Sarpong, S. B., R. A. Wood, T. Karrison, and P. A. Eggleston. 1997. Cockroach allergen Bla g 1 in school dust. *J. Allergy Clin. Immunol.* 99: 486–492.

Schata, M., J. Wolfgang, J. H. Elixmann, and H. F. Linskens. 1989. Allergies to molds caused by fungal spores in air conditioning equipment. *Environ. Int.* 15: 177–179.

Schumacher, M. J., R. D. Griffith, and M. K. O'Rourke. 1988. Recognition of pollen and other particulate aeroantigens by immunoblot microscopy. *J. Allergy Clin. Immunol.* 82: 608–616.

Sears, M. R., G. P. Herbison, M. D. Holdaway, et al. 1989. The relative risks of sensitivity to grass pollen, house dust mite and cat dander in the development of childhood asthma. *Clin. Allergy* 19: 419–424.

Seppanen, O. 1996. Ventilation and air quality. In *Indoor Air '96. Proc. 7th International Conference on Indoor Air Quality and Climate*. vol. 2, eds. K. Ikeda and T. Iwata, pp. 15–32. Tokyo: SEEC Ishibas.

Sinha, R. N., and J. E. van Bronswijk. 1971. Pyroglyphid mites (Acari) and house dust allergy. *J. Allergy Clin. Immunol.* 47: 31–52.

Sly, R. M., and R. O'Donnell. 1997. Stabilization of asthma mortality. *Ann. Allergy Asthma Immunol.* 78: 347–354.

Smith, P. W. 1977. Room humidifiers as a source of Acinetobacter infections. *JAMA* 237: 795.

Smoragiewicz, W., B Cossette, A. Boutard, and K. Krzystyniak. 1993. Trichothecene mycotoxins in the dust of ventilation systems in office buildings. *Int. Arch. Occ. Environ. Health* 65: 113–117.

Solomon, W. R., and H. A. Burge. 1975. *Aspergillus fumigatus* levels in and out of doors in urban air. *J. Allergy Clin. Immunol.* 55: 90–91.

Solomon, W. R. 1988. Aerobiology and Inhalant allergens. In: *Allergy Principles and Practice.* eds. E. Middleton, C. E. Reed, E. F. Ellis, pp. 312–372, St. Louis: Mosby.

Sorenson, W. G., D. G. Frazier, B. B. Jarvis, J. Simpson, and V. Robinson. 1987. Trichothecene mycotoxins in aerosolized conidia of *Stachybotrys atra*. *App. Environ. Microbiol.* 53: 1370–1375.

Spieksma, F. T. M., H. Varekamp, and R. Voorhorst. 1969. *House Dust Atopy and the House Dust Mite.* Leiden: Stafeus.

Sporik, R., J. M. Ingram, W. Price, J. H. Sussman, R. W. Honsinger, and T. A. Platts-Mills. 1995. Association of asthma with serum IgE and skin test reactivity to allergens among children living at high altitude: Tickling the dragon's breath. *Am J. Respir. Crit. Care Med.* 151: 1388–1392.

Staib, F., M. Seibold, and M. Heibenhuber. 1987. Indoor air mycology—Aspergillosis, mucormycosis and cryptococcosis caused by fungal spores from indoor air. In *Indoor Air '87,* eds. B. Seifert, H. Esdorn, M. Fischer, H. Ruden, and J, Wegner, pp. 694–698. Berlin: Institute for Water, Soil and Air Hygiene.

Stern, M. A., U. Allitt, J. M. Corden, and W. M. Millington. 1996. A new continuous volumetric recording indoor air sampler. *J. Allergy Clin. Immunol.* 97(1 part 2): 216.

Strachan, D. P. 1988. Damp housing and childhood asthma: validation of reporting of symptoms. *BMJ* 297: 1223–1226.

Streifel, A. J., D. Vesley, F. S. Rhame, and B. Murray. 1989. Control of airborne fungal spores in a university hospital. *Environ. Int.* 15: 221–227.

Su, H. J., H. A. Burge, and J. D. Spengler. 1989. Microbiological contamination in the residential environment. *Joint Canadian and Pan-American Symposium on Aerobiology and Health*, 7–9 June 1989, Ottawa, Ont., Canada.

Teeuw, K. B., C. M. van den Broucke-Grauls, and J. Verhoef. 1994. Airborne gram negative bacteria and endotoxin in sick building syndrome. A study in Dutch governmental office buildings. *Arch. Internal Med.* 154: 2339–2345.

Thorn, A., M. Lewne, and L. Belin. 1996. Allergic Alveolitis in a school environment. *Scand. J. Work Environ. Health* 22: 311–314.

Tobin, R. S., E. Baranowski, A. P. Gilman, T. Kuipmer-Goodman, J. D. Miller, and M. Giddings. 1987a. Significance of fungi in indoor air: Report of a Canadian working group. In *Indoor Air '87,* eds. B. Seifert, H. Esdorn, M. Fischer, H. Ruden, and J. Wegner, pp. 718–722. Berlin: Institute for Water, Soil and Air Hygiene.

Tobin, R. S., E. Baranowski, A. P. Gilman, T. Kuipmer-Goodman, J. D. Miller, and M. Giddings. 1987b. Significance of fungi in indoor air. *Can. J. Public Health* 78: 21–32.

Tovey, E. R., M. D. Chapman, C. W. Wells, and T. A. Platts-Mills. 1981a. The distribution of dust mite allergen in the houses of patients with asthma. *Am. Rev. Respir. Dis.* 124: 630–635.

Tovey, E. R., M. D. Chapman, and T. A. Platts-Mills. 1981b. Mite faeces are a major source of house dust allergens. *Nature* 289: 592–593.

Turner-Warwick, M. 1978. *Immunology of the Lung.* London: Edward Arnold.

U. S. National Center for Health Statisitcs. 1988. Current estimates from the national Health Interview Survey, United States, 1987. *DHHS Publ.* (PHS) 88-1594. U.S. Dept. Health & Human Services.

Van der Heide, A. J., G. De Monchy, K. De Vries, A. E. Dubois, and H. F. Kauffman. 1997. Seasonal differences in airway hyperresponsiveness in asthmatic patients: Relationship with allergen exposure and sensitization to house dust mites. *Clin. Exper. Allergy* 27: 627–633.

van Wageningen, N., M. Waegemaekers, B. Brunekreef and J. Boleij. 1987. Health complaints and indoor moulds in relation to moist problems in homes. In *Indoor Air '87,* eds. B. Seifert, H. Esdorn, M. Fischer, H. Ruden, and J. Wegner, pp. 723–727. Berlin: Institute for Water, Soil and Air Hygiene.

Verhoeff, A. P., J. H. van Wijnen, E. S. van Reenen-Hoekstra, R. A. Samson, R. T. van Strien, and R. Brunekreef. 1994. Fungal propagules in house dust: II. Relation with residential characteristics and respiratory symptoms. *Allergy* 49: 540–547.

Verhoeff, A. P., and H. A. Burge. 1997. Health risk assessment of fungi in home environments. *Ann. Allergy Asthma Immunol.* 78: 544–556.

Vervloet, D., P. Bongrand, A. Arnaud, Ch. Boutin, and J. Charpin. 1979. Objective immunological and clinical data observed during an altitude cure at Briancon in asthmatic children allergic to house dust and *Dermatophagoides*. *Rev. Fr. Mal. Respir.* 7: 19–27.

Volk, W. A., and M. F. Wheeler. 1980. *Basic Microbiology*, 4th edition, Philadelphia: Lippincott.

Voorhorst, R., F. Th. Spieksma, H. Varekamp, M. J. Leupen, and A. W. Lyklema. 1967. The house dust mite and the allergens it produces. *J. Allergy* 39: 325–339.

Wasserman, S. 1988. Basic mechanisms in asthma. *Ann. Allergy* 116: 477–482.

Weber, A. 1984. Annoyance and irritation by passive smoking. *Prev. Med.* 13: 618–625.

Weill, H., and M. Turner-Warwick. 1981. *Occupational Lung Diseases.* New York: Dekker.

Weinberger, S. E. 1992. *Principles of Pulmonary Medicine.* Philadelphia: Saunders.

Weiss, K. B., P. J. Jergen, and T. A. Hodgson. 1992. An economic evaluation of asthma in the United States. *N. Engl. J. Med.* 326: 862–866.

Wesson, B., and K. O. Schoeps 1996. Microbial volatile organic compounds—what substances can be found in sick buildings? *Analyst* 121: 1203–1205.

WHO. 1983a. Indoor air pollutants: Exposure and health effects. *WHO EURO Reports and Studies* 78. *WHO* European Regional Office, Copenhagen.

WHO. 1983b. *Guidelines on Studies in Environmental Epidemiology.* Geneva: Environmental Health Criteria 27.

WHO. 1986a. Indoor air quality research. Report on a WHO Meeting. *EURO Reports and Studies* 103. *WHO* European Regional Office, Copenhagen.

WHO. 1986b. Dust mite allergens and asthma — A worldwide problem. *WHO Bull.* 66.

WHO. 1990. Biological contaminants in indoor air. *EURO Reports and Studies* 113, 29 August–2 September 1988. Rautavaara.

WHO / EURO. 1982. Legionnaires' disease. *WHO / EURO Reports and Studies* 12. Copenhagen.

WHO / EURO. 1986. Environmental aspects of the control of legionellosis. *Environmental Health Series* 14. Copenhagen.

Wilks, D., M. Farrington, and D. Rubenstein. 1995. *The Infectious Disease Manual.* Cambridge, MA: Blackwell Science.

Wintermeyer, S. F., W. G. Kuschner, H. Wong, A. D'Alessandro, and P. D. Blanc. 1997. Pulmonary responses after wood chip mulch exposure. *J. Occup. Environ.* Med. 39: 308–314.

Woo, A. H., A. Goetz, and V. L. Yu. 1992. Transmission of *Legionella* by respiratory equipment and aerosol generating devises. *Chest* 102: 1586–1590.

Wood, R. A., P. A. Eggleston, P. Lind, L. Ingemann, B. Schwartz, S. Graveson, D. Terry, B. Wheeler, and N. F. Adkinson Jr. 1988. Antigenic analysis of household dust samples. *Am. Rev. Respir. Dis.* 137: 358–363.

Woods, J. E., P. R. Morey, and D. R. Rask. 1989. Indoor air quality diagnostics: qualitative and quantitative procedures to improve environmental conditions. In *Design and Protocol for Monitoring Indoor Air Quality*, ASTM STP 1002, eds. N. L. Nagda, and J. P. Harper, pp. 80–98. Philadelphia: American Society for Testing and Materials.

Yashida, K., T. Hiraoka, M. Ando, K. Uchida, and V. Mohsenin. 1992. *Penicillium decumbens* a new cause of fungal ball. *Chest* 101: 1152–1153.

Yli-Panula, E., and A. Rantio-Lehtimaki. 1996. Grass Pollen Antigenic Activity of settled dust in rural and urban homes. In: *Indoor Air '96 Proc. 7th International Conference on Indoor Air Quality and Climate*, eds. K. Ikeda and T. Iwata. vol. 3, pp. 705–707.

Yoshizawa, S., T. Irie, F. Sugawara, S. Ozawo, Y. Kohsaka, and A. Matsumae. 1987. Microbiological contamination from air conditioning systems in Japanese buildings. In *Indoor Air '87*, eds. B. Seifert, H. Esdorn, M. Fischer, H. Ruden, and J. Wegner, pp. 627– 631. Berlin: Institute for Water, Soil and Air Hygiene.

Zeterberg, J. M. 1973. A review of respiratory virology and the spread of virulent and possibly antigenic viruses via air conditioning systems. *Ann. Allergy*, 31: 228–234 and 291–299.

14 Lead and Compounds

KATHRYN R. MAHAFFEY, Ph.D.
JAMES McKINNEY, Ph.D.
J. ROUTT REIGART, M.D.

Lead has long been recognized to be acutely toxic at high-dose exposure (Aub et al., 1925). Recent findings with respect to understanding the toxicology of lead indicate that lead is capable of producing toxic effects in adults and children at exposures far lower than those producing gross clinical symptoms (Davis and Svengaard, 1987; Lippmann, 1990). Lead exposures that were considered "safe" through the early 1980s are now recognized to produce toxicity. The developing red blood cells, the nervous system, and the kidneys are the organ systems in which these toxic effects have been intensively studied (Skerfving, 1988). Such effects are not identifiable through routine clinical observations of any one patient at one point in time. Subclinical lead toxicity syndrome, which involves multiple organ systems, requires more sophisticated measuring methods than does clinical observation. Subclinical lead toxicity is most readily identified through longitudinal observation. Although the effects, particularly in the neurodevelopmental area are subtle, their impact on a population basis can be substantial as illustrated for lead (Eckerman et al., 1999) or other chemicals (Lester et al., 1998).

Despite this intense study, the mechanism(s) of toxic action of lead at the molecular level is (are) not known. Toxicity may be determined by different routes of administration in single or multiple doses in a variety of animals. Toxicity can be studied mechanistically in two rather different ways. In the first, one would define all those systems that affect the delivery of the toxicant to its site(s) of action. In the second, one would define the site(s) of action of the chemical (i.e., the receptor) and the biological consequences of the interaction of the chemical with the receptor.

Given the wide range of lead exposures that adversely affect health and the number of organ systems involved in this syndrome of lead toxicity, it is important to analyze lead's effects at the subcellular levels. A more general objective of this analysis would be to devise chemical/molecular concepts, involving the interactions of metal ions and their associated ligands with cellular constituents, that could be used for developing a predictive model for metal compound toxicity. This approach basically takes the form of a toxicokinetic model. The biological processes to be examined include absorption, distribution (redistribution), metabolism, elimination, and clearance (normal and enhanced) of lead. The organ systems mediating or associated with toxic/pathogenic states are described where possible at the whole, cellular, and subcellular (biochemical) levels.

Environmental Toxicants: Human Exposures and Their Health Effects, 2/e. Edited by Morton Lippmann.
ISBN: 0-471-29298-2 © 2000 John Wiley & Sons, Inc.

PHYSICAL / CHEMICAL PROPERTIES AND BEHAVIOR OF
LEAD AND ITS COMPOUNDS

Lead is a member of subgroup IVA of the periodic table. It is a typical heavy metal (Greninger et al., 1978); it has a relatively high atomic weight. The valence shell of the lead atom in the ground state has two s and two p electrons. Because lead has four electrons in its outer shell, the element would be expected to show a normal valence $+4$ in its compounds. The two s electrons of lead are reluctant to ionize and are thus sometimes referred to as the inert pair. Lead is considered to have a stable oxidation state (Pb^{2+}) that furnishes a divalent ion. The metabolism of lead in a redox sense would not appear to be an important factor determining its biological / toxicological properties. Bivalent lead has a remarkable tendency to form well-characterized and often highly crystalline basic salts of both anhydrous and hydrated types, for example, white lead, a pigment formerly of great commercial importance. In general, the inorganic chemistry of bivalent lead resembles that of the alkaline earth elements. Several lead salts, including lead carbonate, nitrate, and sulfate, are isomorphous with corresponding strontium and barium compounds. Lead forms highly insoluble salts of phosphate, carbonate, and sulfide. Lead can also form salts with organic acids, which is the basis of certain chelating agents used in lead treatment. Elemental lead would be readily oxidized in biological systems and is therefore not considered a separate form here.

Lead's position in the periodic chart favors the formation of covalent rather than ionic bonds in Pb^{4+} compounds. This expectation is confirmed by the properties of such compounds as lead tetrachloride and tetraacetate. Predominately covalent bonding also exists in the organolead compounds (with up to four Pb–C bonds). An organometallic compound differs fundamentally in both chemical and biological properties from an ionic compound of the same metal. Determining only the total amount of the metal in a biological sample may be very misleading with regard to potential for toxic effects. In general, inorganic lead is far more extensively studied than organometallic lead. Speciation and movement in the environment of lead (and other heavy metals) have been discussed at an international conference (Landner, 1987). The biological effects of organolead compounds were reviewed by Grandjean and Grandjean (1984). Some key differences and similarities in the toxic effects of organic and inorganic lead compounds are described later.

An appreciation of some general features of metal chemistry are of value in understanding specific aspects of lead chemistry (Hanzlik, 1981). One of the most important criteria differentiating metal ions from each other and from electrophilic organic species is the chemistry of their bonding to biological ligands. Metal–ligand bonds can be as strong, in a thermodynamic sense, as bonds formed when a reactive epoxide alkylates a nucleophilic group in DNA or protein. Regardless of the mechanism by which a metal ion enters a biological system, complexation will undoubtedly play a role in both its distribution within and elimination from the organism. Metal's ions are Lewis acids, and one very important determinant of their affinity for ligands is their charge / radius ratios. Increasing the oxidation state of the metal increases its Lewis acidity and its affinity for a given ligand (assuming that it does not ionize the ligand).

In an antagonist sense the relative size of the ion can also be an important consideration. In addition to the energetics of the ligation of ions, one must also consider the energetics of the ionization process itself. In this case complex geometry and ligand exchange rate play an important role. Most metal complexes undergo ligand exchange by processes involving a dissociative rate-limiting step analogous to the Sn 1 solvolysis of alkyl halides. For a given metal the rates are quite sensitive to the nature of the departing ligand and essentially independent of the entering group. The dependence of biological activity on ligand exchange rates is simply an expression of the fact that the complex must be sufficiently inert to survive long enough in vivo to reach critical reactive target molecules and yet be sufficiently labile to react once having reached those sites. A metal-macromolecular interaction may persist long enough to have biological consequences if the equilibrium constant of the rate for dissociation of the complex is very small.

The hard–soft, acid–base dichotomy provides a rationale for many features of the behavior of metal systems in chemistry and biology. This parameter is qualitatively correlated with the charge-size ratio of the ion in that large ions of low ionic charge have easily polarizable or defonnable (i.e., soft) electrostatic fields about them, whereas small highly charged ions with relatively intense electrostatic fields are hard. Flexibility in hard–soft ligand preferences could be an important property underlying the biological activity/ toxicity of metals in living systems. Several of the toxic heavy metal ions (i.e., Pb^{2+}, Hg^{2+}, Th^{1+}, Ni^{2+}, and Sb^{3+}) are classified as soft or have borderline properties in this classification scheme. The ligands can be similarly classified by these hard–soft criteria.

In this regard it is not surprising to find that the rate of transport of a given metal ion across model liquid membranes can be varied by several orders of magnitude simply by altering the anion (ligand) present in the original salt solution (Christensen et al., 1978). Like the other group IVA metals, tin and germanium, lead forms complexes in which the donor atom is chiefly oxygen (Greninger et al., 1978). It also forms stable complexes with sulfur and halogens as the donor. Carbon and nitrogen donors are less common. Lead generally forms complexes with the coordination number six with octahedral geometrical structure; other geometries are less common. On the basis that hard metal ions prefer to bind ligands and vice versa, one might expect lead to bind the halide in the order I > Br > Cl > F. This is consistent with the early use of potassium iodide to enhance lead removal from the body (Aub, 1925).

Another aspect of metal chemistry to consider is the potential of metal compounds to act as initiators or catalysts in vivo (Hanzlik, 1987). It is not difficult to envision that inhibition of enzyme molecules by stoichiometric quantities of tightly bound metal ions could reduce the flow of vital metabolites through a pathway and thus cause toxicity. In addition to stimulating or inhibiting the synthesis of enzymes, as well as the enzyme activities themselves, many simple metal ions and compounds have catalytic activity in their own right. A consideration here is the importance of electrochemical gradients across biological membranes and the potential of a foreign metal ion to act as an "antimetabolite." This could be significant in view of the possible existence of a mechanism for coupling biological oxidation–reduction pathways to ion transport and the control of membrane potential. In many cases apparently nonessential metals are absorbed into an organism and not excreted at all; rather, they are simply concentrated and deposited in granular, insoluble complexes with or without accompanying proteinaceous material.

There are several ways to express the relationship of lead to other metals, both endogenous and foreign. For example, the resemblance of bivalent lead chemistry to that of the alkaline earth metals in general has been previously mentioned. Of particular note here is the similarity to calcium. Lead and calcium both form insoluble carbonates and insoluble phosphates. However, lead phosphate is much more insoluble than lead carbonate, whereas calcium phosphate is more soluble than calcium carbonate. Lead phosphate is one of the few insoluble phosphates that does not react with most chemical reagents. The extreme insolubility of lead phosphate may serve as a driving force for lead to function as a phosphate scavenger in biological systems, which may include inorganic forms of phosphate as well as the various important phosphate esters. The ultimate deposition of the lead in the skeleton in consistent with its chemical relationship to calcium and the formation of highly insoluble salts (Aub, 1925). Strontium, another alkaline earth metal, can also compete with calcium in bone tissue (Smith et al., 1985). This chemical similarity of lead may be related to their ionic radii and stable 2 + oxidation state relative to that of Ca^{2+}.

Intestinal calcium-binding proteins have been shown to bind lead with high affinities and in preference to calcium (Fullmer et al., 1985). These proteins bind several other cations (notably Sr^{2+}, Ba^{2+}, Cd^{2+}) in a fashion apparently related to metal ionic radii relative to calcium.

Another important factor that can determine metal chemistry and biology is the hard–soft, acid–base property (amphoteric nature). In this regard lead is similar to iron, copper, zinc, mercury, and thallium, among others. The amphoteric property, along with redox cycling, can account in large part for the importance of iron in biological systems and its adsorption, storage, and transfer in these systems (Hanzlik, 1981). These effects are attributed to the greater polarizabilities (function of number of electrons) of these cations and the subsequently greater covalent character of the bonds they form with donor ligands relative to that expected for alkaline earth cations of the same size. The situation with Pb^{2+} is quite analogous to that of Th^{1+} (Izatt et al., 1976).

Similarities in size and coordination chemistry may be important factors determining the ability of metals to act antagonistically (Hill and Matrone, 1970). The chemical similarity of lead to certain alkaline earth metals, particularly calcium, and the ability to form highly insoluble salts, particularly of carbonate and phosphate, coupled with increased affinities to biological donors (enriched in oxygen and possibly nitrogen) as a result of favorable polarizabilities could account for much of the relevant biological / toxicological chemistry of lead compounds. In an overall sense we are emphasizing the importance of the ligand–exchange chemistry of divalent lead in the expression of toxicity. Ligands can include simple anions or more complex donors that can form chelates or organic complexes.

The biological activity of a given metal is a consequence of the way in which the metal compound (salts, complexes, etc.) and the cells interact. It is this interaction that is governed by intrinsic chemical properties (modulated by certain physical properties) of both the metal compound and the cell. In addition the extent of cellular interaction can be affected by the same or different chemical properties that determine the in vivo absorption, distribution, and elimination of the compounds.

LEAD IN THE ENVIRONMENT AND HUMAN EXPOSURE

Trace metals such as lead can be present in the environment in a variety of forms (Boline, 1981) which include (1) Free hydrated ions, (2) ion-pair salts / complexes, (3) organic complexes / chelates, (4) undissolved compound, and (5) surface-adsorbed material. Although there may be differences in valence states and associated ligands (including mixed ligands) in these various forms, the metal identity is retained. The chemical reactivity of the metal is a function of the combined properties of the metal and its associated ligands, which can be understood on the basis of physicochemical principles in coordination chemistry. This chemical reactivity can be modulated by physical properties, such as surface properties of the metal compound itself. Under certain physical, chemical, and biological conditions, it is possible for a given metal to assume more than one form, which can permit new pathways of chemical reactivity. It is this same reactive potential that has made certain metals a toxic threat to the environment and to living systems that can concentrate them. The range of chemical properties and reactivities offered by metal compounds of various types is thus considerably greater than that of simple organic compounds. Since the metal is never destroyed, the potential to exert this complex chemistry is always present. Inorganic compounds of lead to which humans are likely to be exposed include the halides and oxides, the sulfides and sulfate, carbonate, and chromate.

With the exception of a few sporadic measurements in human air, marine fish, sediments, birds, and in human brains, there is relatively little information available on organic lead compounds (Jawrerski et al., 1987). It seems that most organic lead compounds in the environment come from the release of organolead compounds such as gasoline additives prior to or during use rather than from inorganic compounds of lead. In areas that have restricted the use of lead-based gasoline additives in the past 15 years, the ratio of inorganic lead compounds can be predicted to increase. Global movement of inorganic lead is of greater concern, and it has been far more extensively studied. The biogeochemical cycling of lead and routes of human exposure have been described (Schlag, 1987). The prime medium for lead transport is air because fine particulates, generated especially by anthropogenic high-temperature sources, may travel long distances before settling out via wet, dry, or cloud deposition. Deposition from air is greatest near a source, but the zone of readily detectable elevated deposition can extend some distance away. Most of the lead particles deposited on soil are retained and eventually become mixed into the surface layer. Lead accumulated at the soil surface may be taken up directly by grazing animals and by soil microorganisms and so enter terrestrial food chains. Direct exposure to children can occur by consumption of dust and dirt during normal hand-to-mouth activity.

Lead in rivers comes from runoff, erosion, and direct deposition from air. Freshwater generally contains more inorganic and organic suspended material than marine water, and this suspended material has a strong tendency to adsorb any dissolved lead. Most of the lead entering the open oceans comes from atmospheric deposition rather than from rivers. The lower concentration of particulate matter is marine waters as well as high salt (chloride, bromide, etc.) concentration would favor a larger proportion of lead in the water column in dissolved form. Deep ocean sediments may represent a sink for lead, since there is no evidence to suggest remobilization. These reservoirs of lead can be quantified in a reasonably straightforward manner, but the rates of transfer within and between the reservoirs are only known qualitatively and semiquantitatively. On a global basis a number of estimates of natural and anthropogenic lead emissions to air and to the oceans have been made (Nriagu and Pacyna, 1988), and all indicate the contribution from the anthropogenic sources is at least one to two orders of magnitude greater than that from natural sources. The history of atmospheric lead deposition in a peat bog in the Jura Mountains of Switzerland documents the rise in deposition of lead attributed to gasoline containing lead additives introduced into Switzerland in 1947 (Shotyk et al., 1998). Samples corresponding to 1991 have shown a decrease in atmospheric lead deposition with a shift in the isotropic ratios toward more radiogenic values (Shotyk et al., 1998) reflecting the phase out of leaded gasoline additives in Europe. The steep increase in global lead emissions begun in the eighteenth century, peaked at around 400,000 tons per year during 1970 to 1980 and has low declined to about 100,000 tons per year (Nriagu, 1998).

Potential exposure through drinking lead-contaminated water has received considerable attention. It has been estimated (apparently without a strong scientific basis) that a typical child not living near point sources or in housing with deteriorating lead paint receives approximately 20% of his/her lead from drinking water (Beechx, 1986). Although exposure to lead through drinking water is undoubtedly occurring, it is difficult to determine the importance of this exposure route to any specific overall toxic insult. This is because of the considerable potential for wide variations in the concentration and bioavailability of lead in water. Additionally the bioavailability of metals in water will depend not only on trace metal solubility but also on many complex chemical equilibria that are affected in various ways by the presence of other trace inorganics and organics in the water (Jackson and Sheiham, 1980). Of course the bioavailability of lead in soils, food, and inhaled air may depend on similar factors that determine the ligand – exchange chemistry once in contact with the biota and aqueous phase. This is an area where metal speciation analysis and solubility modelling would give insight and improved understanding of the potential for toxic insult (Hunt and Creasey, 1980). In fact this type of information would aid in providing a scientific basis for lead and other metal pollutant abatement strategies. It may be possible to control bioavailability of trace metals in water through appropriate manipulation of their solubility and aqueous chemistry (French and Hunt, 1988).

Calculated loading rates of trace metals including lead into environmental compartments have demonstrated that human activities have major impacts on the global and regional cycles of most of the trace elements. (Nriagu and Pacyna, 1988). Other environmental problems such as acid rain (Mohnen, 1988) are contributing to the mobilization and wide distribution of metals in the environment. The greatly increased circulation of toxic metals through the soils, water, and air and their inevitable transfer to the human food chain remain important environmental issues, entailing unknown health risks for future generations. It is also obvious that metals are quite heterogeneous with respect to their release, mobility, and toxicity. Further research will be needed to anticipate all the factors that may change the mobilization, pathways, bioavailability, and effects of lead on a global, regional, and local basis. This may include the development of new and / or improved indicator organisms with specific responses to lead. The adverse health effects of exposure to lead reflect the response of cells following exposure to lead. Transfer of lead from the environment to cells and the subsequent interaction of lead with cell are functions of the physical / chemical properties of lead, some of which were previously described, and of physiological factors inherent to the organism.

The following material is largely descriptive, since the amount of fundamental research that brings together the physical / chemical properties and biological responses is quite limited. By describing the general essence of what is known about the biokinetics of lead in essentially qualitative terms, we may be able to identify patterns that permit us to predict effects of other metals or other responses to lead. It is clear that the human interface with the environment that permits entry / exposure to lead will include the gastrointestinal system, the respiratory system (including the nasal cavity), and the skin.

ABSORPTION

Mechanisms of Gastrointestinal Absorption

The mechanisms of gastrointestinal absorption of lead are only partially understood. Most of the research on mechanisms of gastrointestinal absorption of lead has been carried out in rodents, especially the rat. The more recent findings (Aungst and Fund, 1981; Henning and Cooper, 1988; Fullmer, 1997) emphasize the complexity of the process and the susceptibility of the research findings to factors such as the dose of lead, physiological state of the animals, nutritional condition, and the age of the animal.

The relative importance of the anatomic portion of the gastrointestinal tract where most absorption of lead occurs apparently depends on the animal's age, physiologic state, and dose of lead ingested. Based on data from several types of experiments, there appear to be at least two mechanisms for gastrointestinal lead absorption. One mechanism shows characteristics of energy-dependent, carrier-mediated, active transport (Aungst and Fung, 1981). This process has been reported to be saturable or not, depending at least in part on the dose of lead used in the study (Keller and Doherty, 1980a,b). The absorption mechanism has characteristics of an active transport mechanism because intestinal uptake and flux of lead are dependent on metabolic energy. At a buffer lead concentration on the mucosal side of 0.5 μM, capacity-limited process contributed approximately 200 times more to the mucosal-to-serosal lead flux than did diffusion (Aungst and Fund, 1981). At a lead concentration three orders of magnitude higher (48.3 μM), diffusion still accounted for less than 20% of the flux in Aungst and Fung's experimental work.

Others have concluded that the major control level for gastrointestinal absorption of lead probably resides in the intestinal mucosal cell and that the interrelationships between elements may affect bioavailability at both luminal and mucosal levels. It was further suggested that there are three components to the absorptive phase: uptake by the mucosal cell, transfer through the cell, and movement into the plasma (Ragan, 1983).

Lead absorption also appears to have a concentration-dependent component. In addition to the work of Aungst and Fung cited above, other work includes the in situ studies by Barton et al., (1978a,b), in which the percentage of lead absorbed was dependent on the magnitude of the dose of lead. Dose-dependent lead absorption has been reported in starved (Garber and Wei, 1974) and iron-deficient animals (Hamilton, 1978) but not in fed or iron-replete animals.

Information on the Effects of Age and Lead Absorption

Age substantially influences absorption of lead in human and nonhuman primates. For example, Willes et al. (1977) reported that infant monkeys at 10 and 150 days of age retained 64.5% and 69.8% of an oral dose of ^{210}Pb(NO$_3$)$_2$, whereas adult monkeys retained 3.2% of an oral dose. Similar differences have been observed for humans. Using classic balance study techniques, Kehoe (1962) established that the gastrointestinal absorption of lead by adult males was 5% to 10% of ingested lead. This range of absorption with usual patterns of food intake (i.e., not fasting) has been confirmed to be in the range of 5% to 15% of ingested lead based on studies with short-lived radioisotopes of lead (Hursch and Suomela, 1968) or stable isotopes of lead (Rabinowitz et al., 1975b, 1976). There are very few studies of adult female subjects. Only James et al. (1985) whose subjects (age 26 to 77 years) included females (12 women and 11 men) reported lead absorption from foods and beverages. Unfortunately, the report provided no discussion of whether or not the retention rates of radio-labeled lead differed between male and female subjects.

Uptake rates for children are much less clearly established than those for adults. Children's absorption coefficients were based essentially on two mass balance studies with small numbers of children. Alexander et al. (1974) conducted balance studies in 8 subjects ranging in age from 3 months to 8 years with lead intakes averaging 10.6 µg lead / kg bw / d (body weight / day). Absorption averaged 53% of intake and retention averaged 18% of intake. Zielger et al. (1978) investigated lead absorption by 12 infants ranging in age from 14 to 746 days whose lead intakes were greater than 5 µg / kg bw / d. These two studies are from the 1970s, when exposures to lead were many times higher than current levels. Consequently these fractional absorption estimates may not be directly applicable to current estimates of kinetics. Until additional data at lower exposures are available, it is clearly appropriate to apply much higher fractional absorption estimates to infants.

It is unclear over what age period in childhood the absorption characteristics become more like those of adults than infants. Although specific studies of the fractional absorption of lead by children older than infants are not yet available, some insight can be provided from other studies. Based on analyses of stable lead isotope profiles of a group of nine children who were immigrants from Eastern Europe living in Australia, Gulson et al. (1997) observed that the fractional absorption of ingested lead by children in the 6- to 11-year-old age range is comparable with the absorption patterns observed among adult females in the 29- to 37-year-old age range. Whether or not the 40% to 50% absorption values for ingested lead obtained using subjects who were typically less than 2 years of age apply to children in the 2- to 6-year-old age range remains a question. Lower absorption values for 2- to 6-year-old are supported by the data of Angle et al. (1995) who suggested that absorption of ingested lead among 2- to 3-year-old children was 10% to 15%.

Influence of Nutritional Status and Dietary Factors on Lead Absorption

The influence of nutritional status and dietary factors on blood lead levels and on tissue distributions of lead are much more clearly observed at low levels of environmental lead exposure that are more likely to exist in the late 1990s. Since the mid-1980s, lead exposures have declined markedly in countries that have discontinued the use of lead solder in food and beverage cans and phased out use of lead-based gasoline additives. The beneficial effects of optimal nutrition are enhanced under these lower exposure circumstances (Mahaffey, 1995; Bogden et al., 1997), although the primary approach to reducing effects of lead is to act to limit exposures.

Total Food Intake   Adults in the fasting state have been reported to absorb a substantially greater fraction of lead compared with the fraction absorbed in the nonfasting state (Blake and Mann, 1983). To date, data on comparable information on the effects of fasting state on lead absorption by children or young nonhuman primates do not appear to be available.

Calcium   Dietary calcium can influence gastrointestinal absorption of lead through both acute and long-term effects of low dietary calcium intake. Numerous studies with experimental animals fed low-calcium diets have established that calcium deficiency increased both tissue retention and toxicity of lead (Mahaffey-Six and Goyer, 1970). Long-term calcium deficiency produces a number of physiological adaptations. These include increased concentrations of various binding proteins and the stimulation of endocrine systems and regulatory systems, for example, 1,25-dihydroxycholecalciferol and parathyroid hormone. These secondary changes produced by calcium deficiency also affect the biokinetics of lead.

Overall, calcium deficiency increases lead toxicity. It is currently thought that these changes reflect physiological adaption to low intakes of calcium more than physical competition between calcium and lead for gastrointestinal absorption. However, results of studies with experimental animals show that simultaneous ingestion of lead with reduced concentrations of calcium in the incubation medium (i.e., comparable to a low-calcium meal) enhanced lead absorption. For example, Barton et al. (1978a), using ligated intestinal loop techniques to measure lead absorption, observed that when the concentration of calcium in the incubation medium varied within physiological ranges, lead absorption decreased with increasing calcium concentration. Prior conditioning by low- or high-calcium diets did not significantly alter the rat's lead absorption in vivo. Decreasing lead absorption occurred in rats and chicks (Smith et al., 1980) during studies on the role of vitamin D in lead absorption. Reduced lead uptake from ligated gut loops with addition of calcium to incubation media have been reported by Barltrop and Khoo (1975). Meredith et al. (1977) have shown that oral calcium administered immediately before lead was highly effective in decreasing lead absorption in rats. Increasing dietary calcium intake decreased lead absorption in humans (Zielger et al., 1978; Blake and Mann, 1983; Heard and Chamberlain; 1982).

The mechanisms that produce changes in lead absorption with calcium status are increasingly understood (Fullmer, 1997). In the mid-1980s Aungst and Fung (1985) reported that the apparent systemic availability of 1, 10, and 100 mg/kg oral lead doses were three- to four fold greater in calcium-deficient than in control animals. However, intestinal absorption of 10 kg/mg doses of oral lead was not affected by calcium supplements. These differences were thought to reflect the role of dietary vitamin D (cholecalciferol) and metabolically active vitamin D (1,25-dihydroxycholecalciferol) on lead and calcium absorption. Mykkanen et al. (1982) had reported that in chicks both cholecalciferol and 1,25-dihydroxy vitamin D3 affect both the ^{203}Pb and ^{47}Ca absorptive processes, but the nature of these responses were not identical, suggesting differences in the transport path or the macromolecular interactions of these metal ions during the course of absorption or both. Studies with lead conclusively demonstrated specific, high-affinity binding of lead to several calcium-biding proteins and suggesting that it may be a general property of certain intestinal calcium-binding proteins (Fullmer et al., 1982).

Additional investigation into the time course and dose-response of these interactions has been pursued by Fullmer (1997). By feeding five different levels of calcium and five of lead to chicks, Fullmer determined that lead ingestion and calcium deficiency alone or in combination generally increases serum 1,25-dihydroxy vitamin D levels over most of the range of dietary calcium and lead. In severe calcium deficiency, consumption of lead produced marked decreases in 1,25-dihydroxy vitamin D levels. Overall similarities in the responses of 1,25-dihydroxy vitamin D, intestinal calcium absorption, and calbindin-D indicate that the predominant interaction between lead and calcium is mediated through changes in circulating 1,25-dihydroxy vitamin D concentrations, rather than directly through the intestine. Kidney and bone concentrations of lead also changed in responses to these dietary manipulations providing an indication that additional effects occur not fully dependent on the concentrations of 1,25-dihydroxy vitamin D, although this appears to be the predominant control mechanism for intestinal absorption.

Iron   Iron deficiency increases tissue deposition and toxicity of lead (Mahaffey-Six and Goyer, 1972). Ragan (1983) demonstrated sixfold increases in tissue lead in rats when body iron stores were reduced but before frank iron deficiency developed. Hamilton (1978) and Flanagan et al. (1979) reported significantly increased absorption of lead from the gastrointestinal trace of iron-deficient animals. Based on results obtained by in situ ligated gut loop techniques, Barton et al. (1978b) reported that iron deficiency (secondary to bleeding and to iron-deficient diets) increased lead absorption and that iron loading decreased lead absorption

Ferritin has been shown to bind lead both in vivo and in vitro. In rats fed an iron-deficient diet, the ferritin concentration would be low, permitting increased transfer of lead to blood rather than retention in the small intestine bound to ferritin. Transferrin is increased in iron-deficiency anemia as a result of increased synthesis. Although transferrin binds iron preferentially, transferrin will also transport a number of trivalent and divalent cations such as plutonium, americanium, chromium, cobalt, manganese, and copper, among others. A protein that specifically binds lead, as well as iron, was isolated from both the rat and from human duodenal mucosa (Conrad et al., 1992).

Influence of iron status on lead absorption has also been investigated in human subjects with divergent results (Flannagan, 1979; Watson et al., 1980). To date, it is not clear whether these divergent results reflect the severity of iron deficiency, differences in analytical approaches, or some other undefined factors. Despite the lack of clarity on mechanisms, iron therapy is proving to be a valuable adjunct in treatment of low-level lead toxicity (Granado et al., 1994).

Influence of Chemical Forms of Lead on Gastrointestinal Absorption   The effect of the chemical forms of lead on gastrointestinal absorption of lead can be described in only the most general terms. Lead bound to alkyl compounds is readily absorbed and concentrates in tissues high in lipid such as the brain. The percentage absorption and tissue distribution of alkyl lead differ markedly from those of inorganic lead compounds. Among inorganic lead compounds, particle size of ingested lead plays a major role in determining the fractional absorption. Barltrop and Meek (1979) showed fivefold enhancement in lead absorption by rats when the particle size of lead was reduced from 196 to 6 µm. Healy et al. (1982) reported that lead sulfide, considered one of the least soluble lead compounds, had increased solubility in gastric fluid (apparently as a result of chemical conversion to the most soluble chloride) when the particle size was reduced from 100 to 30 μm (Healy et al., 1982).

Information about the influence of the chemical form of lead on its absorption is frequently complicated by limited information on the experimental conditions, including other factors in the diet, particle size of the inorganic lead source, physiological condition of the animal, and so on. In vitro solubility does not appear to predict the degree of in vivo absorption (Sartorelli et al., 1985). Despite this limitation the use of multiple "in vitro" methods to estimate solubility continues. Interpretation of these in vitro methods is further complicated by organ-to-organ differences in bioaccumulation of lead. To illustrate, immature swine were fed two fully characterized soil samples from a western U.S. Superfund site (Casteel et al., 1997) and the bioavailability ranged from about 50% to 90%, depending on the organ system used to express dose (e.g., blood lead level, liver, or renal lead concentrations).

In mechanistic terms, the absorption of lead is dependent on such factors as chelation, membrane permeability, solubility, and particle size (Brezinski, 1976; Husingh and Husingh, 1974). The coordination chemistry of Pb^{2+} is likely to play an important role in many of these factors. Coordination with proteins may be determining factor for the availability of lead for absorption and transfer across the mucosal cell. It is important to know in which form(s) lead is (are) available and what ligands exist in mucosal cells that may be vehicles for absorption or inhibition. Metals can precipitate or coagulate proteins in solution. Metal salts often show increased solubility in body fluids (Fairhall, 1924); for example, lead carbonate is about 300 times more soluble in serum than in water. Such metal–protein interactions will depend on such factors as the radius, charge, and coordination number of the metal, as well as on factors intrinsic to the proteins, such as size and basicity. In a protein-rich environment, the local metal ion power and complexing ability of the food should be considered.

Absorption via Inhalation   Absorption of lead from the pulmonary system depends, in a major way, on the particle size of the lead source. It is difficult to determine what fraction of lead dust in inhaled air actually gets taken up by alveolar cells or is eventually passed out through the trachea and swallowed with mucus from the trachea or nasal passages. Nevertheless, the pattern of lead in the respiratory tract is affected by the particle size of the inhaled aerosol and the ventilation rate (Chamberlain, 1983). The rate of absorption of lead from the particles deposited also depends on solubility of the chemical species of lead. In humans, absorption of lead from the lung is usually rapid and complete within 24 hours. Apparently even relatively insoluble lead compounds can be taken up directly into the general circulation in this way. Ligand-exchange ability also plays an important role here since it relates to the physiochemical properties of the available lead species and the surface properties of the particles involved.

For occupational exposures, lead dusts in inhaled air are typically of large enough particle size that they are cleared from the airways by mucociliary action. Particles larger than 3 μm in diameter deposit primarily in the nasopharyngeal and tracheobronchial regions of the respiratory tract; they can be transferred by mucociliary transport to the esophagus and swallowed (ACGIH, 1999). All species of lead compounds deposited in the deep lung region (alveoli) are thought to be completely absorbed into the blood stream (Morrow et al., 1980). Because these particles are then swallowed, factors that determine the gastrointestinal absorption of lead will also influence the bioavailability of this source of lead. Depending on the particle size and lead concentration of the source, the digestive tract can be the most important avenue of absorption of lead.

Chemical speciation of lead dusts in occupational settings has shown marked variability in the size of particles generated in primary smelters (Spear et al., 1998). Depending on the process performed (e.g., samples from ore storage, sintering, or blast and dross furnaces), the particle size, mineralogy, and extractability of lead differ substantially. Changes to the ore during processing are thought to influence their biological availability.

Dermal Absorption of Lead Skin absorption is not usually considered a significant mode of uptake of lead (Minot, 1929) unless the lead is present in its more lipid-soluble organic forms such as tetraethyl lead. Florence et al. (1988) demonstrated that inorganic lead can be absorbed through skin and rapidly distributed throughout the body. Of particular note was the finding that the distribution behavior is very different from that of ingested lead. Skin absorption gave rise to increased lead in sweat, although similar increases in blood and urine were not observed.

DISTRIBUTION

Lead is absorbed into the blood plasma, where it rapidly equilibrates with extracellular fluid. More slowly, but within minutes, lead is transferred from plasma into blood cells (Chamberlain, 1985; Simons, 1986). The typical concentration of lead in whole blood is about 10^{-6} M. Because 95% to 98% of the lead is bound in red blood cells, about 10^{-8} M is present in the plasma. If the distribution of lead between plasma and cytosol is analogous to that of calcium (10,000: 1), the cytosolic concentration of lead in exposed individuals should be in the picomolar range. In animal experiments there is no constant relationship between lead concentrations in blood and in soft tissue. There is still controversy (Kazantzis, 1988) as to whether lead in blood represents biologically active lead, and indeed, whether the two are linearly related.

Improved detection limits for analytical methods have increased the ability to determine concentrations of lead present in plasma. Concerns remain, however, that even very slight hemolysis of erythrocytes during the separation process can transfer lead into the plasma fraction. Consequently data on plasma lead concentrations must be treated with caution unless the technique can establish that what is thought to be plasma lead does not simply present in vitro transfer from erythrocytes.

From the blood plasma, the absorbed lead is distributed to different organs, and the liver and kidney attain the highest concentrations. The peripheral nervous system may accumulate considerably more lead than the central nervous system. There is furthermore marked variation in the distribution of lead within various tissues and organs (Barry, 1975; Barry, 1981; Drasch et al., 1987; Drasch, 1974, 1997; Drasch and Ott, 1988). In this context there appear to be several important corollary observations. First, lead appears to accumulate wherever high levels of calcium are found. Therefore the highest concentrations of lead are found in bone and, in particular, in dense cortical bone. Second, within and among soft tissues, the highest concentrations of lead seem to accumulate in those organs and tissues with the highest mitochondrial activity. Likewise, within an organ, the highest concentrations occur in those regions with the highest mitochondrial activity. Examples include the renal tubule and the choroid plexus and cerebellum of the central nervous system.

The skeleton contains more than 90% of the body burden of lead when measured at steady state; however, this pool is not homogeneous (Kehoe, 1961; Chamberlain, 1985; Rabinowitz et al., 1976), nor is it static (Gulson et al., 1995). This association with bone is related to the chemical's similarity to calcium and the formation of insoluble lead phosphate. As described elsewhere in this chapter, there are many bone pools of lead. Bone is a very complex organ with varying density and structure, depending on skeletal site and function. Turnover of tissue lead is high throughout life. Among young adult women between half to three-quarters of blood lead are reported to come from tissue stores (i.e., skeletal) rather than the current environment (Gulson et al., 1995, 1996). Under conditions of physiological stress for calcium (including pregnancy and lactation) release of bone lead becomes even higher (Gulson et al., 1998a,c). Of course, the initial source of the lead is environmental lead that has been accumulated in tissues over previous years. Estimates of the fraction of blood lead from bone were also provided by Smith et al. (1996), who found that the skeleton contributed 40% to 70% of lead in blood among five subjects who had trabecular bone samples obtained at surgery.

Currently there are thought to be three basic types of lead pools: rapidly exchanged lead in very metabolically active portions of bone, trabecular or spongy bone, and dense cortical bone. Lead turnover in these three basic types of pool appears to roughly parallel the relative rates of calcium turnover. A variety of observations have suggested marked variation in distribution and turnover rates within these pools, depending, at least partially, on the particular region of the skeleton studied. It is important to note further that though lead concentration is lower in trabecular bone than in cortical bone, the mass of trabecular bone is, on the average, four times that of cortical bond, and it is approximately four times as labile. Therefore trabecular bone may represent a much more metabolically important pool of lead.

The distribution of lead in tissues reflects a state of constant, dynamic equilibrium. As noted in the section on excretion, many methods of enhancing lead excretion and accompanied by its redistribution within the body (Cory-Slechta et al., 1987, 1988). Clearly, any situation that mobilizes the very large, relatively stable pools of lead within the body, particularly those in bone, will lead to the redistribution of lead to a variety of tissues. This redistribution is thought to explain the frequently noted increased symptomatology in lead-poisoned children during acute illnesses. Redistribution is known to occur during pregnancy and even under usual circumstances to lead to increased risk to the fetus, particularly in women with prior lead poisoning. There is also some evidence that the osteoporosis of aging is accompanied by significant mobilization of lead from bone pools. It is clear that a great deal of additional information is necessary to clarify fully the various physiological and pathological conditions of enhanced mobilization and redistribution of lead.

Excretion

Lead is excreted from the body mainly by urinary and fecal routes. Fecal excretion represents the sum of unabsorbed endogenous lead from saliva, bile, and to a lesser extent other gastrointestinal secretions, plus the unabsorbed portion of inhaled and ingested lead. Somewhat less excretion occurs through sweat and integumentary losses, including skin, hair, and nails. However, these routes are responsible for a small portion of total excretion. Under conditions of relatively constant exposure to low concentrations of lead, a steady-state condition evolves wherein excretion approximates intake (Rabinowitz et al., 1976). Under these conditions approximately 70% of intake is excreted in the urine. Under short-term conditions of low-level increased exposure (Chamberlain, 1985), approximately 60% is retained by the body and 40% is excreted. In one 14-day study with human volunteers receiving single dose of ^{203}Pb, approximately 18% of the dose was excreted while 35% was retained in blood, resulting in a residual of 47% in soft tissues and bone storage. Extrapolation of this result would predict an eventual excretion of approximately 30% and 70% retention of this single dose.

Urinary excretion of lead is quite complex, depending on the situation, but is most likely a function of plasma lead levels. Under most conditions of exposure to low concentrations of lead (e.g., below blood lead concentrations of about 25 µg/dL), the concentration of lead in plasma is very low (about 0.01 µg/dL) and not related to whole blood lead. Above this concentration, plasma lead increases significantly, as does the urinary lead excretion. At blood lead concentrations in the range ($<25\,\mu g/dL$), urinary clearance of lead has been estimated at about 1.1% per day. At blood lead rises above this concentration, the clearance appears to rise in a fashion reasonably related to the increase in plasma lead (Chamberlain, 1985). At very high blood lead concentrations, renal impairment may decrease urinary excretion of lead.

In considering fecal lead excretion, it is important to differentiate between fecal lead that is unabsorbed from ingestion or inhalation and fecal lead that truly represents endogenous fecal excretion of lead. Endogenous excretion was actually measured by Rabinowitz et al. (1976) using stable isotope studies and by Chamberlain (1985) following inhalation and parenteral administration studies of ^{203}Pb. Endogenous excretion is often estimated by comparing renal clearance to apparent total body clearance. All of these estimates suggest a clearance of approximately 0.5% per day at blood lead concentrations $<25\,\mu g/dL$. It appears most likely that this rate of clearance is basically independent of blood lead, so it does not increase significantly with increasing blood or plasma lead. Excretion by all other routes is at a rate of approximately 0.2% per day, and it is again essentially independent of blood lead concentrations. The total for all these routes of excretion is then about 1.8% per day at blood lead concentrations $<25\,\mu g/dL$ and somewhat greater at higher blood levels because of the increase in urine lead excreted at higher concentrations.

A special form of excretion is through breast milk. A variety of studies of maternal breast milk composition indicate breast milk lead concentrations appear to correlate with maternal blood lead concentrations.

One report of plasma lead concentrations in mice (Keller and Doherty, 1980a,b) suggests that breast milk lead concentration is more closely related to plasma lead concentration and is as much as 25 times the plasma lead concentration. This information suggests that at lower blood lead concentration in the mother, breast milk would represent a minor route of excretion and usually a minor exposure route for the infant. At higher blood lead concentrations with increasing plasma lead concentrations, it is possible that a significant amount of lead could be mobilized from the maternal skeleton in the lactating women and that breast milk could represent an important exposure pathway to the breast-feeding infant. Gulson et al. (1998c) have demonstrated with stable isotope methods this mobilization among women with blood lead concentrations less than $10\,\mu g/dL$. Breast milk lead appears to be linearly related to blood lead and has concentrations similar to plasma. For blood lead concentrations in the range of 2 to 34 μ/dL, breast milk contains $<3\%$ of the quantities of lead present in blood. Amounts of lead released from the skeleton show substantial person-to-person variation, suggesting that among women who have had substantial prior lead exposure it is important to assess this exposure source for the infant.

A variety of specific methods have been used to alter clearance of lead. Aub (1925) demonstrated that urinary excretion could be enhanced by acidification, presumably by mobilization of lead from relatively stable pools. After some initial enthusiasm for the therapeutic potential for this intervention, it was abandoned because such therapy often enhanced symptomatology, presumably by redistributing lead to soft tissues. A variety of chelating agents have also been used to enhance clearance of lead. The majority, including ethylene diamine tetraacetic acid (EDTA), dimercaptosuccinic acid, and d-penicillamine, enhance clearance by binding lead and promoting urinary clearance. Dimercaprol is another reasonably effective chelator of lead, but it predominantly enhances biliary excretion of lead.

KINETICS

Basic to the understanding of the effects of lead exposure on animals and humans is an appreciation of the kinetics of lead on living animals. This requires recognition and knowledge of the various phases of lead kinetics, including absorption, distribution, and clearance. Though lead may be present in the body in various ionic forms and compounds, as a material it may not property be considered to be "metabolized" by the body. Rather, it is transported by various more or less metabolically active complexes and compounds. Useful terms to describe this distribution are *lead kinetics* and *biokinetics*.

There have been several divergent approaches to assessing the kinetics of lead in mammals. Of interest is the observation that all of these approaches have produced similar conclusions. The most important of these conclusions is that lead kinetics requires a multicompartment model, with some compartments being very large and relatively stable while others are smaller and comparatively labile. Also it appears most likely that the kinetics of lead at lower concentrations of exposure, may be considered linear, whereas at high concentrations of exposure, they may be nonlinear in nature. This observation has some important implications in consideration of the biological effects of lead at varying levels of exposure.

Approaches used to investigate the biokinetics of lead differ in a number of aspects. Such aspects include

1. Exposure of both experimental animals and human subjects to lead orally or via inhalation, wherein increasing amounts of lead are introduced and the accumulation and excretion of lead are measured by a variety of methods.
2. Introduction of radioactive or stable isotopes of lead in order to determine kinetics without increasing exposure and disturbance of the steady-state situation.
3. Study of the spontaneous clearance of lead in situations where exposure to a high concentration of lead has been terminated.
4. Study of the distribution of lead in various tissues by postmortem examination.

The last approach has been very useful in animal studies but has been little used in studying lead distribution in humans. It is important to remember, in this context, that there is marked interspecies variation in the kinetics of lead because of many factors, including diet, physiology, and relative tissue mass. For these reasons it is clear that all studies of animals, other than humans, should be viewed with great caution when attempting to understand human kinetics. Since the greatest concern is with human exposure, we have emphasized human studies in our considerations.

The earliest studies of lead balance in humans and animals were carried out by Aub (1925). He used several of the above-described approaches in a series of studies that involved exposure of animals to lead by both inhalation and ingestion. Aub concluded from these exposure studies that lead was most readily absorbed from the respiratory tract, particularly by the inhalation of "finely divided particles." Aub noted that lead was somewhat less well absorbed by ingestion. In his animal studies Aub also measured lead concentrations in a variety of tissues after exposure to determine distribution of lead in the body. In addition Aub was able to perform autopsies on human subjects to determine the distribution of lead in the body of lead-exposed patients. He concluded that particularly after lead exposure has been terminated, all of the lead is "permanently" stored in bone. He felt that in this situation lead was harmless to the individual unless there was "recent absorption from an external source or mobilization of a skeletal store." Aub furthermore conducted extensive studies in animals and human subjects of the excretion of lead. He considered spontaneous excretion to be very low and variable, but noted that calcium-deficient diets and administration of acids markedly increased the excretion of lead, particularly if both alterations were performed at the same time.

Subsequent to Aub's studies, a landmark series of experiments were conducted by Kehoe (1961). These experiments involved long-term exposure of human volunteers to lead by inhalation and by ingestion. In all cases the subjects were also observed prior to and subsequent to exposure to lead in order to determine baseline lead balance and balance during a "recovery" stage from lead exposure. Kehoe's studies were summarized by Gross and coworkers (1975), who made several important observations that are relatively consistent with Aub's prior observations. First, there was considerable variability of observations within the subjects during the control period, which appeared to relate, at least in part, to variability in dietary lead exposure. Furthermore these variations in ingested lead (about a mean of approximately 191 µg per day) were paralleled by variations in fecal and urine lead with a net negative lead balance (in most subjects), as calculated by intake versus urine and stool output. It is not clear whether this was a demonstration of a net negative balance or simply was a result of not being able to measure airborne exposures during the control period.

An investigation carried out by Rabinowitz et al. (1976) did much to clarify our understanding of the absorption and distribution of lead in the body. The results of this study have been extensively used by subsequent kineticists, as these are among the most carefully obtained data available. Rabinowitz and colleagues studied "normal" volunteers under standard conditions of diet and activity. These volunteers were fed a low–lead diet supplemented to approximate their usual level of lead intake by addition of ^{204}Pb as a tracer. Lead isotopic distributions in samples were determined by mass spectroscopy. Since this isotope is rare in most usual sources of exposure, it provided a stable tracer for purposes of defining the kinetics of lead in the body. These adult volunteers had prestudy blood lead concentrations of 16 to 25 µg / dL and had intakes of lead between 156 and 215 µg per day during the study, which approximated their prestudy intake. One of the five subjects was studied for 10 days. The other four were studied for longer periods, ranging from 108 to 210 days. The range of absorption was 6.5% to 13.7% of ingested dose. Of this absorbed lead, 54% to 78% was excreted in the urine, with most of the rest being lost through bile and integumentary losses.

The translocation of the tracer lead was best described by a three-compartment kinetic model. The first compartment, which included 1.5 to 2.2 times the amount of lead in blood, contained an average of 1900 µg of lead and was turned over in about 36 days. The second compartment, which comprised most of the soft tissue lead, contained about 600 µg of lead and was turned over every 40 days. These authors noted, however, that the total of less than 3 µg of lead in these two labile pools is much less than the 10 to 30 µg found in autopsy studies, suggesting that most of the soft tissue lead must be in a more stable compartment. The third large and comparatively stable compartment is comprised primarily of bone lead. In these subjects it contained about 200 µg of lead and was turned over approximately every 10^4 days.

Of interest in regard to this pool was the comparison of total lead and tracer lead to total lead ratios in cortical and trabecular bone from the iliac crest. The total concentration of lead in the cortical bone by weight was approximately twice that in trabecular bone. However, the trabecular bone had a two- to threefold greater ratio of tracer to total lead, suggesting that it was turned over much more rapidly than the cortical bone. Of further interest was their calculation, based on these measurements, that the iliac bone received lead three to seven times more rapidly than did the very stable pool as a whole. These observations make it clear that bone cannot be regarded physiologically as a single pool. Furthermore the authors emphasized that all of the pools are in dynamic equilibrium with each other, and therefore alterations in the movement of lead from one to another can cause significant changes in the measured amount. Factors that might cause movement of lead from the large stable pool into blood and hence to target soft tissues are of particular interest.

Steenhout (1982) developed a kinetic model of lead distribution based on observations of lead in teeth in children and adults in three regions of Belgium. Her model is basically consistent with the Rabinowitz model. It suggests that the rate of transfer of lead to teeth is 1.85 ppm y^{-1}/µg (100 mL blood)$^{-1}$. According to the model, lead accumulation in teeth and dense (cortical) bone is linear and continuous over age, suggesting very slow loss from bone of this type [approximately zero to 0.005 ppm y^{-1}/µg (100 mL blood)$^{-1}$]. However, estimates of loss from "porotic" bones, such as ribs and vertebrae, is of the order of 0.06 ppm y^{-1}/µg (100 mL blood)$^{-1}$. She concluded that the apparent nonlinearity of lead transfer in some other studies reflected this relatively rapid loss of lead from such porotic bone. She suggested that her data support the concept that for dense bone, there is no loss of lead with increasing age, and therefore that the osteoporosis of age should not represent a risk for lead mobilization.

Chamberlain (1985) used data from a variety of different data sets, including both the data of others and some data he had developed to assess several aspects of kinetics of lead in humans. He focused primarily on volunteer feeding experiments in order to observe the response of blood lead to either airborne exposure or dietary intake. His discussion concerned largely inorganic lead and relatively short-term studies. He found that lead is absorbed rapidly into plasma and then into extracellular fluid in a matter of minutes, based on experiments with the injection of radioactive lead tracers. He noted that in a time frame measured in tens of minutes, lead in plasma, and lead from extracellular fluid via plasma, becomes largely bound to red blood cells. Approximately 58% of a dose of lead could be identified as bound to red cells after 20 hours.

Chamberlain (1985) found that excretion of lead after a single dose occurs over a month and that lead storage in tissues and bone is measured in months to years. Also he observed that the accumulation and distribution of lead differ in several ways from those of strontium. Most important, the attachment of lead to red cells appears to retard, rather than promote, the distribution to lead to storage sites. Chamberlain's autopsy studies showed that relative to "dose," there is more lead than strontium or calcium in soft tissues. All of the studies he reviewed agreed that the transfer of lead to excreta from blood occurs over a period of approximately one month. Additionally Chamberlain noted that at low-level exposures, urinary excretion is two or more times greater than stool excretion. In discussion of transfer of lead to bone, he analyzed the discrepancies and consistencies among the available data sets. Most important in the context of kinetic modeling is the observation in some data sets that the concentration of lead in trabecular bone is similar to that in cortical bone, whereas in others the concentration in trabecular bone appears much higher than in cortical bone. Some of this discrepancy may be related to the duration of the studies, since short-term (versus longer) studies may show relatively more lead in the presumably more labile trabecular pool. Chamberlain's resorption rates from storage in bone are indirectly inferred based on studies of strontium turnover with the assumption that the rates do not differ significantly for the various trace minerals. In light of his review of differences in blood, plasma, and tissue distribution of strontium and lead, this may not be an entirely valid assumption.

From these studies Chamberlain (1985) suggested a mean life of lead in trabecular bone of 12.5 years and cortical bone of 50 years. His estimate of mean life of lead in soft tissues, derived from autopsy data, is 500 days. The relationship between urinary clearance and blood lead appeared constant in the range of "normal" blood lead but appeared to increase proportionately at blood lead concentrations above 20 to 25 µg/dL. This would result in a decreasing apparent relative uptake with increasing blood lead. Chamberlain reviewed some of the data on intestinal absorption, noting that uptake of soluble lead tracers is markedly affected by a period of fasting, with an average (in several studies) of 8% uptake when lead was taken with a metal and 60% when taken after an overnight fast, if the fast is continued for several hours after the lead ingestion. He noted that the insoluble lead sulfide absorption was less affected by fasting (12% absorbed in fasting vs. 6% with meals). Chamberlain reviewed data showing that addition of calcium and phosphorus salts markedly decreases the absorption of soluble lead. Chemical incorporation of lead with foodstuffs did not alter absorption of lead below the levels observed when it was administered with a metal.

Chamberlain's (1985) discussion of airborne lead exposure centered around three major factors of exposure to inorganic lead only. He did not consider airborne exposure to organic lead. The factors considered were airborne concentration, ventilation rate/volume, and fractional distribution of the aerosols. The particle size in the inhaled aerosol and the "residence time" in the pulmonary region, determined largely by respiratory rate, are unimportant. Of note is that larger particles, deposited higher in the conductive airways, may be returned to the pharynx by mucociliary clearance and thence ingested, reducing this to the problem of ingested inorganic lead. Once retained in the lungs, the lead is essentially completely absorbed into the bloodstream within 24 hours.

A somewhat more complex model of lead distribution was suggested by Bernard (1977). His "reference man" had a total body burden of lead of approximately 120 mg. Of this total burden, approximately 110 mg was in bone and the rest in soft tissues. His model proposed at least two bone pools, a slow pool of cortical bone and a relatively labile pool in trabecular bone. Bernard further proposed two soft tissue pools, one of which is relatively large and slow and another that is quite large and very rapidly turned over. Though this model is logical and based on experimental observations, its actual validity is somewhat subject to question because it is based exclusively on studies in rats and nonhuman primates, which may differ significantly physiologically from humans.

In a more recent study Schutz (1987a) observed the decline of blood lead after the end of occupational exposure. He studied two separate and somewhat different groups. The first was comprised of workers who no longer worked in the lead industry. The second group was made up of workers removed from work because of a rise in blood lead to greater than 3 μmol/L (approximately 60 μg/dL). The first group was older, had longer periods of exposure, and generally had lower mean blood lead concentrations than the second group. In this study the subjects also had bone lead concentrations estimated by use of X-ray fluorescence of the middle phalanx of the left index finger. Schutz determined a satisfactory fit to his data by a two-compartment model. The "fast" compartment had a half-life of approximately 30 days. The "slow" compartment had a half-time of approximately 5.6 years. There was considerable interindividual variation, which he suggested represented "considerable variation in risk at a given exposure level." The "slow" pool was turned over somewhat more rapidly than other reported observations. The bond lead observations by X-ray fluorescence correlated positively with estimates of the slow pool, but the coefficient of correlation was quite low ($r = 0.36$).

Schutz hypothesized that the slow pool may be a combination of two bone pools consisting of trabecular and cortical bone lead. This hypothesis was used to explain why the measurement of bone lead differed somewhat between the two groups. He suggested that this difference may relate to differing proportions of lead in the cortical bone versus trabecular bone, the concept being that long-term exposure would result in higher relative levels in cortical bone than in trabecular bone. If this explanation is correct, it has clear implications in considering widespread application of noninvasive methods of bone lead measurement to research and clinical patient assessment.

The redistribution of pools of lead within the body has been described in a series of reports based on differences in the stable isotope profiles of body lead compartments accumulated in separate geographic locations and during different life periods. Two individuals had been investigated by Manton (1977, 1985) initially describing the process. Research to confirm these changes, as well as determine that they occurred in a number of subjects, was conducted by Gulson et al. who investigated a cohort of adult women who immigrated to Australia from Eastern Europe and Russia during the early 1990s (Gulson et al., 1995, 1997). These subjects accumulated tissue stores of lead in Europe that had a stable isotope ratio distinctly different from that present in Australia. Such differences enabled the investigators through careful, meticulous measurement of the stable isotope ratios through thermal ionization mass spectroscopy to identify the proportion of lead in blood coming from the contemporaneous environment and that mobilized from tissue lead stores accumulated earlier in Europe. Data showed that among these young adult women between 45% and 70% of lead in blood came from long-term tissue stores, presumably bone (Gulson et al., 1995). These proportions occurred at blood lead concentrations averaging under 5 µg/dL with environmental lead exposures characteristic of developed counties that had taken some steps of restrict lead exposures. The objective of the initial study had been to determine the influence of pregnancy and lactation on this mobilization. During pregnancy blood lead concentrations of these subjects increased by about 20% on average with individual changes from minus 14% to 83% (Gulson et al., 1997). Among those subjects whose blood lead increased during pregnancy, the mean increase the mobilization of long-term tissue lead stores varied between 26% and 99%, averaging about 30% (Gulson et al., 1997). Skeletal lead mobilization remained elevated after the pregnancy. Observations of the infants born to these mothers showed that the subjects long-term tissue stores of lead had been transferred to the fetus, and that among those infants who were breast fed additional transfer of lead continued to occur breast feeding (Gulson et al., 1998a,c). The transfer of maternal skeletal lead to the fetus as shown by stable isotope analyses has also been confirmed among nonhuman primates (Franklin et al., 1997).

Barry (1985) measured lead concentrations in the tissues of 129 subjects at autopsy and presented an enormous amount of data on tissue content of lead in this very large series. In accordance with other studies, he noted that the content of lead in bones was much higher than in soft tissues and that the levels of lead in dense bone were much higher than those in more cancellous bone. For example, petrous bone had the highest levels and ribs the lowest (by a ratio of approximately 4 : 1). an observation of importance in understanding the basically nonhomogeneous distribution of lead in bones. Barry noted that in those soft tissues with the higher amounts of lead, male concentrations exceeded female concentrations by about 30%. He stated that soft tissue lead concentrations increased with age only through the second decade of life and thereafter were stable. Children were reported to have soft tissue concentrations similar to adult females but had much lower bone concentrations. He stated that in adults over 90% of the lead was in bone, of which over 70% was in dense bone. Among occupationally exposed adult males, 97% of their total body lead was in bone.

Barry noted that the increasing lead in bone with age, with respect to stable soft tissue levels, is consistent with the hypothesis that lead in bone is not available to soft tissues. He further indicated that the lack of decline in the concentrations of lead in bone in the face of demineralization with increasing age suggested that lead was not mobilizable even under conditions of massive calcium turnover. However, it must be noted that Barry expressed bone lead changes with age only as concentration and not as total lead, and he ignored the fact that demineralized bone would have decreased total mass, so that a constant concentration of lead in bone may reflect a markedly decreased total amount of lead in bone.

Predicting the quantities of lead mobilized from bone requires data on bone lead concentrations for both cortical and trabecular bone. Data sets providing bone lead concentrations among adults and children described above were obtained during time periods in which environmental lead exposures were much higher than currently present in many developed countries. These lower lead exposures result in lower bone lead concentrations. For example, Drasch et al. (1974, 1987, 1997) and Drasch and Ott (1988) reported bone lead concentrations from cases coming to autopsy in Munich between the early 1970s and 1994. These comparisons are for subjects living in the same geographic vicinity in southern Germany. Between 1974 and 1994 trabecular bone lead decreased from 2.5 µg/kg (1974) to 1.7 µg/kg (1984) to 0.7 µg/kg (1994). Compact bone decreased from 5.5 µg/kg (1984) to 2.8 µg/kg (1994). These series are for adults. Changes in bone lead can be anticipated to be even more dramatic among young children, who, unlike adults, do not have the long-term stores of lead accumulated during decades of much higher lead exposures.

Multiple model systems for predicting blood "lead" have been developed over the past two decades. These include those Marcus (1985a–c) in which he used available data sets to derive multicompartment kinetic models for lead. Bert et al. (1989) have developed a compartmental model for adult males, and Leggett (1993) has published an age-specific biokinetic model for lead that was originally developed by the International Commission on Radiological Protection but was expanded to include additional features useful for consideration of lead as a chemical toxicant. Transport of lead between compartments was assumed to follow linear, first-order kinetics provided that the concentrations of lead in red blood cells remained below a nonlinear threshold level, but a nonlinear relation between plasma lead and red blood cell lead is modeled for concentrations above that level. O'Flaherty has published physiologically based models for bone-seeking elements (O'Flaherty, 1993, 1995, 1998). This groups of models utilize information about age dependence of bone formation rate and took into account increasing localization of bone modeling activity with age.

Such models have had varied success in predicting blood lead concentrations. Typically these models are more successful in predicting mean/median blood lead concentrations than in predicting the distribution of blood lead levels. Dose-dependent differences in fractional absorption and distribution of lead complicate application of these models. Person-to-person variability (intensity of hand-to-mouth activity, nutritional status, etc.) also modify the relationship between external (or environmental) and internal (blood or tissue) doses of lead. Among those models that recognize the importance of bone lead contribution to blood lead, the very limited data on contemporary bone lead concentrations is a data gap that remains to be filled.

Workshops have been held attempting to reconcile the differences between modeled distributions of blood lead data and observations from epidemiological studies. The availability of pooled analyses of epidemiological data from childhood lead studies in the United States has identified the loading lead-contaminated dust within the residence as a very strong predictor of blood lead among children (Lanphear et al., 1998). Further the child's age, race, mouthing behaviors, and study-/site-specific factors are influential in predicting blood lead at a given level of lead exposure (Lanphear et al., 1998).

Analysis of all of the available information on the kinetics of lead reveals significant problems in using the presently available models to study lead in the living mammalian subject. It is obvious that all of the models fit observed data sets for lead absorption, distribution, and excretion rather well and often describe observed changes in blood lead quite well. However, current models are inadequate for the purposes of anatomic and physiological description and prediction. This very much limits their usefulness in devising experimental models and in developing clinically useful approaches to diagnosing and managing lead poisoning. For example, the assertion that bone lead is a single homogeneous pool, or two relatively homogeneous pools comprised of cortical and trabecular bone, does not fit the available data. The Rabinowitz models and others derived from his data suggest that the most stable pool, which has been felt to be largely bone, had a mean life of 30 to 50 years (Chamberlain, 1985; Simons, 1988; Kazantzis, 1988; Kehoe, 1961; Rabinowitz et al., 1976; Cory-Slechta et al., 1987). However, when studied directly by bone biopsy (Rabinowitz et al., 1976), the same subjects had trabecular and cortical bone turnover much more rapid than predicted by their models.

The clear conclusion, if both the kinetic model and the biopsy result are accepted as correct, is either that the iliac bone is not part of the stable pool or that there must be exceptionally stable portions of the bone pool that outweigh the relative lability of iliac bone. In either case it is clear that bone is not a single homogeneous pool, nor is either major type of bone, cortical and trabecular, likely to represent a homogeneous pool of lead. This conclusion has obvious implications in assessing both invasive and noninvasive methods of sampling of bone to determine its lead content.

HEALTH EFFECTS

Lead has multiple serious health effects. Its effects at high concentrations include hematological, renal, and neurological impairment. Lead has been shown to result in neurodevelopmental delays with intrauterine lead exposure only sightly above population means. In addition lead appears to cause significant neurophysiological impairment at very low levels. The recognition of what appears to be essentially a no-threshold adverse response to lead emphasize a need for better understanding of the biological mechanisms for these low-level effects. Unfortunately, these mechanisms remain only partially understood at the present time. The various lines of investigation have not yet given a fully acceptable unitary hypothesis for the responses to lead.

The early investigations into lead toxicity focused on the mechanisms for the relatively gross effects of lead noticed at very high levels of exposure. For instance, the study of kidney pathology in lead-exposed animals and humans has demonstrated deposition of lead in the cells of the proximal tubule, particularly in nuclear material (Goyer and Rhyne, 1973). Such studies have also documented mitochondrial degeneration. Although these studies are consistent with the observed proximal tubular dysfunction seen in lead toxicity, they clearly do not fully clarify the mechanism of this toxicity. Likewise studies of the heme biosynthetic pathway, though interesting, reveal certain inconsistencies that remain to be explained (Scott, 1971). Lead certainly inhibits several enzymes in this pathway, particularly porphobilinogen synthetase and heme synthetase. Of these two, heme synthetase is of particular interest, since it is a mitochondrial bound enzyme, suggesting the possibility that lead inhibits this enzyme simply by altering mitochondrial function rather than by specifically altering the enzyme.

The mechanisms for nervous system toxicity remain unclear. There are a number of important insights but not a clear unitary hypothesis. The importance of lead effects on calcium-dependent systems appear to come as close to an overarching explanation as is currently available. Ultimately all lead toxicity may be related to calcium transport or other mechanisms of alteration of functioning of calcium-dependent systems. As noted elsewhere in this chapter, lead accumulates in the nervous system preferentially in areas that are very metabolically active and rich in mitochondria. Furthermore lead has been shown in vitro to be a potent inhibitor of mitochondrial function, possibly by competing with mitochondrial uptake of calcium. Multiple reviews are available on the mechanisms for effects of lead on neural tissue (e.g., see Bressler and Goldstein, 1991; Goldstein, 1993; Winneke et al., 1996; Finkelstein et al., 1998). The relationship between changes in the dopaminergic systems and behavioral changes has been described (Cory-Slechta, 1997). The sensitivity of such changes to lead varies with lead dose, brain region, and developmental state of the subject (Widzowski et al., 1994).

Although the mechanisms through which lead produces adverse effects on neural tissues remain to be fully clarified, there has been an increased understanding, over the past decade, of the adverse effects of levels of lead exposure that had once been considered to be harmless. With additional research on lead, a signature of lead-impaired functions among children has been recognized from investigations in multiple cultures. Four major prospective, longitudinal epidemiology studies have described impaired intellectual functioning in childhood following increases in blood lead over the range of approximately 10 to about 30 μg/dL whole blood, even after control for social and demographic conditions associated with both exposures to lead and with lowered development scores (Bellinger et al., 1986; Dietrich et al., 1993a,b; Baghurst et al., 1992; Wasserman et al., 1997). These studies showed an approximately four- to six-point decrease in subsequent IQ (when measured at about age six or seven years, but not earlier). The signature of changes described by Wasserman et al. (1997) is that perceptual-motor skills are more sensitive to lead exposure than are the language-related aspects of intelligence. Lead is thought to affect visual-motor integration at this range of exposures. (Baghurst et al., 1985; Dietrich et al., 1993b). Despite demonstration of these effects across geographic area, social class, and cultures, it is important to note that these effects were not seen in all studies.

Long-term educational, social, and behavioral consequences of these test-predicted changes have also been identified. Bellinger et al. (1992) reported a higher rate of retention in grade and other general parameters of learning difficulties among the higher blood lead children. Following the same cohort through ages 7 to 11 years, Needleman et al. (1996) identified that lead exposure was associated with an increased risk for antisocial behavior and delinquent behavior at 11 years of age. Similar research is currently underway with the Cincinnati cohort. Long-term effects of increasing blood lead over the range 10 to 30 μg/αL was reported to adversely affect emotional and behavioral development (Burns et al., 1999) when the Port Pirie cohort studies were evaluated at ages 11 to 13 years. Increasing blood level over the range 10 to 20 μg/αl was associated with a three-point decline in mean IQ (Tong et al., 1996) at these ages.

Expanded understanding of the effects of lead on the nervous system of adults is now available. The acute damage of either very high levels of inorganic lead exposure and the neurological consequences of exposure to organic leads have been recognized for decades. Within the past 10 years additional understanding of the adverse effects of levels of lead exposure that were previously not recognized as harmful to the adult has been elucidated. Investigation of the neuropsychological effects of lead among workers whose blood lead concentrations had never been above 2.4 μmols/L (or 50 μg/dL) showed decrements associated with lead in visual-spatial and visual-motor functions, attention, and verbal comprehension (Hanninen et al., 1998). Subjects also showed increased symptoms of impaired well-being as rated by psychological scales and assessments of mood. Blood lead increases in the range of >2.4 μmols/L (50 μg/dL) to approximately 4.9 μmols/L (100 μg/dL) caused long-lasting or possibly permanent impairment of central nervous system function (Hanninen et al., 1998).

Other Effects

The focus of this discussion is on effects of lead occurring at comparatively low exposures. Adverse effects on the renal and reproductive organ systems have been described in almost all earlier reviews of high exposure effects of lead. Acute effects of exposure to high concentrations of lead result in proximal tubule damage manifested by glycosuria and aminoacid uria. Overt nephropathy appears to develop when blood lead levels exceed a threshold of 60 μg/dL (about 2.9 μmol/L) (reviewed by Loghman-Adham, 1997). Early renal tubule dysfunction secondary to far lower levels of lead exposure can now be detected by measurement of urinary excretion of low molecular weight proteins (α_1 and β_2 microglobulins, retinol binding protein) or the lysosomal enzyme NAG, as well as by a number of other brush border proteins (Loghman-Adham, 1997). Changes in urinary or serum markers of function or integrity of specific nephron segments were compared in a cross-sectional study of children (Fels et al., 1998). Children with a mean blood lead concentration of approximately 13 μg/dL had increased excretion rates of prostaglandins and thromboxane B2, epidermal growth factor, β_2-microglobulin, and Clara cell protein compared with children whose mean blood lead averaged less than 4 µg / dL. This pattern of glomerular, proximal, and distal tubular, and interstitial markers was similar to that perviously found among adults; however, they occurred at lower blood lead concentrations than among adults (Fels et al., 1998). The clinical significance of these changes in excretion of low molecular weight proteins and / or lysosomal enzymes is not fully determined.

Investigation of the reproductive effects of lead have most recently focused on male reproductive toxicity (reviewed by Apostoli et al., 1998). Based on review of 32 experimental studies in animals and 22 epidemiological studies and one case report in humans. Apostoli et al. (1998) concluded that when blood lead concentrations exceed 40 µg / dL, there appear to be an associated decrease in sperm count, volume, motility, and morphological alternations with a possible effect on endocrine profile. Dose–response relationships, particularly threshold for effects, remain poorly understood.

Although these effects are documented at high levels as seen in occupational exposures, an additional change in recent years is better documentation of the carcinogenicity of lead to humans. Lead and lead compounds have long been recognized as carcinogenic to animals (IARC, 1987). Data on the carcinogenicity of lead have been reviewed (Vainio, 1997) following publication of two cohort studies among smelter workers (Lundstrom et al., 1997 and by Cocco et al., 1997). Lundstrom et al. found among a cohort of 3979 long-term lead smelter workers at a primary smelter that the lung cancer incidence of the total cohort (standard incidence ratio, SIR: 2.8; 95% confidence interval, CI: 2.1–3.8) and the group with the highest exposure (SIR 3.1, 95% CI: 2.0–4.6) was high. The risk estimate for lung cancer was further evaluated in a subcohort of lead-only workers (SIR 5.1, 95% CI: 2.0–10.5 in the most highly exposed group with a latency period of 15 years). No excesses were observed for other malignancies. In a mortality study of 1388 workers and laborers is production and maintenance departments from an Italian lead-smelting plant described by Cocco et al. (1997), no excess risk of stomach cancer and lung cancer was found, although an increased risk of kidney cancer had previously been reported (Cocco et al., 1996). Vainio (1997) indicated that long-term, high exposure to lead compounds is associated with an increased risk of lung cancer, further concluding that the "weight of evidence is beginning to be convincing enough concerning kidney and even lung cancer" for humans.

BIOMARKERS

An evaluation of potential biomarkers of lead exposure requires the consideration of a variety of specific issues. In common with all toxic exposures is the basic dose–response problem. In any such system, if dose–response characteristics are typical, well defined, and predictable, it makes little difference whether we attempt to measure the dose or prefer to look at a response variable. In the case of a toxicant such as lead, which has many diverse effects, it is usually necessary to define the response variable or variables most important to the investigator.

In the case of mammalian and particularly human studies, it is often useful in such considerations to define the "critical" organ, tissue, or system. This definition presupposes that it is possible to define the most sensitive or most important effect of the toxic agent. In the case of lead toxicity, particularly childhood lead toxicity, the "critical" organ or organ system is most commonly identified as the nervous system. To the extent that the nervous system is accepted as the critical system, measures of lead exposure should ideally define the extent of nervous system exposure. Response variables should be based on nervous system toxicity or should at least correlate strongly with nervous system toxicity. An important correlate of variation in response to a toxic agent such as lead is that it is often more difficult to select a response in an individual than it is for groups of individuals. For this reason measures of dose and response that may be quite useful in epidemiological studies may add little to categorization of diagnosis of the individual subject. An in-depth analysis of analytical methods and considerations in selection of biomarkers, and interpretation of data for sensitive populations (e.g., maternal/fetal pairs, women of childbearing age, infants and young children) was published by the National Research Council's Committee on Measuring Lead in Critical Population (1993).

Lead exposure occurs via multiple routes, at variable doses, with variable absorption depending on route of absorption and other factors described elsewhere in this chapter. Therefore it is very difficult generally to directly specify the "dose" of lead to which a subject is exposed. The exception to this has been studies with stable or radioactive lead tracers, wherein the absorbed dose can be quite carefully calculated by isotope dilution methods (Rabinowitz et al., 1976) or through careful measurement of diverse environmental sources (e.g., see Gulson et al., 1996). With the exception of such tracer methods, measurement of dosage has been generally limited to measurement of lead in relatively easily obtained biological samples. All such methods present difficulties in analytical technique and sample contamination because of the very small amounts of lead typically found in the samples. Although sporadic efforts have been made to use samples such as saliva, hair, and nails to assess exposure or dose, all have been unsatisfactory for general use for one reason or another, and have at best limited applicability.

Urine lead reflects lead in blood in that the stable lead isotope profiles are highly correlated, but concentrations of lead between these two biological fluids are only weakly correlated (Gulson et al., 1998b). Concentrations of lead in urine cannot serve to predict blood lead concentrations, particularly at exposures associated with blood lead values $< 10 \, \mu g/dL$. Measurements of lead in urine may have significant problems for a variety of reasons. First, as noted elsewhere in this chapter, urine lead has a complex relationship to lead dose. Variability in concentration of urine relates to fluid intake. Some, but not all investigators, find the variability of urinary lead excretion during the day to be problematic when expressing lead dose (Gulson et al., 1998b). Variations in concentration of urine, related to fluid intake, and marked variability or urine lead excretion throughout the day, mandate quantitative urine collections, which can be quite difficult in children and experimental animals. A second problem is contamination of the sample with feces or other body products.

A modification of urine lead measurement, often used diagnostically but rather infrequently in research studies, is the measurement of the amount of lead after administration of a chelating agent. Such measurements presumably sample a larger pool of lead than unstimulated urinary lead excretion and have been held to define the "chelatable" pool of lead that should be available for further therapeutic chelation therapy. However, it is clear that the "chelatable" pool varies with the agent used. It is not clear, in any real sense, what the "chelatable" pool represents biologically, or how it can be directly related to response measurements.

Measurement of lead in blood has been widely used, but this has also been widely criticized on both practical and theoretical grounds. Difficulties with contamination and technical aspects of measurement have largely been solved as problems when analyses are carried out by a competent laboratory. In the late 1990s many laboratories can accurately and detect blood lead measurements less than $1 \, \mu g/dL$. In addition lead in blood represents only a small fraction of the body lead burden. However, as it is now recognized, there is extensive turnover of lead in the body, and blood lead can be considered to represent both current and long-term lead exposure (Gulson et al., 1995, 1997, 1998a–c; Smith et al., 1996). It has been hypothesized that lead in plasma is a better measure of lead available for excretion or transport to tissues, particularly neural tissues, and therefore may be the preferable measure of toxic dose of lead. Yet it has been extraordinarily difficult to measure lead in plasma free of contamination, particularly because of the destruction of red cells in preparation of plasma samples. Since more than 95% of lead in blood is in the red cells (de Silva, 1981), even a small measure of contamination from red cells can markedly alter the results of plasma lead measurements.

It is obvious that it is not usually possible to directly sample body tissues other than blood routinely. Furthermore such sampling has seen very limited use. Since lead in the dentine of teeth represents a very stable pool of lead, measurements of lead in the dentine of deciduous teeth has been used for some research on the effects of early lead exposure in children (Needleman et al., 1979). Measurement of bone lead has progressed a great deal in the past decade. Previously occasional bone biopsies had been used to assess the quantity of lead in the more stable and larger pools of lead in the body (Rabinowitz et al., 1976; Aufderheide and Wittmers, 1992). Most direct measures of lead in internal organs and tissues have been done on autopsy subjects (e.g., Barry, 1975, 1981; Drasch et al., 1974, 1987, 1997; Drasch and Ott, 1998).

An area of recent enthusiasm is the noninvasive measurement of lead in tissues, particularly in bone. The human skeleton contains the great majority of body lead burden. The inactivity of the skeletal lead deposits was thought to reflect a very long half-time of lead in bone. The assumption had been that bone was homogeneous as a lead compartment and that the very long half-time would greatly delay transfer of lead from bone back to other tissues. Based on data from stable isotope studies, this is no longer a defensible concept. Current evidence argues that bone is both a set of compartments for lead depositions and a target of lead toxicity itself. Human bone appears to have at least two kinetic compartments for lead. Trabecular (spongy) bone lead is more mobile than lead stored in long, dense, or cortical bone (Skerfving, 1988). Chelatable lead is well correlated with trabecular and less well with cortical bone (Schutz et al., 1987a,b). In adults long-term tissue stores (presumably largely bone) contributed between half and three-fourths of the lead present in blood (Gulson et al., 1995, 1997; Smith et al., 1996). Young children because of constant skeletal turnover secondary to the physiological remodeling process that accompanies somatic growth will recycle lead between bone and other tissue compartments. Rosen et al. (1989) have reported that cortical bone (e.g., tibia) correlated with and was predictive of chelatable lead.

Over the past two decades X-ray fluorescence (XRF) methods have been developed to measure lead in bone noninvasively (Committee on Measuring Lead in Critical Populations, NRC, 1993). Two general groups of XRF techniques exist that sample either the fluorescence emitted by k-shell or by l-shell electrons following radiation from an X-ray machine or other radiation source. Analysis of dosimetry, volume sampled, and precision for these instruments was provided in the National Research Council's report "Measuring Lead Exposure in Infants, Children, and Other Sensitive Populations" (1993). These techniques are now being utilized in a number of epidemiological studies (e.g., see Hu, 1998). These methods have been most successfully applied to groups with high-lead exposures such as groups living in high-lead exposure environments, those occupationally exposed, or lead-poisoned children. A concern is that the quantitation limits and precision of these instruments may be too high for use in a general population (Rosen and Pound, 1998). The rate of improvement in the quantitation limits and precision of these instruments appear to be slower than the decline in bone burden of lead present in many countries.

There is a very wide range of methods that have been employed, with varying success, to define the effects of lead. These range from in vitro biochemical testing to observations and measurement of behavioral attributes of exposed subjects. The vast majority of biochemical measures of lead toxicity in epidemiological studies has been based on the observation that lead inhibits heme synthesis and has been facilitated by readily available blood to study the effects of impaired heme synthesis. In particular, emphasis has been placed on the inhibition of two enzymes in the heme biosynthetic pathway, porphobilinogen synthetase, and heme synthetase (Sassa et al., 1973; Piomelli, 1973). Porphobilinogen synthetase has been measured by activity levels and has been characterized by electrophoresis as to its phenotypic variability (Doss et al., 1982). Heme synthetase, as a mitochondrial bound and dependent enzyme, has been studied primarily be observation of the accumulation of its porphyrin precursors, particularly photo-porphyrin IX. Accumulation of zinc protoporphyrin is strongly and logarithmically correlated with blood lead concentrations in both children (e.g., Piomelli et al., 1973, 1982; Roels et al., 1976) and adults (e.g., Grandjean and Linthrup, 1978; Lilis et al., 1978). Among children the threshold for response is thought to be associated with a blood lead concentration in the range of 15 to 20 µg/dL whole blood (Piomelli et al., 1982; Hammond et al., 1985). Analysis of free erythrocyte protoporphyrin had previously been used in screening children to identify lead poisoning. Because accumulation of protoporphyrin also occurs in iron deficiency, increased FEP is not a change specific to lead. Iron deficiency is sufficiently common among lead-exposed populations that measurement of erythrocyte protoporphyrin distinguishes poorly between iron deficiency and lead excess (Mahaffey and Annest, 1986). This problem, as well as the threshold for change being higher than in the blood lead of concern based on neurobehavioral changes, has resulted in curtailing use of erythrocyte protoporphyrins as a method to screen for lead.

An additional area of biochemical investigation, the examination of levels of neurochemical mediators in blood and urine, has been of interest but as often produced conflicting results in the hands of different investigators. It appears clear, however, in consideration of all areas of biochemical investigation, that these markers have not to date produced reliable and valid measures of response to lead exposure, at least in reference to the neurological effects of lead.

At a more integrated and neurologically relevant levels of response, considerable progress has been made in the area of electrophysiological measures of response. It is clear that peripheral nerve conduction (Seppalainen et al., 1979), as well as visual (Araki et al., 1987) and auditory (Schwartz and Otto, 1987) brainstem responses, are altered at very low levels of lead exposure, again perhaps, at levels below those defined by present biochemical markers of response based on changes in the heme biosynthetic pathway. Epidemiological studies in this area have been quite productive. For example, significant lead-related changes for some visual-evoked potential interpeak latencies were observed (Altmann et al., 1998) in an environmentally exposed population of 6-year-old children having a mean blood lead of 4.2 µg/dL with an 95th percentile value of 8.9 µg/dL (Walkowiak et al., 1998). However, it remains uncertain to what degree such methods will prove useful in defining the degree of toxicity suffered by the individual for purposes of classification and diagnosis. As in many other response variables, it is not clear to what degree they reflect an inadequate ability to define relevant dosage information. Until such understanding improves, their general applicability will be limited.

At still another level of investigation, epidemiological studies based on the effects of high-level integrated functions, including intelligence measures, behavior, and motor functions, have been extraordinarily fruitful. Such studies have done much to substantiate that lead has adverse effects at very low levels of exposure, particularly to the fetus and infant (Needleman et al., 1979; Bellinger et al., 1986, 1987; Baghurst et al., 1992; Dietrich et al., 1990, 1993a; Wasserman et al., 1997). It is now recognized that lead has a signature of changes in that the perceptual-motor skills are more sensitive to lead exposure than are the language-related aspects of intelligence (Wasserman et al., 1997). Lead is thought to affect visual-motor integration at exposure producing blood lead concentrations in the range of 10 to 30 µg/dL (Baghurst et al., 1995; Dietrich et al., 1993b). These studies have confirmed the importance of viewing of nervous system as the critical system in lead exposure and have shown quite clearly the inadequacy of previously available biochemical methods in defining the response to lead at low levels. These studies have thus shown clearly that an improved understanding of the chemical basis for lead toxicity is an absolute necessity for further progress. They have also been important in showing that a large proportion of our population has suffered from lead toxicity. It is also clear, however, that whatever the benefits of such measures are, there is little prospect that they will prove generally useful in the evaluation of individual cases of lead exposure at these levels. It is therefore critical to make further progress in improving other response and dosage methods to aid in providing assistance to the individual while we are attempting to improve the health of the environment and our total population.

SOME CHEMICAL / MOLECULAR CONSIDERATIONS IN LEAD NEUROTOXICITY

Lead compounds may have a variety of targets within the nervous system (Bondy, 1988). Before discussing what some of these targets might be, it is first useful to classify broadly the types of lead compounds that are of environmental concern. As previously pointed out, the inorganic lead compounds are generally of greater environmental concern. A brief discussion of properties of organolead compounds may be helpful in furthering our knowledge about biochemical mechanisms of neurotoxicity for all classes of lead compounds. Consideration of the chemistry of organolead compounds suggests that they differ fundamentally in both chemical and biological properties from ionic compounds of the same metal (Grandjean and Grandjean, 1984). For example, it is well documented that the toxicity of tetraethyl lead results from the breakdown of the compound in the organism to a salt of triethyl lead. The triorganolead compounds form a very distinctive neurotoxic class. Their actions are probably brought about by two rather distinctive chemical properties: one depends on the lipophilic (rather amphoteric) nature of their chlorides and hydroxides and their affinity constants which allow dissociation at the biological concentrations of hydroxyl and chloride ions; the other derives from the potentiality for five-coordinate binding. Therefore it is not surprising that the behavioral toxicity effects of alkyl leads do not closely resemble those of inorganic lead. Some similarities do exist that may be associated with degradation of the alkyl lead to the stage of divalent lead in the organism. Even a small amount of metabolism of this type could become significant because of the much altered tissue distribution of lead as a result of the lipophilic properties of organolead compounds. This suggests that more attention should be paid to the possible complexes of inorganic lead with hydrophobic ligands such as hemic acid. The general lack of involvement/importance of the divalent lead ion in organolead compound toxicity is also supported by the observation that the usual chelators have little effect on intoxication from organolead compounds.

The study of chemical mechanisms of inorganic lead compound toxicity is complicated by a number of factors. As described elsewhere in this chapter, the amount of lead absorbed after its oral administration can vary significantly depending on animal species, age, and diet and on both the chemical and physical form of the inorganic lead compound ingested. For example, in the absence of food in the gut (as during fasting), the lead compound can apparently be more readily acidified and solubilized for tissue uptake. Because of the rather ubiquitous occurrence of lead in the environment and its relatively high toxicity, one must also be concerned about lead contamination of the diet, and even of laboratory reagents (Simons, 1989) used in studies in vitro. Separation of the influence of nutritional status on biokinetics of lead from specific neurotoxic events is another problem that needs more attention.

There are many ostensibly different toxic effects of lead described in the literature. It seems likely that there are only a few triggering events in biological systems that would account for the rather potent neurotoxic effects of lead. There in turn could result in a range of secondary effects. It follows also that the important initiating events will depend in some way on rather distinctive chemical properties of divalent lead, since all other divalent metals produce a toxic syndrome that is qualitatively and/or quantitatively different from that of lead. Considerations of lead chemistry should also permit one to rule out certain possible initiating biochemical pathways. For example, the relatively low affinity of lead for sulfur suggests that interaction with specific sulfur-containing proteins such as metallothionein would not be critical. Carboxyl-oxygen-containing amino acids are more likely points of interactions with proteins, and this possibility is supported by the findings of lead-containing nuclear inclusion bodies in tissues that are rich in acidic amino acids (Choie and Richter, 1972). Since divalent lead is a reasonably stable oxidation state, it seems likely that the divalent lead ion in some way mediates the range of effects seen and that metabolic redox pathways involving tetravalent lead are not important.

The toxic effects of divalent lead may be the result of either physical or chemical change in the biochemical systems with which it interacts. Lead may damage membranes by bringing about change in the ultrastructure of cellular components or by initiating oxidative damage. Membrane damage does appear to be a significant factor in lead toxicity, and myelin-containing membranes seem to be especially sensitive. Membrane damage by peroxidative processes may involve change in calcium homeostasis. Effects of lead on energy production could be related to direct interaction with mitochondrial membranes, altering ion transport, or changes in calcium homeostasis within the cell. A variety of studies have shown that lead accumulates in mitochondria, and this is associated with inhibition of oxidative phosphorylation. Endothelial cells in brain capillaries contain three to five times more mitochondria than do endothelial cells in the vessels of other organs (Oldendorf and Brown, 1975). This difference may reflect the high rate of metabolic activity necessary to maintain the active transport of ions across the blood-brain barrier and may explain the susceptibility of these cells to a wide variety of toxic compounds that cause brain edema. Mitochondria may be a critical subcellular target for the toxic effects of lead.

Inorganic lead has also been shown to compete with some essential divalent metals at several different levels (Chisolm, 1980). These include, in particular, calcium, zinc, copper, and iron. These interactions can occur at several levels, including absorption from the gut, transport across the blood-brain barrier, and at the synapse. For example, active calcium uptake by mitochondria is a critical process required to maintain calcium at very low concentration in the cytosol of cells. Inhibition of the accumulation of calcium by mitochondria may involve a direct blockage of the calcium pumps, but this could also result from depletion of ATP or key intermediates involved in its synthesis, such as inorganic phosphate. No single metal deficiency shows symptoms identical to those seen in lead exposure. The chemistry of lead suggests that a variety of metals are likely to show altered distribution in biological systems in the presence of lead, with some associated biochemical changes. Dietary supplements of various minerals and vitamins do not completely protect against the toxic effects of lead, suggesting also that there are more critical biochemical changes associated with the potent neurotoxic effects of lead.

Other biochemical interactions that may be important in explaining the toxic responses of lead include the possible inhibitory effects of lead on the cholinergic system and activation of catecholaminergic function. This may be related to the calcium agonist property of lead. Lead may be equipotent with calcium in binding to calmodulin. Lead may also be involved in direct reactions carried out by mixed-function oxidases. Complex secondary interactions between organ systems are also a possible factor determining the overall pattern of toxicity. A possible interrelated sequence of events by which lead compounds could cause neurotoxicity, as expressed by behavioral change, has previously been suggested (Bondy, 1988).

What aspects of the chemistry of lead may throw light on the important biochemical / molecular mechanisms of toxicity? The importance of the ligand-exchange chemistry of divalent lead in the overall expression of toxicity has already been pointed out. The relative binding strengths of the various endogenous ligands for lead will determine the fate and distribution of lead in vivo and its competition with other metals such as calcium. Once lead is inside the cells, its eventual fate will be to bind to sites that are stronger than cytosolic pool chelators such as citrate. At slightly acidic pH, at which divalent lead ionic species are likely to be present, phosphate ligands are prime candidates because of the very large association binding constants involved here. The extreme tenacity for phosphate may be the most distinctive feature of lead chemistry relative to other divalent metal ions of the same basic types. Several types of phosphate ligands must be considered, including inorganic orthophosphates, ATP, and the phosphate groups of membrane lipophosphates and phosphorylated proteins. This primary mechanism underlying lead toxicity is compatible with the major reproducible biochemical findings described above, particularly the suggestion that mitochondria (where oxidative phosphorylation takes place) may be a target site in cells. It is of course also compatible with the ultimate localization of the lead in bone as insoluble phosphate salts.

Lead may function as a phosphate scavenger and siphon off minority phosphate species crucial to developing / proliferating cells, especial in neural tissues. If one of the functions of calcium is to store phosphate in the form of calcium phosphate, then lead would be an efficient antagonist for this process. In fact it is, in general, not clear if the effects of lead on calcium homeostasis are the result of direct competition between lead and calcium for binding sites and / or of their differential affinity for phosphate ligands, particularly inorganic phosphate. For example, the report of Markovac and Goldstein (1988) indicating that lead is a potent activator of protein kinase C could be interpreted as a direct effect of lead on protein–phosphorylating–dephosphorylating sequences which do not involve the enzyme at all (a control experiment in the absence of enzyme was apparently not run). Phosphorylating–dephosphorylating sequences are of critical importance to energy transformation in cells and tissues, and this is particularly true of those in the nervous system during rapid growth and maturation.

The possible direct phosphate-deleting effects of lead resemble, in many ways, those seen in poisoning by nitrophenols (Clayton and Clayton, 1981) known to uncouple oxidative phosphorylation (which presumably also reduces the body's reservoirs of high-energy phosphate compounds). Such uncoupling apparently stimulates oxidative metabolism and, in turn, the heat production of the body. Oxygen consumption, body temperature, respiration, and heart rate are all increased. Some similar effects are also associated with the hyperthyroid state (Dratman, 1978). With regard to mechanisms of lead neurotoxicity, it is interesting to note that there is some evidence that hyperthyroidism is associated with reduced catecholamine production rates in both peripheral nerve tissue and the brain. In studies in the rat, McIntosh et al. (1989) reported that the effects of lead on catecholaminergic and cholinergic transmission are regionally specific within the brain, the midbrain, and the diencephalon, showing the greatest degree of change in concentrations of neurotransmitters (dopamine concentrations usually decreased) and activities of rate-limiting enzymes.

Although lead neurotoxicity, poisoning by nitrophenols, and hyperthyroidism involve different triggering mechanisms, these responses may have in common certain secondary effects related to the maintenance of cellular homeostasis and metabolism. The remarkable affinity of lead for phosphate may be the most sensitive primary event to explain the fact that the neurotoxic effects of lead are evident at low concentrations of lead exposure and after only a brief exposure period. This suggests that thyroid status and metabolic state might be important factors to consider in examining correlations between measures of lead exposure and neurotoxicity in human epidemiology studies. There is also the possibility that increased blood lead concentrations could be causally related to increased oxidative metabolism. It should be possible to test this hypothesis at the biochemical levels, perhaps in some cases using the tools now available in molecular biology.

TREATMENT OF LEAD TOXICITY

Metal chelation therapy has been used with some success to treat lead poisoning (Bondy, 1988). Chelators used for this purpose can also remove essential elements, resulting in kidney damage, and most of these drugs tend to have unpleasant side effects. They are also generally useful for acute rather than sustained therapy, and the benefits are usually only transitory, since blood lead can be rapidly replaced from the bone store. In view of the nature of lead chemistry and the possibility that lead is basically functioning as a phosphate scavenger, it is unlikely that a complexing/chelating agent of the usual variety could be found that would be able to compete effectively with phosphate in a ligand-exchange reaction. It may be possible to develop a derivative of phosphate that is sufficiently reactive and excretable to be useful in therapy. On the other hand, soluble forms of phosphate itself might offer some protection against toxic effects, perhaps until lead is deposited in bone. This approach of course does not reduce the body burden of lead, but it may buy time during the process of deposition of lead in bone which at least offers transient sequestering of lead.

The prospects for successful chemical treatment of long-term, low-dose lead toxicity are not promising. Use of chelating agents has been useful for short-term, high-dose exposures. For children use of chelation therapy is recommended (CDC, 1991) only when blood lead levels exceed $45 \mu g / dL$ ($> 2.17 \mu mol / L$). It remains unclear whether or not chelation has sustained benefits for children whose blood lead concentrations are between 25 and $44 \mu g / dL$. Criteria such as the persistence of elevated blood lead levels despite environmental intervention have also been offered as justifications for chelation (American Academy of Pediatrics, 1995). Determining which children may respond to chelation therapy is complex. Markowitz et al. (1997) demonstrated that children with changes in erythrocyte protoporphyrin and hematological index are more likely to respond to chelators with markedly enhanced urinary excretion of lead. Concern has also been raised suggesting that at least some chelators (i.e., succimer) are more effective in removing lead from blood than lead from brain (Pappas et al., 1995; Cory-Slechta, 1988). Smith et al. (1998) cautioned on basing judgements on changes in blood lead concentration on prediction of the impact of chelators on brain lead concentrations. The ratios of change in brain lead and change in blood lead differed over the duration of chelation therapy in rodents.

The usefulness of nutritional therapy is dependent on the timing of their introduction, the severity of lead exposure, and underlying nutritional status. It is clear that marginal nutritional status is associated with increased prevalence of elevated blood lead concentrations. Data from national epidemiological surveys such as the National Health and Nutrition Examination Survey, conducted in the United States during the 1970s through the 1990s, demonstrated that young children from socially disadvantaged, low-income, minority families are more likely to have a greater prevalence of elevated blood lead levels (Mahaffey et al., 1982; Pirkle et al., 1994) and of marginal nutritional status (Life Sciences Research Office, 1996; Mahaffey et al., 1986). Consumption of a higher calcium diet has been shown to be related inversely bone lead among women living in Mexico City (Hernandez-Avila et al., 1996).

The physiological changes that accompany poor nutritional status for calcium and iron result in enhanced absorption of these required elements from the gastrointestinal tract

(Fullmer, 1997; Mahaffey, 1995). Because lead absorption also increases with these physiological changes, improving nutritional status results in reduced future absorption of lead. Some reports indicate reduced blood lead following treatment with iron (Granado et al., 1994). Short-term correction of low calcium intake has not been demonstrated to alter blood lead, but it is clear that skeletal mineral can be mobilized for calcium under conditions of physiological stress and that lead will be released along with calcium during this mineral mobilization (Gulson et al., 1997, 1998a). Whether or not increased calcium intake will reduce this mobilization is a question being addressed in current research.

The best approach to dealing with lead poisoning remains one of preventing exposure. Removal of lead from the environment has been a major success story for some countries through the 1980s and 1990s. Over the past two decades, blood lead levels among U.S. children have been reduced by more than 80%. Between NHANES II (conducted between 1976 and 1980) to Phase I of NHANES III (conducted between 1988 and 1991), the geometric mean blood lead level for all person ages 1 through 74 years declined from 12.8 µg/dL to 2.9 µg/dL. and the prevalence of elevated blood lead levels (i.e., >10 µg/dL) decreased from 77.8% to 4.4% (Mahaffey et al., 1982; Pirkle et al., 1994). Between NHANES III Phase II (1988 through 1991) and Phase III (1991 through 1994), the geometric mean for blood lead levels decreased by 22% (Centers for Disease Control, 1997b). This decline reflects both primary interventions (removal of lead solder from food and beverage cans, and virtual elimination of lead additives from gasoline), and secondary prevention strategies—including public health programs and improved nutrition. Despite this overall success, 4.4% of all children ages 1 through 5 years have blood lead concentrations >10 µg/dL. Elevated blood lead levels are disproportionately high among black children and low-income children. Eleven percent of black children and 8% of low-income children have blood lead concentrations >10 µg/dL. In the United States, the predominant remaining sources of lead exposure for children is lead-based paint in housing, particularly older residences which have an increased likelihood of containing lead-based paints (Jacobs, 1995). Although vigorous national efforts to reduce lead exposure from leaded paint in housing is underway, the problem is a long way from being solved. In the United States, an estimated 890,000 children have blood lead levels high enough (i.e., 10 µg/dL or higher) to cause adverse effects on their ability to learn because of exposure to deteriorating lead-based paint in their homes (CDC, 1997a).

Among the recommended "treatment" activities is identification through screening of cases for environmental/nutritional/pharmaceutical intervention. In 1991 the "case" definition was lowered to define childhood lead poisoning as a blood lead of greater than or equal to 10 µg/dL (0.48 µmol/L) (CDC, 1991; Committee on Environmental Health, American Academy of Pediatrics, 1993). The 1991 guidelines remain in effect (CDC, 1991), however, in a move away from recommendations for universal screening (CDC, 1997), emphasis is now placed on geographic areas with higher prevalence of older housing (i.e., defined as housing where 27% or more built before 1950) or other risk factors that are present (e.g., the child receives services from public assistance programs for the poor, or the child has a sibling or playmate who has had lead poisoning). Part of this change reflects the overall decline in blood lead concentrations in the United States.

Elevated blood lead concentrations are occasionally reported among adults. Use of "folk" remedies, cosmetics, and lead-glazed pottery are typically the source in these isolated cases. The most persistent cause of elevated blood lead concentrations among adults remains occupational exposures. The National Institute for Occupational Safety and Health maintains an Adult Blood Lead Epidemiology and Surveillance Program (ABLES) which monitor laboratory-reported elevated blood lead levels among adults in the United States. Currently these reports include data from 27 states. The cumulative number of reports during all of 1996 was 16,551 adults with blood lead concentrations greater than or

$25\,\mu g\,/\,dL$, with 318 blood lead concentrations greater than or equal to $60\,\mu g\,/\,dL$ (NIOSH, 1998). This pattern continued through 1997 with even higher numbers of elevated blood lead levels reported.

CONCLUSIONS

What are the forms (species) of lead in the environment to which humans are likely to be exposed? This is a question that cannot be answered with certainty, but some things can be said that would have a strong bearing on this question. In general, human lead exposure may be attributed to four components of the human environment: inhaled air, dusts of various types, food, and drinking water. Lead in food is a related to plant and animal exposure to contaminated air, soil, and water, and to products used in processing and storage of foods. Over approximately the past 20 years, lead in foods in many countries has declined dramatically from typically 100 to $200\,\mu g\,/\,day$ (Mahaffey, 1977) to typically less than $5\,\mu g\,/\,day$ (Bolger et al., 1996). This decline resulted from virtual bans on use of lead solders in food and beverage containers, and to more widely practiced limits on use of lead glazes in pottery and food storage containers. Lead contamination of raw food resulting from air and water contamination have also declined.

Lead was emitted into the air from automobiles as lead halides and as double salts with ammonium halides (e.g., $PbBrCl\text{-}2NH_4Cl$). Some organolead vapors (e.g., tetraethyl lead) were also released. In the atmosphere lead is present mainly as a sulfate with minor amounts of halides. Airborne size distribution data indicate that most of the airborne lead mass was found in submicrometer-sized particles. With marked restriction on sales of leaded gasoline additives, lead concentrations in air have also markedly decreased. In areas where lead additives are still permitted in gasoline, these decreases have not occurred.

Lead in water is dependent on the nature of the water and chemical treatments used in purification. In general, the formation of ion pairs, particularly $PbCO_3$, is highly significant in controlling total lead solubility, and lead concentration in water is principally dependent on the carbonate status of the water, determined by pH and alkalinity. Decreases in water lead reflect limitations on use of lead solder, and on public health / environmental health programs that manipulate the pH and alkalinity of water in the distribution system to minimize lead leaching from solder and pipes.

Apart from occupational exposure, the largest remaining source of lead exposure in many countries is lead dusts—particularly those arising from deteriorating lead paints found in a substantial number of old residential units. This source is considered to be the remaining, recalcitrant exposure affecting the health of the most sensitive subpopulation, young children. Major efforts are underway in some countries (e.g., the United States) to improve methods to remove lead from housing in a way that does not increase exposures through release of leaded dusts during the abatement process.

The toxicological properties of lead halides, sulfates, and carbonates may be of particular interest. Organic complexes with natural products such as humic acids may also be important (DeMore and Harrison, 1983).

Many ostensibly different toxic effects of lead have been reported in the literature, but there are likely to be only a few initiating mechanisms associated with a wider range of secondary effects. The most important system affected is the nervous system, and it was suggested that the mitochondria in neuronal cells may be a target site. In terms of developing a predictive model, the effects of lead can be attributed to its overall perturbation of the equilibrium processes in cells involving essential elements and their binding ligands (both inorganic and organic) that support life-giving cellular processes. In the case of lead, the primary element for which lead may act as both an agonist and an antagonist is calcium, and it can be expected that lead also antagonizes many of the ligands that calcium normally controls and regulates. Of particular note in this latter category may be phosphate. For other neurotoxic metals, the same or similar effects may be seen depending on the metal chemistry. For example, it has recently been suggested (Birchall and Chappell, 1988) that the biochemical toxicity of aluminum may be related to the vulnerability of the inositol phosphate system. Because of the wide range of chemical reactivities open to metal compounds, it may be worthwhile to compare overall patterns of divalent metal ion chemistry with each other, as well as with the biochemical toxicological profiles of known toxic divalent metals. This may help in identifying distinctive features or divalent metal ion chemistry associated with specific metal toxicity. In considering metal-organic neurotoxic mixtures, further degrees of mechanistic complexity have to be considered. The organic neurotoxic compounds are likely to operate by fundamentally different biochemical/molecular mechanisms, even though the end result may be the same or similar.

The neurotoxic potential of certain metals, especially lead, has become a paradigm in science. Unfortunately, the biochemical mechanisms that form the basis of the subtle neurotoxic effects of low concentrations of lead in the environment have not been clearly established. The paradigm gains in prominence through the continuation of epidemio-logical studies have shown correlations between subtle neurobehavioral effects in children and small increases in lead concentrations in blood. There are a number of questions concerning the stability of whole-blood lead measurements and the extent to which it represents a measure of the "toxicologically active" lead content of the affected tissue/organs of the body. A major recent change is recognition that the bone compartment of body lead is much more dynamic than previously understood, that it contributes a substantial portion of the lead present in blood. Some of the more important and still limiting factors in understanding the environmental lead toxicity problem include

- A poor understanding of the physical/chemical nature of lead in the environment and its relationship to bioavailability (which may involve both inorganic and organic point sources).
- Lack of definitive biomarkers of especially low lead exposures and/or effects based on fundamental information about biochemical and molecular mechanisms of action.
- Poor understanding of how the biochemical lesions give rise to detectable health effects.
- Individual population sensitivities (e.g., the fetus/neonate and the aged).
- Lack of knowledge of the influence on toxicity of the many other physical/chemical factors (e.g., other metals and organics in mixtures) that occur in combination with lead in the exposure environment.

An underlying deficiency in all of these factors is poor understanding at the molecular level. This is in part because of the wide range of chemical reactivities available to the divalent lead ion in both biological and nonbiological systems. This has complicated attempts to find the one or few biochemical interactions that may be primarily responsible for the neurotoxic effects of lead. This differs from most organic chemicals in our environment that have a much more limited set of reactivities to consider. Examining lead chemistry, in general, and distinctive aspects of lead chemistry in particular, in comparisons with other divalent metal ions, may offer an approach that may be generally applicable to the environmental metal toxicity problem. Since lead is one of the oldest environmental toxicants known that has been extensively studied with only limited success from a mechanistic viewpoint, there is perhaps a need here for some new and creative thinking about how to approach this problem and similar problems involving the potential health effects of other environmental chemicals.

REFERENCES

ACGIH. 1999. *Particle Size-Selective Sampling of Particulate Air Contaminants. Report of an ACGIH Technical Committee.* Cincinnati, OH: American Conference of Governmental Industrial Hygienists.

Alexander, F. W., B. E. Clayton, and H. T. Delves. 1974. *Quart. J. Med. New Series* 43(169): 89–111.

Angle, C. R., W. I. Manton, and Y. L. Stanek. 1995. Stable isotope identification of lead sources in preschool children—The Omaha study. *J. Toxicol. Clin. Toxicol.* 33: 657–662.

Apostoli, P., P. Kiss, S. Porru, J. P. Bonde, M. Vanhoorne and the ASCLEPIOS Study Group. 1998. Male reproductive toxicity of lead in animals and humans. *Occup. Environ. Med.* 55: 364–373.

Araki, S., K. Murata, and H. Aono. 1987. Central and peripheral nervous system dysfunction in workers exposed to lead, zinc, and copper. A follow-up study of visual and somato sensory evoked potentials. *Int. Arch. Occup. Environ. Health* 59: 177–187.

Altmann, L., K. Sveinsson, U. Kramer, M. Weishoff-Houben, M. Turfeld, G. Winneke, and H. Wiegand. 1998. Visual functions in 6-year-old children in relation to lead and mercury levels. *Neurotoxicol. Teratol.* 20: 9–17.

American Academy of Pediatrics/Committee on Environmental Health. 1993. Lead poisoning from screening to prevention. *Pediatr.* 92: 176–183.

Aub, J. C., L. T. Fairhall, A. S. Minot, and R. Reznikuff. 1925. Lead poisoning. In *Medicine*, vol. 4, eds. D. L. Edsall, J. Howland, and A. M. Chesney. Baltimore: Williams and Wilkins.

Apostoli, P., P. Kiss, S. Porru, J. P. Bonde, M. Vanhoorne, and the ASCLEPIOS Study Group. 1998. Male reproductive toxicity of lead in animals and humans. *Occup. Environ. Med.* 55: 364–374.

Aufderheide, A. C., and L. E. Wittmers Jr. 1992. Selected aspects of the spatial distribution of lead in bone. *Neurotoxicology* 13: 809–819.

Aungst, B. J., and H. L. Fung. 1981. Kinetic characterization of *in vitro* lead transport across the rat small intestine. *Toxicol. Appl. Pharmacol.* 61: 39–47.

Aungst, B. J., and H. L. Fung. 1985. Kinetic characterization of *in vitro* lead absorption, distribution and elimination kinetics in rats. *J. Toxicol. Environ. Health* 16: 147–159.

Averill, D. R., Jr., and H. L. Needleman. 1980. Neonatal lead exposure retards cortical synaptogenesis in the rat. In *Low Level Exposure*, ed. H. L. Needleman, New York: Raven Press.

Baghurst, P. A., A. J. McMichael, N. R. Wigg, G. V. Vimpani, E. F. Robertson, R. J. Roberts, and S. O. Tong. 1992, Environmental exposure to lead and children's intelligence at the age of seven years: The Port Pirie Cohort Study. *N. Engl. J. Med.* 327: 1279–1284.

Baghurst, P. A., A. J. McMichael, S. Tong, N. R. Wigg, G. V. Vimpani, and E. F. Robertson. 1995. Exposure to environmental lead and visual-motor integration at age 7 years: The Port Pirie cohort study. *Epidemiol.* 6: 104–109.

Barltrop, D., and H. E. Khoo. 1975. The influence of nutritional factors on lead absorption. *Postgrad. Med. J.* 51: 795–800.

Barltrop, D., and F. Meek. 1979. Effect of particle size on lead absorption from the gut. *Environ. Health* 34: 280–285.

Barry, P. S. 1975. A comparison of concentrations of lead in human tissue. *Br. J. Ind. Med.* 32: 119–139.

Barry, P. S. 1981. Concentrations of lead in tissues of children. *Br. J. Ind. Med.* 38: 61–71.

Barry, P. S. 1985. Multicompartment kinetic models for lead. I. Bone diffusion mode for long time retention. *Environ. Res.* 36: 441–458.

Barton, J. C., M. E. Conrad, L. Harrison, and S. Nuby. 1978a. Effects of calcium on the absorption and retention of lead. *J. Lab. Clin. Med.* 92: 536–543,

Barton, J. C., M. E. Conrad, L. Harrison, and S. Nuby. 1978b. Effects of iron on the absorption and retention of lead. *J. Lab. Clin. Med.* 91: 366–376.

Beechx, R. L. 1986. Lead poisoning in children. *Anal. Chem.* 58: 274–287.

Bellinger, D., A. Leviton, H. L. Needleman, C. Waternaux, and M. Rabinowitz. 1986. Low-level lead exposure and infant development in the first year. *Neurobehav. Toxicol. Teratol.* 8: 151–161.

Bellinger, D., A. Leviton, C. Waterman, L. Needleman, and M. Rabinowitz. 1987. Longitudinal analysis of prenatal and postnatal lead exposure and early cognitive development. *N. Engl. J. Med.* 316: 1037–1043.

Bellinger, D. C., Stiles, K. M., and Needleman, H. L. 1992. Low-level lead exposure, intelligence and academic achievement: a long-term follow-up study. *Pediatr.* 90: 855–871.

Bernard, S. R. 1977. Dosimetric data and metabolic models for lead. *Health Physics* 32: 44–46.

Bert, J. L., L. J. van Dsen and J. R. Grace. 1989. A generalized model for the prediction of lead body burdens. *Environ. Res.* 48: 117–127.

Birchall, J. D., and J. S. Chappell. 1988. Aluminum, chemical physiology, and Alzheimer's disease. *Lancet* 2: 1008–1010.

Blake, K. C. H., and M. Mann. 1983. Effect of calcium and phosphorus on the gastrointestinal absorption of 203 Pb in man. *Environ. Res.* 30: 188–194.

Bogden, J. D., J. M. Oleske, and D. B. Lourie. 1997. Lead poisoning—One approach to a problem that won't go away. *Environ. Health Perspect.* 105: 1284–1287.

Bolger, J. M., N. J. Yess, E. L. Gunderson, T. C. Troxell, and C. D. Carrington. 1996. Identification and reduction of sources of dietary lead in the United States. *Food Addit. Contamin.* 13: 53–60.

Boline, D. R. 1981. Some speciation and mechanistic aspects of trace metals in biological systems. In *Environmental Health Chemistry*, ed. J. D. McKinney. Ann Arbor: Science.

Bondy, S. C. 1988. The neurotoxicity of organic and inorganic lead. In *Metal Neurotoxicity*, eds. S. C. Bondy and K. R. Prasad, Boca Raton, FL: CRC Press.

Bressler, J. P., and G. W. Goldstein. 1991. Mechanisms of lead neurotoxicity. *Biochem. Pharmacol.* 41: 479–484.

Brezinski, D. R. 1976. Review of factors determining solubility and absorption of lead and other trace metals in the gastrointestinal tract. *J. Coatings Technol.* 48: 48–57.

Burns, J. M., P. A. Baghurst, M. G. Sawyer, A. E. McMichael, and S.-L. Tong. 1999. Lifetime low-level exposure to environmental lead and children's emotional and behavioral development at ages 11–13 years. *Am. J. Epidemiol.* 149: 740–749.

Casteel, S. W., R. P. Cowart, C. P. Weiss, G. M. Henningsen, E. Huffman, W. J. Brattin, R. E. Guzman, M. F. Starost, P. T. Payne, S. L. Stockham, S. W. Beeker, J. W. Drexler and J. R. Turk. 1997. Bioavailability of lead to juvenile swine dosed with soil from the Smuggler Mountain NPL site of Aspen, Colorado. *Fundament. Appl. Toxicol.* 36: 177–187.

Centers for Disease Control. 1991. *Preventing Lead Poisoning in Young Children. A Statement by the Centers for Disease Control.* United States Department of Health and Human Service. Atlanta: United States Public Health Service.

Centers for Disease Control. 1997b. Blood lead levels—United States, 1991–1994. Morb. Mor. Weekly Rep. 46: 141–147.

Chamberlain, A. C. 1983. Effect of airborne lead on blood lead. *Atmos. Environ.* 17: 677–692.

Chamberlain, A. C. 1985. Prediction of response of blood lead to airborne and dietary lead from volunteer experiments with lead isotopes. *Proc. Royal Soc. London* B224: 149–182.

Chisolm, J. J. 1980. Lead and other metals–A hypothesis of interactions. In *Lead Toxicity*, eds. R. L. Singhal and J. A. Thomas. Baltimore: Urban and Schwartzenberg.

Choie, D. D., and G. W. Richter. 1972. Lead poisoning: Rapid information of intranuclear inclusion *Science* 177: 1194–95.

Christensen, J. J., J. D. Lamb, S. R. Izatt, S. E. Starr, G. C. Weed, M. S. Astin, B. D. Stitt, and R. M. Izatt. 1978. Effect of anion type on rate of facilitated transport of cations across liquid membranes via neutral macrocyclic carriers. *J. Am. Chem. Soc.* 100: 3219–3220.

Clayton, G. G., and L. E. Clayton. 1981–1982. *Patty's Industrial Hygiene and Toxicology: Toxicology*, 3rd edition, vols. 2A, 2B, 2C. New York: Wiley.

Cocco, P., F. Hua, P. Boffetta, P. Carta, C. Flore, V. Flore, A. Onnis, G. F. Picchiri, and D. Colin. 1997. Mortality of Italian lead smelter workers. *Scand. J. Work Environ. Health* 23: 15–23.

Committee on Measuring Lead in Critical Populations. National Research Council. 1993. *Measuring Lead Exposure in Infants, Children and Other Sensitive Populations.* Washington, DC: National Academy of Sciences Press.

Conrad, M. E., J. N. Umbriet, E. G. Moore, and C. R. Rodning. 1992. Newly identified iron-binding protein in human duodenal mucosa. *Blood* 79: 244–247.

Cory-Slecta, D. 1988. Mobilization of lead over the course of DMSA chelation therapy and long-term efficacy. *J. Pharmacol. Exp. Ther.* 246: 84–91.

Cory-Slechta, D. A. 1997. Relationships between Pb-induced changes in neurotransmitter system function and behavioral toxicity. *Neurotoxicol.* 18: 673–688.

Cory-Slechta, D. A., B. Weiss, and C. Cox. 1987. Mobilization and redistribution of lead over the course of calcium disodium ethylene diamine tetracetate chelation therapy. *J. Pharmacol. Exp. Ther.* 243: 804–813.

Davis, J. M., and D. J. Svendzgaard. 1987. Lead and child development. *Nature* 329: 297–300.

De Mora, S. J. U., and R. M. Harrison. 1983. The physico-chemical speciation of lead in tapwater. *Proc. 4th Heavy Metal Environment International Conference*, vol. 2. Edinburgh, UK: CEP Consultant, Ltd.

DeSilva, P. E. 1981. Determination of lead in plasma and studies on its relationship to lead in erythrocytes. *Br. J. Ind. Med.* 38: 209–217.

Dietrich, K. N., O. G. Berger, P. A. Succop, P. B. Hammond, and R. L. Bornschein. 1993a. The developmental consequences of low to moderate prenatal and postnatal lead exposure: Intellectual attainment in the Cincinnati lead study cohort following school entry. *Neurotoxicol. Teratol.* 15: 37–44.

Dietrich, K. N., O. G. Berger, and P. A. Succop. 1993b. Lead exposure and the developmental status of urban six-year-old children in the Cincinnati Prospective Study. *Pediatr.* 91: 301–307.

Dietrich, K., P.A. Succop, R. L. Bornschein, K. Krafft, O. Berger, P. B. Hammond, and C. R. Buncher. 1990. Lead exposure and neurobehavioral development in later infancy. *Environ. Health Perspect.* 89: 13–19.

Doss. M., U. Becker, E. Sixel, S. Geisse, H. Solcher, G. Kufner, H. Schlegel, and M. Stoeppler. 1982. Persistent protoporphyrinemia in hereditary porphobilinogen under low lead exposure: A new molecular basis for the pathogenesis of lead intoxication. *Klin. Wochenschr.* 60: 599–606.

Dowdle, E. B., E. Wilson, and P. Burger. 1971. Symptomatic porphyria. I. The effects of lead on the synthesis of porphyrin and haem. *S. Afr. Med. J.* 25: 38–45.

Drasch, G. 1974. Untersuchungen zum Bleigehalt menschiecher Knochen. *Arbeitsmed. Socialmez. Praventimed.* 14: 32–34.

Drasch, G. A., J. Bohm, and C. Baur. 1987. Lead in human bones. Investigations on an occupationally non-exposed population in southern Bavaria (FGR). 1. Adults. *Sci. Total Environ.* 64: 303–315.

Drasch, G. A. and J. Ott. 1988. Lead in human bones: Investigations on an occupationally non-exposed population in southern Bavaria (FGR). II. Children. *Sci. Total Environ.* 68: 61–69.

Drasch, G. 1997. Are blood, urine, hair, and muscle valid biomonitors for the internal burden of men with heavy metal mercury, lead and cadmium? *Trace Elem. Electrol.* 14: 116–123.

Dratman, J. B. 1978. The mechanisms of thyrozine action. In *Hormonal Protein and Peptides: Thyroid Hormones*, vol. 6, ed. C. H. Li. New York: Academic Press.

Eckerman, D. A., J. R. Glowa, and W. K. Anger. 1999. Interindividual variability in neurotoxicity. In: *Human Variability in Response to Chemical Exposures*, eds. D. A. Neumann and C. A. Kimmel, pp. 59–86. Boca Raton, FL: CRC Press.

Fairhall, L. T. 1924. The solubility of various lead compounds in blood serum. *J. Biol. Chem.* 60: 481–488.

Fels, L. M., M. Wunsch, J. Baranowski, I. Norska–Borowka, R. G. Price, S. A. Taylor, S. Patel, M. DeBroe, M. M. Elsevier, R. Lauwery, H. Roels, A. Bernard, A. Mutti, E. Gelpi, J. Rosello, and H. Stolte. 1998. Adverse effects of chronic low level lead exposure on kidney function—A risk group study in children. *Nephrol. Dial. Transplant* 13: 2248–2256.

Finklestein, Y., M. E. Markowitz, and J. F. Rosen. 1998. Low-level lead-induced neurotoxicity in children: An update on central nervous system effects. *Brain Res. Rev.* 27: 168–176.

Flannagan, P. R., D. L. Hamilton, J. Haist, and L. S. Valberg. 1979. Interrelationships between iron and lead absorption in iron-deficient mice. *Gastroenterology* 77: 1041–1081.

Florence, T. M., S. G. Lilley, and J. L. Stauber. 1988. Skin absorption of lead. *Lancet* 2: 157–158.

Franklin, C. A., M. J. Inskip, C. L. Baccanale, C. M. Edwards, W. I. Manton, E. Edwards, and E. J. O'Flaherty. 1997. Use of sequentially administered stable lead isotopes to investigate changes in blood lead during pregnancy in a nonhuman primate (Macaca fascicularis). *Fundament. Appl. Toxicol.* 39: 109–119.

French, P., and D. T. E. Hunt 1988. Thermodynamic calculations of dissolved trace metal speciation in river, estuary, and sea waters. *Water Res. Centr. Tech. Rep.* 249: 38.

Fullmer, C. S. 1997. Lead-calcium interactions: Involvement of 1,25-dihydroxyvitamin D. *Environ. Res.* 72: 45–55.

Fullmer, C. W., S. Edelstein, and R. H. Wasserman. 1985. Lead-binding properties of intestinal calcium-binding proteins. *J. Biol. Chem.* 260. 6816–6819.

Garber, B. T., and E. Wei. 1974. Influence of dietary factors on the gastrointestinal absorption of lead. *Toxicol. Appl. Pharmacol.* 27: 685–691.

Goldstein, G. W. 1977. Lead encephalopathy: The significance of lead inhibition of calcium uptake by brain mitochondria. *Brain Res.* 136: 185–188.

Goldstein, G. W. 1993. Evidence that lead acts as a calcium substitute in second messenger metabolism. *Neurotoxicol.* 14: 97–101.

Goyer, R. A., and B. C. Rhyne. 1973. Pathological effects of lead. *Int. Rev. Exp Pathol.* 12: 1–77.

Granado, M. J. R., F. J. A. Guisasola, and A. B. Quirs. 1994. Estuido de la plumbemia en la poblani infantil conferropenia. *Med. Clin. (Barc.)* 102: 210–204.

Grandjean, P., and J. Lintrup. 1978. Erythrocyte Zn-protoporphyrin as an indicator of lead exposure. Scand. *J. Clin. Lab. Invest.* 38: 669–675.

Grandjean, P., and E. C. Grandjean. 1984. *Biological effects of Organolead Compounds.* Boca Raton, FL: CRC Press.

Greninger, D., V. Kolionitsch, and C. K. Kline. 1978. *Lead Chemicals.* New York: Internation Lead and Zinc Organization.

Gross S. B., E. A. Pfitzer, D. W. Yeager, and R. A. Kehoe, 1975. Lead in human tissues. *Toxicol. Appl. Pharmacol.* 132: 628–681.

Gulson, B. L., M. A. Cameron, A. J. Amith, K. J. Mizon, M. J. Korsch, G. Vimpani, A. J. McMichael, D. Pisaniello, C. W. Jameson, and K. R. Mahaffey. 1998b. Blood lead-urine lead relationships in adults and children. *Environ. Res.* 78: 152–160.

Gulson, B. L., C. W. Jameson, K. R. Mahaffey, K. J. Mizon, N. Patison, A. J. Law, M. J. Korsch, and M. A. Salter. 1998c. Relationships of lead in breast milk to lead in blood, urine, and diet of the infant and mother. *Environ. Health Perspect.* 106: 667–674.

Gulson, B. L., K. R. Mahaffey, K. J. Mizon. M. J. Korsch, M. A. Cameron, and G. Vimpani. 1995. Contribution of tissue lead to blood lead in adult female subjects based on stable lead isotope methods. *J. Lab. Clin. Med.* 125: 703–712.

Gulson, B. L., K. R. Mahaffey, C. W. Jameson, M. Vicos, A. J. Law, K. J. Mizon, A. J. M. Smith, and M. J. Korsch. 1997. Dietary lead intakes for mother-child pairs and relevance to pharmacokinetic models. *Environ. Health Perspect.* 105: 1334–1342.

Gulson, B. L., D. Pisaniello, A. J. McMichael, K. R. Mahaffey, C. Luke, K. J. Mizon, M. J. Korsch, R. Ashbolt, G. Vimpani, and D. C. Pederson. 1996. Stable lead isotope profiles in smelter and general urban communities: Comparison of biological and environmental measures. *Environ. Geochem. Health* 18: 147–163.

Gulson, B. L., K. R. Mahaffey, C. W. Jameson, K. J. Mizon, M. J. Korsch. M. A. Cameron, and J. A. Eisman. 1998a. Mobilization of lead from the skeleton during the postnatal period is even larger than during pregnancy. *J. Lab. Clin. Med.* 131: 324–329.

Hamilton, D. L. 1978. Interrelationships of lead and iron retention in iron-deficient mice. *Toxicol. Appl Pharmacol.* 46: 651–661.

Hammond, P. B., R. L. Bornschein, and P. Succop. 1985. Dose-effect and dose-response relationships of blood lead to erythrocyte protoporphyrin in young children. *Environ. Res.* 38: 187–196.

Hanninen, H., A. Aitio, T. Kovala, R. Luukkonen, E. Matikainen, T. Mannelin, J. Erkkila, and V. Riihimaki. 1998. Occupational exposure to lead and neuropsychological dysfunction. *Occup. Environ. Med.* 55: 202–209.

Hanzlik, R. P. 1981. Toxicity and metabolism of metal compounds: Some structure-activity relationships. In *Environmental Health Chemistry*, ed. J. D. Mckinney. Ann Arbor: Science Press.

Healy, M. A., P. G. Harrison, M. Aslam, S. Davis, and C. G. Wilson. 1982. Lead sulphide and traditional preparations: Routes for ingestion and solubility and reactions in gastric fluids. *J. Clin. Hosp. Pharmacol.* 7: 169–173.

Heard, M. J., and A. C. Chamberlain. 1982. Effects of minerals and food on uptake of lead from the gastrointestinal tract in humans. *Human Toxicol.* 1: 411–415.

Henning, S. J., and L. Cooper. 1988. Intestinal accumulation of lead salts and milk lead by suckling rats (42645). *Proc. Soc. Exp. Biol. Med.* 187: 110–116.

Hening, S. J., and L. L. Leeper. 1984. Duodenal uptake of lead by suckling and weanling rats. *Biol. Neonate* 46: 27–35.

Hernandez-Avila, M., T. Gonzalez-Cosio, E. Palazuelos, I. Romieu, A. Aro, E. Fishbein, K. E. Peterson, and H. Hu. 1996. Dietary and environmental determinats of blood and bone lead levels in lactating postpartum women living in Mexico City. *Environ. Health Perspect.* 104: 1076–1082.

Hill, C. H., and G. Matrone. 1970. Chemical parameters in the study of in vivo and in vitro interactions and transition elements. *Fed. Proc.* 29: 1474–1481.

Hu, H. 1998. Bone lead as a new biologic marker of lead dose: Recent findings and implications for public health. *Environ. Health Perspect.* 106 (suppl. 4): 961–967.

Huisingh, D., and J. Huisingh. 1974. Factors influencing the toxicity of heavy metals food. *Ecol. Food Nutr.* 3: 2263–272.

Hunt, D. T. E., and J. D. Creasey. 1980. The calculation of equilibrium trace metal speciation and solubility on aqueous systems by a computer method with particular reference to lead. *Water Res. Cent. Tech. Rep.* 151: 32.

Hursch, J. B., and J. Suomela. 1968. Absorption of 212Pb from the gastrointestinal tract of man. *Acta Radiol.* 7: 108–120.

International Agency of Research on Cancer (IARC). 1987. Overall evaluations of carcinogenicity: An updating of IARC monographs, volumes 1 to 42. *IARC Monographs on the Evaluation of Carcinogenic Risk to Humans*, Suppl. 7, pp. 1–440 Lyon: IARC.

Izatt, R. M., R. E. Terry, B. L. Haymore, L. D. Haven, N. K. Dailey, A. G. Avondet, and J. J. Christensen. 1976. Calorimetric titration study of the interaction of several uni- and bivalent cations with 15-crown-5,18-crown-6, two isomers of dicyclohexo-18-crown-6 in aqueous solutions at 25°C and $u = 0.1$. *J. Amer. Chem. Soc.* 98: 7620–7626.

Jackson, P. J., and I. Sheiham. 1986. Calculations of lead solubility in water. *Water Res. Cent. Tech. Rep.* 152: 43.

Jacobs, D. E. 1995. Lead-based paint as a major source of childhood lead poisoning: A review of the evidence. In *Lead in Paint, Soil, and Dust: Health Risks, Exposure Studies, Control Measures, Measurement Methods, and Quality Assurance*, eds. M. E. Beard and S. D. A. Iska, pp. 175–187. American Society for Testing and Materials: Philadelphia.

James, M., M. E. Hilburn, and J. A. Blair. 1985. Effects of meals and meal times on uptake of lead from the gastrointestinal tract in humans. *Human Toxicol.* 40: 401–407.

Jawrerski, J. F., J. Nriagu, P. Denny, B. T. Hart, M. R. Laskeenn, V. Subramanan, and M. H. Wong. 1987. Group report: Lead. In *Scope 31 / Lead, Mercury, Cadmium and Arsenic in the Environment*, eds. T. C. Hutchinson and K. M. Meemav. New York: Wiley.

Kazantzis, G. 1988. The use of blood in the biological monitoring of toxic metals. In *Biological Monitoring of Toxic Metals*, eds. T. W. Clarkson, L. Friberg, G. F. Nordberg, and P. R. Sager. New York: Plenum Press.

Kehoe, R. A. 1961. The metabolism of lead in man in health and disease. *J. Royal Inst. Public Health Hyg.* 24: 81–97, 129–143, and 177–203.

Keller, C. A., and R. A. Doherty. 1980a. Bone lead mobilization in lactating mice and lead transfer to suckling offspring. *Toxicol. Appl. Pharmacol.* 55: 220–228.

Keller, C. A., and R. A. Doherty. 1980b. Lead and calcium distributions in blood, plasma, and milk of the lactating mouse. *J. Lab. Clin. Med.* 95: 81–89.

Landner, L. 1987. Speciation of metals in water, sediment, and soil systems. In *Lecture Notes in Earth Sciences*, eds. S. Bhattacharji, G. M. Friedman, H. J. Neugebauer, and A. Seilaeher, pp. 179–185, New York: Springer-Verlag.

Lanphear, B. P., T. D. Matte, J. Rogers, R. P. Clickner, B. Dietz, R. L. Bornschein, P. Succop, K. R. Mahaffey, S. Dixon, W. Galke, M. Rabinowitz, M. Farfel, C. Rohde, J. Schwartz, P. Ashley, and D. E. Jacobs. 1998. The contribution of lead-contaminated house dust and residential soil to children's blood lead levels. *Environ. Res.* 79: 51–68.

Leggett. R. W. 1993. An age-specific kinetic model of lead metabolism in humans. *Environ. Health Perspect.* 101: 598–616.

Lester, B. M., L. L. LaGasse, and R. Seifer. 1998. Cocaine exposure and children: The meaning of subtle effects. *Science* 282: 633–634.

Life Science Research Office. 1996. Executive summary from the third report on nutrition monitoring in the United States. *J. Nutr.* 126: iii–x and 1907S–1936S.

Lilis, R., J. Eisinger, W. Blumberg, A. Fischbein, and I. J. Selikoff. 1978. Hemoglobin, serum iron, and zinc protoporphyrin in lead-exposed workers. *Environ. Health Perspect.* 25: 97–102.

Lippmann, M. 1990. Review: 1989 Alice Hamilton Lecture. Lead and human health: Background and recent findings. *Environ. Res.* 51: 1–24.

Loghman-Adham, M. 1997. Renal effects of environmental and occupational lead exposure. Environ. Health Perspect. 105: 928–939.

Lundstrom, N.-G., G. Nordberg, V. Englyst, L. Gehardssen, L. Hagmar, T. Jin, L. Rylander, and S. Walls. 1997. Cumulative lead exposure in relation to mortality and lung caner morbidity in a cohort of primary smelter workers. *Scand. J. Work Environ. Health* 23: 24–30.

Mahaffey, K. R. 1977. Relation between quantities of lead ingested and health effects of lead in humans. *Pediatrics.* 59: 448–455.

Mahaffey, K. R. 1981. Nutritional factors and lead poisoning. *Nutr. Rev.* 39: 353–362.

Mahaffey, K. R. 1995. Nutritional and lead: Strategies for public health. *Environ. Health Perspect.* 103 (suppl. 6): 191–196.

Mahaffey, K. R., J. L. Annest, J. Roberts, and R. S. Murphy. 1982. National estimates of blood lead levels: United States, 1976–1980. Association with selected demographic and socioeconomic factors. *N. Engl. J. Med.* 307: 573–579.

Mahaffey, K. R., and J. L. Annest. 1986. Association of erythrocyte protoporphyrin with blood lead level and iron status in the Second National Health and Nutrition Examination Survey, 1976–1980. *Environ. Res.* 41: 327–338.

Mahaffey, K. R., P. S. Garthside, and C. L. Glueck. 1986. Blood lead and dietary calcium in 2926 1-through 11-year-old black and white children: The second National Health and Nutrition Examination Survey, 1976–1980. *Pediatr.* 78: 257–262.

Mahaffey-Six, K., and R. A. Goyer. 1970. Experimental enhancement of lead toxicity by low dietary calcium. *J. Lab. Clin. Med.* 76: 933–942.

Mahaffey-Six, K., and R. A. Goyer. 1972. The influence of iron deficiency on tissue content and toxicity of ingested lead in the rat. *J. Lab. Clin. Med.* 79: 128–136.

Manton, W. I. 1977. Sources of lead in blood: identification by stable isotopes. *Arch. Environ. Health* 32: 149–157.

Manton, W. I. 1985. Total contribution of airborne lead to blood lead. *Br. J. Ind. Med.* 42: 169–172.

Marcus, A. H. 1985a. Multicompartment kinetic model for lead. I. Bone kinetics and variable absorption in humans without excessive lead exposures. *Environ. Res.* 36: 441–458.

Marcus, A. H. 1985b. Multicompartment kinetic model for lead. II. Linear kinetics and variable absorption in humans without excessive lead exposure. *Environ. Res.* 36: 459–472.

Marcus, A. H. 1985c. Multicompartment kinetic models for lead. III. Lead in blood plasma and erythrocytes. *Environ. Res.* 36: 473–489.

Markovac, J., and G. W. Goldstein, 1988. Picomolar concentrations of lead stimulate brain protein kinase C. *Nature* 334: 71–73.

McIntosh, M. J., P. A. Meredith, M. R. Moore, and A. Goldberg. 1989. Action of lead on neurotransmission in rats. *Xenobiotica* 19: 101–113.

Meredith, P. A., M. R. Moore, and A. Goldberg, 1977. The effects of calcium on lead absorption in rats *Biochem. J.*166: 531–537.

Minot, A. S. 1929. The distribution of lead in the organism after absorption by the lungs and subcataneous tissue. *J. Ind. Hyg.* 6: 137–148.

Mohnen, V. A. 1988. The challenge of acid rain. *Sci. Amer.* 259: 30–38.

Morrow, P. E., H. Beiter, F. Amato, and F. R. Gibb. 1980. Pulmonary retention of lead: An experimental study in man. *Environ. Res.* 21: 373–384.

Mykkanen, H., M. Hannu, and R. H. Wasserman. 1982. Effect of vitamin D on the intestinal absorption of lead-203 and calcium-47 in chicks. *J. Nutr.* 112: 520–527.

National Institute for Occupational Safety and Health. 1998. Adult blood lead epidemiology and surveillance - United States, third quarter, 1997. *Morb. Mort. Weekly Rep.* 47: 77–80.

Needleman, H. L., C. Gunnoe, A. Leviton, R. Reed, H. Peresie, C. Maher, and P. Barrett. 1979. Deficits in psychological and classroom performance of children with elevated dentine lead levels. *N. Engl. J. Med.* 300: 689–695.

Nordberg, G. F., K. R. Mahaffey, and B. A. Fowler. 1991. Introduction and summary. International workshop on led in bone: Implications for dosimetry and toxicology. *Environ. Health Perspect.* 91: 3–7.

Nriagu, J. O. 1998. Tales told in lead. *Science* 281: 1622–1623.

Nriagu, J. O., and J. M. Pacyna. 1988. Quantitative assessment of world wide contamination of air, water and soils by trace metals. *Nature* 333: 134–139.

O'Flaherty, E. J. 1993. Physiologically based models for bone-seeking elements. IV. Kinetics of lead disposition in humans. *Toxicol. Appl. Pharmacol.* 118: 16–29.

O'Flaherty, E. J. 1995. Physiologically based models for bone-seeking elements. V. Lead absorption and deposition in childhood. *Toxicol. Appl. Pharmacol.* 131: 297–308.

O'Flaherty, K. E. 1998; Physiologically based models of metal kinetics. *Crit. Rev. Toxicol.* 28: 271–317.

Oldendorf, W. H., and W. J. Brown. 1975. Greater numbers of capillary endothalial cell mitochondria in brain than in muscle. *Proc. Soc. Exp. Biol. Med.* 149: 736–738.

Paglia, D. E., W. N. Valentin, and J. G. Dahigren. 1975. Effects of low level lead exposures on pyrimidine 5′-nucleotide and other erythrocyte enzymes. Possible role of pyrimidine 5′-nucleotide in the pathogenesis of lead-induced anemia. *J. Clin. Invest.* 56: 1164–1169.

Pappas, J., J. Ahlquist, E. Allen, and W. Banner. 1995. Oral dimercaptosuccinic acid and ongoing exposure to lead: Effects on heme synthesis and lead distribution in a rat model. *Toxicol. Appl. Pharmacol.* 133: 121–129.

Piomelli, S. 1973. A micro method for free erythrocyte porphyrins: The FEP test. *J. Lab. Clin. Med.* 81: 932–940.

Piomelli, S., B. Davidow, V. Guinee, P. Young, and G. Gay. 1973. The FEP [free erythrocyte porphyrin] test: A screening micro-method for lead poisoning. *Pediatr.* 51: 254–259.

Piomelli, S., C. Seaman, D. Zullow, A. Curran, and B. Davidon. 1982. Threshold for lead damage of heme synthesis in urban children. *Proc. Natl. Acad. Sci. USA* 79: 3335–3339.

Pirkle, J. L., J. D. Brody, E. W. Gunter, R. A. Kramer, D. C. Paschal, K. K. Flegal, and T. D. Matte. 1994. The decline in blood lead levels in the United States: the National Health and Nutrition Examination Surveys (NHANES). *J. Amer. Med. Assoc.* 272: 284–291.

Rabinowitz, M. B., J. D. Kopple, and G. W. Wetherill. 1975a. Effect of food intake and fasting on gastrointestinal lead absorption in humans. *Amer. J. Clin. Nutr.* 33: 1784–1788.

Rabinowitz, M. B., G. Wetherill, and J. Kopple. 1975b. Absorption, storage and excretion of lead by normal humans. In *proc. 9th Annual Conference on Trace Substances in Environmental Health*, pp. 361–368. Columbia: University of Missouri.

Rabinowitz, M. B., G. Wetherill, and J. D. Kopple. 1976. Kinetic analysis of lead metabolism in healthy humans. *J. lab. Invest.* 58: 260–270.

Ragan, H. A. 1983. The bioavailability of iron, lead, and cadmium via gastrointestinal absorption: A review. *Sci. Total Environ.* 28: 317–326.

Roels, H. A., R. R. Lauwerys, J. P. Buchet, and M. T. Vrelust. 1976. Response of free erythrocyte porphyrin and urinary delta-aminolevulinic acid in men and women moderately exposed to lead. *Int. Arch. Arbeitsmed.* 34: 97–108.

Rosen, J. F., and J. G. Pounds. 1998. Severe chronic lead insult that maintains body burdens of lead related to those in the skeleton: Observations by Dr. Clair Patterson conclusively demonstrated. *Environ. Res.* 78: 140–151.

Rosen, J. F., M. E. Markowitz, P. E. Bijur, S. T. Jenks, L. Wielopolski, J. A. Kalef-Ezra, and D. N. Slatkin. 1989. L-line X-ray fluorescence of cortical bone lead compared with the CaNa2EDTA test in lead-toxic children. Public health implications. *Proc. Natl. Acad. Sci. USA* 86: 685–689. Correction 86: 7595.

Sartorelli, E., F. Loi, and R. Gori, 1985. Lead silicate toxicity: A comparison among different compounds. *Environ. Res.* 36: 420–425.

Sassa, S., J. L. Granick, S. Granick, A. Kappas, and R. D. Levere. 1973. Studies in lead poisoning. I. Microanalysis of erythrocyte protoporphyrin levels by spectro photometry in the detection of chronic lead intoxication in the subclinical range. *Biochem. Med.* 8: 135–148.

Schlag, R. D. 1987. Lead. In *Genotoxic and Carcinogenic Metals: Environmental and Occupational Occurrence and Exposure*, eds. L. Fishbein, A. Furst, and M. A. Mehlman. Princeton: Princeton Scientific Publishing.

Schutz, A., S. Skerfving, J. Ranstam, and J. O. Christoffersson. 1987a. Kinetics of lead in blood after the end of occupational exposure. *J. Work Environ. Health* 13: 221–231.

Schutz, A., S. Skerfving, and J.-O. Christoffersson. 1987b. Chelatable level versus lead in human trabecular and compact bone. *Sci. Total Environ.* 68: 45–59.

Schwartz, J., and D. Otto. 1987. Blood lead, hearing threshold, and neurobehavioral development in children and youth. *Arch. Environ. Health* 42: 153–160.

Scott, K. M., K. M. Hwang, M. Jurikowitz, and G. P. Brierley. 1971. Ion transfer by heart mitochondria XXIII. The effects of lead on mitochondrial reactions. *Arch. Biochem. Biophys.* 147: 557–567.

Seppalainen, A. M., S. Hernberg, and R. Koch. 1979. Relationship between blood lead levels and nerve conduction velocities. Neurotox. 1: 313–332.

Skerfving, S. 1998. Biological monitoring of exposure to inorganic lead. In *Biological Monitoring of Toxic Metals*, eds. T. W. Clarkson, L. Friberg, G. F. Nordberg, and P. R. Sager, pp. 169–197. New York: Plenum Press.

Shotyk, W., D. Weiss, P. G. Appleby, A. K. Cheburkin, R. Frei, M. Gloor, J. D. Kramers, S. Reese, and W. O. Van Der Knapp. 1998. History of atmospheric lead deposition since 12,370 14C yr BP from a peat bog. Jura Mountains, Switzerland. *Science* 281: 1635–1640.

Simons, T. J. B. 1986. Passive transport and binding of lead by human red blood cells. *J. Physiol.* 378: 267–286.

Simons, T. J. B. 1989. Lead contamination. *Nature* 337: 514.

Smith, C. M., H. F. DeLuca, Y. Tanaka, and K. R. Mahaffey. 1980. Stimulation of lead absorption by vitamin D administration. *J. Nutr.* 108: 843–847.

Smith, G. L., S. B. Rees, and D. R. Williams. 1985. Speciation of strontium on human and bovine milk. *Polyhedron* 4: 713–716.

Smith, D., L. Bayer, B. J. Strupp, 1998. Efficacy of succimer in chelation for reducing brain Pb levels in a rodent model. *Environ. Res.* 78: 168–176.

Smith, D. R., J. D. Osterloh, and A. R. Flegal. 1996. Use of endogenous, stable lead isotopes to determine release of lead from the skeleton. *Environ. Health Perspect.* 104: 60–66.

Somervaille, L. J., D. R. Chettle, M. C. Scott, A. C. Aufderheide, J. E. Waligren, L. E. Wittmers, and G. Rapp. 1986. Comparison of two in vitro methods of bone lead analysis and the implication for in vivo measurements. *Phy. Med. Biol.* 31: 1267–1274.

Spear, T. M., W. Svee, J. H. Vincent, and N. Stanisich. 1998. Chemical speciation of lead dust associated with primary lead smelting. *Environ. Health Perspect.* 106: 565–571.

Steenhout, A. 1982. Kinetics of lead storage in teeth and bones: An epidemiologist's approach. *Arch. Environ. Health.* 37: 224–231.

Tong, S., P. Baghurst, A. McMichael, M. Sawyer, and J. Mudge. 1996. Lifetime exposure to environmental lead and Children's intelligence at 11–13 years: the Port Pirie cohort study. *Br. Med. J.* 312: 1569–1575.

Vainio, H. 1997. Lead and cancer—Association or causation? *Scand. J. Work Environ. Health* 23: 1–3.

Walkowiak, J., L. Altmann, U. Kramer, K. Sveinsson, M. Turfeld, M. Weishoff-Houben, and G. Winneke. 1998. Cognitive and sensorimotor functions in 6-year-old children in relation to lead and mercur-ylevels: adjustment for intelligence and contrast sensitivity in compurterized testing. *Neurotoxicol. Teratol.* 20: 511–521.

Wasserman, G. A., X. Liu, N. J. Lolocono, P. Factor-Litvak, J. K. Kline, D. Popovac. N. Morina, A. Musabergovic, N. Vrenezi, S. Capuni-Paracka, V. Lekic, E. Preteni-Redjepi, S. Hadzialjevic, V. Salkovich, and J. H. Graziano. 1997. Lead exposure and intelligence in 7-year old children: The Yugoslavian prospective study. *Environ. Health Perspect.* 105: 956–962.

Watson, W. S., R. Hume, and M. R. Moore. 1980. Oral absorption of lead and iron. *Lancet* 2: 236–237.

Whetsell, W. O., Jr., S. Sassa, and K. Kappas. 1984. Porpyrin-heme biosynthesis in organotypic cultures of mouse dorsal root ganglia. *J. Clin. Invest.* 74: 600–607.

Widzowski, D. V., J. N. Finkelstein, M. J. Pokora, and D. A. Cory-Slechta. 1994. Time course of postnatal lead-induced changes in dopamine receptors and their relationship to changes in dopamine sensitivity. *Neurotox.* 15(4): 853–865.

Willes, R. F., E. Lok, J. F. Truelove, and A. Sandarum. 1977. Retention and tissue distribution of 210Pb(NO$_3$)$_2$ administered orally to infant and adult monkeys. *J. Toxicol. Environ. Health* 3: 395–406.

Winneke, G., H. Lilienthal, and U. Kramer. 1996. The neurobehavioural toxicology and teratology of lead. *Arch. Toxicol.* 18 (suppl.): 57–70.

Ziegler, E. E., B. B. Edwards, R. L. Jensen, K. R. Mahaffey, and S. J. Fomon. 1978. Absorption and retention of lead by infants. *Pediatr. Res.* 12: 29–34.

15 Man-Made Ionizing Radiation and Radioactivity: Sources, Levels, and Effects

JOHN J. MAURO, Ph.D.
NORMAN COHEN, Ph.D.

SOURCE DOCUMENTS

The characteristics and significance of the sources, levels, and effects of both naturally occurring and man-made ionizing radiation and radioactivity are provided in several authoritative reports published by the National Academy of Sciences (NAS), the National Council on Radiation Protection and Measurement (NCRP), the International Commission on Radiation Protection (ICRP), the United Nations Scientific Committee on the Effects of Atomic Radiation (UNSCEAR), and the International Atomic Energy Agency (IAEA). In addition the U.S. Nuclear Regulatory Commission (NRC), which regulates source, by-product, and special nuclear material, maintains a library of technical reports, regulatory products, and data bases on the commercial nuclear power industry, and the use of radioactive material in education, medicine, and industry. The Office of Radiation and Indoor Air (ORIA) of the U.S. Environmental Protection Agency (EPA) has developed a repository of information, in the form of technical support documents, background information documents, environmental impact statements, and regulatory impact analyses, on radioactivity in the environment. Finally the U.S. Department of Energy (DOE) serves as a national repository of information on all aspects of the use of radioactive materials in research and defense.

In addition to these government funded publications, Merril Eisenbud and Thomas Gesell have published the fourth edition of *Environmental Radioactivity from Natural, Industrial, and Military Sources* (1997), which provides a comprehensive review of many of the topics addressed in this chapter. This chapter summarizes some of this large and continually expanding body of knowledge, collects and supplements these sources of information with new data, and presents this information in a manner that captures the potential magnitude of the exposures to this class of environmental toxicants and its significance in terms of its potential effects on public health and safety. The readers are encouraged to refer to the original source documents cited in this chapter, and their reviews as provided in the UNSCEAR publications and by Eisenbud and Gesell (1997).

Environmental Toxicants: Human Exposures and Their Health Effects, 2/e. Edited by Morton Lippmann.
ISBN: 0-471-29298-2 © 2000 John Wiley & Sons, Inc.

SPECIAL UNITS

The levels of most environmental toxicants are expressed in terms of the mass of the material (e.g., milligrams) per unit measure of the medium in which it is contained (e.g., kilogram of soil, liter of water, or cubic meter of air, or related volumetric concentration (e.g., parts per million). In addition exposure to most toxicants is expressed as the rate of intake of the material per unit time (e.g., milligrams per day) or per unit body weight (e.g., milligrams per day per kilogram). These expressions of levels and exposures are intuitively understandable. However, the units used to characterize the quantities of radioactive material in the environment and exposures of humans and organisms other than human to radiation and radioactive material are unique, and require some discussion prior to addressing the sources, levels, and effects of radioactivity and radiation.

The quantities of radioactive material can be, but are not, expressed in units of mass. Instead, they are expressed in terms of the number of atoms undergoing radioactive transformation (referred to as radioactive decay) per unit time. Units of decay rate instead of mass are used to quantify the amount of radioactive material partly because the effects of radioactive materials are related more to the decay rate of the material than to its mass. For example, one gram of radium-226 (^{226}Ra) has a decay rate of 3.7×10^{10} transformations (also referred to as disintegrations) per second, while one gram of ^{137}Cs has a decay rate of 3.2×10^{12} transformations per second. Since the energy emitted by the radioactive material during radioactive decay is usually of public health concern, and generally not the chemical properties of the radioactive material, it is more convenient to quantify radioactive material according to decay rate. In addition radioactive materials are detected and quantified by their types and amounts of disintegrations and not by their unique chemistry, as is the case for nonradioactive material. For these reasons the quantity of radioactive material is expressed in units of decay rate.

The "Curie," named after the discoverer of radium, Marie Curie, has been the unit most commonly used to define the quantity of radioactive material. It is defined as 3.7×10^{10} disintegrations per second, which corresponds to one gram of ^{226}Ra. Since this is a relatively large quantity of radioactive material from the perspective of environmental radioactivity, it is common to express environmental levels of radioactive material in terms of the picocurie (pCi), where "pico" refers to 10^{-12}. The Curie is being replaced by the "Becquerel," abbreviated Bq and named after Antoine Henri Becquerel, the discoverer of the natural radioactive properties of uranium. The Becquerel has now been formally adopted to quantify environmental levels of radioactivity. A Bq is defined as one disintegration per second (i.e., 1 Ci $= 3.7 \times 10^{10}$ Bq). It is instructive to note that a typical level of naturally occurring ^{226}Ra in soil is approximately 1 pCi/g, which corresponds to 1×10^{-12} g of ^{226}Ra per g of soil, and that a typical level of ^{137}Cs in soil due to weapons testing fallout is about 0.1 pCi/g, which corresponds to 1.1×10^{-15} g of Cs-137 per g of soil. At these extremely low mass concentrations, the potential chemical toxicity of radioisotopes is virtually nonexistent relative to the potential radiological toxicity. An important exception to this general rule is uranium, which can be both chemically and radiologically toxic because of its extremely long half-life.

Exposure to radioactive materials, in addition to being expressed in terms of intake quantities per unit time (e.g., Bq/d), is also expressed in terms of the amount of energy deposited in a unit mass of tissue per unit time due either to the decay of radioactive atoms that have been deposited within tissue (i.e., internal radiation exposure) or to the decay of radioactive atoms that are external to the exposed individual (external radiation exposure). One of the units that is commonly used to express the amount of energy deposited in an absorbing medium (referred to as the absorbed dose), such as tissue, is the rad. The rad is defined as 100 ergs per gram of tissue.[1] For example, it is not uncommon for the decay of a single atom to emit about 1 MeV or 1.6×10^{-6} erg of ionizing radiation. The amount of energy required to break a single chemical bond is about 30 to 40 eV, depending on the molecule (Morgan and Turner, 1973). Hence the disintegration of a single radioactive atom deposited in tissue can result in on the order of 10,000 ionizations. Theoretically a sufficient number of these ionizations can damage or kill a cell or result in chemical changes in biological molecules which can lead to a carcinogenic or mutagenic effect. Because of repair mechanisms, it is not certain whether there exists a dose or dose rate threshold below which no clinical effects of exposure to radiation are expressed. This is an area of active research and debate in the radiobiological and radiation protection sciences. In order to err on the safe side, radiation protection standards and the practice of health physics assume that biological damage is directly related to the amount of energy deposited in living tissue. Notwithstanding the uncertainties in the effects of radiation, it is convenient to express exposure to radiation in units corresponding to deposited energy per unit mass of living tissue (i.e., absorbed dose).

Some sources of radiation exposure are not due to the decay of radioactive atoms but originate from electronic devices, such as X-ray machines. In these cases the source of the radiation is always external to the exposed individual, and radiation exposures are often expressed in terms of the amount of energy deposited in air, namely Roentgens per second (R/s), named after the discoverer of X rays, Wilhelm Konrad Roentgen. As a general rule of thumb, a radiation field in air of 1 R (which is defined as 1 electrostatic unit per cm^3 of air at standard temperature and pressure, or 2.58×10^{-4} C/kg) is equivalent to 1 rad.

Throughout this chapter radiation exposure is expressed in units of rem (Roentgen equivalent man). In addition the expression is further qualified by the term "effective dose equivalent" (EDE). For the purpose of this chapter, the unit "rem/yr EDE" (or mrem/yr EDE) is used to normalize all exposures to the equivalent, in terms of potential adverse health consequences, of 1 rad (i.e., 100 erg/g of tissue) uniform whole-body exposure to either gamma or beta radiation. In this way it does not matter whether the exposures are caused by external or internal radiation, by alpha, beta, or gamma emitters, or by neutrons or if the energy of radioactive decay is deposited uniformly throughout the body or is limited to a given organ. No matter what the form of the exposures, the rem EDE allows the exposures to be intercompared on a potential health equivalent basis. The reader may notice that radiobiology and health physics publications also express the dose equivalent in units of the Sievert (Sv). The Sv = 100 rem, and it was adopted as a means for expressing dose equivalent in standard international (SI) units.

The units used to define the quantity of radioactive material and exposure to radiation and radioactive material have evolved and are undergoing continual refinement to more precisely characterize the interaction of radiation with matter and the biological effects of exposure to ionizing radiation. The International Commission on Radiation Units and Measurement (ICRU)[2] is the standard setting body that establishes the formal definition of radiation units. Brodsky (1978) provides a history of the evolution of radiation units.

SOURCES OF MAN-MADE RADIOACTIVITY AND RADIATION

The actual and/or potential sources of exposures to man-made radioactivity and ionizing radiation can be categorized according to eight sources of exposures, whether the

---

[1] Absorbed dose is also expressed in units of the Gray (Gy) = 1J/kg = 100 rad. This unit, as well as the Sievert (Sv), was developed as a means to express absorbed dose (and absorbed dose equivalent) in standard international (SI) units.

[2] ICRU is located at 7910 Woodmont Avenue, Suite 800, Bethesda, MD 20814-3095 (301-675-2652).

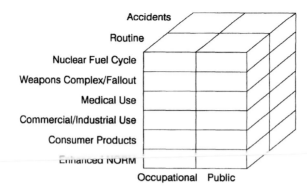

Figure 15-1 Sources and human-made radioactivity and radiation.

exposures occur as a result of normal or accident conditions associated with the source, and whether the persons receiving exposures are members of the general public or radiation workers (Fig. 15-1). In addition there is a consideration (or fourth dimension) of time, whereby the radiation exposures to workers and the public can and have changed over time and are projected to continue to change in the future.

Each source category can cause exposure to the people who work in the industries that are responsible for creating the sources of exposure. In all categories, with the possible exception of the category entitled sources of naturally occurring radioactive materials (enhanced NORM), these individuals are referred to as "radiation workers" and are subject to strict radiation protection controls. Each source category is also responsible, to varying degrees, for exposures to members of the general public. For each source category and for both radiation workers and members of the general public, radiation exposures occur as a result of normal operation of the facility or use of the sources of radioactivity, and also as a result of off-normal conditions and/or accidents.

NUCLEAR FUEL CYCLE

As reported by the Nuclear Regulatory Commission, approximately 22% of the electricity in the United States is being generated by 110 commercial nuclear power reactors in 32 states (NRC, 1997b). Although, for a variety of reasons, no new nuclear plants have been ordered since about the time of the accident at the Three Mile Island-2 site in 1979, there is increasing speculation that circumstances may favor a reconsideration of nuclear power as a viable source of electrical energy. Assuming no major changes in nuclear engineering technology in the immediate future, the light-water fuel cycle will probably continue to dominate the field and therefore generate much of the health-related concern for its potential as a source of radiation exposure for nuclear workers and the general public.

The nuclear fuel cycle (NFC), as discussed here, refers to the totality of those activities surrounding the central defining process of controlled nuclear fission with the ultimate goals of producing energy required for the generation of electricity (see Fig. 15-2). However, the nuclear fuel cycle as described here also applies to the production of radionuclides necessary for a variety of medical and commercial applications, for carrying out scientific research, for creating locomotive power for naval vessels, and for producing nuclear weapons for the military (Cochran and Tsoulfanidis, 1990).

At the outset, it should be noted that the designation "nuclear fuel cycle" may give the incorrect impression of a self-sustaining, closed-loop process. For the U.S. light-water

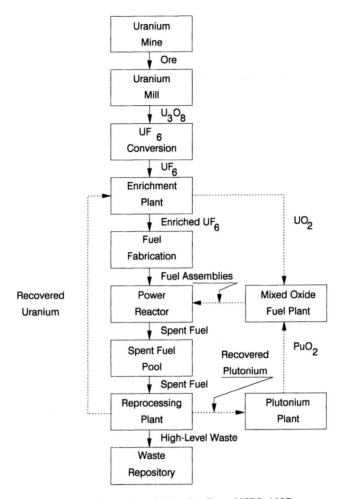

Figure 15-2 Nuclear fuel cycle. (From NCRP, 1987).

reactor program, where recovery of fissionable fuel from spent nuclear fuel elements, namely reprocessing and recycling, are not allowable options, the cycle is left "open." It becomes reasonable therefore to speak of each stage of the fuel cycle as part of "front and back ends" with the operating nuclear fission reactor providing the central focus for both fuel production and waste management planning.

This section briefly summarizes and reviews the various stages of the NFC in general terms, considering each aspect's potential to act as a source of exposure to ionizing radiation. (Each stage of the NFC has some potential for exposing populations to external radiation and to the possible uptake of radionuclides either directly or from related transportation and waste disposal activities.) Thus this review is not intended to be comprehensive in scope, and the reader is directed to the references cited for a more detailed accounting of any of the specific topics.

Exploration and Mining

After exploration for suitable mining areas of naturally high concentrations of uranium ore [for a variety of the most effective uranium exploration techniques (see DOE/NFC, 1990), the only concern noted for possible radiation exposure was the possibility of groundwater contamination resulting from "improperly plugged boreholes" (NCRP, 1987b)], the front end of the cycle begins with the extraction of the ore from the ground. Most often, this process takes place either relatively close to the original surface, namely open pit mining (usually within 120 m of the surface), or from deep within the ground. A third method of uranium mining, "in situ leaching" or solution mining, is gaining popularity as an alternative to underground mining (Cochran and Tsoulfanidis, 1990).

Deep underground hard-rock mining, in particular, is considered a significant potential radiation hazard (although to a far lesser extent at present than in the past when mine ventilation was minimal), primarily because of the inhalation of radon and its short-lived daughters, (decay products). The detrimental health effects to the lungs from this occupational exposure were recognized in the early 1940s (Hueper, 1942; Lorenz, 1944), but it was not until about 1957 (Holaday et al., 1957) that the increased incidence of lung cancer was definitively attributed to high levels of exposure to these particulate radionuclides (Fig. 15-3). Generally speaking, exposures of the nonoccupational public to radioactive emissions resulting from the underground mining of uranium are not considered to represent a significant risk (Blanchard et al., 1982).

Milling and Refining

After mining, the ore (usually containing on the average about $0.1-0.2\%$ U_3O_8 as disseminated pitchblende) is sent to a processing mill where it is first crushed and then ground. A concentration process is begun as part of the milling and refining stage in which uranium is selectively extracted, converted in chemical form, and dried. At the final stages of this process, the chemical composition of uranium is a complex mixture of uranium compounds including diuranates, uranyl sulfates, and U_3O_8, which in combination is generally designated as "yellowcake" (Momeni et al., 1979). The mixture is converted at a chemical refinery to almost pure U_3O_8. In these compounds, uranium still has the isotopic composition given in Table 15-1 for "natural uranium" (U_{nat}).

To define a source term for assessing the ecological and human exposures and doses associated with the releases from the drying and packaging operations, it is first necessary to establish the temporal variability of the release rates as well as the characterization of the effluent by particle size, density, transportability, and bioavailability.

At this stage of the fuel cycle, significant potential for exposure to radiation occurs to both workers and the general public. Occupationally radiation exposure can occur internally from radioisotopes deposited within the body or externally from one or more of the radionuclides of the uranium chain that may be present in radioactive equilibrium (i.e., in equal amounts to uranium activity) in the crushed ore, in concentrates, or in purified products. External exposures result primarily from the more penetrating γ rays, although energetic β^- particles from those nuclides closer to the body will also contribute to the external dose rate. Internal exposures result from the inhalation and/or ingestion of radionuclides, which then proceed to produce a radiological dose resulting from their radioactive decay, leading to energy absorption within specific tissues. The major difference between internal and external exposures is that, with internal exposures, there is the possibility of energy deposition at biologically sensitive sites by highly energetic and damaging α particles. Externally α particles cannot penetrate the dead layer of the skin.

The residual mill tailings are the major waste products that can enter the exposure pathways of the nonoccupational environment, primarily through incorporation into the food web (i.e., ingestion) and by particulate suspension and ^{222}Rn emission (i.e., inhalation). These tailings are comprised predominantly of silica compounds, such as quartz grains, feldspars, rock fragments, and a variety of interstitial clay minerals (NRC/ NAS, 1986), and radionuclides from the uranium decay chain. Of these nuclides, ^{232}Th,

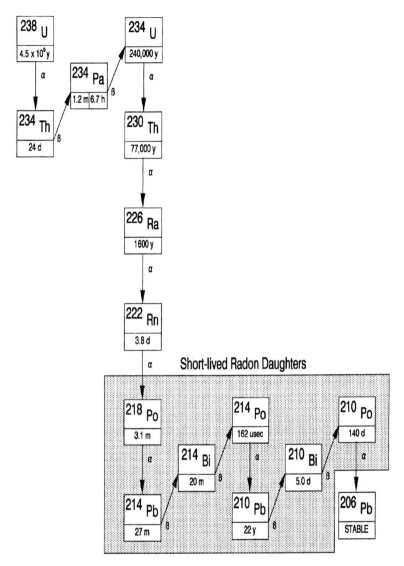

Figure 15-3   Principal decay scheme of the uranium series.

^{226}Ra, and the short-lived decay products of ^{222}Rn (Fig. 15-3) present the greatest risk of radiation exposure.

The most dramatic example of environmental contamination and population exposure to radiation as a result of the existence of mill tailings piles occurred in Grand Junction, Colorado, prior to 1966. Eisenbud and Gesell (1997) report that a number of the local residents of this town used the then readily available uranium mill tailings sands in home construction as backfill and foundations and in concrete mixes. Since the tailing pile sands contained significant concentrations of ^{226}Ra and its decay products, which were left behind after uranium was chemically extracted, a constant flux of ^{222}Rn was produced from whatever home structural material had incorporated the tailings. Consequently, in addition to higher than normal external γ ray exposures to the residents, the excessively elevated airborne concentrations of ^{222}Rn and its short-lived progeny created, in many of

TABLE 15-1 Uranium: Radiological Data

Nuclide	$T_{1/2}$	Series	Nuclide SA ($\mu Ci/mg$)	Natural Abundance (mass %)
^{233}U	1.62×10^5	Neptunium	9.48	—
^{234}U	2.47×10^5	Uranium	6.19	0.0055
^{235}U	7.10×10^8	Actinium	0.00214	0.7
^{238}U	4.50×10^9	Uranium	0.000333	99.3

For U_{nat}	Natural Abundance	SA ($\mu Ci/mg$)	$\mu Ci/mg$ of U_{nat}

Specific activity for U_{nat} and depleted uranium (DU) ($\mu Ci/mg$)

^{138}U	0.993	0.000333	3.31×10^{-4}
^{235}U	0.007	0.00214	0.14×10^{-4}
^{234}U	5.5E-5	6.19	3.40×10^{-4}
			$U_{nat} = 6.86 \times 10^{-4}$

For DU

^{138}U	0.997	0.000333	3.32×10^{-4}
^{235}U	0.003	0.00214	0.06×10^{-4}
^{234}U	3.4×10^{-5}	6.19	2.10×10^{-4}
			$DU = 5.48 \times 10^{-4}$

Nuclide	Activity (%)	
	U_{nat}	DU
^{138}U	48.25	61.18
^{235}U	2.19	1.18
^{234}U	49.56	38.70

Note: U_{nat}, natural uranium; DU, depleted uranium; SA, specific activity.

the homes, a significant risk of bronchial carcinoma from the inhalation of the radon progeny. The magnitude of the problem was greatly reduced by 1978, when more than 700 buildings were renovated at government expense (DOE, 1980).

Since mill tailings can represent a significant source of exposure to radionuclides, the Uranium Mill Tailings Radiation Control Act (UMTRCA) was enacted in 1978. The Act (1) directs the federal government to undertake the elimination of the hazards associated with abandoned inactive tailings piles and (2) clarifies and strengthens the authority of the NRC to insist on proper tailings management by its uranium mill licensees and those states that license such milling operations (NRC/NAS, 1986).

What is termed "uranium refining" is essentially the chemical conversion of the mill concentrates to either uranium metal or intermediate compounds such as UO_3 (orange oxide) or UF_4 (green salt). Once again, these operations have the potential for exposing workers internally to α-emitting uranium dusts and externally to β^- and γ radiations. Eisenbud and Gessel (1997) note that although uranium was released to the environment by the older refineries during World War II, today's more modern plants "are equipped with filtration equipment that effectively removes uranium dust," which, when properly maintained and operated, prevents any significant release to the environment.

Enrichment

The next stage in the process of producing usable nuclear fuel is the final chemical conversion of the refined yellowcake, using hydrofluoric acid and fluorine, to uranium hexafluoride (UF_6) gas. The UF_6 gas is then "enriched." The enrichment process increases the concentration of the fissile uranium isotope ^{235}U from the 0.72% level found in natural uranium to the 2% to 4% needed to sustain a fission reaction with slow neutrons in light-water power reactors and to greater than 90% in some production-type reactors for nuclear weapons manufacture. Since only small quantities of uranium hexafluoride escape to the air or are discharged as liquid waste in the enrichment process by gaseous diffusion, centrifugal techniques, or atomic vapor laser isotope separation (AVLIS), the potential for radiation exposure is considered minimal to both the plant worker and the general public (NCRP, 1987). Furthermore the stringent controls on emissions necessitated by the very high cost of enriched uranium and the antiproliferation safeguards imposed in the name of national security make the possibility of widespread environmental contamination from these plants unlikely (Eisenbud and Gesell, 1997).

Fuel Fabrication

The last step in the production of nuclear reactor fuel (Fig. 15-4) involves the chemical and physical conversion of enriched UF_6 to uranium dioxide UO_2 fuel pellets. The very limited potential for environmental exposure associated with this process is attributed to the minute quantities of radionuclides released to the environment as gaseous, liquid, and solid wastes.

Reactor Operation

Most commercial utility-operated nuclear power reactors in the United States are of the light-water variety in which the uranium fuel is enriched to about 3%, and the water serves as both coolant and moderator. Of the three major categories of radionuclides routinely produced during the normal operation of these reactors (i.e., fission products, actinides, and neutron activation products), fission products (primarily noble gases) are the principal radionuclides that are routinely released to the environment in any significant amount (BNL, 1995). Various federal and state agencies use an extremely effective and stringent system to control and regulate minimal allowable releases of radioactivity to the environment. On behalf of the NRC, Brookhaven National Laboratory publishes an annual report on the quantities of radioactive material released from nuclear power plants (BNL, 1995). These release estimates are used to derive the potential radiation doses to the general public living in the vicinity of the plants (PNL, 1995). In 1989 the EPA published a comprehensive assessment of the potential doses and risks associated with the routine atmospheric releases of radionuclides from nuclear facilities (EPA, 1989). The results revealed that the potential whole body radiation doses to the maximally exposed members of the public generally have been less than 1 mrem/yr (well within the radiation protection standards) and much lower than the variability in doses from natural sources of radiation.

The principal factors that account for the low exposures resulting from normal reactor operation are (1) a multiple barrier system that effectively limits the amounts of radionuclides leaving their points of origin; (2) effective treatment, namely processing technology, for removing activity prior to its release as effluent; and (3) the release into systems that guarantees large dilution factors and minimal environmental transport in both air and water before reaching unrestricted areas.

Estimates of dose have been derived from calculations of normal reactor effluent releases in conjunction with considerations of a variety of pathway parameters leading to ingestion from the food web, inhalation intakes, and / or external radiation exposures. All in all, normal reactor operation and its associated effluent represent the lowest potential for radiation exposure of any of the fuel cycle phases. It has been postulated by Momeni et al. (1979), based on historical experience and estimates from theoretical modeling, that future

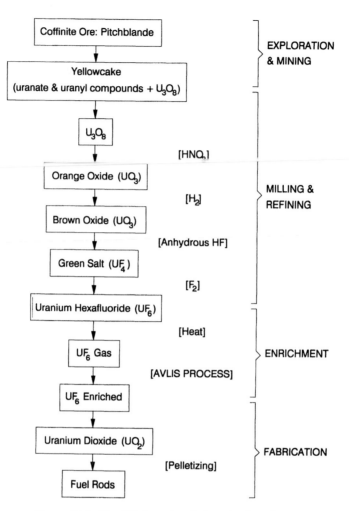

Figure 15-4   Simplified uranium fuel production scheme.

nuclear plants will not produce annual offsite total body exposures of more than 0.05 mSv (5 mrem) to the maximally exposed individual and about 0.02 person-Sv (2 person-rem) to the population within 80 km. Natural background radiation in the United States is currently given as 3.0 mSv / (300 mrem / yr) EDE, with the dose caused by the inhalation of radon and its short-lived decay products accounting for about two-thirds of this total and most of the variability (NCRP, 1987b,c).

It is often assumed that radiation exposures to the general public as a result of any type of reactor accident are always of significant consequence and perhaps even potentially disastrous. However, the extremely low probability of the occurrence of a serious nuclear accident in this country (NRC, 1989), and the experience gained from the Three Mile Island accident, indicate that in terms of the overall population's radiation exposure, reactor accidents have not been as catastrophic as originally feared. No reactor accident in this country has caused quantities of radioactive material to be released that resulted in significant population exposures. The accident that occurred at the Three Mile Island-2 plant in 1979 resulted in the partial destruction of the reactor core. However, the designed safety features prevented all but a very small fraction of the core inventory of radionuclides from escaping into the environment. Furthermore the highest doses to individuals living near the site were generally less than the average natural radiation dose received annually in the United States (Gerusky, 1981).

The Chernobyl accident, at a reactor lacking a containment structure, demonstrates that a serious reactor accident can be disastrous. The Chernobyl-4 reactor accident, which occurred in the former Soviet Union on April 26, 1986, released essentially all of its noble gases, 60% of its radioiodines, 40% of its radiocesium, 10% of its radiotellurium, and about 1% or less of the more refractory radioactive elements (Gudiksen et al., 1989). The geographical and temporal patterns of exposures, the exposure pathways, and the actual and potential health consequences of the accident are extremely complex. The "The Chernobyl Papers" edited by S. E. Merwin and M. I., Balonov (Research Enterprise Publishing Segment, Richland, Washington, 1993) and Eisenbud and Gesell (1997) provide an overview of the accident and its consequences.

Eisenbud and Gesell divide the impacts of the accident into five geographical locations, and summarize the impacts, as follows:

1. On-site personnel
2. Environs within 30 km
3. European portion of the USSR beyond 30 km from the accident
4. European countries outside the USSR
5. North America and Asia

Approximately 1000 cases of acute radiation poisoning occurred, including 28 early deaths, where doses were as high as 1600 rad. During the first year, approximately 200,000 workers were employed in the cleanup. These individuals were estimated to receive an average dose of 20 rem.

The approximately 45,000 persons within 3 km of the reactor, in the town of Pripyat, were exposed to an external radiation field of about 500 to 1500 mR/h prior to being evacuated. Within 10 days, about 135,000 persons were evacuated within a 30 km radius of the accident. The mean whole body dose to the evacuees was estimated to be 1.5 rem. The thyroid doses were estimated to be 100 rem for children and 70 rem for adults.

Beyond 30 km, the principal sources of exposure were ^{137}Cs and radioiodine deposited on the ground and in food. Estimates of the doses to individuals and the collective doses in different regions of the former Soviet Union and Europe are geographically and radioecologically complex, and are the subject of numerous reports, peer-reviewed publications, workshops, and symposia. In North America and Asia the exposures were small because the accident did not contribute to stratospheric fallout.

High-Level Nuclear Waste: Production and Management

When neutrons are captured, uranium atoms are, by virtue of their resulting nuclear instability, split or fissioned into atoms of lower atomic number and mass. The energy generated by the fission process is quantified by the term "burnup," which has units expressed as "megawatt-days per metric ton of fuel." After enough ^{235}U has been so fissioned, "spent" fuel assemblies must be replaced; that is the reactor is refueled. These spent fuel rod assemblies containing fission products, actinides, and other activation products are designated in toto as high-level waste (HLW) (DOE, 1996).

Typically about one-third of the fuel (i.e., uranium enriched to about 3%) of a pressurized water reactor (PWR) and one-fourth of that for a boiling water reactor (BWR) is replaced after every 12 to 18 months of reactor operation. The spent fuel is then stored (usually on site at the present time) under water for cooling and to allow for the initial decay of the relatively short-lived nuclides prior to the fuel rods being shipped to projected storage sites. Under the Nuclear Waste Policy Act of 1982 (Public Law 97-425), the DOE has entered into contracts with all utilities operating nuclear power plants to accept their spent fuel for disposal by 1998. The DOE has missed this deadline. Since these storage sites (the term "waste disposal site" gives an unrealistic impression of permanence) are presently at the investigation and/or construction stage, on-site storage has had to be developed to accommodate present and future generations of spent fuel. As of 1995, 30,000 metric tons of spent fuel is stored at commercial nuclear power reactors. By the year 2005, this amount is expected to increase to 52,000 metric tons (NRC, 1997b).

Engineering characteristics of proposed geological repositories are not described in this chapter, other than to note that design specifications for HLW storage have been set so as to ensure waste isolation for exceedingly long periods of time (greater than 10,000 years after storage), with the goal of preventing accidental fission product release to biosphere transport processes. Regulatory requirements, which are being developed by the EPA in accordance with the Energy Policy Act of 1992, will limit the dose to the general public from HLW received and stored in deep geological repositories to a few mrem/yr to no more than a few tens of mrem/yr. According to the NCRP, "current technology appears to be capable of maintaining doses to a fraction of this requirement" (NCRP, 1987).

The potential for radiation exposure from the storage of HLW results primarily from the occupational handling and preliminary on-site storage of the spent fuel. Radionuclide emissions to the environment as a result of on-site storage (water cooling and shielding) would occur to the air. However, such releases are not expected to result in increases in the measurable level of radiation exposure at unrestricted areas. Worst-case scenarios involving projected breaches in such waste repositories have been modeled by the DOE, and resulting doses to the "maximum individual" have been calculated (DOE, 1979, 1983).

Low-Level Nuclear Waste

As part of routine reactor operation, low-level radioactive waste (LLW) is generated in the form of filters, solidified evaporator bottom, spent resin, and slightly contaminated materials (e.g., used work clothing, papers, gloves, and tools). The LLW is disposed of by burial at land sites designated for this level of activity. In 1995, 690,000 cubic feet of LLW was buried, of which 38% was from reactor operations (NRC, 1997b). Since the geological and hydrological criteria for LLW disposal sites are not as stringent as are those for HLW, there has been considerable controversy about their long-term effects on neighboring residential ground water supplies. The EPA has evaluated the potential doses to members of the general public in the vicinity of a licensed low-level radioactive waste disposal facility and has determined that the doses would be a very small fraction of the radiation protection standards (EPA, 1988e).

Reprocessing

Reprocessing is the chemical extraction and recovery of residual and newly formed fissile material, primarily ^{235}U and ^{239}Pu, from spent reactor fuel for possible recycling, thereby "closing" the nuclear fuel cycle.

There has been only one reprocessing operation for commercial power reactor fuel in the United States, the Nuclear Fuel Services Plant in West Valley, New York, which was closed in 1972. Since there is no commercial reprocessing plant currently operating within the United States excluding those reprocessing nuclear fuels from naval propulsion and special government research and test reactors, estimates of public exposures do not exist except as projected models (NCRP, 1987). Fuel reprocessing is not projected to be a viable component of the fuel cycle in the United States at any time in the foreseeable future.

Since reprocessing, as an alternative to permanent or retrievable storage, is not an allowable option for the commercial United States fuel cycle at this time, it is not considered here as a source of exposure. It is interesting to note, however, that in considering the possibilities of exposure, the regulation preventing reprocessing presents a trade-off of risks between those exposures arising from the need for new uranium mining and enrichment and those exposures from the reprocessing operation itself. An additional risk also results from a decrease in the security of being able to control weapons-grade nuclear material.

Transportation

Routine truck shipments of uranium concentrates are not, under ordinary circumstances, associated with more than negligible radiation exposures to the driver and the general public. It has been reported, for example, that exposure rates in the truck cab and two feet from a loaded trailer rarely reach levels greater than $5 \mu Sv/h$ (0.5 mR/h) (Miller and Scott, 1981). It is conceivable, however, that exposure problems could result after a vehicle accident that causes spillage of the truck contents.

Because of their composition and characteristically greater activity levels, transport of spent fuel (HLW) and other high-level waste could present considerably greater risks of exposure than spills from the transport of low-specific-activity material from the front end of the NFC.

Decommissioning and Decontamination

An additional aspect of the NFC that needs consideration for future exposure prediction is reactor decommissioning. Undoubtedly, many of the older nuclear power plants will be reaching their useful lifetimes within the next 10 to 20 years, and the dismantling of these sites is bound to produce some risk of exposure to radionuclides. The NRC is currently overseeing the decommissioning of 15 nuclear power reactors. In addition the NRC's Site Decommissioning Management Plan lists 28 sites that require special attention to resolve decommissioning policy and regulatory issues. To facilitate decommissioning and license termination, the NRC has issued its final rule on radiological criteria for license termination. The rule requires, in part, that the applicant for a license termination and release of the property for unrestricted use must demonstrate that the radiation exposures associated with the free release of the property would not exceed 25 mrem/yr EDE for all pathways combined, and that the exposures will be as low as reasonably achievable (FR, vol. 62, no. 139, 7/21/97). The U.S. Environmental Protection Agency (EPA) may also develop public health radiation protection criteria for residual radioactivity following cleanup of contaminated lands and facilities. The purpose of such criteria is to assure protection of public health and the environment after nuclear facilities are shut down and decommissioned (Health Physics Society, 1986; EPA, 1993c).

Discussion of Radiation Doses from the Nuclear Fuel Cycle

The nuclear fuel cycle, as defined in this chapter, has been described for the most prevalent commercial fission reactors in the United States namely light-water PWR and BWR facilities. It has also been noted that nuclear energy generates about 20% of the electricity in this country and more than 50% of the electricity production in New England and some parts of the Midwest. Although this is not as high as it is in some European countries (e.g., 74.6% for France, 60.7% for Belgium, and 41.6% for Switzerland), it is a clear indication that nuclear energy continues to exist and can make an even more significant contribution to the future generation of energy in this country. It is essential that the nuclear fuel cycle be considered as a source of possible radiation exposure to U.S. workers and the general public.

Exposures to Radiation Workers   The U.S. Nuclear Regulatory Commission publishes an annual report summarizing the occupational radiation exposure at commercial nuclear power reactors and other facilities (NRC, 1997). Table 15-2 summarizes these exposures for major components of the NFS. The collective exposures to workers has been about 25,000 person rem/yr. Using a risk coefficient of 5×10^{-4} fatal cancers per rem (see the discussion of risk coefficients at the end of this chapter), these exposures may be associated with approximately 10 fatal cancers per year in a worker population of about 150,000 people. This theoretical risk may be compared to the risk of fatal industrial accidents with an overall average of 5 fatalities per 100,000 workers in 1993, and a range of 2 for business services to 155 for fisherman per 100,000 workers in 1993 (DOL, 1995). Hence the theoretical risk of worker fatalities due to radiation exposures at commercial nuclear power plants is comparable to the risks of industrial accidents. Bear in mind that the radiation risks are based on conservative theoretical models relating radiation exposure to risk, while the latter risks are based on actuarial data, namely real verifiable risks.

Exposures to the General Public   Table 15-3, which is taken from a review of the fuel cycle in this country as performed by the National Council on Radiation Protection and Measurements (NCRP, 1987), indicates that based on the radioactive effluents produced by the various stages of the fuel cycle activities, the milling operation is responsible for the greatest potential exposure-dose to regional populations. When expressed on the basis of dose to the maximally exposed individual as a result of airborne radioactive effluent from fuel cycle facilities (Table 15-4), the mining operations are responsible for the highest estimated doses of all NFC stages. In all cases, however, reactor operation represents only a small fraction of the total estimated radiation dose to either an individual worker or the general population. The collective dose to the general public from all commercial reactor operations in 1991 was 88 person rem (PNL, 1995).

TABLE 15-2   Occupational Exposures from Selected Nuclear Fuel Cycle Facilities for 1993 to 1995

Fuel Cycle Category	Calendar Year	Number of monitored Individuals	Number of Workers with Measurable Dose	Collective Dose (person rem)	Average Measurable Dose (rem)
Low-level waste	1993	432	76	21	0.27
disposal	1994	202	83	22	0.27
	1995	212	56	8	0.15
Independent	1993	135	52	14	0.26
spent fuel	1994	158	89	42	0.47
storage	1995	104	49	51	1.04
Fuel fabrication	1993	9649	2611	339	0.13
and processing	1994	3596	2847	1147	0.40
	1995	4106	2959	1217	0.41
Commercial	1993	169,862	86,187	26,365	0.31
light-water	1994	142,707	73,780	21,695	0.29
reactors	1995	133,066	70,986	21,674	0.31
Total	1993			26,739	
	1994			22,906	
	1995			22,950	

Source: NRC (1997).

TABLE 15-3 Summary of Collective Effective Dose Equivalents to Regional Populations Caused by Radioactive Effluents from Fuel Cycle Facilities

Facility	Collective Effective Dose Equivalent (person rem / yr)	Basis of Estimate
Mining		
Open pit—air	1.0	Model mine
Open pit—water	0.2	
Underground—air	10	
Underground—water	21	
Milling	62	Airborne effluent from model mill
Conversion		
Wet	0.4	Plant airborne effluent in 1980
Dry	2.9	
Enrichment	0.002–0.4	3 plants, airborne effluents in 1981
Fabrication	0.01–0.7	7 plants, airborne effluents in 1980
Reactor		
Air	0.003–13	47 plants in 1980
water	0–40	47 plants in 1980
Low-level waste storage	<4	Maxey Flats, estimate

Source: NCRP (1987)

NUCLEAR WEAPONS COMPLEX

The Nuclear Weapons Complex is an industrial complex consisting of a collection of enormous factories devoted primarily to research, development, and production of nuclear weapons. It has resulted in a legacy of radioactive contamination and radiation exposure to radiation workers and the general public that began in the 1940s and continues today. In many respects the nuclear weapons production process is similar to the nuclear fuel cycle; it involves the mining and milling of uranium, uranium enrichment, fuel fabrication, operation of production reactors, and the management of spent fuel, high-level waste, and low-level waste. Some of the important differences between the commercial nuclear fuel cycle and weapons production include the following:

1. The weapons production program continued throughout the cold war, and national security was an important consideration in the management of the program.
2. The program required a large investment in research and development, which greatly exacerbated the potential for worker exposure and environmental contamination.
3. By its very nature, weapons production is associated with the production of large quantities of very long-lived transuranic wastes, which must be isolated from the accessible environment virtually indefinitely.
4. The program required weapons testing, discussed in the next section, which resulted in elevated levels of radiation exposure near the test sites and globally as a result of global fallout, traces of which are still detectable in the environment.
5. Our knowledge of the fate and effects of radioactivity was limited until the program matured, which, in retrospect, resulted in elevated exposures and environmental contamination that could have been minimized or avoided.

TABLE 15-4 Summary of Radiation Doses to the Maximally Exposed Individual Caused by Airborne Radioactive Effluents from Fuel Cycle Facilities

Facility	Effective Dose Equivalent (mrem/yr)	Basis of Estimate
Mining		
Open pit	26	Model mine
Underground	61	Model mine
Milling	0.4 – 200	8 typical mills
Conversion		
Wet	0.8	Plant, calculation
Dry	3.2	Plant, calculation
Enrichment	< 0.1 – 0.4	All 3 plants
Fabrication	< 0.1 – 0.7	All 7 plants
Reactor		
PWR	0.6	Model reactor
BWR	0.1	Model reactor
Low-level waste storage	< 1	Maxey Flats, estimate
Transportation	—	Not reported

Source: NCRP (1987).

With the end of the cold war, an enormous amount of information has become available characterizing the nature and extent of the radioactive contamination at the weapons complex sites and the levels of exposure that have been experienced by both workers and members of the general public as a result of this legacy. Prior to the end of the cold war, most of this information was classified. A better understanding of the legacy is also unfolding as a result of efforts to clean up and release many of these sites for other uses and to better understand past exposures of radiation workers and the general public. Some of the core documents that capture the expanse of this legacy are as follows:

> *Complex Cleanup — The Environmental Legacy of Nuclear Weapons Production*, Congress of the United States, Office of Technology Assessment, 1991.
>
> *Closing the Circle on Splitting of the Atom—The Environmental Legacy of Nuclear Weapons Production in the United States and What the Department of Energy Is Doing about It*, U.S. Department of Energy, Office of Environmental Management, 1996.
>
> *Estimating the Cold War Mortgage—The 1995 Baseline Environmental Management Report*, U.S. Department of Energy, Office of Environmental Management, March 1995.
>
> *Final waste management programmatic environmental impact statement for managing treatment, storage, and disposal of radioactive and hazardous waste*, U.S. Department of Energy, Office of Environmental Management, DOE/EIS-0200-F, May 1997.

Extent of Environmental Contamination from the Weapons Complex

The weapons complex, depicted in Figure 15-5, consists of 137 Department of Energy (DOE) sites in 33 states and 1 territory. The DOE publishes an annual report, *Environmental Management* (DOE, 1996b), which provides an overview of the status of environmental restoration and waste management for these sites. Also DOE publishes an

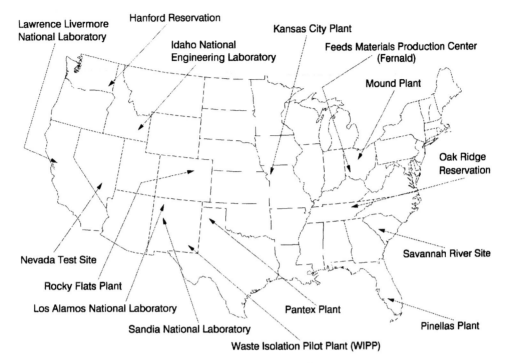

Figure 15-5 Weapons complex.

annual report; the most recent, entitled *Integrated Data Base—1995: U.S. Spent Fuel and Radioactive Waste Inventories, Projections, and Characteristics* (DOE, 1996), describes the quantities of different types of waste attributable to the complex. Table 15-5 presents the projected cumulative inventories of radioactive waste at the DOE complex as of December 31, 1995.

The final disposition of SNF, HLW, LLW, and TRU waste is to isolate the waste from the environment accessible to humans through the use of carefully sited and highly engineered waste isolation systems, which will be effective for as long as the sources of the waste are potentially hazardous. The final disposition of the very large volumes of very low level structure waste is in question at this time because it is not known whether it is in the best interest of public health and safety and the environment to

1. Excavate these large volumes of soil and other bulk material for shipment and disposal at specially sited and designed facilities or at landfills
2. Stabilize the waste in place
3. Establish institutional controls limiting access to the material, or
4. Do nothing to limit exposure of the public, as may be appropriate for extremely low levels of contamination, such as soil contaminated by weapons testing fallout.

The Environmental Protection Agency is studying this issue (EPA, 1994).

Past, Present, and Future Occupational Exposures Attributable to the Weapons Complex and Its Legacy

The Department of Energy periodically prepares a report entitled "DOE Occupational Radiation Exposure." The most recent report is on the World Wide Web and covers the

TABLE 15-5 Types and Quantities of Radioactive Wastes Associated with DOE Weapons Complex and R&D Facilities

Category of Radioactive Waste	Definition	Cumulative Quantities Projected through 2035
Spent nuclear fuel (SNF)	Irradiated fuel discharged from a nuclear reactor.	2,721.56 metric tons heavy metal (MTHM). Information on Curie inventory not available.
High-level waste (HLW)	Waste generated by the chemical reprocessing of spent research and production reactor fuel, irradiated targets, and naval propulsion fuel.	18,948 m^3 of HLW stored as glass in canisters. Peak radionuclide inventory of 425.75 million curies in year 2026.
Low-level waste (LLW)	Radioactive waste not classified as high-level waste, transuranic waste, spent nuclear fuel, or byproduct material (e.g., not uranium or thorium tailings and waste).	5.5 million m^3 projected to be disposed through 2030. 1.55 million Ci inventory in 1995.
Transuranic waste (TRU waste)	Waste containing elements with atomic numbers greater than 92 and half-lives greater than 20 years, in concentrations greater than 100 nCi/g of alpha-emitting isotopes	1.46E5 m^3 of as generated retrievably stored waste (does not include irretrievable TRU waste buried prior to the early 1970s).
Environmental restoration waste	Very large volumes of bulk material containing low levels of radioactivity and which will be generated during the environmental restoration of the sites. Considered a type of LLW. Wastes that are associated with in situ management, where the material is not removed from its location, are not included.	43 million m^3
Large volumes of very low levels of contaminated soil	Soil at DOE sites that contains very low levels of radioactivity and may not be excavated but left in place, perhaps with institutional controls. There may be some overlap with environmental restoration waste.	10^7 to 10^8 $m^{3\ a}$

Source: DOE (1996) except where otherwise indicated.

[a] Estimates of the volume of contaminated soil at DOE sites are provided in a draft EPA report entitled "Radiation Site Cleanup Regulations: Technical Support Document for the Development of Radionuclide Cleanup Levels for Soil," EPA 402-R-96-011, September 1994. This report is part of the docket for EPA's planned cleanup rule (40 CFR 196). Copies of the report are available from EPA Office of Radiation and Indoor Air.

TABLE 15-6   Individual and Collective Doses Received by DOE Employees, Contractors, and Subcontractors

Dose Ranges (rem)	1990	1991	1992	1993	1994
< measurable	71,991	88,444	94,297	102,993	91,121
measurable to <0.1	29,318	25,319	23,896	20,181	21,511
0.1–0.25	3921	3752	3581	2474	2437
0.25–0.5	1683	1447	1252	1013	934
0.5–0.75	566	381	346	195	329
0.75–1	292	187	165	93	99
1–5	289	235	169	89	80
5–10	4	3	4	2	
>10	1	2	1	2	
Total monitored	108,065	119,770	123,711	127,042	116,511
Number with measurable dose	36,074	31,326	29,414	24,049	25,390
% with measurable dose	33	26	24	19	22
Collective dose (person rem)	3,052	2,574	2,295	1,629	1,643
Average measurable dose (rem)	0.085	0.082	0.078	0.068	0.065

Source: From Exhibit 3–4 of DOE (1994).

period from 1992 to 1994. The following table presents the individual and collective doses to DOE workers, contractors, and subcontractors.

As a point of comparison, in 1980, a time when the weapons complex was immersed in cold war activities, there were 40,411 DOE workers, contractors and subcontractors, with detectable levels of radiation exposure. The mean annual individual dose in that population was 160 mrem (EPA, 1984). This corresponds to a collective dose of about 5000 person rem. These doses are relatively small in comparison to the radiation protection standard of 5000 mrem/yr for radiation workers (DOE Order 5480.1A at that time) and the fact that the average member of the general public receives about 360 mrem/yr from exposure to natural background radiation and 40 mrem/yr from diagnostic X-ray examinations (NCRP, 1987b).

Notwithstanding these relatively low overall occupational exposures, it is now believed that there are subgroups within the worker population that may have experienced relatively high levels of exposure. For example, Wiggs et al. (1991) reports on workers at the Mound facility that received elevated internal exposure from Po-210 exceeding 100 rem. The National Institute for Occupational Health and Safety (NIOSH) is investigating these sources of exposures.

Past, Present, and Future Public Exposures Attributable to the Weapons Complex and Its Legacy

Exposures of the general public in the past from weapons complex facilities include exposures associated with routine airborne emissions and episodic events. Because of the size of the DOE facilities, the off-site exposures to the public from routine operations have been small. For example, a compilation of exposure data from airborne emissions for 27 DOE facilities in 1986 revealed organ doses ranging from a fraction of a mrem/yr to a maximum of 25 mrem/yr. The collective organ doses ranged from less than 1 person rem/yr to a maximum of 670 person rem/yr (EPA, 1989).

Notwithstanding these relatively low doses (as compared to natural background and the radiation protection standards) to the members of the public living in the vicinity of DOE facilities, there is increasing concern that many of the weapons complex facilities have had relatively large episodic releases that resulted in significantly elevated exposures of the nearby populations (Miller and Smith, 1996). In response to this concern, the DOE and, more recently the Centers for Disease Control and Prevention (CDC), have implemented several environmental dose reconstruction studies, including dose reconstructions in the vicinity of the Feed Materials Production Center in Fernald, Ohio (Meyer et al., 1996), the Marshall Islands (Simon and Graham, 1996), Oak Ridge National Laboratory (Widner et al., 1996), the Nevada Test Site (Whicker et al., 1996), Rocky Flats (Mongan et al., 1996), and Hanford (Shipler et al., 1996). These dose reconstructions are being performed to help determine whether follow-up epidemiologic studies or other public health activities should be undertaken.

The current exposures to the general public from the weapons complex are small primarily because (1) the physical size of the sites places the public at large distances from the sources of emissions; (2) most of the sites are located in remote areas; and (3) most of the cold war research, development, and production activities have ceased. Each year, each site issues an annual environmental report that presents estimates of the radiation doses to members of the public. For example, each year the Westinghouse Savannah River Company (WSRC) publishes "Savannah River Site—Environmental Report." These annual reports present estimates of releases of radioactivity to the environment, the results of environmental radiological surveillance programs, and estimates of the doses to members of the general public. In the latest annual report for 1996, the WSRC estimated that the dose to the hypothetical maximally exposed member of the public was 0.19 mrem/yr (WSRC, 1997).

Notwithstanding these small doses, there is concern that existing inventories of radioactive material could be inadvertently released or that contamination that has entered the groundwater on site could eventually migrate to wells off site and expose large populations to elevated levels of radioactivity. In addition there is an interest to restore these sites and put them to more productive use. In order to address these concerns, the DOE's Environmental Management program has been established, and funded at a level of about $6 billion per year, to address immediate, urgent risks to human health and the environment and to manage long-term contamination and safety threats. Each site has established a 10-year plan to accomplish its environmental restoration and waste management objectives. These plans are described in detail in an annual DOE report, the most recent of which is "Environmental Management—Progress and Plans of the Environmental Management Program, November 1996, DOE/EM-0317 (DOE, 1996b).

Because of the complex nature of this Environmental Restoration and Waste Management (EM) program, there is concern that decision making will not address the risks to workers, the public, and the environment in a comprehensive, defensible, and consistent manner, which takes into consideration the life-cycle costs and benefits and interrelationships among the various planned EM activities. To address this issue, the DOE is attempting to incorporate risk-based decision making into all plans and budget allocations (DOE, 1995).

LOCAL, TROPOSPHERIC AND GLOBAL FALLOUT

Between 1945 and 1980, 520 atmospheric weapons tests were carried out with a total yield of 545 megatons (MT) equivalent of TNT. The tests were conducted by the United States, the USSR, the United Kingdom, France, and China. These tests introduced radioactive debris into the atmosphere, which resulted in local, tropospheric, and global fallout. Local fallout, which contributed about 12% of the total radioactive fallout, was comprised of relatively large particles that were deposited in the immediate vicinity of the tests and within a few hours following the tests. Tropospheric fallout, which contributed to about

10% of the total fallout, consisted of smaller particles of radioactive debris that was introduced into the troposphere, which extends from ground level to height of about 10 km. Tropospheric fallout occurred within days following the tests and in bands extending tens to hundreds to over 1000 miles downwind in the direction of the prevailing winds (depending on the yield of the device, the elevation of the test, and the prevailing meteorological conditions) and within the latitudes around those at which the tests were conducted. Stratospheric fallout, which contributed about 78% of the total fallout, originated from radioactive debris that was injected into the stratosphere, which extends from a height of about 10 to 30 km. Weapons tests with yields exceeding about 100 kilotons have sufficient energy to inject radioactive debris into the stratosphere. Debris that is introduced into the stratosphere is deposited globally over several months following the detonation. (Eisenbud and Gesell, 1997; UNSCEAR, 1993)

Retrospective dose reconstruction studies have attempted to reconstruct the radiation doses to members of the public living in the vicinity of the Nevada Test Site (Whicker et al., 1996; Thompson and McArthur, 1996) and the Marshall Islands (Simon and Graham, 1996) at the time of, and subsequent to, the tests. The dose reconstruction efforts for both the Marshall Islands and Nevada Test Site make use of radiological surveillance data, meteorological data, land use and demography data, and mathematical models to reconstruct the exposures to members of the nearby populations at the time of the tests and for extended periods following the tests. In addition follow-up epidemiological investigations have attempted to discern a statistically significant increase in adverse health effects in the exposed populations.

A total of 66 tests were conducted in the Bikini and Enewetak Atolls in the Republic of the Marshall Islands (RMI). A definitive reconstruction of the historical internal and external radiation doses to the RMI populace due to fallout has not been published because of the complexity of the dose reconstruction. However, assessments of the doses to individual populations from selected important tests and exposure pathways have been published, along with medical follow-up studies. For example, Cronkite et al. (1997) report on the accidental exposures and the medical follow-up for the Bravo test, which resulted in very high exposures (over 100 rem) to navy personnel and Marshallese inhabitants. These individuals experienced varying degrees of skin burns and symptoms of acute radiation exposure. Latent effects of radiation exposure were also subsequently observed in the exposed populations. The effects included thyroid dysfunction and thyroid cancer. These and other studies are described in the July 1997 issue of Health Physics, which is dedicated to providing an overview of the RMI studies performed to date. In addition the predicted distribution of doses among adult women inhabiting Rongelap Island in 1995 have been reported. The projected doses range up to 200 mrem/yr, with a median between 75 and 100 mrem/yr effective dose equivalent (Simon and Graham, 1996). The purpose of the study was to evaluate the degree to which resettlement of Rongelap Island could result in radiation exposures that exceed the dose action level of 100 mrem/yr above natural background.

An enormous body of literature exists on the environmental radiation exposures from nuclear testing at the Nevada Test Site. The November 1990 issue of Health Physics is dedicated to this subject. The October 1996 issue of Health Physics provides several papers on this subject, and in December 1996 a comprehensive report was published by the University of Nevada, Las Vegas, entitled "Preliminary Risk Assessment DOE Sites in Nevada." Estimates of the time integrated unshielded exposure at 34 locations in the vicinity of the tests range from 0.1 to 23.2 R. (Thompson and McArthur, 1996). Follow-up epidemiologic studies are currently underway (Simon et al., 1995; Till et al., 1995).

Global fallout due to weapons testing has resulted in slightly elevated exposures above background to very large populations located primarily in the 40° to 50° latitude band in the Northern and Southern hemispheres. The time-integrated effective dose from global fallout is estimated to be 370 mrem, and the collective dose is estimated to be 3×10^9 person rem (UNSCEAR, 1993). These values can be placed into perspective, considering that everyone receives approximately 300 mrem/yr EDE from natural background radiation.

In an article in the *Washington Post* dated August 2, 1997, the National Cancer Institute announced the results of a study that revealed that the average cumulative thyroid exposure for all Americans from radioactive iodine in weapons testing fallout was about 2 rads, and more heavily affected areas experienced thyroid doses ranging from 9 to 15 rad. The NCI report estimates that between that 10,000 and 75,000 Americans may develop thyroid cancer during their lifetime because, as children, they were exposed to radioactive iodine fallout from nuclear weapons tests. Notwithstanding these projections, which are based on fallout measurements and theoretical mathematical models which relate radiation exposure to cancer risk, epidemiological investigations were not able to establish an empirically based correlation between areas with predicted high radioiodine exposures and areas with elevated rates of thyroid cancer. These relationships are difficult to establish because predicted increases in the incidence of thyroid cancers are obscured by the large and variable normal incidence of thyroid cancer relative to the predicted effects.

MEDICAL EXPOSURES

The use of radioactive materials, radiation sources, and X-ray machines for medical purposes results in the exposure of the patients under the physicians care, the physicians and medical technicians that administer the care, and, to a limited degree, members of the public exposed to the radioactive waste products generated as a result of medical treatment and to nuclear medicine patients.

Exposure of Patients

NCRP (1989) and UNSCEAR (1993) present overviews of the radiation exposures associated with the diagnostic and therapeutic use of radiation and radioactive materials. The diagnostic use of radiation includes primarily medical and dental X rays and the diagnostic use of radiopharmaceuticals. The therapeutic use of radiation and radioactive materials includes primarily teletherapy, brachytherapy, and the therapeutic use of radiopharmaceuticals. Teletherapy is the use of strong, highly directed external sources of radiation, such as ^{60}Co units, to destroy deep-seated tumors. Brachytherapy is the use of sealed radioactive sources inserted into the body or placed on the surface of the skin to destroy tumors. Therapeutic nuclear medicine is the internal administration of radiopharmaceuticals, such as ^{131}I, to treat various diseases. Diagnostic X rays are the predominate contributor to the collective dose to the general public due to the medical uses of radiation.

UNSCEAR 1993 estimates that there were approximately 800 medical diagnostic X-ray examinations and 402 dental X-ray examinations per year per 1000 people in the United States from 1986 to 1990. The radiation dose per examination varied widely depending on the type of examination. For example, the effective dose equivalent for medical diagnostic examinations ranged from 7 mrem for chest radiography to 460 mrem for lower GI tract examinations. The effective dose equivalent from dental X-ray examinations is relatively small, about 3 mrem per examination. In the United States, the average effective dose equivalent is about 50 mrem per medical (nondental) examination and about 40 mrem/yr per capita. Worldwide, the total collective dose associated with medical X-ray examinations is 1.6×10^8 person rem/yr.

The number of nuclear medicine examination in countries with advanced medical care programs is estimated to be 16.4 per 1000 people, with an average effective dose per examination of 570 mrem, which is about 10 times higher than the average dose per X-ray examination. However, because of the lower frequency of use, the average annual dose per person from nuclear medicine examinations in advanced health care nations is 9.4 mrem (UNSCEAR, 1993).

In countries with advanced health care programs, the frequency of radiotherapy treatments by teletherapy and brachytherapy is estimated to be 2.4 per 1000 people. The doses to individual organs and localized tissues are extremely high (in excess of 1000 rem), and no attempt is made here to estimate the effective dose equivalent per treatment. The worldwide collective dose associated with the therapeutic use of radiation and radioactive materials is estimated to be 1.5×10^8 person rem/yr, or about 80% of the collective doses associated with the diagnostic use of radiation (UNSCEAR, 1993).

NCRP Report No. 100 (NCRP, 1989) reports on exposure of the U.S. population from diagnostic medical radiation and updates some of the information provided in the 1980 survey. The report concludes that the annual per capita effective dose equivalent to the U.S. population from diagnostic X rays is 40 mrem, and that from diagnostic nuclear medicine is 14 mrem, for a total of 54 mrem EDE.

UNSCEAR 1993 estimates that the dose per capita from all sources of medical exposures is 60 mrem/yr and the total, worldwide collective effective dose equivalent is 3.3×10^8 person rem/yr. This is as compared to 1.3×10^9 person rem/yr effective dose equivalent from natural background radiation, including radon. With respect to future trends, it is projected that the total use of diagnostic X radiation will increase because of the increasing proportion of older people in the population and increasing urbanization.

Occupational Exposure to Medical Technicians

NCRP 1989a and EPA 1984 present a compilation of occupational radiation exposures for 1980. The information in these reports is dated and is currently undergoing revision by the EPA. However, the information is useful for providing a general overview of the magnitude of the occupational exposures for medical technicians. Table 15-7 presents the occupational exposure for medical technicians for 1980.

NCRP Report No. 124 (NCRP, 1996) describes the sources and magnitudes of occupational and public exposures from nuclear medicine procedures. Exposures are associated with the receipt and handling of the radioactive material and the practice of

TABLE 15-7 Occupational Radiation Exposures of Medical Technicians in 1980

Occupational Category	Number of Workers (thousands)	Number of Workers Receiving Measurable Dose	Mean Annual Dose (mrem/yr) to Workers with Measurable Exposure	Collective Dose (thousands; person rem/yr)
Dentistry	259	82	70	5.6
Private practice	155	87	180	16
Hospital	126	86	200	17
Vetinary	21	12	110	1.3
Chiropractic	15	6	80	0.5
Podiatry	8	3	30	0.1
Total	584	277		41

Source: From EPA (1984).

nuclear medicine. The annual dose to technical personnel working with the material and the patients (and who are under radiation protection controls) is reported to be about 300 to 500 mrad/yr (a typical range of values for radiation workers). The dose to the members of the public in close contact with a patient being treated with radiopharmaceuticals is estimated to be < 1 mrem / yr to 21 mrem per procedure. The per capita dose to the American public from exposure to patients treated with radiophamaceuticals is considerably less than 1 mrem / yr.

Exposure to General Public from Misplaced Brachytherapy Sources

The New York State Department of Health (New York, 1982) reported on a widespread problem associated with exposure to jewelry containing elevated levels of radioactivity. These exposures occurred as a result of the reuse of "seeds" cut or crimped from hollow gold tubes through which radon had been passed and sealed, and used as implants for the irradiation of diseased tissue. The NYS study surveyed 160,000 pieces of jewelry and found about 170 pieces to be radioactive. Nine individuals were identified who developed squamous cell carcinoma as a result of the long term exposure to the radioactive jewelry. Radon seeds are no longer manufactured in the United States (Lubenau and Nussbaumer, 1986). The mishandling of radium needles, also used as medical implants, has also resulted in environmental contamination and elevated radiation exposures to members of the public (Belanger and Janosik, 1990; Googins, 1990).

Exposure to General Public from Effluents

The medical use of radioisotopes is associated with the discharge of gaseous, liquid, and solid radioactive waste which have some, but limited, potential to cause radiation exposures of members of the general public. The discharges are under the direct regulatory control of the NRC or state authorities.

Of the approximate 3680 hospitals in the United States half handle radiopharmaceuticals for radionuclide imaging and to aid in diagnosis of disease, and a smaller number use radionuclides for therapeutic purposes. Most hospitals are located in highly populated areas. A survey of 100 hospitals revealed that the primary gaseous emissions are ^{133}Xe and ^{131}I, at a typical release rate of 1.0 and 0.01 Ci / yr, respectively. However, larger hospitals report releases several times higher than these typical values (EPA, 1989). The highest radiation doses to members of the general public in the vicinity of the hospitals is estimated to range from < 1 mrem / yr to a high of 8 mrem/yr (EPA, 1993b). Accordingly this source of exposure is relatively small.

Small quantities of radioactive liquid waste may be discharged to sewage under current NRC regulations. There has been concern that these discharges may accumulate in the sludge at sewage treatment plants and result in exposures of members of the public. The work performed to date on this concern indicates that any exposures are extremely small (Shearer et al., 1995; Larsen et al., 1995).

Finally the licensed disposal of the solid radioactive waste produced by the medical community provides a high level of assurance that the exposures to the public will be relatively small. For example, analyses of the performance of low level radioactive waste disposal units have revealed maximum doses less than a few mrem / yr (EPA, 1988e).

INDUSTRIAL USES (OTHER THAN THE NUCLEAR FUEL CYCLE)

Radioactive materials are used in a wide range of industrial applications which are associated with exposures to workers in the industry and members of the public.

TABLE 15-8   Occupational Exposures of Industrial Workers in 1995

Industrial Category	Number of Licensees	Number of Monitored Workers	Workers with Measurable Dose	Average Measurable Dose (mrem/yr)	Collective Dose (person rem/yr)
Industrial radiographers	139	3530	2465	540	1338
Manufacturers and distributors	36	2666	1222	490	595
Total	175	6196	3687	524	1933

Source: NRC (1997).

Worker Exposures

The principal industrial exposures are associated with the use of sealed sources for industrial radiography and the manufacture and distribution of radioisotopes and devices for industrial purposes, research, medical uses, and in commercial products, such as smoke detectors. Table 15-8 presents the occupational exposures for industrial radiographers and manufacturers and distributors for 1995 (NRC, 1997).

Exposures of the General Public

Exposure of the general public as a result of the routine manufacture, use, and disposal of industrial sources is small. However, occasionally, a source will be abandoned, lost, or stolen and create the potential for widespread contamination and exposure of the public. The most serious of these accidents, which involved abandoned teletherapy units, occurred in Juarez, Mexico in 1983 and Goiania, Brazil in 1987. A summary of these accidents is provided by Eisenbud and Gesell (1997). In the Juarez accident, some individuals received doses as high as 700 rem, while several thousand people received some elevated doses. Those individuals that received the higher doses experienced mild symptoms of radiation exposure, but there were no acute radiation exposure fatalities primarily because the exposures were protracted over a period of time. The Goiania accident was more serious in that it resulted in the deaths of four individuals due to acute radiation injury.

Yusko (1995) reports on more recent serious accidents, including exposure to a sealed source in Estonia in 1993, which resulted in a fatality, and exposures in buildings in Taiwan and Japan where the structural reinforcing rods in the concrete contained Co-60 causing exposures in excess of 100 rem.

Misplaced sources are often detected at scrap-handling facilities and steel mills and reported to state authorities. Yusko (1995), who maintains a data base of such reports, found that most incidents are the result of the detection of elevated levels of naturally occurring radioactivity, which have relatively little potential for causing significant exposures (exposures to elevated levels of naturally occurring radioactivity are discussed in the last section of this chapter). However, about one-eighth of the recorded incidents involved sealed sources, primarily of ^{226}Ra, ^{60}Co, and ^{137}Cs which can cause dangerously high exposures, as evidenced by the Juarez, Goiania, Taiwan, and Japan experiences. The number of recorded incidents are increasing, and at the time of the publication of his paper, Yusko recorded over 1200 such incidents.

In response to this serious problem, the Institute of Scrap Recycling Industries (ISRI), the Conference of Radiation Control Program Directors (CRCPD), the Environmental Protection Agency, the Nuclear Regulatory Commission, and other federal agencies and trade organizations have begun aggressively to address this problem (Yusko, 1995).

CONSUMER PRODUCTS

The National Council on Radiation Protection and Measurement has dedicated NCRP Report No. 95 to this topic (NCRP, 1987d). Examples of consumer products that are widely distributed and can result in radiation exposures of members of the general public include

- Smoke detectors
- Airport luggage inspection systems
- Radioluminous products
- Static eliminators
- Televisions and video display terminals
- Plutonium-powered cardiac pacemakers
- Lighting rods
- A wide variety of products that contain discrete[3] enhanced sources of naturally occurring radioactivity

Some of these products are designed and intended to generate a radiation field, while the radioactivity or radiation fields associated with others are an inadvertent by-product of their design and / or operation. Table 15-9 summarizes the individual and collective doses associated with consumer products and other miscellaneous sources, including enhanced sources of discrete naturally occurring radioactivity.

EXPOSURES TO DIFFUSE, ENHANCED SOURCES OF NATURALLY OCCURRING RADIOACTIVE MATERIAL (NORM) AND RADIATION

The average total effective dose equivalent for a member of the population in the United States and Canada from natural background radiation is about 300 mrem/yr (NCRP, 1987b). This includes exposure to cosmic rays, cosmogenic radionuclides produced by the interaction of cosmic rays with atoms in the atmosphere or on the earth, terrestrial radiation from naturally occurring radionuclides in soil and rock, the inhalation of radon and its progeny, and naturally occurring radionuclides deposited internally into the body. This chapter does not address this major source of radiation exposure because it is naturally occurring. However, this chapter is concerned with elevated exposures to background radiation that result from human activities. The sources of these elevated exposures and their magnitude are described in several publications, including UNSCEAR (1993) and Eisenbud and Gesell (1997), and several NCRP reports (NCRP reports no. 77, 93, 94, 95, and 118). In addition, because of the large number of people being exposed to elevated levels of naturally occurring radioactivity resulting from human activities, the Environmental Protection Agency has been investigating this issue (SCA, 1993).

---

[3] Exposure to normally low levels of natural radioactivity can be enhanced through various natural processes and anthropomorphic activities. These enhanced sources of naturally occuring radioactivity are often categorized as discrete and diffuse. Discrete sources are relatively small sources where the atural radionuclide content has been dramatically increased (e.g., in excess of 2000 pCi/g of Ra-226 as compared to natural levels of Ra-226 in soil of about 1pCi / g). Diffuse sources are extremely large volumes of bulk material, such as tailings, and sludge, where the natural radioactivity content has been slightly increased for example, above 5 pCi/g. A distinction is made between discrete and diffuse sources of enhanced NORM because of the significant differences between the two in the nature and extent of the exposures they can cause and the methods by which these exposures may be managed.

TABLE 15-9   Radiation Exposure from Consumer Products

Source	U.S. Population Exposed	Average Annual Effective Dose Equivalent (mrem / yr)	Annual Collective Effective Population Dose Equivalent (person rem/yr)
Electronic products			
Televisions	230,000,000	≪1 mrem	≪28,000
Video display terminals	50,000,000		
Airport luggage inspection	30,000,000	≪1 mrem	60
Luminous watches and clocks and other devices			
H-3 activated watches	10,000,000	< 1 mrem	1520
H-3 activated clocks	750,000		
Pm-147 luminous watches	3,700,000		
Pm-147 luminous clocks	4,400,000		
Static eliminators	40,000	< 1 mrem	13
Electron tubes	230,000,000	≪1 mrem	1000
Smoke detectors	100,000,000	≪1 mrem	800
Check sources	800,000	< 1 mrem	< 800
Dental prosthesis	45,000,000	≪1 mrem	3000
Ophthalmic glass	50,000,000	< 1 mrem	< 20,000
Thorium products and other devices/activities			
Gas mantles	50,000,000	< 1 mrem	8600
Tungsten welding rods	300,000	16 mrem	5000
Fluorescent lamp starters	50,000,000	≪1 mrem	< 1
Aircraft transport of radioactive materials	14,000,000	< 1 mrem	3000
Total		Less than 1 to a few mrem from all sources combined for the vast majority of people	20,000 – 50,000

Source: Data derived from NCRP (1989c).
Note: Diffuse NORM not included.

Table 15-10 presents the sources of enhanced levels of naturally occurring radiation, the levels of exposures to individual, and the collective exposures. A distinction is made here between specific consumer products and electronic devices, as discussed above, and exposure to large volumes of bulk material enhanced in natural radioactivity due to human activities. The management of the very large volumes of this material is being evaluated by the EPA. These evaluations include the life-cycle costs and benefits associated with alternative management strategies, including the no-action alternative.

OVERVIEW OF POTENTIAL HEALTH IMPACTS OF NATURAL AND MAN-MADE SOURCES OF RADIOACTIVITY

The production and use of radioactive materials and a wide variety of human endeavor are associated with increased levels of radiation exposure. Table 15-11 provides an overview of the magnitude of these exposures and compares them to natural background.

TABLE 15-10 Exposures to Enhanced Sources of Naturally Occurring Radioactive Material (NORM) and Radiation-Sources, Quantities, Characteristics, and Exposures

Source	Description	Average Radionuclide Concentration (pCi/g)	Individual Exposures (mrem/yr)	Collective Exposures (person rem/yr EDE)	Reference
Uranium mining overburden	The overburden, low grade ore, and spoils associated with uranium mining contains slightly elevated levels of naturally occurring radioactivity.	About 38 million MT per year are produced containing an average of 25 pCi/g of Ra-226.	*	*	SCA (1993)
Phosphate waste Phosphogypsum Slag Scale	The mining of phosphate rock for phosphate for fertilizers, detergent, and numerous phosphate products generates huge volumes of tailings containing elevated levels of naturally occurring radioactivity.	About 50 million MT per year are produced with average Ra-226 content of about 35 pCi/g and some scale containing over 1000 pCi/g.	*	*	SCA (1993)
Phosphate fertilizers	Fertilizer contains elevated level of naturally occurring radionuclides	About 5 million MT are produced per year containing an average of 8.3 pCi/g of Ra-226.	*	*	SCA (1993)
Coal ash Fly ash Bottom ash and slag	Very large volumes of coal ash are produced each year containing elevated levels of naturally occurring radionuclides.	About 61 million MT are produced per year containing an average of about 3.7 pCi/g of Ra-226.	*	*	SCA (1993)
Oil and gas scale and sludge	Large volumes of scale and sludge are produced in the oil and gas industry.	About 260,000 MT per year are produced with an average Ra-226 concentration of about 90 pCi/g	*	*	SCA (1993)

Source	Description	Quantity/Concentration	Exposure/Dose		Reference
Water treatment Sludges Radium selective resins	Sludges produced in water treatment systems contain elevated levels of naturally occurring radionuclides.	About 300,000 MT are produced per year containing an average Ra-226 concentration of 16 pCi/g. However, radium selective resins can have Ra-226 concentrations as high as 35,000 pCi/g.		*	SCA (1993)
Metal mining and processing Rare earths Zr, Ha, Ti, Sb Large volume industries	The overburden, low-grade ore, and spoils associated with metal mining contain slightly elevated levels of naturally occurring radioactivity.	About 1E9 MT are produced per year containing an average Ra-226 concentration of about 5 pCi/g, with some material containing 900 pCi/g.		*	SCA (1993)
Geothermal energy wastes		About 54,000 MT per year of geothermal waste is produced containing an average Ra-226 concentration of 132 pCi/g.		*	SCA (1993)
Tobacco products	Naturally occurring Pb-210 and Po-210 accumulate on tobacco leaves and are transported to and deposited in the lungs, where they deliver relatively high localized radiation doses.	NA	About 16,000 mrem/yr to lung tissue of smokers[a]	NC	NCRP (1987c)
Air travel	Elevated exposure occurs to pilots, flight attendants, and passengers due to the higher levels of cosmic radiation at high altitudes.	NA	Exposure averages about 0.6 mrem/h of flight at 35,000 ft, and, during solar flares, 10 mrem/h of flight at 41,000 ft. Air crews receive 20–910 mrem/yr.		DOT (1990)

TABLE 15-10 *(Continued)*

Source	Description	Average Radionuclide Concentration (pCi/g)	Individual Exposures (mrem/yr)	Collective Exposures (person rem/yr EDE)	Reference
Building materials	Naturally occurring uranium, thorium, and potassium occur in wall board, cement and other building products.	NC	7 mrem/yr EDE	8.4E5 person rem/yr EDE	NCRP (1987d)
Road construction materials	Travellers are exposed to roadways made of material with elevated levels of natural radioactivity.		4 mrem/yr EDE	2E4 person rem/yr EDE	NCRP (1987d)
Mining and agricultural products	Fertilizer contains elevated levels of naturally occurring radionuclides, and people who handle fertilizer can receive elevated exposures. Also the fertilizer distributed in the environment can increase external and internal exposures from radionuclides in food.		0.5–5 mrem/yr EDE	<2E5 person rem/yr	NCRP (1987d)
Combustible fuels: coal, oil, natural, gas, and LPG	Coal and coal ash can contain elevated levels of natural radionuclides, which are distributed into the environment in the airborne and liquid effluents and in solid wastes. Oil represents a much smaller source of exposure. Natural gas use in the home represents a source of indoor radon, but which is small compared to radon normally present in homes.	About 9 pCi/g of. U-238 in coal fly ash.	<1–1 mrem/yr EDE	About 1E5 person rem/yr	NCRP (1987d)

Note: The asterisk indicates that dose and risk assessments associated with these large volumes of bulk material containing slightly elevated levels of naturally occurring radionuclides, primarily Ra-226, are being performed by EPA. SCA (1993) is a contractor report that is undergoing review and revision as part of the EPA rule-making investigations pertaining to NORM.
[a] NCRP Report No 95 does not convert this lung dose to an effective dose equivalent dose but does report on others that have made the conversion and estimate a dose of 1300 mrem/yr EDE per smoker.

Radiobiologists and epidemiologists have been involved in ongoing studies to determine if these relatively low exposures have an adverse impact on public health, have no impact, or possibly have some net beneficial or hormetic effect on the exposed population. The most authoritative advisory and regulatory bodies on this subject have made the following observations and conclusions regarding exposure to low levels of radiation:

ICRP 1991 cites the following risk coefficients for low dose and low dose rate irradiation:

Exposed Population	Nominal probability coefficients for stochastic effects (Detriment expressed units of 10^{-2} Sv^{-1})[a]			
	Factor Cancer[b]	Non-fatal cancer	Severe hereditary effects	Total
Adult workers	4.0	0.8	0.8	5.6
Whole population	5.0	1.0	1.3	7.3

[a] Rounded values, a Sv is equal to 100 rem.
[b] For fatal cancer, the detriment coefficient is equal to the probability coefficient.

... the use of a nominal value of 5% per Sv for mortality due to leukemia and solid cancers from irradiation at low doses for a population of all ages (4% per Sv for an adult working population) still seems valid to the Committee. (UNSCEAR, 1994).

Of the various types of biomedical effects that may result from irradiation at low doses and low dose rates, alteration of genes and chromosomes remain the best documented.... It is estimated that at least 1 Gy (100 rad) of low dose rate, low LET radiation[4] is required to double the mutation rate in man.... The population-weighted average lifetime excess risk of death from cancer following an acute dose equivalent to all body organs of 0.1 Sv (0.1 Gy of low LET radiation) is estimated to be 0.8%. (NAS, 1990)

... the calculated risk of a premature cancer death attributable to uniform, whole body, low-LET irradiation is about 5.1×10^{-2} Gy^{-1}. The corresponding incidence risk (neglecting nonfatal skin cancer) is about 7.5×10^{-2} Gy^{-1} (EPA, 1994b).

In referring to the data from Japan, the ICRP concludes: Although the study group is large (about 80,000), excess numbers of malignancies, statistically significant at the 95% level, can be found only at doses exceeding 0.2 Sv.... It must also be borne in mind that all the doses to the Japanese study group were incurred at very high dose rates....(ICRP, 1991)

The Committee's estimates of radiation exposure and its estimates of risk of exposure indicate that radiation is a weak carcinogen. About 4% of the deaths due to cancer can be attributed to ionizing radiation, most of which comes from natural sources that are not susceptible to control by man. Nevertheless, it is widely (but wrongly) believed that all the cancer deaths at Hiroshima and Nagasaki are the result of the atomic bombings. The studies in the two cities have included virtually all of the heavily exposed individuals and have shown that of 3,350 cancer deaths, only about 350 could be attributed to radiation exposures from the atomic bombings. (UNSCEAR, 1993)

The collective doses presented in Table 15-11 could be converted to potential fatal cancers by multiplying the collective doses by a nominal risk coefficient of 5×10^{-4} per

---

[4] Footnote added: "Low LET radiation" refers to radiation with a low linear energy transfer to tissue. Different types of radiation (alpha, beta, gamma, x-ray and neutrons) deposit their energy in different patterns. Some deposit energy in highly dense clusters (e.g., alpha particles and neutrons), while others deposit their energy in a less dense pattern (e.g., gamma rays, x-rays, and beta particles). The latter are referred to as low LET radiation, which, for a given amount of energy deposited per gram of tissue, is potentially less harmful than high LET radiation.

TABLE 15-11 Summary of Radiation of Doses from Principal Sources

Source of Exposure	Individual Dose or Dose Rate	Collective Dose	References
Natural background			
Cosmic rays (external)	27 mrem/yr	7.5E7 person rem/yr in U.S. (based on a U.S. population of 250 million people)	NCRP (Report 94)
Terrestrial (external)	28 merm/yr		
Cosmogenic (internal)	1 mrem/yr		
Inhaled (radon, internal)	200 mrem/yr		
Internal terrestrial	40 mrem/yr		
Total	300 mrem/yr		
Commercial nuclear fuel cycle			
Radiation workers	About 300 mrem/yr	About 23,000 person rem/yr in U.S.	NRC (1997), NCRP (1987), PNL (1995)
Members of the general public	<1 to a few mrem/yr from reactor effluents to 61 mrem/yr from mine effluents	75–1800 person rem/yr from all U.S. reactor effluents combined in 1995–1991	
Weapons complex			
Occupational exposure	65 mrem/yr (1994)	1643 person rem/yr (1994)	DOE (1994)
General public (routine emissions)	<1 to 25 mrem/yr organ dose	<1 to 670 person rem/yr depending on site	EPA (1989)
General public (episodic releases)	Under investigation by CDC		
Fallout			
Local at time of test at Republic of the Marshall Islands	Over 100 rem to some individuals	3E9 person rem globally time-integrated	Cronkite et al. (1997), Simon and Graham (1996), Thompson and McArthur (1996), UNSCEAR (1993)
Local at test site at Republic of the Marshall Islands	Up to 200 mrem/yr		
Local at test site Nevada Test Site	0.1 to 23.2 R		
Global	370 mrem time integrated		

Medical exposures

Patients medical diagnostic exposures	60 mrem/yr per caput	UNSCEAR (1993), EPA (1993a)
Occupational exposures	140 mrem/yr	NCRP (1989), EPA (1983)
Public exposure from misplaced sources	Very high potential doses	
Public exposures from routine effluents	<1 to 8 mrem/yr	

Industrial uses

Radiation workers	524 mrem/yr	NRC (1997), Yusko (1995)
General public routine	Negligible	
General public misplaced sources	Potential for very high doses	

Consumer products

Consumers	<1 to a few mrem/yr	NCRP (1987)
NORM	Under study as EPA	

Note: Additional data columns appear as:
- Patients medical diagnostic exposures: 3.3E8 person rem/yr globally
- Occupational exposures: 41,000 person rem/yr in U.S. in 1980
- Radiation workers: 1933 person rem/yr
- Consumers: 20,000 to 50,000 person rem/yr
- NORM: Under study at EPA

TABLE 15-12   Potential Fatal Cancers due to Exposure to Man-made Sources of Radiation

Source	Upper-end Estimate of Fatal Cancers
Actual Incidence of fatal cancer	About 500,000 per year in the U.S. (National Cancer Institute statistics)
Natural background	37,500 per year in U.S.
Nuclear fuel cycle in U.S.	About 10 per year in U.S. (mostly radiation workers)
Weapons complex	About 1 per year in U.S. (predominantly workers)
Fallout	1.5 million time-integrated, global
Medical exposures	165,000 per year globally (due to diagnostic x-rays)
Industrial uses in U.S.	1 per year in U.S. from other than fuel cycle facilities, primarily workers
Consumer products in U.S.	25 per year in U.S. to consumers
Enhanced NORM	Undetermined but relatively large

Note: Except for the actual incidence of fatal cancer, which is based on actuarial data, the estimates of radiogenic fatal cancers are theoretical upper end values that were derived using the collective doses presented in Table 15-11 multiplied by a fatal cancer risk coefficient of 5E-4 risk per person rem.

rem. As such, an upper end estimate of the potential numbers of fatal cancers associated with exposure to man-made radiation is summarized in Table 15-12. These values are compared to the actual number of fatal cancers in the United States from all causes and the theoretical number of fatal cancers from natural background radiation.

REFERENCES

Belanger, W., and V. Jasnosik. 1990. The Lansdown radiation site. In *EPA Workshop on Radioactively Contaminated Sites.* EPA 520/1–90–009. March.

Blanchard, R. L., T. W. Fowler, T. R. Horton, and J. M. Smith. 1982. Potential health effects of radioactive emissions of active surface and underground uranium mines. *Nucl. Saf.* 23: 439–450.

Brodsky, A. 1978. *Handbook of Radiation Measurement and Detection.* Boca Raton, FL: CRC Press, 1978.

Brookhaven National Laboratory. 1995. Radioactive materials released from nuclear power plants. Annual report 1993. Prepared by J. Tichler, K. Doty, and K. Lucadamo, Brookhaven National Laboratory. U.S. Nuclear Regulatory Commission. NUREG/CR-2907, BNL-NUREG-51581, vol. 14. December.

Cochran, R. G., and N. Tsoulfanidis. 1990. *The Nuclear Fuel Cycle: Analysis and Management.* La Grange Park, IL: American Nuclear Society.

Cronkite, E. P., R. A. Conrad, and V. P. Bond. 1997. Historical events associated with fallout from BRAVO Shot-Operation Castle and 25 Y of medical findings, *Health Physics*, 73: 176–186.

DNFSB. 1994a. Defense Nuclear Facilities Safety Board. Recommendation 94-2 to the Secretary of Energy. September 8.

DNFSB. 1994b. Defense Nuclear Facilities Safety Board. Low-level waste disposal policy for Department of Energy Defense Nuclear Facilities. DNFSB/TECH-2. September 14.

DOE. 1979. *Technology for Commercial Radioactive Waste Management, Department of Energy Report DOE/ET-0028.* Springfield, VA: National Technical Information Service.

DOE. 1980. *Grand Junction Remedial Action Program.* DOE/-EV/01621-T1. Washington, DC: Government Printing Office.

DOE. 1983. *Spent Fuel and Radioactive Waste Inventories, Projections and Characteristics.* Department of Energy Report DOE/NE-0017/2. Springfield, VA: National Technical Information Service.

DOE. 1990. *Integrated Data Base for 1990: U.S. Spent Fuel and Radioactive Waste Inventories, Projections, and Characteristics.* DOE/RW-0006 Rev. 6. Washington, DC: Government Printing Office.

DOE. 1988a. U.S. Department of Energy, DOE Order 5820.2A, Radioactive waste management. September 26.

DOE. 1988b. U.S. Department of Energy. Guidance for conduct of waste management systems performance assessment. DOE/LLW-63T. June. Prepared by E G & G Idaho, Inc. under contract to the U.S. DOE Idaho Operations Office.

DOE. 1988c. U.S. Department of Energy. Guidelines for radiological performance assessment of DOE low level radioactive waste disposal units. DOE/LLW-62T, July 1988. Prepared by Marilyn J. Case and Mark D. Otis under contract to the U.S. DOE Idaho Operations Office.

DOE. 1988d. U.S. Department of Energy. Clarification of requirements of DOE Order 5820.2A. DOE Memorandum. February 29.

DOE. 1989a. U.S. Department of Energy. A manual for implementing residual radioactive material guidelines. DOE/CH/8901, June.

DOE. 1989b. U.S. Department of Energy. CERCLA requirements. DOE 5400.4. October 6.

DOE. 1990. U.S. Department of Energy. General environmental protection program. DOE 5400.1, Change 1. June 29.

DOE. 1991. U.S. Department of Energy. Performance assessment review guide for DOE low-level radioactive waste disposal facilities. DOE/LLW-93. October.

DOE. 1993. U.S. Department of Energy. Notice of proposed rulemaking and public hearing, 58 FR 16268, No. 056, March 25. 10 CFR 834. Radiation Protection of the Public and the Environment.

DOE. 1994. U.S. Department of Energy. DOE occupational radiation exposure report, 1992–1994.

DOE. 1995a. U.S. Department of Energy. Risk and the risk debate: Searching for common ground, the first step. Office of Environmental Management. June.

DOE. 1995b. U.S. Department of Energy. Estimating the cold war mortgage. The 1995 Baseline Environmental Management Report. DOE/EM-0230, March.

DOE. 1995c. U.S. Department of Energy. Draft waste management programmatic environmental impact statement for managing treatment, storage, and disposal of radioactive and hazardous waste. DOE/EIS-0200-D. August.

DOE. 1995d. U.S. Department of Energy. Integrated data base —1994: U.S. spent fuel and radioactive waste inventories, projections, and characteristics.

DOE. 1996a. U.S. Department of Energy. Integrated data base —1995: U.S. spent fuel and radioactive waste inventories, projections, and characteristics.

DOE. 1996b. U.S. Department of Energy. Environmental management, progress and plans of the environmental management program. DOE/EM-0317. November.

DOL. 1995. U.S. Department of Labor, Bureau of Labor Statistics. Fatal workplace injuries in 1993: A collection of data and analysis. Report 891. June.

DOT. 1990. U.S. Department of Transportation. Radiation exposure of air carrier crewmembers. Advisory Circular 120–52. March 5.

DOE/NFC. 1990. *Nuclear Fuel Cycle: Current Abstracts.* DOE/NFC-90/12 (PB 90-913412). Washington, DC: Office of Scientific and Technical Information.

Eisenbud, M. and T. Gesell. 1997. *Environmental Radioactivity: From Natural, Industrial and Military Sources,* 4th edition. San Diego, CA: Academic Press, 1997.

EPA. 1984. U.S. Environmental Protection Agency. Occupational exposure to ionizing radiation in the United States. A comprehensive review of the year 1980 and a summary of the trends for the years 1960–1985. EPA 520/1-84-005, September.

EPA. 1987. U.S. Environmental Protection Agency. Guidance on preparing superfund decision documents (ROD guidance). EPA/624/1–87/001.

EPA. 1988a. U.S. Environmental Protection Agency. Guidance for conducting remedial investigations and feasibility studies under CERCLA. EPA/540/G-89/004, OSWER Directive 9355.3-01. October.

EPA. 1988b. U.S. Environmental Protection Agency. Superfund exposure assessment manual. EPA/540/1-88/001, OSWER Directive 9285.5-1. April.

EPA. 1988c. U.S. Environmental Protection Agency. CERCLA compliance with other laws manual. EPA/540/G-89/006. August.

EPA. 1988d. U.S. Environmental Protection Agency. Limiting values of radionuclide intake and air concentration and dose conversion factors for inhalation, submersion, and ingestion. Federal Guidance Report 11, EPA-520/1-88-020. September.

EPA. 1988e. U.S. Environmental Protection Agency. Low-level and NARM radioactive wastes—draft environmental impact statement for proposed rules — Background information document. EPA 520/1-87-012, June.

EPA. 1989a. U.S. Environmental Protection Agency. Risk assessments, environmental impact statement, NESHAPS for radionuclides, background information document. EPA / 520 / 1-89-006. September.

EPA. 1989b. U.S. Environmental Protection Agency. Risk assessment guidance for superfund, vol. 2, Environmental evaluation manual. EPA / 540 / 1-89 / 001.

EPA. 1989c. U.S. Environmental Protection Agency. Ecological assessment of hazardous waste sites: A field and laboratory reference. EPA / 600 / 3-89 / 013.

EPA. 1989d. U.S. Environmental Protection Agency. Risk assessment guidance for superfund, vol. 1. Human health evaluation manual—Part A (HHEM). EPA/540/1-89/002. December.

EPA. 1991a. U.S. Environmental Protection Agency. Role of the baseline risk assessment in Superfund remedy selection decisions. OSWER Directive 9355.0-30. April.

EPA. 1991b. U.S. Environmental Protection Agency. Human health evaluation manual, supplemental guidance: Standard default exposure factors. OSWER Directive 9285.6-03. March 25.

EPA. 1991e. U.S. Environmental Protection Agency. Risk assessment guidance for superfund, vol. 1: Human health evaluation manual—Part B, Development of Risk Based Preliminary Remediation Goals (HHEM), PB92-963333, December.

EPA. 1991d. U.S. Environmental Protection Agency. Risk assessment guidance for superfund, vol. 1. Human health evaluation manual—Part C, Risk evaluation of remedial alternatives (HHEM). PB92-963334. December.

EPA. 1991e. U.S. Environmental Protection Agency. *Health Effects Assessment Summary Tables: FY-1991 Annual.* OERR 9200.6-303(91–1). Washington, DC: Office of Research and Development and Office of Emergency and Remedial Response.

EPA. 1992. U.S. Environmental Protection Agency. Accessing federal data bases for contaminated site cleanup technologies. EPA / 542 / B-92 / 002. August.

EPA. 1993a. U.S. Environmental Protection Agency. External exposure to radionuclides in air, water, and soil. Federal Guidance Report 12. EPA 402-R-93-081. September.

EPA. 1993b. U.S. Environmental Protection Agency. Background information document to support NESHAPS rulemaking on nuclear regulatory commission and agreement state licensees other than nuclear power reactors. EPA 520/1-92. July 20.

EPA. 1993c. U.S. Environmental Protection Agency. Issues paper on radiation site cleanup regulations. EPA 402-R-93-084. September.

EPA. 1994a. U.S. Environmental Protection Agency. Radiation site cleanup regulations: Technical support document for the development of radionuclide cleanup levels for soil. EPA 402-R-96-011. September.

EPA. 1994b. U.S. Environmental Protection Agency. Federal radiation protection guidance for exposure of the general public: Notice. 59 FR 66414, No. 246. December 23.

EPA. 1994c. U.S. Environmental Protection Agency. Estimating radiogenic cancer risk. EPA 402-R-93-076. June.

Gerusky, T. M. 1981. Three Mile Island: Assessment of radiation exposures and environmental contamination. *Ann. NY Acad. Sci.* 365: 54–62.

Googins, S. W. 1990. Radium chemical company site summary. In EPA Workshop on Radioactively Contaminated Sites. EPA 520 / 1-90-009. March.

Gudiksen, P. H., T. F. Harvey, and R. lange. 1989. Chernobyl source term, atmospheric dispersion, and dose estimation. *Health Physics* 57: 697–706. November.

Health Physics Society. 1986. *Proc. 19th Midyear Topical Symposium. Health Physics Considerations in Decontamination and Decommissioning.* CONF-860203. Springfield, VA: National Technical Information Service.

Holaday, D. A., D. E. Rushing, R. D. Coleman, R. E. Woolrich, H. L. Kusnetz, and W. E. Bale. 1957. *Control of Radon and Daughters in Uranium Mines and Calculations on Biologic Effects.* Public Health Service Publ. 494. Washington, DC: Government Printing Office.

Hueper, W. C. 1942. *Occupational Tumors and Allied Diseases.* Springfield, IL: Charles C. Thomas.

ICRP. 1991. International Commission on Radiological Protection. *1990 Recommendations of the International Commission on Radiological Protection.* ICRP-60. Oxford: Pergamon Press.

Larsen, I. L., E. A. Stetar, and K. D. Glass. 1995. In-house screening for radioactive sludge. Rad. Prot. Manag. 12: 29–38.

Larsen, I. L., S. Y. Lee, H. L. Boston, and E. A. Stetar. 1992. Discovery of a Cs-137 hot particle in municipal wastewater treatment sludge. *Health Physics* 62: 235–238.

Lorenz, E. 1944. Radioactivity and lung cancer; a critical review in miners of Schneeberg and Joachimstahl. *J. Natl. Cancer Inst.* 5: 1–15.

Lubenau, J. O. and D. A. Nussbaumer. 1986. Radioactive contamination of manufactured products. *Health Physics* 51: 409–429.

Miller, C. W. and J. M. Smith. 1996. Why should we do environmental dose reconstructions. *Health Physics* 71: 420–424.

Meyer, K. R., P. G. Viollegue, D. W. Schmidt, S. K. Rope, G. G. Killough, B. Schleien, R. G. Moore, M. J. Case, and J. E. Till. 1996. Overview of the Fernald dosimetry reconstruction project and source term estimates for 1951–1988. *Health Physics* 71: 425–437.

Miller, H. T., and L. M. Scott. 1981. Radiation exposures associated with exploration, mining, milling and shipping uranium. In *Radiation Hazards in Mining: Control, Measurement and Medical Aspects,* ed. M. Gomez. Golden, CO: Society of Mining Engineers of American Institute of Mining, Metallurgical and Petroleum Engineers, Inc., New York, NY.

Momeni, M. H., W. E. Kisieleski, D. R. Rayno, and C. S. Sabau. 1979. *Radioisotopic Composition of Yellowcake: An Estimation of Stack Release Rates.* NUREG/CR-1216, ANL/ES-84. Argonne, IL: Argonne National Laboratory.

Mongan, T. R., S. R. Ripple, G. P. Brorby, and D. G. Ditommaso. 1996. Plutonium release from the 1957 fire at Rocky Flats. *Health Physics* 71: 510–521.

Morgan, K. Z., and J. E. Turner. 1973. Principles of radiation protection. Huntington, NY: Robert E. Krieger Publishing.

NAS. 1990. National Academy of Sciences, National Research Council. Health effects of exposure to low levels of ionizing radiation, BEIR V. Washington DC: National Academy Press.

NCRP. 1984. National Council on Radiation Protection and Measurement. Exposures from the uranium series with emphasis on radon and its daughters. NCRP Report 77.

NCRP. 1987a. National Council on Radiation Protection and Measurement. Public radiation exposure from nuclear power generation in the United States. NCRP Report 92.

NCRP. 1987b. National Council on Radiation Protection and Measurement, Ionizing radiation exposure of the population of the United States. NCRP Report 93.

NCRP. 1987c. National Council on Radiation Protection and Measurement. Exposure of the population in the United States and Canada from natural background radiation. NCRP Report 94.

NCRP. 1987d. National Council on Radiation Protection and Measurement. Radiation exposure of the U.S. population for consumer products and miscellaneous sources. NCRP Report 95.

NCRP. 1989a. National Council on Radiation Protection and Measurement. Exposure of the U.S. population from diagnostic medical radiation. NCRP Report 100.

NCRP. 1989b. National Council on Radiation Protection and Measurement. Exposure of the U.S. population from occupational radiation. NCRP Report 101.

NCRP. 1993. National Council on Radiation Protection and Measurement. Radiation protection in the mineral extraction industry, NCRP Report 118.

NCRP. 1996. National Council on Radiation Protection and Measurement. Sources and magnitude of occupational and public exposures from nuclear medicine procedures. NCRP Report 124.

New York. 1982. New York State Department of Health. Report to the governor and legislature: Radioactive gold jewelry. September.

NRC/NAS. 1986. *Uranium Mill Tailings Study Panel: Scientific Basis for Risk Assessment and Management of Uranium Mill Tailings.* Washington, DC: National Academy Press.

NRC. 1982. U.S. Nuclear Regulatory Commission. Site suitability, selection and characterization branch technical position—low-level waste licensing branch. NUREG-0902. April.

NRC. 1988. U.S. Nuclear Regulatory Commission. Standard review plan for the review of a license application for a low-level radioactive waste disposal facility (Revision 1). NUREG-1200-Rev-1. January.

NRC. 1988a. U.S. Nuclear Regulatory Commission. Standard format and content of a license application for a low-level radioactive waste disposal facility (Revision 1). NUREG-1199, Rev. 1. January.

NRC. 1989. Nuclear Regulatory Commission. *Severe Accident Risk: An Assessment of Accident Risks in U.S. Commercial Nuclear Power Plants.* NUREG-1150. Washington, DC: NRC.

NRC. 1989a. U.S. Nuclear Regulatory Commission. Background information for the development of a low-level waste performance assessment methodology. vol. 1–5. Prepared by Sandia National Laboratories for the U.S. Nuclear Regulatory Commission. NUREG/CR-5453. August.

NRC. 1990. U.S. Nuclear Regulatory Commission, NUREG/CR-5532. Performance assessment methodology for low-level waste facilities. Prepared by Sandia National Laboratories for the U.S. NRC. July.

NRC. 1994. U.S. Nuclear Regulatory Commission. 10 CFR 20, et al., Radiological criteria for decommissioning: Proposed rule. 59 FR 43200, No. 161, August 22.

NRC. 1997a. U.S. Nuclear Regulatory Commission. Occupational radiation exposure at commercial nuclear power plants and other facilities. NUREG-0713, vol. 17. January.

NRC. 1997b. U.S. Nuclear Regulatory Commission. Information digest, 1997 edition. NUREG-1350, vol. 9.

Office of Technology Assessment. 1991. *Complex Cleanup: The Environmental Legacy of Nuclear Weapons Production.* Washington, DC: OTA.

PNL. 1995. Pacific Northwest Laboratory. Dose commitment due to radioactive releases from nuclear power plant sites in 1991. Prepared by D.A. Baker of Pacific Northwest Laboratory for the U.S. Nuclear Regulatory Commission. NUREG/CR-2859, PNL-4221, vol. 13, April.

SCA. 1993. Sanford Cohen & Associates and Rogers & Associates Engineering Corporation. Diffuse NORM wastes—Waste characterization and preliminary risk assessment. Prepared for U.S. Environmental Protection Agency, Office of radiation and Indoor Air, Contract 68D20155, Work Assignment 1–16. EPA Work Assignment Manager William E. Russo. May.

Shearer, D. R., P. McCullough, and D. North. 1995. Radioactivity content of sewage and sludge from sewage plants. *Health Physics* 68(6 suppl.): S25.

Shipler, D. B., B. A. Napier, W. T. Farris, and M. D. Freshley, 1996. Hanford environmental dose reconstruction project—an overview. *Health Physics* 71: 532–544.

Simon, S. L., J. E. Till, R. D. Lloyd, R. L. Kerber, D. C. Thomas, S. Preston-Martin, J. L. Lyon. and W. Stevens. 1995. The Utah leukemia case-control study: Dosimetry methodology and results. *Health Physics* 68: 460–471. April.

Simon, S. L. and J. C. Graham 1996. Dose assessment activities in the Republic of the Marshall Islands. *Health Physics* 71: 438–456.

Thompson, C. B., and R. D. McArthur. 1996. Challenges in developing estimates of exposure rate near the Nevada test site. *Health Physics* 71: 470–476.

Till, J. E., S. L. Simon, R. Kerber, R. D. Llyod, W. Stevens, D. C. Thomas, J. L. Lyon, and S. Preston-Martin. The Utah thyroid cohort study: Analysis of the dosimetry results. *Health Physics* 68: 472–483.

UNLV. 1996. University of Nevada, Las Vegas. Preliminary risk assessment DOE sites in Nevada. Harry Reid Center for Environmental Studies. December.

UNSCEAR. 1993. United Nations Scientific Committee on the Effects of Atomic Radiation. Sources and effects of ionizing radiation. United Nations, New York.

UNSCEAR. 1994. United Nations Scientific Committee on the Effects of Atomic Radiation. Sources and effects of Ionizing radiation. United Nations, New York.

Whicker, F.W., T. B. Kirchner, L. R. Anspaugh, and Y. C. Ng. 1996. Ingestion of Nevada test site fallout: Internal Dose Estimates. *Health Physics* 71: 477–486.

Widner, T. E., S. R. Ripple, and J. E. Buddenbaum. 1996. Identification and screening evaluation of key historical materials and emission sources at the Oak Ridge reservation. *Health Physics* 71: 457–469.

Wiggs, L. D., C. A. Cox-DeVore, and G. L. Voelz. 1991. Mortality among a cohort of workers monitored for Po-210 exposure: 1944–1972. *Health Physics* 61: 71–76.

Wood, D. E., et. al. 1993. The U.S. Department of Energy process for performance assessment for disposal of low-level radioactive waste. Presented at '93 International Conference on Nuclear Waste Management and Environmental Remediation, Prague, September. 5–11 NTIS Accession Number: DE93008179 / XAB.

WSRC. 1997 Westinghouse Savannah River Company. Savannah River site environmental report for 1996. WSRC-TR-97-0173.

Yusko, J. G. 1995. Radiation in the scrap recycling stream. *Annual Conference on the Recycle and Reuse of Radioactive Scrap Metal, Beneficial Reuse '95*. Sponsored by the University of Tennessee's Energy, Environment, and Resources Center and Oak Ridge National Laboratory's Center for Risk Management, July 31–August 3, Knoxville, TN.

16 Mercury

JESPER BO NIELSEN, Ph.D.
PHILIPPE GRANDJEAN, M.D., Ph.D.

The toxicity of mercury has been known since antiquity, but its therapeutic effects were also utilized in a variety of drugs. In particular, mercury became an important drug from the sixteenth century when syphilis patients were treated with mercurous chloride (calomel). Such treatments may have cured cases of social disease but inevitably also caused numerous intoxications. Occupational mercury poisoning has been vividly described in the past, for example by Ramazzini, who 300 years ago noted about the mirror makers: "At Venice on the island called Murano where huge mirrors are made, you may see these workmen gazing with reluctance and scowling at the reflection of their own sufferings in their mirrors and cursing the trade they have adopted." A recent update on mercury has been published by the U.S. Environmental Protection Agency (1997), and this source may be consulted for further information and additional references.

CHEMISTRY

Mercury exists in three oxidation states: Hg^0 (metallic), Hg^+ (mercurous), and Hg^{++} (mercuric) mercury. The last named forms a variety of inorganic as well as organometallic compounds. In the case of organometallic derivatives, the mercury atom is covalently bound to one or two carbon atoms, and the organic part of the molecule is often an alkyl group or an alkoxialkyl group. The former compounds are more toxic because they are more easily absorbed and more slowly metabolized. In its elemental form, mercury is a dense, silvery-white, shiny metal, which is liquid at room temperature and boils at 357°C. At 20°C the vapor pressure of the metal is 0.17 Pa (0.0013 mm Hg), and a saturated atmosphere at this temperature contains 14 mg Hg/m³, which is more than 100 times the occupational limit. Mercury compounds differ greatly in solubility. Thus at 25°C the solubilities of metallic mercury, mercurous chloride, and mercuric chloride in water are 60 µg/L, 2 mg/L and 69 g/L, respectively (IARC, 1994). Exact data for the solubility of methyl mercuric chloride in water are lacking but are known to be slightly higher than for mercurous chloride. Certain species of mercury are soluble in nonpolar solvents. These include elemental mercury and the halide compounds of alkylmercurials.

SOURCE

Mercury is emitted to the atmosphere by "degassing" of the earth's surface and by re-evaporation of mercury vapor previously deposited on the earth's surface. Mercury

Environmental Toxicants: Human Exposures and Their Health Effects, 2/e. Edited by Morton Lippmann.
ISBN: 0-471-29298-2 © 2000 John Wiley & Sons, Inc.

is emitted in the form of elemental vapor (Hg^0). The natural emissions are estimated to be between 2700 and 6000 t per year (Lindberg et al., 1987), part of which originates from previous anthropogenic activity. Anthropogenic sources of mercury are numerous and occur worldwide. Mercury is produced by the mining and smelting of cinnabar ore. It is used in chloralkali plants (producing chlorine and sodium hydroxide), in paints as preservatives or pigments, in electrical switching equipment and batteries, in measuring and control equipment (thermometers and other medical equipment), in mercury vacuum instruments, as a catalyst in chemical processes, in mercury quartz and luminescent lamps, in the production and use of high explosives using mercury fulminate, in copper/silver amalgams in dental restoration materials, and as fungicides in agriculture (especially as seed dressings). In total, human activities have been estimated to add 2000 to 4500 t to the total annual release of mercury to the global environment (U.S. DHHS, 1994). However, it should be stressed that there are considerable uncertainties in the estimated fluxes of mercury in the environment and in its speciation. The global cycle of mercury involves the emission of Hg^0 from land and water surfaces to the atmosphere, transport of Hg^0 in the atmosphere on a global scale, possible conversion to unidentified soluble species, and return to land and water by various depositional processes. It should be stressed that despite continued widespread industrial use, the emissions from manufacturing sources accounts only for 10% of the anthropogenic release of mercury to the atmosphere. The predominant source, accounting for some 87% of the total anthropogenic release of mercury, is combustion processes such as coal burning, waste incineration, and emissions from hospitals. For industrial or manufacturing sources the overall consumption of mercury has declined by about 75% within the past decade, and further reductions are expected (U.S. EPA, 1997).

One of the uses of liquid metallic mercury that has escalated during the last decades is informal gold mining. Especially alluvial deposits of fine gold particles may require mercury for efficient extraction. The gold particles are dissolved in the mercury as amalgam, and the mercury is subsequently removed by heating with a gas torch. This use therefore releases elemental mercury into confined and sometimes ecologically sensitive areas. For example, in the Brazilian Amazon Basin alone, the release of elemental mercury from these activities is about 100 t per year. This sort of mining operation occurs in many other countries as well and has previously caused extensive soil contamination in other geographic areas. Thus sites of previous gold mining operations in the United States, such as, Carson River, Nevada, are now recognized as being heavily contaminated with mercury, and the estimated amounts of mercury present in these areas exceeds 6000 t. Other industrial activities have also caused contaminations with elemental mercury, all characterized by the original release into a confined, sometimes remote geographical area. The solubility of mercury from these deposits is generally unknown, and methods to evaluate the bioavailable fraction have only recently been evaluated (Schoof and Nielsen, 1997). Because the mercury probably to a large extent occurs as mercuric salts with low solubility (i.e., sulfides), ecological and health implications should be focused on postdepositional effects due to methylation. The use of mercury-containing sewage sludge is another area of soil contamination of potential importance, where the question of bioavailability is yet unresolved. Thus three dietary studies in which steers were fed diets amended with sewage sludge containing mercury all reported significantly increased concentrations of mercury in kidneys and liver, whereas two studies in which cattle grazed sewage-sludge-treated pastures for long periods failed to demonstrate any significant increase in tissue concentrations of mercury (Schoof and Nielsen, 1997). None of these studies speciated the mercury present in the sludge, but another study suggests that the mercury is predominantly inorganic (Gilmour and Bloom, 1995).

Organomercury compounds are still used as a fungicide on seed grain. Methylmercury was extensively used for this purpose in the past until environmental effects were discovered, and now methoxymethylmercury is the compound preferred, although its use has declined. The paper and pulp industry has previously used these compounds as antislime agents.

The various uses of mercury and mercury compounds result in occupational exposures in a range of occupations. Also the industrial use of mercury may lead to releases to the environment, in particular, through sewage water (IPCS, 1991). Localized problems relating to contamination of river systems and bays have been caused by such contamination from chloralkaline plants, paper and pulp industries, and pesticide factories. In Japan, Minamata Bay became severely contaminated from a factory that used methylmercury as a catalyst in the production of vinyl chloride.

The ultimate deposition of mercury, probably as cinnabar ore, is believed to be in ocean sediments. Part of the inorganic mercury emitted becomes oxidized to Hg^{++} and then methylated or in other ways transformed into organomercurials. The methylation is believed to involve a nonenzymatic reaction between Hg^{++} and a methyl cobalamine compound (analogue of vitamin B_{12}) that is produced by bacteria (Wood and Wang, 1983). This reaction takes place primarily in aquatic systems. The intestinal bacterial flora of various animal species including fish are also, though to a much lower degree, able to convert ionic mercury into methylmercuric compounds (CH_3Hg^+) (Nielsen, 1992). Methylmercury is avidly accumulated by fish and marine mammals and attains its highest concentrations in large predatory species at the top of the aquatic foodchain. By this means it enters the human diet. Certain microorganisms can demethylate CH_3Hg^+; others can reduce Hg^{++} to Hg^0. Thus microorganisms are believed to play an important role in the fate of mercury in the environment and in affecting human exposure.

ENVIRONMENTAL EXPOSURES

Air

In areas of Europe remote from industrial activity, mean concentrations of total mercury in the atmosphere are reported to be in the range of 2 to 3 ng Hg/m^3 in summer and 3 to 4 ng Hg/m^3 in winter (U.S. DHHS, 1997). Mean mercury concentrations in urban air are usually three to fourfold higher (Sweet and Vermette, 1993). Hot spots of mercury concentration exceeding 10,000 ng/m^3 have been reported close to industrial emissions or above areas where mercury fungicides have been used extensively (Fujimura, 1964). Air values may rise to 600 and 1500 ng/m^3 near mercury mines and refineries (IPCS, 1976). Few data are available on the speciation of mercury in the atmosphere, but it is generally assumed that the vapor of metallic mercury is the predominant form (IPCS, 1976; Lindqvist et al., 1979; Matheson, 1979). Mercury has a residence time of 0.4 to 3 years and is therefore at least semiglobally distributed (Lindqvist et al., 1979). A water-soluble form may have a short residence time of only a few weeks, and the same may apply to particulate mercury. Although they contribute only a small fraction of the total atmospheric mercury, they may nevertheless be of importance for the rates of transport and depositional processes.

No data are available on average indoor air pollution due to mercury vapor. Fatalities and severe poisonings have resulted from heating metallic mercury and mercury-containing objects in the home. Some incubators used to house premature infants have been found to contain mercury vapor at levels approaching occupational exposure limits; the source was mercury droplets from broken mercury thermostats. The exposure to mercury vapor released from paint containing mercury compounds used to prolong shelf life of interior latex paint can reach levels of 300 to 1500 ng Hg/m^3 (Beusterien et al.,

1991). Indoor air pollution caused by central-heating thermostats and by the use of vacuum cleaners after thermometer breakage, and the like, also needs attention. Release of mercury from amalgam fillings is otherwise the predominant source of human exposure to inorganic mercury in the general population (Clarkson et al., 1988).

Thus the only prevalent sources of human mercury exposure through inhalation are the general atmosphere and dental fillings. From the atmosphere the daily amount absorbed as a result of respiratory exposure into the bloodstream in adults is about 32 ng Hg in rural areas and about 160 ng Hg in urban areas, assuming rural concentrations of 2 ng/m^3 and urban concentrations of 10 ng/m^3 (absorption rate 80%). Depending on the number of amalgam fillings, the estimated average daily absorption of mercury vapor from dental fillings vary between 3000 and 17,000 ng Hg (IPCS, 1991; Clarkson et al., 1988; Skare and Engqvist, 1994). Tracheal measurements of mercury have found concentrations in range of 1000 to 6000 ng Hg/m^3 during inhalation and less than 1000 ng Hg/m^3 when subjects breathed through their noses (Langworth et al., 1988). However, these figures have been questioned, and recalculations reduce the estimated daily intake from dental fillings to about 2000 ng Hg (Olsson and Bergman, 1992).

Diet (Drinking Water and Food)

Mercury in drinking water is usually in the range of 5 to 100 ng Hg/L, the average value being about 25 ng Hg/L. The forms of mercury in drinking-water are not well studied, but Hg^{++} is probably the predominant species present as complexes and chelates with ligands. The bioaccessibility, namely the extent to which a certain mercury complex is available for absorption at the gastrointestinal mucosal surface, may increase or decrease depending on the ligand and the binding strength between metal and ligand.

Concentrations of mercury in most foodstuffs (IPCS, 1976) are often below the detection limit (usually 20 ng mercury per gram fresh weight). Fish and marine mammals are the dominant sources, mainly in the form of methylmercury compounds (70–90% of the total). The normal concentrations in edible tissues of various species of fish cover a wide range, from 50 to 1400 ng mercury per gram fresh weight depending on factors such as pH and redox potential of the water, species, age, and size of the fish (IPCS, 1990). Large predatory fish, such as pike, trout, and tuna, as well as seals and toothed whales contain the highest average concentrations. Furthermore exposure to organomercurials might occur through the use of mercury-containing skin-lightning cremes and other pharmaceuticals. Thiomersal is sometimes used for preservation of vaccines and immunoglobolins (an amount of 100 μg thiomersal per injection).

Soil

Soil contamination is most often characterized by affecting remote areas with few or no human inhabitants. The bioavailability of the mercury is not known in detail, but it would be expected to be low and not cause direct health effects to humans. However, postdepositional methylation of inorganic mercury and redistribution along water streams above or below soil surface should be taken seriously as well as the potential ecological impact in the contaminated areas.

Relative Significance of Different Routes of Environmental Exposure

Human exposure to the three major forms of mercury present in the environment is summarized in Table 16-1 (based on IPCS, 1991). Although the choice of values given is somewhat arbitrary, the table nevertheless provides a perspective on the relative magnitude of the contributions from various media. Humans may be exposed to additional quantities

TABLE 16-1   Estimated Average Daily Intake (Retention) of Mercury Compounds

Media	Estimated Average Daily Intake (Retention)[a] in ng of Mercury per Day		
	Mercury Vapor	Inorganic Mercury Compounds	Methyl Mercury
Air	40–200[b] (30–160)	0[c]	0[c]
Food			
Marine	0	600[d] (60)	2400[d] (2300)
Non-marine	0	3600 (360)	?
Drinking water	0	50 (5)	0
Dental amalgam	3800–21,000 (3000–17,000)	0	0
Total	3900–21,000 (3100–17,000)	4200 (420)	2400 (2300)

[a] Figures in parentheses are the amounts retained that were estimated from the pharmacokinetic parameters; that is, 80% of inhaled vapor, 95% of ingested methyl mercury, and 10% of inorganic mercury are retained.
[b] Assumes an air concentration of 2 to 10 ng/m^3 and a daily respiratory volume of 20 m^3.
[c] For the purposes of comparison, it is assumed that in the atmospheric concentrations of species of mercury other than mercury vapor are negligible.
[d] It is assumed that 80% of the total mercury in edible fish tissues is methylmercury, and 20% in the form of inorganic mercury compounds. It should be noted that fish intake may vary considerably among individuals and across populations. Certain communities whose major source of protein is fish and marine mammals may exceed this estimated methylmercury intake by an order of magnitude or more.

of mercury occupationally and in heavily polluted areas where additional forms of mercury, such as aryl and alkoxyaryl compounds, are widely used as fungicides.

The intake from drinking water is about 50 ng mercury per day, mainly as Hg^{++}; only a small fraction is absorbed. Intake of fish and fish products, averaged over months or weeks, results in an average daily absorption of methylmercury variously estimated to be between 2000 and 4700 ng mercury (IPCS, 1991). The absorption of inorganic mercury from foodstuffs is difficult to estimate because levels of total mercury are close to the limit of detection in many food items and because the bioavailable fraction is generally not known, since chemical species and ligand binding of mercury have not usually been identified. Based on NHANES III data (>19,000 adults), 85% of Americans consume fish once a month, 40% once a week, and 1% to 2% consume fish or shellfish almost daily.

Total dietary mercury intake has been measured over a number of years for various age groups. The intake of total dietary mercury (ng/day) was measured for various age groups as part of a market basket survey (1984–1986) by the U.S. Food and Drug Administration (IPCS, 1990), and the following total intakes were reported: 310 ng (6–11 months); 900 ng (2 years) and 2000 to 3000 ng in adults. In Belgium two surveys estimated the total mercury intake from all foodstuffs to vary between 6500 and 13,000 ng mercury (Fouassin and Fondu, 1978; Buchet et al., 1983). However, much higher mercury intakes occur in fisheaters.

OCCUPATIONAL EXPOSURES

Occupational exposure is almost exclusively to inorganic mercury and occurs at chloralkali plants, mercury mines, thermometer factories, refineries, and in dental clinics. The latest figures indicate that some 70,000 workers in the United States are annually exposed to mercury, primarily elemental mercury. High mercury concentrations have been described for all these situations, but considerable variations exist according to work environment conditions. Hygiene measures toward reducing the exposures and law enforcement of TLV's have reduced exposure significantly. Serious mercury exposure may occur in connection with gold mining, especially when gold amalgam is heated. In developing countries this process is often carried out in small gold-vending shops with insufficient ventilation.

KINETICS AND METABOLISM

The bioavailability, kinetics, and biotransformation of mercury depend on its chemical and physical form.

Bioavailability

Most experimental studies on the toxicokinetics as well as toxicodynamics of mercuric compounds have used water-soluble salts and administered the compounds orally in solution. The occupational or dietary exposure of humans to mercuric compounds is, however, often a mixed exposure to different species of mercury and with concomitant exposure to potential ligands. Bioavailability is the combination of bioaccessibility and absorption. If the mercuric compounds are bound strongly to ligands in the intestinal tract, they might in some cases not be accessible for the absorptive process, whereas other ligands may even facilitate the absorption. Further, if the mercuric species is insoluble, absorption may be low. Therefore the assessment of hazard or risk must address the question of bioavailability, which may be increased as well as decreased depending on the ligand and mercury species.

Absorption

Elemental Mercury (Hg^0)   Approximately 80% of inhaled mercury vapor is absorbed via the lungs and retained in the body. The amount retained is the same whether inhalation takes place through the nose or the mouth (IPCS, 1976). Elemental mercury is poorly absorbed in the gastrointestinal tract (less than 0.01% in rats), though increased blood levels of mercury has been measured in humans after accidental ingestion of several grams of metallic mercury (IPCS, 1976). Skin absorption is insignificant in relation to human exposure to mercury vapor (Hursh et al., 1989).

Inorganic Mercurous (Hg^+) and Mercuric (Hg^{++}) Mercury   The absorption of inhaled aerosols of inorganic mercury depends on particle size, solubility, and so on (IPCS, 1991). No data have been reported for humans. In dogs, 45% of deposited mercury(II) oxide aerosols were cleared in less than 24 hours, and the remainder cleared with a half-time of 33 days (Morrow et al., 1964). Ten percent to 15% of an oral, nontoxic dose of mercuric mercury are absorbed from the gastrointestinal tract in adults and retained in body tissues, but considerable individual variations may exist. In children the gastrointestinal absorption is probably greater.

Organic Mercury   Human poisoning cases caused by inhalation indicate that a large fraction of these lipophilic compounds are absorbed into the blood. Alkyl mercurials are absorbed almost completely in the gastrointestinal tract and retained in the body. Certain methylmercury compounds are probably absorbed through the skin.

Distribution

Elemental Mercury (Hg^0)   After exposure to mercury vapor the element is found in blood as physically dissolved elemental mercury. Within a few minutes the mercury is oxidized to mercuric mercury in the erythrocytes, a reaction catalyzed by the enzyme catalase. Thus, following short-term exposure to mercury vapor, the maximum concentration of Hg in erythrocytes is seen after less than one hour, whereas plasma levels peak after about 10 hours (Cherian et al., 1978). Before oxidation, Hg^0 readily crosses cell membranes, including the blood–brain barrier and the placental barrier. After oxidation, the Hg^{++} ions (or complexes) are distributed in the body via the blood. The kidneys and the brain are the main deposits of Hg after exposure to mercury vapor, whereas absorbed inorganic mercury salts are mainly deposited in the kidneys.

The uptake and/or elimination of mercury after exposure to mercury vapor can be altered by a moderate intake of alcohol, possibly due to inhibition of catalase. Thus the amount of mercury in red blood cells of humans exposed to mercury vapor was significantly reduced in the humans given alcohol before mercury exposure (Hursh et al., 1980).

Inorganic Mercurous (Hg^+) and Mercuric (Hg^{++}) Mercury The kidneys are the predominant site of inorganic mercury accumulation. However, after oral exposure accumulation also occurs in the cells of the mucous membranes of the gastrointestinal tract, though a significant part of this accumulation is later eliminated due to cell shedding and therefore never reaches the general circulation. Mercuric mercury in blood is divided between erythrocytes and plasma in about equal amounts. In erythrocytes, mercury is probably to a large extent bound to sulfhydryl groups on the haemoglobin molecule and possibly also to glutathione. The distribution between different plasma-protein fractions varies with dose and time after exposure.

Mercuric mercury crosses the blood–brain and placental barriers only to a limited extent. However, mercuric mercury does accumulate in the placenta, fetal membranes, and amniotic fluid. The rate of uptake from blood and different organs varies widely, so does the rate of elimination from different organs. Thus the distribution of mercury within the body and within organs varies widely with dose and time lapse after absorption. However, under all conditions the dominating mercury pool in the body after exposure to mercuric mercury is the kidney. Inorganic divalent mercury can induce metallothionein, and a large proportion of the mercury in the kidneys is soluble and bound to metallothionein.

Organic Mercury Methylmercury is distributed via the bloodstream to all tissues in the body. The pattern of tissue distribution is much more uniform than after inorganic mercury exposure, except in red cells, where the concentration is 10 to 20 times greater than the plasma concentration. Methylmercury readily crosses the blood–brain and placental barriers. In the fetus methylmercury is accumulated and concentrated especially in the brain. As with other forms of mercury, the kidneys retain the highest tissue concentration, though the total amount of mercury deposited in muscles might be higher. Experimental studies has demonstrated that the kinetics and disposition of methylmercury depend on gender (Nielsen and Andersen, 1994). At the end of the initial phase of distribution, approximately 1% of the body's methylmercury is found in one liter of blood in the human adult weighing 70 kg (IPCS, 1990). The brain–blood concentration ratio is about 5 : 1. Methylmercury accumulates in hair in the process of formation of hair strands. The hair–blood concentration ratio is approximately 250 : 1 in humans at the time of incorporation into hair. Methylmercury undergoes biotransformation to inorganic mercury by demethylation, particularly in the gut. The fraction present as inorganic mercury depends on the duration of exposure to methylmercury and the time after cessation of exposure.

Elimination

Elemental Mercury (Hg^0) After short-term exposure to mercury vapor, about one-third of the absorbed mercury will be eliminated in unchanged form through exhalation, whereas the remaining mercury predominantly will be eliminated as mercuric mercury through feces (Hursh et al., 1976). A recent study on 10 occupationally exposed dentists and dental nurses demonstrate, assuming first-order kinetics for the clearance of urinary mercury obtained from mercury vapor, a median half-time of 41 days (Skare and Engqvist, 1990). Blood levels can serve as indicators of recent mercury vapor exposure, though speciation must be carried out in order to eliminate possible influence of dietary intake of mercury from marine sources.

Inorganic Mercurous (Hg$^+$) and Mercuric (Hg^{++}) Mercury   Excretion of absorbed inorganic mercury is mainly via urine and feces, the rates by each pathway being roughly equal. The whole-body half-time in adults is about 40 days. The elimination of inorganic mercury follows a complicated pattern with biological half-times that differ according to the tissue and the time after exposure. Hence there are at present no general and suitable indicator media that will reflect concentrations of inorganic mercury in the critical organs, the brain, or kidney under different exposure conditions (IPCS, 1991). One important consequence is that concentrations of mercury in urine or blood may be low quite soon after exposure has ceased, despite the fact that concentrations in the critical organs may still be high.

Organic Mercury   Excretion of methylmercury is predominantly via the feces. Methylmercury is slowly demethylated in the gut, and most, if not all, of the mercury excreted is in the inorganic form. Enterohepatic recirculation probably explains the absence of methylmercury in the feces. The whole-body half-time of methylmercury is usually between 70 and 80 days, but substantial differences occur. The half-time in the brain is roughly the same as that in the whole body, whereas the half-time in the blood compartment is somewhat less. Further laboratory animal studies involving tracer techniques have shown that following acute dosage with methylmercury, blood mercury concentrations will initially reflect organ concentrations reasonably well, but with time, an increasing fraction of the body burden will be in the brain, muscles, and kidney (Nielsen and Andersen, 1992). Sex differences in whole-body clearance and tissue distribution of intestinally absorbed methylmercury have been demonstrated in rodents (Thomas et al., 1986; Nielsen and Andersen, 1994). In particular, a sex-related difference has been observed in the ratio between concentrations of mercury in blood and in potential target organs.

The blood concentration might be a useful indicator of the body burden of mercury, although the erythrocyte mercury concentration is more specific for methyl mercury exposure. Thus, if exposure to mercury vapor or other inorganic mercury compounds is suspected, mercury should be speciated or a serum sample analyzed. Mercury in hair, when measured along the length of a hair strand, has also been used as an indicator of past blood levels. However, hair mercury concentrations may be augmented by the binding of exogenous mercury to the surface. Concomitant oral exposure to inorganic mercury adds more to the concentration in blood than in hair.

HEALTH EFFECTS

Acute and Local Effects

Acute poisoning by mercury vapor may cause a severe airway irritation, chemical pneumonitis, and pulmonary edema in severe cases. Ingestion of inorganic compounds may cause gastrointestinal corrosion and irritation, such as vomiting, bloody diarrhea, and stomach pains. Shock and acute kidney dysfunction with uremia may ensue. Cutaneous exposure to mercury compounds may result in local irritation, and mercury compounds are among the most common allergens in patients with contact dermatitis.

Chronic and Systemic Effects

Chronic intoxication may develop already a few weeks after the onset of a mercury exposure. More commonly, however, the exposure has lasted for several months or years. The symptoms depend on the degree of exposure and the kind of mercury in question. The symptoms may involve the oral cavity, the peripheral and central nervous system, and the kidneys. As the elemental mercury present in vapor is oxidized to mercuric mercury in the blood, the nonneurotoxic effects of absorbed mercury vapor and other inorganic mercury compounds will be similar.

Elemental Mercury (Hg⁰)   Severe exposure to inorganic mercury causes an inflammation of gingiva and oral mucosa which become tender and bleed easily. Salivation is increased, most obviously so in subacute cases. Often the patient complains of a metallic taste in the mouth. Especially when oral hygiene is bad, a grey border is formed on the gingival edges.

In exposures to mercury vapor, the central nervous system is the critical organ, and the classic triad of symptoms includes erethism, intention tremor, and the gingivitis described above. The fine intention tremor of fingers, eyelids, lips, and tongue may progress to spasms of arms and legs. A jerky micrographia is typical as well. The changes in the central nervous system result in psychological effects known as erethism: restlessness, irritability, insomnia, concentration difficulties, decreased memory and depression, sometimes in combination with shyness, unusual psychological vulnerability and anxiety. Newer studies suggest that early stages of erethism may occur, and this psychasthenic-vegetative syndrome has been dubbed "micro mercurialism." The main symptoms appear to be decreased memory, dizziness, and irritability. Similar nonspecific symptoms are described by patients who attribute their ill health to mercury from their dental fillings. Although slight adverse effects are difficult to rule out in susceptible subjects, little evidence is presently available to support this notion (Friberg and Schrauzer, 1995). Induction of minimal tremor by mercury vapor have been reported at urinary excretion levels of 50 µg/L (0.25 µmol/L) and above.

A recent study on monkeys suggested that mercury exposure from amalgam may enrich the intestinal flora with mercury-resistant bacterial species, which in turn also become resistant to antibiotics (Lorscheider et al., 1995). The human health implication of this observation in monkeys is presently unclear, although antibiotic resistance is a problem of increasing importance.

Limited information is available on effects of mercury vapor on early stages of the human life cycle. Effects on pregnancy and birth in women occupationally exposed to mercury vapor have been reported, but insufficient details were available to evaluate dose-response relationships. In children, "pink disease" may occur, as described below.

Inorganic Mercurous (Hg⁺) and Mercuric (Hg⁺⁺) Mercury   The target organ following long-term exposure causing no acute toxicity are the kidneys. In general, the early renal effects of mercury appear to be reversible after cessation of exposure.
Nephrotoxic effects include proximal tubular damage, as indicated by an increased excretion of small proteins in the urine, for example β_2-micro globulin. Glomerular damage seems to be caused by an autoimmune reaction to mercury complexes in the basal membrane, and mercury-related cases of nephrotic syndrome have been traced to this pathogenesis (Kazantzis et al., 1962). Increased circulating antiglomerular basement membrane antibodies have been demonstrated in 8 out of 131 occupationally exposed

males (Roels et al., 1985), and another study demonstrated correlations between increased levels of IgA and IgM and exposure to inorganic mercury (Bencko et al., 1990). However, no dose–effect relationship was established, and in both studies an unknown fraction of the study population had relatively high exposures. A study on 36 chloralkali workers with a mean urinary mercury of 13 µg/g did not show any effects on white blood cells, immunoglobulins, or autoantibodies (Langworth et al., 1993). Nevertheless, as the knowledge from animal studies demonstrate that immunological effects exist and are genetically determined (Druet, 1994; Hultman and Eneström, 1987), an immunotoxic effect of low doses of inorganic mercury in susceptible individuals cannot be excluded based on the limited number of exposed workers investigated.

In children, a different syndrome is seen, the so-called "pink-disease" or acrodynia, diagnosed most frequently in children treated with teething powders which contained calomel and also occasionally seen in children who had inhaled mercury vapor, such as from broken thermometers (Agocs et al., 1990). A generalized eruption develops, and the hands and feet show a characteristic, scaly, reddish appearance. In addition the children are irritable, sleep badly, fail to thrive, sweat profusely, and have photophobia. This condition was extremely common until 30 years ago, when the etiology was finally found and teething powders were phased out.

Organic Mercury   Intoxications with alkoxialkyl or aryl compounds are similar to intoxications with inorganic mercury compounds, because these organomercurials are relatively unstable. Alkyl mercury compounds, such as methylmercury, result in a different syndrome. The earliest symptoms in adults are paresthesias in the fingers, the tongue, and the face, particularly around the mouth. Later on, disturbances occur in the motor functions, resulting in ataxia and dysphasia. The visual field is decreased, and in severe cases the result may be total blindness. Similarly impaired hearing may progress to complete deafness. This syndrome has been caused by methylmercury-contaminated fish in Japan and by methylmercury-treated grain used for baking or animal feed in Iraq and elsewhere.

Children are more susceptible to the toxic effects of methylmercury than are adults, and congenital methylmercury poisoning may result in a cerebral palsy syndrome, even though the mother remains healthy or suffers only minor symptoms due to the exposure (Davis et al., 1994). In populations with a high consumption of fish or marine mammals, methylmercury intakes may approach the levels which resulted in such serious disease in Japan and Iraq. Recent evidence has suggested that prenatal exposure to methylmercury may result in neuropsychological deficits that are detectable at age 7 years of age (Grandjean et al., 1997).

The earliest effects due to methylmercury, such as paresthesias, appear to occur when blood concentrations in adults are above 200 µg/L (1 µmol/L), but an uncertainty factor of perhaps 10 should be applied to take into account possible individual susceptibility and the increased vulnerability of the fetus. Developmental delays appear to be related to maternal hair mercury concentrations above 3 µg/g (Grandjean et al., 1997), that is, a maternal blood concentration of 12 µg/L.

Sufficient evidence exists that methylmercury chloride is carcinogenic to experimental animals. In the absence of comprehensive epidemiological data, methylmercury is considered a possible human carcinogen (class 2B) (IARC, 1994). The U.S. EPA has classified both inorganic mercury compounds and methylmercury as possible human carcinogens.

Prevention

Biological monitoring is very useful in the diagnosis of mercury exposure and in the control of occupational exposure levels. In the blood, inorganic mercury has a half-life of about 30 days, and methylmercury has a half-life about twice as long. Unfortunately, blood levels do not reflect mercury retained in the brain where mercury after vapor inhalation has a half-life of several years. Urine levels are usually preferred as an indicator of occupational exposures.

WHO has recommended that long-term mercury vapor exposures should be limited to a time-weighted average limit of 25 $\mu g/m^3$, a value that has also been adopted in the current (1999) ACGIH limits. The corresponding TWA for inorganic mercury should be 50 $\mu g/m^3$. A limit of 50 μg mercury/g creatinine (28 $\mu mol/mol$ creatinine) has been recommended for urinary mercury excretion (IPCS, 1991). The current occupational exposure limit is 100 $\mu g/m^3$ as a ceiling value for inorganic mercury (OSHA, 1992), which is equivalent to the recommendation from NIOSH (U.S. DHHS, 1992). A RfD for inorganic mercury of 0,3 $\mu g/kg$-d has recently been verified by U.S. EPA. The critical effect serving as basis for the RfD is kidney toxicity due to an autoimmune disease caused by accumulation of IgG antibodies in the glomerular region of the kidneys (U.S. EPA, 1997).

Methylmercury is incorporated in hair, and hair mercury analyses, have proved very useful for screening and quite reliable as indicators of individual exposures during the past months. Methylmercury toxicity has been seen at hair levels above 50 $\mu g/g$ (0.25 $\mu mol/g$). WHO recommends that hair mercury concentrations be kept below 10 to 20 ppm (0.05–0.10 $\mu mol/g$) to protect the fetus. Using an uncertainty factor of 10, the U.S. EPA recommends a reference dose based on a hair concentration of 1.1 $\mu g/g$, equivalent to 4.5 $\mu g/L$ blood. WHO has recommended a provisional tolerable weekly intake (PTWI) level for mercury at 300 μg, of which no more than 200 μg may be methylmercury (IPCS, 1976). Recent official numbers from the United States on methylmercury exposure describes that 9% of the general population exceeds the RfD as does 7% of women in the childbearing age (U.S. EPA, 1997). Concentration limits have been proposed for various fish products, especially for tuna, swordfish, and shark. A level of 0.5 mg/kg or 1.0 mg/kg is frequently used. Although these limits may be appropriate for individuals who only occasionally eat seafood, they may not at all protect people who eat fish every day. The current occupational exposure limit is 10 $\mu g/m^3$ as a TWA value for organic (alkyl) mercury (OSHA, 1992; ACGIH, 1997).

Preventive measures should include the limitation of mercury released from industrial operations to the environment. One of the important nonindustrial sources is discarded batteries (for cameras and watches) and thermometers. Some countries have instituted a practice of collecting and recycling the mercury from such consumer products. If mercury is used for fungicidal treatment of grain, the grain should be dyed red to indicate that it is unsuitable for human consumption. Mercury exposures from dental amalgam fillings should be minimized, but alternative restorative materials should only be used if their safety and durability are known to be superior to amalgam.

REFERENCES

ACGIH. 1999. American Conference of Governmental Industrial Hygienists. Threshold limit values for chemical substances and physical agents and biological exposure indices for 1999. Cincinnati, OH.

Agocs, M. M., R. A. Etzel, R. G. Parrish, D. C. Paschal, P. R. Campagna, D. S. Cohen, E. M. Kilbourne, and J. L. Hesse. 1990. Mercury exposure from interior paint. *N. Engl. J. Med.* 323: 1096–1101.

Bencko, V., V. Wagner, M. Wagnerova, and V. Ondrejcak. 1990. Immunological profiles in workers occupationally exposed to inorganic mercury. *J. Hygiene, Epidemiol. Microbiol. Immunol.* 34: 9–15.

Beusterien, K. M., R. A. Etzel, M. M. Agocs, G. M. Egeland, E. M. Socie, M. A. Rouse, and B. K. Mortensen. 1991. Indoor air mercury concentrations following application of interior latex paint. *Arch. Environ. Contam. Toxicol.* 21: 62–64.

Buchet, J. P., R. Lauwerys, A. Vandervoorde, and J. M. Pycke. 1983. Oral daily intake of cadmium, lead, manganese, chromium, mercury, calcium, zinc, and arsenic in Belgium: A duplicate meal study. *Food Chem. Toxicol.* 21: 19–24.

Cherian, M. G., J. B. Hursh, T. W. Clarkson, and J. Allen. 1978. Radioactive mercury distribution in biological fluids and excretion in human subjects after inhalation of mercury vapour. *Arch. Environ. Health* 33: 109–114.

Clarkson, T. W., J. B. Hursh, P. R. Sager, and T. L. M. Syversen. 1988. Mercury. In *Biological Monitoring of Toxic Metals, eds.* T. W. Clarkson, L. Friberg, G. F. Nordberg, and P. Sager. pp. 199–246. New York: Plenum.

Davis, L. E., M. Kornfeld, H. S. Mooney, K. J. Fiedler, K. Y. Haaland, W. W. Orrison, E. Cercichiari, and T. W. Clarkson. 1994. Methylmercury poisoning. Long-term clinical, radiological, toxicological, and pathological studies of an affected family. *Ann. Neurol.* 35: 680–688.

Druet, P. 1994. Metal-induced autoimmunity. *Arch. Toxicol.* 16(suppl.): 185–191.

Fouassin, A., and M. Fondu. 1978. Evaluation de la teneur moyenne en mercure de la ration alimentaire en Belgique. *Archives Belges de Medecine Sociale, Hygiene, Medecine du Travail et Medecine Legale* 36: 481–490.

Friberg, L., and G. N. Schrauzer, eds. 1995. *Status quo and Perspectives of Amalgam and Other Dental Materials.* Stuttgart: Georg Thieme.

Fujimura, Y. 1964. Studies on the toxicity of mercury (Hg Series No. 7). II. The present status of mercury contamination in the environment and foodstuffs. *Jap. J. Hygiene* 18: 402–411.

Gilmour, C. C., and N. S. Bloom. 1995. A case study of mercury and methylmercury dynamics in a Hg-contaminated municipal wastewater treatment plant. *Water Air Soil Pollut.* 80: 799–803.

Grandjean, P., P. Weihe, R. F. White, F. Debes, S. Araki, K. Yokoyama, K. Murata, N. Sørensen, R. Dahl, and P. J. Jørgensen. 1997. Cognitive deficit in 7-year-old children with prenatal exposure to methylmercury. *Neurotox. Teratol.* 19: 417–428.

Hultman, P., and S. Eneström, 1987. The induction of immune complex deposits in mice by peroral and parenteral administration of mercuric chloride; strain dependent susceptibility. Clinical Experim. Immunol. 67: 283–292.

Hursh, J. B., T. W. Clarkson, M. G. Cherian, J. V. Vostal, and R. V. Mallie. 1976. Clearance of mercury (Hg-197, Hg-203) vapor inhaled by human subjects. *Arch. Environ. Health* 31: 301–309.

Hursh, J. B., T. W., Clarkson, E. Miles, and L. A. Goldsmith, 1989. Percutaneous absorption of mercury vapor by man. *Arch. Environ. Health* 44: 120–127.

Hursh, J. B., M. R. Greenwood, T. W. Clarkson, J. Allen, and S. Demuth. 1980. The effect of ethanol on the fate of mercury vapor inhaled by man. *J. Pharmacol. Experim. Therapeutics* 214: 520–527.

IARC. 1994. *Mercury and Mercury Compounds.* IARC Monographs on the Evaluation of Carcinogenic Risk to Humans, vol. 58. Lyon: IARC.

IPCS. 1976. International Programme on Chemical Safety. *WHO Task Group on Environmental Health Criteria for Mercury.* EHC 1. Geneva: WHO.

IPCS. 1990. International Programme on Chemical Safety. *WHO Task Group on Environmental Health Criteria for Methylmercury.* EHC 101. Geneva: WHO.

IPCS. 1991. International Programme on Chemical Safety. *WHO Task Group on Environmental Health Criteria for Inorganic Mercury.* EHC 118. Geneva: WHO.

Kazantzis, G., K. F. R. Schiller, A. W. Asscher, and R. G. Drew. 1962. Albuminuria and the nephrotic syndrome following exposure to mercury and its compounds. *Quart. J. Med.* 31: 403–418.

Langworth, S., C.-G. Elinder, and K. G. Sundqvist 1993. Minor effects of low exposure to inorganic mercury on the human immune system. *Scand. J. Work Environ. Health* 19: 405–413.

Langworth, S., C.-G. Elinder, and A. Åkesson. 1988. Mercury exposure from dental fillings. II. Release and absorption. *Swed. Dental J.* 12: 71–72.

Lindberg, S., P. Stokes, E. Goldberg, and C. Wren. 1987. Group report: Mercury. In *Lead, Mercury, Cadmium and Arsenic in the Environment*, eds. T. W. Hutchinson, and K. M. Meena, pp. 17–34. New York: Wiley.

Lindqvist, O., A. Jernelov, K. Johansson, and R. Rodhe. 1979. *Mercury in the Swedish Environment: Global and Local Sources*, pp. 1–105 Sweden Report 1816. Solna: National Swedish Environmental Protection Board.

Lorscheider, F. L., M. J. Vimy, A. O. Summers, and H. Zweirs. 1995. The dental amalgam mercury controversy—inorganic mercury and the CNS; genetic linkage of mercury and antibiotic resistances in intestinal bacteria. *Toxicol.* 97: 19–22.

Matheson, D. H. 1979. Mercury in the atmosphere and in precipitation. In *The Biogeochemistry of Mercury in the Environment*, ed. J. O. Nriagu, pp. 113–129. Amsterdam Elsevier.

Morrow, P. E., F. R. Gibb, and L. Johnson. 1964. Clearance of insoluble dust from the lower respiratory tract. *Health physics* 10: 543–555.

Nielsen, J. B., 1992. Toxicokinetics of mercuric chloride and methylmercuric chloride in mice. *J. Toxicol. Environ. Health* 37: 85–122.

Nielsen, J. B. and O. Andersen. 1992. Time dependent disposition of mercury after oral dosage. In *Metal Compounds in Environment and Life*, eds. E. Merian and W. Haerdi, pp. 341–348 Science and Technology Letters, Middlesex, U.K.

Nielsen, J. B., and O. Andersen. 1994. Evaluation of mercury in hair, blood and muscle as biomarkers for methylmercury exposure in male and female mice. *Arch. Toxicol* 68: 317–321.

Olsson, S., and M. Bergman. 1992. Daily dose calculations from measurements of intra-oral mercury vapor. *J. Dental Res.* 71: 414–423.

OSHA. 1992. Occupational Safety and Health Administration. Air contaminants. Washington D.C.: U.S. Department of Labor.

Roels, H., J.-P. Gennart, R. Lauwerys, J.-P. Buchet, J. Malchaire, and A. Bernard. 1985. Surveillance of workers exposed to mercury vapour: Validation of a previously proposed biological threshold limit value for mercury concentration in urine. *Am. J. Ind. Med.* 7: 45–71.

Schoof, R., and J. B. Nielsen. 1997. Evaluation of methods for assessing the oral bioavailability of inorganic mercury in soil. *Risk Anal.* 17: 545–555.

Skare, I., and A. Engqvist. 1990. Urinary mercury clearance of dental personnel after a long term intermission in occupational exposure. *Swed. Dental J.* 14: 255–259.

Skare, I., and A. Engqvist. 1994. Human exposure to mercury and silver released from dental amalgam restorations. *Arch. Environ. Health* 49: 384–394.

Sweet, C. W., and S. J. Vermette. 1993. Sources of toxic trace elements in urban air in Illinois. *Environ. Sci. Technol.* 27: 2502–2510.

Thomas D. J., H. L. Fisher, M. R. Sumler, P. Mushak, and L. L. Hall. 1986. Sexual differences in the distribution and retention of organic and inorganic mercury in methyl mercury-treated rats. *Environ. Res.* 41: 219–234.

U.S. DHHS. 1992. Department of Health and Human Services, NIOSH (National Institute for Occupational Safety and Health). NIOSH recommendations for occupational safety and health — compendium of policy documents and statements. Cincinnati, OH.

U.S. DHHS. 1994. ATSDR (Agency for Toxic Substances and Disease Registry). Toxicological profile for mercury (update), TP-93/10, Atlanta, GA.

U.S. DHHS. 1997. ATSDR. Toxicological profile for mercury (update), Atlanta, GA.

U.S. EPA. 1997. Environmental Protection Agency. Mercury study report to congress. Washington, D.C.

Wood, J. M., and H. K. Wang. 1983. Microbial resistance to heavy metals. *Environ. Sci. Technol.* 17: 82a–90a.

17 Microwaves and Electromagnetic Fields

DAVID H. SLINEY, Ph.D
FRANCIS COLVILLE

Few occupational or environmental exposures have received more press than electromagnetic fields. Alleged health hazards include "possible carcinogenicity," teratogenic effects, and a host of stress-type syndromes. However, when most scientific panels meet to recommend exposure control standards, much of the supporting epidemiological and laboratory data are found to be nonexistent, very weak, or inconclusive. Present standards are based on well-recognized biological effects of induced currents or heating in exposed biological tissue. Thermal effects dominate at high frequencies and induced current effects dominate at lower frequencies.

Occupational exposure limits (OELs) or guidelines for electromagnetic (EM) fields have been promulgated by different professional, governmental, and standards organizations over the past 30 years. Most attention has focused on the microwave (0.3–300 GHz) region of the spectrum. Initially the primary attention paid to this health issue was limited to the communications industry and military establishments. This was true worldwide. However, with the rapidly expanding use of microwave cooking ovens in the 1970s and portable cellular devices in the 1990s, many other organizations became interested in the question of potential health hazards from EM fields (Schwan, 1982; NCRP, 1993; Harlen, 1982; ICNIRP, 1998).

The possibility of occupational health hazards associated with the use of radio-frequency (RF) inductive heaters and heat sealers led standards-setting groups to reexamine the frequency range below 100 MHz. Their concern was focused on the well-known ability of devices at these low frequencies to produce localized heating in biological tissue. For example, RF medical diathermy is a widely used therapeutic modality. Through coupling of RF energy (usually at 13.5 MHz and 27 MHz), it produces a significant temperature rise directly into a selected region of the body (Hill, 1989).

Coincidentally the EM bioeffects community's interest grew in the specific absorption rate (SAR) of the human body, particularly as affected by its size relative to the wavelength of the incident EM energy. This is known as the "resonance" absorption phenomenon. The practical extent of the frequency region for this to occur is 30 to 70 MHz (for a standing adult). This resonance region of enhanced absorption of EM energy shifts slightly to shorter wavelengths for a seated adult or a child. In addition there is a growing concern today about possible adverse effects of exposure to even lower-frequency EM energy—

Environmental Toxicants: Human Exposures and Their Health Effects, 2/e. Edited by Morton Lippmann.
ISBN: 0-471-29298-2 © 2000 John Wiley & Sons, Inc.
Note: The opinions or assertions herein are those of the authors and do not necessarily reflect the official position of the Department of the Army or Department of Defense.

that associated with video display units, electric blankets, and power transmission lines. This has raised the question of the need for standards down to the 50/60 Hz region even though thermal damage mechanisms have not been suggested at these frequencies. Limits are also proposed, or being considered, at even lower frequencies (below 10 Hz) to prevent induced pseudodirect currents in the body. At these frequencies the body can misinterpret them as direct currents and interact adversely with the very low direct-current levels functioning in the neurological circuits of the central nervous system. The exposure limits (ELs) being considered in the extremely low frequency (ELF) region (see Table 17-1) are several orders of magnitude higher than those based on thermal effects at 10 kHz. As a result of the interest in lower-frequency exposures, concerns that had once been limited to occupational exposure have expanded to environmental exposure. Thus some groups have demanded environmental exposure limits (EELs) (Bernhardt, 1979, 1986).

Previously most EM standards-setting committees groups in the United States and around the world had concentrated their attention on the regions above 10 kHz. The consensus was that the SAR of biological tissue was so low that bioeffects would not be of concern at lower frequencies. Currently the issue has increasingly focused on much lower frequencies (Schwan, 1982; NCRP, 1993; Harlen, 1982; UNEP/WHO/IRPA, 1993).

The issue of potential adverse health effects of EM fields has sometimes been clouded by special interests concerned with community appearance. The siting of large structures such as microwave communication, radar, and high-voltage power lines and cellular phone towers has been their main concern. Their effort has been to block the construction of what were deemed "unsightly" structures. Cellular phone towers are presently being installed in both residential and business localities. Some community groups and legal counsel have sought to convince authorities that the mere possibility of adverse health effects should prohibit construction near inhabited areas, even when present exposure standards would not be exceeded. In such instances, lawyers and journalists began to debate the scientific conclusions of specific biological studies, often without the rigor or balance that is customary in normal scientific analysis. The challenge for the health professional to maintain a balanced judgment.

BACKGROUND

Prior to discussing ELs for EM fields, it is necessary to briefly review the physical units and quantities used to express such limits. Electromagnetic waves are periodic and are characterized by their frequency and their wavelength. Frequency is the wave's rate of

TABLE 17-1 Electromagnetic Energy Bands and Their Associated Frequency and Wavelength Ranges

Bands	Frequency	Wavelength(m)
(ELF) Extremely low frequency	1–30 Hz	10^8–10^7
(SLF) Superlow frequency	30–300 Hz	10^7–10^6
(ULF) Ultralow frequency	300 Hz–3 kHz	10^6–10^5
(VLF) Very low frequency	3–30 kHz	10^5–10^4
(LF) Low frequency	30–300 kHz	10^4–10^3
(MF) Medium frequency	300 kHz–3 MHz	10^3–100
(HF) High frequency	3–30 MHz	100–10
(VHF) Very high frequency	30–300 MHz	10–1
(UHF) Ultrahigh frequency	300 MHz–3 GHz	1–0.1
(SHF) Superhigh frequency	3–30 GHz	10^{-1}–10^{-2}
(EHF) Extremely high frequency	30–300 GHz	10^{-2}–10^{-3}

generation, and wavelength is the distance from the start of one cycle to the start of another. Frequency is generally expressed in hertz (Hz, cycles per second). The Greek symbol λ (lambda) represents the wavelength, normally in meters (m). The relationship of the frequency and wavelength for all EM waves is dependent on the speed of light, such that frequency (f in hertz) multiplied by the wavelength (λ in meters) is equal to the speed of light (c in meters per second):

$$f\lambda = c \quad \text{or} \quad f = \frac{c}{\lambda} \quad \text{or} \quad \lambda = \frac{c}{f}.$$

The EM spectrum is divided into several regions exhibiting common properties. Each region is designated in terms of wavelength or frequency band. Each band in the EM spectrum is additionally identified by name, as shown in Table 17-1 for frequencies less than 300 GHz (Dolezalek, 1990).

Electromagnetic field intensities are characterized in two ways, either as power density (power per unit area) or as a field strength component (voltage or current per unit length). The most conventional unit for expressing power density is milliwatts per centimeter squared (mW/cm^2), and for field strength it is volts per meter (V/m) for an electric (**E**) field and amperes per meter (A/m) for the magnetic (**H**) field. The selection of a measurement quantity is determined by the kind of EM field that is being measured and its location in space.

If the EM field is coupled to a free radiating wave, then the E and H field vectors of the radiating wave are at right angles to each other and at right angles to the direction of propagation (so-called transverse EM propagation mode, TEM). In this region, fields decrease proportionately with distance following the inverse square law. With a TEM wave, the **E** and **H** field vectors are constantly related by the impedance of the propagation medium (120π or 377 ohms [Ω] for free space). For this reason the **E** or **H** field vectors can be measured to characterize the EM energy at the wave front. Normally the E field is measured, and because we know that $\mathbf{E}/\mathbf{H} = 377\,\Omega$, the power ($\mathbf{E} \times \mathbf{H}$) can be automatically calculated and presented on a meter as power density. In the radiating field condition, either field strength component or the power density can be determined by a simple field component measurement. Power density for the radiating field condition may be calculated from the output power, radiating frequency, the antenna gain, and the distance to the point of interest. In the radiating field region, EM energy transfer into the tissue is based on the power density of the wave front and the cross-sectional area of the tissue exposed (ANSI, 1992; Johnson and Jasik, 1984).

Situations in which the **E** and **H** fields are not related by a constant factor require independent measurements of both the **E** and **H** fields. The measurement of only one field vector cannot characterize the EM energy available at that point in space. This most often occurs in the region close to an antenna element or an open transmission line. This area is called the reactive near-field region (usually closer than λ/2π from such a source). In this reactive near field region, energy transfer occurs by a mechanism called capacitive or inductive coupling. In the reactive near field region both the **E** and **H** fields must be measured to determine exposure levels.

PHILOSOPHICAL APPROACHES

Occupational exposure limits are intended for a narrow segment of the population who are involved in working with equipment or machinery that produce EM energy. Some examples of this type of workforce include military personnel, police officers who use radar guns, and medical technicians who use diathermy devices. In the United States, OEL and EEL guidelines for EM fields were first developed by the American National Standards Institute (ANSI) and the Institute for Electrical and Electronic Engineers (IEEE) in ANSI/IEEE C95.1 (1992). The American Conference of Governmental Industrial Hygienists (ACGIH, 1997) have also adopted the ANSI/IEEE OEL guidelines for inclusion in their standard. The International Commission on Non-Ionizing Radiation Protection (ICNIRP), a successor to the International Radiation Protection Association's International Non-Ionizing Radiation Committee (IRPA/INIRC), has developed OEL and EEL guidelines that differ slightly from the ANSI/IEEE standards. The biological data base required to derive the ELs was the same for the occupational and environmental conditions. The differences in the standards and guidelines is based on the level of awareness of the population to the EM energy around them. OELs are invoked on personnel who are aware of the potential for EM exposure as a concomitant of employment or others who have to pass through an EM area. EELs address the general population, those individuals who have no knowledge or awareness of being in an EM environment.

In considering the need for an exposure standard or guideline for the **E** or **H** fields of ELF to VLF EM fields, one must first question whether sufficient knowledge of potential injury thresholds exist. The promulgation of an EL standard suggests that even more knowledge is available than for a guideline. Additionally promulgation of a standard often curtails much support of further biological studies necessary to determine thresholds of injury and interaction mechanisms. The opponents of standard setting have argued that history can show that premature standards stifle the technological and bioelectromagnetic studies that lead to the understanding of injury thresholds and mechanisms.

In the HF frequency region there has been a lack of knowledge about any interaction mechanisms other than thermal for biological systems. Aside from such thermal effects and RF shock and burns, any other potentially adverse effect is purely speculative and subject to review on the basis of additional research. At these frequencies even extremely high external fields induce only minute electrical currents within the body. The magnitude of these currents can be calculated (Bernhardt, 1986); however, the biological effects, either helpful or adverse, of such currents are still being debated.

It is worth noting that some early OEL proposals for static magnet fields originated from engineers and scientists who were attempting to allay concerns about potential hazards. They proposed working levels that could readily implemented in industry and the military environments without disrupting current workforce operations (Sliney, 1985).

Alternatively, in some socialist countries such as the former Soviet Union (FSU), the dynamics of standards setting led to more conservative OELs. Among the several reasons it has been alleged that very conservative levels were supported by workers' organizations in order to obtain extra benefits if they worked in "hazardous environments." Different philosophies of setting standards in the East and West also explain much of the historical basis for the variation in recommended OELs and EELs despite the use of the same biological data base (GOST, 1982; ACGIH, 1990; Sliney et al., 1985; Minnin, 1962; Magnuson et al., 1964). For example, it has been argued that the Soviets had set OELs at which no known biological effects of potential concern existed, and generally it was well below any adverse effect levels. Indeed, it was argued that the Soviets in practice allowed exposure above their guidelines, since they knew that it was not seriously hazardous (Sliney et al., 1985; Minin, 1962; Magnuson et al., 1964). By contrast, the United States and most Western countries had set limits closer to known thresholds for injury. Exceeding a threshold exposure level will more likely result in injury. Hence more serious protective efforts than those in the East were made in the West to limit exposures levels to below the EL (Sliney et al., 1985; Minnin, 1962). It is important to add, however, that the ELs in the West do not actually border the threshold of known injury level but are usually severalfold, even 10-fold, lower than any known risk of adverse health effect. Health scientists from different countries differ on these interpretations, but it is well to remember that one may be comparing "apples with oranges" when simply comparing numerical values of OELs or EELs published by different countries.

At an international symposium devoted to the setting of OELs (Copenhagen, Denmark, 23–26 April 1985), the philosophies of setting health standards were reviewed. Although most of the presentations at that symposium related to setting limits for airborne chemical contaminants, the proceedings of that symposium are worthwhile to review to obtain a broad perspective on this issue (ACGIH, 1985).

STANDARDS DEVELOPMENT

Over the past decade, a quest for orderliness and completeness led the standards-setting community to extend earlier RF limits into the HF to VLF region and even the ELF and SLF frequency region. The SARs are generally considered insignificant at these frequency regions without direct contact with a current-carrying conductor. There were few or no biological data on which to base a standard in these frequency regions (ICNIRP, 1998; ACGIH, 1997). Some industrial and user groups, however, favored EL development for HF to VLF regions in order to calm the concerns from users who had argued, "if there are no standards for safe exposure, then any exposure should be considered potentially hazardous." These proponents for standards felt that any limit could be lived with and would be better than allowing a void to exist.

The OELs for lower frequencies required separate treatments of the **E** fields and the **H** fields, since almost all potential exposures of individuals were within the reactive field where a simple power-density specification was not meaningful (Schwan, 1982; Harlen, 1982; ICNIRP, 1998; ACGIH, 1997).

During the past 15 to 20 years, standards committees of governmental and professional organizations (e.g., the Committee on Threshold Limit Valued [TLVs] for Physical Agents of ACGIH) have periodically reviewed the state of knowledge regarding the biological effects of ULF, SLF, and ELF fields and pulsed **E** or **H** fields with an eye toward establishing EL guidelines and relevant control measures. However, until this decade all these groups consistently came to the conclusion that there was an absence of scientific information pointing to pathological or other adverse effects on which to base such OELs or EEL (Harlen, 1982; ICNIRP, 1998; ACGIH, 1999; Repacholi, 1985; Sliney, 1985). Even at the very lowest frequencies (less than 10 Hz), adverse physiological effects of currents induced in the human body are believed to occur only at levels higher than those ever likely to be experienced in a realistic environment (Bernhardt, 1979, 1986).

ACGIH proposed revised EM TLVs in 1982 that extended for the first time into the VLF region, and TLVs for the ELF region were first proposed in 1990. These TLVs extended down to 1 Hz, and this low-frequency extension was prompted primarily by what the Committee considered to be unwarranted concerns about health hazards from VDTs. It was felt that TLVs based on theoretical biophysical principles and limited biological data would be well above those produced by most electrical and electronic equipment and thereby put to rest many unwarranted concerns. The biophysical principle used was to keep TLVs low enough at the frequencies involved so that the induced currents would be lower than those that exist naturally in the body. This same principle was used initially to set the thermal SAR limit at higher frequencies. That earlier application of the principle fixed a standard (0.4 W/kg SAR) that is still considered to incorporate an adequately be conservative safety factor 30 years later (ACGIH, 1982). In 1980 and 1983, ACGIH published a statement that insufficient knowledge existed to set guidelines for exposure to static or slowly varying **H** fields, but in 1987 and 1990, ACGIH published Notices of Intent to Establish TLVs for both ELF and static **H** fields. These guidelines have been only slightly modified since then.

TABLE 17-2   ANSI/IEEE and ACGIH Occupational Exposure Limits

Frequency Range (MHz)	Electric Field Strength (E) (V/m)	Magnetic Field Strength (H) (A/m)	Power Density (S) E-Field, H-Field (mW/cm^2)	Averaging Time (min)
0.003–0.1	614	163	$(100, 1{,}000{,}000)^2$	6
0.1–3.0	614	$16.3/f$	$(100, 10{,}000/f^2)^2$	6
3–30	$1842/f$	$16.3/f$	$(900/f^2, 10{,}000/f^2)$	6
30–100	61.4	$16.3/f$	$(1.0, 10{,}000/f^2)^2$	6
100–300	61.4	0.163	1.0	6
300–3000			$f/300$	6
3000–15,000			10	6
15,000–300,000			10	$616{,}000/f^{1.2}$

Note: (1) f is frequency in MHz. (2) These plane wave equivalent power densities values are commonly used as a convenient comparison with OELs at higher frequencies and are displayed on some measuring instruments.

Today there is little movement to revise standards in the microwave and other higher-frequency RF bands, but there remains continued discussion with regard to limits below 20 kHz.

CURRENT OELs AND EELs FOR RF RADIATION

Tables 17-2 and 17-3 show the principal, well-known EM OELs published in the U.S. literature. Tables 17-4 and 17-5 show the EM EELs for the United States. The difference between the two ELs is the level of awareness of the personnel. Figure 17-1 provides the log-log representation of the OELs and EELs of ACGIH, ANSI/IEEE, and ICNIRP

TABLE 17-3   ICNIRP Occupational Exposure Limits

Frequency Range (MHz)	Electric Field Strength (E) (V/m)	Magnetic Field Strength (H) (A/m)	Power Density (S) E-Field, H-Field (W/m^2)
Up to 1 Hz	—	1.63×10^5	—
1–8 Hz	20,000	$1.63 \times 10^5/f^2$	—
8–25 Hz	20,000	$2 \times 104/f$	—
0.025–0.82 kHz	$500/f$	$20/f$	—
0.82–65 kHz	610	24.4	—
0.065–1 MHz	610	$1.6/f$	—
1–10 MHz	$610/f$	$1.6/f$	—
10–400 MHz	61	0.16	10
400–2000 MHz	$3f^{1/2}$	$0.008f^{1/2}$	$f/40$
2–300 GHz	137	0.36	50

Note: (1) f as indicted in the frequency range column. (2) For frequencies between 100 kHz and 10 Ghz. S, E, and H are averaged over a 6 minutes period. (3) For frequencies exceeding 10 GHz. S, E, H are to be averaged over any $68/f^{1.05}$ min period (f in GHz).

TABLE 17-4   ANSI/IEEE and ACGIH Environmental Exposure Limits

Frequency Range (MHz)	Electric Field Strength (E) (V/m)	Magnetic Field Strength (H) (A/m)	Power Density (S) E-Field, H-Field (mW/cm^2)	Averaging Time $\|E\|^2$, S	$\|H\|^2$
0.003–0.1	614	163	$(100, 1{,}000{,}000)^2$	6	6
0.1–1.34	614	$16.3/f$	$(100, 10{,}000/f^2)^2$	6	6
1.34–3.0	$823.8/f$	$16.3f$	$(180/f^2, 10{,}000/f^2)^2$	$f^2/0.3$	6
3–30	$823.8/f$	$16.3/f$	$(180/f^2, 10{,}000/f^2)^2$	30	6
30–100	27.5	$158.3/f^{1.668}$	$(0.2, 940{,}000/f^{3.336})^2$	30	$0.0636f^{1.337}$
100–300	27.5	0.0729	0.2	30	30
300–3000			$f/1500$	30	
3000–15,000			$f/1500$	$90\,000/f$	
15,000–300,000			10	$616\,000/f^{1.2}$	

Note: (1) f is frequency in MHz. (2) These plane wave equivalent power densities values are commonly used as a convenient comparison with OELs at higher frequencies and are displayed on some measuring instruments.

expressed as equivalent far-field (radiating field) power densities. Figures 17-2 and 17-3 provide the log-log representations as a function of frequency of the **E** field and the **H** field, respectively. The low-frequency region (less than 3 MHz) in Figure 17-1 has rather large ELs for all three standards. This is due to the poor absorption efficiency of the human body at low frequencies. As stated earlier, most of the energy is sensed as a form of neurological stimulation. The region between approximately 30 MHz and 3GHz define the SAR boundaries. This is the frequency band where the human body most efficiently absorbs EM energy. Therefore the ELs in this region are significantly lower to compensate for this condition. In the region above approximately 3 GHz, most thermal energy is deposited on or near the skin. There is very little penetration of EM energy into the body. The ANSI/ IEEE, ACGIH, and the ICNIRP all have about the same ELs in the middle (SAR) region. In the upper-frequency region, the ANSI/IEEE and the ACGIH both have adopted the same EM ELs, while the ICNIRP EL is set at half of the ANSI/ACGIH ELs. The ANSI/ IEEE and ACGIH EELs are set at one-fifth the OELs. This is an additional level of protection provided the general population. It is not based on any additional scientific

TABLE 17-5   ICNIRP Environmental Exposure Limits

Frequency Range (MHz)	Electric Field Strength (E) (V/m)	Magnetic Field Strength (H) (A/m)	Power Density (S) E-Field, H-Field (W/m^2)
Up to 1 Hz	—	3.2×10^4	—
1–8 Hz	10,000	$3.2 \times 10^4/f^2$	—
8–25 Hz	10,000	$4000/f$	—
0.025–0.8 KHz	$250/f$	$4/f$	—
0.8–3 KHz	$250/f$	5	—
3–150 KHz	87	5	—
0.15–1 MHz	87	$0.73/f$	—
1–10 MHz	$87/f^{1/2}$	$0.73/f$	—
10–400 MHz	28	0.073	2
400–2000 MHz	$1.375f^{1/2}$	$0.0037f^{1/2}$	$f/200$
2–300 GHz	61	0.16	10

Note: (1) f as indicted in the frequency range column. (2) For frequencies between 100 kHz and 10 GHz. S, **E**, and **H** are averaged over a 6 minute period. (3) For frequencies exceeding 10 GHz. S, **E**, **H** are to be averaged over any $68/f^{1.05}$ min period (f in GHz).

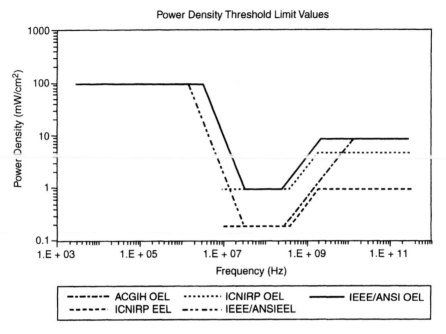

Figure 17-1   OEL / EEL power density limits.

studies or investigations, but on the premise that the general population requires an extra margin of safety due to their lack of EM awareness. The ANSI / IEEE, ACGIH, and ICNIRP guidelines all provide an important caveat, that higher levels are permitted if one wishes to go to the trouble of calculating the actual SAR and showing that an individual is

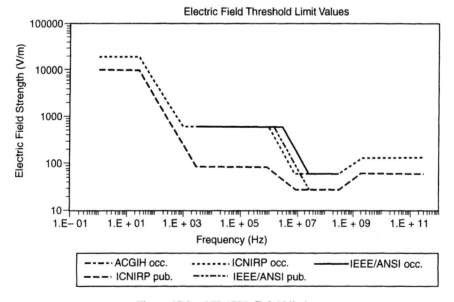

Figure 17-2   OEL / EEL **E** field limits.

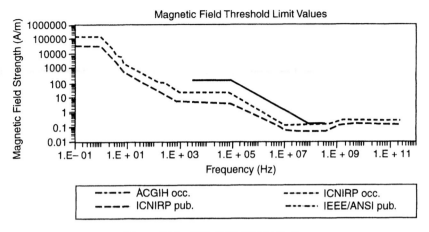

Figure 17-3 OEL / EEL **H** field limits.

actually absorbing less than an average SAR of 0.4 W/kg. This permits a user to follow much less stringent limits; however, safety procedures must be followed to limit "startle reaction" to RF or shock from large ungrounded metal structures such as truck or school bus bodies immersed in the field (ACGIH, 1997; Repacholi, 1985; DIN, 1984; ICNIRP, 1998).

LOWEST FREQUENCIES

All of the initial EM standards concentrated on the microwave radiation frequencies where biological effects could be clearly demonstrated at a result of overt heating of tissue (Schwan, 1982). As time passed, OELs at lower frequencies were promulgated. Concerns about potential adverse effects from RF heat sealers forced most groups to recommend standards or guidelines in the frequency range down to 10 MHz or lower, and essentially all standards reach down to 100-300 KHz (ACGIH 1997; ICNIRP 1998).

As seen in Figure 17-2, the EELs are more stringent for the **E** field because the **E**-field-induced currents were thought to account for more absorbed power than the **H** field at lower frequencies (Bernhardt, 1979, 1986; NRPB, 1988; ICNIRP, 1998; Ghandi et al., 1980; Deno, 1974). This distinction was also made by ANSI / IEEE.

The limits at 100 KHz — the lowest frequency at which most limits are given — can vary by orders of magnitude among the standards. This can be explained by the significant lack of biological data showing any adverse effect on which to base a limit more realistically. At frequencies below 100 KHz, there is virtually no absorption of energy in the human body. This led to the ever-ascending OEL and EEL of the standards; however, concerns about "startle-reaction" RF shocks led ANSI / IEEE and ACGIH to place a cap on their ELs (ANSI / IEEE, 1992; ACGIH, 1997).

The new ICNIRP standard (ICNIRP, 1998), as shown in Tables 17-3 and 17-5, are the result of certain modifications of the IRPA / INIRC (1984) and IRPA / INIRC (1988) standards. Although the basic limits of an SAR or 0.4 W/kg over the whole body was retained, the SAR limit is now 2 W per 0.1 kg for partial-body exposure of the extremities (hands, feet, etc.). All SAR values are averaged over any 6 minutes. These partial-body SAR limits overcome the possibly excessive SARs that could occur for exposures in small regions (wrists or ankles) of the body. Below 10 MHz it is found that the EM **H** field limit between 0.1 and 10 MHz now remains at the same value.

U.S. GOVERNMENT ACTIVITIES

In 1996 the Federal Communications Commission (FCC) circulated proposed EM ELs to other governmental agencies and outside scientific experts for comments. These proposals were somewhat different and in some cases more conservative than those used by ANSI/ IEEE, ACGIH, or OSHA. Both OSHA and ACGIH had adopted the ANSI/IEEE standards. The written reviews included considerable criticism from various governmental agencies including the Department of Defense (DOD), which had already adopted the ANSI/IEEE standard. The FCC draft standard included parts of the ANSI/IEEE standard along with parts of the National Council on Radiation Protection standard. The primary objections to this FCC standard was that is lacked completeness, and it was not a general consensus standard. Despite its shortcomings the FCC guidelines were accepted and released on August 1, 1996. Since these guidelines were accepted by the FCC and published in the Federal Register, there is expected to be increased pressure on the National Telecommunications and Information Administration (NTIA) to require other federal agencies to comply with the new FCC guidelines.

ALTERNATIVES TO OELs: DO THEY EXIST?

Some occupational health professionals argue that there appears to be little or no reason for concern regarding conventional occupational exposure to most EM transmitter sources operating in the HF bands (other than RF heat sealers). They question whether there is any justification for protective measures. In the absence of knowledge, one can always encourage avoidance of needless exposure and then use protective measures to reduce human exposure where practical and where little added cost is involved. The problem with this approach is that a controversy ensures as to what is practical, realistic, and reasonable in terms of added cost. One needs only observe the impact of recent developments from a similar approach tried in the field of ionizing radiation protection to see the potential problem.

In the ionizing radiation protection field, the idealistic philosophy of "as low as reasonably achievable," or ALARA, was inserted into regulations. Many legal and regulatory controversies ensued. The ALARA principle unsettled the orderliness provided by the existence of a fixed-value EL. The fundamental problem is that almost anything is achievable by engineering means and enough financial support; however, everyone differs with regard to what is "reasonable." The lesson here is that idealistic goals should not be regulated.

For the reasons illustrated above, many health professionals welcomed the promulgation of VLF to HF OELs as an alternative to reduce the level of controversy, even though little scientific basis for the standard truly existed. When control measures are employed, most are inexpensive. An exception has been on naval vessels where many antenna exist near walkways. It is worth noting that in order to reduce electromagnetic interference (EMI), other electronic means such as shielding and signal reduction have often been employed in the past, independent of any motivation for reducing potential health hazards.

EPIDEMIOLOGICAL STUDIES

As noted earlier, there has been a degree of controversy surrounding the interpretation of epidemiological studies, which appeared to relate the incidence of childhood cancer and other cancers with low-frequency (60 Hz) EM fields. One of the most widely referenced early studies suggesting this correlation was that of Wertheimer and Leeper (1979). This study was highly criticized and a re-evaluation at the same location with an eye toward reducing confounders still showed a weaker correlation with increased cancer risk (Savitz et. al., 1988). The critics argued that many other factors (confounders) may explain these and other findings, for instance heavier roadway traffic densities near the same areas where wiring codes would indicate higher currents. A more recent study by the National Research Council (NRC, 1998) revisited the controversy of power lines causing certain types of cancers. The NRC concluded that there is no clear, convincing evidence to show that residential exposures to electric and magnetic fields (EMFs) are a threat to human health. The NRC also tried to duplicate the 1979 findings linking EMFs with childhood leukemia. Although the NRC found a weak but statistically significant correlation between childhood leukemia (which is rare) and electrical wire configurations, it could not determine if the correlation was based on another confounder or on EMF. It has never been demonstrated that this apparent association was caused by exposure to electromagnetic fields. Controversy can be expected to continue with epidemiological studies such as those that appeared to show correlations between illness and exposure despite a lack of theoretical basis for linking a given disease with EM fields (Lin et al., 1985; Logue et al., 1985).

Even the studies themselves concluded that the correlation was uncertain (Wertheimer and Leeper, 1979; Fulton et al., 1980; Juutilainen et al., 1990). Most studies like these are limited by their exposure assessment and control of factors other than EM fields as a cause for cancer. Using similar controls and configurations as those that find possible correlations, other studies have found "no relationship between leukemia and power lines" (Fulton et al., 1980). Although conclusions as to whether EM fields have adverse or positive health effects have not been achieved, studies do support the need for more research, both epidemiological and theoretical (Savitz et al., 1988; Monson, 1990; Juutilainen et al., 1990).

PROTECTIVE MEASURES

Protective measures for industrial and scientific EM exposure control can be conveniently separated into three categories: the use of engineering, installation, or system-design controls to keep the exposure threat away from people; the use of range controls, namely the principle of using separation or distance to keep the people away from the threat; and the use of administrative controls to ansure that all of the EM control measures are understood and observed. A fourth category of exposure control involves the issue of personal protective equipment such as special garments, goggles, or face masks to protect those who must enter intense fields (e.g., to replace aircraft warning lights on active broadcast towers or to repair on-line military broadcast antennas). These have been tried in the past (e.g., Czerski et al., 1974) but are generally too cumbersome for continuous use or have proved ineffective against the pervasiveness of the EM fields at the lower-frequency (broadcast) portion of the spectrum.

Insulated gloves or similar outer clothing can protect against EM shock such as from physical contact with an active emitter or physical contact with a metallic body (fence, tower, vehicle, etc.) carrying induced EM energy from high-power sources. Such insulated protection is commonly used around antennas and open transmission lines. The effect of damaging levels of induced currents in metallic surgical and dental implants or implanted electronic devices (cardiac pacemakers, etc.) is also important to consider in assessing the need for "control measures."

ENGINEERING / INSTALLATION / DESIGN CONTROLS

The most dependable control measures for protecting against exposure are those that isolate the EM energy from people. In the original design of a device that incorporates an

EM source, interlocks can be included to control the direction and intensity of radiation. Also components should be selected (e.g., coaxial cable versus waveguide) that reduce the possibility of inadvertently leaking EM energy into areas that might be occupied. Installation control involves mounting radiating systems on inaccessible places like towers or rooftops. Electromechanical limit switches should be designed into the EM beam-directing mechanisms of radar systems to ensure that the energy does not radiate into occupied places. Careful design of industrial RF heat sealers can greatly reduce potential exposure to the operator.

Another engineering control method involves the use of metal enclosures (e.g., a Faraday cage) to reduce stray **E** fields around sources that emit EM energy. External enclosures of ferromagnetic materials can also "capture" magnetic flux lines and reduce external magnetic flux densities around some low-frequency equipment. Such shielding measures applied to large equipment are expensive and are primarily designed to reduce the effects of EM interference (EMI) on sensitive industrial, scientific, or medical instrumentation. Some basic form of such shielding, usually at the component level, is required for all electronic devices that produce EM emissions (computers, TVs, radios, remote controllers, etc.) to ensure that normal EM emissions from such devices are not a source of EMI to other nearby electronic systems. These EMI controls are mandated by the Federal Communications Commission (FCC), and although they are not designed for personnel exposure control, these controls do provide assurance that the device does not and will not exceed certain FCC-approved EM emission levels during its lifetime.

Responding to the heightened concerns among VDT users regarding EM exposure, some computer manufacturers have included magnetic shielding in their VDT designs, stating that it was a business decision rather than one based on any serious concern of actual existing health threats. These shields are supposed to reduce EM levels even lower than the levels required by FCC.

Some electric blanket manufacturers have redesigned the heating-wire routing in their products to minimize stray **H** fields, also for business reasons. The modifications are designed to position the wires so that the alternating EM fields' negative minimum and positive maximum cancel one another. This results in local minima that approach zero field strength within the exposure area. Recent studies have been inconclusive concerning adverse effects of electric blanket exposure. Any EL considered for their frequency region have recommended controls for exposure levels greater than those produced by electric blankets. However, the public's perceived threat of EM fields from electric blankets is economically real for manufacturers (Florig and Hoburg, 1990; Verreault et al., 1990).

RANGE CONTROLS

If the EM energy cannot be kept entirely away from occupied areas through engineering / design / installation means, then ways must be found to keep the people away from the source. Because there is always a decrease in EM energy level as the separation (distance or range) from the source is increased, the exposure control can be accomplished by keeping the people far enough away from the source so that the EM level is below the OEL or EEL. Fences or other barricades can be erected to prevent personnel entry into areas where the EM levels exceed the OELs or EELs. Simple warning signs are adequate if the EM levels are only marginally excessive. "Walk-through" areas can be designated (painted on roofs or decks, walkways, etc.) around certain EM sources, where the maximum exposure will not be an "overexposure" if the time spent in the overexposure zone is controlled (thus walk-through, as opposed to areas where stopping or other delay is permitted). Warning lights, buzzers, horns, and the like, are also effective in alerting people to the need for control and the necessary distances around high-power sources that need to be controlled.

Administrative Controls

As the name suggests, this category is always a necessary part of exposure control. The types of administrative controls include all of the management, information, and documentation features of the protection program. Some key elements are the inventory of all controlled items, a list of people who are known to be at risk of overexposure, the record of all required personnel controls, the standing operating procedures specified for controlling each source, identification of the persons responsible for administering the programs, and procedures to follow in case of a suspected overexposure. Individuals with special needs, such as those with medical conditions or electronic implants, must be identified and warned about any threat to them from entry into areas of high EM field strengths. Special initial and routine EM safety briefings should be required to inform all appropriate persons of the exposure threats and the control programs. Normally records need to be kept of persons attending such briefings and of the material covered.

In the end there can be no substitute for properly informing and training those personnel who must work around sources of potential EM overexposure, whether whole systems or portions of systems, such as antennas, transmission lines, and transmitters. The need for all controls intensifies in proportion to the degree of the overexposure threat.

CONCLUSIONS

Final comprehensive standards for controlling either occupational or general public exposure in all frequency bands of EM energy are not considered likely at this time. Reasonable agreement (within an order of magnitude) exists for exposure control in the microwave frequency region, at least for short-term exposures. Only interim guidelines are realistic regarding possible adverse health effects associated with exposure to VLF and ELF fields. There are still too many unanswered questions for the standards-setting community to define a level and say definitively that above that level some or all effects are adverse, or even that below that level all effects are not adverse. Even the choice of parameters to be controlled is uncertain, whether it should be **E** or **H** field strength, duration of exposure, kinds of exposure (short pulse, continuous wave, pulse trains, peak field limits, duty cycle limits, etc.), or combinations of some or all of these.

The guidelines proposed at this time are based on dependable physiological principles. These guidelines are acceptable in present-day occupational and environmental settings; that is, the interim guidelines can be enforced without requiring significant change in most installations. These guidelines should be applied and monitored continually against ongoing developments in the bioelectromagnetics research and epidemiological communities. Unless some special need exists for relief in the OEL guidelines (e.g., to permit "hot" work on 60 Hz high-voltage transmission lines), change in the direction toward more relaxed limits should not be encouraged. If, on the other hand, scientific research and credible epidemiology demonstrate a need for a more conservative standard, then that change should be made at that time.

U.S. governmental ELs have been proposed by the EPA and NIOSH, but because of some controversies, these proposed standards may not become official or binding in the near future, if ever. Even without such standards, practical applications and exposure situations (radar and communications operators, and certainly VDT users) for actual human exposure levels are very low. By comparison with RF levels used in biological experiments, one can safely assure the user that there are no known adverse effects from such uses based on the available biomedical knowledge and benefit-versus-risk estimates (Cox, 1980; Weiss and Peterson, 1979; Wolbarsht et al., 1979; Stuckly et al., 1983).

GLOSSARY

EEL. Environmental exposure limits, which are for areas where access is not controlled to exclude persons less than 140 cm (55 inches) in stature — common ground where any individual may be found. The RF exposures in these areas do not exceed the permissible exposure limits. Generally, these locations represent living quarters, workplaces, or public access areas where personnel would not expect to be exposed to levels of RF and energy.

E Field. Electric field, a fundamental component of electromagnetic waves that exists when there is a voltage potential difference between two points in space.

Electric field strength (E). Magnitude of the electric field expressed in volts per meter (V / m).

EM radiation (fields). Electromagnetic radiation, the propagation of energy in the form of varying electric and magnetic fields through space at the velocity of light.

H Field. Magnetic field, a fundamental component of electromagnetic waves produced by a moving electric charge.

Magnetic field strength (H). Strength of the magnetic field expressed in amperes per meter (A / m).

OEL. Occupational exposure limits, which are for areas where access is controlled for the purpose of excluding entry of persons less than 140 cm (55 inches) in stature. At these locations, RF exposures may be incurred by workers who knowingly accept potential exposure as a condition of employment or duties, by individuals who knowingly enter areas where RF exposure is to be expected, and through incidental exposure during transient passage in areas where analysis shows that exposure levels may be above those set but not above the permissible exposure limit.

Overexposure. Any human exposure to RFR that exceeds the established permissible exposure limit (PEL).

Permissible exposure limit (PEL). The maximum level expressed as root mean square or peak electric and magnetic field strengths, as plane-wave equivalent power densities or induced body and contact currents, with added safety factor values, to which an individual may be exposed without expectation of any harmful effects.

RF. Radio frequency. Although the RF spectrum is formally defined in terms of frequency as extending from 0 to 3000 GHz, commonly it is electromagnetic energy in the frequency region useful for radio transmission. The present practical limits of radio frequency are roughly 10 KHz to 300 GHz.

SAR. Specific absorption rate, the time rate at which RFR energy is imparted to an element of biological body mass. Average SAR in a body is the time rate of total energy absorption divided by the total mass of the body. SAR is usually expressed in units of watts per kilogram (W/kg). Specific absorption (SA) refers to amount of energy absorbed over the exposure time and is usually expressed in units of Joules / cm^2.

REFERENCES

ACGIH. 1985. American Conference of Governmental Industrial Hygienists. *Proc. International Sympo-sium on Setting Occupational Exposure Limits, Annals of the ACGIH*, vol. 12. Cincinnati, OH: ACGIH.

ACGIH. 1992. American Conference of Governmental Industrial Hygienists. *Documentation for Threshold Limit Values (TLV's) for Chemical Substances and Physical Agents in the Work Environment with Intended Changes*, Cincinnati, OH: ACGIH.

ACGIH. 1999. American Conference of Governmental Industrial Hygienists. *Threshold Limit Values and Biological Exposure Indices for 1999*. Cincinnati, OH: ACGIH.

ANSI. 1982. American National Standards Institute. *American National Standard C95.1, Safety Levels with Respect to Human Exposure to Radio Frequency Electromagnetic Fields (300 KHz–100 GHz)*. New York: ANSI.

ANSI. 1991. American National Standards Institute. *American National Standard Safety IEEE Standard for Levels with Respect to Human Exposure to Radio Frequency Electromagnetic Fields, 3 KHz to 300 GHz*. New York: ANSI.

Austria (Austrian Standards Institute). 1990. *Mikrowellen und Hochfrequenzfelder Zulassige Expositionswert*. Vienna: Osterreichisches Normungsinstitut.

Bernhardt, J. 1979. The direct influence of electromagnetic fields on nerve and muscle cells of man within the frequency range of 1 Hz to 30 MHz. *Rad. Environ. Biophys.* 16: 309–320.

Bernhardt, J. 1986. Assessment of experimentally observed bioeffects in view of their clinical relevance and the exposure at work places. In *Proc. Symposium on the Biological Effects of Static and Extremely Low Frequency Magnetic Fields*, eds. A. Kaul and J. Bernhardt. Munich: MMV Medizin Verlag.

Blank, M., ed. 1995. *Electromagnetic Fields: Biological Interactions and Mechanisms*, Washington, DC: American Chemical Society Press.

Cox, E. A. 1980. Radiation emissions from visual display units. In *Health Hazards of VDUs?* Loughborough, England: HUSAT Research Group.

Czerski, P., K. Ostrowski, M. L. Shore, C. Silverman, M. J. Suess, and B. Waldeskog, eds. 1974. *Biological effects and Health Hazards of Microwave Radiation, Proc. International Symposium*, Warsaw, 15–18 October 1973. Warsaw: Polish Medical Publishers.

Deno, D. W. 1974. Calculating electrostatic effects of overhead transmission lines. *IEEE Trans. Power Appl. Sys.* 93: 1458–1471.

Deutsche Institut für Normeln (DIN). 1984. *Hazards for Electromagnetic Fields, Protection of Persons in the Frequency Range from 10 KHz to 300 Ghz, vol. 2. DIN 578.848. Berlin: DIN (German Standards Institute).*

Dolezalek, H. 1990. Classification of electromagnetic radiation. *In CRC Handbook of Chemistry and Physics*, 71st edition. Boca Raton, FL: CRC Press.

Florig, H. K., and J. f. Hoburg. 1990. Power-frequency magnetic fields from electric blankets. *Health Phys.* 58: 493-502.

FRG. 1986a. Federal Republic of Germany. *Hazards from Electromagnetic Fields: Protection of Persons in the Frequency Range from 0 Hz to 3000 Ghz* (in German). New DIN BDE No. 0848, August. Berlin: Beuth, Verlag, Deutsche Norm.

FRG. 1986b. Federal Republic of Germany. *Safety at Electromagnetic Fields: Limits of Field-Strength for the Protection of Persons in the Frequency Range from 30 kHz to 3000 Ghz* (in German). New DIN BDE No. 0848, Part 4. Berlin: Beuth, Verlag, Deutsche Norm.

Fulton, J. P., C. S. Cobb, L. Preble, L. Leone, and E. Forman. 1980. Electrical wiring configurations and childhood leukemia in Rhode Island. *Am. J. Epidemiol.* 11: 292–296.

Ghandi, O. P., I., Chatterjee, D. Wu, and Y.-G. Gu. 1980. Likelihood of high rates of energy deposition in the human legs at the ANSI recommended 3-30 MHz RF safety levels. *Proc. IEEE* 68: 104–113.

Germany. 1990. *Sicherheit in elektromagnetichen Feldern*. Frankfurt: Institut für Rundfunktechnik.

GOST. 1882. State Standards Institute. *Occupational Safety Standards System: Electromagnetic Fields of Radiofrequency, General Safety Requirements*. GOST-12, 1006-76, Moscow: State Standards Institute (originally issued in 1976 and amended in 1982).

Harlen, F. 1982, Criteria for setting exposure limits for RF and MW. *Gig. Ital. Med. Lab.* 4: 39–48.

Hill, C. R. 1989. *Physical Principles of Medical Ultrasonics*. New York: Ellis Horwood.

IRPA. 1988a. Guidelines on limits of exposure to radiofrequency electromagnetic fields in the frequency range from 100 kHz to 300 GHz. *Health Phys.*, 54: 115–123.

IRPA. 1988b. Alleged radiation risks form visual display units. *Health Phys.*, 54: 231–232.

IRPA. 1990. *Electromagnetic Fields in the Range of 300 Hz to 300 GHz.* Environmental Health Criteria Document 16, rev. version, Geneva: 1990.

ICNIRP. 1998. International Commision on Non-Ionizing Radiation Protection. Health issues related to the use of hand-held radiotelephones and base transmitters. *Health Phys.* 70: 587–593.

ICNIRP. 1998. Guidelines for limiting exposures to time-varying electric, magnetic, and electromagnetic fields (up to 300GHz). *Health Phys.* 74: 494–522.

ICNIRP/WHO. 1998. *Risk Perception, Risk Communication and Its Application to EMF Exposure. Munchen: Markl-Druck*

ITU. 1982. *Radio Regulations.* Geneva: General Secretariat of the International Telecommunication Union.

Japan. 1990. *Outline of Japanese Radio Frequency Protection Guide, Organization of Deliberations.* Tokyo: Telecommunications Technology Council of the Minister of Posts and Telecommunications.

Johnson, R. C., and H. Jasik. 1984. *Antenna Engineering Handbook*, 2nd edition. New York: McGraw-Hill.

Juutilainen, J., E. Laara, and E. Pukala. 1990. Incidence of leukaemia and brain tumours in Finnish workers exposed to ELF magnetic fields. *Int. Arch. Occup. Environ. Health*, 62: 289–295.

Kandioan, A. G., ed. 1993. *Reference Data for Radio Engineers.* 8th edition. Indianapolis: Howard W. Sams.

Lin, R. S., P. C. Dischinger, J. Conde, and K. P. Farrell. 1985. Occupational exposure to electromagnetic fields and the occurrence of brain tumors, *J. Occup. Med.* 27: 413–419.

Logue, J. N., S. Hamburger, P. M. Silverman, and R. P. Chiacchierini. 1985. Congenital anomalities and paernal occupational exposure to shortwave, microwave, infrared, and acoustic radiation. *J. Occup. Med.* 27: 451–452.

Magnuson, H. J., D. W. Fassett, H. W. Gerarde, V. K. Rowe, M. S. Henry, Jr. F. Smyth, and H. E. Stokinger. 1964. Industrial toxicology in the Soviet Union — Theoretical and applied. *Am. Ind. Hyg. Assoc. J.* 25: 185–197.

McKinlay, A.F., J. B. Anderson, J. H. Bernhardt, M. Grandolfo, K.-A. Hossmann, K. H. Mild, A. J. Swerdlow, M. Van Leeuwen, L. Verschaeve, and B. Veyret. 1996. *Radiotelephones and Human Health—Proposal for a European Commission Expert Group.* Brussels: European Commission Directorate General XIII.

Minnin, B. A. 1962. *Microwaves and Human Safety* (in Russian). Moscow: Radio Publication (Available in translation as Report JPR-655506-1 and 0- from NTIS, Springfield, VA).

Monson, R. R. 1990. Editorial commentary: Epidemiology and exposure to electromagnetic fields. *Am. J. Epidemiol.* 131: 774–775.

National Academy of Science/National Research Council. 1996. *Possible Health Effects of Exposure to Residential Electric and Magnetic Fields.* Washington, DC: National Academy Press.

National Council on Radiation Protection and Measurements (NCRP). 1993. *A Practical Guide to the Determination of Human Exposure to Radiofrequency Fields.* NCRP Report 119. Washington, DC: NCRP.

NRPB. 1982. National Radiological Protection Board. *Proposals for the Health Protection of Workers and Members of the Public against the Dangers of Extra Low Frequency, Radiofrequency and Microwave Radiations*, Harwell, U. K. : NRPB.

NRPB. 1986. National Radiological Protection Board. Advice on the protection of workers and members of the general public from the possible hazards of electric and magnetic fields with frequencies below 300 GHz: A consultative document. NRPB, Harwell, U.K.

NRPB. 1988. National Radiological Protection Board. *Guidance on Standards: Guidance as to Restriction on Exposures to Time Varying, Electromagnetic Fields and the 1988 Recommendation of the International Non-ionizing Radiation Committee.* Harwell, U.K.: NRPB.

NRPB. 1994a. National Radiological Protection Board. Health effects related to the use of visual display units. Report by the Advisory Group on Non-ionising Radiation, Chilton, U.K., National Radiological Protection Board, NRPB Documents 5(2).

NRPB. 1994b. National Radiological Protection Board. Electromagnetic fields and the risk of cancer. Supplementary report by the Advisory Group on Non-ionising Radiation of 12 April 1994. *Rad. Protect. Bull.* 154: 10–12.

Polk, C., and E. Postow. 1998. *Biological Effects of Electromagnetic Fields,* 2nd edition. Boca Raton, FL: CRC Press.

Repacholi, M. R. 1985. Limits of human exposure to magnetic fields. In *Proc. Symposium on the Biological Effects of Static and Extremely Low Frequency Magnetic Fields*, eds. A. Kaul and J. Bernhardt. Munich: MMV Medizin Verlag.

Repacholi, M. R. 1998. Low-level exposure to radiofrequency fields: Health effects and research needs. *Bioelectromagnetics* 19: 1–19.

Savitz, D.A., H. Wachtel, F. A. Barnes, E. M. John, and J. G. Tvrdik. 1988. Case-control study of childhood cancer and exposure to 60-Hz magnetic fields, *Am. J. Epidemiol.* 128: 21–38.

Schwan, H. P. 1982. Physical properties of biological matter: Some history, principles, and applications. *Bioelectromagnetics* 3: 3–14.

Sliney, D. H. 1985. Does the basis for a standard exist? In *Proc. Symposium on the Biological Effects of Sattic and Extremely Low Frequency Magnetic Fields*, eds. A. Kaul and J. Bernhardt. Munich: MMV Medizin Verlag.

Sliney, D. H., J. L. Wolbarsht, and A. M. Mue.1985. Editorial: Differing radiofrequency standards in the microwave region-implications for future research. *Health Phys.* 49: 677–683.

Stuchly, M. A., D. W. Lecuyer, and R. D. Mann. 1983. Extremely low frequency electromagnetic emissions from video display terminals and other devices. *Health Phys.* 45: 713–722.

Tenforde, T. S. 1996. Interaction of ELF magnetic fields with living systems, In *Biological Effects of Electromagnetic Fields*, eds. C. Polk, and E. Postow, pp. 185–230. Boca Raton, FL: CRC Press.

Ueno, S. 1996, *Biological Effects of Magnetic and Electromagnetic Fields*. New York, Plenum Press.

UNEP/WHO/IRPA. 1993. United Nations Environmental Programme/World Health Organization/ International Radiation Protection Association. *Electromagnetic Fields (300Hz to 300GHz)*. Geneva: World Health Organization; Environmental Health Criteria 137.

USSR. 1984b. *Temporary Safety Standards and Regulations on Protection of the General Public against the Effects of Electromagnetic Fields Generated by Radio-Transmitting Equipment* (in Russian). Ct. 2963-84. Moscow: USSR, Ministry of Public Health.

USSR. 1986a. Standard of the Soviet Council for Mutual Economic Assistance. Protection of workers against radiofrequency electromagnetic fields (in Russian). ST-SEV 5801-86. Moscow.

USSR. 1986b. USSR standard for occupational exposure, Amendment 1 of 1 January 1982 to State Standard 12.0.006-76. Moscow.

USSR. 1987. Health Recommendations for the General Public Referring to Exposure Limits to Electromagnetic Fields of Different Frequencies Emitted by TV Stations (in Russian). Moscow: USSR Ministry of Public Health.

Verreault, R., N. S. Weiss, K. A. Hollenbach, C. H. Strader, and J. R. Daling. 1990. Use of electric blankets and risk of testicular cancer. *Am. J. Epidemiol.* 131: 159–162.

Weiss, M. W., and P. C. Peterson. 1979. Electromagnetic radiation emitted from video computer teminals. *Am. Ind. Hyg. Assoc. J.* 40: 300–309.

Wertheimer, N., and E. Leeper. 1979. Electrical wiring configurations and childhood cancer. *Am. J. Epidemiol.* 109: 273–284.

Wolbarsht, M. L., F. A. O'Foghludha, D. H. Sliney, A. H. Guy, A. A. Smith, and G. A. Johnson. 1979. Electromagnetic emission from visual display units: A nonhazard. *Proc. Soc. Photo-Opt. Instrum. Eng.* 229: 185–195.

18 Nitrogen Oxides

RICHARD B. SCHLESINGER, Ph.D.

Oxides of nitrogen can exist in the atmosphere as gases/vapors or as particles. The former includes nitric oxide (NO), nitrogen dioxide (NO_2), nitrous oxide (N_2O), and possibly nitrogen trioxide (NO_3), dinitrogen trioxide (N_2O_3), dinitrogen tetroxide (N_2O_4) and dinitrogen pentoxide (N_2O_5), while the latter includes nitrate (NO_3^-) salts. Components that may exist in either state are nitric acid (HNO_3) and nitrous acid (HONO). Because these various chemical species may occur together and many are chemically interconvertible, the generic designation of NO_x is often used to describe their combined presence in air.

Nitric oxide and nitrogen dioxide are the most important of the NO_x in terms of public health concern because they can exist in the atmosphere in significant concentrations and they are quite chemically reactive. Although nitrous oxide is also ubiquitous, as the product of natural biological processes in soil, it is not involved in chemical reactions in polluted air. Most other NO_x, if found at all, are present at very low concentrations. However, two other NO_x species of interest from a health standpoint are nitric acid and inorganic nitrates.

SOURCES OF NO_x

Nitrogen oxides can be produced by natural sources such as forest fires, organic decay, and lightning. Anthropogenic emissions, which annually average about 20 million metric tons (U.S. EPA, 1993), derive from high-temperature combustion processes of both mobile and stationary sources. The major mobile source is motor vehicles, while the major stationary source is electric power generation using fossil fuels, with industrial combustion processes a close second.

During combustion, nitrogen derived from the combustion air and/or the fuel being consumed reacts with atmospheric oxygen. Although most of the resulting NO_x produced is initially in the form of NO, this is generally rapidly oxidized to NO_2. The conversion rate depends on a number of factors, including the concentration of NO, temperature of the combustion process, and distance from the emission zone. Several reaction pathways are possible. Although simple oxidation involving molecular oxygen (O_2) is the primary one for NO_2 production in combustion gas effluents, it does not play a major role in the ambient atmosphere because transformations via other pathways occur at faster rates. Thus, for example, in polluted air containing many reactive substances, irradiation by sunlight catalyzes photochemical reactions, leading to the rapid formation of NO_2.

The acidic component of the ambient atmosphere in the western part of the United States can contain significant amounts of nitric acid (Aris et al., 1993; Pierson and

Environmental Toxicants: Human Exposures and Their Health Effects, 2/e. Edited by Morton Lippmann.
ISBN: 0-471-29298-2 © 2000 John Wiley & Sons, Inc.

Brachaczek, 1988). Because of its high saturation vapor pressure, HNO_3 generally exists as a vapor under most ambient conditions, for example within photochemical smog, where levels generally peak during daytime hours (Ellestad and Knapp, 1988). Within acidic fogs, however, HNO_3 may be found in the particulate state (Jacob et al., 1985).

Nitric acid is a product of the photo-oxidation cycle of polluted air, and along with nitrous acid, it derives from primary emissions released by mobile sources. The major production pathway involves reaction between the hydroxyl radical ($OH\cdot$), formed within the smog cycle, with NO_2. Other routes, which are potentially important at night, involve reactions between N_2O_5 with water or nitrate radicals with volatile organics, or production in droplets containing both hydrogen ion (H^+) and nitrate (NO_3^-).

Another inorganic nitrogenous acid which may occur in some atmospheres is nitrous acid (HNO_2). This can be found in ambient air as a primary product from combustion sources and as a secondary product of photochemical smog reactions. It is also an indoor pollutant produced by reaction between NO_2 and H_2O.

Nitrate salts may be formed in the atmosphere via various pathways, many of which involve HNO_3. For example, ammonium nitrate results from the homogeneous reaction between nitric acid and atmospheric ammonia. Nitrates may also be formed by heterogeneous reactions involving NO_2 or NO and water droplets, or HNO_3 vapor and dust or sea salt particles.

NITROGEN DIOXIDE

Exposure

Atmospheric Concentrations   The outdoor NO_2 concentration in urban areas is generally characterized by two daily peaks related to motor vehicle traffic patterns in the morning and afternoon. In areas having significant stationary sources, the pattern is characterized by a baseline NO_2 level, superimposed upon which are higher spikes occurring on an irregular basis. In those areas not affected by significant local sources, NO_2 has little variation on an hourly basis throughout the day, unless there is transport of NO_2 into the region.

Annual average outdoor concentrations of NO_2 in most regions of the country range from 0.015 to 0.035 ppm; levels in nonmetropolitan or rural areas tend toward the low end, while those in major urban areas tend toward the high end (U.S. EPA, 1993). Some metropolitan areas, notably those in southern California, may have annual averages exceeding 0.06 ppm. Short-term levels in major urban regions are generally ≤ 0.17 ppm as a 24 hour average and ≤ 0.3 ppm as a 1 hour average. However, short-term peaks in many regions can exceed 0.5 ppm. In most areas of the United States NO_2 levels are highest in the summer. However, southern California is characterized by elevated NO_2 throughout the year.

Nitrogen dioxide is widespread indoor air pollutant in homes, deriving from indoor combustion sources such as gas-fired ranges, kerosene heaters, and improperly or unvented gas space heaters. Nitrogen oxides are also major components of smoke derived from the burning of tobacco products. Cigarette smoke contains high levels of NO, which is oxidized to NO_2 as the smoke ages. The indoor– outdoor concentration ratio for NO_2 in the absence of significant indoor sources is 0.5 to 0.6 but is often > 1 when such sources are present (Berglund, 1993).

Indoor levels vary widely depending on the strength of the sources and the degree of ventilation. Furthermore, because combustion from indoor sources tends to be episodic, fairly high short-term peaks are possible. Daily (24 h average) levels of NO_2 in homes using gas-fired ranges or heaters are 0.05 to 0.5 ppm, but short-term peaks can exceed 1 ppm (U.S. EPA, 1993; Spengler and Cohen, 1985; Goldstein et al., 1988).

A recently documented source of significant short-term indoor exposure to NO_2, especially for children, derives from the fuel-operated resurfacing equipment used in enclosed ice skating rinks. Levels exceeding 2 ppm have been measured over 1 to 2 hour periods at these sites (Berglund et al., 1994; Brauer and Spengler, 1994; Lee et al., 1994).

Exposure Assessment Based on the preceding discussion, it is evident that exposure to nitrogen oxides can occur in numerous settings, which include residential areas, transportation vehicles, and the outdoor atmosphere. The integrated exposure is therefore the sum of the individual exposures over all possible time intervals and for all of these different environments. Such exposure can be assessed either by direct methods, which include biomarkers and personal monitoring, or by indirect methods, which involve measurement of pollutant levels at monitoring sites and the use of mathematical models for the estimation of actual individual or population exposures.

There is currently no accepted biomarker for exposure to NO_2. Some suggestions are urinary hydroxyproline excretion (Adgate et al., 1992), the NO-heme protein complex in bronchial lavage (Maples et al., 1991), and 3-nitrotyrosine in urine (Oshima et al., 1990). However, because of their lack of sensitivity and/or specificity, there is still no useful marker for environmental NO_2 exposure.

Personal monitoring to provide a direct measure of NO_2 exposure has involved the use of passive samplers (Palmes et al., 1976; Yanagisawa and Nishimura, 1982). However, these have been used largely for exposure assessment only in certain microenvironments and have not been commonly used to monitor total personal exposure in all environments. The available data from such monitoring indicates that outdoor measures of NO_2 levels, while related to and contributing to total exposure, are poor predictors of total personal exposures for most people. Since indoor concentrations are often greater than those outdoors, indoor exposure is commonly the main contributor to total exposure (Keller et al., 1979; Spengler et al., 1983), and actual personal exposures to NO_2 may differ from what has been assumed based on ambient outdoor air measures (Linaker et al., 1996). Thus, indoor residential levels are generally a much better predictor of personal exposure, explaining over 50% of the variation in such exposure. However, it should be borne in mind that this is a generalization, and there are likely to be selected groups of people for which indoor levels are not a good predictor of total exposure due to greater percentages of time spent in other significant NO_x containing environments.

Indirect methods of NO_2 exposure assessment have employed various degrees of outdoor monitoring within specific environments and the use of questionnaires to estimate an individual or population exposure. Total personal exposures have been indirectly assessed by use of these microenvironmental measurements in combination with mathematical modeling involving time/activity patterns. However, as noted above, outdoor NO_2 levels may be weak predictors of total exposure due to significant time spent indoors, although this may not be the case in areas where there are high outdoor ambient levels.

Exposure Limits There are various ambient and occupational exposure limits for NO_x. These are listed in Table 18-1.

Dosimetry

The exposure route for NO_2 is inhalation. A large percentage of NO_2, up to 90% of the amount inspired during normal respiration, can be removed from inhaled air within the human respiratory tract (Wagner, 1970). Estimates of regional uptake for the upper

TABLE 18-1   Exposure Limits for Nitrogen Oxides

Nitric Oxide	
TLV[a]	25 ppm
PEL[b]	25 ppm
REL[c]	25 ppm
IDLH[d]	100 ppm

Nitrogen Dioxide	
IPCS[e]	0.021 ppm (40 µg/m^3)
NAAQS[f]	0.053 ppm
WHO[g]	0.105 ppm (200 µg/m^3)
PEL[h]	1 ppm
REL[i]	1 ppm
EEGL[j]	1 ppm
TLV[a]	3 ppm
STEL[k]	5 ppm
IDLH[d]	50 ppm

[a] Threshold limit value (ACGIH; time-weighted average for an 8 h work day and a 40 h work week).
[b] Permissible exposure limit (OSHA; time-weighted average for an 8 h work day).
[c] Recommended exposure limit (NIOSH; time-weighted average for an 8 h work day).
[d] Immediately dangerous to life and health (NIOSH; 30 min average).
[e] IPCS EHC guideline (annual average).
[f] National ambient air quality standard (U.S. EPA; annual average).
[g] WHO guideline (1 h).
[h] Permissible exposure limit (OSHA; ceiling for 15 min exposure).
[i] Recommended exposure limit (NIOSH; ceiling for 15 min exposure).
[j] Emergency exposure guidance level (NAS; 1 h exposure).
[k] Short-term exposure limit (ACGIH; ceiling for 15 min exposure).

respiratory tract (airways proximal to the trachea), based on laboratory animal studies, ranged from 28% to 90% of the amount inhaled (Cavanagh and Morris, 1987; Dalhamn and Sjoholm, 1963; Yokoyama, 1968; Vaughan et al., 1969; Kleinman and Mautz, 1989), while that for the lungs ranged from 36% to 90% of the amount entering the trachea (Postlethwait and Mustafa, 1981; Kleinman and Mautz, 1989).

Specific ventilatory factors influence the extent of NO$_2$ uptake. Thus more NO$_2$ will be absorbed in the upper respiratory tract during nasal breathing than during oral breathing (Kleinman and Mautz, 1989), implying that the latter would allow a greater percentage of inhaled NO$_2$ to enter the lungs. Increased ventilation, such as due to exercise, may alter regional gas distribution from that occurring at rest by reducing NO$_2$ uptake in the upper respiratory tract and tracheobronchial tree, and thus increasing the amount of NO$_2$ delivered to and absorbed in the respiratory region (Miller et al., 1982; Overton, 1984; Kleinman and Mautz, 1989; Wagner, 1970; Mohsenin, 1994).

Within the lungs, inhaled NO$_2$ is absorbed throughout the entire tracheobronchial tree and respiratory region, although the major dose to tissue is delivered at the junction between the conducting and respiratory airways (Miller et al., 1982; Overton, 1984). But regardless of the site of initial contact with airway surfaces, the primary determinant of NO$_2$ uptake is surface reactivity, that is direct interaction with airway lining fluid and/or cellular components (Postlethwait and Bidani, 1990).

Unreacted NO$_2$ does not penetrate through the airway epithelium, but the specific substrates with which it initially interacts have not been elucidated with certainty. They likely include oxidizable chemical species, such as amino acids, proteins, and unsaturated fatty acids (Hood et al., 1993), resulting in the production of nitrite ion or various radicals (Postlethwait and Mustafa, 1981; Saul and Archer, 1983; Postlethwait and Bidani, 1989, 1990) which can then interact with the epithelium or rapidly pass into the bloodstream and undergo other chemical reactions in extrapulmonary sites, for example, oxidation to nitrate by interaction with hemoglobin in red blood cells (Parks et al., 1981; Oda et al., 1981; Kosaka et al., 1979; Case et al., 1979). On the other hand, simple dissolution of NO_2 in airway fluids could result in production of nitric and nitrous acids, with any subsequent toxicity likely due to the hydrogen or nitrite ions (Goldstein et al., 1977, 1980). It is, however, likely that both oxidative and nonoxidative mechanisms are involved in the toxicity of NO_2. Furthemore antioxidants present within airway lining fluid can react with deposited NO_2, potentially modulating its toxicological impact (Kelly et al., 1996).

Epidemiology

Epidemiological studies have attempted to assess the potential role of exposure to NO_2 in producing adverse human health effects. While early studies related health endpoints to outdoor concentrations, the current trend is to provide better measures of actual personal exposures which, as previously noted, can be reflections of strong indoor sources. Although some epidemiological studies are weakened by a lack of reliable estimates of actual NO_x exposure conditions, inadequate sample size, inadequate compensation for the effects of covariates (e.g., cigarette smoking and ozone) and / or misclassification of health endpoints, they do provide a linkage between chronic laboratory animal studies and long-term exposure of humans.

Ambient NO_2 has been related to increased mortality in some analyses (e.g., Wietlisbach et al., 1996; Sunyer et al., 1996; Anderson et al., 1996). However, most studies used index of respiratory illness and / or changes in pulmonary mechanical function to assess the health consequences of exposure. Examples of results obtained in such studies are discussed below.

One of the first studies to examine acute respiratory illness and pulmonary function in relation to ambient NO_2 levels reported some decrement in lung function of children in areas characterized by high NO_2 compared to low NO_2 and a higher rate of illness in the families in the high NO_2 areas (Shy et al., 1970a, b). However, technical and methodological flaws resulted in a lack of reliability of these relationships. In a series of epidemiological surveys conducted in a number of cities in the United States selected to represent a range of outdoor air quality (Harvard 6-Cities Air Pollution Health Study), grade school age children within each community were followed for several years by reporting on questionnaires and by annual measurements of pulmonary function. Outdoor NO_2 levels were measured at various sites within each community, and indoor levels were also measured in selected households. While results of this study from 1974 to 1977 on over 8000 children aged 6 to 10 years indicated a significant increase in the rate of respiratory illness before age two in homes with gas-fired compared to those with electric stoves (Speizer et al., 1980), a later examination of the same communities over a longer time period did not show any NO_2-related increase in respiratory illness (Ware et al., 1984). A further analysis of over 5000 children aged 7 to 11 years during the period 1983 to 1986 noted marginal significance for physician-diagnosed respiratory illness prior to age two in homes using gas-fired stoves compared to those using electric stoves (Dockery et al., 1989).

When pulmonary mechanical indices were evaluated in the above children (Ware et al., 1984), gas stove use was associated with significant reductions in parameters of expiratory flow (FEV_1, FVC) in a first examination, but no such relationship was found in a subsequent evaluation. Other studies have shown no NO_2-associated effect on pulmonary function endpoints in children (Vedal et al., 1987; Scarlett et al., 1996).

It is possible that certain subpopulations are more susceptible to effects of NO_2 than are others. A borderline significant effect was noted between peak flow reduction in healthy children residing in homes having gas stoves, while a much stronger association was noted in asthmatics (Lebowitz et al., 1985). Children with asthmatic symptoms appeared to be more susceptible to reduced lung function when outdoor average NO_2 concentrations exceeded a certain level (0.02 ppm), but no such effect was found with children having no asthmatic symptoms (Moseler et al., 1994). The issue of special sensitivity of asthmatics to NO_2 is addressed further in subsequent sections of this chapter.

In a study examining respiratory symptoms in adult women and children aged 13 years and younger (Berwick et al., 1984), indoor NO_2 levels were measured in most the homes. Children under the age of 7 exposed to ≥ 0.016 ppm were found to be at an increased risk of upper and lower respiratory tract symptoms compared to those who were not so exposed. No increased risk was found in older children or adults. This study was, however, characterized by a lack of consistency across age groups, perhaps due to a small sample size. In a later study (Samet et al., 1993) no association was found between indoor levels of NO_2 and either the incidence or duration of respiratory illness in infants examined during their first 18 months of life, but this may have been due to the very low exposures to NO_2 in this study.

A relationship between outdoor levels of NO_2 and common respiratory symptoms (cough, sore throat, etc.) in children up to 5 years of age was noted in one study (Gnehm et al., 1988), while another found an association between NO_2 exposure and wheeze in females, but not in males, aged 4 months to 4 years (Pershagen et al., 1995). Braun-Fahrlander et al. (1992) examined symptoms in children in relation to outdoor and indoor levels of NO_2. While the incidence of symptoms was not associated with either indoor or outdoor levels, the duration of increased symptoms was associated with outdoor concentration.

In studies of the effect of NO_2 on respiratory health in 6 to 9 year-old children, personal exposures to NO_2 were measured, as were indoor levels in the home (Houthuijs et al., 1987; Brunekreef et al., 1987). The prevalence of lung disease was found to be associated with the presence of unvented gas water heaters, with weekly average exposures estimated at 0.021 ppm. On the other hand, Dijkstra et al. (1990) found no association between respiratory symptoms with indoor NO_2 measurements in homes. Koo et al. (1990) used personal samplers to monitor NO_2 exposure in children aged 7 to 13 in Hong Kong. No association was noted between exposure levels (means ranged from 0.013–0.023 ppm for a 1 wk period) and respiratory symptoms, such as wheeze, running nose, or cough.

The effects of both indoor and outdoor air pollution on respiratory illness in a cohort of primary school children indicated a gradient of increased respiratory symptoms with increasing indoor levels of NO_2 in homes with gas stoves, although no actual measurements of NO_2 were made (Melia et al., 1977). A later assessment also indicated some increase in relative risk in homes with gas stoves, but this was not a consistent finding (Melia et al., 1979). In this case levels of NO_2 measured in bedrooms of homes having gas stoves ranged from 0.003 to 0.017 ppm. In another study of children aged 5 to 6 years, no significant relationship was noted between levels of NO_2 and the prevalance of respiratory illness (Melia et al., 1982); levels of NO_2 in the bedrooms of homes with gas stoves were 0.005 to 0.029 ppm. Other attempts to relate gas stove use in homes to acute respiratory illness, respiratory symptoms, or index of reduced lung function for various age populations have had mixed results, with some studies reporting no association and others reporting some relationship (Keller et al., 1979; Comstock et al., 1981; Schenker et al., 1983; Dodge, 1982; Ekwo et al., 1983).

Exposure to NO_2 may result in extrapulmonary responses. For example, daily outdoor concentrations of NO_2 were associated with emergency room admissions due to cerebrovascular disease and short-term ischemic attacks (Ponka and Virtanen, 1996).

It should be evident from the preceding discussion that it is not possible to provide any definitive conclusion regarding adverse health effects of NO_2 based on the epidemiological data base. There have been both positive and negative findings at various levels of NO_2 exposure and with various degrees of precision in measuring actual exposure levels. Some results are suggestive that an increase in acute respiratory illness, especially in younger children, may be associated with chronic exposure, although the extent of any effect or excess risk is small.

Toxicology

A significant fraction of the NO_2 toxicological database involves experimental exposures to concentrations $> 5\,ppm$. While such studies may help elucidate mechanisms of toxicity, they are of limited use in attempts to determine the public health significance from actual atmospheric exposure. Thus, in this chapter, generally only studies using $\leq 5\,ppm$ will be discussed. However, when necessary to help explain mechanisms, references to effects at higher levels will be made.

Studies in Laboratory Animals   The largest data base concerning the biological effects of NO_2 is that derived from laboratory animals. Since the mechanisms underlying many responses are similar across species, effects in these animals may have implications for humans. It should be borne in mind, however, that the exposure concentrations needed for comparable response likely differs between species.

Effects on the Respiratory Tract   The major target for inhaled NO_2 is the respiratory tract and various interactions between NO_2 and this organ system have been studied.

Pulmonary Defense Mechanisms—Particle Clearance   Mucociliary transport provides a first line of defense against prolonged retention of deposited particles in the tracheobronchial tree. Acute (1–2 h) exposures to NO_2 at levels $\leq 10\,ppm$ did not alter mucociliary transport rate from the tracheobronchial tree of laboratory animals (Schlesinger, 1989a), but humans exposed for 20 minutes to 1.5 to 3.5 ppm NO_2 did show a reduction of mucociliary activity measured 45 minutes following exposure (Helleday et al., 1995). Rats exposed for 6 weeks to 6 ppm NO_2 showed a transient depression in mucociliary activity (Giordano and Morrow, 1972), while rabbits exposed for 2 h/d for 14 days to 0.3 or 1 ppm did not show altered tracheobronchial mucociliary transport (Schlesinger et al., 1987). Thus the available data suggest that with either single or short-term repeated exposures, higher than ambient levels are needed to alter tracheobronchial mucociliary transport. While the mechanisms underlying any such changes are not certain, they may involve NO_2-induced effects on ion transport across the airway epithelium (Robison and Kim, 1995) or on ciliary activity (Ohashi et al., 1993).

Particle clearance from the respiratory (alveolated) region of the lungs has also been assessed following exposures to NO_2. Rats exposed to 1, 15, and 24 ppm showed a decrease in clearance after 22 daily exposures to 15 and 24 ppm, but accelerated clearance after exposures to 1 ppm (Ferin and Leach, 1977). Rabbits exposed for 2 hours to 0.3, 1, 3, or 10 ppm showed accelerated clearance at all concentrations, while repeated 2 h/d exposures for 14 days to 1 or 10 ppm NO_2 resulted in clearance patterns similar to those with single exposures at the same concentration (Vollmuth et al., 1986). Ferrets exposed to either 0.5 or 10 ppm NO_2 for 4 h/d, 5 d/wk for 8 or 15 weeks showed a reduction in clearance measured 12 weeks after the start of either exposure regime (Rasmussen et al. 1994).

Pulmonary Defense Mechanisms—Alveolar Macrophage Function Alveolar macrophages play a central role in the defense of the lungs, and alterations in numbers and functional properties of these cells may affect susceptibility to disease or injury. Macrophage numbers increased with continuous exposure of rats to 17 ppm, but not with 2 ppm (Stephens et al., 1972), and after 7 days of continuous exposure of rats to 4 ppm (Mochitate et al., 1986). However, no change in cell number was found following exposure of rabbits to 0.3 or 1 ppm NO_2 for 2 h/d for 13 days (Schlesinger, 1987). A subpleural accumulation of alveolar macrophages was found in rats exposed for 7 h/d, 5 d/wk for 15 weeks to 5 ppm NO_2, but not to 1 ppm (Gregory et al., 1983). Rombout et al. (1986) noted some increase, by 2 days, in the number of macrophages in terminal bronchioles and adjacent alveoli in the lungs of rats exposed continuously to 5 ppm NO_2; this was not seen with 1 or 2.5 ppm. Others have noted concentration-related increases in macrophage numbers with exposure to 5 to 40 ppm for 2 days to 15 weeks (Kleinerman et al., 1982; DeNicola et al., 1981; Busey et al., 1974; Wright et al., 1982; Foster et al., 1985).

Various functional properties of macrophages essential to adequate defense, such as surface attachment, mobility, and phagocytosis, have been assessed following exposure to NO_2. Schlesinger (1987) exposed rabbits to 0.3 or 1 ppm for 2 h/d and found no effect on attachment, but a depression of mobility at day 3 in the 0.3 ppm group. Macrophages obtained from baboons exposed to 2 ppm for 8 h/d, 5d/wk for 6 months showed reduced responsiveness to migration inhibitory factor, a lymphokine that mediates cell movement (Greene and Schneider, 1978).

Suzuki et al. (1986) found depressed phagocytic activity in macrophages obtained from rats exposed for 10 days to 4 or 8 ppm NO_2, while Lefkowitz et al. (1986) noted no change in such activity in macrophages from mice exposed for 7 days to 5 ppm. The phagocytic activity of rabbit macrophages was reduced by in vivo exposure to 0.3 ppm, but was enhanced with exposure to 1 ppm by 3 days, and returned to control values by 7 days and remained there through 13 days of exposure (Schlesinger, 1987). An exposure-concentration dependent difference in the direction of phagocytic response seems to be a characteristic of NO_2. Thus Schlesinger (1989a) found a reduction in phagocytic activity of macrophages recovered immediately after a 2 hour exposure of rabbits to 1 ppm NO_2; with 10 ppm, no change was seen immediately after exposure, but activity was increased 24 hours postexposure. Ehrlich et al. (1979) found exposure of mice to 0.5 ppm NO_2 for 3 h/d, 5 d/wk for 2 months to depress phagocytosis, while Sone et al. (1983) showed enhanced phagocytosis in macrophages obtained from rats exposed to 40 ppm for 4 h/d for 7 days. The reason for such differences in direction of response are unknown.

Macrophages are a source of various biological mediators, and their ability to produce these may be compromised by pollutant exposure. The eicosanoids are a class of mediators produced in response to a wide variety of cellular perturbation and having various effects on airway physiology and the immune system. Alveolar macrophages obtained from rats exposed to 0.5 ppm NO_2 for 0.5 to 10 d exhibited complex responses related to the production of eicosanoids (Robison et al., 1993). An initial depression of production was followed by recovery for some of these mediators, but not others, with increasing exposure duration. The complexity of response was also noted in a study of rat alveolar macrophages acutely exposed in vitro to 0.1 to 20 ppm NO_2 (Robison and Forman, 1993). Low concentrations (up to 5 ppm) had small effects on basal synthesis of eicosanoids but amplified response to stimulated production of eicosanoids, while high concentrations (20 ppm) showed the reverse pattern of response.

Pulmonary Defense Mechanisms—Resistance to Infectious Agents Nitrogen dioxide may impair the ability to resist infectious agents. Mice exposed continuously to 0.5 ppm NO_2 showed increased mortality to *K.pneumonia* after 3 months of exposure (Ehrlich and Henry, 1968), while 0.05 ppm for 24 h/d for 15 days did not change bacterial resistance

(Gardner et al., 1982). The finding of increased susceptibility does, however, depend upon the specific organism being used. Thus, while exposure of mice for 3 h/d for 3 months to 0.5 ppm increased mortality to *Streptococcus sp.* (Ehrlich et al., 1979), exposure to 0.5 to 1.5 ppm NO_2 continuously for 3 months produced no effect on mortality due to *K.pneumoniae* (McGrath and Oyervides, 1985); on the other hand, exposure to 5 ppm for 3 days did result in enhanced mortality.

A number of infectivity studies involved exposure to a baseline NO_2 concentration upon which spikes to a higher level were superimposed to mimic ambient exposures. The relative effect of such spikes is not always clear but seems to depend on both spike duration and time between spikes. Miller et al. (1987) noted that mortality due to infection was greater in a spike regimen (to 0.8 ppm) than in the baseline-exposed group (0.2 ppm). Others have found that both the number and amplitude of spikes are of importance in increasing mortality (Gardner et al., 1979; Graham et al., 1987). In fact, effects from such exposure excusions may approach those due to more continuous exposure to a lower concentration. This is consistent with the notion that, in general, brief exposures to high NO_2 levels are more hazardous than are longer duration exposures at lower concentrations (Lehnert et al., 1994).

The effect of NO_2 on mortality due to bacterial infection appears to increase with both exposure duration (T) and peak concentration (C), although the latter seems to have more influence than the former for fixed $C \times T$ values (Gardner et al., 1979). Any differences between intermittent and continuous exposure also seem to disappear as the number of days of exposure increases (Gardner et al., 1979). Other studies suggest that as concentration increases, a shorter exposure time is needed for intermittent and continuous exposure regimes to produce similar degrees of effect (Ehrlich and Henry, 1968; Ehrlich, 1979). Mortality is also proportional to exposure duration if the bacterial challenge is given immediately after exposure, but it may not be when the challenge is given much later (Gardner et al., 1982). For example, no effect of 3.5 ppm NO_2 for 2 hours was seen in mice when bacteria were administered 27 hours after exposure, while increased mortality was evident when administration was immediately after NO_2 inhalation (Ehrlich, 1980). Effects of 25 ppm for 2 hours on mice were seen only when the microbial challenge was given within 72 hours after NO_2 exposure (Purvis and Ehrlich, 1963). These results suggest that a critical time frame exists between NO_2 and bacterial challenge after which NO_2 exposure will not affect resistance.

The mechanism(s) underlying any NO_2-induced change in host resistance to bacteria are not known. However, since exposure levels that alter resistance do not affect physical clearance processes (discussed above and Parker et al., 1990), the response to NO_2 may be due to impaired intracellular killing of microbes, perhaps reflecting macrophage dysfunction. For example, macrophages are a source of numerous biochemical mediators that are directly involved in antibacterial action, for example, the superoxide anion, and a depression in superoxide production has been noted following NO_2 exposure in some studies (Amoruso et al., 1981; Suzuki et al., 1986; Robison et al., 1993), generally at higher than ambient levels. However, human alveolar macrophages exposed in vitro to 0.1 to 0.5 ppm NO_2 for 30 to 120 minutes showed increased reactive oxygen intermediate production in a dose-dependent fashion (Kienast et al., 1994).

The effects of NO_2 on viral infectivity have also been examined. Exposures to 0.5 ppm or greater on a continuous basis likely increase susceptibility, while at higher concentrations the exposure duration needed for any effect is lowered (Ito, 1971; Rose et al., 1988).

Environmental stresses may enhance the lethality of infectious agents over and above that due solely to NO_2 exposure. These may include exercise (Illing et al., 1980), elevated temperature (Gardner et al., 1982) and the presence of other pollutants (discussed below).

Histopathology   Exposure to NO_2 may produce structural alterations in the respiratory tract (Evans et al., 1975; Rombout et al., 1986; DeNicola et al., 1981; Kubota et al., 1987; Stephens et al., 1972). The anatomic region most sensitive to NO_2 is the area encompassing the terminal and respiratory bronchioles and adjacent alveolar ducts and alveoli and the primary cellular targets within this region are the ciliated cells of the bronchiolar epithelium and the type 1 cells of the alveolar epithelium.

Acute exposure to NO_2 results in hypertrophy and hyperplasia of alveolar type 1 cells, followed by cell death and desquamation and proliferation of and replacement by type 2 cells. The end result can be a thickened air-blood barrier. The bronchiolar response is characterized by hypertrophy and hyperplasia of epithelial cells, loss of secretory granules and surface protrusions of Clara cells, and loss of ciliated cells, or cilia. With chronic exposure, many of these same changes are seen, but there is increased cilia loss over larger areas of epithelium and in more proximal airways, and the structure of the remaining cilia may be altered.

The temporal progression of NO_2 induced lesions has best been described in the rat. The earliest alterations resulting from concentrations ≥ 2 ppm occur within 24 to 72 hours of continuous exposure with repair of injured tissue and replacement of destroyed cells beginning within 24 to 48 hours of continuous exposure. Division of type 2 cells is observed within 12 hours after initial NO_2 exposure, the rate becoming maximal by about 48 h and decreasing to pre-exposure levels by about 6 d, even with continued exposure. In some cases the resolution of NO_2-induced morphologic changes may be complete after exposures end; on the other hand, some lesions may resolve while others remain, even when exposure continues (Rombout et al., 1986; De Nicola et al., 1981; Kubota et al., 1987).

Chronic exposure to NO_2 may result in alterations in lung architecture resembling emphysema-like disease, such as enlargement of airspaces, an increase in mean linear intercept (a measure of the distance between alveolar walls), and a reduction in the internal surface area of the alveolar region. However, the relationship between exposure and the development of emphysema remains unclear. A problem in evaluating reported emphysematic changes in animal models is the definition of the disease, which has changed over the years and which has been defined differently by various professional groups (NIH, 1985). While long-term exposure to high NO_2 concentrations (> 10 ppm) are required to produce clearly definable emphysemalike changes (e.g., Barth et al., 1995), there is evidence that lower NO_2 levels may result in emphysema, emphysema-like changes, or altered alveolar dimensions if present in complex mixtures of NO_x (Hyde et al., 1978) or administered during lung development (Rasmussen and McClure, 1992). However, clear evidence of changes characteristic of human emphysema, namely alveolar septal degeneration, enlarged airspaces, and associated functional changes, is absent, especially with exposure at low levels. While the older literature suggests that chronic exposure to NO_2 at high levels may lead to emphysema, more recent work has suggested rather that such exposure actually results in centriacinar fibrosis (Crapo et al., 1984; Last et al., 1993).

While the extent and degree of morphologic alterations induced by NO_2 appear to be related to exposure concentration, little is known about effects of other modifying factors, such as exposure duration or the temporal pattern of exposure. The contribution of exposure time in the histopathologic response to acute inhalation was examined in rats (Stavert and Lehnert, 1988). The most pronounced effects were found with the highest NO_2 concentration in any particular set of exposures where the product of concentration and time was equivalent, indicating that concentration played a more important role than did exposure time in tissue injury. This is consistent with the relative roles of C and T in infectivity, discussed previously. Another study (Rombout et al., 1986) assessed the concentration–time response relation for intermittent and continuous exposures and likewise concluded that concentration played a more important role in inducing morphologic lesions than did exposure duration, as long as the product of $C \times T$ was constant. The effect of concentration was found to be greater with intermittent than with continuous exposure, and the onset of response was also delayed with intermittent compared to continuous exposure. The morphological effects of exposure patterns involving transient spikes were examined in a number of studies (Gregory et al., 1983; Miller et al., 1987; Crapo et al., 1984; Chang et al. 1986). Results are equivocal, and it is not clear whether these peaks significantly contributed to morphological damage in excess of that due to integral exposure.

Despite the fact that there is a fairly extensive data base concerning morphologic effects of NO_2 in animal models, it is still quite difficult to establish a threshold exposure condition for this endpoint. This is due to the great complexity of changes occurring with exposure, as well as to large interspecies differences in response. For example, the rat appears to be less sensitive to NO_2 compared to other species, such as the guinea pig or monkey. Furthermore different cell types show differential sensitivity to NO_2. In general, morphological alterations, some of which may be persistent, are found with chronic exposure to concentrations < 1 ppm. However, long-term exposure to levels ≥ 2 ppm are generally required to produce more extensive or permanent changes.

An added complication in evaluating morphologic effects is that they may depend on the age of the animals at the time of exposure (Stephens et al., 1982; Azoulay-Dupuis et al., 1983; Chang et al., 1986; Kyono and Kawai, 1982). Neonates, specifically prior to weaning, seem to be relatively resistant to NO_2, with sensitivity increasing with age until adulthood. However, the response in animals of different ages is similar in terms of the cell types affected, the nature of the damage incurred, and repair capacity. Age-related differences occur in the extent of damage and in the time required for repair, this latter taking longer in older animals. The reasons for age differences in sensitivity are not known but may reflect diet and variable sensitivity of target cells during different growth phases (Stephens et al., 1982; Hahn, 1979).

Of importance in assessing the morphological effects of NO_2 is consideration of individuals with compromised lung function, such as those with respiratory disease. There is, however, a very limited data base in laboratory animals with preexisting chronic disease. No effect of NO_2 exposure on pneumoconiosis development in guinea pigs was found in one study (Gross et al., 1968). Two studies assessed whether prolonged exposure to NO_2 would alter the progression or severity of preexisting emphysema (produced by elastase instillation). NO_2 did not potentiate preexisting emphysema in rats (Stavert et al., 1986) but may have done so in hamsters (Lafuma et al., 1987).

It is also possible that acute lung disease may affect NO_2 toxicity. Fenters et al. (1973) challenged squirrel monkeys with an influenza virus at various times during continuous exposure to 1 ppm NO_2 for 16 months, and compared the response to that seen in animals not challenged but similarly exposed. Only the virus-challenged animals showed effects of NO_2, namely slight emphysemalike changes, and thickening of the bronchial and bronchiolar epithelium. This suggests that the presence of acute lung disease may have affected NO_2 toxicity.

Biochemistry   Exposure to NO_2 can result in damage to the cell membrane, and fairly low inhaled exposure levels have been associated with such alterations. For example, lipid peroxidation was noted in rats exposed to 0.04 ppm for 9 months (Sagai et al., 1984). However, extended exposures at low levels may be needed for such effects, since rats and guinea pigs exposed to 0.4 ppm NO_2 for 24 h/d for only 2 weeks showed no change in the level of lipid peroxides in the lungs (Ichinose and Sagai, 1989).

NO_2 exposure may also result in oxidation of protein or protein components. (Freeman and Mudd, 1981; Prutz et al., 1985). Of importance in the pathogenesis of chronic lung disease is effects on lung structural proteins, such as elastin and collagen. Thickened collagen fibrils were noted in the lungs of monkeys exposed to 3 ppm for 4 h/d for 4 days (Bils, 1976). Increased rates of lung collagen synthesis, a possible marker for development of fibrosis, has been noted in NO_2 exposed rats (Last et al., 1983; Last and Warren, 1987). A decrease in elastin may be associated with the development of emphysema, but there are few data following exposure using levels of relevance to actual ambient conditions. Chronic exposure at high levels, about 10 ppm, are needed to increase collagen deposition within the lungs (Rasmussen, 1994). Experiments at high concentrations (Kleinerman et al., 1985; Kleinerman and Ip, 1979) suggest that NO_2 may reduce elastin content via an increase in the activity of neutrophil elastase, the enzyme responsible for elastin breakdown.

Other NO_2-induced biochemical effects related to proteins involve changes in activity of various pulmonary enzymes (Takahashi et al., 1986; Ichinose and Sagai, 1982; Azoulay-Dupuis et al., 1983; Elsayed and Mustafa, 1982). For example, glutathione (GSH) is a reducing compound found in the lungs, and NO_2 exposure has been reported to alter the activity of enzymes that regulate its levels, or to affect the lung content of glutathione itself. Suppressed GSH-peroxidase activity has been noted, for example, in mice exposed continuously for 17 months to 1 ppm, but not to 0.5 ppm (Ayaz and Csallany, 1978), while an increase in GSH-reductase activity was noted in mice exposed to 6 ppm for 4 h/d for 30 days (Csallany, 1975) or in rats exposed to 6.2 (and not 1 or 2.3 ppm) for 4 days (Chow et al., 1974). High NO_2 exposure levels are thus apparently needed for changes in GSH metabolism.

The biochemical response to NO_2 may be modulated by dietary factors, in particular, levels of certain antioxidant vitamins. For example, increases in the lavage content of proteins and lipids were noted in vitamin C depleted guinea pigs exposed to 1 ppm NO_2 for 72 hours, but not in normal controls (Selgrade et al., 1981); similarly depleted guinea pigs exposed for 1 wk to 0.4 ppm showed an increase in lavage protein content, an indicator of serum transudation and possible membrane damage (Sherwin and Carlson, 1973). Another possible modulator of effect is vitamin E. Changes in protein content and enzyme activity in lung homogenates from rats exposed for 7 days to 3 ppm were found to be more severe in those animals which were deficient in this vitamin (Elsayed and Mustafa, 1982).

The lungs participate in the metabolism of various xenobiotics, and it is possible that inhaled pollutants may alter their ability to handle these materials. However, if NO_2 does alter xenobiotic metabolism, it is only at high exposure levels. Thus exposure of rats continuously to 4 ppm NO_2 for up to 2 months produced no change in the cytochrome P-450 content of the lungs, although some other xenobiotic metabolizing enzymes were decreased by this exposure (Takahashi and Miura, 1989).

Pulmonary Function   The effects of NO_2 on pulmonary mechanics have been studied in laboratory animals using standard indexes of pulmonary function, with mixed results. Hamsters exposed to 2 ppm for 8 h/d, 5 d/wk for 8 weeks exhibited an increase in tidal volume, but no change in compliance or vital capacity (Lafuma et al., 1987). Exposure of mice to 0.2 ppm NO_2 for 23 h/d, 7 d/wk for up to 52 weeks resulted in no change in pulmonary mechanics (Miller et al., 1987); however, when 1 hour spikes to 0.2 ppm twice daily for 5 d/wk were superimposed upon this baseline, a significant decrease in end-expiratory volume and vital capacity, as well as a trend toward increased residual volume, were found. Stevens et al. (1988) exposed neonate and 7-week-old mice continuously for 1, 3, or 6 weeks to baseline levels of 0.5, 1 or 2 ppm NO_2 upon which were superimposed twice daily 1 hour spikes (5 d/wk) to 1.5, 3, or 6 ppm, respectively. The two higher levels produced increased vital capacity and compliance by 3 weeks only in the neonates, but the effect resolved by 6 weeks. Furthermore adult animals showed a reduction in compliance after 6 weeks of exposure to 2 ppm. Suzuki et al. (1982) noted a concentration-related increase in respiratory rate in mice exposed to 5–20 ppm NO_2 for 24 hour; exposure to 5 ppm also resulted in a decrease in arterial CO_2 tension (Pa_{CO_2}), suggesting hyperventilation.

Bronchoprovocation challenge testing is often used to assess nonspecific airway hyperresponsivity. Silbaugh et al. (1981) examined the effects of histamine aerosol on guinea pigs exposed to NO_2 for 1 hour at 7 to 146 ppm. While a concentration-related increase in sensitivity to histamine was noted when the latter was inhaled 10 minutes after NO_2 exposure (but not 2 or 19 h after exposure) the response became significant only when NO_2 levels were > 25 ppm. A more recent study involving long-term exposures (Kobayashi and Miura, 1995) involved exposure of guinea pigs to 0.06, 0.5, 1, 2, or 4 ppm NO_2 for 24 h/d for 6 or 12 weeks. Airway responsiveness to histamine and specific airway resistance were assessed on the last day of each exposure. Exposure to 2 and 4 ppm by 6 weeks of exposure resulted in increased airway responsiveness, while exposure to the same concentration resulted in increased resistance by 12 weeks of exposure.

Tepper et al. (1993) performed a long-term exposure of rats to NO_2. Animals were exposed to NO_2 having a 0.5 ppm background with 1.5 ppm peaks (2 h) for up to 78 weeks. No exposure related changes in nitrogen washout, compliance, lung volume or CO diffusion capactiy was noted, but at 78 weeks there was some reduction in a measure of forced expiratory flow rate. However, the authors indicated that the change was borderline and suggested that long-term exposure to high ambient urban levels did not lead to any dysfunction suggestive of degenerative lung disease. The overall database suggests that NO_2 at realistic levels in terms of ambient exposure has not been shown to significantly alter pulmonary mechanics or bronchial responsivity in animal models, consistent with results of controlled clinical studies in humans.

Extrapulmonary Effects

Immune Response   A number of studies have examined the effects of NO_2 on specific parameters of both humoral and cellular immunity. While immune suppression has clearly been shown to follow exposure to levels of NO_2 above 5 ppm, as evidenced by various endpoints including the response of T-cells, antibodies, or production of interferon (e.g., Holt et al., 1979; Valand et al., 1970; Fujimaki and Shimizu, 1981; Campbell and Hilsenroth, 1976), there are only a few reports of response to lower levels. These studies suggest that short-term repeated exposures may result in reductions in counts of lymphocytes in the lungs or spleen, or a depression in antibody responsivity to particular antigens.

Mice exposed for 7 h/d, 5 d/wk for 7 weeks to 0.25 ppm NO_2 showed reduced total T-lymphocyte numbers in the spleen, with concomitant reductions in certain subpopulations of these cells, for example helper cells (Richters and Damji, 1988). Exposure of mice for 3 months to 0.5 ppm NO_2 resulted in a depressed responsiveness of both T- and B-lymphocytes in spleen (Maigetter et al., 1978). No effect on the cell-mediated immune system was found in mice exposed for 24 hours to 5 ppm NO_2 (Lefkowitz et al., 1986), nor to 1.6 ppm for 4 weeks (Fujimaki et al., 1982).

Mice exposed to 0.4 or 1.6 ppm NO_2 for 4 weeks showed depressed primary antibody responsivity to sheep red blood cells in vitro (Fujimaki et al., 1982), while mice exposed to 4 ppm NO_2 continuously for up to 56 days showed no change in the antibody response to T-cell-dependent and independent antigens in spleen (Fujimaki, 1989). In another study mice were vaccinated with influenza virus after they had undergone 3 months of continuous exposure to 0.5 or 2 ppm NO_2 with daily spikes (1 h) of 2 ppm for 5 d/wk. Both concentrations resulted in a reduction in mean serum neutralizing antibody titers (Ehrlich et al., 1975). Guinea pigs exposed to 1 ppm for 6 months showed a reduction in all immunoglobulin fractions (Kosmider et al., 1973). On the other hand, Balchum et al.

(1965) noted an increase in serum antibody titers against lung tissue in guinea pigs exposed to 5 ppm NO_2 for 4 h/d after 160 hours of exposure, and further increases as exposure duration increased. Enhanced immune function may be just as detrimental as suppressed function, through overstimulation of response and hypersensitivity.

As with other endpoints, the effects of NO_2 upon the immune system appear to be related to various exposure parameters. While some studies show no effect, others show enhancement or depression of immune parameters, depending on the exposure concentration, the length of exposure, and the animal species used. In addition the direction of change appears to depend on exposure concentration. For example, humoral response in monkeys chronically exposed to NO_2 was enhanced at a low concentration (1 ppm) but suppressed at a higher level (5 ppm) (Fenters et al., 1971, 1973).

Exposure to NO_2 may affect allergic response. Rats exposed to 5 ppm for 3 hours after sensitization with house dust mite antigen had higher levels of serum IgE and local respiratory tract IgA, IgG, and IgE antibodies than did controls (Gilmour, 1995). The exposed animals also had increased lymphocyte activity in the spleen and local lymph nodes and showed an increase in respiratory tract inflammatory cells. This suggests that NO_2 may enhance immune responsiveness and increase the severity of pulmonary inflammation in sensitized lungs and may, thus, play some role in the exacerbation of immune-mediated respiratory disease.

Other Effects   Exposure to NO_2 may affect target sites beyond the lungs. Endpoints that have been shown to be altered include body weight, blood cell counts, blood cell membrane and serum chemistry, liver and kidney function, and the nervous system, such as brain protein enzymes and neuromotor function (e.g., Graham et al., 1982; Tabacova et al., 1985; Freeman et al., 1966; Wagner et al., 1965; Case et al., 1979; Kaya et al., 1980, Kaya and Miura, 1982; Mochitate et al., 1984; Kosmider et al., 1973; Miller et al., 1980; Takahashi et al., 1986; Sherwin and Layfield, 1974). However, the data are conflicting, and because of this, the ability to relate reported changes to human health effects is severely limited.

Genotoxicity/Carcinogenicity   Exposure to NO_2 even at high levels does not seem to be genotoxic or teratogenic in appropriate assay systems (Kripke and Sherwin, 1984; Gooch et al., 1977). While a study did note an increase in the rate of DNA strand breaks in hamster cells exposed in vitro to 10 ppm for 20 minutes, while 5 ppm for up to 30 minutes had no such effect (Görsdorf et al., 1990), in vivo exposure of mice to 20 ppm for up to 23 hours did not result in any genotoxicity (Victorin et al., 1990). This apparent conflict in response may be due to repair mechanisms operating in vivo that are not operative in in vitro assays.

The ability of NO_2 to act as a carcinogen or co-carcinogen is unclear, but there is no direct evidence that NO_2 exposure results in the development of tumors. Some concern is, however, based on the fact that exposure can result in nitrite in blood, and this in turn may produce carcinogens, such as nitrosamines, after further reactions in the body. Although there have been no long-term carcinogenesis bioassays performed with NO_2, one chronic inhalation study, in which mice were exposed to 1, 5, and 10 ppm NO_2 for 6 h/d, 5 d/wk for 6 months, suggested a small increase in tumor (pulmonary adenoma) frequency and incidence in the highest-dose group (Adkins et al., 1986). However, such data must be interpreted with caution, and the relationship between cancer development in mice and that in humans is not clear.

Although not likely a carcinogen itself, NO_2 may modulate tumorogenic processes in the lungs (Witschi, 1988). For example, in conjunction with a specific carcinogen, NO_2 exposure may be involved in the pathogenesis of small cell carcinoma (Witschi, 1988), especially since it has been shown to modulate the number of neuroendocrine cells, the precursor cells for this disease (Kleinerman et al., 1981; Palisano and Kleinerman, 1980). As another example, an enhancement of tumor colonization in the lungs of mice injected with melanoma cells was noted after exposure to NO_2 at 0.4 or 0.8 ppm for 8 h/d, 5 d/wk for 10 to 12 weeks (Richters and Kuraitis, 1981). This could be due to injury of lung capillary endothelium by NO_2, facilitating metastases of blood-borne cancer cells to the lungs (Richters and Richters, 1989), or to suppression of immune system components (discussed above). However, as with other endpoints, the data base regarding the role of NO_2 in carcinogenic processes is conflicting. For example, NO_2 has been shown to actually enhance the cytotoxic response of macrophages (Sone et al., 1983), which implies greater anti-tumor defense capabilities. Thus the role for NO_2 in cancer etiology, if any, requires further study.

Controlled Studies with Humans By their nature, studies with human volunteers can only be used to evaluate transient effects of acute exposure. They have generally used changes in standard pulmonary mechanical indexes as markers of response; a few studies, however, have employed other endpoints, which include bronchoprovocation challenge testing, clearance of inhaled aerosols, and analysis of biochemical and cellular components of bronchopulmonary lavage. Various subject groups have been examined. These include healthy individuals with no history of respiratory disease, allergy, and so on as well as people with allergies or a history of asthma or chronic obstructive pulmonary disease (COPD).

Acute exposures (up to about 2 h) to NO_2 at levels ≤ 1 ppm have not resulted in any significant changes in pulmonary mechanics in normal, healthy adult subjects at rest (Beil and Ulmer, 1976; Bylin et al., 1985; Hazucha et al., 1982; Koenig et al., 1985; Bascom et al., 1996). Although there have been some reports of altered mechanics at this level, there is no consistent pattern of response. Regarding higher levels, the study of Beil and Ulmer (1976) involving 2 hour exposures to 1, 2.5, 5, and 7.5 ppm indicated a change in total respiratory resistance occurring at ≥ 2.5 ppm, although the effects were quite small. Von Nieding et al. (1973) noted a decrease in diffusing capacity (DL_{co}) with a 15 minute exposure to 5 ppm. Finally no changes in lung mechanical function were found with exposure to 2 ppm for 2 hours, or for 2 h/d for 3 days (Mohsenin, 1988; Goings et al., 1989).

It is possible that some variability in response may be due to biochemical differences between individuals, perhaps related to diet. Mohsenin (1987a) exposed normal adults, some of whom had received vitamin C prior to exposure, to 2 ppm NO_2 for 1 hour, and measured airway responsiveness. An increased responsiveness seen in the untreated subjects was not found in those receiving the vitamin. Vitamin C is an antioxidant, and the apparent protective effect found in this study is consistent with results of toxicologic studies previously discussed.

Exposure to ≤ 1 ppm NO_2 in conjunction with various degrees of exercise have also resulted in inconsistent effects on the lung function of healthy people; most of the studies showed no effects that could be unequivocally attributed to NO_2 (Folinsbee et al., 1978; Frampton et al., 1989a; Hackney et al., 1978; Kerr et al., 1979; Morrow and Utell, 1989). Reduced compliance was noted following exposure for 2 hours at 0.5 ppm (Kulle, 1982), but the meaning of this with a lack of other lung mechanical changes was not clear. Linn et al. (1985a) found no change in resistance or spirometry with exposure at 4 ppm for 75 minutes.

Increased airway responsivity in healthy subjects has been noted following a 2 hour exposure to 7.5 ppm (Beil and Ulmer, 1976), with 1 hour to 2 ppm (Mohsenin, 1988), and with 3 hours (with intermittent exercise) to 1.5 ppm (Frampton et al., 1989a). Again, however, the results are not consistent with other studies at similar concentrations and exposure durations finding no change (e.g., Kulle and Clements, 1987). Exposures at ≤ 0.6

ppm have not produced any change in responsivity at all (Morrow and Utell, 1989; Frampton et al., 1989a; Bylin et al., 1985; Hazucha et al., 1983).

Particular subsegments of the population may be especially susceptible to the effects of NO_2. As noted in some epidemiological studies, one such group is asthmatics. A number of studies have been performed with exposure levels ranging from 0.1 to 4 ppm for durations ranging up to 4 hours, usually with exercise; effects on various aspects of lung mechanical function, such as spirometry or airway resistance, have ranged from none to slight, and all with much inconsistency (e.g., Avol et al., 1988; Bauer et al., 1986; Ahmed et al., 1982; Hazucha et al., 1982, 1983; Bylin et al., 1985; Koenig et al.. 1985, 1987; Kerr et al., 1979; Rubinstein et al.. 1990; Morrow and Utell, 1989; Roger et al.. 1990; Kleinman et al., 1983; Linn et al., 1985a, 1986; Mohsenin, 1987b; Salome et al., 1996, Morrow et al., 1992). In a unique study Goldstein et al. (1988) measured pulmonary function in adult asthmatics in their home and also monitored indoor NO_2 levels. The results suggested that average exposures to > 0.3 ppm produced a decline in certain pulmonary function measures, but inconsistent effects were seen at lower exposure levels. Finally, when there is any response, it may only occur with exercise. Exposure to 0.3 ppm for 30 minutes produced no change in pulmonary mechanics indexes in resting asthmatics, but effects were noted when exercise was incorporated into the exposure protocol (Bauer et al., 1986).

The most sensitive pulmonary mechanical response to NO_2 in people with airway disease appears to involve changes in airway responsiveness. However, there is much variabilty in results from different studies and also an apparent lack of a dose–response relationship. While some studies have indicated increased responsiveness due to NO_2 exposures at 0.14 to 0.5 ppm (Bauer et al., 1986; Bylin et al., 1988; Kleinman et al., 1983; Mohsenin, 1987b; Salome et al., 1996; Strand et al., 1996), others have indicated no such effects at similar levels (Hazucha et al., 1983; Roger et al., 1990; Linn et al., 1986; Orehek et al., 1981; Avol et al., 1988; Bylin et al., 1988), and exposure to a much higher level (3 ppm) has also produced no effect (Linn et al., 1986). Any NO_2-induced increased responsiveness may occur with a several hour delay following expsoure in asthmatics (Strand et al., 1996).

While the mechanism of any NO_2-induced hyperresponsiveness is not known, it may involve alterations in the metabolism of endogenous bronchoconstrictors (Hoshi et al., 1996) or activation of specific cells within the airways (Ohashi et al., 1993). Mild asthmatics and normals were exposed to 1 ppm NO_2 (with intermittent exercise) for 3 hours, followed by bronchopulmonary lavage 1 hour postexposure. While no change in differential cell counts was noted in either group, the asthmatics showed changes in lung eicosanoids not seen in normals, suggesting that NO_2 could activate cells compatible with airway inflammation (Jorres et al., 1995).

While asthmatics or allergic individuals may not show enhanced response directly to NO_2, exposure may alter their response to antigens. Humans having a history of allergic rhinitis were exposed to 0.4 ppm NO_2 for 6 hours, followed by challenge with an allergen (Wang et al., 1995). There was some evidence that NO_2 primed eosinophils for subsequent activation by the allergen. Mild asthmatics were exposed to 0.1 or 0.4 ppm NO_2 for 1 hour followed by exposure to house dust mite antigen challenge to see the effect of NO_2 on response to allergen (Tunnicliffe et al., 1994). Asthmatic response was assessed by changes in FEV_1. An increase in response to antigen challenge was noted only following exposure to the higher NO_2 level.

Another possibly sensitive subsegment of the population is people with COPD, that is chronic bronchitis and emphysema. Increased airway resistance has been found in individuals with COPD after exposure to 1.6 ppm in conjunction with exercise (von Nieding and Wagner, 1979), while a decrease in forced vital capacity (FVC) was noted following exposure to 0.3 ppm for 4 hours with intermittent exercise (Morrow and Utell, 1989), and a decrease in FEV_1 was noted following exposure for 1 hour to 0.3 ppm

(Vagaggini et al., 1996). On the other hand, no changes in airway resistance in chronic bronchitics exposed to 0.5 ppm for 2 hours with exercise, nor in spirometry of COPD patients exposed to 0.5 to 2 ppm for 1 hour, also with exercise, have been noted (Kerr et al., 1979; Linn et al., 1985b).

Thus the data base is currently not sufficiently robust to allow determination of the specific exposure conditions, namely concentration, duration, and ventilation, for threshold effects on lung function in healthy humans with acute exposure. Pulmonary mechanics may in fact not provide very sensitive indexes of response in such people. On the other hand, functional changes may occur in individuals with asthma and/or COPD following exposure to lower levels of NO_2 than affect normals. Again, however, the results are inconsistent. Results of one study examining pulmonary functional indexes with asthmatics have not been confirmed by a subsequent one, or responses of a particular subject group are not always reproducible (Orehek et al., 1976; Hazucha et al., 1983; Bauer et al., 1985; Bromberg, 1988). There is some evidence that especially sensitive subgroup(s) may exist within the asthmatic population (Bauer et al., 1986; Morrow and Utell, 1989). That is, the variability in responses noted above may be the result of differences in the severity or type of asthma in the subjects examined within one, or between, studies. Asthmatics also exhibit a wide range of response to external stimuli, so some variability may merely be due to an interindividual variation in response to NO_2. The lowest concentration that does result in observed effects on airway responsivity in exercising asthmatics is in the 0.2 to 0.5 ppm range; in normals, levels of 5 ppm may cause bronchoconstriction, but minimum levels of 1 to 2 ppm are needed for changes in pulmonary functional parameters. Most mild asthmatics are not sensitive to NO_2 at less than or equal to 0.6 ppm, at least in terms of changes in pulmonary mechanics, while nonspecific airway responsiveness in mild asthmatics may be increased at levels > 0.1 ppm.

Controlled clinical studies have examined other aspects of pulmonary biology after exposure to NO_2. Humans exposed for 20 minutes to 1.5 to 3.5 ppm NO_2 did show a reduction of mucociliary activity measured 45 minutes following exposure (Helleday et al., 1995). The effects on infectivity of an attenuated influenza virus in healthy humans was assessed by Kulle and Clements (1987); NO_2 exposure levels were 1 to 3 ppm. There were no overall statistically significant changes in infectivity rates, although they were elevated in some of the NO_2 exposed groups. In another study (Goings et al., 1989) there was also suggestive evidence that exposure for 2 h/d for 3 days to 1 or 2 ppm NO_2 increased susceptibility to respiratory viruses in healthy adults. Frampton et al. (1989b) examined the effect of NO_2 exposure in vivo on the ability of alveolar macrophages to inactivate influenza virus in vitro. Healthy humans were exposed either to 0.6 ppm for 3 hours, or to 0.05 ppm for 3 hours with three, 15 minute spikes to 2 ppm. There appeared to be less effective inactivation of the virus by macrophages harvested from the humans exposed to 0.6 ppm, but the results just missed statistical significance ($p = 0.07$). No effects were noted in the individuals exposed to the lower concentration with the 2 ppm spikes. There also seemed to be a trend of increased production of interleukin-1 (IL-1) by macrophages from some individuals, namely those whose cells tended to have reduced viral inactivation activity. Effects on IL-1 were also examined by Pinkston et al. (1988), with exposure of macrophages harvested by lavage to 5 to 15 ppm NO_2 for 3 hours. No change in cell viability nor in release of IL-1 was noted. In any case, increased infectivity in NO_2 exposed laboratory animals together with the above suggestive findings in humans indicate that NO_2 may indeed alter host defense in humans. Further work is needed, especially with larger sample sizes and better-defined human populations.

Some biochemical effects of inhaled NO_2 have been examined in controlled clinical studies. In vitro exposure of human blood to high levels (> 6 ppm) of NO_2 has been shown to result in production of methemoglobin (metHb) (Chiodi et al., 1983), but Chaney et al.

(1981) found no such change in normal humans exposed for 2 hours to 0.2 ppm. A reported elevation of glutathione in these exposed subjects was not supported by the results of Posin et al. (1978), who found no effect following exposure to 1 ppm. The results of some of these studies are clouded by the lack of any consistent dose-response relationship.

Exposure to 4 ppm NO_2 for 20 minutes resulted in an inflammatory response in healthy individuals, as evidenced by changes in lymphocyte counts in lavage fluid obtained 4 to 24 hours after exposure (Sandström et al., 1990). This is, however, not a consistent finding in humans (e.g., Mohsenin and Gee, 1987), possibly due to differences in experimental protocols, such as the times at which lavage was performed after exposure. Thus exposure to 0.3 ppm for 1 hour with exercise produced no acute inflammation in the proximal airways of normals, asthmatics or people with COPD (Vagaggini et al., 1996). On the other hand, it should be noted that exposures of laboratory animals to NO_2 at levels up to 8 ppm for up to 10 days did not produce evidence of acute inflammation (Schlesinger et al. 1987; Gregory et al. 1983; Mochitate et al., 1986; Suzuki et al., 1986). Perhaps NO_2 is not very effective in eliciting an inflammatory response at ambient levels with short-term exposure.

Nitrogen dioxide exposure has been associated with development of emphysema in animal models. A component of the lung defense against proteolysis is α-1-protease inhibitor. Mohsenin and Gee (1987) noted a decrease in levels of this enzyme in the lavage fluid of subjects exposed to 3 to 4 ppm for 3 hours. However, the investigators noted that the extent of the decrease was not associated with any increased risk of emphysema. On the other hand, exposure of normal humans for 3 hours (with intermittent exercise) to 1.5 ppm, or for 3 hours to 0.05 ppm with three 2 ppm peaks, did not result in any change in activity of α-1-protease inhibitor in lavage fluid (Johnson et al., 1990). A 3 hour exposure to 0.6 ppm resulted in an increase in levels of another anti-protease (α-2-macroglobulin) in lung lavage (Frampton et al., 1989c). In another study of potential lung damage, normal humans exposed to 0.6 ppm NO_2 for 4 h/d for 3 days showed no effect on the excretion of hydroxyproline, a marker for connective tissue injury (Muelenaer et al., 1987). Effects of repeated exposures, which would more likely be involved in disease development, on these endpoints are unknown.

NITRIC OXIDE

Exposure

Maximum hourly average NO concentrations range from 0.17 to 1 ppm in metropolitan areas while annual averages are in the range of 0.01 to 0.06 ppm (U.S. EPA, 1993). Rural areas show maximum hourly averages of 0.01 to 0.4 ppm and annual averages of 0.005 to 0.009 ppm. Indoor concentrations are not commonly measured, and thus data are limited. Levels associated with gas cooking may reach daily mean peaks of 0.4 ppm (Keller et al., 1979) but generally are about 0.1 ppm.

Dosimetry and Toxicology

The lower aqueous solubility of NO compared to NO_2 may result in greater amounts of the former reaching the respiratory region (Yoshida and Kasama, 1987). This NO will then diffuse rapidly, at a somewhat faster rate than does NO_2 (Chiodi and Mohler, 1985), through pulmonary tissue with little reaction, but it is not transported to any great extent through the vasculature due to its rapid interaction with oxyhemoglobin, as discussed further below. While the direct toxicity of NO is low, indirect toxicity can result from its reaction with superoxide to produce peroxynitrite, a potent oxidant.

Nitric oxide entering the bloodstream binds to hemoglobin (Hb), producing nitrosylhemoglobin (NOHb). The affinity of Hb for NO is very high, much higher even than that for O_2. The NOHb formed is rapidly oxidized to methemoglobin (MetHb) in the presence of O_2. The MetHb is subsequently reduced into ferrous Hb by MetHb-reductase, an enzyme present in red blood cells. Despite the affinity for hemoglobin, in vivo exposure to NO at levels ranging from 2 to 10 ppm have shown that the amount of NOHb in blood was such that any reduction of oxygen transport was not lethal nor damaging to organs sensitive to O_2 depletion (e.g., Oda et al., 1980a, 1976; Azouley et al., 1977). Thus it appears that as long as the activity of MetHb-reductase is maintained, the conversion of NOHb to MetHb should mitigate any potential toxicity due to NO-related oxygen transport effects.

Nitric oxide is synthesized endogenously in the cells of many tissues. Low concentrations of NO are produced by constitutive enzymes, while higher concentrations are formed by enzymes that increase in amount through their induction upon exposure to certain cytokines or other mediators. Since endogeneous NO is involved in numerous processes, such as nervous system signaling, regulation of pulmonary and systemic vascular resistance, and mediation of immune defenses, the impact of inhaled, exogenous NO, especially at low concentrations, is often difficult to evaluate.

Nitric oxide appears to stimulate guanylate cyclase, which in turn leads to its various biological effects. Furthermore NO can react with thiol-associated iron in enzymes, which is a mechanism for cytotoxicity. It can also react with superoxide, producing peroxynitrite which can then react with proteins (Ischiropoulos et al., 1992). Many of these effects have been noted in vitro and offer potential explanations for effects of NO on host defenses. Whether they can explain any effects of NO inhalation exposure is not clear. There is, however, indication that at least for some endpoints, effects of endogeneous NO can be mimicked by exposure to exogeneous NO (Gustafsson, 1993). It has been suggested, for example, that the vasodilatory response of the bronchial and pulmonary vascular systems to cigarette smoke is due to NO in the smoke (Alving et al., 1992). Furthermore individuals with depressed endogenous NO may be more sensitive to inhaled NO.

The specific substrates and reactions that mediate NO toxicity are not clear. Some studies indicate that the toxic effects of NO are different from the membrane damage due to NO_2. For example, NO may target fibroblasts that are responsible for the maintenance and repair of the alveolar interstitium (Mercer et al., 1995). Any respiratory tract morphologic responses to NO are similar to those found with NO_2, except that NO levels needed to produce them in most studies were higher, that is ≥ 2 ppm with continuous exposure (Azoulay et al., 1977; Oda et al., 1980a; Hugod, 1979; Holt et al., 1979; Oda et al., 1976). While little NO appears to react with lung tissue at exposure concentrations found in ambient outdoor or indoor air, with most diffusing into the blood, chronic exposure of rats to 0.5 ppm (with spikes to 1.5 ppm) produced interstitial lung damage (Mercer et al., 1995). Recent work suggests that NO may actually be more potent than NO_2 for some morphological injury, such as effects in interstitial spaces of alveolar septa (Mercer et al., 1995).

Studies of physiological effects of inhaled NO are sparse, and exposure levels used were quite high. Murphy (1964) found no change in pulmonary mechanical function of guinea pigs exposed for 4 hours to NO at 16 or 50 ppm. Holt et al. (1979) examined immunological endpoints in mice exposed to 10 ppm NO for 2 h/d, 5 d/w up to 30 weeks. Leukocytosis was evident by 5 week of exposure, while a decrease in mean hemoglobin content of red blood cells was found by 30 weeks. The ability of spleen cells to mount a graft compated to host reaction was stimulated by 20 weeks of exposure but suppressed by 26 weeks. When the ability of mice to reject virus-induced tumors was assessed, less of the NO-exposed animals survived tumor challenge compared to control; this suggests that NO, at high levels, may have affected immunologic competence. In this regard mice were exposed continuously to 2 ppm NO for 6 hours up to 4 weeks, to assess the effect on resistance to bacterial infection (Azouley et al., 1981). There was some indication that NO-exposed females, but not males, showed a significant increase in mortality and a significant decrease in survival time. Finally NO does not appear to be genotoxic (Görsdorf et al., 1990).

There is only one report of controlled exposure of humans to NO (Kagawa, 1982). Following a 2 hour exposure to 1 ppm, there appeared to be some variability in pulmonary function response among subjects, but only one of a large battery of tests showed statistical significance; it is likely that this effect, if not due to chance, has little biological significance. On the other hand, vasodilation is a sensitive target for NO, and pulmonary vasodilation has been noted with acute exposure to 5 to 10 ppm in normal animals and humans (Gustafsson, 1993).

In summary, a large fraction of inhaled NO reaches the respiratory region of the lungs, where it rapidly diffuses into blood and reacts with hemoglobin; little NO directly interacts with lung tissue, especially at ambient concentrations. Despite any binding with hemoglobin, anoxia of O_2-sensitive organs does not seem to occur, at least with NO exposure levels ≤ 10 ppm.

NITRIC / NITROUS ACID

Exposure

There are few data for ambient HNO_3 levels and those that are available suggest much variability. For example, levels in southern California were found to range from 0.5 to 4.8 $\mu g / m^3$ (0.02–0.19 ppm) [averaging 1.8 $\mu g/m^3$ (0.07 ppm)] in one city, while in another area they ranged from 0.8–56 $\mu g/m^3$ [0.03–0.22 ppm, averaging 17 $\mu g/m^3$ (0.066 ppm)] (Munger et al., 1990). On the other hand, levels (24 h avg.) in a rural area of North Carolina ranged from 0.8 to 2.1 $\mu g/m^3$ (0.03–0.08 ppm) (Shaw et al., 1982). Indoor levels of nitric acid have been reported to range up to about 0.001 ppm (Brauer et al., 1991). Indoor levels of nitrous acid can reach 0.1 ppm when gas stoves and unvented kerosene heaters are used (Beckett et al., 1995), while outdoor (short-term) levels of 0.007 to 0.016 ppm have been reported in southern California (Winer and Bierman, 1991).

Dosimetry and Toxicology

The dosimetry of inhaled HNO_3 is unknown. However, because of its very high water solubility and vapor state, inhaled HNO_3 should undergo significant removal in the upper respiratory tract. It has also been suggested that inhaled vapor phase HNO_3 may be converted into or deposited onto small particles within the humid atmosphere of the respiratory tract, thus facilitating its transport to and deposition within the deep lung (Chen and Schlesinger, 1996). By contrast, HNO_3 in fog droplets that are inhaled deposits by impaction in large airways.

The current data base concerning potential health effects from exposure to HNO_3 is limited. In one study, both normal and allergic sheep (i.e., those having airway responses similar to those occurring in humans with allergic airway disease) were exposed for 4 hours to 1.6 ppm (42.7 $\mu g/m^3$) HNO_3 vapor (Abraham et al., 1982). A decrease in specific pulmonary flow resistance, compared to preexposure control values, in both groups of sheep was noted, indicating that there was no bronchoconstriction. However, allergic sheep showed increased airway responsiveness, both immediately and 24 hours after HNO_3 exposure. Although there was no significant change in responsiveness in the normal group as a whole, two of the animals showed an increase in responsiveness to bronchoconstrictor challenge (carbachol) after HNO_3 exposure. According to the investigators, this suggested that some individuals in a normal population may be more sensitive than are others.

Allergic adolescent asthmatic human subjects were exposed for 40 minutes during rest and moderate exercise to 0.05 ppm (1.3 $\mu g/m^3$) HNO_3. An increase in total respiratory resistance and a decrease in forced expiratory volume were noted (Koenig et al., 1989). In another report Koenig (1989) examined exercising adolescent asthmatics exposed to 0.057 (1.5 $\mu g/m^3$) ppm HNO_3 vapor for 45 minutes. Small, but not statistically significant, decreases in forced expiratory volume and expiratory flow rates were found. Particulate HNO_3 has also been found to enhance bronchoconstriction in humans produced by exposure to hypoosmolar aerosols (Balmes et al., 1988).

Aris et al. (1993) measured pulmonary functional parameters (specific airway resistance, SRaw, FEV_1, FVC) and lavage indexes (total and differential cell counts, LDH, fibronectin, total protein) in healthy subjects exposed for 4 hours (including moderated exercise) to 500 $\mu g/m^3$ HNO_3 vapor. Lavage was performed 18 hours postexpsoure. No HNO_3-related effects on any of the measured endpoints were found.

Heat shock proteins (HSP) have been correlated with environmental stress and pathophysiological conditions. Stress induced HSP 70 in rat lungs was examined following inhalation exposure to 4 h/d, 3 d/wk for 40 weeks to 50 $\mu g/m^3$ HNO_3 (Wong et al., 1996). HNO_3 was found to elevate lung stress inducible HSP above baseline control levels.

Schlesinger et al. (1994) exposed rabbits for 4 h/d, 3 d/wk for 4 weeks to HNO_3 vapor at 0, 50, 150, and 450 $\mu g/m^3$. Exposure was followed by assays of biochemical markers in lavage fluid, pulmonary macrophage function, and in vitro bronchial responsivity to smooth muscle constrictor challenge. Nitric acid had no effect on viability or numbers of cells recovered, nor on lactate dehydrogenase or total protein in lavage. All acid concentrations reduced both basal levels and stimulated production of superoxide anion by macrophages, while the release/activity of tumor necrosis factor by stimulated macrophages was reduced following exposure to ≥ 150 $\mu g/m^3$ HNO_3. Bronchi from rabbits exposed to ≥ 150 $\mu g/m^3$ HNO_3 exhibited reduced smooth muscle responsivity in vitro compared to control.

Nitric acid-induced alterations in both conducting and respiratory airways were also noted by Mautz et al. (1993), who observed changes in breathing pattern, alveolar macrophage receptor binding capacity, and alveolar morphometry in rats exposed to 50, 170, and 470 $\mu g/m^3$ HNO_3 for 4 h/d, 3 d/wk for 4 weeks. Further evidence for penetration of HNO_3 into the deep lung was provided by Nadziejko et al. (1992), who noted reduced production of superoxide anion by macrophages harvested from rats exposed to 250 $\mu g/m^3$ for 4 h/d for 4 days. Similar to results of Schlesinger et al. (1994), Nadziejko et al. (1992) found no effects of acid exposure on total numbers of cells recovered by lavage, differential counts, nor in total soluble protein in lavage fluid.

Healthy adults exposed, with some exercise, to HNO_2 for 3.5 hours at 0.077 and 0.395 ppm showed a decrease in specific airway conductance compared to air exposure (Rasmussen et al., 1995). Mildly asthmatic adults exposed to 0.65 ppm HNO_2 for 3 hours with exercise periods showed a decrease in FVC which began during the exposure period. Respiratory symptoms indicative of irritation were also associated with the acid exposure (Beckett et al., 1995).

INORGANIC NITRATES

There are limited data on ambient levels of particulate inorganic nitrates (NO_3^-). Maximum (24 h avg.) ambient concentrations are generally well below 10 $\mu g/m^3$, although certain regions having persistent smog problems, such as southern California, may show peaks between 20 and 35 $\mu g/m^3$ (Pierson and Brachaczek, 1988; Ellestad and Knapp, 1988; Shaw et al., 1982).

The toxicologic data base supporting any health effects from inhaled nitrates is also sparse. Sackner et al. (1976) exposed anesthetized dogs to sodium nitrate ($NaNO_3$) at 740 or 4000 $\mu g/m^3$ for 7.5 minutes. No effects on pulmonary function were found. Ehrlich (1979) examined the effect of 3 hour exposures to various nitrate salts (1290–4500 $\mu g/m^3$) on resistance to respiratory bacterial infection in mice. Only zinc nitrate [$Zn(NO_3)_2$] resulted in any significant mortality increase, the extent of which seemed to be exposure concentration related. However, since the response was similar to that seen with zinc sulfate ($ZnSO_4$), the effect was likely due to the zinc ion (Zn^{+2}) rather than to the NO_3^-.

Charles and Menzel (1975) examined the effects of nitrate on the release of histamine by guinea pig lung fragments; response to some pollutants may be a function of their ability to elicit biologic mediators. Histamine was released in proportion to the concentration of salt present. However, the response was not totally due to NO_3^-; ammonium (NH_4^+) ion was also a possible contributor. The relation of this to actual in vivo exposures is, however, not clear. Other in vitro studies suggest that NO_3^- may affect red blood cells by altering the transport of calcium across the cell membrane (Kunimoto et al., 1984).

Some controlled clinical studies have been conducted with NO_3^- aerosols (Kleinman et al., 1980; Sackner et al., 1979; Stacy et al., 1983; Utell et al., 1979, 1980). Concentrations ranged from 200 to 7000 $\mu g/m^3$, and pulmonary function was the endpoint. The only effects noted were decreases in airway conductance and partial-expiratory flow-volume curves in subjects with influenza exposed for 16 minutes to 7000 $\mu g/m^3$ of $NaNO_3$ aerosol (Utell et al., 1980). This was not seen in normals or asthmatics (Utell et al., 1979). Since this concentration is well above ambient levels, there are likely no adverse effects, as far as lung function is concerned, from current levels of NO_3^- aerosols, even in presumably more sensitive asthmatics.

MIXTURES OF NITROGEN OXIDES

Actual environmental exposures are generally not to one, but to a mixture of different pollutants, and such combinations may behave differently than would be expected from consideration of the action of each constituent separately. In many cases the toxicologic assessment of mixtures containing NO_x involved exposures to only two pollutants, so the role played by each may be clear. However, there is a fairly large data base that involved mixtures of more than two components, often with no single pollutant test as a control; in this case the contribution of each individual agent to overall response was often obscure. In some cases, however, the NO_x may have varied between exposure groups or was present in one group and not in another, so its relative influence could be assessed.

Toxicology

The largest toxicological data base for binary mixtures involves the combination of NO_2 plus ozone (O_3). These studies indicate that depending on the biological endpoint, various interactions, or none at all, may occur with simultaneous exposure to these two pollutants. Some biochemical responses to NO_2/O_3 mixtures involve synergism (Mustafa et al., 1984) which could be due to the production of reaction products in the exposure atmosphere, while other biochemical responses to NO_2/O_3 mixtures may be additive or even antagonistic (Lee et al., 1990; Takahashi and Miura, 1989).

Interactions involving NO_2 and O_3 in relation to infectivity were generally noted to be additive (Goldstein et al., 1974; Ehrlich et al., 1977), with each pollutant contributing to the observed response when its concentration reached the threshold at which it would have affected bacterial resistance when administered alone.

The extent of interaction may also depend on the concentration of the pollutants in the mixture atmosphere. In one study (Rajini et al., 1993) rats were exposed to mixtures of O_3 and NO_2 as follows: 0.2 ppm O_3 with 3.6 ppm NO_2 for 24 h; 0.2 ppm O_3 with 7.2 ppm NO_2 for 12 h; 0.6 ppm O_3 with 10.8 ppm NO_2 for 8 h; and 0.8 ppm O_3 with 14.4 ppm NO_2 for 6 h. Exposure was for 3 days and biological assays were performed 7 days from the first exposure. Labeling indexes in peripheral airways were increased in all animals exposed to all mixtures, while alveolar labeling indexes were increased only in 0.8/14.4 ppm exposed animals. The response to the mixtures was greater than the calculated sum of responses to the two individual gases only for the three highest dose rates in the larger airways and only for the highest dose rate in peripheral airways. On the other hand and with a different endpoint, in vitro exposures of human red blood cells to a combination of 3.6 to 102 ppm NO_2 and 2 to 41 ppm O_3 were examined by Goldstein (1976), and MetHb, GSH, and malonaldehyde (a marker of membrane lipid peroxidation) were assessed. In general, the response to concentrations in the midrange was additive. However, at low concentrations of O_3 and NO_2 (e.g., 2.2 ppm O_3 and 3.6 ppm NO_2), there was a greater than additive increase in lipid peroxide formation, while at higher concentrations (e.g., 41 ppm O_3 and 102 ppm NO_2), the effect was less than additive.

The studies above involved simultaneous exposure to both NO_2 and O_3 gas. However, actual exposures often have temporal variations, and exposure to one agent may then alter the response to another subsequentally inhaled. For example, Yokoyama et al. (1980) exposed rats for 14 or 30 consecutive days to either NO_2 (5.4 ppm) or O_3 (1 ppm) for 3 hours, or to NO_2 for 3 hours followed by O_3 for 3 hours. Histologically the lungs of the animals exposed to both NO_2 and O_3 appeared similar to those exposed to O_3 alone. However, a slight degree of epithelial necrosis in some bronchi not found with either NO_2 or O_3 alone was seen in the animals exposed to both pollutants. In addition damage at the bronchiolo-alveolar junction appeared to be somewhat more marked in animals exposed to both gases than in those exposed to O_3 alone. This study suggests that sequential exposures may produce responses that are not greatly different from those due to O_3 alone; that is NO_2 pre-exposure did not markedly alter the response from subsequent exposure to O_3.

Fukase et al. (1978) exposed mice for 7 days to 3 to 15 ppm NO_2 for 3 hours, followed by 1 ppm O_3 for 3 hours. An additive effect on the level of GSH was found. Watanabe et al. (1980) also examined levels of GSH in mice exposed for 7 days to 3 hours daily of 30 ppm NO_2 followed by 3 hours daily of 1 ppm O_3; in this case the exposure produced a response that was less than that obtained by summing the responses to each pollutant if given separately. This likely occurred because the level of GSH obtained with 30 ppm NO_2 had reached a plateau, and subequent exposure to O_3 could not increase it any further. In the Goldstein (1976) study above, O_3 was found to potentiate the methemoglobinemic effect of NO_2 especially when O_3 preceeded NO_2; this was suggested to be due to interference by O_3 with the normal process whereby MetHb is reduced to ferrous Hb.

The simulation of ambient pollutant scenarios involving NO_2 and O_3 has also been performed by examining the effects of a continuous baseline exposure to one concentration, with superimposed short-term peaks to a higher level. Using bacterial infectivity as the endpoint, Ehrlich et al. (1979) exposed mice for 1 to 6 months (24 h/d, 7 d/wk) to a baseline concentration of 0.1 ppm NO_2, upon which were superimposed 3 h/d, 5 d/wk peak exposures to 0.5 ppm NO_2, or a combination of 0.5 ppm NO_2 and 0.1 ppm O_3. A similar increase in percentage mortality was found by 6 months in all groups, with no evidence that exposure to the NO_2/O_3 peaks altered the response. In another experiment, mice were re-exposed for 14 days (after 1–3 mo of initial pollutant exposure and after bacterial challenge) to the same pollutant concentrations as above, and mortality examined. Animals pre-exposed for a least 2 months either to NO_2/O_3 peaks over the air baseline or to NO_2/O_3 peaks over the 0.1 ppm NO_2 baseline, showed significant reductions in survival time. Although no conclusions were drawn as to the efficacy of the mixture, the investigators noted that the sequence of peak exposure was important in altering resistance to infection. Other studies also indicate that response may depend on the specific pattern of exposure to NO_2 and other co-pollutants (Ehrlich, 1983; Gardner et al., 1982).

Some limited data exist for combinations of NO_2 with gases other than O_3. In two reported long-term studies with SO_2, neither SO_2 nor NO_2 given alone, or together, produced any response on morphology in the rat (Azoulay et al., 1980), nor on pulmonary mechanics in the guinea pig (Antweiler and Brockhaus, 1976). However, in the morphologic study, the concentrations used (2 ppm NO_2, 2 ppm SO_2) were relatively low, while in the other, which involved NO_2 at 4 to 6 ppm and SO_2 at 3 to 4 ppm, the respiratory mechanical endpoints were likely not very sensitive to pollutant-induced change.

Schlesinger et al. (1994) exposed rabbits were exposed for 4 h/d, 3 d/wk for 4 weeks to a mixture of 50 $\mu g/m^3$ HNO_3 vapor $+0.15$ ppm O_3. Although exposure to the HNO_3/O_3 mixture resulted in no interaction for most endpoints, antagonism was noted for stimulated superoxide production by macrophages, while synergism was noted for spontaneous superoxide production and bronchial responsivity. Exposure to the mixture resulted in a total abrogation of reponse to spasmogens noted with acid alone in most bronchi examined and a marked attenuation in others. Nadziejko et al. (1992) exposed rats for 4 hours to 0.6 ppm O_3 plus 1000 $\mu g/m^3$ HNO_3, or for 4 h/d for 4 days to 0.15 ppm O_3 plus 250 $\mu g/m^3$ HNO_3. While most responses were additive, antagonism was noted following the single exposure regime for neutrophil counts and protein in lavage fluid.

Heat shock proteins are correlated with environmental stress and pathophysiological conditions and the ability of air pollutants to induce them is not clear. Wong et al. (1996) examined stress induced HSP 70 in rat lungs following inhalation exposure to 4 h/d, 3d/wk for 40 weeks to 50 $\mu g/m^3$ HNO_3, to 0.15 ppm O_3 and mixture of acid and ozone. Both O_3 and HNO_3 elevated lung stress inducible HSP above control levels. The combined exposure showed an elevation that was greater than that for the air control, but less than the effects of either O_3 or HNO_3 alone.

Another type of interaction that may occur in ambient air is that between NO_2 and particles. These latter may be inert, such as carbon, or toxicologically active, such as acid sulfate droplets. Particle interaction may result in gas adsorption, and subsequent transport after inhalation to sites in the lungs where the NO_2 normally would not deposit in concentrated amounts. This is a possible scenario with inert particles (Boren 1964). More chemically active particles may potentiate the response to NO_2 by producing local changes in the lungs that enhance the action of NO_2.

Last et al. (1983) exposed rats to 5 to 25 ppm NO_2 alone, or in combination with 5 mg/m^3 ammonium sulfate [$(NH_4)_2SO_4$], for up to 7 days and examined the rate of collagen synthesis by lung minces. There was an approximate doubling of synthesis rate when the mixture was employed compared to NO_2 alone. However, examination of responses at individual NO_2 concentrations showed that the mixture increased synthesis rate (above NO_2 alone) only when NO_2 levels were > 10 ppm. On the other hand, there was no difference in the level of pulmonary edema between animals exposed to NO_2 alone or to NO_2 in combination with $(NH_4)_2SO_4$. In a subsequent study, Last and Warren (1987) exposed rats to 5 ppm NO_2 alone, or in combination with either 1 mg/m^3 H_2SO_4 or sodium chloride (NaCl), for up to 7 days. A synergistic interaction was found when either aerosol was used with NO_2 when collagen synthesis rate was measured. Reduction of the NO_2 level to 2 ppm, when combined with H_2SO_4, also resulted in a synergistic increase in collagen synthesis rate (Last, 1989). Protein content of the lavage fluid (an index of lung damage) showed evidence of synergism at 1 days with H_2SO_4, or 3 days with NaCl. The investigators suggested that the interaction with NaCl was due to the formation of acids from nitrosyl chloride (NOCl), following its hydrolysis after deposition in the lung. The

NOCl was formed from the reaction between NO_2 with NaCl. Similarly potentiation with the acid sulfate aerosols could also be due to localized effects following their deposition. It has been proposed that these aerosols would produce a shift in local pH within the alveolar milieu, which would in turn result in a change in the reactivity or residence time of reactants involved in oxidant-induced pulmonary effects (Last et al., 1984).

Furiosi et al. (1973) exposed rats and monkeys continuously to a combination of 2 ppm NO_2 and 0.33 mg/m^3 NaCl. The histological response after 14 months of exposure in monkeys (i.e., respiratory bronchiolar epithelial hypertrophy) was similar in groups exposed to NO_2 alone or with NaCl. Hematologic changes (polycythemia) in monkeys after 18 months, and rats after 6 months, were similar for groups exposed to NO_2 with or without NaCl. Thus in this study the NaCl did not potentiate response to NO_2. Perhaps the endpoints were not sensitive to the effects of any reaction products between NO_2 and NaCl, or the concentration of NaCl was too low to allow production of significant amounts of any secondary products.

The effects on particle clearance mechanisms of exposure to mixed atmospheres of NO_2 and H_2SO_4 have been examined by Schlesinger and Gearhart (1987) and Schlesinger et al. (1987). In the former study, rabbits were exposed for 2 h/d for 14 days to 0.3 ppm or 1 ppm NO_2, to 0.5 mg/m^3 H_2SO_4, or to mixtures of the low and high NO_2 concentrations with acid. Inhaled singly, both concentrations of NO_2 accelerated particle clearance from the respiratory region, while H_2SO_4 retarded it, compared to control. Exposure to the combination of 0.3 ppm NO_2 plus H_2SO_4 resulted in a response that was not different from that due to the acid alone. However, exposure to 1 ppm NO_2 plus H_2SO_4 resulted in a clearance pattern that differed from either NO_2 or H_2SO_4 but was more similar to that due to the latter.

Schlesinger et al. (1987) exposed rabbits, as above, and examined mucociliary clearance from the tracheobronchial tree. Exposure to NO_2 did not alter clearance, while H_2SO_4 produced a retardation. The combination of 0.3 ppm NO_2 with H_2SO_4 resulted in speeding of clearance, while no change from control was seen with the mixture employing 1 ppm NO_2 with acid.

Schlesinger (1987) also exposed rabbits to the same NO_2/H_2SO_4 atmospheres as above, and recovered cells from the lungs by lavage 24 hours after 2, 6, or 13 exposures. Exposure to 1 ppm NO_2 with acid resulted in an increase in neutrophil count, indicating an inflammatory response, at all time points (not seen with either pollutant alone), and an increase in phagocytic activity of macrophages after two or six exposures. On the other hand, exposure to 0.3 ppm NO_2 with acid resulted in depressed phagocytic activity and cell mobility. A comparison of responses due to exposure to the mixture with those due to either pollutant alone showed that the effects of the combined atmospheres were either additive or synergistic, depending on the specific endpoint being examined.

A few studies have examined the response to inhalation of simple mixtures containing NO. Watanabe et al. (1980) exposed mice for 3 h/d, for 7 days to NO (10 ppm) plus O_3 (1 ppm); they observed an increase in the level of lung GSH, but this was attributed solely to the O_3. Azoulay et al. (1980) exposed rats to NO (2 ppm) with SO_2 (2 ppm) for 13 weeks; no change in blood-O_2 affinity, MetHb level, red blood cell count, or lung histology was seen with the mixtures, or with either pollutant given alone.

Although many studies have examined the response to NO_2 or NO in combination with only one additional pollutant, the atmospheres in most environments are a complex mix of many materials. While a number of studies have attempted to determine the effects of multicomponent atmospheres containing NO_x, the exact role it plays in the responses is not always clear. For example, Kleinman et al. (1985a) exposed rats for 4 hours to atmospheres consisting of a combination of O_3 (0.6 ppm), NO_2 (2.5 ppm), SO_2 (5 ppm), and particles. The latter consisted of 1 mg/m^3 of either H_2SO_4 or $(NH_4)_2SO_4$. The respiratory region of the lungs was examined for morphological effects. A confounding factor in these studies was the production of nitric acid in atmospheres containing O_3 and NO_2, and nitrate in those containing O_3 and $(NH_4)_2SO_4$ but not NO_2. Nevertheless, a significant enhancement of tissue damage was produced by exposure to atmospheres containing H_2SO_4 or HNO_3, compared to those containing $(NH_4)_2SO_4$. In addition there was a suggestion that the former atmospheres resulted in a greater area of the lung becoming involved in lesions, which were characterized by a thickening of alveolar walls, cellular infiltration into the interstitium, and an increase in free cells within the alveoli. Furthermore exercise seemed to potentiate the histological response to those complex mixtures containing the strong acids (Kleinman et al., 1989).

One of the more common complex mixtures that has been examined is automobile exhaust. In many cases it was irradiated to produce a reactive mixture that is a model for photochemical smog. Coffin and Bloomer (1967) exposed mice for 4 hours to such an irradiated atmosphere to assess effects on bacterial resistance. Levels of NO_2 were 0.1 to 0.85 ppm, NO, 0.02 to 0.15 ppm. Exposure was found to result in an increase in percentage mortality, but the investigators were not able to clearly ascribe the results to any one pollutant. However, they noted that exposure levels of NO_2 were less than those that were known to alter resistance when the gas was given alone, and thus they suggested that the effect of the exhaust mixture was due to other oxidants, such as O_3. Similarly Stupfel et al. (1973) exposed rats to exhaust mixtures for 6 h/d, 5 d/wk for 2.5 months to 2 years, followed by morphologic analysis. The atmosphere contained carbon dioxide (CO_2), aldehydes, carbon monoxide (CO), and NO_x (at either 0.2 or 23 ppm). Only the mixture with the higher NO_x concentration resulted in any significant response, namely a decrease in body weight and increase in spontaneous tumors. However, the latter effect was ascribed to the hydrocarbon component of the exhaust mixture. Finally Cooper et al. (1977) exposed rats continuously for 38 or 88 d to three auto exhaust atmospheres that differed in their component concentrations; all contained H_2SO_4, SO_2, and CO, as well as NO (7.1–10.8 ppm) and NO_2 (0.3–5.1 ppm). All exposures resulted in a significant depression of spontaneous locomotor activity not seen with exposure to either H_2SO_4 or CO alone; the investigators concluded that this response was due to either the hydrocarbon or NO_x components of the mixture.

The results of a long-term exposure of dogs to automobile exhaust have been described (Stara et al., 1980). Animals were exposed for 68 months (16 h/d) to various atmospheres that included raw exhaust, irradiated exhaust, or two mixtures of NO_x—one with a high NO_2 and low NO level (0.64 ppm NO_2, 0.25 ppm NO) and one with low NO_2 and high NO (0.14 ppm NO_2, 1.67 ppm NO). Numerous pulmonary function, hematologic, and histologic endpoints were examined after various times of exposure. No alterations in DL_{co}, dynamic compliance, or total expiratory resistance to flow after 18 months of exposure was noted (Vaughan et al., 1969). However, by 36 months, a significant number of animals exposed to high NO_2/low NO had an abnormally lower DL_{co} (as a ratio of total lung capacity, TLC) (Lewis et al., 1974). Additional changes were observed after 61 months of exposure; in the dogs breathing low NO_2/high NO or raw exhaust, residual volume was increased compared to animals exposed to control or high NO_2/low NO. The common factor causing this effect appeared to be the higher concentration of NO. A significant number of dogs exposed to high NO_2/low NO had a lower mean DL_{co}/TLC ratio, and a lower peak flow rate, compared to control. The investigators attributed the change in DL_{co} to an alteration in the alveolo-capillary membrane. No significant changes were noted in hematocrit, blood viscosity, nor level of MetHb after 48 months of exposure in any group (Bloch et al., 1973).

After all exposures terminated, the animals were maintained for 2 years before pulmonary function measurements were performed again (Gillespie et al., 1975). In all pollutant-exposed dogs, TLC was increased relative to control. Those animals that received the NO_2/NO mixtures also exhibited modest increases in inspiratory volume and vital capacity. When biochemical parameters were evaluated 2.5 to 3 years after the end of all exposures, those groups exposed to irradiated exhaust or high NO_2/low NO showed a rise in lung prolylhydroxylase (an enzyme involved in collagen synthesis) (Orthoefer et al., 1976). In addition a correlation was found between lung weight and hydroxyproline content in animals exposed to the NO_x atmospheres.

Lung morphology was evaluated 2.5 to 3 years after exposures ended (Hyde et al., 1978). Increased lung volumes, and decreases in surface density of alveoli and volumetric density of parenchymal tissue, were found in the high NO_2/low NO group. Alveoli were enlarged in both the high NO_2 and high NO groups. In the high NO_2 but not in the high NO group, there was cilia loss and hyperplasia of nonciliated bronchiolar cells. In the high NO group, there were also lesions in the interalveolar pores. In the most severely affected lungs of dogs in the high NO_2 group, morphological changes considered to be analogous to centrilobular emphysema were present. Since the morphologic measurements were made after a considerable holding period, it cannot be determined with certainty whether these disease processes abated or progressed during this time. In any case it is clear that the long-term exposures produced some persistent damage.

Controlled Clinical Studies

A few controlled clinical studies have been reported using mixtures containing NO_2. Pulmonary mechanics were examined in various studies using NO_2 at 0.5 to 0.6 ppm and with O_3 at 0.3 to 0.5 ppm (Adams et al., 1987; Folinsbee, 1981; Drechsler-Parks, 1987; Hackney et al., 1975a, b). Results indicated that the effects of the mixture could be attributed solely to the O_3.

Adolescent asthmatics were exposed for 90 min/d, with some exercise, on two consecutive days (Koenig et al., 1994) to 0.12 ppm O_3 plus 0.3 ppm NO_2. No pollutant-related changes with the mixture or either alone in (pulmonary function) or airway responsiveness were found. Aris et al. (1993) acutely exposed normal humans to 500 g/m³ HNO_3 with 0.2 ppm O_3 and concluded that there was no interaction between the two pollutants in regards to pulmonary function, including airway resistance or various indexes related to an inflammatory response.

Linn et al. (1980) exposed normal volunteers to 0.5 ppm NO_2 and 0.5 ppm SO_2 for 2 hours with intermittent exercise. No effects on lung function were found. Kleinman et al. (1985b) added NaCl aerosol to the above atmosphere and also found no effects on pulmonary function, although the mixture with the particles resulted in some increase in symptoms over that seen with the particles alone. A small increase in symptoms was also noted with the simple mixture exposure. No effect on pulmonary function was found in humans exposed for 2 hours, with intermittent exercise, to 0.15 ppm of both NO_2 and SO_2 (Kagawa, 1986). It appears that much higher levels are needed for any response, since additive effects of NO_2 and SO_2 on airway resistance were found when exposures were to 4 to 5 ppm (Abe, 1967).

It is possible that pre-exposure to one pollutant can affect response to another subsequently inhaled. Healthy adults were exposed to 0.6 ppm NO_2 for 2 hours followed 3 hours later by a 2 hours exposure to 0.3 ppm O_3 (Hazucha et al., 1994). The control was air followed by ozone. There was intermittent exercise. Exposure to NO_2 alone did not alter FEV_1 but enhanced O_3-induced spirometric changes.

SUMMARY AND CONCLUSIONS

A large data base exists concerning biological responses resulting from the inhalation of NO_x. However, comparisons of animal studies with controlled human exposures or epidemiologic studies are difficult, since the assays used in these different types of evaluations are not always directly comparable. One group of the response indexes that has been examined in all of these studies is pulmonary mechanics. However, changes in pulmonary function may not be very sensitive to NO_2 due to the tendency of such tests to reflect changes in the large airways, while the major targets for NO_2 are the smaller conducting airways and respiratory region. In any case there is little evidence that exposure of normal humans or laboratory animals to ≤ 1 ppm NO_2 affects standard pulmonary mechanics responses. Even exposure to higher levels has resulted in inconsistent results. Airway responsiveness may be increased in normal human subjects but generally only with exposures at > 1 ppm NO_2. Epidemiological data are not sufficient to determine whether there are any long- or short-term effects of NO_2 on pulmonary function, although this is not surprising given the results of the laboratory studies.

Asthmatics may represent a population subgroup showing susceptibility to NO_2. However, even among asthmatics, responses were not always consistent or reproducible, and those that have occurred involved increased airway responsiveness rather than changes in standard pulmonary function indexes. Surprisingly effects noted in some studies at ≤ 1 ppm NO_2 have not always been found with higher levels (up to 3 ppm), and this apparent lack of dose–response is of concern in evaluating the health significance of NO_2 exposure. While it is possible that differences in the degree of asthma severity in the subjects used in the various studies may have accounted for some of this discrepancy, it does seem that mild asthmatics are not generally sensitive to NO_2 concentrations < 0.6 ppm when examining pulmonary function and airway responsiveness. The data base for pulmonary function effects in COPD patients is similarly confusing, with some studies showing effects and others none at NO_2 exposure levels < 2 ppm. Nevertheless, while controlled clinical studies do not unequivocally indicate any enhanced susceptibility to NO_2 among mild asthmatics or people with COPD, there is indication that some asthmatics may respond at lower exposure concentrations than do healthy individuals. This is, however, based on endpoints that may not be the most sensitive markers of NO_2 exposure.

Various biological responses not generally examined in humans have been assessed in animal models, and these indicate effects due to NO_2 that may have potential health significance. This includes NO_2-related alterations in various host defense parameters, such as mucociliary clearance, pulmonary macrophage and immunologic function, and susceptibility to respiratory infection. Tracheobronchial mucus transport rates remain unaltered by single exposures up to 10 ppm or short-term repeated exposures to ≤ 1 ppm, while respiratory region clearance may be affected by short-term repeated exposures at < 1 ppm. Morphological changes in macrophages begin to occur at 0.5 ppm, while functional activity has been affected by short-term repeated exposures to 0.3 ppm. As a likely consequence of altered defenses, animals may be less able to cope with respiratory infection. Nitrogen dioxide levels as low as 0.5 ppm will increase bacterial infectivity if exposure is prolonged. Clear, direct suppressive effects on humoral or cellular immunity have been noted only with exposure to > 5 ppm NO_2, with lower levels possibly resulting in some depression or activation of immune system components. Limited results from controlled clinical studies suggest that some similar responses may be occurring in humans.

Additional evidence for human health effects resulting from NO_2 exposure comes from epidemiological examinations of acute respiratory illness, especially since this is supported by toxicological studies on host defense mechanisms and a limited number of clinical studies. A major problem with many epidemiological studies is that they did not adequately measure actual personal NO_2 exposures. However, those that did provide relatively reliable estimates of NO_2, either by direct measure or by suitable surrogates, are somewhat suggestive of some increased risk or susceptibility to lower and/or upper respiratory tract infection in young children associated with long-term NO_2 exposure.

However, this conclusion is by no means definitive. Furthermore the effects of short-term NO_2 exposure on acute respiratory illness are not clear.

Animal models have been extensively used in studying effects of NO_2 on pulmonary morphology. The target site is consistently the area around the terminal/respiratory bronchiolar junction and associated alveoli, and the cells that are most sensitive are the ciliated cells of the bronchiolar epithelium and the type 1 cells of the alveolar epithelium. Neonates seem to be more resistant than adults to these morphological effects. Acute exposure to < 5 ppm can produce hyperplasia and hypertrophy of bronchiolar and alveolar cells, and proliferation of type 2 cells. Long-term exposure to 0.3 to 0.5 ppm can result in similar lesions, although chronic exposures to ≥ 2 ppm are generally needed to produce extensive and permanent pulmonary structural changes. Some changes may resolve even with continued exposure. Although the data base does not currently allow for determination of the lowest NO_2 level and shortest exposure duration that will produce clear and permanent morphological effects, the concentrations that do seem to result in such changes are well above those currently found in most outdoor or indoor environments.

The primary target organ for NO_2 is the respiratory tract, but there may be some extrapulmonary effects of exposure as well. This could involve changes in body weight, blood cell count, and liver enzymes. Conclusions as to the possible health significance of these cannot as yet be made. Furthermore there is no support for any teratogenic or genotoxic potential for NO_2, nor for any direct carcinogenic action. Although NO_2 may modulate pulmonary cancer originating elsewhere, the data base is weak in this regard and needs much further support.

Quite a few questions regarding health effects from exposure to NO_2 remain unanswered. For example, there is no complete picture of the transition between acute and chronic effects nor is the extent of reversibility of effects resolved, especially with short-term peak exposures. High concentrations of NO_2 (≥ 5 ppm) are associated with structural and physiological changes in the respiratory tract. However, the extent to which these may occur at levels more relevant to either outdoor or indoor exposures is not clear. Furthermore the relationship between biological responses and specific exposure patterns, namely constant low-level versus low baseline plus higher spikes, is also not clear. The latter scenario may be more relevant to indoor exposure, and the former to most outdoor exposures. The contribution of differing biochemical mechanisms, namely acid versus oxidative, in the expression of NO_2 toxicity is not fully understood. Observations that the direction of change in various biological endpoints seems to depend on exposure concentration may reflect differences in underlying mechanisms of action.

Thus, while toxicologic studies may provide indications of possible mechanisms of action leading to adverse health effects, controlled clinical and epidemiologic studies have not as yet resulted in a consistent pattern of responses that could be used to allow an unequivocal conclusion as to the potential effects on human health of ambient exposure to NO_2.

ACKNOWLEDGMENT

The author's work is part of a Center Program supported by the National Institute of Environmental Health Sciences (ES00260).

REFERENCES

Abe, M. 1967. Effects of mixed NO_2–SO_2 gas on human pulmonary functions. *Bull. Tokyo Med. Dent. Univ.* 14: 415–433.

Abraham, W. M., C. S. Kim, M. M. King, W. Oliver Jr., and L. Yerger. 1982. Effects of nitric acid on carbachol reactivity of the airways in normal and allergic sheep. *Arch. Environ. Health* 37: 36–40.

Adams, W. C., K. A. Brookes, and E. S. Schelegle. 1987. Effects of NO_2 alone and in combination with O_3 on young men and women. *J. Appl. Physiol.* 62: 1698–1704.

Adgate, J. L., H. F. Reid, R. Morris, R. W. Helms, R. A. Berg, P-C. Hu, et al. 1992. Nitrogen dioxide exposure and urinary excretion of hydroxyproline and desmosine. *Arch. Environ. Health* 47: 376–384.

Adkins, B., Jr., E. W. Van Stee, J. E. Simmons, and S. L. Eustis. 1986. Oncogenic response of strain A/J mice to inhaled chemicals. *J. Toxicol. Environ. Health* 17: 311–322.

Ahmed, T., B. Marchette, I. Danta, S. Birch, R. L. Dougherty, R. Schreck, and M. A. Sackner. 1982. Effect of 0.1 ppm NO_2 on bronchial reactivity in normals and subjects with bronchial asthma. *Am. Rev. Respir. Dis.* 125 (suppl.): 152S.

Alving, K., C. Fornhem, E. Weitzbergm, and J. M. Lundberg. 1992. Nitric oxide mediates cigarette smoke-induced vasocilatory responses in the lung. *Acta Physiol. Scand.* 146: 407–408.

Amoruso, M. A., G. Witz, and B. D. Goldstein. 1981. Decreased superoxide anion radical production by rat alveolar macrophages following inhalation of ozone or nitrogen dioxide. *Life Sci.* 28: 2215-2221.

Anderson, H., R., A. Ponce de Leon, J. M. Bland, J. S. Bower, and D. P. Strachan. 1996. Air pollution and daily mortality in London: 1987–92. *Br. Med. J.* 312: 665–669.

Antweiler, H., and A. Brockhaus. 1976. Respiratory frequency, flowrate and minute volume in non-anaesthetised guinea-pigs during prolonged exposure to low concentrations of SO_2 and NO_2. *Ann. Occup. Hyg.* 19: 13–16.

Aris, R., D. Christian, I. Tager, L. Ngo, W. E. Finkbeinger, and J. R. Balmes. 1993. Effects of nitric acid gas alone or in combination with ozone on healthy volunteers. *Am. Rev. Respir. Dis.* 148(4 Pt. 1): 965–973.

Avol, E. L., W. S. Linn, R. C. Peng, G. Valencia, D. Little, and J. D. Hackney. 1988. Laboratory study of asthmatic volunteers exposed to nitrogen dioxide and to ambient air pollution. *Am. Ind. Hyg. Assoc. J.* 49: 143–149.

Ayaz, K. L., and A. S. Csallany. 1978. Long-term NO_2 exposure of mice in the presence and absence of vitamin E: II. Effect of glutathione peroxidase. *Arch. Environ. Health* 33: 292–296.

Azoulay, E., G. Bouley, and M. C. Blayo. 1981. Effects of nitric oxide on resistance to bacterial infection in mice. *J. Toxicol. Environ. Health* 7: 873–882.

Azoulay, E., P. Soler, J. Moreau, and M. C. Blayo. 1980. Effects of low-concentration NO_x SO_2 gas mixtures on lung structure and blood-oxygen affinity in rats. *J. Environ. Pathol. Toxicol.* 4: 399–409.

Azoulay, E., P. Soler, M. C. Blayo, and F. Basset. 1977. Nitric oxide effects on lung structure and blood oxygen affinity in rats. *Bull. Eur. Physiopath. Respir.* 13: 629–644.

Azoulay-Dupuis, E., M. Torres, P. Soler, and J. Moreau. 1983. Pulmonary NO_2 toxicity in neonate and adult guinea pigs and rats. *Environ. Res.* 30: 322–339.

Balchum, O. J., R. D. Buckley, R. Sherwin, and M. Gardner. 1965. Nitrogen dioxide inhalation and lung antibodies. *Arch. Environ. Health* 10: 274–277.

Balmes, J. R., J. M. Fine, D. Christian, T. Gordon, and D. Sheppard. 1988. Acidity potentiates bronchoconstriction induced by hypoosmolar aerosols. *Am. Rev. Respir. Dis.* 138: 35–39.

Barth, P. J., B. Muller, U. Wagner, and A. Bittinger. 1995. Quantitative analysis of parenchymal and vascular alterations in NO_2-induced lung injury in rats. *Eur. Respir. J.* 8: 1115–1121.

Bascom, R., P. A. Bromberg, D. L. Costa, et al. 1996. Health effects of outdoor air pollution. *Am. J. Respir. Crit. Care Med.* 153: 477–498.

Bauer, M. A., M. J. Utell, P. E. Morrow, D. M. Speers, and F. R. Gibb. 1985. Route of inhalation influences airway responses to 0.3 ppm nitrogen dioxide in asthmatic subjects. *Am. Rev. Respir. Dis.* 131: A171.

Bauer, M. A., M. J. Utell, P. E. Morrow, D. M. Speers, and F. R. Gibb. 1986. Inhalation of 0.30 ppm nitrogen dioxide potentiates exercise-induced bronchospasm in asthmatics. *Am. Rev. Respir. Dis.* 134: 1203–1208.

Beckett, W. S., M. B. Russi, A. D. Haber, R. M. Rivkin, J. R. Sullivan, Z. Tameroglu, V. Mohsenin, and B. R. Leaderer. 1995. Effect of nitrous acid on lung function in asthmatics: A chamber study. *Environ. Health Perspect.* 103: 372–375.

Beil, M., and W. T. Ulmer. 1976. Wirkung von NO_2 in MAK-Bereich auf Atemmechanik und bronchiale Acetylcholinempfindlichkeit bei Normalpersonen (Effect of NO_2 in workroom concentrations on respiratory mechanics and bronchial susceptibility to acetylcholine in normal persons). *Int. Arch. Occup. Environ. Health* 38: 31–44.

Berglund, M. 1993. Exposure. *Scand. J. Work Environ. Health* 19: 14–20.

Berglund, M., L. Braback, G. Bylin, J. O. Jonson, and M. Vahter. 1994. Personal NO_2 exposure monitoring shows high exposure among ice skating school children. *Arch. Environ. Health* 49: 17–24.

Berwick, M., R. T. Zagraniski, B. P. Leaderer, and J. A. Stolwijk. 1984. Respiratory illness in children exposed to unvented combustion sources. In *Indoor Air*, vol. 2, eds. B. Berglund, T. Lindvall, J. Sundell, pp. 255–260. Stockholm: Swedish Council for Building Research.

Bils, R. F. 1976. The connective tissues and alveolar walls in the lungs of normal and oxidant-exposed squirrel monkeys. *J. Cell Biol.* 70: 318.

Bloch, W. N., Jr., S. Lassiter, J. F. Stara, and T. R. Lewis. 1973. Blood rheology of dogs chronically exposed to air pollutants. *Toxicol. Appl. Pharmacol.* 25: 576–581.

Boren, H. G. 1964. Carbon as a carrier mechanism for irritant gases. *Arch. Environ. Health* 8: 119–124.

Brauer, M., and J. D. Spengler. 1994. Nitrogen dioxide exposures inside ice skating rinks. *Am. J. Public Health* 84: 429–433.

Brauer, M., P. Koutrakis, G. J. Keeler, and J. D. Spengler. 1991. Indoor and outdoor concentrations of inorganic acidic aerosols and gases. *J. Air Waste Manage. Assoc.* 41: 171–181.

Braun-Fahrlander, C., U. Ackermann-Liebrich, J. Schwartz, H. P. Gnehm, M. Rutishauser, and H. U. Wanner. 1992. Air pollution and respiratory symptoms in preschool children. *Am. Rev. Respir. Dis.* 145: 42–47.

Bromberg, P. A. 1988. Asthma and automotive emissions. In *Air Pollution, the Automobile and Public Health*, eds. A. Y. Watson, R. R. Bates, and D. Kennedy, pp. 465–498. Washington, DC: National Academy Press.

Brunekreef, B., P. Fischer, D. Houthuijs, B. Remijn, and J. Boleij. 1987. Health effects of indoor NO_2 pollution. In *Indoor Air '87*, vol. 1, eds. B. Seifert, H. Esdorn, M. Fischer, H. Rueden, and J. Wegner, pp. 304–308. Berlin: Institute for Water, Soil and Air Hygiene.

Busey, W. M., W. B. Coate, and D. W. Badger. 1974. Histopatholic effects of nitrogen dioxide exposure and heat stress in cynomolgus monkeys. *Toxicol. Appl. Pharmacol.* 29: 130.

Bylin, G., G. Hedenstierna, T. Lindvall, and B. Sundin. 1988. Ambient nitrogen dioxide concentrations increase bronchial responsiveness in subjects with mild asthma. *Eur. Respir. J.* 1: 606–612.

Bylin, G., T. Lindvall, T. Rehn, and B. Sundin. 1985. Effects of short-term exposure to ambient nitrogen dioxide concentrations on human bronchial reactivity and lung function. *Eur. J. Respir. Dis.* 66: 205–217.

Campbell, K. I., and R. H. Hilsenroth. 1976. Impaired resistance to toxin in toxoid-immunized mice exposed to ozone or nitrogen dioxide. *Clin. Toxicol.* 9: 943–954.

Case, G. D., J. S. Dixon, and J. C. Schooley. 1979. Interactions of blood metalloproteins with nitrogen oxides and oxidant air pollutants. *Environ. Res.* 20: 43–65.

Cavanagh, D. G., and J. B. Morris. 1987. Mucus protection and airway peroxidation following nitrogen dioxide exposure in the rat. *J. Toxicol. Environ. Health* 22: 313–328.

Chaney, S., W. Blomquist, P. DeWitt, and K. Muller. 1981. Biochemical changes in humans upon exposure to nitrogen dioxide while at rest. *Arch. Environ. Health* 36: 53–58.

Chang, L.-Y., J. A. Graham, F. J. Miller, J. J. Ospital, and J. D. Crapo. 1986. Effects of subchronic inhalation of low concentrations of nitrogen dioxide. I. The proximal alveolar region of juvenile and adult rats. *Toxicol. Appl. Pharmacol.* 83: 46–61.

Charles, J. M., and D. B. Menzel. 1975. Ammonium and sulfate on release of histamine from lung fragments. *Arch. Environ. Health* 30: 314–316.

Chen, L. C., and R. B. Schlesinger. 1996. Considerations for the respiratory tract dosimetry of inhaled nitric acid vapor. *Inhal. Toxicol.* 8: 639–654.

Chiodi, H., and J. G. Mohler. 1985. Effects of exposure of blood hemoblogin to nitric oxide. *Environ. Res.* 37: 355–363.

Chiodi, H., C. R. Collier, and J. G. Mohler. 1983. *In vitro* methemoglobin formation in human blood exposed to NO_2. *Environ. Res.* 30: 9–15.

Chow, C. K., C. J. Dillard, and A. L. Tappel. 1974. Glutathione peroxidase system ad lysozyme in rats exposed to ozone or nitrogen dioxide. *Environ. Res.* 7: 311–319.

Coffin, D. L., and E. J. Blommer. 1967. Acute toxicity of irradiated auto exhaust: Its indication by enhancement of mortality from streptococcal pneumonia. *Arch. Environ. Health* 15: 36–38.

Comstock, G. W., M. B. Meger, K. J. Helsing, and M. J. Tockman. 1981. Respiratory effects of household exposures to tobacco smoke and gas cooking. *Am. Rev. Respir. Dis.* 124: 143–148.

Cooper, G. P., J. P. Lewkowski, L. Hastings, and M. Malanchuk. 1977. Catalytically and noncatalytically treated automobile exhaust: Biological effects in rats. *J. Toxicol. Environ. Health* 3: 923–934.

Crapo, J. D., B. E. Barry, L.-Y. Chang, and R. R. Mercer. 1984. Alterations in lung structure caused by inhalation of oxidants. *J. Toxicol. Environ. Health* 13: 301–321.

Csallany, A. S. 1975. The effect of nitrogen dioxide on the growth of vitamin E deficient, vitamin E supplemented and DPPD supplemented mice. *Proc. Fed. Am. Soc. Exp. Biol.* 34: 913.

Dalhamn, T., and J. Sjoholm. 1963. Studies on SO_2, NO_2 and NH_3: Effect on ciliary activity in rabbit trachea of single *in vitro* exposure and resorption in rabbit nasal cavity. *Acta Physiol. Scand.* 58: 287–291.

DeNicola, D. B., A. H. Rebar, and R. F. Henderson. 1981. Early damage indicators in the lung. V. Biochemical and cytological response to NO_2 inhalation. *Toxicol. Appl. Pharmacol.* 60: 301–312.

Dijkstra, L., D. Houthuijs, B. Brunekreef, I. Akkerman, and J. S. M. Boleij. 1990. Respiratory health effects of the indoor environment in a population of Dutch children. *Am. Rev. Respir. Dis.* 142: 1172–1178.

Dockery, D. W., F. E. Speizer, D. O. Stram, J. H. Ware, J. D. Spengler, and B. G. Ferris Jr. 1989. Effects of inhalable particles on respiratory health of children. *Am. Rev. Respir. Dis.* 139: 587–594.

Dodge, R. 1982. The effects of indoor pollution on Arizona children. *Arch. Environ. Health* 37: 151–155.

Drechsler-Parks, D. M. 1987. Effect of nitrogen dioxide, ozone, and peroxyacetyl nitrate on metabolic and pulmonary function. Report 6. Cambridge, MA: Health Effects Institute.

Ehrlich, R. 1979. Interaction between environmental pollutants and respiratory infections. In *Proc. of the Symposium on Experimental Models for Pulmonary Research*, eds. D. E. Gardner, E. P. C. Hu, and J. A. Graham, pp. 145–163. EPA-600/9-79–022. Research Triangle Park, NC: U.S. EPA.

Ehrlich, R. 1980. Interaction between environmental pollutants and respiratory infections. *Environ. Health Perspect.* 35: 89–100.

Ehrlich, R. 1983. Changes in susceptibility to respiratory infection caused by exposures to photochemical oxidant pollutants. In *International Symposium on the Biomedical Effects of Ozone and Related Photochemical Oxidants*, eds. S. D. Lee, M. G. Mustafa, and M. A. Mehlman, pp. 273–285. Princeton: Princeton Scientific.

Ehrlich, R., and M. C. Henry. 1968. Chronic toxicity of nitrogen dioxide: I. Effect on resistance to bacterial pneumonia. *Arch. Environ. Health* 17: 860–865.

Ehrlich, R., E. Silverstein, R. Maigetter, J. D. Fenters, and D. Gardner. 1975. Immunologic response in vaccinated mice during long-term exposure to nitrogen dioxide. *Environ. Res.* 10: 217–223.

Ehrlich, R., J. Findlay, and D. E. Gardner. 1979. Effects of repeated exposures to peak concentrations of nitrogen dioxide and ozone on resistance to streptococcal pneumonia. *J. Toxicol. Environ. Health* 5: 631–642.

Ehrlich, R., J. C. Findlay, J. D. Fenters, and D. E. Gardner. 1977. Health effects of short-term inhalation of nitrogen dioxide and ozone mixtures. *Environ. Res.* 14: 223–231.

Ekwo, E. E., M. W. Weinberger, P. A. Lachenbruch, and W. H. Huntley. 1983. Relationship of parental smoking and gas cooking to respiratory disease in children. *Chest* 84: 662–668.

Ellestad, T. G., and K. T. Knapp. 1988. The sampling of reactive atmospheric species by transition-flow reactor. Application to nitrogen species. *Atmos. Environ.* 22: 1595–1600.

Elsayed, N. M., and M. G. Mustafa. 1982. Dietary antioxidants and the biochemical response to oxidant inhalation. I. Influence of dietary vitamin E on the biochemical effects of nitrogen dioxide exposure in rat lung. *Toxicol. Appl. Pharmacol.* 66: 319–328.

Evans, M. J., L. J. Cabral, R. J. Stephens, and G. Freeman. 1975. Transformation of alveolar type 2 cells to type 1 cells following exposure to NO_2. *Exp. Mol. Pathol.* 22: 142–150.

Fenters, J. D., J. D. Findlay, C. D. Port, R. Ehrlich, and D. L. Coffin. 1973. Chronic exposure to nitrogen dioxide: Immunologic, physiologic, and pathologic effects in virus-challenged squirrel monkeys. *Arch. Environ. Health* 27: 85–89.

Fenters, J. D., R. Ehrlich, J. Findlay, J. Spangler, and V. Tolkacz. 1971. Serologic response in squirrel monkeys exposed to nitrogen dioxide and influenza virus. *Am. Rev. Respir. Dis.* 104: 448–451.

Ferin, J., and L. J. Leach. 1977. The effects of selected air pollutants on clearance of titanic oxide particles from the lungs of rats. In *Inhaled Particles IV,* ed. W. H. Walton, pp. 333–341. New York: Pergamon Press.

Folinsbee, L. 1981. Effects of ozone exposure on lung function in man: A review. *Rev. Environ. Health* 3: 211–240.

Folinsbee, L. J., S. M. Horvath, J. F. Bedi, and J. C. Delehunt. 1978. Effect of 0.62 pm NO_2 on cardiopulmonary function in young male nonsmokers. *Environ. Res.* 15: 199–205.

Foster, J. R., R. C. Cottrell, I. A. Herod, H. A. C. Atkinson, and K. Miller. 1985. A comparative study of the pulmonary effects of NO_2 in the rat and hamster. *Br. J. Exp. Pathol.* 66: 193–204.

Frampton, M. W., F. R. Gibb, D. M. Speers, P. E. Morrow, and M. J. Utell. 1989a. Effects of NO_2 exposure on pulmonary function and airway reactivity. *Am. Rev. Respir. Dis.* 139: A124.

Frampton, M. W., A. M. Smeglin, N. J. Roberts Jr., J. N. Finkelstein, P. E. Morrow, and M. J. Utell. 1989b. Nitrogen dioxide exposure *in vivo* and human alveolar macrophage inactivation of influenza virus *in vitro. Environ. Res.* 48: 179–192.

Frampton, M. W., J. N. Finkelstein, N. J. Roberts, A. M. Smeglin, P. E. Morrow, and M. Utell. 1989c. Effects of nitrogen dioxide exposure on bronchoalveolar lavage proteins in humans. *Am. J. Respir. Cell Mol. Biol.* 1: 499–505.

Freeman, B. A., and J. B. Mudd. 1981. Reaction of ozone with sulfhydryls of human erythrocytes. *Arch. Biochem. Biophys.* 208: 212–220.

Freeman, G., N. J. Furiosi, and G. B. Haydon. 1966. Effects of continuous exposure of 0.8 ppm NO_2 on respiration of rats. *Arch. Environ. Health* 13: 454–456.

Fujimaki, H. 1989. Impairment of humoral immune responses in mice exposed to nitrogen dioxide and ozone mixtures. *Environ. Res.* 48: 211–217.

Fujimaki, H., and F. Shimizu. 1981. Effects of acute exposure to nitrogen dioxide on primary antibody response. *Arch. Environ. Health* 36: 114–119.

Fujimaki, H., F. Shimizu, and K. Kubota. 1982. Effect of subacute exposure to NO_2 on lymphocytes required for antibody response. *Environ. Res.* 29: 280–286.

Fukase, O., K. Isomura, and H. Watanabe. 1978. Effects of exercise on mice exposed to ozone. *Arch. Environ. Health* 33: 198–201.

Furiosi, N. J., S. C. Crane, and G. Freeman. 1973. Mixed sodium chloride aerosol and nitrogen dioxide in air: Biological effects on monkeys and rats. *Arch. Environ. Health* 27: 405–408.

Gardner, D. E., F. J. Miller, E. J. Blommer, and D. L. Coffin. 1979. Influence of exposure mode on the toxicity of NO_2. *Environ. Health Perspect.* 30: 23–29.

Gardner, D. E., F. J. Miller, J. W. Illing, and J. A. Graham. 1982. Non-respiratory function of the lungs: Host defenses against infection. In *Air Pollution by Nitrogen Oxides, Proc. US-Dutch International Symposium,* eds. T. Schneider, and L. Grant, pp. 401–415. Maastricht, The Netherlands: Elsevier.

Gillespie, J. R., J. D. Berry, and J. C. Stara. 1975. Pulmonary function changes in the period following termination of air pollution exposure in beagles. *Am. Rev. Respir. Dis.* 113 (suppl.): 92.

Gilmour, M. I. 1995. Interaction of air pollutants and pulmonary allergic responses in experimental animals. *Toxicology* 105: 335–342.

Giordano, A. M., Jr., and P. E. Morrow. 1972. Chronic low-level nitrogen dioxide exposure and mucociliary clearance. *Arch. Environ. Health* 25: 443–449.

Gnehm, H. E., U. Ackerman, C. Braun, M. Rutishauser, and H. U. Wanner. 1988. Significant association of respiratory symptoms in small children with outdoor NO_2 air pollution. *Pediatr. Res.* 23: 291A.

Goings, S. A. J., T. J. Kulle, R. Bascom, L. R. Sauder, D. J. Green, J. R. Hebel, and M. L. Clements. 1989. Effect of nitrogen dioxide exposure on susceptibility to influenza A virus infection in healthy adults. *Am. Rev. Respir. Dis.* 139: 1075–1081.

Goldstein, B. D. 1976. Combined exposure to ozone and nitrogen dioxide. *Environ. Health Perspect.* 13: 107–110.

Goldstein, E., D. Warshauer, W. Lippert, and B. Tarkington. 1974. Ozone and nitrogen dioxide exposure: Murine pulmonary defense mechanisms. *Arch. Environ. Health* 28: 85–90.

Goldstein, E., F. Goldstein, N. F. Peek, and N. J. Parks. 1980. Absorption and transport of nitrogen oxides. In *Nitrogen Oxides and Their Effects on Health*, ed. S. D. Lee, pp. 143–160. Ann Arbor, MI: Ann Arbor Sciences.

Goldstein, E., N. F. Peek, N. J. Parks, H. H. Hines, E. P. Steffey, and B. Tarkington. 1977. Fate and distribution of inhaled nitrogen dioxide in rhesus monkeys. *Am. Rev. Respir. Dis.* 115: 403–412.

Goldstein, I. F., K. Lieber, L. R. Andrews, F. Kazembe, G. Foutrakis, P. Huang, and C. Hayes. 1988. Acute respiratory effects of short-term exposures to nitrogen dioxide. *Arch. Environ. Health* 43: 138–142.

Gooch, P. C., H. E. Luippold, D. A. Creasia, and J. G. Brewen. 1977. Observations on mouse chromosomes following nitrogen dioxide inhalation. *Mutat. Res.* 48: 117–120.

Görsdorf, S., K. E. Appel, C. Engeholm, and G. Obe. 1990. Nitrogen dioxide induces DNA single-strand breaks in cultured Chinese hamster cells. *Carcinogenesis* 11: 37–41.

Graham, J. A., D. B. Menzel, F. J. Miller, J. W. Illing, and D. E. Gardner. 1982. Effect of ozone on drug-induced sleeping time in mice pretreated with mixed-function oxidase inducers and inhibitors. *Toxicol. Appl. Pharmacol.* 62: 489–497.

Graham, J. A., D. E. Gardner, E. J. Blommer, D. E. House, M. G. Menache, and F. J. Miller. 1987. Influence of exposure patterns of nitrogen dioxide and modifications by ozone on susceptibility to bacterial infectious disease in mice. *J. Toxicol. Environ. Health* 21: 113–125.

Greene, N. D., and S. L. Schneider. 1978. Effects of NO_2 on the response of baboon alveolar macrophages to migration inhibitory factor. *J. Toxicol. Environ. Health* 4: 869–880.

Gregory, R. E., J. A. Pickrell, F. F. Hahn, and C. H. Hobbs. 1983. Pulmonary effects of intermittent subacute exposure to low-level nitrogen dioxide. *J. Toxicol. Environ. Health* 11: 405–414.

Gross, P., R. T. P. deTreville, M. A. Babyak, M. Kaschak, and E. B. Tolker. 1968. Experimental emphysema: Effect of chronic nitrogen dioxide exposure and papain on normal and pneumoconiotic lungs. *Arch. Environ. Health* 16: 51–58.

Gustafsson, L. E. 1993. Experimental studies on nitric oxide. *Scand. J. Work Environ. Health* 19: 44–49.

Hackney, J. D., F. C. Thiede, W. S. Linn, E. E. Pedersen, C. E. Spier, D. C. Law, and D. A. Fischer. 1978. Experimental studies on human health effects of air pollutants. IV: Short-term physiological and clinical effects of nitrogen dioxide exposure. *Arch. Environ. Health* 33: 176–181.

Hackney, J. D., W. S. Linn, J. G. Mohler, E. E. Pedersen, P. Breisacher, and A. Russo. 1975a. Experimental studies on human health effects of air pollutants. II: Four-hour exposure to ozone alone and in combination with other pollutant gases. *Arch. Environ. Health* 30: 379–384.

Hackney, J. D., W. S. Linn, D. C. Law, S. K. Karuza, H. Greenberg, R. D. Buckley, and E. E. Pedersen. 1975b. Experimental studies on human health effects of air pollutants. III: Two-hour exposure to ozone alone and in combination with other pollutant gases. *Arch. Environ. Health* 30: 385–390.

Hahn, P. 1979. Nutrition and metabolic development in mammals. In *Nutrition: Pre- and Postnatal Development*, ed. M. Winick, pp. 1–40. New York: Plenum Press.

Hazucha, M. J., J. F. Ginsberg, W. F. McDonnell, E. D. Haak Jr., R. L. Pimmel, D. E. House, and P. A. Bromberg. 1982. Changes in bronchial reactivity of asthmatics and normals following exposures to 0.1 ppm NO_2. In *Air Pollution by Nitrogen Oxides*, eds. T. Schneider and L. Grant, pp. 387–400. Amsterdam: Elsevier.

Hazucha, M. J., J. F. Ginsberg, W. F. McDonnell, E. D. Haak Jr., R. L. Pimmel, S. A. Salaam, D. E. House, and P. A. Bromberg. 1983. Effects of 0.1 ppm nitrogen dioxide on airways of normal and asthmatic subjects. *J. Appl. Physiol.* 54: 730–739.

Hazucha, M. J., L. J. Folinsbee, E. Seal, and P. A. Bromberg. 1994. Lung function response of healthy women after sequential exposures to NO_2 and O_3. *Am. J. Respir. Crit. Care Med.* 150: 642–647.

Helleday, R., D. Huberman, A. Blomberg, N. Stjernberg, and T. Sandstron. 1995. Nitrogen dioxide exposure impairs the frequency of the mucociliary activity in healthy subjects. *Eur. Respir. J.* 8: 1664–1668.

Holt, P. G., L. M. Finlay-Jones, D. Keast, and J. J. Papadimitrou. 1979. Immunological function in mice chronically exposed to nitrogen oxides (NO_x). *Environ. Res.* 19: 154–162.

Hood, D. B., P. Gettins, and D. A. Johnson. 1993. Nitrogen dioxide reactivity with proteins: Effects on activity and immunoreactivity with alpha-1-proteinase inhibitor and implications for NO_2-mediated peptide degradation. *Arch. Biochem. BIophys.* 304: 17–26.

Hoshi, H., K. Yamauchi, K. Sekizawa, Y. Ohkawara, H. Iijima, E. Sakurai, K. Maeda, S. Okinaga, I. Ohno, M. Honma, G. Tamura, Y. Tanno, T. Watanabe, H. Sasaki, and K. Shirato K. 1996. Nitrogen dioxide exposure increases airway contractile response to histamine by decreasing histamine N-methyltransferase activity in guinea pigs. *Am. J. Respir. Cell Mol. Biol.* 14: 76–83.

Houthuijs, D., B. Remijn, B. Brunekreef, and R. de Koning. 1987. Exposure to nitrogen dioxide and tobacco smoke and respiratory health of children. In *Indoor Air '87*, vol. 1, eds. B. Seifert, H. Esdorn, M. Fischer, H. Rueden, and J. Wegner, pp. 463–467. Berlin: Institute for Water, Soil and Air Hygiene.

Hugod, C. 1979. Ultrastructural changes of the rabbit lung after a 5 ppm nitric oxide exposure. *Arch. Environ. Health* 34: 12–17.

Hyde, D., J. Orthoefer, D. Dungworth, W. Tyler, R. Carter, and H. Lum. 1978. Morphometric and morphologic evaluation of pulmonary lesions in beagle dogs chronically exposed to high ambient levels of air pollutants. *Lab. Invest.* 38: 455–469.

Ichinose, T., and M. Sagai. 1982. Studies on biochemical effects of nitrogen dioxide. III: Changes of the antioxidative protective systems in rat lungs and of lipid peroxidation by chronic exposure. *Toxicol. Appl. Pharmacol.* 66: 1–8.

Ichinose, T., and M. Sagai. 1989. Biochemical effects of combined gases of nitrogen dioxide and ozone. III: Synergistic effects on lipid peroxidation and antioxidative protective systems in the lungs of rats and guinea pigs. *Toxicology* 59: 259–270.

Illing, J. W., F. J. Miller, and D. E. Gardner. 1980. Decreased resistance to infection in exercised mice exposed to NO_2 and O_3. *J. Toxicol. Environ. Health* 6: 843–851.

Ischiropoulos, H., L. Zhu, and J. S. Beckman. 1992. Peroxy-nitrite formation from macrophage-derived nitric oxide. *Arch. Biochem. Biophys.* 298: 446–451.

Ito, K. 1971. Effect of nitrogen dioxide inhalation on influenza virus infection in mice (in Japanese). *Nippon Eiseigaku Zasshi* 26: 304–314.

Jacob, D. S., J. W. Waldman, J. W. Munger, and M. R. Hoffman. 1985. Chemical composition of fogwater collected along the California coast. *Environ. Sci. Technol.* 19: 730–736.

Johnson, D. A., M. W. Frampton, R. S. Winters, P. E. Morrow, and M. J. Utell. 1990. Inhalation of nitrogen dioxide fails to reduce the activity of human lung alpha-1-proteinase inhibitor. *Am. Rev. Respir. Dis.* 142: 758–762.

Jorres, R., D. Nowak, F. Grimminger, W. Seeger, M. Oldigs, and H. Magnussen. 1995. The effect of 1 ppm nitrogen dioxide on bronchoalveolar lavage cells and inflammatory mediators in normal and asthmatic subjects. *Eur. Respir. J.* 8: 416–424.

Kagawa, J. 1982. Respiratory effects of 2-hr exposure to 1.0 ppm nitric oxide in normal subjects. *Environ. Res.* 27: 485–490.

Kagawa, J. 1986. Experimental studies on human health effects of aerosol and gaseous pollutants. In *Aerosols: Research, Risk Assessment and Control Strategie*, eds. S. D. Lee, T. Schneider, L. D. Grant, and P. J. Verkerk, pp. 683–697. Chelsea, MI: Lewis Publishers.

Kaya, K., and T. Miura. 1982. Effects of nitrogen dioxide on fatty acid compositions of red cell membranes, sera, and livers in rats. *Environ. Res.* 27: 24–35.

Kaya, K., T. Miura, and K. Kubota. 1980. Effects of nitrogen dioxide on red blood cells of rats: Changes in components of red cell membranes during *in vivo* exposure to NO_2. *Environ. Res.* 23: 397–409.

Keller, M. D., R. R. Lanese, R. I. Mitchell, and R. W. Cote. 1979. Respiratory illness in households using gas and electricity for cooking. I: Survey of incidence. *Environ. Res.* 19: 495–503.

Kelly, F. J., A. Blomberg, A. Frew, S. T. Holgate, and T. Sandstron. 1996. Antioxidant kinetics in lung lavage fluid following exposure of humans to nitrogen dioxide. *Am. J. Respir. Crit. Care Med.* 154 (6 part): 1700–1705.

Kerr, H. D., T. J. Kulle, M. L. McIlhany, and P. Swidersky. 1979. Effects of nitrogen dioxide on pulmonary function in human subjects: An environmental chamber study. *Environ. Res.* 19: 392–404.

Kienast, K., M. Knorst, S. Lubjuhn, J. Muller-Quernheim, and R. Ferlinz. 1994. Nitrogen dioxode-induced reactive oxygen intermediates production by human alveolar macrophages and peripheral blood mononuclear cells. *Arch. Environ. Health* 49: 246–250.

Kleinerman, J., A. M. Marchevsky, and J. Thornton. 1981. Quantitative studies of APUD cells in airways of rats. The effects of diethylnitrosamine and NO$_2$. *Am. Rev. Respir. Dis.* 124: 458–462.

Kleinerman, J., and M. P. C. Ip. 1979. Effects of nitrogen dioxide on elastin and collagen contents of lung. *Arch. Environ. Health* 34: 228–232.

Kleinerman, J., M. P. C. Ip, and J. Sorensen. 1982. Nitrogen dioxide exposure and alveolar macrophage elastase in hamsters. *Am. Rev. Respir. Dis.* 125: 203–207.

Kleinerman, J., R. E. Gordon, M. P. C. Ip, and A. Collins. 1985. Structure and function of airways in experimental chronic nitrogen dioxide exposure. In *Indoor Air and Human Health*, eds. R. B. Gammage, and S. V. Kaye, pp. 297–301. Chelsea, MI: Lewis Publishers.

Kleinman, M. T., and W. J. Mautz. 1989. Upper airway scrubbing at rest and exercise. In: *Susceptibility to Inhaled Pollutants*, eds. M. J. Utell, and R. Frank, pp. 100–110. ASTM STP 1024. Philadelphia: American Society for Testing and Material.

Kleinman, M. T., R. F. Phalen, W. J. Mautz, R. C. Mannix, T. R. McClure, and T. T. Crocker. 1989. Health effects of acid aerosols formed by atmospheric mixtures. *Environ. Health Perspect.* 79: 137–145.

Kleinman, M. T., W. J. Mautz, T. R. McClure, R. Mannix, and R. F. Phalen. 1985a. Comparative effects of acidic and non-acidic multicomponent atmospheres on the lungs of rats exposed by inhalation. Presented at 78th Annual Meeting of the Air Pollution Control Association, June, Detroit, MI. Paper 85–29.3 Pittsburgh: Air Pollution Control Association.

Kleinman, M. T., R. M. Bailey, J. D. Wynot, K. R. Anderson, W. S. Linn, and J. D. Hackney. 1985b. Controlled exposure to a mixture of SO$_2$, NO$_2$, and particulate air pollutants: Effects on human pulmonary function and respiratory symptoms. *Arch. Environ. Health* 40: 197–201.

Kleinman, M. T., R. M. Bailey, W. S. Linn, K. R. Anderson, J. D. Whynot, D. A. Shamoo, and J. D. Hackney. 1983. Effects of 0.2 ppm nitrogen dioxide on pulmonary function and response to bronchoprovocation in asthmatics. *J. Toxicol. Environ. Health* 12: 815–826.

Kleinman, M. T., W. S. Linn, R. M. Bailey, M. P. Jones, and J. D. Hackney. 1980. Effect of ammonium nitrate aerosol on human respiratory function and symptoms. *Environ. Res.* 21: 317–326.

Kobayashi, T, and T. Miura. 1995. Concentration- and time-dependent increase in specific airway resistance after induction of airway hyperresponsiveness by subchronic exposure of guinea pigs to nitrogen dioxide. *Fundam. Appl. Toxicol.* 25: 154–158.

Koenig, J. Q. 1989. Paper 89–92.4. Presented at 82nd Annual Meeting of Air and Waste Management Association. Anaheim, CA, June, 1989.

Koenig, J. Q., D. S. Covert, and W. E. Pierson. 1989. Effects of inhalation of acidic compounds on pulmonary function in allergic adolescent subjects. *Environ. Health Perspect.* 79: 173–178.

Koenig, J. Q., D. S. Covert, M. S. Morgan, M. Horike, N. Horike, S. G. Marshall, and W. E. Pierson. 1985. Acute effects of 0.12 ppm ozone or 0.12 ppm nitrogen dioxide on pulmonary function in healthy and asthmatic adolescents. *Am. Rev. Respir. Dis.* 132: 648–651.

Koenig, J. Q., D. S. Covert, S. G. Marshall, G. van Belle, and W. E. Pierson. 1987. The effects of ozone and nitrogen dioxide on pulmonary function in healthy and asthmatic adolescents. *Am. Rev. Respir. Dis.* 136: 1152–1157.

Koenig, J. Q., D. S. Covert, W. E. Pierson, Q. S. Hanley, V. Rebolledo, K. Dumler, and S. E. McKinney. 1994. Oxidant and acid aerosol exposure in healthy subjects and subjects with asthma. Part I: Effects of oxidants, combined with sulfuric acid or nitric acid, on the pulmonary function of adolescents with asthma. Health Effects Institute Research Report 70. HEI, Cambridge, MA.

Koo, L. C., J. H. C. Ho, C-Y. Ho, H. Matsuki, H. Shimizu, T. Mori, and S. Tominaga. 1990. Personal exposure to nitrogen dioxide and its association with respiratory illness in Hong Kong. *Am. Rev. Respir. Dis.* 141: 1119–1126.

Kosaka, H., K. Imaizumi, K. Imai, and I. Tyuma. 1979. Stoichiometry of the reaction of oxyhemoglobin with nitrate. *Biochim. Biophys. Acta* 581: 184–188.

Kosmider, S., A. Misiewicz, E. Felus, M. Drozdz, and K. Ludyga. 1973. Experimentelle und klinische Untersuchungen ueber den Einfluss der Stickstoffoxyde auf die Immunitaet (Experimental and clinical studies on the effects of nitrogen oxides on immunity). *Int. Arch. Arbeitsmed.* 31: 9–23.

Kripke, B. J., and R. P. Sherwin. 1984. Nitrogen dioxide exposure—influence on rat testes. *Anesth. Analg.* 63: 526–528.

Kubota, K., M. Murakami, S. Takenaka, K. Kawai, and H. Kyono. 1987. Effects of long-term nitrogen dioxide exposure on rat lung: Morphological observations. *Environ. Health Perspect.* 73: 157–169.

Kulle, T. J. 1982. Effects of nitrogen dioxide on pulmonary function in normal healthy humans and subjects with asthma and bronchitis. In *Air Pollution by Nitrogen Oxides*, eds. T. Schneider, and L. Grant, pp. 477–486. Amsterdam: Elsevier.

Kulle, T. J., and M. L. Clements. 1987. Susceptibility to virus infection with exposure to nitrogen dioxide. Health Effects Institute. Research Report 15.Cambridge, MA.

Kunimoto, M., H. Tsubone, N. Tsujii, K. Mochitate, K. Kaya, N. Shimojo, and T. Miura. 1984. Effects of nitrate and nitrite, chemical intermediates of inhaled nitrogen dioxide, on membrane components of red blood cells of rats. *Toxicol. Appl. Pharmacol.* 74: 10–16.

Kyono, H., and K. Kawai. 1982. Morphometric study on age-dependent pulmonary lesions in rats exposed to nitrogen dioxide. *Ind. Health* 20: 73–99.

Lafuma, C., A. Harf, F. Lange, L. Bozzi, J. L. Poncy, and J. Bignon. 1987. Effect of low-level NO$_2$ chronic exposure on elastase-induced emphysema. *Environ. Res.* 43: 75–84.

Last, J.A. 1989. Effects of inhaled acids on lung biochemistry. *Environ. Health Perspect.* 79: 115–119.

Last, J. A., and D. L. Warren. 1987. Synergistic interaction between nitrogen dioxide and respirable aerosols of sulfuric acid or sodium chloride on rat lungs. *Toxicol. Appl. Pharmacol.* 90: 34–42.

Last, J. A., D. M. Hyde, and D. P. Y. Chang. 1984. A mechanism of synergistic lung damage by ozone and a respirable aerosol. *Exp. Lung Res.* 7: 223–235.

Last, J. A., J. E. Gerriets, and D. M. Hyde. 1983. Synergistic effects on rat lungs of mixtures of oxidant air pollutants (ozone or nitrogen dioxide) and respirable aerosols. *Am. Rev. Respir. Dis.* 128: 539–544.

Last, J. A., T. R. Gelzleichter, K. E. Pinkerton, R. M. Walker, and H. Witschi. 1993. A new model of progressive pulmonary fibrosis in rats. *Am. Rev. Respir. Dis.* 148: 487–494.

Lebowitz, M. D., C. J. Holberg, B. Boyer, and C. Hayes. 1985. Respiratory symptoms and peak flow associated with indoor and outdoor air pollutants in the southwest. *J. Air Pollut. Control Assoc.* 35: 1154–1158.

Lee, J. S., M. G. Mustafa, and A. A. Afifi. 1990. Effects of short-term, single and combined exposure to low level NO$_2$ and O$_3$ on lung tissue enzyme activities in rats. *J. Toxicol. Environ. Health* 29: 293–305.

Lee, K., Y. Yanagisawa, J. D. Spengler, and S. Nakai. 1994. Carbon monoxide and nitrogen dioxide exposures in indoor ice skating rinks. *J. Sports Sci.* 12: 279–283.

Lefkowitz, S. S., J. J. McGrath, and D. L. Lefkowitz. 1986. Effects of NO$_2$ on immune responses. *J. Toxicol. Environ. Health* 17: 241–248.

Lehnert, B. E., D. C. Archuleta, T. Ellis, W. S. Session, N. M. Lehnert, L. R. Gurley, and D. M. Stavert. 1994. Lung injury following exposure of rats to relatively high mass concentrations of nitrogen dioxide. *Toxicology* 89: 239–277.

Lewis, T. R., W. J. Moorman, Y.-Y. Yang, and J. F. Stara. 1974. Long-term exposure to auto exhaust and other pollutant mixtures: Effects on pulmonary function in the beagle. *Arch. Environ. Health* 29: 102–106.

Linaker, C. H., A. J. Chauhan, H. Inskip, A. J. Frew, A. Sillence, D. Coggon, and S. T. Holgate. 1996. Distribution and determinants of personal exposure to nitrogen dioxide in school children. *Occup. Environ. Med.* 53: 200–203.

Linn, W. S., J. C. Solomon, S. C. Trim, C. E. Spier, D. A. Shamoo, T. G. Venet, E. L. Avol, and J. D. Hackney. 1985a. Effects of exposure to 4 ppm nitrogen dioxide in healthy and asthmatic volunteers. *Arch. Environ. Health* 40: 234–239.

Linn, W. S., D. A. Shamoo, C. E. Spier, L. M. Valencia, U. T. Anzar, T. G. Venet, E. L. Avol, and J. D. Hackney. 1985b. Controlled exposure of volunteers with chronic obstructive pulmonary disease to nitrogen dioxide. *Arch. Environ. Health* 40: 313–317.

Linn, W. S., D. A. Shamoo, E. L. Avol, J. D. Whynot, K. R. Anderson, T. G. Venet, and J. D. Hackney. 1986. Dose–response study of asthmatic volunteers exposed to nitrogen dioxide during intermittent exercise. *Arch. Environ. Health* 41: 292–296.

Linn, W. S., M. P. Jones, R. M. Bailey, M. T. Kleinman, C. E. Spier, D. A. Fischer, and J. D. Hackney. 1980. Respiratory effects of mixed nitrogen dioxide and sulfur dioxide in human volunteers under simulated ambient exposure conditions. *Environ. Res.* 22: 431–438.

Maigetter, R. Z., J. D. Fenters, J. C. Findlay, R. Ehrlich, and D. E. Gardner. 1978. Effect of exposure to nitrogen dioxide on T and B cells in mouse spleens. *Toxicol. Lett.* 2: 157–161.

Maples, K. R., T. Sandström, Y-F. Su, and R. F. Henderson. 1991. The nitric oxide/heme protein complex as a biological marker of exposure to nitrogen dioxide in humans, rats and *in vitro* models. *Am. J. Respir. Cell Mol. Biol.* 4: 538–543.

Mautz, W. J., M. T. Kleinman, C. Bufalino, and W. Cheng. 1993. Effects of episodic exposure to nitric acid on pulmonary structure and function in the rat. *Toxicologist* 13: 150.

McGrath, J. J., and J. Oyervides. 1985. Effects of nitrogen dioxide on resistance of *Klebsiella pneumoniae* in mice. *J. Am. Coll. Toxicol.* 4: 227–231.

Melia, R. J. W., C. D. V. Florey, and S. Chinn. 1979. The relation between respiratory illness in primary schoolchildren and the use of gas for cooking. I: Results from a national survey. *Int. J. Epidemiol.* 8: 333–339.

Melia, R. J. W., C. D. V. Florey, R. W. Morris, B. D. Goldstein, H. H. John, D. Clark, I. B. Craighead, and J. C. Mackinlay. 1982. Childhood respiratory illness and the home environment. II: Association between respiratory illness and nitrogen dioxide, temperature and relative humidity. *Int. J. Epidemiol.* 11: 164–169.

Melia, R. J. W., C. V. Florey, D. G. Altman, and A. V. Swan. 1977. Association between gas cooking and respiratory disease in children. *Br. Med. J.* 2: 149–152.

Mercer, R. R., D. L. Costa, and J. D. Crapo. 1995. Effects of prolonged exposure to low doses of nitric oxide or nitrogen dioxide on the alveolar septa of the adult rat lung. *Lab. Invest.* 73: 20–28.

Miller, F. J., J. A. Graham, J. A. Raub, J. W. Illing, M. G. Menache, D. E. House, and D. E. Gardner. 1987. Evaluating the toxicity of urban patterns of oxidant gases. II: Effects in mice from chronic exposure to nitrogen dioxide. *J. Toxicol. Environ. Health* 21: 99–112.

Miller, F. J., J. A. Graham, J. W. Illing, and D. E. Gardner. 1980. Extrapulmonary effects of NO_2 as reflected by pentobarbital-induced sleeping time in mice. *Toxicol. Lett.* 6: 267–274.

Miller, F. J., J. H. Overton, E. T. Myers, and J. A. Graham. 1982. Pulmonary dosimetry of nitrogen dioxide in animals and man. In *Air Pollution by Nitrogen Oxides*, eds. T. Schneider, and L. Grant, pp. 377–386. Amsterdam: Elsevier.

Mochitate, K., K. Kaya, T. Miura, and K. Kubota. 1984. *In vivo* effects of nitrogen dioxide on membrane constituents in lung and liver of rats. *Environ. Res.* 33: 17–28.

Mochitate, K., Y. Takahashi, T. Ohsumi, and T. Miura. 1986. Activation and increment of alveolar macrophages induced by nitrogen dioxide. *J. Toxicol. Environ. Health* 17: 229–239.

Mohsenin V. 1994. Human exposure to oxides of nitrogen at ambient and supra-ambient concentrations. *Toxicology* 89: 301–312.

Mohsenin, V. 1987a. Effect of vitamin C on NO_2-induced airway hyperresponsiveness in normal subjects: A randomized double-blind study. *Am. Rev. Respir. Dis.* 136: 1408–1411.

Mohsenin, V. 1987b. Airway responses to nitrogen dioxide in asthmatic subjects. *J. Toxicol. Environ. Health* 22: 371–380.

Mohsenin, V. 1988. Airway responses to 2.0 ppm nitrogen dioxide in normal subjects. *Arch. Environ. Health* 43: 242–246.

Mohsenin, V., and J. B. L. Gee. 1987. Acute effect of nitrogen dioxide exposure on the functional activity of α-1-protease inhibitor in bronchoalveolar lavage fluid of normal subjects. *Am. Rev. Respir. Dis.* 136: 646–650.

Morrow, P. E., M. J. Utell, M. A. Bauer, et al. 1992. Pulmonary performance of elderly normal subjects and subjects with chronic obstructive pulmonary disease exposed to 0.3 ppm nitrogen dioxide. *Am. Rev. Respir. Dis.* 145: 291–300.

Morrow, P. E., and M. J. Utell. 1989. Responses of susceptible subpopulations to nitrogen dioxide. Research Report 23. Health Effects Institute, Cambridge, MA.

Moseler, M., A. Hendel-Kramer, W. Karmaus, J. Forster, K. Weiss, R. Urbanek, and J. Kuehr. 1994. Effect of moderate NO_2 air pollution on the lung function of children with asthmatic symptoms. *Environ. Res.* 67: 109–124.

Muelenaer, P., H. Reid, R. Morris, L. Saltzman, D. Horstman, A. Collier, and F. Henderson. 1987. Urinary hydroxyproline excretion in young male exposed experimentally to nitrogen dioxide. In *Indoor Air '87*, vol. 2, eds., B. Seifert, H. Esdorn, M. Fischer, H. Rieden, and J. Wegner, pp. 97–103. Berlin: Institute for Water, Soil and Air Hygiene.

Munger, J. W., J. Collett Jr., B. Danbe Jr., and M. R. Hoffman. 1990. Fogwater chemistry at Riverside California. *Atmos. Environ.* 24B: 185–205.

Murphy, S. D. 1964. A review of effects on animals of exposure to auto exhaust and some of its components. *J. Air Pollut. Contr. Assoc.* 14: 303–308.

Mustafa, M. G., N. M. Elsayed, F. M. von Dohlen, C. M. Hassett, E. M. Postlethwait, C. L. Quinn, J. A. Graham, and D. E. Gardner. 1984. A comparison of biochemical effects of nitrogen dioxide, ozone, and their combination in mouse lung. I: Intermittent exposures. *Toxicol. Appl. Pharmacol.* 72: 82–90.

Nadziejko, C. E., L. Nansen, R. C. Mannix, M. T. Kleinman, and R. F. Phalen. 1992. Effect of nitric acid vapor on the response to inhaled ozone. *Inhal. Toxicol.* 4: 343–358.

National Institutes of Health. 1985. The definition of emphysema: Report of a National Heart, Lung, and Blood Institute, Division of Lung Diseases Workshop. *Am. Rev. Respir. Dis.* 132: 182–185.

Oda, H., H. Nogami, S. Kusumoto, T. Mukajima, and A. Kurata. 1980. Lifetime exposure to 2.4 ppm nitric oxide in mice. *Environ. Res.* 22: 254–263.

Oda, H., H. Nogami, S. Kusumoto, T. Nakajima, A. Kurata, and K. Imai. 1976. Long-term exposure to nitric oxide in mice. *J. Jap. Soc. Air Pollut.* 11: 150–160.

Oda, H., H. Tsubone, A. Suzuki, T. Ichinose, and K. Kubota. 1981. Alterations of nitrite and nitrate concentrations in the blood of mice exposed to nitrogen dioxide. *Environ. Res.* 25: 294–301.

Ohashi, Y., Y. Nakai, Y. Sugiura, Y. Ohno, and H. Okamoto. 1993. Nitrogen dioxide induced eosinophilia and mucosal injury in the trachea of the guinea pig. *J. Oto-Rhino-Laryngol.* 55: 36–40.

Orehek, J., F. Grimaldi, E. Muls, J. P. Durand, A. Viala, and J. Charpin. 1981. Response bronchique aux allergenes apres exposition controlee au dioxyde d'azote (Bronchial response to allergens after controlled NO_2 exposure). *Bull. Eur. Physiopath. Respir. Clin. Respir. Physiol.* 17: 911–915.

Orehek, J., J. P. Massari, P. Gayrard, C. Grimaud, and J. Charpin. 1976. Effect of short-term, low-level nitrogen dioxide exposure on bronchial sensitivity of asthmatic patients. *J. Clin. Invest.* 57: 301–307.

Orthoefer, J. G., R. S. Bhatnagar, A. Rahman, Y. Y. Yang, S. D. Lee, and J. F. Stara. 1976. Collagen and prolylhydroxylase levels in lungs of beagles exposed to air pollutants. *Environ. Res.* 12: 299–305.

Oshima, H., M. Friesen, I. Brouet, and H. Bartsch. 1990. Nitrotyrosine as a new marker for endogenous nitrosation and nitration of products. *Food Chem. Toxicol.* 28: 647–652.

Overton, J. H., Jr. 1984. Physicochemical processes and the formulation of dosimetry models. In *Fundamentals of Extrapolation Modeling of Inhaled Toxicants: Ozone and Nitrogen Dioxide*, eds. F. J. Miller, and D. B. Menzel, pp. 93–114. Washington, DC: Hemisphere Publishing.

Palisano, J. R., and J. Kleinerman. 1980. APUD cells and NEB in hamster lung: Methods, quantitation and response to injury. *Thorax* 35: 5–11.

Palmes, E. D., A. F. Gunnison, J. DiMattio, and C. Tomczyk. 1976. Personal sampler for nitrogen dioxide. *Am. Ind. Hyg. Assoc. J.* 37: 570–577.

Parker, R. F., J. K. Davis, G. H. Cassell, H. White, D. Dziedzic, D. K. Blalock, R. B. Thorp, and J. W. Simecka. 1990. Short-term exposure to nitrogen dioxide enhances susceptibility to murine respiratory Mycoplasmosis and decreases intrapulmonary killing of *Mycoplasma pulmonis*. *Am. Rev. Respir. Dis.* 140: 502–512.

Parks, N. J., K. A. Krohn, C. A. Mathis, J. H. Chasko, K. R. Greiger, M. E. Gregor, and N. F. Peek. 1981. Nitrogen-13-labeled nitrate: Distribution and metabolism after intratracheal administration. *Science* (Washington, DC) 212: 58–61.

Pershagen, G. E. Rylander, S. Norberg, M. Eriksson, and S. I. Nordvall. 1995. Air pollution involving nitrogen dioxide exposure and wheezing bronchitis in children. *Int. J. Epidemiol.* 24: 1147–1153.

Pierson, W. R., and W. W. Brachaczek. 1988. Coarse- and fine-particle atmospheric nitrate and HNO$_3$(g) in Claremont, California, during the 1985 nitrogen species methods comparison. *Atmos. Environ.* 22: 1665–1668.

Pinkston, P., A. Smeglin, N. J. Roberts Jr., F. R. Gibb, P. E. Morrow, and M. J. Utell. 1988. Effects of *in vitro* exposure to nitrogen dioxide on human alveolar macrophage release of neutrophil chemotactic factor and interleukin-1. *Environ. Res.* 47: 48–58.

Ponka, A., and M. Virtanen. 1996. Low-level air pollution and hospital admissions for cardiac and cerebrovascular diseases in Helsinki. *Am. J. Public Health* 86: 1273–1280.

Posin, C., K. Clark, M. P. Jones, J. V. Patterson, R. D. Buckley, and J. D. Hackney. 1978. Nitrogen dioxide inhalation and human blood biochemistry. *Arch. Environ. Health* 33: 318–324.

Postlethwait, E. M., and A. Bidani. 1989. Pulmonary disposition of inhaled NO$_2$-nitrogen in isolated rat lungs. *Toxicol. Appl. Pharmacol.* 98: 303–312.

Postlethwait, E. M., and A. Bidani. 1990. Reactive uptake governs the pulmonary air space removal of inhaled nitrogen dioxide. *J. Appl. Physiol.* 68: 594–603.

Postlethwait, E. M., and M. G. Mustafa. 1981. Fate of inhaled nitrogen dioxide in isolated perfused rat lung. *J. Toxicol. Environ. Health* 7: 861–872.

Prütz, W. A., H. Mönig, J. Butler, and E. J. Land. 1985. Reactions of nitrogen dioxide in aqueous model systems: Oxidation of tyrosine units in peptides and proteins. *Arch. Biochem. Biophys.* 243: 125–134.

Purvis, M. R., and R. Ehrlich. 1963. Effect of atmospheric pollutants on susceptibility to respiratory infection. II: Effect of nitrogen dioxide. *J. Infect. Dis.* 113: 72–76.

Rajini, P., T. R. Gelzleichter, J. A. Last, and H. Witschi. 1993. Alveolar and airway cell kinetics in the lungs of rats exposed to nitrogen dioxide, ozone and a combination of the two gases. *Toxicol. Appl. Pharmacol.* 121: 186–192.

Rasmussen, R.E., and T. R. McClure. 1992. Effect of chronic exposure to NO$_2$ in the developing ferret lung. *Toxicol. Lett.* 63: 253–260.

Rasmussen, R. E., R. C. Mannix, M. J. Oldham, and R. F. Phalen. 1994. Effects of nitrogen dioxide on respiratory tract clearance in the ferret. *J. Toxicol. Environ. Health* 41: 109–120.

Rasmussen, R. E. 1994. Localization of increased collagen in ferret lung tissue after chronic exposure to nitrogen dioxide. *Toxicol. Lett.* 73: 241–248.

Rasmussen, T. R., M. Brauer, and S. Kjaergaard. 1995. Effects of nitrous acid exposure on human mucous membranes. *Am. J. Respir. Crit. Care Med.* 151: 1504–1511.

Richters, A., and K. Kuraitis. 1981. Inhalation of NO$_2$ and blood borne cancer cell spread to the lungs. *Arch. Environ. Health* 36: 36–39.

Richters, A., and K. S. Damji. 1988. Changes in T-lymphocyte subpopulations and natural killer cells following exposure to ambient levels of nitrogen dioxide. *J. Toxicol. Environ. Health* 25: 247–256.

Richters, A., and V. Richters. 1989. Nitrogen dioxide (NO$_2$) inhalation, formation of microthrombi in lungs and cancer metastasis. *J. Environ. Pathol. Toxicol. Oncol.* 9: 45–51.

Robison, T. W., and H. J. Forman. 1993. Dual effect of nitrogen dioxide on rat alveolar macrophage arachidonate metabolism. *Exp. Lung Res.* 19: 21–36.

Robison, T. W., and K. J. Kim. 1995. Dual effect of nitrogen dioxide on barrier properties of guinea pig tracheobronchial epithelial monolayers cultured in an air interface. *J. Toxicol. Environ. Health* 44: 57–71.

Robison, T. W., J. K. Murphy, L. L. Beyer, A. Richters, and H. J. Forman. 1993. Depression of stimulated arachidonate metabolism and superoxide production in rat alveolar macrophages following *in vivo* exposure to 0.5 ppm NO$_2$. *J. Toxicol. Environ. Health* 38: 273–292.

Roger, L. J., D. H. Horstman, W. F. McDonnell, H. Kehrl, P. J. Ives, E. Seal, R. Chapman, and E. Massoro. 1990. Pulmonary function, airway responsiveness, and respiratory symptoms in asthmatics following exercise in NO$_2$. *Toxicol. Ind. Health* 6: 155–171.

Rombout, P. J. A., J. A. M. A. Dormans, M. Marra, and G. J. van Esch. 1986. Influence of exposure regimen on nitrogen dioxide-induced morphological changes in the rat lung. *Environ. Res.* 41: 466–480.

Rose, R. M., J. M. Fuglestad, W. A. Skornik, S. M. Hammer, S. F. Wolfthal, B. D. Beck, and J. D. Brain. 1988. The pathophysiology of enhanced susceptibility to murine cytomegalovirus respiratory infection during short-term exposure to 5 ppm nitrogen dioxide. *Am. Rev. Respir. Dis.* 137: 912–917.

Rubinstein, I., B. G. Bigby, T. F. Reiss, and H. A. Bousley. 1990. Short-term exposure to 0.3 ppm nitrogen dioxide does not potentiate airway responsiveness to sulfur dioxide in asthmatic subjects. *Am. Rev. Respir. Dis.* 139: 381–385.

Sackner, M. A., R. D. Dougherty, and G. A. Chapman. 1976. Effect of inorganic nitrate and sulfate salts on cardiopulmonary function. *Am. Rev. Respir. Dis.* 113 (suppl): 89.

Sackner, M. A., R. D. Dougherty, G. A. Chapman, S. Zarzecki, L. Zarzemski, and R. Schreck. 1979. Effects of sodium nitrate aerosol on cardiopulmonary function of dogs, sheep, and man. *Environ. Res.* 18: 421–436.

Sagai, M., T. Ichinose, and K. Kubota. 1984. Studies on the biochemical effects of nitrogen dioxide. IV: Relation between the change of lipid peroxidation and the antioxidative protective system in rat lungs upon life span exposure to low levels of NO_2. *Toxicol. Appl. Pharmacol.* 73: 444–456.

Salome, C. M., N. J. Brown, G. B. Marks, A. J. Woolcock, G. M. Johnson, P. C. Nancarrow, S. Quigley, and J. Tiong. 1996. Effect of nitrogen dioxide and other combustion products on asthmatic subjects in a home-like environment. *Eur. Respir. J.* 9: 910–918.

Samet, J. M., W. E. Lambert, B. J. Skipper, A. H. Cushing, W. C. Hunt, S. A. Young, L. C. McLaren, M. Schwab, and J. D. Spengler. 1993. Nitrogen dioxide and respiratory illness in infants. *Am. Rev. Respir. Dis.* 148: 1258–1265.

Sandström, T., M. C. Anderson, B. Kolmodin-Hedman, N. Stjernberg, and T. Angström. 1990. Bronchoalveolar mastocytosis and lymphocytosis after nitrogen dioxide exposure in man: A time-kinetic study. *Eur. Respir. J.* 3: 138–143.

Saul, R. L., and M. C. Archer. 1983. Nitrate formation in rats exposed to nitrogen dioxide. *Toxicol. Appl. Pharmacol.* 67: 284–291.

Scarlett, J. F., K. J. Abbott, J. L. Peacock, D. P. Strachan, and H. R. Anderson. 1996. Acute effects of summer air pollution on respiratory function in primary school children in southern England. *Thorax* 51: 1109–1114.

Schenker, M. B., J. M. Samet, and F. E. Speizer. 1983. Risk factors for childhood respiratory disease: The effect of host factors and home environmental exposures. *Am. Rev. Respir. Dis.* 28: 1038–1043.

Schlesinger, R. B. 1987. Intermittent inhalation of nitrogen dioxide: Effects on rabbit alveolar macrophages. *J. Toxicol. Environ. Health* 21: 127–139.

Schlesinger, R. B. 1989. Comparative toxicity of ambient air pollutants: Some aspects related to lung defense. *Environ. Health Perspect.* 81: 123–128.

Schlesinger, R. B., and J. M. Gearhart. 1987. Intermittent exposures to mixed atmospheres of nitrogen dioxide and sulfuric acid: Effect on particle clearance from the respiratory region of rabbit lungs. *Toxicology* 44: 309–319.

Schlesinger, R. B., H. A. N. El-Fawal, J. T. Zelikoff, J. E. Gorczynski, T. McGovern, C. E. Nadziejko, and L. C. Chen. 1994. Pulmonary effects of repeated episodic exposures to nitric acid vapor alone and in combination with ozone. *Inhal. Toxicol.* 6: 21–41.

Schlesinger, R. B., K. E. Driscoll, and T. A. Vollmuth. 1987. Effect of repeated exposures to nitrogen dioxide and sulfuric acid mist alone or in combination on mucociliary clearance from the lungs of rabbits. *Environ. Res.* 44: 294–301.

Selgrade, M. J. K., M. L. Mole, F. J. Miller, G. E. Hatch, D. E. Gardner, and P. C. Hu. 1981. Effect of NO_2 inhalation and vitamin C deficiency on protein and lipid accumulation in the lung. *Environ. Res.* 26: 422–437.

Shaw, R. W., Jr., R. K. Stevens, J. Bowermaster, J. W. Tesch, and E. Tew. 1982. Measurements of atmospheric nitrate and nitric acid: The denuder difference experiment. *Atmos. Environ.* 16: 845–853.

Sherwin, R. P., and D. A. Carlson. 1973. Protein content of lung lavage fluid of guinea pigs exposed to 0.4 ppm nitrogen dioxide: Disc-gel electrophoresis for amount and types. *Arch. Environ. Health* 27: 90–93.

Sherwin, R. P., and L. J. Layfield. 1974. Proteinuria in guinea pigs exposed to 0.5 ppm nitrogen dioxide. *Arch. Environ. Health* 28: 336–341.

Shy, C. M., J. P. Creason, M. E. Pearlman, K. E. McClain, F. B. Benson, and M. M. Young. 1970a. The Chattanooga school children study: Effects of community exposure to nitrogen dioxide. I. Methods, description of pollutant exposure and results of ventilatory function testing. *J. Air Pollut. Control Assoc.* 20: 539–545.

Shy, C. M., J. P. Creason, M. E. Pearlman, K. E. McClain, F. B. Benson, and M. M. Young. 1970b. The Chattanooga school study: Effects of community exposure to nitrogen dioxide. II: Incidence of acute respiratory illness. *J. Air Pollut. Control Assoc.* 20: 582–588.

Silbaugh, S. A., J. L. Mauderly, and C. A. Macken. 1981. Effects of sulfuric acid and nitrogen dioxide on airway responsiveness of the guinea pig. *J. Toxicol. Environ. Health* 8: 31–45.

Sone, S., L. M. Brennan, and D. A. Creasia. 1983. *In vivo* and *in vitro* NO$_2$ exposures enhance phagocytic and tumoricidal activities of rat alveolar macrophages. *J. Toxicol. Environ. Health* 11: 151–163.

Speizer, F. E., B. Ferris Jr., Y. M. M. Bishop, and J. Spengler. 1980. Respiratory disease rates and pulmonary function in children associated with NO$_2$ exposure. *Am. Rev. Respir. Dis.* 121: 3–10.

Spengler, J. D., and M. A. Cohen. 1985. Emissions from indoor sources. In *Indoor Air and Human Health*, eds. R. B. Gammage, and S. V. Kaye, pp. 261–278. Chelsea, MI: Lewis Publishers.

Spengler, J. D., C. P. Duffy, R. Letz, T. W. Tibbitts, and B. G. Feris Jr. 1983. Nitrogen dioxide inside and outside 137 homes and implications for ambient air quality standards and health effects research. *Environ. Sci. Technol.* 17: 164–168.

Stacy, R. W., E. Seal Jr., D. E. House, J. Green, L. J. Roger, and L. Raggio. 1983. A survey of effects of gaseous and aerosol pollutants on pulmonary function of normal males. *Arch. Environ. Health* 38: 104–115.

Stara, J. F., D. L. Dungworth, J. G. Orthoefer, and W. S. Tyler, eds. 1980. Long-term effects of air pollutants: In *Canine Species*. Environmental Criteria and Assessment Office, Report. EPA-600/8-80-014. Cincinnati, OH: U.S. Environmental Protection Agency. Available from: NTIS, Springfield, VA; PB81-144875.

Stavert, D. M., and B. E. Lehnert. 1988. Concentration versus time is the more important exposure variable in nitrogen dioxide-induced acute lung injury. *Toxicologist* 8: 140.

Stavert, D. M., D. C. Archuleta, L. M. Holland, and B. E. Lehnert. 1986. Nitrogen dioxide exposure and development of pulmonary emphysema. *J. Toxicol. Environ. Health* 17: 249–267.

Stephens, R. J., C. Tallent, C. Hart, and D. S. Negi. 1982. Postnatal tolerance to NO$_2$ toxicity. *Exp. Mol. Pathol.* 37: 1–14.

Stephens, R. J., G. Freeman, and M. J. Evans. 1972. Early response of lungs to low levels of nitrogen dioxide: Light and electron microscopy. *Arch. Environ. Health* 24: 160–179.

Stevens, M. A., M. G. Menache, J. D. Crapo, F. J. Miller, and J. A. Grahan. 1988. Pulmonary function in juvenile and young adult rats exposed to low-level NO$_2$ with diurnal spikes. *J. Toxicol. Environ. Health* 23: 229–240.

Strand, V., P. Salomonsson, J. Lundahl, and G. Bylin. 1996. Immediate and delayed effects of nitrogen dioxide exposure at an ambient level on bronchial responsiveness to histamine in subjects with asthma. *Eur. Respir. J.* 9: 733–40.

Stupfel, M., M. Magnier, F. Romary, M.-H. Tran, and J.-P. Moutet. 1973. Lifelong exposure to SPF rats to automotive exhaust gas: Dilution containing 20 ppm of nitrogen oxides. *Arch. Environ. Health* 26: 264–269.

Sunyer, J., J. Castellsague, M. Saez, A. Tobias, and J. M. Anto. 1996. Air pollution and mortality in Barcelona. *J. Epidemiol. Comm. Health* 50(suppl) 1: 76–80.

Suzuki, A. K., H. Tsubone, and K. Kubota. 1982. Changes of gaseous exchange in the lung of mice acutely exposed to nitrogen dioxide. *Toxicol. Lett.* 10: 327–335.

Suzuki, T., S. Ikeda, T. Kanoh, and I. Mizoguchi. 1986. Decreased phagocytosis and superoxide anion production in alveolar macrophages of rats exposed to nitrogen dioxide. *Arch. Environ. Contam. Toxicol.* 15: 733–739.

Tabacova, S., B. Nikiforov, and L. Balabaeva. 1985. Postnatal effects of maternal exposure to nitrogen dioxide. *Neurobehav. Toxicol. Teratol.* 7: 785–789.

Takahashi, Y., and T. Miura. 1989. Effects of nitrogen dioxide and ozone in combination on xenobiotic metabolizing activities of rat lungs. *Toxicology* 56: 253–262.

Takahashi, Y., K. Mochitate, and T. Miura. 1986. Subacute effects of nitrogen dioxide on membrane constituents of lung, liver, and kidney of rats. *Environ. Res.* 41: 184–194.

Tepper, J. S., D. L. Costa, D. W. Winsett, M. A. Stevens, D. L. Doerfler, and W. P. Watkinson. 1993. Near-lifetime exposure of the rat to a simulated urban profile of nitrogen dioxide: Pulmonary function evaluation. *Fundam. Appl. Toxicol.* 20: 88–96.

Tunnicliffe, W. S., P. S. Burge, and J. G. Ayres. 1994. Effect of domestic concentrations of nitrogen dioxide on airway responses to inhaled allergen in asthmatic patients. *Lancet* 344: 1733–1736.

U.S. EPA. 1993. United States Environmental Protection Agency. Air quality criteria for oxides of nitrogen. EPA/600/8–91/049aF. Washington, DC.

Utell, M. J., A. J. Swinburne, R. W. Hyde, D. M. Speers, F. R. Gibb, and P. E. Morrow. 1979. Airway reactivity to nitrates in normal and mild asthmatic subjects. *J. Appl. Physiol.* 46: 189–196.

Utell, M. J., A. T. Aquilina, W. J. Hall, D. M. Speers, R. G. Douglas Jr., F. R. Gibb, P. E. Morrow, and R. W. Hyde. 1980. Development of airway reactivity to nitrates in subjects with influenza. *Am. Rev. Respir. Dis.* 121: 233–241.

Vagaggini, B., P. L. Paggiaro, D. Giannini, A. D. Franco, S. Cianchetti, S. Carnevali, M. Taccola, E. Bacci, L. Bancalari, F. L. Dente, and C. Giuntini. 1996. Effects of short term NO_2 exposure on induced sputum in normal, asthmatic and COPD subjects. *Eur. Med. J.* 9: 1852–1857.

Valand, S. B., J. D. Acton, and Q. N. Myrvik. 1970. Nitrogen dioxide inhibition of viral-induced resistance in alveolar monocytes. *Arch. Environ. Health* 20: 303–309.

Yanagisawa, Y., and H. Nishimura. 1982. A badget-type personal sampler for measurement of personal exposure to NO_2 and NO in ambient air. *Environ. Int.* 8: 235–242.

Vaughan, T. R., Jr., L. F. Jennelle, and T. R. Lewis. 1969. Long-term exposure to low levels of air pollutants. Effects on pulmonary function in the beagle. *Arch. Environ. Health* 19: 45–50.

Vedal, S., M. B. Schenker, A. Munoz, J. M. Samet, S. Batterman, and F. E. Speizer. 1987. Daily air pollution effects on children's respiratory symptoms and peak expiratory flow. *Am. J. Public Health* 77: 694–698.

Victorin, K., L. Busk, H. Cederberg, and J. Magnusson. 1990. Genotoxic activity of 1,3 butadiene and nitrogen dioxide and their photochemical reaction products in Drosophila and in the mouse bone marrow micronucleus assay. *Mutat. Res.* 228: 203–209.

Vollmuth, T. A., K. E. Driscoll, and R. B. Schlesinger. 1986. Changes in early alveolar particle clearance due to single and repeated nitrogen dioxide exposures in the rabbit. *J. Toxicol. Environ. Health* 19: 255–266.

von Nieding, G., and H. M. Wagner. 1979. Effects of NO_2 on chronic bronchitics. *Environ. Health Perspect.* 29: 137–142.

von Nieding, G., H. Krekeler, R. Fuchs, M. Wagner, and K. Koppenhagen. 1973. Studies of the acute effects of NO_2 on lung function: Influence on diffusion, perfusion and ventilation in the lungs. *Int. Arch. Arbeitsmed.* 31: 61–72.

Wagner, H.-M. 1970. Absorption of NO and NO_2 in MIK and MAK concentrations during inhalation. *Staub. Reinhalt. Luft* (Engl.) 30: 25–26.

Wagner, W. D., B. R. Duncan, P. G. Wright, and H. E. Stokinger. 1965. Experimental study of threshold limit of NO_2. *Arch. Environ. Health* 10: 455–466.

Wang, J. H., J. L. Devalia, J. M. Duddle, S. A. Hamilton, and R. J. Davies. 1995. Effect of six-hour exposure to nitrogen dioxide on early-phase nasal response to allergen challenge in patients with a history of seasonal allergic rhinitis. *J. Allergy Clin. Immunol.* 96 (5 PT 1): 669–676.

Ware, J. H., D. W. Dockery, A. Spiro, III, F. E. Speizer, and B. G. Ferris Jr. 1984. Passive smoking, gas cooking, and respiratory health of children living in six cities. *Am. Rev. Respir. Dis.* 129: 366–374.

Watanabe, H., O. Fukase, and K. Isomura. 1980. Combined effects of nitrogen oxides and ozone on mice. In *Nitrogen Oxides and Their Effects on Health*, ed. S. D. Lee, pp. 181–189. Ann Arbor, MI: Ann Arbor Science.

Wietlisbach, V, C. A. Pope 3rd, and U. Ackermann-Liebrich. 1996. Air pollution and daily mortality in three Swiss urban areas. *Sozial- und Praventivmedizin.* 41: 107–115.

Winer, A. M., and H. W. Biermann. 1991. Measurements of nitrous acid, nitrate radicals, formaldehyde and nitrogen dioxide for the Southern California Air Quality Study by differential optical absorption spectroscopy. In *Conference on Chemical Sensing of the Environment: Measurement of Atmospheric Gases*, January. Los Angeles, CA. *Proc. SPIE-Int. Soc. Opt. Eng.* 1433: 44–55.

Witschi, H. 1988. Ozone, nitrogen dioxide and lung cancer: A review of some recent issues and problems. *Toxicology* 48: 1–20.

Wong, C. G., M. Bonakdar, W. J. Mautz, and M. T. Kleinman. 1996. Chronic inhalation exposure to ozone and nitric acid elevates stress-inducible heat shock protein 70 in the rat lung. *Toxicology* 107: 111–119.

Wright, E. S., M. J. Vang, J. N. Finkelstein, and R. D. Mavis. 1982. Changes in phospholipid biosynthetic enzymes in type II cells and alveolar macrophages isolated from rat lungs after NO_2 exposure. *Toxicol. Appl. Pharmacol.* 66: 305–311.

Yokoyama, E. 1968. Effects of acute controlled exposure to NO_2 on mechanics of breathing in health subjects. *Koshu Eiseiin Kenkyu Hokoku* 17: 337–346.

Yokoyama, E., I. Ichikawa, and K. Kawai. 1980. Does nitrogen dioxide modify the respiratory effects of ozone? In *Nitrogen Oxides and Their Effects on Health*, ed. S. D. Lee, pp. 217–229. Ann Arbor, MI: Ann Arbor Science.

Yoshida, K., and K. Kasama. 1987. Biotransformation of nitric oxide. *Environ. Health Perspect.* 73: 201–206.

19 Noise: Its Effects and Control

DANIEL L. JOHNSON, Ph.D.

Unlike most other environmental toxicants, human exposure to sound can be both beneficial and detrimental. The fact that what is pleasant sound to some can be undesirable noise to others emphasizes the point that control of noise will always be somewhat of a compromise. Using the definition of noise as "unwanted sound," the only way to completely erase noise exposure for all people is to not have sound at all! Humanity would lose one of its greatest senses. So we should not try to completely eliminate noise but to reduce and control it so that it is not a predominant part of what adversely affects a person's life. This is the challenge for all involved in controlling noise.

It should also be made clear that, when discussing certain aspects of the effects of noise, such as noise-induced hearing loss, noise exposure will include both wanted and unwanted sound. The ear does not discriminate whether a damaging sound is from a jackhammer or a rock concert.

With these thoughts in mind, the effects part of this chapter is organized into two major sections. The first section covers direct physical effects of noise, of which noise-induced hearing loss is the predominant consideration. The second section covers the general effects of noise as shown by annoyance or interference of activities such as speech or sleep. The control of noise is broken down into public awareness, noise control at the source, voluntary standards, government regulations, and new technology. Before discussing the effects and control of noise, a brief description of human hearing and the measurement of sound are in order.

HUMAN AUDITORY SYSTEM

The human auditory system is normally described as being capable of hearing between frequencies of 20 to 20,000 Hz (cycles/s) and between levels of 0 decibels (dB), corresponding to a pressure of 20 micropascals, to the threshold of pain at 140 dB (ANSI S3.6-1996). While for many environmental noises this description is adequate, there are cases where a more general description is needed. The total range of human hearing and sensation is shown in Figure 19-1. A typical human can hear, or at least sense, sound between 1 and 100,000 Hz (100 kHz) (Yeowart et al., 1968; Lenhart etal., 1991). Of course, the sound pressure levels (SPL) at the very low infrasound frequencies (< 20 Hz) and at the very high ultrasound frequencies (> 20 kHz) must be much higher than the SPL at a more sensitive frequency such as 1000 Hz. The most sensitive frequency is at 4000 Hz. The auditory threshold for the median of a population is $- 6$ dB. There are individuals that can hear up to 20 dB better than the median. Thus a very sensitive individual in a very quiet

Environmental Toxicants: Human Exposures and Their Health Effects, 2/e. Edited by Morton Lippmann.
ISBN: 0-471-29298-2 © 2000 John Wiley & Sons, Inc.

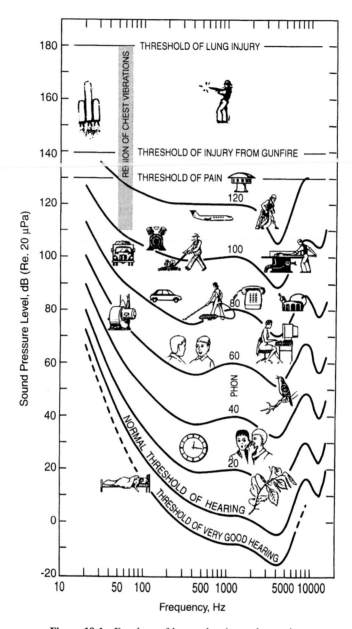

Figure 19-1 Envelope of human hearing and sensation.

environment might hear a sound as low as $-26\,\mathrm{dB}$ (ANSI S3.6-1996). It is the hearing at this very sensitive frequency that normally is the most susceptible to damage from excess noise.

A pure tone at $1000\,\mathrm{Hz}$ will become very obnoxious or even painful at levels between 120 and $140\,\mathrm{dB}$. As the frequency of a sound becomes greater or smaller than $1000\,\mathrm{Hz}$, the auditory threshold becomes greater. For instance, the mean threshold of audibility for $10\,\mathrm{Hz}$ is $80\,\mathrm{dB}$ (Yeowart and Evans, 1974) and for $16\,\mathrm{kHz}$ it is $44\,\mathrm{dB}$ (ANSI S3.6-1996). At the low infrasonic frequencies, sounds lose their tonal characteristics and are perceived more like rumbles (Nixon and Johnson, 1973; Von Bekesy, 1936). As the frequency of the sound becomes lower yet, a person is more likely to sense the vibration of the eardrum (or tympanic membrane) as well as a pressure buildup behind the eardrum (Slarve and Johnson, 1975). In addition, at very low frequencies, discomfort or pain may not occur until the SPL's exceed 180 to 190 dB (3 to 10 psi or 20 to 68 kPa) (Johnson, 1997). At 190 dB, the threshold of eardrum rupture is reached. At the ultrasonic region, even some deaf individuals can sense ultrasound when the head is directly stimulated (Lenhart et al., 1991).

While it is useful to understand that there are sounds that may cause environmental problems outside that of normal hearing, most environmental problems will be from sound with frequencies well inside the frequency range of 20 Hz to 20 kHz. Even with these sounds, there is a strong effect of frequency, and the common way of dealing with this is to use an A-weighting frequency network (ANSI S1.4-1983 (R 1994)). A-weighting de-emphasizes both low and high frequencies as shown in Figure 19-2. A-weighting is derived from an equal loudness curve in which the sound pressure level is about 40 dB (more specifically, the 40 phon curve shown in Figure 19-1). Fortunately, A-weighting has been found to be a good indicator for the evaluation of the effects of noise-induced hearing loss (NIHL), speech interference, and community noise in general (EPA, 1974). Therefore A-weighting has become almost universally accepted as the unifying approach for the frequency content of noise. Keep in mind, however, that the noise control engineers may use a more precise approach for frequency weighting when attempting to reduce the noise of a certain product or environment. For instance, aircraft certification uses a loudness descriptor, perceived noise (PNdB) (ANSI S3.4-1980 (R 1992)). A precise description of the effect of noise on speech would use the speech interference level (SIL) (ANSI S3.14-1977 (R 1986)). Finally, an acoustician designing a room may refer to noise rating (NR) or noise criteria (NC) curves (ANSI S12.2-1995). These are more precise measures for room acoustics.

It should be recognized that the effort to minimize noise by a more precise measure, such as perceived noise in decibels (PNdB) used for aircraft certification would enhance the utility of A-weighting. For example, PNdB has a correction for pure tones. Because of this, an aircraft manufacturer will try to suppress the tonal components of an aircraft. This then will result in A-weighting becoming more representative of the true impact of the noise, even though this measure has no correction for pure tones.

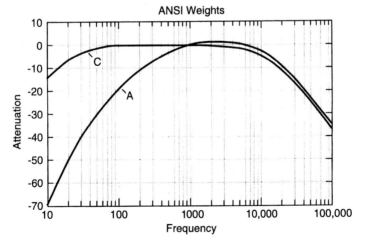

Figure 19-2   A-weighting and C-weighting curves.

Another necessary factor in dealing with environmental noise is the variability of the sound level with time. The commonly accepted method is to use an energy average. This average has been called by many names, but the preferred nomenclature is given in ANSI S1.1/1994: a time-average sound level or time interval equivalent continuous A-weighted sound pressure level, abbreviated TAV and TEQ, with symbols L_{AT} and L_{Aeqt}.

The equation for this measure is

$$L_{AT} = 10 \lg\left\{ \left(\frac{1}{T}\right) \frac{\int_\theta^T p_A^2(t)dt}{p_0^2} \right\}$$

$$= L_{AeqT}$$

Where p_A is the instantaneous A-weighted sound pressure as a function of time (t), p_0 is the reference sound pressure of $20\,\mu p_A$ and T is the stated time period. The unit is the decibel. This rather long expression is often shortened in speech by saying the letters of the symbol, for example, "Leq." For evaluation of noise-induced hearing loss, this measure is usually considered over an 8 hour time period.

For community noise, this measure for a 24 hour day is broken up into day and night average sound level abbreviations DL and NL (symbols L_d and L_n, respectively). The daytime measure is the time-average sound level between 0700 and 2200 hours. The nighttime measure is the time-average sound level between 2200 and 0700 hours. Ten decibels are then added to the nighttime measure. The combined values of DL and DN are called the day–night average sound level abbreviation DNL, and symbol is L_{dn}. Again, in speech the symbol for this measure is often pronounced "Ldn."

The approach of using logarithms for averaging sounds is well accepted and has proved to be a practical expedient in evaluating the overall impact of noise. However, it does not always work well for individual situations. The following illustration should help the reader to understand how this energy average works.

Consider a sound source that produces an A-weighted sound pressure level of 100 dB for a minute every other minute. The background level is 30 dB. Over an hour, the $L_{Aeq(h)}$ becomes equal to 97 dB. If the background level were raised to 70 dB, the overall level, $L_{Aeq(h)}$, would still be 97 dB. Not until the background level approaches 90 dB does the overall $L_{Aeq(h)}$ become larger than 97 dB. Of course, if the background level were also 100 dB, the $L_{Aeq(h)}$ would also be 100 dB. This example illustrates the emphasis that the louder sound levels receive by use of the energy average. Most of the time, this is the more appropriate way to assess sound exposure, but the reader is left to imagine individual cases where there would be an impact of a background level of 70 dB instead of 30 dB.

MEASUREMENT OF SOUND

In order to properly evaluate environmental noise, it needs to be measured. There are many textbooks and standards on sound measurement and the details of such information will not be repeated here. In general, published standards are referenced for those needing more specific information.

The basic measures, A-weighted sound level and the A-weighted average sound level, over a period of time are provided by the use of a sound level meter or an integrating sound level meter. Specifications of such meters are provided by ANSI S1.4-1983 (R 1994) American National Standard Specifications for Sound Level Meters and IEC 804 (1985). These meters are available from many manufacturers, so the user needs only to verify that the manufacturer assures that the appropriate standards are met. The use of such meters requires field calibration by a calibrator. Such calibration should meet the specification of ANSI S1.40-1984 (R 1994).

ANSI S1.13-1995, American National Standard Measurement of Sound Pressure Levels in Air, covers the general use of the sound measurement equipment.

For community noise specifically, there are four standards that are appropriate: ANSI S12.9-1988/Part 1 (R 1993), Quantities and Procedures for Description and Measurement of Environmental Sound; ANSI S12.9-1992/Part 2 and ANSI S12.9-1993/Part 3, short-term Measurements with an Observer Present; and ANSI S12.9-1996/Part 4, Noise Assessment and Prediction of Long-Term Community Response.

For the measurement of occupational noise exposure, the procedures outlined in ANSI S12.19-1996, ANSI S3.44-1996, or ISO 1999 are appropriate. For sound exposures such as infrasound and ultrasound, $\frac{1}{3}$-octave band analysis may be needed. This capability can be part of a sound level meter (SLM) or a real-time analyzer (RTA).

DIRECT PHYSICAL EFFECTS

Noise-Induced Hearing Loss

For the purposes of noise-induced hearing loss (NIHL), the term "noise" is used to denote both wanted sound and unwanted sound, since either can damage hearing. NIHL has undoubtedly occurred throughout human history. With the advent of gunpowder and modern industrial processes, NIHL began to be recognized. However, before 1950 reliable dose–effect data were not available. Before World War II there was also a lack of uniformity in instrumentation and related scales. Studies from various parts of the world often yielded different results.

Currently American, European, and international standards relating to noise measurement and hearing acuity measurements are in reasonable agreement. An international standard, ISO-R-1999 (1990), provides the method for predicting NIHL from noise exposure. A complete description of NIHL for various exposure levels and times can be calculated. An example of the data in this standard is provided in Table 19-1.

Table 19-1 provides the differences in hearing levels for better hearing at the 90th percentile, at the median, and at the poorer hearing 10th percentile, due to noise exposure. These statistical differences are between a population not exposed to occupational noise and a population exposed to a measurable occupational noise. Figure 19-3 illustrates the use of the values of Table 19-1 to predict a statistical distribution of hearing levels. There are several observations that can be made.

First, the part of the population distribution starting with the worst hearing changes the most. In other words, the 10th percentile point of a noise-exposed population changes

TABLE 19-1   NIPTS in dB Averaged Across Audiometric Test Frequencies 0.5, 1, 2, and 3 kHz

Exposure Time	10 Years			20 Years			30 Years			40 Years		
						Fractiles						
L_{A8hn}	0.9	0.5	0.1	0.9	0.5	0.1	0.9	0.5	0.1	0.9	0.5	0.1
85	0.5	1.0	1.5	1.0	1.3	2.0	1.0	1.3	2.3	1.0	1.8	2.3
90	1.0	2.5	4.8	2.3	3.5	6.0	2.8	4.0	6.8	3.3	4.5	7.3
95	2.3	5.8	10.8	5.0	7.8	13.5	6.3	9.5	15.0	7.3	10.3	16.5
100	4.5	11.0	21.0	9.5	15.5	26.5	12.5	18.0	29.8	14.5	20.0	32.5

Source: Average of NIPTS values from Tables F1 to F4 of ANSI S3.44-1996.

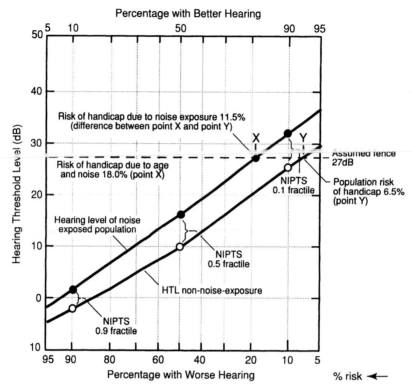

Figure 19-3 Example of hearing risk assessment: noise exposure level $L_{ex,8h} = 90$ dB for 30 years exposure with HTLA data from data base A. From Fig. E-1, ANSI S3.44-1996.

more from noise exposure than the better hearing median. This is the result of adding a distribution of noise-induced hearing loss to a normal distribution of hearing. It does not mean that individuals with poorer hearing are more susceptible to more loss.

Second, as an amplification of the preceding thought, the predictions of NIHL (also called noise-induced permanent threshold shift, or NIPTS) in Table 19-1 are for populations, not individuals. For an individual with a hearing loss, there is no certain method for separating the noise component from the aging component.

Third, as the combined effects of noise and aging approach approximately 70 to 80 dB, a limit as to the amount of noise-induced hearing loss that can occur seems to be reached.

Finally, Table 19-1 is for sounds that are generally broadband (contain many frequencies) and are not greatly fluctuating in intensity. A noise with one or two tones could be more hazardous, and the L_{Aeq} values might need to be adjusted 5 dB downward. On the other hand, an intermittent noise with many quiet periods (periods below 75 dB) might well be 5 dB less hazardous.

For the most part, the major threat to hearing comes from occupational noise exposure and from recreational noise exposure. Attending rock concerts and race tracks and using firearms, chainsaws, fireworks, and the like, without hearing protection are a few examples of potentially harmful nonoccupational noise.

Generally, environmental noises are not a problem with respect to hearing loss. For example, even around a very busy airport, aircraft flyovers are broadband, are interrupted, and just do not have the energy necessary to significantly harm the auditory system. Annoyance, of course, is a separate problem.

Nonauditory Stress

A commonly held view is that noise exposure can adversely affect physical and mental health. Noise exposure not only interferes with various activities such as speech and sleep, which causes stress, but noise may directly affect psychological and physiological processes (Shaw, 1996). However, at this time, there is no clear causal link between nonauditory disease and noise. While there are many cases in which workers exposed to noise have higher blood pressure levels than normal, these same workers are also exposed to the stresses of a typical industrial setting, such as dust, vibration, time constraints, and safety hazards. For this reason the U.S. Environmental Protection Agency (EPA) "levels" document concluded that "If noise control sufficient to protect persons from ear damage and hearing loss were instituted, then it is highly unlikely that the noises of lower level and duration resulting from this effect could directly induce non-auditory disease." For this reason, noise-induced hearing loss was considered the controlling nonauditory effect (EPA 550/9-74-004).

Sound-Induced Vibration

The resonance of the chest to low frequency is in the range of 50 to 60 Hz, although the resonance of a very large person may be somewhat lower and the resonance of a very small person may be higher (Johnson, 1997). While many discotheques and other types of musical entertainment clubs use this effect as part of the musical experience, the occurrence of such effects on an unwilling population is generally completely unacceptable.

Vibration effects first occur at low-frequency sound levels above 105 dB. The ACGIH TLV document (1999) states that any nonimpulsive level from 1 to 100 Hz as unacceptable if above 145 dB, even if such exposure is desired. For unwanted exposure to such low-frequency sounds, a sound that can be sensed will probably be a problem and efforts should be made to control the exposure at the source.

GENERAL EFFECTS OF NOISE

In 1973 the U.S. EPA published the "Levels Document" (EPA 550/9-74-004). This document, required by the Noise Control Act of 1972, provided information to protect the public health and welfare with an adequate margin of safety. In this document, the concept of the day–night sound level was promoted. Two major methods for assessing noise exposure were also put forth. The first was the annoyance or complaint frequency demonstrated by the exposed population. The second was the activity interference, such as speech or sleep interference, caused by noise. These two methods will frame the two sections of this chapter.

Annoyance / Community Response

In 1978 a paper by Schultz demonstrated the value of day–night average sound level for predicting the annoyance of a community as a result of noise from a variety of sources including railroads, highways, aircraft, and industrial sites (Schultz, 1978). An updated version of this overall annoyance response is shown in Figure 19-4 (Shaw, 1996). From such data the EPA "Levels" document suggested that a DNL of 55 dB be identified as the maximum sound level for residential noise, as measured outside the home, if the public health and welfare are to be maintained with an adequate margin of safety. Unfortunately, traffic noise will cause this level to be exceeded in most urban areas. It was estimated for

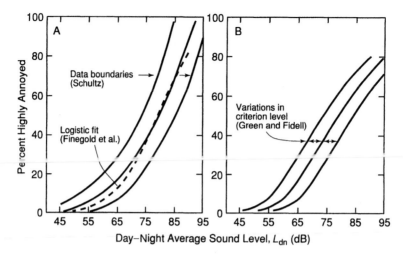

Figure 19-4 Various presentations of the relationship between "percent highly annoyed" and day–night average sound level L_{dn}. Boundaries in panel *a* encompass 90% of the 161 data points from 12 "clustering survey" data sets analyzed by Schultz in 1978. The solid centerline shows the fitted curve. The broken line in panel *a* shows logistic fit to 400 data points from 28 survey data sets according to Finegold et al. and based on data from Fidell et al. Panel *b* indicates typical variations in the "annoyance criterion level," based on data from 34 survey data sets (453 data points), according to the Green-Fidell probabilistic model. The central curve in Panel B is positioned to fit their average criterion level. (From Shaw, 1996)

residential noise exposure that over 100 million people are exposed to more than 55 dB, 33 million to more than 65 dB, and 3 million to more than 75 dB (EPA 550/9-74-009). A distribution of the number of people exposed to various average day–night levels in the United States is shown in Figure 19-5. Note the dominance of road traffic noise. The Office of Housing and Urban Development (HUD) came up with guidelines on new developments that were intended to cover residential noise exposure. Basically they only supported developments in which the exposure was 65 dB or lower. Such actions are a step in the right direction, but they will not solve the problem until quieter transportation vehicles (cars, trucks, aircraft, etc.) are produced.

Other guidelines for compatibility of land use are available such as ANSI S12.40-1990. Such guidelines are best used with master planning by local activities such that present or future land use can be evaluated. In Figure 19-6 are provided some of the components of Table A-1 of S12.40-1990. Note that residential single family, which assumes outdoor use, has the most restrictive requirements. As outdoor use becomes less important, the yearly day–night average sound level (DNL) will be greater. Where there is no outdoor use, noise control by sound insulation becomes a viable option. This is why hotel, motels, and transient lodging may be compatible with higher DNL's. Of course one should always be aware of exceptions. For instance, a resort hotel based on outside activity should be treated like a single-family residence.

While the yearly DNL is a practical and useful measure for environmental noise, specific noise exposures might require additional analysis and review (seasonal variations in land use, seasonal variations in sound exposure, interaction between noise occurrences, etc.; ANSI S12.9-1996/Part 4). In addition a new standard has been published that provides adjustments for certain types of environmental noise. These special noise categories are impulsive noises (subdivided into regular impulsive, highly impulsive, and high-energy impulsive), noises with rapid onset rate, tonal noise, and noise with strong low-frequency content (ANSI S12.9-1996/Part 4).

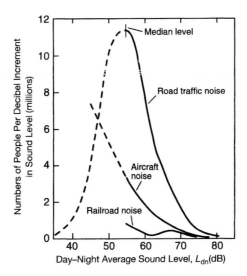

Figure 19-5   Population of the United States distributed by the day–night average outdoor sound levels to which various numbers were exposed in 1980 (nominal population: 20 million). Smooth curves have been fitted to tabulated estimates of the numbers of people exposed *t* various levels to noise from (*a*) air carrier aircraft noise, (*b*) traffic on urban and rural roads, and (*c*) railroads, rail rapid transit systems, and rail yards (see also Galloway et al). Broken lines are hypothetical extrapolations. (From Shaw, 1996)

The amount of correction for such special noise on the yearly DNL may be as much as 12 dB. The need for such special adjustments would most likely occur for residential areas near outdoor firing ranges, quarries, military bases with training missions requiring explosives, military operating areas with sonic booms or low-level military overflights, and wind power production devices.

The yearly DNL can be measured or predicted through computer modeling. Contours of equal yearly DNL can be drawn around a noise source such as an airport, and the total number of highly annoyed residents can be predicted using the demographics of the area and a relationship shown in Figure 19-4. The impact of noise changes then can be presented in the overall change in total number expected to be highly annoyed.

Activity Interference

The second environmental impact of noise is the interference of activities such as speech, music, and sleep. The advantage of viewing noise by activity interference, in addition to annoyance, is that such interference occurs regardless of the exposed person's attitude about the noise or sound. For instance, participants in a discotheque will find it difficult to communicate regardless what their feelings are about the music. In addition sound insulation, such as could be placed around classrooms, is more likely to be effective in reducing speech interference.

Speech interference is the effect that is easiest to quantify. Figure 19-7 from the EPA "Levels Document" shows the effect of a noise background on the distance two persons can carry on a conversation. The curves are adjusted such that as the background noise rises, the voice effort is also increased. Nevertheless, at some point it becomes impossible to communicate. Also shown on this figure is the predicted effect of a mildly impaired person with a high-frequency noise hearing loss, such as occurs at 3 and 4 kHz from noise exposure. Smoorenburg (1991) and Suter (1978) have shown that the speech level must be

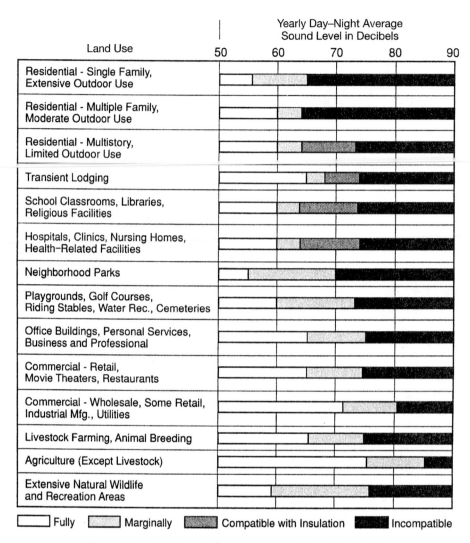

Figure 19-6   Guidelines for land use. Adapted from S12.40-1990.

as much as 6 dB dB greater for such persons for the same noise level. Using 6 dB as a nominal value, a legend for mildly hearing-impaired persons is also presented in Figure 19-7. This figure is but one way to show the additional problems individuals with noise-induced hearing loss have with a noise exposure. Note that for the same degree of speech intelligibility, people engaged in conversation either have to talk louder or get closer when one of them has noise-induced hearing loss.

Sleep interference is a more difficult problem to analyze because individuals do adapt to sleep-interrupting noise. This is why laboratory studies will often show completely different results from field studies (Pearsons, 1995). This is best illustrated by some published relationships between noise exposure and sleep interference. Figure 19-8 gives the relationship proposed by some members of the Federal Interagency Committee on Noise (FICON) based on laboratory studies (FICON, 1992).

ANSI has set up a working group to review this issue, and they expect to propose the use of field studies. The proposed curve will be like the Pearson's curve shown in Figure

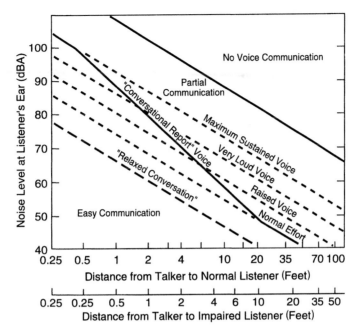

Figure 19-7 Maximum distances outdoors over which conversation is considered to be satisfactorily intelligible in steady noise. With one or both of the conversationalists with noise-induced hearing loss in which the signal to noise must be 6 dB or greater, the distance between the conversationalist needs to be halved. (From EPA levels document, 1974)

19-8 (Pearsons, 1996). While the curve of the field studies shows less effect, it demonstrates an important problem in that not all individuals of an exposed population will adapt.

CONTROL OF NOISE

Noise can be controlled in a variety of ways. Laws, voluntary standards, proper design of the sources, proper community planning, and public awareness are just some of the approaches. The more important approaches to control noise will be discussed in further detail.

Public Awareness

Awareness that noise is a problem and can sometimes be avoided is an important step in controlling noise. The inner ear can be protected by either avoiding excessive noise (e.g., rock concerts and firearms) or wearing hearing protection when participating in such noisy events. There are plugs that are designed to attenuate rather evenly across frequencies in order to not unduly interfere with the enjoyment of the music. Unfortunately, these are not universally accepted and one is likely to see only a few participants at a noisy recreational event wearing them. At shooting ranges, however, the wearing of hearing protection is more common than not. This is a step in the right direction, since the nonoccupational noise exposures are at least as important as the occupational noise exposures. In the workplace, the individual needs to follow the guidance that he / she should be getting from management. If such guidance appears to be inadequate, a complaint to the proper government authority is not out of line.

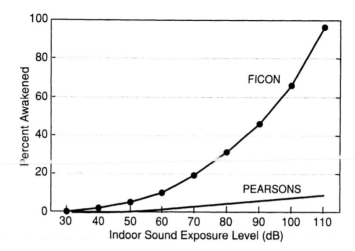

Figure 19-8   Dose–response curve adopted by FICON (1992) compared to curves considered by ANSI working group S12-37 (Pearsons, 1996). Sleep disturbance is in a home environment and the event occurs within 5 minutes of awakening, which is defined by the sleeper pushing a button upon awakening.

For nonhearing loss concerns, the aware individuals can do much. First, they can avoid living in areas with noise problems. They will avoid living next to an airport or busy highway. If a noise source tries to move next to them, they will be active in preventing such a move, requiring the noise source to reduce the noise impact to acceptable levels or providing compensation. They will also support their local government zoning activities. They will also try to buy quieter products. Aware teachers will ensure that their classrooms are quiet enough for all their students. Aware listeners will not accept not understanding what is said.

In summary, noise is best controlled by an aware society that wants it controlled.

Noise Control at the Source

The best and most efficient method for controlling noise is at the source. The most efficient action has undoubtedly been the various programs of government and aircraft industry to reduce jet engine noise. Significant progress has been made over the years as shown in Figure 19-9. Note the 20-dB drop from the levels produced by the early jet aircraft versus those by the current generation of aircraft. The National Aeronautics and Space Administration still has a goal to reduce the levels associated with the 1992 technology by another 10 dB (Stephen and Cozier, 1996).

Success for the control of other noise sources has not been as good. However, the European Union has taken the lead by mandating low-noise requirements in the 1989 EEC Machinery Safety Directive (Brooks, 1996). In the world market this action is predicted to provide an incentive for all manufacturers to try to reduce the noise from their products, although it is expected European manufacturers will take the lead.

Voluntary Standards

Standards serve to harmonize the way noise is measured and its effects assessed throughout the world. While these standards do not set limits on noise exposure, they serve as the framework for setting limits. They also serve to provide reliable methods for evaluating how well noise control efforts are progressing. This effort is increasing. In ISO,

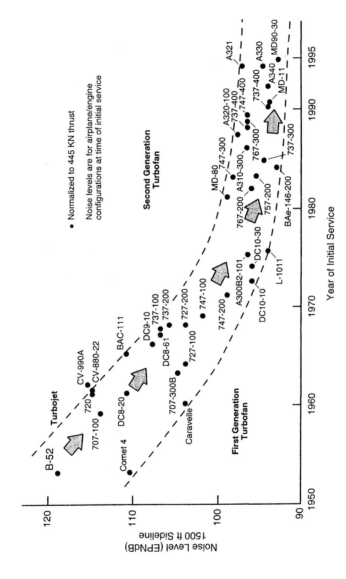

Figure 19-9 Progress in noise reduction. (From Stephens and Crazier, 1996)

651

the number of work efforts was 17 in 1970 as compared to over 80 in 1994 (Schomer, 1996). The 80 are too many to list, but a sample of the broad range of topics are as follows: 17-4869, hearing protector; 0-6393, earth-moving machinery; 20-8297, determination of sound power levels of multisource industrial plants for evaluation of sound pressure levels in the environment (Schomer, 1996).

Government Regulations

Ultimately it is necessary for some public authority to decide how much noise is too much. For noise-induced hearing loss, most developed countries now have statutory regulations for work-related exposures. These vary from the typical 85 dBA 8 hours Leq based on a 3-dB trading relation to the more lenient 90 dBA 8 hours Leq based on the 5 dB trading relation of the Occupational Safety and Health Administration (OSHA) in the United States.

For community noise, the lead has come from the more industrialized countries. Especially noteworthy is the effort of the European Common Market countries. By setting noise standards on many products, domestic U.S. manufacturers now have a goal if they expect to compete in the world market.

In the United States, the EPA's Office of Noise Abatement and Control (ONAC) might have led the way. When the Reagan administration succeeded in eliminating funding for ONAC, other U.S. government agencies took the lead in mandating controls; the most important among these is the Federal Aviation Administration (FAA). Initially applicable to aircraft manufactured after 1973, the FAA set noise standards for the certification of new aircraft (Stephens and Crazier, 1996). The standards, which are dependent on the weight of the aircraft, have become more restrictive over time and have led to categories of stage 1, stage 2, stage 3, and stage 4. The stage 3 aircraft can be as much as 15 dB quieter than a stage 2 aircraft, and it is expected that only stage 3 aircraft will be allowed at major airports by the year 2000 (Stephens and Crazier, 1996). Other countries have followed the U.S. lead to restrict the earlier aircraft from landing at their airports. Thus this program has helped control aircraft noise worldwide.

New Technology

The ability to control noise can be enhanced by technological breakthroughs. Perhaps the most important achievement recently has been noise cancellation. The advent of the microchip has allowed development of feasible active-noise-control devices in which the noise is measured and a canceling signal produced. These devices work best for noise signals below 1000 Hz, and they have proved effective for various low-frequency noise sources such as exhaust systems. Where the active-noise-control device cannot directly reduce the noise, such as rotor noise from a helicopter, the device can be placed in a hearing protector. Noise canceling earmuffs have indeed proved effective for helicopter crews, as well as for anyone else in noise that is dominated by low frequency sound.

Another recent development is the recognition and increased use of "sound quality". Engineers are recognizing that just reducing the intensity of product noise is not as effective as making the noise both more pleasing and less intense. The concept of making noise more acceptable by use of "listener panels" or other techniques cannot but help to improve our acoustic environment.

SUMMARY

In summary, the battle against environmental noise will probably never be completely won, but progress has been and will continue to be made. The need for some governmental group to provide leadership will remain necessary. In addition the general public must increase their awareness that noise can be and should be controlled.

REFERENCES

ACGIH (American Conference of Governmental Industrial Hygienists). 1999. TLVs and BEIs. Cincinnati, OH.

ANSI (American National Standards Institute). 1996. *American National Standard Specification for Audiometers. ANSI S3.6-1996.* New York: ANSI.

ANSI (American National Standards Institute). 1986. *American National Standard for Rating Noise with Respect to Speech Interference. ANSI S3.14-1977 (R 1986).* New York: ANSI.

ANSI (American National Standards Institute). 1992. *American National Standard Procedure for the Computation of Loudness of Noise. ANSI S3.4-1980 (R 1992).* New York: ANSI.

ANSI (American National Standards Institute). 1992. *American National Standard Quantities and Procedures for Description and Measurement of Environmental Sound, Part 1: Measurement of Long-Term, Wide-Area Sound. ANSI S12.9-1992/Part 2.* New York: ANSI.

ANSI (American National Standards Institute). 1993. *American National Standard Quantities and Procedures for Description and Measurement of Environmental Sound, Part 1. ANSI S12.9-1988/Part 1 (R 1993).* New York: ANSI.

ANSI (American National Standards Institute). 1993. *American National Standard Quantities and Procedures for Description and Measurement of Environmental Sound, Part 3: Short-Term Measurements with an Observer Present. ANSII S12.9-1993/Part 3.* New York: ANSI.

ANSI (American National Standards Institute). 1994. *American National Standard Acoustical Terminology. ANSI S.1-1994.* New York: ANSI.

ANSI (American National Standards Institute). 1994. *American National Standard Specification for Acoustical Calibrators. ANSI S1.40-1984 (R 1994).* New York: ANSI.

ANSI (American National Standards Institute). 1995. *American National Standard Criteria for Evaluating Room Noise. ANSI S12.2-1995.* New York: ANSI.

ANSI (American National Standards Institute). 1995. *American National Standard Measurement of Sound Pressure Levels in Air. ANSI S1.40-1984 (R 1994).* New York: ANSI.

ANSI (American National Standards Institute). 1996. *American National Standard Quantities and Procedures for Description and Measurement of Environmental Sound. Part 4: Noise Assessment and Prediction of Long-Term Community Response.* New York: ANSI.

ANSI (American National Standards Institute). 1996. *American National Standard Determination of Occupational Noise Exposure and Estimation of Noise-Induced Hearing Impairment. ANSI S3.44-1996.* New York: ANSI.

ANSI (American National Standards Institute). 1996. *American National Standard Sound Level Descriptors for Determination of Compatible Land Use. ANSI S12.40-1990 (R 1996) (Revision of ANSI S3.23-1980).* New York: ANSI.

ANSI (American National Standards Institute). 1996. *American National Standard Specification for Audiometers. ANSI S3.6-1996.* New York: ANSI.

ANSI (American National Standards Institute). 1996. *American National Standard Measurement of Occupational Noise Exposure. ANSI S12.19-1996.* New York: ANSI.

Brooks, B. M., T. J. DuBois, G. C. Maling, and L. C. Sutherland. 1996. A global vision for the noise control market place. *Noise Control Eng. J.* 44: 153–160.

EPA (U. S. Environmental Protection Agency). 1974. Information on levels of environmental noise requisite to protect the public health and welfare with an adequate margin of safety. EPA 550/9-74-004. Washington, DC.

FICON (Federal Interagency Committee on Noise). 1992. *Final Report: Airport Noise Assessment Methodologies and Metrics.* Washington, DC: FICON.

IEC (International Electrotechnical Commission). 1985. *Integrating-Averaging Sound Level Meters. IEC 804.* New York: IEC.

ISO (International Organization for Standardization). 1990. *Acoustics: Determination of Occupational Noise Exposure and Estimate of Noise-Induced Hearing Impariment. ISO 1999.2.* Geneva: ISO.

Johnson, D. L. 1997. Blast overpressure studies. Task Order 1: Firing from a bunker simulator study. Task Order 4: Nonlinear plug study. Final report contract DAMD17-93-C-3101, submitted to U.S. Army Medical Research and Materiel Command, Fort Detrick, Frederick, MD.

Lenhart, M. L., Skeilett, R., Wang, P. and Clarke, A. M. 1991. Human ultrasonic speech preception. *Science* 253: 82–85.

Nixon, C. W., and D. L. Johnson. 1973. Infrasound and Hearing. *Proc. International Conference on Noise as a Public Health Hazard, Dubrovnik, Yugoslavia, May 1973*, pp 329–347. EPA Document 550/9-73-008.

Pearsons, K. i. 1996. Recent field studies in the United States involving the disturbance of sleep from aircraft noise. *Proceedings of Internoise 96, Liverpool, Eng.* Inst. Noise Control Eng., pp. 2271–2275.

Fidell, S., D. S. Barber, and T. J. Schultz, 1991. Updating of dosage-effect relationship for the prevalence of annoyance due to general transportation noise. *J. Acoust. Soc. Am.* (89): 221–233.

Finegold, L. S., C. S. Harris, and H. E. vonGierke. 1994. Community annoyance and sleep disturbance: Updated criteria for assessing the impacts of general transportation noise on people. *Noise Control Eng. J.* 42(1): 25–30.

Galloway, W. J., K. Eldred, and M. A. Simpson. 1974. Population distribution of the United States as a function of outdoor noise level, prepared by Bolt, Beranek, and Newman (EPA-550/0-74-009) for U.S. EPA, Washington, D.C.

Pearsons, K. D., Barber, B. Tabachnic, and S. Fidell. 1995. Predicting noise-induced sleep disturbance, *J. Acoust. Soc. Am.*, 97: 331–338.

Schomer, P. D. 1996. 25 years of progress in noise standardization. *Noise Control Eng. J.* 44: 141–148.

Schultz, T. J. 1978. Synthesis of social surveys on noise annoyance. *J. Acoust. Soc. Am.* 64: 377–405.

Shaw, E. A. G. 1996. Noise environments outdoors and the effects of community noise exposure. *Noise Control Eng. J.* 44: 109–119.

Smoorenburg, G. F. 1991. Speech reception in quiet and in noisy conditions by individuals with noise-induced hearing loss in to their tone audiogram. *J. Acoust. Soc. Am.* 91: 421–437.

Stephens, D. G., and F. W. Cazier Jr. 1996. NASA noise reduction program for advanced subsonic transports. *Noise Control Eng. J.* 44: 135–140.

Suter, A. H. 1978. The ability of mildly hearing-impaired individuals to discriminate speech in noise. U. S. Environmental Protection Agency. EPA 550/9-78-100.

von Bekesy, G. 1936. Reported in *Experiments in Hearing*, ed. E. G. Wever, pp. 257–267. New York: McGraw-Hill.

Whittle, S. J., S. J. Collins, and D. W. Robinson. 1972. The audibility of low frequency sounds. *J. Sound Vib.* 21: pp. 431–448.

Yeowart, N. S., M. Bryan, and W. Tempest. 1968. Low frequency noise thresholds. *J. Sound Vib.* 9: 447–453.

Yeowart, N.S. and M. J. Evans. 1974. Threshold of audibility for very low frequency pure tones. *J. Acoust. Soc. Am.* 55: 814–818.

20 Ozone

MORTON LIPPMANN, Ph.D.

In 1851, soon after its initial laboratory synthesis, Schonbein recognized ozone (O_3) as a powerful lung irritant (Bates, 1989). The Occupational Safety and Health Administration's permissible exposure limit (PEL) for O_3 is 100 parts per billion (ppb), equivalent to $235\,\mu g/m^3$, as a time-weighted average for 8 h/d, along with a short-term exposure limit of 300 ppb for 15 minutes (USDOL, 1989). The American Conference of Governmental Industrial Hygienists (ACGIH, 1997) threshold limit value (TLV) for occupational exposure is 100 ppb as an 8 hour time-weighted average for light work, 80 ppb for moderate work, and 50 ppb for heavy work.

Health effects among the general community were first reported among high school athletes in California, in terms of lesser performance on high-exposure days (Wayne et al., 1967). The initial primary (health-based) National Ambient Air Quality Standard (NAAQS) established by the Environmental Protection Agency (EPA) in 1971 was 0.80 ppb of total oxidant as a one hour maximum not to be exceeded more than once per year. The NAAQS was revised in 1979 to 120 ppb of O_3 as a one hour maximum not to be exceeded more than four times in three years. The revision was based on clinical studies by DeLucia and Adams (1977), showing that exercising asthmatic adults exposed for one hour to 150 ppb in a test chamber had increased cough, dyspnea, and wheezing, along with small but nonsignificant reductions in pulmonary function (U.S. EPA, 1986). A small margin of safety was applied to protect against adverse effects not yet uncovered by research and effects whose medical significance is a matter of disagreement.

EPA initiated a review of the 1979 NAAQS in 1983, and completed a Criteria Document for Ozone in 1986 and updated it in 1992 (U.S. EPA, 1992). However, the Agency did not decide to either retain the 1979 standard or promulgate a new one until it was compelled to do so by a August 1992 court order. In response, the EPA decided, in March 1993, to maintain the existing standard and to proceed as rapidly as possible with the next round of review. This expedited review was completed with the publication of both a new criteria document (U.S. EPA, 1996a) and staff paper (U.S. EPA, 1996b) in 1996. In July of 1997 the EPA administrator promulgated a revised primary O_3 NAAQS of 80 ppb as an 8 hour time-weighted average daily maximum, with no more than four annual exceedances, and averaged over three years (Federal Register 1997, 62:38762–38896). The reason for the switch from one allowable annual exceedance to four was to minimize the designation of NAAQS nonattainment in a community that was triggered by rare meteorological conditions especially conducive to O_3 formation. The goal was to have a more stable NAAQS that allowed for extremes of annual variations of weather. The switch to an 8 hour averaging time was in recognition that ambient O_3 in much of the United States has broad daily peaks, and that human responses are more closely related to total

Environmental Toxicants: Human Exposures and Their Health Effects, 2/e. Edited by Morton Lippmann.
ISBN: 0-471-29298-2 © 2000 John Wiley & Sons, Inc.

daily exposure than to brief peaks of O_3 exposure. The 1997 NAAQS represents about a 10% reduction in permissable O_3 exposure, since the 120 ppb, 1 hour average, 1 exceedance NAAQS was approximately equivalent to an 8 hour average, 4 exceedance NAAQS at a concentration a bit below 90 ppb in average stringency in the United States as a whole.

The effects of concern with respect to acute response in the population at large are reductions in lung function and increases in respiratory symptoms, airway reactivity, airway permeability, and airway inflammation. For persons with asthma, there are also increased rates of medication usage and restricted activities. Margin-of-safety considerations include (1) the influence of repetitive elicitation of such responses in the progression of chronic damage to the lung of the kinds seen in chronic exposure studies in rats and monkeys and (2) evidence from laboratory and field studies that ambient air copollutants potentiate the responses to O_3. The bases for these concerns are discussed later in this chapter.

Ozone is almost entirely a secondary air pollutant, formed in the atmosphere through a complex photochemical reaction sequence requiring reactive hydrocarbons, nitrogen dioxide (NO_2), and sunlight. It can only be controlled by reducing ambient air concentrations of hydrocarbons, NO_2, or both. Both NO and NO_2 are primary pollutants, known collectively as NO_x. In the atmosphere, NO is gradually converted to NO_2. Motor vehicles, one of the major categories of sources of hydrocarbons and NO_x, have been the target of control efforts, and major reductions ($> 90\%$) have been achieved in hydrocarbon emissions per vehicle. However, there have been major increases in vehicle miles driven. Reductions in NO_x from motor vehicles and stationary-source combustion have been much smaller. The net reduction in exposure has been modest at best, with some reductions in areas with more stringent controls, such as California, and some increases in exposure in other parts of the United States. In 1988 there were record high levels of ambient O_3 with exceedance of the 120 ppb limit in 96 communities containing over 150 million people. Since then, there has been a gradual decrease of ambient O_3 in most of the United States, as indicated in Figure 20-1.

We know a great deal about O_3 chemistry and have developed highly sophisticated O_3 air quality models (Seinfeld, 1988). Unfortunately, the models, and their applications in control strategies have clearly been inadequate in terms of community compliance with the NAAQS. We also know a great deal about some of the health effects of O_3. However, much of what we know relates to transient, apparently reversible effects that follow acute exposures lasting from 5 minutes to 6.6 hours. These effects include changes in lung capacity, flow resistance, epithelial permeability, and reactivity to bronchoactive challenges; such effects can be observed within the first few hours after the start of the exposure and may persist for many hours or days after the exposure ceases. Repetitive daily exposures over several days or weeks can exacerbate and prolong these transient effects. There has been a great deal of controversy about the health significance of such effects and whether such effects are sufficiently adverse to serve as a basis for the O_3 NAAQS (Lippmann, 1988, 1991, 1993).

Decrements in respiratory function such as forced vital capacity (FVC) and forced expiratory volume in the first second of a vital capacity maneuver (FEV_1) fall into the category where adversity begins at some specific level of pollutant-associated change. However, there are clear differences of opinion on what the threshold of adversity ought to be. Some degree of consensus was achieved on this issue at public meetings of the Clean Air Scientific Advisory Committee (CASAC) that reviewed draft Staff Papers prepared by the EPA Office of Air Quality Planning and Standards (OAQPS) as part of the process by which EPA prepares new and revised NAAQS. The 1989 Staff Paper (U.S. EPA, 1989) included a table (Table 20-1) in which the responses were categorized as mild, moderate, severe, and incapacitating. The judgment was that mild responses are not adverse, but the

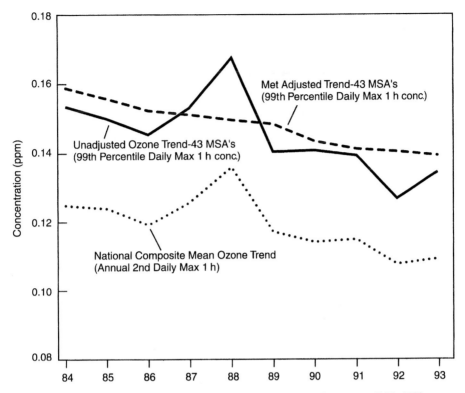

Figure 20-1   Trend of ozone concentrations in U.S. metropolitan areas, 1984–1993.

other categories were. The 1989 Staff Paper made the explicit distinction that more than one response had to be in the moderate or greater range to cross the threshold for adversity, except as it applies to children since children do not normally exhibit symptoms when exposed to O_3 that affects their lung function to a similar degree to that seen in symptomatic adults. The 10% threshold applied to asthmatic individuals. Thus protection of the more sensitive members of the population from a 10% change would ensure that the bulk of the population would have fewer responses.

The 1996 O_3 Staff Paper (U.S. EPA, 1996b) made numerous elaborations on these gradations, and focused them on persons with impaired respiratory symptoms because NAAQS are generally set to protect sensitive subgroups of the population. These more elaborate gradations are presented in Tables 20-2 and 20-3 for healthy persons and persons with impaired respiratory symptoms, respectively.

With respect to adversity, the 1996 Staff Paper concluded that responses listed as large or severe were clearly adverse. For responses listed as moderate, it was concluded that they could be considered adverse if there were repetitive exposures.

Although we know a great deal about the transient effects following single exposures to O_3, our current knowledge about the chronic health effects of O_3 is much less complete. As discussed in the latter part of this chapter, the chronic effects include alterations in lung function or structure. Such effects may result from cumulative damage and/or from the side effects of adaptive responses to repetitive daily or intermittent exposures. This review does not discuss the effects of O_3 or its metabolites on nonrespiratory tissues. It also does not discuss the health effects of increased ultraviolet radiation resulting from the depletion of stratospheric O_3.

TABLE 20-1   Gradation of Individual Physiological Response to Acute O$_3$ Exposure

	Gradation of response			
	Mild	Moderate	Severe	Incapacitating
Change in spirometry FEV1, FVC	5–10%	10–20%	20–40%	>40%
Duration of effect	Complete recovery in <30 min	Complete recovery in <6 h	Complete recovery in 24 h	Recovery in >24 h
Symptoms	Mild to moderate cough	Mild to moderate cough, pain on deep inspiration, shortness of breath	Repeated cough, moderate to severe pain on deep inspiration, shortness of breath, breathing distress	Severe cough, pain on deep inspiration, shortness of breath, obvious distress
Limitation of activity	None	Few individuals choose to discontinue activity	Some individuals choose to discontinue activity	Many individuals choose to discontinue activity

Source: U.S. EPA (1989).

TABLE 20-2 Gradation of Individual Responses to Short-Term Ozone Exposure in Healthy Persons

Functional Response	None	Small	Moderate	Large
FEV$_1$	Within normal range ($\pm 3\%$)	Decrements of 3% to $\leq 10\%$	Decrements of $> 10\%$ but $< 20\%$	Decrements of $\geq 20\%$
Nonspecific bronchial responsiveness	Within normal range	Increases of $<100\%$	Increases of $\leq 300\%$	Increases of $> 300\%$
Duration of response	None	$<4\,$h	>4 but $\leq 24\,$h	$>24\,$h
Symptomatic Response	Normal	Mild	Moderate	Severe
Cough	Infrequent cough	Cough with deep breath	Frequent spontaneous cough	Persistent uncontrollable cough
Chest pain	None	Discomfort just noticeable on exercise or deep breath	Marked discomfort on exercise or deep breath	Severe discomfort on exercise or deep breath
Duration of response	None	$<4\,$h	>4 but $\leq 24\,$h	$>24\,$h
Impact of Various Functional and/or Symptomatic Responses	Normal Functional and/or Symptomatic Responses	Small Functional and/or Mild Symptomatic Responses	Moderate Functional and/or Symptomatic Responses	Large Functional and/or Severe Symptomatic Responses
Interference with normal activity	None	None	A few sensitive individuals likely to limit activity	Many sensitive individuals likely to limit activity

Source: U.S. EPA (1996b).

TABLE 20-3 Gradation of Individual Responses to Short-Term Ozone Exposure in Persons with Impaired Respiratory Systems

Functional Response	None	Small	Moderate	Large
FEV_1 change	Decrements of <3%	Decrements of 3% to ≤10%	Decrements of >10% but <20%	Decrements of ≥20%
Nonspecific bronchial responsiveness	Within normal range	Increases of <100%	Increases of ≤300%	Increases of >300%
Airway resistance (SR_{aw})	Within normal range (±20%)	SR_{aw} increased <100%	SR_{aw} increased up to 200% or up to 15 cm H_2O/s >4 but ≤24 h	SR_{aw} increased >200% or more than 15 cm H_2O/s >24 h
Duration of response	None	<4 h	>4 but ≤24 h	>24 h
Symptomatic Response	Normal	Mild	Moderate	Severe
Wheeze	None	With otherwise normal breathing	With shortness of breath	Persistent with shortness of breath
Cough	Infrequent cough	Cough with deep breath	Frequent spontaneous cough	Persistent uncontrollable cough
Chest pain	None	Discomfort just noticeable on exercise or deep breath <4 h	Marked discomfort on exercise or deep breath >4 but ≤24 h	Severe discomfort on exercise or deep breath >24 h
Duration of response	None	<4 h	>4 but ≤24 h	>24 h
Impact of Various Functional and/or Symptomatic Responses	Normal Functional and/or Symptomatic Responses	Small Functional and/or Mild Symptomatic Responses	Moderate Functional and/or Symptomatic Responses	Large Functional and/or Severe Symptomatic Responses
Interference with normal activity	None	Few individuals likely to limit activity	Many individuals likely to limit activity	Most individuals likely to limit activity
Medical treatment/self medication	No change	Normal medication as needed	Increased frequency or additional medication use	Increased likelihood of physician or ER visit

Source: U.S. EPA (1996b).

660

This chapter provides a critical review of the health effects data and their significance to public health in relation to the populations exposed. The judgments made have been influenced by my participation in public CASAC reviews of EPA documents, but they differ in some cases from those of the EPA and of others on the CASAC panels.

BACKGROUND

Sources and Distribution of O_3 in Ambient Air

Ozone in ambient air is attributable to several different sources. One is the intrusion of stratospheric O_3, especially in the spring when the stratospheric-tropospheric air exchange is greatest. The other sources are driven by complex photochemical reaction sequences requiring input of organic vapors, nitrogen oxides (NO_x), and actinic radiation. Reactive organic vapors such as olefinic hydrocarbons, formaldehyde, and m-xylene, which are largely products of anthropogenic activities, are highly efficient contributors to O_3 formation. On the other hand, methane, a major product of natural biogenic decay and a relatively nonreactive hydrocarbon, can also contribute to O_3 formation. Actually the background concentration of methane has been rising throughout this century as a result of increasingly intensive agriculture and animal husbandry. The coincident increase in continental background O_3, from 10 to 20 ppb (Altshuller, 1987) to the current level of about 40 ppb, may be due to the rising background of both methane and NO_x. The NO_x concentrations have grown continuously throughout the twentieth century as fossil fuel usage has increased. The increase in NO_x may also account for a greater rate of O_3 formation by photochemical reactions with isoprene and terpenes emitted by trees.

As noted by Altshuller (1987), the role of NO_x in tropospheric O_3 formation is especially critical. Unless NO_x concentrations exceed about 0.02 to 0.03 ppb, photochemical O_3 loss exceeds photochemical O_3 production. There are remote regions of the troposphere where the NO_x concentrations may be below such values. On the other hand, NO_x concentrations in the rural planetary boundary layer over the United States usually exceed 1 ppb. He also noted that NO_x concentrations of 5 to 10 ppb are typical of rural areas within more heavily populated areas in the United States and western Europe. Empirical estimates based on O_3 and NO_x measurements at a site at 3 km elevation, Niwot Ridge, Colorado, indicate in summer that 17 ± 3 ppb of O_3 is formed per 1 ppb of NO_x at NO_x concentrations below 1 ppb. At lower elevation rural sites elsewhere in the United States, where NO_x concentrations were within the 1 to 10 ppb range, 5 to 7 ppb of O_3 was estimated to be formed per 1 ppb of NO_x reacted.

Since O_3 is highly reactive, its concentration at ground level drops markedly in the evening. On the other hand, it can remain at elevated concentrations in the ambient air above the mixing layer. This elevated reservoir of O_3 can then contribute to elevated ground level O_3 on the following day as air mixing increases. This contributes to multiday summer episode exposures. Rao (1988) has shown that the likelihood of O_3 >80 ppb continuing for three days or longer, once it has been in existance for one day, is high in the northeastern United States. This is illustrated in Figure 20-2 for a typical year (1981) and a relatively high O_3 exposure year (1983).

The peak concentrations of O_3 reached during a specific day at a specific location are determined largely by the baseline level in the air aloft, the photochemical production rate during the day, and the concentration of O_3 scavenging chemicals such as nitric oxide (NO) and ethylene. The peak O_3 concentration depends on the ambient ratio of reactive organic gases (ROG) to NO_x concentrations. As noted by Seinfeld (1988), when [ROG]/[NO_x] is approximately 5 to 6, the two species have about an equal chance of reacting with hydroxy radical (OH). If this ratio is much larger than 5 to 6, there is a shortage of NO that

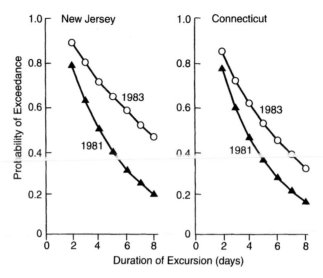

Figure 20-2 Frequency functions of duration of O_3 concentrations in excess of 80 ppb over New Jersey and Connecticut for two years. From Rao (1988).

can be oxidized to NO_2, and O_3 production is controlled by the amount of NO_x available. In this region, decreasing NO_x leads to a decrease in the peak O_3. On the other hand, when $[ROG]/[NO_x]$ is on the order of 5 or less, the ready availability of NO_x make O_3 formation dependent on ROG. NO will scavenge O_3 faster than it reacts with RO_2, and also NO_2 will react with OH to give nitric acid. Decreasing NO_x can lead to an increase in peak O_3 as the efficiency of O_3 formation increases.

The daily formation of O_3, in the absence of a substantial baseline level from the air aloft or upwind, leads to a relatively sharp daily peak in concentration, with a major part of the effective exposure taking place over a relatively few hours. In recent years this type of exposure pattern has become relatively rare. In heavily populated areas, such as the eastern United States and western Europe, we typically have a daily plateau of exposure after about 10 a.m. in which the maximum 8 hour exposure is about 90% of the maximum 1 hour exposure (Rombout et al., 1986). This type of exposure pattern is consistent with the hypothesis that relatively little of the exposure on a typical high exposure summer day is attributable to local sources or amenable to local source control. Rather, the local generation of O_3 represents a bump on a broad daily hump arising from a series of upwind sources and photochemistry. The size of the bump depends on the concentration of precursor reactants in the incoming air and the local increments of reactants. The broad humps can be attributed to the sum of the contributions of stratospheric O_3 injections and O_3 formed upwind and retained aloft for one or many days.

The nature of contemporary O_3 exposure is illustrated for a rural area of western Massachusetts in Figure 20-3, showing both locally generated midday peaks and late afternoon peaks from upwind population centers superimposed on a broad daily plateau (Lioy and Dyba, 1989). It clearly shows that the O_3 exposure problem affects broad areas of the country and that it is not just an urban problem as widely believed.

Ozone Exposures and Dosimetry

For O_3, the only significant exposure route is inhalation, and exposure can be defined as the concentration at the nose and mouth. There have been few personal measurements of O_3,

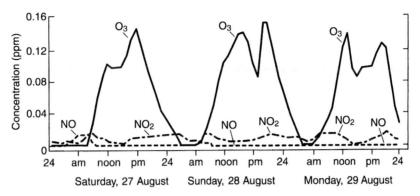

Figure 20-3   Three day sequence of hourly O_3 concentrations at Montague, MA SURE station showing locally generated midday peaks and long-range-transport late peaks. From EPA (1986).

and it is generally assumed that the concentrations we breathe are the same as those measured at central monitoring sites. However, this assumption has limited validity. For the time we spend outdoors, we must recognize that local concentrations are reduced in the vicinity of heavy vehicular traffic due to scavenging by NO. On the other hand, less trafficked areas downwind of the monitor may have a higher O_3 concentration because of the enrichment of the air mass with motor vehicle exhaust precursor chemicals and active photochemistry. Thus outdoor O_3 concentrations can be either higher or lower than those measured at monitoring sites.

Indoor concentrations of O_3 are almost always substantially lower than those outdoors because of efficient scavenging by indoor surfaces and the lack of indoor sources. The only common indoor sources are copying machines and electrostatic air cleaners. Since most people spend more than 80% of their time indoors, their O_3 exposures are much lower than estimates based on outdoor concentrations.

Ozone exposures are only one determinant of O_3 dose. Dose is also determined by the volumes of air inhaled and the pattern of uptake of O_3 molecules along the respiratory tract. When people work or exercise outdoors and increase their rate of ventilation, the contribution of outdoor exposure to total dose of O_3 becomes an even greater determinant of total O_3 dose. The dose to target tissues in the respiratory acini (the region from the terminal bronchioles through the alveolar ducts) increases more with exercise than does total respiratory tract dose, since O_3 penetration increases with tidal volume and flow rate.

Gerrity et al. (1988) measured the efficiency of O_3 removal from inspired air by the extrathoracic and intrathoracic airways in 18 healthy, nonsmoking, young male volunteers. Removal efficiencies were measured at O_3 concentrations of 100, 200, and 400 ppb for nose only, mouth only, and oronasal breathing at 12 and 24 breaths/min. The mean extrathoracic removal efficiency for all measurements was $39.6 \pm 0.7\%$, and the mean intrathoracic removal efficiency was $91.0 \pm 0.5\%$. Although significant effects of concentration, breathing frequency, and mode of breathing on removal efficiency were found, they were relatively small.

Gerrity et al. (1995) followed up their O_3 uptake studies using a bronchoscope to sample air at various lung depths in 10 healthy nonsmokers. The distal end of a bronchoscope was sequentially positioned at the bronchus intermedius (BI), main carina (CAR), upper trachea, and above the vocal cords. O_3 concentration was measured continuously at each site using a rapid-responding O_3 analyzer. The subjects breathed through a mouthpiece at 12 breaths/min. Integration of the product of the flow and O_3 concentrations during inspiration and expiration provided the O_3 mass passing each anatomic location during each phase of respiration. On inspiration the uptake efficiencies of O_3 by structures between the mouth and each location were 0.176 ± 0.037 (SE), 0.271 ± 0.024, 0.355 ± 0.030, and 0.325 ± 0.031 for above the vocal cords, upper trachea, CAR, and BI, respectively. A significant effect of location on uptake was found by analysis of variance.

The tissues within the respiratory acini of humans, rabbits, guinea pigs, and rats receive the highest local dose from inhaled O_3 according to the models developed by Miller and colleagues (Miller et al., 1978b; Overton and Miller, 1987; Hatch et al., 1989), with the dose in humans being about twice that in rats for the same exposure (Gerrity and Wiester, 1987) and children having somewhat greater doses than adult humans (Overton and Graham, 1989). This comparative dosimetry is consistent with the greater effects of O_3 on lung function seen in humans than in rats (Costa et al., 1989).

Populations of Concern

In general, the NAAQS have been established to protect against adverse health effects in the most sensitive subpopulation that is identifiable (Lippmann, 1987). For example, cardiovascular patients were of paramount concern in establishing the NAAQS for carbon monoxide (CO), which binds to hemoglobin and further reduces their already limited capacity to oxygenate the blood. Asthmatics were of special concern in establishing the sulfur dioxide (SO_2) NAAQS because the concentrations required to produce comparable levels of bronchoconstriction were about an order of magnitude lower than for normal people and because of the potential for a disabling or fatal bronchospasm being initiated by a transient high concentration of SO_2.

In the case of O_3, no special functional responsiveness has yet been clearly demonstrated among the potentially more sensitive groups with preexisting disease (Lippmann, 1989a, 1993). Thus consideration is being given to healthy people who exercise regularly outdoors as a primary population of concern on the basis of their higher O_3 exposures and doses. The EPA Staff Papers (U.S. EPA, 1989, 1996b) have also identified people with asthma as a population of concern on the basis of reports of symptomatic responses, increased rates of visits to clinics, and hospital admissions at very low ambient concentrations.

Responses of Concern

As has been previously noted, O_3 in ambient air has been associated with a variety of transient effects on the respiratory airways. Among the best documented of these changes is a dose-related decrement in indexes of forced expiratory flow capacity, which is reproducible in individuals and highly variable among the population. Increased rates of symptoms, clinic visits, and hospital admissions are other responses of concern with respect to acute exposures.

More persistent physiological decrements associated with structural alterations of lung airways could also be considered to be adverse effects if they occurred in humans as a result of repetitive O_3 exposures. Although human evidence is currently lacking, such effects have been produced in laboratory animals following chronic exposures. Thus these effects are also of concern for human populations with high levels of chronic exposure (Lippmann, 1989a, 1993).

Study Options

In the discussion of the health effects data base that follows, it will help to keep things in perspective if we can appreciate the strengths and limitations of the various kinds of studies that generated the data.

Controlled Human Exposures

There is a very large data base from studies in which selected human volunteers were exposed to O_3 in purified lab air for specific time intervals. Most studies involve a series of such exposures in random order in which there are exposures at one or more concentrations as well as a sham exposure to purified air. Many of them involved prescribed periods and intensities of exercise during the exposure interval. The most commonly measured effects were changes in forced expiratory flow rates and volumes and / or changes in airway resistance and compliance (Lippmann, 1988; U.S. EPA, 1986, 1996a).

A broad variety of other function tests require the inhalation of special breathing mixtures and hence more elaborate controls and protocol reviews. These include the inhalation of (1) a single breath of pure oxygen (O_2) for the nitrogen washout test of small airway function (Buist and Ross, 1973), (2) 0.3% CO to determine diffusing capacity at the alveolocapillary membrane (Crapo, 1986), and (3) low-density inert gases such as helium (He) and high-density gases such as sulfur hexafluoride (SF_6) to measure inhomogeneities in flow distribution (Scott and Van Liew, 1983). Large-scale spatial inhomogeneities in ventilation can be detected using radioactive xenon (Xe) and external γ-emission imaging equipment such as the Anger camera (Robertson et al., 1969).

Functional tests made before and after administration of bronchoactive agents can also be of diagnostic value. These can include bronchodilators such as isoproterenol, epinephrine, and atropine to measure reversible bronchoconstriction. They also include bronchoconstrictors such as histamine, carbachol, methacholine, cold air, and sulfur dioxide to detect airway hyperresponsiveness.

Other tests of demonstrated utility and / or with potential for supplying important diagnostic information can also be applied. The permeability of the respiratory epithelium can be determined from the externally measured rate of clearance from the lung of γ-emitting [^{99m}Tc] tagged diethylenetriaminepentaacetate (DTPA), which is inhaled as a droplet aerosol (Oberdorster et al., 1986).

Inert, insoluble, nonhygroscopic, γ-tagged aerosols can be used to measure the regional deposition and clearance rates for inhaled particles. Thoracic retention of such aerosols after one day is considered to represent deposition in the nonciliated alveolar lung spaces, while the difference between the retention measured immediately after the particle inhalation and that at one day represents the aerosol that deposited on the conductive airways of the tracheobronchial tree (Lippmann, 1977). By appropriate control of particle size and respiratory parameters, the deposition efficiency data can be used to characterize airway obstruction (Chan and Lippmann, 1980). The rate and pattern of mucociliary particle clearance can be determined from serial measurements of thoracic retention during the first day, and the much slower rate of particle clearance from the gas-exchange region can be determined from serial retention measurements made after the first day (Albert et al., 1969).

The advantages of controlled human exposure studies are (1) the opportunity to carefully select and characterize the subjects, whether they are healthy normals, atopics and asthmatics, smokers, and so forth; (2) the willingness and ability of most volunteer subjects to perform various levels and durations of exercise during the exposures; (3) the ability to deliver and monitor the preselected challenge atmospheres during the exposure; (4) the ability of the subjects to reproducibly perform respiratory maneuvers required for some functional assays affected by the exposures and to provide information on mild symptomatic responses; and (5) avoidance of the need to make interspecies extrapolations in evaluating human exposure–response relationships.

The limitations of controlled human exposures are as follows: (1) Ethical constraints limit the challenges and effects assays that can be performed. In effect, we are limited to challenges that produce only transient functional changes. The most invasive assay that has been used involves analyses of the contents of lung lavage. (2) The numbers of repetitive challenges and assays are limited by subject tolerance and cooperation. (3) The number of subjects that can be studied is limited by the generally large costs of performing the studies and / or by the availability of sufficient numbers of subjects with the desired characteristics.

In summary, controlled human exposure studies are most useful for studying the nature and extent of transient functional changes resulting from one or a few brief controlled exposures. They can provide information on chronic pollutant effects only to the extent that prior exposures affect the transient response to single exposure challenges. Furthermore interpretation of the results of such tests is limited by our generally inadequate ability to characterize the nature and / or magnitude of the prior chronic exposures.

Natural Human Exposures

There is a substantial data base emerging from studies in my laboratory of the responses of natural populations to acute exposures to air pollutants (Lippmann et al., 1989b; Spektor et al., 1991; Thurston et al., 1997). Studying natural populations for evidence of acute health effects associated with exposures to ambient air pollutants is a challenging task. Among the more difficult challenges are (1) identifying an accessible population at risk whose relevant exposures can be defined and adequately characterized, (2) specifying measurable indexes of responses that may be expected to occur as a result of the exposures of interest, (3) collecting an adequate amount of suitable quality-assured data on exposure and responses at times when exposures of magnitudes sufficient to elicit measurable responses actually occur, and (4) collecting sufficient data on identifiable host characteristics and environmental exposures to other agents that may influence the response variables and confound any of the hypothesized pollutant exposure–response relationships that may be present. In addition one must also account for the usual operational problems encountered in performing population studies, especially studies in the field, such as maintaining (1) the motivation and skills of the field personnel for collecting reliable data, (2) the cooperation of the subjects in producing reliable data, and (3) access to sufficient numbers of subjects with the preselected characteristics in each category as may be needed.

The basic design premise in each of the NYU field studies was to maximize the signal-to-noise ratio for the pollutant exposure versus response relationships. The noise on the response side of the relationships has been the focus of much work by others, and guidance on these aspects is available from the American Thoracic Society (1985). Accordingly our focus was primarily on the reduction of the noise in the exposure variables. The summer haze is regional in scale and enriched in secondary air pollutants such as O_3 and sulfuric acid (H_2SO_4), both of which form gradually during daylight hours in air masses containing diluted primary pollutants transported over long distances from industrial, power plant, and motor vehicle sources, especially SO_2, nitrogen dioxide (NO_2), and hydrocarbons (HC). We therefore studied populations in communities remote from local sources of air pollution, primarily in wooded regions where ammonia (NH_3) sources, which would rapidly neutralize the H_2SO_4, would also be minimal.

For our studies in 1980 (Lippmann et al., 1983), 1982 (Lioy et al., 1985), 1984 (Spektor et al., 1988a), 1988 (Spektor et al., 1991) and 1991–93 (Thurston et al., 1997), we selected populations of children attending summer camp programs for three main reasons: (1) cigarette smoking and occupational exposure to lung irritants would not be confounding factors, (2) the program of camp activities insured that they would be out of doors and physically active during the daytime periods when O_3 and H_2SO_4 exposures would be highest, and (3) the cooperation of the camp staff provided effective access to the children on a daily basis for the administration of functional tests and symptom questionnaires. Exposures to O_3 and H_2SO_4 are almost always higher outdoors than indoors, and as regional-scale secondary pollutants, their concentrations do not vary greatly from site to site within the camp's activity areas or from those measured at nearby samplers or monitors. In addition there was little variation of activity level among the children in the camp program.

Our 1985 summer study (Spektor et al., 1988b) on the effects of the summer haze pollutants on respiratory function in healthy nonsmoking adults engaged in a regular program of outdoor exercise had a similar absence of confounding exposure factors as well as similar exposures to the ambient secondary air pollutants. Each of the adult volunteers maintained a constant daily level and duration of exercise, but they differed widely from one to another in these important variables. This increased the variability of the response among the population but also provided a means of studying the influence of these variables on the responses.

For studies of acute responses to the inhalation of secondary air pollutants, which are distributed relatively uniformly over large geographic areas, it is not possible to identify a nonexposed or control population. On the other hand, the concentrations of the secondary pollutants have large temporal variations. There are both diurnal variations, with peak concentrations generally occurring in the afternoon, and day-to-day variations in concentration associated with the trajectory of the air mass over pollutant precursor source areas, atmospheric stability, intensity of incident solar radiation, temperature, and humidity. Thus the volunteer subjects are exposed to different concentration profiles each day. By using repetitive measures of response, one can correlate variations in response with variations in exposure within the group.

In summary, natural human exposure studies are most useful for studying the magnitude and extent of the acute responses to naturally occurring pollutants among people engaged in normal outdoor recreational activities. They provide little information on the possible influence of prior chronic exposures on acute responses to the exposure of the day or immediately preceding days. Also, since the ambient mixture contains varying amounts of a variety of pollutants, it may sometimes be difficult to apportion the responses to one or more of the pollutants or to other, uncontrolled variables such as temperature, humidity, and each individual's precise level of exercise or ventilation.

Population-Based Studies of Chronic Health Effects

Since neither controlled human exposure studies in the laboratory nor natural human exposure studies in the field can provide any direct information on chronic effects of prolonged human exposures to O_3, the only way to get such information is to use the conventional epidemiological approach of comparing data on function, symptom frequency, lost activity days, hospital admissions, clinic visits, medical diagnoses, and so on, with estimates of chronic exposure intensity. There are many factors confounding the effects indexes of concern in such studies. The characteristics of the populations under study are highly variable in terms of age, sex, smoking history, cohabitation with smokers, health status, disease history, occupational exposures, hobby activities that generate air pollutants, use of unvented stoves and heaters at home, and the like. Also their exposures to outdoor pollutants such as O_3 are difficult to quantitate and are influenced by their proximity to the monitor that provides their exposure index, the time they spend outdoors, and whether this includes hours when O_3 is high as well as the amount and duration of vigorous exercise during periods of high exposure.

Because of the large number of possible confounders and the difficulty of properly classifying exposures, very large populations must be studied in order to find significant associations between exposures and effects. Any statistically significant effects that are attributed to O_3 would tend to be underestimated because of the influence of the confounders. Alternatively, they could be spurious if the effects are really caused by variables that are colinear with O_3.

In summary, epidemiological studies offer the prospect of establishing chronic health effects of long-term O_3 exposure in relevant populations and offer the possibility that the analyses can show the influence of other environmental factors on responses to O_3 exposure. On the other hand, the strengths of any of the associations may be difficult to establish because of the complications introduced by uncontrolled cofactors that may confound or obscure the underlying causal factors.

Controlled Exposures of Laboratory Animals

The most convenient and efficient way to study mechanisms and patterns of response to inhaled O_3, and of the influence of other pollutants and stresses on these responses is by controlled exposures of laboratory animals. One can study the transient functional responses to acute exposures and establish the differences in response among different animal species and between them and humans similarly exposed. One can also look for responses that require highly invasive procedures or serial sacrifice and gain information that cannot be obtained from studies on human volunteers. Finally one can use long-term exposure protocols to study cumulative responses and the pathogenesis of chronic disease in animals. Other advantages of studies on animals are the ability to examine the presence of and basis for variations in response that are related to age, sex, species, strain, genetic markers, nutrition, the presence of other pollutants, and so on. As in controlled human exposure studies, the concentrations and duration of the exposure can be tightly controlled, as can the presence or absence of other pollutants and environmental variables. Another important advantage of controlled animal studies is that relatively large numbers of individuals can be simultaneously exposed, creating the possibility of detecting responses that only affect a limited fraction of the population.

Among the significant limitations to the use of exposure–response data from animal studies in human risk assessments is our quite limited ability to interpret the animal responses in relation to likely responses in humans who might be exposed to the same or lower levels. Controlled chronic exposure protocols can be very labor intensive and expensive, which tends to limit the number of variables that can effectively be examined in any given study.

Controlled Exposures In vitro

For studies focused on the biochemical mechanisms of epithelial cells' responses to O_3, cells can be harvested from humans or animals and exposed to O_3 in vitro. Techniques have been developed for reasonably realistic O_3 exposures to cells and cell cultures in vitro (Valentine, 1985) for characterizing the release of eicosanoids from such cells (Leikauf et al., 1988) and for examining cell function (Driscoll et al., 1987). The main advantage of in vitro studies is their efficiency and relatively low cost. Interspecies comparisons of cellular response can often be made, and relatively few animals can provide much study material. However, our ability to interpret the results of in vitro assays in relation to likely effects in humans in vivo is limited, even when the studies are done with human cells. The cellular response in vitro may differ from that of the same cells in vivo, and the in vivo controls on cellular metabolism and function, which may play a significant role in the overall response, are absent.

EFFECTS OF SINGLE EXPOSURES TO OZONE

There has been a very large, and perhaps excessive, focus on the health effects of a single day's maximum hourly exposure to ambient O_3. The 1971 and 1979 NAAQS for photochemical oxidants were based on the maximum 1 hour concentrations as the relevant index of exposure, and this in turn focused most of the earlier clinical research on exposure protocols involving either 1 or 2 hours of exposure. However, effects can be produced with exposures as short as 5 minutes (Fouke et al., 1988) and effects can become progressively larger as exposures at a given concentration are extended out to 6.6 hours (Folinsbee et al., 1988, 1994; Horstman et al., 1990). This section examines the complex of effects that result from single exposures of < 8 hours duration. The effects that successive days of exposure or long-term chronic exposures produce are discussed later in this chapter.

Respiratory Mechanical Function Responses

There are more data on respiratory function responses than on any of the other coincident responses to short-term O_3 inhalation. Such functional responses can be obtained with noninvasive, readily performed protocols and can be detected at levels of exposure as low as or lower than any of the other well established assays. The major debate about very small but statistically significant decrements in function from such studies is how to interpret their health significance (Lippmann, 1988).

It is well established that the inhalation of O_3 causes concentration-dependent mean decrements in exhaled volumes and flow rates during forced expiratory maneuvers, and that the mean decrements increase with increasing depth of breathing (Hazucha, 1987). There is a wide range of reproducible responsiveness among healthy subjects (McDonnell et al., 1985a; Weinmann et al., 1995; Frampton et al., 1997), and functional responsiveness to O_3 is no greater, and usually lower, among cigarette smokers (Kagawa, 1984; Shephard et al., 1983; Frampton et al., 1997), older adults (Drechsler-Parks et al., 1987; Reisenauer et al., 1988; McDonnell et al., 1993, 1995), asthmatics (Koenig et al., 1987; Linn et al., 1980), and patients with chronic obstructive pulmonary disease (COPD) (Linn et al., 1983; Solic et al., 1982). An exception is that patients with allergic rhinitis had greater changes in airway resistance (McDonnell et al., 1987).

A prospective confirmation of reduced responsiveness to O_3 among asymptomatic cigarette smokers was produced by Emmons and Foster (1991). They measured respiratory function before and after 2 hours of O_3 at 400 ppb with light exercise in 18 smokers before they stopped smoking and again after 6 months of not smoking. None were responsive to O_3 exposure before smoking cessation. During smoking cessation, their mean baseline FEF_{25-75} was raised from 3.02 to 4.08 L/s. For the nine subjects re-exposed to O_3 6 months later, the exposure reduced their mean FEF_{25-75} from 3.86 to 2.99 L/s. The subjects with the greatest improvement in FEF_{25-75} after withdrawal had the largest acute decrements after O_3 exposure. Smoking cessation did not significantly increase FVC or FEV_1, and O_3 exposure after smoking cessation did not produce significant decrements in these respiratory function parameters.

Weinmann et al. (1995) showed that O_3-induced changes in FEF_{25-75} were unexplained by, and followed a different time course than O_3-induced changes in FVC. Their analysis indicated that intrinsic narrowing of the small airways may be significant indicator of the functional response.

While the results of some laboratory studies have indicated that responses in young females was greater than those in young males (Messineo and Adams, 1990), the largest study of both males and females did not find gender-related differences in responsiveness to O_3 among either black or white adults (Seal et al., 1993).

The first indications that the effects of O_3 on respiratory function accumulate over more than 1 hour were the observations of McDonnell et al. (1983) and Kulle et al. (1985) in chamber exposures to O_3 in purified air for 2 hours with the volunteer subjects engaged in vigorous intermittent exercise. Significant function decrements observed after 2 hours of exposure were not present at measurements made after 1 hour.

Spektor et al. (1988a) noted that children at summer camps with active outdoor recreation programs had greater decrements in lung function than children exposed to O_3 at comparable concentrations in chambers for 1 or 2 hours (see Table 20-4). Furthermore their activity levels, although not measured, were known to be considerably lower than those of the children exposed in the chamber studies while performing very vigorous exercise. Since it is well established that functional responses to O_3 increase with levels of physical activity and ventilation (Hazucha, 1987), the greater responses in the camp children had to be caused by other factors, such as greater cumulative exposure, or by the potentiation of the response to O_3 by other pollutants in the ambient air. Cumulative daily exposures to O_3 were generally greater for the camp children, since they were exposed all day long rather than for a 1 or 2 hours period preceded and followed by clean air exposure.

Similar considerations apply to the studies of Kinney et al. (1988) and Hoek et al. (1993) of school children. In the Kinney et al. study in Kingston and Harriman, TN, lung function was measured in school on up to six occasions during a 2 month period in the late winter and early spring. Child-specific regressions of function versus maximum 1 hour O_3 during the previous day indicated significant associations between O_3 and function, with coefficients similar to those seen in the summer camp studies of Lippmann et al. (1983), Spektor et al. (1988a, 1991), Higgins et al. (1990), and Hoek et al. (1993). Since children in school may be expected to have relatively low activity levels, the relatively high response coefficients may be related to potentiation by other pollutants or to a low level of seasonal adaptation. Kingston-Harriman is notable for its relatively high levels of aerosol acidity. As shown by Spengler et al. (1989) Kingston-Harriman has higher annual average and higher peak acid aerosol concentrations than other cities studied, namely Steubenville, Ohio; St. Louis, Missouri; and Portage, Wisconsin. Alternatively, the relatively high-response coefficients could have been caused by the fact that the measurements were made in the late winter and early spring. Linn et al. (1988) have shown evidence for a seasonal adaptation, and children studied during the summer may not be as responsive as children measured earlier in the year. This study will be discussed further under "Effects of Multiple-Day and Ambient Episode Exposures."

In a study of children with moderate to severe asthma at a summer camp in the Connecticut River Valley (Thurston et al., 1997), the association between decrements in peak expiratory flow rates associated with ambient O_3 concentrations were similar in magnitude to those reported by the same group of investigators for healthy children at other northeastern U.S. summer camps (Spektor et al., 1988a, 1991). However, the level of physical activity of the asthmatic children, and hence their O_3 intake, was much lower. Also the asthmatic children have less reserve functional capacity. Thus the level of health concern for such comparable functional decrements is much greater.

Other recent studies of the effects of O_3 on lung function in children in natural settings have also demonstrated O_3-related functional decrements. Braun-Fahrländer et al. (1994) showed O_3-related reductions in PEFR among 9 to 11-year-old Swiss children following 10 minutes of heavy exercise at peak O_3 concentrations below 80 ppb. Neas et al. (1995) demonstrated O_3-related reductions in PEFR between morning and evening in fourth and fifth grade children in Uniontown, Pennsylvania, in relation to 12 hour average O_3 below 88 ppb. Castillejos et al. (1995) studied the change in lung function following exercise out of doors for 7 1/2 to 11-year-old children in Mexico City who were repeatedly exposed to high ambient levels of O_3 and PM. They had O_3-related decrements in FVC, $FEV_{1.0}$, FEF_{25-75} and $FEV_{1.0}/FVC$ when the peak 1 hour O_3 exceeded 150 ppb.

Field studies of functional responses of adults engaged in recreational activities outdoors in the presence of varying levels of O_3 have also been performed. Spektor et al. (1988b) made pre- and postexercise respiratory function measurements on 30 young adults who were engaged in daily outdoor exercise for about one-half hour per day in an area with regional summer haze but no local point sources. The magnitudes of the functional

TABLE 20-4 Mean Functional Changes per 1 ppb O$_3$ in Adults and Children after Exercise: Comparison of Results from Field and Chamber Exposure Studies with O$_3$ ≤ 180 ppb

Study	Number of Subjects and Gender	Age Range	Activity level (minute ventilation) (L)	Exposure (Exercise) Time (min)	O$_3$ Conc. (ppb)	Mean Rate of Functional Change			
						FVC (mL/ppb)	FEV$_1$ (mL/ppb)	PEFR (mL/s/ppb)	FEF$_{25-75}$ (mL/s/ppb)
Adults									
Folinsbee et al. (1988)	10M	18–33	Moderate (40)	395 (300)	120[b]	-3.8	-4.5	—	-5.0
Gibbons and Adams (1984)	10F	22.9 ± 2.5[a]	High (55)	60 (60)	150[b]	-1.1	-1.0	—	-0.6
Avol et al. (1984)	42M, 8F	26.4 ± 6.9[a]	High (57)	60 (60)	153[c]	-1.2	-1.3	—	—
McDonnell et al. (1983)	22M	22.3 ± 3.1[a]	High (65)	120 (60)	120[b]	-1.5	-1.5	—	-2.9
	20M	23.3 ± 3.2[a]	High (65)	120 (60)	180[b]	-1.4	-1.3	—	-3.0
	20M	25.3 ± 4.1[a]	High (68)	120 (60)	150[b]	-1.8	-1.6	—	-2.1
Kulle et al. (1985)	24M	18–33	High	120 (60)	160[b]	-0.5	-0.2	-1.1	-1.1
Linn et al. (1988)	20M, 10F	22–44	Varied (78.6 ± 34.8[a])	29.3 ± 9.2[a]	21–124[c]	-0.7	-0.6	-9.2	-6.0
Spektor et al. (1988b)	7M, 13F	22–40	(64.6 ± 10.0[a])	26.7 ± 8.7[a]	21–124[c]	-2.1	-1.4	-13.7	-9.7
Children									
Lioy et al. (1985)	17M, 22F	7–13	Low	150–550	20–145[c]	-0.1	-0.3	-3.0	-0.6
Kinney et al. (1988)	94M, 60F	10–12	Low	1440	7–78[c]	-0.9	-1.0[d]	—	-1.9
Lippmann et al. (1983)	34M, 24F	8–13	Moderate	150–550	46–110[c]	-1.1	-0.8	—	—
Spektor et al. (1988a)	53M, 38F	7–13	Moderate	150–550	19–113[c]	-1.0	-1.4	-6.8	-2.5
Avol et al. (1985)	33M, 33F	8–11	Moderate (22)	60 (60)	113[c]	-0.3	-0.3	-0.4	—
Avol et al. (1985)	46M, 13F	12–15	High (32)	60 (60)	150[b]	-0.7	-0.8	-1.6	-0.7
McDonnell et al. (1985b)	23M	8–11	Very high (39)	150 (60)	120[b]	-0.3	-0.5	-1.8	-0.6

[a] Mean ± SD.
[b] Ozone concentration within purified air.
[c] Ozone concentration within ambient mixture.
[d] FEV$_{0.75}$.

671

decrements per unit of ambient O_3 concentration were similar to those observed in volunteers exposed while exercising vigorously for one or two hours in controlled chamber exposure studies. Functional decrements in proportion to relatively low ambient O_3 concentrations have also been reported for joggers in Houston, Texas (Selwyn et al., 1985), competitive cyclists in the Netherlands (Brunekreef et al., 1994), hikers on Mount Washington in New Hampshire (Korrick et al., 1998) and agricultural workers in British Columbia (Brauer et al., 1996).

The observations from the field studies in the children's camps stimulated Folinsbee et al. (1988) at the EPA Clinical Studies Laboratory in Chapel Hill, North Carolinan, to undertake a chamber exposure study of 10 adult male volunteers involving 6.6 hours of O_3 exposure at 120 ppb. Moderate exercise was performed for 50 min/h for 3 hours in the morning and again in the afternoon. They found that the functional decrements become progressively greater after each hour of exposure, reaching average values of about 400 mL for forced vital capacity (FVC) and about 540 mL for forced expiratory volume in 1 second (FEV_1) by the end of the day. The effects were transient in that there were no residual functional decrements on the following day. The decrements in FEV_1 after 6.6 hours of exposure at 120 ppb averaged 13.6% and were comparable to those seen previously in the same laboratory on similar subjects following 2 hours of intermittent heavier exercise (68 L inhaled per minute for a total exercise time of 60 minutes) at an interpolated concentration of about 220 ppb. Assuming that the rate of ventilation was 10 L/min between exercise periods, the total amount of O_3 inhaled during 2 hours of intermittent heavy exercise at 220 ppb (430 $\mu g/m^3$) would be [60 min $\times$ 0.068 m^3/min $+$ 60 min $\times$ 0.010 m^3/min] $\times$ 430 $\mu g/m^3$ = 2.01 mg O_3. The corresponding amount of O_3 inhaled during 6.6 hours of intermittent moderate exercise at 120 ppb would be [300 min $\times$ 0.040 m^3/min + 100 min $\times$ 0.010 m^3/min] $\times$ 235 $\mu g/m^3$ = 3.06 mg O_3. Thus the effect accumulates with time, but there appears to be a temporal decay of effect going on at the same time. Follow-up studies in the same laboratory by Horstman et al. (1990) were done on 21 adult males with 6.6 hour exposures at 80, 100, and 120 ppb. The exposures at 120 ppb produced very similar responses, for example, a mean FEV_1 decline of 12.3%, whereas those at 80 and 100 ppb showed lesser changes that also became progressively greater after each hour of exposure (Figure 20-4).

A further follow-up study using the same exposure protocol on 38 additional healthy young men was done by McDonnell et al. (1991) at 80 ppb. There was a mean FEV_1 decline of 8.4%, which was similar to that seen by Horstman et al. (1990) at that concentration.

The time scale for effective O_3 dose in relation to functional response was explored further by Hazucha et al. (1992) in exposures of 23 healthy young adults lasting 8 hours, with 30 minutes of exercise (at 40 L/min) at the beginning of each hour. The O_3 concentration rose from 0 to 240 ppb over the first 4 hours and dropped back to 0 over the second 4 hours. The functional responses were compared to both sham exposures and constant 120 ppb exposures in the same subjects. By 4 hours the FEV_1 changes from both O_3 exposures were similar, and the largest decrement in FEV_1, which occurred after 6 hours of exposure, was about twice as large as that after 5 to 8 hours of constant exposure at 120 ppb. The peak response faded by the end of 8 hours, and was not significantly greater than that produced by the constant 120 ppb exposure at the eighth hour.

Another study looking at the integral effects of temporally varying exposures with the same integral exposure was performed by McKittrick and Adams (1995). Twelve aerobically trained young adult men were exposed while exercising at 60 L/min to either 1 hour at 300 ppb O_3 followed by 1 hour of clean air; intermittent half hours at 300 ppb and 0 ppb, or intermittent quarter hours at 300 and 0 ppb. The FEV_1 decrements at the end of exposure to O_3 were essentially the same, −17.6, −17.0, and −17.9%.

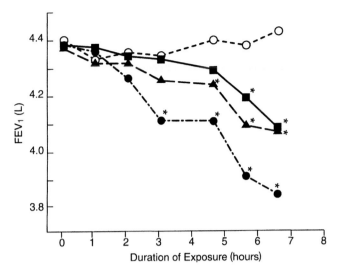

Figure 20-4   Mean FEV_1 after each 50 min of exercise during exposures to O_3 at 0 (open circles), 80 ppb (squares), 100 ppb (triangles), and 120 ppb (solid circles). Asterisks indicate significant reduction in FEV_1 from corresponding values at 0 ppb. From Horstman et al. (1990).

Larsen et al. (1991) modeled the data of Horstman et al. (1990) using multiple linear regression on the mean responses at each hour for all three concentrations but excluding those with FEV_1 decreases of less than 0.5%. With O_3 concentration and duration of exposure as the only two independent variables, the model explained 95% of the variance of the dependent variable Z, a Gaussian transform of the percentage decrease in FEV_1. In this model the exponent of the exposure duration is 0.754. This further demonstrates that exposure time is almost equally important to exposure concentration in cumulative response when concentrations are in the range of normal peak ambient levels.

Further evidence of the time scale for the biological integration of O_3 exposure can be deduced from the rate at which the effects dissipate. This kind of data was produced by Folinsbee and Hazucha (1989) in a study in which 18 young adult females were exposed to 350 ppb O_3 for 70 minutes, including two 30 minute periods of treadmill exercise at 40 L / min. Their mean decrement in FEV_1 at the end of the exposure was 21%. After 18 hours, their mean decrement was 4%, whereas at 42 hours it was 2%.

The time scale for the biological integration of the effects of a single O_3 exposure has also been examined in studies on laboratory animals. Costa et al. (1989) exposed F-344 rats for 2, 4, or 8 hours to O_3 at 100, 200, 400, and 800 ppb. Lung function was measured immediately after exposure, and bronchoalveolar lavage (BAL) was performed immediately and 24 hours later. Functional decrements increased with the product ppb-h, leveling off at > 6000, whereas BAL proteins increased rapidly for ppb-h > 4000. In another test series involving 6.6 hours of exposure with 8% CO_2 to stimulate respiration, rats exposed to 500 ppb O_3 had functional decrements closely matching those seen in humans at 120 ppb. Thus, rats can provide a good test model for the observed human responses to O_3, even though they are a less sensitive species than humans. The lesser responses to a given O_3 concentration reported here are consistent with the lesser retention of O_3 by rats, as discussed previously.

This issue was further addressed by Highfill et al. (1992) through an examination of relationships between concentration (C) and exposure time (T) and the impact of changes in the $C \times T$ product on toxic responses. Using protein concentration of bronchoalveolar lavage fluid (BALP) as an index of O_3-induced lung damage, models were developed from a matrix of C (0.0, 0.1, 0.2, 0.4, and 0.8 ppm) and T (2, 4, and 8 h) values in rat and guinea pig. Equal $C \times T$ products with different levels of C and T were incorporated into the protocol. Polynomial and exponential least-squares models were developed, and the log-normal linear model (Larsen et al., 1991) was evaluated for the rat and guinea pig data. For equal $C \times T$ products the results showed similar BALP responses at low $C \times T$ products. Calculations from the data and the models showed that (1) the models were consistent with reported experiments (Hatch et al. 1986), (2) exercising humans were more responsive to O_3 exposure (without adjustments for ventilation rates) than were either rats or guinea pigs as measured by changes in BALP (Koren et al., 1989), and (3) the exponential model provided more generality than Haber's law by providing estimates of BALP levels for various $C \times T$.

The large interindividual variability of O_3-induced functional responses that is illustrated in Figure 20-5 is not yet understood, and functional responses in individuals do not correlate well with the other responses that will be discussed below. Using the large data base accumulated over a 10 year period at the EPA Clinical Studies Laboratory in Chapel Hill, North Carolina, McDonnell et al. (1993) found that O_3 concentration explained 31% of the variance in FEV_1 responses, and subject age explained another 4%. The modeled influence of age is illustrated in Figure 20-6.

Upon further modeling of this large dataset, McDonnell et al. (1997) reported that a sigmoid-shaped model was consistent with previous observations of O_3 exposure–response (E–R) characteristics and accurately predicted the mean response with independent data. They did not find that response was more sensitive to changes in C than in V_E, nor did they find convincing evidence of an effect of body size on response, but response to O_3 decreased with age.

Using the data collected in 68 individuals exposed two or more times for 6.6 hours, McDonnell et al. (1995a) found that 47% of those exposed to 120 ppb had an FEV_1 decrement of 10% or greater. These analyses helped to demonstrate that the respiratory function effects can accumulate over many hours, and that an appropriate averaging time for transient functional decrements caused by O_3 is ≥ 6 hours. This was a major factor for the change in the averaging time for the primary O_3 NAAQS from 1 to 8 hours. Another factor was the recognition that O_3 exposures in ambient air can have broad peaks with 8 hour averages equal to about 90% of the peak 1 hour averages (Rombout et al., 1986).

There is evidently a large genetic component to this variability. Kleeberger (1995) and Kleeberger et al. (1997) have explored the contribution of genetic background to the pathogenesis of airway responses to air pollutants. Kleeberger (1995) demonstrated a strong genetic influence on responsiveness to O_3 using inbred mice strains, and the follow-up study with NO_2, another ambient air oxidant, examined the genetic basis for differences in response to the two agents. In Kleeberger et al. (1997) they determined significant genetic contributions in susceptibility to lung injury and inflammation induced by single and repeated acute exposures to NO_2, and whether similar genetic factors control susceptibility to O_3. Nine strains of inbred mice (male, 5–6 wk) were studied. Each was exposed for 3 hours to filtered air (controls) or 15 ppm NO_2, and cellular inflammation, epithelial injury, and cytotoxicity were measured 2, 6, and 24 hours thereafter. NO_2 exposure caused significant increases in cytotoxicity and lavageable macrophages, epithelial cells, polymorphonuclear leukocytes, and protein in all strains. Interstrain variation in each of these effects indicated that genetic background contributed a significant portion of the variance in responses to this oxidant. Two strains that were differentially susceptible to 3 hours exposure to 15 ppm NO_2 [C57BL / 6J (B6), C3H / HeJ (C3)] were also exposed for 6 h/d to 10 ppm NO_2 on 5 consecutive days. Each of the responses to NO_2 was completely adapted after 5 days in resistant C3 mice. Only the lavageable total protein response was adapted in susceptible B6 mice. To determine whether mechanisms of susceptibility to NO_2 and O_3 were the same, each strain was

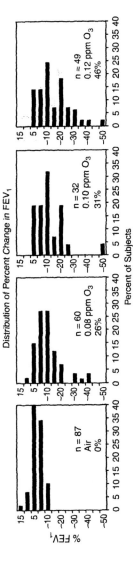

Figure 20-5 Percentage change in FEV_1 in healthy nonsmokers following 6.6 hours exposures to clean air and O_3 at 80, 100, and 120 ppb during exercise lasting 50 minutes of each hour for studies performed at EPA's Clinical Research Laboratory at Chapel Hill, North Carolina. Each box shows the number of subjects studied and the percentage of subjects with reductions in FEV_1 that were greater than 10%.

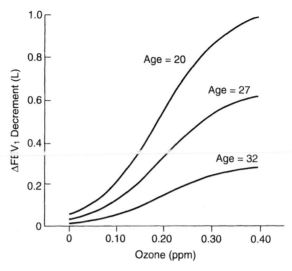

Figure 20-6 Predicted mean decrements in forced expiratory volume in L(ΔFEV$_1$) following 2 hours exposures to ozone while undergoing heavy intermittent exercise for three ages. (Note: To convert ΔFEV$_1$ to % ΔFEV$_1$, multiply by 22.2%.) From McDonnell et al. (1993).

exposed for 3 hours to filtered air or 2 ppm O$_3$, and inflammation was assessed 6 and 24 hours thereafter. Strain distribution patterns for responses to each oxidant were not significantly concordant and indicated that susceptibility mechanisms were different. Results of these studies suggest that there is a strong genetic component to NO$_2$ susceptibility that is partially adaptable and significantly different from O$_3$ susceptibility.

Although there is a great deal of knowledge about O$_3$ exposure-respiratory function response in humans, as summarized above, we still know very little about the mechanisms responsible for the responses. Other irritants, such as SO$_2$, NO$_2$, and H$_2$SO$_4$, produce greater responses among asthmatics than among healthy subjects, but this is not true for O$_3$, as indicated previously. For other irritants, functional responses correlate with responsiveness to bronchoconstrictor challenge. For example, Utell et al. (1983) found a high correlation between reactivity to inhaled carbachol and responsiveness to inhaled H$_2$SO$_4$ in asthmatics ($r = 0.90$, $p < 0.001$), whereas Horstman et al. (1986) reported that methacholine (MCh) reactivity and SO$_2$ response were significantly but weakly correlated ($r = 0.31$). Although both functional decrements and bronchial responsiveness are produced by O$_3$ exposure, Folinsbee et al. (1988) and Horstman et al. (1990) found no apparent relationship between these responses for individual subjects. On the other hand, Aris et al. (1991) screened 39 healthy, nonsmoking volunteers for their functional responsiveness to 3 hours of exposure to 200 ppb O$_3$ at a ventilatory rate of 40 L / min and found that the MCh responsiveness of 10 O$_3$-sensitive subjects (PC$_{100}$ = 3.0 ± 0.8) was significantly greater than that of 10 O$_3$-nonsensitive subjects (PC$_{100}$ = 18.7 ± 4.5).

Beckett et al. (1985) examined the effect of atropine, a muscarinic receptor blocker, on responses to exposure to 400 ppb O$_3$. Atropine pretreatment prevented the significant increase in airway resistance with O$_3$ exposure and partially blocked the decrease in forced expiratory flow rates but did not prevent a significant fall in FVC, changes in respiratory frequency and tidal volume, or the frequency of reported respiratory symptoms. These results suggest that the increase in pulmonary resistance during O$_3$ exposure is mediated by a parasympathetic mechanism and that changes in other measured variables are mediated, at least partially, by mechanisms not dependent on muscarinic cholinergic receptors of the parasympathetic nervous system.

Gong et al. (1988) studied the contribution of β-adrenergic mechanisms to the acute airway responses to O_3 in a study in which symptoms, pulmonary function, exercise performance, and postexposure histamine bronchoprovocation were studied in 15 nonasthmatic athletes exposed to 210 ppb O_3 during heavy continuous exercise, with mean minute ventilation $(V_E) \geq 80$ L/min for 60 minutes, followed by a maximal sprint (peak $V_E > 140$ L/min) until exhaustion. Each subject was exposed randomly to either 210 ppb O_3 or filtered air (FA) during the four single-blinded exposure sessions. Albuterol pretreatment resulted in modest but significant bronchodilation as compared to placebo. However, albuterol did not prevent O_3-induced respiratory symptoms, decrements in FVC, FEV_1, and maximum midexpiratory flow rate (FEF_{25-75}), and positive histamine challenges as compared to that with placebo and O_3. There were no statistically significant differences in the metabolic data or ride times across all drugs and exposures, although the peak V_E was significantly lower with O_3 than FA (142.3 vs. 150.7 L/min, respectively) regardless of drug. The results indicate that acute pretreatment with inhaled albuterol is unable to prevent or ameliorate O_3-induced symptoms and alterations in pulmonary function and exercise performance. The contribution of β-adrenergic mechanisms in the acute airway responses to O_3 appears to be minimal.

In their study on bronchial hyperresponsiveness, consequent to O_3 exposure, Seltzer et al. (1986) found significant increases in the concentration of prostaglandins E_2 and F_{2a} and thromboxane B_2 in bronchoalveolar lavage fluid. Prostaglandins E_2 and F_{2a} have been found to stimulate pulmonary neural afferents that initiate several responses characteristic of acute O_3 exposure (Coleridge et al., 1976; Roberts et al., 1985) These findings suggest that the release of prostaglandins in the lung consequent to acute O_3 exposure may be involved in routinely observed pulmonary function decrements and perhaps in altered exercise ventilatory pattern and reported subjective symptomology.

Schelegle et al. (1987) studied whether O_3-induced pulmonary function decrements could be inhibited by the prostaglandin synthetase inhibitor, indomethacin, in healthy human subjects. College-age males completed six 1 hour exposure protocols consisting of no-drug, placebo, and indomethacin pretreatments, with filtered air and O_3 (350 ppb) exposures within each pretreatment. Exposures consisted of 1 hour exercise on a bicycle ergometer with work loads set to elicit a V_E of 60 L/min. Significant differences were found for comparisons of no drug versus indomethacin and of placebo versus indomethacin. These findings suggest that cyclooxygenase products of arachidonic acid, which are sensitive to indomethacin inhibition, play a prominent role in the development of pulmonary function decrements consequent to acute O_3 exposure. In a similar study Ying et al. (1990) administered indomethacin for 4 days to 14 young adult male nonsmokers prior to 2 hour O_3 exposures with intermittent exercise at 400 ppb to determine if it would alter their O_3 responsiveness as well as their lung function. Only seven of the subjects had detectable serum levels of indomethacin and significant responses to methacholine on the sham-exposure day. For these seven, the indomethacin attenuated the O_3-induced decrements in lung function but did not attenuate the O_3-induced responsiveness to methacholine. They concluded that the O_3-induced decrements in respiratory function are mediated by cyclooxygenase products but that the O_3-induced increase in airway reactivity occurs by some other mechanism.

Ozone-induced bronchial hyperresponsiveness in dogs is inhibited by neutrophil depletion (O'Byrne et al., 1984a) and indomethacin pretreatment (O'Byrne et al., 1984b), suggesting that neutrophils that infiltrate the airway after acute O_3 exposure (O'Byrne et al., 1984b; Holtzman et al., 1979) are the cells that release the cyclooxygenase products responsible for O_3-induced bronchial hyperreactivity. However, neutrophil infiltration is a relatively late effect (i.e., occurring > 6 hour postexposure) and is not likely to account for the immediate responses. In a follow-up study (Jones et al., 1990), thromboxane antagonists were given to the dogs to further determine the role of thromboxane in O_3-

induced airway hyperresponsiveness. The antagonists did not inhibit the response, indicating that thromboxane does not have an important role in causing O_3-induced airway hyperresponsiveness.

Leikauf et al. (1988) investigated the hypothesis that oxidant damage to the tracheal epithelium may result in elaboration of various eicosanoids. To examine eicosanoid metabolism after exposure to 100 ppb to 10.0 ppm ozone, epithelial cells derived from bovine trachea were isolated and grown to confluency. Bovine tracheal cells in culture expressed differentiated features characterstic of epithelial cells, including a plasma membrane with a specialized polar morphology, an extensive network of filaments that were connected through intercellular junctional complexes, and keratin-containing monofilaments as determined by indirect immunofluorescent localization. Monolayers were alternately exposed to ozone and culture medium for 2 hour in a specially designed in vitro chamber using a rotating inclined platform (Valentine, 1985). Eicosanoid products were measured by the release of ^{3}H-labeled products from cells incubated with [^{3}H]arachidonic acid for 24 hours before exposure and by the release of immunoreactive products into the cell supernatant. Both methods revealed ozone-induced increases in cyclooxygenase and lipoxygenase product formation with significant increases in prostaglandins E_2, $F_{2\alpha}$, 6-keto $F_{1\alpha}$, and leukotriene B_4. Release rates of immunoreactive products were dose-dependent, and ozone concentrations as low as 100 ppb produced an increase in prostaglandin $F_{2\alpha}$. Thus ozone can augment eicosanoid metabolism in airway epithelial cells.

The mechanism by which the release of cyclooxygenase products in the lung leads to pulmonary function decrements in humans upon O_3 exposure remains undefined. Available data indicate that O_3-induced pulmonary function decrements and ventilatory pattern changes are neurally mediated (Lee et al., 1979; Hazucha et al., 1989). Hazucha et al. (1989) concluded that O_3 inhalation stimulates airway receptors, which leads to an involuntary inhibition of full inspiration, reduction in FVC, and a concomitant decrease in maximal expiratory flow rates in humans. The observation that cyclooxygenase products stimulate neural afferents in the lung (Coleridge et al., 1976; Roberts et al., 1985), combined with the observation of reduced O_3-induced pulmonary function decrements after indomethacin pretreatment, suggests that cyclooxygenase products released consequent to O_3-induced tissue damage stimulate neural afferents in the lung, which results in the observed pulmonary function decrements.

Effects on Aerosol Dispersion

As discussed above, acute exposures of humans to low levels of ozone cause decreases in lung function. However, such changes do not elucidate the potential for the acute small airways responses that do not produce measurable changes in conventional respiratory function indexes. In order to study the potential effects of ozone on small airways in humans, Keefe et al. (1991) employed a test of aerosol dispersion. Twenty-two healthy nonsmoking male volunteers were exposed to 400 ppb O_3 for 1 hour while exercising at 20 L/min/m^2 body surface area (BSA). Prior to and immediately following exposure, tests of spirometry (FVC, FEV$_1$, and FEF$_{25-75}$) and plethysmography (R$_{aw}$ and sR$_{aw}$) were performed. Subjects also performed an aerosol dispersion test before and after exposure. Each test involved a subject inhaling 5 to 7 breaths of a 300 mL bolus of a 0.5 μm triphenyl phosphate (TPP) aerosol injected into a 2 L tidal volume. The bolus was injected into the tidal breath at three different depths: at depth A after 1.6 L of clean air from functional residual capacity (FRC), at depth B after 1.2 L, and at depth C after 1.2 L but with inhalation beginning from residual volume (RV). The primary measure of bolus dispersion was the expired half-width (HW). Changes in pulmonary function following ozone exposure were consistent with previous findings. When corrected for exercise, FVC,

FEV_1, and FEF_{25-75} all significantly declined ($p < 0.001$, $p < 0.002$, and $p < 0.03$, respectively) with nonsignificant increases in R_{aw} and sR_{aw}. The HW significantly increased following ozone exposure relative to air exposure at all depths (17 mL, $p < 0.05$ at depth A, 56 mL, $p < 0.001$ at depth B, and 53 mL, $p < 0.005$ at depth C). The HW was only weakly correlated with spirometric measures, accounting for less than 25% of the variance. Half-width was not correlated with R_{aw} or sR_{aw}. They concluded that the changes in aerosol dispersion seen with O_3 exposure were related to changes in turbulent mixing and / or regional time constants in the small airways, thus implying a possible O_3 effect in that region of the lung as well as effects in the larger airways that produce the respiratory function decrements.

Symptomatic Responses

Respiratory symptoms have been closely associated with group mean pulmonary function changes in adults acutely exposed in controlled exposures to O_3 and in ambient air containing O_3 as the predominant pollutant. However, Hayes et al. (1987) found only a weak to moderate correlation between FEV_1 changes and symptoms severity when the analysis is conducted using individual data.

In controlled 2 hour O_3 exposures, McDonnell et al. (1983) reported that some heavily exercising adult subjects experienced cough, shortness of breath, and pain on deep inspiration at 120 ppb O_3, although the group mean response was statistically significant for cough only. Above 120 ppb O_3, respiratory and nonrespiratory symptoms have included throat dryness, chest tightness, substernal pain, cough, wheeze, pain on deep inspiration, shortness of breath, dyspnea, lassitude, malaise, headache, and nausea.

The prolonged exposure studies involving 6.6 hours of exposure at concentrations between 80 and 120 ppb also produced significant increases in respiratory symptoms including cough and pain on deep inspiration (Koenig et al., 1987; Linn, 1980). Linder et al. (1988) reported that brief exposures (16–28 min) to 120 to 130 ppb O_3 at high ventilatory rates (30–120 L / min) produced symptoms of irritation and cough in young adults.

Although O_3 causes symptomatic responses in adults at current peak levels, there is a large set of data indicating that such responses do not occur in healthy children (Avol et al., 1985, 1987). Children (ages 8–11) exposed for 2.5 hours at 120 ppb O_3 while intermittently exercising ($V_E = 39$ L / min) showed small but statistically significant decreases in FEV_1 but showed no changes in frequency or severity of cough compared to controls (McDonnell et al., 1985a,b). Similarly adolescents (ages 12–15) continuously exercising ($V_E = 31-33$ L / min) during exposure to 144 ppb mean O_3 in ambient air showed no changes in symptoms despite statistically significant decrements in group mean FEV_1 (4%), which persisted at least 1 hour during postexposure resting (Avol et al., 1985).

These laboratory results are consistent with the results obtained in a series of field studies of healthy children at summer camps, which failed to find any symptomatic responses despite the occurrence of relatively large decrements in function that were proportional to the ambient O_3 concentrations (Spektor et al., 1988a). Also, in a follow-up study by Hoek and Brunekreef (1995) of a general population sample of 300 children aged 7 to 11 who had shown functional responses to O_3 in ambient air, there were no responses in terms of symptoms based on diaries maintained by their parents. In panels of 300 healthy children in the Harvard six-cities study, diaries of respiratory symptoms were kept over one year. In single pollutant models for the April–August period, there was a significant association between O_3 and the incidence of cough that was independent of other measured pollutants (Schwartz et al., 1994).

For a group of 143 children aged 7 to 9 years old in Mexico City who were repeatedly exposed to high concentration of O_3 and PM, Castillejos et al. (1992) reported that mean

O_3 in the previous 48 hours was associated with a child's report of cough or phlegm, while mean O_3 in the previous day or week did not. For a panel of 71 asthmatic 5 to 7-year-old children in Mexico City, respiratory symptoms (coughing, phlegm production, wheezing, and difficulty breathing) and the frequency of lower respiratory illness on the same day were associated with both O_3 and PM_{10} (Romieu et al., 1996). In the study of children with moderate to severe asthma in the Connecticut River Valley, where O_3 exposures were much lower than those in Mexico City, Thurston et al. (1997) found that respiratory symptoms were significantly associated with O_3.

Several other epidemiology studies have provided evidence of qualitative associations between ambient oxidant levels > 0.10 ppm and symptoms in children and young adults, such as throat irritation, chest discomfort, cough, and headache (Hammer et al., 1974; Makino and Mizoguchi, 1975). Thus symptoms reported in individuals exposed to O_3 in purified air are similar to those found for ambient air exposures except for eye irritation, a common symptom associated with exposure to photochemical oxidants, which has not been reported for controlled exposures to O_3 alone. Other oxidants, such as aldehydes and peroxyacetyl nitrate (PAN), are primarily responsible for eye irritation and are generally found in atmospheres containing higher ambient O_3 levels (Altshuller, 1977; National Research Council, 1977).

There have been several studies reporting associations between ambient photochemical oxidant pollution and exacerbation of asthma (Schoettlin and Landau, 1961; Whittemore and Korn, 1980; Holguin et al., 1985), but the role of O_3 specifically and the nature of the exposure–response relationships remain poorly defined.

Respiratory symptoms in healthy young adult females (100 student nurses) in Los Angeles, in relation to ambient pollution levels, were monitored by Hammer et al. (1974). They found associations between photochemical oxidants and respiratory symptoms. However, that analysis ignored smoking and serial correlation in the data, used linear regression to model the probability of a respiratory incident, ignored other potentially colinear air pollutants, and assumed that a pollutant would have the same impact on starting an episode of symptoms as on prolonging the episode. Because of limited computational facilities at the time, the data on individual subjects were collapsed to rates per day.

Schwartz and Zeger (1990) reexamined the original diaries from this study, which contained smoking and allergy histories as well as symptom reports that had never been analyzed. Diaries were completed daily and collected weekly for as long as 3 years. Air pollution was measured at a monitoring location within 2.5 miles of the school. Incidence and duration of a symptom were modeled separately. Photochemical oxidants (74 ppb) were associated with increased risk of chest discomfort (OR = 1.17, $p < 0.001$) and eye irritation (OR = 1.20, $p < 0.001$).

Ostro et al. (1993) recorded the respiratory symptoms in 321 nonsmoking adults residing in southern California. Participants recorded the daily incidence of several respiratory symptoms over a 6 month period between 1978 and 1979. Ambient concentrations of O_3, $SO_4^=$, and other air pollutants were measured. Using a logistic regression model, the authors found a significant association between the incidence of lower respiratory tract symptoms and 7 hour O_3 (OR = 1.32, 95% CI 1.14–1.52, for a 100 ppb change), and $SO_4^=$ (OR = 1.30, 95% CI 1.09–1.54, for a 10 μg/m^3 change), but they found no association with the coefficient of haze, a more general measure of particulates. The existence of a gas stove in the home was also associated with lower respiratory tract symptoms (OR = 1.23, 95% CI 1.03-1.47). The effects of O_3 were greater in the subpopulation without a residential air conditioner. In addition O_3 had a greater effect among individuals with a preexisting respiratory infection.

Morbidity Associations between ambient air pollutants and respiratory morbidity were examined by Ostro and Rothschild (1989) using the Health Interview Survey (HIS), a large cross-sectional data base collected by the National Center for Health Statistics. They attempted to determine the separate health consequences of O_3 and particulate matter using six separate years of the HIS. The results, using a fixed-effects model that controls for intercity differences, indicate an association between fine particulate pollutants and both minor restrictions in activity and respiratory conditions severe enough to result in work loss and bed disability in adults. Ozone, on the other hand, was associated only with the more minor restrictions.

Bates and Sizto (1989) examined associations between ambient air pollutants and hospital admissions for respiratory disease in southern Ontario. They found a consistent association in summer between hospital admissions for respiratory disease and daily levels of SO_4^{2-}, O_3, and temperature but no association for a group nonrespiratory conditions. Multiple regression analyses showed that all environmental variables together accounted for 5.6% of the variability in respiratory admissions and that when temperature was forced into the analysis first, it accounted for only 0.89% of the variability. It was found that daily SO_4^{2-} data collected at one monitoring site in the center of the region were not correlated with respiratory admissions, whereas the SO_4^{2-} values collected every sixth day, on different days of the week, at 17 stations in the region had the highest correlation with respiratory admissions. They concluded that probably neither O_3 nor SO_4^{2-} alone is responsible for the observed associations with acute respiratory admissions but that either some unmeasured species (of which H_2SO_4 is the strongest candidate) or some pattern of sequential or cumulative exposure was responsible for the observed morbidity.

The Bates and Sizto (1989) study stimulated a series of additional studies as summarized in Table 20-5. Burnett et al. (1994) also employed the Ontario acute care hospital database to analyze the effects of air pollution on hospital admissions, but their analysis considered all of Ontario and analyzed the data from each individual hospital, rather than aggregating the counts by region. Slow-moving temporal cycles, including seasonal and yearly effects, were removed, and day-of-week effects were controlled prior to the analysis. Poisson regression techniques were employed because of the low daily admission counts at individual hospitals. O_3 displayed a positive association with respiratory admissions in 91% of the 168 hospitals, and 5% of summertime (May–August) respiratory admissions (mean = 107/d) were attributed to O_3 (mean = 50 ppb). Positive associations were found in all age groups (0 to 1, 2 to 34, 35 to 64, and 65 +). A parallel analysis of nonrespiratory admissions showed no such associations. These results are illustrated in Figure 20-7.

Thurston et al. (1994) focused their analysis of respiratory hospital admissions in the Toronto metropolitan area during the summers (July–August) of 1986 to 1988, when they directly monitored for strong particulate acidity (H^+) pollution on a daily basis at several sites in that city. Long-wave cycles, and their associated autocorrelations, were removed. Strong and significant positive associations with asthma and respiratory admissions were found for both O_3 and H^+, and somewhat weaker significant associations with $SO_4^=$, $PM_{2.5}$, PM_{10}, and TSP, as measured at a central site in downtown Toronto. No such associations were found for SO_2 or NO_2, nor for any pollutant with nonrespiratory control admissions. Temperature was only weakly correlated with respiratory admissions and became nonsignificant when entered in regressions with air pollution indexes. Simultaneous regressions and sensitivity analyses indicated that O_3 was the summertime haze constituent of greatest importance to respiratory and asthma admissions, although elevated H^+ was suggested as a possible potentiator of this effect. During multipollutant, simultaneous regressions on admissions, O_3 was consistently the most significant. Of the particle metrics, only H^+ remained statistically significant when entered into the admissions regressions simultaneously with O_3. Sensitivity analyses also showed that dropping all days with 1 hour O_3 above 120 ppb (2 of a total 117 days) did not significantly change the O_3 coefficients. The simultaneous O_3, H^+, and temperature model indicated

TABLE 20-5 Summary of Effect Estimates for Ozone in Recent Studies of Respiratory Hospital Admissions

Location	Reference	Respiratory Admission Category	Effect Size ($\pm$SE) [Admissions/100 ppb O_3/d/10^6 persons]	Relative Risk (95% CI)[a] RR of 100 ppb O_3, 1-h max]
New York City, NY[b]	Thurston et al. (1992)	All	1.4 ($\pm$0.5)	1.14 (1.06 to 1.22)
Buffalo, NY[b]	Thurston et al. (1992)	All	3.1 ($\pm$1.6)	1.25 (1.04 to 1.46)
Ontario, Canada[b]	Burnett et al. (1994)	All	1.4 ($\pm$0.3)	1.10 (1.06 to 1.14)
Toronto, Canada[b]	Thurston et al. (1994)	All	2.1 ($\pm$0.8)	1.36 (1.13 to 1.59)
Montreal, Canada[c]	Delfino et al. (1994a)	All	1.4 ($\pm$0.5)	1.22 (1.09 to 1.35)
Birmingham, AL[d]	Schwartz (1994a)	Pneumonia in elderly	0.73 ($\pm$0.54)	1.11 (0.97 to 1.26)
Birmingham, AL[d]	Schwartz (1994a)	COPD in elderly	0.83 ($\pm$0.33)	1.13 (0.92 to 1.39)
Detroit, MI[d]	Schwartz (1994b)	Pneumonia in elderly	0.82 ($\pm$0.26)	1.22 (1.12 to 1.35)
Detroit, MI[d]	Schwartz (1994b)	COPD in elderly	0.90 ($\pm$0.41)	1.25 (1.07 to 1.45)
Minneapolis, MN[d]	Schwartz (1994c)	Pneumonia in elderly	0.41 ($\pm$0.19)	1.117 (1.03 to 1.39)
Minneapolis, MN[d]	Schwartz (1994c)	COPD in elderly	[e]	[e]

[a] One-way ($\beta \pm 1.65$ SE).
[b] One hour daily maximum ozone data employed in analysis.
[c] Eight hour daily maximum ozone data employed in analysis.
[d] Twenty-four hour daily average ozone data employed in analysis (1 h/24 h average ratio = 2.5 assumed to compute effects and RR estimates).
[e] Not reported (nonsignificant).

682

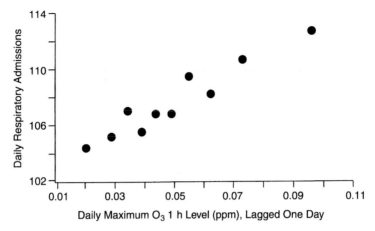

Figure 20-7   Average number of adjusted respiratory admissions among all 168 hospitals by decile of the daily 1 hour maximum ozone level (ppm), lagged 1 day. From Burnett et al. (1984).

that $21 \pm 8\%$ of all respiratory admissions during the three summers were associated with O_3 air pollution, on average, and that admissions rose an estimated $37 \pm 15\%$ above that otherwise expected on the highest O_3 day (0.159 ppm). Moreover, despite differing health care systems, the Toronto regression results for the summer of 1988 were remarkably consistent with previously reported results for that same summer in Buffalo, New York (Thurston et al., 1992).

Delfino et al. (1994a) studied daily urgent hospital admissions for respiratory and other illnesses at 31 hospitals in Montreal, Canada, during the warm periods of the year between 1984 and 1988. Respiratory admissions were considered as a whole and split into asthma and nonasthma categories, using definitions compatible with those previously used by Bates and Sizto (1989) and by Thurston et al. (1994). Both 1 hour and 8 hours maximum O_3 concentrations were considered in the analyses, as well as weather variables (temperature and relative humidity) and PM measurements (Delfino et al., 1994b). Day-of-the-week and autocorrelation effects were addressed. For the months of July and August a significant association was found between all respiratory admissions and both 8 hour daily maximum O_3 ($p \leq 0.01$) and 1 hour daily maximum O_3 ($p \leq 0.03$) 4 days prior to admission, despite the low O_3 concentrations (90th percentile $= 60$ ppb O_3). No significant correlations were found between O_3 and nonrespiratory, control admissions.

Lipfert and Hammerstrom (1992) re-analyzed the Bates and Sizto (1989) hospital admissions data set for 79 acute-care hospitals in southern Ontario, incorporating more elaborate statistical methods and extending the data set through 1985. Long-wave influences, autoregression, and day-of-week effects were controlled. Despite possible model overspecification (e.g., the inclusion of wind speed), summer haze pollutants (i.e., O_3, $SO_4^=$, SO_2) were found to have significant effects on hospital admissions. By contrast, pollution associations with hospital admissions for accidental causes became nonsignificant in these models. The pollutant mean effect accounted for 19% to 24% of all summer respiratory admissions.

Burnett et al. (1997) extended their study of the effects of O_3 on hospitalization for respiratory disease compared to hospital admissions for 16 cities across Canada representing 12.6 million people from 1981 to 1991. There were 720,519 admissions for which the principle diagnosis was a respiratory disease. After controlling for SO_2, NO_2, CO, soiling index, and dew point, the daily high hour concentration of O_3 recorded one day previous to the date of admission was positively associated with respiratory admissions in the April to December period but not in the winter months. The association between O_3 and respiratory hospitalizations varied among cities, with relative risks ranging from 1.000 to 1.088 after simultaneous covariate adjustment. PM and CO were also positively associated with respiratory hospitalizations.

Thurston et al. (1992) analyzed admissions to acute care hospitals in three New York State metropolitan areas during the summers of 1988 and 1989. Environmental variables considered included daily 1 hour maximum O_3 and 24 hours average $SO_4^=$ and acid aerosol (H^+) concentrations, as well as daily maximum temperature recorded at central sites in each community. Long-wave periodicities in the data were prefiltered using sine and cosine waves. Day-of-week effects were controlled via regression. The strongest O_3-respiratory admissions associations were found during the period of high pollution in the summer of 1988 and in the most urbanized communities considered (i.e., Buffalo and New York City). After controlling for temperature effects via simultaneous regression, the summer haze pollutants (i.e., $SO_4^=$, H^+, O_3) remained significantly related to total respiratory and asthma admissions. However, these pollutants' high intercorrelation prevented the clear discrimination of a single pollutant as the causal agent. Depending on the index pollutant, the admission category, and the city considered, it was found that summer haze pollutants accounted for approximately 5% to 20% of June through August total respiratory and asthma admissions, on average, and that these admissions increased approximately 30% above average on the highest pollution days.

White et al. (1994) reported daily emergency room visit records from June through August 1990 at a large inner city hospital in Atlanta, Georgia. Daily counts of visits for asthma or reactive airway disease by patients 1 to 16 years of age (mean = 6.6/d) were related to daily levels of O_3, SO_2, PM_{10}, pollen, and temperature. Seasonality likely was reduced by the study period selection. Day-of-week and temperature effects were controlled as part of a Poisson model. The model yielded a 1.42 admissions rate ratio ($p = 0.057$, 95% CI = 0.99 to 2.0) for the number of asthma visits following days with O_3 levels equal to or exceeding a 1 hour maximum of 0.11 ppm, which is consistent with the relative risk values reported by Thurston et al. (1992, 1994).

In a study of Birmingham, Alabama, data, Schwartz (1994a) separately examined O_3 and PM_{10} influences on hospital admissions by the elderly for pneumonia (mean = 5.9/d) and COPD (mean = 2.2/d) causes from 1986 to 1989. Poisson regression analyses were employed, controlling for time trends, seasonal fluctuations, and weather, but day-of-week effects were not addressed. Weather was controlled by including dummy variables for seven (unspecified) temperature and dew point range categories in the regression. Base model results (excluding winter months) yielded a 2 day lag relative risk (RR) estimate of 1.14 for pneumonia admissions from a 50 ppb increase in 24 hour average O_3 (95% confidence interval, CI = 0.94 to 1.38). Excluding days exceeding 120 ppb yielded similar results (RR = 1.12, CI = 0.92 to 1.37). For COPD, the basic model yielded a RR = 1.17 (CI = 0.86 to 1.60), whereas excluding days above 120 ppb similarly gave RR = 1.18 (CI = 0.86 to 1.62).

Schwartz (1994b) analyzed O_3 and PM_{10} air pollution relationships with daily hospital admissions of persons 65 years or older in the Detroit, Michigan, metropolitan statistical area from 1986 to 1989. Daily counts for pneumonia (mean = 15.7/d), asthma (mean = 0.75/d), and all other COPDs (mean = 5.8/d) were regressed on the pollution variables and various seasonal, trend, and temperature dummy variables, using Poisson modeling. Day-of-week effects were not addressed. O_3 was analyzed with respect to both its daily 24 hour average and 1 hour maximum. Autoregressive analyses and residuals plots indicated no remaining autocorrelation in the model. Both O_3 and PM_{10} were significant in simultaneous pollutant models for pneumonia and COPD but not for asthma (which was ascribed to the low daily counts for this category). Based on the regression coefficients and data presented, it can be estimated that the mean effect for O_3 (11.6%) was double that for PM_{10} (5.7%) in the pneumonia model but comparable for COPD (12.2% for O_3 versus 10.2% for PM_{10}).

Schwartz (1994c) evaluated the associations of both PM_{10} and O_3 with respiratory hospital admissions by the elderly in Minneapolis-St. Paul, Minnesota, from 1986 to 1989, using Poisson modeling methods. Although no association was found for COPD in the elderly, O_3 did make a significant independent contribution to hospital admissions by the elderly for pneumonia (mean = 6.0/d), even after controlling for weather and PM_{10}.

In summary, the Schwartz studies of the elderly suggest that a large portion of the O_3 effects on total respiratory hospital admissions are contributed by COPD and pneumonia cases in the elderly. Based on results presented by Thurston et al. (1992, 1994), the other major contributor is asthma admissions, which are usually more prevalent in younger age groups.

The results of the hospital admission studies are summarized in Table 20-5. They indicate that ambient O_3 often has a significant effect on hospital admissions for respiratory causes, ranging in these studies from 1 to 3 total respiratory admissions/day/ 100 ppb O_3/10^6 persons, or from a 1.1 to 1.36 relative risk/100 ppb O_3.

A variety of recent population studies have analyzed associations between ambient O_3 and emergency room (ER) admissions. Cody et al. (1992) analyzed central New Jersey hospital ER visits to the high O_3 season (May–August). Their intial correlational analysis yielded negative associations between hospital visits and both temperature and O_3, which suggests that within-season long-wave effects existed. However, the authors conducted subsequent regressions of respiratory visits on both temperature and O_3 simultaneously, yielding a significant positive coefficient for O_3 and a negative coefficient for temperature, which suggests that the inclusion of temperature may have indirectly accounted for the long-wave cycle, allowing the positive short wave O_3-visit relationship to be seen. Day-of-week influence were considered but found to be unimportant for these ER visit data. No such pollution-hospital visit relationship was found for finger cut (i.e., control disease) visits.

Weisel et al. (1995) examined central New Jersey hospital ER visits for asthma (mean = 5.4/d) during the high O_3 season (May through August) for 1986 through 1990. Using a stepwise regression analysis, a significant positive coefficient for O_3 and a negative coefficient for morning temperature was found. Other environmental factors considered, including rate of temperature change, RH, every-sixth-day sulfates, NO_2, SO_2, and visibility (an index of fine particles, FPs), were not found to be correlated with asthma visits.

Stieb et al. (1996) examined the relationship of asthma ER visits to daily concentrations of O_3 and other air pollutants in Saint John, New Brunswick, Canada. Data on ER visits with a presenting complaint of asthma ($n = 1987$) were abstracted for the period 1984 to 1992 (May–September). Air pollution variables included O_3, SO_2, NO_2, $SO_4^=$, and TSP; weather variables included temperature, dewpoint, and relative humidity. Daily ER visit frequencies were filtered to remove day-of-week and long wave trends, and filtered values were regressed on air pollution and weather variables for the same day and the three previous days. The mean daily 1 hour O_3 maximum concentration during the study period was 41.6 ppb. A positive, statistically significant ($p < 0.05$) association was observed between O_3 and asthma ER visits two days later, and the strength of the association was greater in nonlinear models. The frequency of asthma ER visits was 33% higher (95% CI, 10–56%) when the daily 1 hour O_3 maximum exceeded 75 ppb (the 95th percentile). The O_3 effect was not significantly influenced by the addition of weather or other pollutant variables into the model or by the exclusion of repeat ER visits.

Yang et al. (1997) examined the association between air pollution and the ER visits for asthma in Reno, Nevada, for the period 1992 to 1994. All three hospitals in the region were included, and there was a total of 1593 ER visits for asthma during this period. The air pollution variables were collected from seven monitoring stations, including PM-10, O_3, and CO. Levels of pollution were moderately elevated (the average concentrations of PM-

10, CO, and O_3 were $38.0\,\mu g\,/\,m^3$, 4.55 ppm, and 51.0 ppb, respectively). Weighted least-squares (WLS) regression and autoregressive integrated moving average (ARIMA) time-series analyses were applied and compared. After adjusting for such factors as day of the week, seasonal variation, and weather, both modeling methods showed that the daily 1 hour maximum O_3 concentration was a significant predictor of asthma ER visits. Total asthma visits increased 33.7% (95% CI, range 6.0–61.5%) for each 100 ppb increase in the O_3 level. No association of the concentration of other measured pollutants with daily asthma ER visits was found.

Another index of respiratory morbidity that has been studied is clinic visits. Hernandez-Garduno et al. (1997) monitored patient visits for upper respiratory tract infections in Mexico City at five clinics, and collected data on levels of O_3, NO_2, CO, SO_2, and climatological variables. Correlations of filtered data revealed an association between NO_2 and O_3 and an increase in visits to clinics because of respiratory problems. Autoregressive analysis indicated that pollutant levels / respiratory visits associations remained significant even after simultaneous inclusion of temperature, suggesting that air pollution was associated with 10% to 16% of the clinic visits. High levels of O_3 and NO_2 increased the total number of clinic visits to between 19% and 43% above average. The other pollutants and the control group did not demonstrate significant associations. Overall, these results are consistent with an O_3 effect on asthma morbidity.

Another index of respiratory morbidity in asthmatics is physician authorized medication usage. In their study of children with moderate to severe asthma at a summer camp in the Connecticut River valley, Thurston et al. (1997) found that the camp physician authorized supplemental medication to children in the group at a rate proportional to the ambient O_3 concentration.

Mortality   Kinney and Ozkaynak (1991) examined a 10-year record of daily mortality data from Los Angeles County. They demonstrated assocations between short-term variations in total mortality (excluding accidents and suicides) and O_3, controlling for temperature. Similar results were detected for cardiovascular mortality. They were obtained by fitting multiple linear regression models with mortality as the outcome variable and up to seven environmental variables as regressors. A parsimonious three-variable model (NO_2, 1 day lagged O_3, and temperature) explained 4% of the short-term variation in total mortality. Temperature and O_3 had the strongest association with mortality.

However, in a follow-up study that included PM_{10} as an additional variable in a multiple regression analysis, Kinney et al. (1995) reported that the association between O_3 and daily mortality disappeared when PM-10 was added to the model. These results suggest that the relationship, if any, between O_3 and daily mortality is weaker than that involving PM-10 and, further, that the univariate O_3 effect may have been due to O_3 acting as a PM-10 surrogate. The results of this follow-up study indicated that CO had an independent association with mortality that was of similar strength to that of PM-10. Similar findings were reported for Mexico City by Borja-Aburto et al. (1997). O_3 was significantly associated with daily mortality when considered alone. However, when a multiple regression analysis with TSP, SO_2, and O_3 was performed, only TSP remained significant.

On the other hand, many other recent studies that have examined the possible influence of O_3 on daily mortality have reported independent effects of O_3 in multiple regression analyses. Sartor et al. (1995, 1997) found that O_3 affected mortality during the summer of 1994 for both all ages, and for the elderly in Belgium and that temperature potentiated the response to O_3. Verhoeff et al. (1996), examined daily mortality in Amsterdam, the Netherlands, for 1986 to 1992, and reported that O_3 lagged two days was positively associated with mortality, along with current day black smoke (BS) and PM_{10}. There was no association with SO_2 or CO. Anderson et al. (1996) studied air pollution and daily mortality in London, England, during 1987 to 1992. They reported that both same day O_3 and BS were independently associated with all cause mortality, which was greater on warm days, and independent of the effects of other pollutants. O_3 was also significantly associated with cardiovascular and respiratory disease mortality.

Touloumi et al. (1997) performed a combined analysis of daily mortality for six western and central European cities participating in the Air Pollution and Health: A European Approach (APHEA) project. They reported that a $50\,\mu g/m^3$ increase in daily 1 hour maximum O_3 concentration was associated with a 2.9% increase in the number of deaths, and the effect was independent of the BS concentration change and consistent across the cities.

Abstracts of daily mortality studies from Toronto, Canada, Brisbane, Australia, and Rotterdam, the Netherlands, have also reported associations between daily mortality and O_3. Collectively all of this recent research appears to indicate that O_3 can affect daily mortality, but that the effect of coexposures to PM have a somewhat greater impact.

Effects on Athletic Performance

It has been more than three decades since epidemiological evidence suggested that the precentage of high school track team members failing to improve performance increased with increasing oxidant concentrations the hour before a race (Wayne et al., 1967). The effects may have been related to increased airway resistance or to associated discomfort, which may have limited motivation to run at maximal levels. Controlled exposure studies of heavily exercising competitive runners have demonstrated decreased function at 200 to 300 ppb (Savin and Adams, 1979; Adams and Schelegle, 1983). At 210 ppb O_3, Folinsbee et al. (1984) reported symptoms as well in seven distance cyclists exercising heavily ($V_E = 81\,L/min$).

Recent studies have shown reduced performance at lower O_3 concentrations. Schelegle and Adams (1986) exposed 10 young male adult endurance athletes to 120, 180, and 240 ppb O_3 while they exercised at a mean V_E of $54\,L/min$ for 30 minutes, followed by a mean V_E of $120\,L/min$ for an additional 30 minutes. Although all 10 completed the protocol for filtered air exposure, 1, 5, and 7 of them could not complete it for the 120, 180, and 240 ppb exposures. Linder et al. (1988) also found that maximum performance time was reduced for their 16 to 28 min progressive maximum exercise for V_E of 30 to $120\,L/min$ in young adults when O_3 was present. For example, performance was reduced 11% in females exposed to 130 ppb O_3.

There are animal models for decreased performance during O_3 exposure. Tepper et al. (1985) exposed rats and mice for 6 hours to O_3 at 80, 120, 250, or 500 ppb while housed in running wheels. Running in both species decreased in a concentration-related manner during exposure to O_3, with the decrease being greater with increasing time of exposure. The decrease in running activity produced by O_3 persisted for several hours after exposure. At comparable concentrations, activity in rats decreased more than in mice.

Effects on Airway Reactivity

Exposure to O_3 can also alter the responsiveness of the airways to other bronchoconstrictive challenges as measured by changes in respiratory mechanics. For example, Folinsbee et al. (1988) reported that airway reactivity to the bronchoconstrictive drug methacholine for the group of subjects as a whole was approximately doubled following 6.6 hour exposures to 120 ppb O_3. Airway hyperresponsiveness (to histamine) had previously been demonstrated, but only at O_3 concentrations ≥ 400 ppb (Seltzer et al., 1986; Holtzman et al., 1979). On an individual basis, Folinsbee et al. (1988) found no apparent relationship between the O_3-associated changes in methacholine reactivity and those in FVC or FEV_1. On the other hand, Aris et al. (1991) reported a closer relationship, more similar to reported responses to inhaled H_2SO_4 aerosol, where changes in function correlated closely to changes in reactivity to carbachol aerosol, a bronchonconstrictive drug (Utell et al., 1983). The O_3-associated changes in bronchial reactivity may predispose individuals to bronchospasm from other environmental agents such as acid aerosol and naturally occurring aeroallergens.

The follow-up tests by Horstman et al. (1990), involving 6.6 hour exposures to 80, 100, and 120 ppb, produced 56%, 89%, and 121% increases in methacholine responsiveness, respectively. Increased responsiveness to methacholine was also seen in the Folinsbee and Hazucha (1989) study with 1 hour at 350 ppb. An increased responsiveness to histamine was seen by Gong et al. (1988) in one of 17 competitive cyclists exposed at 120 ppb for 1 hour at V_E of 89 L/min followed by 3 to 4 minutes at 150 L/min. At 200 ppb, responsiveness increased in 9 of the 17 subjects. McDonnell et al. (1987) found increased histamine responsiveness in 26 young adult males with allergic rhinitis after O_3 at 180 ppb during 2 hours of exercise at 64 L/min. Jorres et al. (1996) exposed 24 subjects with mild stable allergic asthma, 12 subjects with allergic rhinitis without asthma, and 10 healthy subjects to 250 ppb O_3 or filtered air (FA) for 3 hours with intermittent exercise. They determined the concentration of methacholine (PC20FEV$_1$) and the dose of allergen (PD20FEV$_1$) producing a 20% fall in FEV$_1$. In the subjects with asthma, FEV$_1$ decreased by $12.5 \pm 2.2\%$, PC20FEV$_1$ of methacholine by 0.91 ± 0.19 doubling concentrations and PD20FEV$_1$ of allergen by 1.74 ± 0.25 doubling doses after O_3 compared with sham exposure to filtered air (FA). The changes in lung function, methacholine, and allergen responsiveness did not correlate with each other. In the subjects with rhinitis, mean FEV$_1$ decreased by 7.8% and 1.3% when O_3 or FA, respectively, were followed by allergen inhalation.

The basis for the effect of O_3 on airway reactivity was examined by Gordon et al. (1981) in guinea pigs exposed for 1 hour to either 100 or 800 ppb O_3. Both exposures significantly inhibited lung cholinesterase activity as compared to levels in unexposed animals.

The O_3-induced responsiveness may be centered in the peripheral lung and be retained long after the O_3 exposure ceases on the basis of a study by Beckett et al. (1988). They exposed the peripheral lungs of anesthetized dogs to 1000 ppb O_3 for 2 hours using a wedged bronchoscope technique. A contralateral sublobar segment was simultaneously exposed to air as a control. In the O_3-exposed segments, collateral resistance (R_{cs}) was increased within 15 minutes and remained elevated about 150% throughout the 2 hour exposure period. Fifteen hours later, the baseline R_{cs} of the O_3-exposed sublobar segments was significantly elevated, and these segments demonstrated increased responsiveness to aerosolized acetylcholine (100 and 500 μg/mL). There were no differences in neutrophils, mononuclear cells, or mast cells (numbers or degree of mast cell degranulation) between O_3- and air-exposed airways at 15 hours. The small airways of the lung periphery thus are capable of remaining hyperresponsive hours after cessation of localized exposure to O_3, but this does not appear to be dependent on the presence of inflammatory cells in the small airway wall.

Effects on Airway Permeability

Kehrl et al. (1987) studied the effects of inhaled O_3 on respiratory epithelial permeability in healthy, nonsmoking young men. They were exposed for 2 hours to purified air and 400 ppb ozone while performing intermittent treadmill exercise at 67 L/min. Specific airway resistance (SR$_{aw}$) and FVC were measured before and at the end of exposures. Seventy-five minutes after the exposures, the pulmonary clearance of a radioisotope-labeled organic molecule, namely [^{99m}Tc]DTPA, was measured as an index of epithelial permeability. Ozone exposure caused respiratory symptoms in all 8 subjects and was associated with a $14 \pm 2.8\%$ (mean $\pm$ S.E.) decrement in FVC ($p < 0.001$) and a $71 \pm 22\%$

increase in SR_{aw} ($p = 0.04$). Compared with the air exposure day, 7 of the 8 subjects showed increased [^{99m}Tc]DTPA clearance after the O_3 exposure, with the mean value increasing from $0.59 \pm 0.08\%$ to $1.75 \pm 0.43\%$/min ($p = 0.03$). Thus O_3 exposure sufficient to produce decrements in the respiratory function of human subjects also causes an increase in permeability. An increased permeability could facilitate the uptake of other inhaled toxicants and/or the release of inflammatory cells such as neutrophils onto the airway surfaces.

Foster and Stetkiewicz (1996) studied the influence of O_3 on lung permeability in nine healthy subjects at 18 to 20 hours after 2 hour exposures at 150 and 350 ppb. Permeability was measured in terms of the clearance rate of a water soluble aerosol containing ^{99m}Tc-labeled DTPA (diethylamine pentaacetic acid). Based on a sequence of γ-camera measurements of ^{99m}Tc clearance from the lungs, they concluded that ^{99m}Tc-DTPA clearance from the lung periphery and apexes was significantly increased by O_3, but changes in clearance for the base of the lung were not significant. The FEV_1 at the late time after O_3 was slightly but significantly reduced (-2.1%) from pre-exposure levels. There was no relationship between the functional changes observed acutely after exposure to O_3 and subsequent changes in ^{99m}Tc-DTPA clearance or FEV_1 observed at the late period. These results suggest that epithelial permeability of the lung is altered 18 to 20 hours post-O_3; this injury is regional, and the lung base appears to have a different time course of response or is in an adapted state with respect to O_3 exposure.

In laboratory tests in rats, Bhalla et al. (1987) reported that exposure to resting rats to 800 ppb O_3 increased tracheal and bronchoalveolar permeability to DTPA at 1 hour after the exposure. Bronchoalveolar but not tracheal permeability remained elevated 24 hours after the exposure. Exercise during exposure to O_3 increased permeability to both tracers in the tracheal and the bronchoalveolar zones and prolonged the duration of increased permeability in the tracheal zone from 1 to 24 hours and that in the bronchoalveolar zone from 24 to 48 hours. Exposure at rest to 600 ppb O_3 plus 2500 ppb NO_2 significantly increased bronchoalveolar permeability at 1 and 24 hours after exposure, although exposure at rest to 600 ppb O_3 alone increased bronchoalveolar permeability only at 1 hour after exposure. Exposure to O_3 and NO_2 during exercise led to significantly greater permeability to DTPA than did exercising exposure to O_3 alone. Nitric acid vapor was formed in the $O_3 + NO_2$ atmosphere, suggesting that acidic components in the atmospheres produced effects that were additive on the effect of O_3 in producing both increase and prolongation of permeability in tracheal and bronchoalveolar zones of the respiratory tract.

Guth et al. (1986) examined changes in apparent lung permeability in rats by measurement of recovery of labeled bovine serum albumin in lung lavage fluid after intravenous injection at the end of the O_3 exposure. Their permeability index increased in an exposure-concentration-dependent manner after 6 or 24 hours of exposure to O_3 at or above levels of 400 ppb. It was also increased after 2 days of exposure to 200 ppb of O_3. Abraham et al. (1984) measured changes in airway permeability of tritiated histamine in sheep after exposure to O_3. Measurements made 24 hours after a 2 hour exposure to 500 ppb showed increased permeability. This persistently increased permeability is consistent with the observations of Bhalla et al. (1987) in rats.

Effects on Airway Inflammation

Seltzer et al. (1986) showed that O_3-induced airway reactivity to methacholine is associated with neutrophil influx into the airways and with changes in cyclooxygenase metabolites of arachidonic acid. For 2 hour exposures to O_3 at 400 ppb with intermittent exercise, the BAL fluid had increased prostaglandins E_2 and $F_{2\alpha}$ and thromboxane B_2 3 hours after the O_3 exposure.

Reports of Koren et al. (1989) and Devlin et al. (1991) also described inflammatory and biochemical changes in the airways following O_3 exposure. In the initial studies, subjects were exposed to 400 ppb for 2 hours while performing intermittent exercise at a ventilation of 70 L/min in order to examine cellular and biochemical responses in the airways. The BAL was performed 18 hours after the O_3 exposure. An 8.2-fold increase in polymorphonuclear leukocytes (PMNs or neutrophils) was observed after ozone exposure, confirming the observations of Seltzer et al. (1986). Twofold increases in protein, albumin, and IgG were indicative of increased epithelial permeability, as previously suggested by the [^{99m}Tc]DTPA clearance studies of Kehrl et al. (1987). In addition to confirmation of the Kehrl et al. (1987) findings, Koren et al. (1989) provided evidence of stimulation of fibrogenic processes including increases in fibronectin ($6.4 \times$), tissue factor ($2.1 \times$), factor VII ($1.8 \times$), and urokinase plasminogen activator ($3.6 \times$). There was a twofold increase in the level of prostaglandin E_2 and a similar elevation of the complement component C3a. Levels of leukotrienes C_4 and B_4 were not affected.

Devlin et al. (1991) reported that a significant inflammatory response, as indicated by increased levels of PMN, was also observed in BAL fluid from subjects exposed to either 80 or 100 ppb O_3 for 6.6 hours. As illustrated in Figure 20-8, the 6.6 hours at 100 ppb O_3 produced a 3.8-fold increase in PMNs at 18 hours after the exposure, whereas the 6.6 hours at 80 ppb produced a 2.1-fold increase. The amounts of O_3 inhaled in the 80 and 100 ppb protocols were about 2.0 and 2.5 µg, and about 3.6 µg in the 400 ppb protocol. Thus the effect of concentration was apparently somewhat greater than that of exposure duration. The significant increase in PMNs at a concentration as low as 80 ppb suggests that lung inflammation from inhaled O_3 has no threshold down to ambient background O_3 levels.

The above studies indicate that the inflammatory process caused by O_3 exposure is promptly initiated (Seltzer et al., 1986) and persists for at least 18 hours (Koren et al., 1989). The time course of this inflammatory response and the O_3 exposures necessary to initiate it, however, have not yet been fully elucidated. Furthermore these studies demonstrate that cells and enzymes capable of causing damage to pulmonary tissues were increased, and the proteins that play a role in the fibrotic and fibrinolytic processes were elevated as a result of ozone exposure.

Scannell et al. (1996) studied a group of 18 asthmatic subjects to O_3 using the same exposure protocol previously used by the same investigators for 81 healthy subjects. They reported no significant differences in lung function responses and a trend toward higher airway resistance ($p < 0.13$). By contrast, the asthmatic subjects had significantly greater ($p < 0.05$) O_3-induced increases in inflammatory endpoints (% neutrophils and total protein) in bronchoalveolar lavage fluid (BAL) as compared to 20 of the normal subjects who also underwent bronchoscopy.

Prolonged inflammatory processes following repetitive exposures to O_3 in ambient air were reported by Kinney et al. (1996) in terms of reduced release of reactive oxygen species, increased levels of LDH, IL-8, and PGE_2 in the BAL.

Interpretation of the nature and significance of the inflammatory responses following short-term O_3 exposures is difficult without knowledge of the cumulative effects that may be triggered by repetitive episodes of lung inflammation. The relation of the inflammatory reponses, if any, to the well-studied respiratory function responses also remains unknown. We do know that these responses are poorly correlated. Balmes et al. (1996) tested the hypothesis that changes in lung function induced by O_3 are correlated with indexes of respiratory tract/injury inflammation. They exposed 20 healthy subjects, on separate days, to O_3 (0.2 ppm) and filtered air for 4 hours during exercise. Symptom questionnaires were administered before and after exposure, and pulmonary function tests (FEV_1, FVC, and SR_{aw}) were performed before, during, and immediately after each exposure. Fiberoptic bronchoscopy, with isolated left main bronchus proximal airway lavage (PAL) and bronchoalveolar lavage (BAL; bronchial fraction, the first 10 ml of fluid recovered) of the

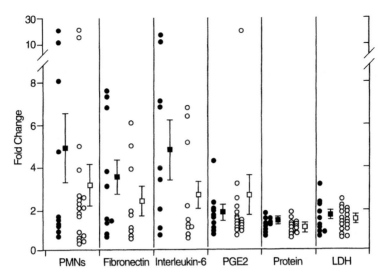

Figure 20-8 Range of subject response 18 hours after 6.6 hours of O_3 exposure at 100 ppb (closed circles) or 80 ppb (open circles). Squares indicate the mean changes ($\pm$ SE). From Devlin et al. (1991).

right middle lobe, was performed 18 hours after each exposure. The PAL, bronchial fraction, and BAL fluids were analyzed for the following endpoints: total and differential cell counts, and total protein, fibronectin, interleukin-8 (IL-8), and granulocyte-macrophage colony-stimulating factor (GM-CSF) concentrations. The study population was divided into two groups, least sensitive ($n = 12$; mean O_3-induced change in $FEV_1 = -7.0\%$) and most sensitive ($n = 8$; mean O_3-induced change in $FEV_1 = -36.0\%$). They found a highly significant O_3 effect on SR_{aw} and lower respiratory symptoms for all subjects combined but no significant differences between the least- and most-sensitive groups. Ozone exposure increased significantly percent neutrophils in PAL; percent neutrophils, total protein, and IL-8 in bronchial fraction ($p < 0.001$, $p < 0.001$, and $p < 0.01$, respectively); and percent neutrophils, total protein, fibronectin, and GM-CSF in BAL for all subjects combined. There were no significant differences, however, between least- and most-sensitive groups. Thus levels of O_3-induced symptoms and respiratory tract injury / inflammation were not correlated with the magnitude of decrements in FEV_1 and FVC.

A similar conclusion was drawn by Torres et al. (1997), who studied whether individuals who differed in lung-function responsiveness to O_3, or in smoking status, also differed in susceptibility to airway inflammation. Healthy subjects were selected on the basis of responsiveness to a classifying exposure to 220 ppb O_3 for 4 hours with exercise (responders, with a decrease in $FEV_1 > 15\%$; and non-responders, with a decrease in $FEV_1 > 5\%$). Three groups were studied: nonsmoker-nonresponders ($n = 12$), nonsmoker-responders ($n = 13$), and smokers ($n = 13$, 11 nonresponders and 2 responders). Each subject underwent two exposures to O_3 and one to air, separated by at least 3 weeks; bronchoalveolar and nasal lavages were performed on three occasions: immediately (early) and 18 hours (late) after O_3 exposure, and either early or late after air exposure. Recovery of PMNs increased progressively in all groups, and by up to 6-fold late after O_3 exposure. IL-6 and IL-8 increased early (by up to 10-fold and up to 2-fold, respectively), and correlated with the late increase in PMN. Lymphocytes, mast cells, and eosinophils also increased late after exposure. Thus O_3-induced airway inflammation was independent of smoking status or airway responsiveness to O_3.

Inflammatory reactions occur in the nasal passages as well as in the lungs. Graham et al. (1988) exposed 41 subjects to either filtered air or 500 ppb O_3 for 4 hours on two consecutive days. Nasal lavages were taken before and immediately following each exposure and 22 hours after the last exposure. Lavage PMN counts increased significantly ($p = 0.005$) in the O_3-exposed group, with 3.5-, 6.5-, and 3.9-fold increases over the air-exposed group at the post-1, pre-2, and post-2 time points, respectively. Graham and Koren (1990) compared the cellular changes detected in nasal lavage (NL) with those detected in the bronchoalveolar lavage (BAL) taken from the same individual. A group of 10 subjects was exposed to either filtered air or 400 ppb O_3, with exercise, for 2 hours. The NL was done prior to, immediately following, and 18 hour postexposure; the BAL was done only at 18 hour postexposure. A significant increase in PMNs was detected in the NL immediately postexposure to O_3 (7.7-fold increase, $p = 0.003$) and remained elevated in the 8 hour post-O_3 NL (6.1-fold increase, $p < 0.001$). A similar increase in PMNs was detected in the BAL 18 hours after exposure to O_3 (6.0-fold increase, $p < 0.001$). The albumin levels in the NL and BAL were also similarly increased 18 hours after O_3 (3.9-fold and 2.2-fold, respectively). Although a qualitative correlation in the mean number of PMNs existed between the upper and lower respiratory tract after O_3, comparison of the NL and BAL PMNs from each individual showed a significant quantitative correlation for the air data ($r = 0.741$, $p = 0.014$) but not for the O_3 data ($r = 0.408$, $p = 0.243$).

The utility of this approach at low ambient levels of O_3 was demonstrated by Frischer et al. (1993). They studied nasal airways inflammation after O_3 exposure in 44 children by repeated nasal lavages from May to October 1991. During this time period five to eight lavages were performed for each child. On 14 days following "high" O_3 (> 90 ppb) 148 nasal lavages were performed, and on 10 days following "low" O_3 (< 70 ppb) 106 nasal lavages were performed. A significant increase of PMN counts from low to high O_3 days was observed. Concomitant with a decrease of O_3 in the fall mean PMN counts showed a downward trend. Humoral markers of inflammation were also measured. A significant increase was observed for eosinophilic cationic protein and myeloperoxidase. Thus O_3 at ambient concentrations initiated a reversible inflammatory response of the upper airways in normal children.

Peden et al. (1995) studied the role that O_3 may play in the exacerbation of airway disease in asthmatics, either by priming the airway mucosa such that cellular responses to allergen are enhanced or by exerting an intrinsic effect on airway inflammation. The effect of exposure to 400 ppb O_3 on nasal inflammation was examined in 11 allergic asthmatics sensitive to *Dermatophygoides farinae*. This study design emphasized the effect of O_3 exposure on the late-phase reaction to allergen using eosinophil influx and changes in eosinophil cationic protein as principal endpoints. By employing a "split-nose" design, in which allergen was applied to only one side of the nose while saline was applied to the contralateral side, both the effect of O_3 on nasal inflammation due to allergen challenge as well as its direct action on non-allergen-challenged nasal tissues was examined. They found that O_3 exposure had both a priming effect on allergen-induced responses as well as an intrinsic inflammatory action in the nasal airways.

Studies in laboratory animals have examined the roles of O_3 concentration and exposure time on biochemical and cellular responses. Rombout et al. (1989) exposed mice and rats to 380, 750, 1250, and 2000 ppb O_3 for 1, 2, 4, and 8 hours and measured BAL protein with both daytime and nighttime exposures. Observation times extended from 1 to 54 hours. The responses varied with O_3 concentration, duration of exposure, time after the start of the exposure, and minute volume, with time of exposure having a greater than proportional influence. For 4 and 8 hour exposures, the protein content of BAL peaked at 24 hours and remained at elevated levels even at 54 hours. As indicated previously, Devlin et al. (1991) found increased BAL protein in humans 18 hours after an exposure to 100 ppb O_3 for 6.6 hours.

Bhalla and Young (1992) studied the sequenc of changes in lung epithelial permeability, free cells in the airways, prostaglandin E_2 (PGE_2) levels, PMN flux, and alveolar lesions in rats exposed to 0.8 ppm ozone (O_3) for 3 hours and then studied at 4 hour intervals up to 24 hour postexposure. Protein content of the BAL increased immediately after O_3 exposure and returned to control levels by 16 hour postexposure. Albumin concentration in the BAL increased more gradually, and the albumin concentrations at 20 and 24 hour postexposure were still higher than the control levels. While the total protein in the BAL could be attributed to tissue injury and increased transmucosal transport, the albumin primarily reflected elevated transport from the serum. Total cells in the BAL decreased immediately after the O_3 exposure but returned to near normal levels by 4 hours. PGE_2 levels did not change significantly after O_3 exposure. PMNs in the lung sections increased in number with time, peaked at 8 hours, and returned to normal levels by 16 hours following O_3 exposure. The data suggest that the permeability changes may be produced by the direct toxic effects of O_3 on the airway epithelia, but the PMNs contribute to the injury process, especially at the later stages. Lung lesions, represented by the thickening of the alveolar septae and increased cellularity, were present at 12 hour postexposure and increased with time, thus coinciding with declining permeability at the later stages. The morphological changes lag behind the functional perturbations and appear to represent a phase of functional recovery.

The weight of the evidence from these results, showing both functional and biochemical responses in humans and laboratory animals which accumulate over multiple hours and persist for many hours or days after exposure ceases, is clear and compelling. Both functional changes and inflammatory processes were shown to occur in humans following exposures to 100 ppb O_3 for 6.6 hours, whereas higher concentrations were required to elicit comparable responses in rats. Thus the rat data, which provide evidence of other effects as well, appear to provide conservative indications of effects in humans.

Effect of Single- and Multiday Exposures on Particle Clearance

Foster et al. (1987) studied the effect of 2 hour exposures to 200 or 400 ppb O_3 with intermittent light exercise on the rates of tracheobronchial mucociliary particle clearance in healthy adult males. The 400 ppb O_3 exposure produced a marked acceleration in particle clearance from both central and peripheral airways, as well as a 12% drop in FVC. It is of interest that the 200 ppb O_3 exposure produced a significant acceleration of particle clearance in peripheral airways but failed to produce a significant reduction in FVC, suggesting that significant changes in the ability of the deep lung to clear deposited particles take place before significant changes in respiratory function take place.

The effects of O_3 on mucociliary particle clearance have also been studied in rats and rabbits. Rats exposed for 4 hours to O_3 at concentrations in the range of 400 to 1200 ppb exhibited a slowing of particle clearance at ≥ 800 ppb but not at 400 ppb (Frager et al., 1979; Kenoyer et al., 1981). Rabbits exposed for 2 hours at 100, 250, and 600 ppb O_3 showed a concentration-dependent trend of reduced clearance rate with increasing concentrations, with the change at 600 ppb being about 50% and significantly different from control (Schlesinger and Driscoll, 1987). It is not known why the animal tests show only retarded mucociliary clearance in response to O_3 exposure whereas the human tests show accelerated clearance. In corresponding tests with other irritants, namely, H_2SO_4 aerosol and cigarette smoke, both humans and animals have exhibited accelerated clearance at lower exposures and retarded clearance at higher exposures (Lippmann et al., 1987).

Phipps et al. (1986) examined the effects of acute exposure to O_3 on some of the factors that affect mucociliary transport rates in studies in which sheep were exposed to 500 ppb O_3 for 2 hours on two consecutive days. The exposures produced increased basal secretion of sulfated glycoproteins but had no effect on ion fluxes. Histological examination indicated a moderate hypertrophy of submucosal glands in the lower trachea, and they concluded that the exposure caused airway-mucus hypersecretion.

Studies of the effects of O_3 on alveolar macrophage-mediated particle clearance during the first few weeks have also been performed in rats and rabbits. Rats exposed for 4 hours to 800 ppb O_3 had accelerated particle clearance (Frager et al., 1979). Rabbits exposed to 100, 600, or 1200 ppb O_3 once for 2 hours had accelerated clearance at 100 ppb and retarded clearance at 1200 ppb. Rabbits exposed for 2 h / d for 13 consecutive days at 100 or 600 ppb O_3 had accelerated clearance for the first 10 days, with a greater effect at 600 ppb (Driscoll et al., 1986).

The responses of the alveolar macrophages to these exposures was examined by Driscoll et al. (1987). A single exposure to 100 ppb resulted in increased macrophage numbers at 7 days, and repeated exposures resulted in an increase in macrophages and neutrophils on days 7 and 14. Macrophage phagocytosis was depressed immediately and 24 hours after acute exposure to 100 ppb and at all times after exposure to 1200 ppb. Repeated exposures to 100 ppb produced reductions in the numbers of phagocytically active macrophages on days 3 and 7, with a return to control levels by day 14. Substrate attachment by macrophages was impaired immediately after exposure to 1200 ppb. The results of these studies demonstrated significant alterations in the numbers and functional properties of alveolar macrophages as a result of single or repeated exposure to 100 ppb ozone, a level frequently encountered in areas of high photochemical air pollution.

Effects of Single and Multiday Exposures on Lung Infectivity

Both in vivo and in vitro studies have demonstrated that O_3 can affect the ability of the immune system to defend against infection. Increased susceptibility to bacterial infection has been reported in mice at 80 to 100 ppb O_3 for a single 3 hour exposure (Coffin et al., 1967; Ehrlich et al., 1977; Miller et al., 1978a). Related alterations of the pulmonary defenses caused by short-term exposures to O_3 include impaired ability to inactivate bacteria in rabbits and mice (Coffin et al., 1968; Coffin and Gardner, 1972; Goldstein et al., 1977; Ehrlich et al., 1979) and impaired macrophage phagocytic activity, mobility, fragility, and membrane alterations and reduced lysosomal enzymatic activity (Witz et al., 1983; Dowell et al., 1970; Hurst and Coffin, 1971; Hurst et al., 1970; Goldstein et al., 1971a,b; McAllen et al., 1981; Amoruso et al., 1981). Some of these effects have been shown to occur in a variety of species including mice, rats, rabbits, guinea pigs, dogs, sheep, and monkeys.

Other studies indicate similar effects for short-term and subchronic exposures of mice to O_3 combined with pollutants such as SO_2, NO_2, H_2SO_4, and particles (Gardner et al., 1977; Aranyi et al., 1983; Ehrlich, 1980; Grose et al., 1980a,b; Phalen et al., 1980). Similar to the human pulmonary function response to O_3, activity levels of mice exposed to O_3 have been shown to play a role in determining the lowest effective concentration that alters the immune defenses (Illing et al., 1980). In addition the duration of exposure must be considered. In groups of mice exposed to 200 ppb O_3 for 1, 3, or 6 hours, superoxide anion radical production decreased 8%, 18%, and 35%, respectively, indicating a progressive decrease in bacteriocidal capacity with increasing duration of exposure (Amoruso and Goldstein, 1988).

The major limitation of this large body of data on the influence of inhaled O_3 on lung infectivity is that it requires uncertain interspecies extrapolating in order to estimate the possible effects of O_3 on infectivity in humans.

Gilmour and Selgrade (1993) compared the pulmonary defenses of rats and mice against streptococcal infection following O_3 exposures. In mice, 3 hour O_3 exposures at

400 ppb resulted in bacterial proliferation and PMN influx in the lungs and excess mortality. By contrast, the rats had only a transient impairment of microbial inactivation. These results indicate that caution is needed in translating the results from either species to predictions of human responses.

Genotoxic Effects

The 1996 EPA Criteria Document (U.S. EPA, 1996a) reviewed the genotoxic effects of ozone in detail. The available reported data is summarized here as follows:

- The data on the genotoxicity of O_3 are both weakly positive and negative.
- The in vitro studies are mechanistically interesting, but there were difficulties in the design of many of these studies. First, the concentrations used were typically orders of magnitude greater than those found in ambient air. Second, extrapolation of in vitro exposure concentrations to human exposure dose requires special methods that were not used in these studies. Third, direct exposure of isolated cells to O_3 is somewhat artifactual because it bypasses host defenses and also results in chemical reactions between O_3 and culture media to generate chemical species that may not be produced in vivo. For these reasons the relevance and predictive value of in vitro studies to human health are questionable. The most relevant data on the genotoxicity of O_3 should therefore be obtained from in vivo studies.
- The earlier studies in whole animal carcinogenesis bioassays must be considered ambiguous at this time (Witschi, 1988, 1991). The earlier negative animal carcinogenesis studies, the negative carcinogenicity results in inhalation carcinogenesis studies in F344/N male and female rats, the ambiguous data in male $B6C3F_1$ mice, and the weak carcinogenicity of O_3 in female $B6C3F_1$ mice indicate that O_3 is carcinogenic only in female $B6C3F_1$ mice at high concentrations (1.0 ppm). The weak carcinogenicity of O_3 in female mice, the weak/ambiguous results in male mice, and the negative results in male and female F344/N rats point to, at best, a weak carcinogenicity of O_3 at very high concentrations.

Effects of Other Pollutants on Responses to Ozone

A study that addressed the issue of the potentiation of the characteristic functional response to inhaled O_3 by other environmental cofactors was performed in Tuxedo, New York (Spektor et al., 1988b). It involved healthy adult nonsmokers engaged in a daily program of outdoor exercise with exposures to an ambient mixture containing low concentrations of acidic aerosols and NO_2 as well as O_3. Each subject did the same exercise each day, but exercise intensity and duration varied widely between subjects, with minute ventilation ranging from 20 to 153 L, with an average of 79 L, and with duration of daily exercise ranging from 15 to 55 minutes, with an average of 29 minutes. Respiratory function measurements were performed immediately before and after each exercise period. The O_3 concentrations during exercise ranged from 21 to 124 ppb. All measured functional indexes showed significant ($p < 0.01$) O_3-associated mean decrements. As shown in Table 20-4, the functional decrements were similar, in proportion to lung volume, to those seen in children engaged in supervised recreational programs in summer camps. They were as large (FEV_1) as or much larger [FVC, FEF_{25-75}, peak expiratory flow rate (PEFR)] than those seen in controlled 1 and 2 hour exposures in chambers. For the subgroup with the most comparable levels of physical activity, the responses in the field study were even greater. Since the ambient exposures of the adults exercising out of doors were for about one-half hour, as compared to the 1 or 2 hour exposures in the chamber studies, it was concluded that ambient cofactors potentiate the responses to O_3. Thus the results of the exposures in chambers to O_3 in purified air underestimate the O_3-associated responses that occur among populations engaged in normal outdoor recreational activity and exposed to O_3 in ambient air in the northeastern United States.

The apparent potentiation of O_3-induced functional decrements seen by Spektor et al. (1988b) in rural New York was not seen by Avol et al. (1984) in a study in southern California in which 42 healthy young men and 8 healthy young women were exposed for 1 hour to ambient air containing an average of 153 ppb O_3 while exercising heavily in a chamber. The functional decrements were slightly but not significantly smaller than those produced in the same subjects on another day when they were exposed to 160 ppb O_3 in purified air. The ambient air in southern California has much higher NO_2 concentrations and much lower acid aerosol concentrations than the ambient air in the northeastern United States. Thus it appears that the H^+ content of aerosols is a more likely causal factor for the potentiation seen by Spektor et al. (1988b) than is NO_2.

However, it must be noted that the Spektor et al. (1988b) study on exercising adults, and earlier studies on children at summer camps (Lioy et al., 1985; Spektor et al., 1988a), were not able to demonstrate the specific effect of any of the measured environmental variables, including heat stress and acid aerosol concentration, on the O_3-associated responses. The inability to show the individual effects of other environmental cofactors on the response to ambient O_3 may result from inadequate knowledge on the appropriate biological averaging time for these other factors. However, in the study of functional responses of children to ambient pollution in Mendham, New Jersey, a week-long baseline shift in PEFR was associated with both O_3 and H_2SO_4 exposures during a 4 day pollution episode that preceded it (Lioy et al., 1985). A similar response to a brief episode with elevated O_3 and a much higher peak 4 hour concentration of H_2SO_4 (46 $\mu g/m^3$) was seen among girls attending a summer camp in 1986 at Dunnville, Ontario, Canada, on the northeast shore of Lake Erie (Raizenne et al., 1989).

Several controlled human exposure studies in chambers have not demonstrated synergism in functional response between O_3 and NO_2 (Koenig et al., 1988) or between O_3 and H_2SO_4, although Stacy et al. (1983) did report that the mean responses to 400 ppb O_3 and 100 $\mu g/m^3$ H_2SO_4 after 2 hours of exposure at rest were -9.0% for FVC and -11.5% for FEV_1, compared to corresponding values of -5.7% and -7.7% for O_3 alone, -1.4%, and -1.2% for sham exposure, and $+0.9\%$ and $+0.9\%$ for H_2SO_4 alone. One possible reason why these mean differences, which appear to indicate an enhancement of the O_3 response by H_2SO_4, were not statistically significant is the very high variability of the sham exposure results. By contrast, Koenig et al. (1990) did demonstrate that prior exposure to O_3 at 120 ppb with intermittent exercise for 45 minutes potentiated the subsequent respiratory function response to a 15 minute exposure to SO_2 at 100 ppb. More recently Frampton et al. (1995) exposed 30 healthy and 30 asthmatic volunteers to either 100 $\mu g/m^3$ H_2SO_4 or NaCl for 3 hour followed 24 hours later by 3 hours exposures to O_3 at either 80, 120, or 180 ppb. For the healthy group, no convincing symptomatic or physiologic effects of exposure to either the aerosol or O_3 on lung function were found. For the asthmatic group, pre-exposure to H_2SO_4 altered the pattern of response to O_3 in comparison with NaCl pre-exposure, and appeared to enhance the small mean decrements in FVC that occurred in response to 180 ppb O_3. Individual responses among asthmatic subjects were quite variable, some demonstrating reductions in FEV_1 of more than 35% following O_3 exposure. Analysis of variance of changes in FVC revealed evidence for interactions between aerosol and O_3 exposure both immediately after ($p = 0.005$) and 4 hours after ($p = 0.030$) exposure. Similar effects were seen for FEV_1. When normal and asthmatic subjects were combined, four-way analysis of variance revealed an interaction between O_3 and aerosol for the entire group ($p = 0.0022$) and a difference between normal and asthmatic subjects ($p = 0.0048$). There was no significant effect of exposures on symptoms for either normal or asthmatic subjects.

Pollutant interactions that potentiate the characteristic O_3 response have also been reported for other effects in controlled exposure studies in animals. Osebold et al. (1980) exposed antigenically sensitized mice to 500 ppb O_3 for 3 days, with and without concurrent exposure to 1 mg / m^3 of submicrometer H_2SO_4 droplets. There was an increase in atopic reactivity that was greater than that for each pollutant alone. Lee et al. (1990) exposed 3-month-old male rats to filtered room air (control) or 1.20 ppm (2256 µg / m^3) NO_2, 300 ppb (588 µg / m^3) O_3, or a combination of the two oxidants continuously for 3 days. They studied a series of parameters in the lung, including lung weight and enzyme activities related to NADPH generation, sulfhydryl metabolism, and cellular detoxification. The results showed that relative to control, exposure to NO_2 caused small (nonsignificant) changes in all the parameters; O_3 caused significant increases in all the parameters except for superoxide dismutase; and a combination of NO_2 and O_3 caused increases in all the parameters, and the increases were greater than those caused by NO_2 or O_3 alone. Statistical analysis of the data showed that the effects of combined exposure were synergistic for 6-phosphogluconate dehydrogenase, isocitrate dehydrogenase, glutathione reductase, and superoxide dismutase activities; they were additive for glutathione peroxidase and disulfide reductase activities but not different from those of O_3 exposure for other enzyme activities.

Kleinman et al. (1989) reported that lesions in the gas-exhange region of the lung of rats exposed to O_3 were greater in size in rats exposed to mixtures containing O_3 with either H_2SO_4 or NO_2. Graham et al. (1987) reported a synergistic interaction between O_3 and NO_2 in terms of mortality in mice challenged with streptococcal infection either immediately or 18 hours after pollutant exposure. Last (1989) reported synergistic interaction in rats, in terms of a significant increase in lung protein content, following 9 day exposures at 200 ppb O_3 with 20 or 40 µg / m^3 H_2SO_4, and a nonsignificant increase for 9 days at 200 ppb O_3 with 5 µg / m^3 H_2SO_4.

In summary, single O_3 exposures to healthy nonsmoking young adults at concentrations in the range of 80 to 200 ppb have produced a complex array of pulmonary responses including decreases in respiratory function and athletic performance and increases in symptoms, airway reactivity, neutrophil content in lung lavage, and rate of mucociliary particle clearance. As shown in Table 20-4, the responses to O_3 in purified air in chambers occur at concentrations of 80 or 100 ppb when the exposures involve moderate exercise for 6 hours or more and require concentrations of 180 or 200 ppb when the duration of exposure is 2 hours or less. On the other hand, mean FEV_1 decrements $> 5\%$ have been seen at 100 ppb of O_3 in ambient air for children at summer camps and for adults engaged in outdoor exercise for only one-half hour. The apparently greater responses to O_3 in ambient air may result from the presence of, or prior exposures to, acidic aerosol, but further investigation of this tentative hypothesis is needed.

More research is also needed to establish the interrelationships between small transient functional decrements, such as FEV_1, PEFR, mucociliary clearance rates, as well as changes in symptoms, performance, reactivity, permeability and neutrophil counts. The latter may be adverse in themselves or may be more closely related to the accumulation or progression of chronic lung damage. If transient changes in readily measured functions, such as FEV_1 or PEFR, are closely correlated with other, more significant health effects, then they could be established as useful surrogates in large-scale laboratory, field, and epidemiologic research as well as further retrospective analyses of published data on human exposure–response.

Finally we need more investigation of the mechanisms underlying the pulmonary responses to inhaled O_3. Our current understanding of the mechanisms has been summarized by Bates (1989, 1995). He notes that after ozone exposure, the inspiratory capacity is first reduced as a consequence of a lower maximal negative intrapleural pressure on taking a full inspiration. Maximal inspiratory and expiratory mouth pressures are not affected. He emphasizes that the FEV_1/FVC ratio is not initially affected after ozone exposure, which is to say that the FVC and FEV_1 initially fall together. He postulates that stimulation of the C-fiber system in the lung must lead to a "braking" effect on the inspiratory muscles as a first consequence of ozone exposure, and this probably occurs as a result of induced inflammation. The increased respiratory rate after ozone exposure, the increased lung permeability, the increased airway reactivity, and the fact that β blockers do not prevent the changes induced by ozone all support this hypothesis. A similar mechanism was invoked by Lee (1990) for the inhibitory effect of the gas phase of cigarette smoke on breathing. He showed that the effect could be largely prevented in rats by the administration of dimethylthiourea, a hydroxyl radical scavenger. The reduced response after repeated exposures might result from a thicker lining of mucus over the surface of the airway or from actual cell replacement after exposure.

EFFECTS OF MULTIPLE-DAY AND AMBIENT EPISODE EXPOSURES

Since single exposures lasting for an hour or more at current peak ambient O_3 levels produce measurable biological responses in healthy humans, and since there is a high probability that one high-O_3 day will be followed by several more high-O_3 days (Rao, 1988), it is important to know the extent to which the effects accumulate or progress over multiple days. This section reviews the fairly substantial data base on functional adaptation to repetitive exposures and the more limited data base on biochemical and structural changes that such exposures produce. It should be noted that the data on functional adaptation is largely, but not exclusively, based on studies in human volunteers, whereas the data base on biochemical and structural changes caused by O_3 is based entirely on studies in laboratory animals. Data on exposures lasting more than two weeks are discussed in the section on "Chronic Effects of Ambient Ozone Exposures."

It is well established that repetitive daily exposures, at a level that produces a functional response upon single exposure, result in an enhanced response on the second day, with diminishing responses on days 3 and 4 and virtually no response by day 5 (Farrell et al., 1979; Folinsbee et al., 1980; Hackney et al., 1977).

Brookes et al. (1989) found enhanced responses on the second day of successive exposures of exercising young adult males to 350 ppb O_3 for 1 hour as well as an enhanced response to 250 ppb when the previous day's exposure was to 350 ppb. In older adults (60–89 years) successive days of 2 hour exposures to 450 ppb O_3 with light exercise led to small functional decrements on the first 2 days but no changes on successive days (Bedi et al., 1989).

For repeated 6.6 h/d exposures to 120 ppb O_3, the peak functional response occurs on the first day, with progressively lesser responses after the second, third, and fourth days of exposure. However, for these same subjects, their responsiveness to methocholine challenge peaked on the second day, and remained elevated throughout all five days of exposure (Folinsbee et al., 1994). The persistent elevation of airway responsiveness is one reason to discount the view of some people that the functional adaptation phenomenon indicates that transient functional decrements are not an important health effect. Additional evidence comes from research in animals showing that persistent damage to lung cells accumulates even as functional adaptation takes place.

This kind of functional adaptation to exposure disappears about a week after exposure ceases (Horvath et al., 1981; Kulle et al., 1982). The adaptation phenomenon has led some people to conclude that transient functional decrements are not important health effects. On the other hand, recent research in animals has shown that persistent damage to lung cells accumulates even as functional adaptation takes place. Tepper et al. (1989) exposed rats to 350, 500, or 1000 ppb O_3 for 2.25 hours on five consecutive days. Carbon dioxide (8%) was added to the exposure during alternate 15 minute periods to stimulate breathing and thereby increase O_3 uptake and distribution. The consequences of exposure on pulmonary function, histology, macrophage phagocytosis, lavagable protein, differential cell counts, and lung tissue antioxidants were assessed. Tidal volume, frequency of breathing, inspiratory time, expiratory time, and maximal tidal flows were affected by O_3 during days 1 and 2 at all O_3 concentrations. By day 5, these O_3 responses were completely adapted at 350 ppb, greatly attenuated at 500 ppb, but showed no signs of adaptation in the group exposed to 1000 ppb. Unlike the pulmonary function data, light microscopy indicated a pattern of progressive epithelial damage and inflammatory changes associated with the terminal bronchiole region. Over the 5 day testing period, a sustained 37% increase in lavagable protein and 60% suppression of macrophage phagocytic activity were observed with exposure to 500 ppb. There were no changes in differential cell counts. Lung glutathione was initially increased but was within the control range on days 4 and 5. Lung ascorbate was significantly elevated above control on days 3 to 5. These data suggest that attenuation of the pulmonary functional response occurs, while aspects of the tissue response reveal progressive damage.

Van Bree et al. (1989) reported the influence of exposure time per day and number of exposure days on biochemical and cellular changes in the lung. Seven day exposures at 800 ppb produced a loss of normal cilia, a hypertrophic response of Clara cells, and an increase in P-450 isoenzyme activity, whereas 4 day exposures produced increases in protein, G6PDH and $GSHP_4$. In rats exposed for 2, 4, 8, or 16 days at 400 ppb O_3 for 4, 8, or 24 h / d, the quantity of antioxidant in whole-lung tissue was influenced about twice as much by the exposure duration per day as by the number of exposure days. Finally, in rats exposed to 400 ppb O_3 for 12 hours at either daytime or night time, the effects at night, when they were active, were much greater; once again showing the influence of physical activity on responses to O_3.

Further indications that functional adaptation, as measured in the days and weeks following exposure, is not fully protective against the development of pathological changes have been provided by a study reported by Farman et al. (1997). This was follow-up study of one by Last et al. (1993) that showed that rats exposed to 800 ppb O_3 and 14.4 ppm NO_2 for 6 hours daily developed progressive bronchiolitis and pulmonary fibrosis after about 8 to 10 weeks of exposure, with a high level of mortality. To begin to understand what processes are occurring during the approximately 2 to 2.5 month long period of lesion development, they studied the time course of evolution of fibrotic lesions in rats exposed to O_3 and NO_2. Rats were sampled weekly for 9 weeks from the onset of exposure, and biochemical and histopathological evaluations were performed. They also quantified the reparative potential of the airway epithelium after 4 and 8 weeks of exposure by in vivo labeling with bromodeoxyuridine (BrdU). Histopathological evaluation indicated a triphasic response temporally: inflammatory and fibrotic changes increased mildly for the first 3 weeks of exposure, stabilized or apparently decreased during weeks 4 to 6, and demonstrated severe increases over weeks 7 to 9. Biochemical quantification of lung 4-hydroxyproline (collagen) content showed a pattern consistent with the histopathology: no significant differences from controls for the first 3 weeks of exposure, significant increases in collagen content after 4 to 5 weeks of exposure, and a stabilization of lung collagen content after 6 weeks of exposure. In vivo determination of cumulative labeling indexes showed normal (or slightly decreased) repair of the small airway and alveolar epithelium after 4 weeks of exposure, with significantly diminished reparative capacity after 8 weeks. The diminished reparative capacity of the bronchiolar and alveolar epithelium may be causally linked with the rapid, progressive fibrosis that occurs in this model after about 7 to 8 weeks of exposure to O_3 plus NO_2. However, it should be noted that this progression of responses may not be relevant to lower level of exposures, since the Last et al. (1993) paper reported no long-term effects in the rats exposed to 200 ppb O_3 plus 3.6 ppm NO_2 for 90 days.

The effects of multiday O_3 exposures of laboratory animals on particle clearance from the lungs and on lung infectivity were reviewed previously. They also show that O_3-induced transient effects often become greater with repetitive exposures.

Effects in humans of a multiday episode-type exposure to O_3 in ambient air were described by Lioy et al. (1985). During a study focused on daily variations in lung function among 39 children attending a summer day camp in Mendham, New Jersey, a summer haze episode occurred in which the daily 1 hour peak O_3 concentrations exceeded 120 ppb on four consecutive days, with the highest concentration being 185 ppb. During the week following the episode, there were consistent deviations in function from the concentration compared to peak flow regressions for the individual children, indicating a persistent loss of lung function during that time. In a subsequent reanalysis of the data from this study, Lioy and Dyba (1989) suggested that the persistence of the reduced function during the week following the episode was more likely due to the cumulative daily exposure than by the daily peak concentrations. In any case, the exposure episode was apparently responsible for an approximately 1 week long shift in the function base line, suggesting that epithelial cell death and regeneration were involved and not just a reflex airway constriction.

In summary, successive days of exposure of adult humans in chambers to O_3 at current high ambient levels lead to a functional adaptation in that the responses are attenuated by the third day and are negligible by the fifth day. On the other hand, a comparable functional adaptation in rats does not prevent the progressive damage to the lung epithelium. Daily exposures of animals also increase other responses in comparison to single exposures, such as a loss of cilia, a hypertrophic response of Clara cells, alterations in macrophage function, and alterations in the rates of particle clearance from the lungs.

For children exposed to O_3 in ambient air there was a week long baseline shift in peak flow following a summer haze exposure of 4 days' duration with daily peak O_3 concentrations ranging from 125 to 185 ppb. Since higher concentrations used in adult adaptation studies in chambers did not produce such effects, it is possible that baseline shifts require the presence of other pollutants in the ambient air. A baseline shift in peak flow in camp children was also reported by Raizenne et al. (1989) following a brief episode characterized by a peak O_3 concentration of 143 ppb and a peak acidic aerosol concentration of 559 nmoles / m^3.

Chronic Effects of Ambient Ozone Exposures

The chronic effects data base includes a quite limited amount of information on human effects and a more substantial volume of data on effects seen in laboratory animals undergoing chronic exposures.

Controlled Laboratory Exposure Studies: Human Responses

A study by Linn et al. (1988) in southern California provided evidence for a seasonal adaptation of lung function. In this study a group of subjects selected for their relatively high functional responsiveness to O_3 had much greater functional decrements following 2 hours of exposure to O_3 at 180 ppb with intermittent exercise in a chamber in the spring than they did in the following autumn or winter, although their responses in the following spring were equivalent to those in the preceding spring. These findings suggest that some of the variability in acute response coefficients reported for earlier controlled human exposures to O_3 in chambers could have been related to seasonal variations in responsiveness, which, in turn, may be related to a long-term adaptation to chronic O_3 exposure.

Epidemiological Studies

Epidemiologic studies of populations living in southern California suggest that chronic oxidant exposures do affect baseline respiratory function. Detels et al. (1987) compared respiratory function at two times 5 years apart in Glendora (a high-oxidant community) and in Lancaster (a lower-oxidant community, but not low by national standards). Baseline function was lower in Glendora, and there was a greater rate of decline over 5 years. Table 20-6 shows a comparison of the annual change in lung function in Lancaster and Glendora from the Detels et al. (1987) study with that reported for Tucson, Arizonas, by Knudson et al. (1983) for a comparable population of Caucasian nonsmokers. The second-highest 1 hour O_3 concentrations in Tucson in all of 1981, 1982, and 1983 were 100, 120, and 110 ppb (U.S. EPA, 1986). In Lancaster there were 58 days in 1985 with 1 hour O_3 maxima greater than 120 ppb, whereas in Azusa, adjacent to Glendora, there were 117 days in 1985 with 1 hour O_3 maxima greater than 120 ppb (Air Resources Board, 1988). Thus the three different rates of function decline in Table 20-6 appear to suggest an exposure–response relationship with potentially significant health importance. Kilburn et al. (1985) reported that nonsmoking and ex-smoking wives of Long Beach shipyard workers had significantly lower values of FEV_1, midexpiratory flow, terminal expiratory flow, and carbon monoxide diffusing capacity than those in a matched population from Michigan. The oxidant exposures in Long Beach and Michigan are not known; those in Long Beach are similar to those in Lancaster, whereas those in Michigan are generally much lower. While both of these epidemiological studies had some serious methodologic deficiencies, they warrant citation in this discussion because they suggest effects that are consistent with the findings in the chronic animal exposure studies; namely they suggest premature aging of the lung in terms of lung function which might be expected on the basis of the cumulative changes in lung structure seen in the animals undergoing chronic exposure protocols.

Some more recent cross-sectional studies also suggest O_3-related decrements in respiratory function. In one, Stern et al. (1994) examined differences in the respiratory health status of school children, aged 7 to 11 years, who resided in 10 rural Canadian communities in areas of moderate and low exposure to regional $SO_4^=$ and O_3 pollution. Five of the communities were located in central Saskatchewan, a low-exposure region, and five were located in southwestern Ontario, an area with moderately elevated exposures resulting from long-range atmospheric transport of polluted air masses. Summertime 1 hour daily O_3 maxima means were 69.0 ppb in Ontario and 36.1 ppb in Saskatchewan.

TABLE 20-6 Annual change in lung function in various studies of ozone exposure

Population	FEV_1 (ml)	FVC (ml)	FEF_{25-75} (ml/s)	$\dot{V}_{50}$ (ml/s)	$\dot{V}_{75}$ (ml/s)	1 h $O_3 > 120$ ppb (d/y)
Males						
Tucson (86)[a]	− 29	− 30	− 36	− 37	− 23	∼ 1[d]
Lancaster (153)[b]	− 46	− 51	− 47	− 65	− 44	− 58
Glendora (168)[b]	− 48	− 60	− 89	− 112	− 69	+ 117[e]
Females						
Tucson (176)[c]	− 19	− 17	− 31	− 24	− 25	∼ 1[d]
Lancaster (286)[b]	− 33	− 38	− 53	− 77	− 41	+ 58
Glendora (325)[b]	− 44	− 44	− 97	− 109	− 76	+ 117[e]

[a] White, non–Mexican-American, > 25 years of age who never smoked (Detels et al., 1987).
[b] White non-Spanish surnames only, 19 to 59 years, who never smoked. Test results were between baseline and retest 5 years later. None had changed, their job or residence because of a respiratory problem (Knudsen et al., 1983).
[c] White, non–Mexican-American, aged > 20 but < 70 years, who never smoked (Detels et al., 1987).
[d] Second highest 1 hour ozone levels for 1981, 1982, and 1983 were 0.10, 0.12, and 0.11 ppm.
[e] Data for Azusa (about 3 mi from Glendora).

Concentrations of $SO_4^=$ were three times higher in Ontario than in Saskatchewan; there were no significant differences in levels of PM_{10} or particulate nitrates. Levels of SO_2 and NO_2 were low in both regions. After controlling for the effects of age, sex, parental smoking, parental education, and gas cooking, no significant regional differences were observed in symptoms. Children living in Ontario had statistically significant ($p < 0.01$) mean decrements of 1.7% in FVC and 1.3% in $FEV_{1.0}$ compared with Saskatchewan children, after adjusting for age, sex, weight, standing height, parental smoking, and gas cooking, but there were no statistically significant regional differences in the pulmonary flow parameters. The differences could have been due to exposures to either O_3 or $SO_4^=$, or their combination.

Another, more definitive, study by Kunzli et al. (1997) regressed mid- and end-expiratory flows ($FEF_{25-75\%}$, $FEF_{75\%}$) against effective exposure to O_3. A convenience sample of 130 UC Berkeley freshmen, ages 17 to 21, participated twice in the same tests (residential history, questionnaire, pulmonary function), 5 to 7 days apart. Students had to be life-long residents of northern (SF) or southern (LA) California. Monthly ambient 8 hour O_3 concentrations were assigned based on the lifetime residential history and nearby monitoring data for O_3.

For a 20 ppb increase (interquartile range) in 8 hour O_3, FEF 75% decreased, 14% (95% CI: 1.0–28.3%) of the population mean FEF 75%. The effect on FEF 25–75% was 7.2% of the mean. Negative confounding factors were region (SF vs. LA), gender, and ethnicity. Lifetime 8 hour average O_3 ranged from 16 to 74 ppb with little overlap between regions. There was no evidence for different O_3 effects across regions. Effects were independent of lifetime mean PM_{10}, NO_2, temperature, or humidity. Effects on FEV1 tended to be negative, whereas those for FVC, although negative in some models, where inconsistent and small. The strong relationship of lifetime ambient O_3 on mid- and end-expiratory flows of college freshmen and the lack of association with FEV1 and FVC are consistent with biologic models of chronic effects of O_3 in the small airways.

The effects of chronic exposure to O_3 and PM on the development of chronic disease was followed for 10 years in a prospective cohort study by Abbey et al. (1995) in 6340 nonsmoking Seventh-Day Adventists living in California. Ambient air monitoring data were available for O_3, TSP, $SO_4^=$, NO_2, and SO_2. No significant associations were found for NO_2 or SO_2. O_3 was significantly associated with increasing severity of asthma, and with the development of asthma in males. Measured TSP and $SO_4^=$, and estimated $PM_{2.5}$ and PM_{10}, were associated with the development of airway obstructive disease, chronic bronchitis, and asthma, and these were not confounded by the presence of the gaseous pollutants.

In terms of the effect of O_3 on longevity, the limited evidence available to date is largely negative. Mendelsohn and Orcutt (1979), in a study utilizing the Public Use Sample containing data on 2 million individuals in the United States obtained both death certificate data and air pollution network data in eight regions of the United States Highly significant and consistent associations with mortality were found for $SO_4^=$. Significant, but weaker and less consistent, associations were seen for SO_2 and CO. No significant associations were seen for O_3 or NO_2.

The only other multipollutant study of annual mortality rates was the six-cities study of Dockery et al. (1993). In this prospective cohort study of 8111 adults who were studies over a period of 14 to 16 years, highly significant and consistent mortality effects were seen for $PM_{2.5}$ and $SO_4^=$, with smaller effects indicated for TSP, SO_2, and NO_2. The variations in O_3 were too small across the six cities for effects to be detected.

Further evidence for chronic effects of O_3 were recently reported by Schwartz (1989) based an analysis of pulmonary function data in a national population study in 1976 to 1980, namely the second National Health and Nutrition Examination Survey (NHANES II). Using ambient O_3 data from nearby monitoring sites, he reported a highly significant

O_3-associated reduction in lung function for people living in areas where the annual average O_3 concentrations exceeded 40 ppb.

An autopsy study of 107 lungs from 14 to 25-year-old accident victims in Los Angeles County by Sherwin and Richters (1991) reported that 27% had what were judged to be severe degrees of structural abnormalities and bronchiolitis not expected for such young subjects, while another 48% of them had similar, but less severe, abnormalities. In the absence of corresponding analyses of lungs of comparable subjects from communities having much lower levels of air pollution, the possible association of the observed abnormalities with chronic O_3 exposure remains speculative. Some of the abnormalities observed could have been due to smoking and/or drug abuse, although the authors noted that published work on the association between smoking and small airway effects showed lesser degrees of abnormality (Cosio et al., 1980).

Although the results of these studies autopsy are strongly suggestive of serious health effects, they have been found wanting for standards setting by EPA staff (U.S. EPA, 1989). The basis for the skepticism of the findings lies in the uncertainty about the exposure characterization of the populations and the lack of control of possibly important confounding factors. Some of these limitations are inherent in large-scale epidemiologic studies. Others can be addressed in more carefully focussed study protocols.

Controlled Laboratory Exposure Studies: Animal Responses

As previously discussed, the highest O_3 dose is received at the acinus, where the terminal bronchioles lead into alveolar ducts, and a series of studies has shown that the effects of inhaled O_3 on lung structure is also greatest in this region. Using morphometric techniques selectively focused on this limited region of the lung, Barry et al. (1985) showed that significant changes occurred in the alveoli just distal to the terminal bronchioles in rats exposed for 12 h/d for 6 or 12 weeks to 120 or 240 ppb O_3. In both juvenile and adult rats there were significant increases in the numbers of alveolar type I and type II epithelial cells and alterations in the interstitium and endothelium. From physiological studies of rats that were simultaneously exposed, Raub et al. (1983) reported that there were significant increases in the vital capacity and end-expiratory volume that suggested alterations in distensibility of the lung tissue.

In a study focused on the effects of the 6 week exposures at 250 ppb on the terminal bronchioles, Barry et al. (1988) reported that exposure to O_3 produced alterations in the surface characteristics of ciliated and nonciliated (Clara) cells in both groups of rats. There were significant losses (20–30%) of the surface area contributed by ciliated cells, the luminal surface of Clara cells was decreased by 16% to 25%, and the number of brush cells per square millimeter of terminal bronchiolar basement membrane was also decreased. Thus the normal structure of terminal bronchiolar epithelial cells was significantly altered. No statistically significant interactions between the effects of O_3 and animal age at the beginning of the exposure were found.

The series of inhalation studies in which rats were exposed to O_3 at constant concentrations of either 120 or 250 ppb for 12 h/d for 6 weeks were extended to include tests in which there was a daily cycle with a baseline of 60 ppb for 13 hours with a 5 d/wk broad peak for 9 hours averaging 180 ppb and containing a 1 hour maximum of 250 ppb for a period of 3 or 12 weeks. Combining the results of these tests with the 6 week studies, Huang et al. (1988) and Chang et al. (1991) reported that hyperplasia of type I alveolar cells in the proximal alveoli was linearly related to the cumulative O_3 exposure in the four groups. Thus there is no threshold for cumulative lung damage, and any future standard to protect against chronic health damage from O_3 should have a seasonal or annual averaging time.

Rats exposed for 6 weeks to clean air or to O_3 using the daily cyclic exposure regimen used by Huang et al. (1988) were exposed once for 5 hours to an asbestos aerosol by

Pinkerton et al. (1989). When they were sacrificed 30 days later, the fiber count in the lungs of the O_3-exposed animals was three times greater than in the sham-exposed animals. Thus subchronic O_3 exposure can increase the effective dose of insoluble particles which may have toxic and/or carcinogenic effects.

In rats exposed for 12 months by Grose et al. (1989) to the daily cycle used by Huang et al. (1988), an increase in the rate of lung nitrogen washout was observed. Residual volume and total lung capacity were reduced. Glutathione peroxidase and reductase activities were increased, but pulmonary superoxide dismutase was unchanged. α-Tocopherol levels were decreased in lung lavage supernatant and unchanged in lavaged cells, while ascorbic acid and lavage fluid protein were increased. Immunological changes were not observed. Thus 12 months of exposure to O_3 caused (1) functional lung changes indicative of a "stiffer" lung, (2) biochemical changes suggestive of increased antioxidant metabolism, and (3) no observable immunological changes.

In a follow-up study in which the same exposure cycle was extended for up to 78 weeks, Tepper et al. (1991) found small, but statistically significant, changes in breathing patterns and mechanisms in unanesthetized, restrained rats at weeks 1, 3, 13, 52, and 78 during postexposure challenge with 0%, 4%, and 8% carbon dioxide (CO_2). The data indicate that O_3 exposure caused an overall increase in expiratory resistance (R_e), but particularly at 78 weeks. The spontaneous frequency of breathing and CO_2-induced hyperventilation were also reduced. The decrease in frequency was dependent on a significant increase in the inspiratory time relative to control without a change in expiratory time. However, light microscopic evaluation of the lung did not reveal any lesions associated with O_3 exposure.

Chang et al. (1992) extended the analyses of animals exposed for 78 weeks to electron microscopic morphometry. Samples from proximal alveolar regions and terminal bronchioles were obtained by microdissection. Analysis of the proximal alveolar region revealed a biphasic response. Acute tissue reactions after 1 week of exposure included epithelial inflammation, interstitial edema, interstitial cell hypertrophy, and influx of macrophages. These responses subsided after 3 weeks of exposure. Progressive epithelial and interstitial tissue responses developed with prolonged exposure and included epithelial hyperplasia, fibroblast proliferation, and interstitial matrix accumulation. The epithelial responses involved both type I and type II epithelial cells. Alveolar type I cells increased in number, became thicker, and covered a smaller average surface area. These changes persisted throughout the entire exposure and did not change during the recovery period, indicating the sensitivity of these cells to injury. The main response of type II epithelial cells was cell proliferation. The accumulation of interstitial matrix after chronic exposure consisted of deposition of both increased amounts of basement membrane and collagen fibers. Interstitial matrix accumulation underwent partial recovery during follow-up periods in air; however, the thickening of the basement membrane did not resolve. Analysis of terminal bronchioles showed that short-term exposure to O_3 caused a loss of ciliated cells and differentiation of preciliated and Clara cells. The bronchiolar cell population stabilized on continued exposure; however, chronic exposure resulted in structural changes, suggesting injury to both ciliated and Clara cells. Thus chronic exposure to low levels of O_3 caused epithelial inflammation and interstitial fibrosis in the proximal alveolar region and bronchiolar epithelial cell injury.

Studies at relatively low O_3 concentrations have also been done in monkeys. Hyde et al. (1989) exposed them to O_3 for 8 h/d for 6 or 90 days to 150 or 300 ppb. Responses included ciliated cell necrosis, shortened cilia, and secretory cell hyperplasia with less stored glycoconjugates in the nasal region. Respiratory bronchiolitis observed at 6 days persisted to 90 days of exposure. Even at the lower concentration of 150 ppb O_3, nonciliated bronchiolar cells appeared hypertrophied and increased in abundance in respiratory bronchioles.

For some chronic effects, intermittent exposures can produce greater effects than those produced by a continuous exposure regime which results in higher cumulative exposures. For example, Tyler et al. (1988) exposed two groups of 7-month-old male monkeys to 250 ppb O_3 for 8 h/d either daily or, in the seasonal model, on days of alternate months during a total exposure period of 18 months. A control group breathed only filtered air. Monkeys from the seasonal exposure model, but not those exposed daily, had significantly increased total lung collagen content, chest wall compliance, and inspiratory capacity. All monkeys exposed to O_3 had respiratory bronchiolitis with significant increases in related morphometric parameters. The only significant morphometric difference between seasonal and daily groups was in the volume fraction of macrophages. Even though the seasonally exposed monkeys were exposed to the same concentration of O_3 for only half as many days, they had larger biochemical and physiological alterations and equivalent morphometric changes as those exposed daily. Lung growth was not completely normal in either exposed group. Thus long-term effects of oxidant air pollutants that have a seasonal occurrence may be more dependent on the sequence of polluted and clean air than on the total number of days of pollution, and estimations of the risks of human exposure to seasonal air pollutants from effects observed in animals exposed daily may underestimate long-term pulmonary damage.

The preceding chronic animal exposure studies were performed at concentrations that occur frequently in ambient air, at least in southern California. Thus the effects observed may be considered directly relevant to human health, especially in view of our knowledge that humans receive even greater local doses of O_3 in the vicinity of the acinus than do rats.

A number of other interesting chronic exposure studies have been done in animals with O_3 concentrations in the range of 300 to 1000 ppb. Those that appear to provide useful insights into mechanisms of toxic action will also be briefly reviewed.

Sherwin and Richters (1985) exposed newborn Swiss-Webster mice to intermittent 300 ppb O_3 for 7 h/d, 5 d/wk for 6 weeks. Using computer-assisted image-analysis quantitation, data obtained on numbers and areas of lactate dehydrogenase stained type II cells, and also area, perimeters, and linear intercepts of the alveolar wall indicated that O_3 exposure increased cell and wall measurements. In contrast to results previously reported for adult animals (Sherwin et al., 1983), there was a greater increase in mean type II cell area than in numbers of type II cells. The increase in cell area at the expense of cell number may largely be a result of cell pairing or multicell clustering, events that would mask type II cell hyperplasia. Effects on the type II cell population implicate damage to the type I alveolar lining cells. The increases in alveolar wall measurements that were found in both the adult and developing mouse lung imply an alteration of the lung scaffolding, and raising the question of impaired regeneration of the epithelial lining.

The results of a chronic exposure study in rats by Gross and White (1987) illustrate the importance of exposure pattern on the magnitude of the response. They exposed F-344 rats to 500 ppb O_3 for 20 h/d, 7 d/wk for 52 weeks and produced only mild functional changes (functional residual capacity, residual volume, and DL_{CO}), which returned to normal during 3 months of recovery. Grose et al. (1989), using a 23 hours exposure ranging from 60 ppb to a peak 1 hour maximum of 250 ppb for 5 d/w produced comparable functional changes at 1 year. Thus, as in the comparison of Tyler et al. (1988) in monkeys, intermittent exposures, modeled after realistic human exposure conditions, can produce much greater responses per unit dose than continuous exposure at high concentration. These results suggest that the damage results, at least in part, from the repeated attempts to adapt to the irritant challenge as well as to the direct effects of the irritant exposure.

To characterize the response of respiratory bronchioles (RBs) to chronic high ambient levels of O_3, Moffatt et al. (1987) exposed bonnet monkeys 8 h/d for 90 days to 400 or 640 ppb O_3. Morphologic changes in respiratory bronchiolar epithelium and interstitium were evaluated quantitatively at both the light and transmission electron microscopic levels. Significant changes in RB following exposure included (1) a thicker wall and a narrower lumen, (2) a thicker epithelial compartment and a much thicker interstitial compartment, (3) shifts in epithelial cell populations with many more nonciliated bronchiolar epithelial cells and fewer squamous type I epithelial cells, (4) larger nonciliated bronchiolar epithelial cells with a larger compliment of cellular organelles associated with protein synthesis, (5) greater amounts of both interstitial fibers and amorphous ground substance, (6) greater numbers of interstitial smooth muscle cells per epithelial basal lamina surface area, and (7) greater volumes of interstitial smooth muscle, macrophages, mast cells, and neutrophils per epithelial basal lamina surface area. These observations imply that chronic O_3 exposure causes a concentration-dependent reactive peribronchiolar inflammatory response and an adaptive response consisting of hypertrophy and hyperplasia of the nonciliated bronchiolar cell.

Fujinaka et al. (1985) quantitated the response of RB epithelium and peribronchiolar connective tissue (PCT) to chronic exposure to high ambient levels of O_3. Adult male bonnet monkeys were exposed 8 hours daily for 1 year to either 640 ppb or filtered air. Blocks of tissue selected throughout the lung and from first-generation RBs following airway microdissection had the following significant exposure-related changes: greater volume of RB in the lung, smaller diameter of RB lumen, thicker media and intima of peribronchiolar arterioles, thicker RB epithelium, and thicker PCT. Cellular numerical density increased in cuboidal bronchiolar cells and decreased in type I pneumocytes. Cell volume increases occurred in cuboidal bronchiolar, ciliated, and type 2 cells. PCT changes included more amorphous extracellular matrix, neutrophils, and lymphocytes/plasma cells. It was concluded that centriacinar changes caused by exposure to long-term high ambient O_3 in bonnet monkeys results in narrowing of RBs primarily by peribronchiolar inflammation (inflammatory cells, fibers, amorphous matrix) and secondarily through hyperplasia of cuboidal bronchiolar cells.

The effects of chronic O_3 exposure on lung collagen crosslinking were investigated by Reiser et al. (1987) in two groups of juvenile cynomolgus monkeys exposed to 610 ppb for 8 h/d for 1 year. One group was killed immediately after the exposure period; the second exposed group breathed filtered air for 6 months after the O_3 exposure before being killed. Previous studies of these monkeys had revealed that lung collagen content was increased in both exposed groups (Last et al., 1984). In this study, specific collagen crosslinks were quantified in order to determine whether the excess collagen in the lungs of these animals was structurally normal or abnormal. The changes in collagen crosslinking observed in the group killed at the termination of exposure were characteristic of those seen in lung tissue in the acute stage of experimental pulmonary fibrosis. Although the changes seen in the postexposure group suggest that the lung collagen being synthesized at the time the animals were killed was normal, "abnormal" collagen synthesized during the period of O_3 exposure was irreversibly deposited in the lungs. This study suggests that long-term exposure to relatively low levels of O_3 may cause irreversible changes in lung collagen structure.

Barr et al. (1988) exposed rats to either filtered air or 950 ppb O_3 8 hours daily for 90 days and examined the centriacinar region of lungs morphologically and morphometrically. The volume of proximal bronchiole, terminal bronchiole, respiratory bronchiole (RB), and combined alveolar duct/sac within the lung was estimated. Bronchioles dissected from preselected regions of the right middle lobe were studied by transmission electron microscopy. From these dissected airways, four subregions of the centriacinus were then examined: (1) terminal bronchiole, (2) RB, (3) centriacinar alveolar duct wall, and (4) centriacinar alveolar septa. After chronic O_3 exposure, there was a decrease in terminal bronchiole luminal diameter but no change in total terminal bronchiole volume. The most notable change was a 3.4-fold increase in RB volume. They concluded that RB is formed from the centriacinar alveolar duct. Morphologic parameters supporting this conclusion included the presence of fused basement membrane beneath reactive bronchiolar epithelium in the RB, the presence of similar basal laminar changes in both the RB and proximal alveolar duct septal tips, and the observation that most severe epithelial damage and inflammation occurred in the most proximal alveolar duct rather than in the terminal bronchiole. The focus of the severe injury within the acinus shifts distally as RB segments are formed. Hence most of the damage occurs at the tips of alveolar septa at the RB alveolar duct junction.

The issue of the effects of chronic O_3 exposure during childhood on lung development was investigated by Tyler et al. (1987) in studies in 28-day-old rats exposed to filtered air or to 640 or 960 ppb O_3, 8 h/night, for 42 nights. A second control group was fed ad libitum and exposed to only filtered air. Half the rats were studied at the end of the 42 night exposures, the rest after a 42 day postexposure period during which all rats were fed ad libitum and breathed filtered air. Rats examined at the end of the exposure period had larger saline and fixed lung volumes. These larger lungs had greater volumes of parenchyma, alveoli, and respiratory bronchioles. Some of these changes persisted throughout a 42 day postexposure period. Thus O_3 inhalation by young rats alters lung growth and development in ways likely to be detrimental, and those changes persist after O_3 inhalation stops.

There has long been interest in the possible role of O_3 in lung cancer because of its radiomimetic properties. A comprehensive review of these issues is presented in the 1996 EPA Criteria Document (U.S. EPA, 1996a). There is, to date, no epidemiological or experimental evidence to support the hypothesis that O_3 is a pulmonary carcinogen. There are data showing that O_3 increases the incidence of lung tumors in strain A mice, but the tumor yield can be either increased or decreased depending on the exposure protocol. Also the proliferation of pulmonary neuroendricrine cells, the precursor cells for small-cell lung cancer, can be altered by O_3 exposure. While there is little evidence to implicate O_3 as a pulmonary carcinogen, it might modify and influence the carcinogenic process in the lung.

In summary, chronic exposures to ambient air appear to produce a functional adaptation that persists for at least a few months after the end of the O_3 season but dissipates by the spring. Several population-based studies of lung function indicate that there may be an accelerated aging of the lung associated with living in communities with persistently elevated ambient O_3, but the limited ability to accurately assign exposure classifications of the various populations in these studies makes a cautious assessment of these data prudent.

The plausibility of accelerated aging of the human lung from chronic O_3 exposure is greatly enhanced by the results of a series of recent chronic animal exposure studies in rats and monkeys, (especially those in rats of Huang et al., 1988, and Grose et al., 1989, using a daily cycle with a 180 ppb average over 9 hours superimposed on a 13 hour base of 60 ppb, and those in monkeys of Hyde et al., 1989. and Tyler et al., 1988, using 8 h/d of 150 and 250 ppb. The persisent cellular and morphometric changes produced by these exposures in the terminal bronchioles and proximal alveolar region and the functional changes consistent with a stiffening of the lung reported by Raub et al. (1983) and Tyler et al. (1988) are certainly consistent with the results of the epidemiological studies.

SUMMARY AND CONCLUSIONS

The apparently reversible effects that have followed acute exposures lasting from 5 minutes to 6.6 hours include changes in lung capacity, flow resistance, epithelial permeability, and reactivity to bronchoactive challenges. These effects may persist for many hours or days after the exposure ceases. Repetitive daily exposures over several days or weeks can exacerbate and prolong these effects.

Most of the data available on transient functional effects of O_3 were obtained from controlled human exposure studies and field studies of limited duration. Such studies can provide information on chronic pollutant effects only to the extent that prior exposures affect the transient response to single-exposure challenges. Furthermore interpretation of the results of such tests is limited by our generally inadequate ability to characterize the nature and/or magnitude of the prior chronic exposures. Most of the limited data we have on the effects of chronic O_3 exposures on humans come from epidemological studies.

Epidemiological studies offer the prospect of establishing chronic health effects of long-term O_3 exposure in relevant populations and offer the possibility that the analyses can show the influence of other environmental factors on responses to O_3 exposure. On the other hand, the strengths of any of the associations may be difficult to firmly establish because of the complications introduced by uncontrolled cofactors which may confound or obscure the underlying causal factors.

The most convenient and efficient way to study mechanisms and patterns of response to inhaled O_3 and of the influence of other pollutants and stresses on these responses is by controlled exposures of laboratory animals. One can study the transient functional responses to acute exposures and establish the interspecies differences in response among different animal species and between them and humans similarly exposed. One can also look for responses that require highly invasive procedures or serial sacrifice and gain information that cannot be obtained from studies on human volunteers. Finally one can use long-term exposure protocols to study cumulative responses and the pathogenesis of chronic disease in animals. Other advantages of studies on animals are the ability to examine the presence and basis for variations in response that are related to age, sex, species, strain, genetic markers, nutrition, the presence of other pollutants, and so on.

Among the significant limitations to the use of exposure–response data from animal studies in human risk assessments is our quite limited ability to interpret the responses in relation to likely responses in humans who might be exposed to the same or lower levels. Controlled chronic exposure protocols can be very expensive, limiting the number of variables that can effectively be examined in any given study.

For studies focused on the biochemical mechanisms of epithelial cells' responses to O_3, cells can be harvested from humans or animals and exposed to O_3 in vitro. Interspecies comparisons of cellular response can often be made, and relatively few animals can provide much study material. However, our ability to interpret the results of in vitro assays in relation to likely effects in humans in vivo is quite limited, even when the studies are done with human cells. The cellular response in vitro may differ from that of the same cells in vivo, and the in vivo controls on cellular metabolism and function, which may play a significant role in the overall response, are absent.

In terms of functional effects, we know that single O_3 exposures to healthy nonsmoking young adults at concentrations in the range of 80 to 200 ppb produce a complex array of pulmonary responses including decreases in respiratory function and athletic performance, and increases in symptoms, airway reactivity, neutrophil content in lung lavage, and rate of mucociliary particle clearance. Responses to O_3 in purified air in chambers occur at concentrations of 80 or 100 ppb when the exposures involve moderate exercise over 6 hours or more and require concentrations of 180 or 200 ppb when the duration of exposure is 2 hours or less. On the other hand, mean FEV_1 decrements $> 5\%$ have been seen at 100 ppb of O_3 in ambient air for children at summer camps and for adults engaged in outdoor exercise for only one-half hour. The apparently greater responses to O_3 in ambient air may be related to the presence of, or prior exposures to, acidic aerosol, but further investigation of this hypothesis is needed.

Further research is also needed to establish the interrelationships between small transient functional decrements, such as FEV_1, PEFR, and mucociliary clearance rates,

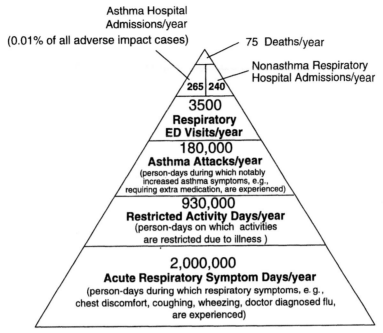

Asthma Hospital
Admissions/year
(0.01% of all adverse impact cases)   75 Deaths/year

Nonasthma Respiratory
Hospital Admissions/year

265 | 240

3500
Respiratory
ED Visits/year

180,000
Asthma Attacks/year
(person-days during which notably
increased asthma symptoms, e.g.,
requiring extra medication, are experienced)

930,000
Restricted Activity Days/year
(person-days on which activities
are restricted due to illness)

2,000,000
Acute Respiratory Symptom Days/year
(person-days during which respiratory symptoms, e. g.,
chest discomfort, coughing, wheezing, doctor diagnosed flu,
are experienced)

*Figure section sizes not drawn to scale.

Figure 20-9   Pyramid summarizing the adverse effects of ambient O_3 in New York City that can be averted by reduction of mid-1990s levels to those meeting the 1997 NAAQS revision. Data assembled by Dr. George D. Thurston for testimony to the U.S. Senate Committee on Public Works.

which may not in themselves be adverse effects, and changes in symptoms, performance, reactivity, permeability, and neutrophil counts. The latter may be more closely associated with adversity in themselves or in the accumulation or progression of chronic lung damage.

Successive days of exposure of adult humans in chambers to O_3 at current high ambient levels leads to a functional adaptation in that the responses are attenuated by the third day, and are negligible by the fifth day. On the other hand, a comparable functional adaptation in rats does not prevent the progressive damage to the lung epithelium. Daily exposures of animals also increase other responses in comparison to single exposures, such as a loss of cilia, a hypertrophic response of Clara cells, alterations in macrophage function, and alterations in the rates of particle clearance from the lungs.

The clearest evidence that current ambient levels of O_3 are closely associated with health effects in human populations comes from epidemiological studies focused on acute responses. The 1997 revision to the O_3 NAAQS relied heavily for its quantitative basis on a study of emergency hospital admissions for asthma in New York City (Thurston et al., 1992) and its consistency with other time-series studies of hospital admissions for respiratory diseases in Toronto, all of southern Ontario, Montreal, Detroit, and Buffalo, New York. However, other acute responses, while less firmly established on quantitative bases, are also occurring. In order to put them in perspective, Thurston (1997) prepared a graphic presentation showing the extent of related human responses based on the exposure–response relationships established in a variety of studies reviewed earlier in this chapter. This is shown, for New York City, in Figure 20-9. It estimates the extent of the human health responses to ambient ozone exposures in New York City that could be avoided by full implementation of the new O_3 NAAQS of 80 ppb averaged over 8 hours.

The extent of effects avoided on a national scale would be much larger. However, the extent of health responses have not been estimated, and they would require knowledge of current (1997) O_3 levels and populations at risk in other parts of the country.

Chronic human exposures to ambient air appear to produce a functional adaptation that persists for at least a few months after the end of the O_3 season but dissipates by the spring. Several population-based studies of lung function indicate that there may be an accelerated aging of the lung associated with living in communities with persistently elevated ambient O_3, but the limited ability to accurately assign exposure classifications of the various populations in these studies makes a cautious assessment of these provocative data prudent.

The plausibility of accelerated aging of the human lung from chronic O_3 exposure is greatly enhanced by the results of a series of chronic animal exposure studies in rats and monkeys. There is little reason to expect humans to be less sensitive than rats or monkeys. On the contrary, humans have a greater dosage delivered to the respiratory acinus than do rats for the same exposures. Another factor is that the rat and monkey exposures were to confined animals with little opportunity for heavy exercise. Thus humans who are active outdoors during the warmer months may have greater effective O_3 exposures than the test animals. Finally humans are exposed to O_3 in ambient mixtures. The potentiation of the characteristic O_3 responses by other ambient air constituents seen in the short-term exposure studies in humans and animals may also contribute toward the accumulation of chronic lung damage from long-term exposures to ambient air containing O_3.

The lack of a more definitive data base on the chronic effects of ambient O_3 exposures on humans is a serious failing that must be addressed with a long-term research program. The potential impacts of such exposures on public health deserve serious scrutiny and, if they turn out to be substantial, strong corrective action. Further controls on ambient O_3 exposure will be extraordinarily expensive and will need to be very well justified.

In summary, this review has shown that (1) the control of ambient O_3 to levels within the current NAAQS presents an intractable problem; (2) the current NAAQS contains little, if any, margin of safety against effects considered to be adverse; and (3) a large fraction of the U.S. population resides in communities that exceed the O_3 NAAQS. Thus it is important that health scientists and control agency personnel understand the nature and extent of human exposures and the effects they produce in order to communicate health risks effectively to the public and to help to prioritize feasible options for reducing exposures.

ACKNOWLEDGMENTS

This research is part of a Center program supported by Grant ES 00260 from the National Institute of Environmental Health Sciences. The author thanks Dr. Richard B. Schlesinger for his careful review and thoughtful comments.

REFERENCES

Abbey, D. E., M. D. Lebowitz, P. K. Mills, F. F. Petersen, W. L. Beeson, and R. J. Burchette. 1995. Long-term ambient concentrations of particulates and oxidants and development of chronic disease in a cohort of nonsmoking California residents. *Inhal. Toxicol.* 7: 19–34.

Abraham, W. M., J. C. Delehunt, L. Yerger, B. Marchete, and W. Oliver Jr. 1984. Changes in airway permeability and responsiveness after exposure to ozone. *Environ. Res.* 34: 110–119.

ACGIH. 1997. *Threshold Limit Values and Biological Exposure Indices for 1997.* Cincinnati OH: American Conference of Governmental Industrial Hygienists.

Adams, W. C., and E. S. Schelegle. 1983. Ozone and high ventilation effects on pulmonary function and endurance performance. *J. Appl. Physiol. Respir. Environ. Exercise Physiol.* 55: 805–812.

Air Resources Board. 1988. *Effects of Ozone on Health. Technical Support Document.* Sacramento, CA: Air Resources Board.

Albert, R. E., M. Lippmann, and W. Briscoe. 1969. The characteristics of bronchial clearance in humans and the effects of cigarette smoking. *Arch. Environ. Health* 18: 738–755.

Altshuller, A. P. 1977. Eye irritation as an effect of photochemical air pollution. *J. Air Pollut. Control Assoc.* 27: 1125–1126.

Altshuller, A. P. 1987. Estimation of the natural background of ozone present at surface rural locations. *J. Air Pollut. Control Assoc.* 37: 1409–1417.

American Thoracic Society. 1985. Guidelines as to what constitutes an adverse respiratory health effect, with special reference to epidemiologic studies of air pollution. *Am. Rev. Respir. Dis.* 131: 666–668.

Amoruso, M. A., and B. D. Goldstein. 1988. Effect of 1, 3, and 6 hour ozone exposure on alveolar macrophages superoxide production. *Toxicologist* 8: 197.

Amoruso, M. A., G. Witz, and B. D. Goldstein. 1981. Decreased superoxide anion radical production by rat alveolar macrophages following inhalation of ozone or nitrogen dioxide. *Life Sci.* 12: 2215–2221.

Anderson, H. R., A. Ponce de Leon, M. J. Bland, J. S. Bower, and D. P. Strachan. 1996. Air pollution and daily mortality in London: 1987–1992. *Brit. Med. J.* 312: 665–669.

Aranyi, C., S. C. Vana, P. T. Thomas, J. N. Bradof, J. D. Fenters, J. A. Graham, and F. J. Miller. 1983. Effects of subchronic exposure to a mixture of O_3, SO_2, and $(NH_4)_2SO_4$ on host defenses of mice. *J. Toxicol. Environ. Health* 12: 55–71.

Aris, R., D. Christian, D. Sheppard, and J. R. Balmes. 1991. The effects of sequential exposure to acidic fog and ozone on pulmonary function in exercising subjects. *Am. Rev. Respir. Dis.* 143: 85–91.

Avol, E. L., W. S. Linn, D. A. Shamoo, C. E. Spier, L. M. Valencia, T. G. Venet, S. C. Trim, and J. D. Hackney. 1987. Short-term respiratory effects of photochemical oxidant exposure in exercising children. *J. Air Pollut. Control Assoc.* 37: 158–162.

Avol, E. L., W. S. Linn, D. A. Shamoo, L. M. Valencia, U. T. Anzar, and J. D. Hackney. 1985. Respiratory effects of photochemical oxidant air pollution in exercising adolescents. *Am. Rev. Respir. Dis.* 132: 619–622.

Avol, E. L., W. S. Linn, T. G. Venet, D. A. Shamoo, and J. D. Hackney. 1984. Comparative respiratory effects of ozone and ambient oxidant pollution exposure during heavy exercise. *J. Air Pollut. Control Assoc.* 34: 804–809.

Balmes, J. R., L. L. Chen, C. Scannell, I. Tager, D. Christian, P. Q. Hearne, T. Kelly, and R. M. Aris. 1996. Ozone-induced decrements in FEV_1 and FVC do not correlate with measures of inflammation. *Am. J. Respir. Crit. Care Med.* 153: 904–909.

Barr, B. C., D. M. Hyde, C. G. Plopper, and D. L. Dungworth. 1988. Distal airway remodeling in rats chronically exposed to ozone. *Am. Rev. Respir. Dis.* 137: 924–938.

Barry, B. E., F. J. Miller, and J. D. Crapo. 1985. Effects of inhalation of 0.12 and 0.5 ppm ozone on the proximal alveolar region of juvenile and adults rats. *Lab. Invest.* 53: 692–704.

Barry, B. E., R. R. Mercer, F. J. Miller, and J. D. Crapo. 1988. Effects of inhalation of 0.25 ppm ozone on the terminal bronchioles of juvenile and adult rats. *Exp. Lung Res.* 14: 225–245.

Bates, D. V. 1989. Ozone-myth and reality. *Environ. Res.* 50: 230–237.

Bates, D. V. 1995. Ozone: A review of recent experimental, clinical and epidemiological evidence, with notes on causation. *Can. Respir. J.* 2: 25–31 and 161–171.

Bates, D. V., and R. Sizto. 1989. The Ontario air pollution study: Identification of the causative agent. *Environ. Health Perspect.* 79: 69–72.

Beckett, W. S., W. F. McDonnell, D. H. Horstman, and D. E. House. 1985. Role of the parasympathetic nervous system in acute lung response to ozone. *J. Appl. Physiol.* 59: 1879–1885.

Beckett, W. S., A. N. Freed, C. Turner, and H. A. Menkes. 1988. Prolonged increased responsiveness of canine peripheral airways after exposure to O_3. *J. Appl. Physiol.* 64: 605–610.

Bedi, J. F., S. M. Horvath, and D. M. Drechsler-Parks. 1989. Adaptation by older individuals repeatedly exposed to 0.45 parts per million ozone for two hours. *J. Air Pollut. Control Assoc.* 39: 194–199.

Bhalla, D. K., and C. Young. 1992. Effects of acute exposure to O_3 on rats: Sequence of epithelial and inflammatory changes in the distal airways. *Inhal. Toxicol.* 4: 17–31.

Bhalla, D. K., R. C. Manniz, S. M. Lavan, R. F. Phalen, M. T. Kleinman, and T. T. Crocker. 1987. Tracheal and bronchoalveolar permeability changes in rats inhaling oxidant atmospheres during rest of exercise. *J. Toxicol. Environ. Health* 22: 417–437.

Borja-Aburto, V. H., D. P. Loomis, S. I. Bangdiwala, C. M. Shy, and R. A. Rascon-Pacheco. 1997. Ozone, suspended particulates, and daily mortality in Mexico City. *Am. J. Epidemiol.* 145: 258–268.

Brauer, M., J. Blair, and S. Vedal. 1996. Effect of ambient ozone exposure on lung function in farm workers. *Am. J. Respir. Crit. Care Med.* 154: 981–987.

Braun-Fahrlander, C., N. Kunzli, G. Domenighetti, C. F. Carell, and U. Ackermann-Liebrich. 1994. Acute effects of ambient ozone on respiratory function of Swiss schoolchildren after a 10-minute heavy exercise. *Pediat. Pulmonul.* 17: 169–177.

Brookes, K. A., W. C. Adams, and E. S. Schelegle. 1989. 0.35 ppm O_3 exposure induces hyperresponsiveness on 24-h reexposure to 0.20 ppm O_3. *J. Appl. Physiol.* 66: 2756–2762.

Brunekreef, B., G. Hoek, O. Breugelmans, and M. Leentvaar. 1994. Respiratory effects of low-level photochemical air pollution in amateur cyclists. *Am. J. Respir. Crit. Care Med.* 150: 962–966.

Buist, A. S., and B. B. Ross. 1973. Quantitative analysis of the alveolar plateau in the diagnosis of early airway obstruction. *Am. Rev. Respir. Dis.* 108: 1078–1085.

Burnett, R. T., J. R. Brook, W. T. Yung, R. E. Dales, and D. Krewski. 1997. Association between ozone and hospitalization for respiratory diseases in 16 Canadian cities. *Environ. Res.* 72: 24–31.

Burnett, R. T., R. E. Dales, M. E. Raizenne, D. Krewski, P. W. Summers, G. R. Roberts, M. Raad-Young, T. Dann, and J. Brook. 1994. Effects of low ambient levels of ozone and sulfates on the frequency of respiratory admissions to Ontario hospitals. *Environ. Res.* 65: 172–194.

CASAC. 1989. *Review of the NAAQS for Ozone. EPA-SAB-CASAC-89-1092.* Washington DC: U.S. EPA.

Castillejos, M., D. R. Gold, A. I. Damokosh, P. Serrano, G. Allen, W. F. McDonnell, D. W. Dockery, S. R. Velasco, M. Hernandez, and C. Hayes. 1995. Acute effects of ozone on the pulmonary function of exercising schoolchildren from Mexico City. *Am. J. Respir. Crit. Care Med.* 152: 1501–1507.

Chan, T. L., and M. Lippmann. 1980. Experimental measurements and empirical modelling of the regional deposition of inhaled particles in humans. *Am. Ind. Hyg. Assoc. J.* 41: 399–409.

Chang, L., F. J. Miller, J. Ultman, Y. Huang, B. L. Stockstill, E. Grose, J. A. Graham, J. J. Ospital, and J. D. Crapo. 1991. Alveolar epithelial cell injuries by subchronic exposure to low concentrations of ozone correlate with cumulative exposure. *Toxicol. Appl. Pharmacol.* 109: 219–234.

Chang, L.-Y., Y. Huang, B. L. Stockstill, J. A. Graham, E. C. Grose, M. G. Menache, F. J. Miller, D. L. Costa, and J. D. Crapo. 1992. Epithelial injury and interstitial fibrosis in the proximal alveolar regions of rats chronically exposed to a simulated pattern of urban ambient ozone. *Toxicol. Appl. Pharmacol.* 115: 241–252.

Cody, R. P., C. P. Weisel, G. Birnbaum, and P. J. Lioy. 1992. The effect of ozone associated with summertime photochemical smog on the frequency of asthma visits to hospital emergency departments. *Environ. Res.* 58: 184–194.

Coffin, D. L., and D. E. Gardner. 1972. Interaction of biological agents and chemical air pollutants. *Ann. Occup. Hyg.* 15: 219–235.

Coffin, D. L., D. E. Gardner, R. S. Holzman, and F. J. Wolock. 1968. Influence of ozone on pulmonary cells. *Arch. Environ. Health* 16: 633–636.

Coffin, D. L., E. J. Blommer, D. E. Gardner, and R. Holzman. 1967. Effect of air pollution on alteration of susceptibility to pulmonary infection. In *Proc. 3rd Annual Conference on Atmospheric Contamination in Confined Spaces.* Report AMRL-TR-67-200. Wright-Patterson Air Force Base, OH; Aerospace Medical Research Laboratories. (Available from NTIS, Springfield, VA, AD-835008.)

Coleridge, H. M., J. C. G. Coleridge, K. H. Ginzel, D. G. Baker, R. B. Banzett, and M. A. Morrison. 1976. Stimulation of "irritant" receptors and afferent C-fibres in the lungs of prostaglandins. *Nature* 264: 451–453.

Cosio, M. G., K. A. Hole, and D. E. Niewohner. 1980. Morphologic and morphometric effects of prolonged cigarette smoking on the small airways. *Am. Rev. Respir. Dis.* 122: 265–271.

Costa, D. L., G. E. Hatch, J. Highfill, M. A. Stevens, and J. S. Tepper. 1989. Pulmonary function studies in the rat addressing concentration vs. time relationships for ozone. In *Atmospheric Ozone Research and Its Policy Implications*, eds. T. Schneider, S. D. Lee, G. J. R. Wolters, and L. D. Grant. Nijmegen, the Netherlands: Elsevier.

Crapo, R. O. 1986. Single breath carbon monoxide diffusing capacity. *ATS News* (spring).

Delfino, R. J., M. R. Becklake, and J. A. Hanley. 1994a. The relationship of urgent hospital admissions for respiratory illnesses to photochemical air pollution levels in Montreal. *Environ. Res.* 67: 1–19.

Delfino, R. J., M. R. Becklake, and J. A. Hanley. 1994b. Estimation of unmeasured particulate air pollution for an epidemiological study of daily respiratory morbidity. *Environ. Res.* 67: 20–38.

DeLucia, A. J., and W. C. Adams. 1977. Effects of O_3 inhalation during exercise on pulmonary function and blood biochemistry. *J. Appl. Physiol.* 43: 75–81.

Detels, R., D. P. Tashkin, J. W. Sayre, S. N. Rokaw, A. H. Coulson, F. J. Massey, and D. H. Wegman. 1987. The UCLA population studies of chronic obstructive respiratory disease. 9. Lung function changes associated with chronic exposure to photochemical oxidants; a cohort study among never-smokers. *Chest* 92: 594–603.

Devlin, R. B., W. F. McDonnell, R. Mann, S. Becker, D. E. House, D. Schreinemachers, and H. S. Koren. 1991. Exposure of humans to ambient levels of ozone for 6.6 hours causes cellular and biochemical changes in the lung. *Am. J. Respir. Cell Mol. Biol.* 4: 72–81.

Dockery, D. W., C. A. Pope, III, X. Xu, J. D. Spengler, J. H. Ware, M. E. Fay, B. G. Ferris Jr., and F. E. Speizer. 1993. An association between air pollution and mortality in six U.S. Cities. *N. Engl. J. Med.* 329: 1753–1759.

Dowell, A. R., L. A. Lohrbauer, D. Hurst, and S. D. Lee. 1970. Rabbit alveolar macrophage damage caused by *in vivo* ozone inhalation. *Arch. Environ. Health* 21: 121–127.

Drechsler-Parks, D. M., J. F. Bedi, and S. M. Horvath. 1987. Pulmonary function responses of older men and women to ozone exposure. *Exp. Gerontol.* 22: 91–101.

Driscoll, K. E., T. A. Vollmuth, and R. B. Schlesinger. 1986. Early alveolar clearance of particles in rabbits undergoing acute and subchronic exposure to ozone. *Fundam. Appl. Toxicol.* 7: 264–271.

Driscoll, K. E., T. A. Vollmuth, and R. B. Schlesinger. 1987. Acute and subchronic ozone inhalation in the rabbit: Response of alveolar macrophages. *J. Toxicol. Environ. Health* 21: 27–43.

Ehrlich, R. 1980. Interaction between environmental pollutants and respiratory infections. *Environ. Health Perspect.* 35: 89–100.

Ehrlich, R., J. C. Findlay, and D. E. Gardner. 1979. Effects of repeated exposures to peak concentrations of nitrogen dioxide and ozone on resistance to streptococcal pneumonia. *J. Toxicol. Environ. Health* 5: 631–642.

Ehrlich, R., J. C. Findlay, J. D. Fenters, and D. E. Gardner. 1977. Health effects of short-term inhalation of nitrogen dioxide and ozone mixtures. *Environ. Res.* 14: 223–231.

Emmons, K., and W. M. Foster. 1991. Smoking cessation and acute airway response to ozone. *Arch. Environ. Health* 46: 288–295.

Farman, C. A., K. E. Pinkerton, P. Rajini, H. Witschi, and J. A. Last. 1997. Evolution of lung lesions in rats exposed to mixtures of ozone and nitrogen dioxide. *Inhal. Toxicol.* 9: 647–677.

Farrell, B. P., H. D. Kerr, T. J. Kulle, L. R. Sauder, and J. L. Young. 1979. Adaptation in human subjects to the effects of inhaled ozone after repeated exposure. *Am. Rev. Respir. Dis.* 119: 725–730.

Folinsbee, L. J., and M. J. Hazucha. 1989. Persistence of ozone-induced changes in lung function and airway responsiveness. In *Atmospheric Ozone Research and Its Policy Implications*, eds. T. Schneider, S. D. Lee, G. J. R. Wolters, and L. D. Grant. Nijmegen, the Netherlands: Elsevier.

Folinsbee, L. J., D. H. Horstman, H. R. Kehrl, S. Harder, S. Abdul-Salaam, and P. J. Ives. 1994. Respiratory responses to repeated prolonged exposure to 0.12 ppm ozone. *Am. J. Respir. Crit. Care Med.* 149: 98–105.

Folinsbee, L. J., J. F. Bedi, and S. M. Horvath. 1980. Respiratory responses in humans repeatedly exposed to low concentrations of ozone. *Am. Rev. Respir. Dis.* 121: 431–439.

Folinsbee, L. J., J. F. Bedi, and S. M. Horvath. 1984. Pulmonary function changes in trained athletes following 1-hour continuous heavy exercise while breathing 0.21 ppm ozone. *J. Appl. Physiol. Respir. Environ. Exercise Physiol.* 57: 984–988.

Folinsbee, L. J., W. F. McDonnell, and D. H. Horstman. 1988. Pulmonary function and symptom responses after 6.6 hour exposure to 0.12 ppm ozone with moderate exercise. *J. Air Pollut. Control Assoc.* 38: 28–35.

Foster, W. M., and P. T. Stetkiewicz. 1996. Regional clearance of solute from the respiratory epithelia: 18–20 hr postexposure to ozone. *J. Appl. Physiol.* 81: 1143–1149.

Foster, W. M., D. L. Costa, and E. G. Langenback. 1987. Ozone exposure alters tracheobronchial mucociliary function in humans. *J. Appl. Physiol.* 63: 996–1002.

Fouke, J. M., R. A. Delemos, and E. R. McFadden Jr. 1988. Airway response to ultra short-term exposure to ozone. *Am. Rev. Respir. Dis.* 137: 326–330.

Frager, N. B., R. F. Phalen, and J. L. Kenoyer. 1979. Adaptation to ozone in reference to mucociliary clearance. *Arch. Environ. Health* 34: 51–57.

Frampton, M. W., P. E. Morrow, A. Torres, C. Cox, K. Z. Voter, and M. J. Utell. 1997. Ozone responsiveness in smokers and nonsmokers. *Am. J. Respir. Crit. Care Med.* 155: 116–121.

Frampton, M. W., P. E. Morrow, C. Cox, P. C. Levy, J. J. Condemi, D. Speers, F. R. Gibb, and M. J. Utell. 1995. Sulfuric acid aerosol following by ozone exposure in healthy and asthmatic subjects. *Environ. Res.* 69: 1–14.

Frischer, T. M., J. Kuehr, A. Pullwitt, R. Meinert, J. Forster, M. Studnicka, and H. Koren. 1993. Ambient ozone causes upper airways inflammation in children. *Am. Rev. Respir. Dis.* 148: 961–964.

Fujinaka, L. E., D. M. Hyde, C. G. Plopper, W. S. Tyler, D. L. Dungworth, and L. O. Lollini. 1985. Respiratory bronchiolitis following long-term ozone exposure in bonnet monkeys: A morphometric study. *Exp. Lung Res.* 8: 167–190.

Gardner, D. E., F. J. Miller, J. W. Illing, and J. M. Kirtz. 1977. Increased infectivity with exposure to ozone and sulfuric acid. *Toxicol. Lett.* 1: 59–64.

Gerrity, T. R., and M. J. Wiester. 1987. Experimental measurements of the uptake of ozone in rats and human subjects. Preprint 87-99.3. 1987 Annual Meeting of the Air Pollution Control Association, New York, June.

Gerrity, T. R., F. Biscardi, A. Strong, A. R. Garlington, J. S. Brown, and P. A. Bromberg. 1995. Bronchoscopic determination of ozone uptake in humans. *J. Appl. Physiol.* 79: 852–860.

Gerrity, T. R., R. A. Weaver, J. Berntsen, D. E. House, and J. J. O'Neil. 1988. Extrathoracic and intrathoracic removal of O_3 in tidal-breathing humans. *J. Appl. Physiol.* 65: 393–400.

Gilmour, M. I., and M. K. Selgrade. 1993. A comparison of the pulmonary defenses against streptococcal infection in rats and mice following O_3 exposure. *Toxicol. Appl. Pharmacol.* 123: 211–218.

Goldstein, B. D., S. J. Hamburger, G. W. Falk, and M. A. Amoruso. 1977. Effect of ozone and nitrogen dioxide on the agglutination of rat alveolar macrophages by concanavalin A. *Life Sci.* 21: 1637–1644.

Goldstein, E., W. S. Tyler, P. D. Hoeprich, and C. Eagle. 1971a. Ozone and the antibacterial defense mechanisms of the murine lung. *Arch. Intern. Med.* 128: 1099–1102.

Goldstein, E., W. S. Tyler, P. D. Hoeprich, and C. Eagle. 1971b. Adverse influence of ozone on pulmonary bactericidal activity of murine lungs. *Nature* 229: 262–263.

Gong, H., Jr., J. F. Bedi, and S. M. Horvath. 1988. Inhaled albuterol does not protect against ozone toxicity in nonasthmatic athletes. *Arch. Environ. Health* 43: 46–53.

Gordon, T., B. F. Taylor, and M. O. Amdur. 1981. Ozone inhibition of tissue cholinesterase in guinea pigs. *Arch. Environ. Health* 36: 284–288.

Graham, D. E., and H. S. Koren. 1990. Biomarkers of inflammation in ozone-exposed humans: Comparison of the nasal and bronchoalveolar lavage. *Am. Rev. Respir. Dis.* 142: 152–156.

Graham, D., F. Henderson, and D. House. 1988. Neutrophil influx measured in nasal lavages of humans exposed to ozone. *Arch. Environ. Health* 43: 228–233.

Graham, J. A., D. E. Gardner, E. J. Blommer, D. E. House, M. G. Menache, and F. J. Miller. 1987. Influence of exposure patterns of nitrogen dioxide and modifications by ozone on susceptibility to bacterial infectious disease in mice. *J. Toxicol. Environ. Health* 21: 113–125.

Grose, E. C., D. E. Gardner, and F. J. Miller. 1980a. Response of ciliated epithelium to ozone and sulfuric acid. *Environ. Res.* 22: 377–385.

Grose, E. C., J. H. Richards, J. W. Illing, F. J. Miller, D. W. Davies, J. A. Graham, and D. E. Gardner. 1980b. Pulmonary host defense responses to inhalation of sulfuric acid and ozone. *J. Toxicol. Environ. Health* 10: 351–362.

Grose, E. C., M. A. Stevens, G. E. Hatch, R. H. Jaskot, M. J. K. Selgrade, A. G. Stead, D. L. Costa, and J. A. Graham. 1989. The impact of a 12 month exposure to a diurnal pattern of ozone on pulmonary function, antioxidant biochemistry and immunology. In *Atmospheric Ozone Research and Its Policy Implications*, eds. T. Schneider, S. D. Lee, G. J. R. Wolters, and L. D. Grant, Nijmegen, the Netherlands: Elsevier.

Gross, K. B., and H. J. White. 1987. Functional and pathologic consequences of a 52 week exposure to 0.5 ppm ozone followed by a clean air recovery period. *Lung* 165: 283–295.

Guth, D. J., D. L. Warren, and J. A. Last. 1986. Comparative sensitivity of measurements of lung damage made by bronchoalveolar lavage after short-term exposure of rats to ozone. *Toxicology* 40: 131–143.

Hackney, J. D., W. S. Linn, J. G. Mohler, and C. R. Collier. 1977. Adaptation to short-term respiratory effects of ozone in men exposed repeatedly. *J. Appl. Physiol.* 43: 82–85.

Hammer, D. I., V. Hasselblad, B. Portnoy, and P. F. Wehrle. 1974. Los Angeles student nurse study: Daily symptom reporting and photochemical oxidants. *Arch. Environ. Health* 28: 255–260.

Hatch, G. E., H. Koren, and M. Aissa. 1989. A method for comparison of animal and human alveolar dose and toxic effect of inhaled ozone. *Health Phys.* 57(suppl. 1): 37–40.

Hatch, G. E., R. Slade, A. G. Stead, and J. A. Graham. 1986. Species comparison of acute inhalation toxicity of ozone and phosgene. *J. Toxicol. Environ. Health* 19: 43–53.

Hayes, S. R., M. Moezzi, T. S. Wallsten, and R. L. Winkler. 1987. *An Analysis of Symptom and Lung Function Data from Several Human Controlled Ozone Exposure Studies (Draft Final Report)*. San Rafael, CA: Systems Applications, Inc.

Hazucha, M. J. 1987. Relationship between ozone exposure and pulmonary function changes. *J. Appl. Physiol.* 62: 1671–1680.

Hazucha, M. J., D. V. Bates, and P. A. Bromberg. 1989. Mechanism of action of ozone on the human lung. *J. Appl. Physiol.* 67: 1535–1541.

Hazucha, M. J., L. J. Folinsbee, and E. Seal, Jr. 1992. Effects of steady-state and variable O_3 concentration profiles on pulmonary function. *Am. Rev. Respir. Dis.* 146: 1487–1493.

Hernandez-Garduno, E., J. Perez-Neria, A. M. Paccagnells, M. A. Pina-Garcia, M. Mungufa-Castro, M. Catalan-Vazquez, and M. Rojas-Ramos. 1997. Air pollution and respiratory health in Mexico City. *J. Occup. Environ. Med.* 39: 299–307.

Higgins, I. T. T., J. B. D'Arcy, D. I. Gibbons, E. L. Avol, and K. B. Gross. 1990. Effect of exposures to ambient ozone on ventilatory lung function in children. *Am. Rev. Respir. Dis.* 141: 1136–1146.

Highfill, J. W., G. E. Hatch, R. Slade, K. M. Crissman, J. Norwood, R. B. Devlin, and D. L. Costa. 1992. Concentration-time models for the effects of ozone on bronchoalveolar lavage fluid protein from rats and guinea pigs. *Inhal. Toxicol.* 4: 1–16.

Hoek, G., and B. Brunekreef. 1995. Effect of photochemical air pollution on acute respiratory symptoms in children. *Am. J. Respir. Crit. Care Med.* 151: 27–32.

Hoek, G., P. Fischer, B. Brunekreef, E. Lebret, P. Hofschreuder, and M. G. Mennen. 1993. Acute effects of ambient ozone on pulmonary function of children in the Netherlands. *Am. Rev. Respir. Dis.* 147: 111–117.

Holguin, A. H., P. A. Buffler, C. F. Contant Jr., T. H. Stock, D. Kotchmar, B. P. Hsi, D. E. Jenkins, B. M. Gehan, L. M. Noel, and M. Mei. 1985. The effects of ozone on asthmatics in the Houston area. *Trans. Air Pollut. Control Assoc.* 4: 262–280.

Holtzman, M. J., J. H. Cunningham, J. R. Sheller, G. B. Irsigler, J. A. Nadel, and H. Boushey. 1979. Effect of ozone on bronchial reactivity in atopic and nonatopic subjects. *Am. Rev. Respir. Dis.* 120: 1059–1067.

Horstman, D. H., L. J. Folinsbee, P. J. Ives, S. Abdul-Salaam, and W. F. McDonnell. 1990. Ozone concentration and pulmonary response relationships for 6.6-hour exposures with five hours of moderate exercise to 0.08, 0.10, and 0.12 ppm. *Am. Rev. Respir. Dis.* 142: 1158–1163.

Horstman, D., L. J. Roger, H. Kehrl, and M. Hazucha. 1986. Airway sensitivity of asthmatics to sulfur dioxide. *Toxicol. Ind. Health* 2: 289–298.

Horvath, S. M., J. A. Gliner, and L. J. Folinsbee. 1981. Adaptation to ozone: Duration of effect. *Am. Rev. Respir. Dis.* 123: 496–499.

Huang, Y., L. Y. Chang, F. J. Miller, J. A. Graham, J. J. Ospital, and J. D. Crapo. 1988. Lung injury caused by ambient levels of oxidant air pollutants: Extrapolation from animal to man. *Am. J. Aerosol Med.* 1: 180–183.

Hurst, D. J., and D. L. Coffin. 1971. Ozone effect on lysosomal hydrolases of alveolar macrophages *in vitro*. *Arch. Intern. Med.* 127: 1059–1063.

Hurst, D. J., D. E. Gardner, and D. L. Coffin. 1970. Effect of ozone on acid hydrolases of the pulmonary alveolar macrophage. *J. Reticuloendothel. Soc.* 8: 288–300.

Hyde, D. M., C. G. Plopper, J. R. Harkema, J. A. St. George, W. S. Tyler, and D. L. Dungworth. 1989. Ozone-induced structural changes in monkey respiratory system. In *Atmospheric Ozone Research and Its Policy Implications*, eds. T. Schneider, S. D. Lee, G. J. R. Wolters, and L. D. Grant, Nijmegen, the Netherlands: Elsevier.

Illing, J. W., F. J. Miller, and D. E. Gardner. 1980. Decreased resistance to infection in exercised mice exposed to NO_2 and O_3. *J. Toxicol. Environ. Health* 6: 843–851.

Jones, G. L., C. G. Lane, and P. M. O'Byrne. 1990. Effect of thromboxane antagonists on ozone-induced airway responses in dogs. *J. Appl. Physiol.* 69: 880–884.

Jorres, R., D. Nowak, H. Magnussen, P. Speckin, and S. Koschyk. 1996. The effect of ozone exposure on allergen responsiveness in subjects with asthma or rhinitis. *Am. J. Respir. Crit. Care Med.* 153: 56–64.

Kagawa, J. 1984. Exposure-effect relationship of selected pulmonary function measurements in subjects exposed to ozone. *Int. Arch. Occup. Environ. Health* 53: 345–358.

Keefe, M. J., W. D. Bennett, P. DeWitt, E. Seal, A. A. Strong, and T. R. Gerrity. 1991. The effect of ozone exposure on the dispersion of inhaled aerosol boluses in healthy human subjects. *Am. Rev. Respir. Dis.* 144: 23–30.

Kehrl, H. R., L. W. Vincent, R. J. Kowalsky, D. H. Horstman, J. J. O'Neil, W. H. McCartney, and P. A. Bromberg. 1987. Ozone exposure increases respiratory epithelial permeability in humans. *Am. Rev. Respir. Dis.* 135: 1174–1178.

Kenoyer, J. L., R. F. Phalen, and J. R. Davis. 1981. Particle clearance from the respiratory tract as a test of toxicity: Effect of ozone on short and long term clearance. *Exp. Lung Res.* 2: 111–120.

Kilburn, K. H., R. Warshaw, and J. C. Thornton. 1985. Pulmonary functional impairment and symptoms in women in the Los Angeles harbor area. *Am. J. Med.* 79: 23–28.

Kinney, P. L., and H. Ozkaynak. 1991. Associations of daily mortality and air pollution in Los Angeles County. *Environ. Res.* 54: 99–120.

Kinney, P. L., D. M. Nilsen, M. Lippmann, M. Brescia, T. Gordon, T. McGovern, H. El-Fawal, D. B. Devlin, and W. N. Rom. 1996. Biomarkers of lung inflammation in recreational joggers exposed to ozone. *Am. J. Respir. Crit. Care Med.* 154: 1430–1435.

Kinney, P. L., J. H. Ware, and J. D. Spengler. 1988. A critical evaluation of acute ozone epidemiology results. *Arch. Environ. Health* 43: 168–173.

Kinney, P. L., K. Ito, and G. D. Thurston. 1995. A sensitivity analysis of mortality/PM-10 associations in Los Angeles. *Inhal. Toxicol.* 7: 59–69.

Kleeberger, S. R. 1995. Genetic susceptibility to ozone exposure. *Toxicol. Lett.* 82/83: 295–300.

Kleeberger, S. R., L.-Y. Zhang, and G. J. Jakab. 1997. Differential susceptibility to oxidant exposure in inbred strains of mice: Nitrogen dioxide versus ozone. *Inhal. Toxicol.* 9: 601–621.

Kleinman, M. T., R. F. Phalen, W. J. Mautz, R. C. Mannix, T. R. McClure, and T. T. Crocker. 1989. Health effects of acid aerosols formed by atmospheric mixtures. *Environ. Health Perspect.* 79: 137–145.

Knudson, R. J., M. D. Lebowitz, C. J. Holberg, and B. Burrows. 1983. Changes in the normal maximal expiratory flow-volume curve with growth and aging. *Am. Rev. Respir. Dis.* 127: 725–734.

Koenig, J. Q., D. S. Covert, M. S. Smith, G. van Belle, and W. E. Pierson. 1988. The pulmonary effects of ozone and nitrogen dioxide alone and combined in healthy and asthmatic subjects. *Toxicol. Ind. Health* 4: 521–532.

Koenig, J. Q., D. S. Covert, S. G. Marshall, G. van Belle, and W. E. Pierson. 1987. The effects of ozone and nitrogen dioxide on pulmonary function in healthy and in asthmatic adolescents. *Am. Rev. Respir. Dis.* 136: 1152–1157.

Koenig, J. Q., D. W. Covert, Q. S. Hanley, G. vanBelle, and W. E. Pierson. 1990. Prior exposure to ozone potentiates subsequent response to sulfur dioxide in adolescent asthmatic subjects. *Am. Rev. Respir. Dis.* 141: 377–380.

Koren, H. S., R. B. Devlin, D. E. Graham, R. Mann, M. P. McGee, D. E. Horstman, W. J. Kozumbo, S. Becker, D. E. House, W. F. McDonnell, and P. A. Bromberg. 1989. Ozone-induced inflammation in the lower airways of human subjects. *Am. Rev. Respir. Dis.* 139: 407–415.

Korrick, S. A., L. M. Neas, D. W. Dockery, D. R. Gold, G. A. Allen, L. B. Hill, K. O. Kimball, B. A. Rosner, and F. E. Speizer. 1998. Effects of ozone and other pollutants on the pulmonary function of adult hikers. *Environ. Health Perspect.* 106: 93–99.

Kulle, T. J., L. R. Sauder, H. D. Kerr, B. P. Farrell, M. S. Bermel, and D. M. Smith. 1982. Duration of pulmonary function adaptation to ozone in humans. *Am. Ind. Hyg. Assoc. J.* 43: 832–837.

Kulle, T. J., L. R. Sauder, J. R. Hebel, and M. D. Chatham. 1985. Ozone response relationships in healthy nonsmokers. *Am. Rev. Respir. Dis.* 132: 36–41.

Kunzli, N., F. Lurmann, M. Segal, L. Ngo, J. Balmes, and I. B. Tager. 1997. Association between lifetime ambient ozone exposure and pulmonary function in college freshmen—Results of a pilot study. *Environ. Res.* 72: 8–23.

Larsen, R. I., W. F. McDonnell, D. H. Horstman, and L. J. Folinsbee. 1991. An air quality data analysis system for interrelating effects, standards, and needed source reductions: Part 11. A lognormal model relating human lung function decrease to O_3 exposure. *J. Air Waste Manage. Assoc.* 41: 455–459.

Last, J. A., K. M. Reiser, W. S. Tyler, and R. B. Rucker. 1984. Long-term consequences of exposure to ozone: I. Lung collagen content. *Toxicol. Appl. Pharmacol.* 72: 111–118.

Last, J. A. 1989. Effects of inhaled acids on lung biochemistry. *Environ. Health Perspect.* 79: 115–119.

Last, J. A., T. R. Gelzleichter, K. E. Pinkerton, R. M. Walker, and H. W. Witschi. 1993. A new model of progressive pulmonary fibrosis in rats. *Am. Rev. Respir. Dis.* 148: 487–494.

Lee, J. S., M. G. Mustafa, and A. A. Afifi. 1990. Effects of short-term, single and combined exposure to low-level NO_2 and O_3 on lung tissue enzyme activities in rats. *J. Toxicol. Environ. Health* 29: 293–305.

Lee, L. Y. 1990. Inhibiting effect of gas phase cigarette smoke on breathing: Role of hydroxyl radical. *Respir. Physiol.* 82: 227–238.

Lee, L. Y., C. Dumont, T. D. Djokie, T. E. Menzel, and J. A. Nadel. 1979. Mechanism of rapid shallow breathing after ozone exposure in conscious dogs. *J. Appl. Physiol.* 46: 1108–1114.

Leikauf, G. D., K. E. Driscoll, and H. E. Wey. 1988. Ozone-induced augmentation of eicosanoid metabolism in epithelial cells from bovine trachea. *Am. Rev. Respir. Dis.* 137: 435–442.

Linder, J., D. Herren, C. Monn, and H. U. Wanner. 1988. Die Wirkung von Ozon auf die korperliche Leistungsfahigkeit (The effect of ozone on physical activity). *Schweiz. Z. Sport-med.* 36: 5–10.

Linn, W. S., D. A. Shamoo, T. G. Venet, C. E. Spier, L. M. Valencia, U. T. Anzar, and J. D. Hackney. 1983. Response to ozone in volunteers with chronic obstructive pulmonary disease. *Arch. Environ. Health* 38: 278–283.

Linn, W. S., E. L. Avol, D. A. Shamoo, R. C. Peng, L. M. Valencia, D. E. Little, and J. D. Hackney. 1988. Repeated laboratory ozone exposures of volunteer Los Angeles residents: An apparent seasonal variation in response. *Toxicol. Ind. Health* 4: 505–520.

Linn, W. S., M. P. Jones, E. A. Bachmeyer, C. E. Spier, S. F. Mazur, E. L. Avol, and J. D. Hackney. 1980. Short-term respiratory effects of polluted air: A laboratory study of volunteers in a high-oxidant community. *Am. Rev. Respir. Dis.* 121: 243–252.

Lioy, P. J., and R. V. Dyba. 1989. The dynamics of human exposure to tropospheric ozone. In *Atmospheric Ozone Research and Its Policy Implications*, eds. T. Schneider, S. D. Lee, G. J. R. Wolters, and L. D. Grant, Nijmegen, the Netherlands: Elsevier.

Lioy, P. J., T. A. Vollmuth, and M. Lippmann. 1985. Persistence of peak flow decrement in children following ozone exposures exceeding the national ambient air quality standard. *J. Air Pollut. Control Assoc.* 35: 1068–1071.

Lipfert, F. W., and T. Hammerstrom. 1992. Temporal patterns in air pollution and hospital admissions. *Environ. Res.* 59: 374–399.

Lippmann, M. 1977. Regional deposition of particles in the human respiratory tract. In *Handbook of Physiology, Section 9, Reactions to Environmental Agents*, eds. D. H. K. Lee, H. L. Falk, and S. D. Murphy, Bethesda: American Physiological Society.

Lippmann, M. 1987. Role of science advisory groups in establishing standards for ambient air pollutants. *Aerosol Sci. Tech.* 6: 93–114.

Lippmann, M. 1988. Health significance of pulmonary function tests. *J. Air Pollut. Control Assoc.* 38: 881–887.

Lippmann, M. 1989a. Effects of ozone on respiratory function and structure. *Annu. Rev. Public Health* 10: 49–67.

Lippmann, M. 1989b. Effective strategies for population studies of acute air pollution health effects. *Environ. Health Perspect.* 81: 115–119.

Lippmann, M. 1991. Morbidity associated with air pollution. In *The Handbook of Environmental Chemistry*. Volume 4: Part C: *Air Pollution*, ed. O. Hutzinger, pp. 31–71. Heidelberg: Springer Verlag.

Lippmann, M. 1993. Health effects of tropospheric ozone: Implications of recent research findings to ambient air quality standards. *J. Exp. Anal. Environ. Epidemiol.* 3: 103–129.

Lippmann, M., J. M. Gearhart, and R. B. Schlesinger. 1987. Basis for a particle size-selective TLV for sulfuric acid aerosols. *Appl. Ind. Hyg.* 2: 188–199.

Lippmann, M., P. J. Lioy, G. Leikauf, K. B. Green, D. Baxter, M. Morandi, B. Pasternack, D. Fife, and F. E. Speizer. 1983. Effects of ozone on the pulmonary function of children. *Adv. Mod. Environ. Toxicol.* 5: 423–446.

Makino, K., and I. Mizoguchi. 1975. Symptoms caused by photochemical smog. *Nippon Koshu Eisei Zasshi* 2: 421–430.

McAllen, S. J., S. P. Chiu, R. F. Phalen, and R. E. Rasmussen. 1981. Effect of *in vivo* ozone exposure on *in vitro* pulmonary alveolar macrophage mobility. *J. Toxicol. Environ. Health* 7: 373–381.

McDonnell, W. F., D. H. Horstman, M. J. Hazucha, E. Seal, E. D. Haak, S. A. Salaam, and D. E. House. 1983. Pulmonary effects of ozone exposure during exercise: Dose–response characteristics. *J. Appl. Physiol.* 54: 1345–1352.

McDonnell, W. F., D. H. Horstman, S. Abdul-Salaam, and D. E. House. 1985a. Reproducibility of individual responses to ozone exposure. *Am. Rev. Respir. Dis.* 131: 36–40.

McDonnell, W. F. III, R. S. Chapman, M. W. Leigh, G. L. Strope, and A. M. Collier. 1985b. Respiratory responses of vigorously exercising children to 0.12 ppm ozone exposure. *Am. Rev. Respir. Dis.* 132: 875–879.

McDonnell, W. F., D. H. Horstman, S. Abdul-Salaam, L. J. Raggio, and J. A. Green. 1987. The respiratory responses of subjects with allergic rhinitis to ozone exposure and their relationship to nonspecific airway reactivity. *Toxicol. Ind. Health* 3: 507–517.

McDonnell, W. F., H. R. Kehrl, S. Abdul-Salaam, P. J. Ives, L. J. Folinsbee, R. B. Devlin, J. J. O'Neil, and D. H. Horstman. 1991. Respiratory response of humans exposed to low levels of ozone for 6.6 hours. *Arch. Environ. Health* 46: 145–150.

McDonnell, W. F., K. E. Muller, P. A. Bromberg, and C. M. Shy. 1993. Predictors of individual differences in acute response to ozone exposure. *Am. Rev. Respir. Dis.* 147: 818–825.

McDonnell, W. F., P. W. Stewart, S. Andreoni, and M. V. Smith. 1995. Proportion of moderately exercising individuals responding to low-level, multi-hour ozone exposure. *Am. J. Respir. Crit. Care Med.* 152: 589–596.

McDonnell, W. F., P. W. Stewart, S. Andreoni, E. Seal, Jr., H. R. Kehrl, D. H. Horstman, L. J. Folinsbee, and M. V. Smith. 1997. Prediction of ozone-induced FEV$_1$ changes: Effects of concentration, duration, and ventilation. *Am. J. Respir. Crit. Care Med.* 156: 715–722.

McKittrick, T., and W. C. Adams. 1995. Pulmonary function response to equivalent doses of ozone consequent to intermittent and continuous exercise. *Arch. Environ. Health* 50: 153–158.

Mendelsohn, R., and G. Orcutt. 1979. An empirical analysis of air pollution dose–response curves. *J. Environ. Econ. Management* 6: 85–106.

Messineo, T. D., and W. C. Adams. 1990. Ozone inhalation effects in females varying widely in lung size: Comparison with males. *J. Appl. Physiol.* 69: 96–103.

Miller, F. J., D. B. Menzel, and D. L. Coffin. 1978b. Similarity between man and laboratory animals in regional pulmonary deposition of ozone. *Environ. Res.* 17: 84–101.

Miller, F. J., J. W. Illing, and D. E. Gardner. 1978a. Effects of urban ozone levels on laboratory-induced respiratory infections. *Toxicol. Lett.* 2: 163–169.

Moffatt, R. K., D. M. Hyde, C. G. Plopper, W. S. Tyler, and L. F. Putney. 1987. Ozone-induced adaptive and reactive cellular changes in respiratory bronchioles of bonnet monkeys. *Exp. Lung Res.* 12: 57–74.

National Research Council. 1977. Toxicology. In *Ozone and Other Photochemical Oxidants*. Washington, DC: National Academy of Sciences, Committee on Medical and Biologic Effects of Environmental Pollutants.

Neas, L. M., D. W. Dockery, P. Koutrakis, D. J. Tollerud, and F. E. Speizer. 1995. The association of ambient air pollution with twice daily peak expiratory flow rate measurements in children. *Am. J. Epidemiol.* 141: 111–122.

O'Bryne, P. M., E. H. Waters, B. D. Gold, H. A. Aizawa, L. M. Fabbri, S. E. Alpert, J. A. Nadel, and M. J. Holtzman. 1984a. Neutrophil depletion inhibits airway hyperresponsiveness induced by ozone exposure. *Am. Rev. Respir. Dis.* 130: 214–219.

O'Byrne, P. M., E. H. Waters, H. Aizawa, L. M. Fabbri, M. J. Holtzman, and J. A. Nadel. 1984b. Indomethacin inhibits the airway hyperresponsiveness but not the neutrophil influx induced by ozone in dogs. *Am. Rev. Respir. Dis.* 130: 220–224.

Oberdorster, G., M. J. Utell, P. E. Morrow, R. W. Hyde, and D. A. Weber. 1986. Bronchial and alveolar absorption of inhaled ^{99m}Tc-DTPA. *Am. Rev. Respir. Dis.* 134: 944–950.

Osebold, J. W., L. J. Gerschwin, and Y. C. Zee. 1980. Studies on the enhancement of allergic lung sensitization by inhalation of ozone and sulfur acid aerosol. *J. Environ. Pathol. Toxicol.* 3: 221–234.

Ostro, B. D., and S. Rothschild. 1989. Air pollution and acute respiratory morbidity: An observational study of multiple pollutants. *Environ. Res.* 50: 238–247.

Ostro, B. D., M. J. Lipsett, J. K. Mann, A. Krupnick, and W. Harrington. 1993. Air pollution and respiratory morbidity in Southern California. *Am. J. Epidemiol.* 137: 691–700.

Overton, J. H., and F. J. Miller. 1987. Modelling ozone absorption in lower respiratory tract. Paper presented at 1987 Annual Meeting of Air Pollution Control Association, New York, June.

Overton, J. H., and R. C. Graham. 1989. Predictions of ozone absorption in human lungs from newborn to adult. *Health Phys.* 57 (Supp. 1): 29–36.

Peden, D. B., R. W. Setzer Jr., and R. B. Devlin. 1995. Ozone exposure has both a priming effect on allergen-induced responses and an intrinsic inflammatory action in the nasal airways of perennially allergic asthmatics. *Am. J. Respir. Crit. Care Med.* 151: 1336–1345.

Phalen, R. F., J. L. Kenoyer, T. T. Crocker, and T. R. McClure. 1980. Effects of sulfate aerosols in combination with ozone on elimination of tracer particles inhaled by rats. *J. Toxicol. Environ. Health* 6: 797–810.

Phipps, R. J., S. M. Denas, M. W. Siekzak, and A. Wanner. 1986. Effects of 0.5 ppm ozone on glycoprotein secretion, ion and water fluxes in sheep trachea. *J. Appl. Physiol.* 60: 918–927.

Pinkerton, K. E., A. R. Brody, F. J. Miller, and J. D. Crapo. 1989. Exposure to low levels of ozone results in enhanced pulmonary retention of inhaled asbestos fibers. *Am. Rev. Respir. Dis.* 140: 1075–1081.

Raizenne, M. E., R. T. Burnett, B. Stern, C. A. Franklin, and J. D. Spenger. 1989. Acute lung function responses to ambient acid aerosol exposures in children. *Environ. Health Perspect.* 79: 179–185.

Rao, S. T. 1988. Prepared discussion: Ozone air quality models. *J. Air Pollut. Control Assoc.* 38: 1129–1135.

Raub, J. A., F. J. Miller, and J. A. Graham. 1983. Effects of low level ozone exposure on pulmonary function in adult and neonatal rats. *Adv. Mod. Environ. Toxicol.* 5: 363–367.

Reisenauer, C. S., J. Q. Koenig, M. S. McManus, M. S. Smith, G. Kusic, and W. E. Pierson. 1988. Pulmonary response to ozone exposures in healthy individuals aged 55 years or greater. *J. Air Pollut. Control Assoc.* 38: 51–55.

Reiser, K. M., W. S. Tyler, S. M. Hennessy, J. J. Dominguez, and J. A. Last. 1987. Long-term consequences of exposure to ozone. I. Structural alterations in lung collagen of monkeys. *Toxicol. Appl. Pharmacol.* 89: 314–322.

Review of the National Ambient Air Quality Standards for Ozone-Preliminary Assessment of Scientific and Technical Information. 1996. OAQPS Staff Paper, June. EPA publication 452/R-96-007.

Roberts, A. M., H. D. Schultz, J. F. Green, D. J. Armstrong, M. P. Kaufman, H. M. Coleridge, and J. C. G. Coleridge. 1985. Reflex tracheal contraction evoked in dogs by bronchodilator prostaglandins E_2 and I_2. *J. Appl. Physiol.* 58: 1823–1831.

Robertson, P. C., N. R. Anthonisen, and D. Ross. 1969. Effect of inspiratory flow rate on regional distribution of inspired gas. *J. Appl. Physiol.* 26: 438–443.

Rombout, P. J. A., L. vanBree, S. H. Heisterkamp, and M. Marra. 1989. The need for an eight hour standard. In *Atmospheric Ozone Research and Its Policy Implications*, eds. T. Schneider, S. D. Lee, G. J. R. Wolters, and L. D. Grant. Nijegen, the Netherland: Elsevier.

Rombout, P. J. A., P. J. Lioy, and B. D. Goldstein. 1986. Rationale for an eight-hour ozone standard. *J. Air Pollut. Control Assoc.* 36: 913–917.

Romieu, I., F. Meneses, S. Ruiz, J. J. Sienta, J. Huerta, M. C. White, and R. A. Etzel. 1996. Effects of air pollution on the respiratory health of asthmatic children living in Mexico City. *Am. J. Respir. Crit. Care Med.* 154: 300–307.

Sartor, F., C. Demuth, R. Snacken, and D. Walckiers. 1997. Mortality in elderly and ambient ozone concentration during the hot summer, 1994, in Belgium. *Environ. Res.* 72: 109–117.

Sartor, F., R. Snacken, C. Demuth, and D. Walckiers. 1995. Temperature, ambient ozone levels, and mortality during summer, 1994, in Belgium. *Environ. Res.* 70: 105–113.

Savin, W., and W. Adams. 1979. Effects of ozone inhalation on work performance and VO_2 max. *J. Appl. Physiol.* 46: 309–314.

Scannell, C., L. Chen, R. M. Aris, I. Tager, D. Christian, R. Ferrando, B. Welch, T. Kelly, and J. R. Balmes. 1996. Greater ozone-induced inflammatory responses in subjects with asthma. *Am. J. Respir. Crit. Care Med.* 154: 24–29.

Schelegle, E. S., and W. C. Adams. 1986. Reduced exercise time in competitive simulations consequent to low level ozone exposure. *Med. Sci. Sports Exercise* 18: 408–414.

Schelegle, E. S., W. C. Adams, and A. D. Siefkin. 1987. Indomethacin pretreatment reduces ozone-induced pulmonary function decrements in human subjects. *Am. Rev. Respir. Dis.* 136: 1350–1354.

Schlesinger, R. B., and K. E. Driscoll. 1987. Mucociliary clearance from the lungs of rabbits following single and intermittent exposures to ozone. *J. Toxicol. Environ. Health* 20: 125–134.

Schoettlin, C. E., and E. Landau. 1961. Air pollution and asthmatic attacks in the Los Angeles area. *Public Health Rep.* 76: 545–548.

Schwartz, J. 1989. Lung function and chronic exposure to air pollution: A cross-sectional analysis of NHANES II. *Environ. Res.* 50: 309–321.

Schwartz, J. 1994a. Air pollution and hospital admissions for the elderly in Birmingham, Alabama. *Am. J. Epidemiol.* 139: 589–598.

Schwartz, J. 1994b. Air pollution and hospital admissions for the elderly in Detroit, Michigan. *Am. J. Respir. Crit. Care Med.* 150: 648–655.

Schwartz, J. 1994c. PM_{10}, ozone, and hospital admissions for the elderly in Minneapolis, MN. *Arch. Environ. Health* 49: 366–374.

Schwartz, J., and S. Zeger. 1990. Passive smoking, air pollution, and acute respiratory symptoms in a diary study of student nurses. *Am. Rev. Respir. Dis.* 141: 62–67.

Schwartz, J., D. W. Dockery, L. M. Neas, D. Wypij, J. H. Ware, J. D. Spengler, P. Koutrakis, F. E. Speizer, and B. G. Ferris Jr. 1994. Acute effects of summer air pollution on respiratory symptom reporting in children. *Am. J. Respir. Crit. Care Med.* 150: 1234–1242.

Scott, W. R., and H. D. Van Liew. 1983. Measurement of lung emptying patterns during slow exhalations. *J. Appl. Physiol.* 55: 1818–1824.

Seal, E, Jr., W. F. McDonnell, D. E. House, S. A. Salaam, P. J. Dewitt, S. O. Butler, J. Green, and L. Raggio. 1993. The pulmonary response of white and black adults to six concentrations of ozone. *Am. Rev. Respir. Dis.* 147: 804–810.

Seinfeld, J. H. 1988. Ozone air quality models: A critical review. *J. Air Pollut. Control Assoc.* 38: 616–645.

Seltzer, J., B. G. Bigby, M. Stulbarg, M. J. Holtzman, and J. A. Nadel. 1986. O_3-induced changes in bronchial reactivity to methacholine and airway inflammation in humans. *J. Appl. Physiol.* 60: 1321–1326.

Selwyn, B. J., T. H. Stock, R. J. Hardy, F. A. Chan, D. E. Jenkins, D. J. Kotchmar, and R. S. Chapman. 1985. Health effects of ambient ozone exposure in vigorously exercising adults. In *Evaluation of the Scientific Basis for Ozone/Oxidants Standards: Proc. APCA International Specialty Conference* (TR4), ed. S. D. Lee, pp. 281–296. Pittsburgh, PA: Air Pollution Control Association.

Shephard, R. J., B. Urch, F. Silverman, and P. N. Corey. 1983. Interaction of ozone and cigarette smoke exposure. *Environ. Res.* 31: 125–137.

Sherwin, R. P., and V. Richters. 1985. Effect of 0.3 ppm ozone exposure on type II cells and alveolar walls of newborn mice: An image-analysis quantitation. *J. Toxicol. Environ. Health* 16: 535–546.

Sherwin, R. P., and V. Richters. 1991. Centriacinar region (CAR) disease in the lungs of young adults: A preliminary report. In *Tropospheric Ozone and the Environment* (TR-19), eds. R. L. Berglund, D. R. Lawson, and D. J. McKee, pp. 178–196. Pittsburgh, PA: Air and Waste Management Association.

Sherwin, R. P., V. Richters, and D. Okimoto. 1983. Type 2 pneumocyte hyperplasia in the lungs of mice exposed to an ambient level (0.3 ppm) of ozone. *Adv. Mod. Environ. Toxicol.* 5: 289–297.

Solic, J. J., M. J. Hazucha, and P. A. Bromberg. 1982. The acute effects of 0.2 ppm ozone in patients with chronic obstructive pulmonary disease. *Am. Rev. Respir. Dis.* 125: 664–669.

Spektor, D. M., G. D. Thurston, J. Mao, D. He, C. Hayes, and M. Lippmann. 1991. Effects of single- and multi-day ozone exposures on respiratory function in active normal children. *Environ. Res.* 55: 107–122.

Spektor, D. M., M. Lippmann, P. J. Lioy, G. D. Thurston, K. Citak, D. J. James, N. Bock, F. E. Speizer, and C. Hayes. 1988a. Effects of ambient ozone on respiratory function in active normal children. *Am. Rev. Respir. Dis.* 137: 313–320.

Spektor, D. M., M. Lippmann, G. D. Thurston, P. J. Lioy, J. Stecko, G. O'Connor, E. Garshick, F. E. Speizer, and C. Hayes. 1988b. Effects of ambient ozone on respiratory function in healthy adults exercising outdoors. *Am. Rev. Respir. Dis.* 138: 821–828.

Spengler, J. D., G. J. Keeler, P. Koutrakis, P. B. Ryan, M. Raizenne, and C. A. Franklin. 1989. Exposures to acidic aerosols. *Environ. Health Perspect.* 79: 43–51.

Stacy, R. W., E. Seal Jr., D. E. House, J. Green, L. J. Roger, and L. Raggio. 1983. A survey of effects of gaseous and aerosol pollutants on pulmonary function of normal males. *Arch. Environ. Health* 38: 104–115.

Stern, B. R., M. E. Raizenne, R. T. Burnett, L. Jones, J. Kearney, and C. A. Franklin. 1994. Air pollution and childhood respiratory health: Exposure to sulfate and ozone in 10 Canadian rural communities. *Environ. Res.* 66: 125–142.

Stieb, D. M., R. T. Burnett, R. C. Beveridge, and J. R. Brook. 1996. Association between ozone and asthma emergency department visits in Saint John, New Brunswick, Canada. *Environ. Health Perspect.* 104: 1354–1360.

Tepper, J. S., B. Weiss, and R. W. Wood. 1985. Alterations in behavior produced by inhaled ozone or ammonia. *Fundam. Appl. Toxicol.* 5: 1110–1118.

Tepper, J. S., D. L. Costa, J. R. Lehmann, M. F. Weber, and G. E. Hatch. 1989. Unattenuated structural and biochemical alterations in the rat lung during functional adaptation to ozone. *Am. Rev. Respir. Dis.* 140: 493–501.

Tepper, J. S., M. J. Wiester, M. F. Weber, S. Fitzgerald, and D. L. Costa. 1991. Chronic exposure to a stimulated urban profile of ozone alters ventilatory responses to carbon dioxide challenge in rats. *Fundam. Appl. Toxicol.* 17: 52–60.

Thurston, G. D. 1997. Testimony submitted to U.S. Senate Committee on Environment and Public Works, Subcommittee on Clean Air, Wetlands, Private Property, and Nuclear Safety. February 1977.

Thurston, G. D., K. Ito, C. G. Hayes, D. V. Bates, and M. Lippmann. 1994. Respiratory hospital admissions and summertime haze air pollution in Toronto, Ontario: Consideration of the role of acid aerosols. *Environ. Res.* 65: 271–290.

Thurston, G. D., K. Ito, P. L. Kinney, and M. Lippmann. 1992. A multi-year study of air pollution and respiratory hospital admissions in three New York State metropolitan areas: Results for 1988 and 1989 summers. *J. Expo. Anal. Environ. Epidemiol.* 2: 429–450.

Thurston, G. D., M. Lippmann, M. B. Scott, and J. M. Fine. 1997. Summertime haze air pollution and children with asthma. *Am. J. Respir. Crit. Care Med.* 155: 654–660.

Torres, A., M. J. Utell, P. E. Morrow, K. Z. Voter, J. C. Whitin, C. Cox, R. J. Looney, D. M. Speers, Y. Tsai, and M. W. Frampton. 1997. Airway inflammation in smokers and nonsmokers with varying responsiveness to ozone. *Am. J. Respir. Crit. Care Med.* 156: 728–736.

Touloumi, G., K. Katsouyanni, D. Zmirou, J. Schwartz, C. Spix, A. Ponce de Leon, A. Tobias, P. Quennel, D. Rabczenko, L. Bacharova, L. Bisanti, J. M. Vonk, and A. Ponka. 1997. Short-term effects of ambient oxidant exposure on mortality: A combined analysis within the APHEA project. *Am. J. Epidemiol.* 146: 177–185.

Tyler, W. S., N. K. Tyler, J. A. Last, M. J. Gillespie, and T. J. Barstow. 1988. Comparison of daily and seasonal exposures of young monkeys to ozone. *Toxicology* 50: 131–144.

Tyler, W. S., N. K. Tyler, J. A. Last, T. J. Barstow, D. J. Magliano, and D. M. Hinds. 1987. Effects of ozone on lung and somatic growth: Pair fed rats after ozone exposure and recovery periods. *Toxicology* 46: 1–20.

U.S. DOL. 1989. Air contaminants; Final Rule. 29CFR, Part 1910. *Federal Register* 54: 2332–2983.

U.S. EPA. 1986. *Air Quality Criteria for Ozone and Other Photochemical Oxidants*, Vol. 2. EPA/600/8-84/020F, ECAO. NTIS, Springfield, VA.

U.S. EPA. 1989. *Review of the National Ambient Air Quality Standards for Ozone—Assessment of Scientific and Technical Information.* OAQPS Staff Paper. EPA-450/2-92/001. NTIS Springfield, VA.

U.S. EPA. 1992. *Summary of Selected New Information on Effects of Ozone on Health and Vegetation: Supplement to 1986 Air Quality Criteria for Ozone and Other Photochemical Oxidants.* EPA/600/8-88/105F, ECAO. NTIS, Springfield, VA.

U.S. EPA. 1996a. *Air Quality Criteria for Ozone and Other Photochemical Oxidants.* EPA publication 600/P-93/004F. Research Triangle Park, NC: U.S. Environmental Protection Agency.

U.S. EPA. 1996b. *Review of National Ambient Air Quality Standards for Ozone-Assessment of Scientific and Technical Information.* OAQPS Staff Paper. EPA-452/A-96-007. Research Triangle Park, NC. U.S. EPA-OAQPS.

Utell, M. J., P. E. Morrow, D. M. Speers, J. Darling, and R. W. Hyde. 1983. Airway responses to sulfate and sulfuric acid aerosols in asthmatics. *Am. Rev. Respir. Dis.* 128: 444–450.

Valentine, R. 1985. An *in vitro* system for exposure of lung cells to gases: Effects of ozone on rat macrophages. *J. Toxicol. Environ. Health* 16: 115–126.

Van Bree, L., P. J. A. Rombout, I. M. C. M. Rietjens, J. A. M. A. Dormans, and M. Marra. 1989. Pathobiochemical effects in rat lung related to episodic ozone exposure. In *Atmospheric Ozone Research and Its Policy Implications*, eds. T. Schneider, S. D. Lee, G. J. R. Wolters, and L. D. Grant. Nijmegen, the Netherlands: Elsevier.

Verhoeff, A. P., G. Hoek, J. Schwartz, and J. H. vanWijnen. 1996. Air pollution and daily mortality in Amsterdam. *Epidemiology* 7: 225–230.

Wayne, W. S., P. F. Wehrle, and R. E. Carroll. 1967. Oxidant air pollution and athletic performance. *JAMA* 199: 901–904.

Weinmann, G. G., S. M. Bowes, M. W. Gerbase, A. W. Kimball, and R. Frank. 1995. Response to acute ozone exposure in healthy men. *Am. J. Respir. Crit. Care Med.* 151: 33–40.

Weisel, C. P., R. P. Cody, and P. J. Lioy. 1995. Relationship between summertime ambient ozone levels and emergency department visits for asthma in central New Jersey. *Environ. Health Perspect.* 103: 97–102.

White, M. C., R. A. Etzel, W. D. Wilcox, and C. Lloyd. 1994. Exacerbations of childhood asthma and ozone pollution in Atlanta. *Environ. Res.* 65: 56–68.

Whittemore, A., and E. Korn. 1980. Asthma and air pollution in the Los Angeles area. *Am. J. Public Health* 70: 687–696.

Witschi, H. 1988. Ozone, nitrogen dioxide and lung cancer: A review of some recent issues and problems. *Toxicology* 48: 1–20.

Witschi, H. 1991. Effects of oxygen and ozone on mouse lung tumorigenesis. *Exp. Lung Res.* 17: 473–483.

Witz, G., M. A. Amoruso, and B. D. Goldstein. 1983. Effect of ozone on alveolar macrophage function: Membrane dynamic properties. *Adv. Mod. Environ. Toxicol.* 5: 263–272.

Yang, W., B. L. Jennison, and S. T. Omaye. 1997. Air pollution and asthma emergency room visits in Reno, Nevada. *Inhal. Toxicol.* 9: 15–29.

Ying, R. L., K. B. Gross, T. S. Terzo, and W. L. Eschenbacher. 1990. Indomethacin does not inhibit the ozone-induced increase in bronchial responsiveness in human subjects. *Am. Rev. Respir. Dis.* 142: 817–821.

21 Pesticides

PHILIP J. LANDRIGAN, M.D., M.Sc.
LUZ CLAUDIO, Ph.D.
ROB MCCONNELL, M.D.

Synthetic pesticides are a diverse group of chemical compounds, most of them derived from petroleum, that are used to control insects, unwanted plants, fungi, rodents, and other pests. (Hayes and Laws, 1991). Pesticides are used in an extraordinarily wide range of settings. By controlling agricultural pests, they have contributed to dramatic increases in crop yields and in the quantity and variety of the crops (National Research Council, 1993). In the home they control mice, termites, and rodents. In gardens and lawns as well as along highways and under power line right-of-ways, synthetic pesticides control the growth of unwanted plants. There are also naturally occurring pesticides produced by plants and other organisms; these compounds are discussed in the Chapter 11.

Approximately 600 pesticide active ingredients, including insecticides, herbicides, rodenticides, and fungicides, are currently registered for use with the U.S. Environmental Protection Agency (EPA). These compounds are mixed with each other and also blended with "inert" ingredients to produce more than 20,000 commercial pesticide products. EPA estimates that in 1993 domestic users in the United States spent $8.5 billion for 1.1 billion pounds of pesticide active ingredients (Schierow, 1996).

Agriculture is the major consumer of pesticides, accounting for 75% of use by volume. Industrial, commercial, and governmental users (18%) and home and garden users (7%) account for the remainder. Herbicides for weed control account for the largest volume of agricultural pesticide use (59%), and they are applied primarily on corn and soybeans. Insecticides are the next major category of agricultural pesticides (21% of volume), and they are used primarily on corn, cotton, and soybeans. (Schierow, 1996).

Because they convey benefits as well as risks, pesticides pose a perennial problem for public policy and regulation (National Research Council, 1993). Pesticides are specifically designed to be toxic to certain species, and that toxicity is the basis of their utility (Hayes and Laws, 1991). But many pesticides are also toxic to species beyond those targeted. Consequently pesticides have caused severe damage to ecosystems. Also many pesticides are known to be toxic to humans, and others are suspected of human toxicity. They can produce a wide range of adverse effects on human health, including acute and chronic injury to the nervous system, lung damage, injury to the reproductive organs, dysfunction of the immune and endocrine systems, birth defects, and cancer. Children, by virtue of their patterns of exposure and their inherent biological vulnerability, are especially susceptible to the health effects of pesticides (National Research Council, 1993).

Recognition of the toxicity of pesticides has stimulated enactment of a vast body of protective laws and regulations in nations around the world. It has also fostered

Environmental Toxicants: Human Exposures and Their Health Effects, 2/e. Edited by Morton Lippmann.
ISBN: 0-471-29298-2 © 2000 John Wiley & Sons, Inc.

development of a series of ever newer and less toxic pesticides. These actions have helped to control the toxic hazards of pesticides; the National Academy of Sciences estimates that since 1954, a 90% reduction in the toxicity of pesticides applied to food crops in the United States (National Research Council, 1996).

EVOLVING PATTERNS OF PESTICIDE USE

The era of modern pesticides began in the nineteenth century when sulfur compounds were developed as fungicides. In the late nineteenth century, arsenical compounds were introduced to control the insects that attack fruit and vegetable crops; for example, lead arsenate was used widely on apples and grapes. All of these substances were acutely toxic (Schierow, 1996).

In the 1940s, the chlorinated hydrocarbon pesticides, most notably DDT (dichlorodiphenyltrichloroethane), were introduced. For a time DDT and similar chemicals were used extensively in agriculture and in the control of malaria and other insectborne diseases. Because they had little or no immediate toxicity, they were widely hailed and initially were believed to be safe (Wargo, 1996).

In 1962, with the publication of Rachel Carson's *Silent Spring*, the potential of the chlorinated hydrocarbon pesticides for long-term toxicity and for accumulation in the food chain became evident. It was shown, for example, that DDT caused reproductive failure in eagles and ospreys, species that had accumulated large doses of DDT because of their position high in the food chain. In 1972 DDT was banned in the United States by the newly created EPA. Application has continued, however, in many nations and especially in less developed countries (World Health Organization, 1992).

Today the principal classes of insecticides in use in most industrialized countries are organophosphates, carbamates, and pyrethroids. Unlike the chlorinated hydrocarbons, these compounds are short-lived in the environment and do not bioaccumulate. However, some of them can affect the nervous system, causing serious acute and chronic toxicity (Blondell, 1997). Others are known or suspected to be carcinogens, reproductive toxins or toxic to the endocrine system (Costa, 1997; Zahm, Ward, and Blair, 1997).

Insecticide use has declined in recent years, reflecting in part the adoption of integrated pest-management systems. Such programs emphasize the use of nonchemical means of pest control to replace and complement pesticide use. In agriculture, for example, integrated pest management may involve crop rotation and the use of resistant plant strains. In homes and buildings such programs incorporate the cleanup of food residues, the sealing of foundation cracks, and good maintenance (Benbrook, 1996). Unlike insecticides, fungicides have continued in steady use, and herbicide use has increased substantially.

Export to developing nations of highly toxic pesticides that are manufactured in the industrially developed nations, but banned for use there, is a major unresolved issue in pesticide regulation. EPA estimates that over 400 million pounds of banned pesticides are exported each year from the United States, almost one-third of domestic pesticide production and 10% of world consumption; this trade is valued annually at approximately $2 billion (Schierow, 1996). Toxic pesticides exported to the third world can return to the developed nations on imported foodstuffs, a phenomenon termed the "circle of poison" (World Health Organization, 1992).

EXPOSURE

Exposure to pesticides may be percutaneous, by inhalation, or by ingestion. Exposure may occur in the workplace, via the diet, in the yard or home, and in the community. In assessing exposure, it is important to understand that persons may simultaneously be exposed to multiple pesticides by several of these routes, and that the effects of these multiple exposures may be additive or even synergistic (National Research Council, 1996).

Occupational Exposure

Occupational exposure to pesticides occurs among manufacturers and formulators; during transport and storage; among mixers, loaders, and applicators working in fields, greenhouses, parks, and residential buildings; among vector control and structural applicators; and among farmworkers entering fields or greenhouse workers handling foliage previously sprayed by pesticides (Blondell, 1997; McConnell, 1994). Crop duster aviation mechanics have been reported to be at high risk for pesticide poisoning. Other groups occasionally exposed include emergency crews or sewer workers involved in cleanup. In developed countries the largest exposed group consists of building maintenance workers who apply insecticides in public and private housing, schools, hospitals, and commercial structures.

Environmental Exposure

Environmental exposure to pesticides occurs from consumption of contaminated water, ingestion of residues in food, inhalation of airborne drift, exposure to contaminated dust in the home, or from exposure to improperly disposed hazardous waste. Seasonal contamination of drinking water by herbicides is reported each spring in the American midwest, a pattern that coincides with annual application of these compounds before spring planting. Although nonoccupational exposure is usually low level, numerous episodes of acute illness have resulted from environmental exposure to pesticides (National Research Council, 1993). Also, intentional ingestion of pesticides is a frequent means of suicide.

Pediatric Exposures

Children are a group at particular risk of exposure to pesticides (National Research Council, 1993). Diet is a major route of children's exposure. Children may also be exposed to pesticides applied in homes or schools, on lawns, and in gardens. Children employed in agriculture or living in migrant farm worker camps are at particularly high risk of exposure to pesticides and of suffering acute pesticide intoxication (McConnell, 1994).

Children's tissues and organs are rapidly developing, and at various stages in early development, these growth processes create windows of great vulnerability to pesticides and other environmental toxicants. An analysis undertaken by the National Academy of Sciences (National Research Council, 1993) has established that the unique vulnerability of infants and children to pesticides and other environmental toxicants is based on the following four factors:

- Children have greater exposures to environmental toxicants than adults. Pound for pound of body weight, children drink more water, eat more food, and breathe more air than adults. For example, children in the first six months of life consume seven times as much water per unit body weight as does the average American adult. In consequence, children are more heavily exposed than adults to toxicants in air, food, and water. Two behavioral characteristics of infants and children further magnify their exposures: (1) their normal hand-to-mouth activity and (2) their play close to the ground. Lastly dermal absorption by young children to certain environmental toxicants such as pesticides is higher than in adults because of their greater surface area relative to body weight and greater skin permeability.

- Children's metabolic pathways, especially in the first months after birth, are immature compared to those of adults. In some instances, children are actually better able than adults to cope with environmental toxicants because, for example, they are unable to metabolize toxicants to their active form (Kimmel, 1992). More commonly, however, children are less able to detoxify chemicals such as organophosphate pesticides and thus are more vulnerable to them (Mortensen et al., 1996; Bearer, 1995; Peto et al., 1996).
- Infants and children are growing and developing, and their delicate developmental processes are easily disrupted. Many organ systems in infants and children—the nervous system in particular—undergo extensive growth and development throughout the prenatal period and the first months and years of extrauterine life. If cells in an infant's brain are destroyed by pesticides, lead, or mercury, or if reproductive development is diverted by endocrine disrupters, the resulting dysfunction can be permanent and irreversible. (National Research Council, 1993).
- Because children have more future years of life than most adults, they have more time to develop chronic disease that may be initiated by early exposures. Exposures sustained early in life, including prenatal exposures, appear more likely to lead to disease than similar exposures encountered later. Also deficits sustained early may persist lifelong (National Research Council, 1993).

Surveys of foods commonly consumed by children have shown that a high proportion contain pesticide residues and that these foods frequently contain residues of multiple pesticides (Wiles and Campbell, 1993).

These observations on children's exposures to pesticides in food were further extended by a 1995 study which found that 16 different pesticides were present in some of the baby foods most commonly sold in the United States (Wiles and Davies, 1995). These pesticide residues included eight that have been shown to be toxic to the nervous system, five that affect the endocrine system, and eight that are potential carcinogens.

EPIDEMIOLOGY OF ACUTE PESTICIDE POISONING

Data on pesticide poisonings are sparse, and there is serious underreporting of even acute, life-threatening episodes (Blondell, 1997). The best information on occupational pesticide poisoning in the United States comes from California where physicians are required under law to report all incidents of pesticide poisoning. In the mid-1990s the average annual number of occupational pesticide poisoning cases reported in California was approximately 1500, of which 54% occurred in agriculture (Blondell, 1997). Organophosphates were the class of compounds most frequently involved. Extrapolating California data to the nation, it has been estimated that there are between 10,000 and 20,000 cases of physician-diagnosed pesticide poisonings in the United States per year (U.S. EPA, 1992).

Data on nonoccupational pesticide poisonings in the United States are collected by the Consumer Product Safety Commission based on a statistical sample of emergency rooms in 6000 selected hospitals across the United States; these data are sumarized by Blondell (1997). From 1990 to 1992 there were an estimated 20,000 emergency room visits resulting from pesticide exposure. Incidence was disproportionately high in children, who accounted for 61% of cases.

Pesticides: Epidemiology in the Third World

Although only 25% of the 3 million tons of pesticides produced yearly worldwide are used in developing countries, pesticide consumption in these countries continues to increase,

TABLE 21-1   Pesticide Residues on Fruits and Vegetables Heavily Consumed by Young Children

Supermarket Warehouse Data 1990–1992

Food	Number of Samples	Number with One or More Pesticides Detected	Percentage with One or More Pesticides Detected	Number of Different Pesticides Detected
Apples	542	425	78%	25
Bananas	368	134	36%	9
Broccoli	63	16	25%	9
Cantaloupes	225	78	35%	19
Carrots	252	125	50%	12
Caulifower	65	26	40%	13
Celery	114	85	75%	13
Cherries	90	72	80%	13
Grapes	313	192	61%	22
Green beans	249	95	38%	20
Leaf lettuce	201	136	68%	22
Oranges	237	190	80%	25
Peas	191	87	46%	19
Peaches	246	194	79%	20
Pears	328	240	73%	11
Potatoes	258	120	47%	17
Spinach	163	88	54%	19
Strawberries	168	138	82%	17
Tomatoes	395	203	51%	22
Total	4,468	2,644	59%	81

Source: Environmental Working Group (Wiles and Campbell, 1993). Compiled from U.S. EPA. Office of Planning, Policy, and Evaluation, Pesticide Food Residue Database, Anticipated Pesticide Residues in Food.

especially in Africa and Latin America (McConnell, 1994). Ninety percent of the estimated 3 million yearly poisonings worldwide and more than 99% of the 220,000 deaths occur in the developing countries. In surveys of agricultural workers in several Asian countries and of cotton workers in Mexico, 3% to 7% and 13% to 15%, respectively, reported poisoning in the previous year. In addition, pesticide poisoning may be more likely to be underdiagnosed in these nations than in the developed countries (Jeyaratnam, 1990).

Serious epidemics of pesticide poisoning have occurred in the developing world. Examples of major outbreaks of pesticide-associated disease include an estimated 60,000 illnesses and 2000 to 2500 deaths from exposure to methyl isocyanate used as an intermediary in insecticide manufacture in Bhopal, India (Melius, 1998), and an epidemic of acute parathion poisoning in Jamaica (with 17 deaths) caused by consumption of contaminated, imported wheat flour (Diggoty et al., 1977).

TOXICITY OF PESTICIDES

Because the chemistry of pesticides is highly diverse, pesticides are capable of causing a wide range of health effects. Depending on the pesticide or combination of pesticides to which an individual or a population is exposed, these effects can involve virtually every organ system in the body. Pesticides can produce acutely toxic effects, delayed effects, and chronic effects. Also some pesticides are developmental toxicants, and others are carcinogens and reproductive toxicants. This review will summarize data on the toxic effects of the major classes of agents.

Insecticides: Cholinesterase Inhibitors

This class includes both the organophosphates and the carbamates.

Acute Clinical Effects   The toxicites of organophosphates and carbamates are similar, and both inhibit neuronal acetylcholinesterase (Costa, 1997). Acute poisonings by organophosphates and carbamates account for the majority of systemic pesticide poisoning cases seen each year in the United States (Blondell, 1997). Inhibition of acetylcholinesterase results in increase in acetylcholine with resultant overstimulation of the postsynaptic receptors in the cholinergic nervous system. These effects can be differentiated toxicologically into (1) overstimulation of the central nervous system, (2) overstimulation of the nicotinic receptors (skeletal muscle and autonomic ganglia), and (3) overstimulation of the muscarinic receptors (secretory glands and postganglionic fibers in the parasympathetic nervous system). The nicotinic effects generally appear later and only in the more severe cases.

Headache, anxiety, and sleep disturbance, often accompanied by salivation and anorexia, are common early symptoms of mild overexposure to cholinesterase inhibitors (McConneell, 1994). Chest tightness is a symptom of moderately severe poisoning after dermal exposure, but it can be an early symptom if there is significant exposure via the respiratory tract. Seizures and impaired consciousness occur in the most severe cases. Death can follow respiratory arrest. Other reported acute effects include myopathy (including myocardiopathy), hypothermia, liver dysfunction, brady- or tachyarrhythmias, leukocytosis, and acute psychosis.

Delayed or Chronic Effects of Exposure to Organophosphates   Chronic low-level exposure to organophosphates may result in weakness and malaise, often accompanied by headache and light-headedness, but without other specific symptoms. Also several additional complications may occur in patients poisoned with organophosphates as follows (McConnell, 1994):

1. *Psychosis.* There have been case reports of acute and persistent psychotic illness associated with poisoning by organophosphates.
2. *Intermediate syndrome.* A recently reported (and rare) so-called intermediate syndrome, characterized by the paralysis of the proximal musculature and muscles of respiration and of cranial motor nerves, occurs 1 to 4 days after acute poisoning. Although the mechanism of this intermediate syndrome is not known, it is not thought to result from inhibition of acetylcholinesterase.
3. *Organophosphate-induced delayed polyneuropathy (OPIDP).* This distal dying-back axonopathy is characterized clinically by cramping muscle pain in the legs, often followed by paresthesia and motor weakness. The onset occurs 10 days to 3 weeks after severe poisoning (Lotti, 1992). There may be marked foot drop and weakness of the distal upper extremities. The pathophysiology of the disease probably requires the inhibition and subsequent aging of a poorly characterized intraneuronal esterase known as neuropathy target esterase (NTE), which is distinct from acetylcholinesterase (Costa, 1997).

Pyreththrum and Pyreththroids

In the mid-1800s pyrethrum extracts of chrysanthemum flowers (containing pyrethrin and other active ingredients) were found to be effective insecticides (Hayes and Laws, 1991). They are relatively less toxic than other commonly used insecticides. Pyrethrum may cause asthma or allergic rhinitis, and contact dermatitis is frequent.

The pyrethroid insecticides, in use today are all synthetic, although they are closely related chemically to the naturally occurring pyrethrins. They are more stable in the natural environment than the natural compounds, and are used in agriculture and in household pest control. Ingestion of large doses of pyrethroids causes salivation, nausea, vomiting, diarrhea, irritability, tremor, incoordination, seizures, and death. Toxicity is thought to be mediated through delay in the closing of sodium channels after discharge of an action potential, which results in repetitive neuronal discharge (Narahashi, 1985).

Organochlorine Insecticides

This class includes DDT, lindane, and the cyclodienes: aldrin, dieldrin, endrin, and heptachlor. Most use of these chemically diverse insecticides has been banned or restricted in the developed world because they persist in the environment and concentrate in the food chain, damaging wildlife (Blondell, 1997). Fat levels of DDT in human surveys have decreased markedly since DDT was banned in the United States in 1973. In the third world high concentrations of DDT in the fat and milk of humans and cows continue to be found.

Acute Effects   Dermal absorption of the cyclodienes, chlordecone, and lindane is high. Because acute toxicity is high for chlordecone, endrin, aldrin, and dieldrin, these account for most occupational poisonings within this class. Most other acute poisonings result from ingestion. Acute toxicity reflects poorly understood neuronal hyperactivity in the central nervous system. Sudden seizures (especially from aldrin, dieldrin, endrin, lindane, and toxaphene) may occur up to 48 hours after exposure and may be relatively intractable. Headache, nausea, dizziness, incoordination, confusion, tremor, and paresthesia are common. Tremor is characteristic of poisoning with DDT and chlordecone. Abnormal liver enzyme levels and renal tubular abnormalities may be seen.

Chronic Effects   Epidemic occupational chlordecone (Kepone) poisoning in a manufacturing facility in Virginia was characterized by anxiety and tremor, opsoclonus, personality change, oligospermia, pleuritic and joint pains, weight loss, and liver disease. The effects were chronic. In addition, two workers' wives were poisoned by contact with contaminated work clothes, and a portion of the Chesapeake Bay was polluted by discharge from the plant (Cannon et al., 1978).

Almost all organochlorine insecticides have been found to be carcinogenic in at least one species of rodent. Idiosyncratic cases of aplastic anemia have been reported anecdotally in association with exposure to organochlorines, especially to chlordane and lindane (McConnell, 1994).

Herbicides   Herbicides are the most important class of pesticides in the United States today in terms of market share. Their use in agriculture and elsewhere is increasing steadily. This diverse class includes atrazine; 2,4-D; 2,4,5-T; glyphosate; and paraquat. Most of these compounds, paraquat excepted, have low acute toxicity. Some herbicides are important groundwater contaminants and are animal carcinogens, including, for example, alachlor and atrazine.

Bipyridils (Diquat and Paraquat)

High acute toxicity, lack of an effective antidote, and ready availability (because of low cost and herbicidal efficacy) have contributed to the notoriety of paraquat.

Acute Effects   Painful burns and bleeding of the gastrointestinal tract are common following acute exposure. Approximately 20% of ingested paraquat is absorbed systemically, where it may cause acute hepatic necrosis and renal disease.

The most distinctive aspect of paraquat poisoning is delayed pulmonary toxicity. Paraquat is concentrated from the systemic circulation into the lungs, where pulmonary edema may develop 2 to 4 days after ingestion. The mortality rate of pulmonary toxicity induced by paraquat is greater than 50% in most case series. The lethal dose in 50% of rabbits dosed dermally is only 4.5 mg / kg / d. Occupational poisoning resulting from dermal absorption is more likely to occur in developing countries, where applicators may carry and mix concentrated paraquat in leaky backpack sprayers. Splashes of paraquat may cause corneal opacification; nosebleeds, rashes, burns, and loss of fingernails are common local effects (McConnell, 1994).

Chronic Effects   Pulmonary fibrosis has been reported among survivors of paraquat poisoning. Paraquat is structurally similar to 1-methyl-4-phenyl-1,2,3,6-tetrahydropyridine (MPTP), an illicit drug produced as a heroin substitute that caused an outbreak of acute-onset Parkinson's disease. Although it has been argued that paraquat does not cross the blood-brain barrier, ecologic studies and one case-control study suggest an association between herbicide exposure and Parkinson's disease (Costa, 1997). This issue requires further study.

Chlorophenoxy Herbicides (2,4-D,2,4-DP,2,4-DB,2,4,5-T, and MCPA) and Polychlorinated Dibenzo-Dioxins (PCDD)

Chlorophenoxy herbicides have been used widely in the United States and elsewhere against broad-leaved plants. During the Vietnam War, 2,4-D and 2,4,5-T were applied together by American troops for deforestation and to destroy food crops in a formulation known as Agent Orange.

2,4,5-T, which is no longer marketed in many of the industrialized countries, becomes contaminated in its manufacture with dioxins, of which the most toxic and intensely studied is the tetrachlorinated 2,3,7,8-tetrachloro-dibenzodioxin isomer, TCDD. In workers chronically and heavily exposed to TCDD, an increased incidence of cancer has been observed. The largest published cohort study of heavily exposed herbicide production workers demonstrated an association between exposure, non–Hodgkin's lymphoma and soft tissue sarcoma (Fingerhut, Halperin, and Marlow, 1991).

To assess the hazards of exposure to dioxin in Agent Orange among Vietnam War Veterans, the U.S. National Academy of Sciences convened an expert panel in 1991. After evaluating the epidemiological and toxicological data, this committee concluded on the basis of the studies cited above (Fingerhut, Halpesin, and Marlow, 1991) that there was strong evidence for a positive association between herbicide exposure in Vietnam and soft-tissue sarcoma, non-Hodgkin's lymphoma, and Hodgkin's disease. The committee also concluded that there was strong evidence for a link between Agent Orange and the skin condition chloracne (characterized by eruptions produced by exposure to chlorine) and for a link between exposure to 2,4,5-T and the metabolic disease porphyria cutanea tarda (a liver ailment that also produces skin lesions). In addition the committee found weaker evidence of association between exposure to herbicides and cancer of the lungs, larynx, and trachea, as well as prostate cancer and multiple myeloma.

(Further discussion of the toxicity and epidemiology of dioxins and related compounds is presented in Chapter 8.)

FUNGICIDES

This class includes hexachlorobenzene, mancozeb, maneb, methyl mercury, pentachlorophenol, and zineb. Fungicides applied to seeds, crops, and gardens encompass a wide variety of classes of chemicals, including copper, cadmium, organomercury and organotin compounds, substituted benzene, dithiocarbamates and thiophthalimides.

The dimethyldithiocarbamates ziram, ferbam, and thiram inhibit acetaldehyde dehydrogenase and have a disulfiram (Antabuse) effect. There have been reports of illness consistent with disulfiram reactions (nausea, vomiting, headache, diaphoresis, thirst, chest pain, and vertigo) among thiram-exposed workers who subsequently consumed ethanol. Ziram and ferbam are irritants, and hemolysis occurred in one case of ziram poisoning. All dithiocarbamates are metabolized to carbon disulfide, which may explain similarities in the symptoms of poisoning.

The ethylenebisdithiocarbamates (maneb, mancozeb, and zineb) are metabolized to ethylene thiourea, a potent animal carcinogen. This metabolite may also account for the antithyroid effects that occur in animals dosed with these compounds. Ethylene thiourea may concentrate on cooked food previously treated with ethylenebisdithiocarbamates. Maneb is of interest because it contains manganese, which produces a condition similar to Parkinson's disease (National Research Council, 1992).

Although little used now in the United States, alkyl mercury has resulted in occupational poisoning in seed treating facilities and has produced epidemics of poisoning and death, including catastrophic fetotoxicity among farm families in New Mexico (Pierce, Thompson, and Likosky, 1972) and Iraq (Marsh et al., 1980) who consumed treated seed grain or meat from animals that had consumed mercury-treated grain. Acute poisoning is manifested by headache, metallic taste, paresthesia, tremor, incoordination, slurred speech, constricted visual fields, hearing loss, loss of position sense, and spasticity. Among survivors, permanent neurologic effects are common.

Consumption of hexachlorobenzene-treated seed grain resulted in thousands of cases of poisoning that resembled porphyria cutanea tarda in Turkey in the 1950s. Hexachlorobenzene is a potent inhibitor of uroporphyrinogen decarboxylase, resulting in increases in photosensitive porphyrins. Bullous dermatitis, liver damage, hypertrichosis, and arthritis were permanent in many cases. Acutely, hexachlorobenzene levels can be measured in blood, and metabolites can be measured in urine.

Pentachlorophenol, used to treat lumber, is well absorbed through the skin. It produces an uncoupling of oxidative phosphorylation from oxidative metabolism with resultant hyperthermia (McConnell, 1994). Numerous occupational deaths have occurred from overexposure. Symptoms include fever, thirst, sweating, weakness, tachycardia, other arrhythmias, and tachypnea. Restlessness, anxiety, and dizziness reflect injury to the central nervous system.

FUMIGANTS AND NEMATOCIDES

Fumigants and nematocides are a chemically diverse group of pesticides, characterized by vapor pressures that are sufficiently high at room temperature to create airborne concentrations that cause acute toxicity. Inhalation is the principal route of absorption.

Acute Effects

Many fumigants cause acute pulmonary edema and central nervous system depression.

Methyl bromide vapors cause respiratory irritation, pulmonary edema, anorexia, nausea, vomiting, headache, visual disturbances, agitation, dizziness, tremor, incoordination, myoclonus, and muscle weakness. Liquid methyl bromide will cause severe skin burns and is absorbed dermally.

Aluminum phosphide (phosphine) slowly releases phosphine upon contact with water in air; the release is more rapid in a moist environment. Phosphine is a mucous membrane and respiratory irritant that produces nausea, vomiting, diarrhea, headache, vertigo, fatigue, paresthesia, cough, dyspnea, chest tightness, and pulmonary edema. Nephro-, hepato-, cardio-, and central nervous system toxicity are common. Patients may smell of rotten fish or garlic. Deaths have occurred among people living near recently fumigated granaries, as a result of early re-entry into fumigated structures and aboard grain-hauling ships (Wilson et al., 1980).

Chronic Effects

Survivors of acute poisoning with methyl bromide may be left with organic brain damage, seizures, and personality disorders. Ethylene dibromide is a potent animal carcinogen, and in the occupational setting, a human spermatotoxin; residues have been found in food. As a fumigant it is no longer used in the United States.

DBCP causes decreased sperm counts and testicular atrophy (Babich, 1981). In 1977 almost one-half of a group of poorly protected production workers exposed to DBCP in a plant in California were demonstrated to be azospermic or oligospermic. Recovery was better among initially oligo- than among azospermic workers (Whorton et al., 1979). DBCP is an animal carcinogen. It has been removed from the continental U.S. market.

OTHER PESTICIDES

In the United States, N,N-diethyltoluamide (DEET) is the most commonly used insect repellent. Repellents are purposely applied topically or to clothing. Severe irritation of the eyes, irritation of the skin, and exacerbation of preexisting skin disease has been reported. Application of DEET formulations with high concentrations (more than 75% active ingredient) in tropical climates has resulted in severe dermatitis in antecubital and popliteal fossae. It is rapidly absorbed dermally and by ingestion. Behavioral effects have been demonstrated in chronic feeding studies in rats, and several idiosyncratic cases of encephalopathy and death have been reported among children heavily treated with DEET. In one study of exposed workers, there was an increased prevalence of symptoms associated with impaired cognitive function and sleep disturbances and a trend toward poorer objectively measured neurobehavioral performance among highly exposed workers. (McConnell, Fidler, and Chrislip, 1986).

INERT INGREDIENTS

Pesticidal active ingredients represent only a portion of most pesticide formulations. In most countries, the remainder of the formulation is listed on the label as "inert ingredients," namely solvents, emulsifiers, spreaders, stickers, penetrants, anticaking agents, and other chemicals used in formulating the pesticide product.

The term "inert"is misleading and reflects only the lack of toxicity of these agents to pests; some inert ingredients are known or suspected to be human toxicants. Volatile mixtures of aliphatic and aromatic hydrocarbons are the most common inert ingredients. Some hydrocarbon agents used to facilitate the penetration of active ingredients to the interior of plants (penetrants) may be skin and eye irritants. The identity of these ingredients, some of which have acute and chronic toxicities are available in most jurisdictions only at the discretion of the manufacturer (Vacco, 1996).

EPA categorizes inert ingredients into four groups: (1) substances known to cause long-term health damage and to harm the environment, (2) substances suspected of causing such health and environmental effects, (3) chemicals of unknown toxicity, and (4) chemicals of minimal concern.

PESTICIDES AND ENDOCRINE/REPRODUCTIVE TOXICITY

Concern has arisen in recent years that certain pesticides may have adverse effects on the endocrine system. It has been found, for example, that certain organochlorine pesticides such as DDT can interfere with the effects of estrogen. Indeed, it was the study of estrogenic effects of DDT in eagles and ospreys that led to Rachel Carson's original recognition of the ecotoxicology of the persistent chlorinated hydrocarbon compounds (Carson, 1962).

The estrogenic and antiestrogenic properties of pesticides may be examined in cell culture models such as normal human mammary epithelial cells and human breast cancer cells. When these cells are exposed to an estrogenic substance, they divide and grow more rapidly, and these effects can be quantified. Many pesticides have been found to be estrogenic, including dieldrin, toxaphene, chlordane, DDT and endosulfan (Soto, Chung, and Sonnenschein, 1994).

In fetal life, even low-dose exposure to endocrine disrupting pesticides can have devastating effects because hormones play critical roles in the early development of the immune, nervous, and reproductive systems. The developmental effects of exposure to endocrine disrupters will vary depending on age at exposure and sex. It has been proposed that increased exposure to these agents may be the cause of an observed doubling in the incidence of undescended testes in male infants which has been reported to have occurred since 1960. Effects have also been documented in the sexual development of wildlife in areas where there are elevated levels of pesticides such as DDT in the environment (Guillette et al., 1994).

The Food Quality Protection Act of 1996 (see below) now requires that pesticides be tested for potential endocrine toxicity. The EPA must therefore design a new screening protocol for testing pesticides for endocrine disrupting potential, implement this protocol and make recommendations for setting safety standards based on these tests. Design of the protocol proceeds as of this writing.

Legislative Framework

The regulation of pesticides has hinged historically upon an assumed need to balance the economic benefits of these compounds against the risks associated with their use (Wargo, 1996). That is the principle that underlies the Federal Insecticide, Fungicide and Rodenticide Act (FIFRA) of 1947, the first federal statute controlling pesticide use in the United States. This law, which has undergone several revisions, regulated pesticides on the basis that they would not cause "unreasonable adverse effects." Unreasonable adverse effects were defined in the statute as "any unreasonable risk to man or the environment taking into account the economic, social and environmental costs and benefits of its use." As this statement implies, some adverse effects were considered reasonable under FIFRA when weighed against potential economic benefits (Schierow, 1996).

In 1958, because of rising concern about the health effects of pesticides in foods, and particularly concern about the potential of some agents to cause cancer, Congress passed the Delaney Clause as an amendment to the Federal Food, Drug, and Cosmetic Act. This clause banned from processed foods any pesticide that had been shown to cause cancer in humans or animals.

The Delaney Clause was from the beginning, highly controversial. Representatives of the pesticide and food industries argued that it is too inflexible, since it totally prohibited in processed food even the smallest amounts of carcinogenic chemicals. Environmentalists, however, considered the Delaney Clause a bulwark of public health and environmental protection.

A policy dilemma posed by the Delaney Clause was that it established a standard for pesticides in processed foods that was much stricter than that established for pesticides in raw foods—this has been termed the "Delaney paradox" (National Research Council, 1987). To cope with this paradox, the EPA for many years did not strictly enforce the Delaney Clause and allowed very low, or "de minimis," levels of pesticides in processed foods—levels that in the Agency's opinion posed no more than a "minimal risk" to health. In 1992, however, the U.S. Court of Appeals ruled that this approach contravened the intent of the Delaney Clause and thus was not legal. This decision set the stage for passage in 1996 of the Food Quality Protection Act (FQPA), the major statute regulating pesticides in the United States today.

The central premise of the Food Quality Protection Act of 1996 is that there must be "a reasonable certainty that no harm will result from aggregate exposure to the pesticide chemical residue, including all anticipated dietary exposures and all other exposures for which there is reliable information." In terms of public health, this is unquestionably a more protective standard than the previous risk–benefit standard based "no unreasonable adverse effect."

The intellectual foundation for FQPA was provided by a landmark report released in 1993 by the National Academy of Sciences, which found that the then current laws and regulations did not adequately protect children from the risks of pesticides in foods (National Research Council, 1993). The report recommended that Congress enact legislation that would specifically consider the effects of pesticide residues on children's health. Following that guidance, the new law requires that:

- Regulation of pesticides be based on health effects.
- One uniform health-based standard be applied to pesticide residues in both processed and raw foods.
- The latest scientific data be used for the assessment of health risks.
- The regulation of "reduced risk" pesticides be streamlined.
- Pollution prevention be promoted through integrated pest management practices.

Four provisions in FQPA are aimed specifically at increasing protection for infants and children. Accordingly, the Environmental Protection Agency is directed to:

1. Consider children's sensitivities and unique exposure patterns to pesticides in setting pesticide standards.
2. Explicitly determine that tolerance levels are safe for children.
3. Adopt an additional safety factor of up to 10-fold to account for uncertainty in the data base relative to children, and to reflect children's greater exposure and greater susceptibility to pesticides, unless there is reliable evidence that a different factor should be used.
4. Consider sources of pesticide exposure in addition to diet when performing risk assessments and in setting tolerances.

CONCLUSION: ISSUES FOR THE FUTURE

Achieving full implementation of the Food Quality Protection Act (FQPA). A major provision of the Food Quality Protection Act, noted above, is a requirement that a third 10-

fold safety factor be applied in setting tolerances for pesticide residues in food to protect children against noncarcinogenic effects of pesticide exposure. Traditionally two 10-fold safety factors have been employed in setting standards: The first of these factors is used to account for the extrapolation from animal species to human, and the second to account for variation among humans. The new, third factor was recommended by the National Academy of Sciences committee in their report *Pesticides in the Diets of Infants and Children* (National Research Council, 1993). It is based in part on the increased biological susceptibility of children as compared to adults, and to an even greater extent on the substantial differences in exposure that have been demonstrated to exist between children and adults.

The third 10-fold safety factor is intended in the law as a "default provision" that will automatically be utilized unless "reliable data" exist to show that there is no difference in susceptibility between children and adults. The term "reliable data" is not defined in the law.

A critical decision now confronting EPA is to define "reliable data" under FQPA. The traditional toxicologic tests that have been used to assess differences in susceptibility between adult and young animals are relatively insensitive (Tilsons, 1995). They tend not to show differences in susceptibility between infants and adults even when such differences may exist, unless the differences lead to gross anatomical defects (Rodier, 1995). Relying on such traditional tests, the EPA failed to apply a third 10-fold safety factor in more than two-thirds of the first 80 pesticides to come before the Agency for re-assessment of tolerance in 1996 and 1997. Concern exists in the environmental community that even chemicals such as lead and PCBs, which are known to be functional neurotoxins but which do not cause anatomical birth defects, would be judged "innocent" in this schema.

This is an issue that will require close and continual scrutiny in the years ahead. Others are:

- *Addressing pesticide export issues.* Earlier in this chapter the concept of the "circle of poison" was discussed; this phenomenon refers to the export from the developed nations of hazardous pesticides that are banned for use followed by the subsequent return of those highly toxic pesticides on food grown in developing nations and imported by the industralized world. Legislative pressure to resolve this problem has surfaced periodically in the past. To date, this legislative concern has not resulted in passage of protective legislation. However, it seems likely that renewed legislative concern over this major unresolved issue will rise again.

- *Ending DDT manufacture.* DDT and other highly persistent and bioaccumulative pesticides continue to be manufactured and used in certain developing nations. A major international effort seeks to bring this manufacture to an end. An economic issue that must be addressed is that the chlorinated hydrocarbon compounds are relatively less expensive to manufacture than the organophosphates, carbamates, and other newer generation pesticides that have been introduced as substitutes. On the other hand, the increasing resistance of insects to DDT and other traditional pesticides may force this transition.

- *Risk assessment versus pollution prevention.* Risk assessment has for the past 20 years been the predominant paradigm utilized by regulatory agencies to control exposure to pesticides. While it has had its successes, it is an inherently slow process that typically proceeds by considering only one chemical compound at a time. Moreover a perennial problem is that pesticides under assessment typically remain on the market until the assessment is completed.

A more effective paradigm for controlling exposure to pesticides consists of pollution prevention. Under this approach numerical targets are set for reducing pesticide use over a span of years. The principal approach to use reduction in most instances is integrated pest management. A study undertaken by the Congressional Office of Technology Assessment has demonstrated that IPM can potentially reduce the use of pesticides by as much as 50%.

REFERENCES

Babich, A., and D. L. Davis. 1981. Dibromochloropropane (DBCP): A review. *Sci. Total Environ.* 17: 207–221.

Bearer, C. 1995. How are children different from adults? *Environ. Health Perspect.* 103 (suppl 6): 7–12.

Benbrook, C. 1996. *Pest Management at the Crossroads.* Yonkers. NY. Consumers Union.

Blondell, J. 1997. Epidemiology of pesticide poisonings in the United States, with special reference to occupational cases. *Occup. Med.—State of the Art Rev.* 12: 209–220.

Cannon, S.B., J. M. Veazey, R. S. Jackson, V. M. Burse, C. Hayes, W. E. Straub, and P. J. Landrigan. 1978. Epidemic kepone poisoning in chemical workers. *Am. J. Epid.* 107: 529–537.

Carson, R. 1962. *Silent Spring.* Cambridge, MA: Riverside Press.

Costa, L. 1997. Basic toxicology of pesticides. *Occup. Med.—State of the Art Rev.* 12: 251–268.

Diggory, P., P. J. Landrigan, K. P. Latimer, A. C. Ellington, R. D. Kimbrough, J. A. Liddle, A. F. Cline, and A. L. Smrek. 1977. Fatal parathion poisoning caused by contamination of flour in international commerce. *Am. J. Epidemiol.* 106: 145–153.

Fingerhut, M.A., W. E. Halperin, and D. A. Marlow. 1991. Cancer mortality in workers exposed to 2,3,7,8-tetrachlorodibenzo-p-dioxin. *N. Engl. J. Med.* 324: 212–218.

Guillette, L.J., Jr., T. S. Gross, G. R. Masson, J. M. Matter, H. F. Percival, and A. R. Woodward. 1994. Developmental abnormalities of the gonad and abnormal sex hormone concentrations in juvenile alligators from contaminated and control lakes in Florida. *Environ. Health Perspect.* 102: 680–688.

Hayes, W. J., and E. R. Laws. 1991. *Handbook of Pesticide Toxicology.* San Diego, CA: Academic Press.

Jeyaratnam, J. 1990. Acute pesticide poisoning: A major global health problem. *World Health Stat. Q.* 43: 139–144.

Kimmel, C. 1992. Animal models for assessing developmental toxicity. In *Similarities and Differences between Children and Adults.* pp. 43–65. Washington, DC: ILSI Press.

Lotti, M. 1992. The pathogenesis of organophosphate neuropathy. *Crit. Rev. Toxicol.* 21: 465–487.

Marsh, D. O., G. J. Myers, T. W. Clarkson, L. Amin-Zaki, S. Tikriti, and M. Majud. 1980. Fetal methyl mercury poisoning: Clinical and toxicological data on 29 cases. *Ann. Neurol.* 7: 348–353.

McConnell, R. 1994. Pesticides and Related Compounds. In *Textbook of Clinical Occupational and Environmental Medicine,* eds. L. Rosenstock and M. Cullen. Philadelphia: Saunders.

McConnell, R., A. Fidler, and D. Chrislip. 1986. *Health Hazard Evaluation Report. Everglades National Park, Everglades, Florida.* HETA 83-085-1757. Cincinnati, OH: National Institute for Occupational Safety and Health.

Melius, J.M. 1998. The Bhopal disaster. In Environmental and Occupational Medicine, 3rd edition, ed. W. N. Rom. Boston: Little, Brown.

Mortensen, S. R., S. M. Chanda, M. J. Hooper, and S. Padilla. 1996. Maturational differences in chlorpyrifos-oxonase activity may contribute to age-related sensitivity to chlorpyrifos. *J. Biochem. Toxicol.* 11: 279–287.

Narahashi, T. 1985. Nerve membrane ionic channels as the primary target of pyrethroids. *Neurotoxicology* 2: 3–22.

National Research Council. 1987. *The Delaney Paradox.* Washington, DC: National Academy Press.

National Research Council. 1992. *Environmental Neurotoxicology.* Washington, DC: National Academy Press.

National Research Council. 1993. *Pesticides in the Diets of Infants and Children.* Washington, DC: National Academy Press.

National Research Council. 1996. *Carcinogens and Anticarcinogens in the Diet.* Washington, DC: National Academy Press.

Peto, R., R. Gray, P. Brantom, and P. Grasso. 1991. Dose and time relationships for tumor induction in the liver and esophagus of 4080 inbred rats by chronic ingestion of N-nitrosodiethylamine or N-nitrosodimethinalmine. *Cancer Res.* 51: 6452–6469.

Pierce, P. E., J. F. Thompson, and W. H. Likosky. 1972. Alkyl mercury poisoning in humans: A report of an outbreak. *JAMA* 220: 1439–1442.

Rodier, P. M. 1995. Developing brain as a target of toxicity. *Environ. Health Perspect.* 103: 73–76.

Schierow, L. J. 1996. *Pesticide Policy Issues.* Washington, DC: The Library of Congress, Congressional Research Service, Environment and Natural Resources Policy Division (IB95016).

Schuman, S. H., and W. Simpson Jr. 1997. A clinical historical overview of pesticide health issues. *Occup. Med.—State of the Art Rev.* 12: 203–207.

Soto, A. M., K. L. Chung, and C. Sonnenschein. 1994. The pesticides endosulfan, toxaphene, and dieldrin have estrogenic effects on human estrogen-sensitive cells. *Environ. Health Perspect.* 102: 380–383.

Tilson, H. A. 1995. The concern for developmental neurotoxicology: Is it justified and what is being done about it? *Environ. Health Perspect.* 103 (suppl 6): 147–151.

U.S. Environmental Protection Agency. 1992. *Regulatory Impact Analysis of Worker Protection Standards for Agricultural Pesticides.* Washington, DC: EPA.

Vacco, D. C. 1996. *The Secret Hazards of Pesticides: Inert Ingredients.* Albany, NY: New York Department of Law, Environmental Protection Bureau.

Wargo, J. 1996. *Our Children's Toxic Legacy.* New Haven: Yale University Press.

Whorton, D., T. H. Milby, R. M. Krauss, and H. A. Stubbs. 1979. Testicular function in DBCP exposed pesticide workers. *J. Occup. Med.* 21: 161–166.

Wiles, R., and C. Campbell.,1993. *Pesticides in Children's Food.* Washington, DC: Environmental Working Group.

Wiles, R., and E. Davies. 1995. *Pesticides in Baby Food.* Washington, DC: Environmental Working Group.

Wilson, R., F. H. Lovejoy, R. J. Jaeger, and P. J. Landrigan. 1980. Acute phosphine poisoning aboard a grain freighter: epidemiologic, clinical, and pathological findings. *JAMA* 244: 148–150.

World Health Organization. 1992. *Our Planet, Our Health.* Geneva: WHO.

Zahm, S. H., M. H. Ward, and A. Blair. 1997. *Pesticides and cancer. Occup. Med.—State of the Art Rev.* 12: 269–289.

22 Radon and Daughters

NAOMI H. HARLEY, Ph.D.

EFFECTS OF RADON EXPOSURE

Beginning in 1984 (NCRP, 1984), the evidence from underground mines relating radon exposure and lung cancer led to concern that indoor domestic radon exposure may produce significant lung cancer in the population. Most domestic exposure is lower than that in mines; however, some homes display concentrations similar to or even higher than those in mines.

The pooling of 11 major epidemiological studies in underground mines from 9 countries, now show conclusively that exposure to radon and its short-lived decay products cause lung cancer in excess of that expected from smoking (NIH, 1994). There is peripheral information that other hazardous airborne substances, although present, do not appear to influence lung cancer induction. The ores mined in these follow-up studies include uranium, lead, and fluorspar. Radon was clearly the primary carcinogen, with a clear dose–response relationship in essentially all of the 11 underground cohorts.

Most countries with significant health programs have now completed environmental surveys of radon concentrations. There are 34 countries with surveys that show the average levels in homes to be about $40 \, \mathrm{Bq \, m^{-3}}$ ($1 \, \mathrm{pCi \, L^{-1}}$) with a few percent of homes showing measured concentrations over $740 \, \mathrm{Bq \, m^{-3}}$ ($20 \, \mathrm{pCi \, L^{-1}}$).

Some differences do exist between radon exposure in the home and in an underground mine, and this is described in detail in later sections. Generally, miners were exposed to concentrations about 100 times that found in the average home, the exposures were for relatively few years (from 3 to about 20), whereas home exposure is over full lifetime, aerosol characteristics differ somewhat, and breathing rates in homes are lower than in an occupational setting. It is probable that no additional mining populations will be added to the data base, and that this work is finished excepting for longer-term follow-up of the miners.

The present ^{222}Rn epidemiology is directed toward domestic case control studies to demonstrate whether extrapolations of risk from the mining epidemiology apply directly to indoor environmental exposure. Pooling of the domestic studies should provide some support to the extrapolation but this work will not be complete until year 2000. The existing domestic case control studies have not shown any statistically significant increase in lung cancer due to environmental exposure.

The major confounder in assessing lung cancer risk is smoking. This is because of the high background lung cancer rate in all populations due to smoking. The risk from smoking and ^{222}Rn exposure is about two times greater than the risk from ^{222}Rn exposure alone. The difficulty in assessing the combined effects of smoking and radon is given emphasis.

Environmental Toxicants: Human Exposures and Their Health Effects, 2/e. Edited by Morton Lippmann.
ISBN: 0-471-29298-2 © 2000 John Wiley & Sons, Inc.

Although pooling of the domestic studies may increase the power or ability to detect an effect, it is unlikely that there will be sufficient precision to provide a risk model. The best that is expected from pooling is general agreement with the extrapolations from mining studies and a trend toward higher lung cancer with higher lifetime exposures.

The difference in exposure rate and duration between mining studies and home exposure precludes direct comparisons. Thus it is necessary to base environmental risk estimates on predictive or projection models. Beginning in 1984, projection models for domestic risk were developed. Initially three models based on the mining epidemiology were accepted (NCRP, 1984; ICRP, 1987; NRC, 1988).

At present, the most widely accepted risk projection model is that developed from the pooling of the 11 underground mining cohorts. This is a conservative model, and it generally overestimates lung cancer risk (NIH, 1994; NRC, 1999a).

The animal studies have been supportive of the human epidemiology, and they are considered briefly.

This chapter describes the background information concerning exposures in the mines, indoor and outdoor environmental radon concentrations, differences in lung dosimetry between mining and environmental populations, and the predictive risk model from the pooled miner follow-up studies that permit estimates of risk in environmental situations.

UNITS OF RADON EXPOSURE

The conventional units for exposure to airborne radioactivity are Bq m^{-3} (or historically pCi L^{-1}). In the case of radon exposure, it is actually the solid, short-lived alpha-emitting products of radon, ^{218}Po and ^{214}Po, (^{214}Po is supported by ^{214}Pb and ^{214}Bi) which deposit in the bronchial airways and deliver the carcinogenic dose to target stem cells lining the airways in the thin layer of epithelial tissue (NCRP, 1984a, 1987a, b; NRC, 1988; NIH, 1994; NRC, 1999a).

These short-lived decay products (T$_{1/2}$ 30 minutes) are never in equilibrium or steady state with the parent ^{222}Rn gas (T$_{1/2}$ 3.8 days) in practical situations. This is because the solid decay products readily plate out or attach to available surfaces as they are formed. Radon gas must be present to maintain the mixture of short-lived decay products and measurement of a particular nuclide becomes an issue. To circumvent this problem, mining exposures were documented in terms of the working level (WL) which was easy to measure in the mines using a short alpha count of a 5 minute filtered air sample (NCRP, 1988), thus measuring the mixture of decay products. The working level is the total decay energy of any combination of the short-lived daughters in 1 liter of air resulting in the release of 1.3×10^5 Mev of alpha energy. The working level could be calculated easily as a direct multiple of the alpha count.

Cumulative exposure was recorded for workers in units of the working level month (WLM) which was exposure in WL times the number of work months (170 hours equals a work month). One WL is equal to 3700 Bq m^{-3} (100 pCi L^{-1}) at equilibrium; however, equilibrium with the decay products is never attained. The exact relationship between WL and the short-lived decay products is

$$WL = 0.00103(^{218}Po) + 0.00507(^{214}Pb) + 0.00373(^{214}Bi), \qquad (1)$$

where ^{218}Po, ^{214}Bi, etc. = concentration of the decay product in pCi L^{-1}, or

$$WL = 2.78 \times 10^{-5}(^{218}Po) + 1.37 \times 10^{-4}(^{214}Pb) + 1.01 \times 10^{-4}(^{214}Bi),$$

where ^{218}Po, ^{214}Bi, etc. = concentration of the decay product in Bq m−3,

$$WLM = WL(hours\ exposed\ /170). \tag{2}$$

The relationship between radon concentration and the short-lived daughters in WL depends mainly on the ventilation rate and the atmospheric particle concentration in the space considered. The daughters can be removed by plate-out on walls or any surface and the plate-out is enhanced by air movement or ventilation. The concentration of submicrometer particles or condensation nuclei is important because the freshly formed decay products quickly attach to these particles. Their motion is now controlled by the larger-sized particle, which inhibits diffusion and plate-out.

In mines, homes, and outdoors the approximate relationship between radon and decay products is

$$1\ WL = 300\ pCi\ L^{-1}\ ^{222}Rn \qquad (mine),$$
$$1\ WL = 250\ pCi\ L^{-1} \qquad (home),$$
$$1\ WL = 150\ pCi\ L^{-1} \qquad (outdoors).$$

A simple way of expressing the relationship between the parent ^{222}Rn and the daughter products is in terms of the fractional equilibrium, F. This is

$$F = \frac{100(WL)}{pCi\ L^{-1}\ ^{222}Rn} \tag{3}$$

For the cases above F would be 0.33, 0.40, and 0.67 for mines, homes, and outdoors, respectively.

OUTDOOR RADON

Uranium-238 is a trace element in all materials native to the earth. Radon-222 is the gaseous decay product of ^{226}Ra, which in turn is a member of the ^{238}U series. The half-life of ^{222}Rn is sufficiently long (3.82 d) so that it can escape from the surface of most substances with an efficiency of a few percent. Therefore ^{222}Rn exists in all atmospheres on the planet. The decay scheme for the ^{238}U series is shown in Figure 22-1 (NCRP, 1988). The radioactive ^{232}Th series also has a gaseous isotope of radon, ^{220}Rn, thoron in the older terminology. However, the half-life of ^{220}Rn is so short (55 s), that environmental concentrations are generally much lower than ^{222}Rn, and demonstrable health effects have never been shown. For these reasons this chapter will stress ^{222}Rn with only minor consideration of ^{220}Rn.

Some long-term outdoor measurements of ^{222}Rn are available. Fisenne (1988, 1996; NCRP, 1987a) has reported ^{222}Rn concentrations in New York City and Chester, New Jersey. These are shown in Figure 22-2. Harley (1997) has measured outdoor concentrations in a suburban New Jersey location for 7 years, and these data are shown in Figure 22-3. Harley (1990) summarized the long-term outdoor data in the published literature, and these data are shown in Table 22-1.

The U.S. Environmental Protection Agency (EPA) assessed outdoor or ambient ^{222}Rn for the purpose of assessing guidelines for indoor ^{222}Rn and ^{222}Rn released from groundwater use in homes. Their published outdoor concentrations state by state for all of the United States shown in Table 22-2.

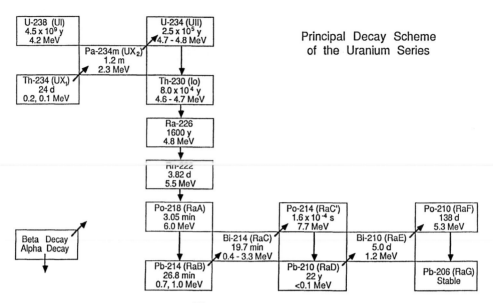

Figure 22-1 ^{238}U primordial series decay scheme.

Average outdoor ^{222}Rn is thus seen to average $10\,\mathrm{Bq\,m^{-3}}$ $(0.2\,\mathrm{pCi\,L^{-1}})$ for locations where no elevated sources are present. In the western United States the potential for mineralized uranium deposits occurs, so local outdoor concentrations could increase. However, despite the occurrence of significant horizontal transport of ^{222}Rn, measurements at a particular site do not exclusively measure ^{222}Rn emanated locally. Average wind speed at ground level is $5\,\mathrm{km/h}$ and this brings ^{222}Rn from significant distances to the site of measurement (Harley, 1990).

Large short-term differences can exist in outdoor ^{222}Rn concentration depending on local circumstances. For example, in Figure 22-2, data from Chester, New Jersey, show 9 years of data where annual averages have a range of only 30%. If hourly data were compared, differences of a factor of 10 can be observed (NCRP, 1987). Radon

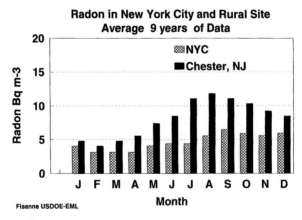

Figure 22-2   Outdoor ^{222}Rn concentration measured by Fisenne (1988) at Chester, New Jersey (9 year agerage) and New York City (4 year average).

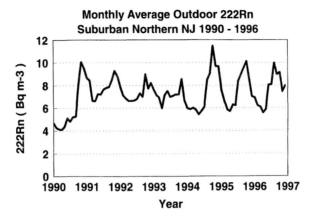

Figure 22-3 Monthly average outdoor ^{22}Rn concentration for seven years at a northern New Jersey suburban site in Bergen County (Harley and Chittaporn, 1997).

concentration is highest during the night and lowest in late afternoon. A nighttime inversion occurs (air temperature increasing rather than decreasing with height) as the soil surface cools by radiative heat transfer resulting in very stable air. There is little upward dilution of radon emanating from the soil surface, and resulting high surface ^{222}Rn.

Solar heating at the soil surface during the day causes large turbulent (eddy) diffusion in the atmosphere and dilution of the radon emanating from the soil surface. Vertical wind profiles also mix ^{222}Rn to great altitude. Radon originating at the soil surface is transported to various heights in the atmosphere depending on these factors, which are not constant. Therefore models of ^{222}Rn with height cannot be precise.

Figure 22-4 shows the measured falloff of radon concentration with height. A rough generality for greater heights is that the radon is reduced from ground level concentration by 2 for each 1000 meters.

Very little ^{226}Ra exists in seawater, and therefore ^{222}Rn over the oceans should be low if no nearby land source can be accessed by wind transport. Table 22-3 (Harley, 1990) is a summary of ^{222}Rn measured over oceans. It can be seen that the Mediterranean is the exception (4 Bq m^{-3}) to the average values of 0.1 Bq m^{-3} because wind transport from land is significant.

Harley (1974) modeled global ^{222}Rn concentration based on an average emanation from soil of 20 Bq m^{-2} s^{-1} (0.5 pCi m^{-2} s^{-1}), the land and water areas of the globe and a half-depth in the atmosphere of 700 meters. The estimate of ground level concentration was 8 Bq m^{-3} (0.2 pCi L^{-1}), which is in good agreement with measurements.

The lung cancer risk from exposure to outdoor radon can be estimated from current models. This is only possible assuming a linear, no-threshold model for carcinogenesis. This is done in the section on risk models. This estimate is not of particular significance because outdoor radon is a small fraction of exposure indoors and is, at most, 30% of the total exposure (Harley et al., 1991). For this reason outdoor ^{222}Rn is often neglected when estimating health effects from lifetime exposure.

INDOOR RADON

Indoor radon was first measured in the United States by Glauberman and Breslin (1957), and in Sweden by Hultqvist (1956). Hultqvist found a few homes with concentrations up to 800 Bq m^{-3} (20 pCi L^{-1}), but the significance of the early measurements was not known.

TABLE 22-1   Average Outdoor Radon Concentrations from Extended Measurements. Range in Parentheses

Location	Method	pCi m^{-3}	Reference
Manila	Charcoal ion chamber	70	Wright and Smith (1915)
New York City	13 L ion chamber	54 (10–120)	Hess (1953)
Chicago	Charcoal scintillation cell	(50–1600)	Moses et al. (1963)
Netherlands	Karlsruhe alpha track	90	Put and DeMeijer (1988)
Chester, NJ	Continuous two		Fisenne (1988)
1977	filter	230	
1978		230	
1979		190	
1980		240	
1981		220	
1982		220	
1983		250	
1984		200	
1985		200	
New York City	Continuous two filter		Fisenne (1996)
1983		125	
1984		115	
1985		130	
1986		135	
1987		80	
1988		90	
Northern NJ	Continuous radon monitor		Harley (1977)
1986		200	
1987		200	
1988		180	
1989		140	
1990		160	
1991		210	
1992		200	
1993		200	
1994		150	
1995		210	
1996		220	

Source: From Harley (1990), with additions.

This was because quantitative risk estimates for lung cancer in underground miners were not yet available.

Beginning in mid-1975, several studies of indoor radon appeared in the literature (Rundo, 1979; George and Breslin, 1980; Sachs et al., 1982; Nero et al., 1983). These indicated that measurements of ^{222}Rn concentrations in a sample of homes were distributed lognormally. The geometric mean ^{222}Rn concentration was generally 60 Bq m^{-3} (1.5 pCi L^{-1}) with a geometric standard deviation of 2.0 to 2.5.

In December 1984, upon discovery that a home occupied by the now famous Watras family had ^{222}Rn concentrations of 110,000 Bq m^{-3} (3000 pCi L^{-1}), the Pennsylvania Department of Environmental Resources moved the family (NCRP, 1989; Reilly, 1990). Stanley Watras, an engineer at a nuclear power facility, showed significant external contamination of his clothing that was not related to any workplace exposure. Investigation showed that the radioactive contamination was derived from home. The short-lived decay products of ^{222}Rn formed in air deposit on any surface, including people

TABLE 22-2   EPA National Ambient Radon Survey

State	^{222}Rn (pCi/L)	State	^{222}Rn (pCi/L)
AK: Juneau	0.25	NC: Charlotte	0.31
AR: Little Rock	0.46	ND: Bismark	0.52
AZ: Phoenix	0.53	NE: Llncoln	0.52
CA: Los Angeles	0.39	NH: Concord	0.37
CO: Denver	0.43	NJ: Trenton	0.42
CT: Hartfford	0.46	NM: Santa Fe	0.16
DE: Newcastle	0.35	NV: Las Vegas	0.22
FL: Miami	0.33	NY: New York City	0.31
GA: Atlanta	0.48	OH: Toledo	0.38
HI: Honolulu	0.19	OK: Oklahoma Ci	0.41
IA: Iowa City	0.49	OR: Portland	0.33
ID: Idaho Falls	0.44	PA: Hassirburg	0.49
IL: Chicago	0.57	RI: Providence	0.28
IN: Indianapolis	0.45	SC: Columbia	0.56
KY: Frankfort	0.45	SD: Plctre	0.52
KS: Topeka	0.53	TN: Nashville	0.46
LA: Metairie	0.25	TX: Austin	0.43
MA: Lawrence	0.37	UT: Salt Lake City	0.31
MD: Baltimore	0.48	VA: Lynchburg	0.46
GA: Augusta	0.45	VT: Montpelier	0.39
MI: Lansing	0.36	WA: Spokane	0.51
MN: Minneapolis	0.35	WI: Madison	0.4
MO: Jefferson Cit	0.59	WV: Charleston	0.42
MS: Jackson	0.37	WY: Chenyanne	0.32
MT: Helena	0.48		

and clothing. Lung cancer risk estimates for exposure to environmental concentrations were available at this time (NCRP, 1984a, b), and the family was moved because of the public health implications. This incident was a watershed for environmental ^{222}Rn in that it was clear that homes could attain ^{222}Rn concentrations equal to the highest historical values observed in mines. Surveys have now been carried out in the living space of homes in 34 countries. These are summarized in Figure 22-5.

In the United States, a stratified random sample of 5,694 dwellings was conducted by the EPA to determine average exposure. Over 15,000 alpha track detectors were placed in all levels of the homes for 1 year. The measured median concentration in the United States was 25 Bq m^{-3} (0.67 pCi L^{-1}) with an average of 46 Bq m^{-3} (1.25 pCi L^{-1}). About 6% of homes had measured concentrations greater than 150 Bq m^{-3} (4 pCi L^{-1}).

Individuals, for example, Dr. Bernard Cohen of the University of Pittsburgh, have programs to measure ^{222}Rn for various scientific purposes. Dr. Cohen has measured ^{222}Rn in 175,000 homes as of the writing of this chapter and obtained data in living areas for most of the counties in the United States (Cohen, 1992). Nero (1986) utilized published data to arrive at an estimate of the typical distribution of ^{222}Rn exposures in living areas. Many surveys, such as the state surveys supported by EPA, measure ^{222}Rn in the basement, if a basement is available. Basement measurements are not indicative of actual exposure and overestimate actual exposure, on average, by factor of 2.

In a study conducted near Chicago of 52 homes and 88 occupants, there was found to be a consistent relationship between first-floor living levels and actual personal exposure (Harley et al., 1991). The personal exposure was on average 0.71 of the measured first-floor concentration with good correlation ($R^2 = 85\%$). Exposure outside the home in public places and offices is generally lower than home exposure and near outdoor levels

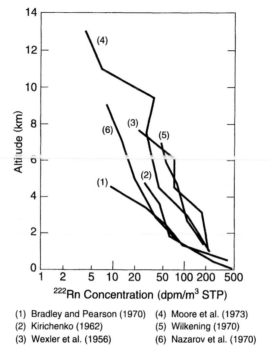

(1) Bradley and Pearson (1970)   (4) Moore et al. (1973)
(2) Kirichenko (1962)   (5) Wilkening (1970)
(3) Wexler et al. (1956)   (6) Nazarov et al. (1970)

Figure 22-4   Profiles of ^{222}Rn in the lower atmosphere at measured by 6 different investigators. From NCRP (1988).

due to differences in construction. Correlation of personal exposure with basement ^{222}Rn measurements was poor.

Thus, from information available to date, it appears that the average indoor exposure in the United States (and the world) is about 40 Bq m^{-3} (1 pCi L^{-1}). The number of lung cancers estimated from the average population exposure is 9,000 to 15,000 per year in the United States (NCRP, 1984a; NAS, 1988; Lubin and Boice, 1989; NIH, 1994; NRC, 1997).

The average individual is calculated to have a risk of about 1 in 400 of dying from ^{222}Rn- induced lung cancer. Of importance is the distribution of exposures, with perhaps 5% the population having exposures of greater than 150 Bq m^{-3} (> 4 pCi L^{-1}) as estimated by the various individuals and organizations (NCRP, 1984b; Nero, 1986; NRC, 1988; NIH, 1994; NRC, 1999a).

Using the variables known to control ^{222}Rn entry into a building, models can adequately predict the variability of indoor concentrations (Harley and Chittaporn, 1993). The major variables are (1) the baseline ^{222}Rn concentration established by diffusion, radium

TABLE 22-3   Radon Concentration over the Oceans

Ocean	^{222}Rn Concentration (pCi m^{-3})	Range	Reference
Mediterranean	100	30–200	Servant (1966)
North Atlantic	6	0–280	
South Atlantic	1.5	0–2.9	
Antarctic	0.8	0–4	

Source: J. Harley (1990).

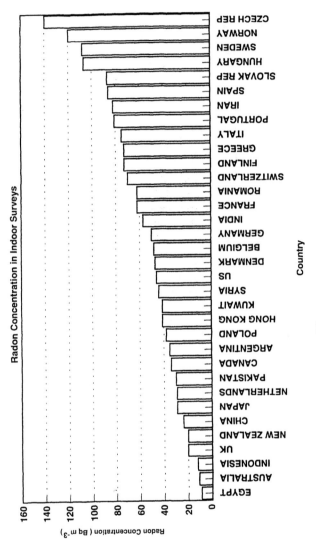

Figure 22-5 Indoor ^{222}Rn concentration reported in country surveys.

749

concentration of soil, and soil temperature; (2) indoor/outdoor temperature difference, which in turn causes a differential pressure known as the *stack effect*; (3) the air exchange rate in the home, and (4) barometric pressure changes. To a lesser extent, wind and rain affect the indoor concentration. With a few basic measurements in a home, the variability can be modeled; however; it is not as yet possible to predict the concentration in a home without a measurement.

The source of indoor ^{222}Rn is the ^{226}Ra-bearing soil under any home. A clear decrease in ^{222}Rn concentration can be seen with height above ground level, with an average of 2 for the ratio of basement to first-floor concentrations (Cohen, 1992). The only exception to the soil as a source of ^{222}Rn is in high-rise apartments. In this case the soil is too remote to be a source for apartments above about the third floor, and construction materials, such as wallboard play a role as well as outdoor ^{222}Rn exchanging with indoor air, dominate the source. Harley (1991) summarized the data for high-rise apartments and showed the average indoor concentration to be a factor of 2 higher than outdoor concentration.

Detailed knowledge of the geological properties of a particular region could help to identify geographic areas of potentially high indoor radon in single-family dwellings. There is an attempt being made to determine the 100,000 highest concentration homes in the United States, but lack of funding has impeded this program. In general, ^{222}Rn is measured in homes at a real estate transaction and is mandatory in some states. Radon-resistant construction is emerging as a priority to prevent new homes from attaining unacceptable concentrations.

Groundwater as a Source of Indoor ^{222}Rn

In some cases indoor ^{222}Rn is increased substantially by the use of groundwater. Radon, like any gas, is somewhat soluble in water. Well or groundwater in close contact with rock and soil can exhibit typical concentrations of ^{222}Rn range from 20 to 200 Bq l^{-1}. Some wells in the state of Maine, for example, have measured ^{222}Rn concentrations of 3.7×10^4 Bq l^{-1} (10^6 pCi l^{-1}) (Hess et al., 1985, 1987). Surface water, namely from reservoirs, is very low in ^{222}Rn concentration because the gas is readily removed by surface agitation.

The dose to internal organs from drinking water with even high concentrations is very low. (Harley and Robbins, 1994). However, the ^{222}Rn released to indoor air through normal use, such as showering, can increase the overall indoor concentration significantly depending on the groundwater concentration (Hess et al., 1985, 1987; Chittaporn and Harley, 1994; NRC, 1999b). Airborne ^{222}Rn and decay products derived from water cannot be distinguished from ^{222}Rn entering the dwelling from the usual soil source. Estimates of the contribution of groundwater to indoor air usually apply a 1/10,000 factor; that is 10,000 units (pCi l^{-1} or Bq l^{-1}) in groundwater will yield on average 1 unit in indoor air.

On October 1, 1997, the Swedish government on request of the National Food Administration, set a limit for ^{222}Rn in public water supplies of 100 Bq l^{-1} (2700 pCi l^{-1}). The water must be remediated if the concentration is >100 Bq l^{-1}, and public drinking water cannot be delivered for use if the concentration exceeds 1000 Bq l^{-1}.

The U.S. EPA has the authority to set a ^{222}Rn limit for drinking water supplied for public use (> 25 households). Since ^{222}Rn is a known carcinogen, this limit can be set to zero. However, since zero concentration is not attainable by any present technology, EPA has proposed a limit of 300 pCi l^{-1}, on the basis of the practical detection limit for the measurement of ^{222}Rn in water. There is considerable pressure to increase this proposed limit because of the high cost of remediating water to this limit and because of the negligible health consequences implied from air concentrations of ^{222}Rn associated with water use near this limit. The final EPA decision is expected in 1999.

UNDERGROUND MINE RADON EPIDEMIOLOGY

The pooling of the follow-up studies of 11 underground miner cohorts provide the best data to date with which to project the lung cancer risk at domestic concentrations. The excess risk in miners was observed at high exposures, and it is extrapolated to the risk at environmental ^{222}Rn concentrations (NIH, 1994; NRC, 1999a). The underground mining populations are from China, Czechoslovakia, Canada, Colorado, New Mexico, France, Australia, and Sweden.

Although the results from 11 studies are pooled, it is clear that the exposure assessments for the various cohorts are of extremely varied quality. In the Eldorado mine (Canada, Beaverlodge mine), for example, it is clear that exposures in mines other than the Beaverlodge contribute to lung cancer in these miners. The additional exposure is not documented in the miner's work records (Chambers, 1990). In the Australian Radium Hill cohort (Woodward et al., 1991), the authors state that increased rate of lung cancer in this workforce may be due wholly or partly to factors other than radiation. Cigarette smoking is potentially the most important confounding factor.

It remains, however, that lung cancer above that expected from smoking alone is reported in all of these mines, and radon and radon daughter exposure is the primary carcinogen, which is shown by the clear dose-response relationship.

The detailed information concerning the eleven mining cohorts can be found in NIH 1994 and NRC, 1999a. Miners were exposed for a period of from 3 to over 20 years. Radon exposures were made in most of the mines after 1950. However, the measurements were generally sparse, and the data on individuals and sometimes entire mines had to be interpolated. In all mines the weakest part of the study is the poor quality of the exposure estimate.

In the case of the Swedish Malmberget iron mines, exposure measurements were not begun until 1972, although workers had underground history beginning in 1930 (Radford and Renard, 1984). Efforts have been made to reconstruct exposure data from mine ventilation records, but this is difficult and fraught with inaccuracies.

The excess relative risk of lung cancer per WLM exposure (ERR/WLM) for these 11 cohorts are shown in Figure 22-6 (NIH, 1994). The observed lung cancer as a function of

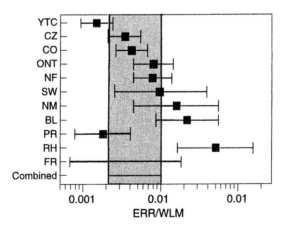

Figure 22-6 Estimates of excess relative risk of lung cancer per WLM exposure and 95% confidence limits for each of the pooled 11 underground mining cohorts. From NIH (1994). (Yunnan Province, China, Czechoslovakia, Colorado, Ontario, Canada, Newfoundland, Sweden, New Mexico, Beaverlodge, Canada, Port Radium, Canada, Radium Hill, Australia, France)

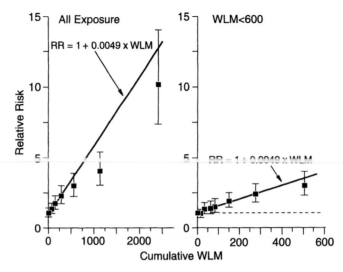

Figure 22-7 Relative Risk (RR) of lung cancer as a function of cumulative exposure (WLM) for all 11 underground mining cohorts combined. The equation is the fitted linear excess RR. From NIH (1994).

cumulative exposure in WLM for the pooled data from all 11 cohorts is shown in Figure 22-7 (NIH, 1994).

One of the best mining populations for establishing risk from environmental radon is probably the Colorado Plateau uranium miner follow-up. This is the only study so far to have essentially complete smoking information on each miner. Other studies rely on a small subgroup within the cohort for smoking information. The Colorado uranium miner follow-up does not show excess lung cancers until a cumulative exposure of 120 WLM.

Unfortunately, complete information to address risk from environmental radon exposure is lacking in the miner studies. Home exposures at an average of $150\,\mathrm{Bq\,m^{-3}}$ $(4\,\mathrm{pCi\,L^{-1}})$ yield a lifetime exposure of about 50 WLM. An important mining study of Ontario uranium miners showing excess lung cancer risk, has documented such low exposures, with exposures in the study at a range of 33 to 74 WLM to indicate the associated uncertainty (Muller et al., 1983).

For the purpose of extrapolating lung cancer risk from high radon levels, the concentrations known to cause lung cancer are less than an order of magnitude higher than typical environmental exposures. If a threshold for lung cancer exists, it is very near the environmental exposures.

ENVIRONMENTAL EPIDEMIOLOGY

Lung cancer excess (above that expected from smoking) in the underground miner populations has been demonstrated conclusively. Combining this and the knowledge that some homes have radon and daughter concentrations above those found in historical mines, it is virtually certain that environmental radon is responsible for some lung cancer in the general population.

There are more than 20 environmental epidemiological studies of radon exposure to determine whether health effects can be documented directly (Neuberger, 1989, 1996; DOE, 1989; Borek and Johnson, 1988). Most studies show either a slight positive or negative correlation between measured radon in the home and lung cancer mortality. The majority of studies are ecological exercises that relate lung cancer mortality in a region with indoor radon concentration. In some cases the radon is not measured but estimated as high or low depending on the type of house. The ecological studies are unsatisfying because no attempt is made to determine actual exposure to individuals in the area of study, and no correction can be made for smoking, the strongest confounder for lung cancer.

The exception to this is the ecological study of Dr. Bernard Cohen of the University of Pittsburgh. He has measured over 170,000 homes, accounting for nearly every county in the United States. These data show a strong negative correlation with 1970 to 1979 lung cancer mortality statistics by county (Cohen, 1987, 1990). Data are not available to adequately adjust his data for the effect of smoking. Harley (1989) has provided a crude means to do this, and the trend is reduced markedly. However, such a persistent negative trend in the Cohen publications, suggesting higher radon concentrations associated with less smoking, is interesting. The reason for this is not clear but the negative correlation in his data is so prominent that it should be pursued to some resolution.

An example of a case control study with good exposure assessment, is the New Jersey study of Schoenberg et al. (1990). They analyzed data for 400 lung cancer cases and 400 controls. The individuals had to be living in their present residence for at least 10 years in order to comply with the study design. Radon measurements were made in the current residence on most living levels and measurements of historical exposure in past residences were also performed.

The major correlation found was with smoking and lung cancer. No statistically significant lung cancer excess was found for exposures over $150 \, \mathrm{Bq \, m^{-3}}$ ($4 \, \mathrm{pCi \, L^{-1}}$). Because of the small number of cases with home exposure $>150 \, \mathrm{Bq \, m^{-3}}$, the trend toward higher relative risk with increasing exposure was tested and found statistically significant. Thus, although statistically weak, it suggests that environmental exposure is linked to excess lung cancer.

A significant contribution of this study was that high-quality radon measurements were performed. Significant resources were committed to quality control samples consisting of paired samples, blanks, and positive controls. Radon measured in basements was several-fold higher than in first-floor living levels, as expected. The investigators cautioned that basement concentrations should not be used as indicators of exposure, although they often are.

The largest case control study to date was performed in Sweden (Pershagen et al., 1994). There were 1360 cases and 2847 controls. The exposure was assessed with 3 month measurements during the heating season, retrospectively assessing homes lived in for more than 2 years since 1947 up to 3 years prior to diagnosis of cancer. The lung cancer excess was not statistically significant even for smokers or nonsmokers with over $400 \, \mathrm{Bq \, m^{-3}}$ ($>10 \, \mathrm{pCi \, L^{-1}}$) in the home for over 32 years.

A meta analysis was performed using results from eight published domestic studies. The lung cancer excess is not statistically significant but the trend with increasing concentration in the homes was significant (Lubin and Boice, 1997). The graph of the 8 studies from Lubin and Boice (1997) is shown in Figure 22-8.

All that can be said about domestic risk, at present, is that it is low and difficult if not impossible to detect given the high background lung cancer mortality in the populations studied. Although a pooling of the largest case-control studies from all countries will be performed by the year 2000, it is unlikely to provide quantitative domestic risk estimates because of the poor precision of the studies. It is more likely that further numerical risk estimates for lung cancer from ^{222}Rn and decay product exposure will rely on projection models based on the underground mining experience.

The difficulty in pooling the domestic studies is described by Neuberger et al. (1996).

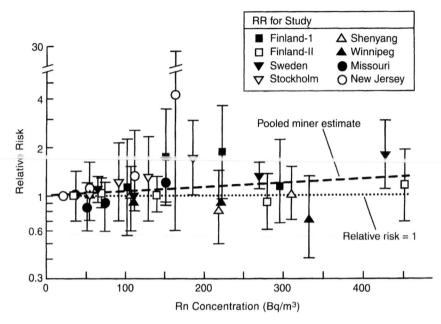

Figure 22-8 Relative Risk (RR) from eight lung cancer case-control studies of domestic radon exposure. Dashed line is the extrapolation of the RR from underground miners. From Lubin and Boice (1997).

LUNG DOSIMETRY

Lung cancer due to radon exposure is actually due to the inhalation of the particulate short-lived daughters of radon ^{218}Po, ^{214}Pb, and ^{214}Bi– ^{214}Po (the half-life of ^{214}Po is so short that it is always in steady-state equilibrium with ^{214}Bi). As each ^{218}Po atom is formed from the decay of ^{222}Rn, it grows by condensation of water and other molecules such as SO_2 to a few nanometers diameter. In ordinary indoor atmospheres there are abundant submicrometer-sized particles (1000–50,000 cm^{-3} in the 50–200 nanometer size range) present from various sources such as energy use and influx of outdoor aerosol. Subsequent to formation from ^{222}Rn, most atoms of ^{218}Po rapidly attach to this larger sized (termed normal, ambient aerosol). As the ^{218}Po atom decays through the chain—^{214}Pb to ^{214}Bi– Po—these subsequent radioactive atoms (mostly) remain on the carrier aerosol particle. The ^{218}Po and some ^{214}Pb not attached to the carrier aerosol are called the *unattached* or *ultrafine fraction*, while the decay products attached to the carrier aerosol are called the *attached fraction* of ^{222}Rn daughters (NCRP, 1988).

In homes there are normally fewer aerosol particles than in underground mines. Therefore the fraction of the radioactivity that is unattached is larger in homes than in mines because there is a greater probability for attachment to particles in mines.

Inhaled decay products of radon are primarily on the 50–200 nm diameter carrier particles. A varying percentage (from a few to over 50%) of the ^{218}Po radioactivity exist as the original ultrafine particle of a few nanometers size. The actual size of the ultrafine aerosol depends on the trace gas composition as well as on other factors that are not well identified at present. The greater the concentration of carrier aerosol, the less unattached is the fraction of ^{218}Po. This is because rapid diffusion of the ultrafine species allows interaction with the larger aerosol particles; the interaction will remove the ultrafine particle to become part of the larger particle size population.

Polonium-218 emits an alpha particle, and it is possible that the recoil energy is large enough to dislodge or free the daughter ^{214}Pb atom from the larger particle to which it is attached so that it is in the ultrafine or unattached form. Also some unattached ^{218}Po atoms can decay to ^{214}Pb before attachment to larger particles and contribute to airborne unattached ^{214}Pb. The ratio of unattached ^{214}Pb/^{218}Po is considered to be 1/10 for dosimetric modeling purposes.

As this mixed size aerosol of unattached and attached ^{218}Po/^{214}Po aerosol is inhaled and exhaled, radon decay products are deposited by diffusional deposition on the airway lumen. All of these aerosol particles are too small for sedimentation or impaction to play a significant role in airway deposition. The primary carcinogenic dose is then delivered by alpha particles from the decay of ^{218}Po and ^{214}Po residing on the bronchial airways. These alpha particles easily reach the target cells in bronchial epithelium (basal and/or mucous cells) as their ranges in tissue are 47 and 70 μm. Figure 22-9 shows a section of human bronchial epithelium with the target basal and mucous cells identified (Robbins, 1990). The stem cells are the only targets for carcinogenesis because they are capable of division to maintain and replace terminally differentiated epithelial cells which are normally lost throughout life. The lifespan of most terminally differentiated epithelial cells is about four months.

The inhalation and deposition of any particulates on the bronchial airways is accompanied by mucociliary clearance of particles up the tree to the pharynx. This is the major defense of the lung against inhaled material deposited in the conducting airways. A steady-state activity through inhalation, deposition, and clearance is attained for each of the radioactive daughter products, ^{218}Po, ^{214}Pb, and ^{214}Bi/^{214}Po.

Diffusion deposition onto the airway wall increases as the particle diameter decreases. Therefore the steady-state radioactivity on the bronchial tree is considerably higher for small-sized aerosol particles. For example, open flame burning or space heating with a kerosene heater can produce an aerosol with a median diameter of 30 nm or a factor of about 4 smaller than that considered in a normal room aerosol, namely 120 nm in diameter (Tu and Knutson, 1988).

Diffusion deposition on the bronchial airways has now been measured exhaustively in casts of the human lung. The deposition is well described by the equations below (Cohen and Asgharian, 1990) and varies as

$$n_{\mathrm{d}} = a(\Delta)^{b}, \tag{4}$$

where a and b are constants and

$\Delta = \pi L D/(4Q)$,
$L =$ airway length,
$D =$ diffusion coefficient,
$Q =$ flow rate.

This compensating factor, inverse proportionality with flow rate, along with the higher values of unattached fraction in the home versus mines, actually leads to similar values of the dose conversion factor in both homes and mines. This is an important feature because it implies that the risk estimates obtained from mining exposures may be transported to environmental situations, assuming other factors to be equal.

There are actually three factors operating in the comparative dosimetry of mines versus homes that equalize the dose. These are (1) similarity in particle size spectra in mines and homes (George and Hinchliffe, 1972; George and Breslin, 1980); (2) the breathing rate under working conditions in a mine is higher than in homes, leading to somewhat higher

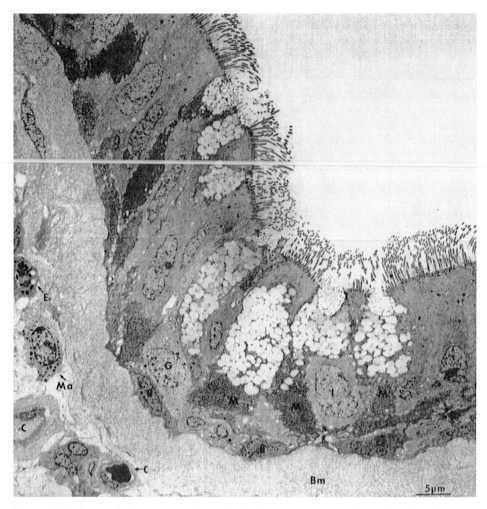

Figure 22-9   A transmission electron micrograph of a bronchus from the uninvolved portion of the lung of a 69-year-old male smoker with adenocarcinoma. Among the citiated cells of the epithelial lining are mucous (M), basal (B) intermediate/indeterminate (I), and granulated endocrine or APUD (amine precursor uptake and decarboxylation) (G) cells. Beneath the thick basement membrane (Bm) is an incomplete layer of fibroblasts, one of which is sectioned through its nucleus (F). Within the connective tissue of the lamina propria are capillaries (C), a mast cell (Ma) and an eosinophil (E). Magnification = 2500 × . Bar = 5 μm.

dose per unit exposure than in homes; and (3) the unattached fraction of the radioactivity is higher in homes and lower in mines.

Figure 22-10 shows the complete modeled relationship between alpha dose to cells in bronchial epithelium located at a mean depth of 27 μm below the epithelial surface and the median particle size of a carrier aerosol (geometric standard deviation of 2). The depth of stem cells in the bronchial airways has been studied extensively by Robbins; it is reported in Harley et al. (1996). The model calculations are shown for different breathing rates and unattached fractions in Figure 22-10. The central value of the dose conversion factor for typical aerosol particle diameters is 6 mGy/WLM (0.6 rad/WLM) and for the ultrafine species (a few to 50 nm) 20 mGy/WLM (2 rad/WLM).

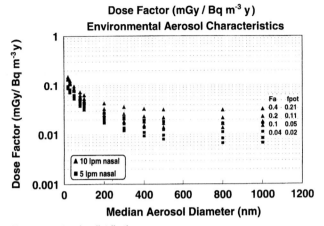

Figure 22-10   Dose conversion factor (mGy/Bq m^{-3} y) for basal cell nuclei in bronchial epithelium for two nasal breathing rates and four values of the unattached fraction of ^{218}Po. Dose factor shown as a function of the median aerosol particle size inhaled.

The dose for different ratios of individual decay products, expressed in terms of potential energy (WLM), is essentially the same. Thus disequilibrium of the daughters in an atmosphere does not lead to significantly different bronchial dose for the same total potential energy (WL or WLM) content.

There are only a few moderately large-scale studies of the particle size of indoor aerosols (George and Breslin, 1980; Reineking and Porstendorfer, 1986; Reineking et al., 1990; Hopke et al., 1995). Because the dose for the same radioactivity content in an atmosphere is so dependent on particle size, there is a great need for more detailed information concerning the indoor aerosol. This is an area that needs considerable work if the uncertainty associated with estimating lung cancer risk from indoor radon exposure is to be reduced. In addition to ^{222}Rn dosimetry, a study of the indoor aerosol particle size and composition is important because of the poorly understood increase in respiratory disease.

LUNG CANCER MODELS FOR HUMANS

There are at present three models for transporting lung cancer risk from the underground mining studies to exposure in the environment. These are the historic National Council on Radiation Protection and Measurements (NCRP, 1984), the National Research Council, Biological Effects of Ionizing Radiation (BEIR IV), and the National Cancer Institute model (NIH, 1994) derived from the pooling of 11 underground mining studies. The BEIR VI model is essentially the same as the NIH 1994 model. Although the exposure data are universally weak in all of the mine epidemiological follow-up studies, they are the only human data available to estimate lung cancer risk and some generalizations are possible and necessary to quantitate this risk.

NCRP Model

The National Council on Radiation Protection and Measurements was the first to propose a model for environmental lung cancer risk based on the miner data (NCRP, 1984a). The model was cognizant of the fact that miners exposed for the first time at more than age 40 appeared to have a higher lifetime risk of lung cancer than miners exposed for the first time in their 20s. Because age, as such, was not thought to confer greater risk for lung cancer, this effect was assumed to be due to a reduction in risk with time. Thus earlier exposure was assumed to diminish because of cell death or repair of cells transformed by earlier exposure. This half-life for repair (or loss) was assumed to be 20 years.

One key factor noted by NCRP was that lung cancer is a rare disease before age 40, regardless of the population considered. A miner exposed at young ages did not generally appear as a lung cancer case until the usual cancer ages were attained (50–70).

This would account for an apparent increase in lifetime lung cancer risk at older ages because there would be a shorter time for the loss of transformed cells to occur compared with a person exposed at young age. Miners were exposed, on average, for less than 10 years in the Colorado, Ontario, and Czech cohorts. The total time for follow up was 20 or more years so that the apparent reduction of risk with time from exposure could be observed.

The NCRP model took the form of an exponential reduction with time from exposure, with the stipulation that there was a minimum latent period (the time between exposure and a frank cancer) of 5 years. Also, lung cancer could not appear before age 40. This model is known as a modified absolute risk model. Risk is expressed following exposure without regard to other risks of lung cancer such as smoking, but risk is modified by time from exposure.

Mathematically the risk is expressed for each year's exposure by,

$$R(t, T) = CE\sigma \left[\exp\left(-0.0345(t - T)\right] \frac{L}{L_0}, \tag{5}$$

$$\sigma = \begin{cases} 0 & \text{if} \quad t < 40, \\ 1 & \text{if} \quad t >= 40, \end{cases}$$

$$\text{for} \quad (t - T) \geq 5,$$

where

$R(t, T) =$ lung cancer mortality at age t, from an exposure at age T.

$C =$ risk coefficient, lung cancer rate per year per WLM exposure,

$E =$ exposure in one year's time in WLM,

$L/L_0 =$ life table correction for other causes of death (persons alive at age t, divided by persons alive at age T per 100,000 born).

To express lifetime risk (LR) following a single exposure, it is necessary to sum the risk in equation (5) over the number of years of life following exposure, taken as age of exposure to age 85:

$$\text{LR}(T) = \sum_{T}^{85} R(t, T). \tag{6}$$

The lifetime risk, TR, from continuous exposure was expressed as the sum of lifetime risk for a single years exposure, equation (6), over the total exposure interval considered:

$$\text{TR} = \sum_{t_0}^{85} \text{LR}(T), \tag{7}$$

where $t_0 =$ age at first exposure.

TABLE 22-4   Lung Cancer Risk for Whole-Life Exposure to 150 Bqm^{-3} (4 pCi/L), Predicted by Various Models of Domestic Exposure

Model [a]	Lifetime Risk (%)	Model Type	Comment
NCRP (1984a)	0.9	Modified absolute risk. Two-parameter model	Risk decreases with time since exposure
ICRP (1987)	1.6	Constant relative risk	
ICRP (1987)	1.1	Constant additive risk	
ICRP (1993)	1.0	Single value risk per WLM	Adopted lifetime risk per WLM exposure
BEIR IV (NRC 1988)	2.5	Modified relative risk. Two time windows, Two-parameter model	Risk decreases with time since exposure
NIH (1994) [a]	3.2	Modified relative risk. Three time windows and exposure rate. Three-parameter model.	Risk decreases with time since exposure and decreases with very high exposures
BEIR VI (NRC 1999a)	3.6	Modified relative risk. Three time windows and exposure rate. Three-parameter model.	Risk decreases with time since exposure and decreases with very high exposures
Meta analysis 8 domestic Case Control (Lubin and Boice, 1997)	1.2	Observed mortality	Linear regression fit to data from 8 domestic studies

[a] Lifetime risks for the NIH and BEIR VI model are calculated by the authors for a lifetime equal to 110 years.
[b] Actual exposure are assumed to be equal to 1 WLM/y in order to equate to mining conditions.

At the time the model was developed, there was not enough information on the risk of smoking and ^{222}Rn exposure combined to separate an additional effect from this carcinogen. It was stated that the risk coefficient C could be modified when sufficient data were available. Numerical values of lifetime risk for different exposure protocols are shown in Table 22-4.

BEIR IV Model

The National Research Council, BEIR IV Committee, produced a report on the Health Risks of Radon and other Internally Deposited Radionuclides (NRC, 1988). The Committee was given the raw data or selected parts of the original data from four mining cohorts, the United States (Colorado), Canadian (Ontario and Eldorado), and Malmberget (Swedish). Reanalysis was performed using the program AMFIT developed for analysis of the Japanese A-bomb survivor data. The program estimates parameters based on Poisson regression.

Using AMFIT, the data were analyzed using both internal and external cohorts for a control population. The BEIR IV committee stated that a relative risk model fit the observed mortality well. The relative risk model assumes that radon exposure increases the known baseline age-specific lung cancer mortality rate in the population by a constant fraction per WLM exposure.

However, in all cohorts, there was an obvious reduced lung cancer mortality with time from exposure. The relative risk model was modified to reduce risk with time since exposure. The BEIR IV Committee called their modified relative risk model a *time since exposure model* (TSE).

Smoking was examined as a confounder. The only study with complete smoking history on the miners is the Colorado study. The effect was tested using a hybrid relative risk model which incorporated a mixing parameter for smoking. A parameter value of zero fit an additive effect of smoking and ^{222}Rn interaction, while a value of 1 fit a multiplicative model best. A maximum log-likelihood test was applied to the data. It was found that the best parameter fit was between 0 and 1, indicating the combined risk, but it was more than additive and less than multiplicative. That is, the lifetime risk of lung cancer from radon exposure did not simply add to the lifetime risk of lung cancer from smoking. Neither did the risks multiply. The risk of radon and smoking appeared to be between these two extremes.

However, in the final BEIR IV model, the risks of radon and smoking was treated as though they were multiplicative because there was no methodology to treat the hybrid model. The TSE model was given the mathematical form

$$r(a) = r_0(a)[1 + 0.025\,\gamma\,(a)(\text{WLM}_1 + 0.5\text{WLM}_2)], \tag{8}$$

where

$r(a)$ = age specific lung cancer mortality rate,
$r_0(a)$ = baseline age specific lung cancer mortality rate,
$\gamma(a)$ = 1.2 for age < 55 = 1.0 for age 55–64 = 0.4 for age ≥ 65,
WLM_1 = WLM incurred between 5 and 15 years before age a,
WLM_2 = WLM incurred 15 or more years before age a.

The exposure data for the Eldorado cohort were not considered carefully by the BEIR IV committee. A reported Eldorado mining exposure of 1 WLM gave a 50% excess lung cancer mortality, clearly an erroneous value. It is known that the miners had prior exposure in other mines, but this additional exposure was not added to the Eldorado exposure (Chambers, 1990). The exaggerated risk per WLM in this study for the 1 WLM exposure cohort is significant in controlling the overall BEIR IV model. This exposure category included a large number of person years; therefore, when combining the four cohorts to yield a "best estimate" of the relative risk coefficient, the 1 WLM group and its erroneously high risk carried a substantial weight. If this data point were omitted, as it should have been, the risk coefficient in the model would be about half the calculated value or 0.015/WLM instead of 0.025/WLM, as used in the final BEIR IV model. This was a serious error by the BEIR IV committee and requires correction in any future models using the Eldorado cohort. Thus, considering all of the inaccuracies incorporated into the BEIR IV model, the calculated risk estimates for both smokers and nonsmokers at environmental exposures are overestimates. The values of lifetime risk as calculated by the BEIR IV TSE model are shown in Table 22-4.

ICRP Model

The International Commission on Radiation Protection (ICRP, 1987) developed their models for environmental risk based on both a constant relative risk model and a constant absolute risk model. The ICRP assumed that the risk expressed over the years cancer occurs would be enhanced if exposure occurred in childhood. They assumed that the risk was three times as great for exposure from ages 0 to 20 than for exposure over age 20. There is no justification for this assumption, and later information suggests that children may be at less risk than adults because of the reduction in risk with time from exposure. This is discussed further in the section on childhood exposure.

The constant absolute or constant relative risk model is no longer considered to be an appropriate model for lung cancer. Although not biologically correct, risk estimates calculated using this model are within a factor of 3 of those from other models. Values of lifetime risk for the ICRP model are shown in Table 22-4.

NIH MODEL

The National Cancer Institute coordinated an effort to pool the epidemiological data from 11 underground mining studies. The pooled results are reported in NIH (1994), which gives the most complete analysis of the health detriment to underground miners. The analysis was published in the document *Radon and Lung Cancer Risk: A Joint Analysis of 11 Underground Miners Studies* (NIH, 1994). This work brought together the investigators from each of the 11 mining groups, and their data were analyzed jointly to provide the best information for estimating the lung cancer risk from exposure to ^{222}Rn and decay products. There were 2701 lung cancer deaths among 68,000 miners accumulating about 1.2 million person-years of exposure.

In all of the 11 cohorts the excess relative risk (ERR) of lung cancer (the fractional increase in lung cancer) was linearly related to the cumulative exposure estimated in working level months (WLM). Thus although other carcinogens may be present in mine atmospheres, a clear relationship was associated exposure to ^{222}Rn decay products.

The Colorado uranium miner data from NIH (1994) is shown as a typical example of the 11 cohorts (Fig. 22-11). The ERR/WLM for all of the studies is shown in Figure 22-6.

One important aspect of the data shown in Figure 22-11 is that the ERR at high exposures tends to flatten out. This observation is erroneously called the inverse exposure effect. It is usually stated that the lung cancer risk per unit exposure increases for low exposures compared with high exposures. The flattening of the response curve is likely the result of cell killing due to multiple traversals of cell nuclei. Therefore the effect is a reduced response at high exposure, not an increased response at low exposure.

This confused terminology has caused considerable misinterpretation with the implication that domestic exposure can somehow be more dangerous than mine exposure.

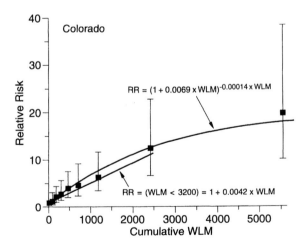

Figure 22-11 Relative Risk (RR) for the Colorado underground uranium miner cohort for exposures less than 5500 WLM. Linear and power function fitted to excess. Note the reduced risk at very high exposures. From NIH (1994).

This is not true, and it has been demonstrated that no additional risk above the linearity showed in all cohorts is present in domestic exposures. In fact, no domestic study has as yet shown a statistically significant excess of lung cancer. This is described later in the section on domestic case control studies.

The main features of the lung cancer risk model derived from the jointly analyzed data are as follows:

1. There is a reduction in risk subsequent to cessation of mining. This is called the time since exposure (TSE Factor) effect.
2. There appears to be no clear effect of age at start of exposure; that is the age at start of mining is not a factor. However, the age attained after start of mining is a factor, and there is decreased risk with older age subsequent to exposure (AGE Factor).
3. Longer duration (DUR Factor), or lower ^{222}Rn concentration (WL Factor), gives rise to larger risk. Since this is the way the model parameters are derived, it is the reason for the so-called inverse exposure effect.

The two models derived from the joint analysis are considered equally likely as a fit to the observations.

A striking feature of the data is the time since exposure effect, with three time windows modeled for the joint analysis, versus two time windows modeled in the BEIR IV report when four cohorts were available for analysis.

TSE/AGE/WL

$$RR = 1 + \beta \times (w_{5-14} + \theta_2 w_{15-24} + \theta_3 w_{25+}) \times \phi_{age} \times \gamma_{WL},$$

where

$w_{5-14}, w_{15-24} =$ exposure in WLM 5 to 14 and 15 to 24 years prior to the end of mining,
$\beta = 0.0611,$
$\theta_2 = 0.81,$
$\theta_3 = 0.40,$

$$\phi_{age} = \begin{cases} 1 & \text{for age} < 55, \\ 0.65 & 55 < \text{age} < 65, \\ 0.38 & 65 < \text{age} < 75, \\ 0.22 & 75 < \text{age}, \end{cases}$$

$$\gamma_{WL} = \begin{cases} 1.0 & \text{WL} < 0.5, \\ 0.51 & 0.5 < \text{WL} < 1.0, \\ 0.32 & 1.0 < \text{WL} < 3.0, \\ 0.27 & 3.0 < \text{WL} < 5.0, \\ 0.13 & 5.0 < \text{WL} < 15.0, \\ 0.10 & 15 < \text{WL}. \end{cases}$$

TSE/AGE/DUR Model

$$RR = 1 + \beta \times (w_{5-14} + \theta_2 w_{15-24} + \theta_3 w_{25+}) \times \phi_{age} \times \gamma_{DUR},$$

where

$$\beta = 0.0611,$$
$$\theta_2 = 0.81,$$
$$\theta_3 = 0.40,$$

$$\phi_{\text{age}} = \begin{cases} 1 & \text{for age} < 55, \\ 0.57 & 55 < \text{age} < 65, \\ 0.34 & 65 < \text{age} < 75, \\ 0.28 & 75 < \text{age}, \end{cases}$$

$$\gamma_{\text{DUR}} = \begin{cases} 1.0 & \text{DUR} < 0.5, \\ 3.17 & 3.17 < \text{DUR} < 15, \\ 5.27 & 5.27 < \text{DUR} < 25, \\ 9.08 & 9.08 < \text{DUR} < 35, \\ 13.6 & 35 < \text{DUR}. \end{cases}$$

The combined effect of smoking and ^{222}Rn exposure could not be determined quantitatively. The pooled analysis showed a linear increase in risk of about a factor of 2 for smokers over never smokers, in agreement with the graph in Figure 22-12.

The NIH report summarized the calculated deaths in the U.S population from the assumed exposure of 45 Bq m^{-3} (1.2 pCi l^{-1}). Their calculated value was 15,000 deaths per year with 10,000 deaths in smokers and 5,000 in nonsmokers. The BEIR VI report changed these values slightly.

BEIR VI

The National Research Council revised and updated the BEIR IV report (Biological Effects of Ionizing Radiation) published in 1988. This report was published in 1999

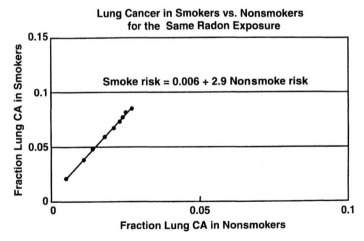

Figure 22-12 Lung cancer risk for smokers versus nonsmokers. Points plotted for cumulative exposures of 0–500 WLM, 0–1000 WLM, 0–1500 WLM, and so on, up to 0–4500 WLM in the Colorado cohort of underground uranium miners (3360 miners; see text).

(NRC, 1999a). The model to project lung cancer from ^{222}Rn decay product exposure is essentially identical to that reported in NIH (1994). The BEIR VI committee analyzed the same 11 underground mining cohort data with slight modification, and updating of the data, so the models produce similar results.

The BEIR VI committee found that the risk at the lower mining exposures could be used to estimate environmental risk. At very high exposures the risk decreases as discussed earlier. Thus there is no projected increase in risk per unit exposure for lower home ^{222}Rn exposure over that observed at higher mine ^{222}Rn concentrations.

Two types of models were used similar to the NIH report. One model was an exposure/age/duration model and the other an exposure / age / concentration model. The two models predict 15,400 and 21,800 lung cancer deaths per year, respectively, in the United States from ^{222}Rn exposure in the home. An uncertainty analysis suggested the number of calculated cases could range from 3,000 to 33,000. The long-term follow-up of the mining populations was strongly recommended.

CHILDHOOD EXPOSURE

It is apparent that leukemia and breast cancer are elevated for radiation exposure in childhood versus exposure as an adult. Concern has been expressed that the same might be true for lung cancer derived from exposure to radon and its decay products at early ages. There is a suggestion in the literature that the alpha dose per unit exposure is somewhat larger at about 10 years because of the smaller dimensions of the child's bronchial tree with breathing rates similar to those of an adult (Harley, 1984a).

Some human data are available for occupational exposure to elevated radon in childhood. Lubin et al. 1990 analyzed data from tin mines in the Yunnan province, China. Thirty-seven percent of exposed workers started employment under the age of 13. For this group the risk coefficient was 1.2%/WLM, while for those first employed over age 18 the risk coefficient was 2.9%/WLM. Although this difference was not statistically significant, the results suggest that children are not a particularly sensitive population. Tentatively a lower risk coefficient for children compared with that for adults reported by Lubin et al. (1990), suggests that the reduction in lung cancer risk with time since exposure is also effective in children. The fact that lung cancer does not appear at a significant rate in any population before the age of 40 permits a substantial time interval for risk reduction in the exposed child.

ANIMAL STUDIES

The animal studies have been supportive of the human data on lung cancer related to radon exposure. Studies with SPF Wistar rats at Battelle Pacific Northwest Laboratories and with SPF Sprague Dawley rats at COGEMA laboratories in France have produced lung tumors at total exposures as low as 200 and 20 to 50 WLM, respectively (NCRP, 1984a, 1989).

Detailed tracheobronchial dosimetry in the rat lung shows that the alpha dose per unit exposure in the rat and the human are similar (Harley, 1988). The dose conversion factor for both are 5 mGy / WLM. However, the distribution of tumors differs in that the rat has a predominance of tumors that are in the distal airways, essentially in the pulmonary parenchyma, while in humans the tumors appear in the upper or proximal airways. The reason for this is not known; however, there are significant differences between cell types and cell turnover rates in the rat and human bronchial airways.

In the distal airways of the rat, Clara cells predominate, and there are no basal cells. In the human, basal cells persist down to the distal airways (bronchioles). The reason that no human tumors occur in the distal airways but are preferentially found in the most proximal airways (airway branching generations 1 to about 10) is not known (Saccomanno et al., 1996). Cellular turnover rates most likely play a key role. One biological model of ^{222}Rn-related lung cancer showed that the reduced number of stem cells with age may be responsible for the time since exposure decrease in lung cancer observed (Harley et al., 1996).

SMOKING AND RADON

One of the most critical issues concerning lung cancer and radon exposure concerns the effect of cigarette smoking on carcinogenesis. Underground miners were mostly smokers in all the cohorts studied. In smoking miners there is a significant excess of lung cancer above that expected due to smoking alone. Regardless of the type of mine exposure, the increased or excess lung cancer is linearly related to total or cumulative radon exposure (NIH, 1994; NRC, 1999a). This is convincing evidence that radon decay products are the major carcinogen even if there is the potential for a minor influence of other inhaled agents.

There are some nonsmokers in the exposed mining populations (Radford and Renard, 1984; Samet et al., 1984; Roscoe et al., 1989, 1995; Sevc et al., 1988). Nonsmoking miners also have increased risk of lung cancer following radon exposure. However, the risk per unit exposure appears to differ somewhat depending on the study. Radford and Renard (1984) found the absolute excess risk in lung cancer per year per WLM exposure to be similar for smokers and nonsmokers, while the relative risk (observed/expected risk for the population of either smokers or nonsmokers) for nonsmokers was considerably higher (11/1). This relationship suggested that the lung cancer risk from radon acts independently of the smoking risk. Since the baseline risk for nonsmokers is about 1/10, that for smokers the higher relative risk for nonsmokers yields the same number of absolute excess lung cancers for a given exposure in both groups.

Contradictory evidence exists in the Colorado uranium miner follow-up. In this group the ratio of observed to expected lung cancers was about 2/1 for smokers/nonsmokers having the same exposure. The NAS BEIR IV, NIH 1994, and BEIR VI reports all state that the data were better fit by a relative or multiplicative risk model than an absolute additive model.

The type of model underlying the estimation of projection of effects to the environment is critical. If the increase in lung cancer per unit exposure is the same for smokers and nonsmokers, and a relative risk model applies, then the number of lung cancers in a group of smokers will be much greater than for the same size group of nonsmokers because of the large difference in baseline cancer mortality. This can be seen mathematically in the NRC or NIH models.

Lubin and Boice (1989), using the NRC BEIR IV model, estimate that 13,000 deaths per year occur from environmental radon exposure and that these are apportioned 9000 smokers versus 4000 nonsmokers. The NCRP model, on the other hand, which does not differentiate between smokers and nonsmokers, estimated that 9000 deaths per year occur.

The difference between smokers and nonsmokers in the Colorado mining population can be seen in Figure 22-12. This plot shows the lung cancer mortality as of the time of last follow-up (1982) for smokers versus nonsmokers. Figure 22-12 shows the relationship for the whole cohort of 3360 miners, 760 of whom were nonsmokers. Each plotted point is the fraction of smoking or nonsmoking miners with lung cancer in the cumulative exposure categories of up to 500 WLM, up to 1000 WLM, up to 1500 WLM amd so on.

A similar plot showing a breakdown by birth year had little effect on the slope of the lines. Thus in this analysis the effect of smoking appears to confer a greater risk for the same ^{222}Rn decay product exposure. The slope in Figure 22-12 indicates that for the same total exposure, smokers are about 2.9 times as likely to die of lung cancer than a nonsmoker.

SUMMARY

There is a large body of evidence demonstrating that ^{222}Rn and its short-lived daughters are the carcinogens responsible for lung cancer in underground miners in excess of that expected due to smoking. The studies with documented exposure and mortality data show that for exposures as low as 50 WLM, excess lung cancer is observed. This exposure is approximately the same as lifelong exposure in a home with a ^{222}Rn concentration at the current EPA guideline of $4\,\mathrm{pCi\,L^{-1}}$. The only difference between the mining and home exposures is that in underground mines the exposure was generally for a short period of time (< 20 years), whereas in the home it takes a lifelong to accumulate the same total exposure. The dose to the target cells in bronchial airways implicated in lung cancer is the same per unit exposure in both homes and mines.

It is thus reasonable to believe that environmental exposure to ^{222}Rn should be reduced, especially in homes with high concentrations. Smoking miners are at greater risk of lung cancer, by about a factor of 2, than nonsmoking miners given the same total exposure. This is likely true for environmental exposure, and stopping the use of tobacco is strongly encouraged. Good radon-resistance construction practices in new homes, and the identification and remediation of existing homes with high radon concentration, should reduce the risk for the long term.

REFERENCES

Axelson, O., and L. Sundell. 1978. Mining, lung cancer and smoking. *Scand. J. Work. Environ. Health* 46: 46–52.

Borak, T. B., and J. A. Johnson. 1988. Estimating the risk of lung cancer from inhalation of radon daughters indoors: Review and evaluation EPA 600/6-88/008. Environmental Monitoring Systems Laboratory, Las Vegas.

Chambers, D. B., L. M. Lowe, P. M. Reilly, and P. Duport. 1990. Effects of exposure uncertainty on estimation of radon risks. Presented at the 29th Hanford Symposium on Health and the Environment— Indoor Radon and Lung Cancer: Reality or Myth. Columbus, OH: Battelle Press. pp. 987–1012.

Chittaporn, P., and N. H. Harley. 1994. Water use contribution to indoor ^{222}Rn. *Health Phys.* S29: 529.

Cohen, B. L. 1987. Tests of the linear no-threshold dose response relationship for high LET radiation. *Health Phys.* 52: 629–636.

Cohen, B. L. 1990. A test of the linear-no threshold theory of radiation carcinogenesis. *Environ. Res.* 193: 193–220.

Cohen, B. L. 1992. A compilation and integration of studies of radon levels in U.S. homes by states and counties. *Crit. Rev. in Environ. Control* 22: 243–364.

Cohen, B. S., and B. Asgharian. 1990. Deposition of ultrafine particles in the upper airways: An empirical analysis. *J. Aerosol Sci.* 21: 789–797.

DOE/CEC 1989. International Workshop on Residential Radon Epidemiology. CONF-8907178. Springfield, VA: NTIS.

Edling, C. 1982. Lung cancer and smoking in a group of iron ore miners, *Am. J. Indust. Med.* 3: 191–199.

U.S. EPA. 1992. National Radon Survey Summary Report. U.S. Environmental Protection Agency EPA 402-R-92-011.

Fisenne, I. M. 1988. Radon-222 measurements at Chester, NJ, through July 1986. 1985–1986 Biennial Report of the EML Regional Baseline Station at Chester, NJ. Environmental Measurements Laboratory Report EML-504. New York.

Fisenne, I. M., and H. W. Keller. 1996. Continuous indoor and outdoor measurements of [222]Rn in New York City: City as a source. *Environ. International* 22: S131–138.

George, A. C., and A. J. Breslin. 1980. The distribution of ambient radon and radon daughters in residential buildings in the New Jersey–New York area, eds. T. F. Gesell, W. M. Lowder. Natural Radiation Environment III CONF-780422. Washington DC: DOE.

George, A. C., and L. Hinchliffe. 1972. Measurements of uncombined radon daughters in uranium mines. *Health Phys.* 23: 791–803.

Glauberman, H., and A. J. Breslin. 1957. Environmental radon concentrations U.S. Atomic Energy Commission, Health and Safety Laboratory Report NYO-4861. New York: HASL.

Harley, J. H. 1974. *Environmental Radon*, eds. R. E. Stanley, and A. A. Moghissi. In *Noble Gases*. CONF-730915 Washington DC: EPA.

Harley, J. H. 1990. Radon is out. Presented at the 29th Hanford Symposium on Health and the Environment—Indoor Radon and Lung Cancer: Reality or Myth. Columbus, OH: Battelle Press.

Harley, N. H. 1984. Comparing radon daughter dose: Environmental versus underground exposure. *Rad. Prot. Dosimetry* 20: 371–379.

Harley, N. H. 1988. Radon daughter dosimetry in the rat tracheobronchial tree. *RPD* 457.

Harley, N. H. 1989. Lung cancer risk from exposure to environmental radon. 3rd International Conference on Anticarcinogenesis and Radiation Protection, Dubrovnik.

Harley, N. H. 1991. Radon levels in a high-rise apartment. *Health Phys.* 61: 263–265.

Harley, N. H. 1991. A Personal and home [222]Rn and gamma-ray exposure measured in 52 dwellings@. *Health Phys.* 61: 737–744.

Harley, N. H., and E. S. Robbins. 1994. A biokinetic model for [222]Rn gas distribution and alpha dose in humans following ingestion. *Environ. International* 20: 605–610.

Harley, N. H., B. S. Cohen, and E. S. Robbins. 1996. The variability in radon decay product bronchial dose. *Environ. International* 22: S959–964.

Harley, N. H., O. A. Meyers, P. Chittaporn, and E. S. Robbins/ 1996. A biological model for lung cancer risk from [222]Rn exposure. *Environ. International* 22: S 977–989.

Harley, N. H. 1997. Outdoor radon measurements at two New Jersey sites. *Health Physics* (submitted).

Hess, C. T., M. A. Vietti, and D. T. Mager. 1987. Radon from drinking water: Evaluation of water borne transfer into house air. *Environ. Geochem. Health* 8: 68.

Hess, C. T., J. K. Korsah, and C. J. Einloth. 1985. Radon in houses due to radon in potable water. In *Radon and Its Decay Products*, ed. P. Hopke. ACS Symposium. p. 553, Washington, DC: American Chemical Society.

Hess, V. F. 1953. Radon, thoron and their decay products in the atmosphere, *J. Atmos. Terrest. Phys.* 3: 172–177.

Hopke, P. K, B. Jensen, C. S. Li, N. Montassier, P. Wasoliek, A. Cavallo, K. Gatsby, R. Socolow, and A. C. James. 1995. Assessment of the exposure to and dose from radon and decay products in normally occupied homes. *Environ. Sci. and Technol.* 29: 1359–1364.

Hornung, R. W., and T. J. Meinhardt. 1987. Quantitative risk assessment of lung cancer in U.S. uranium miners. *Health Phys.* 52: 417–430.

Hosler, C. R. 1968. Urban-rural climatology of atmospheric radon concentrations. *J. Geophys. Res.* 1155.

Howe, G. R., R. C. Nair, H. B. Newcombe, A. B. Miller, and J.D. Abbatt. 1986. Lung cancer mortality (1950–1980) in relation to radon daughter exposure in a cohort of workers at the Eldorado Beaverlodge uranium mine. *J. Nat. Cancer Inst.* 77: 357–362.

Howe, G. R., R. C. Nair, H. B. Newcombe, A. B. Miller, J. D. Burch, and J. D. Abbatt. 1987. Lung cancer mortality (1950–1980) in relation to radon daughter exposure in a cohort of workers at Eldorado Port Radium uranium mine. *J. Nat. Cancer Inst.* 79: 1255–1260.

Hultqvist, B. 1956. Studies on naturally occurring ionizing radiations—Thesis (in English), *Kgl. Svenska Vetenkaps Handl.* 3 (series 4).

ICRP. 1987. *Lung Cancer Risk from Indoor Exposures to Radon Daughters International Commission on Radiological Protection Publication 50*. Oxford: Pergamon Press.

Lubin, J. H., and J. D. Boice. 1989. Estimating Rn-induced lung cancer in the United States. *Health Physics* 57: 417–427.

Lubin, J. H., and J. D. Boice. 1997. Lung cancer risk from residential radon meta-analysis of eight epidemiologic studies. *J. Nat. Cancer Inst.* 89: 49–57.

Lubin, J. H., Q. You-Lin, P. R. Taylor, Y. Shu-Xiang, A. Schatzkin, M. Bao-Lin, R. Jian-Yu, and X. Xiang-Zhen. 1990. Quantitative evaluation of the radon and lung cancer association in a case control study of Chinese tin miners. *Cancer Res.* 50: 174–180.

Lundin, F. E., J. K. Wagoner, and V. E. Archer. 1971. Radon daughter exposure and respiratory cancer: Quantitative and temporal aspects. *National Institute for Occupational Safety and Health and National Institute for Environmental Health Sciences Joint Monograph.* Springfield, VA: NTIS.

Morrison, H. I., R. M. Semenciw, Y. Mao, and D. T. Wigle. 1988. Cancer mortality among a group of fluorspar miners exposed to radon progeny. *Am. J. Epidemiol.* 128: 1266–1275.

Moses, H., H. F. Lucas, and G. A. Zerbe. 1963. The effect of meteorological variables upon radon concentration three feet above the ground. *JAPCA* 13: 12–19.

Muller, J., R. Kusiak, and A. C. Ritchie. 1989. Factors modifying lung cancer risk in Ontario uranium miners, 1955–1981. Ontario Ministry of Labour Report. Ministry of Labour, Toronto.

Muller, J., R. A. Kusiak, G. Suranyi, and A. C. Ritchie. 1986. Study of mortality of Ontario gold miners, 1955–1977. Ontario Ministry of Labor, Toronto.

Muller, J., W. C. Wheeler, J. F. Gentleman, G. Suranyi, and R. A. Kusiak. 1983. Study of mortality of Ontario miners. Ontario Ministry of Labor, Toronto.

NCRP. 1984a. Evaluation of occupational and environmental exposures to radon and radon daughters in the United States. National Council on Radiation Protection and Measurements Report 78. NCRP, Bethesda, MD.

NCRP. 1984b. Exposures from the uranium series with emphasis on radon and its daughters. National Council on Radiation Protection and Measurements Report 77. NCRP, Bethesda, MD.

NCRP. 1987a. Exposure to the population in the United States and Canada from natural background radiation. National Council on Radiation Protection and Measurements Report 94. NCRP, Bethesda, MD.

NCRP. 1987b. Ionizing radiation exposure of the population of the United States. National Council on Radiation Protection and Measurements Report 93. NCRP, Bethesda, MD.

NCRP. 1988. Measurement of radon and radon daughters in air. National Council on Radiation Protection and Measurements Report 97. NCRP, Bethesda, MD.

NCRP. 1989. Radon. *Proc. 24th Annual Meeting of the National Council on Radiation Protection and Measurements.* Bethesda, MD: NCRP.

NRC. 1988. *Health Risks of Radon and Other Internally Deposited Alpha-Emitters.* National Academy of Sciences Report BEIR IV. Washington, DC: National Academy Press.

NRC. 1999a. *Health Effects of Exposure to Radon.* BEIR VI. Board on Radiation Effects Research. Commission on Life Sciences. National Research Council. Washington, DC: National Academy Press.

NRC. 1999b. *Risk Assessment of Radon in Drinking Water.* Board on Radiation Effects Research. National Research Council. Washington DC: National Academy Press.

Nero, A. V. 1983. Indoor radiation exposures from Rn-222 and its daughters: A view of the issue. *Health Phys.* 45: 277–288.

Nero, A. V., M. B. Schwehr, W. W. Nazaroff, and K. L. Revzan. 1986. Distribution of airborne radon-222 concentrations in U.S. homes. *Science* 234: 992–996.

Neuberger, J. S. 1989. Worldwide studies of household radon exposure and lung cancer. Final Report to the U.S. Department of Energy, Office of Health and Environmental Research. (U.S. DOE, Washington, DC.

Neuberger, J. S., N. H. Harley, and B. C. Kross. 1996. Residential radon exposure and lung cancer potential for pooled or meta analysis. *J. Clean Technol. Environ. Occup. Med.* 5: 207–221.

Pershagen, G., G. Ackerblom, O. Axelson, B. Clavensjo, L. Damber, G. Desai, A. Enflo, F. LaGarde, H. Mellander, M. Svartengren, and G. A. Swedjemark. 1994. Residential radon exposure and lung cancer in Sweden. *N. Eng. J. Med.* 330: 159–164.

Put, L. W., and R. J. deMeijer. 1988. Variation of time-averaged indoor and outdoor radon concentrations with time, location and sampling height. *Rad. Prot. Dosimetry* 317.

Radford, E. P., and K. G. S. Renard. 1984. Lung cancer in Swedish iron miners exposed to low doses of radon daughters. *New Eng. J. Med.* 310: 1485–1494.

Reilly, M. A. 1990. The index house: Pennsylvania radon research and demonstration project, Pottstown, PA 1986–1988. In *Environmental Radon Occurrence and Control*, eds. S. K. Majumdar, R. F. Schmaltz, and E. W. Miller, pp. 26–38. Philadelphia: Pennsylvania Academy of Sciences.

Reineking, A., G. Butterweck, J. Kesten, and J. Porstendorfer. 1990. Unattached fraction and size distribution of aerosol-attached radon and thoron daughters in realistic living atmospheres and their influence on radiation dose eds. F. Cross. pp. 129–147. Presented at the 29th Hanford Symposium on Health and the Environment- Indoor Radon and Lung Cancer: Reality or Myth. Columbus, OH: Battelle Press.

Reineking, A., and J. Porstendorfer. 1986. High-volume screen diffusion batteries and alpha-spectroscopy for measurement of the radon daughter activity size distributions in the environment. *J. Aerosol Sci.* 17: 873–879.

Robbins, E. S. 1990. Cellular morphometry in human bronchial epithelium. Private communication.

Roscoe, R. J., K. Steenland, W. E. Halperin, J. J. Beaumont, and R. J. Waxweiler. 1989. Lung cancer mortality among nonsmoking uranium miners exposed to radon. *JAMA* 262: 629.

Roscoe, R. J., J. A. Deddens, A. Salvan, and T. M. Schnorr. 1995. Mortality among Navajo uranium miners *Am. J. Public Health* 85: 535–540.

Rundo, J., F. Markun, and N. J. Plondke. 1979. Observation of high concentrations of radon in certain houses. *Health Phys.* 36: 729–730.

Ruzer, L. S., A. V. Nero, and N. H. Harley. 1995. Assessment of lung deposition and breathing rate in underground miners in Tadjikistan. *Rad. Prot. Dosimetry* 58: 261–268.

Sachs, H. M., T. L. Hernandez, and J. W. Ring. 1982. Regional geology and radon variability in buildings. *Envir. Intern.* 8: 97.

Saccomanno, G., O. Auerbach, M. Kuschner, N. H. Harley, R. Y. Michaels, M. W. Anderson, and J. J. Bechtel. 1996. A comparison between the localization of lung tumors in uranium miners and in nonminers from 1947 to 1991. *Cancer* 77: 1278–1283.

Samet, J. M. 1989. Epidemiological studies of lung cancer in underground miners. Proceedings No. 10. NCRP, 30.

Samet, J. M., O. M. Kutvirt, R. J. Waxweiler, and C. R. Key. 1984. Uranium mining and lung cancer in Navaho men. *N. Engl. J. Med.* 310: 1481–1484.

Samet, J.M., D. R. Pathak, M. V. Morgan, M. C. Marbury, C. R. Key, and A. A. Valdivia. 1989. Radon progeny exposure and lung cancer risk in New Mexico U miners: A case control study. *Health Physics*, 56: 415–420.

Schoenberg, J. B., J. B. Klotz, H. B. Wilcox, G. P. Nicholls, M. T. Gil-del-Real, A. Stemhagen, and T. J. Mason. 1990. Case-control study of residential radon and lung cancer among New Jersey women *Cancer Res.* 50: 6520–6524.

Servant, J. 1966. Temporal and spatial variations of the concentration of the short-lived decay products of radon in the lower atmosphere. *Tellus* 663.

Sevc, J., E. Kunz, and V. Placek. 1976. Lung cancer in uranium mines and long-term exposure to radon daughters. *Health Phys.* 20: 433–437.

Sevc, J., E. Kunz, V. Placek, and A. Smid. 1984. Comments on lung cancer risk estimates. *Health Phys.* 46: 961–964.

Sevc, J., E. Kunz, L. Tomasek, V. Placek, and J. Horacek 1988. Cancer in man after exposure to Rn daughters. *Health Phys.* 54: 27–46.

Tirmarche, M., J. Brenot, J. Piechowski, J. Chameaud, and J. Pradel. 1985. The present state of an epidemiological study of uranium miners in France. In *Occupational Radiation Safety in Mining, vol. 1*, ed. H. Stocker, pp. 344–349, Toronto.

Tu, K. W., and E. O. Knutson. 1988. Indoor outdoor aerosol measurements for two residential buildings in New Jersey. *Aerosol Sci. Tech.* 9: 71–82.

Whittemore, A. S. and A. McMillan. 1983. Lung cancer mortality among U.S. uranium miners. *J. Natl. Cancer Inst.* 71: 489–499.

Woodward, A., D. Roder, A. J. McMichael, P. Crouch, and A. Mylvaganam. 1991. Radon daughter exposures at the Radium Hill uranium mine and lung cancer rates among former workers, 1952–1987. *Cancer Causes Control* 2: 213–220.

Wright, J. R., and O. F. Smith. 1915. The variation with meteorological conditions of the amount of radon emanation in the atmosphere, in the soil gas and in the air exhaled from the surface of the ground in Manila. *Phys. Rev.* 5: 459.

23 Sulfur Oxides: Acidic Aerosols and SO₂

MORTON LIPPMANN, Ph.D.

A variety of gaseous and particulate chemicals in the ambient air are acidic, and some of them are known to have produced health effects in exposed populations. The best documented of the effects in laboratory studies are attributable to strong acids in aerosol form, namely sulfuric acid (H_2SO_4) and ammonium bisulfate (NH_4HSO_4) (U.S. EPA, 1989). Strong acids that are present in the atmosphere as vapors, such as anhydrous nitric acid (HNO_3) and hydrochloric acid (HCl), have not been shown to produce measurable health effects at commonly encountered ambient air levels, although one controlled laboratory study did report a bronchoconstrictive response in adolescent asthmatics at 50 parts per billion by volume (ppb) HNO_3 (Koenig et al., 1989). Among the weak acids, sulfur dioxide (SO_2) and its hydrolysis products have been associated with both acute bronchoconstriction and elevated morbidity and mortality rates. With respect to these elevated rates, SO_2 may have been a surrogate for its oxidation products and other particulate pollutants that often coexist with SO_2. Nitrogen dioxide (NO_2) is both an oxidant and a source of hydrogen ion (H^+) upon hydrolysis on airway surfaces. Some of the health effects associated with NO_2 may therefore be caused by its acidity (U.S. EPA, 1993). In any case the health effects associated with ambient exposures to nitrogen oxides are much harder to document and appear to be of less public health concern than those associated with exposures to the sulfur oxides.

Other airborne acids include hydroxymethanesulfonate, a reaction product of SO_2 and formaldehyde (HCHO), as well as a variety of organic acids. However, these acids have not, to date, been associated with measurable health effects at ambient environmental levels. Leung and Paustenbach (1990) have proposed occupational exposure guidelines for 13 organic acids based on their irritancy as predicted by their dissociation constants.

This chapter summarizes and discusses the health effects attributable to SO_2 and acidic aerosols at concentrations that have been monitored or measured in community and industrial atmospheres. The role of acidic aerosols in the health effects associated with ambient air particulate matter (PM) is also discussed in Chapter 2. This chapter does not discuss effects associated with exposures to these or other acidic pollutants at much higher concentrations because of their lack of relevance to the subject at issue: the health effects of atmospheric acidity.

Environmental Toxicants: Human Exposures and Their Health Effects, 2/e. Edited by Morton Lippmann.
ISBN: 0-471-29298-2 © 2000 John Wiley & Sons, Inc.

SOURCES AND EXPOSURES

Sources of Sulfur Oxides

Most of the sulfur in fossil fuel is converted into SO$_2$ in the combustion zone, and it is vented to the atmosphere with the other products of combustion. A small fraction of the sulfur, generally less than 10%, is emitted as sulfuric acid (H$_2$SO$_4$), with some of it forming a surface film on ultrafine-sized mineral ash particles. When the discharge point is a tall stack, most of the SO$_2$ escapes local deposition on terrestrial surfaces and is gradually (1–10%/h) converted into SO$_3$, a highly hygroscopic vapor. The SO$_3$ rapidly combines with water vapor to produce an ultrafine droplet aerosol of H$_2$SO$_4$. The H$_2$SO$_4$ is then gradually neutralized by ammonia, first to the strong acid ammonium bisulfate (NH$_4$HSO$_4$) and then to ammonium sulfate [(NH$_4$)$_2$SO$_4$), a nearly neutral salt. Rates of ammonia neutralization vary widely, depending on emission rates from ground-based sources. Rates are high over cities and agricultural areas, low over forests, and virtually nil over deep water bodies.

The ratios between SO$_2$, H$_2$SO$_4$, and total particulate sulfate (SO$_4^{2-}$) in the atmosphere are highly variable in space and time. While ambient concentration data are relatively plentiful for SO$_2$ and, to less extent, for SO$_4^{2-}$, they are, unfortunately, very sparse for H$_2$SO$_4$ and NH$_4$HSO$_4$, the strong acid aerosols that may account for much of the mortality and morbidity historically associated with mixtures of SO$_2$ and particulate matter (PM). SO$_2$ is a very poor surrogate index for ambient concentrations of acid aerosols, but SO$_4^{2-}$ can often serve as an excellent surrogate in some parts of the United States.

One of the few significant indoor sources of SO$_2$ and H$_2$SO$_4$ is the unvented kerosene space heater. The sulfur content of kerosene is generally within the ASTM D-3699 standard of 0.04%. Leaderer et al. (1990) studied pollutant emissions from four portable kerosene space heaters using kerosene containing 0.039% sulfur. The heaters were operated in a 34 m^3 room at 1.4 air changes per hour. Background chamber pollution levels were low. On a mass balance basis, sulfate accounted for 2–26% of the sulfur in the fuel, with the balance emitted as SO$_2$. Sulfate concentrations ranged from 33 to 693 µg/ m^3, and acidic particulates, as H$_2$SO$_4$, ranged from 1.3 to 75 µg/m^3. Since the sulfur content of kerosene has been reduced since 1990, these concentrations may represent upper limits.

Exposures to Sulfur Oxides

Current U.S. ambient air levels of SO$_2$ are generally well within the current primary National Ambient Air Quality Standard (NAAQS) of 80 µg/m^3 for an annual average and 365 µg/m^3 for a 24 hour maximum. There is an additional special concern for asthmatics' peak exposures to SO$_2$ while performing outdoor exercise. It has been estimated that the size of the asthmatic population with peak 5 to 10 minute exposures at concentrations > 0.2 ppm (520 µg/m^3) during light to moderate exercise, who may exhibit a bronchoconstrictive response, varies from 5000 to 50,000.

For acidic aerosols there is a very limited ambient concentration data base. The latest EPA Criteria Document for PM (U.S. EPA, 1996a) summarized the available data from research investigations. Levels of acidic aerosol in excess of 20–40 µg/m^3 (as H$_2$SO$_4$) have been observed for time durations ranging from 1 to 12 hours. These were associated with high but not necessarily the highest atmospheric SO$_4^{2-}$ levels. Exposures (concentration-time product) of 100 to 900 µg/m^3-h were calculated for the acid events that were monitored. In contrast, earlier London studies indicated that acidity in excess of 100 µg/m^3 (as H$_2$SO$_4$) were present in the atmosphere, and exposures >2000 µg/m^3-hr were possible.

The first data on annual average acidic aerosol concentrations in contemporary U.S. communities were reported by Spengler et al. (1989). In the four eastern U.S. communities studied, the annual average ranged up to $1.8\,\mu g/m^3$ (as H_2SO_4).

Brauer et al. (1989) measured exposures to acidic and basic vapors and aerosols with a personal annular denuder/filter pack sampler and compared the results to those measured at a centrally located monitoring site in the metropolitan Boston, Massachusetts, area. Personal exposures to aerosol H^+ were only slightly lower than the concentrations at the central monitor, and personal SO_4^{2-} and NH_4^+ were similar to central site values. By contrast, SO_2 and HNO_3 were much lower for personal exposures than at the central site.

Meteorology and regional transport are extremely important to acid sulfate concentrations. Keeler et al. (1991) measured elevated levels of ambient H^+ simultaneously during a regional episode at multiple sites located from Tennessee to Connecticut, and Lamborg et al. (1992) measured H^+ concentrations to investigate the behavior of regional and urban plumes advecting across Lake Michigan. Their results suggested that aerosol acidity is maintained over long distances (up to 100 km or more) in air masses moving over large bodies of water. Lee et al. (1993) reported that H^+ and $SO_4^=$ concentrations measured in Chicago over a year were similar to levels measured in St. Louis. In an analysis of acid sulfate concentrations measured at Pittsburgh, State College, and Uniontown, Pennsylvania, Liu et al. (1996) reported high correlations for H^+ between all three locations. The three locations are separated by large distances (approximately 60–240 km) and have vastly different population densities. The conversion of SO_2 to acidic aerosols takes place as the prevailing winds carry the precursors from the source region in the midwest, northeast to the northeastern United States and southwestern Canada. This type of northeasterly wind flow occurs on the backside (western side) of mid-latitude anticyclones (high-pressure systems).

Highest atmospheric acidity was associated with (1) slow westerly winds traversing westward SO_2 source areas, (2) local stagnation, or (3) regional transport around to the back side of a high-pressure system. Low acidity was associated with fast-moving air masses and with winds from the northerly directions; upwind precipitation also played a moderating role in air parcel acidity. Much of the SO_2 and aerosol H^+ appeared to have originated from coal-fired power plants.

Size distributions of aerosol H^+ and $SO_4^=$ were alike, with MMAD about 0.7 μm, in the optimum range for efficient light scattering and inefficient wet/dry removal. Thus light scattering and visual range degradation were attributable to the acidic $SO_4^=$ aerosol. With inefficient removal of aerosol H^+ strong acids may be capable of long-distance transport in the lower troposphere. Water associated with the acidic aerosol was shown to account for much of the light scattering.

A study of acid aerosols and ammonia (Suh et al., 1992) found no significant spatial variation of H^+ at Uniontown, Pennsylvania, a suburb of Pittsburgh. Measurements at the central monitoring site accounted for 92% of the variability in outdoor concentrations measured at various homes throughout the town. There was no statistical difference ($p > 0.01$) between concentrations of outdoor H^+ among five sites (a central site and four satellite sites) in Newtown, Connecticut (Thompson et al., 1991). However, there were differences in peak values that were probably related to the proximity of the sampling sites to ammonia sources. These studies suggest that long-term averages should not substantially differ across a suburban community, although peak values may differ significantly.

In small suburban communities outdoor concentrations of H^+ are fairly uniform, suggesting that minor differences in population density do not significantly affect outdoor H^+ or NH_3 concentrations (Suh et al., 1992). In urban areas, however, both H^+ and NH_3 exhibit significant spatial variation. Waldman et al. (1990) measured ambient concentrations of H^+, NH_3, and $SO_4^=$ at three locations in metropolitan Toronto. The sites, located up to 33 km apart, had significant differences in outdoor concentrations of H$^+$. Waldman and coworkers reported that the sites with higher NH$_3$ measured lower H$^+$ concentrations.

An intensive monitoring study was conducted during the summers of 1992 and 1993 in Philadelphia (Suh et al., 1995). Twenty-four hour measurements of aerosol acidity (H$^+$) sulfate and NH$_3$ were collected simultaneously at 7 sites in metropolitan Philadelphia and at Valley Forge, 30 km northwest of the city center. The researchers reported that SO$_4^=$ was evenly distributed throughout the measurement area but H$^+$ concentrations varied spatially within metropolitan Philadelphia. This variation was related to local NH$_3$ concentrations and varied spatially within metropolitan Philadelphia. This variation was related to local NH$_3$ concentrations and the local population density (Fig. 23-1). The amount of NH$_3$ available to neutralize H$^+$ increased with population density, resulting in lower H$^+$ concentrations in more densely populated areas. The extent of the spatial variation in H$^+$ concentrations did not appear to depend on the overall H$^+$ concentration. It did, however, show a strong inverse association with local NH$_3$ concentrations.

An analysis of results from Harvard's 24 city study (Thompson et al., 1991; Spengler et al., 1996), which measured acid aerosols concentrations at 8 different small cities across North America each year during a three year period, revealed that the summer H$^+$ mean concentrations were significantly higher than the annual means at all sites. The results showed that at the sites with high H$^+$ concentrations, approximately two-thirds of the aerosol acidity occurred from May through September (Fig. 23-2). Little or no seasonal variation was observed at sites with low acidity. These findings were supported by those of Thurston et al. (1992a) in which H$^+$ concentrations measured at Buffalo, Albany, and

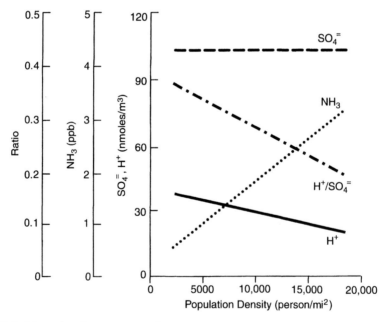

Figure 23-1 Mean air pollutant concentrations for days when winds were from the southerly direction, plotted versus population density. The solid line represents H$^+$ concentrations, the long dashed line represents SO$_4^{2-}$ concentrations, the dashed and dotted line represents the ratio of H$^+$ to SO$_4^{2-}$ levels, and the dotted line represents NH$_3$ concentrations. All data collected in Philadelphia during the summers of 1992 and 1993. (Source: Adapted from Suh et al., 1995)

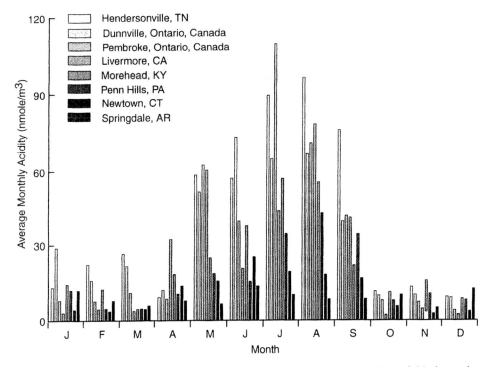

Figure 23-2 Average monthly aerosol strong acidity for year 1 sites of the Harvard 24 city study. (Source: Thompson et al., 1991)

White Plains, New York, were found to be highest during the summertime. Thurston and coworkers also reported that moderate concentrations of H^+ could occur during nonsummer months.

Evidence exists of a distinct diurnal pattern in outdoor H^+ concentrations. Wilson et al. (1991) examined concentration data for H^+, NH_3, and $SO_4^=$ from the Harvard 24 city study for evidence of diurnal variability (Fig. 23-3). This investigation found a distinct diurnal pattern for H^+ concentrations and the $H^+/SO_4^=$ ratio, with daytime concentrations being substantially higher than nighttime levels. Both H^+ and $SO_4^=$ concentrations peaked between noon and 6:00 p.m. No such diurnal variation was found for NH_3. Wilson and coworkers concluded that the diurnal variation in H^+ and $SO_4^=$ was probably due to atmospheric mixing. Air containing high concentrations of H^+ and $SO_4^=$ mixes downward during daylight hours when the atmosphere is unstable and well-mixed. During the night, ammonia emitted from ground-based sources neutralizes the acid in nocturnal boundary layer, the very stable lower part of the atmosphere, but a nocturnal inversion prevents the ammonia from reacting with the acid aerosols aloft. Then in the morning, as the nocturnal inversion dissipates, the acid aerosols mix downward again as the process begins anew. Spengler et al. (1986) also noted diurnal variations in sulfate and sulfuric acid concentrations and suggested atmospheric dynamics as the cause. The diurnal variation in $SO_4^=$ has been observed by other workers and discussed in terms of atmospheric dynamics by Wolff et al. (1979) and Wilson and Stockberger (1990).

A recent summary of intercommunity differences in strong acid aerosol concentrations in the Harvard 6 city and multicity studies, and in the New York University studies in three New York State communities was provided by Ozkaynak et al. (1996).

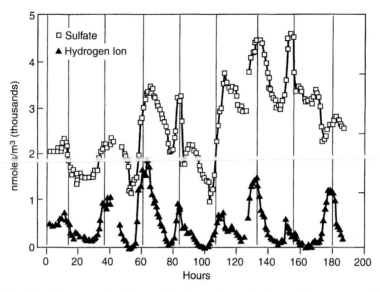

Figure 23-3 Diurnal pattern of sulfate and hydrogen ion at Harriman, Tennessee, weekly pattern. (Source: Wilson et al., 1991).

HEALTH EFFECTS

Health Effects of SO₂

Dosimetry of Inhaled SO₂   As a water-soluble acidic vapor, SO₂ is highly efficiently captured in the upper respiratory tract during inhalation, and virtually none penetrates to the lungs during normal, quiescent breathing. However, during vigorous physical activity there is less residence time in the upper airways, and in humans, a shift to oronasal breathing involving partial flow through the less efficient oral passages. Under exercise conditions, some inhaled SO₂ can penetrate to the smaller conductive airways of the lungs and perhaps beyond them. Skornik and Brain (1990) showed that hamsters exposed to SO₂ while running had reduced pulmonary macrophage endocytosis of particles in comparison to sham-exposed animals.

Acute Bronchoconstrictive Effects of SO₂ in Humans   When asthmatics and others with hyper-reactive airways are exposed to SO₂ at 0.25 to 0.50 ppm and higher while exercising, the most striking acute response is rapid bronchoconstriction (airway narrowing), usually evidenced in increased airway resistance, decreased expiratory flow rates, and the occurrence of symptoms such as wheezing and shortness of breath. Similar responses can be produced in healthy persons but require exposure concentrations about an order of magnitude higher and outside the range of ambient levels.

The penetration of SO₂ to sensitive portions of respiratory tract is largely determined by the efficiency of the oral or nasal mucosa in absorbing SO₂, which in turn depends on the mode of breathing (nasal, oral, or oronasal) and the rate of airflow. Controlled SO₂ exposure studies on asthmatics show that at comparable SO₂ concentrations, bronchoconstrictive effects increase with increased ventilation rates and with the relative contribution of oral ventilation to total ventilation (Bethel et al., 1983; Roger et al., 1985). Increased oral ventilation not only allows more direct penetration of SO₂ but may also result in airway drying and changes in surface liquids, affecting SO_2 absorption and penetration. Evaporation of airway surface liquid and perhaps convective cooling of the airways caused by cold dry air can act as direct bronchoconstrictive stimuli in asthmatics (Deal et al., 1979; Strauss et al., 1977; Anderson, 1985). The combined effect of SO_2 and cold, dry air further exacerbates the asthmatic response (Bethel et al., 1984; Sheppard et al., 1984; Linn et al., 1985). The bronchoconstrictive effects of SO_2 are reduced under warm, humid conditions (Linn et al., 1985). In order to determine whether bronchoconstriction induced by SO_2 can be predicted by the airway response to inhaled histamine, Magnussen et al. (1990) exposed 46 patients with asthma to air or 0.5 ppm SO_2 on two days. The exposure protocol consisted of 10 minutes of tidal breathing followed by 10 minutes of isocapnic hyperventilation at a rate of 30 L/min. Airway response was measured before (baseline) and after hyperventilation in terms of specific airway resistance, SR_{AW}. Exposure to air increased baseline mean SR_{AW} by 45%. Exposure to SO_2 with hyperinflation increased mean baseline SR_{AW} by 163%. When evaluated individually, 26 and 34 of the 46 patients showed an airway response to hyperventilation of air and SO_2, respectively. Airway response to histamine was determined as the histamine concentration necessary to increase specific airway resistance by 100%. The airway response after SO_2 and histamine showed a weak but significant correlation ($R = -0.48$), whereas the responses to hyperventilation and SO_2 did not correlate. Thus the mechanisms by which histamine and SO_2 exert their bronchomotor effects are different, and the risk of SO_2-induced asthmatic symptoms can be poorly predicted by histamine responsiveness.

The response to inhaled SO_2 can also be exacerbated by prior exposure to ozone (O_3). Koenig et al. (1990) exposed eight male and five female adolescent asthmatics during intermittent exercise to a sequence of atmospheres, with 45 minutes to one followed by 15 minutes to the other. The combinations were (1) air—100 ppb SO_2; (2) 120 ppb O_3—120 ppb O_3; and (3) 120 ppb O_3—100 ppb SO_2. Air-SO_2 and O_3-O_3 did not cause significant changes in function. By contrast, O_3-SO_2 produced significant changes, namely an 8% decline in FEV_1, a 19% increase in total flow resistance, and a 15% decrease in V_{max50}.

By contrast, Rubinstein et al. (1990) found that prior 30 minute exposures to nitrogen dioxide (NO_2) at 0.3 ppm did not potentiate the responses of asthmatics to subsequent 1 hour exposures SO_2 at concentrations of 0.25 to 4 ppm.

The time required for SO_2 exposure to elicit significant bronchoconstriction in exercising asthmatics is brief. Exposure durations as short as 2 minutes at 1.0 ppm have produced significant responses (Horstman et al., 1988). Little enhancement of response is apparent on prolonged exposure beyond 5 minutes, although some suggestion of an increase is seen with continuous exercise between 10 and 30 minutes (Kehrl et al., 1987). Following a single SO_2 exposure during exercise, airway resistance in asthmatics appears to require a recovery period of 1 to 2 hours (Hackney et al., 1984).

The magnitude of response induced by any given SO_2 concentration is variable among individual asthmatics. Exposures to SO_2 concentrations of 0.25 ppm or less, which do not induce significant group mean increases in airway resistance, do not cause symptomatic bronchoconstriction. On the other hand, exposures to 0.40 ppm SO_2 or greater (combined with moderate to heavy exercise), which induce significant group mean increases in airway resistance, cause substantial bronchoconstriction in some individual asthmatics. This bronchoconstriction is often associated with wheezing and the perception of respiratory distress, sometimes necessitating the discontinuance of the exposure and the provision of medication. The significance of these observations is that some SO_2-sensitive asthmatics are at risk of experiencing symptomatic bronchoconstriction requiring termination of activity and/or medical intervention when exposed to SO_2 concentrations of 0.40 to 0.50 ppm ($1040-1300\,\mu g/m^3$) or greater when this exposure is accompanied by at least moderate activity. These concentrations can occur downwind of point sources as 10 minute averages.

Various studies have examined exposure–response relationships over various concentration and ventilation ranges. Some examined the influence of various subject-related and environmental factors. Since the individual studies used different conditions of airway entry, ventilation rate, concentration, and so on it is difficult to compare directly the results from different investigations. An approach used by Kleinman (1984) and Linn et al. (1983) normalizes studies according to effective oral dose rate. They showed that reasonably consistent results are derived from the various controlled SO_2 asthmatic studies when adjustments are made for differences in ventilation rates and oral/nasal breathing patterns.

Associations between Ambient SO_2 and Rates of Mortality and Morbidity   Evidence for effects of SO_2 other than short-term bronchoconstriction is less direct. There is a considerable body of epidemiological evidence demonstrating statistically significant associations between SO_2 and rates of mortality and morbidity. However, it is less likely that SO_2 was a causal factor than that it was serving as a surrogate exposure index for other pollutants in the sulfur oxide–particulate complex deriving from fossil fuel combustion.

Mortality   After exhaustive review of the London mortality data from 1958 to 1972, the U.S. EPA (1986) concluded

1. Markedly increased mortality occurred, mainly among the elderly and chronically ill, in association with black smoke (BS) and SO_2 concentrations above $1000\,\mu g/m^3$, especially during episodes when such pollutant elevations occurred for several consecutive days.
2. The relative contributions of BS and SO_2 cannot be clearly distinguished from those of each other, nor can the effects of other factors be clearly delineated, although it appears likely that coincident high humidity (fog) was also important (possibly in providing conditions leading to formation of H_2SO_4 or other acidic aerosols).
3. Increased risk of mortality is associated with exposure to BS and SO_2 levels in the range of 500 to $1000\,\mu g/m^3$, clearly at concentrations in excess of 700 to $750\,\mu g/m^3$.
4. Less certain evidence suggests possible slight increases in the risk of mortality of BS levels below $500\,\mu g/m^3$, with no specific threshold levels having yet been demonstrated or ruled out at lower concentrations of BS (e.g., at $150\,\mu g/m^3$), nor potential contribution of other plausibly confounding variables having yet been fully evaluated.

Other studies examined pollutant/mortality relationships in New York City, Pittsburgh, and Athens, Greece. The Ozkaynak and Spengler (1985) reanalysis of 14 years of New York City data (1963–76) found significant associations between excess daily mortality and airborne particulate matter (PM), SO_2, and temperature. Differences in the rate of change of SO_2 and PM indicators during the study period allowed estimation of their separate effects. In joint regression analysis across all years, PM indicators (coefficient of haze and visibility extinction coefficient) together accounted for significantly greater excess mortality than did SO_2.

For Pittsburgh, Mazumdar and Sussman (1983) found a significant association between PM and excess deaths but no effect of SO_2. On the other hand, Hatzakis et al. (1986) found an association with SO_2, but not with smoke measurements, in Athens, Greece.

Morbidity   The studies of Lawther and colleagues (Lawther, 1958; Lawther et al., 1970) showed associations between 24 hour average concentrations of SO_2 of about $0.18\,ppm$

($500\,\mu g/m^3$), in association with BS of about $250\,\mu g/m^3$, and a worsening of health status among chronic bronchitis patients in London in the 1950s and 1960s.

Schenker et al. (1983) reported that wheeze was more prevalent in nonsmoking women living downwind from mine-mouth coal-burning electric utility plants than among women in control communities with less exposure to the effluents. There was a significant association with SO_2, the only effluent measured, and the highest exposure group had 24 hour and annual average SO_2 levels that were between 100% and 125% of the U.S. standards.

Bates and Sizto (1983) reported that daily rates of hospital admissions for respiratory diseases in southern Ontario during the summer were associated with ambient levels of SO_2 with 24 and 48 hour lags. However, subsequent analyses of data from this population showed that there were stronger associations with the sulfate content of the aerosol than with gaseous pollutants such as SO_2 or ozone (O_3) (Bates and Sizto, 1987).

For an acidic pollution episode in January 1985 in the Ruhr district in West Germany in which average concentrations of SO_2 and suspended particles were 800 and $600\,\mu g/m^3$, Wichmann et al. (1989) reported significant increases in deaths, hospital admissions, outpatient visits, and ambulance deliveries to hospitals in comparison to those in a less polluted control area.

Baskurt et al. (1990) studied the hematogical and hemorheological effects of an air pollution episode in Ankara, Turkey, using SO_2 as a surrogate of the pollution mixture. The blood measurements were made on 16 young male military students. The mean SO_2 levels at a station proximal to the campus where the students lived were $188\,\mu g/m^3$ and $201\,\mu g/m^3$ during first and second blood measurements, respectively. During the period between the two measurements, the mean sulfur dioxide level was $292\,\mu g/m^3$. Significant erythropoiesis was indicated by increased erythrocyte counts and hemoglobin and hematocrit levels. Methemoglobin percentage was increased to $2.37 \pm 0.47\%$ (mean $\pm$ standard error) from $0.51 \pm 0.23\%$. Sulfhemoglobinemia was present in six subjects after the period of pollution, but it was not present in any student prior to this period. Significant increases in erythrocyte deformability indexes were observed after the period of pollution, namely from 1.13 ± 0.01 to 1.21 ± 0.02, implying that erythrocytes were less flexible, which might impair tissue perfusion.

Other short-term responses to PM–SO_2 mixtures have been seen in children. Repeated measurements of lung function by Dockery et al. (1982) in schoolchildren in Steubenville, Ohio, in 1978–1980 showed statistically significant but physiologically small and apparently reversible declines of FVC and $FEV_{0.75}$ levels to be associated with short-term increases in PM and SO_2. The highest 24 hour average PM and SO_2 concentrations were 422 and $455\,\mu g/m^3$, respectively. The small, reversible decrements persisted for up to 3 to 4 weeks after episodic exposures.

A study of the association between episodic exposures to particulate matter and SO_2 and pulmonary function in children was conducted in the Netherlands by Dassen et al. (1986) producing results similar to those of Dockery et al. (1982). Pulmonary function values measured during an air pollution episode in which both 24 hour average PM and SO_2 levels reached 200 to $250\,\mu g/m^3$ were significantly lower (3–5%) than baseline values measured 1–2 months earlier in the same group of Dutch school children. Lung function parameters that showed significant declines included FVC and FEV_1 as well as measures of small airway function. Declines from baseline were observed 2 weeks after the episode in a different subset of children, but not after 3.5 weeks in a third subgroup.

Studies of associations between chronic exposure to SO_2 and PM and long-term changes in respiratory function in children have also been performed. Arossa et al. (1987) reported on the changes in baseline lung function between 1981 and 1983 in 1880 schoolchildren living in or near Turin, Italy. During that interval, annual average SO_2 in central Turin decreased from about $200\,\mu g/m^3$ to about $110\,\mu g/m^3$, and total suspended particulate matter dropped from about 150 to about 100 µg/m^3. During the same period SO$_2$ in a suburban area declined from nearly 70 to about 50 µg/m^3. A group of 162 children from the suburban area served as controls. In the first survey, FEV$_1$, FEF$_{25-75}$, and MEF$_{50}$ of children from urban areas were significantly lower, while in the second survey they were not significantly different from those of the controls. The slopes over time of FEV$_1$, FEF$_{25-75}$, and MEF$_{50}$, adjusted for sex and anthropometric variables, were closely related to the decrease of pollutant concentrations, suggesting that the decrease of air pollution produced an improvement of baseline lung function.

Summary of Health Effects of SO$_2$ In summary, the more quantitative epidemiological evidence from London suggests that effects may occur at SO$_2$ levels at or above 0.19 ppm (500 µg/m^3), 24 hour average, in combination with elevated particle levels. Additional evidence suggests the possibility of short-term, reversible declines in lung function at SO$_2$ levels above 250 to 450 µg/m^3 (0.10–0.18 ppm). These effects could be due to SO$_2$ alone, formation of sulfuric acid or other irritant aerosols, other particles, or peak SO$_2$ values well above the daily mean, but the relative roles of these factors cannot be determined at this time. We do know that the capacity of fog particles to "carry" untransformed SO$_2$ is limited. Thus, it appears more likely that the role of SO$_2$, in the presence of smoke, involved transformation products such as acidic fine particles.

The statistically significant associations between annual average levels of SO$_2$ and chronic disease endpoints do not have any credible mechanistic basis and will not be reviewed here. To an even greater extent than the more acute response associations, they are likely to be artifacts of co-linear associations between SO$_2$ and fine particles from combustion processes.

Health Effects of Acidic Aerosols

Deposition, Growth, and Neutralization within the Respiratory Tract   The deposition pattern within the respiratory tract is dependent on the size distribution of the droplets. Acidic ambient aerosol typically has a mass median aerodynamic diameter (MMAD) of 0.3 to 0.6 µm, while industrial aerosols can have an MMAD as large as 14 µm (Williams, 1970). With hygroscopic growth in the airways, submicrometer-sized droplets can increase in diameter by a factor of 2 to 4 and still remain within the fine particle range which deposits preferentially in the distal lung airways and airspaces. As droplet sizes increase above about 3 µm MMAD, deposition efficiency within the airways increases, with more of the deposition taking place within the upper respiratory tract, trachea, and larger bronchi (Lippmann et al., 1980). For larger droplets the residence time in the airways is too short for a large growth factor.

Some neutralization of inhaled acidic droplets can occur before deposition, due to the normal excretion of endogenous ammonia into the airways (Larson et al., 1977). Once deposited, free H$^+$ reacts with components of the mucus of the respiratory tract, changing its viscosity (Larson et al., 1977). Unreacted H$^+$ diffuses into surrounding tissues. The capacity of the mucus to react with H$^+$ is dependent on the H$^+$ absorption capacity, which is reduced in acidic saturated mucus as found in certain disease states, such as asthma (Holma, 1985).

Effects on Experimental Animals

Short-Term Exposures   Respiratory Mechanical Function Alterations of pulmonary function, particularly increases in pulmonary flow resistance, occur after acute exposure. Reports of the irritant potency of various sulfate species are variable, due in part to differences in animal species and strains, and also to differences in particle sizes, pH, composition, and solubility (U.S. EPA, 1986). H_2SO_4 is more irritating than any of the sulfate salts in terms of increasing airway resistance. For short-term (1 h) exposures, the lowest concentration of H_2SO_4 shown to increase airway resistance was $100\,\mu g/m^3$ (in guinea pigs). The irritant potency of H_2SO_4 depends in part on droplet size, with smaller droplets having more effect (Amdur et al., 1978).

Animal inhalation studies by Amdur and colleagues are of interest to this discussion because they demonstrate that effects produced by single exposures at very low acid concentrations can be persistent (Amdur et al., 1986). They exposed guinea pigs by inhalation for 3 hours to the diluted effluent from a furnace that simulates a model coal combuster. Pulverized coal yields large particle mineral ash particles and an ultrafine $(< 0.1\,\mu m)$ condensation aerosol. The core of the ultrafine particles consists of oxides of Fe, Ca, and Mg, covered by a layer containing Na, As, Sb, and Zn. The Zn is important because it generally has the highest concentration on the surface of the solidified particle. As the particles cool further, there is surface formation and/or condensation of a layer of H_2SO_4.

In the initial experiments, the model aerosol was a mixture containing SO_2, ZnO, and water vapor, and there was a single 3 hour exposure to a mixture containing 1 ppm SO_2 and $5\,mg/m^3$ of ZnO passed through a humid furnace. The amount of H_2SO_4 on the surface of the ZnO particles was about $40\,\mu g/m^3$. In control studies neither 1 ppm of SO_2 nor 5 mg/m^3 of ZnO alone produced any significant responses. There were also no significant responses to the mixture in the absence of water vapor and passage through the furnace. However, the humid mixture, passed through the furnace, where it acquired a surface coating of H_2SO_4, produced significant decrements in lung diffusing capacity (DL_{co}). At 1 hour after exposure, there was an increase in lung permeability. At 12 hours after exposure, there were distention of perivascular and peribronchial connective tissues, and an increase in lung weight. The alveolar interstitium also appeared distended. At 72 hours after exposure, total lung capacity (TLC), vital capacity (VC), and functional residual capacity (FRC) had returned to baseline levels, but DL_{co} was still significantly depressed. Based on prior experience with pure SO_2 and pure H_2SO_4 exposures in the guinea pig model, Amdur et al. (1986) concluded that the humid furnace effluent effect was an acid aerosol effect because of its persistence.

In subsequent tests, 3 hour exposures to the acid-coated ZnO aerosol were given on five successive days. Significant depressions of DL_{co} were produced on the second and subsequent days for $30\,\mu g/m^3$ of H_2SO_4, while $20\,\mu g/m^3$ produced significant depressions on the fourth and fifth days. The most sensitive response was a change in airway reactivity, where a significant response was produced by a single 1 hour exposure to $20\,\mu g/m^3$ H_2SO_4 as a surface coating on the ZnO (Amdur, 1989a,b).

The persistent changes in function and morphological changes following exposure to very low levels of acidic aerosol suggest that repetitive exposures could lead to chronic lung disease. However, the implications of these changes in guinea pigs to human disease remain highly speculative.

Particle Clearance Function Donkeys exposed by inhalation for 1 hour to 0.3 to $0.6\,\mu m$ H_2SO_4 at concentrations ranging from 100 to $1000\,\mu g/m^3$ exhibited slowed bronchial mucociliary clearance function at concentrations $\geqslant 200\,\mu g/m^3$, whereas, as shown in Figure 23-4, rabbits undergoing similar exposures exhibited an acceleration of clearance at concentrations between 100 and $300\,\mu g/m^3$, and a progressive slowing of clearance at $\geqslant 500\,\mu g/m^3$ (Schlesinger, 1985).

Schlesinger (1989) examined the relative roles of concentration (C) and daily exposure (T) on H_2SO_4-induced changes in particle clearance from the gas-exchange region of rabbit lungs. Exposures were for 1 to 4 h/d for 14 days at concentrations ranging from 250 to $1000\,\mu g/m^3$. In a follow-up study Schlesinger (1990) extended the concentrations

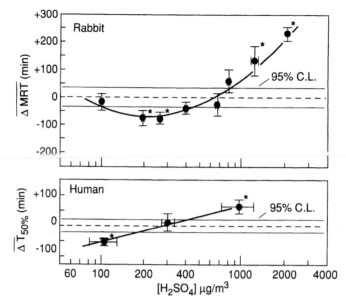

Figure 23-4   Exposure-dependent changes in characteristic bronchial mucociliary clearance times in rabbits (mean residence time) and humans (clearance half-time) from 1 hour exposures to submicrometer-sized H$_2$SO$_4$ aerosols. Each point represents the average for the group, with the vertical bars indicating ± 1 SE. The horizontal bands represent the mean ± 1 SE of the measurements for the sham-exposure controls. Asterisks indicate a significant change ($p < 0.05$) at an individual concentration (paired t test, one-tailed). (Reproduced from Lippmann, 1986).

downward to 50 μg/m^3. The results are summarized in Figure 23-5. The acceleration in clearance produced by 4 hours at 50 μg/m^3 is essentially the same as that produced by 2 hours at 100 μg/m^3 and 1 hour at 250 μg/m^3, indicating that cumulative exposure, rather than concentration, governs the response, at least within the ranges of concentration and time evaluated. The results are similar to those for mucociliary clearance in the sense that relatively low levels of exposure produce an acceleration of clearance, but clearance retardation occurs at higher levels of exposure.

Cellular Function   Schlesinger et al. (1990) examined the comparative effects of exposure to the two main ambient acidic sulfates, sulfuric acid (H$_2$SO$_4$) and ammonium bisulfate (NH$_4$HSO$_4$), using the phagocytic activity of alveolar macrophages as the endpoint. Rabbits were exposed to 250–2000 μg/m^3 H$_2$SO$_4$ (as SO$_4^{2-}$) and 500 to 4000 μg/m^3 NH$_4$HSO$_4$ (as SO$_4^{2-}$) for 1 h/d for 5 days; bronchopulmonary lavage was then performed for recovery of free lung cells. Phagocytosis, measured by uptake of opsonized latex spheres in vitro, was altered by exposure to H$_2$SO$_4$ at concentrations $\geqslant 500$ μg/m^3 and to NH$_4$HSO$_4$ at $\geqslant 2000$ μg/m^3. Assessment of results in terms of the calculated hydrogen ion concentration in the exposure atmosphere showed that identical levels of H$^+$ produced different degrees of response depending on whether the exposure was to H$_2$SO$_4$ or NH$_4$HSO$_4$. On the other hand, macrophages incubated in acidic environments in vitro responded similarly, regardless of whether H$_2$SO$_4$ or NH$_4$HSO$_4$ was used to adjust the pH. Thus the response may relate more to the local pH change in the vicinity of the depositing droplet than to the total H$^+$ delivered.

Pollutant Interactions   Osebold et al., (1980) exposed antigenically sensitized mice to 500 ppb O$_3$ for 3 days, with and without concurrent exposure 1 mg/m^3 of submicrometer

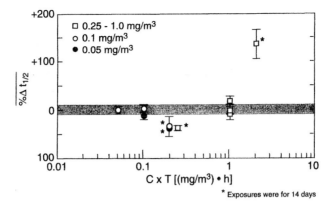

* Exposures were for 14 days

Figure 23-5 Mean percentage change in half-time $(\%\overline{\Delta t_{1/2}})$ of clearance of tracer particles from the respiratory region of the lungs following exposure to H_2SO_4, as a function of the product of exposure concentration (C) and exposure time (T) ($n = 5$ rabbits for each point). Positive changes indicate slowing of clearance; negative changes indicate speeding. Shading represents 95% confidence interval for $(\%\overline{\Delta t_{1/2}}) = 0$ (based on sham-control exposures). Data for 0.25 to $1.0\,mg/m^3$ are from Schlesinger (1989); $^*p < 0.05$ compared to control.

H_2SO_4 droplets. There was an increase in atopic reactivity that was greater than that for each pollutant alone. Kleinman et al. (1989) reported that lesions in the gas-exchange region of the lung of rats exposed to O_3 were greater in size in rats exposed to mixtures containing H_2SO_4 or NO_2 as well as O_3. Last (1989) reported significant increases in lung protein content in rats exposed for 9 days to 200 ppb O_3 plus $20\,\mu g/m^3$ H_2SO_4 over those in rats exposed to 200 ppb O_3 alone, as well as a trend toward increased protein in rats exposed to 200 ppb O_3 and $5\,\mu g/m^3$ H_2SO_4.

Subchronic Exposures

PARTICLE CLEARANCE FUNCTION   Donkeys exposed for 1 h/d (5 d/wk) for 6 months to an aerosol (0.3–0.6 μm) of H_2SO_4 at a concentration of $100\,\mu g/m^3$ developed highly variable clearance rates, and a persistent shift from baseline rate of bronchial mucociliary clearance during the exposures and for 3 months after the last exposure. Two animals had much slower clearance than their baseline during the 3 months of follow-up, but two had faster than baseline rates (Schlesinger et al., 1979). Rabbits exposed for 1 h/d (5 d/wk) for 4 weeks to 0.3 μm H_2SO_4 at $250\,\mu g/m^3$ developed variable mucociliary clearance rates during the exposure period, and their clearance during a 2 week period following the exposures was substantially faster than their baseline rates (Schlesinger et al., 1983). For a group of rabbits undergoing daily exposures via the nose at $250\,\mu g/m^3$ for 1 year, Figure 23-6 shows that bronchial mucociliary clearance was consistently slowed after the first few weeks and became even slower during a 3 month period following the end of acid exposures (Gearhart and Schlesinger, 1988).

During the course of a one year series of 1 h/d, 5 d/w nasal exposures to submicrometer H_2SO_4 at $250\,\mu g/m^3$, groups of rabbits were exposed on three occasions to ^{85}Sr-tagged latex aerosols for determination of the rates of clearance from the nonciliated alveolar region (Schlesinger and Gearhart, 1986). The latex aerosols were inhaled on days 1, 57, and 240 following the start of the H_2SO_4 exposures, and particle retention was followed for 14 days after each latex administration. As compared to baseline rates of clearance in control animals, early alveolar clearance was accelerated to a similar degree in all three tests performed during the chronic H_2SO_4 exposures.

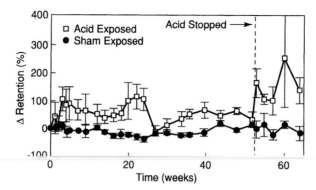

Figure 23-6 Mean change in percentage retention of tracer particles ($\pm$ SD) during intermittent exposure to H$_2$SO$_4$ in acid- and sham-exposed animals from that established in preexposure control tests. (Reproduced from Lippmann et al., 1987)

AIRWAY HYPERRESPONSIVENESS   The effects of daily 1 hour exposures of rabbits to 250 µg/m^3 of H$_2$SO$_4$ on bronchial responsiveness was assessed at the end of 4, 8, and 12 months by administration (i.v.) of doubling doses of acetylcholine and measurement of pulmonary resistance (R_L), as shown in Figure 23-7 (Gearhart and Schlesinger, 1986). Dynamic compliance (C_{dyn}) and respiratory rate (f) were also measured following agonist challenge. Those animals exposed for 4 months showed increased sensitivity to acetylcholine (i.e., the dose required to produce a 150% increase in R_L), and there was an increase in reactivity (i.e., the slope of dose vs. change in R_L) by 8 months, with a leveling off of the response after this time. No changes in C_{dyn} or f were noted at any time. Thus repeated exposures to H$_2$SO$_4$ resulted in the production of hyperresponsive airways in previously healthy animals. This has implications for the role of nonspecific irritants in the pathogenesis of airway disease.

HISTOLOGY   In the study of Schlesinger et al. in which rabbits were exposed to 250 µg/m^3 for 4 weeks and sacrificed 2 weeks later, histological examination showed increased numbers of secretory cells in distal airways and thickened epithelium in airways

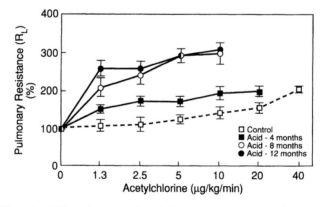

Figure 23-7 Effect of serial bronchoprovocation challenges on pulmonary resistance (R_L). The abscissa is expressed in terms of doubling doses of acetylcholine. Data are expressed as the group mean ($\pm$ SE) percentage of baseline R_L at each dose ($n = 12$ for control; $n = 4$ for each acid group). (Reproduced from Gearhart and Schlesinger, 1986)

extending from midsized bronchi to terminal bronchioles (Schlesinger et al., 1983). There were no corresponding changes in the trachea or other large airways. In the follow-up study, in which rabbits received daily exposures for 1 year via the nose at 250 µg / m³, the secretory cell density was elevated in some lung airways at 4 months and in all lung airways at 8 months (Gearhart and Schlesinger, 1986, 1988; Schlesinger and Gearhart, 1986). At 12 months the increased density remained in small and midsized airways, but not large airways. Partial recovery was observed at 3 months after the last exposure.

In a study in which dogs were exposed daily for 5 years to 1100 µg / m³ SO₂ plus 90 µg / m³ H₂SO₄ and then allowed to remain in unpolluted air for 2 years, there were small changes in pulmonary functions during the exposures, which continued following the termination of exposure. Morphometric lung measurements made at the end of a 2 year postexposure period showed changes analogous to an incipient stage of human centrilobular emphysema (Stara et al., 1980).

Effects on Humans

Acute Effects: Controlled Exposures

RESPIRATORY MECHANICAL FUNCTION   Sulfuric acid and other sulfates have been found to affect both sensory and respiratory function in humans. Respiratory effects from exposure to H₂SO₄ (350–500 µg / m³) have been reported to include increased respiratory rates and tidal volumes (Amdur et al., 1952; Ericsson and Camner, 1983). However, other studies of pulmonary function in nonsensitive healthy adult subjects indicated little effect on pulmonary mechanical function when subjects were exposed to submicrometer H₂SO₄ at 10 to 1000 µg / m³ for 10 to 120 minutes. In one study the bronchoconstrictive action of carbachol was potentiated by 0.8 µm H₂SO₄ and other sulfate aerosols, more or less in relation to their acidity (Utell et al. 1984). Asthmatics are substantially more sensitive in terms of changes in pulmonary mechanics than healthy people, and vigorous exercise potentiates the effects at a given concentration. The lowest-demonstrated-effect level was 68 µg / m³ of 0.6 µm H₂SO₄ via mouthpiece inhalation in exercising adolescent asthmatics (Koenig et al., 1989) with somewhat greater responses at 100 µg / m³ (Koenig et al., 1983a). The effects disappeared within about 15 minutes. In adult asthmatics undergoing exposure to 0.8 µm H₂SO₄ for 2 hours, the lowest-observed-effect level was 75 µg / m³ (Bauer et al., 1988). Spengler et al. (1989) concluded that these results are consistent when the exposure metric is total amount of H₂SO₄ inhaled rather than the concentration of H₂SO₄.

By contrast, Avol et al. (1990) found no significant functional responses to H₂SO₄. They exposed 32 asthmatic volunteers, 8 to 16 years of age, in a chamber to clean air and to sulfuric acid aerosol at a "low" concentration (46 ± 11 µg / m³; mean ± SD) and at a "high" concentration (127 ± 21 µg / m³). Acid aerosols had mass median aerodynamic diameters near 0.5 µm with geometric standard deviations near 1.9. Temperature was 21°C, and relative humidity was near 50%. Subjects were exposed with unencumbered oronasal breathing for 30 minutes at rest plus 10 minutes at moderate exercise (ventilation rate about 20 L / min m² of body surface). A subgroup (21 subjects) were exposed similarly to clean air and to "high" acid (134 ± 20 µg / m³) with 100% oral breathing. Increased symptoms and bronchoconstriction were found after exercise under all exposure conditions. For the group, symptom and lung function responses were not statistically different during control and during acid exposures with unencumbered breathing or with oral breathing.

Aris et al. (1990) exposed nonsmoking adult volunteers in chambers for 1 hour to fogs containing hydroxymethanesulfonate (HMSA), the bisulfate adduct of formaldehyde, and a common constituent of California acid fogs. The droplet size was 7 µm, the HMSA concentration was $260\,\mu g\,/\,m^3$, and the H$_2$SO$_4$ content of the aerosol was $1.1\,\mu g\,/\,m^3$. A control exposure was to H$_2$SO$_4$ only. Both acid fogs produced slight increases in respiratory symptoms, but no changes in airway resistance. Thus HMSA did not produce a specific bronchoconstrictor effect at a concentration about three times times greater than the highest ambient measurements.

The effects of acid fog droplets on respiratory function and symptoms have been studied by Avol et al. (1988). They exposed both normal and mild asthmatic adult volunteers for 60 minutes to $8\,\mu m$ MMAD fog droplets containing 0, 150, and $680\,\mu g\,/\,m^3$ of H$_2$SO$_4$, with alternating 10 minute periods of rest and heavy exercise. Both normals and asthmatics reported more symptoms with increasing concentration, and the asthmatics showed an increase in airway resistance at the higher acid concentration. There were no significant differences in either forced expiratory function or airway reactivity to methacholine between the sham and acid exposures.

Linn et al. (1989) exposed both healthy and asthmatic volunteers for 1 hour with intermittent exercise to H$_2$SO$_4$ at $2000\,\mu g\,/\,m^3$, with droplet sizes of 1, 10, and $20\,\mu m$. Healthy subjects had no significant changes in lung function or bronchial reactivity to methacholine (MC), but did show irritant symptoms with the 10 and $20\,\mu m$ aerosols. By contrast, the asthmatics had significant decreases in function, increases in airway resistance, and increases in symptoms for all three droplet sizes.

Raizenne et al. (1996) examined the effects of exposure to acidic air pollution on respiratory function among 8 to 12-year-old children living in 22 communities in the United States and Canada. Air quality and meteorology were measured in each community for the year preceding the pulmonary function tests. Forced vital capacity (FVC) and forced expiratory volume in 1 second (FEV$_{1.0}$) of 10,251 white children, adjusted for age, sex, height, weight, and sex-height interaction, were examined. A $52\,nmol\,/\,m^3$ difference in annual mean particle strong acidity was associated with a 3.5% (95% CI, 2.0–4.9) decrement in adjusted FVC and a 3.1% (95% CI, 1.6–4.6) decrement in adjusted FEV$_{1.0}$. The FVC decrement was larger, although not significantly different, for children who were lifelong residents of their communities (4.1%, 95% CI, 2.5–5.8). The relative odds for low lung function (i.e., measured FVC less than or equal to 85% of predicted), was 2.5 (95% CI, 1.8–3.6) across the range of particle strong acidity exposures. These data suggested that long-term exposure to ambient particle strong acidity may have a deleterious effect on lung growth, development, and function.

Particle Clearance Function   In healthy nonsmoking adult volunteers exposed to $0.5\,\mu m$ H$_2$SO$_4$ at rest at $100\,\mu g\,/\,m^3$ for 1 hour there, was an acceleration of bronchial mucociliary clearance of tracer particles ($7.6\,\mu m$), which deposited primarily in the larger bronchial airways, and a slowing of clearance when the exposure was raised to $1000\,\mu g\,/\,m^3$ (Fig. 23-4 and 23-8) (Leikauf et al., 1981). For tracer particles ($4.2\,\mu m$), which deposited primarily in midsized to small conducting airways, there was a small but significant slowing of clearance at $100\,\mu g\,/\,m^3$ H$_2$SO$_4$ and a greater slowing at $1000\,\mu g\,/\,m^3$ (Leikauf et al., 1984). These changes are consistent with the greater deposition of acid in midsized to smaller airways. Exposures to $100\,\mu g\,/\,m^3$ for 2 hours produced slower clearance than the same exposure for 1 hour, indicating a cumulative relationship to dose (Spektor et al., 1989).

The results of these studies were used by Yu et al. to construct a model for the effects of surface deposition of acidic droplets on mucus transport velocity along the tracheobronchial airways (Yu et al., 1986). Based on this model, mucus velocities are increased when less than about $10^{-7}\,g\,/\,cm^2$ of H$_2$SO$_4$ is deposited, while clearance is retarded when the acid deposition exceeds this limit.

The effects of a 1 hour inhalation of submicrometer sulfuric acid (H$_2$SO$_4$) aerosols via nasal mask on tracheobronchial mucociliary particle clearance and respiratory mechanics

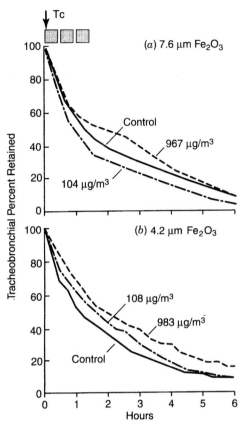

Figure 23-8 Tracheobronchial retention of ^{99m}Tc-tagged Fe_2O_3 microspheres in healthy adult volunteers as a function of time after a 1 minute tagged aerosol inhalation for particles with aerodynamic diameter of (a) 7.6 μm or (b) 4.2 μm. Submicrometer-sized droplets of H_2SO_4 are inhaled via nasal mask during three 20 minute intervals as indicated by cross-hatched boxes. The solid line indicates retention for sham exposure, the long dash-dot line for about 100 μg/m^3 H_2SO_4, and the short dash line for about 1000 μm/m^3 H_2SO_4. (Reproduced from Leikauf et al., 1984)

were studied by Spektor et al. (1985) in subjects with histories of asthma. A brief inhalation of tagged aerosol preceded the 1 hour H_2SO_4 or a sham exposure. Respiratory function was measured before and 15 minutes and 3 hours after the H_2SO_4 or sham exposure. After exposure to 1000 μg/m^3 of H_2SO_4, the six subjects not on routine medication exhibited a transient slowing of mucociliary clearance and also decrements in specific airway conductance (SG_{aw}), forced expiratory volume in 1 second (FEV_1), midmaximal expiratory flowrate (MMEF), and flow rate at 25% of total lung capacity (V_{25}) ($p < 0.05$) in both sets of measurements. The four asthmatics on daily medication exhibited stepwise mucociliary clearance that was too variable to allow detection of any H_2SO_4 effect on clearance. Mucociliary clearance rates in both groups in the sham exposure tests were significantly slower than those of healthy nonsmokers studied previously by Leikauf et al. (1984) using the same protocols. The extent of mucociliary clearance slowing following the 1000 μg/m^3 exposure in the nonmedicated subjects was similar to that in the healthy nonsmokers. This similar change, from a reduced baseline rate of clearance, together with the significant change in respiratory function, indicate that asymptomatic asthmatics may respond to H_2SO_4 exposures with functional changes of greater potential health significance than do healthy nonsmokers.

Effects: Ambient Air Exposures   There are numerous studies of associations between sulfur oxide pollutants such as SO_2 and SO_4^{2-} and various health effect indexes in polluted communities. As discussed earlier in the section on SO_2, the associations have generally been stronger with the concentrations of indexes of particulate pollution such as black smoke (BS) and suspended particulate matter (PM) than with SO_2 in those cases where attempts were made to determine the separate contributions.

Association with Aerosol Acidity   The earliest direct association between measured acidity and human health was Gorham's highly significant ($p < 0.01$) correlation between mortality rates for bronchitis in 53 U.K. metropolitan areas from 1950 to 1954 and the pH of winter precipitation in these areas (Gorham, 1958). There was also a correlation with SO_4^{2-} at the 5% level of significance. When multiple regression analyses were performed, pH remained significant at the 1% levels, but SO_4^{2-} lost its statistical significance.

An association based on some limited, but direct measurements was reported by Kitagawa who identified sulfuric acid as the probable causal agent for approximately six hundred cases of acute respiratory disease in the Yokkaichi area in central Japan between 1960 and 1969 (Kitagawa, 1984). The patients' residences were concentrated within 5 km of a titanium dioxide plant with a 14 m stack which emitted from 100,000 to 300,000 kg/mo of H_2SO_4 from 1961 to 1967. The average concentration of SO_3 in February 1965 in Isozu, a village 1 to 2 km from the plant, was $130 \, \mu g/m^3$, equivalent to $159 \, \mu g/m^3$ of H_2SO_4. Kitagawa estimated that the peak concentrations might be up to 100 times as high with a north wind. Electrostatic precipitators were installed to control aerosol emissions in 1967, and after 1968 the number of newly found patients with "allergic asthmatic bronchitis" or "Yokkaichi asthma" gradually decreased. Although Kitagawa's quantitative estimates of exposure to H_2SO_4 and the criteria used to describe cases of respiratory disease may differ from current methods, the unique aspect of this report is the identification of H_2SO_4 as the likely causal agent for an excess in morbidity.

In an independent analysis of mortality from asthma and chronic bronchitis associated with changes in sulfur oxide air pollution in Yokkaichi from 1963 to 1983, Imai et al. correlated mortality with sulfation index (lead peroxide candle measurements), and focused on reductions in SO_x emissions from a petroleum refinery in the harbor area in 1972 (Imai et al., 1986). Thus it is not clear, from their analysis, what the SO_2 or H_2SO_4 exposures to the population from these emissions were. In any case, mortality rates for bronchial asthma were significantly elevated in Yokkaichi from 1967 to 1970, and the mortality rates due to chronic bronchitis were significantly elevated from 1967 to 1970 and from 1971 to 1974. There was a greater lag between the reduction in SO_x pollution and reduction in mortality rate for chronic bronchitis than for bronchial asthma.

While sulfuric acid aerosol was believed, by some, to be a likely causal factor for excess mortality and morbidity during and following the December 1952 smog episode in London, the only air quality available for that time were for BS and SO_2. During the late 1950s, a monitoring method was developed by Commins and Waller (1963) to measure H_2SO_4 in urban air, and they used it to make daily measurements of H_2SO_4 at St. Bartholomew's Hospital in central London during the December 1962 episode. As shown in Chapter 2 (Fig. 2-10), the airborne H_2SO_4 rose rapidly during the 1962 episode, with a greater relative increase than that for black smoke (BS) or SO_2.

Using the method of Commins and Waller (1963), daily measurements of aerosol strong acid (H^+) were made at a central London site (St. Bartholomew's Medical School) between 1965 and 1972. The December 1962 London fog episode was the last to produce a clearly evident increase in the number of daily deaths, albeit a much smaller one than

December 1952. The U.K. Clean Air Act of 1954 had led to the mandated use of smokeless fuels and annual mean smoke levels had declined by 1962, to about one-half of the 1958 level. The annual average SO_2 concentrations had not declined by 1962 but dropped off markedly thereafter, along with a further marked decline in BS levels. For the period between 1964 and 1972, the measured levels of H_2SO_4 followed a similar pattern of decline. The daily concentration data have been correlated with concurrent daily records of mortality in several studies. Based on an initial time-series analysis of the winter data (Thurston et al., 1989), H^+ appeared to be more strongly associated with total daily mortality than either BS or SO_2. However, a more detailed analysis of the full-year data set by Ito et al. (1993), involving statistical "pre-whitening," did not indicate that H^+ had a greater degree of association with daily mortality than BS or SO_2. In the Ito et al. (1993) analysis, temperature had the greatest influence in all seasons, and all three of the pollution variables (same day and lagged one or two days) were significantly associated with daily mortality. However, there were limitations imposed on the analysis in terms of the limitation of the H^+ data to only one monitoring site, the limited precision of the measurement of H^+, and the selection of filters for controlling the confounding long-wave influences.

In a further exploratory further analysis of the central London data set, Lippmann and Ito (1995) developed an alternate approach for separating the effects of season and temperature on daily mortality from those of pollution. They analyzed the data for each season separately, and within each season they restricted analyses to those days in which ambient temperature had little, if any, influence on mortality. Regressions were performed for BS, SO_2, and aerosol H^+. For the winter period (November–February) mortality was most closely correlated with H^+, while for the rest of the year, it was most closely correlated with SO_2. In all seasons the correlation was poorest for BS. The results for winter and summer are illustrated in Figures 23-9 and 23-10.

A more recent report of a direct association between measured levels of ambient acidic aerosol concentration and human health effects was that of Ostro et al. (1989, 1991). They correlated data on aerosol H^+, SO_4^{2-}, NO_3^-, and FP, as well as gaseous SO_2 and CO with daily symptom, medication usage, and other variables for a panel of about 200 adults with moderate to severe asthma in Denver, Colorado, between November 1987 and March 1988. The H^+ concentrations ranged from 2 to 41 neq/m^3 (0.04 to 0.84 µg/m^3 of H_2SO_4 equivalent), and they were significantly related to both the proportion of the survey respondents reporting a moderate or worse overall asthma condition, and the proportion reporting a moderate or worse cough. Of all the pollutants considered, H^+ displayed the strongest association with asthma and cough. The magnitudes of the effects were compared by computing elasticities, or the percent change in the health effect due to a given percent change in the pollutant. Using asthma as an example, the results indicate elasticities with respect to SO_4^{2-}, FP, and H^+ of 0.060, 0.055, and 0.096, respectively (Ostro et al., 1989). This indicates that a 10% change in the concentrations of H^+ could increase the proportion reporting a moderate or worse asthma condition by 0.96%.

In their follow-up report on this study, Ostro et al. (1991) examined evidence for lagged effects. They concluded that contemporaneous measures of H^+ concentration provided the best associations with asthma status and that meteorological variables were not associated with the health effects reported. Ostro et al. also examined the effects of exposure to H^+, adjusting for time spent outdoors, level of activity, and penetration of acid aerosol indoors. Based on the adjusted exposures, the effect of H^+ on cough increased 43%, suggesting that dose–response estimates that do not incorporate behavioral factors affecting actual H^+ exposures may substantially underestimate the impact of the pollution.

In more recent years a number of morbidity studies have utilized daily measurements of H^+ concentrations. In terms of hospital admissions, the data summarized in Table 2-5

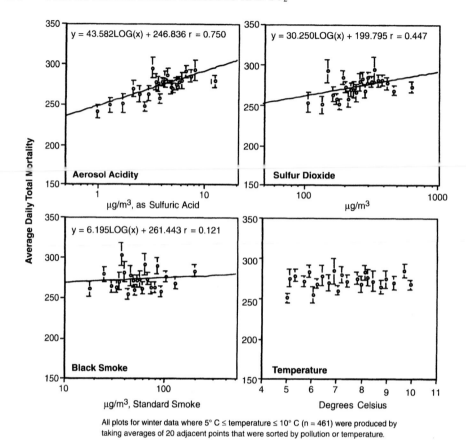

All plots for winter data where 5° C ≤ temperature ≤ 10° C (n = 461) were produced by taking averages of 20 adjacent points that were sorted by pollution or temperature.

Figure 23-9   Mortality in London: 1965–1972, winter days with temperatures between 5 and 10°C. (From Lippmann and Ito, 1995)

suggest that the strongest association that can be seen with a measured component of PM was with the hydrogen content of the aerosol (in those studies where H$^+$ data were available), and also that SO$_4^=$ was significantly associated with hospital admissions in all of the studies for which it was available.

In the 6 city study (Speizer, 1989; Damokosh et al., 1993) aerosol H$^+$ had a closer association with parent-reported bronchitis symptoms in children than any of the other PM or gas-phase components. This was also true in the Harvard-Health Canada study in 22 North American towns (Dockery et al., 1996), and in this study aerosol H$^+$ was also the most closely related pollutant to baseline lung function (Raizenne et al., 1996). While pulmonary function differences in the 6 city study were not statistically significant, the direction and magnitude of the differences were consistent with the results reported by Raizenne et al. (1996).

In a supplemental acute-response study in Uniontown, PA, one of the 22 communities in the Harvard-Health Canada study, Neas et al. (1995) had a stratified sample of 83 children report twice daily peak expiratory flow rate (PEFR) measurements on 3582 child-days during the summer of 1990. Upon arising and before retiring, each child recorded PEFR and the presence of cold, cough, or wheeze symptoms. The session-specific average deviation was then calculated across all of the children. A 12 hour H$^+$ exposure to a 125 nmol/m^3 increment was associated with a -2.5 L/min deviation in the group mean

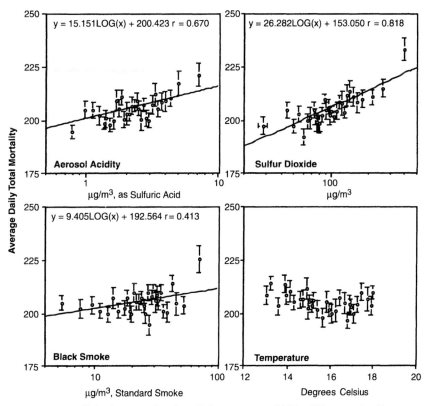

All plots for summer data where 13° C ≤ temperature ≤ 18° C (n = 610) were produced by
taking averages of 20 adjacent points that were sorted by pollution or temperature.

Figure 23-10   Mortality in London: 1965–1972, summer days with temperatures between 13 and 18°C.
(From Lippmann and Ito, 1995)

PEFR (95% CI) -4.2 to -0.8) and with increased cough incidence (odds ratio
(OR) $= 1.6$, 95% CI, 1.1 to 2.4).

Studnicka et al. (1995) studied three consecutive panels of children participating in a
summer camp in the Austrain Alps. For 47, 45, and 41 subjects, daily FEV_1, FVC, and
peak PEFR were recorded. Fifteen percent, 11%, and 5% of participants, respectively,
reported current asthma medication. Mean levels of ambient pollutants were approximately 15% higher for the first panel than for the other two panels, but the H^+ component
was twice as high for panel 1. The maximum H^+ exposure during panel 1 was 84 nmol / m^3
(4 µg / m^3 H_2SO_4 equivalent). For FEV_1 in panel 1, a significant decrease of -0.99 ml per
nmol / m^3 H^+ ($p = 0.01$) was observed. For panel 2, the FEV_1/H^+ coefficient was found to
be similar (-0.74 ml per nmol / m^3 H^+; $p = 0.28$), while for panel 3 it was in the opposite
direction (0.10 ml per nmol / m^3 H^+; $p = 0.83$). The decrease in FEV_1 observed in panel 1
was more pronounced when the mean exposure during the previous 4 days was considered
(-2.99 ml FEV_1 per nmol / m^3 H^+; $p = 0.004$).

Thurston et al. (1997) studied 52, 58, and 56 children (ages 7 to 13) attending a summer
"asthma camp" in the Connecticut River Valley; they were observed during the last week
of June in 1991, 1992, and 1993, respectively. Most of the subjects had moderate to severe
asthma. Daily records were kept of the environmental conditions, as well as of subject
medication use, lung function, and respiratory symptoms. H^+ and $SO_4^=$ were found to be

significantly and consistently correlated with acute asthma exacerbations and chest symptoms. Lung function decrements were consistently associated with O_3 but not with $SO_4^=$ and H^+.

Table 2-6 summarizes associations reported between acidic PM concentrations and respiratory symptoms and respiratory function in some recent studies, as well as showing the relative strengths of association among the pollutant variables measured. It indicates that in those studies where H^+ was measured, it was generally more highly correlated with the effects than the other measured PM constituents.

The prospective cohort mortality study of Dockery et al. (1993) reported that H^+ correlated less well with mortality than $PM_{2.5}$ or $SO_4^=$, but they only had 9 to 12 months of H^+ data in each city, compared to 14 to 16 years of data on the other pollutant variables, and many of the daily concentrations of H^+ were below the detection limit. A similar limitation was present in the analysis of Dockery et al. (1992) of air pollution and daily mortality rates.

Associations with Sulfate Ion In a study of children with mild asthma in Sokolov, Czech Republic, who were exposed to much higher $SO_4^=$ concentrations, Peters et al. (1997) analyzed the role of medication use. Children ($n = 82$) recorded PEFR symptoms and medication use in a diary. Linear and logistic regression analyses estimated the impact of concentrations of $SO_4^=$ with diameters less than 2.5 µm, adjusting for linear trend, mean temperature, weekend (v. weekday), and prevalence of fever in the sample. Fifty-one children took no asthma medication, and only 31 were current medication users. For the nonmedicated children, weak associations between a 5 day mean of $SO_4^=$ and respiratory symptoms were observed. Medicated children, in contrast, increased their bega-agonist use in direct association with an increase in 5 day mean of $SO_4^=$, but medication use did not prevent decreases in PEFR and increases in the prevalence of cough.

One other recent cross-sectional study also suggests $SO_4^=$ related decrements in respiratory function. Stern et al. (1994) examined differences in the respiratory health status of school children, aged 7 to 11 years, who resided in 10 rural Canadian communities in areas of moderate and low exposure to regional $SO_4^=$ and O_3 pollution. Five of the communities were located in central Saskatchewan, a low-exposure region, and five were located in southwestern Ontario, an area with moderately elevated exposures resulting from long-range atmospheric transport of polluted air masses. Summertime 1 hour daily O_3 maxima means were 69.0 ppb in Ontario and 36.1 ppb in Saskatchewan. Concentrations of $SO_4^=$ were three times higher in Ontario than in Saskatchewan; there were no significant differences in levels of PM_{10} or particulate nitrates. Levels of SO_2 and NO_2 were low in both regions. After controlling for the effects of age, sex, parental smoking, parental education, and gas cooking, no significant regional differences were observed in symptoms. However, children living in Ontario had statistically significant ($p < 0.01$) mean decrements of 1.7% in FVC and 1.3% in $FEV_{1.0}$ compared with Saskatchewan children, after adjusting for age, sex, weight, standing height, parental smoking, and gas cooking, but there were no statistically significant regional differences in the pulmonary flow parameters. The differences could have been due to exposures to either O_3 or $SO_4^=$, or their combination.

The use of historic $SO_4^=$ data for retrospective epidemiology studies has been complicated by the need to account for "sulfate artifact." This is the $SO_4^=$ fraction of the analysis attributable to the collection, by glass fiber filters, of SO_2 vapor and its transformation on the filter to $SO_4^=$. Glass fiber filters were commonly used in sampling networks operated to determine compliance with the now obsolete NAAQS for TSP. Chow (1995) estimated that the positive SO_2-driven artifact could add several µg/m^3 to the reported mass while Lipfert (1994) estimated it to be about 5 µg/m^3, with the level varying with location and season. The basicity of the filter, the ambient SO_2 concentration, and ambient temperature are the key variables. The extent of the artifact is determined by regressing the daily $SO_4^=$ as measured on a TSP filter against the $SO_4^=$ measured in the same day on a quartz fiber or Teflon membrane filter, which does not collect artifact $SO_4^=$. Some retrospective epidemiology studies relying on historic $SO_4^=$ measured on glass fiber filters have made corrections to the $SO_4^=$ data based on local calibrations of the extent of the artifact. Burnett et al. (1994) have described the procedures they used to make this correction for their time-series analyses.

Despite there being some artifact $SO_4^=$ formation, sulfate ion concentrations have generally correlated better with indexes of both mortality and morbidity in populations than have other frequently measured PM indexes, such as TSP, BS, CoH, and PM_{10}. Lippmann (1989) proposed that $SO_4^=$ is the best surrogate for H^+ exposure, the latter being the most likely causal factor for the observed associations between PM and chronic mortality. The hypothesis, illustrated in Figure 23-11, was based on an annual mortality analysis by Ozkaynak and Thurston (1987). Some of the scatter in this figure can be attributed to intercommunity differences in population density and local sources of ammonia (Thurston et al., 1994b; Suh et al., 1995; Ozkaynak et al., 1996). In any case, there has been a reluctance on the part of many to accept the $SO_4^=$ mortality association as likely to be causal on the basis of ecological analyses such as those of Ozkaynak and Thurston (1987), or the earlier analyses of Lave and Seskin (1977). Many skeptics felt that the results could have been due to confounding by differences among the communities in smoking, occupations, ethnicity, and so on. However, these studies are of current interest in relation to the results of more recent prospective cohort studies of associations between $SO_4^=$ and mortality and morbidity that are discussed in the next section.

Dockery et al. (1993) reported on a 14 to 16 year mortality follow-up of 8111 adults in six U.S. cities in relation to average ambient air concentrations of total particle mass, fine particle mass ($PM_{2.5}$), fine particle $SO_4^=$, O_3, SO_2, and NO_2. Aerosol acidity (H^+) data were available for only about one year in each city, while concentration data were available for the other pollutant variables for most or all of the 14 to 16 years. The

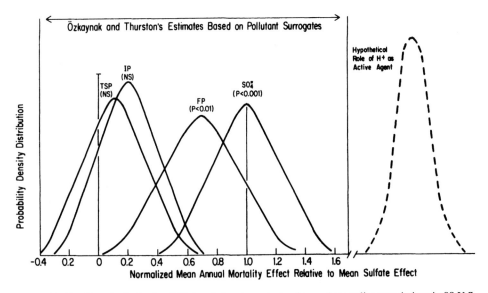

Figure 23-11 Hypothetical role of H^+ in relation to analysis of annual mortality associations in 98 U.S. Standardized Metropolitan Statistical Areas (SMSA) (Source: Ozkaynak and Thurston, 1987)

mortality rates were adjusted for cigarette smoking, education, body mass index and other influential factors not associated with pollution. As shown in Figure 2-14, the pollutant variables that correlated best with total mortality (which was mostly attributable to cardiopulmonary mortality) were PM$_{2.5}$ and SO$_4^=$. The overall mortality rate ratios were expressed in terms of the range of air pollutant concentrations in the six cities. The rate ratios for both PM$_{2.5}$ and SO$_4^=$ were 1.26 (1.08–1.47) overall, and 1.37 (1.11–1.68) for cardiopulmonary. The mean life-shortening was in the range of 2 to 3 years.

Pope et al. (1995) linked ambient air pollution data from 151 U.S. metropolitan areas in 1980 with individual risk factor on 552,138 adults who resided in these areas when enrolled in a prospective study in 1982. Deaths were ascertained through December 1989. Exposure to SO$_4^=$ and PM$_{2.5}$ pollution was estimated from national data bases. The relationships of air pollution to all-cause, lung cancer, and cardiopulmonary mortality was examined using multivariate analysis which controlled for smoking, education, and other risk factors. An association between mortality and particulate air pollution was observed. Adjusted relative risk ratios (and 95% confidence intervals) of all-cause mortality for the most polluted areas compared with the least polluted equaled 1.15 (1.09–1.22) and 1.17 (1.09–1.26) when using SO$_4^=$ and PM$_{2.5}$, respectively. Particulate air pollution was associated with cardiopulmonary and lung cancer mortality but not with mortality due to other causes. The mean life-shortening in this study was between 1.5 and 2 years. Figure 23-12 shows the range of values for the adjusted mortality rates in the various communities versus annual average SO$_4^=$ concentrations. The results appear, both by inspection and analysis, to be quite similar to those found in the previous studies of Ozkaynak and Thurston (1987) and Lave and Seskin (1970). The Pope et al. (1995) results thus indicate that the concerns raised about the credibility of the earlier results, due to their inability to control for potentially confounding factors such as smoking and socioeconomic variables, can be eased, and the findings of Pope et al. (1995) are consistent with the prior findings of Ozkaynak and Thurston (1987) and Lave and Seskin (1970).

The findings of Dockery et al. (1993) and Pope et al. (1995), in prospective cohort studies, indicate that mean lifespan shortening is of the order of two years. This implies

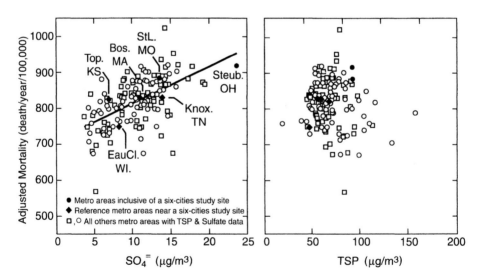

Figure 23-12   Age-, sex-, and race-adjusted population-based mortality rates for 1980 plotted against mean sulfate air pollution levels for 1980. Data from metropolitan areas that correspond approximately to areas used in prospective cohort analysis. (Adapted from Pope, 1995)

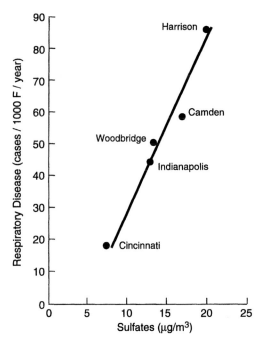

Figure 23-13 Incidence of respiratory disease lasting more than 7 days in women (mean of 3 years) versus concentration of suspended particulate sulfates in the city air at test sites. (From Dohan and Taylor, 1960)

that many individuals in the population have lives shortened by many years, and that there is excess mortality associated with fine particle exposure greater than that implied by the cumulative results of the time-series studies of daily mortality.

An early morbidity study by Dohan et al. (1962) compared the incidence of respiratory disease lasting more than seven days in women workers at assembly plants in five U.S. cities in relation to $SO_4^=$ concentrations in those cities (Fig. 23-13).

An important recent study addressed morbidity in a large number of individuals also adjusted for individual risk factors. Ostro (1990) examined lost-time due to respiratory causes in relation to ambient particulate matter. The study was based on interview data on a random sample of U.S. households in 25 communities in the national Health Interview Survey (HIS) of 1979 to 1981. The lost-time was most closely related to $SO_4^=$. As shown in Figure 23-14, the associations, in terms of exposure–response slopes and scatter, were similar in nature to those seen for mortality in Figure 23-12.

Several groups of investigators have reported significant associations between ambient air SO_4^{2-} and hospital admissions for respiratory diseases as shown in Table 2-5. Burnett et al. (1995) extended their analyses to carefully address the associations between SO_4^{2-} and cardiac disease and to assess whether there were variations in these associations. Respiratory admissions in his Ontario population exceed those for cardiac disease in the winter, but the numbers are more equal in the summer. Also summer admissions may be confounded by their associations with O_3, while winter admissions are not. Table 23-1 shows that adjustments for O_3 and temperature decrease, but do not eliminate, statistically significant associations with respiratory disease and increase the excess for cardiac disease. It also shows that there is very little seasonal variation in the excess disease associated with $SO_4^=$ in ambient air.

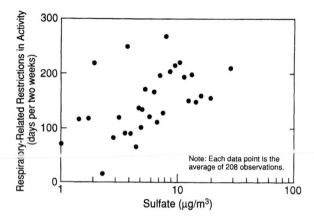

Figure 23-14   Association between respiratory-related restricted activity and sulfates, controlling for covariates. (From Ostro, 1990)

Implications of the Effects of Acidic Aerosols on Respiratory Function in the Exacerbation of Asthma and Chronic Bronchitis

The studies of Utell and colleagues demonstrate that brief exposures to acidic aerosols reduce airway conductance in healthy humans, and that asthmatic subjects are more sensitive than healthy individuals (Utell et al., 1982, 1984). The lowest concentration that produced a significant response in the group as a whole was $450 \, \mu g / m^3$. Koenig et al. reported a 40% increase in total airway resistance in a group of exercising asthmatic adolescents when they were exposed to $100 \, \mu g / m^3$ of H$_2$SO$_4$ (Koenig et al., 1983a), and lesser but still significant effects at $68 \, \mu g / m^3$ (Koenig et al., 1989). The responses were similar to those reported by Koenig and colleagues for the same protocols and kinds of subjects for exposure to 0.5 ppm of SO$_2$ ($1300 \, \mu g / m^3$) (Koenig et al., 1981, 1983b). Thus, when SO$_2$ is oxidized and hydrolyzed, the resulting H$_2$SO$_4$ is 10 to 20 times more potent. While the average increases in airway resistance were small because the populations studied were small, some subjects had much greater than the average responses. Also the populations were carefully selected and did not include the more unstable and potentially more reactive asthmatics in the population.

Moderate exercise appears to enhance the response, by increasing the dose of irritant delivered to epithelial surfaces. With increasing exercise, more pollutant is inhaled. The

TABLE 23-1   Percentage of Excess Hospital Admissions Associated with SO$_4^=$ in Ontario, 1983–1988

Category of Population	Respiratory	Cardiac
All	3.7 (2.5–4.9)	2.8 (1.8–3.8)
Males	4.0 (2.4–5.5)	3.4 (1.8–5.0)
Females	3.3 (1.5–5.0)	2.0 (0.2–3.7)
>65	3.7 (1.8–5.7)	3.5 (1.9–5.0)
April.–September[a]	3.2 (1.6–4.7)	3.2 (1.4–5.0)
October–March[a]	2.8 (0.3–5.3)	3.4 (0.7–6.1)

Source: Adapted from Burnett (1995).

Note: Excess for a change from 0 to $13 \, \mu g / m^3$ of SO$_4^=$ based on linear-quadratic regression model; mean (95% confidence interval).

[a]Adjusted for influences of O$_3$, O$_3^2$, temp, and temp^2.

greater inspiratory flow rates also act to increase the percentage of the highly soluble SO_2 vapor that can penetrate beyond the upper airways into those bronchial airways where reflex responses are most likely to be initiated. The greater flow rate also produces a thinner boundary layer around the airway bifurcations, enhancing "hot spots" of deposition of particles and vapors from the airstream. Thus exercise results in increased deposition in this region for the submicrometer sized H_2SO_4 droplets that would have minimal deposition in such airways at lower flow rates.

The irritant dose delivered to the larger bronchial airways is greater in asthmatics and bronchitics than in healthy individuals because the former groups have airways with smaller diameters. This may account for some, or perhaps all, of the greater responsiveness of asthmatics to inhaled irritants. They may also have a greater responsiveness at the sites of deposition to the delivered dose, but this has not been clearly established in in vivo tests. Clearly, an irritant-induced narrowing of the conducting airways of the lung can increase the surface deposition of subsequently inhaled irritant, resulting in further airway constriction.

The subjective responses to inhaled acid aerosols may include a feeling of chest tightness, and the work of breathing is increased. For individuals with chronic respiratory disease, any increment of work in breathing may be considered an adverse effect. For asthmatic individuals, the major concern is the induction of bronchospasm. The few clinical laboratory studies on carefully selected asthmatics cannot be expected to generate data on the exact conditions that provoke bronchospasm and acute respiratory insufficiency. It would be highly desirable to have an animal model for bronchial asthma so that this important issue could be systematically studied.

Implications of the Effects of Acidic Aerosols on Mucociliary Clearance in the Pathogenesis of Chronic Bronchitis

Schlesinger et al. (1983) studied the effects of concentration and duration of exposure to submicrometer-sized H_2SO_4 aerosols on tracheobronchial and alveolar rates of particle clearance in rabbits and found that the effects increased with duration and concentration. Spektor et al. (1989) reported a similar finding for tracheobronchial particle clearance in humans.

The altered clearance rates during and after the exposure period may be an adaptive response of the mucociliary system to acid exposures. On the other hand, they may be early stages in the progression toward more serious dysfunctions, such as those found in chronic bronchitis, which may result from continued irritant exposures.

A mechanistic basis for the linkage between chronic exposure to H_2SO_4 and the pathogenesis of chronic bronchitis lies in the series of studies involving chronic exposures of animals and persistent histological alterations in lung structure. As noted by Lippmann et al. (1987), these structural changes in the rabbit model have correlates in terms of clearance function changes. The mucociliary changes in turn are indicative of changes in mucus secretion leading to mucus stasis, a hallmark of bronchitic disease.

The animal studies can be related to human responses in two ways. One is the concordance in functional and morphometric responses of animals to H_2SO_4 and cigarette smoke, a known causal factor for human chronic bronchitis. The other is that humans, rabbits, and donkeys all have essentially the same transient mucociliary clearance function responses to single 1 hour exposures to H_2SO_4. The fact that daily 1 hour H_2SO_4 exposures in rabbits and donkeys produce persistent changes in clearance function makes it highly likely that humans would also show these effects if similarly exposed. Furthermore a comparison of the human and rabbit responses to single exposures indicates that humans respond at lower concentrations than do rabbits (Schlesinger, 1986).

The effects of H$_2$SO$_4$ on the airways are very likely to be cumulative during each exposure day, at least in part. Thus, the daily 1 hour exposures at 250 µg / m^3 in the rabbits may be equivalent to < 50 µg / m^3 for a 7 to 8 hour day and to a still lower concentration for equivalent effects in humans. On the other hand, the effects produced by the 1 year series of exposures in the rabbits were less severe than the condition corresponding to a clinical diagnosis of chronic bronchitis in humans.

Unfortunately, there are few data concerning the response of the human mucociliary clearance system under prolonged insult by potentially harmful pollutants such as H$_2$SO$_4$. The most direct evidence for an association between chronic bronchitis and exposure to H$_2$SO$_4$ comes from occupational exposures, but these were at high levels. Williams observed an excess incidence of chronic bronchitis in workers occupationally exposed to H$_2$SO$_4$ levels above 1 mg / m^3 (probable diameter = 14 µm); however, the excess was actually in increased incidence of episodes in affected workers rather than an increase in the number of workers affected (Williams, 1970).

Although available evidence suggests that exposure to H$_2$SO$_4$ may exacerbate disease, it has not been clearly established that it can initiate it. Some limited evidence indicates that it can. For example, in two previously healthy human subjects, Sim and Pattle (1957) found the development of what appeared to be long-lasting symptoms of bronchitis as a result of repeated exposure to H$_2$SO$_4$ lasting 1 hour and given no more than twice a week, with at least 24 hour between exposures. Concentrations were, however, high, ranging from 3 to 39 mg / m^3.

The suggestion for a role of H$_2$SO$_4$ in the development of chronic bronchitis is given added strength when results of studies of submicrometer H$_2$SO$_4$ or whole fresh cigarette smoke exposures, both conducted at New York University Medical Center with laboratory animals and humans, are compared (Lippmann et al., 1982). Cigarette smoke is an agent known to be involved in the etiology of human chronic bronchitis, and as shown in Figure 23-15, the effects of smoking two cigarettes on the mucociliary clearance of tracer particles are essentially the same in humans and donkeys in terms of a transient acceleration of clearance in single low-dose exposures. Both agents produce a transient slowing of mucociliary particle clearance following single high-dose exposures (Lippmann et al., 1982). Furthermore alterations in clearance rates persist for several months followed multiple exposures to both agents (Figs. 23-6 and 23-16). Thus, although direct evidence for an association between intermittent low-level exposures to H$_2$SO$_4$ and chronic bronchitis is lacking, the similarity in response between H$_2$SO$_4$ and cigarette smoke exposures suggests that such an association is likely.

Human chronic bronchitis is a clinically diagnosed disease, but one that is characterized by certain morphological changes associated with these clinical symptoms (Lourenco, 1969; Reid, 1963; Mitchell, 1967; Suhs et al., 1969; Jefferey, 1982). One of the basic stigmata is an increase in the number and/or size of epithelial mucus secretory cells in both proximal bronchi as well as in peripheral airways where such cells are normally absent or few in number; this change is accompanied by an increase in the volume of secretion (Reid, 1963). In the subchronic rabbit studies as well as the chronic studies, an increase in epithelial secretory cell proportions in smaller airways was noted (Schlesinger et al., 1983; Gearhart and Schlesinger, 1989).

The appearance of persistently increased secretory cell number in peripheral airways as a result of H$_2$SO$_4$ is a finding of major importance, since excessive mucus production in small airways, which is consistent with an increase in the propagation of secretory cells, may be an early feature in the pathogenesis of bronchitis (Hogg et al., 1968). Furthermore it demonstrates an underlying histological change consistent with the observed physiological effects of the H$_2$SO$_4$, namely altered mucociliary clearance.

In addition to a change in the relative number of secretory cells in different airway levels of acid-exposed rabbits, two other changes were noted after H$_2$SO$_4$ exposures.

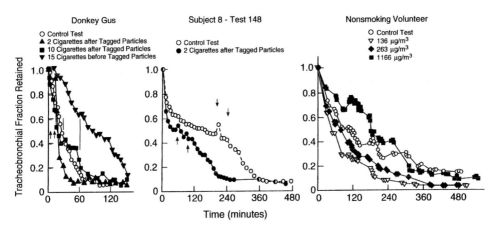

Figure 23-15 (*a*) Tracheobronchial particle retention versus time for donkey Gus in a control test, and in tests involving exposure to whole fresh cigarette smoke from the indicated number of cigarettes. (*b*) Tracheobronchial particle retention versus time for a 38-year-old nonsmoking man for two tagged aerosols inhaled 2.5 hours apart on the same day. Smoke from two cigarettes, which was inhaled beginning about 1 hour after the inhalation of the second tagged aerosol, accelerated the clearance of both. (Reproduced from Lippmann et al., 1982).

There was an increase in epithelial thickness and a decrease in airway diameter. A significant increase in epithelial thickness of small bronchi and bronchioles occurred in rabbits exposed orally at approximately $250\,\mu g/m^3$ and nasally at approximately $500\,\mu g/m^3$. In addition, in the oral exposure series, the lumen diameter of the smallest airways was significantly less than in the sham controls.

In human chronic bronchitis and in experimental bronchitis in laboratory animals, an initial change in secretory cell number or size is followed by intrabronchial narrowing, especially in small bronchi and bronchioles; in part due to a thickening of the bronchial wall (Matsuba and Thurlbeck, 1973; McKenzie et al., 1969).

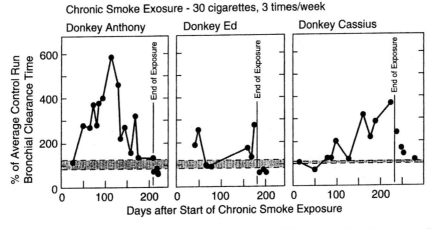

Figure 23-16 Effect of exposures to the whole fresh smoke from 30 cigarettes, three times per week, on the mean residence time for tagged particles on the tracheobronchial airways in three donkeys. The dashed lines indicate the range of the three control tests for each animal, which preceded the smoke exposures. (Reproduced from Lippmann et al., 1982).

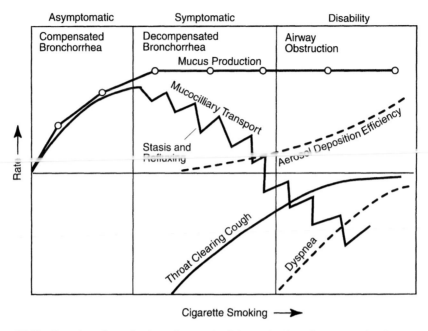

Figure 23-17   Tentative scheme for the pathogenesis of obstructive lung disease resulting from exposure to inhaled irritants. (Reproduced from Albert et al., 1973)

In summary, the first stage of effect of acid exposure may be a change in secretory cell proportions in the airways, and thickening of the epithelium may occur later. Thus the studies of Schlesinger et al. (1983) and Gearhart and Schlesinger (1989) provide further support for the role of H_2SO_4 in the pathogenesis of chronic bronchitis via effects on the mucociliary clearance system. However, the progression of clearance dysfunction in the pathogenesis of chronic bronchitis is not known.

The Albert et al. (1973) schema describing the pathogenesis of chronic bronchitis in man from cigarette smoking is illustrated in Figure 23-17. It may also apply to repeated exposures to other irritants such as H_2SO_4. According to this schema, irritant inhalation initially results in a tendency toward some acceleration of clearance, since excess mucus is produced but mucosal damage has not occurred. The H_2SO_4 dose delivered to the rabbit in nasal breathing at $250\,\mu g/m^3$ may have been enough to initiate this first stage. An increase in the number of airways containing epithelial secretory cells is consistent with increased mucus production. However, the degree of clearance rate change could vary with the individual rabbit and with the time after exposure at which the clearance was measured. This may account for the fact that a significant acceleration was often observed when clearance was measured immediately after H_2SO_4 exposure, whereas retardation was more commonly observed when clearance was measured 1 day after the last H_2SO_4 exposure (Gearhart and Schlesinger, 1988).

In the next stage of the Albert et al. (1973) schema, a further increase in the level of secretion, coupled with some mucosal damage, results in an overloading of transport mechanisms; the result is a retardation of clearance. Such a retardation was observed in the study by Schlesinger et al. (1979) involving 6 months of daily 1 hour H_2SO_4 exposures at $100\,\mu g/m^3$ in donkeys, and in the study of Gearhart and Schlesinger (1988) involving daily 1 hour H_2SO_4 exposures in rabbits for 1 year.

Since H_2SO_4 produces essentially the same sequence of effects on mucociliary bronchial clearance as cigarette smoke following both short-term and chronic exposures, it may be capable of contributing to the development of bronchitis. But the question still remains whether variable clearance rates and persistant clearance rate changes merely predispose to chronic bronchitis or are the actual initiating events in a pathogenic sequence leading to its development. Furthermore the response of the mucociliary clearance system observed in the rabbits may be adaptive rather than pathological. Many irritants may stimulate clearance at low doses or after exposure for a short time and then retard it at higher doses or with prolonged exposures (Wolff et al., 1981). An increase in secretory cell proportions is consistent with hypersecretion. Thus low-level exposures may initially increase secretion, which can be coped with, and may even be protective. However, pathological changes appear when adaptive capacity is overloaded. Thus, with increasing exposure time or dose, the degree of enhanced secretion may be too great, resulting in overwhelming of clearance and leading to retardation and, eventually, bronchitis (Schlesinger et al., 1983).

Airborne Acidity and Cancer

There is a possibility that exposure to acidic aerosols may play a role in carcinogenesis. Soskolne et al. (1989) published a review that examined a broad array of epidemological and toxicological literature. They concluded that there was support for the hypothesis that acidic pollutants contribute to carcinogenesis in humans. They examined possible biologic mechanisms for such a contribution, including pH modulation of toxicity of xenobiotics and pH-induced changes of cells involving mitotic and enzyme regulation.

The strongest epidemiological evidence for an effect of acid mists on lung cancer comes from a follow-up study through 1986 of 1165 steelworkers exposed to acid mists at steel-pickling operations at concentrations on the order of $200 \mu g/m^3$ (droplet size not specified). The results are summarized in Table 23-2. Since the H_2SO_4 concentrations in ambient air are about two orders of magnitude lower, there is no strong evidence at this time to link ambient air exposures to carcinogenesis. Public health authorities should consider the Soskolne et al. hypothesis as a margin-of-safety factor in the establishment of air quality guidelines and/or standards based on the more clearly established health effects associated with exposure to acidic aerosols.

Summary of Health Effects of Acidic Aerosols

The human health effects of major concern with respect to the inhalation of acidic aerosols are bronchospasm in asthmatics and chronic bronchitis in all exposed persons. The former relates to acute exposure, whereas the latter can be related more closely to chronic or

TABLE 23-2   Lung Cancer and Acid Mists

	Standardized Mortality Ratio [a]	
Disease	Overall	20 Years Since First Exposure
Lung cancer (without adjustment for smoking, $n = 1156$)	1.55 (1.12–2.11)	1.72 (1.21–2.39)
Lung cancer (with adjustment for smoking, $n = 752$)	1.36 (0.97–1.84)	1.50 (1.05–2.27)
Heart disease ($n = 1156$)	0.92 (0.77–1.09)	
All causes ($n = 1156$)	0.92 (0.83–1.01)	

Source: Steenland and Beaumont (1989).

Note: The cohort was 1156 male steelworkers. Exposure was to an average H_2SO_4 concentration of $0.2 mg/m^3$ based on 49 air samples collected in the late 1970s. Average duration of employment (and exposure) was 8.8 years.

[a] (With 95% confidence intervals)

cumulative exposures. In either case the effects are produced by droplets depositing on the surface of the conductive airways of the lungs.

Studies related to the provocation of bronchospasm show evidence for increased airway resistance in exercising mild to moderate asthmatics. Koenig and colleagues (1983a, 1989) reported increased airway resistance following H$_2$SO$_4$ exposures for 30 minutes at rest and 10 minutes of exercise for adolescents at 68 or 100 μg/m^3 (0.6 m diameter droplets). Bauer et al. (1988) saw similar effects in adults exposed for 2 hours at 75 μg/m^3 while exercising or for 16 minutes at 450 μg/m^3 while at rest (0.8 μm). Koenig et al. (1989) also showed that the effects previously seen at 68 μg/m^3 were increased when there was coexposure to 0.1 ppm (260 μg/m^3) of SO$_2$.

Evidence for synergism is also to be found in the work of Amdur and Chen (1989), who showed that sulfuric acid (1 hour at 20 μg/m^3) on ultrafine ZnO particles that simulate coal combustion effluent, when present in a mixture with SO$_2$, produces increased lung reactivity responses about 10-fold greater than those produced by pure droplets of H$_2$SO$_4$ of comparable size.

A causal basis for the historic association between acidic aerosols and the prevalence of bronchitis in humans has been established, at least in part, by the acute and chronic exposure studies in which rates of particle clearance from the lungs have been measured. The short-term effects are cumulative over at least several hours, and total exposures at the equivalent of current peak ambient levels produce similar transient changes in mucociliary clearance rates in rabbits, donkeys, and humans. Repetitive daily exposures of rabbits and donkeys, at comparable rates of exposure, produce both transient and persistent clearance abnormalitites that are essentially the same as those produced by whole fresh cigarette smoke, a known causal factor for chronic bronchitis in humans.

Conclusive evidence for human health responses to ambient acidic aerosols is lacking, and inferences have had to be drawn from associations between health and SO$_4^{2-}$. Of particular interest are the studies of Dockery et al. (1982) and Dassen et al. (1986) showing the effects of episodic overexposures to ambient mixtures containing concentrations of SO$_2$ and PM close to current U.S. standards. These exposures produced an apparent continuum of response, with a substantial fraction (perhaps 25% or more) of children having at least a small loss of lung function persisting for at least several weeks. A smaller percentage may have persistent functional decrements exceeding 10%. At concentrations that are about twice the current U.S. standards, an episode in western Germany in 1985 produced increases in deaths, hospital admissions, outpatient visits, and ambulance deliveries to hospitals (Wichmann et al., 1989).

More direct semiquantitative evidence for a causal role for acidic aerosols comes from the studies of Kitagawa (1984) and Thurston et al. (1989). Kitagawa showed an association between acid aerosols and morbidity in Japan, and Lippmann and Ito (1995) showed that total daily mortality in London in the period 1965 to 1972 was more closely associated with daily measured acid aerosol than with BS or SO$_2$.

Epidemiological studies that directly address the role of acidic aerosols on human health are beginning to produce results. The reports of Raizenne et al. (1996) and Ostro et al. (1989, 1991) are both encouraging and dismaying. They are encouraging in that they directly address serious public health concerns. The initial findings are, however, quite disturbing. Dockery et al. (1996) showed that the prevalence of bronchitic symptoms in schoolchildren varies from about 3.5% to 10% as annual average H$^+$ concentrations (expressed as H$_2$SO$_4$ equivalent) varied from 0.4 to 1.8 μg/m^3. Ostro et al. (1989, 1991) reported that responses among adult asthmatics were more closely associated with H$^+$ than with any other pollution variable for concentrations (expressed as H$_2$SO$_4$ equivalent) ranging from 0.04 to 0.84 μg/m^3. These are commonly encountered levels in the United States. and well below historic ambient levels in the United States. and Europe. More direct measurement data need to be made and coupled to health effects studies. The implications of the preliminary data to public health and, ultimately, to the health costs of fossil fuel consumption need to be much better documented.

ACKNOWLEDGMENTS

This research was supported, in part, by a Cooperative Agreement with the EPA (CR818325 and 822050), and by Grant ES 04612 from the National Institute of Environmental Health Sciences (NIEHS). It is part of a Center Program supported by Grant ES 00260.

REFERENCES

Albert, R. E., M. Lippmann, H. T. Peterson Jr., J. M. Berger, K. Sanborn, and D. E. Bohning. 1973. Deposition and clearance of aerosols. *Arch. Intern. Med.* 131: 115–127.

Amdur, M. O. 1989. Sulfuric acid: The animals tried to tell us. *Appl. Ind. Hyg.* 4: 189–197.

Amdur, M. O., and L. C. Chen. 1989. Furnace generated acid aerosols: Speciation and pulmonary effects. *Environ. Health Perspect.* 79: 147–150.

Amdur, M. O., A. F. Sarofim, M. Neville, R. J. Quann, J. F. McCarthy, J. F. Elliot, H. F. Lam, A. E. Rogers, and M. W. Connor. 1986. Coal combustion aerosols and SO_2: An interdisciplinary analysis. *Environ. Sci. Technol.* 20: 138–145.

Amdur, M. O., L. Silverman, and P. Drinker. 1952. Inhalation of H_2SO_4 mist by human subjects. *Arch. Ind. Hyg. Occup. Med.* 6: 305–313.

Amdur, M. O., M. Dubriel, and D. Creasia. 1978. Respiratory response of guinea pigs to low levels of sulfuric acid. *Environ. Res.* 15: 418–423.

Anderson, S. D. 1985. Issues in exercise-induced asthma. *J. Allergy Clin. Immunol.* 76: 763–772.

Aris, R., D. Christian, D. Sheppard, and J. R. Balmes. 1990. Acid fog-induced bronchoconstriction. *Am. Rev. Respir. Dis.* 141: 546–551.

Arossa, W., S. Spinaci, M. Bugiani, P. Natale, C. Bucca, and G. deCandussio. 1987. Changes in lung function of children after an air pollution decrease. *Arch. Environ. Health* 42: 170–174.

Avol, E. L., W. S. Linn, D. A. Shamoo, K. R. Anderson, R. C. Peng, and J. D. Hackney. 1990. Respiratory responses of young asthmatic volunteers in controlled exposures to sulfuric acid aerosol. *Am. Rev. Respir. Dis.* 142: 343–348.

Avol, E. L., W. S. Linn, L. H. Wightman, J. D. Whynot, K. R. Anderson, and J. D. Hackney. 1988. Short-term respiratory effects of sulfuric acid in fog: A laboratory study of healthy and asthmatic volunteers. *J. Air Pollut. Control Assoc.* 38: 258–263.

Baskurt, O. K., E. Levi, S. Caglayan, N. Dikmenoglu, and M. N. Kutman. 1990. Hematological and hemorheological effects of air pollution. *Arch. Environ. Health* 45: 224–228.

Bates, D. V., and R. Sizto. 1983. Relationships between air pollutant levels and hospital admissions in southern Ontario. *Can. J. Public Health* 74: 117–122.

Bates, D. V., and R. Sizto. 1987. Air pollution and hospital admissions in southern Ontario: The acid summer haze effect. *Environ. Res.* 43: 317–331.

Bauer, M. A., M. J. Utell, D. M. Speers, F. R. Gibb, and P. E. Morrow. 1988. Effects of near ambient levels of sulfuric acid aerosol on lung function in exercising subjects with asthma and COPD. *Am. Rev. Respir. Dis.* 137: A167.

Bethel, R. A., D. J. Erle, J. Epstein, D. Sheppard, J. A. Nadel, and H. A. Boushey. 1983. Effect of exercise rate and route of inhalation on sulfur-dioxide-induced bronchoconstriction in asthmatic subjects. *Am. Rev. Respir. Dis.* 128: 592–596.

Bethel, R. A., D. Sheppard, J. Epstein, E. Tam, J. A. Nadel, and H. A. Boushey. 1984. Interaction of sulfur dioxide and cold dry air in causing bronchoconstriction in asthmatic subjects. *J. Appl. Physiol. Respir. Environ. Exercise Physiol.* 57: 419–423.

Brauer, M., P. Koutrakis, and J. D. Spengler. 1989. Personal exposures to acidic aerosols and gases. *Environ. Sci. Technol.* 23: 1408–1412.

Burnett, R. T., R. E. Dales, M. E. Raizenne, D. Krewski, P. W. Summers, G. R. Roberts, M. Raad-Young, T. Dann, and J. Brook. 1994. Effects of low ambient levels of ozone and sulfates on the frequency of respiratory admissions to Ontario hospitals. *Environ. Res.* 65: 172–194.

Burnett, R. T., R. E. Dales, M. E. Raizenne, D. Krewski, R. Vincent, T. Dann, and J. Brook. 1995. Associations between ambient particulate sulfate and admissions to Ontario hospitals for cardiac and respiratory diseases. *Am. J. Epidemiol.* 142: 15–22.

Chow, J. C. 1995. Critical review: Measurement methods to determine compliance with ambient air quality standards for suspended particles. *J. Air Waste Manage. Assoc.* 45: 320–382.

Commins, B. T., and R. E. Waller. 1963. Determination of particulate acid in town air. *Analyst* 88. 364–367.

Damokosh, A. I., J. D. Spengler, D. W. Dockery, J. H. Ware, and F. E. Speizer. 1993. Effects of acidic particles on respiratory symptoms in 7 U.S. Communities. *Am. Rev. Respir. Dis.* 147: A632.

Dassen, W., B. Brunekreef, G. Hoek, P. Hofschreuder, B. Staatsen, H. deGroot, E. Schouten, and K. Biersteker. 1986. Decline in children's pulmonary function during an air pollution episode. *J. Air Pollut. Control Assoc.* 36: 1223–1227.

Deal, E. C., E. R. McFadden, R. H. Ingram, and J. J. Jaeger. 1979. Hyperpnea and heat flux: Initial reaction sequence in exerciseinduced asthma. *J. Appl. Physiol.* 46: 476–483.

Dockery, D. W., J. Cunningham, A. I. Damokosh, L. M. Neas, J. D. Spengler, P. Koutrakis, J. H. Ware, M. Raizenne, and F. E. Speizer. 1996. Health effects of acid aerosols on North American children: Respiratory symptoms. *Environ. Health Perspect.* 104: 500–505.

Dockery, D. W., C. A. Pope, III, X. Xu, J. D. Spengler, J. H. Ware, M. E. Fay, B. G. Ferris Jr., and F. E. Speizer. 1993. An association between air pollution and mortality in six U.S. cities. *N. Engl. J. Med.* 329: 1753–1759.

Dockery, D. W., J. H. Ware, B. G. Ferris Jr., F. E. Speizer, N. R. Cook, and S. M. Herman. 1982. Change in pulmonary function in children associated with air pollution episodes. *J. Air Pollut. Control Assoc.* 32: 937–942.

Dockery, D. W., J. Schwartz, and J. D. Spengler. 1992. Air pollution and daily mortality: Associations with particulates and acid aerosols. *Environ. Res.* 59: 362–373.

Dohan, F. C., G. S. Everts, and R. Smith. 1962. Variations in air pollution and the incidence of respiratory disease. *J. Air Pollut. Control Assoc.* 12: 418–436.

Ericsson, G., and P. Camner. 1983. Health effects of sulfur oxides and particulate matter in ambient air. *Scand. J. Work Environ. Health* 9(S3): 1–52.

Gearhart, J. M., and R. B. Schlesinger. 1986. Sulfuric acid-induced airway hyperresponsiveness. *Fundam. Appl. Toxicol.* 7: 681–689.

Gearhart, J. M., and R. B. Schlesinger. 1988. Response of the tracheobronchial mucociliary clearance system to repeated irritant exposure: Effect of sulfuric acid mist on function and structure. *Exp. Lung Res.* 14: 587–605.

Gearhart, J. M. and R. B. Schlesinger. 1989. Sulfuric acid-induced changes in the physiology and structure of the tracheobronchial airways. *Environ. Health Perspect.* 79: 127–137.

Gorham, E. 1958. Bronchitis and the acidity of urban precipitation. *Lancet* 2: 691–693.

Hackney, J. D., W. S. Linn, R. M. Bailey, C. E. Spier, and L. M. Valencia. 1984. Time course of exercise-induced bronchoconstriction in asthmatics exposed to sulfur dioxide. *Environ. Res.* 34: 321–327.

Hatzakis, A., K. Katsouyanni, A. Kalandidi, N. Day, and D. Trichopoulos. 1986. Short-term effects of air pollution on mortality in Athens. *Int. J. Epidemiol.* 15: 73–81.

Hogg, J. C., P. T. Macklem, and W. M. Thurlbeck. 1968. Site and nature airway obstruction in obstructive lung disease. *N. Engl. J. Med.* 278: 1355–1360.

Holma, B. 1985. Influence of buffer capacity and pH-dependent rheological properties of respiratory mucus on health effects due to acidic pollution. *Sci. Total Environ.* 41: 101–123.

Horstman, D. H., E. Seal Jr., L. J. Folinsbee, P. Ives, and L. J. Roger. 1988. The relationship between exposure duration and sulfur dioxide-induced bronchoconstriction in asthmatic subjects. *Am. Ind. Hyg. Assoc. J.* 49: 38–47.

Imai, M., K. Yoshida, and M. Kitabatake. 1986. Mortality from asthma and chronic bronchitis associated with changes in sulfur oxides air pollution. *Arch. Environ. Health* 41: 29–35.

Ito, K., G. D. Thurston, C. Hayes, and M. Lippmann. 1993. Associations of London, England, daily mortality with particulate matter, sulfur dioxide, and acidic aerosol pollution. *Arch. Environ. Health* 48: 213–220.

Jefferey, P. K. 1982. The effects of irritation on the structure of bronchial epithelium. In *The Lung in the Environment*, eds. G. Bonsignore, and G. Cummings, pp. 303–313. New York: Plenum Press.

Keeler, G. J., J. D. Spengler, and R. A. Castillo. 1991. Acid aerosol measurements at a suburban Connecticut site. *Atmos. Environ.* Part A 25: 681–690.

Kehrl, H. R., L. J. Roger, M. J. Hazucha, and D. H. Horstman. 1987. Differing response of asthmatics to SO$_2$ exposure with continuous and intermittent exercise. *Am. Rev. Respir. Dis.* 135: 350–355.

Kitagawa, T. 1984. Cause analysis of the Yokkaichi asthma episode in Japan. *J. Air Pollut. Control Assoc.* 34: 743–746.

Kleinman, M. T. 1984. Sulfur dioxide and exercise: Relationships between response and absorption in upper airways. *J. Air Pollut. Control Assoc.* 34: 32–37.

Kleinman, M. T., R. F. Phalen, W. J. Mautz, R. C. Mannix, T. R. McClure, and T. T. Crocker. 1989. Health effects of acid aerosols formed by atmospheric mixtures. *Environ. Health Perspect.* 79: 137–145.

Koenig, J. Q., D. S. Covert, and W. E. Pierson. 1989. Effects of inhalation of acidic compounds on pulmonary function in allergic adolescent subjects. *Environ. Health Perspect.* 79: 173–178.

Koenig, J. Q., D. S. Covert, Q. S. Hanley, G. van Belle, and W. E. Pierson. 1990. Prior exposure to ozone potentiates subsequent response to sulfur dioxide in adolescent asthmatic subjects. *Am. Rev. Respir. Dis.* 141: 377–380.

Koenig, J. Q., W. E. Pierson, and M. Horike. 1983a. The effects of inhaled sulfuric acid on pulmonary function in adolescent asthmatics. *Am. Rev. Respir. Dis.* 128: 221–225.

Koenig, J. Q., W. E. Pierson, M. Horike, and R. Frank. 1981. Effects of inhaled SO$_2$ plus NaCl aerosol combined with moderate exercise on pulmonary function in asthmatic adolescents. *Environ. Res.* 25: 340–348.

Koenig, J. Q., W. E. Pierson, M. Horike, and R. Frank. 1983b. A comparison of the pulmonary effects of 0.5 ppm versus 1.0 ppm sulfur dioxide plus sodium chloride droplet in asthmatic adolescents. *J. Toxicol. Environ. Health* 11: 129–139.

Lamborg, C., G. J. Keeler, and G. Evans. 1992. *Atmospheric Acidity Measurements during the Lake Michigan Urban Air Toxics Study*. Research Triangle Park, NC: U.S. Environmental Protection Agency, Atmospheric Research and Exposure Assessment Laboratory; EPA Report No. EPA/600/A-92/250. Available from: NTIS, Springfield, VA; PB93-121069.

Larson, T. V., D. S. Covert, R. Frank, and R. J. Charlson. 1977. Ammonia in the human airways: Neutralization of inspired acid sulfate aerosols. *Science* 197: 161–163.

Last, J. A. 1989. Effects of inhaled acids on lung biochemistry. *Environ. Health Perspect.* 79: 115–119.

Lave, L. B., and E. P. Seskin. 1970. Air pollution and human health. *Science* 169: 723–733.

Lawther, P. J. 1958. Climate, air pollution and chronic bronchitis. *Proc. R. Soc. Med.* 51: 262–264.

Lawther, P. J., R. E. Waller, and M. Henderson. 1970. Air pollution and exacerbations of bronchitis. *Thorax* 25: 525–539.

Leaderer, B. P., P. M. Boone, and S. K. Hammond. 1990. Total particle, sulfate, and acidic aerosol emissions from kerosene space heaters. *Environ. Sci. Technol.* 24: 908–912.

Lee, H. S., R. A. Wadden, and P. A. Scheff. 1993. Measurement and evaluation of acid air pollutants in Chicago using an annular denuder system. *Atmos. Environ.* Part A 27: 543–553.

Leikauf, G. D., D. M. Spektor, R. E. Albert, and M. Lippmann. 1984. Dose dependent effects of submicrometer sulfuric acid aerosol on particle clearance from ciliated human lung airways. *Am. Ind. Hyg. Assoc.* 45: 285–292.

Leikauf, G., D. B. Yeates, K. A. Wales, R. E. Albert, and M. Lippmann. 1981. Effects of sulfuric acid aerosol on respiratory mechanics and mucociliary particle clearance in healthy nonsmoking adults. *Am. Ind. Hyg. Assoc. J.* 42: 273–282.

Leung, H. W., and D. J. Paustenbach. 1990. Organic acids and bases: Review of toxicological studies. *Am. J. Ind. Med.* 18: 717–735.

Linn, W. S., D. A. Shamoo, K. R. Anderson, J. D. Whynot, E. L. Avol, and J. D. Hackney. 1985. Effects of heat and humidity on the responses of exercising asthmatics to sulfur dioxide exposure. *Am. Rev. Respir. Dis.* 131: 221–225.

Linn, W. S., E. L. Avol, K. R. Anderson, D. A. Shamoo, R. C. Peng, and J. D. Hackney. 1989. Effect of droplet size on respiratory responses to inhaled sulfuric acid in normal and asthmatic volunteers. *Am. Rev. Respir. Dis.* 140: 161–166.

Linn, W. S., T. G. Venet, D. A. Shamoo, L. M. Valencia, U. T. Anzar, C. E. Spier, and J. D. Hackney. 1983. Respiratory effects of sulfur dioxide in heavily exercising asthmatics: A dose-response study. *Am. Rev. Respir. Dis.* 127: 278–283.

Lipfert, F. W. 1994. Filter artifacts associated with particulate measurements: Recent evidence and effects on statistical relationships. *Atmos. Environ.* 28: 3233–3249.

Lippmann, M. 1989. Background on health effects of acid aerosols. *Environ. Health Perspect.* 79: 3–6.

Lippmann, M., and K. Ito. 1995. Separating the effects of temperature and season on daily mortality from those of air pollution in London: 1965–1972. *Inhal. Toxicol.* 7: 85–97.

Lippmann, M., D. B. Yeates, and R. E. Albert. 1980. Deposition, retention, and clearance of inhaled particles. *Br. J. Ind. Med.* 37: 337–362.

Lippmann, M., J. M. Gearhart, and R. B. Schlesinger. 1987. Basis for a particle size-selective TLV for sulfuric acid aerosols. *Appl. Ind. Hyg.* 2: 188–199.

Lippmann, M., R. B. Schlesinger, G. Leikauf, D. Spektor, and R. E. Albert. 1982. Effects of sulphuric acid aerosols on respiratory tract airways. *Ann. Occup. Hyg.* 26: 677–690.

Liu, L. J. S., R. Burton, W. E. Wilson, and P. Koutrakis. 1996. Comparison of aerosol acidity in urban and semi-rural environments. *Atmos. Environ.* 30: 1237–1245.

Lourenco, R. V. 1969. Distribution and clearance of aerosols. *Am. Rev. Respir. Dis.* 101: 460–461.

Magnussen, H., R. Jorres, H. M. Wagner, and G. von Nieding. 1990. Relationship between the airway response to inhaled sulfur dioxide, isocapnic hyperventilation, and histamine in asthmatic subjects. *Int. Arch. Occup. Environ. Health* 62: 485–491.

Matsuba, K., and W. M. Thurlbeck. 1973. Disease of the small airways in chronic bronchitis. *Am. Rev. Respir. Dis.* 107: 552–558.

Mazumdar, S., and N. Sussman. 1983. Relationships of air pollution to health: Results from the Pittsburgh study. *Arch. Environ. Health* 38: 17–24.

McKenzie, H. I., M. Glick, and K. G. Outhred. 1969. Chronic bronchitis in coal miners: Antemortem/post-mortem correlations. *Thorax* 24: 527–535.

Mitchell, R. S. 1967. Clinical and morphologic correlations in chronic airway obstruction. *Am. Rev. Respir. Dis.* 97: 54–62.

Neas, L. M., D. W. Dockery, P. Koutrakis, D. J. Tollerud, and F. E. Speizer. 1995. The association of ambient air pollution with twice daily peak expiratory flow rate measurement in children. *Am. J. Epidemiol.* 141: 111–122.

Osebold, J. W., L. J. Gershwin, and C. Z. Yuan. 1980. Studies on the enhancement of allergic lung sensitization by inhalation of ozone and sulfuric acid aerosol. *J. Environ. Pathol. Toxicol.* 3: 221–234.

Ostro, B. 1990. Associations between morbidity and alternative measures of particulate matter. *Risk Anal.* 10: 421–427.

Ostro, B. D., M. J. Lipsett, M. B. Wiener, and J. C. Selner. 1991. Asthmatic responses to airborne acid aerosols. *Am. J. Public Health* 81: 694–702.

Ostro, B., M. Lipsett, M. Wiener, and J. C. Selner. 1989. A panel study of the effect of acid aerosols on asthmatics. Paper presented at Annual Meeting of the Air and Waste Management Association, Anaheim, CA, June.

Ozkaynak, H., and G. D. Thurston. 1987. Associations between 1980 U.S. mortality rates and alternative measures of airborne particle concentration. *Risk Anal.* 7: 449–460.

Ozkaynak, H., and J. D. Spengler. 1985. Analysis of health effects resulting from population exposures to acid precipitation precursors. *Environ. Health Perspect.* 63: 45–55.

Ozkaynak, H., J. P. Xue, H. Zhou, J. D. Spengler, and G. D. Thurston. 1996a. Intercommunity differences in acid aerosol (H^+/SO_4^{2-}). *J. Expos. Anal. Environ. Epidemiol.* 6: 35–55.

Peters, A., D. W. Dockery, J. Heinrich, and H. E. Wichmann. 1997. Medication use modifies the health effects of particulate sulfate air pollution in children with asthma. *Environ. Health Perspect.* 105: 430–435.

Pope, C. A., III, M. J. Thun, M. Namboodiri, D. W. Dockery, J. S. Evans, F. E. Speizer, and C. W. Heath Jr. 1995. Particulate air pollution is a predictor of mortality in a prospective study of U.S. adults. *Am. J. Respir. Crit. Care Med.* 151: 669–674.

Raizenne, M., L. M. Neas, A. I. Damokosh, D. W. Dockery, J. D. Spengler, P. Koutrakis, J. Ware, and F. E. Speizer. 1996. Health effects of acid aerosols on North American children: Pulmonary function. *Environ. Health Perspect.* 104: 506–514.

Reid, L. 1963. An experimental study of the hypersecretion of mucus in the bronchial tree. *Br. J. Exp. Pathol.* 44: 437–445.

Roger, L. J., H. R. Kehrl, M. Hazucha, and D. H. Horstman. 1985. Bronchoconstriction in asthmatics exposed to sulfur dioxide during repeated exercise. *J. Appl. Physiol.* 59: 784–791.

Rubinstein, I., B. G. Bigby, T. F. Reiss, and H. A. Boushey Jr. 1990. Short-term exposure to 0.3 ppm nitrogen dioxide does not potentiate airway responsiveness to sulfur dioxide in asthmatic subjects. *Am. Rev. Respir. Dis.* 141: 381–385.

Schenker, M. B., J. M. Samet, F. E. Speizer, J. Gruhl, and S. Batterman. 1983. Health effects of air pollution due to coal combustion in the Chestnut Ridge region of Pennsylvania: Results of cross-sectional analysis in adults. *Arch. Environ. Health* 38: 325–330.

Schlesinger, R. B. 1985. Effects of inhaled acids on respiratory tract defense mechanisms. *Environ. Health Perspect.* 63: 25–38.

Schlesinger, R. B. 1986. The effects of inhaled acids on lung defenses. In *Aerosols*, eds. S. D. Lee, T. Schneider, L. D. Grant, and P. J. Verkerk. Chelsea, MI: Lewis Publishers.

Schlesinger, R. B. 1989. Factors affecting the response of lung clearance systems to acid aerosols: Role of exposure concentration, exposure time, and relative activity. *Environ. Health Perspect.* 79: 121–126.

Schlesinger, R. B. 1990. Exposure-response pattern for sulfuric acid-induced effects on particle clearance from the respiratory region of rabbit lungs. *Inhal. Toxicol.* 2: 21–27.

Schlesinger, R. B., and J. M. Gearhart. 1986. Early alveolar clearance in rabbits intermittently exposed to sulfuric acid mist. *J. Toxicol. Environ. Health* 17: 213–220.

Schlesinger, R. B., B. D. Naumann, and L. C. Chen. 1983. Physiological and histological alterations in the bronchial mucociliary clearance system of rabbits following intermittent oral or nasal inhalation of sulfuric acid mist. *J. Toxicol. Environ. Health* 12: 441–465.

Schlesinger, R. B., M. Halpern, R. E. Albert, and M. Lippmann. 1979. Effect of chronic inhalation of sulfuric acid mist upon mucociliary clearance from the lungs of donkeys. *J. Environ. Pathol. Toxicol.* 2: 1351–1367.

Sheppard, D., W. L. Eschenbacher, H. A. Boushey, and R. A. Bethel. 1984. Magnitude of the interaction between the bronchomotor effects of sulfur dioxide and those of dry (cold) air. *Am. Rev. Respir. Dis.* 130: 52–55.

Sim, V. M., and R. E. Pattle. 1957. Effect of possible smog irritants on human subjects. *JAMA* 165: 1908–1913.

Skornik, W. A., and J. D. Brain. 1990. Effect of sulfur dioxide on pulmonary macrophage endocytosis at rest and during exercise. *Am. Rev. Respir. Dis.* 142: 655–659.

Soskolne, C. L., G. Pagano, M. Cipollaro, J. J. Beaumont, and G. G. Giordano. 1989. Epidemiologic and toxicologic evidence for chronic health effects and the underlying biologic mechanisms involved in sublethal exposures to acidic pollutants. *Arch. Environ. Health* 44: 180–191.

Speizer, F. E. 1989. Studies of acid aerosols in six cities and in a new multicity investigation: Design issues. *Environ. Health Perspect.* 79: 61–67.

Spektor, D. M., B. M. Yen, and M. Lippmann. 1989. Effect of concentration and cumulative dose of inhaled sulfuric acid on lung clearance in humans. *Environ. Health Perspect.* 79: 167–172.

Spektor, D. M., G. D. Leikauf, R. E. Albert, and M. Lippmann. 1985. Effects of submicrometer sulfuric acid aerosols on mucociliary transport and respiratory mechanics in asymptomatic asthmatics. *Environ. Res.* 37: 174–191.

Spengler, J. D., G. A. Allen, S. Foster, P. Severance, B. Ferris Jr. 1986. Sulfuric acid and sulfate aerosol events in two U.S. cities. In: *Aerosols: Research, Risk Assessment and Control Strategies. Proc. 2nd U.S.–Dutch International Symposium*, May 1985, Williamsburg, VA, eds. S. D. Lee, T. Schneider, L. D. Grant, and P. J. Verkerk, pp. 107–120. Chelsea, MI: Lewis Publishers.

Spengler, J. D., G. J. Keeler, P. Koutrakis, P. B. Ryan, M. Raizenne, and C. A. Franklin. 1989. Exposures to acidic aerosols. *Environ. Health Perspect.* 79: 43–51.

Spengler, J. D., P. Koutrakis, D. W. Dockery, M. Raizenne, and F. E. Speizer. 1996. Health effects of acid aerosols on North American children. Air pollution exposures. *Environ. Health Perspect.* 104: 492–499.

Stara, J. F., D. L. Dungworth, J. G. Orthoefer, and W. S. Tyler. 1980. *Long-Term Effects of Air Pollutants in Canine Species.* EPA-600/8-80-014. Research Triangle Park, NC: U.S. Environmental Protection Agency.

Steenland, K., and J. Beaumont. 1989. Further follow-up and adjustment for smoking in a study of lung cancer and acid mists. *Am. J. Ind. Med.* 16: 347–354.

Stern, B. R., M. E. Raizenne, R. T. Burnett, L. Jones, J. Kearney, and C. A. Franklin. 1994. Air pollution and childhood respiratory health: Exposure to sulfate and ozone in 10 Canadian rural communities. *Environ. Res.* 66: 125–142.

Strauss, R. H., E. R. McFadden Jr., R. H. Ingram Jr., and J. J. Jaeger. 1977. Enhancement of exercise-induced asthma by cold air. *N. Engl. J. Med.* 297: 743–747.

Studnicka, M. J., T. Frischer, R. Meinert, A. Studnicka-Benke, K. Hajek, J. D. Spengler, and M. G. Neumann. 1995. Acidic particles and lung function in children. A summer camp study in the Austrian Alps. *Am. J. Respir. Crit. Care Med.* 151: 423–430.

Suh, H. H., G. A. Allen, P. Koutrakis, and R. M. Burton. 1995. Spatial variation in acidic sulfate and ammonia concentrations within Metropolitan Philadelphia. *J. Air Waste Manage. Assoc.* 45: 442–452.

Suh, H. H., J. D. Spengler, and P. Koutrakis. 1992. Personal exposures to acid aerosols and ammonia. *Environ. Sci. Technol.* 26: 2507–2517.

Suhs, R. H., J. L. Lumeng, and M. H. Leppe. 1969. An experimental immunologic approach to the induction and perpetuation of chronic bronchitis. *Arch. Environ. Health* 18: 564–573.

Thompson, K. M., P. Koutrakis, M. Brauer, J. D. Spengler, W. E. Wilson, and R. M. Burton. 1991. Measurements of aerosol acidity: Sampling frequency, seasonal variability, and spatial variation. Presented at the 84th Annual Meeting of the Air and Waste Management Association, June, Vancouver, BC, Canada. Paper 91–89.5. Air and Waste Management Association, Pittsburgh, PA.

Thurston, G. D., K. Ito, M. Lippmann, and C. Hayes. 1989. Re-examination of London mortality in relation to exposure to acidic aerosols during 1962–1973 winters. *Environ. Health Perspect.* 79: 73–82.

Thurston, G. D., J. E. Gorczynski, P. Jaques, J. Currie, and D. He. 1992a. An automated sequential sampling system for particulate aerosols: Description, characterization, and field sampling results. *J. Exposure Anal. Environ. Epidemiol.* 2: 415–428.

Thurston, G. D., K. Ito, P. L. Kinney, and M. Lippmann. 1992b. A multi-year study of air pollution and respiratory hospital admissions in three New York State metropolitan areas: Results for 1988 and 1989 summers. *J. Expos. Anal. Environ. Epidemiol.* 2: 429–450.

Thurston, G. D., J. E. Gorczynski, J. H. Currie, D. He, K. Ito, J. Hipfner, J. Waldman, P. J. Lioy, and M. Lippmann. 1994a. The nature and origins of acid summer haze air pollution in Metropolitan Toronto, Ontario. *Environ. Res.* 65: 254–270.

Thurston, G. D., K. Ito, C. G. Hayes, D. V. Bates, and M. Lippmann. 1994b. Respiratory hospital admissions and summertime haze air pollution in Toronto, Ontario: Consideration of the role of acid aerosols. *Environ. Res.* 65: 271–290.

Thurston, G. D., M. Lippmann, M. Scott, and J. M. Fine. 1997. Summertime haze pollution and children with asthma. *Am. J. Respir. Crit. Care Med.* 155: 654–660.

U.S. EPA. 1986. *Second Addendum to Air Quality Criteria for Particulate Matter and Sulfur Oxides (1982).* EPA/600/8-86/020F. Washington, DC: Office of Health and Environmental Assessment.

U.S. EPA. 1989. *An Acid Aerosols Issue Paper.* EPA/600/8-88/005F. Research Triangle Park, NC: Environmental Criteria and Assessment Office, U.S. EPA.

Utell, M. J., P. E. Morrow, and R. W. Hyde. 1982. Comparison of normal and asthmatic subjects' response to sulfate pollutant aerosols. *Ann. Occup. Hyg.* 26: 691–697.

Utell, M. J., P. E. Morrow, and R. W. Hyde. 1984. Airway reactivity to sulfate and sulfuric acid aerosols in normal and asthmatic subjects. *J. Air Pollut. Control Assoc.* 34: 931–935.

Waldman, J. M., P. J. Lioy, G. D. Thurston, and M. Lippmann. 1990. Spatial and temporal patterns in summertime sulfate aerosol acidity and neutralization within a metropolitan area. *Atmos. Environ.* Part B 24: 115–126.

Wichmann, H. E., W. Mueller, P. Allhoff, M. Beckmann, N. Bochter, M. J. Csicsaky, M. Jung, B. Molik, and G. Schoeneberg. 1989. Health effects during a smog episode in West Germany in 1985. *Environ. Health Perspect.* 79: 89–99.

Williams, M. K. 1970. Sickness, absence and ventilatory capacity of workers exposed to sulphuric acid mist. *Br. J. Ind. Med.* 27: 61–66.

Wilson, W. E. and L. Stockburger. 1990. Diurnal variations in aerosol composition and concentration. In: *Aerosols: Science, Industry, Health and Environment*, eds. S. Masuda, and K. Takahashi, pp. 962–965. Oxford, Pergamon.

Wilson, W. E., P. Koutrakis, and J. D. Spengler. 1991. Diurnal variations of aerosol acidity, sulfate, and ammonia in the atmosphere. Presented at the 84th Annual Meeting and Exhibition; June; Vancouver, BC, Canada. Air and Waste Management Association, Pittsburgh, PA. Paper No. 91-89.9.

Wolff, G. T., P. R. Manson, and M. A. Ferman. 1979. On the nature of the diurnal variation at rural sites in the Eastern United States. *Environ. Sci. Technol.* 13: 1271–1276.

Wolff, R. K., J. L. Mauderly, and J. A. Pickrell. 1981. Chronic bronchitis and asthma: Biochemistry, rheology and mucociliary clearance. In *Lung Connective Tissue: Location, Metabolism and Response to Injury*, ed. J. A. Pickrell, pp. 169–183. Boca Raton, FL: CRC Press.

Yu, C. P., J. P. Hu, B. M. Yen, D. M. Spektor, and M. Lippmann. 1986. Models for mucociliary particle clearance in lung airways. In *Aerosols*, eds. S. D. Lee, T. Schneider, L. D. Grant, and P. J. Verkerk, pp. 569–578. Chelsea, MI: Lewis Publishers.

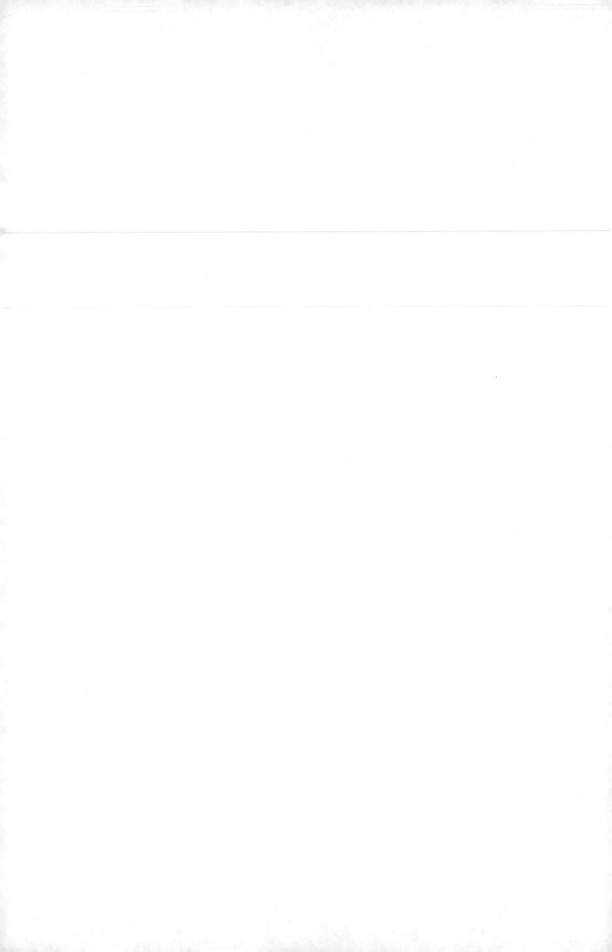

24 Trace Elements: Aluminum, Arsenic, Cadmium, and Nickel

MAX COSTA, Ph.D.

Although there are numerous metals and trace elements of toxicological concern, there is insufficient space in this chapter to thoroughly discuss all of them. Additionally human exposure to certain toxic metals is more prevalent and/or imparts more serious health damage than exposures to others. Consequently this chapter is limited to a discussion of the toxicology of aluminum, arsenic, cadmium, and nickel. There are chapters on chromium, lead and mercury elsewhere in the text. The metals and their compounds discussed in this chapter are relatively abundant in the environment, as well as of considerable toxicological concern. They are considered in terms of their toxicology and their essentiality. This is followed by discussions of their environmental sources and routes of exposure. Discussion of their uptake, distribution, and toxicological effects is also included. Specific consideration is given to the carcinogenic and teratogenic effects of these metals as well as the genotoxicity and mutagenicity of each metal and its compounds.

ALUMINUM

Aluminum (Al) is the third most common element encountered in nature, accounting for about 7.5% of the lithosphere (Cotton and Wilkinson, 1980). It does not naturally occur in the free state; it is usually found combined with oxygen, silicon, and fluorine in minerals comprising igneous, metamorphic, and sedimentary rocks (Carson et al., 1986). The primary industrial source of Al is bauxite, a mixture of hydrated aluminum oxides containing impurities of various other metal oxides such as iron, silicon, titanium, gallium, and indium. Other industrial sources from which Al is extracted are cryolite and aluminum fluoride. The commercial use of Al is dictated by its physical and chemical properties, which include a low specific gravity, high tensile strength, ductility, malleability, corrosion resistance, and high electrical conductivity (Cotton and Wilkinson, 1980). In industry, Al is most important in electrical equipment, transport, and construction, and is familiar in its uses in beverage containers, household utensils, and appliances. Aluminum compounds are widely used in the processing, packaging, and preservation of food products and additionally as food additives. Aluminum sulfate is widely used as a flocculant for sedimenting particles in the treatment of drinking water. Further uses for Al compounds include preventive therapy for hyperphosphatemia in patients with renal disease and silicosis (Norseth, 1979). Other pharmaceutical and therapeutic uses of Al compounds are

Environmental Toxicants: Human Exposures and Their Health Effects, 2/e. Edited by Morton Lippmann.
ISBN: 0-471-29298-2 © 2000 John Wiley & Sons, Inc.

as antacids, antidotes, antiperspirants, and as an adjuvant for vaccines, toxoids, and Al-penicillin.

Essentiality

Aluminum is not classified as an essential trace element, but its nonessentiality has been difficult to prove because the high Al concentrations in the earth's crust make the preparation of Al-deficient animal feeds difficult (Sorensen et al., 1974). However, the nonessential nature of Al for humans is suggested by the ultimate net loss of Al when it is administered to humans (Venugopal and Luckey, 1978). An attempt to induce Al-deficient diseases in rats fed an "Al-deficient diet" led to the conclusion that if Al were an essential element, the required dietary intake for human would be very low (1 mg/d) (Hove et al., 1938).

Environmental Sources and Exposure

Exposure to Al compounds mainly arises from two sources: occupational contact and dietary ingestion. Epidemiological studies of occupational exposure to Al have not provided specific information that adequately defines or quantitates the nature of chemical exposure. This stems from an inadequate appreciation of the multiple variations in the physical and chemical forms of Al. Monitoring is further complicated by the number of other pollutants released during production processes. During electrolysis of alumina (Al_2O_3) from molten cryolite ($NaAlF_3$), gaseous fluoride, carbon monoxide (CO), carbon dioxide (CO_2), and sulfur dioxide (SO_2) are released, as well as particulate fluoride (Moller and Gudjonsson, 1932). Chronic exposure to fluoride can result in a condition known as skeletal fluorosis. Similarly plant workers exposed to metalworking fluids and abrasives are at risk not only from Al exposure but also from nitrosamines (Fan et al., 1977). In addition a large number of toxic compounds are released during certain Al-refining processes, including the well-known carcinogen benzopyrene (Kreyberg, 1959) and to crystalline silicon dioxide, exposure to which can result in pulmonary silicosis (IARC, 1983). Although it is difficult to assess precisely the toxicological impact of Al exposure in aluminum refineries due to concomitant exposure to other contaminants, one study has shown a direct association between exposure to Al and altered pulmonary function (Townsend et al., 1985).

Concentrations of airborne Al in reduction plants varies from 0.18 to 975 mg/m^3 (IARC, 1983). These levels are extremely high in comparison with the normal mean atmospheric Al concentrations of 0.5 and 10 μg/m^3 in suburban and urban areas, respectively (Sorensen et al., 1974). In water, Al concentrations also vary considerably for fresh water and saltwater, with typical readings being 300 ng/m^3 and 2 mg/m^3, respectively (Bowen, 1979; Kabata-Pendias and Pendias, 1984). The OSHA permissible exposure limit (PEL) is 15 mg/m^3 (total) and 5 mg/m^3 (respirable). The ACGIH (1999) Threshold Limit Values (TLVs) are 10 mg/m^3 for the metal and aluminum oxide; 5 mg/m^3 for pyro powders and welding fumes; and 2 mg/m^3 for soluble salts and alkyl compounds. Elevated Al contamination has been considered to be one of the main cause of death in fish, especially in lakes polluted by acid rain (Hutchinson, 1983). Acidification results in the leaching of Al from lakebed sediments and the surrounding rocks. As a result of environmental pollution, certain plants have been shown to contain more than 100 ppm soluble Al (Shackette et al., 1977). Some edible plants have been shown to contain 200 to 1500 ppm Al in their ash.

Since Al compounds are widely used in the food industry, the content of Al in food products can range from 150 to 1000 ppm in ash (Shackette et al., 1977), whereas most unprocessed food items contains less than 10 ppm (Norseth, 1979). Although the use of Al in the processing and storage of food increases its relative concentration, this elevation is not toxicologically significant (Maitson, 1981). The total daily intake of Al is estimated at 80 mg/d; however, large interindividual variations depend on diet (Greger, 1987). Pharmaceutical products, such as the Al-based antacids used in the treatment of gastric ulcers, can increase this intake to greater than 500 mg Al/d (Sorensen et al., 1974). The dietary intake may further be increased by cooking and storing food in aluminum pans or trays. However, most food accumulates less than 2 mg Al/g of food (Ondreicka et al., 1971; Greger et al., 1985). Aluminum absorption by food cooked and stored in these trays is influenced by several factors such as pH, the length of the cooking period, and use of new pans. Acidic and basic foods, as well as the presence of fluoride in the cooking water, will increase the Al content of food cooked in these pans (Poe and Leberman, 1949). Concern about the presence of Al in nutritional formulas and parenteral solutions has been raised (Baydar et al., 1997). Aluminum levels in nutritional formulas range from 87.6 to 961.2 ng/ml and from 58.4 to 1232.0 ng/ml in parenteral solutions (Baydar et al., 1997).

Uptake and Distribution

Absorption of Al from the gastrointestinal tract into the bloodstream has been discussed in relation to the use of $Al(OH)_3$ for the treatment of hyperphosphatemia in patients with renal failure (Clarkson et al., 1972). About 15% of the dose is absorbed in these patients, with lower values observed in healthy subjects. In adults, the absorption of Al from the gut has been estimated to be between 0.05% and 0.3% based on the urinary excretion (Ganrot, 1986). Following absorption from either the gastrointestinal or the respiratory tract, distribution of Al occurs to all major organs. In occupationally exposed individuals, the lungs invariably show the highest concentrations of Al, ranging from 200 to 300 mg/g; 10% of this value was frequently observed in the other organs examined (Norseth, 1979). This is most probably due to the inhalation route of exposure. In animal studies, high Al concentrations in food did not result in increased Al levels in the lungs of rats, although there was a substantial increase in the measurable levels in the liver, brain, testes, and blood (Ondreicka et al., 1966).

Patients with renal distress often exhibit an accumulation of Al during dialysis, although there is an absence of any symptoms of encephalopathy. In these patients, the mean concentration of Al has been reported to be 1.6 times normal lung burdens, 4 times normal cerebral gray matter levels, 35 times normal bone levels, 40 times normal liver levels, and 64 times the normal splenic levels (Alfrey, 1980). Although dialysis patients display the highest Al concentration in their spleens, patients without renal failure but receiving total parenteral feeding have their greatest accumulation of Al in the brain. Certain disease states, such as Alzheimer's disease, are thought to influence the concentration of Al in the brain and in other major organs (Markesbery et al., 1981; Crapper et al., 1973; Perl and Brody, 1980; Perl et al., 1982).

The normal half-time of Al in man is about 8 hours (Sjorgen et al., 1985), but this may be prolonged in those subjected to chronic exposure. For example, welders exposed to welding fumes containing Al may retain some of the inhaled metal fumes for an extended period of time (i.e., >12 h) (Sjorgen et al., 1985; Mussi et al., 1984). This may be related to the delayed clearance of Al particles from the lungs. In experimental animals, the half-time of Al varies, with values of 120 to 240 minutes in the rabbit (Yokel and McNamara 1985), 80 to 90 minutes in the rat (Wachi and Aikawa 1975), and 280 minutes in the dog (Henry et al., 1984). The typically small amount of Al absorbed from the lungs and from ingestion is excreted primarily in the urine and to a lesser extent via the bile. The majority of unabsorbed dietary Al is excreted as insoluble $Al(PO_4)$ in the feces (Norseth, 1979).

Aluminum is also excreted via transplacental passage and during lactation. As a result the developing fetus and the breast-fed infant are exposed to Al. However, the extent of Al exposure in these fetuses and neonates has not been assessed. A study of the toxicity of Al in rabbits revealed no obvious signs of overt toxicity in the offspring and the suckling pups, but there was a reduction in weight gain in the group that had received a high transplacental dose (Yokel, 1984).

Toxicological Effects

Orally administered Al can be considered to be relatively nontoxic in comparison with the other possible routes of exposure. For example, the LD_{50} of $Al_2(SO_4)_3$ in intraperitoneally exposed mice is $0.14\,g/kg$ compared with $6.2\,g/kg$ when administered orally (Krasovski et al., 1979). In these studies the doses employed are very large compared with the dietary intake of Al in order to achieve a level of metal that allows for detection in the animal tissues. Similarly the use of such high doses are required to induce harmful effects; these high doses do not reflect those that are measured and encountered in even the most severe public or occupational exposures (Ondreicka et al., 1971). It has been shown from these experimental studies that Al significantly binds to phosphate ions in the gastrointestinal tract, leading to phosphate deficiency and overall interference with phosphate metabolism (Leonard and Gerber, 1988). Parenteral and oral dosing of rats with large concentrations of Al salts such as the hydroxide, chloride, or sulfate forms, caused lethargy, anorexia, and ultimately death (Berlyne et al., 1970). Long-term feeding of rats with $AlCl_3$ (100–200 mg/kg) caused growth retardation and disturbed carbohydrate and phosphate metabolism. From these and other studies (Sorensen et al., 1974; Thurston, et al., 1972), it was concluded that the toxicity of Al is chiefly due to its effects on calcium and phosphate homeostasis. However, the possibility of Al toxicity due to interactions with other essential trace metals such as zinc and magnesium (Harrison et al., 1972) cannot be excluded.

Phosphate depletion also occurs among chronic users of large doses of Al-based antacids (Dent and Winter, 1974). In addition large doses of antacids may contribute to an onset of encephalopathy, a condition that can also occur in renal patients treated prophylactically with antacids but in the absence of dialysis. Blood and peritoneal dialysis with fluids containing Al at concentrations near the normal serum levels have been reported to progressively cause a usually fatal dialysis encephalopathy (dementia) (Alfrey et al., 1976). An increased body load of Al may also occur after prolonged continuous intravenous feeding of solutions containing Al even in the absence of renal failure. Accumulation of Al in bone often results in and is accompanied by most of the problems mentioned above (Dent and Winter, 1974). Neurotoxicity, especially of the Alzheimer type, has been associated with Al accumulation (Crapper et al., 1973) as has been a blood disorder, although the latter condition is less frequently observed. Increased serum Al concentrations have also been associated with jaundice (Andersen et al., 1979), and this may be due to decreased biliary excretion of Al in these patients. However, studies have demonstrated successful removal of Al by hemodialysis from patients with hyperaluminemia; the plasma ultrafiltratable fraction being 8% to 15% (Graf et al., 1981; Burnatowska-Hledin et al., 1985). Desferrioxamine has also been used to remove Al from bones of some uremic patients (Malluche et al., 1984).

Conditions such as pulmonary fibrosis, alveolar proteinosis, and encephalopathy have been associated with occupational exposure to Al (Schauer, 1948; Dinman, 1987, 1988). Bronchial asthma, as well as dyspnea, wheezing, and coughing have also been observed (IARC, 1983). The onset of these symptoms may, however, be linked with the inhalation of a complex mixture containing other airborne pollutants besides Al. Among workers occupationally exposed to Al, the mortality rate increases substantially. For example, in men working in the prebake process for 20 years, the standardized mortality ratio (SMR) for asthma was 260.2 based on seven deaths observed (IARC, 1983). Potroom employees and carbon workers in the Soderberg process had an increased mortality from emphysema, with observed SMR values of 194 and 267, respectively (Rockette and Arena, 1983).

As a hard trivalent metal ion, Al^{-3} binds strongly to oxygen donor ligands such as citrate and phosphate. Al is bound to the protein transferrin which plays a major role in Al transport in the serum (Harris et al., 1996). Recent studies have suggested that the biochemical mechanisms of Al neurotoxicity may be involved in affecting the GTPase activity of the *ras* p21 protein. GTPase activity was inhibited 60% in the presence of $100\,\mu M\,Mg^{2+}$ and 2.9×10^{-10} M Al^{+3} (Landino and MacDonald, 1997). Genetic studies demonstrated that the mode of Al-induced inhibition *ras* p21 GTPase activity changed from competitive to mixed noncompetitive as the number of p21 turnovers increased. Further dissection of the *ras* p21 cycles showed that Mg^{2+}-dependent GDP/GTP exchange was the Al^{+3} sensitive step (Landino and MacDonald, 1997). Some studies have shown that Al may produce oxidative injury by oral exposure with a decrease in thiols, glutathione reductase, and adenosine triphosphatase observed in brain homogenates (Katyal et al., 1997).

Carcinogenic and Teratogenic Effects

Aluminum has been found to cause cancer in a few experimental animal studies, although most of these failed to demonstrate a carcinogenicity attributable solely to Al compounds administered by various routes. Sarcomas were induced in 45% of NIH black rats given subcutaneous implants of 0.5 mm thick Al foil (O'Gara and Brown, 1967), whereas Al fibers having a median diameter of 3.5 mm were noncarcinogenic in these rats following intrapleural or intraperitoneal administration (Stanton, 1974; Pigott and Ishmael, 1981). This demonstrates the importance of the physical characteristics of Al in relation to its carcinogenicity (Krueger et al., 1984).

The possible use of Al compounds as chemotherapeutic agents in human cancer has been suggested. Aluminum nitrate ($Al(NO_3)_3 9H_2O$) administered at doses of 50 to 400 mg / kg caused a reduction in the growth of intraperitoneally transplanted Walker 256 carcinosarcomas in female Sprague-Dawley rats (Adamson et al., 1975; Hart and Adamson, 1971); the optimal dose was calculated to be 150 mg / kg. However, this compound exhibited little activity against the P388 leukemia cells and none against L1210 leukemia, K1964 leukemia, or YPC-1 plasma cells, or even Ehrlich ascites carcinoma cells. The differences in activity have been associated with differential uptake of the Al salts by these cells (Adamson et al., 1975). When mice were pretreated with $AlCl_3$ prior to administration of dimethylnitrosamine, the number of developing nodules decreased in comparison with controls given dimethylnitrosamine only (Yamane and Ohtawa, 1979). These results suggest that the antitumor activity of Al is not influenced by the anionic nature of its salts because the nitrate, chloride, and sulfate forms all possessed the same activity (Hart and Adamson, 1971). Rather than affecting the tumor cells directly, Al compounds might alter the host's ability to resist the abnormally growing cells. For example, exposure to $Al(OH)_3$ has been associated with alterations of the immune response in animals (Pauwels et al., 1979).

The absence of positive epidemiological evidence suggests that Al exposure does not represent a carcinogenic hazard to humans. The data on mortality (Milham, 1979) among workers suggests that some of the observed lymphatic, hematopoietic (especially malignant lymphomas), and lung cancers in these workers may be of occupational origin. However, these conclusions have not been proved statistically (Leonard and Gerber, 1988). Another study of worker mortality from malignant neoplasms of the bladder and/or lung found correlations with the number of years of exposure to coal-tar pitch volatiles (Gibbs and Horowitz, 1979). Still, the excess risk of bladder cancer among these workers

(Theriault et al., 1981; Armstrong et al., 1988; Silverstein et al., 1988; Andersen et al., 1982) cannot be considered as evidence of Al-induced carcinogenesis. The causes appeared to be related mainly to the duration of worker exposure to aromatic substances present in the coal-tar pitch volatiles. Similarly increased incidences of stomach cancer have been reported among workers exposed to Al-bearing abrasive materials (Silverstein et al., 1988), but this has not been confirmed (Edling et al., 1987).

Teratogenesis studies with experimental animals have demonstrated that Al compounds display embryotoxic properties depending on a number of factors such as dose and route of administration as well as the stage of embryogenesis at the time of treatment (Leonard and Gerber, 1988). These embryotoxic effects could be related to the Al-induced increase in protein synthesis and the decrease in ribosomal RNA content. This may be caused by Al binding to nuclear chromatin or by interference with microtubular polymerization (Deboni et al., 1974). In addition Al is known to alter phosphate and calcium metabolism, highly active processes during the critical stages of embryogenesis, thereby affecting fetal development.

Aluminum has been shown to cause fetal malformation when injected (3–18 mg AlCl$_3$/egg) into the air sac of chicken eggs after 0, 1, 2, and 3 days of incubation (Galini and Chatzinoff, 1981). Dose-dependent decreases in the percentage of surviving embryos were observed in all groups, but a greater sensitivity was exhibited in those injected at day 2 or 3 of incubation irrespective of the dose. Furthermore Al has been shown to cause hemorrhage and intrauterine bleeding into the eggshells of the Al-contaminated wild Passerine bird (Nyholm, 1981). Phosphate deficiency may also be responsible for the failure of the clotting mechanism frequently observed following prenatal exposure (Ondreicka, Gunter, and Kortus, 1966; Ondreick, Kortus, and Gunter, 1971; Wide, 1984).

Aluminum can also cross the placental barrier, although it has been shown that the placenta restricts Al accumulation in the rat fetus (McCormack, 1978). This is supported by the lack of adverse effects in the offspring of the mother treated orally with Al (Ondreicka et al., 1966). Similarly a single intraperitoneal dose of 40 mg / kg AlCl$_3$ did not influence weight gain or perinatal death, whereas chronic treatment at 75, 100, or 200 mg / kg resulted in a higher incidence of maternal and fetal death, as well as dose-related decreases in the birth weight (Bennett et al., 1975). Gross fetal abnormalities were observed in the group receiving 100 mg / kg.

The teratogenic effects of Al and its compounds has not been established in humans. A small study involving 22 women monitored the effects of chronic usage of Al-based antacids during pregnancy. The results suggested that such treatments did not cause hyperaluminumemia in the newborn (Weberg et al., 1985).

Genotoxicity and Mutagenicity

Aluminum and its compounds have not been designated as genotoxic agents, although Al$_2$(SO$_4$)$_3$ has been shown to decrease DNA synthesis without affecting replication fidelity (Sirover and Loeb, 1976). In bacteria, Al is generally nonmutagenic. The use of the Rec-assay failed to show that Al possesses mutagenic activity in the *Bacillus subtilis* strain employed in the assay (Nishioka, 1975). Moreover Al$_2$O$_3$, AlCl$_3$, and Al$_2$(SO$_4$)$_3$ at concentrations of 1 to 10 mM were negative in the Rec-assay with the *B. subtilis* H17 *rec* + and M45 *rec* − strains (Kada et al., 1980; Kanematsu et al., 1980). Reverse mutations also were not induced in the *Salmonella typhimurium* TA102 strain at doses ranging from 10 to 100 nM AlCl$_3$ per plate (Marzin and Hung, 1985); however, the Ames assay is notoriously poor as a tool for accurately assessing metal mutagenicity and many carcinogenic metals are not very mutagenic in any assay (Farrell and Costa, 1997).

Several studies have shown that Al is nonmutagenic in both in vitro and in vivo assays. In mammalian cells, Al compounds such as AlCl$_3$ and Al$_2$(SO$_4$)$_3$ at the high concentration of 0.9 mM failed to cause morphological transformations of Syrian hamster embryo cells or to enhance their transformation by Simian adenovirus SA7 (Di Paolo and Casto, 1979; Casto et al., 1979). The mutagenic activity of dimethylnitrosamine was increased by Al_2O_3 treatment of Chinese hamster ovary cells and monitoring mutations in the hypoxanthine-guanine phosphoribosyl transferase locus; these increases were not significantly above the background level (Tan and Abraham, 1981). Doses of $AlCl_3$ from 500 to 620 µg / ml failed to induce forward mutations at the thymidine kinase locus in the L5178Y mouse lymphoma assay (Oberley et al., 1982).

Numerous studies have shown that Al can inhibit cell division and produce chromosomal aberrations in plants. Inhibition of cell division in the root-tip of the meristem has been associated with Al exposure (Clarkson, 1965). Similarly growth in *Allium cepa* roots was inhibited, with mitoses disappearing as early as 6 to 8 hours after exposure to 10^{-4} and 10^{-3} M $Al_2(SO4)_3$ (Horst et al., 1983). It has been suggested that Al blocks cell division by interacting with phosphate, or by inhibiting the uptake and transport of Ca, or by interfering with spindle formation. It has also been suggested that Al can bind directly to DNA (Wojciechowska and Kocik, 1983). Each of these mechanisms could exist, since the results demonstrate that while Al is bound to the peptic substances in the cell walls, some can also enter the protoplast and associate with nucleic acids and most soluble phosphates (Leonard and Gerber, 1988). Furthermore high concentrations of Ca were shown to suppress Al toxicity, confirming that the decrease in root elongation produced by $Al_2(SO_4)_3$ was a result of an inhibition in DNA synthesis.

Chromosomal aberrations such as fragmentation, micronuclei formation, and binuclear cell development have been reported in Al-treated plant cells (Wojciechowska and Kocik, 1983; Matsumato et al., 1976). The occurrence of these anomalies does not necessarily imply that Al and its compounds have clastogenic properties, since these may also be related to their inhibiting action on microtubular polymerization (Leonard and Gerber, 1988). Chromosomal aberrations have been observed in peritoneal cells from mammals such as rats, mice, and Chinese hamsters (Nashed, 1975), as well as in the spermatocytes of grasshoppers (Manna and Mukherjee, 1966), after in vivo treatment with Al salts. Aberrations also occurred in the hematopoietic bone-marrow cells of rats treated with $AlCl_3$ (Manna and Das, 1972); these included gaps, breaks, and translocations, in addition to ring formations.

The negative results for Al compounds in most short-term mutagenic assays appears to be in agreement with their noncarcinogenic activity. The major health concern in the Al industry should not be directed toward Al itself but rather should emphasize the other substances generated during processing such as aromatic compounds, SO_2, tar, and particularly fluoride.

In conclusion, Al can be considered as relatively nontoxic and noncarcinogenic in humans. However, necessary precautions must be taken into consideration when dealing with patients at high risk for developing Al toxicity, such as the renally impaired, the elderly, and premature infants and exposure to readily bioavailable forms of Al salts (i.e., citrate) should be avoided because of its neurotoxic effects at high doses.

ARSENIC

Introduction

Arsenic (As) is widely distributed in nature and is classified as a metalloid, since it occurs in both the solid and liquid states (Carson et al., 1986). Although found in minerals such as arsenopyrites (FeAsS), realgar (As_2S_2), orpiment (As_2S_3), and arsenolite (As_2O_3), As is obtained primarily as a by-product from smelting copper, lead, zinc, gold, and other ores (Carson et al., 1986). It is released into the environment as a pollutant from several industrial processes and is predominantly released during the generation of power from coal-fired furnaces. Arsenic compounds have been widely used in agricultural and silvicultural products, and small quantities of organic As compounds can be found in feed additives for livestock. The latter are employed to stimulate host immune systems and assure rapid disease-free growth. In addition As is used as an alloy for hardening lead, in the manufacturing of glass, and gallium arsenite is used in electrical devices. Formerly As was extensively used in medicine for the treatment of dermatoses and syphilis (Fowler et al., 1979). In general, exposure to As is mainly through ingestion of food containing inorganic and organic arsenicals and in the drinking water. Symptoms associated with As toxicity include hyperkeratosis, blackfoot disease, myocardial ischemia, liver dysfunction, epithelima, and several cancers. The carcinogenicity and toxicity of As mainly result from exposure to trivalent As [As(III)] rather than to its pentavalent state [As(V)] or organic arsenicals, which are among the least toxic; As(III) is overall most toxic.

Essentiality

Arsenic has been considered as an essential trace element for the normal growth and development of experimental animals (Schwarz, 1977; Anke et al., 1980). A study using goats fed a diet deficient in As showed a substantial increase in the mortality rate (77%) as compared with a rate of 13% in the control group (Anke et al., 1980). The newborn of As-deficient goats weighed significantly less than those of the control group. After weaning, 60% of the As-deficient kids died within 140 days after birth. In addition As deficiency has been shown to influence a number of physiological parameters in female goats resulting in decreased fertility, an increased spontaneous abortion rate, and a decreased hematocrit. Similar observations were encountered in a study utilizing minipig models (Anke et al., 1976). Arsenic deficiency in rats influenced their physical appearance (e.g., roughening of the fur) and resulted in a decreased hematocrit as well as increased erythrocyte osmotic fragility. Necropsies of these rats revealed black, enlarged spleens containing more than a 50% iron content (Nielsen et al., 1975). Since As-deficiency influences the physiological development of these animals, it has been suggested that the minimum requirement for normal growth is 0.5 µg As/g body weight (Schwarz, 1977).

Environmental Sources and Exposure

Occupational exposure to inorganic As compounds occurs mainly among workers in smelting plants and those engaged in the production and use of As-containing pesticides. Airborne As concentrations in smelting plants can range from 0.01 to 0.075 µg/m^3, although these values may exceed 1 µg/m^3 near the emission source (Goyer, 1986). The OSHA permissible exposure limit (PEL) is 10 µg/m^3 for inorganic As (Cant and Legendre, 1982) as is the ACGIH threshold limit volume (TLV) (ACGIH, 1999). Atmospheric As may also be increased through the burning of coal and wood treated with As-containing preservatives. On average, coal has been shown to contain 5 ppm As, although concentrations as high as 100 ppm have been measured (Nashed, 1975).

In tap water, the level of arsenic is usually below 0.01 ppm, but levels exceeding 0.05 ppm have been found in Nova Scotia. These levels resulted from the high As content of the bedrock (Goyer, 1986). Higher concentrations have been measured in mineral spring water taken from various geographical locations such as Japan, Argentina, and Taiwan, with observed values of 1.7, 3.4, and 1.8 ppm As, respectively (Goyer, 1986). A further increase in the level of As in water may occur through industrial pollution and by the use of geothermal energy (Pershagen, 1981).

Extensive use of As-containing pesticides and other agricultural products in the past led to high As concentrations in the soil, consequently leading to outbreaks of As poisoning.

The latter were attributable to As-contaminated wine, bread, and beer produced from As-tainted grapes and grains grown on these soils (Fowler, 1977; Crecelius, 1977). In addition the use of pesticides has resulted in As levels in tobacco up to 40 ppm (Holland and Acerodo, 1966). More recently, however, there has been a gradual decline in the levels of As found in foods due to the restricted use of As-containing products by farmers. Most foodstuffs, with the exception of fish, contain on average 1 ppm As (Leonard and Lauwerys, 1980). Arsenic concentrations in fish usually range from 1 to 10 ppm, but this value may be as high as 100 ppm in certain shellfish (NAS, 1977; Luten et al., 1982). Because of the high concentration of As, particularly in seafood, the U.S government has defined the upper permissible limit of contamination to be 2.6 ppm As (Wesley and Kunis, 1981). Even with these restrictions, presently the estimated average daily intake of As as a food impurity is 900 µg As/d.

Formerly, As compounds were extensively and somewhat indiscriminately used in medicine. These compounds were used in the treatment of nutritional diseases such as anemia and pellagra, as well as for other diseases such as asthma, rheumatism, neuralgia, cholera, malaria, skin diseases (i.e., psoriasis), and syphilis (Leonard and Lauwery, 1980). Fowler's solution, containing 7.6 g/L arsenite (AsO_2^-), was widely prescribed and in some incidences doses were as high as 3 g As/d (Fowler et al., 1979). In most countries the use of Fowler's solution has been banned. Fowler's solution was applied topically, but As can be absorbed through the skin. Solutions containing organic As are still prescribed for humans mainly as antiparastic medications.

Since acute and chronic toxicity of As depend on its chemical and physical state, it is important to consider As speciation in assessing environmental levels. However, organic arsenicals, such as arsenobetaine and arsenocholine are found to accumulate in fish and shellfish but are generally regarded as nontoxic because the As is not bioavailable (Garcia-Vargas and Cebrián, 1996). Elemental As is nontoxic, even if eaten in substantial amounts. The most common inorganic arsenical in the air is arsenic trioxide, whereas a variety of inorganic arsenates and arsenites occur in water, soil, and food (Garcia-Vargas and Cebrián, 1996). There are noted differences in toxicity of these compounds, with trivalent arsenites being much more toxic than pentavalent arsenates (Garcia-Vargas and Cebrián, 1996). Environmental exposures should consider the speciation of the As compound.

Uptake and Distribution

The absorption of As is highly dependent on its chemical and physical form. For those exposed to airborne As as the trivalent As_2O_3, deposition in air passages and absorption from the lung is dependent on the particle size (Fowler et al., 1979). The major risk of exposure to As is not by inhalation but rather by ingestion. Both human and animal data indicates that approximately 80% of a dose of As(III) is absorbed from the gastrointestinal tract. A similar value is observed for As(V) in animals, but similar data are lacking for humans (Fowler et al., 1979). Organic As compounds, such as those found in seafood, are taken up actively (99%) in both human and animal models, while only 15 to 20% of arsenilic acid (used as a livestock feed additive) is absorbed from the gut (Dutkiewicz, 1977; Munro, 1976). In the case of the airborne pollutant As_2O_3, intestinal absorption following expectoration is dependent on a number of factors such as particle size and gastric juice pH (Fowler et al., 1979). In addition As may be dermally absorbed as demonstrated by the occurrence of systemic toxicity following accidental topical exposure to arsenic acid and arsenic trichloride (Garb and Hine, 1977).

The distribution of As upon ingestion and inhalation is dependent on its oxidation state. Trivalent As is transported via the bloodstream to major organs such as the liver and kidneys. Accumulation of As occurs in the brain, heart, uterus, and in the skin, as well as in bone and muscle (Fowler et al., 1979). Data regarding the distribution of As(V) in humans is lacking; however, a few animal studies have shown minor differences in distribution between the two oxidation states. In mice, the retention of As(III) was 2 to 3 times higher than that of AS(V) (Tam et al., 1979; Vahter and Norin, 1980). In addition As(III) is methylated to a greater extent than As(V), and this may contribute to the differences in retention in certain organs such as the liver, gall bladder, and the skin (Vahter and Norin, 1980; Vahter, 1981). This methylation process may also explain the reduced renal clearance of As(III). Recent thinking suggests that methylation of arsenite makes these species more water soluble, less lipid soluble, and enhances excretion (Aposhian, 1996). Arsenic, especially as As(V), has also been shown to readily cross the blood brain barrier, yet there is virtually no accumulation in the brain due to its rapid clearance (Vahter, 1981).

Most of the absorbed As is eliminated within a few days, mainly via the urine. The major urinary metabolites of As are dimethylarsinic acid and methylarsonic acid with small quantities of inorganic As(III) and As(V). The presence of As(V) in urine following administration of As(III) suggests that the latter form oxidizes to the pentavalent state (Bencko et al., 1976). However, it is uncertain whether these oxidation reactions are general metabolic processes or occur primarily in the kidney. In fact, it is thought that most of the arsenate is converted to arsenite in the body, since cellular and blood components create a reducing environment. The values obtained for the half-times of As(III) and its metabolites were 10 and 30 hours, respectively (Crecelius, 1977). Unlike the methylated forms of As, organoarsenicals normally present in seafood exhibited a shorter half-time of 20 hours. These compounds are not broken down to inorganic As in the body; thus the majority of As present in the urine is organically bound. It has also been suggested that the high As concentrations in seafood may enhance the overall elimination of As from the body. Other routes of elimination, although less important, are via the skin, hair, nails, and sweat. An enterohepatic circulation has also been demonstrated (Klaassen, 1974). A small amount of the unabsorbed As is excreted in the feces.

Transfer of As across the placenta has been shown in hamsters injected intravenously with a high dose of (20 mg/kg) $NaAsO_2$ (Ferm, 1977). Further studies that measured tissue As levels in the fetus and neonates of exposed dams demonstrated that total As levels were accumulative and increased with the period of gestation (Goyer, 1986). However, a more recent study showed that As levels in cord blood were similar to those measured in maternal blood (Kagey et al., 1977).

Toxicological Effects

The different retention levels of As(III) and As(V) may also explain the differences in their toxicities. Trivalent As is significantly more toxic than As(V) or the organic arsenicals. The comparatively lower toxicity of the organic compounds is consistent with their rapid clearance from the body. The cellular mechanisms of toxicity for As(III) also differs from those for As(V) (Fowler, 1977). Trivalent As reacts with cellular sulfydryl groups and inhibits cellular respiration via the tricarboxylic acid cycle through its interaction with the sulfhydryl agent lipoic acid. In fact arsenite (As^{+3}) has a very high affinity for vicinyl sulfhydryl groups on proteins. The ability of As^{+3} to inhibit ATP production suggests that organ functions will cease rapidly, especially in the event of acute poisoning. In contrast, As(V) exerts its toxic effects by uncoupling mitochondrial oxidative phosphorylation by acting like inorganic phosphate. The complexes formed are unstable arsenate esters that spontaneously decompose in a process known as arsenolysis. Much of As^{+5} will be converted to As^{+3}, but in the conversion process, As^{+3} will probably be bound to the reductant and may be less active (i.e., glutathione–As^{+3} complexes).

Most reported incidences of As poisoning do not attempt to differentiate between toxicity associated with either the trivalent or the pentavalent form of As. Symptoms of acute exposure include severe inflammation of the gastrointestinal tract. These can be accompanied by secondary electrolyte disturbances, cardiac dysfunction, coma, and even death, as a result of cardiac failure (Fowler et al., 1979). Other evident features include facial edema, anorexia, anemia, upper respiratory distress, skin lesions, neurotic signs, and hepatomegaly. Sensory loss in the peripheral nervous system is the most common neurological effect of acute As exposure, and usually manifests itself 1 to 2 weeks postexposure (Fowler et al., 1979; Wesley and Kunis, 1981). Supportive treatment includes dialysis and administration of chelating antidotes such as BAL (British antilewisite). In many circumstances techniques such as hemodialysis and hemoperfusion have not been effective in the removal of As from the blood (Smith and Wombolt, 1981). In humans, the fatal dose of ingested As_2O_3 ranges from 70 to 180 mg (Vallee et al., 1960).

In contrast, symptoms of chronic As inhalation may be manifested by lesions of the skin and mucous membranes, as well as alterations of the nervous and respiratory systems, and ultimately, lung cancer (Fowler, 1977). Arsine gas (AsH_3), a potent hemolytic agent, is of particular concern in the metal-refining industry. Acute exposure to this gas causes nausea, headaches, anemia, decreased hemoglobin levels, and hemoglobinuria; coppery pigmentation of the skin occurs within a few hours of arsine poisoning. Renal failure is the ultimate cause of death in such cases.

Chronic exposure to As via the drinking water can also occur in the general population, especially to individuals living in areas of high As content in the soil and air. In such cases the most frequently reported symptoms include hyperkeratosis, white striae of the cutica, cardiovascular irregularities, myocardial ischemia, hypertension, liver dysfunction, hematological changes, blackfoot disease, Raynaud's syndrome, skin epithelima, and other cancers (Fowler et al., 1979).

Carcinogenic and Teratogenic Effects

Based on the earlier investigations, the carcinogenicity of As has not been established in experimental animals (Leonard and Lauwery, 1980; Paroni et al., 1963; Milner, 1969; Hueper and Payne, 1962). These studies, which were performed predominately during the early 1960s, may be inadequate to define the role of As in carcinogenesis. An experiment with mice and rats which were chronically exposed for a period of two years to As via their drinking waters showed that the animals suffered from As intoxication but did not demonstrate increased rates of cancer as compared with controls (Hueper and Payne, 1962). However, lung carcinomas were induced in Syrian golden hamsters by intratracheal instillation of AsO_3 alone and in combination with benzo(a)pyrene (BP) (Pershagen et al., 1984). The incidences of pulmonary adenomas, papillomas, and adenomatoid lesions were significantly higher in the As group than in the control group. It was suggested that the positive interactions between As and BP, in relation to adenomatous lung carcinomas, may be of importance for synergism between As and smoking observed in smelter workers. The positive results in this study may be related to the use of carbon dust as a carrier, since it has been shown to increase retention of both BP and As in the lung (Henry et al., 1973). Lung adenomas were also observed in separate studies on Syrian golden hamsters following instillation of either AsO_3 (Ishinishi et al., 1983) or calcium sulfate (Pershagen and Bjorklund, 1985), while AsS_3 produced inconclusive results. In addition pulmonary tumors and/or carcinomas were induced in experimental animals following intratracheal instillation of AsO_3 (Ishinishi et al., 1977, 1980). Bronchial carcinomas, predominantly adenocarcinomas, were induced in 60% of rats given a single instillation of a mixture containing calcium arsenate, calcium oxide, and copper sulfate (Ivankovic et al., 1979). However, interpretation of these results are difficult, since the control animals received instillation of saline only. Subcutaneous injection of $NaAsO_2$ during pregnancy increased the incidences of lymphocytic leukemia and malignant lymphomas in female Swiss mice and their offspring (Oswald and Goerttler, 1971). The incidences of these cancers in dams were further increased by additional postnatal injection of the compound. Embryonic cells appear to be sensitive to arsenic carcinogenesis, since morphological transformation of Syrian hamster cells was induced by As in vitro (Wang and Rossman, 1996).

Epidemiological studies have demonstrated that inorganic As is carcinogenic in humans. Increased incidences of respiratory cancer have been documented for occupationally exposed individuals in smelting and chemical industries (Hill and Faning, 1948; Kurastsune et al., 1975; Wester et al., 1981; Ott et al., 1974; Satterlee, 1960), with similar incidences of lung cancer among agricultural workers exposed to As-containing pesticides and in those medically treated with As compounds (Goldman, 1964; Cuzick et al., 1982; Minkowitz, 1964). A strong correlation exists between As therapy and bronchial carcinoma (Minkowitz, 1964; Robson and Jelliffe, 1963; Novey and Martel, 1969); for example, asthmatic patients treated with As therapy may develop Bowen's disease, which has the clinical characteristic of chronic precancerous dermatosis and multiple epitheliomatosis (Novey and Martel, 1969). Cases of skin cancer, hyperpigmentation, and keratosis have predominated in areas where the drinking water contains 0.8 to 2.6 ppm As (Yeh, 1973; Chen et al., 1985). In addition As-contaminated drinking water and wine, as well as treatments with Fowler's solution, have been associated with the development of liver angiosarcoma (Regelson et al., 1968; Roth, 1958; Stone, 1965). Other malignancies associated with As exposure include neoplasms of the lymphatic and hematopoietic tissues and cancers of the gastrointestinal tract (Ott et al., 1974).

Mortality rates of workers engaged in the production of arsenical pesticides showed a twofold increase in deaths due to lung cancer (Hill and Fanning, 1948). Similarly a three fold increase in the rate of mortality due to respiratory cancer was observed among workers in copper smelting plants (Pinto et al., 1977). Increases in the mortality rates resulting from neoplasms of lymphatic and hematopoietic tissues were observed among As-exposed workers in other plants (Ott et al., 1974).

The contradiction in these results between humans and experimental animals suggests that As is a co-carcinogen and not a primary carcinogen (Leonard and Lauwery, 1980). It has been shown that As(V) suppresses host-resistance factors and this could help in the survival of tumors arising from other agents (Stone, 1965). Inhibition of DNA repair may also be involved (Rossman et al., 1977). Recent studies suggest that arsenite inhibits the DNA repair ligase component of DNA repair and modulates excision repair as well. The latter process appears to be more sensitive to arsenite while the former effects may not be mediated directly by arsenite (Farrell and Costa, 1997; Wang and Rossman, 1996). The influence of SO_2 and other unidentified chemicals which are associated with As exposure must also be accounted for when assessing the role of As in cancers in industrially exposed workers. It has been proposed that long-term As exposure could result in a depletion of selenium (Se) from the body, thereby increasing the susceptibility to cancer (Oswald and Goerttler, 1971; Neubauer, 1946). A study has shown that As exerts its antagonist effects on Se by its decreasing retention and toxicity (Levander and Bauman, 1966), which may be related to increased clearances via the bile (Levander and Argrett, 1969).

The teratogenic effects of As have not been studied extensively in mammals. One study based on ewes that were fed $NaAsO_2$ showed a reduction in the size of the offspring (James et al., 1966). Another study showed that intravenous administration of this compound to pregnant golden hamsters on the eighth day of gestation resulted in fetal exencephaly (Ferm and Carpenter, 1968). Other malformations include genitourinary abnormalities, cleft palate, microanophthalmia, and ear deformities during the critical stages of development (Hood and Bishop, 1972). Malformations were also seen in the pups when 45 mg/kg Na_2HAsO_4 was administered intraperitoneally to dams during any of the days 6 to 12 of gestation. However, following treatment with 25 mg/kg, incidences of fetal resorption or malformations were not significantly different from those of the control group (Hood and Piken, 1972). All of these teratogenic effects were increased when the dams were pretreated with BAL (Hood and Piken, 1972) and were decreased following treatment with Se which protected the pups against the effects of As (Holmberg and Ferm, 1969).

Although the teratogenicity of As has been established in experimental animals, its teratogenic effects have not been demonstrated in humans.

Genotoxicity and Mutagenicity

Studies have demonstrated genotoxic properties of As in many bacterial cells. Sodium arsenite has been shown to inhibit a *rec A*-dependent repair pathway in UV-irradiated *Escherichia coli* (Rossman et al., 1975). These results were entirely based on the analysis of survival data in several strains of *E. coli* such as WP2 (wild-type) and several DNA repair mutants such as WP2-*uvrA*, WP6 *(poly A)*, and WP10 *(rec A$^-$)*. Following UV irradiation, all of the strains except the *rec A* deficient mutant showed a decrease in survival. A similar study showed that nonlethal doses of NaAsO$_2$ dose-dependently inhibited the formation of single-stranded DNA in WP2 and WP6 *E. coli* mutant strains following UV irradiation (Fong et al., 1980). Since the level of ATP in the treated WP2 cells had also decreased, it was suggested by the authors that inhibition of DNA strand-break formation may be mediated through the low ATP levels in irradiated cells. Similar results were obtained for the wild-type WP2 As-treated, irradiated cells. Although these studies indicate an inhibition of DNA synthesis, the accuracy of DNA synthesis *in vitro* has been shown to be unaffected by As (Tkeshelashvili, 1980).

Arsenic salts and some organoarsenicals, such as arsenic dimethyldithio-carbamate, have been shown to cause damage to DNA as demonstrated by the *B. subtilis* Rec-assay (Nishioka and Takaga, 1975; Shirasu et al., 1976). Positive results were also obtained for NaAsO$_2$, As$_2$O$_5$, AsCl$_3$, and As$_2$O$_3$ in this assay (Nishioka, 1975; Nakumura and Sayato, 1981). In contrast, negative results were obtained with other organic arsenicals in the same assay, such as sodium methyl arsonate and calcium methyl arsonate (Shirasu et al., 1976). In addition the effects of sodium methyl arsonate and methyl arsonic acid were evaluated in *S. typhiurium*, by measuring the frequency of reversion to histidine independence; both agents yielded negative results (Andersen et al., 1972). Unlike their effects in the Rec-assay, NaAsO$_2$ and Na$_2$HAsO$_4$ were incapable of inducing mutations at the Na$^+$,K$^+$-ATPase and HPRT gene loci in Chinese hamster V79 cells (Rossman et al., 1980). Similarly a negative response with NaAsO$_2$ was obtained at the thymidine kinase locus in the mouse lymphoma (L5178Y) assay (Oberley et al., 1982; Amacher and Paillet, 1980).

Most As compounds are powerful clastogenic agents in many types of cells. However, compounds containing AsO$_4^{3-}$ are significantly less clastogenic than those containing AsO$_2$. The efficiency of various arsenicals in inducing chromosomal aberrations (Nakumura and Sayato, 1981) have been reported to be As$_2$O$_3$ > AsCl$_3$ > NaAsO$_2$ > Na$_2$HAsO$_4$ > H$_3$AsO$_4$ = As$_2$O$_5$. The dose response on a µg As/g basis for the total aberration frequency was linear for both As(III) and As(V). Mitotic inhibition and chromosomal aberrations have been observed in maize tips and in *Allium cepa* cells treated with organic arsenicals (El-Sadek, 1972; Nygren, 1949). Chromosomal and spindle aberrations have also been observed in mouse fibroblastic cells treated with As compounds (King and Lunford, 1950). The clastogenic properties of NaAsO$_2$ has been demonstrated in vivo in laboratory animals; however, it could not produce heritable damage in these hosts. This has been demonstrated using a single dose of 250 mg As/kg which failed to increase the numbers of dominant lethals (Sram and Beneko, 1974). In addition acute dosing of these animals did not produce chromosomal damage in their germ cells. The results of an in vivo micronucleus test in mice indicates, however, that AsO$_2$, at doses that allow survival of the animals up to 30 hours following treatment, is clastogenic to the mammalian somatic cells.

Some observations have also been made on cultured somatic cells from individuals exposed to As for medical and professional reasons. An elevated frequency of sister chromatid exchange has been reported in lymphocytes of patients treated with As and those with blackfoot disease (Crossen, 1983; Nordenson and Beckman, 1982; Wen et al., 1981). In cultured human lymphocytes, chromosomal rearrangement and breaks were produced by low concentrations of $KAsO_2$ (10–50 µM) (Oppenheim and Fishbein, 1965). Significant increases in chromosomal aberrations were observed in cultured leukocytes after exposure to $NaAsO_2$ or Na_2HAsO_4; similar results were achieved in fibroblasts treated with $NaAsO_2$. Recent studies suggest that As may be carcinogenic due to its ability to enhance the methylation of the promoter for the tumor suppressor gene p53 (Mass, 1997). Loss of function of tumor suppressor genes is considered an important event in carcinogenesis and loss of transcription of p53 by enhanced DNA methylation will be inherited through cell divisions.

In summary, the toxicity and carcinogenicity of As is complicated by the different oxidation states of the metal. Although As is a powerful clastogen, it is nonmutagenic in many mammalian cell systems. The carcinogenicity of As in humans may not be dependent on interactions with any one specific region of DNA to yield mutations. It may, however, be related to the clastogenic activities which give rise to chromosomal rearrangements and breaks as well as deletions of important genes, namely tumor suppressor gene(s).

CADMIUM

Cadmium (Cd) is closely related to zinc (Zn) in its chemical properties and is found as a contaminant of many Zn-containing minerals (Cotton and Wilkinson, 1980; Carson et al., 1986). While Cd is obtained primarily as the commercial by-product of the refinement of zinc- and other metal-bearing ores, mineral ores of Cd such as greenockite (CdS) do exist. The major uses of Cd are in electroplating metals to inhibit corrosion, and as pigments and heat stabilizers for plastics production. Cadmium alloys are commonly used in soldering, brazing, as well as in Ni–Cd batteries. Cadmium contamination of the air and water is mainly produced by mine runoff, and as waste release from metal smelteries and other industries that utilize Cd in alkaline batteries, paints, and plastics. The use of Cd-containing fertilizers in agriculture, either as synthesized products or as a natural organic sludge obtained from sewage plants, along with metal-bearing pesticides, all potentially contribute to further environmental contamination. The major routes of exposure for Cd intoxication include inhalation and ingestion (Goyer, 1986; Lee and White, 1980). Symptoms of acute toxicity with the former pathway include pulmonary edema and pneumonitis, whereas powerful emetic effects are produced upon ingestion (Carson et al., 1986). The effects from chronic exposure to Cd-containing materials include lung fibrosis, emphysema, and bronchitis. Cancers of the prostate and lung have been observed in individuals following low-level long-term exposure to Cd compounds.

Essentiality

Cadmium is considered to be nonessential to humans, but some evidence of essentiality has been demonstrated in experimental animals. A study with rats fed a Cd-deficient diet showed that the animals weighed considerably less than those in the control group (Schwarz, 1977). Cadmium supplementation resulted in a dose-dependent increase in body weight and length, and an overall improved physical appearance. Furthermore studies demonstrate that Zn-containing enzymes such as tryptophan oxygenase and delta-aminolevulinate dehydrogenase are activated by Cd in vitro (Vallee and Ulmer, 1972).

However, Cd incorporation into Zn-bearing carboxy peptidase B resulted in no augmentation of activity. Although these and other enzymes are now known to accommodate the presence of Cd ions, it is not considered an essential element.

Environmental Sources and Exposures

Cadmium is referred to as the "dissipated element" with regards to the environment. In industry, 17,000 tons of Cd are used annually, of which only 5% is recovered (De Voogt et al., 1980). Air concentrations as high as 4000 to 5000 $\mu g/m^3$ were detected at certain industrial sites such as battery manufacturing plants (Adams et al.,1969); however, airborne Cd is currently restricted to levels below 0.02 $\mu g/m^3$ (Goyer, 1986). These restricted levels are high compared to the atmospheric concentrations in rural and urban areas, where typically observed values are 0.001 to 0.005 and 0.05 to 0.06 $\mu g/m^3$, respectively (Friberg et al., 1979). The OSHA permissible exposed limit is currently 5 $\mu g/m^3$ and the TLV (ACGIH, 1999) is 10 $\mu g/m^3$ (total) and 2 $\mu g/m^3$ (respirable).

In areas not affected by Cd-utilizing or -generating industries, the normal concentration of Cd in water is less than 1 ng/L, although values as high as 10 ng/L have been reported in both natural and drinking water (Friberg et al., 1974). An increase in the amount of Cd contamination in water may be due to either industrial discharge of untreated waste, or leaching from the metal and plastic pipes used for distribution. The accepted upper limit of the Cd concentration in drinking water is 5 ng/L (De Voogt et al., 1980).

Cadmium concentrations in soil from unpolluted areas have been reported to be less than 1 ppb (De Voogt et al., 1980). Both air- and waterborne Cd can cause an increase in Cd concentrations normally found in soil. Relatively high soil concentrations have been reported in residential, agricultural, and industrial regions, with observed values of 0.41, 0.57, and 0.66 ppm, respectively (Kneip et al., 1970). Relatively higher levels have been measured in areas suspected of heavy metal contamination such as some rice fields in Japan, which were shown to contain 1 to 69 ppm Cd (Goyer, 1986). Further contamination of the soil and water table results from the use of Cd-containing fertilizer and pesticides. The use of commercial phosphate fertilizers containing less than 20 ppm Cd have been shown to increase the Cd content in soil (Andersen and Hahlin, 1981). This may be reflected in the progressive increase in the metal concentration found in barley grain over a 5 year period. Commercially produced sewage sludge has been shown to contain 1500 ppm Cd in dry material (Pahren et al., 1979). The liberal use of this "natural" fertilizer readily deposits greater quantities of Cd in shortest periods of time.

High soil and water concentrations can lead to significant accumulation of Cd in food. Products such as meat, fruit, and fish (except shellfish) usually contain between 1 to 50 ppb Cd (Goyer, 1986). Grains have been shown to contain 10 to 150 ppb Cd (Goyer, 1986); with meats, the greatest concentrations are found in offals such as liver and kidney. Shellfish such as mussels, scallops, and oysters are another major source of dietary Cd. Overall, the total daily intake of Cd from shellfish is generally estimated to be less than 100 $\mu g/d$, whereas in certain polluted areas (e.g., Japan), the estimated value may be as high as 150 $\mu g/d$ (Kjellstrom, 1979; Underwood, 1977).

Another means of nonoccupational exposure to Cd is through smoking. It has been shown that one cigarette may contain up to 1 to 2 μg Cd, of which 10% is inhaled (Friberg et al., 1974; Lewis et al., 1972). Therefore smoking 20 cigarette per day will probably lead to inhalation of 2 to 4 μg of Cd daily.

Uptake and Distribution

Absorption of Cd from the respiratory tract has been estimated to be in the range of 10% to 50%, depending on the particle size and chemical nature of the aerosol (Friberg et al.,

1974). On the other hand, absorption from the gastrointestinal tract is only about 5% to 8% (Poe and Leberman, 1949). Absorption has been shown to be enhanced by certain dietary deficiencies of calcium (Ca), iron (Fe), or protein. In experimental animals, absorption was found to be increased to > 10% following consumption of a diet deficient in Ca and/or protein (Friberg et al., 1974). Low dietary Ca has been shown to stimulate synthesis of Ca-binding proteins which may enhance Cd absorption. Similarly women with low serum ferritin levels showed a twofold increase in their Cd-absorption rate (Flanagan et al., 1978). Zinc, on the other hand, decreased Cd absorption secondarily to the stimulation of metallothionein production (Goyer, 1986).

Following absorption from the gastrointestinal or respiratory tract, Cd is transported via the blood either bound to erythrocytes or to other high molecular weight plasma proteins such as albumin; a small fraction of Cd is transported by metallothionein. Cadmium is distributed to all the major organs, but the liver and kidneys (i.e., renal cortex) are the main storage sites. Cadmium is stored to a lesser extent in the pancreas, salivary glands, skeletal muscle, and testes (Friberg et al., 1974). Since Cd is extensively stored in the kidney, urinary excretion is very slow, with the biological half-time estimated to be as long as 10 to 30 years (Friberg et al., 1974). A small percentage of Cd bound to metallothionein is known to leave the liver cells, and at high levels, Cd metallothionein complexes are more destructive to the kidney than nonprotein bound Cd (Dorian et al., 1995; Liu et al., 1996). For adults living in unpolluted areas, the amount excreted daily via the urine is usually below 2 µg Cd/day, although there are large interindividual variations. This value may further increase proportionally with age; Cd measured in the urine is often used as an indicator of total body burdens in individuals without renal dysfunction (Kjellstrom and Nordberg, 1978). The nonabsorbed fraction of Cd, which constitutes approximately 95% of the daily intake, is excreted via the feces. The small quantities of Cd originating from mucociliary clearance of Cd stored in the pulmonary system are primarily excreted via the bile.

Other minor routes for the removal of absorbed Cd are limited to females. The levels of Cd excreted during lactation usually contain less than 1 ppb Cd in the milk (Schroeder and Balassa, 1961). While this metal is known to cross the placental barrier, the placenta itself is known to synthesize metallothionein and so may protect the fetus by acting as barrier to maternal Cd (Kowal et al., 1979).

Toxicological Effects

The major toxic effects of Cd in humans are dependent on the two primary routes of exposure: inhalation and ingestion. Following acute inhalation to CdO fumes, the first signs of toxicity usually appear after 4 to 10 hours with symptoms such as dyspnea, coughing, and tightness of the chest, and there may be later development of pulmonary edema and possibly bronchopneumonia (Carson et al., 1986; Lee and White, 1980). Pulmonary edema is the immediate cause of death of acutely exposed individuals. In contrast, the effects from acutely ingested Cd-containing products are more immediate and usually appear within 15 to 30 minutes (Stokinger, 1981). These include persistent vomiting, increased salivation, choking, abdominal pains, tenesmus, diarrhea, and headaches, which may be followed by renal failure and cardiopulmonary collapse.

Chronic inhalation of Cd produces a variety of effects such as emphysema, liver damage, anemia, proteinuria, and renal tubular damage (Goyer, 1986; Lee and White, 1980; Friberg et al., 1974). The effects on proximal renal tubular function are manifested by increased Cd in the urine, proteinuria, amino aciduria, glucosuria, and decreased renal tubular resorption of phosphate. The latter phenomenon may lead to kidney stones and osteomalacia (Lee and White, 1980; Winter, 1982). The chronic ingestion of Cd can also result in a painful degenerative disease called *Itai-Itai*. This condition was first reported in

Japan, predominantly in older women on Ca-deficient diets consuming Cd-tainted rice. A variety of skeletal effects can be manifested including pain in the back and extremities, difficulty in walking, pseudofractures, and osteomalacia; most of these are probably secondary to the derangement of mineral metabolism in the kidney, although some direct effects of Cd on bone cells have been noted in the literature (Blumental et al., 1995; Wilson et al., 1996). Anemia is also known to occur as result of prolonged exposure to Cd, and appears to be more associated with the Fe deficiency than with direct Cd toxicity to the bone marrow (Lee and White, 1980; Friberg et al., 1974). Other toxic effects due to chronic exposure are Cd-induced suppression of testicular function (Stokinger, 1981), with cardiovascular diseases accompanied by hypertension (Schroeder and Balassa, 1961). Rather striking testicular toxicity can be induced by injection of water-soluble Cd salts to rats. However, this does not occur if given by oral route, since with a slower infusion of the same dose, there is more time for Cd to induce metallothionein. A number of mechanisms for the pathogenesis of Cd-induced hypertension have been suggested, including increased renal sodium retention, direct vasoconstriction, hyperanemia, and increased cardiac output.

Carcinogenic and Teratogenic Effects

The carcinogenicity of Cd has been demonstrated in experimental animals. Sarcomas developed in 25% of a group of rats injected subcutaneously over a period of two years with $CdSO_4$ (Levy et al., 1973), but no signs of prostate tumors were detected. Similarly administration of Cd compounds by gavage to rats and mice for a period of two years also failed to produce tumors of the prostrate or other major organs (Levy et al., 1973; Levy and Clack, 1975). However, studies have shown that the chloride, sulfate, and acetate salts of Cd did induce lung cancer in rats and mice following inhalation, but not after exposure via diet or gavage (Kazantzis, 1984; Takenakas et al., 1983). Based on these three sets of studies, the failure of ingested Cd to induce cancer formation in vivo may be the result of poor absorption of Cd compounds from the gut.

Other inhalation studies have shown that $CdCl_2$ produced a dose-dependent increase in the incidence of primary lung carcinomas in Wistar rats (Takenakas et al., 1983; Oldiges et al., 1984). However, CdO instilled intratracheally in rats at doses equivalent to 75% of the oral LD_{50} did not increase the incidences of tumors (Sanders and Mahaffey, 1984); while only 5% of the rats developed lung cancer, there was a significant increase in mammary tumors.

Despite the evidence dealing with the carcinogenic potency of Cd in experimental animals, its carcinogenicity in humans is not well defined. However, IARC has classified Cd and its compounds as a Group 1 human carcinogen (IARC, 1993). A number of epidemiological studies have been conducted with regard to cancer morbidity and mortality resulting from Cd exposure. An increased risk of prostate cancer was observed in battery workers exposed to fumes containing Ni–Cd oxides (Potts, 1965). A more comprehensive study involving 248 workers at the same plant, exposed for a minimum period of one year, showed an eightfold increase in deaths from prostate cancer (Kipling and Waterhouse, 1967). In another study a significant increase in mortality from lung cancer was observed in occupationally exposed workers (Lemen et al., 1976); however, the importance of the contribution from Cd is uncertain, since these workers were also exposed to As and data on their smoking history was lacking. A recent study showed a Cd-specific mortality (SMR of 280) among workers in Cd production plants mainly resulting from respiratory cancers (Thun et al., 1985). This study also showed that the increase in mortality from lung cancer paralleled an increased cumulative exposure to Cd. The data that confirmed that Cd was a human carcinogen were derived from epidemiological studies limited only to exposure via Cd inhalation (as Cd oxide) (Oberdorster, 1986).

However, a comparison of these results with the animal studies indicate that rats are more sensitive to the carcinogenic effects of inhaled Cd than are humans.

In animal studies the teratogenic effects of Cd were observed when large doses of $CdCl_2$ (2–28 mg /kg) were administered subcutaneously; these doses caused severe hemorrhagic ganglionic lesions in neonatal rats and rabbits (Gabbiani et al., 1967). Damage to the cerebrum and cerebellum were found in these newborns, but these changes were not observed in the exposed adult animals. A reduction in pup body weights were noted after the dams were exposed to 3 mg / m^3 $CdSO_4$ (Cvetkova, 1970). These pups also had an increased mortality rate during the first 10 days after birth. In mice, Cd produced toxic effects on the placenta, induced necrotic changes, and caused a higher incidence of embryonic death (Chiquoine and Suntseff, 1965). Cadmium has also been shown to cause malformations in Golden hamster newborns from dams treated with 2 mg / kg $CdSO_4$ on day 8 of gestation (Holmberg and Ferm, 1969). The results showed that with exposed dams, 53% of the fetuses were malformed and 73% were ultimately resorbed. The types of malformations frequently observed included encephalocele, exencephaly, and cleft lip.

The teratogenic effects of Cd are not well established in humans, although a study showed weight reduction in the newborns of mothers working in alkaline battery factories or Zn smelting plants (Cvetkova, 1970). In addition signs of rhinitis and delayed development of teeth were observed in the children of Zn smelting plant workers.

Genotoxicity and Mutagenicity

Cadmium has been shown to modify the metabolism of nucleic acids both by direct interaction with bases and by interference with their synthesis. Both an enhancement and an inhibition of polynucleotide synthesis have been observed in studies with microorganisms, plants, and mammalian cells (Kazantzis, 1984). Divalent Cd ions effectively inhibit DNA synthesis at doses lower than those that inhibit RNA synthesis. In addition inhibition of human DNA polymerase has been demonstrated in vitro (Sirover and Loeb, 1976). A decrease in the fidelity of DNA synthesis has been shown using $CdCl_2$ and $Cd(CH_3COO^-)_2$ in a cell-free system, resulting in increased basepair mismatch (Sunderland et al., 1974; Moselt et al., 1988). Thymidine incorporation into liver, testicular, and thymic (re: lymphocyte) DNA were decreased following Cd treatment of several animal models (Cohen et al., 1990). Single-strand breaks, as well as a disruption of the structure of isolated helical double-stranded DNA (as indicated by the decrease in melting temperature) resulted from the exposure of intact hepatocytes to Cd.

Cadmium has given negative results in a number of experiments using standard bacterial assays for genotoxicity including the *S. typhimurium* histidine reversion assay and the forward mutation system with *E. coli* (Marzin and Hung, 1985). However, the *B. subilitis* Rec assay, which measures repairable DNA damage in recombination deficient and recombination competent strains, gave weak positive results with the $CdCl_2$, $CdSO_4$, and $Cd(NO_3)_2$ (Kanematsu et al., 1980). Cadmium also gave mixed results in two different mammalian cell lines used to detect mutagenicity. Mutants were induced by Cd at the thymidine kinase locus in L5178Y/TK$^{+/-}$ mouse cells but not in the C3H mouse cell HGPRT assay (Oberley et al., 1982; Umeda and Nishimura, 1979).

A number of studies investigating the ability of $CdCl_2$ to induce dominant lethal mutations in mice were unsuccessful. Negative results have also been observed in heritable translocation assays, in spermatocytes (Gilliavod and Leonard, 1975), and in the micronucleus assay (Bruce and Heddle, 1979). However, female rodents exposed to $CdCl_2$ in vivo showed aneuploidy and Cd accumulation in the ovaries (Shimada et al., 1976; Watanabe et al., 1979), whereas males treated with the same compound showed no increases in sperm head abnormalities (Gilliavod and Leonard, 1975).

Dose-dependent chromosomal aberrations have been observed in a number of plant species. However, both negative and positive results have been reported with $CdCl_2$ in *Drosophila melanogaster* and *Poecilocerus pictus* respectively, although in the latter the results may have been artifactual (Friberg et al., 1974; Degraeve, 1981). Cadmium chloride also gave negative results in cultured mouse carcinoma cells (Umeda and Nishimura, 1979), whereas $CdSO_4$ produced aberrations in cultured Chinese hamster fibroblasts (Rohr and Bauchinger, 1976). Negative results were also obtained in cultured human lymphocytes following treatment with $CdCl_2$ (DeKnudt and Deminalti, 1978), although CdS was clastogenic (Shiraishi et al., 1972).

An increase in the numbers of chromosomal aberrations were noted in the peripheral leukocytes from seven patients with Itai-Itai disease (Shiraishi and Yosida, 1972). In contrast, a separate study demonstrated an insignificant increase in the numbers of aberrations in the peripheral leukocytes from these patients or Swedish Cd workers (Bui et al., 1975). A more recent investigation demonstrated a significant difference in the numbers of chromosome aberration between Cd-polluted and nonpolluted areas (Tang et al., 1990; Buichinger et al., 1976). The frequency of aberration correlated with the Cd urine concentration (Buichinger et al., 1976).

Enhancement of viral transformation of Syrian hamster embryo cells following exposure to $CdCl_2$ and $Cd(CH_3COO^-)_2$ have been reported (Casto et al., 1979). Transformations were also obtained in these cells without the virus intermediary and $Cd(CH_3COO^-)_2$ was found to be equipotent as sodium dichromate in producing these effects. Furthermore transformations were observed following transplacental exposure to these agents (Di Paolo and Casto, 1979). Cd is structurally similar to Zn, and Zn exposure can ameliorate the carcinogenic effects of Cd (Waalkes and Misra, 1996). Additionally Cd can antagonize or enhance the carcinogenic effects of organic chemicals. Since Cd is a very toxic and reactive molecule, and can deplete reduced glutathione, it may be inducing oxidative stress in cells secondary to antioxidant enzyme inhibition and depletion of reduced GSH (Waalkes and Misra, 1996). Cd^{2+} has been shown to inhibit DNA repair (Hartwig, 1994; Hartwig et al., 1994).

In summary, the results from in vitro and in vivo chromosome studies using rodent and human somatic cells indicate that Cd is a weak clastogen. The mutagenic potential of Cd has been difficult to assess; however, Cd can be considered a weak mutagen based on the results from the prokaryotic mutation studies. The weakly positive mutagenicity and clastogenicity and carcinogenic activity make Cd a potential health risk to humans in both the natural and industrial environments. While all of these effects are evidenced in the long term, the acute toxic effects from Cd make it noteworthy as a rapid acting poison following accidental exposure.

NICKEL

Nickel (Ni) is widely distributed in nature, constituting about 0.008% of the earth's crust and 8.5% of the earth's core (Carson et al., 1986). The most abundant ores are the oxides and sulfides of Ni; these minerals also contain other metals such as Co, Cu, Au, Hg, and Pt. The chemical composition of the ores dictates their respective smelting and refining processes, although a widely used procedure involves either roasting to form the oxide (NiO) or conversion to volatile nickel carbonyl ($Ni(CO)_4$), which produces nickel metal by reduction. Another process used for isolating purified Ni is electrolytic refining. The main use of Ni is in the steel industry, with further applications as alloys, chemical catalysts, in electroplating metals, and for the production of ceramics, pigments, Ni–Cd batteries, and coins (to replace silver) (Carson et al., 1986). In addition, Ni-containing compounds, such as ferrite, are used in the electronics industry. The release of Ni particles into the atmosphere is mainly as a pollutant from industrial processes and through the combustion of fossil fuels. Exposure to Ni is primarily in the industrial setting; however, Ni metal and most of its derivatives (except $Ni(CO)_4$) have little overt toxicity. Acute inhalation of $Ni(CO)_4$ produces irritating effects on pulmonary tissues which develops into life-threatening pulmonary edema. Other symptoms of Ni toxicity particularly associated with Ni alloys include various types of dermatosis such as contact and atopic dermatosis. Cancer of the nasal cavity and lung has also been associated with prolonged occupational exposure to certain Ni compounds.

Essentiality

Nickel has been implicated as an essential trace metal in experimental animals. Studies on rats, goats, and fowl demonstrated that a Ni deficiency resulted in retarded growth, skeletal malformations, anemia, and biochemical disorders of carbohydrate, lipid, and/or iron metabolism (Neilsen and Ollerich, 1974; Kirshgessener and Schnegg, 1976; Schnegg and Kirchgessener, 1975a,b). Nickel has been shown to be an essential constitituent for plant growth and functionality and for certain bacterial enzymes and metabolic cofactors including ureases, hydrogenases, dehydrogenases, and F_{430} coenzymes (a microbacterial analogue to vitamin B_{12}) (Dixon et al., 1980). The role of Ni as an essential constituent in mammalian enzymes has not been established (Thauer et al., 1980), although changes in Ni distribution in humans have been associated with several pathological states (Mertz, 1970). The daily requirement of Ni in growing cattle has been estimated to be $> 500\,\mu g\,Ni/d$. Nutritional requirements of Ni have not been established for humans, although the predicted daily requirement is probably greater than $> 200\,\mu g\,Ni/d$ for adult humans based on the dietary intake of 100 to $500\,\mu g\,Ni/d$ (Anke et al., 1984).

Environmental Sources and Exposure

Exposure to Ni occurs primarily in industries involved with refining of Ni ores and processing of the metal into Ni alloys. Different levels of exposure occur depending on the process involved; average airborne concentrations were $1.3\,mg/m^3$ in roasting and smelting plants, whereas the exposure level was $0.4\,mg/m^3$ in the electrolysis sector (Bencko, 1983). Atmospheric Ni concentrations in large cities and industrialized areas have been estimated to be in the range of 120 to $170\,ng/m^3$. These values are extremely high compared with atmospheric Ni concentrations in rural and suburban areas of 6 and $17\,ng\,Ni/m^3$, respectively (Norseth and Piscator, 1979). In some suburban areas airborne Ni concentrations have been shown to increase to $25\,ng/m^3$ during the winter due to the increased consumption of oils and coal for heat and power production. Nickel occurs in both oil and coal at levels up to 20 ppm Ni (Bencko, 1983). The release of Ni into air may also occur as a result of the incineration of solid waste containing nickel-cadmium batteries.

A natural source of atmospheric Ni are windblown dusts containing particles from the natural weathering of rocks and soils, and from volcanic emissions; high levels of Ni are readily found in igneous rocks. Direct leaching of Ni from rocks and sediments may give rise to high Ni concentrations in water. Nickel concentrations in deep-sea waters usually range from 0.1 to 0.5 ppb, while surface waters contain on average 15 to 20 ppb Ni (Norseth and Piscator, 1979). Drinking water normally contains less than 10 ppb Ni; however, concentrations as high as 75 ppb Ni have been measured (NAS, 1979). The latter may be due to either Ni contamination of the water supply or as a result of leaching from Ni-containing pipes or Ni-plated faucets. High concentrations (200 ppb Ni) have been measured in water from areas within the vicinity of active mining (McNeely et al., 1972). The Occupational Safety and Health Administration's (OSHA) permissible exposure limit

(PEL) is 1 mg/m^3; the American Conference of Governmental Industrial Hygienst's (ACGIH, 1999) threshold exposure values (TEVs) are 1.5 mg/m^3 for the metal, 0.2 mg/m^3 (water insoluble compounds) and 0.1 mg/m^3 (water soluble compounds).

A wide range of Ni concentrations (3–1000 ppm Ni) has been found in soils depending on the overall mineral content of the topsoil (NAS, 1979). As with other metals, uptake of Ni from the soil can cause accumulation of the metal in the roots, leaves, and seeds of many plants. Nickel concentrations in grains ranged from 0 to 6.45 ppm Ni, while vegetables and fruits were shown to contain 0 to 2.56 ppm Ni (Pennington and Jones, 1987). In general, Ni levels in most foods, except nuts and legumes, range from 0.7 to 33.6 ppm Ni; for nuts and legumes, levels were estimated to be 228 and 128 ppm Ni, respectively. Nickel is also present in tobacco, with concentrations in cigarettes of 1.1 to 3.1 μg Ni/cigarette, of which 10% to 20% are inhaled (Norseth and Piscator, 1979).

The chance for some human exposure to Ni is high at all times due to the preponderance of Ni-containing materials. Nickel is present in stainless steel, in Ni-plated materials including coins and jewelry, and in many other commonly used objects. Small residual quantities of Ni are also present in soaps, fats, and oils due to the use of Ni catalysts in the manufacturing process. Iatrogenic exposure to Ni also occurs from implantation of surgical and dental prostheses as well as from contaminated medications, intravenous fluids, and extracorporeal dialysis due to spoiled dialysis fluids (Sunderman, 1986).

Uptake and Distribution

In the occupational setting, inhalation is the major route for Ni absorption. As with As, uptake of Ni into the bloodstream is largely dependent on the physical properties of the Ni-bearing particle such as size, shape, density, hygroscopicity, and electrical charge. However, there is no data from either animal or human studies that can be used to estimate Ni absorption following inhalation. A large number of animal studies have investigated Ni clearance from the lungs following intratracheal instillation or exposure to aerosols. For example, when mice were exposed to NiCl$_2$ aerosol (64.4 mg/m^3) for a 2 hour period, 28% of the dose still remained in the lung after 4 days of exposure (Graham et al., 1978). In a separate study, 80% of an inhaled NiO aerosol was retained in the lungs of Syrian golden hamsters regardless of the total dose or length of exposure (Wehner and Craig, 1972). Mice intratracheally instilled with ^{63}Ni$_3$S$_2$ showed a 10% dose retention in the lungs 35 days after exposure (Valentine and Fisher, 1984). In contrast, it is thought that at least 50% of a dose of Ni(CO)$_4$ is absorbed from the lungs after inhalation (200 mg Ni/L, 15 min), since 26% of this dose was excreted within 4 days and about the same amount was estimated to be exhaled (Sunderman and Selin, 1968).

Less is known about Ni absorption from the gastrointestinal tract. Most Ni compounds, in particular the Ni-containing dusts, are characterized by a low water solubility. However, studies with animals and humans have shown that at least 10% of a dose of soluble Ni salt is absorbed from the gut (NAS, 1979). Another study estimated that absorption of Ni from the gut is approximately 3% based on the urinary excretion of Ni (Horak and Sunderman, 1973). A similar value was indicated following a single oral dose of NiSO$_4$·6H$_2$O (5.6 mg Ni), although higher values were obtained in fasting volunteers (Cronin et al., 1980). Water-soluble Ni salts may be absorbed from the skin, since hepatic and testicular lesions were observed in rats following high dermal exposure (Mathur et al., 1977). In humans, dermal uptake has been estimated at between 55% and 75% of an applied NiSO$_4$ dose within 24 hours of treatment (Norgaard, 1955). More recent confirmatory studies of the dermal uptake are not available.

Following absorption from either the gastrointestinal or respiratory tracts, Ni is transported via the bloodstream bound mainly to albumin. A major fraction of Ni is also bound to μ-macroglobulin nickeloplasmin; however, Ni content is not readily exchanged.

Therefore this protein does not appear to play an important role in the extracellular transport of Ni (Sarker, 1984). Nickel is also known to bind to transferrin, μ-macroglobulin, and gamma-globulin. Distribution of Ni occurs to all organs, with the highest concentrations found in the kidney (Parker and Sunderman, 1974). Other major sites of retention include the pituitary gland, liver, and lungs. Following exposure to $Ni(CO)_4$, 50% of the body Ni burden is in the viscera and blood, with 30% in body fat and muscle, and 15% in the bone and connective tissues (Sunderman and Selin, 1968). In humans, the total body burden has been estimated to be 0.5 mg Ni, based on a 35% retention of Ni following inhalation at 0.4 and 0.2 μg Ni / d among dwellers in urban and rural areas, respectively. Nickel is primarily excreted in the urine, with small amounts in the bile, and approximately 90% of the unabsorbed fraction excreted in the feces (Sunderman and Selin, 1968; Nomoto and Sunderman, 1970); other routes of excretion include saliva and sweat. Nickel also crosses the placental barrier as has been demonstrated by the accumulation of Ni in the fetuses of exposed mothers (Schroeder et al., 1964; Schneider et al., 1980).

Toxicological Effects

Nickel alloys and Ni compounds are a major cause of dermatoses (including contact and atopic dermatosis). This effect, however, is not limited to occupationally exposed individuals but also occurs in the general population, particularly in women, as a result of Ni-sensitization among individuals exposed to Ni-containing objects such as coins and jewelry. Nickel dermatosis often begins as an erythema of the hand, with the skin gradually becoming eczematous tending to a generalized lichenification (Sunderman, 1986). A study showed that 17 of 28 patients that had ingested 2.5 mg Ni (as $NiSO_4$) developed aggravated chronic dermatitis and nine of these patients recovered when their dietary Ni intake was reduced (Kaaber et al., 1978).

Nickel-induced allergies have also been associated with dental prostheses (Sunderman, 1986). In addition nickel intoxication has been documented in 23 patients during extracorporeal hemodialysis due to contaminated dialysis fluid (Webster et al., 1980). Spoilage of these fluids occurred as a result of leaching from the Ni-plated heating tanks used for their preparation. Symptoms included nausea, vomiting, weakness, headaches, and palpitations, and these dissipated within a few hours after cessation of hemodialysis. In addition hypernickelemia has been reported in patients with acute renal failure; the hypernickelemia may contribute to the onset of dialysis-associated hypersensitivity, encephalopathy, and artheriosclerosis (Hopfer et al., 1984; Savory et al., 1984). To overcome this clinical problem, it was suggested that the permissible upper limit for Ni should be no more than 5 μg / L in common dialysis fluids and 10 μg / L for solutions containing amino acids and albumin (Sunderman, 1983). High Ni blood concentrations have also been observed in patients with acute myocardial infarction and unstable angina pectoris (Leach et al., 1984). Administration of Ni-contaminated intravenous fluids to patients with myocardial infarction could result in hazardous consequences due to an increased coronary artery resistances associated with Ni.

Nickel compounds are known to produce a number of other toxicological effects. Asthma has been associated with inhalation of Ni-containing mists in the Ni-plating industry (McConnell et al., 1973) and in hypersensitive patients due to nonoccupational exposure (Arvidsson and Bogg, 1959). Hypertrophic rhinitis and nasal sinusitis have been reported to occur in workers in Ni refineries and electrolysis plants. These conditions are frequently accompanied by nasal polyposis and perforation of the nasal septum, as well as pulmonary irritations.

In contrast to inorganic Ni compounds, exposure to $Ni(CO)_4$ can result in acute poisoning. Nickel carbonyl, a colorless volatile liquid, is produced as an intermediate product during Ni-refining (Monds process). Inadvertent formation of $Ni(CO)_4$ also occurs during chemical processes that use Ni catalysts, such as petroleum refining, coal gasification, and hydrogenation of fats (Sunderman, 1986). Initial exposure to $Ni(CO)_4$ produces nausea, vertigo, headaches, dyspnea, and chest pain; these symptoms disappear a few hours after removal from the exposure (Sunderman, 1981a). However, after a latency period of 12 to 36 hours, and in some unusual cases 5 days, severe pulmonary symptoms develop with coughing, tachycardia, cyanosis, and profound weakness. Diffuse interstitial pneumonitis accompanied by either a cerebral hemorrhage or pulmonary edema are the most likely cause of death 4 to 13 days after exposure. Any recovery from the cases of acute poisoning is very slow due to pulmonary insufficiency (Sunderman, 1971). The measurement of blood Ni concentration immediately following exposure to $Ni(CO)_4$ provides a guideline as to the severity of the poisoning and the choice of appropriate supportive therapy. Sodium diethyldithiocarbonate is the preferred drug, although other chelating agents such as D-penicillamine and triethylenetetramine are effective in some cases. There is a danger of Ni redistribution to other organs such as the brain with diethyl diethiocarbonate, and it should be used cautiously. As opposed to the case of $Ni(CO)_4$, acute Ni poisoning is rare; however, the major signs of intoxication include gastroenteritis, colic, anemia, and cachexia (Raithel and Schaller, 1981). Neurological symptoms such as tremor, chorea, and convulsions are also associated with acute Ni poisoning. Only one fatality from acute Ni poisoning has been reported involving a 2-year-old girl who ingested approximately 15 g $Ni(SO_4)_2$ (Daldrup et al., 1983). Nickel is known to affect Mg^{2+} and Ca^{2+} dependent processes, and thus it has a wide spectrum of toxic action (Costa, 1991).

Carcinogenicity and Teratogenic Effects

Nickel compounds are potent carcinogens in experimental animal models. Metastasizing pulmonary tumors were induced in rats following inhalation of $NiCO_4$ (Sunderman and Donnelly, 1965; Sunderman et al., 1959) or Ni_3S_2 dust (Ottolenghi et al., 1975). Nickel subsulfide (0.97 mg Ni/m^3) caused hyperplasia, metaplasia, adenomas, and adenocarcinomas of the lung, equally in both male and female Fisher 344 rats. Anaplasia and adenocarcinomas of the lungs were induced in guinea pigs by inhalation of Ni-containing dust (Hueper, 1958). A significant increase in mouse lung adenomas was also observed following intraperitoneal injection of $Ni(CH_3COO^-)_2$ (Stoner et al., 1976). However, these Ni-induced tumors in the strain A mouse could be prevented by co-administration of Ca^{2+} and Mg^{2+} at a molar ratio of $> 1 : 1$ against the $Ni(CHCOO^-)_2$ (Poirer et al., 1984). Similarly Mn^{2+} ions suppressed Ni_3S_2-induced rhabdomyosarcomas in rats (Smialowicz et al., 1987).

A recent two year inhalation carcinogen bioassay has been conducted with Ni_3S_2, green high temperature NiO, and water-soluble Ni sulfate hexahydrate in rats and mice. There was a dose-dependent increase in tumor incidence in rats by Ni_3S_2 and by NiO but $NiSO_4$ hexahydrate failed to increase the incidence of tumors in rats or mice. There was no increase in tumor incidence in mice exposed by inhalation to Ni_3S_2 and green high temperature NiO (Dunnick et al., 1995).

Besides inhalation-related cancers, malignant neoplasms could be induced by Ni compounds at the site of exposure. Sarcomas were induced in rats and hamsters by intramuscular injection of the sandwich compound nickellocene and by solution of poorly soluble Ni_3S_2 dust (Lau et al., 1972; Haro et al., 1968). In other studies rhabdomyosarcomas were induced in rats with Ni dust or with Ni_3S_2, and with NiO dust in both rats and mice (Heath and Daniles, 1964). Nearly all routes of Ni_3S_2 exposure, except via oral dosing, produced various types of malignant tumors in the test animals at the site of administration (Sunderman et al., 1978). However, repeated dosing with a water-soluble

Ni compound by intramuscular injection failed to induce any tumors (Kasprzak, 1994). A study of mice exposed to Ni (0.5 ppm) in their drinking water for 36 months demonstrated no significant increase in tumor formation as compared with the control group (Schroeder et al., 1964). Negative results were also obtained in Syrian golden hamsters treated with Ni_3S_2 after painting the agent on the mucosa of each cheek three times per week (Sunderman et al., 1978). However, regardless of the results from these studies, it was suggested that Ni_3S_2 was the most potent carcinogen in experimental animal models.

Epidemiological studies have also demonstrated an association between the incidences of respiratory cancer with the industrial exposure to Ni-containing aerosols and dusts (IARC, 1976, 1990). A 5-fold increase in the incidence of lung cancer was observed among workers in Ni refineries, with a 150-fold increase in the incidence of nasal cancer as compared with the general population (Doll et al., 1977). Further studies also showed an increase in mortality among refinery workers due to lung and/or sinonasal cancers (Magnus et al., 1982; Enterline and Marsh, 1982). However, an increased risk of respiratory cancer was not observed among workers involved with different sectors of Ni refinery (Godbold and Tompkin, 1979; Cuckle et al., 1980; Cox et al., 1981). These workers were exposed to various types of Ni compounds such as metallic Ni and water-soluble Ni compounds such as $NiSO_4$. Besides lung and nasal cancer, an increased risk of gastric and renal cancers was observed among these occupationally exposed individuals in Ni electroplating and electrolytic refining plants (Sunderman, 1981b; McEwan, 1978). Originally it was thought that $Ni(CO)_4$ was the primary carcinogen, since the earlier studies were carried out in Ni refineries employed in the Mond process. However, epidemiological studies in Ni refineries not employing the Mond process also demonstrated an increased risk of cancer in the employees, suggesting that Ni_3S_2 was also a potent carcinogen. Carcinogenic activity has since also been implicated for both NiO and $NiSO_4$ and has been confirmed for each by experimental animal studies (Dunnick et al., 1995).

The teratogenicity of Ni compounds is well established in experimental animals. The embryotoxic and teratogenic effects have been related to altered maternal hyperglycemia, which altered the supply of glucose to the fetus (Mas et al., 1985). A study showed a reduction in the mean number of live pups delivered by dams exposed to $^{63}NiCl_2$ (12 or 16 mg Ni / kg) on day 8 or 18 of gestation. In addition a reduction in fetal weight was observed on day 20 of gestation and in weanling pups 4 or 8 weeks olds (Sunderman et al., 1978). Another study with three consecutive generations of rats administered Ni salts (0.5 ppm) in their drinking demonstrated an increased number of neonatal deaths and runts in all three generations, as well as increased female to male ratio by the third generation (Schroeder and Mitchener, 1971). Similarly intravenous administration of $Ni(CH_3COO^-)_2$ to hamsters (2 to 30 mg / kg body weight [0.5 to 7 mg Ni / kg]) on day 8 of gestation increased the number of fetal resorptions, overall embryo mortality, as well as the incidence of unspecified congenital malformations (Ferm, 1972). In addition malformations were observed from dams exposed to 1.2 to 6.9 mg Ni / kg as $NiCl_2$ intraperitoneal doses to groups of mice on days 7 to 11 of gestation (Lu et al., 1976, 1979). Malformations included anencephaly, cerebral hernia, open eyelids, cleft palate, micromelia, ankylosis of the extremity, club foot, and skeletal anomalies. The highest incidences of malformations were observed when Ni was injected on day 8 or 9 of gestation (Lu et al., 1979). More recent investigations demonstrated that the pregnant rats were more susceptible to Ni (as $NiCL_2$ 1,2,4 mg / kg i.p.) compared with the control group, as was evident by the decrease in LD_{50} (Mas et al., 1985). Furthermore the teratogenic effects were demonstrated when Ni was administrated to dams during organogenesis.

Although the teratogenic effects of Ni have been demonstrated in experimental animal models, the doses employed are high and may not relate to the human exposure. However, there is no information on either the reproductive effects or teratogenic effects of Ni in humans.

Genotoxicity and Mutagenicity

The genotoxicity of Ni compounds have been studied extensively (Costa, 1991). While carcinogenic Ni compounds can produce some DNA strand breaks and some crosslinking of proteins to DNA particularly in heterochromatin, they are not very genotoxic. However, the greatest genotoxic effect of Ni compounds is the selective damage that Ni produces to heterochromatin. Since heterochromatin contains genetically inactive DNA, the selective damage that Ni produces to this region may explain why carcinogenic Ni compounds are not very mutagenic in mutation assays, which require an actively expressed target gene.

Nickel salts such as $NiCl_2$ and $Ni(CO)_4$ have been shown to react with DNA and alter the constitution and function of nucleic acids. Nickel chloride has been shown to increase base misincorporation during replication thereby impairing the fidelity of DNA synthesis in in vitro systems (Sirover and Loeb, 1976; Miyaki et al., 1979). In addition to these in vitro observations, exposure to Ni compounds affects DNA structure and biochemistry in situ. Exposure of rats to $Ni(CO)_4$ was shown to inhibit DNA and RNA synthesis in the liver, lungs, and kidneys (Beach and Sunderman, 1970; Hui and Sunderman, 1980; Sunderman and Esfahani, 1968; Witschi, 1972). In addition DNA–protein crosslinks were induced by $NiCO_3$–$2Ni(OH)_2$ (nickel carbonate) in the kidneys of exposed rats (Ciccarelli and Wetterhahn, 1982).

Nickel is clearly not an active mutagen in assays with bacterial cells. Nickel sulfate ($NiSO_4$) at a concentration of $300\,\mu g / L$ was nonmutagenic in the T_4-bacteriophage assay (Corbett et al., 1970). Similarly water-soluble $NiCl_2$, NiO, and Ni_2O_3 produced negative results in the *B. subtilis* Rec-assay; with the water insoluble compounds this may be due to a lack of Ni uptake by bacteria, since they cannot phagocytize (Nishioka, 1975; Kanematsu et al., 1980). A negative response was also obtained with $NiCl_2$ in the *E. coli* WP fluctuation assay (Green et al., 1976; Arlauskas 1985) and in the Ames assay (Arlauskas et al., 1985; Tso and Fung, 1981). Although metal ions alone yield negative responses, Ni (maximum effective dose was $500\,\mu M$ Ni / plate) was shown to act synergistically with 9-aminoacridine in inducing bacterial mutagenesis (in the Ames assay) (Ogawa et al., 1987). Similar cooperative interactions between Ni and alkylating agents that induce mutagenesis were shown in both *E. coli* and *S.thphimurium* (Dublins and LaVelle, 1986). In these studies, base-pair substitution was enhanced several-fold by Ni as compared with the alkylating agent by itself, and this effect in *E. coli* was dependent on both DNA polymerase I or II and SOS functions. By contrast, positive results were obtained with $NiCl_2$ in a homoserine-dependent strain of *Corynebacterium sp.* 887 using a simplified fluctuation test as well as a cloning method and in *E. coli* (repair-deficient strains) using a killing assay (Pikalet and Necksek, 1983; Tweats et al., 1981). $NiSO_4$ was only weakly positive in the production of gene conversions at the *try5* locus and negative in the production of reverse mutations at the *ilvI* locus in *Saccharomyces cerevisiae* (Singh, 1984).

Nickel produces weak genotoxic and mutagenic effects in vitro in mammalian cells. Nickel chloride produced an insignificant (2 to 4-fold) increase in 8-azaguanine resistance in cultured Chinese hamster (CH) cells (Miyaki et al., 1979). However, conflicting results are commonly obtained with Ni agents in these assays. A different study achieved positive results at the same locus with $NiCl_2$ in cultured Chinese hamster ovary cells (Hsie et al., 1979). These authors mentioned that such results needed further confirmation, since mutation assays are influenced by subtle changes in ionic composition of the media and the physiological state of the cells during the treatment. Furthermore a dose-dependent increase in the number of mutants at the thymidine kinase locus was obtained for mouse lymphoma cells (Amacher and Paillet, 1980). Nickel sulfide (NiS) and Ni_3S_2 produced weak positive results in CH cells at the HGPRT locus; however, a relatively stronger mutagenic response was obtained with Ni_3S_2 (Costa et al., 1980).

The clastogenic and mitostatic properties of Ni compounds have also been demonstrated in many cell types. In *Allium cepa*, $NiCl_2$ induced scattered c-mitosis with chromosomes either evenly scattered in the cytoplasm or c-mitosis with partial spindle leading to chromosomes stuck on the equatorial plate (Fishesjo, 1988). This effect has not been associated with any other metal studied. Abnormal arrangement of chromatin in dividing cells and supernumerary micronuclei as well as grossly deformed cells were produced in *Vicia faba* in vitro following treatment with $Ni(NO_3)_2$, $NiCl_2$, or $NiSO_4$ (Komczynski et al., 1963). Similar effects have been observed in cultured mammalian cells with these agents. Aberrations and abnormal mitotic figures were induced by NiS (1.0 ng/ml) in cultured embryonic rat muscle cells (Swierenga and Basrur, 1968). In addition aberrations were induced by $NiCl_2$, $Ni(CH_3COO)_2$, $K_2Ni(CN)_4$, and $NiSO_4$ in FM3A mouse mammary carcinoma cells (Umeda and Nishimura, 1979). All of these compounds produced a variety of chromosomal breaks, with chromatid gaps predominating. In contrast, NiS induced damage primarily to the heterochromatic region of the chromosomes (Costa et al., 1988), particularly to the heterochromatic X chromosome from Chinese hamster ovary cells (Conway et al., 1987). A relatively large number of sister chromatid exchange (SCE) was induced by NiS, whereas $NiCl_2$ produced a much lower incidence of dicentrics and had no significant effect on the X chromosome in the same system. However, negative results were obtained with metallic Ni and NiO in cultured human leukocytes (Kato et al., 1976). Sister-chromatid exchanges were also not induced by NiO and Ni_3S_2 in cultured human lymphocytes (Waksvik et al., 1984), although chromatid gaps were induced by these compounds as well as with $NiCl_2$ and $NiSO_4$ in this same system (Waksvik et al., 1984; Larramendy et al., 1981).

Despite the clastogenic property of Ni compounds, structural chromosomal aberrations were not found in rat bone marrow cells following in vivo treatment with 3 or 6 mg Ni/kg as $NiSO_4$ (Mathur et al., 1978). Negative results were also obtained with $NiCl_2$ and $Ni(NO_3)_2$ in the micronucleus test using mouse bone-marrow cells and in the dominant mutation lethal assay (DeKnudt and Leonard, 1982). A similar result was obtained with $Ni(NO_3)_2$ in a different dominant lethal assay (Jacquet and Mayencem, 1982). However, positive results were produced with $Ni(CO)_4$ in the same assay, suggesting that this salt could also induce chromosomal aberrations in male germ cells (Sunderman et al., 1981b).

In cell transformation assays, positive results were obtained in cultured C3H10T$_{1/2}$ Cl8 mouse cells with Ni_3S_2 and in Syrian hamster embryo cells with either Ni_3S_2 or $NiSO_4$ (Nishioka, 1975; Waksvik et al., 1984). Nickel also enhanced viral transformations and potentiated benzo(a)pyrene-induced transformations (Rivedel and Sanner, 1981). Following pretreatment with benzo(a)pyrene, $NiSO_4$ also increased the incidence of chromosomal aberrations. In addition amorphous NiS, a compound similar to Ni_3S_2, was shown not to induce transformations and this was deemed to be related to the different physical properties of the two compounds (Costa and Mollenhauer, 1980). Subsequent studies attributed these differences to the inability of amorphous compounds to be internalized by cells, a property which appeared to be influenced by a combination of surface charge and solubility (Costa et al., 1981a,b).

The strong activity exhibited by crystalline nickel subsulfide and relatively weak activity exhibited by soluble Ni salts is clearly related to the ability of the Ni ion to reach the nucleus and interact with chromatin (Costa, 1991; Farrell and Costa, 1997). There is very little Ni inside the cell following the treatment of cultured cells with water-soluble Ni salts, while cells treated with crystalline nickel subsulfide have very high concentrations found in the nucleus (Abbracchio et al., 1982). Additionally, once a particle is phagocytized, it is dissolved inside the cell. This dissolution process yields very high concentrations of intracellular Ni that have been calculated to be in the millimolar to molar range (Abbracchio et al., 1982). High intracellular soluble Ni levels that result from dissolution of particles allows Ni to enter the nucleus, where it interacts selectively with heterochromatin (Patierno et al., 1985). This interaction with heterochromatin causes a change in the DNA methylation state of genes, producing hypermethylation of genes bordering heterochromatin (Klein et al., 1991; Lee et al., 1995). This effect is exemplified in a model system where a marker gene has been placed in two different positions in transgenic cell lines. When the marker gene was placed near heterochromatin, it was selectively inactivated by hypermethylation in response to treatment with crystalline nickel subsulfide; however, when placed away from heterochromatin, it was not responsive to crystalline nickel subsulfide induced inactivation (Lee et al., 1995). A new mechanism by which Ni may be producing cancers involves its ability to condense chromatin and induce DNA hypermethylation which will turn off the expression of genes. Some of these genes will be important in cancer induction (Farrell and Costa, 1997). Water-soluble Ni^{2+} has also been shown to inhibit DNA repair (Hartwig et al., 1994; Dally and Hartwig, 1997). This effect may also be operative in the mechanism of Ni^{2+} carcinogenesis.

REFERENCES

Abbracchio, M. P., J. Simmons-Hansen, and M. Costa. 1982. Cytoplasmic dissolution of phagocytized crystalline nickel sulfide particles: A prerequisite for nuclear uptake of nickel. *J. Toxicol. Environ. Health* 9: 663–676.

ACGIH, 1999. TLVs and BEIs, Cincinnati, American Conference of Governmental Industrial Hygienists.

Adams, R. G., J. G. Harrison, and P. Scott. 1969. The development of cadmium-induced proteinuria, impaired renal function, and ostemalacia in alkaline battery workers. *J. Med.* 38: 425–434.

Adamson, R. H., G. P. Canollos, and S. M. Sieber. 1975. Studies on the antitumor activity of gallium nitrate (NSC-15200) and other group IIIA metal salts. *Cancer Chemother Reports* 59: 599–610.

Alfrey, A. C. 1980. Aluminum metabolism in uremia. *Neurotoxicology* 1: 43–45.

Alfrey, A., G. Le Grende, and W. Kaehny. 1976. The dialysis encephalopathy syndrome: Possible aluminum intoxication. *New Eng. J. Med.* 294: 184–188.

Amacher, D. E., and S. C. Paillet. 1980. Induction of trifluorothymidine resistant mutants by metal ions in $L5178/TK^{+/-}$ cells. *Mut. Res.* 78: 279–288.

Andersen, A., and M. Hahlin. 1981. Cadmium effects from phosphorous fertilization in field experiments. *Swedish J. Agr. Res.* 11: 2.

Andersen, H., B. E. Dahlberg, K. Magnus, and A. Wannag. 1982. Risk of cancer in the Norwegian aluminum industry. *Br. J. Cancer* 29: 295–298.

Andersen, K. J., E. G. Leighty, and M. T. Takahaski. 1972. Evaluation of herbicides for possible mutagenic properties. *J. Agr. Food Chem.* 20: 647–656.

Andersen, K. J., K. Nordgaard, K. Julshumn, and H. Schjoensby. 1979. Increased serum aluminum in patients with jaundice. *New Eng. J. Med.* 301: 718–729.

Anke, M., B. Groppel, M. Grun, A. Hennig, and D. Meissner. 1980. The influence of arsenic deficiency on growth reproductiveness, life expectancy and health of goats. *Spurenelement Symp.* pp. 25–32.

Anke, M., B. Groppel, H. Kronemann, and M. Grun. 1984. Nickel—An essential element. In *Nickel in the Human Environment*, ed. F. W. Sunderman Jr., pp. 339–365. IARC Scientific Publication 53. Lyon: International Agency for Research on Cancer.

Anke, M., A. Hennig, M. Grun, M. Parteschefeld, B. Groppel, and H. Ludke. 1976. Arsenic—A new essential trace element. *Arch. Tierernahrung* 26: 742–743.

Aposhian, H. V. 1996. Arsenic toxicology: does methylation of arsenic species have an evolutionary significance? In *Metal Ions in Biology and Medicine*, ed. P. Collery, J. Corbell, J. L. Domingo, J.-C.

Etienne, and J. M. Llobet, pp. 399–401. *Proc. 4th International Symposium on Metal Ions in Biology and Medicine.* Eurotext, France: John Libbey.

Arlauskas, A., R. S. U. Baker, A. M. Bonin, R. K. Tandon, P. T. Crisp, and J. Ellis. 1985. Mutagenicity of metal ions in bacteria. *Environ. Res.* 36: 379–388.

Armstrong, B., C. Tremblay, and G. Theriault. 1988. Compensating bladder cancer victims employed in aluminum reduction plants. *J. Occup. Med.* 30: 771–775.

Arvidsson, H., and A. Bogg. 1959. Transitory pulmonary infilterations (Leoffler's syndrome) in acute generalized dermatitis. *Acta. Derm. Venerol.* 39: 30–34.

Baydar, T., A. Aydin, S. Duru, A. Isimer, and G. Sahin. 1997. Aluminum in enteral nutrition formulas and parenteral solutions. *J. Toxicol. Clin. Toxicol.* 35: 277–281.

Beach, D. J., and F. W. Sunderman Jr. 1970. Nickel carbonyl inhibition of RNA synthesis by chromatin-RNA polyermase complex from hepatic nuclei. *Cancer Res.* 30: 48–50.

Bencko, V. 1983. Nickel: a review of its occupational and environmental toxicology. *J. Hyg. Epidemiol. Microbiol. Immunol.* 27: 237–247.

Bencko, V., B. Benes, and M. Cikrt. 1976. Biotransformation of As(III) to As(VI) and arsenic tolerance. *Arch. Toxicol.* 36: 159–162.

Bennett, R. W., T. V. N. Persaud, and K. L. Moore. 1975. Experimental studies on the effects of aluminum on pregnancy and fetal development. *Anat. Anz. Bd.* 138: 365–378.

Berlyne, G. M., J. Benari, D. Pest, J. Weinberg, J. Stern, G. R. Gilmore, and R. Levine. 1970. Hyperaluminaemia from aluminum resins in renal failure. *Lancet* 2: 494–496.

Bowen, H. J. M., ed. 1979. *Environmental Chemistry of the Elements.* London: Academic Press.

Bruce, W., and J. Heddle. 1979. The mutagenic activity of 61 agents as determined by micronucleus, *Salmonella*, and sperm abnormality assays. *J. Genet. Cytol.* 21: 319–334.

Bui, T. H., J. Lindsten, and G. F. Nordberg. 1975. Chromosome analysis of lymphocytes from cadmium workers and Itai-Itai patients. *Environ. Res.* 9: 187–195.

Buichinger, M., E. Schnud, H. Einbrodt, and J. Dresp. 1976. Chromosome aberrations in lymphocytes after occupational exposure to lead and cadmium. *Mut. Res.* 40: 57–62.

Burnatowska-Hledin, M. A., G. H. Mayor, and K. Law. 1985. Renal handling of aluminum in rats clearance and micropuncture studies. *Am. J. Physiol.* F249: F192–197.

Cant, S. A., and L. A. Legendre. 1982. Assessment of occupational exposure to arsenic, copper, and lead in a Western copper smelter. *Am. Ind. Hyg. Assoc. J.* 43: 223–226.

Carson, B. L., H. V. Ellis, and J. L. McCann. 1986. *Toxicology and Biological Monitoring of Metals in Humans: Including Feasibilty and Need.* Chelsea, MI: Lewis Publishers.

Casto, B. C., J. Meyer, and J. A. Di Paolo. 1979. Enhancement of viral transformation for evaulation of the carcinogenic or mutagenic potential of inorganic metal salts. *Cancer Res.* 39: 193–198.

Chen, Y. J., Y. C. Chuang, T. M. Lin, and H. Y. Wu. 1985. Malignant neoplasms among residents of a blackfoot disease-endemic area of Taiwan: high-arsenic artensian well water and cancers. *Cancer Res.* 45: 5895–5899.

Chiquoine, A. D., and V, Suntseff. 1965. Sensitivity of mammals to cadmium necrosis of the testes. *J. Reprod. Fertil.* 10: 455–457.

Ciccarelli, R. B., and K.E. Wetterhahn. 1982. Nickel distribution and DNA lesions induced in rats tissue by the carcinogen nickel carbonate. *Cancer Res.* 42: 3544–3549.

Clarkson, D. T. 1965. Effect of aluminum and some other trivalent metal cations on cell division in the roots apices of *Allium cepa. Ann. Bot.* 29: 309–315.

Clarkson, E. M., V. A. Luch, W. V. Hynson, R. R. Bailey, J. B. Eastwood, J. S. Woodhead, V. R. Clements, J. L. H. O'Riordan, and H. E. De Wardener. 1972. The effect of alumimium hydroxide on calcium phosphorous and aluminium balances, the serum parathyroid hormone concentration and the aluminium content of bone in patients with chronic renal failure. *Clin. Sci.* 43: 519–531.

Cohen, M., D. Latta, T. Coogan, and M. Costa. 1990. The reactions of metals with nucleic acid. In *Biological Effects of Heavy Metals, Mechanisms of Metal Carcinogenesis*, vol. 2, ed. E. Foulkes, pp. 19–77. Boca Raton, FL: CRC Press.

Conway, K., X. W. Wang, L. S. Xu, and M. Costa. 1987. Effects of magnesium on nickel-induced genotoxicity and cell transformation. *Carcinogenesis* 8: 1115–1121.

Conway, K., and M. Costa. 1989. The involvement of heterochromatic damage in of nickel-induced transformation. *Biol. Trace Elem. Res.* 21: 437–444.

Corbett, T. H., C. Heidelberger, and W. F. Dove. 1970. Determination of the mutagenic activity to bacteriophage T4 of carcinogenic and noncarcinogenic compounds. *Mol. Pharmacol.* 6: 667–679.

Costa, M. 1991. Molecular mechanisms of nickel carcinogenesis. *Ann. Rev. Pharmacol. Toxicol.* 31: 321–337.

Costa, M., and H. H. Mollenhaur. 1980. Phagocytosis of nickel subsulfide particles during the early stages of neoplastic transformation in tissue culture. *Cancer Res.* 40: 2688–2694.

Costa, M., M. P. Abbrachio, and J. Simmons-Hansen. 1981a. Factors influencing the phagocytosis, neoplastic transformation, and cytotoxicity of particulate nickel compounds in tissue culture systems. *Toxicol. Appl. Pharmacol.* 60: 313–323.

Costa, M., J. Simmons-Hansen, C. W. N. Bedrossian, J. Bonura, and R. M. Caprioli. 1981b. Phagocytosis, cellular distribution, and carcinogenic activity of particulate nickel compounds in tissue cultures. *Cancer Res.* 41: 2868–2976.

Costa, M., M. K. Jones, and O. Lindberg. 1980. Metal carcinogenesis in tissue culture systems. In *Inorganic Chemistry in Biology and Medicine*, ed. A. C. Martell, pp. 45–73. ACS Symposium, Serial 140. Washington, DC: American Chemical Society.

Cotton, F. A., and G. Wilkinson. 1980. *Advanced Inorganic Chemistry, a Comprehensive Text*, 4th edition. New York: Wiley.

Cox, J. E., R. Doll, W. A. Scott, and S. Smith. 1981. Mortality of nickel workers: Experience of men working with metallic nickel. *Br. J. Ind. Med.* 38: 235–239.

Crapper, D. R., S. S. Krishnan, and A. J. Dalton. 1973. Brain aluminum distribution in Alhzeimer's disease and experimental neurofibillary degeneration. *Science* 111: 511–513.

Crecelius, E. A. 1977. Changes in the chemical specification of arsenic following ingestion by man. *Environ. Health Perspect.* 19: 147–150.

Crecelius, E. A. 1977. Arsenic and arsenate levels in wine. *Bull. Environ. Contam. Toxicol.* 18: 227–230.

Cronin, E., A. D. DiMichiel, and S. S. Brown. 1980. Oral challenge in nickel sensitive women with hand eczema. In *Nickel Toxicology*, eds. S. S. Brown, and F. W. Sunderman Jr., pp. 149–152. New York: Academic Press.

Crossen, P. E. 1983. Arsenic and SCE in human lymphocytes. *Mut. Res.* 119: 415–419.

Cuckle, H., R. Doll, and L. G. Morgan. 1980. Mortality study of men working with soluble nickel compounds. In *Nickel Toxicology*, eds. S. S. Brown, and F. W. Sunderman Jr., pp. 11–14. New York: Academic Press.

Cuzick, J., S. Evans, M. Gillman, and D. A. Price Evans. 1982. Medicinal arsenic and internal malignancies. *Br. J. Cancer* 45: 904–911.

Cvetkova, R. P. 1970. Materials on the study of the influence of cadmium compounds on the generative function. *Gig. Tr. Prof. Zabol.* 14: 31–35.

Daldrup, T., K. Haarhoff, and S. C. Szathmary. 1983. Teodliche nickelsulfate-intoxikation. *Berichte Zur. Gerichlichen Medizin* 41: 141–144.

Dally, H., and A. Hartwig. 1997. Induction and repair inhibition of oxidative DNA damage by nickel (II) and cadmium (II) in mammalian cells. *Carcinogenesis* 18(5): 1021–1026.

De Voogt, P., B. Van Hattum, J. F. Feenstra, and J. W. Copius Peereboom. 1980. Exposure and health effects of cadmium. *Toxicol. Environ. Chem. Rev.* 3: 89–109.

Deboni, V., J. W. Scott, and D. R. Crapper. 1974. Intracellular aluminum binding: A histochemical study. *Histochemistry* 40: 31–37.

Degraeve, N. 1981. Carcinogenic, teratogenic and mutagenic effects of cadmium. *Mut. Res.* 86: 115–135.

DeKnudt, G., and A. Leonard. 1982. Mutagenicity test with nickel salts in the male mouse. *Toxicology* 25: 289–292.

DeKnudt, G. H., and M. Deminalti. 1978. Chromosome studies in human lymphocytes after in vitro exposure to metal salts. *Toxicology* 10: 67–75.

Dent, C. E., and C. S. Winter. 1974. Osteomalacia due to phosphate depletion from excessive aluminum hydroxide ingestion. *Br. Med. J.* 1: 551.

Di Paolo, J. A., and B. C. Casto. 1979. Quantitative studies of in vitro morphological transformation of Syrian hamster cells by inorganic metal salts. *Cancer Res.* 39: 1008–1013.

Dinman, B. D. 1988. Alumina-related pulmonary disease. *J. Occup. Med.* 30: 328–335.

Dinman, B. D. 1987. Aluminum in the lung: the pyropowder conundrum. *J. Occup. Med.* 29: 869–886.

Dixon, N. E., C. Gazzola, C. J. Asher, D. S. W. Lee, R. L. Blakely, and B. Zerner. 1980. Jack bean urase (EC 3.5.1.5). II. The relationship between nickel enzymatic activity and the abnormal ultraviolet spectrum. The nickel content of jack beans. *Can. J. Biochem.* 58: 474–480.

Doll, R., J. G. Mathews, and L. G. Morgan. 1977. Cancer of the lung and nasal sinuses in nickel workers: a reassessment of the period risk. *Br. J. Ind. Med.* 34: 102–105.

Dorian, C., V. H. Gattone, and C. D. Klaassen. 1995. Discrepancy between the nephrotoxic potencies of cadmium-metallothionein and cadmium chloride and the renal concentration of cadmium in the promixal convoluted tubules. *Toxicol. Appl. Pharmacol.* 130: 161–168.

Dublins, J. S., and J. M. LaVelle. 1986. Nickel (II) genotoxicity: potentation of mutagenesis of simple alkylating agents. *Mut. Res.* 162: 187–199.

Dunnick, J. K., M. R. Elwell, A. E. Radovsky, J. M. Benson, F. F. Hahn, K. J. Nikula, E. B. Barr, and C. H. Hobbs. 1995. Comparative carcinogenic effects of nickel subsulfide, nickel oxide, or nickel sulfate hexahydrate on chronic exposures in the lung. *Cancer Res.* 55: 5251–5256.

Dutkiewicz, T. 1977. Experimental studies on arsenic absorption routes in rats. *Environ. Health Perspect.* 19: 173–177.

Edling, C., B. Jarvhilm, L. Andersson, and O. Axelson. 1987. Mortality and cancer incidence among workers in an abrasive manufacturing industry. *Br. J. Ind. Med.* 44: 57–59.

El-Sadek, L. M. 1972. Mitotic inhibition and chromosomal aberrations induced by some arylarsenic and its compounds in root-tips of maize. *Eygpt J. Genet. Cytol.* 1: 218–224.

Enterline, P. E., and G. M. Marsh. 1982. Mortality among workers in a nickel refinery and alloy manufacturing plant in West Virginia. *J. Natl. Cancer Inst.* 68: 925–933.

Fan, T. Y., J. Morrison, R. R. Rounbehler, D. H. Fine, W. Miles, and N. P. Sen. 1977. N-Nitrosodiethanolamine in synthetic cutting fluids: a part-per-hundred impurity. *Science* 196: 70–71.

Farrell, R. P., and M. Costa. 1997. Carcinogenic inorganic chemicals. In *Comprehensive Toxicology, Chemical Carcinogens and Anticarcinogens*, vol. 12, eds. G. T. Bowden and S. M. Fischer, pp. 225–253. Oxford: Elsevier Science Ltd. Pergamon.

Ferm, V. H. 1972. The teratogenic effects of metals on mammalian embryo. *Adv. Terat.* 5: 51–75.

Ferm, V. H. 1977. Arsenic as a teratogenic agent. *Environ. Health Perspect* 19: 215–217.

Ferm, V. H., and S. Carpenter. 1968. Malformations induced by sodium arsenate. *J. Reprod. Fertil.* 17: 199–201.

Fishesjo, G. 1988. The *Allium* test—An alternative in environmental studies: The relative toxicity of metal ions. *Mut. Res.* 197: 243–260.

Flanagan, P. R., J. Mclellan, J. Haist, G. Cherian, M. J. Chamberlain, and L. S. Valberg. 1978. Increased dietary cadmium absorption in mice and human subjects with iron deficiency. *Gastroenterology* 74: 841–846.

Fong, K., F. Lee, and R. Bockrath. 1980. Effects of sodium arsenite on single-strand DNA break formation and post-replication repair in *E. coli* following UV irradiation. *Mut. Res.* 70: 151–156.

Fowler, B. A. 1977. Toxicology of environmental arsenic. In *Toxicology of Trace Elements*, eds. R. A. Goyer and M. A. Mehlman, pp. 79–122. New York: Hemisphere.

Fowler, B., N. Ishinishi, K. Tsuchiya, and M. Vahter. 1979. Arsenic. In *Handbook on the Toxicology of Metals*, eds. L. Friberg, G. F. Nordberg, and V. B. Vouk, pp. 1721–1723. New York: Elsevier North-Holland Biomedical Press.

Friberg, L., T. Kjellstrom, G. Nordberg, and M. Piscator. 1979. Cadmium. In *Handbook on The Toxicology of Metals*, eds. L. Friberg, G. F. Nordberg and V. B. Vouk, pp. 355–381. New York: Elsevier.

Friberg, L., M. Piscator, G. F. Nordberg, and T. Kjellstrom. 1974. *Cadmium in the Environment.* Boca Raton, FL: CRC Press.

Gabbiani, G., D. Baic, and C. Dezil. 1967. Toxicity of cadmium for the central nervous system. *Exp. Neurol.* 18: 154–160.

Galini, S. H., and M. Chatzinoff. 1981. Aluminum poisoning and chick embyro-genesis. *Environ. Res.* 24: 1–5.

Ganrot, P. D. 1986. Metabolism and possible health effects of aluminium. *Environ. Health Perspect.* 63: 363–441.

Garb, L. G., and C. H. Hine. 1977. Arsenical neuropathy: Residual effects following acute exposure. *J. Occup. Med.* 19: 567–568.

Garcia-Vargas, G. G., and M. E. Cebrián. 1996. Health effects of metals. In *Toxicology of Metals*, ed. L. W. Chang, pp. 422–438. Boca Raton, FL: CRC Lewis Publishers.

Gibbs, G. W., and I. Horowitz. 1979. Lung cancer mortality in aluminum reduction plant workers. *J. Occup. Med.* 21: 347–353.

Gilliavod, N., and A. Leonard. 1975. Mutagenicity test with cadmium in the mouse. *Toxicology* 5: 43–47.

Godbold, J. H., and E. A. Tompkin. 1979. A long-term mortality study of workers occupationally exposed to metallic nickel at the Oak Ridge gaseous diffusion plant. *J. Occup. Med.* 21: 799–805.

Goldman, A. L. 1964. Lung cancer in Bowen's disease. *Am. Rev. Resp. Dis.* 108: 1205–1207.

Goyer, R. A. 1986. Toxicity of metals. In *Toxicology*, eds. C. D. Klaassen, M. O. Amdur, and J. Doull, pp. 588–591. New York: Macmillan.

Graf, H., H. K. Stummvolt, V. Meisinger, J. Kovarik, A. Wolf, and W. F. Pinggera. 1981. Aluminum removal by hemodialysis. *Kidney Intl.* 19: 589–592.

Graham, J. A., F. J. Mitter, M. J. Daniels, E. A. Payne, and D. E. Gardener. 1978. Influence of cadmium, nickel, and chromium on primary immunity in mice. *Environ. Res.* 16: 77–87.

Green, M. H. L., W. J. Muriel, and B. A. Bridges. 1976. Use of a simplified fluctuation test to detect low levels of mutagens. *Mut. Res.* 38: 33–41.

Greger, J. L., W. Goetz, and D. Sullivan. 1985. Aluminum levels in food cooked and stored in aluminum pans, trays, and foil. *J. Fed. Prot.* 48: 772–777.

Greger, J. L. 1987. Aluminum and tin. *World Rev. Nutr. Diet* 54: 255–285.

Haro, R. T., A. Furst, W. W. Payne, and H. Falh. 1968. A new nickel carcinogen. *Proc. Am. Assoc. Cancer Res.* 9: 28.

Harris, W. R., G, Berthon, J. P. Day, C. Exley, T. P. Flaten, W. F. Forbes, T. Kiss, C. Orvig, and P. F. Zatta. 1996. Speciation of aluminum in biological systems. *J. Toxicol. Environ. Health* 48: 543–568.

Harrison, W. H., E. Codd, and R. M. Gray. 1972. Aluminum inhibition of hexakinase. *Lancet* 2: 277.

Hart, M. M., and R.H. Adamson. 1971. Antitumor activity of salts of inorganic group IIIA metals; aluminum, gallium, indium, and thallium. *Proc. Natl. Acad. Sci. USA.* 68: 1623–1626.

Hartwig, A. 1994. Role of DNA repair inhibition in lead- and cadmium-induced genotoxicity: A review. *Environ. Health Perspect.* 102 (suppl. 3): 45–50.

Hartwig, A., I. Kruger, and D. Beyersmann. 1994. Mechanisms in nickel gentoxicity: The significance of interactions with DNA repair. *Toxicol. Lett.* 72: 353–358.

Hartwig, A., L. H. Mullenders, R. Schlepegrell, U. Kasten, and D. Beyersmann. 1994. Nickel (II) interferes with the incision step in nucleotide excision repair in mammalian cells. *Cancer Res.* 54: 4045–4051.

Heath, J. C., and M. R. Daniels. 1964. The production of malignant tumors by nickel in the rat. *Br. J. Cancer* 18: 261–264.

Henry, D. A., W. G. Goodman, R. K. Nudelman, N. C. Di-Dimenico, A. C. Alfrey, T. Statopolsky, M. Stanley, and J. W. Coburn. 1984. Parenteral administration in the dog: I. Plasma kinetics, tissue levels, calcium metabolism and parathyroid hormone. *Kidney Int.* 25: 362–369.

Henry, M. C., C. D. Port, R. R. Bates, and D. G. Kaufman. 1973. Respiratory tract tumors in hamsters induced by benzopyrene. *Cancer Res.* 33: 1585–1597.

Hill, A. B., and E. L. Faning. 1948. Studies on the incidences of cancer in a factory handling inorganic compounds of arsenic: I. Mortality experience in the factory. *Br. J. Ind. Med.* 5: 1–6.

Holland, R. H., and A. R. Acerodom. 1966. Current status of arsenic in American cigarettes. *Cancer* 19: 1248.

Holmberg, R. E., and V. H. Ferm. 1969. Interrelationships of selenium, cadmium and arsenic in mammalian teratogenesis. *Arch. Environ. Health* 18: 873–877.

Hood, R. D., and S. L. Bishop. 1972. Teratogenic effects of sodium arsenate in mice. *Arch. Environ. Health* 24: 62–65.

Hood, R. D., and C. T. Piken. 1972. BAL alleviation of arsenate-induced teratogenesis in mice. *Teratology* 6: 235–238.

Hopfer, S. M., J. V. Linden, C. Cristomo, F. Catanaotto, M. Galen, and F. W. Sunderman Jr. 1984. Hypernickelemia in hemodialysis patients. *Ann. Clin. Lab. Sci.* 14: 412–413.

Horak, E., and F. W. Sunderman Jr. 1973. Fecal nickel excretion by healthy adults. *Clin. Chem.* 19: 429–430.

Horst, W. J., A. Wagner, and H. Marschner. 1983. Effects of aluminum on root growth, cell division rate and mineral element content in root of *Vigna unquiculata* genotypes. *Z. Pflanzenphysiol.* 109: 95–103.

Hove, E., C. A. Elvehejm, and E. B. Hart. 1938. Aluminum in the nutrition of the rat. *Am. J. Physiol.* 123: 640–643.

Hsie, A. W., N. D. Johnson, D. B. Couch, S. San Jr., P. O'Neill, J. D. Hoeschele, R. O. Rahn, and N. L. Forbes. 1979. Quantitative mammalian cell mutagenesis and a preliminary study of the mutagenic potential of metallic compounds. In *Trace Metals in Health and Disease*, ed. N. Kharsch, pp. 55–69. New York: Raven Press.

Hueper, W. C., and W. W. Payne. 1962. Experimental studies in metal carcinogenesis: chromium, nickel, iron, and arsenic. *Arch. Environ. Health* 5: 445–462.

Hueper, W. C. 1958. Experimental studies in metal carcinogenesis: IV. Pulmonary lesions in the guinea pig and rats exposed to prolonged inhalation of powdered metallic nickel. *AMA Arch. Pathol.* 65: 600–607.

Hui, G., and F. W. Sunderman Jr. 1980. Effects of nickel compounds on incorporation of ^{3}H-tymidine into DNA in rat liver and kidney. *Carcinogenesis* 1: 297–304.

Hutchinson, T. C. 1983. A historical perspective on the role of aluminium in toxicity of acidic soils and lake wastes. In *Heavy Metals in the Environment*, pp. 17–27. International conference, Heidelberg.

IARC. 1976. IARC Monographs on the Evaluation of Carcinogenic Risk of Chemicals to Man, vol. 11, pp. 77–112. Lyon: International Agency for Research on Cancer.

IARC. 1983. *Polynuclear Aromatic Compounds, Part 3: Industrial Exposure in Aluminium Production, Coal Gasification, Coke Production, and Iron and Steel Founding. Aluminum Production*, vol. 34: 37–64. IARC Monographs on the Evaluation of the Carcinogenic Risk of Chemicals to Humans. Lyon: Internationl Agency for Research on Cancer.

IARC. 1990. *Chromium, Nickel and Welding*, IARC Monographs on the Evaluation of Carcinogenic Risks of Chemicals to Humans. IARC Monographs on the Evaluation of Carcinogenic Risk of Chemicals to Humans. vol. 49, 677 pp. Lyon: International Agency for Research on Cancer.

IARC. 1993. *Cadmium and Cadmium Compounds*, vol. 58, pp. 119–237. IARC Monographs on the Evaluation of Carcinogenic Risks to Humans. Lyon: International Agency for Research on Cancer.

Ishinishi, N., Y. Kodama, K. Nabutomom and A. Hisanaga. 1977. Preliminary experimental study on carcinogenicity of arsenic trioxide in rat lung. *Environ. Health Perspect.* 19: 191–196.

Ishinishi, N., M. Mizunoe, T. Inamasu, and A. Hisanaga. 1980. Experimental study on carcinogenicity of beryllium oxide and arsenic trioxide to the lung of rats by intratracheal instillation. *Fukuoka Acta Med.* 71: 19–21.

Ishinishi, N., A. Yamamato, A. Hisanaga, and T. Inamasu. 1983. Tumorigenicity of arsenic trioxide to the lung in Syrian golden hamster by intermittent instillations. *Cancer Lett.* 21: 141–147.

Ivankovic, S., G. Eisenbrand, and R. Preussmann. 1979. Lung carcinoma induction in BD rats after a single intratracheal instillation of an arsenic-containing pesticide mixture formerly used in vineyards. *Int. J. Cancer* 24: 786–789.

Jacquet, P., and A. Mayencem. 1982. Application of the in vitro embryo culture to the stage of mutagenic effects in nickel in male germ cells. *Toxicol. Lett.* 11: 193–197.

James, L. F., V. A. Lazer, and W. Binno. 1966. Effects of sublethal doses of certain minerals on pregnant ewes and fetal development. *Am. J. Vet. Res.* 27: 132–145.

Kaaber, K., N. K. Veinin, and J. C. Tjell. 1978. Low nickel diet in the treatment of patients with chronic nickel dermatitis. *Br. J. Derm.* 98: 197–201.

Kabata-Pendias, A., and H. Pendias, eds. 1984. *Trace Elements in Soils and Plants*. Boca Raton, FL: CRC Press.

Kada, T., K. Harano and Y. Shirasu. 1980. Screening of environmental chemical mutagen by the Rec-assay system with *Bacillus subtilis*. In *Chemical Mutagens: Principles and Methods for Their Detection*, vol. 6, eds. A. Hollaender, and F. J. de Serres, pp. 149–173. New York: Plenum Press.

Kagey, B. T., J. G. Burngarner, and J. P. Creason. 1977. Arsenic levels in maternal-fetal tissue sets. In *Trace Substances in Environmental Health XI*, ed. O. D. Hemphill, pp. 252–256. Columbia: University of Missouri Press.

Kanematsu, N., M. Hara, and T. Kada. 1980. Rec-assay and mutagenicity studies on metal compounds. *Mut. Res.* 77: 109–116.

Kasprzak, K. S. 1994. Lack of carcinogenic activity of promptly soluble (hydrated) and sparingly soluble (anhydrous) commercial preparations of nickel (II) sulfate in the skeletal muscle of male F334.NCR rats. *Toxicologist* 14: 339.

Kato, R., A. Nakamara, and T. Sewai. 1976. Chromosome breakage associated with organic mercury in human leukocytes in vitro and in vivo. *Japan. J. Hum. Genet.* 20: 256–257.

Katyal, R., B. Desigan, C. P. Sodhi, and S. Ojha. 1997. Oral aluminum administration and oxidative injury. *Biol. Trace Element Res.* 57: 125–130.

Kazantzis, G. 1984. Mutagenic and carcinogenic effects of cadmium. *Toxicol. Environ. Chem.* 8: 267–278.

King, H., and R. J. Lunford. 1950. The relation between the constitution of arsenicals and their action on cell division. *J. Chem. Soc.* 8: 2086–2088.

Kipling, M. D., and J. A. H. Waterhouse. 1967. Cadmium and prostate cancer. *Lancet* 1: 730.

Kirshgessener, M., and A. Schnegg. 1976. Nickel content of milk from lactating rats fed varying nickel levels. *Archiv. für Tierernahrung* 11: 774–776.

Kjellstrom, T. 1979. Exposure and accumulation of cadmium in populations from Japan, the United States, and Sweden. *Environ. Health Persp.* 28: 169–197.

Kjellstrom, T., and G. F. Nordberg. 1978. A kinetic model of cadmium metabolism in the human being. *Environ. Res.* 16: 248–269.

Klaassen, C. D. 1974. Biliary excretion of arsenic in rats, rabbits, and dog. *Toxicol. Appl. Pharmacol.* 29: 447–457.

Klein, C. B., K. Conway, X. W. Wang, R. K. Bhamra, X. Lin, M. D. Cohen, L. Annab, J. C. Barrett, and M. Costa. 1991. Senescence of nickel-transformed cells by an X chromosome: possible epigenetic control. *Science* 251: 796–799.

Kneip, T. J., M. Eisenbud, C. D. Strehlow, and P. C. Freudenthal. 1970. Airborne particulates in New York City. *J. Air. Pollut. Control Assoc.* 20: 144–149.

Komczynski, L., H. Nowak, and L. Rejniak. 1963. Effect of cobalt, nickel, and iron on mitosis in the roots of the broad bean (*Vicia faba*). *Nature* 198: 1016–1067.

Kowal, N. E., D. E. Johnson, D. F. Kaemer, and H. E. Pahren. 1979. Normal levels of cadmium in diet, urine, blood, and tissues of inhabitants of the United States. *J. Toxicol. Environ. Health* 5: 995–1012.

Krasovski, G. N., L. Vasukovich, and O. G. Chariev. 1979. Experimental study of biological effects of lead and aluminum following oral administration. *Environ. Health Perspect.* 30: 47–58.

Kreyberg, L. 1959. 3,4-Benzopyrene in industrial air pollution: some reflexions. *Br. J. Cancer* 13: 618–622.

Krueger, G. L., T. K. Morris, R. R. Suskind, and E. M. Widner. 1984. The health effects of aluminum compounds in mammals. *CRC Crit. Rev. Toxicol.* 13: 1–24.

Kurartsune, M., S. Tokudome, T. Shirakusa, M. Yoshida, Y. Tomumitsu, T. Hayano, and M. Seita. 1975. Occupational lung cancer among smelters. *Int. J. Cancer* 13: 552–558.

Landino, L. M., and T. L. MacDonald. 1997. Inhibition of the GDP.GTP exchange reaction of *ras* p21 by aluminum ion. *J. Inorgan. Biochem.* 66: 99–102.

Larramendy, M. L., N. C. Popescu, and J. A. DiPaolo. 1981. Induction by inorganic metal salts of sister chromatid exchanges and chromosome aberrations in human and Syrian hamster cell strains. *Environ. Mutag.* 3: 589–606.

Lau, T. J., R. L. Hackett, and F. W. Sunderman Jr. 1972. The carcinogenicity of intravenous carbonyl in rats. *Cancer Res.* 32: 2253–2258.

Leach, C. N., Jr., J. Linden, S. M. Hopfer, C. Chrisostomo, C., and F. W. Sunderman Jr. 1984. Serum nickel concentrations in patients with unstable angina and myocardial infarction. *Ann. Clin. Lab. Sci.* 14: 414–415.

Lee, J. S., and K. L. White. 1980. A review of the health effects of cadmium. *Am. J. Ind. Med.* 1: 307–317.

Lee, Y. W., C. B. Klein, B. Kargacin, K. Salnikow, J. Kitahara, K. Dowjat, A. Zhitkovich, N. Y. Christie, and M. Costa. 1995. Carcinogenic nickel silences gene expression by chromatin condensation and DNA methylation: A new model for epigenetic carcinogens. *Mol. Cell. Biol.* 15(5): 2547–2557.

Lemen, R., J. S. Lee, J. K. Wagoner, and H. P. Blejer. 1976. Cancer mortality survey workers exposed to cadmium. *Ann. N.Y. Acad. Sci.* 271: 273–276.

Leonard, A., and G. B. Gerber. 1988. Mutagenicity, carcinogenicity, and teratogenicity of aluminum. *Mut. Res.* 196: 247–257.

Leonard, A., and R. R. Lauwerys. 1980. Carcinogenicity, teratogenicity and mutagenicity of arsenic. *Mut. Res.* 75: 49–62.

Levander, O. A., and L. C. Argrett. 1969. Effects of arsenic, mercury, thallium and lead on selenium metabolism in rats. *Toxicol. Appl. Pharmacol.* 14: 308–314.

Levander, O. A., and C. A. Bauman. 1966. Selenium metabolism. VI. Effect of arsenic on the excretion of selenium in the bile. *Toxicol. Appl. Pharmacol.* 9: 308–314.

Levy, L. S., F. J. C. Roe, D. Malcolm, G. Kazantzis, J. Clack, and H. S. Platt. 1973. Absence of prostate changes in rats exposed to cadmium. *Ann. Occup. Hyg.* 16: 111–118.

Levy, L. S., and J. Clack. 1975. Further studies on the effect of cadmium on the prostate gland. I. Absence of prostatic changes in rats given oral cadmium sulfate for two years. *Ann. Occup. Hyg.* 17: 205–211.

Lewis, G. P., L. Loughlin, W. Jusko, and S. Hartz. 1972. Contribution of cigarette smoking to cadmium accumulation in man. *Lancet* 1: 291–292.

Liu, J., Y. Liu, A. E. Michalska, K. H. Choo, and C. D. Klaassen. 1996. Metallothionein plays less of a protective role in cadmium-metallothionein-induced nephrotoxicity than in cadmium chloride-induced hepatotoxicity. *J. Pharmacol. Exper. Therapeut.* 276: 1216–1223.

Lu, C. C., N. Matsumoto, and S. Iijama. 1976. Placental transfer of $NiCl_2$ to fetus in mice. *Teratology* 14: 245.

Lu, C. C., N. Matsumoto, and S. Iijama. 1979. Teratogenic effects of nickel chloride on embryonic mice and its transfer to embryonic mice. *Teratology* 19: 137–142.

Luten, J. B., G. Riekwel-Booy, and A. Rauchbaar. 1982. Occurrence of arsenic in plaice (*Pleuronectes platessa*): nature of organoarsenic compounds present and its excretion by man. *Environ. Health Perspect.* 45: 165–170.

Magnus, K., A. Andersen, and A. C. Hogetveit. 1982. Cancer of respiratory organs among workers at a nickel refinery in Norway. Second report. *Int. J. Cancer* 30: 681–685.

Maitson, P. 1981. Aluminium. *Fran Kokkarl Var Foda* 33: 231–236.

Malluche, H. H., A. Smith, K. Abreo and M. C. Faugene. 1984. The use of desferrioxamine in the management of aluminum accumulation in bones in patients with renal failure. *N. Engl. J. Med.* 311: 140–144.

Manna, G. K., and R. K. Das. 1972. Chromosome aberrations in mice induced by aluminium chloride. *Nucleus* 15: 180–186.

Manna, G. K., and A. K. Mukherjee. 1966. Spermatocyte chromosome aberrations in two species of grasshopper in two different ionic activities. *Nucleus* 9: 119–120.

Markesbery, W. R., W. D. Ehmann, T. I. M. Hossain, M. Alauddin and D. T. Goodin. 1981. Instrumental neutron activation analysis of brain aluminum in Alhzeimer's disease and aging. *Ann. Neurol.* 10: 511–516.

Marzin, D. R., and V. P. Hung. 1985. Study of the mutagenicity of metal derivatives with *Salmonella typhimurium*. *Mut. Res.* 155: 49–51.

Mas, A., D. Holt, and M. Webb. 1985. The acute toxicity and teratogenicity of nickel in pregnant rats. *Toxicology* 35: 47–57.

Mass, M. J. 1997. CpG methylation inactivates the transcriptional activity of the promoter of the human p53 tumor suppressor gene. *Biochem. Biophys. Res. Commun.* 235: 403–406.

Mathur, A. K., K. K. Datta, S. K. Tandon, and T. S. Dikshith. 1977. Effect of nickel sulfate on male rats. *Bull. Environ. Contam. Toxicol.* 17: 241–248.

Mathur, A. K., T. S. Dikshith, L. S. Lal, and S. K. Tandon. 1978. Distribution of nickel and cytogenetic changes in poisoned rats. *Toxicology* 10: 105–113.

Matsumato, H., E. Hirasawa, E. Torikai, and E. Takahashi. 1976. Location and absorption of aluminum in pea root and its binding to nucleic acids. *Plant Cell Physiol.* 17: 127–137.

McCormack, K. M., L. D. Ottosen, G. H. Mayor, V. L. Sanger, and J. B. Hook. 1978. The teratogenic effects of aluminum in rats. *Teratology* 17: 50.

McConnell, L. H., J. N. Fink, D. P. Schlueter, M. G. Schmidt Jr. 1973. Asthma caused by nickel sensitivity. *Ann. Inter. Med.* 78: 888–890.

McEwan, J. C. 1978. Five year reviews of sputum cytology in workers at a nickel sinter plant. *Ann. Clin. Lab. Sci.* 86: 503.

McNeely, M. D., F. W. Nechay, and F. W. Sunderman Jr. 1972. Measurements of nickel in serum and urine as indices of environmental exposure to nickel. *Clin.Chem.* 18: 992–995.

Mertz, M. 1970. Some aspects of nutritional trace element research. *Fed. Proc.* 29: 1482–1488.

Milham, S. 1979. Mortality in aluminum reduction plant worker. *J. Occup. Med.* 21: 475–480.

Milner, J. E. 1969. The effects of ingested arsenic on methylcholanthrene-induced tumours in mice. *Arch. Environ. Health* 18: 7–11.

Minkowitz, S. 1964. Multiple carcinoma following ingestion of medical arsenic. *Ann. Int. Med.* 41: 296–299.

Miyaki, M., N. Akamatsu, T. Ono, and H. Kayama. 1979. Mutagenicity of metal cations in cultured cells from Chinese hamster. *Mut. Res.* 68: 259–263.

Moller, P. F. G., and S. V. Gudjonsson. 1932. Massive fluorosis of bones and ligaments. *Acta Radiol.* 13: 269–294.

Moselt, A. F. W., W. Leene, C. de Groot, J. B. A. Kipp, M. Evers, A. M. Roelofsen, and K. S. Bosch. 1988. Differences in immunological susceptibility to cadmium toxicity between two strains as demonstrated with cell biological methods. *Toxicology* 48: 127–139.

Munro, I. C. 1976. Naturally occurring toxicants in food and their significance. *Clin. Toxicol.* 9: 647–663.

Mussi, I., G. Calzaferri, M. Buratti, and L. Alessio. 1984. Behaviour of plasma and urinary aluminum levels in occupationally exposed subjects. *Int. Arch. Occup. Environ. Health* 54: 155–161.

NAS. 1977. Medical and Biological Effects of Environmental Pollutants: Arsenic. National Academy of Science, Washington, DC.

NAS. 1979. Nickel. National Research Council, National Academy of Sciences, Committee on Medical and Biologic Effects of Environment Pollutants, Washington, DC.

Nashed, N. 1975. Preparation of peritoneal cell metaphases of rats, mice and Chinese hamsters after mitogenic stimulation with magnesium sulfate and/or aluminium hydroxide. *Mut. Res.* 30: 407–416.

Neilsen, F. H., and D. A. Ollerich. 1974. Nickel: a new essential trace element. *Fed. Proc.* 33: 1767–1774.

Neubauer, O. 1946. Arsenical cancer. A review. *Br. J. Cancer* 1: 192–196.

Nielsen, F. H., S. H. Givand, and D. R. Myron. 1975. Evidence of a possible requirement for arsenic by the rat. *Fed. Proc.* 34: 923.

Nishioka, H. 1975. Mutagenic activities of metal compounds in bacteria. *Mut. Res.* 31: 185–189.

Nishioka, H., and K. Takaga. 1975. Mechanism of mutation induction by metal compounds in bacteria. III. Metabolic activation. *Japan. J. Genet.* 50: 485–486.

Nomoto, S., and F. W. Sunderman Jr. 1970. Atomic absorption spectometry of nickel in serum, urine and other biological materials. *Clin. Chem.* 16: 477–485.

Nordenson, A., and L. Beckman. 1982. Occupational and environmental risks in and around a smelter in northern Sweden. VII. Reanalysis and follow-up of chromosomal aberrations of workers exposed to arsenic. *Hereditas* 96: 175–181.

Norgaard, O. 1955. Investigation with radioactive Ni[57] into the resorption of nickel through skin in normal and in nickel hypersensitive persons. *Acta. Derm. Venereol.* 35: 111–117.

Norseth, T. 1979. Aluminum. In *Handbook on the Toxicology of Metals*, eds. L. Friberg, G. F. Nordberg, and V. B. Vouk, pp. 275–281. New York: Elsevier\ North-Holland Biomedical Press.

Norseth, T., and M. Piscator. 1979. Nickel. In *Handbook on the Toxicology of Metals*, ed. Lars Friberg, Gunnar F. Nordberg, and Velimir B. Vouk, pp. 541–553. Amsterdam: Elsevier/North-Holland Biomedical Press.

Novey, H. S., and S. H. Martel. 1969. Asthma, arsenic and cancer. *J. Allergy* 44: 315–319.

Nygren, A. 1949. Cytological studies on the effects of 2,4-D, MCPA and 2,4,5-T on *Allium cepa*. *Ann. Rev. Agr. Coll.* 16: 723–728.

Nyholm, N. E. 1981. Evidence of involvement of aluminum in causation of defective formation of eggshells and of impaired breeding in wild passerine bird. *Environ. Res.* 26: 363–374.

O'Gara, R. W., and J. M. Brown. 1967. Comparison of the carcinogenic actions of subcutaneous implants of iron and aluminium in rodents. *J. Natl. Cancer Inst.* 38: 947–957.

Oberdorster, G. 1986. Airborne cadmium and carcinogenesis of respiratory tract. *Scand. J. Work Environ. Health* 12: 523–537.

Oberley, T. J., C. E. Piper, and D. S. Mc Donald. 1982. Mutagenicity of metal salts in the L5178Y mouse lymphoma assay. *J. Toxicol. Environ. Health* 9: 367–376.

Ogawa, H. I., S. Tsurata, Y. Niyiatani, H. Mino, K. Sakata, and Y. Kato. 1987. Mutagenicity of metal salts in combination with 9-aminoacridine in *Salmonella typhimurium*. *Jap. J. Genet.* 62: 159–162.

Oldiges, H., D. Hochrainer, S. H. Takenaka, G. Oberdorster, and H. Konig. 1984. Lung carcinomas in rats atfer low level cadmium inhalation. *Toxicol. Environ. Chem.* 9: 401–419.

Ondreicka, R., E. Gunter, and J. Kortus. 1966. Chronic toxicity of aluminum in rats and mice and its effects on phosphorous metabolism. *Br. J. Ind. Med.* 23: 305–312.

Ondreicka, P., J. Kortus, and E. Gunter. 1971. Aluminum; its absorption, distribution and effects on phosphorous metabolism. In *Intestinal Absorption of Metal Ions, Trace Metals and Radionucleotide*, ed. W. E. Skoryna, pp. 293–305. Oxford: Permagon Press.

Oppenheim, P. P., and W. N. Fishbein. 1965. Induction of chromosome breaks in cultured normal human luekocytes by potassium arsenite, hydroxyurea and its related compounds. *Cancer Res.* 25: 980–985.

Oswald, H., and K. Goerttler. 1971. Arsenic-induced leucosis in mice after displacental and postnatal application. *Verh. Deut. Ges. Pathol.* 55: 289–293.

Ott, M. G., B. B. Holder, and H. L. Gordon. 1974. Respiratory cancer and occupational exposure to arsenicals. *Arch. Environ. Health* 29: 250–255.

Ottolenghi, A. D., J. K. Haseman, W. W. Payne, H. L. Falk, and H. N. MacFarl. 1975. Inhalation studies on nickel sulfide in pulmonary carcinogenesis of rats. *J. Natl. Cancer Inst.* 54: 1165–1172.

Pahren, H. R., J. B. Lucas, A. Ryan, and K. K. Dotson. 1979. Health risks associated with land application of municipal sludge. *J. Water Pollut. Control Fed.* 52: 1588–1598.

Parker, K., and F. W. Sunderman Jr. 1974. Distribution of [63]Ni in tissues following intravenous injection of [63]NiCl. *Res. Commun. Chem. Pathol. Pharmacol.* 7: 755–762.

Paroni, G., G. J. van Esch, and V. Saffioti. 1963. Carcinogenesis test of two inorganic arsenicals. *Arch. Environ. Health* 7: 668–674.

Patierno, S. R., M. Sugiyama, J. P. Basilion, and M. Costa. 1985. Preferential DNA-protein crosslinking by $NiCl_2$ in magnesium-insoluble regions of fractionated Chinese hamster ovary cell chromatin. *Cancer Res.* 45: 5787–5794.

Pauwels, R., H. Bazin, B. Platteau, and M. Van der Straeten. 1979. The influence of different adjuvants on the production of IgE and IgE antibodies. *Ann. Immunol.* 1306: 49–53.

Pennington, J. A. T., and J. W. Jones. 1987. Molybdenum, nickel, cobalt, vanadium, and strontium in total diets. *Am. Diet. Assoc. Res.* 87: 1644–1650.

Perl, D. P., and A. R. Brody. 1980. Alhzeimer's disease: X-ray spectometric evidence of aluminum accumulation in neurofibrillary tangle bearing neurons. *Science* 208: 297–299.

Perl, D. P., D. C. Gujdusik, R. Y. Garruto, R. T. Yanagihara, and C. J. Gibbs. 1982. Intraneuronal aluminum accumulation in amyotropic lateral sclerosis and Parkinson-dementia in Guam. *Science* 217: 1053–1055.

Pershagen, G. 1981. The carcinogenicity of arsenic. *Environ. Health Perspect.* 40: 93–100.

Pershagen, G., and N. Bjorklund. 1985. On the pulmonary tumorigenicity of arsenic trisulfide and calcium arsenate in hamsters. *Cancer Lett.* 25: 99–104.

Pershagen, G., G. Nordberg, and N. Bjorklund. 1984. Carcinomas of the respiratory tract in hamsters given arsenic trioxide and/or benzo(a)pyrene by the pulmonary route. *Environ. Res.* 34: 227–241.

Pigott, R., and J. Ishmael. 1981. An assessment of the fibrogenic potential of two refractory fibres by intraperitoneal ingestion in rats. *Toxicol. Lett.* 8: 153–163.

Pikalet, P., and J. Necksek. 1983. The mutagenic activity of nickel in *Corynebacterium Sp. Folia Microbiol.* 28: 17–21.

Pinto, S. S., P. E. Enterline, N. Henderson, and M. O. Varner, 1977. Mortality experience to a measured arsenic trioxide exposure. *Environ. Health Perspect.* 19: 127–130.

Poe, C. F., and J. M. Leberman. 1949. The effects of acid food on aluminum cooking utensils. *Food Tech.* 149: 71–74.

Poirer, L. A., J. C. Theisse, A. J. Lyle, and M. Shimkin. 1984. Inhibition by magnesium and calcium acetates of lead subacetate- and nickel acetate-induced lung tumors in strain A mice. *Cancer Res.* 44: 1520–1522.

Potts, C. L. 1965. Cadmium proteinuria—The health of battery workers exposed to cadmium oxide dust. *Ann. Occup. Hyg.* 8: 55–61.

Raithel, H. J., and K. H. Schaller. 1981. About the toxicity and carcinogenicity of nickel and its compounds: A review of the current knowledge. *Zentrazlbl. Bakteriol. Hyg.* 173: 63–91.

Regelson, W., U. Kim, J. Ospina, and J. F. Holland. 1968. Hemangioclothelial sarcoma of liver from chronic intoxication by Fowler's solution. *Cancer* 12: 514–522.

Rivedel, E., and T. Sanner. 1981. Metal salts as promoter of in vitro morphological transformation of hamster embryo cells initated by benzo(a)pyrene. *Cancer Res.* 41: 2950–2953.

Robson, A. O., and A. J. Jelliffe. 1963. Medical arsenic poisoning and lung cancer. *Br. Med. J.* 2: 207–209.

Rockette, K., and V. C. Arena. 1983. Mortality studies on aluminum reduction plants workers; Potroom and carbon department. *J. Occup. Med.* 25: 249–259.

Rohr, G., and M. Bauchinger. 1976. Chromosome analyses in cell cultures of the Chinese hamster after application of cadmium sulfate. *Mut. Res.* 40: 125–130.

Rossman, T., M. S. Meyn, and W. Troll. 1975. Effects of sodium arsenite on the survival of UV-irradiated *E. coli*: Inhibition of a rec A-dependent function. *Mut. Res.* 30: 157–162.

Rossman, T. G., M. S. Meyn, and W. Troll. 1977. Effects of arsenite on DNA repair in *Escherichia coli. Environ. Health Perspect.* 19: 229–233.

Rossman, T. G., D. Stone, M. Molina, and W. Troll. 1980. Absence of arsenite mutagenicity in *E. coli* and Chinese hamster cells. *Environ. Mut.* 2: 371–379.

Roth, F. 1958. Bronchial cancer in vintners exposed to arsenic. *Virchow Arch. Path. Anat.* 331: 119–137.

Sanders, C. L., and J. A. Mahaffey. 1984. Carcinogenicity of single and multiple intratracheal instillations of cadmium oxide in rats. *Environ. Res.* 33: 227–233.

Sarker, B. 1984. Nickel metabolism. In *Nickel in the Human Environment*, ed. F. William Sunderman Jr., pp. 367–384. IARC Scientific Publication, 53, Lyon: International Agency for Research on Cancer.

Satterlee, H. S. 1960. The arsenic poisoning epidemic of 1900: Its relation to lung cancer in 1960. An excerise to retrospective epidemiology. *N. Engl. J. Med.* 263: 674–684.

Savory, J., S. Brown, R. Bertholf, R. Ross, M. G. Savory, and M. R. Wells. 1984. Serum and lymphocyte nickel and aluminum concentrations in patients with extracorporeal hemodialysis. *Ann. Clin. Lab. Sci.* 14: 413–414.

Schauer, C. G. 1948. Pulmonary changes encountered in employees engaged in the manufacture of aluminum abrasives: Clinical and roetgenologic aspects. *J. Occup. Med.* 5: 718–728.

Schnegg, A., and M. Kirchgessener. 1975a. Essentiality of nickel for growth of animals. *Z. Tierphysiol. Tierernah. Futtermittelkunde* 36: 63–74.

Schnegg, A., and M. Kirchgessener. 1975b. Changes in the hemoglobin content, erythrocyte count and hematocrit in nickel deficiency. *Nutr. Metab.* 19: 268–278.

Schneider, H. J., M. Anke, and G. Klinger. 1980. The nickel status of human beings. In *3 Spurelement-Symposium Nickel, Leipzig*, ed. M. Anke, H. J. Schneider, and C. Bruckner, pp. 277–283. Jena, DDR: Karl-Marx-Universitat and Freidrich-Schiller-Universitat.

Schroeder, H. A., and J. J. Balassa. 1961. Hypertension induced in rats by small doses of cadmium. *Am. J. Physiol.* 202: 515–518.

Schroeder, H. A., and M. Mitchener. 1971. Trace effects of trace elements on the production of mice and rats. *Arch. Environ. Health* 23: 102–106.

Schroeder, H. A., J. J. Balassa, and W. H. Vinton. 1964. Chromium, lead, cadmium, nickel and titanium in mice. Effect on mortality, tumors, and tissue levels. *J. Nutr.* 83: 239–250.

Schwarz, K. 1977. Essentiality versus toxicity of metals. In *Clinical Chemistry and Chemical Toxicology of Metals*, ed. S. S. Brown, pp. 3–22. New York: Elsevier.

Shackette, H. T., J. A. Erdman, T. F. Harm, and C. S. E. Papp. 1977. Trace elements in plant food stuff. In *Toxicity of Heavy Metals in the Environment*, ed. F. W. Oehme, pp. 25–68. New York: Dekker.

Shimada, T., T. Watanabe, and A, Endo. 1976. Potential mutagenicity of cadmium in mammalian oocyte chromosomes. *Mut. Res.* 40: 389–396.

Shiraishi, Y., and T. H. Yosida. 1972. Chromosomal abnormalities in cultured leucocyte cells from Itai-Itai disease patients. *Proc. Jap. Acad. Sci.* 48: 248–251.

Shiraishi, Y., H. Kurahashi, and T. H. Yoshida. 1972. Chromosomal aberrations in cultured human leucocytes induced by cadmium sulfide. *Proc. Jap. Acad. Sci.* 48: 133–146.

Shirasu, Y., M. Moriya, K. Kato, A. Furuchashi, and T. Kada. 1976. Mutagenicity screening of pesticides in the microbial system. *Mut. Res.* 40: 19–30.

Silverstein, M., R. Park, M. Marmor, N. Maizlish, and F. Mirer. 1988. Mortality among workers exposed to metal-working fluids and abrasives. *J. Occup. Med.* 30: 706–714.

Singh, I. 1984. Induction of gene conversion and reverse mutation by manganese sulfate and nickel sulphate in *Saccharomyes cerevisiae. Mut. Res.* 137: 47–49.

Sirover, M. A., and L. A. Loeb. 1976. Infidelity of DNA synthesis in vitro: Screening for potential metal mutagens or carcinogens. *Science* 194: 1434–1436.

Sjorgen, B., V. Lidum, M. Hakanssen, and L. Hedstrom. 1985. Exposure and urinary excretion of aluminum during welding. *Scand. J. Work Env. Health* 11: 39–43.

Smialowicz, R. J., R. R. Rogers, M. M. Riddle, R. W. Luebke, and L. D. Fogleson. 1987. Effects of manganese, calcium, magnesium, and zinc on nickel-induced suppression of murine natural killer cell activity. *J. Toxicol. Environ. Health* 20: 67–80.

Smith, S. B., and D. G. Wombolt. 1981. Results of hemoperfusion in the treatment of acute arsenic ingestion. *Clin. Exper. Dialysis Aphersis.* 5: 399–401.

Sorensen, J. R. J., I. R. Campbell, L. B. Tepper, and R. D. Ling. 1974. Aluminium in the environment and human health. *Environ. Health Perspect.* 8: 3–95.

Sram, R. J., and V. Beneko. 1974. A contribution evaluation of the genetic risk of exposure to arsenic. *Cesh. Hyg.* 19: 308–315.

Stanton, M. F. 1974. Fiber carcinogenesis: is asbestos the only hazard? *J. Intl. Cancer Inst.* 38: 633–634.

Stokinger, H. E. 1981. The metals. In *Patty's Industrial Hygiene and Toxicity*, 3rd edition., eds. G. D. Clayton and F. E. Clayton, pp. 1493–2060. New York: Wiley Interscience.

Stone, O. J. 1965. The effect of arsenic on inflammation, infection, and carcinogenesis. *Tex. State J. Med.* 65: 40–43.

Stoner, G. D., M. B. Shimkin, M. C. Troxell, T. L. Thompson, and L. S. Terry. 1976. Test for carcinogenicity of metallic compounds by pulmonary tumor response in strain A mice. *Cancer Res.* 36: 1744–1747.

Sunderland, D. J. B., B. K. Tsang, Z. Merali, and R. L. Singhal. 1974. Testicular and prostatic cyclic AMP metabolism following chronic cadmium treatment and subsequent withdrawal. *Environ. Physiol. Biochem.* 4: 205–217.

Sunderman, F. W., Jr. 1971. The treatment of acute nickel carbonyl poisoning with sodium diethyldithio-carbamate. *Ann. Clin. Res.* 3: 182–185.

Sunderman, F. W., Jr. 1981a. Nickel. In *Disorders of Mineral Metabolism*, Vol. 1, ed. F. Bronner, and J. W. Coburn, pp. 201–232. New York: Academic Press.

Sunderman, F. W., Jr. 1981b. Recent research on nickel carcinogenesis. *Environ. Health Perspect.* 40: 131–141.

Sunderman, F. W., Jr. 1983. Potential toxicity from nickel contamination of intravenous fluids. *Ann. Clin. Lab. Sci.* 13: 1–4.

Sunderman, F. W., Jr. 1986. Sources of exposure and biological effects of nickel. In *Environmental Carcinogens—Selected Methods of Analysis*, eds. I. K. O'Neill, P. Schuller, and L. Fishbein, pp. 79–92. Lyon: International Agency for Research on Cancer Publication 71.

Sunderman, F. W., Jr., and A. J. Donnelly. 1965. Studies of nickel carcinogenesis: metastasizing pulmonary tumors in rats induced by inhalation of nickel carbonyl. *Am. J. Pathol.* 46: 1027–1042.

Sunderman, F. W., Jr., and M. Esfahani. 1968. Nickel carbonyl inhibition of RNA polymerase activity in hepatic nuclei. *Cancer Res.* 28: 2565–2567.

Sunderman, F. W., Jr., and C. E. Selin. 1968. Nickel poisoning. XI. Implication of nickel as a pulmonary carcinogen in tobacco smoke. *Toxicol. Appl. Pharmacol.* 12: 207–218.

Sunderman, F. W., Jr., A. J. Donnelly, B. West, and J. F. Kincaid. 1959. Nickel poisoning. XI. Carcinogenesis in rats exposed to nickel carbonyl. *AMA Arch. Ind. Health* 20: 36–41.

Sunderman, F. W., Jr., R. M. Maenza, P. R., Allpass, J. M. Mitchel, I. Damjanev, and P. J. Oldblatt. 1978. Carcinogenicity of nickel subsulphide in Fischer rats and Syrian hamster after administration by various routes. In *Inorganic and Nutritional Aspects of Cancer*, ed. G. N. Schrauzer, pp. 57–67. New York: Plenum Press.

Sunderman, F. W., Jr., S. K. Shen, J. M. Mitchell, P. R. Allpass, and I. Damjanov. 1978. Embryotoxicity and fetal toxicity of nickel in rats. *Toxicol. Appl. Pharmacol.* 43: 381–390.

Sunderman, F. W., Jr., S. K. Shen, M. C. Reid, and P. R. Allpass. 1980. Teratogenicity and embryotoxicity of nickel carbonyl in Syrian hamsters. In *3 Spurelement-Symposium Nickel, Leipzig*, eds. M. Anke, H. J. Schneider, and C. Bruckner, pp. 301–307. Jena, DDR: Karl-Marx-Universitat and Freidrich-Schiller-Universitat.

Swierenga, S. H. H., and P. K. Basrur. 1968. Effect of nickel on cultured rat embryo muscle cells. *Lab. Invest.* 19: 663–674.

Takenakas, S., H. Oldiges, H. Konig, D. Hochrainer, and G. Oberdorster. 1983. Carcinogenicity of cadmium chloride aerosols in Wistar rats. *J. Natl. Cancer Inst.* 70: 367–371.

Tam, G. K. H., S. M. Charbonnau, F. Bryce, C. Pomroy, and E. Sandi. 1979. Metabolism of inorganic arsenic (^{74}As) in humans following oral ingestion. *Toxicol. Appl. Pharmacol.* 50: 319–322.

Tan, E.-L., and W. H. Abraham. 1981. Effect of calcium phosphate and alumina C_ gels on the mutagenicity and cytotoxicity of dimethylnitrosamine as studied in CHO/HGPRT system. *Mut. Res.* 84: 147–156.

Tang, X., X. Chen, J. X. Zhang, and W. Qin. 1990. Cytogenetic investigations in lymphocytes of people living in cadmium-polluted areas. *Mut. Res.* 241: 243–249.

Thauer, R. K., G. Diekert, and P. Schonheit. 1980. Biological role of nickel. *Trends Biochem. Sci.* 5: 304–306.

Theriault, G., L. De Guire, and S. Cordier. 1981. Reducing aluminum: an occupation possibily associated with bladder cancer. *Can. Med. Assoc. J.* 124: 419–422.

Thun, M. T., T. M. Schnorr, A. B. Smith, W. E. Halperin, and R. A. Lemen. 1985. Mortality among a cohort of U.S. cadmium production workers—An update. *J. Natl. Cancer Inst.* 74: 325–333.

Thurston, H., G. R. Gilmore, and J. D. Swales. 1972. Aluminum retention and toxicity in chronic renal failure. *Lancet* 1: 881–883.

Tkeshelashvili, L. K., C. V. Shearman, R. A. Zakour, R. M. Koplitz, and L. A. Loeb. 1980. Effects of arsenic, selenium, and chromium on the fidelity of DNA. *Cancer Res.* 40: 2455–2460.

Townsend, M. C., P. E. Enterline, N. B. Sussman, T. B. Bonney, and L. L. Rippey. 1985. Pulmonary function in relation to total dust exposure at a bauxite refinery and alumina-based chemical product plants. *Am. Rev. Resp. Dis.* 132: 1174–1180.

Tso, W. W., and W. P. Fung. 1981. Mutagneicity of metallic cation. *Toxicol. Lett.* 8: 195–200.

Tweats, D. J., M. H. L. Green, and M. J. Muriel. 1981. A differential killing assay for mutagens and carcinogens based on an improved repair-deficient strain of *Escherichia coli*. *Carcinogenesis* 2: 189–194.

Umeda, M., and M. Nishimura. 1979. Inducibility of chromosomal aberrations by metal compounds in cultured mammalian cells. *Mut. Res.* 67: 221–229.

Vahter, M. 1981. Biotransformation of trivalent and pentavalent inorganic arsenic in mice and rats. *Environ. Res.* 25: 286–293.

Vahter, M., and H. Norin. 1980. Metabolism of [74]As-labelled trivalent and pentavalent inorganic arsenic in mice. *Environ. Res.* 21: 446–457.

Valentine, R., and G. L. Fisher. 1984. Pulmonary clearance of intratracheally administered [63]Ni$_3$S$_2$ in strain A/J mice. *Environ. Res.* 34: 328–334.

Vallee, B. L., and D. D. Ulmer. 1972. Biochemical effects of mercury, cadmium, and lead. *Ann. Rev. Biochem.* 41: 91–130.

Vallee, B. L., D. D. Ulmer, and W. E. C. Wacker. 1960. Arsenic toxicology and biochemistry. *AMA Arch. Indust. Health* 21: 132–151.

Venugopal, B., and T. D. Luckey. 1978. *Metal Toxicity in Mammals*, vol 2, 238 pp. New York: Plenum Press.

Wachi, M., and K. Aikawa. 1975. Serum aluminium assay by flameless atomic spectroscopic method and oral absorption of some aluminum compounds by rats. *Oyo Yakuri* 10: 359–363.

Waksvik, H., M. Boysen, and A. C. Hogetveit. 1984. Increased incidence of chromosomal aberrations in peripheral lymphocytes of retired nickel workers. *Carcinogenesis* 5: 1525–1527.

Waalkes, M. P., and R. R. Misra. 1996. Cadmium carcinogenicity and genotoxicity. In *Toxicology of Metals*, ed. L. W. Chang, pp. 231–243. Boca Raton, FL: CRC Lewis Publishers.

Wang, Z., and T. G. Rossman. 1996. The carcinogenicity of arsenic. In *Toxicology of Metals*, ed. L. W. Chang, pp. 221–229. Boca Raton, FL: CRC Lewis Publishers.

Watanabe, T., T. Shimada, and A. Endo. 1979. Mutagenic effects of cadmium on mammalian oocyte chromosomes. *Mut. Res.* 67: 349–356.

Weberg, R., A. Berstod, B. Ladehaug, and Y. Thomassen. 1985. Are aluminum containing antacids during pregnancy safe? *Acta. Pharmacol. Toxicol.* 59: 63–65.

Webster, J. D., T. F. Parker, A. C. Alfrey, W. R. Smythe, H. Kubo, G. Neal, and A. Hull. 1980. Acute nickel intoxication by dialysis. *Ann. Inter. Med.* 92: 631–633.

Wehner, A. P., and D. K. Craig. 1972. Toxicology of inhaled NiO and CoO in Syrian golden hamster. *Am. Ind. Hyg. Assoc. J.* 33: 145–155.

Wen, W. N., T. L. Liev, H. J. Chang, S. W. Wuu, M. L. Yau, and K. Y. Jan. 1981. Baseline and sodium arsenite-induced sister chromatid exchange in cultured lymphocytes from patients with blackfoot disease and healthy persons. *Human Genet.* 59: 201–203.

Wesley, G., and A. Kunis. 1981. Arsenic neuropathy. *Illinois Med. J.* 160: 396–398.

Wester, P. O., D. Brune, and G. Nordberg. 1981. Arsenic and selenium in lung, liver, and kidney tissues from dead smelter workers. *Br. J. Ind. Med.* 38: 179–184.

Wide, M. 1984. Effects of short-term exposure to five industrial metals on the embryonic and fetal development of mouse. *Environ. Res.* 33: 47–53.

Wilson, A. K., E. A. Cerny, E. D. Smith, A. Wagh, and M. H. Bhattacharyya. 1996. Effects of cadmium on osteoclast formation and activity in vitro. *Toxicol. Appl. Pharmacol.* 140: 451–460.

Winter, H. 1982. The hazard of cadmium in man and animals. *J. Appl. Toxicol.* 2: 61–67.

Witschi, H. P. 1972. A comparative study of in vivo RNA and protein synthesis in rat liver and lung. *Cancer Res.* 32: 1685–1694.

Wojciechowska, B., and H. Kocik. 1983. Effect of AlCl$_2$ and SO$_4$ on root meristem of *Vicia faba L. Acta. Soc. Bot. Pol.* 52: 185–195.

Yamane, Y., and M. Ohtawa. 1979. Possible mechanism of suppressive action of aluminium chloride on lung carcinogenesis in mice induced by 4-nitro-quinoline 1-oxide: II. Effects of aluminium chloride on metabolism of 4-nitroquinoline 1-oxide. *Gann* 70: 147–152.

Yeh, S. 1973. Skin cancer in chronic arsenicalism. *Human Pathol.* 4: 469–485.

Yokel, R. A. 1984. Toxicity of aluminum exposure during lactation to the maternal and suckling rabbits. *Toxicol. Appl. Pharmacol.* 75: 35–43.

Yokel, R. A., and P. J. McNamara. 1985. Aluminum bioavailability and disposition in adults and immature rabbits. *Toxicol. Appl. Pharmacol.* 77: 344–352.

25 Ultraviolet Radiation

COLIN M. H. DRISCOLL, Ph.D.
NIGEL A. CRIDLAND, D. Phil.

Ultraviolet radiation (UVR) falls within the nonionizing radiation region of the electromagnetic spectrum (Fig. 25-1) and lies within the range of wavelengths 100 nm (which corresponds to a photon energy of approximately 12 eV) to 400 nm. The short wavelength limit of the UVR region is often taken as the boundary between the ionizing radiation spectrum (wavelengths < 100 nm) and the nonionizing radiation spectrum. For considerations of human health, UVR can be subdivided into three spectral regions (CIE, 1987), namely UVA (315–400 nm), UVB (280–315 nm), and UVC (100–280 nm). UVR with wavelengths less than 180 nm is strongly absorbed in air and common materials, and the direct potential radiation hazards to health arise from UVR with wavelengths greater than 180 nm. The eyes and the skin are the organs principally at risk from UVR because of its limited penetration in human tissue (WHO, 1994).

This chapter considers the biological mechanisms leading to health effects to the eye, the skin, and the immune system. It then considers populations at special risks, and the guidelines applicable to the control of UVR exposure and occupational protection measures. UVR sources are reviewed in the context of natural and artificial exposures, and in a section on risk assessment and education policy, approaches to minimize UVR-induced skin and eye damage are presented. A final section provides a review of techniques for evaluating UVR exposures, including methods for personal dosimetry.

RADIATION EMISSIONS

The sun is the principal source of UVR exposure for most people. Individual habits in terms of exposures to sunlight are considered most important in assessing personal risks from UVR exposure (NRPB, 1995). In addition, with depletion of the UVR-protective stratospheric ozone layer, people and the environment might be exposed to higher intensities of solar UVR.

For some individuals UVR from artificial sources could also contribute significantly to their total exposure. Such sources include sunbeds used for cosmetic tanning, high-intensity industrial sources, such as welding and xenon arcs, and irradiance devices used for medical therapy.

Emissions from many artificial sources can occur throughout the UVR spectrum. However, the solar UVR spectrum at the earth's surface does not extend below about 290 nm, due to absorption of UVB/C by stratospheric ozone and scattering and absorption processes in the atmosphere. Below 315 nm, the intensity of solar radiation decreases

Environmental Toxicants: Human Exposures and Their Health Effects, 2/e. Edited by Morton Lippmann.
ISBN: 0-471-29298-2   © 2000 John Wiley & Sons, Inc.

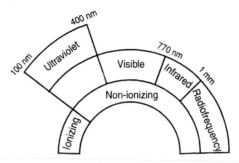

Figure 25-1   Electromagnetic spectrum.

rapidly, contributing less that 1.5% to the total solar radiation reaching the earth's surface. A summary of quantities and units used to describe UVR is given in Table 25-1.

UVR-induced biological effects depend on the wavelengths of the radiation. It is necessary for a proper determination of hazard to have spectral emission data. These consist of spectral irradiance ($W\,m^{-2}\,nm^{-1}$) measurements or calculations of emissions from the source. The total irradiance ($W\,m^{-2}$) is obtained by summing over all wavelengths emitted. The biological or hazard weighted irradiance ($W\,m^{-2}$ effective) is determined by multiplying the spectral irradiance at each wavelength by the biological or hazard weighting factor (which quantifies the relative efficacy at each wavelength for causing the effect) and summing over all wavelengths. This simple summation assumes that there are no synergistic interactions between the spectral components.

Biological or hazard weighting factors are obtained from action spectra. An action spectrum is a graph of the reciprocal of the radiant exposure required to produce the given effect at each wavelength. All the data in such curves are normalized to the datum at the most efficacious wavelength(s). By summing the biologically effective irradiance over the exposure period, the biologically effective radiant exposure ($J\,m^{-2}$ effective) can be calculated. For example, for UVR-induced erythema, the action spectrum adopted by the International Commission on Non-Ionizing Radiation Protection (ICNIRP), International Commission on Illumination (CIE), the International Electrotechnical Commission (IEC), and various national bodies is a composite curve obtained by statistical analysis of many research results on the minimum radiant exposure of UVR at different wavelengths necessary to just cause erythema (McKinlay and Diffey, 1987) (Fig. 25-2).

The most commonly used quantity for describing the erythemal potential of an exposure to UVR is the number of minimum erythemal doses (MEDs) represented by the exposure. A MED is the radiant exposure of UVR that produces a just perceptible erythema on a previously unexposed skin. It corresponds to a radiant exposure of monochromatic radiation at the maximum spectral efficacy for erythema (around 300 nm) of approximately 150 to $2000\,J\,m^{-2}$ effective, depending on skin type (Table 25-2).

TABLE 25-1   Radiometric Quantities and Units

Quantity	Unit
Radiant energy	joule (J)
Radiant flux	watt (W)
Irradiance	watt per square metre ($W\,m^{-2}$)
Effective irradiance	$W\,m^{-2}$ eff
Radiant exposure	joule per square metre ($J\,m^{-2}$)
Effective radiant exposure	$J\,m^{-2}$ eff

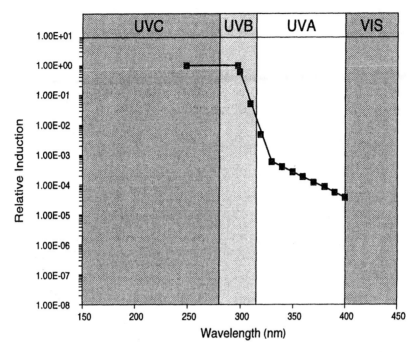

Figure 25-2   Reference erythema action spectrum (Adopted from McKinlay and Diffey, 1987)

$200\,\mathrm{J\,m^{-2}}$ effective is often used as the value of 1 MED for comparative safety purposes for white skin, which is twice the value of the standard erythema dose (SED) recently introduced by the Commission Internationale de l'Éclairage (CIE, 1996).

PATHWAYS FOR HUMAN EXPOSURE

The penetration of the body by UVR is limited and consequently the resulting adverse health effects are effectively limited to just two target organs, the skin and the eye. The

TABLE 25-2   Information on Human Skin Type

Skin Type	Unexposed Skin Color	UVR Sensitivity	Minimum Erythemal UVR Dose ($\mathrm{J\,m^{-2}}$ eff)	Sunburn / Tanning History
I	White	Very sensitive	150–300	Always burns easily, never tans
II	White	Very sensitive	250–350	Always burns easily, tans minimally
III	White	Sensitive	300–500	Burns moderately, tans gradually (light brown)
IV	Light brown	Moderately sensitive	450–600	Burns minimally, tans well always (moderate brown)
V	Brown	Minimally sensitive	600–1000	Rarely burns, tans profusely (dark brown)
VI	Chocolate brown, black	Insensitive	1000–2000	Never burns, deeply pigmented (black)

Source: Adapted from Pathak (1983).

human eye is a roughly spherical organ, deeply set in a bony orbital cavity. The bony ridge above the eyes provides protection from both mechanical injury and overhead sunlight. Hence many UVR-induced ocular conditions are mainly related to high levels of reflected solar radiation. On the other hand, damage to skin results principally from exposure to direct sunlight. Exposure of skin may be significantly modified by wearing clothes, which generally provide a high degree of protection. Thus parts of the body that are not normally clothed, such as the face and hands, tend to receive much higher cumulative exposures, and are consequently subject to more damage. There may, however, be an important exception to this, since malignant melanoma appears to be associated with intermittent intense exposure of normally unexposed skin.

BIOLOGICAL MECHANISMS LEADING TO HEALTH EFFECTS

The biological effects of UVR have been extensively reviewed (e.g., IARC, 1992; WHO, 1994; NRPB, 1995; Saunders et al., 1997). The summary of biological effects presented here has been drawn extensively from Saunders et al. (1997). Acute exposure to UVR may produce deterministic effects such as increased pigmentation, skin reddening (erythema), swelling (edema), and corneal sensitivity (photokeratitis). In addition chronic exposure can induce degenerative changes such as wrinkling and elastosis of the skin, and cataract formation in the eyes; retinal degeneration is also associated with solar exposure. Chronic exposure may also elicit stochastic effects including both melanoma and nonmelanoma skin cancers. The induction of antigen-specific immunosuppression, which may occur following acute exposure, could be relevant to skin carcinogenesis and infectious disease. Such effects, however, are not established in human populations.

While human volunteer studies are of most relevance to human health effects, they are limited by ethical considerations, and it is necessary to consider data from studies on other animals where the human data are inadequate. It is, however, essential to exercise due caution when extrapolating data from animals to humans. This is especially so in the case of UVR, where target cells may be shielded by overlying cells or tissue. For example, in the case of skin, target cells in the basal and suprabasal layers are shielded by overlying layers, particularly the stratum corneum. This is approximately ten cell layers thick in humans, but only one to two cell layers thick in mice, suggesting that mice will be much more sensitive, an effect likely to be more pronounced at shorter wavelengths where the radiation is generally more strongly absorbed by overlying cells. Similarly for the eye, differences in size and structure will affect the penetration of damaging UVR in a wavelength dependant manner, making it difficult to extrapolate rodent data to humans. The adaptation of the rodent eye to a nocturnal habit further limits its usefulness, as an animal model in this context.

Ocular Effects

The eye (see Fig. 25-3) is adapted to focus visible radiation but will also focus other optical radiations including UVR, and the consequent increase in irradiance within the eye increases its sensitivity to the harmful effects of exposure. For the purposes of discussing these effects, the eye may be conveniently divided into three compartments, the anterior eye, the lens, and the posterior eye. The anterior eye is composed of the conjunctiva and cornea, the aqueous humour, and the iris. The cornea absorbs UVR strongly, particularly at shorter wavelengths, with over 90% of incident radiation below 300 nm absorbed. Transmission of UVA by the human lens is greatest in young people, falling from about 75% under the age of 10 years to around 20% in adults. There is a small peak in transmission between 310 and 340 nm, and a further increase between 380 and 400 nm;

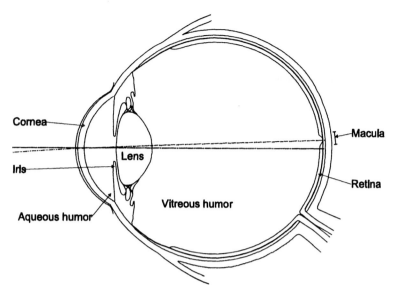

Figure 25-3   Structure of the human eye. (Adopted from Davson, 1967)

maximum transmittance at 320 nm is similar to that at 400 nm. The human lens absorbs strongly throughout the UVA and blue light regions. As the wavelength of the radiation increases, progressively more penetrates to the posterior eye, and in particular to the retina. Here the effect of focusing by the optical components of the eye is most marked and results in an increase in irradiance of over 10^5-fold. The combination of carotenoid and other pigments and a highly oxygenated environment, particularly in the central macula, can result in damage as a consequence of the photosensitized generation of reactive oxygen species.

Acute Effects   Acute overexposure to UVR can induce photokeratitis and photo-conjunctivitis, inflammatory responses of the cornea and conjunctiva, respectively. Photokeratitis is a painful condition said to give the sensation of sand in the eyes. Symptoms typically occur around 6 to 12 hours after exposure and usually start to ease after about 24 hours, although the exact time course depends on the severity of the exposure. Photoconjunctivitis exhibits a similar time course, but the symptoms may be less obvious, as the conjunctiva is less richly innervated than the cornea.

Action spectra for photokeratitis have been determined in rabbits, primates, and humans (Pitts et al., 1977), and all show maximum sensitivity at around 270 nm, where the threshold value for humans is about $40 \, \mathrm{J \, m^{-2}}$. Photoconjunctivitis exhibits a similar action spectrum, but with lower thresholds below 310 nm; at 270 nm the threshold value is around $30 \, \mathrm{J \, m^{-2}}$ (Cullen and Perera, 1994).

Prolonged viewing of the sun may produce solar retinitis, a form of photochemical damage to the retina that results from the action of both UVR and blue light; similar injuries can occur following prolonged exposure to welding arcs (Romanchuk et al., 1978). Thresholds for photochemical damage may be exceeded within 90 seconds (even with a constricted pupil) when gazing directly at the sun (Sliney and Wolbarsht, 1980), and the risk of damage may be increased through the use of poorly designed sunglasses that filter out long wavelength visible radiation, but transmit UVA and blue light. Moreover the risk is generally higher in the young, due to the greater UVR transmittance of the young lens and the greater sensitivity of the young retina (Sliney, 1986; Boettner and Wolter,

1962). A degree of recovery from this type of damage may be possible, although this depends on the severity of the injury.

Chronic Exposures Repeated exposure to high levels of solar UVR is associated with the development of climatic droplet keratopathy (CDK), pterygium and, to a lesser extent, pinguecula. CDK is a condition that involves the accumulation of translucent yellow deposits in the cornea, which spread from the periphery toward the center (Gray et al., 1992). The deposits are thought to be derived from plasma proteins that diffuse into the normal cornea and are then photochemically degraded following excessive exposure to UVR. Progressive accumulation of these deposits in later life can lead to significant visual disability, and people leading an outdoor life, especially in areas with high levels of reflected UVR, are particularly at risk. Pterygium are wing-shaped overgrowths of the conjunctiva that arise on the nasal side of the cornea and spread over the corneal surface. In severe cases these overgrowths may obstruct vision. Like CDK, pterygium appears to be associated with an outdoor life in areas with high levels of UVR, particularly UVA and UVB (Taylor et al., 1989). Pinguecula, which are fleshy lesions of the conjunctiva, have no effect on vision.

Cataracts are opacities of the lens and may be classified into cortical, nuclear, and anterior or posterior subcapsular on the basis of anatomical location. They arise as a consequence of disruption of the highly ordered structure of the lens fibers and damage to crystallins, the major lens proteins. Animal studies provide clear evidence of anterior cortical cataract induction by both acute and chronic exposure to UVB, although the former required extremely high irradiances. The experimental evidence for cataract induction by UVA is weaker. Similarly epidemiological studies of human populations suggest that cumulative exposure to solar UVR is an important cause of cortical cataracts, and that UVB is the main causative agent. However, most of these data were obtained from studying populations of highly exposed men, and it is unclear whether UVR is an important risk factor for cataracts in general populations (NRPB, 1995).

Chronic exposure to solar radiation, and in particular to UVA and blue light, has been associated with the development of age-related macular degeneration (ARMD), a major cause of blindness in the developed world (Mainster, 1978; Young, 1988), although it is generally accepted that the aetiology of this condition is multifactorial. ARMD results from damage to the macula, the cone-rich central part of the retina, which is responsible for high visual acuity and color vision. Fair-skinned, blue-eyed individuals appear to be more at risk than those with dark eyes (Young, 1988).

Non-malignant Skin Effects

It is generally considered that most of the UVR incident on the skin is absorbed by the epidermis, with penetration into the dermis increasing markedly only at longer wavelengths. However, recent data indicate that penetration, at least to the basal layer of the epidermis, remains high at wavelengths as short as 300 nm, and this suggests that most of the UVR present in sunlight should show significant penetration (Chadwick et al., 1995).

Acute Exposure With the exception of vitamin D synthesis, the acute responses of skin to UVR may be broadly divided into inflammatory responses (sunburn), which include erythema and edema, reparative responses, and protective responses, which include not only the familiar tanning response but also thickening of the epidermis and stratum corneum.

One of the most obvious, and therefore most intensively studied, consequences of acute overexposure to UVR is sunburn, which is characterized by erythema and blistering. Erythema, or reddening of the skin, results from increased blood volume in the superficial and deep vascular plexi of the dermis (Gange and Parrish, 1983), and it is thought to be a consequence of localized release of eicosanoids, particularly prostaglandins. Histological examination has revealed that this is associated with intracellular edema, cytolysis, and most prominently, the presence of sunburn cells. These cells can appear as early as one hour after exposure, are eliminated within a few days, and probably arise from basal keratinocytes as a consequence of apoptosis. The nature of the erythemal response is spectrally dependent, with longer wavelength UVA radiation penetrating further and thereby producing more severe damage to the dermis, which may include vascular damage (Hruza and Pentland, 1993). A reference erythemal action spectrum (Fig. 25-2) has been derived from a statistical analysis of post-1945 data derived mostly from studies on volunteers with skin types I and II (McKinlay and Diffey, 1987). This has been adopted by the International Commission on Illumination (CIE), the International Commission on Non-Ionizing Radiation Protection (ICNIRP), and the International Electrotechnical Commission (IEC) for spectral weighting and evaluation of effective irradiances of sources. Recent work has indicated that while this action spectrum accurately predicts the response of human skin at shorter wavelengths, it may underestimate the effectiveness of long wavelength UVA (Diffey, 1994; Anders et al., 1995).

In mice, the most commonly used species for studying skin photobiology, edema is probably a more sensitive response to UVR than erythema, but it has a similar action spectrum to erythema in humans (Cole et al., 1983). This action spectrum (Cole et al., 1986a) has been superseded by that derived by de Gruijl et al., 1993.

The other well-characterized effect of acute overexposure is altered skin pigmentation, or tanning. Normal skin color is primarily determined by the nature, amount, and distribution of melanin in the keratinocytes of the epidermis. Melanin is an extremely dense, virtually insoluble polymer that occurs in at least two forms; brown eumelanin predominates in darkly pigmented skins, while reddish pheomelanin is found in lighter skin types. Melanin is synthesized in specialized cells called *melanocytes*, packaged into melanosomes, and exported to neighboring keratinocytes. Exposure to UVR transiently increases the level of pigmentation in the skin, and this is known as *facultative* or *inducible skin color* to distinguish it from that of unexposed skin, which is referred to as *constitutive skin color*. Inducible pigmentation occurs in two phases, immediate pigment darkening and delayed tanning.

Immediate pigment darkening (IPD) begins during exposure to UVR, and reaches a maximum immediately afterward. It is characteristically short-lived, and may fade within minutes or days depending on the constitutive skin color and the dose of UVR. It is thought that IPD results from the oxidation and redistribution of melanin already present in the skin, and occurs mainly as a result of exposure to UVA and possibly visible light.

Delayed tanning, or melanogenesis, does not become visible until about 72 hours after exposure, and results from increases in both the number and activity of melanocytes. The action spectrum for melanogenesis is broadly similar to that for erythema, although wavelengths shorter than 290 nm are less effective for the former (Parrish et al., 1982). Melanogenesis is often thought of as a protective response, but it is in reality relatively ineffective, providing sun protection factors that range from about 1 (skin type II) to 4 (skin types V and VI).

Chronic Exposure   With the exception of skin cancers, which will be discussed separately, the most important consequences of excessive chronic exposure of the skin to UVR are photoaging and solar keratoses.

Severely photoaged skin is characterized by dryness, wrinkling, and telangiectasia, or dilated blood vessels. It has a leathery, yellowed appearance, together with areas of irregular pigmentation known as solar lentigines or sunburn freckles. Comparison of exposed and unexposed skin on the same individuals indicates that photoaging of skin is different from chronological aging. Histologically, photoaged skin is characterized by the presence, in the dermis, of tangled, degraded elastic fibers that eventually degenerate into an amorphous mass (Oikarinen, 1990; Oikarinen et al., 1991). This is associated with degeneration and loss of collagen fibers, and a marked increase in proteoglycans and glycosaminoglycans, the "ground substance" of the dermal matrix. There is an increase in the number of inflammatory cells, particularly mast cells, and photoaged skin thus has the appearance of being chronically inflamed. Damage to the microcirculation, which results in the formation of telangiectasias, may become severe, with almost complete destruction of the horizontal superficial plexus. Although normally associated with excessive exposure to UVR, recent evidence suggests that changes associated with photoageing may result from even suberythemal doses. In particular, suberythemal UVA (30–50 kJ m^{-2}) produces both dermal and epidermal damage (Lowe et al., 1995), while suberythemal UVB (30–50 J m^{-2}) induces the activity of metalloproteinases that can degrade both collagen and elastin (Fisher et al., 1996).

The mouse is probably the most frequently used model system for studies of photoaging, and despite considerable differences in skin structure, the changes observed appear to be broadly consistent with those in human skin. Mice have been used to determine action spectra for a variety of endpoints associated with photoaging, including collagen damage, elastosis, epidermal thickening, dermal cellularity, dermal inflammation, and skin wrinkling; almost all were broadly similar with peak effectiveness observed around 290 to 300 nm, and sharp decline in the UVA region (Bissett et al., 1989). In contrast, the action spectrum for skin sagging appears to be very broad with maximum effectiveness observed around 340 nm. It has been suggested that pig skin more closely resembles human skin and that it may therefore be a better model. Certainly chronic exposure to broadband UVR at suberythemal doses induces similar changes to those observed in photoaged human skin (Fourtanier and Berrebi., 1989).

Chronic exposure to UVR is associated with the development of small scaly, erythematous lesions called solar keratoses. They consist of benign proliferations of epidermal keratinocytes, and are common on exposed body sites in older Caucasians living in areas of high ambient solar irradiance. They are considered to be pre-malignant lesions, with the potential to progress to squamous cell carcinoma, although it appears that the probability of an individual lesion progressing is low. Moreover many may actually regress if appropriate sun avoidance is adopted (Marks et al., 1986). Nevertheless, they usually occur as multiple lesions and their number on the skin is strongly associated with the risk of nonmelanoma skin cancer (Kricker et al., 1991).

Skin Cancer

The most serious health effects in humans for which exposure to UVR is a recognized risk factor are the cutaneous malignancies (skin cancers). They can be divided into two main types, nonmelanoma skin cancer and the malignant melanomas.

Nonmelanoma Skin Cancer   Although the nonmelanoma skin cancers (NMSC) are relatively common in white populations, they are rarely fatal, accounting for around 10% of registered malignancies in the United Kingdom, but under 0.5% of cancer deaths. There are two main types of NMSC, basal cell carcinomas (BCC), which account for around three-quarters of cases, and the less frequently observed squamous cell carcinomas (SCC). The former appear typically as raised translucent nodules, which develop slowly over a period of months or even years on the face, head, and neck, and have a relentless capacity for local spread and destruction. Squamous cell carcinomas, which develop from slightly more differentiated epidermal cells, appear as persistent red crusted lesions on sun-exposed skin, most commonly on the face and scalp.

Overall, the findings from both descriptive and analytical epidemiological studies support the hypothesis that NMSC aetiology is related to cumulative dose of solar radiation exposure (NRPB, 1995). The evidence suggests that SCC is more strongly related to UVR exposure than is BCC. Furthermore there is evidence that therapeutic treatment with a combination of psoralen and UVA contributes to the risk of SCC and, to a much lesser extent, BCC.

Most recent studies of photocarcinogenesis have used the hairless mouse model, employing either the albino (Skh:h-1) strain, or the lightly pigmented (Skh:h-2) strain. Tumors have been induced following repeated exposure of these strains to simulated solar radiation and broadband UVR, as well as to radiations in each of the UVC, UVB, and UVA regions of the spectrum. The tumors induced are usually SCC, often preceded and accompanied by papillomas; keratoacanthomas, and similar benign epidermal neoplasms found in humans have also been reported. However, the most common human malignant skin tumor, basal cell carcinoma, is rarely observed, having been identified in only a few studies with nude mice and one or two early studies with rats (IARC, 1992). Hence the validity of the hairless mouse as a model of human skin carcinogenesis must be open to question. The induction of squamous cell carcinoma in hairless mice provides most of the recent quantitative data available on experimental photocarcinogenesis in vivo. However, extrapolation to humans is not straightforward, since mouse skin differs from human skin in several respects. Mouse skin is much thinner, for example, and daily doses of UVR required for skin tumorigenesis in mice are usually well below those present outdoors, and most experiments have been conducted with UVB doses lower than those required to elicit acute reactions, such as erythema, in mice.

The wavelength dependence of UVR-induced carcinogenesis is crucial to accurate risk assessment. Clearly an action spectrum for skin cancer can only be obtained from animal models such as the hairless mouse, and this effectively restricts the data to squamous cell carcinomas. The best spectrum currently available is the SCUP (Skin Cancer Utrecht–Philadelphia) action spectrum (de Gruijl et al., 1993) derived by combining data on chronic UVR-induced tumors from experiments carried out at the University of Utrecht (de Gruijl and van der Leun, 1992) and at the former Skin and Cancer Hospital in Philadelphia (Cole et al., 1986). It is based on data from a total of 1100 hairless albino Skh:h-1 mice exposed each day to radiation from one of 14, mainly broadband, sources; in general, the use of narrowband sources presents logistical problems. Exposures in the UVA and UVB regions were below thresholds for acute effects, whereas UVC exposures exceeded them. The SCUP action spectrum (Fig. 25-4) extends between 270 and 400 nm but is best defined between 280 and 340 nm, with increased uncertainty outside this region.

The interpretation of action spectra could be complicated by the possibility that UVR of different wavelengths, might interact in the induction of skin tumors in a more complex way than simple addition. This has been the subject of much debate and investigation and remains controversial (IARC, 1992). Difficulties with interpretation arise from differing spectral content of various sources of UVR, uncertainties in measurement, exposure to insufficient doses of UVA, and differences in epidermal transmission, absorption and photoproduct formation across the UVR spectrum; it has also been suggested that UVB may be a more effective initiator, and UVA a more effective promoter (e.g., Kelfkens et al., 1992). Overall (IARC, 1992), it appears that the interactions of UVR from different wavelength ranges when given simultaneously, prior to, or immediately after each other are either unproved or small.

Malignant Melanoma   Although it is much less common than nonmelanoma skin cancer, cutaneous malignant melanoma (CMM) is the main cause of skin cancer death, particularly in young people; between the ages of 20 and 39, CMM accounts for 1 in 12

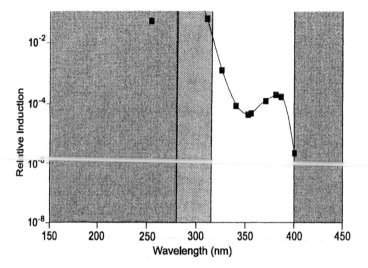

Figure 25-4   SCUP action spectrum for mouse carcinogenesis.

cancers and 1 in 25 deaths. There are four main clinical pathological types. Superficial spreading melanomas are by far the most common and are typically seen on the leg in women and the trunk in men. Nodular melanomas may be seen on any site, and like superficial spreading melanomas are associated with intense intermittent exposure to UVR. Lentigo maligna melanomas are found on sun-exposed skin in the elderly and are associated with cumulative exposure. Acral (or acral lentiginous) melanomas are found on the palms of the hands and soles of the feet and do not appear to be associated with exposure.

The incidence of CMM has increased substantially in white populations for several decades. The major risk factor appears to be exposure to solar radiation, with cumulative dose probably the main cause for melanomas of the head and neck (NRPB, 1995). Intense short-term exposure of untanned skin appears likely to be a major factor for intermittently exposed sites, although there is insufficient evidence on which to assess the contribution of solar radiation to cancers of rarely exposed sites. In addition there is some evidence that exposures during childhood and adolescence may be of special importance. The evidence that exposure to sunlamps and sunbeds may contribute to melanoma risk is suggestive but not definitive (NRPB, 1995).

A higher incidence is seen in people with large numbers of naevi (moles), atypical naevi, light skin, red or blond hair, blue eyes, a tendency to freckle, and a tendency to sunburn and not to tan on sun exposure. In a small number of cases ($< 5\%$) there is a strong family history of disease.

Despite many concerted attempts, malignant melanomas have not been experimentally induced by UVR in any placental mammals, although pigmented melanomalike tumors have been induced in mice by a combination of UVR and chemical carcinogens (see below). At present, the best animal models for UVR-induced melanoma are the South American opossum, *Monodelphis domestica*, and certain hybrid fish (platyfish and swordtail fish hybrids). However, melanomas induced in these animals are histologically different to human malignant melanomas. Hybrids of the fish *Xiphophorus maculatus* and *X. Couchianus* have been used to determine an action spectrum for melanoma induction (Setlow et al., 1993). The effectiveness of UVR in inducing melanoma appeared to decrease by less than two orders of magnitude between 302 and 435 nm, which contrasts strongly with action spectra for DNA damage and suggests the presence of an efficient sensitizer in the target melanocytes. However, these fish represent a specialized genetic model in which melanoma can be induced by inactivation of a single gene that may not be relevant to exposed human populations.

Mechanisms of UVR-Induced Carcinogenesis   Experimental protocols that involve sequential application of different carcinogens provide a means to investigate mechanistic aspects of carcinogenesis. This approach has been extremely informative in relation to skin carcinogenesis induced by exposure to chemical carcinogens and has been central to the development of the multistage model of carcinogenesis. It is currently believed that there are at least three main stages of carcinogenesis, initiation, promotion, and progression. Initiating events are thought to result from stable changes in the genetic information (DNA) carried by an affected cell. Initiation can occur following a single exposure to the initiating agent and is irreversible. Promotion is usually a more extended process than initiation, requiring prolonged or repeated exposure and may be at least partially reversible if the promoting agent is withdrawn. Promoting agents often induce hyperplasia, and it is thought that this increased proliferation permits initiated cells to multiply and form a clone of cells expressing an altered phenotype. However, while clonal expansion of initiated cells may be required for promotion, it is not sufficient; agents that are capable of promoting carcinogenesis following a single application of an initiating agent usually induce additional changes in a process sometimes termed conversion. These may include stable genetic changes and probably result from oxidative stress. The third stage of carcinogenesis, progression is the process by which initiated and promoted cells acquire increasingly malignant phenotypes. These changes are associated with increasing genetic instability, loss of growth control, and ultimately acquisition of invasive characteristics.

Since exposure to UVR alone is sufficient to induce tumors, it may be classified as a complete carcinogen (IARC, 1992). This implies that exposure to UVR has an effect on both of the first two stages of carcinogenesis, initiation and promotion. This conclusion is supported by evidence from traditional two-stage experimental carcinogenesis protocols.

Studies designed to evaluate the action of UVR as a tumor initiator have employed a protocol involving irradiation of mice, followed by repeated application of known chemical tumor promoters such as phorbol esters. Irradiation has usually involved a single exposure to UVR, although in some cases the exposure has been fractionated over a period of days or even weeks; fractionation, particularly over a long period, may complicate interpretation of the results. In general, the results of these studies have shown that both UVC (Pound, 1970) and broadband UVB (Epstein and Roth, 1968; Stenbäck, 1975) radiations are effective initiating agents. In addition to studies designed to assess whether UVR can act as a tumor initiating agent, there have been a number of studies that have investigated whether known or suspect tumor-promoting agents can enhance tumor formation in mouse skin initiated with UVR. One agent that was found to promote UVR-initiated skin tumors was methyl ethyl ketone peroxide, a compound widely used in the polymer industry (Logani et al., 1984); the mechanism of action of this compound appeared to involve oxidative stress. In contrast, there was no evidence for promotion of UVR-initiated skin tumors by benzoyl peroxide, a known skin tumor promoter that is used in the treatment of acne and also has applications in the polymer industry (Epstein, 1988; Iverson, 1986, 1988).

Possible promoting actions of UVR have been investigated by painting mouse skin with the chemical initiator 7,12-dimethylbenz[a]anthracene (DMBA) prior to repeated exposure to UVR. In general, such studies have shown that the combination of chemical initiation, and either UVB or UVA is more effective at inducing tumors than treatment with DMBA alone (Epstein and Epstein, 1962; Epstein, 1965; Epstein et al., 1967; Husein et al., 1991). Interestingly, when pigmented mice were used in these studies it was found

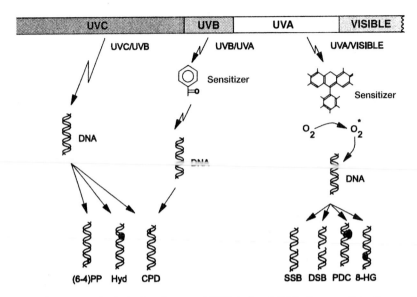

Figure 25-5   Summary of principal pathways of UVR-induced DNA damage. Only those pathways producing the most common photoproducts at each wavelength are shown: (6-4) PP, (6-4) photo-products; Hyd, pyrimidine hydrates; CPD, cyclobutane pyrimidine dimers; SSB, single-strand breaks; DSB, double strand breaks; PDC, protein-DNA crosslinks; 8-HG, 8-hydroxyguanine.

that both UVB and UVA promoted the development of chemically induced pigmented lesions, including melanomalike tumors (Epstein et al., 1967; Husein et al., 1991). A recent novel approach has been used to demonstrate that UVB also promotes chemically initiated SCCs in human skin grafted onto immunocompromised mice. However, human skin was much less susceptible than the surrounding mouse skin (Soballe et al., 1996).

UVR Induced DNA Damage   The transition from a normal cell to a malignant one is a complex process involving a number of changes, many of which involve the induction of mutations as a consequence of genetic damage. UVR is an effective DNA damaging agent (Cridland and Saunders, 1994), although the nature of the damage is wavelength dependant (Fig. 25-5). UVB and UVC radiations are absorbed directly by the bases of DNA resulting in electronic excitation and the formation of photoproducts. The most common photoproducts are those formed between adjacent pyrimidines and include cyclobutane pyrimidine dimers and, less frequently, pyrimidine (6-4) pyrimidone adducts or "(6-4) photoproducts." There has been much debate about the relative importance of these two photoproducts, and overall the available data suggest that they are probably of roughly equal importance. Action spectra for photoproduct formation have been determined in vitro, in cultured cells and in skin (Fig. 25-6).

Above about 300 nm, the absorption of DNA, and consequently the formation of pyrimidine photoproducts, falls rapidly. However, the presence of photosensitizing chemicals that can absorb UVR and transfer the energy to DNA may extend photoproduct formation to longer wavelengths. Sensitized DNA damage may occur either by direct energy transfer from an excited sensitizer to DNA, or through the generation of a chemically reactive intermediate, although the latter mechanism is probably the most important and certainly predominates at longer wavelengths (Tyrrell and Keyse, 1990). Typically the intermediates formed are activated oxygen species, and such reactions are termed *photodynamic*; the energy required to form these species is very low and corresponds to wavelengths extending into the infrared region. The most important

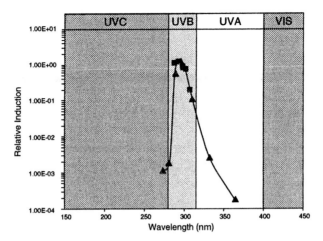

Figure 25-6   Action spectrum for cyclobutane pyrimidine dimer formation in epidermal DNA. (■ data from Ley et al., 1983; ▲, data from Freeman et al., 1989)

intermediate is probably singlet oxygen ($^1O_2$), and this appears to react principally with guanine to form products such as 8-hydoxyguanine (Epe, 1991; Piette, 1991), which appears to be mispaired with adenine leading to the mutation of G:C base-pair to a T:A. Unfortunately, there are, as yet, few data to resolve the question of 8-hydroxyguanine formation in vivo following exposure to long wavelength UVR, although broadband UVR irradiation increased its rate of formation in initiated mouse keratinocytes exposed in vitro. Breaks in the sugar-phosphate backbone of one (single-strand breaks or SSBs) or both (double-strand breaks or DSBs) of the DNA strands are produced following irradiation at both short and long wavelengths. However, SSBs are produced much less efficiently than CPDs at short wavelengths, and only constitute a major type of photodamage at wavelengths in the UVA and visible regions (Moan and Peak, 1989). Double-strand breaks are likely to show a similar wavelength dependence, although they are produced at a lower frequency than single-strand breaks. The biological importance of both types of lesion is unclear. The third major lesion which is produced by indirect sensitization is the DNA–protein crosslink (DPC) (Moan and Peak, 1989; Cridland and Saunders, 1994). Cellular DNA is intimately associated with protein to form chromatin, and reactions between excited bases and susceptible protein components in close proximity have been well established for some time. It is considered that these lesions may be biologically important at longer wavelengths.

A number of compounds can act to sensitize UV-induced DNA damage. Cellular constituents capable of behaving in this way include riboflavin, bilirubin, porphyrins, nicotinamide coenzymes, and rare thiolated bases (Tyrrell and Keyse, 1990; Cridland and Saunders, 1994); some steroids, quinones, and carotenoids may exhibit similar properties. Synthetic chemicals that may act as photosensitizers include dyes, drugs, both oral and topical, antibiotics, ketones, polycyclic aromatic hydrocarbons, and some cosmetic and sunscreen preparations (Hawk, 1984; Cridland and Saunders, 1994; Saunders et al., 1997). In addition natural products such as chlorophyll may also act as sensitizers.

Immune System Effects

Immunological responses protect individuals from infectious disease caused by invading microorganisms such as viruses, bacteria, and various single celled or multicellular organisms. Responses can also be elicited by noninfectious foreign substances that enter the body, such as bacterial toxins, foreign proteins, and various organic and inorganic chemicals. In addition tumor cells may express on their surfaces molecules that can induce immunological responses against them, although, in general, for a number of different reasons, most tumors elicit only weak immune reponses (Saunders et al., 1997).

UVR exerts its effect on the immune system via its interaction with the skin. This is a major site of entry of foreign antigens into the body and is an active participant in immunological defence; the dermis and epidermis contain cell populations able to initiate and support appropriate immunological responses. Many skin cells, especially the keratinocytes, secrete cytokines which are important mediators in the control of immune and inflammatory responses. Effective immune responses additionally depend on the clonal expansion and activation of appropriate antigen-specific lymphocytes. Antigen presenting cells are particularly important in this context, and the epidermal Langerhans cells are the major antigen-presenting cells in the skin. Langerhans cells process antigen encountered in the skin and migrate via lymphatic vessels to the regional lymph node where they "present" the antigen to helper T lymphocytes, activating those specific to the antigen. Activated helper T cells undergo clonal expansion and differentiation, releasing cytokines that further activate cell types involved in the immune response. In general, the first application of an antigen results in sensitization, a process in which the immune system becomes poised to respond; a second, later, application of the antigen elicits a much stronger immune response from previously activated antigen-specific lymphocytes such as memory T cells, the predominant dermal T cell.

The effects of UVR on the immune system, and the mechanisms that underlie them, have been reviewed widely (Kripke, 1993; Noonan and De Fabo, 1993; Cridland and Saunders, 1994; Vermeer and Hurks, 1994; Krutman and Elmets, 1995; Ullrich, 1995; Saunders et al., 1997). Animal and human studies have shown that the major effect of exposure to UVR on immune system responses is to suppress T-cell-mediated responses such as delayed-type (type IV) hypersensitivity (DTH), the primary defence mechanism against intracellular bacteria and protozoa, and the anti-viral and anti-tumour activities of cytolytic T cells and natural killer cells. This is believed to be a consequence of profound changes to the populations of epidermal antigen presenting cells and changes in cytokine secretion. These are thought to result in the inactivation of the helper T-cell subset which stimulates the T-cell-mediated responses. Nevertheless, activation of the helper T-cell subset mediating antibody responses such as immediate hypersensitivity appears to be retained.

One form of DTH that has been the subject of considerable investigation in relation to UVR effects is contact hypersensitivity (CHS), which is characterized by an eczematous reaction at the point of contact with the allergen; CHS is a significant cause of morbidity among employees in industries that use highly reactive chemicals such as nickel, chromate, and rubber (chemical) accelerators. Volunteer studies have shown that exposure to UVR sufficient to induce erythema, followed by chemical sensitization on either exposed or unexposed skin, can result in a marked, dose-dependent suppression of the CHS response to a subsequent challenge. Individual responses to UVR are, however, quite variable, and there is evidence to suggest that the susceptibility of the immune system to UVR exists as a balanced polymorphism within the human population; it is possible that UVR sensitivity may be an additional risk factor for skin cancer. Moreover there is some evidence that the CHS response to previously encountered antigens may actually be enhanced following exposure to UVR.

Pathogenic organisms differ greatly in their patterns of host invasion, in colonization, and in the nature of the antigenic signal that they generate, and not surprisingly, they are able to elicit a very diverse number of immune responses involving both antibody-mediated and cell-mediated effector mechanisms. Exposure to UVR has been shown to down-regulate T-cell-mediated tuberculin-type DTH responses, characterized by an area of hardening and swelling, following intradermal challenge by a variety of pathogens (or antigenic preparations), mostly associated with intracellular skin infection. These include bacteria such as the leprosy and tuberculosis bacilli, protozoan parasites such as *Leishmania* and viruses such as the cold sore virus herpes simplex (HSV). Suppression of DTH responses to leprosy antigens, and reactivation of latent HSV infection following UVR exposure was seen in human studies.

Support for some role of the immune system in tumor eradication in humans includes the occurrence of spontaneous tumor regression, the observation of lymphoid infiltration in many tumors (although this is not clearly related to patient prognosis) and a higher incidence of certain types of tumor in immune-suppressed (e.g., transplant) patients. Strongly immunogenic tumors include the skin cancers induced by UVR and lymphocytic infiltration, and more rarely, spontaneous regression, have been observed. Moreover the risk of skin cancer, especially squamous cell carcinoma, is elevated in immunosuppressed patients, particularly those living in areas of high insolation. Although animal studies have provided good evidence that UVR-induced immunosuppression plays a role in the growth of SCC, there is no animal model for basal cell carcinoma and the evidence concerning melanomas induced by exposure to a combination of chemicals and UVR is less clear.

POPULATIONS AT SPECIAL RISK

Ocular Damage

A number of people have a greater sensitivity to UVR-induced damage to the retina as a consequence of increased transmission through the anterior eye. In addition there is a potential for overexposure as a consequence of clinical examinations and through accidental exposure to laser radiation.

Children and Young People   The risk of retinal damage is higher in the young because their lenses transmit more UVR and blue light. This is an area of particular concern as neonates and infants may be exposed to high blue light radiances in neonatal intensive-care units.

Aphakes   Those who have had the lens of the eye removed during cataract surgery are also a high risk group for retinal injury. Replacement by a polymethyl methacrylate (PMMA) lens implant does not provide the same protection for the retina that results from the presence of the natural lens (Mainster, 1978; West et al., 1989). It is therefore important to incorporate appropriate filters for retinal protection, and these should reduce transmission of blue light as well as UVR.

Ophthalmic Patients   Patients undergoing ophthalmic examination with the slit-lamp microscope or indirect ophthalmascope may be exposed to high irradiances of visible radiation. In practice, extremes of exposure are probably avoided by the lack of a focused image and by constant movement of the source, but there is a need for practioners to exercise care, especially in anaesthetized patients whose eyes are immobilized (NRPB, 1995).

Laser Workers   Accidental injuries may occur in those working with high-power lasers, particularly during alignment procedures or as a result of reflections from neighboring surfaces (Sliney and Wolbarsht, 1980). In addition bystanders observing laser ocular surgery may suffer injury as a result of reflections from contact lens used to direct radiation into the patient's eyes.

Skin Effects

Skin phenotype is probably the most important factor determining sun sensitivity in the general population. In addition there are small numbers of people with clinical conditions that result in extreme sun sensitivity, while exposure to photosensitizing chemicals from a variety of sources can greatly modify the response to UVR.

Phenotype   Certain phenotypic traits such as pale skin, red or blond hair, and blue eyes are clearly associated with sun sensitivity and a tendency to burn easily and to tan poorly. In addition to predisposing to the acute effects of overexposure, such characteristics also carry an elevated risk of UV-induced skin cancers; for malignant melanoma, a tendency to freckle, large numbers of naevi and atypical naevi, are also risk factors.

Clinical Conditions   A number of genetic disorders also predispose to sun sensitivity. For example, oculocutaneous albinism is an uncommon autosomal recessively inherited disorder of melanin synthesis that results in reduced or absent melanin pigmentation in the skin, hair, and eyes. Patients suffer an increased frequency of sunburn, actinic damage and NMSC but appear to have a low incidence of malignant melanoma.

Predictably, genetic disorders that affect DNA repair also affect sun sensitivity. The best characterized of these is probably xeroderma pigmentosum, a rare autosomal condition characterized by sun-sensitivity, an abnormal erythemal response, and changes in chronically exposed skin including the development of pigmented macules, achromic spots, telangiectasia, BCC, SCC, and malignant melanoma. Two other rare recessive disorders of DNA repair, Cockayne syndrome and trichothiodystrophy, result in increased sun sensitivity but interestingly do not appear to confer an elevated risk of skin cancer.

Other clinical conditions associated with increased sun sensitivity include lupus erythematosus and the porphyria group of disorders. Patients typically exhibit acute and prolonged UVR-induced erythema and even blistering following exposure to levels of UVR that would not affect most people.

Exposure to Photosensitizers   Exposure to photosensitizing chemicals may result in increased sun sensitivity, and these responses may be conveniently divided into phototoxic and photoallergic reactions (Saunders et al., 1997). Phototoxic reactions usually involve reactive oxygen species that damage cells in the exposed tissue; phototoxic reactions may be observed in both the skin and the eye. There are three main types of phototoxic response. The first is an immediate burning sensation with erythema and urticaria (wheal and flare); the second is a delayed reaction resembling sunburn (erythema and edema). A third type of reaction involves increased pigmentation, which is often delayed in onset, and confined to the exposed area.

Photoallergic reactions are those in which an immune mechanism can be demonstrated. Rather than an exaggerated sunburn, the clinical reaction more usually consists of an eczematous eruption or discrete papules and plaques. Because photoallergy depends on individual immunologic reactivity, it occurs in only a small minority of exposed individuals. Moreover the dose–response relationship is less evident than in phototoxic reactions, and small quantities of chemical or radiation may be adequate to elicit a response.

In a minority of people, a photoallergic reaction persists after exposure to the photosensitizer has stopped. Whereas photocontact dermatitis is usually UVA induced, the action spectrum for persistent light reactivity alters to include UVB, and the patient may be unable to tolerate even minimal exposure to sunlight. This syndrome of persistent light reactivity is now thought to be a form of chronic actinic dermatosis, an acquired idiopathic disorder. Other idiopathic dermatoses include solar urticaria, an immediate (type I) hypersensitivity which may occasionally be photosensitized by topical chemicals and drugs, and polymorphic light eruption, the commonest of these disorders for which, however, there is no evidence of prior chemical photosensitization.

Photosensitizing chemicals may be present in coal tar extracts and their derivatives, plant extracts, pharmaceuticals, and cosmetics (Saunders et al., 1997). Thus they may be encountered in a variety of situations, including the home (Harber and Levine, 1969), manufacturing industry (Crow et al., 1961), agricultural industry (Birmingham et al., 1961), and during recreational activities (Hjorth and Möller, 1976).

APPLICABLE STANDARDS AND EXPOSURE GUIDELINES

Protection standards and exposure guidelines with respect to occupational exposure to UVR sources address principally the acute effects of exposure. The reason is the lack of quantitative data on the chronic effects of UVR exposure.

Exposure criteria for coherent sources of UVR (lasers) are published by the American Conference of Governmental Industrial Hygienists (ACGIH, 1997) and by the International Electrotechnical Commission in the standard IEC 825: 1984/90 (IEC, 1984, 1990). UVR laser technology and applications are not covered here, but they have been comprehensively reviewed (Elliot, 1995).

The most comprehensive occupational exposure guidelines for noncoherent sources of UVR are those published by the International Non-Ionizing Radiation Committee (INIRC) of the International Radiation Protection Association (IRPA, 1985, 1989) and by ACGIH (ACGIH, 1997). Both sets of guidelines define similar exposure criteria for UVR. A statement in support of the IRPA guidelines has been published by the International Commission on Non-Ionizing Radiation Protection (ICNIRP, 1996). The recommendations of IRPA are representative of the advice of an international committee of experts. The INIRC/IRPA membership during the preparation of the 1985 INIRC guidelines was drawn from the United States, the United Kingdom, France, Australia, Denmark, Germany, Poland, and the Netherlands.

INIRC/IRPA and subsequently ICNIRP have undertaken responsibility for the development of health criteria documents on nonionizing radiation. This has been carried out in cooperation with the Environmental Health Division of the World Health Organization (WHO) and forms part of the WHO Health Criteria Program, which has been funded by the United Nations Environmental Program (UNEP). The criteria are intended to be used as the scientific data bases for the development of exposure limits and codes of practice.

The INIRC/IRPA guidelines on limits of exposure to sources of noncoherent UVR are based on the available scientific data, and no consideration is given to economic impact or other nonscientific priorities. The stated intention of the guidelines is to serve as guidance to the various international and national bodies or individual experts who are responsible for the development of regulations, recommendations or codes of practice to protect workers and the general public from the potentially adverse effects of UVR. The guidelines define occupational exposure limit values (ELVs) below which it is expected that nearly all people may be repeatedly exposed without adverse effect. The criteria for limiting exposure to sources of noncoherent UVR are summarized in Table 25-3.

The ELVs are intended for use in the control of exposure to both pulsed and continuous noncoherent sources where the exposure duration is not less than 0.1 µs. They are used to evaluate potentially hazardous exposure from, for example, arcs, gas and vapor discharges, fluorescent lamps, incandescent sources, and solar radiation. The ELVs are below the levels often used for the UVR exposure of patients required as part of medical treatment and below the levels for elective cosmetic purposes. The limits apply to exposure directed

TABLE 25-3 Summary of Exposure Limit Values (ELVs) for the Skin and the Eye

Wavelength (nm)	ELV	Protection
180–400 (UVR)	$30\,\mathrm{J\,m^{-2}}$ eff (within 8 h)	Skin and eye
315–400 (UVA)	$10^4\,\mathrm{J\,m^{-2}}$ (within 8 h)	Eye

Source: IRPA (1991) and NCNIRP (1996).

perpendicular to those surfaces of the body facing the source of UVR, measured with an instrument having a cosine angular response. The measured irradiance (W m^{-2}) and the radiant exposure (J m^{-2}) should be averaged over the area of a circular measurement aperture not greater than 1 mm in diameter.

Where required (by regulations) the ELVs should be considered absolute limits for the eye but only as advisory for the skin due to the wide range of susceptibility to skin injury depending on skin type. The values were developed by considering lightly pigmented populations (white Caucasian) with greatest sensitivity and genetic predisposition to sunburn. ACGIH (1997) indicates that conditioned (tanned) individuals can tolerate skin exposure in excess of the exposure limits without erythemal effects, but that conditioning may not protect individuals against skin cancer. For certain sources the threshold for erythema may be exceeded in certain people without exceeding the exposure limit. Therefore all exposures should be reduced as far as is reasonably practicable.

The ELVs do not apply to UVR exposure of photosensitive individuals nor to individuals concomitantly exposed to photosensitizing agents. The values are not intended to protect neonates and separate weighting functions for aphakes (persons whose natural lens has been surgically removed) are presented in the wavelength range 305 to 400 nm of the UVR spectrum by ACGIH (1997).

Many unfiltered or uncontrolled industrial optical radiation sources have the potential to produce emissions that exceed recommended ELVs under certain conditions. However, because of the limited penetration of ultraviolet radiation in materials, all practices involving artificial ultraviolet radiation sources can have any potential exposures to workers reduced to acceptably low levels by the use of suitable control measures. These are listed in Table 25-4.

Shielding of the source by engineering controls is difficult in some processes, such as arc welding and outdoor work in the sun, so personal protection measures are needed to comply with the guidelines.

Sources of Ultraviolet Radiation

The Sun The main source of UVR is the sun, and individual habits with respect to sun exposure are important in assessing personal risk associated with UVR exposure.

The broad spectrum and intensity of UVR from the sun are due to the high temperature at its surface and its size. Solar UVR undergoes absorption and scattering as it passes through the earth's atmosphere, with absorption by molecular oxygen and ozone being the most important processes (Fig. 25-7). The ozone layer prevents almost all UVR of

TABLE 25-4 Protection against UVR Exposure

Protective Measure	Controls
Engineering	enclosures, interlocks, screens, viewing panels, nonreflective surfaces
Administrative	Restriction of access, warning signs, training, reduction of exposure using distance and time
Personal	Eyewear, clothing, gloves, face masks, skin screens

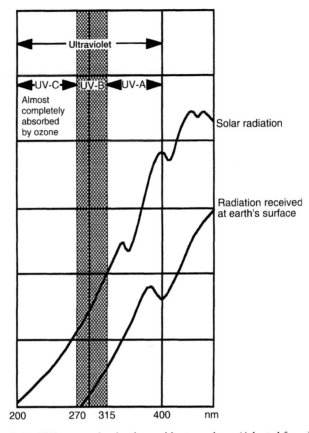

Figure 25-7   Solar UVR attenuation by the earth's atmosphere. (Adopted from UNEP, 1987)

wavelengths $\lambda < 290$ nm and a substantial fraction (in excess of 90% of the total energy) of 290 to 315 nm from reaching the earth's surface. Thus the terrestrial environment is exposed to UVR between 290 and 400 nm.

The sun approximates to a "black-body" emitter with a temperature of about 5900 K. The solar radiation reaching the top of the earth's atmosphere is affected by the solar output and the earth–sun distance. Variations in solar output are much smaller than the variations caused by atmospheric attenuation factors. The mean solar irradiance just outside the earth's atmosphere is approximately 1370 W m^{-2} (the so-called solar constant). The spectral distribution is summarized in Table 25-5, but will vary with the exact distance of the earth from the sun at a particular time. The extreme values associated

TABLE 25-5   **Spectral Distribution of Solar Radiation prior to Attenuation by the Earth's Atmosphere**

Wavelength Band	Irradiance (W m^{-2})	Percentage of Total
UVC	6.4	0.5
UVB	21.1	1.5
UVA	85.7	6.3
Total UV	113.2	8.3
Visible and IR	1254	91.7

Source: Frederick et al. (1989).

with this variation are approximately $\pm 3.3\%$ above and below the annual mean and occur in January and July, respectively.

The total solar UVR reaching the earth's surface, termed *global UVR*, can be divided into two components: direct and diffuse. Global UVR reaching a horizontal surface is the quantity most often measured. On average, this comprises about 98% UVA and 2% UVB. However, the exact amount and spectral distribution of solar UVR irradiance reaching the earth's surface depends on a number of factors (WHO, 1994), including

- Wavelength of the UVR
- Solar zenith angle, which depends on latitude, date of the year, and time of day
- Solar source spectrum incident at the top of the atmosphere
- Ozone column thickness and vertical distribution
- Molecular absorption and scattering (including localized gaseous pollutants)
- Aerosol absorption and scattering (including anthropogenic aerosols)
- Absorption, scattering, and reflection by clouds
- Reflectance characteristics (albedo) of the ground
- Shadowing by surrounding objects
- Altitude above sea level

In January (in the Northern Hemisphere) or July (in the Southern Hemisphere) when the solar elevation is low, direct UVR travels a longer path through the atmosphere and a large amount of scattering occurs. In addition much of the resultant scattered UVR propagates downward to the earth's surface at angles to the horizontal that are larger than the solar elevation, hence traveling a shorter and less absorptive path. This results in large ratios of scattered to direct UVR. During the summer the ratio of diffuse to direct UVR is smaller.

The maximum erythemally effective UVB irradiances are shown in Table 25-6 for the Northern Hemisphere as a function of latitude and time of year at sea level (Driscoll, 1992). There are strong seasonal and latitudinal variations in UVB. Under cloudless skies the UVB is more intense in summer and at all times of year is greater at lower latitudes. Approximately 50% of the daily UVR is received during the middle four hours around noon when the sun is high in the sky (Sliney, 1987). The number of MEDs in a three hour exposure period centered around 12 GMT is shown for the Northern Hemisphere as a function of latitude and time of year in Table 25-7. Data for the Southern Hemisphere can be derived from these tables by advancing the data sets by six months so that June's data becomes those of December, and vice versa.

The presence of cloud cover, air pollution, haze, or even scattered clouds, plays a significant role in attenuating UVR. UVB and UVA irradiances are reduced due to scattering by water droplets and/or ice crystals in the clouds. Clouds can block a significant portion of the UVR that would have otherwise reached the surface. Cloud cover and type are highly variable. The transmission of UVR radiation through clouds depends on cloud height, type, and optical density. The resultant effect on UVR transmission is difficult to assess particularly in the case of partial cloudiness. The effect of cloudiness on the solar irradiation of a horizontal plane can be approximated by

$$F = 1 - 0.056\,C,$$

where C is the total cloud index in tenths of sky covered from 0 to 10, 10 being complete sky cover. Thus, on this analysis for complete cloud cover, the transmitted UVR irradiance would decrease to 44% and for half cloud cover to 72% of the incident value. However, in

TABLE 25-6   Maximum Erythemally Effective UV-B Irradiances for the Northern Hemisphere

	Jan.	Feb.	Mar.	Apr.	May	Jun.	Jul.	Aug.	Sep.	Oct.	Nov.	Dec.
0	229	251	260	229	210	207	214	233	278	248	226	221
5	212	232	242	235	214	213	220	241	258	227	207	206
10	203	220	229	248	226	225	232	255	244	215	198	175
15	155	199	201	227	221	226	234	240	223	198	155	135
20	127	183	191	215	234	239	247	227	212	184	127	111
25	95	134	165	185	203	227	219	200	194	143	101	84
30	79	110	157	176	192	215	208	190	186	117	85	56
35	42	80	114	146	160	188	182	166	148	93	50	31
40	28	61	93	139	152	178	172	158	121	73	33	21
45	16	33	66	105	126	158	153	128	93	42	21	13
50	12	22	54	85	119	150	145	104	77	28	15	8
55	6	14	33	65	92	130	114	81	48	18	8	4
60	4	10	21	53	75	105	93	67	31	12	5	2
65	0	6	14	35	59	85	76	42	21	7	2	0
70	0	3	10	23	48	70	62	29	15	4	0	0
75	0	0	6	15	30	53	39	20	9;	0	0	0
80	0	0	3	11	20	33	26	14	5	0	0	0
85	0	0	2	7	14	23	18	9	2	0	0	0
90	0	0	0	4	10	16	13	5	0	0	0	0

Note: Maximum erythemally effective UV-B irradiances (m W m^{-2} eff) are calculated as a function of latitude (%) and time of year (21st of each month).

extreme cases cloud cover has been shown to decrease the measured UVR irradiance by over 90%. Estimates of the average reduction of UVB due to clouds (relative to cloudless skies) based on satellite measurements of backscattered solar UVR are 30% at 60 degrees latitude, 10% at 20 degrees latitude, and 20% at the equator (WHO, 1994).

Increased levels of solar UVR due to stratospheric ozone layer depletion may have serious consequences for living organisms. A 10% reduction in stratospheric ozone could lead to as much as a 15% to 20% increase in UVR effective exposure at the earth's surface depending on the state of the troposphere and the biological process being considered.

Artificial Sources Ultraviolet radiation from artificial sources may contribute significantly to certain people's exposure. UVR sources used for specific applications are shown in Table 25-8. It should be noted that a particular application may have the option of using a number of sources, and conversely a particular type of source may be used in a variety of applications. It is therefore important to obtain information about source characteristics when considering the particular applications of UVR sources. However, there is only a limited amount of measurement data published for the wide range of optical radiation sources currently available, and further measurement studies are required to enlarge the data bank. This may require suitable measurements of the source emissions to be obtained. A general assessment of compliance with the relevant exposure guidelines in terms of the exposure limit values (ELVs) is also given for each unshielded source in Table 25-8 and more specific measurement data for a range of sources are given in Table 25-9.

Incandescent Lamps When a material is heated, a large number of energy transitions occur within the molecules of the material, and optical photons are emitted. An idealized (most efficient) radiator of such radiation is termed a *black-body*. The total radiant power and its spectral distribution depend only on the temperature of the black-body. In practice, no real material emits radiation with a black-body spectrum. However, tungsten

TABLE 25-7   Number of Minimum Erythemal Doses (MEDs) in a 3 h Exposure Period for a Sensitive Skin Type for the Calculated Maximum Erythemally Effective UV-B Irradiances Given in Table 25-6

	Jan.	Feb.	Mar.	Apr.	May	Jun.	Jul.	Aug.	Sep.	Oct.	Nov.	Dec.
0	12	14	14	12	11	11	12	13	15	13	12	12
5	11	13	13	13	12	12	12	13	14	12	11	11
10	11	12	12	13	12	12	13	14	13	12	11	9
15	8	11	11	12	12	12	13	13	12	11	8	7
20	7	10	10	12	13	13	13	12	11	10	7	6
25	5	7	9	10	11	12	12	11	10	8	5	5
30	4	6	8	10	10	12	11	10	10	6	3	3
35	2	4	6	8	9	10	10	9	8	5	3	2
40	2	3	5	8	8	10	9	9	7	4	2	1
45	1	2	4	6	7	9	8	7	5	2	1	1
50	1	1	3	5	6	8	8	6	4	2	1	0
55	0	1	2	4	5	7	6	4	3	1	0	0
60	0	1	1	3	4	6	5	4	2	1	0	0
65	0	0	1	2	3	5	4	2	1	0	0	0
70	0	0	1	1	3	4	3	2	1	0	0	0
75	0	0	0	1	2	3	2	1	0	0	0	0
80	0	0	0	1	1	2	1	1	0	0	0	0
85	0	0	0	0	1	1	1	0	0	0	0	0
90	0	0	0	0	1	1	1	0	0	0	0	0

Note: For sensitive skin types, 1 MED $= 200 \, \mathrm{J \, m^{-2}}$ eff.

TABLE 25-8   Nonlaser Ultraviolet Radiation Sources and Some of Their Applications

Source Type	Subgroup	Typical Applications	ELVs exceeded[a]
Incandescent	Tungsten	General, display, and emergency lighting	No
	Tungsten halogen	Spotlights, heating, and floodlighting	Yes
Solid state lamps	LEDs, electro-luminescent lamps	Display, panel indicators, night lights	No
Open arcs	Various	Welding	Yes
Gaseous discharge	Low-pressure Na	General and industrial lighting	No
	Low-pressure Hg	General lighting horticultural and germicidal, sunbeds	Yes
	UVA black-light Hg	Fluorescence, medical	Possibly
	High-pressure Na	Floodlighting	No
	High-pressure Hg	Industrial, printing, curing, commercial lighting	Yes
	Special high-intensity discharge (HID)	Polymerization, reprography, sunlamps	Yes
	High-pressure Hg / Xe	Photochemical and projection	Yes
	Xenon	Projection and photography	Yes
	Pulsed Xe	Printing	Yes

[a] Indications whether the relevant ELVs can or are likely to be exceeded for unshielded sources.

TABLE 25-9 Summary of Available Optical Radiation Data

Lamp[a]	UVR ELVs[b]	Typical Application[c]
Xenon short arc	6700	Solar simulators, searchlights, cinema projectors, spotlights
HID (high-intensity discharge) medium pressure Hg, metal halide 400 W	10	400 W—highway, industrial 3000 W—photochemical, Photoresist and UVR ink and paint Drying and UVR curing
HID (Hg and metal halide)	Up to 240	Printing, graphics arts (at entry and exit slits of print machine)
Low-pressure Hg 30 W	5760 750 380	Germicidal—15 W at 0.2 m 30 W at 0.5 m 15 W at 1 m
Medium-pressure Hg 275 W	4800	Sunlamp
Tungsten halogen 1 kW	20	Stage lighting
High-pressure Hg (400 W at 2 m)	< 1 to 12 < 1 to 3900	Lighting—with outer envelope —without outer envelope
Medium-pressure Hg clear 400 W	10	Lighting
Medium-pressure Hg fluorescent 400 W	10	Lighting
High-pressure Na 150 W (HID)	0	Roadway lighting

Source: Adapted from Sliney and Wolbarsht (1980) and McKinley et al. (1988).

[a] For base lamps at 0.5 m.

[b] Number of ELVs possible in an 8 hour working day.

[c] The typical applications listed are illustrations of the uses of the lamps, but may not be representative of the data shown in columns 2 and 3, which are reported values appropriate to the bare lamps. In most applications, the ELVs will not exceed 1 due to adequate shielding of the lamps.

at high temperatures (such as used for the filaments of incandescent lamps) and molten metals approximate to a black-body.

The incandescent lamp is the oldest type of lamp still in common use. Its emission results from a tungsten filament which generally is heated to between 2700 and 3000 K with powers up to 500 W. In applications where more power, or a physically smaller source is required, tungsten (quartz) halogen lamps are often used. The combination of filament temperatures which are likely to be in the range 2900 to 3450 K and quartz bulbs results in a significantly higher level of emission of potentially harmful UVR compared with "ordinary" tungsten filament lamps. Where such lamps are used in luminaires when exposure of people at close distances for long times is possible, consideration should be given to the incorporation of appropriate UVR absorption filters in the luminaire. Details of emissions measured from some desktop luminaires are given in Table 25-10.

Incandescent lamps, other than tungsten halogen, normally have sufficiently thick glass envelopes to completely preclude a UVR hazard. Tungsten halogen lamps are used in agricultural applications, such as in plant cultivation and stock raising, and in industrial applications, such as ink and paint drying. If they are not enclosed or filtered, they can represent a potential UVR hazard, as can unfiltered tungsten halogen lamps used for stage, display, and heating applications.

Electrical (Gaseous) Discharge Optical radiation can be generated by electrical excitation of a low-pressure gas or vapor. A current is passed through a gas (or gases) ionized to produce electrons and positive ions. A fluorescent lamp discharge is a typical

TABLE 25-10 Summary of Measurement Data for Ultraviolet Radiation from Desktop Luminaires

Type of Lamp[a]	Effective Irradiance[b] (mW m_{eff}^{-2})		Illuminace (lux)[b]
	ACGIH[c]	Erythema[d]	
Desktop tungsten halogen 20 W	6.1	10.1	1400
Desktop tungsten halogen 20 W	2.2	3.3	7600
Desktop tungsten halogen 20 W	25.0	41.0	14000
Desktop tungsten halogen 50 W	2.2	3.8	1600
"Cool white" general lighting fluorescent lamp 100 W	0.20	0.28	500

Source: McKinlay et al. (1989) and Whillock et al. (1988).

[a] Incorporating tungsten halogen lamps and from general lighting fluorescent lamps.
[b] All tungsten halogen lamp measurements at 0.3 m from lamps.
[c] ACGIH occupational hazard weighted irradiance. The exposure limit is equivalent to 8 hour exposure to 1 mW m_{eff}^{-2}.
[d] International Commission on Illumination reference action spectrum (see McKinlay and Diffey, 1987).

example. The energetic electrons that produce the ionization also excite the electrons of the gas atoms that subsequently de-excite resulting in the emission of characteristic radiations. The emission at 253.7 nm from mercury vapor is used as a source of excitation of the phosphors of low-pressure fluorescent lamps. By raising the pressure of the discharge to a few atmospheres, the emission lines increasingly broaden, eventually effectively forming a continuum. In some cases the 253.7 nm line emission will be self-absorbed by the vapor of the discharge.

Low-Pressure Gas-Discharge Lamps   In low-pressure gas-discharge lamps the filling gas is usually an inert gas. The commonest type of low-pressure (nonphosphor) discharge lamp is the "neon" lamp. Low-pressure discharge lamps (mercury, sodium) with glass envelopes will absorb UVB/C, and only lamps with quartz envelopes can transmit significant UVB/C. Of the common low-pressure lamps, only unfiltered mercury lamps can create a severe UVR hazard. For example, low-pressure mercury (quartz) germicidal lamps (with up to 95% of the radiant energy being emitted at 253.7 nm) are used for sterilization in hospital hallways, intensive-care wards, operating room suites, water and food sterilization, chromatographic analysis, document and mineral identification, biological laboratory hoods, and so on. Where possible, germicidal lamps should be contained within a shielded enclosure with a clearly displayed warning notice. Because tubular germicidal lamps fit into and operate with standard bi-pin lighting fitments, care must be taken not to accidentally interchange germicidal for lighting tubes. Other uses of low-pressure discharge lamps that may represent a UVR hazard include sunbeds in horticulture.

Fluorescent Lamps   The most common application of the low-pressure discharge is in fluorescent lamps. The fluorescent lamp operates by means of a discharge between two electrodes through a mixture of mercury vapor and a rare gas, usually argon. Light is produced by conversion of 253.7 nm mercury emission radiation to longer wavelength radiations by means of a phosphor coating on the inside of the wall of the lamp. Lamps are available with many different phosphors and envelopes to produce a wide range of spectral emissions covering the visible, UVA, and UVB regions. While the continuum emissions of fluorescent lamps are characteristic of the phosphors, the narrow peak spectral emissions are dominated by the characteristic line emission spectrum of the low-pressure mercury vapor discharge.

TABLE 25-11 Measurements of UVR from Compact Fluorescent Lamps, Normalized to an Illuminance of 500 lux

Lamp Type	UVA mW m^{-2}	UVB W m^{-2}
Luma (7W) LC7	4.7×10^4	0
Luma (7W) LC7 with diffuser	197	0
Osram (11W) Dulux EL	3.8×10^4	0.1
Philips (9W) SL9	3.7×10^4	0
Sylvania (13W) Lynx CFD	4.3×10^4	30.81
Thorn (16W) 2D	5.4×10^4	2.48
Tungsram (16W) Globulux	663	0

Source: Whillock et al. (1990).

General Lighting Fluorescent Lamps Fluoresent lamps are available in a range of physical sizes, powers, and phosphors. The range of phosphors includes a large selection of "near white" and "special color" lamps.

Data from a study of the amount of UVR emitted by white fluorescent lamps used in the United Kingdom for general lighting purposes indicated that people exposed for 1500 h per year would receive only 2 to 5 minimum erythemal doses (MEDs) per year (Whillock et al., 1988). These data differ somewhat from those obtained from measurements on general lighting lamps used in the United States where with some super high output lamps the levels of UVR emissions were higher (Cole et al., 1986). During the past few years the further development and improved design of general lighting fluorescent lamps has been evident in the production of compact fluorescent lamps. These lamps are essentially low-wattage, small-diameter fluorescent tubes folded in a compact form. Measurements from compact fluorescent lamps, normalised to an illuminance of 500 lux, are presented in Table 25-11. The effect of various diffusers/controllers on the emissions from a white fluorescent lamp are given in Table 25-12.

High-Pressure Discharge Lamps High-pressure discharge lamps (mercury, sodium) are widely used for industrial and commercial lighting, streetlighting, display lighting, and floodlighting. The general construction of high-pressure mercury lamps is a fused silica (quartz) discharge tube containing the mercury/argon vapor discharge mounted inside an outer envelope of soda-lime or borosilicate glass. The outer glass envelope effectively absorbs UVR; consequently the quantity of potentially harmful UVR emitted by such lamps depends critically on the integrity of this envelope (FDA, 1988), although, even when intact, secondary filtration may also be required.

The family of "metal halide" lamps encompasses a number of different types of high-intensity mercury lamps whose discharges all contain additives. The additives are most

TABLE 25-12 Measurements of UVR Irradiance from Various Diffusers/Controllers with a White Fluorescent Lamp as the Source

Diffuser Type	UVA mW m^{-2}	UVB mW m^{-2}	UVR$_{eff}$ (ACGIH weighted) mW m$_{eff}^{-2}$
Bare lamp	22.32	3.45	5.9×10^{-2}
Clear acrylic	16.35	2.91	4.8×10^{-2}
Clear styrene	2.87	0	0
Opal styrene	0.92	3×10^{-3}	2×10^{-5}
Opal polycarbonate	0.20	1.2×10^{-2}	9×10^{-5}

Source: McKinlay et al. (1988).

TABLE 25-13   UV Irradiances Measured at 1 m from Typical Graphics Arts Metal Halide Mercury Lamps

Lamp Type	Power (W)	UVC (W m^{-2})	UVB (W m^{-2})	UVA (W m^{-2})
HPA 400	400	0.5	3.2	9.0
HPA 1000	930	2.3	9.0	23.0
HPA 2000	1750	4.5	19.0	48.0

Source: McKinlay et al., (1988).

typically metal halides chosen to produce either a strongly colored emission (usually a single halide), to produce a more broadly spectrally uniform emission (multi-halide) or to enhance the UVR (most often UVA) emission. Compared with "ordinary" mercury high-intensity discharge lamps, the luminous efficacies of metal halide lamps are high. Special HID mercury and metal halide lamps are used for photopolymerization, drying of inks and resins, reprography, projection and studio lighting, graphic arts, and commercial and domestic sunlamps, and they emit large amounts of UVR (Table 25-13). HID lamps require a UVR hazard evaluation and units employing them should be interlocked to prevent exposure of workers and have appropriate warning signs.

High-pressure sodium lamps are similar in construction to but generally have a smaller diameter than high-pressure mercury lamps. The inner tube is made from polycrystalline alumina and the outer envelope from borosilicate glass. The emissions are characteristic of the sodium vapor and as the vapor pressure is raised the emissions broaden across the visible spectrum.

Black (UVA) Lamps   Black (UVA) lamps are high- or low- pressure mercury discharge tubes (e.g., used with fluorescent powders in many nondestructive testing applications, forensic, philatelic, and mineralogical studies and for special effects in display and entertainment or in medical facilities). They use a nickel/cobalt oxide (Woods's glass) envelope, and the glass is almost entirely opaque to light. The phosphor chosen for these lamps emits around 370 nm in the UVA. They are not normally considered hazardous. Problems can arise (1) when the lamp envelope insufficiently filters the actinic UVR lines of the mercury spectrum (297, 303, 313 nm) or actinic UVR leaks out of cooling louvers or cracks in the instrument housing and (2) when photosensitive people use these lamps (e.g., a worker taking a medication that sensitizes skin to UVA and sunlight may develop a skin reaction to black light exposure).

Arc Lamps   The UVR emissions from carbon and short-arc lamps (high-pressure xenon, mercury) can be very high and exposure to such sources may require an extensive hazard evaluation. Carbon arcs are commonly used in welding processes. High-pressure xenon lamps are used, for example, as solar simulators and in projection units and searchlights. Low-pressure and pulsed xenon lamps are often used in printing. Effective controls are required in the use of these lamps.

Where an optical source of very high radiance is required and of small size, a very high pressure arc lamp may be used. These have a filling gas of mercury vapor, mercury vapor plus xenon gas, or xenon gas. Metal halide types are also available. Two physical types are commonly used: the compact (or short) arc and the linear arc. Typical applications of compact arcs include projectors, searchlights, and solar radiation simulators.

The spectral emission of xenon lamps, which at wavelengths shorter than infrared, closely matches that of a black-body radiator at about 6000 K enables their use as solar radiation simulators. Their emission spectrum is continuous from the UVR through to the infrared region. Emission peaks in the infrared principally between 800 and 1000 nm may

TABLE 25-14 UVR Emission Data at 1 m from Electric Welding Arcs

Process/Base Metal / Gas	Arc Gap mm	Current A	UVR ELVs[a]
TIG / steel /Ar	1.6	50–300	30–1000
TIG / steel / He	1.6	40–450	400–4500
TIG / steel /Ar	3.2	50–300	30–1200
TIG /Al /Ar	3.1	50–265	30–600
MIG / MAG / steel / CO_2	—	90–150	490–1300
MIG / MAG / steel / O_2 + Ar	6.4–9.5	150–350	6500–23000
MIG / MAG /Al /Ar	6.4–9.5	130–300	2000–12500
FCAW/steel / CO_2	—	175–350	210–3000
PAC / steel / N_2	6.4–19	300–1000	440–2800
PAW / steel /Ar	4.8	260	1000
MMA / steel / none	3.2	100–200	400–4400

Source: Adapted from McKinlay et al. (1988).

Key: TIG (tungsten inert gas), MIG / MAG (metal inert / active gas),
FCAW (flux core arc welding), PAC / W (plasma arc cutting / welding),
MMA (manual metal arc).
[a] Number of ELVs in an 8 hour working period.

be effectively removed by filtration. The luminance of compact xenon arcs may approach that of the sun (approximately 10^9 cd m^{-2}) and in some lamps with greater than 10 kW rating the luminance of the brightest spot may exceed 10^{10} cd m^{-2}.

Gas and Arc Welding   Because of their comparatively low operating temperature, the optical radiation hazards associated with gas welding processes are minimal. The use of standard welding filters necessary for comfort of viewing will prevent injury.

In comparison with gas-welding processes, the emissions of optical radiations from arc welding are very high, and many data on the optical radiation emissions associated with a variety of electric arc welding processes have been published (Sliney and Wolbarsht, 1980) (Table 25-14). Long-term viewing of a welding arc is unlikely, but not unknown. Under these conditions retinal photochemical injury is possible. Accidental exposure is limited by the aversion response and retinal injury should not occur within this time. The aversion response might not protect the eye from photokeratitis. Exposed skin may develop ultraviolet-induced erythema. Clearly a combination of personal protection for the operator and the use of containment screens to prevent exposure of others is necessary.

RISK ASSESSMENT AND EDUCATION POLICY

Risk assessments for long-term health effects can only be made with respect to the induction of nonmelanoma skin cancers (NMSC) due to a lack of data on the risks of other long-term biological effects in humans.

Epidemiological studies (Fears et al., 1977; Slaper et al., 1987) have shown that the cumulative incidence (*I*) of nonmelanoma skin cancer can be expressed by the equation:

$$I = \gamma A H^2 a^5,$$

where *I* is the total number of cases per 10^5 of population up to age *a* years, γ is the genetic susceptibility of the population, *H* is the annual carcinogenic-effective dose (expressed in MEDs, (minimal erythemal doses) at the skin surface, and *A* is the fraction of exposed skin.

TABLE 25-15 Approaches to Minimize UVR-Induced Skin and Eye Damage

1. Do not try to get a UVR-induced tanned skin. There is no such thing as a safe or healthy tan, not naturally, nor artificially induced.
2. Take sensible precautions to avoid sunburn, particularly in children.
3. Limit unprotected personal exposure to the sun, particularly during the four hours around noon.
4. Seek shade wherever possible, but remember that sunburn can occur even in partial shade or under cloudy skies, particularly in summer.
5. Remember that sunburn can occur while swimming and is more likely when there is a high level of reflected UVR, such as from snow and sand.
6. Wear suitable head wear, such as a wide-brimmed hat, to reduce exposure to the face, head, and neck.
7. Cover exposed skin with clothing giving good UVR protection, such as long-sleeved shirts and loose clothing with a close weave.
8. Sunglasses should be worn that are designed to exclude both direct and peripheral exposure of the eye.
9. Apply sunblocks, or broadband sunscreens with high sun protection factors (generally 15 or above), to exposed or uncovered skin. Apply generously and reapply frequently.
10. Remember that certain prescribed drugs, medicines, cosmetics, and plant materials can make people more sensitive to sunlight.

For a worker (at age 60 years) occupationally exposed to predominantly UVB radiation and receiving over 40 years the ELV for skin exposure for each 8 h working day, the additional risk of induction of NMSC would be about a factor of 3.

There are various practical protection measures to reduce personal exposure to solar UVR. These include good information and education policy regarding the hazards of sun exposure (Table 25-15). The Global Solar UV Index (referred to subsequently as UV index) has been introduced as a means of providing standardized information to the public about the levels of solar UV radiation to which they may be exposed, wherever they may go in the world. It is part of an integrated public health program of informing the public about the potential detrimental effects from sun exposure. Although ideally such an index should address both skin and ocular hazards of sun exposure, the current UV index addresses only the acute effects on skin.

Techniques for Evaluating Actual or Potential Exposures

Determination of the biologically effective irradiance can be achieved by measuring the spectral distribution with a spectroradiometer and then calculating the weighted integral or by direct measurement using a broad-band radiation detector whose sensitivity varies with wavelength according to the prescribed weighting function. Personal monitoring is often the preferred measurement method to evaluate adequately individual exposures and to establish appropriate protective measures. By this method the fraction and distribution of the daily radiant exposure (J m^{-2} effective) can be assessed for people particularly at risk.

A spectroradiometer measures irradiance within a narrow bandwidth, centerd at a wavelength, which is selected by the operator, and is continuously variable. The basic components, as shown in Figure 25-8 which illustrates the principles of operation, are input optics, monochromator, and detector.

Optical radiation is collected by the input optics, which should possess a 2π field of view and a cosine-weighted angular response. Two types of input optics achieve these requirements. A transmission diffuser at the entrance slit of the spectroradiometer can produce an approximate cosine response. Alternatively, an integrating sphere with a small entrance aperture and an internal diffuse coating, such as MgO or BaSO$_4$, with a high UVR

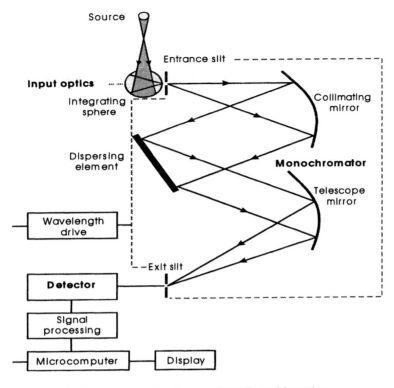

Basic components of a spectroradiometric system

Figure 25-8   Basic components of a spectroradiometer.

reflectance can produce a cosine-weighted response. A second aperture in the integrating sphere provides input for the optical radiation via an entrance slit to a monochromator.

The entrance slit of the monochromator is at the focal point of a collimating mirror and optical radiation is reflected from the mirror as a parallel beam incident on a ruled diffraction grating. A second mirror collects optical radiation from the grating at a particular angle (hence wavelength) and focuses it onto the exit slit of the monochromator. High-performance spectroradiometers, used for determining low irradiances of UVR, require low stray radiation levels and use a double grating monochromator. The emerging wavelength is altered by angular rotation of the diffraction grating. An appropriate detector, such as a photomultiplier tube or occasionally a photodiode, is mounted at the exit slit of the monochromator. The signal from the detector is integrated for a pre-selected time and then is transferred to a microcomputer for storage and display. The wavelength drive and output integration are synchronized to provide a spectral scan of irradiance in equal wavelength intervals throughout a given optical spectrum.

The optical radiation flux passing through the exit slit depends on factors such as angular dispersion and the square of the bandwidth. For a small entrance slit the bandwidth ($\Delta\lambda$) is equal to the width of the exit slit divided by the linear dispersion, and the intensity distribution across the exit slit corresponds to the wavelength distribution of the source. When the widths of the entrance and exit slits are comparable, a triangular distribution across the exit slit results, with the $\Delta\lambda$ defined at full width half height. This can lead to inaccuracies in measurement, particularly when the spectral irradiance varies rapidly with wavelength, such as with the solar spectrum below 305 nm.

When the monochromator slit widths are sufficiently narrow, the detected output signal $S(\lambda)$ is related to the measured spectral irradiance $E(\lambda)$ through the equation

$$S(\lambda) = E(\lambda) R(\lambda),$$

where $R(\lambda)$ is the spectral responsivity, determined by measuring the response of the spectroradiometer to a source, such as a tungsten halogen or deuterium lamp, of known spectral irradiance and traceable to national standards. The biologically effective irradiance E_{eff} is obtained by summing over all wavelengths emitted by a source using the equation

$$E_{eff} = \sum_{\lambda} E(\lambda)B(\lambda)\Delta\lambda \quad (\text{Wm}^{-2} \text{ effective})$$

where $B(\lambda)$ is the appropriate biological weighting function (i.e., the relative biological effectiveness of optical radiation of wavelength λ in producing a given biological effect) and $\Delta\lambda$ is the wavelength interval.

The UVR spectral measuring capabilities of Brewer spectrophotometers (used for ozone column measurements) can be exploited to measure the solar spectral irradiance in the wavelength region 290 to 325 nm, although these instruments do have limitations in precision below 310 nm.

Spectroradiometers are capable of high precision in the measurement of spectral irradiance, but they are expensive. Less precise estimates of $E(\lambda)$ or E_{eff} are achievable with less expensive broad-band instruments, which integrate spectral irradiance over a range of wavelengths. Physical phenomena used in two measurement methods are either thermal, where energy absorption results in a measurable temperature change in a detector, or photoelectric, which involves a conversion of UVR into an electrical signal.

Thermal detectors have a uniform response within their region of operation and are particularly useful for the absolute determination of irradiance and as such are often used as calibration instruments. There are two types of thermal detector for operation with UVR:

1. A thermopile, which depends on the Seebeck effect, whereby a voltage is generated when heat is applied to the junction of two dissimilar metals
2. A pyroelectric detector, which depends on a voltage generated by a temperature change via a change in electrical polarization in a crystal, such as lithium tantalate.

A fused silica window is used in a thermopile for UVR operation, and the instrument will operate with a near-flat response over the wavelength range 180 nm to 3.4 μm. Heat losses in a thermopile can result in nonlinearity in response, particularly at high irradiances (e.g., greater than around 300 W m^{-2}). Thermopiles should not be used for irradiances greater than 2000 W m^{-2}. Pyroelectric detectors have a faster response than a thermopile and a typical irradiance range of 10^{-4} to 10^{6} W m^{-2}.

There is a range of devices employing photoelectric detectors for UVR measurement. Some of these devices provide a measurement of $E(\lambda)$, and some with the addition of optical filters provide an assessment of E_{eff}. The photoelectric detectors used in such devices include photomultiplier tubes, vacuum photodiodes, silicon photodiodes, and GaAsP photodiodes.

Three commonly used devices, which employ this technology for health hazard assessment and environmental monitoring in the UVR spectral region, are the direct reading radiometer, the filtered UVR meter, and the Robertson-Berger (R-B) meter. The

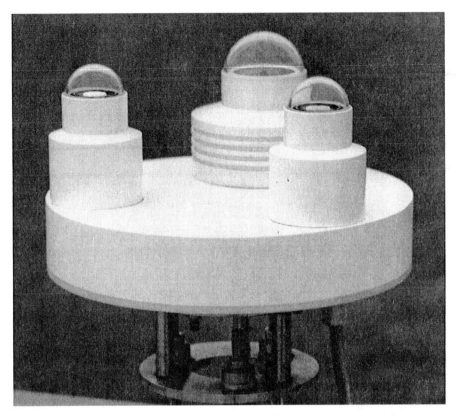

Figure 25-9 NRPB solar measurement system incorporating an R-B meter. (From Dean et al., 1991)

detecting head of a typical direct reading radiometer incorporates a quartz wide angle diffuser, an interference filter, a blocking filter and a "solar blind" vacuum photodiode. Different detector heads are available for the assessment of different biological effects. Filtered UVR meters, which incorporate a diffuser and filters to provide measurements of global UVB at 306 nm and UVA at 360 nm, have been used in Sweden since 1989 (Wester, 1983).

The R-B meter design of detector (Berger, 1976) is available commercially, and is used as the erythemally weighted UVR detector elements in solar radiation measurement systems (Fig. 25-9). The detector is housed in an aluminium cylinder with a Vycor quartz dome to seal the input. UVR incident upon the dome passes through a UG11 black glass filter, which absorbs visible and infrared radiation. This is then wavelength shifted by a magnesium tungstate phosphor deposited on a Corning 4010 green filter, which absorbs UVR and the small amount of red light transmitted by the UG11 filter. The emission from the fluorescing phosphor in the wavelength range of 400 to 600 nm is detected by a side window vacuum photodiode with an S4 bialkali photocathode. The relative spectral response of the R-B detector is an acceptable approximation to the spectral efficacy curve for UVR-induced erythema in human skin. Desiccants are used to control condensation and humidity in the housing. Temperature coefficients of between 0.3% and 0.8%$°C^{-1}$ have been reported in the older design of R-B (model 500), mainly due to the temperature sensitivity of the phosphor in the temperature range of 20° to 40°C.

Broad-band instruments employing diffusers and filters for measurement in the UVA are also commercially available.

Personal monitoring may be the preferred measurement method in order to adequately evaluate individual exposures and to establish appropriate protective measures. By this method the fraction and distribution of the daily radiant exposure ($J\,m^{-2}$ effective) from an optical radiation source, such as the sun, can be assessed for people particularly at risk. Sometimes the principles (e.g., the weighted response characteristic) of the broad-band radiation detector are employed in a personal detector, but there are a range of other physical, chemical and biological options (Moseley, 1988).

The biologically effective UVR dose applied to the body over a time interval T (s) is defined as

$$D = \sum_t \sum_\lambda E(\lambda, t)\, B(\lambda) \Delta\lambda \Delta t,$$

where $E(\lambda, t)$ is the spectral irradiance and $B(\lambda)$ is the appropriate biological weighting factor at wavelength λ.

Changes in the optical properties of photosensitive films to incident UVR can be used in UVR personal and environmental dosimetry. These dosemeters provide a simple means of integrating UVR exposure continuously, and because they are cheap and compact, they can be used for environmental measurements at many locations inaccessible to bulky instrumentation.

The UVR absorption of polysulphone film increases when exposed to UVR of wavelength less than 330 nm. The increased absorbance is proportional to the UVR dose. The spectral response characteristics of 1 μm thick film matches closely the erythema action spectrum for wavelengths in the range 300 to 315 nm (Diffey, 1982). The spectral response of the more commonly used 40 μm thick film deviates from the erythema action curve, which can lead to significant errors if uncorrected.

CR39 (Allyl diglycol carbonate) plastic has a response which approximates to the reference erythema action spectrum (Wong et al., 1992). After exposure to UVR, the plastic is etched in a concentrated caustic solution at an elevated temperature of 80°C for 3 hours and then rinsed and dried. The change in absorbance in the exposed dosemeter is measured. The sensitivity of the dosemeter can be changed by the concentration of the etching solution and by the wavelength at which the absorbance is measured (400 nm for D less than $3000\,J\,m^{-2}$ eff and at 700 nm for higher doses). Overall measurement uncertainties of 20% have been reported.

A number of other personal UVR devices, including personal sun alarms, UVR sensitive stick-on tapes, sun sensors, timers, and small monitors can be bought at relatively low cost. Many of these are very poor indicators of UVR dose, have a restricted angular response, and are no substitute for common sense in the sun. Other devices, such as photoluminescent and thermoluminescent dosemeters and diazo film, have been reported (WHO, 1979).

SUMMARY

Many optical radiation sources emit UVR, often as an unwanted side-product, requiring filtration to eliminate unnecessary exposure. The major source of personal exposure is from the sun, although under certain conditions exposure from artificial sources (e.g., sunbeds, arcs, and medical procedures) can be significant.

The major target organs are the eyes and the skin. The ocular effects of acute overexposure include photokeratitis and photoconjunctivitis, inflammation of the cornea and conjunctiva, respectively, and solar retinitis, photochemical damage to the retina. Chronic overexposure may contribute to corneal injuries such as climatic droplet keratopathy and pterygium, lens opacities or cataracts, and age-related macular degeneration, a retinal condition that is a major cause of blindness in the developed world.

Acute overexposure of the skin may result in sunburn, characterized by erythema, edema, and in severe cases, blistering; the response to skin damage includes skin thickening and increased pigmentation. Chronic overexposure results in photoaging of exposed skin and the development of solar keratoses, benign proliferations of epidermal keratinocytes that are considered to be premalignant lesions; chronic overexposure to UVA may result in increased skin fragility.

The most serious health effect of chronic overexposure is the development of skin cancer. There are two main types, the nonmelanoma skin cancers, comprising basal cell carcinomas and squamous cell carcinomas, and the cutaneous malignant melanomas. Cumulative dose is a major factor determining risk for the nonmelanoma skin cancers. Although much less common than nonmelanoma skin cancers, malignant melanoma is the main cause of skin cancer death, particularly in the young. The most common type of this cancer, superficial spreading melanoma, is associated with intense intermittent exposure.

Phenotype is an important risk factor for the development of skin cancers, with light skin, red or blond hair, blue eyes, a tendency to burn easily and to tan poorly all associated with increased risk. A tendency to freckle, large numbers of naevi, and atypical naevi, are all additional risk factors for malignant melanoma.

Guidelines exist that provide exposure limits to UVR, and these are based on avoidance of acute damage to the skin and eyes. However, they do not apply to long-term damage, since there is currently insufficient information to derive appropriate limits. Moreover these guidelines do not apply to medical and elective cosmetic exposures.

Since UVR has limited penetration in human tissue, it should be possible to limit overexposure by a suitable coordinated protection program, requiring easily understandable advice and personal protection measures. Good education policy is the key to reducing people's overall exposure to UVR. An educational efforts to address the health effects issues raised by exposure to UVR should be combined with a comprehensive range of effective personal protective measures and reliable measurement data pertaining to both global, occupational, and personal exposures, particularly from the sun. In addition there is need to develop inexpensive and reliable integrating personal dosimetry methods that allow UVR baseline measurement data to be compared with UVR doses at specific body locations.

REFERENCES

ACGIH. 1997. *Threshold Limit Values for Chemical Substances and Physical Agents and Biological Exposure Indices.* Cincinnati, OH: The American Conference of Governmental Industrial Hygienists.

Anders, A., H.-J. Altheide, M. Knälmann, and H. Tronnier. 1995. Action spectrum for erythema in humans investigated with dye lasers. *Photochem. Photobiol.* 61: 200–205.

Berger, D. S. 1976. The sunburning ultraviolet meter. Design and performance. *Photochem. Photobiol.* 24: 587–593.

Birmingham, D. J., M. M. Key, G. E Tubich, and V. B. Perone. 1961. Phototoxic bullae among celery harvesters. *Arch Dermatol.* 83: 73–87.

Bissett, D. L., D. P. Hannon, and T. V. OR. 1989. Wavelength dependence of histological, physical, and visible changes in chronically UV-irradiated hairless mouse skin. *Photochem. Photobiol.* 50: 763–769.

Boettner, E. A., and J. R. Wolter. 1962. Transmission of the ocular media. *Invest. Ophthalmol.* 1: 776–783.

CIE. 1987. *International Lighting Vocabulary,* vol. 3, p. 51. CIE Publ. No 17.4; p. 3, Geneva: Bureau Central de la Commission Electrotechnique Internationale.

CIE. 1996. *Standard Erythema Dose.* Draft standard DS 007.1/E. Paris: Commission Internationale de l'Eclairage.

Chadwick, C. A., C. S. Potten, O. Nikaido, T. Matsunaga, C. Proby, and A. R. Young. 1995. The detection of cyclobutane thymine dimers, (6-4) photolesions and the Dewar photoisomers in sections of UV-irradiated human skin using specific antibodies, and the demonstration of depth penetration effects. *J. Photochem. Photobiol. B: Biol.* 28: 163–170.

Cole, C. A., R. E. Davies, P. D. Forbes, and L. C. D'Alosio. 1983. Comparison of action spectra for acute cutaneous responses to ultraviolet radiation: Man and albino hairless mouse. *Photochem. Photobiol.* 37: 623–631.

Cole, C. A., P. D. Forbes, R. E. Davies, and F. Urbach. 1986a. *Effect of Indoor Lighting on Normal Skin.* New York: New York Academy of Sciences.

Cole, C. C., P. D. Forbes, and R. E. Davies. 1986b. An action spectrum for UV photocarcinogenesis. *Photochem. Photobiol.* 43: 275–284.

Cridland, N. A., and R. D. Saunders. 1994. *Cellular and Molecular Effects of UVA and UVB.* NRPB-R269. London: HMSO.

Crow, K. D. 1961 Photosensitivity due to pitch. *Br. J. Dermatol.* 73: 220–232.

Cullen A. P., and S. C. Perera. 1994 Sunlight and human conjunctival action spectrum. *SPEI Proc.*, 2134B: 24–30.

Davson, H. Ed. 1967. *The Eye Vegetative Physiology and Biochemistry*, vol. 1. New York: Academic Press.

Dean S. F., A. I. Rawlinson, A. F. McKinlay, A. J. Pearson, M. J. Whillock, and C. M. H. Driscoll. 1991. NRPB solar radiation measurement system *Radiol. Prot. Bull.* 124: 6.

de Gruijl, F. R., and J. C. van der Leun. 1992. Action spectra for carcinogenesis. In *Biological Responses to Ultraviolet A Radiation. Proc. 2nd International Conference: Biological Effects of UVA Radiation*, San Antonio, June, 1991, ed. F. Urbach, pp 91–97. Overland Park: Valdenmar.

de Gruijl, F. R., H. J. C. M, Sterenborg, P. D. Forbes, R.E. Davies, C. Cole, G. Kelfkens, H. van Weelden, H. Slaper, and J. C. van der Leun. 1993. Wavelength dependence of skin cancer induction by ultraviolet irradiation of albino hairless mice. *Cancer Res.* 53: 53–60.

Diffey, B. L. 1982. Ultraviolet radiation in medicine. *Medical Physics Handbook 11* Bristol (UK): Adam Hilger.

Diffey, B. L. 1994. Observed and predicted minimal erythema doses: a comparative study. *Photochem. Photobiol. 60*: 380–382.

Driscoll, C. M. H. 1992. Solar UV trends and distributions. *Radiol. Prot. Bull.* 137: 7–13.

Elliot, D. J. 1995, *Ultraviolet laser technology and applications.* San Diego: Academic Press.

Epe, B. 1991. Genotoxicity of singlet oxygen. *Chem.-Biol. Interactions* 80: 239–260.

Epstein, J. H. 1965. Comparison of the carcinogenic and cocarcinogenic effects of ultraviolet light on hairless mice. *J. Nat. Cancer Inst.* 34: 741–745.

Epstein, J. H. 1988. Photocarcinogenesis promotion studies with benzoyl peroxide (BPO) and croton oil. *J. Invest. Dermatol.* 91: 114–116.

Epstein, J. H., and W. L. Epstein. 1962. Cocarcinogenic effect of ultraviolet light on DMBA tumour initiation in albino mice. *J. Invest. Dermatol.* 39: 455–460.

Epstein, J. H., and H. L. Roth. 1968. Experimental ultraviolet light carcinogenesis. *J. Invest. Dermatol.* 50: 387–389.

Epstein, J. H., W. L. Epstein, and T. Nakai. 1967. Production of melanomas from DMBA- induced "blue nevi" in hairless mice with ultraviolet light. *J. Nat. Cancer Inst.* 39: 19–30.

Fears T. R., J. Scotto, M. A. Schneiderman. 1977. Mathematical models of age and ultraviolet effects on the incidence of skin cancer among whites in the United States, *Am. J. Epidemiol.* 105: 420–427.

Fisher, G. J., S. C. Datta, H. S. Talwar, Z.-Q. Wang, J. Varni, S. Kang, and J. J. Voorhees. 1996. Molecular basis of sun-induced premature skin ageing and retinoid antagonism. *Nature* 379: 335–339.

Fourtanier, A., and C. Berrebi. 1989. Minature pig as an animal model to study photoaging. *Photochem. Photobiol.* 50: 771–784.

Frederick, J. E., H. E. Snell, and E. K. Haywood. 1989. Solar ultraviolet radiation at the earth's surface. *Photochem. Photobiol.* 50: 443–450.

Freeman, S. E., H. Hacham, R. W. Gange, D. J. Maytum, J. C. J. C. Sutherland, and B. M. Sutherland. 1989. Wavelength dependence of pyrimidine dimer formation in DNA of human skin irradiated *in situ* with ultraviolet light. *Proc. Nat. Acad. Sci. USA* 86: 5605–5609.

Gange, W. R., and J. A. Parrish. 1983. Acute effects of ultraviolet radiation upon the skin. In *Photoimmunology*, eds. J. A. Parrish, M. L. Kripke, and W. L. Morison. pp. 77–94. New York: Plenum Press.

Gray, R. H., G. J. Johnson, and A. Freedman. 1992. Climatic droplet keratopathy. *Survey Ophthalmol.* 36: 241–253.

Harber, L. C., and G. M. Levine. 1969. Photosensitivity dermatitis from household products. *General Practice* 39: 95–100.

Hawk, J. L. M. 1984. Photosensitising agents used in the United Kingdom. *Clin. Exp. Dermatol.* 9: 300–302.

Hjorth, N., and H. Möller. 1976. Phototoxic textile dermatitis ("bikini dermatitis"). *Arch. Dermatol.* 112: 1445–1447.

Hruza, L. L., and A. P. Pentland. 1993. Mechanisms of UV-induced inflamation. *J. Invest. Dermatol.* 100: 35S–41S.

Husein, Z., M. A. Pathak, T. Flotte, and M. M. Wick. 1991. Role of ultraviolet light in the induction of melanocytic tumours in hairless mice following 7, 12-dimethylbenz(a)anthracene application and ultraviolet irradiation. *Cancer. Res.* 51: 4964–4970.

IARC. 1992. International Agency for Research on Cancer. *Solar and Ultraviolet Radiation*, vol. 55. IARC Monographs on the Evaluation of Carcinogenic Risks to Humans. Lyon: IARC.

ICNIRP. 1996. Guidelines of UV radiation exposure limits. International Commission on Non- Ionizing Radiation Protection (ICNIRP) Statement. *Health Phy.* 71: 978.

IEC. 1984. *Radiation Safety of Laser Products, Equipment Classification, Requirements and User's Guide.* Publication 825. Geneva: International Electrotechnical Commission.

IEC. 1990. *Modification 1.* Publication 825. Geneva: International Electrotechnical Commission.

IRPA. 1985. Guidelines on limits of exposure to ultraviolet radiation of wavelengths between 180 nm and 400 nm (incoherent optical radiation). The International Non-Ionizing Radiation Committee (INIRC) of the International Radiation Protection Association (IRPA). *Health Phy.* 49: 331–340.

IRPA. 1989. Proposed change to the IRPA 1985 Guidelines on limits of exposure to ultraviolet radiation. The International Non-Ionizing Radiation Committee (INIRC) of the International Radiation Protection Association (IRPA). *Health Phy.* 56: 971–972

IRPA. 1991. Guidelines on limits of exposure to ultraviolet radiation of wavelengths between 180 nm and 400 nm (incoherent optical radiation). *In IRPA Guidelines on Protection against Non-ionizing Radiation*, eds. A. S. Duchene, J. R. A. Lakey, and M. H. Repacholi. pp. 42–52. New York: Pergamon Press.

Iverson, O. H. 1986. Carcinogenesis studies with benzoyl peroxide (Panoxyl gel 5%). *J. Invest. Dermatol.* 86: 442–448.

Iverson, O. H. 1988. Skin tumourigenesis and carcinogenesis studies with 7,12-dimethylbenz(α)anthracene, ultraviolet light, benzoyl peroxide (Panoxyl gel 5%) and ointment gel. *Carcinogenesis* 9: 803–809.

Kelfkens G., F. R. de Gruijl, and J. C. van der Leun. 1992. Carcinogenesis by short- and long wave ultraviolet-A; papilloma versus squamous cell carcinomas. In: *Biological Responses to Ultraviolet A Radiation. Proc. 2nd International Conference: Biological Effects of UVA Radiation*, San Antonio, June, 1991, ed. F. Urbach, pp. 285–294. Overland Park: Valdenmar.

Kricker, A., B. K. Armstrong, D. R. English, and P. J. Heenan. 1991. Pigmentary and cutaneous risk factors for non-melanocytic skin cancer—a case-control study. *Int. J. Cancer* 48: 650–662.

Kripke, M. L. 1993. Immunosuppressive action of UV radiation. In *The Dark Side of Sunlight*, ed., F. R. De Gruijl, pp. 77–86. Utrecht University.

Krutman, J., and Elmets, C. A. eds. 1995. *Photoimmunology.* Oxford: Blackwell Science.

Ley, R. D., M. J. Peak, and L. L. Lyon. 1983. Induction of pyrimidine dimers in epidermal DNA of hairless mice by UVB: an action spectrum. *J. Invest. Dermatol.* 80: 188–191.

Logani, M. K., P. D. Sambuco, P. D. Forbes, and R. E. Davies. 1984. Skin-tumour promoting activity of methyl ethyl ketone peroxide—A potent lipid peroidizing agent. *Food. Chem. Toxic.* 22: 879–882.

Lowe, N. J., D. P. Meyers, J. M. Wieder, D. Luftman, T. Borget, M. D. Lehman, A. W. Johnson, and I. R. Scott. 1995. Low doses of repetative ultraviolet A induce morphologic changes in human skin. *J. Invest. Dermatol.* 105: 739–743.

Mainster, M. A. 1978. Spectral transmittance of intraocular lenses and retinal damage from intense light sources. *Am. J. Ophthalmol.* 85: 167–170.

Marks, R., P. Foley, G. Goodman, B. H. Hage, and T. S. Slewood. 1986. Spontaneous remission of solar keratoses: the case for conservative management. *Br. J. Dermatol.* 115: 649–655.

Moan, J., and M. J. Peak. 1989. Effects of UV radiation on cells. *J. Photochem. Photobiol. B: Biol.* 4: 21–34.

McKinlay, A. F., and B. L. Diffey. 1987. A reference action spectrum for ultraviolet induced erythema in human skin. *CIE J.* 1: 17–22.

McKinlay, A. F., F. Harlen, and M. J. Whillock. 1988. *Hazards of Optical Radiation. A Guide to Sources, Uses and Safety.* Philadelphia: Adam Hilger.

McKinlay, A. F., M. J. Whillock, and C. C. E. Meulemans. 1989. Ultraviolet radiation and blue light emissions from spotlights incorporating tungsten halogen lamps. Report R228. Chilton, National Radiological Protection Board (NRPB).

Moseley, H. 1988. Non-ionising radiation. In *Medical Physics Handbook 18*, ch. 8, Bristol and Philadelpha: Adam Hilger.

Noonan, F. P., and E. C. De Fabo. 1993. UV-induced immunosuppression. In *Environmental UV Photobiology*, eds. A. R. Young, L. O. Björn, J. Moan, and W. Nultch, pp. 113–148. New York: Plenum Press.

NRPB. 1995. Health effects from ultraviolet radiation. *Documents of the NRPB*, vol 6, no 2. Oikarinen, A. 1990. The aging of skin: Chronoageing versus photoageing. *Photodermatol. Photoimmunol. Photomed.* 7: 3–4.

Oikarinen, A., J. Peltonen, and M. Kallioinen. 1991. Ultraviolet radiation in skin ageing and carcinogenesis: The role of retinoids for treatment and prevention. *Ann. Med.* 23: 497–505.

Pathak, M. A., and D. L. Fanselow. 1983. Photobiology of melanin pigmentation: dose / response of skin to sunlight and its content, *J. Am. Acad. Dermatol.* 9: 724–733.

Parrish, J. A., K. F. Jaenicke, and R. R. Anderson. 1982. Erythema and melanogenesis action spectra of normal human skin. *Photochem. Photobiol.* 36: 187–191.

Piette, J. 1991. Biological consequences associated with DNA oxidation mediated by singlet oxygen. *J. Photochem. Photobiol. B: Biol.* 11: 241–260.

Pitts, D. G., A. P. Cullen, and P. D. Hacker. 1977. Ocular effects of ultraviolet radiation from 295 to 365 nm. *Invest. Ophthalmol. Vis. Sci.* 16: 932–939.

Pound, A. W. 1970. Induced cell proliferation and the initiation of skin tumour formation in mice by ultraviolet light. *Pathology* 2: 269–275.

Romanchuk, K. G., V. Pollak, and R. J. Schneider. 1978. Retinal burn from a welding arc. *Can. J. Ophthalmol.* 13: 120–122.

Saunders, R. D., N. A. Cridland, and C. I. Kowalczuk. 1997. Animal and human responses to UVA and UVB. NRPB-R297. London HMSO.

Setlow, R. B., E. Grist, K. Thompson, and A. Woodhead. 1993. Wavelengths effective in the induction of malignant melanoma. *Proc. Nat. Acad. Sci. USA.* 90: 6666–6670.

Sliney, D. H. 1986. Physical factors in cataractogenesis: Ambient ultraviolet radiation and temperature. *Invest. Ophthalmol. Vis. Sci.* 27: 781–790.

Sliney, D. H., and M. Wolbarsht. 1980. *Safety with Lasers and Other Optical Sources: A Comprehensive Handbook.* New York: Plenum Press.

Soballe, P. W., K. T. Montone, K. Satyamoorthy, M. Nesbit, and M. Herlyn. 1996. Carcinogenesis in human skin grafted to SCID mice. *Cancer Res.* 56: 757–764.

Stenbäck, F. 1975. Ultraviolet light irradiation as initiating agent in skin tumour formation by the two-stage method. *Eur. J. Cancer*, 11: 241–246.

Slaper, H., and J. C. van der Leun. 1987. Quantitative modelling of skin cancer incidence. In: *Human Exposure to Ultraviolet Radiation: Risks and Regulations*, eds W. F. Passchier and B. F. M. Bosnjakovic, pp. 155–171. Amsterdam: Elsevier.

Sliney, D. H. 1987. Estimating the solar ultraviolet radiation exposure to an intraocular lens implant. *J. Cataract. Refract. Surg.* 13: 296–301.

Taylor, H. R., S. K. West, F. S. Rosenthal, B. Munoz, H. S. Newland, and E. A. Emmett. 1989. Corneal changes associated with chronic UV irradiation. *Arch. Ophthalmol.* 107: 1481–1484.

Tyrrell, R. M., and S.M. Keyse. 1990. New trends in photobiology (invited review): The interaction of UVA radiation with cultured cells. *J. Photochem. Photobiol. B: Biol.* 4: 349–361.

Ullrich, S. E. 1995. Modulation of immunity by ultraviolet radiation: key effects on antigen presentation. *J. Invest. Dermatol.* 105: 30S–36S.

UNEP. 1987. The ozone layer. United Nations Environment Program. *UNEP/GEMS Environmental Library*, No 2. Nairobi: UNEP.

Vermeer, M., and H. Hurks. 1994. The clinical relevance of immunosup pression by UV radiation *J. Photochem. Photobiol. B: Biol.* 24: 149–154.

West, S. K., F. S. Rosenthal, S. B. Bressler, S. B. Munoz, S. L. Fine, and H. R. Taylor. 1989. Exposure to sunlight and other risk factors for age related macular degeneration. *Arch. Ophthalmol.* 107: 875–879.

Wester, U. 1983. Solar ultraviolet radiation—A method for measuring and monitoring. Report RI 1983-02. *Swedish Radiation Protection Institute*, Box 60204, Stockholm.

Whillock, M. J., I. Clark, A. F. McKinlay, C. Todd, and S. Mundy. 1988. Ultraviolet radiation levels associated with the use of fluorescent general lighting, UVA and UVB lamps in the workplace and home. Report R221. Chilton, National Radiological Protection Board (NRPB).

Whillock, M. J., A. F. McKinlay, J. Kemmlert, and R. G. Forsgren. 1990. Ultraviolet radiation emissions from miniature (compact) fluorescent lamps. *Lighting Res. and Technol.* 23: 125–128.

WHO. 1979. Ultraviolet Radiation. *Environmental Health Criteria 14*. Geneva. World Health Organization.

WHO. 1994. Ultraviolet Radiation. *Environmental Health Criteria 160*. Geneva. World Health Organization.

Wong C. F., R. A. Fleming, S. J. Carter, I. T. Ring, and D. Vishvakarman. 1992. Measurement of human exposure to ultraviolet-B solar radiation using a CR-39 dosimeter. *Health Phys.* 63: 457.

Young, R W. 1988. Solar radiation and age-related macular degeneration. *Surv. Ophthalmol.* 32: 252–269.

26 Volatile Organic Compounds and the Sick Building Syndrome

LARS MØLHAVE, Ph.D.

TOXIC EFFECTS

Volatile Organic Compounds

Volatile organic compounds (VOC) are frequent air pollutants in nonindustrial environments. A working group of WHO categorized the entire range of organic indoor pollutants into four groups, as indicated in Table 26-1 (WHO, 1989). No sharp limits exist between categories, which were defined by boiling-point ranges. The VOC category was defined by a boiling-point range with a lower limit between 50°C and 100°C and an upper limit between 240°C and 260°C, where the higher values refer to polar compounds (WHO, 1989).

Health

Health has been defined by WHO (1961) as "a state of complete physical, mental, and social well-being and not merely the absence of disease or infirmity." The toxic effects of VOCs may be divided into those common to most compounds and special effects caused by individual compounds. The special effects of individual compounds may be effects such as cancer or allergy that have been associated with specific volatile organic compounds or more commonly seen effects caused by an unusually high potential of some compounds. Reviews of such special effects are found in textbooks (Andrews and Snyder, 1980). A review of indoor air quality (IAQ) related health effects is found in Berglund et al. (1992).

Genotoxic effects or toxic effects on the immune system are severe for the few unlucky occupants affected by them, but they are, from what we know, rare VOC effects in normal indoor environments. For this reason they are not discussed further in this chapter. Such low-level VOC effects may evade recognition if their prevalence is too small to allow a statistically significant association in a population of the size found in most normal nonindustrial buildings.

PREVALENCE OF EXPOSURES TO VOLATILE ORGANIC COMPOUNDS

Exposures to VOC in Nonindustrial Buildings

Building and furniture materials are known to emit VOCs. Ventilation transports outdoor pollutants to the indoor environment. The ventilation system may be a source of VOCs

Environmental Toxicants: Human Exposures and Their Health Effects, 2/e. Edited by Morton Lippmann.
ISBN: 0-471-29298-2   © 2000 John Wiley & Sons, Inc.

TABLE 26-1 Classification of Indoor Organic Pollutants

Description	Abbreviation	Boiling-point range ($^\circ$C)[a]
Very volatile (gaseous) organic compounds	VVOC	< 0 to 50–100
Volatile organic compounds	VOC	50–100 to 240–260
Semivolatile organic compounds	SVOC	240–260 to 380–400
Organic compounds associated with particulate matter or particulate organic matter	POM	> 380

Source: WHO (1989).
[a] Polar compounds appear at the higher of the range.

(Mølhave and Thorsen, 1991). Any human activity is a potential source of such volatile organic compounds. Maintenance, cleaning, and cooking create their own sources. Human metabolism and human activities such as smoking are other sources of gases and vapors. To these sources may be added copy machines, printing machines, glue, spray cans, and so on.

From a number of early small-scale studies, it became evident that the concentration of many organic compounds in indoor air exceeds that in the outdoor air. A review lists 307 VOCs identified in indoor air in different countries (Berglund et al., 1986). A WHO report (WHO, 1989) on VOCs indoors summarized the concentrations found in four major European studies. These studies (Krause et al., 1987; De Bortoli et al., 1986; Lebret et al., 1986; Wallace, 1987) were used to construct one data set for each component, representative of an average home. The data set includes percentiles of the concentration distribution for individual compounds (WHO, 1989).

TABLE 26-2 Total Concentrations of Volatile Organic Compounds (mg/m^3) Reported for Nonindustrial Atmospheric Environments

Environment	Uninhabited		Inhabited	
	New	Old	New	Old
Dwellings	0.48–18.7[a]	0.24–0.52[b]	12.9[c]	0.02–1.7[d]
				0.25[e l m]
Offices	[o]	[o]	[o]	0.09–1.51[p]
				1.05[f]
				0.4–1.6[nq]
Schools	[o]	0.01[g l]	0.86[i l m]	0.13–0.18[g l]
		0.05[h l m]		0.14[h l m]
				0.29–0.50[i k l m]
				0.22–0.31[l m]

[a] Mølhave et al. (1979).
[b] Mølhave and Andersen (1980).
[c] Frederiksson (1979).
[d] Mølhave and Møller (1979).
[e] Berglund et al. (1981).
[f] Mølhave et al. (1982).
[g] Wang (1975).
[h] Johansson (1978).
[i] Berglund et al. (1982).
[j] Johansson et al. (1978).
[k] Johansson et al. (1979).
[l] Sum of selected compounds.
[m] Johansson (1982).
[n] Estimated value.
[o] No information.
[p] Mølhave et al. (1982).
[q] Misch et al. (1982).

TABLE 26-3 Total Concentrations of Volatile Organic Compounds (mg/m^3) Measured in Occupied Nonindustrial Indoor Environments

Environment	No Complaints or Information	Complaints
Dwellings	0.02–1.7 [b]	1.05 [d]
		0.25[ckl]
		12.9[a]
Offices	—	0.09–1.51[d]
		0.4–1.6
		0.29–0.50[ijkl]
Schools	0.86[hkl]	
	0.22–0.31[hkl]	
	0.14[gkl]	
	0.13–0.18[fk]	
Weighted average	0.36($n = 47$)	1.31($n = 24$)

[a] Frederiksson (1979).
[b] Mølhave and Møller (1979).
[c] Berglund et al. (1981).
[d] Mølhave et al. (1982).
[e] Miksch et al. (1982).
[f] Wang (1975).
[g] Johansson (1978).
[h] Berglund et al. (1982).
[i] Johansson et al. (1978).
[j] Johansson et al. (1979).
[k] Sum of selected compounds.
[l] Johansson (1982).

These and a few other publications have been reviewed (Mølhave, 1986). Table 26-2 shows the total concentrations (TVOC) reported by Mølhave (1986) for a few other buildings than the average home (Mølhave et al., 1982; Miksch et al., 1982). The measurement sites have been divided into dwellings, offices, and schoolrooms. The concentrations in older houses (range 0.02–1.7 mg/m^3) seem to be about 1/10 that found in new houses, where the range of concentrations is from 0.5 mg/m^3 to 19 mg/m^3. Corresponding occupational total concentrations will typically be in the range of 0.1 to 1 times their respective occupational threshold limit values (TLVs), which are about 40 to 400 mg/m^3 (ACGIH, 1997). The question therefore is whether the nonindustrial concentrations are so low that the VOCs have no effect by themselves or do not interact with other factors to result in noticeable effects.

In 8 of the 12 measurements reported by Johansson (1982), human reactions were described. These 8 measurements are shown in Table 26-3. The concentrations in houses with indoor climate problems are in the range from 0.09 to 13 mg/m^3, whereas the concentration in houses where no problems were reported is from 0.02 to 1.7 mg/m^3.

The reported concentrations are improperly documented and may represent biased sampling. Further the number of houses and the measurements are treated nonsystematically and are therefore insufficient for one to draw any conclusions. The concentrations do, however, indicate that exposure to volatile organic compounds is generally higher in problem houses than in houses without problems, and complaints seem to arise when the concentrations exceed 1.7 mg/m^3.

In summary, about 50 to 300 volatile organic compounds are usually found in air samples from nonindustrial environments. Each compound seldom exceeds a concentration of about 50 mg/m^3, which is 100 to 1000 times lower than relevant occupational threshold limit values (TLVs) (ACGIH, 1999). An upper extreme average total concentration of all VOCs in most occupied homes seems to be 20 mg/m^3. The total concentration of all VOCs is, however, usually well below 1 mg/m^3, which is only 0.2% of the TLV for toluene. Toluene is one of the most frequently found compounds and in relatively high concentrations.

The Concept of Total Volatile Organic Compounds

At present there is no standardized way to summarize the combined effects of the many different compounds in the atmosphere. Addition of the masses of the various molecules has been suggested (Mølhave, 1986; Mølhave and Nielsen, 1992) as a total VOC (TVOC) indicator. This measure is easily obtained through chemical analysis. From a biological point of view, molar concentrations (number of molecules per cubic meter, in ppm of ppb) may be more relevant. Mathematical functions based on combinations of other variables such as type of radicals, vapor pressure, or polarity of the compounds have also been suggested as indicators.

For practical and analytical reasons, identification and quantification of each of the hundreds of compounds in normal indoor air is impossible in most cases. The TVOC therefore is often measured on a flame ionization detector calibrated against toluene (or any other normally occurring organic compound). The use of flame ionization detectors (FID) and photo ionization detectors (PID) is discussed by Gammage (1986), and Mølhave and Nielsen (1992) explains the necessary calibration procedures. The EU-ECA discourage the use of simple integrating instruments (EU-ECA, 1997).

This simplification of the TVOC concept is based on limited experimental evidence (Mølhave and Nielsen, 1992). It must be noted that the TVOC concept has not yet been thoroughly tested in practice, as a health risk indicator and, it therefore is still a postulate.

A standardized method for measuring TVOC has been proposed by an EU working group (EU-ECA, 1997). A Nordic consensus group (Andersson, 1997) discussed the use of this method and concluded that the literature is inconclusive with respect to the use of TVOC for risk estimates, since insufficient data are available to establish threshold limit values/guidelines based on TVOC.

A working group at the ASTM conference "Healthy Buildings 97" also discussed the use of TVOC and concluded that despite its obvious limitations and imperfections TVOC will be used in the future as an aid in limiting the concentrations of pollutants indoors. TVOC should, however, be used in the recommended standardized way and as a screening tool only. The group concluded that TVOC should be reported together with a list of all identified VOC compounds. It should not be used as the only tool in making definitive conclusions about indoor air quality.

HEALTH AND VOLATILE ORGANIC COMPOUNDS

Sick Building Syndrome

An international working group under WHO noted in 1982 that many of the indoor climate problems dealt with in the literature seem to describe buildings with the same types of problems (WHO, 1982). These buildings are characterized by the same set of frequently appearing complaints and symptoms. The group suggested that the term *sick building syndrome (SBS)* be used for this set of symptoms, which appears as part of Table 26-4.

In the literature the symtoms listed in Table 26-4 and similar symptoms have been used to define other syndromes, which in many cases appear to be synonyms for the sick building syndrome. These synonyms include the building disease, building illness syndrome, building-related illness, or tight office building syndrome. The WHO definition of the SBS was the first attempt to combine these syndromes into one general definition. Table 26-5 summarizes the definition of the SBS (WHO, 1982, 1984; Mølhave, 1986, 1990).

The WHO group stated that more than 30% of all new buildings seem to be affected by these indoor climate problems, which, further, seem to have no evident cause (WHO,

TABLE 26-4   Five Categories of Symptoms Exemplified by Some Complaints Reported by Occupants Supposed to Suffer from the Sick Building Syndrome

Sensory irritation in eyes, nose, and throat
Pain, sensation of dryness, smarting feeling, stinging, irritation, hoarseness, voice problems
Neurological or general health symptoms
Headache, sluggishness, mental fatigue, reduced memory, reduced capability to concentrate, dizziness, intoxication, nausea and vomiting, tiredness
Skin irritation
Pain, reddening, smarting or itching sensations, dry skin
Nonspecific hypersensitivity reactions
Running nose and eyes, asthmalike symptoms among nonasthmatics, sounds from the respiratory system
Odor and taste symptoms
Changed sensitivity of olfactory or gustatory sense, unpleasant olfactory or gustatory perceptions

Source: WHO (1982).

1982). In these buildings, no excessive air pollution (e.g., formaldehyde) or defects in the technical installations or in the construction were evident.

The symptoms included in the syndrome may be observed in any group of persons, but "sick buildings" are characterized by a large fraction of the occupants having the symptoms. The syndrome therefore seems to be a normal reaction of a normal population to an unfavorable indoor climate. The syndrome does not seem to be restricted to a minority reacting because of an unusually high sensitivity. The WHO group suggested the possibility that the SBS symptoms have a common causality and mechanism (WHO, 1982).

No investigation of the content of this postulated SBS has yet been reported in which a well-defined spectrum of symptoms was used. In general, the descriptions of the symptoms in the literature are anecdotal and unsystematic. Therefore the existence of SBS is still a postulate.

Multiple Chemical Sensitivity

As stated by Ashford et al. (1994), most physicians generally acknowledge the existence of a small fraction of their patients with unexplainable symptoms and signs of unexplainable dysfunctions which may or may not be related to their environment.

TABLE 26-5   Summary of the Sick Building Syndrome

1. The five categories of symptoms shown in Table 26-1 cover the major complaints in the building.
2. Irritation of mucous membranes in eye, nose, and throat is among the most frequent symptoms.
3. Other symptoms, such as from lower airways or from internal organs, should be infrequent.
4. A large majority of occupants report symptoms.
5. The symptoms appear especially frequent in one building or in part of it.
6. No evident causality can be identified in relation either to exposures or to occupant sensitivity.

Source: WHO (1982, 1984) and Mølhave (1986, 1990).

Because of the diversity of the health effects reported by such patients most physicians abstain from classifying these as manifestations of a single disease.

However, exposures to low levels of chemicals in industrial workplaces, in indoor environments, through consumer products, or pharmaceuticals have been suggested as causative agents for some of these health effects and have given rise to a public health concern most often called multiple chemical sensitivity (MCS). The history of MCS has been summarized by Shorter (1997).

The term *multiple chemical sensitivity* and a multitude of synonyms were first coined in the United States, but it now is used also in Europe (NAC, 1992; Ashford et al., 1994; Shorter 1997). Descriptions of the observations and the nature of this controversial syndrome differ at the two sides of the Atlantic Ocean. No generally agreed definition exists, and no firm scientific basis has yet been established for the syndrome. Multiple chemical sensitivity could be called a phenomenon rather than an illness (Levy, 1997).

Most authors seem to refer to an intolerance or hyperresponsiveness to exposures to low levels of chemicals at home, during work, or in the course of their life activities. Sensitization and subsequent responses are supposedly not associated with exposures to one specific chemical but to the mere presence of chemicals as such. When exposed, the affected persons report a variety of symptoms in several organs or body systems in addition to allergy and asthma, and the "diagnosis" is often made by the patient, usually alone or with the help of clinical ecologists. Since MCS seen to affect few individual occupants with unusual high sensitivity, MCS must be different from SBS, which affects large fractions of building occupants.

No single widely accepted test of physiological function has been shown to correlate with MCS symptoms presented by patients and medical diagnosis, and treatments are still to be considered experiments.

PREVALENCE OF THE SICK BUILDING SYNDROME

Field Investigations

The SBS symptoms referred to by different authors are nonspecific and undefined in most publications. In addition exposures are poorly measured. Therefore a scientifically performed comparison of the prevalence of symptoms found in different reports of field investigations is generally not possible. To review the available publications on investigations of SBS symptoms, these symptoms were instead classified according to the five categories of symptoms mentioned in Table 26-5 (Mølhave, 1991).

Indoor climate reactions classified as SBS according to Tables 26-4 and 26-5 were found in 11 of 13 investigations identified (Mølhave, 1991). Most of these investigations dealt with comparison of a building with manifest indoor climate reactions among its occupants to a control building without such problems. Two publications dealt with the frequencies of symptoms among the normal populations of randomly selected buildings. These publications were used as references for comparison with the frequencies of symptoms among occupants who seem to suffer from SBS. Further reference was made to a major questionnaire investigation among the Danes.

Table 26-6 summarizes the 13 investigations and shows the range of peak frequencies of symptoms reported within each of the five categories of symptoms shown in Table 26-5. This table is explained in detail elsewhere (Mølhave, 1991). No definitive conclusion regarding the SBS and its symptoms is possible from the unsystematic investigations summarized in Table 26-6. Nevertheless, some tendencies are seen in the scant material. The main conclusion is that if a SBS exists, it probably includes sensory irritation and headache. In six of the supposed sick buildings, information was given about both

TABLE 26-6 Ranges of Percentage of Complainers in Buildings with Occupants Apparently Suffering from the Sick Building Syndrome

	Sick buildings	Control buildings	Random buildings	Number of Significant Differences [a]	Number of Investigations
Sensory irritation	35–90	0–36	8–56	5	11
Neurological symptoms	31–100	0–45	20–56	3	9
Skin irritation	5–38	2–22	2–25	1	5
Unspecific reaction	4–41	4–24	2–21	1	3
Odor and taste	(0) [b]	(25) [b]	[c]	0	1

Source: Mølhave (1991).

Note: The frequencies are compared to frequencies in control buildings without complaints and in randomly selected buildings. The symptoms have been grouped according to the five categories of symptoms described in Tables 26-4 and 26.5.

[a] Between sick buildings and control buildings.
[b] Estimated values.
[c] No information.

irritation and headache, and in all six cases the symptom frequencies were highest in the supposed sick buildings. Further these six investigations included five of the six cases where a significant difference was found between buildings with and without indoor climate problems. This supports the hypothesis that these two symptoms are part of an SBS.

It is not possible from the available literature to evaluate the revalence of other symptoms for the SBS, although odor and taste symptoms appear in so few publications that their relevance for the SBS is unlikely. These two symptoms, however, may be included in other occupant complaints such as bad air quality or stuffiness.

Controlled Experiments

Occupational threshold limit values are normally based on evidence from exposures to concentrations that are much higher than those found in the indoor environment. Furthermore such experiments often focus on health effects that are much more severe than the relatively harmless comfort-reducing mucous membrane irritation.

Only a few relevant controlled experiments are therefore available for extrapolation to the low concentration range. The question is still open whether concentrations of volatile organic compounds in the nonindustrial indoor air are sufficiently below the threshold for comfort-reducing irritation and other symptoms included in the sick building syndrome.

To test if low exposure levels of VOCs may cause discomfort, four controlled exposure experiments were established in climate chambers in Denmark (Mølhave, et al. 1986, 1991; Kjœrgaard et al., 1989; 1991). A more recent experiment in the United States replicated the first of these Danish experiments (Otto et al., 1991). The exposure in four of these experiments consisted of a mixture of the same 22 compounds in the same relative concentrations. Only the total concentration of VOC was changed. These experiments have been summarized (Mølhave, 1991), and Table 26-7 brings together the conclusions of the five exposure experiments and the review of 13 field investigations mentioned

TABLE 26-7   Effects on Human Health and Well-being Caused by Exposure to VOC in the Indoor Climate

Effect	VOC Exposure (mg/m^3)			Cofactors	
	0–2.9	3–25	> 25	Exposure Duration and Carryover	Subject Sensibility
Sensory irritation	1/1/4	5/0/1	2/0/4	1/2/3	1/1/4
Olfaction	2/0/4	5/0/1	2/0/4	2/1/3	1/1/4
Toxic irritation (tissue changes)	1/1/4	5/0/1	2/0/4	1/1/4	2/0/4
Weak neurological	1/1/4	5/0/1	2/0/4	1/0/5	0/1/5
Lung and lower airway	0/0/6	0/0/6	1/0/5	0/0/6	1/0/5
Allergy, etc.	0/0/6	0/0/6	0/0/6	0/0/6	0/0/6
Systemic and organ	0/0/6	0/0/6	0/0/6	0/0/6	0/0/6

Source: Mølhave (1991).

Note: Six investigations (5 exposure experiments and a review of 13 field investigations) are summarized. The numbers show the numbers of these studies indicating positive or negative effects or the effects not investigated (positive/negative/not investigated).

previously. The table shows how many of the six data sets indicated positive or negative findings at different VOC levels in relation to five main types of effects.

The five exposure experiments provide no consistent information about lung function or allergic or systemic effects at any exposure levels and, except for olfaction, no effects at exposure levels below 3 mg/m^3. At present the response of the olfactory sense seems to be the most sensitive indicator of VOC exposure.

Investigations of sensory irritation, olfaction, skin irritation, and weak neurological effects caused by exposure levels of 3 mg/m^3 and higher have indicated effects in all experiments dealing with such exposure levels. Further, in Table 26-7, the possibility of cofactor interaction is indicated for the two groups of factors: (1) effect of exposure duration, adaptation, and carryover effects from one exposure episode to the next; and (2) personal factors, for example, relating to a subject's sensitivity. No conclusion can be made about the influence of cofactors. In the few investigations dealing with cofactors, both positive and negative indications were found. The information, however, indicates that future research with more sensitive experimental designs and analytical methods may better reveal such effects.

DOSE–RESPONSE FOR HEALTH EFFECTS CAUSED BY LOW LEVEL VOC EXPOSURE

Little is known about the effects of low-level VOC exposures characteristic of nonindustrial environments. Evidence from experiments and investigation indicates (Mølhave, 1990) that the most frequent effects of VOC exposure at low level fall into three classes: (1) perception of the environmental exposure caused by acute stimulations of sense, (2) perception or observation of acute or subacute inflammatorylike reactions, mostly in the exposed tissues, and (3) subacute environmental stress reactions caused by the perceptions (Mølhave, 1990). The primary effects are stimulation of sensory nerve endings and initiation of weak inflammatory tissue reactions. The secondary acute effects are perceptions of the tissue reactions, reflexes initiated by the primary perception of

TABLE 26-8   Three classes of Human Responses to VOCs in Normal Indoor Air

Primary effects	Secondary effects
Acutely perceived deterioration of the quality of the environment	
Recognition of the environmental exposures (odors)	Related reflexes in eyes, upper or lower airways
Stinging, itching, or tingling feeling from tissues (irritation)	Changed mucosal secretion (changed tearfilm stability; changed cell counts in eye liquids)
Reduced air quality (need more ventilation)	Difficulties in breathing
	Activities to change the environment
Acute or subacute reactions in skin or mucous membranes similar to beginning inflammatory reactions	
Dilatation of peripheral vessels	Pain
Stinging, itching, or tingling feeling (irritation)	Changed skin temperature (face and body, subjective temperature)
Subacute and weak stress-like reactions ("environmental stress")	
Discomfort, complaints (headache, drowsiness)	Complications in other body functions and psychological effects such as mood changes and absenteeism
	Changes composition of eye and nose liquids
	Changed odor threshold
	Changed performance

Note: Primary reactions are observed at acute low-level exposures. Secondary effects are observed after prolonged or more intense exposures.

exposures or changed sensitivity of the senses from the tissue changes. Subacute effects may also occur. They are environmental stress reactions or more severe skin reaction. The three types of effects expected to follow from low-level exposure to VOC according to this model are summarized in Table 26-8.

The intensity of each of the symptoms may be modified by additional factors such as age, smoking habits, and gender. The number of symptoms observed and their intensity may further have a feedback effect on people's behavior, causing them, for example, to modify their environment or to focus on certain symptoms and thus suppress others. As a consequence each subject may react differently to the mixed exposure and exhibit only a few of the spectrum of symptoms observed in the exposed population.

The effects associated with VOC exposures in this model are nonspecific and may be caused by other environmental exposures than chemicals. For example, physical exposures such as temperature or biological inert dust may cause a similar spectrum of symptoms. A discussion of the relationship between VOCs and the different symptoms listed in Table 26-8 must consider not only the VOC exposure levels but also the levels of other contributing exposures.

In consequence field conditions reveal three exposure ranges of VOCs to be of interest. They are defined by the relative contribution of VOCs to the effects or symptoms observed. Below the lowest threshold (the no-effect level) no effect is expected to follow from exposure to VOCs despite the simultaneous exposure to other exposure factors. Above the upper threshold (the effect level) an effect of VOCs is always seen, even when all other factors are controlled and acceptable. Between the two thresholds a correlation may or may not occur between exposure and effects of VOCs depending on interactions with other exposure factors and the potency of the compounds in the mixture of VOC. In this exposure range complaints do not necessarily disappear if one exposure factor (e.g., the VOCs) is identified and removed from the environment.

Measurable group responses were found in the controlled exposure experiments summarized above. They follow a gradient from sensory effects (for example, an odor at about 3 mg/m^3)– to indications of subacute stress reactions at about 25 mg/m^3. Regular toxic health effects such as inflammatory tissue changes or neurotoxic effects such as intoxication in the normal unsensitized population may be expected at higher exposures (> 25 mg/m^3). This exposure range, however, is outside the scope of this review.

From the field investigations it appears that although the symptoms observed are not systematically described, they are more frequent among those exposed than among the nonexposed. It was found that complaints seem to be present when the concentrations exceed 1.7 mg/m^3. Below 1.7 mg/m^3 complaints may occur if other types of simultaneous exposures are present (Mølhave, 1986). The concentrations reported from field investigations are improperly documented, and they may be biased. The exposure range of 0.19 to 0.66 mg/m^3 was estimated in the Danish Town Hall Study for the lower, no-effect threshold (Zweers et al., 1990). This range corresponds to the range of lower limit of concentrations in buildings with complaints (Mølhave, 1986). It is at present the best first estimate of the lower exposure limit for no effects of VOC, but it should, at this level of documentation, only be used for screening purposes.

Laboratory experiments indicate that the main effects can be experimentally reproduced and that they acutely follow exposure. No field investigations have been reported tests of the effects of elimination or modification of VOC exposure. Postexposure measurements during the controlled experiments indicate, however, that the effects are reversible and disappear shortly after exposure (Mølhave et al., 1991).

Exposures in most field investigations are multifactorial, since factors other than VOC exposure may exceed their no-effects levels and most of the effects reported in field investigations may have more than one cause. It is therefore not surprising that the effects of VOC exposures in field investigations occur at lower exposure levels than in controlled experiments where most other factors are supposed to be below their no-effect levels. In the experiments the exposure times were less than 3 hours, which, from field experience, seem too short to cause severe subacute effects at low-exposure levels. More research is needed to test for subacute effects at prolonged exposures.

In conclusion, there is no evidence to contradict the proposed causal link between low-level exposure to VOC and the effects shown in Table 26-8. On the contrary, evidence from both field investigations and controlled exposure experiments supports causality. The field investigations and controlled experiments, as concluded by the Nordic consensus group (Andersson et al., 1997), are, however, still too few to allow a final conclusion.

GUIDELINES FOR VOLATILE ORGANIC COMPOUNDS IN NONINDUSTRIAL INDOOR ENVIRONMENTS

Principles for Establishment of Guidelines

Two different methods are used in the evaluation of indoor air. The first involves a quantitative evaluation of the risks of adverse irreversible health effects (e.g., asphyxiation by CO or lung cancer associated with radon) or the risks of reversible or irreversible changes in the body's physiological functions (e.g., nervous system effects). This is the traditional occupational or environmental evaluation of health risks, which is done according to standard toxicological principles including risk estimates and cost–benefit analysis. This is the background for air quality guidelines, for ambient air standards for air pollutants, and for TLVs and occupational exposure standards for light levels and sound levels; it is based on lists of high-risk compounds.

The second method involves qualitative evaluations of the atmospheric environment and is, in many respects, a new concept for regulation, since qualitative aspects are often neglected in discussions of indoor air quality. Air deodorants, painting, wallpapers, and music are liked by some persons and disliked by others. Indeed, generally accepted principles for regulation of the quality of the indoor environment with respect to odor, sound, and color may be impossible to achieve if they are at all desirable.

Some general principle IAQ guideline for setting can, however, be drawn for future regulations of VOCs in the indoor environment, including building codes, acoustics, and lightning, besides the principles used for setting TLV levels.

The first is a basic consideration of the building's occupants, since the indoor environment often supports a range of human activities, habits, and preferences. Complaints and a decrease in productivity will automatically follow outside this range, for example, if the occupants must read in a dark room, are disturbed by loud intermittent noise, or must work in bright light causing reflections on their computer monitors.

Activity patterns in homes are generally different from those in offices. They include recreation, rest and sleep, and other activities which are not usually found in offices. Further the occupants of homes may be more sensitive than the working population, since they could include the sick, the young, and the elderly.

The second consideration is based on the assumption that humans do not feel well if they do not have full use of their senses to perceive information about their environment and to monitor the activities. The ideal indoor environment therefore is one that does not interfere with the occupants use of their senses nor hinder them in attending to their daily activities. The occupants should be able to discriminate among environmental signals undisturbed by unwanted information, or environmental noise. This means that environmental noise should be damped, for example, the sound of a typing machine when in an office or the neighbor's radio when at home. The environment should facilitate private conversation or concentration on one's own activities. In short, the idea is to optimize the signal-to-noise ratio by allowing the wanted signals to propagate and damping unwanted sensory signals.

This principle reflects the different needs of occupants and their different optimal environments. The signals that carry information to one person relevant to his activity may for another person create sensory noise. Therefore the signal-to-noise ratio differ from person to person.

In summary, indoor air quality is acceptable if no unacceptable health risk exists and if all chemical sources can be easily detected by the occupants and the unwanted sources can be removed.

A Tentative Guideline for VOCs in Nonindustrial Environments

Investigations of VOCs have encountered major limitations. Presently there is no acceptable basis for setting official recommendations or guidelines (Andersson et al., 1997), though discussion of some possible guidelines has been initiated (Mølhave, 1998). There are indications that VOCs are responsible for some of the discomfort from indoor odors and irritative symptoms in eyes, nose, and throat, and headache due to indoor air quality. The effects on the senses may be reflected in human productivity and performance. However, such effects have not yet been positively identified.

Most indoor environments in nonindustrial buildings are air polluted with 10 to 100 VOCs. Each pollutant is generally present in concentrations ranging from ng to few hundred micrograms. The list of indoor compounds, when identified, may exceed 1000 compounds. So far toxicity of the VOCs in the low exposure range is unknown, and their possible interactions cannot be predicted with the existing knowledge.

Lacking guidelines for indoor air quality, practitioners have had to use simple approximations in evaluating air quality. One of these is the Total Volatile Organic Compound indicator (TVOC), which is the sum of the individual concentrations of all VOC present. TVOC has been discussed by several international working groups (EU-ECA, 1997; Andersson et al., 1997) as described above. TVOC should only be used to screen potentially unacceptable exposures to VOC and should not be used to arrive at definitive conclusions.

Tentative screening values for VOCs in nonindustrial environments have been suggested (Mølhave, 1991). Presently the available epidemiological studies and the exposure experiments indicate that if specific potential irritants can be eliminated from an indoor environment (which they seldom can), exposures to VOCs below about $0.2 \, mg/m^3$ are unlikely to have irritation effects. The ambient air levels are generally below that level, which for screening purposes may be used as a first estimate of a lower limit for possible effects of VOCs.

At concentrations higher than about $3 \, mg/m^3$, complaints often occur, which has been the case in most investigated buildings where occupants complain symptoms. Controlled exposure experiments using a mixture 22 VOCs show odors to be significant at $3 \, mg/m^3$. At $5 \, mg/m^3$ in these exposure experiments, objective effects are indicated in addition to general irritant discomfort. Exposures for 50 minutes to $8 \, mg/m^3$ have resulted in significant irritation of mucous membranes in the eyes, nose, and throat.

Few acceptable exposure levels are given in the literature that allow us to estimate the threshold for a headache. Concentrations below $3 \, mg/m^3$ were found, in field investigations, to produce a significant difference in the frequency of a headache in problem buildings and in control buildings. A strong headache was found in only one exposure experiment which involved $25 \, mg/m^3$. The lower threshold in field investigations may reflect the interaction of other exposures or the effect of longer exposure durations. Therefore, based on the present information, the threshold for a headache and other weak neurotoxic effects caused by exposure of less than a few hours' duration are expected to be between 3 and $25 \, mg/m^3$. These conclusions are based on prevalent effects of VOC on otherwise healthy subjects. Risk groups may respond more strongly. Future investigations involving larger groups of people may reveal other effects, allergic or carcinogenic, associated with low-level exposures to VOCs. These effects, however, have not been demonstrated so far for the type and concentration of VOCs found in indoor air.

A tentative dose–response relationship for discomfort resulting from exposure to VOCs is shown in Table 26-9. The table, which should only be used for screening purposes,

TABLE 26-9   Tentative Dose–Response for Discomfort Resulting from Exposure to Solventlike Volatile Organic Compounds

Total Concentration (mg/m^3)	Irritation and Discomfort	Exposure Range
< 0.20	No irritation or discomfort	Comfort range
0.20–3.00	Irritation and discomfort possible if other exposures interact	Multifactorial exposure range
3.0–25	Exposure effect and probable headache possible if other exposures interact	Discomfort range
> 25	Additional neurotoxic effects other than headache may occur	Toxic range

Source: Mølhave (1991)

Note: VOCs with a normal range of biological activity. The table should only be used for screening purposes.

indicates a possible no-effect level at about 0.2 mg/m^3. A multifactorial exposure range may exist from 0.2 to 3 mg/m^3 where odor, irritation, and discomfort due to VOC exposure may depend on the types of compounds present and whether other exposures contribute to the etiology. Above about 3 mg/m^3, responses to VOC exposure are likely, and in exposures above 25 mg/m^3 there can be expected toxic effects.

REFERENCES

American Conference of Governmental Industrial Hygienists (ACGIH). 1999. *TLVs: Threshold Limit Values and Biological Exposure Indices for 1999.* Cincinnati, OH: ACGIH.

Andersson, K., J. V. Bakke, O. Björseth, C. G. Bornhehag, G. Clausen, J. K. Hongslo, M. Kjellman, S. K. Kjærgaard, F. Levy, L. Mølhave, S. Skerfving, J. Sundell. 1997. TVOC and health in non-industrial indoor environments. Report from a Nordic scientific consensus meeting at Långholmen in Stockholm, 1996. *Indoor Air* 7: 78–91.

Andrew, L. S., and R. Snyder. 1980. Toxic effects of solvents and vapors. In *Casarett and Doull's Toxicology. The Basic Science of Poisons*, eds. L. J. Casarett and J. Doull. New York: Macmillan.

Ashford, N., B. Hewinzow, K. Lütjen, C. Maruoli, L. Mølhave, B. Mönch, S. Papadopoulos, K. Rest, D. Rosdahl, P. Siskos, and E. Volonakis. 1994. Chemical sensitivity in selected European countries: An explorative study. Report from Ergonomia Ltd, Athens, Greece. Commission of the European Union, DG-V. Agreement SOC 93 2027 48 05E01 (93CVVF1-613-0).

Berglund, B., I. Johansson, and T. Lindvall. 1981. *Underlag för Ventilationsnormer. ETAPP II* (Ventilation Requirements, in Swedish). Stockholm: National Institute of Environmental Medicine.

Berglund, B., I. Johansson, and T. Lindvall. 1982. A longitudinal study of air contaminants in a newly built preschool. *Environ. Int.* 8: 111–116.

Berglund, B., U. Berglund, and T. Lindvall. 1986. Assessment of discomfort and irritation from the indoor air. p. 138–149. In *Proc. IAQ-86.* Managing Indoor Air for Health and Energy Conservation, Atlanta: American Society of Heating Refrigerating and Air Conditioning Engineers.

Berglund, B., B. Brunekreef, H. Knöppel, T. Lindvall, M. Maroni and L. Mølhave. 1992. Effects of indoor air pollution on human health. *Indoor Air* 2: 2–25.

De Bortoli, A, H. Knöppel, E. Pecchio, and A. Peil. 1986. Concentrations of selected organic pollutants in the indoor and outdoor air in northern Italy. *Environ. Int.* 12: 343–356.

(EU-ECA) Berglund, B., G. Clausen, J. De Ceaurriz, A. Kettrup, T. Lindvall, M. Maroni, L. Mølhave, T. C. Pickering, U. Risse, H. Rothweiler, B. Seifert and M. Younes. 1997. Total organic compounds (TVOC) in indoor air quality investigations. Report 19 of the European collaborative action "Indoor Air Quality and Its Impact on Man." *EU-Report EUR 17675 EN.* Joint Research Center, Ispra, Italy.

Frederiksson, K. 1979. Gifter i Bostadsluft (Indoor air pollution, in Swedish). *Hälovårdskontakt* 3: 14–19.

Gammage, R. B. 1986. *Volatile Organic Compounds. AIHA Indoor Environmental Quality.* Reference Manual (DE-AC05-840R-21400). Oak Ridge, TN: Health and Safety Research Division, Oak Ridge National Laboratory.

Johannsson, I. 1978. Determination of organic compounds in indoor air with potential reference to air quality. *Atmos. Environ.* 12: 1371–1377.

Johansson, I. 1982. Kemiska Luftförreningar Inomhus. *En litteraturs Sammentätllning (Chemical Indoor Air Pollution, a Swedish Review).* Stockholm: National Institute of Environmental Medicine.

Johansson, I., S. Petterson, and T. Rehn. 1978. Gas chromatographic analysis of room air in recently built preschools (in Swedish). *VVSJ* 49: 51–55.

Johansson, I., S. Petterson, and T. Rehn. 1979. Indoor air pollutants (in Swedish). *VVSJ* 50: 6–7.

Kjærgaard, S. K., L. Mølhave, and O. F. Pedersen. 1989. Human reactions to indoor air pollutants: *n*-Decane. *Environ. Int.* 15: 473–482.

Kjærgaard, S. K., L. Mølhave, and O. F. Pedersen. 1991. Human reactions to a mixture of indoor air volatile organic compounds. *Atmos. Environ.* 24A: 1417–1426.

Krause, C., W. Mailahn, R. Nagel, C. Schulz, B. Seifert, and D. Ulrich. 1987. Occurrence of volatile organic compounds in the air of 500 homes in the Federal Republic of Germany. In *Indoor Air 87'*, eds. B. Seifert, H. Esdron, M. Fischer, H. Füden, and J. Wegner. Berlin: Institute of Water, Soil and Air Hygiene.

Lebret, E., J. Van de Wiel, H. P. Bos, D. Noij, and J. S. M. Boleij. 1986. Volatile organic compounds in Dutch homes. *Environ. Int.* 12: 323–332.

Levy, F. 1997. Clinical features of multiple chemical sensitivity. *Scand. J. Work. Environ. Health* 23 (suppl. 3): 69–73.

Miksch, R. R., C. D. Hollowell, and H. E. Schmidt. 1982. Trace organic chemical contaminants in office spaces. *Environ. Int.* 8:129–137.

Mølhave, L. 1986. Indoor air quality in relation to sensory irritation due to volatile organic compounds. Publication 2954 *ASHRAE Trans.* 92: 306–316.

Mølhave, L. 1990. Volatile organic compounds, indoor air quality and health. In *Indoor Air '90: Proc. 5th International Conference on Indoor Air Quality and Climate, Toronto.* 1990, ed. D. Walkinshaw, vol 5, pp. 15–33. Ottawa: Canada Mortgage and Housing Corporation.

Mølhave, L. 1991. Human response to volatile organic compounds as air pollutants in normal buildings. *J. Exposure Anal. Environ. Epidemiol.* 1: 63–81.

Mølhave, L. 1998. Principles for evaluation of health and comfort hazards caused by indoor air pollution. *Indoor Air.* 8(Suppl. 4): 17–25.

Mølhave, L., and I. Andersen. 1980. Forureningskomponenter i indeluften i "Nulenergihuset" ved DTH (Air pollution in an experimental house, in Danish). *Varme* 45: 121–125.

Mølhave, L., and J. Møller. 1979. The atmospheric environment in modern Danish dwellings – Measurements in 39 flats. In *Indoor Climate*, eds. P. O. Fanger and O. Valbjørn. Copenhagen: Danish Building Research Institute.

Mølhave, L., and M. Thorsen. 1991. A model for investigations of ventilation systems as sources for volatile organic compounds in indoor climate. *Atmos. Environ.* 25A: 241–249.

Mølhave, L., and G. D. Nielsen. 1992. The TVOC indicator of human response to low level exposures to volatile organic compounds (VOC). *Indoor Air* 2:65–77.

Mølhave, L., J. Møller, and I. Andersen. 1979. Luftens indhold af gasser, dampe og støv i nyere boliger (Indoor air pollution in home, in Danish). *Ugesk. Læger* 141: 956–961.

Mølhave, L., I. Andersen, G. R. Lundqvist, P. A. Nielsen, and O. Nielsen. 1982. *Afgasning fra Byggematerialer – forekomst og Hygiejnisk Vurdering* (Emission of Air Pollutants from Building Materials, in Danish with English summary). SBI-Report 137. Copenhagen: Danish Institute of Building Research.

Mølhave, L., B. Bach, and O. F. Pedersen. 1986. Human reactions to low concentrations of volatile organic compounds. *Environ. Int.* 12: 167–175.

Mølhave, L., J. G. Jensen, and S. Larsen. 1991. Subjective reactions to volatile organic compounds as air pollutants. *Atmos. Environ.* 25A:1283–1293.

(NAS) National Research Council. 1992. Multiple Chemical Sensitivities. Addendum to Biological Markers in Immunotoxicology. National Research Council. Washington DC: National Academy Press.

Otto, D. A., L. Mølhave, G. Rose, H. K. Hudnell and D. House. 1991. Neurobehavioral and sensory irritant effects of controlled exposure to a complex mixture of volatile organic compounds. *Neurotoxicol. Teratol.* 12: 649–652.

Shorter, E. 1997. Multiple chemical sensitivity: Pseudo disease in historical perspective. *Scand. J. Work Environ. Health* 23 (suppl. 3): 35–42.

Wallace, L. 1987. *The Total Assessment Methodology (TEAM) Study: Summary and Analyses,* vol. 1. Washington, DC: U.S. Environmental Protection Agency.

Wang, T. C. 1975. A study of bioeffluents in a college classroom. *ASHRAE Trans.* 81: 32–44.

World Health Organization (WHO). 1961. *Constitution of the World Health Organization: Basic Documents,* 15th edition. Geneva: WHO.

World Health Organization (WHO). 1982. *Indoor Air Pollutants, Exposure and Health Effects Assessment.* Euro-Reports and Studies 78: Working Group Report. Copenhagen: WHO Regional Office for Europe.

World Health Organization (WHO). 1984. *Indoor Air Quality Research*. Euro-Reports and Studies 103. Copenhagen: WHO Regional Office for Europe.

World Health Organization (WHO). 1989. *Indoor Air Quality: Organic Pollutants*. Report on a WHO Meeting, Euro-Reports and Studies 111. Copenhagen: WHO Regional Office for Europe.

Zweers, T., P. Skov, O. Valbjørn, and L. Molhave. 1990. The effect of ventilation and air pollution on perceived indoor air quality in five town halls. *Energy Bldgs.* 14: 175–181.

27 Perspectives on Individual and Community Risks

ARTHUR C. UPTON, M.D.

Humankind has always faced certain dangers. Risk is an inescapable fact of life. However, enlightened societies have traditionally sought to minimize avoidable risks. The greatly increased life expectancy now enjoyed by populations in the industrialized world attests to the success with which modern civilization has been able to reduce certain risks to human health and safety.

This chapter reviews environmental risks to human health from two standpoints: the risk to the individual and the risk to the community. Considered in this context are scientific bases for assessing such risks, the relative magnitudes of different environmental risks as evaluated by knowledgeable experts, the contrasting perspectives in which risks may be perceived by different members of the public, difficulties in risk communication that complicate societal efforts to protect health and the environment, and options for reducing risks at the individual and community levels.

NATURE OF RISK

Probability of Effect

Risk is commonly defined as "hazard, peril, or exposure to loss or injury." The term *environmental risk to health* is taken herein to mean the probability of an adverse effect on human health resulting from exposure to a particular environmental agent or combination of agents. Such a risk may be expressed in various ways, depending on the context in which it is considered, for example: (1) average annual risk per individual; (2) average lifetime risk per individual; (3) average number of individuals affected annually in a given population; or (4) average loss of life expectancy in affected individuals.

For certain types of health effects, such as pollutant-induced cancers, the risk may also be expressed either as an absolute risk (i.e., absolute increase in the number or probability of such growths) or as a relative risk (i.e., a relative increase in the background frequency of such growths). Depending on the baseline frequency, or background rate, a small increase in relative risk may be equivalent to a large increase in the number of individuals affected. Conversely, merely a few additional cases of an otherwise rare disorder may result in a large increase in the relative risk, and thus in a high attributable risk, of the disorder (Table 27-1).

Environmental Toxicants: Human Exposures and Their Health Effects, 2/e. Edited by Morton Lippmann.
ISBN: 0-471-29298-2 © 2000 John Wiley & Sons, Inc.

TABLE 27-1   Different Ways in Which the Carcinogenic Effects of 1 Sv Acute Whole Body Ionizing Radiation May Be Expressed in the Individual or in the Community

	Type of cancer	
	Fatal Leukemia	Other Fatal Cancer
Risk to the individual		
Increase in relative risk (%)	400	30
Annual risk of death ($\times 10^{-4}$)	2.3	7.5
Lifetime risk of death ($\times 10^{-3}$)	10	60
Attributable risk (%)	57	8
Years of life lost per excess death	25	13
Years of life lost per exposed person	0.3	0.8
Risk to a population of 100,000		
Increase in relative risk (%)	400	30
Annual excess deaths	23	75
Lifetime excess deaths	1000	6000
Attributable risk (%)	57	8
Person-years of life lost	25,000	80,000
Year of life lost per exposed person	0.3	0.8

Sources: UNSCEAR (1988) and NAS (1990); based on data for atomic bomb survivors (Shimizu et al., 1988).

Severity of Effect

The importance attached to a given risk depends on the severity as well as the frequency of the effect in question. Determinants of severity include such factors as the extent to which the effect is or is not symptomatic, painful, disfiguring, incapacitating, reversible, progressive, lethal, and so on, these being the properties that determine its impact on the affected individual and on his or her loved ones, descendants, coworkers, neighbors, and community. In the broadest context, the measures of severity therefore have many ramifications, including esthetic, psychosocial, ethical, and economic impacts, as well as impacts on health per se (Hammond and Coppock, 1990; Arrow et al; 1996).

Psychosocial and Cultural Factors Influencing the Perception of Risk

Apart from objective measures of the frequency and severity of environmental risks to health, other qualitative characteristics, such as those listed in Table 27-2, can be important in determining how the risks are perceived (Raynor and Cantor, 1987; Fischoff et al; 1997; Omenn and Faustman, 1997). Nonscientists often not only fail to understand the technical basis for evaluating a given risk but actually distrust and reject it (Plough and Krimsky, 1987; Fischoff et al; 1997). It has been suggested therefore that the definition of an environmental risk needs to be broadened to include its nontechnical aspects that may be of concern to the public, that is, its "outrage" factors (Fig. 27-1). The importance of such nontechnical factors is illustrated by the marked degree to which public perceptions of a given risk may differ from those of informed experts (Table 27-3).

IDENTIFICATION AND QUANTIFICATION OF RISKS

Assessment of an environmental risk to human health involves a sequence of interrelated steps (Omenn and Faustman, 1997), beginning with identification of the causative agent or exposure situation, and culminating in an evaluation of the number of persons who are ultimately affected and the severity of their effects (Fig. 27-2).

TABLE 27-2 Psychosocial and Cultural Characteristics Affecting the Perception of Risk

Characteristics That Increase Acceptability of Risk	Characteristics That Decrease Acceptability of Risk
Voluntary	Involuntary
Familiar	Unfamiliar
Immediate impact	Remote impact
Detectable by individual	Nondetectable by individual
Controllable by individual	Uncontrollable by individual
Fair	Unfair
Noncatastophic	Catastrophic
Well understood	Poorly understood
Natural	Artificial
Trusted source	Untrusted source
Visible benefits	No visible benefits

Sources: Slovic et al. (1979) and Plough and Krimsky (1987).

Hazard Identification

The first of the above steps, hazard identification, consists of identifying potentially harmful agents to which persons may be exposed, regardless of the level of exposure. For this purpose, reliance has traditionally been placed primarily on clinical and epidemiological evidence. For most environmental agents of interest, however, toxicity to humans cannot be evaluated adequately from the limited clinical and epidemiological data that are available (NAS, 1984, 1994). Instead, the evaluation must depend on other toxicological approaches, including systematic analysis of pertinent molecular structure–activity relationships, results of in vitro short-term tests, and biological activity in short-term or long-term whole-animal bioassays (e.g., Tennant et al; 1987; Ashby and Tennant, 1988; ICPEMC, 1988; Omenn and Faustman, 1997). Principles and procedures for utilizing such methods in predicting toxicity to humans have been developed, but the diversity of toxic reactions caused by different agents is so large, and the variations in reactivity among different species so great, that the reliability of this approach is limited (e.g., Lave et al; 1988; NAS, 1994). For most of the chemicals in commercial production, moreover, the available toxicological data do not suffice to enable adequate evaluation (Fig. 27-3).

Dose – Response Analysis

In the second of the above steps, dose–response analysis, the mathematical relationship between the dose of the agent of interest and any health effects that it may cause is evaluated in order to estimate the nature and magnitude of risks attributable to the agent at

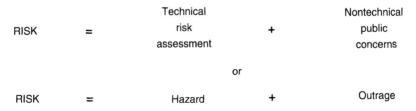

Figure 27-1 Holistic definition of risk. (Sources: Adapted from Allen 1992, and from Sandman 1985.

TABLE 27-3 'Perceived' Compared with 'Real' Risks Associated with 30 Widespread Activities and Technologies

Activity or Technology	Technical Estimates (deaths/year)[a]	Geometric Mean Fatality Estimates, Average Year		Geometric Mean Multiplier, Disastrous Year	
		LOWV[b]	Students[c]	LOWV[b]	Students[c]
Smoking	150,000	6,900	2,400	1.9	2.0
Alcoholic beverages	100,000	12,000	2,600	1.9	1.4
Motor vehicles	50,000	28,000	10,500	1.6	1.8
Handguns	17,000	3,000	1,900	2.0	2.0
Electric power	14,000	660	500	1.9	2.4
Motorcycles	3,000	1,600	1,600	1.8	1.6
Swimming	3,000	930	370	1.6	1.7
Surgery	2,800	2,500	900	1.5	1.6
X rays	2,300	90	40	2.7	1.6
Railroads	1,950	190	210	3.2	1.6
General (private) aviation	1,300	550	650	2.8	2.0
Large construction	1,000	400	370	2.1	1.4
Bicycles	1,000	910	420	1.8	1.4
Hunting	800	380	410	1.8	1.7
Home appliances	200	200	240	1.6	1.3
Fire fighting	195	220	390	2.3	2.2
Police work	160	460	390	2.1	1.9
Contraceptives	150	180	120	2.1	1.4
Commercial aviation	130	280	650	3.0	1.8
Nuclear power	100[d]	20	27	107.1	87.6
Mountain climbing	30	50	70	1.9	1.4
Power mowers	24	40	33	1.6	1.3
School and college football	23	39	40	1.9	1.4
Skiing	18	55	72	1.9	1.6
Vaccinations	10	65	52	2.1	1.6
Food coloring	[e]	38	33	3.5	1.4
Food preservatives	[e]	61	63	3.9	1.7
Pesticides	[e]	140	84	9.3	2.4
Prescription antibiotics	[e]	160	290	2.3	1.6
Spray cans	[e]	56	38	3.7	2.4

Source: Slovic et al. (1979).

[a] Based on assessments by technical experts.
[b] League of Women Voters.
[c] College students.
[d] Geometric mean of estimates, which ranged from 16 to 600 per year.
[e] Estimates were unavailable.

the levels of exposure encountered in practice. Since ambient exposure levels are typically many times lower than the levels at which any toxic effects may have been documented previously, formulation of the desired risk estimate often requires extrapolation over a broad range of doses and/or animal species, necessitating the use of a dose–response model which may be of uncertain validity (Omenn and Faustman, 1997).

Although thresholds are known to exist for many, if not most, types of toxic reactions, no threshold is known or presumed to exist for the mutagenic and carcinogenic effects of cetain toxicants (OSTP, 1985). For such agents an appropriate dose–response model must therefore be employed in estimating for exposed populations the magnitude of any risks whose selection is fraught with uncertainty (NAS, 1994). Again, the problem is

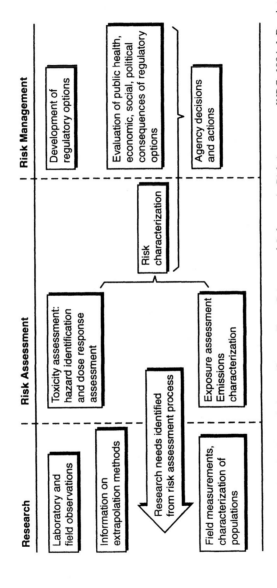

Figure 27-2 Risk assessment relies on evaluation techniques. (Source: From *Science and Judgment in Risk Assessment [NRC, 1994a]*. Reprinted with permission.)

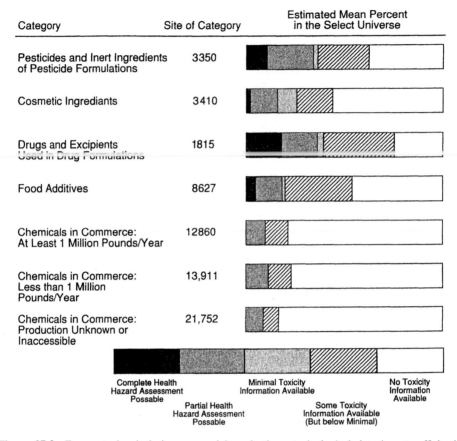

Figure 27-3 For most chemicals in commercial productions, toxicological date is not sufficiently available for adequate evaluation.

complicated by a paucity of relevant dose–response data. Even in the relatively few instances where human data are available to provide anchor points from which to extrapolate, the data do not suffice to define the dose–response relationship in the low-dose domain. In the use of dose–response data from laboratory animals, moreover, there is uncertainty both about the choice of the model for extrapolation to low doses and of the model for extrapolation to the human species (Zeise et al; 1987; Lave et al; 1988).

Another major source of uncertainty stems from the fact that in the human environment, agents are usually, if not always, encountered in combination with untold numbers of other agents, rather than in the pure form in which they have been studied in most clinical or toxicological experiments. Because synergistic or other complex interactions among agents may occur under such conditions, the combined effects of mixtures of agents can seldom be confidently predicted from what is known about the toxicological effects of any given agent acting alone (NAS, 1988; Mauderly, 1993).

Exposure Assessment

The third of the above steps, exposure assessment, consists in evaluating the extent to which persons are, or are likely to be, exposed to a particular environmental agent or combination of agents. For the most part, assessments of exposure have relied thus far largely on data from unvalidated exposure models or from the monitoring of relevant exposure media (air, water, soil, food, etc.). Monitoring of human beings themselves has been limited, in part because of the lack of suitably sensitive, reliable, and practicable methods and measures of exposure. Recent advances in analytical techniques, however, and in the development of biomolecular markers such as DNA adducts (NAS, 1987), give promise of future improvements in this area.

Risk Characterization

In the fourth of the above steps, risk characterization, the information generated in the first three steps is integrated to derive an estimate of the numbers of persons who may be affected and the types and severities of their effects. To the extent that the information obtained in each of the preceding steps is constrained by uncertainty, the final characterization of risk derived in the fourth step will, of course, be constrained correspondingly. Because of the complexity, data requirements, and cost of each step in the process, as well as the uncertainties inherent therein, detailed and comprehensive attempts at risk characterization have been made for relatively few environmental problems to date (e.g., U.S. EPA, 1987). Examples illustrating some of the uncertainties involved in such assessments are shown in Tables 27-4 and 27-5.

RISK COMMUNICATION

Bridging Different Cultures

People respond to risks as they perceive them (Fischoff et al; 1997). Hence, since experts trained and experienced in evaluating risks often fail to communicate their assessments adequately to the public, efforts to protect health and the environment are sometimes misdirected (NAS, 1996).

As noted above, perceptions of risk involve nontechnical considerations ("cultural rationality") as well as technical considerations ("technical rationality"). Hence, in order to communicate effectively about the nature and magnitude of a given risk, both types of considerations (Table 27-6) must be taken into account. Because the nontechnical considerations are rooted in cultural, anthropological, and ethical traditions, they vary among different groups in society (Fischoff et al; 1997; NAS, 1989). For communicating a given risk to all audiences, no single message is therefore likely to be adequate.

Furthermore, for optimal effectiveness in risk communication, the process should involve a two-way, iterative exchange of information between the technical risk assessor and any stakeholders who may be directly or indirectly affected. Ideally such an exchange should begin as early as possible in the process of risk assessment so that those who may bear the risks can participate fully in the derivation of the assessment itself. Trust between all who are involved is also critical to the success of risk communication, and it is best fostered through the mutual exchange of information in an open, participatory, consensual process (Sandman, 1992; NAS, 1996).

Treatment of Uncertainty

In contrast to other risks in daily life (e.g., various types of accidents whose frequencies are well documented in recorded statistics), many environmental risks to health are not known precisely and can be estimated only on the basis of unproved assumptions and extrapolations. As noted above, such assessments are complicated at virtually every step by large uncertainties in (1) the numerical values of measurements or other quantities

TABLE 27-4   Cancer Risk Rankings Assigned to Various Environmental Problems in EPA's "Unfinished Business" Report

Environmental Problem	Rank Order	Estimated U.S. Yearly Number of Cancers
Category 1 (high risk)		
Exposure of workers to chemicals	1	250 from only four of the many carcinogens in question; risks to individuals may be high
Indoor radon	1 (tied)	5000–20,000 (of lung); risks to individuals may be high
Pesticide residues in foods	3	6000 based on assessment of only seven of 200 potentially oncogenic pesticides)
Indoor air pollution (nonradon)	4	3500–6500 (primarily from tobacco smoke); risks to individuals may be high
Exposure to consumer products	4 (tied)	100–135 from only four of the more than 10,000 chemicals in consumer products
Other hazardous air pollutants	6	2000 from only 20 of the many pollutants in air; risks to individuals may be high
Category 2 (medium tohigh) risk		
Depletion of stratospheric ozone	7	Possibly 10,000 annually by the year 2100
Hazardous waste sites (inactive)	8	More than 1000
Drinking water	9	400–1000
Application of pesticides	10	100 in small population exposed; risks to individuals can be high
Radiation	11	360 (largely from building materials); risks to individuals can be high
Other pesticide risks	12	150 (estimate highly uncertain)
Hazardous waste sites (active)	13	Probably fewer than 100; risks to individuals can be high
New toxic chemicals	15	No quantitative estimate possible; risks judged to be moderate
Category 3 (low to medium risk)		
Municipal waste	16	40 (excluding municipal surface impoundments)
Contaminated sludge	17	40 (mostly from incineration and sludge)
Mining waste	18	10–20 (largely from arsenic); risks to individuals can be high
Storage tank releases	19	Less than one
Non-point-source discharges to surface water	20	No quantitative estimate, but judge to be the most serious surface water category
Other groundwater contamination	21	Less than one
Criteria air pollutants	22	Carcinogenicity questionable but exposure extensive
Category 4 (low risk)		
Direct point discharges to surface water	23	No quantitative estimate (excluding drinking water)
Indirect point-source discharges to surface water	24	No quantitative estimate
Accidental release—toxicants	25	No quantitative estimate
Accidental release—oil spills	26	No quantitative estimate
Category 5 (unranked)		
Biotechnology	—	No estimate
CO_2 and global warming	—	No estimate
Other air pollutants	—	No estimate

Source: U.S. EPA (1987).

TABLE 27-5   Estimated Risks of Human Bladder Cancer From Daily Ingestion of 0.12 g Saccharin, Based on Extrapolation from Oncogenic Effects Observed in the Rat

Method of High-to-Low-Dose Extrapolation	Liftetime Cases per Million Exposed	Cases per Million per Year
Rat dose adjusted to human dose by surface area rule		
Single-hit model	1200	840
Multistage model (with quadratic term)	5	3.5
Multihit model	0.001	0.0007
Mantel-Bryan probit model	450	315
Rat dose adjusted to human dose by mg chemical per Kg		
Body weight per day equivalence		
Single-hit model	200	147
Multihit model	0.001	0.0007
Mantel-Bryan probit model	21	14.7
Rat dose adjusted to human dose by mg chemical per Kg		
Body weight per lifetime		
Single-hit model	5200	3640
Multihit model	0.001	0.0007
Mantel-Bryan probit model	4200	2940

Source: NAS/NRC (1978).

affecting the risks; (2) the modeling of exposure and/or toxic responses; (3) temporal, spatial, and interindividual differences in exposure and/or susceptibility; and (4) the comparison of societal and personal measures of risk. To the extent that these sources of uncertainty limit the reliability of a risk assessment, each must be made explicit if the comprehensibility, credibility, and utility of the assessment are not to be jeopardized (Finkel, 1990; Morgan and Henrion, 1990; NAS, 1994).

TABLE 27-6   Comparison of Factors Relevant to the Cultural Rationality, as Opposed to the Technical Rationality, of Risk

Technical Rationality	Cultural Rationality
Trust in scientific methods, explanations, democratic process	Trust in political culture and evidence
Appeal to authority and expertise	Appeal to folk wisdom, peer groups, and traditions
Boundaries of analysis are narrow and reductionist	Boundaries of analysis are broad and include the use of analogy and historical precedent
Risks are depersonalized	Risks are personalized
Emphasis on statistical variation and probability	Emphasis on the impacts of risk on the family and community
Appeal to consistency and universality	Focus on particularity; less concerned about consistency of approach
Where there is controversy in science, resolution follows expertise, status	Popular responses to science; the differences do not follow the prestige principle
Those impacts that cannot be measured are less relevant	Unanticipated or unarticulated risk are relevant

Source: Plough and Krimsky (1987).

Placing Risks in Proper Perspective

Because the perception of risk is a complex process, risk is difficult to communicate in a way that places it in proper perspective (e.g., NAS, 1989; Zeckhauser and Viscusi, 1990; Fischoff et al; 1997). Comparisons of quantitative risk estimates, such as have often been presented for the purpose (e.g., Tables 27-7 and 27-8), or attempts to weight risks solely on the basis of their impacts on life expectancy (e.g., Cohen and Lee, 1979), on the quality of life (e.g., ICRP, 1977), or on their economic costs (e.g., Arrow et al; 1996) are likely to be inadequate by themselves (Slovic et al; 1981; NAS, 1989). Instead, the strategy for risk communication must take into account the known dynamics of risk perception, which involve the following principles: (1) unfamiliar risks tend to be less acceptable than familiar risks, (2) involuntary risks are less acceptable than voluntary risks, (3) risks controlled by others are less acceptable than risks that are under one's own control, (4) inapparent and undetectable risks are less acceptable than risks that are apparent and detectable, (5) risks that are perceived to be unfair are less acceptable than risks that are perceived to be fair, (6) risks that do not permit individual protective action are less acceptable than risks that do, (7) dramatic and dreadful risks are less acceptable than undramatic and commonplace risks, (8) unpredictable risks are less acceptable than predictable risks, (9) cross-hazard comparisons tend to be unacceptable, and (10) risk estimation is inherently of less interest to people than risk reduction, and neither is likely to be of interest in the absence of real concern about the risk, or risks, in question (Sandman, 1985; Fischoff et al., 1997).

RISK REDUCTION

While the acceptability of a given risk may vary widely among different individuals, for the reasons stated above, regulatory agencies are guided by the prevailing views of society at large in setting standards to protect human health (Rodricks, 1992). Under the Clean Air

TABLE 27-7   Situations or activities Involving a One-in-a-Million Risk of Death

Exposure of Activity	Cause of Death
Smoking 1.4 cigarettes	Cancer, heart disease
Drinking $\frac{1}{2}$ L of wine	Cirrhosis of the liver
Spending 1 h in a coal mine	Black lung disease
Spending 3 h in a coal mine	Accident
Living 2 days in New York or Boston	Air pollution
Traveling 6 min by canoe	Accident
Traveling 10 mi by bicycle	Accident
Traveling 300 mi by car	Accident
Flying 1000 mi by jet	Accident
Flying 6000 mi by jet	Cancer caused by cosmic radiation
Living 2 mo in Denver	Cancer caused by cosmic radiation
Living 2 mo in an average masonry building	Cancer caused by natural radioactivity
One chest X ray	Cancer caused by radiation
Living 2 mo with a cigarette smoker	Cancer, heart disease
Eating 40 tablespoons of peanut butter	Liver cancer caused by aflatoxin B_1
Drinking Miami drinking water for i year	Cancer caused by chloroform
Drinking 30 12-ox cans of diet soda	Cancer caused by saccharin
Living 5 years at the boundary of a nuclear plant	Cancer caused by radiation
Eating 100 charcoal-broiled steaks	Cancer caused by benzopyrene

Source: Wilson (1979).

TABLE 27-8   Ranking the Risks from Possible Carcinogens on the Basis of Their Estimated Potencies

Hazard index: HERP (%)[a]	Daily human exposure[b]	Carcinogen Dose per 70 kg Person	Potency of Carcinogen: TD 50 (mg/kg)	
Environmental pollution				
0.001*	Tap water, 1 L	Chloroform, 83 µg (U.S. avg)	(119)	90
0.004*	Well water, 1 L contaminated (worst well in Silicon Valley)	Trichloroethylene, 280 µg	(−)	941
0.0004*	Well water, 1 L contaminated, Woburn	Trichloroethylene, 267 µg	(−)	941
0.0002*		Chloroform, 12 µg	(119)	90
0.0003*		Tetrachloroethylene, 21 µg	101	(126)
0.008*	Swimming pool, 1 h (for child)	Chloroform, 250 µg (Avg. pool)	(119)	90
0.6	Conventional home air (14 h/d)	Formaldehyde, 2.2 mg	1.5	(44)
0.004		Benzene, 155 µg	(157)	53
2.1	Mobile home air (14 h/d)	Formaldehyde, 2.2 mg	1.5	(44)
Pesticide and other residues				
0.0002*	PCOs: daily dietary intake	PCDs, 0.2 µg (U.S. avg)	1.7	(9.6)
0.0003*	DDE/DT: daily dietary intake	DDE, 2.2 µg (U.S. avg)	(−)	13
0.0004*	EDB: daily dietary intake (from grains and grain products)	Ethylene dibromide, 0.42 µg (U.S. avg)	1.5	(5.1)
Natural Pesticides and dietary toxins				
0.03	Bacon, cooked (100 g)	Dimethylnitrosamine, 0.3 µg	(0.2)	0.2
0.006		Diethylnitrosamine, 0.1 µg	0.002	(+)
0.003	Sake (250 ml)	Urethane, 43 µg	(41)	22
0.003	Comfrey herb tea, 1 cup	Symphytine, 38 µg (750 µg of pyrrolizidine alkaloids)	1.9	(?)
0.003	Peanut butter (32 g; one sandwich)	Aflatoxin, 64 ng (U.S. avg, 2 ppb)	0.003	(+)
0.06	Dried squid, broiled in gas oven (54g)	Dimethylnitrosamine, 7.9 µg	(0.02)	0.2
0.007	Brown mustard (5 g)	Allyl isothiocyanate, 4.6 mg	96	(−)
0.1	Basil (1 g of dried leaf)	Estragole, 3.8 mg	(?)	52
2.8*	Beer (12 oz, 354 ml)	Ethyl alcohol, 18 ml	9110	(?)
4.7*	Wine (250 ml)	Ethyl alcohol, 30 ml	9110	(?)
Food additives				
0.06*	Diet cola	Saccharin 95 mg	2143	(−)
Drugs				
[0.3]	Phenacetin pill (avg dose)	Phenacetin, 300 mg	1246	(2137)
16*	Phenobarbital, one sleeping pill	Phenobarbital, 60 mg	(+)	5.5
17*	Clofibrate (avg daily dose)	Clofibrate, 2000 mg	169	(?)
Occupational exposure				
5.8	Formaldehyde: Avg daily intake	Formaldehyde, 6.1 mg	1.5	(44)
140	EDB: Avg daily intake (high exposure)	Ethylene dibromide, 150 mg	1.5	(5.1)

Source: Ames et al. (1987)

[a] Possible hazard: the amount of rodent carcinogen indicated under carcinogen dose is divided by 70 kg to give milligram per kilogram equivalent of human exposure, and this human dose is given as the percentage of TD_{50} in the rodent (in milligrams per kilogram) to calculate the human-exposure/rodent potency index (HERP).

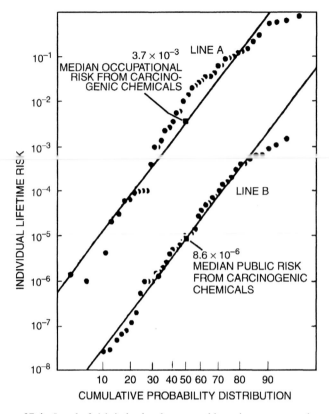

Figure 27-4   Level of risk judged to be acceptable varies among carcinogens.

Act, for example, EPA sought to limit the permissable levels of carcinogenic contaminants in air sufficiently to prevent the attributable lifetime risks of cancer in members of the public from exceeding 10^{-6}, a level of risk that was judged to be acceptably protective for the purpose (Travis, 1989). It is clear, however, that the level of risk that is judged to be acceptable has varied among different carcinogens, depending on specific circumstances (Fig. 27-4). For occupationally exposed workers, moreover, whose choice of employment is more or less voluntary, the attributable risks implied by existing regulatory limits for carcinogens are appreciably higher than those which are considered acceptable for members of the public at large (e.g., Fig. 27-4).

Measures for reducing environmental risks may involve substantial economic costs and/or the substitution of other undesirable risks. For this reason, as discussed in the next chapter, the relative costs and benefits of alternate risk management strategies must be compared with one another to decide on the most appropriate approach for reducing a given risk (Davies, 1996). Included among the criteria to be considered in such comparative risk assessments are both the risk to society and the risk to the individual, since the acceptability of a given risk generally varies inversely with the number of victims affected (e.g., Fig. 27-5).

Options for Risk Reduction at the Individual and Community Levels

Options for reducing environmental risks to human health may include measures for intervening at any point in the sequence of steps typically involved in the process by which a potentially hazardous agent is produced, is released, is transported through the

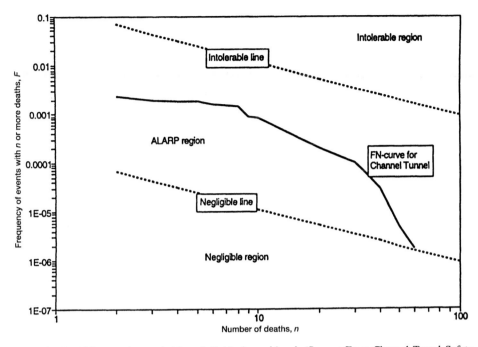

Figure 27-5 Risk to society and risk to individual considered. (Source: From Channel Turnel Safety Case (1994).

environment, reaches a susceptible individual, is taken up by the individual, and subsequently gives rise to a reaction adversely affecting the health of the individual and/or his/her offspring (Fig. 27-6). Some options are not possible without action at the community level, whereas others lie within the power of the individual acting alone. All options, however, depend to varying degrees on understanding each of the risks in question and on having the skills needed to reduce them. Research and education in the relevant

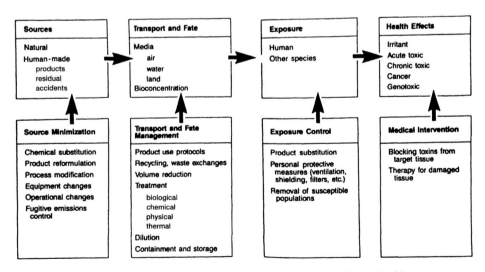

Figure 27-6 Options for reducing environmental risks to human health.

aspects of environmental health and safety are, therefore, essential for arriving at sound policies for risk reduction at the individual and the community levels (Tones, 1997).

At the community level, the options for risk reduction encompass a broad range of activities, including (1) support of research for identifying potentially hazardous agents, elucidating their toxicity and modes of action, and defining their relevant dose–effect relationships; (2) systematic monitoring of the extent to which individuals or populations may be exposed to harmful agents via air, water, soil, food, or other media, and proper assessment of the magnitude of any risks that may result from such exposures; (3) identification of individuals or groups at unusually increased risk because of heightened susceptibility and/or level of exposure; (4) formulation and enforcement of standards and regulations for limiting the exposure of individuals or populations to potentially harmful agents, along with engineering measures for controlling the production and/or release of potentially toxic agents, as discussed in the next chapter; (5) planning ahead to cope with emergencies that may result from the accidental release of hazardous agents; (6) maintaining in readiness the organizational capability needed to cope with environmental emergencies; (7) mounting programs of public and professional education in environmental risk reduction (including information clearinghouses, workshops, telephone hot lines, internet web pages, etc.) (U.S. EPA, 1990; Griffith and Saunders, 1997; Omenn and Faustman, 1997; Presidential Commission, 1997).

At the individual level, the options for risk reduction include (1) staying abreast of relevant information received via the media and/or communications from health authorities, environmental protection agencies, and other sources; (2) modifying one's own behavior, diet, and lifestyle to minimize risks to oneself and to others; (3) carefully observing any special precautions that may be called for to protect oneself and one's fellow workers against hazardous agents in the workplace; and (4) joining with others in efforts to promote collective awareness of environmental risks and to reduce such risks (Griffith and Saunders, 1997).

REFERENCES

Allen, F. W. 1992. Differing views of risk: The challenge for decision makers in a democracy. In: *Management of Hazardous Agents: Social, Political, and Policy Aspects*, Vol 2, eds. D.C. Levine and A.C. Upton, pp 81–94. Westport: Praeger.

Ames, B. N., R. Magaw, and L. S. Bold, 1987. Ranking possible carcinogenic hazards. *Science* 236: 271–280.

Andrews, R. N. L., and A. G. Turner. 1987. Controlling toxic chemicals in the environment. In eds. *Toxic Chemicals, Health, and the Environment*, L. B. Lave and A. C. Upton, Baltimore: Johns Hopkins University Press. pp. 5–37.

Arrow, K.J., M. L. Cropper, G. C. Eads, R. W. Hahn, L. B. Lave, R. G. Noll, P.R. Portney, M. Russell, R. Schmalensee, V. K. Smith, and R. N. Stavins. 1996. *Is there a role for Benefit-Cost Analysis in Environmental, Health, and Safety Regulation. Science* 272: 221–222.

Ashby, J., and R. Tennant. 1988. Chemical structure, *Salmonella* mutagenicity, and extent of carcinogenicity as indicators of genotoxic carcinogens among 222 chemical tests in rodents by the U.S. NCI/NTP. *Mutat. Res.* 204: 17–115. Eurotunnel 1994. The Channel Tunnel: A Safety Case. Folkestone, Eurotunnel.

Davies, J. C. ed. 1996. *Comparing Environmental Risks*. Washington, DC, Resources for the Future.

Evans, A. W., and N. Q. Verlander. 1997. What is wrong with criterion FN-lines for judging the tolerability of risk. *Risk Anal.* 17: 157–168.

Finkel, A. M. 1990. *Confronting Uncertainty in Risk Management*. Washington, DC: Center for Risk Management, Resources for the Future.

Fischoff, B., A. Bostrom, and M. J. Quadrel. 1997. Risk perception and communication. In: *Oxford Textbook of Public Health,* eds. R. Detels, W. Holland, J. McEwen, and G. S. Omenn, eds. pp. 987–1002. New York: Oxford University Press.

Gold, L. S., C. B. Sawyer, R. Magaw, G. M. Backman, M. DeVeciana, R. Levinson, N. K. Hooper, W. R. Havender, L. Bernstein, R. Peto, M. C. Pike, and B. N. Ames. 1984. A carcinogenic potency database of the standard results of animal bioassays. *Envir. Health Perspect.* 58: 9–319.

Gold, L. S., M. DeVeciana, G. M. Backman, R. Magaw, P. Lopipero, M. Smith, M. Blumenthal, R. Levinson, L. Bernstein, and B. N. Ames. 1986. Chronological supplement to the carcinogenic potency database: Standardized results of animal bioassays published through December 1982. *Environ. Health Perspect.* 67: 161–200.

Gold, L. S., T. H. Slone, G. M. Backman, R. Magaw, M. DaCosta, P. Lopipero, M. Blumenthal, and B. N. Ames. 1987. Second chronological supplement to the carcinogenic potency database: Standardized results of animal bioassays published through December 1984 and by the National Toxicology Program through May 1986. *Environ. Health Perspect.* 74: 237–329.

Griffith, R. and P. Saunders. 1997. Reducing environmental risk. In: *Oxford Textbook of Public Health,* eds. R. Detels, W. Holland, J. McEwen, and G. S. Omenn, pp. 1601–1620. New York: Oxford University Press.

Hammond, P. B. and R. Coppock, eds. 1990. *Valuing Health Risks, Costs, and Benefits for Environmental Decision Making.* Washington, DC: National Academy Press.

International Commission on Radiological Protection. 1977. Problems involved in developing an index of harm. ICRP Publication 27. *Annals of the ICRP,* 1(4).

International Commission on Protection against Environmental Mutagens and Carcinogens. 1988. Testing for mutagens and carcinogens: The role of short-term genotoxicity assays. *Mutat. Res.* 205: 3–12.

Lave, L. B., F. K. Ennever, H. S. Rosenkranz, and G. S. Omenn. 1988. Information value of the rodent bioassay. *Nature* 336: 631–633.

Mauderly, J. L. 1993. Toxicological approaches to complex mixtures. *Environ. Health Perspect. Suppl.* 101: 155–164.

Morgan, M. G. and M. Henrion. 1990. *Uncertainty: A Guide to Dealing with Uncertainty in Quantitative Risk and Policy Analysis.* New York: Cambridge University Press.

National Academy of Sciences/National Research Council. 1978. *Saccharin: Technical Assessment of Risks and Benefits. Part I of a 2-part Study of the Committee for a Study of Saccharin and Food Safety Policy, Panel I: Saccharin and Its Impurities.* Washington, DC: National Academy Press.

National Academy of Sciences/National research Council. 1983. *Risk Assessment in the Federal Government: Managing the Process.* Washington, DC: National Academy Press.

National Academy of Sciences/National Research Council. 1984. *Toxicity Testing: Strategies to Determine Needs and Priorities.* Washington, DC: National Academy Press.

National Academy of Sciences/National Research Council. 1987. Biological markers in environmental health research. Report of the National Research Council Committee on Biological Markers. *Environ. Health Perspect.* 74: 3–9.

National Academy of Sciences/National Research Council. 1988. *Complex Mixtures: Method for In vivo Toxicity Testing.* Washington, DC: National Academy Press.

National Academy of Sciences/National Research Council. 1989. *Improving Risk Communication.* Washington, DC: National Academy Press.

National Academy of Sciences/National Research Council. 1990. *Effects of Exposure to Low Levels of Ionizing Radiation. BEIR V.* Washington, DC: National Academy Press.

National Academy of Sciences/National Research Council. 1994. *Science and Judgement in Risk Assessment.* Washington, DC: National Academy Press.

National Academy of Sciences/National Research Council. 1996. *Understanding Risk: Informing Decisions in a Democratic Society.* Washington, DC: National Academy Press.

Office of Science and Technology Policy. 1985. Chemical carcinogens: A review of the science and its associated principle. *Fed. Register* 50: 10371.

Omenn, G. S., and E. M. Faustman. 1997. Risk Assessment, risk communication, and risk management. In: *Oxford Textbook of Public Health*, eds. R. Detels, W. Holland, J. McEwen, and G. S. Omenn, pp. 969–986. New York: Oxford University Press.

Peto, R., M. C. Pike, L. Bernstein, L. S. Gold, and B. N. Ames. 1984. A proposed general convention for the numerical description of the carcinogenic potency of chemicals in chronic-exposure animal experiments. *Environ. Health Perspect.* 58: 1–8.

Plough, A. and S. Krimsky. 1987. The emergence of risk communication studies social and political context. *Sci. Technol. Hum. Values* 12: 4–10.

Presidential/Congressional Commission on Risk Assessment and Risk Management. 1997. *Risk Assessment and Risk Management in Regulatory Decision Making*. Washington, DC.

Raynor, S., and K. Cantor. 1987. How fair is safe enough? The cultured approach to societal technology choice. *Risk Anal.* 7: 3–9.

Rodricks, J. V. 1992. *Calculated Risks: Understanding the Toxicity and Human Health Risks of Chemicals in Our Environment*. Cambridge: University of Cambridge Press.

Sandman, P. M. 1985. Getting to maybr: Some communication aspects of siting hazardous waste facilities. *Seton Hall Legis. J.* 9: 442–465.

Shimizu, Y., H. Kato, and W. J. Schull. 1990. Studies of the mortality of A-bomb survivors. 9. Mortality 1950–1985: Part 2. Cancer mortality based on the recently revised doses (DS86). *Radiat. Res.* 121: 120–141.

Slovic, P. B., B. Fischoff, and S. Lichtenstein. 1979. Rating the risks: *Environment* 21: 14–20, 36–39.

Slovic, P. B., B. Fischoff, and S. Lichtenstein. 1981. Perceived risk: Psychological factors and social implications. *Proc. R. Soc. Lond.* A376: 17–34.

Tennant, R. W., B. H. Margolin, M. D. Shelby, E. Zeiger, J. K. Haseman, J. Spalding, W. Caspary, M. Resnick, S. Staciewicz, B. Anderson, and R. Minor. 1987. Prediction of chemical carcinogenicity in rodents from in vitro genetic toxicity assays. *Science* 236: 933–941.

Tones, K. 1997. Health education, hehaviour change, and the public health. In: *Oxford Textbook of Public Health*, eds. R. Detels, W. Holland, J. McEwen, and G. S. Omenn, pp. 783–814. New York: Oxford University Press.

Travis, C. C., S. R. Pack, and H. A. Hattmer-Frey. 1989. Is ionizing radiation regulated more stringently than chemical carcinogens? *Health Phys.* 56: 527–531.

United Nations Scientific Committee on the Effects of Atomic Radiation (UNSCEAR). 1988. *Sources, Effects, and Risks of Ionizing Radiation. Report to the General Assembly, Official Records*. New York: United Nations.

United States Environmental Protection Agency. 1987. *Unfinished Business: A Comparative Assessment of Environmental Problems*. Washington, DC: U.S. EPA.

United States Environmental Protection Agency. 1990. *Reducing Risk: Setting Priorities and Strategies for Environmental Protection*. Washington, DC: U.S. EPA.

Wilson, R. 1979. Analyzing the risks of daily life. *Technol. Rev.* 81: 41–46.

Zeckhauser, R. J. and W. K. Viscusi. 1990. Risk within reason. *Science* 248: 559–564.

Zeise, L. R., R. Wilson, and A. C. Crouch. 1987. The dose–response relationship for carcinogens: A review. *Environ. Health Perspect.* 73: 259–306.

28 Reducing Risks: An Environmental Engineering Perspective

RAYMOND C. LOEHR, Ph.D.

Concern about environmental risks, particularly those affecting human health, can be traced to the earliest human records (Graham, 1994; Paustenbach, 1989). However, it was not until the twentieth century that there was a concerted focus on the protection of humans from the adverse effects of chemicals at work, from industrial emissions, from commerce, and in the environment. The general approach to risk assessment evolved over time and recognizes that adverse impacts on human health are related to both the toxicity of a chemical and the degree of exposure.

A definition of environmental risk and perspectives on individual and community risks have been provided in Chapter 27. The purpose of this chapter is to build on that information and to provide a perspective of the use of risk assessment and risk management by environmental engineers to protect human health and the environment.

HISTORICAL PERSPECTIVE

Initial public environmental engineering concerns were related to water supply and wastewater disposal. In ancient times human waste disposal was an individual problem and ample space existed for such disposal without nuisance or harm to others. As the population in the ancient world grew, communities developed bathrooms. Early in the Roman Republic, the main drain of Rome, the renowned Cloaca Maxima, was built to provide human waste and storm sewer service for the Roman Forum and part of the city (Fuhrman, 1984). The sewer also assisted with malaria control.

In the United States, the beginnings of the environmental engineering profession can be traced to the Sanitary Commission of Massachusetts around 1850. That Commission issued a report emphasizing the relationship between water supply, sewers, and human health. Thereafter the profession focused on construction of sewers and physical structures to alleviate poor sanitary conditions and to transport wastes to streams and rivers. That began the period of modern environmental engineering that continues through today. This has included understanding the science of water- and vector-borne diseases, treatment of drinking water and wastewater, improvements in sanitation, and treatment of wastes.

Eventually it was recognized that simply transporting wastes to streams and rivers was not enough to protect human health and the environment. Human epidemics, such as those caused by cholera, as well as fish kills resulted. To cope with these problems, wastewater began to be treated to remove detrimental constituents and to achieve a quality of treated

Environmental Toxicants: Human Exposures and Their Health Effects, 2/e. Edited by Morton Lippmann.
ISBN: 0-471-29298-2 © 2000 John Wiley & Sons, Inc.

TABLE 28-1 llustrative Federal Environmental Legislation

Date	Legislation	Primary Item Controlled
1899	Rivers and Harbors Act	Pollution of navigable waters
1948	Federal Water Pollution Control Act	Water pollution
1965	Solid Waste Disposal Act	Solid wastes
1967	Clean Air Act	Air pollution
1972	Marine Protection, Research and Sanctuaries Act	Ocean disposal of wastes
1974	Safe Drinking Water Act	Drinking water
1976	Resource Conservation and Recovery Act (RCRA)	Hazardous wastes
1976	Toxic Substances Control Act	New products
1977	Clean Water Act	Water pollution
1980	Comprehensive Environmental Response, Compensation and Liability Act (CERCLA or Superfund)	Abandoned hazardous waste sites
1990	Pollution Prevention Act	Industrial wastes

Note: There have been amendments to all such federal legislation.

effluent that could be discharged without causing human health or environmental problems. The first processes were simple primary treatment units to remove solids. Later secondary, tertiary, and toxic removal processes were used. Thus began the "end-of-pipe" approach to waste treatment, which is common throughout the world.

The environmental engineering profession has broadened its activities beyond water supply and municipal wastewater disposal. It now covers industrial and hazardous waste management, air pollution abatement and control, remediation of contaminated soils and sludges, solid waste disposal, groundwater treatment and site remediation, waste minimization and pollution prevention, and geoenvironmental engineering. The profession has grown to meet the needs of society.

Since the 1960s extensive and detailed policies have been put into place to control almost every environmental problem. These policies have been supported by legislation, regulations, and guidance developed by government at all levels and have led to very real public benefits.

An early set of federal regulations was included in the Rivers and Harbors Act of 1899. That Act protected water quality in navigable waterways. Over the years legislation was enacted to control various contaminants and to assure clean water, clean air and a quality environment. Some of the major pieces of legislation are noted in Table 28-1. In addition numerous amendments to the Acts and many lesser pieces of legislation were enacted to protect human health and the environment.

Existing environmental legislation is characterized as "command-and-control" legislation. Each piece of legislation states a required action and establishes general and specific goals. Such legislation has not been comprehensive and focuses on one problem or medium (water, air, solid waste) at a time.

The pace of federal environmental legislation increased dramatically in the past three decades. In addition numerous state and county governments enacted environmental protection regulations. Such laws require regulatory agencies to:

- Identify environmental, health, and safety hazards.
- Establish limits on emissions and releases of various substances from industrial facilities, waste sites, and motor vehicles.
- Establish limits on permissible human exposure to substances in food, drinking water, air, and in the workplace.
- Oversee the cleanup of present and past industrial facilities and waste sites.

These activities frequently are accomplished by a regulatory process which depends in part on risk assessment. Although some environmental, health, and safety laws consider "risk" as a basis for regulation, risk assessment is not specifically mandated by most laws enacted to protect the public and environment. Rather, risk assessment is a process that has been developed over time to assist regulators in establishing a basis for implementing their statutory responsibilities.

POLLUTION CONTROL PROGRESS

The existing environmental legislation has been directed at curbing damages from gross air and water pollution and hazardous wastes. Early symbols of environmental degradation included a burning Cuyahoga River, a dying Lake Erie, a smog-choked Los Angeles, a Pittsburgh so dark from air pollution at noon that the street lights had to be turned on, massive fish kills, and acids in stacks from factories pitting paint on cars parked nearby. With these problems etched in public consciousness, the public required that the quality of the environment be improved.

Considerable control of environmental problems has occurred in the past 30 years. Streams and lakes are cleaner, and fish have returned. Technological controls regulate hazardous wastes, landfills, incineration, and waste treatment facilities. Abandoned hazardous waste sites are being remediated and emissions of lead, air pollution particulates, and volatile organics have decreased dramatically.

Setting priorities was not an issue in the early years. The problems and apparent culprits seemed obvious. The Congress, the public, and the regulatory agencies agreed on the severity of environmental problems facing the nation and what needed to be done to correct them. With such consensus, environmental legislation was passed, regulations promulgated, and efforts and resources were focused on massive cleanup and control programs.

Over time, the increasing environmental legislation and limited financial and personnel resources strained the ability of regulatory agencies. Industry felt the same demands and constraints. It became clear that the United States could not meet all of the social, economic, security, and environmental concerns that arise. Resource constraints have become a reality for the foreseeable future.

Continuing and future environmental problems need a different regulatory approach, one that relies less on command-and-control regulations. Such an approach would make greater use of all tools available to reduce environmental risk.

ENVIRONMENTAL RISK ASSESSMENT AND MANAGEMENT

Overview

Environmental risks have changed over time. In the early 1900s, lead arsenate was the principal insecticide sprayed on fruits and potatoes to control insects, medicinals were unreliable, industrial towns were black with soot as were people's lungs, and workers labored at their own peril (Lowrance, 1976). The principal fatal diseases were pneumonia, influenza and tuberculosis. More than 13% of all American children died before their first birthday.

Many steps have been taken to reduce these risks and other risks, which at one time were low in priority, are now of concern. However, both personal and societal risks are inherent in human activity, and there can be no hope of reducing all risks to zero. As noted (Chapter 27), risk is an inescapable fact of life.

Actually, it is not risk per se that is of concern to the public. Involuntary risk is the major concern. Opinions of acceptable risk depend on the degree of choice to decline a risk. Of particular concern are cancer, lingering and painful death, and debilitating sicknesses.

The use of risk assessment provides information to policy makers, regulatory agencies, and other risk managers so that the most appropriate decisions can be made. Since the 1970s, the use of risk assessment for this purpose has increased. A risk assessment provides the bridge between scientific information and risk management and puts the words toxicity, hazard, and risk into perspective (Paustenbach, 1989).

Risk assessment is a valuable tool to gauge the existence and severity of potential risks to human health and the environment, although it rarely provides definitive answers. However, risk assessment can frame the debate about whether particular potential risks should be regulated and who should bear the costs of regulation.

The concept of environmental risk and risk assessment, together with the related terminology and analytical methodologies, allows disparate environmental problems to be discussed with a common language. It also allows different environmental problems to be compared in common terms, allows different risk reduction options to be evaluated from a common basis, and allows the development of environmental policies in a consistent and systematic way. It is in this context that environmental risk assessment is used by environmental engineers.

The commonly accepted definitions of risk assessment and risk management are those suggested by the National Research Council (NRC, 1983):

- *Risk assessment*: the characterization of potential adverse health effects of human exposures to environmental hazards; the assessment includes characterization of the uncertainties inherent in the process of inferring risk
- *Risk management*: the process of evaluating alternative regulatory actions and selecting among them; the selection process requires the use of value judgments on such issues as the acceptability of risk and the reasonableness of the costs of control

Until the early 1990s the concepts of the risk assessment paradigm and the use of risk assessment as part of the environmental decision-making process were viewed by environmental engineers as an esoteric practice. While possibly valuable, it was considered on the fringes of environmental engineering and hazardous waste management practice. Emphasis was placed on meeting specific regulatory requirements, which commonly were based on worst-case assumptions used to assure maximum protection of human health.

Today (late 1990s), risk assessment is an important component of many environmental engineering and waste management projects. Specific state and federal guidance is available, and it is an integral part of major environmental legislation, such as CERCLA and the Clean Air Act Amendments.

Risk Assessment Process

The risk assessment process can be divided into four major steps: hazard identification, exposure assessment, dose–response assessment, and risk characterization (NAS, 1983). Risk assessment is followed by risk management if the estimated risk is indicated to be unacceptable. Thus risk assessment considers how risky the situation or exposure is. Risk management considers what to do about the risk; that is, how to reduce or remove it, if it is deemed unacceptable. These steps are discussed in detail in Chapter 27 of this book, in Paustenbach (1989), and in the NRC Report (1983).

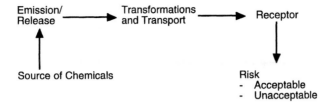

Figure 28-1   Conceptual risk assessment paradigm.

The values of the risk assessment process are many. Perhaps the most important is that it provides a consistent, disciplined approach to organize scientific information so that the relevant items are considered. In doing so, it helps identify the uncertainties involved in the data and the assumptions that are involved. It helps indicate the timeframes involved, and who or what is affected. It also helps identify strategies and priorities such as where in the process risk management decisions can be most effective. Overall, it helps educate all involved about the factors, exposures, effects, and relative risks that exist at a site or for a particular situation.

Currently the concepts of risk-based corrective action and risk-based decision making are being widely applied to determine the most appropriate actions to be used at specific sites to protect human health and the environment. These concepts are discussed in subsequent sections of this chapter.

Before doing so, the following example may help put the use of the risk assessment process for environmental decision making into perspective. A simplistic risk assessment paradigm is shown in Figure 28-1.

For a situation to pose a threat to human health and the environment, there must be a source of contamination. One or more chemicals must be released from that source. Once released, the chemicals must be transported to a receptor such as a human, plant, or an object. During the transport, there may be transformations that alter the form or speciation of the chemical, which in turn may make the chemical more or less mobile or toxic. If the chemical can contact a sensitive area of a receptor, and create exposure, there could be a negative impact. The environmental risk associated with that negative impact can be calculated, and this risk may be considered acceptable or unacceptable.

The environmental risks caused by an actual chemical or mixture of chemicals in the environment are determined by environmental scientists, toxicologists, and medical doctors. The risk assessment process has been formalized and is used increasingly by the U.S. Environmental Protection Agency (EPA) and state regulatory agencies as part of environmental decision making. Early examples of formal guidelines that have been issued by EPA include those for carcinogenicity, mutagenicity, chemical mixtures, developmental toxicants, and estimating exposure (U.S. EPA, 1984; 1987)

Risk Management from an Environmental Engineering Perspective

An environmental engineer uses the knowledge from the risk assessment process to identify locations and situations by which the identified risks can be reduced. For instance, in terms of the paradigm in Figure 28-1, possible options are noted in Table 28-2. These options can be schematically included in the risk assessment paradigm in Figure 28-2. The interaction between risk assessment and risk management is shown in Figure 28-3, which also indicates some of the nonengineering factors that are involved in a risk management decision.

For a real-world situation there are many risk management options that can be considered. The challenge for the environmental engineer, for a specific problem, is to

TABLE 28-2   Examples Environmental Engineering Options to Reduce Environmental Risks

- Removing the source of contamination in soils and allowing natural environmental assimilative processes to control any remaining chemicals and those that have been released.
- Changing the chemical or manufacturing process that is emitting chemicals of concern, thus decreasing or eliminating the chemical causing the risk. This is the cornerstone of the pollution prevention approach now widely used by industry.
- Changing the form of the chemical, either at the source or after release. This can be done by modifying the pH of the media containing the chemical, or adding other chemicals that will immobilize the chemical of concern by solidification-stabilization.
- Intercepting and treating emitted and released chemicals of concern before they reach a receptor. Examples include in situ and ex situ biological and chemical treatment processes.
- Preventing released chemicals of concern from reaching a receptor. Capturing a chemical of concern at the source and in situ slurry walls are two such possibilities.
- Separating the receptor from the chemical of concern. Providing alternative drinking water and food supplies and purchasing property and moving residents are possibilities.

develop cost-effective technical solutions that will protect human health and the environment.

The cost implications of conducting a site-specific risk assessment are not trivial. Consider the following example which resulted at an actual site where alternatives for remediation were evaluated. The detailed site remedial investigation studies indicated that the life-cycle remediation costs were related to the required cleanup levels (Table 28-3). A risk-based site-specific evaluation determined that a cleanup level of 400 ppm for the chemical of concern was protective of human health. In the absence of the risk-based evaluation, a lower default cleanup level would have been required, resulting in a considerably larger site remediation cost.

Paustenbach (1989, p. 92) also provided a pertinent example of the relationship between the cost of remediation and cleanup levels. In that example, the estimated costs of soil removal and destruction for various soil clean-up levels of dioxin were shown. The cost was indicated to be about $17 million for a clean-up level of about one ppb dioxin to less than $1 million for a cleanup level of 100 ppb dioxin in the soil.

Evaluations of the risk associated with specific chemicals at a site can help identify the site specific cleanup levels that are protective of human health and the environment.

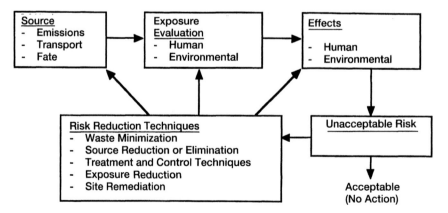

Figure 28-2   Risk assessment and illustrative engineering risk management approaches.

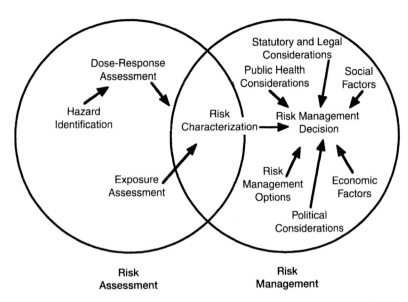

Figure 28-3 Conceptual interaction between risk assessment and risk management. (Source: adapted from NRC, 1983)

Comparative Risk Analyses

The resource considerations related to reducing environmental risks were stated clearly by EPA in 1984 (U.S. EPA, 1984, p. 23):

> One can argue about how much should be spent on environmental protection, but at some point everyone must accept that the commitment of resources for any social purpose has a finite limit. If the number of potential risk targets is very large in comparison to the number we can realistically pursue, which seems now to be the case, then some rational method of choosing which risks to reduce and deciding how far we should try to reduce them is indispensable.
>
> It is important to keep in mind that while individual risk management decisions may be seen as balancing risk reduction against resources, the system as a whole is designed to balance risk against risk. In other words, it is essential that we address the worst and most controllable risks first; failure to do so means that the total amount of harm that we prevent is smaller than the amount we might have prevented. Making incorrect priority choices, saving one where we might have saved two, represents a profound failure of the Agency's basic mission.

The ideas and concepts in the above statement have been recognized broadly, and have stimulated many of the approaches now being used to ensure that (1) the focus is on the

TABLE 28-3 Example of Relationship of Cleanup Action Levels to Remediation Life-Cycle Costs

Assumed Cleanup Action Level (ppm of Chemical in Soil)	Total Estimated Remediation Site-Specific Life-Cycle Costs ($ millions)
10	1375
50	163
180	69
400	30

TABLE 28-4   **Recommendations from the EPA Report on Reducing Risk**

---

1. Target environmental protection efforts on the basis of opportunities for the greatest risk reduction.
2. Attach as much importance to reducing ecological risk as to reducing human health risk.
3. Improve data and analytical methodologies that support the assessment, comparison, and reduction of different environmental risks.
4. Reflect risk-based priorities in strategic planning processes.
5. Reflect risk-based priorities in the budget process.
6. Promote nationally and make greater use of all the tools available to reduce risk.
7. Emphasize pollution prevention as the preferred option for reducing risk.
8. Increase efforts to integrate environmental considerations into broader aspects of public policy in as fundamental a manner as are economic concerns.
9. Work to improve public understanding of environmental risks and train a professional workforce to help reduce them.
10. Develop improved analytical methods to value natural resources and to account for long-term environmental effects in economic analyses.

Source: Adapted from: U.S. EPA (1990).

larger environmental risks, and (2) cost-effective environmental risk reduction strategies are utilized.

The EPA continued to explore approaches to use the concept of relative risk for environmental decision making. In 1990 the EPA administrator called for a national debate on environmental directions and policies (Reilly, 1990). What stimulated that call and the debate was the U.S. EPA Science Advisory Board Report, Reducing Risk (U.S. EPA, 1990). The 10 summary recommendations of the report are noted in Table 28-4. The recommendations emphasized targeting environmental protection efforts on the basis of environmental risk and risk reduction opportunities. They called for risk-based priorities in national planning and budgeting and for emphasis on pollution prevention rather than on end-of-pipe treatment. Efforts to better educate the public about actual risks also were recommended.

The Reducing Risk report and its recommendations have been discussed widely, and they have had an impact on national environmental policy. For example, specific guidance on risk characterization for risk managers and assessors was provided by EPA (Habicht, 1992). The EPA also began to develop risk-based priorities for its activities and began budgetary decisions using the concept of risk as a basis. In addition the U.S. General Accounting Office (1991) has called for actions similar to those in Reducing Risk.

Many entities are using comparative risk analyses to determine the greater environmental risks and to develop strategies to address those risks (U.S. EPA, 1992). Some three dozen states, cities, tribes, and regions have been engaged in some form of comparative risk projects (Minard, 1995). Such comparative risk reports are available to all relevant state agencies, members of the state legislatures, the EPA, and other interested parties. Each project produced useful tools for environmental planning to manage important environmental risks. The strength of the comparative risk evaluation process is its capacity to frame important public policy questions and to engage people in a productive attempt to answer them. Comparative risk has added depth to policy debates and helped decision makers set priorities.

In addition to the activities at the EPA and in the states and regions that increased the emphasis on risk assessments and comparative risk analyses, there were several Presidential Executive Orders and similarly broad actions that provided impetus to the use of risk assessments for environmental decision making. Such actions are noted in Table 28-5.

TABLE 28-5   Illustrative Broad Actions Related to Risk Assessment and Environmental Decision Making

- **Executive Order 12498.** This 1985 Executive Order explicitly included risk assessment in the regulatory review process and required that regulatory agencies comply with the principle that "[r]egulations that seek to reduce health or safety risks should be based upon scientific risk-assessment procedures, and should address risks that are real and significant rather than remote or hypothetical." (Federal Register, 1985)
- **Interagency Risk Assessment Coordination.** In 1990 the Federal Coordinating Council on Science, Engineering and Technology (FCCSET), developed two groups to address risk assessment issues from an interagency perspective: (1) the Ad hoc Working Group on Risk Assessment, and (2) the Subcommittee on Risk Assessment.
- **Executive Order 12866.** This 1993 Executive Order indicated additional policy concerning regulatory review. Agencies were explicitly directed to consider the degree and nature of risks posed by various substances or activities within their respective jurisdictions. (Federal Register, 1993)
- **Science and Judgment in Risk Assessment.** This report critiqued the EPA approach to characterizing human cancer risks from exposure to chemicals. The report found that the general approach of EPA to assessing risk was fundamentally sound and made a number of recommendations for improvement (National Academy of Sciences, 1994).
- **Commission on Risk Assessment and Risk Management.** The committee was formed to make a full investigation of the policy implications and appropriate uses of risk assessment and risk management in regulatory programs under various federal laws to prevent cancer and other chronic human health effects which may result from exposure to hazardous substances. The Commission Report contained a Risk Management Framework and six recommendations to implement the framework (Presidential Commission, 1997).

APPLICATIONS AND USE

Risk assessment evaluations have been applied in many situations for environmental management decisions. Risk to human health and the environment is becoming the overriding criteria for evaluating and prioritizing waste management and site remediation options. This is a result of the following: (1) environmental engineers and regulators better understand the limits of existing technologies, (2) the sciences of risk assessment and modeling now can be used to measure and compare the benefits of possible options, and (3) many studies have documented that all sites and situations do not require treatment or removal to the same generic standard.

The following sections illustrate the use of risk assessment evaluations for different environmental situations and decisions. These include an overview of the risk assessment process as used to evaluate site-specific risks, Superfund remediations, sewage sludge application to land, and contaminated sediments. Also included is discussion of the risk-based corrective action approach now used widely for environmental management decisions and the risk reduction program developed by the state of Texas for environmental decisions.

Overview

There are many uses of a site-specific risk assessment (Table 28-6). From an engineering and environmental decision standpoint, an environmental risk assessment can be conducted in a forward or a reverse mode. In the forward mode, using the items in Figure 28-1, data about the chemical at the source and transformation and transport knowledge are used to assess the risk to a site-specific human or ecological receptor from a defined source, such as a leaking fuel tank, a spill, or a gaseous emission.

TABLE 28-6   Examples of Uses of a Risk Assessment for Environmental Engineering Purposes

- Determines the need for remedial action at contaminated sites
- Helps set priorities and establish the urgency to remediate sites
- Determines site-specific, health-based cleanup levels
- Provides a position from which the concerned parties can negotiate cleanup levels
- Allows the use of less expensive remedial alternatives, while still being protective of human health and the environment
- Helps identify suitable locations for waste management facilities, such as municipal incinerators and landfills
- Supports litigation involving chemical emissions and exposures
- Helps meet mandates of federal or state environmental regulations

In the reverse mode, one would work backward from a known receptor and, using protective health or ecological criteria, calculate soil, groundwater, or emission levels that would have to exist to be protective of human health and the environment. This reverse approach can be used to determine remediation or emission levels that would have to be achieved. An example of health criteria used in this approach could be drinking water criteria for humans.

Risk assessments commonly are conducted at several levels, with a screening level assessment being done first. The screening level risk assessment should estimate the risk using a conservative set of assumptions. Only if the estimated risk determined from the screening assessment appears to be unacceptable is it necessary to conduct a more detailed risk assessment. This is referred to as the *tiered approach to risk assessment*, and it is part of all currently used risk assessments.

The basic steps of a site specific risk assessment are indicated in Table 28-7. The detail and accuracy of the information needed, the time needed to complete the risk assessment evaluation, and the cost of the evaluation are different in each tier of the evaluation. The screening level evaluation requires the least amount of information, since many conservative assumptions are involved. The cost of a risk assessment evaluation can increase by a factor of 5 to 10 when the evaluation moves from a screening level to a detailed evaluation.

The specifics of a risk assessment plan will be different for each site. The general characteristics of a risk assessment process are indicated in Table 28-8.

Superfund

From an environmental engineering standpoint, the risk assessments associated with remediation decisions for Superfund sites represent one of the more detailed and comprehensive evaluations. The details of a Superfund risk assessment are well developed and standardized (U.S. EPA, 1988, 1989a,b,c, 1991a,b). The following is a summary of the Superfund site risk assessment steps and process.

The major decisions made at a Superfund site are based on answers to several questions: How serious are the problems at the site? Should something be done at this site? What should be done? And, when has enough been done?

The Comprehensive Environmental Response, Compensation, and Liability Act (CERCLA, also known as Superfund) was passed by Congress in 1980 and amended in 1986. Superfund allows the EPA to reduce the risks from inadequate waste management approaches. Written by the EPA, the National Contingency Plan (NCP) is the regulation to implement and carry out Superfund law so that it protects the health of both people and the environment.

TABLE 28-7   Basic Steps in a Site-Specific Risk Assessment

- Prepare a risk assessment plan for the site or situation
- Identify available data, data needs, and data gaps
- Define data quality objectives
- Prepare a sampling plan
- Identify chemicals of concern and assess toxicology
- Identify current and potential future receptor(s)
- Define exposure pathways
- Estimate exposure point concentrations
- Estimate applied or absorbed dose
- Characterize health risks and uncertainties
- Identify and state key assumptions

Different risk assessment approaches are applied in evaluating possible effects of Superfund sites on human health and the environment. Neither the EPA nor the Superfund program has one standardized environmental evaluation methodology because there are so many different aspects of the environment — individuals, species, ecosystems, natural resources, endangered species, — that may need to be evaluated. As a result the Superfund program has identified an orderly process for environmental evaluation.

Risk assessment for a Superfund site is a four-step process. The first step, data collection and evaluation, identifies contaminants present in the environmental media— soil, groundwater, surface water, air, fish—of the site. The second step, toxicity assessment, uses the results of prior research and testing to decide which of the contaminants found on site might pose a health threat.

TABLE 28-8   Characteristics of Risk Assessment Process for Environmental Engineering Purposes

Develop reasonable exposure scenarios

Current site and surrounding land use
Future reasonable site and surrounding land use
Real and possible hypothetical pathways from source to receptor

Evaluate multiple exposure pathways

Air
Soil
Groundwater
Surface water

Evaluate multiple exposure routes

Ingestion
Inhalation
Dermal

Involve multidisciplinary expertise

Quantify environmental multimedia fate and transport
Understand and apply toxicological principles
Understand site-specific environmental chemistry
Interpret multimedia field data
Involve statistical analysis of the data
Develop risk communication skills

The third step, exposure assessment, defines which pathways (e.g., using the groundwater for drinking and showering or surface water in relation to eating the fish) might bring the contaminants in contact with people. The final step, risk characterization, brings information from the first three steps together to determine the potential severity of health threats from the site.

Figure 28-4 indicates the basic steps of the Superfund site evaluation process and the role of risk assessment in that process. As indicated, the detailed risk assessment evaluation occurs at the remedial investigation/feasibility study (RI/FS) stage in the process. However, a screening level risk assessment occurs earlier in the hazard-ranking system (HRS) scoring. The HRS analysis is structured by assessment principles to determine whether conditions warrant placing a site on the National Priorities List (NPL) and using federal funds to continue with the rest of the site evaluation process.

However, most of the formal risk assessment activities occur after a site is placed on the NPL. These activities

- Help develop preliminary remediation goals during project scoping and their modification during the feasibility study (FS).
- Develop the baseline risk assessment during the remediation investigation (RI).
- Evaluate the effectiveness of remedial alternatives in the FS report; in the Record of Decision (ROD) to relate target cleanup concentrations to health risks; and during remedial action to monitor progress toward "acceptable risk"

The baseline risk assessment of the RI is the central risk evaluation activity in the Superfund program, and it is a four-step risk assessment paradigm, involving data evaluation, exposure assessment, toxicity assessment, and risk characterization.

To initiate the baseline risk assessment of the RI, information on the site's history and data gathered during the pre-remedial program or during a recent site visit are assembled

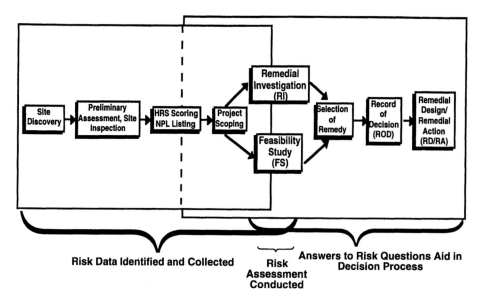

Figure 28-4   Major steps in the Superfund site evaluation process. (Source: Adapted from U.S. EPA, 1991b.)

and used to guide the remedial investigation. A critical step is identifying contaminants of significant toxicity and all exposure pathways of concern. In addition to the media paths — soil, air, and drinking water — other paths such as the eating of contaminated food or recreation may be important. Knowing toxicity and exposures to be evaluated leads directly to a sampling strategy (e.g., identifying "hot spots," gathering sufficient data for reasonable maximum exposure (RME) determinations), appropriate analytical methods (e.g., requesting special analytical services for detection at low concentration), and related data quality objectives (DQOs) for sampling and analysis.

The exposure assessment looks for pathways of exposure to particular types of people on or near the site, since the activities of the people determine the exposure. The baseline risk assessment considers both present exposures and those that might result from current or probable future land use. For each exposure pathway, the risk assessor must decide five basic variables to use in estimating exposure: (1) exposure point concentrations, (2) contact rate, (3) exposure frequency and duration, (4) body weight for humans, and (5) exposure averaging time.

What is determined is the RME. This is to be the highest exposure that is reasonably expected to occur at a site, considering land use, intake variables, and pathway combinations. The intent is to estimate a conservative exposure case that is still within the range of possible exposures. The result is that people at or near sites will be protected, but cleanups will not be driven by assumed exposures outside the range of possibility.

Toxicity assessments are the next step in the process, and they are done using available information and the advice of toxicologists. In addition to estimating quantitative toxicity values for carcinogens, toxicologists make qualitative evaluations of the sum total of all studies using a given substance. These are weight-of-evidence classifications. EPA has standardized this approach in a five-class grouping. In general, multiple well-designed studies, studies showing adverse effects in several species of animals, and evidence of adverse effects in humans provide greater weight-of-evidence of information. The Superfund risk assessor uses this classification in the risk characterization aspects of the risk assessment.

Once the exposure and toxicity assessments are complete, the risk assessor must characterize the risks. A schematic of these steps is provided in Figure 28-5. These steps are crucial for communicating both to individuals who must decide what actions to take at a site and to those who may live at or near the site.

Excess lifetime carcinogen risks to individuals of less than 10^{-4} (1 in 10,000) do not require remedial actions at Superfund sites. Actions may be taken to reduce risks below 10^{-4}. If the baseline risk assessment shows risks greater than 10^{-4} to individuals, then initial cleanup target concentrations corresponding to 10^{-6} risk are chosen.

For chemicals that show noncancer risks from chronic (long-term) exposures, the risk assessor estimates a hazard index (HI). HI values greater than 1 are an indication of the need to look closely at possible need for remedial action.

A key component of the risk characterization is the uncertainties involved, namely the assumptions made, the variations of factors used, and the possible ranges of impacts or effects. Such information is important to subsequent decisions about the degree of actual risk that is involved, the type of remediation that is needed and the cleanup levels that are to be achieved.

Remedial alternatives are evaluated against nine criteria (Table 28-9). The remedy selected in the Record of Decision (ROD) is the one that best satisfies the criteria. Risk assessment can address several of these criteria:

- Overall protection of human health and the environment is a threshold criterion that the selected remedy must satisfy. Risk analyses for long-term and short-term effectiveness demonstrate this "protectiveness."

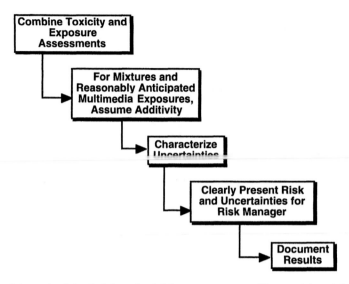

Figure 28-5 Schematic of the final Superfund risk assessment steps. (Source: Adapted from U.S. EPA, 1991b)

- A risk assessment that relates concentrations of chemicals expected after remediation to residual risks remaining at the site provides a measure of long-term effectiveness.
- A remedy that presents no unacceptable risks during the remedial action meets the short-term effectiveness criterion. Risk assessment can evaluate activities at the site that may release contaminants, create new pathways of exposure, or even new chemicals.

Every ROD should, at a minimum, identify the contaminants posing risks, target concentrations for cleanup, points of compliance for cleanup in each medium, and the risks that will remain after completion of the remedy if cleanup goals are achieved.

Every attempt is made to have a Superfund risk assessment and the remediation decision-making process be straightforward, and progress logically. In practice, each site is unique, data are incomplete, uncertainties can be large, and professional judgment and interpretation are involved. However, the risk assessment evaluation is an extremely important part of the decision process and is the key to environmentally sound and protective site-specific decisions.

TABLE 28-9 Criteria Used to Determine Superfund Site Remediation Alternatives

- Overall protection of human health and the environment
- Compliance with other regulations
- Long-term effectiveness and permanence
- Reduction of toxicity, mobility, or volume
- Short-term effectiveness
- Implementability
- Cost
- State acceptance
- Community acceptance

Source: Adapted from U.S. EPA (1991b).

Other Applications

The incorporation of risk assessment in Superfund decisions represents the most standardized environmental engineering application of the process. However, many other applications have occurred in recent years. Two examples of these application are noted below.

Wastewater Treatment Solids   The risk assessment requirements developed for the wastewater solids regulations (Code of Federal Regulations, 1993) protect the public from exposure to hazardous substances, yet they are less restrictive than the requirements developed for Superfund. These regulations establish requirements for the final use or disposal of sewage sludge (biosolids) when the biosolids are (1) applied to land to condition the soil or to fertilize crops or other vegetation grown in the soil, (2) placed on a surface disposal site for final disposal, or (3) used in a biosolids incinerator. Many of these requirements were based on the results of an extensive multimedia risk assessment.

The risk assessment developed for these regulations was to protect against "reasonably anticipated adverse affects to human health and the environment." Fourteen pathways of potential exposure to the human population were evaluated. Based on the risk assessment, limitations were developed on the concentrations of contaminants in biosolids. The intent was to avoid even a minimal potential of harm to the public.

Most aspects of these risk assessment analyses, such as toxicity characterization and exposure assessment, parallel Superfund risk assessments. However, some of the worst-case assumptions required under Superfund risk assessments are not required under the biosolids regulations. The biosolids risk assessment was judged as fully protective of human health and the environment without relying on multiple worst-case assumptions.

The maximum exposed individual (MEI) approach was not used for the biosolids risk assessment. Instead, the risk for a highly exposed individual (HEI) was evaluated. In contrast to the MEI, the HEI is based on many, but not all, of the worst-case assumptions prevalent in the Superfund program. For example, it was assumed that not all of an individual's diet consists of products grown on biosolids-amended soils. The HEI approach was stated as being conservative in a highly mobile society.

These risk assessments also do not assume that all of a hazardous substance is in its most toxic form as the Superfund risk assessments typically do. Additional safety margins were included to ensure that the risk calculated for biosolids will not increase over time. The risk-based concentrations of lead allowed in the land applied biosolids were decreased to reduce risks to children.

Contaminated Sediments   More recently risk analysis has been recommended for the management of contaminated sediments (National Research Council, 1997). A specific methodology or series of steps was not provided. However, it was noted that contaminated marine sediments can pose risks to public health and the environment, and that sound decisions about health and ecological risks must be based on formal assessments of those risks. Cost-effective contaminated sediments management requires the application of risk analysis — the combination of risk assessment, risk management, and risk communication.

At present, risk analysis is not applied comprehensively in contaminated sediments management. Risks are usually assessed only at the beginning of the decision-making process to determine the severity of the in-place contamination. The risks associated with removing and relocating the sediments, or the risks remaining after the implementation of solutions, are not evaluated. It was indicated that the expanded application of risk analysis would both inform decision makers in specific situations and provide data that could be used in the selection and evaluation of sediment management techniques and remediation technologies.

Summary These examples—Superfund, biosolids, and contaminated sediments—indicate the diverse media and situations to which risk assessment is being applied and contemplated for environmental decision making. The examples also indicate the extent to which risk assessment is being used by environmental engineers and regulators. It has been broadly used in one situation—Superfund—and has yet to be used (but recommended) for contaminated sediments.

For real-world environmental problems, the use of risk assessment is a dynamic evolving approach. The increased use of this approach will benefit from a methodology that can be applied to many situations rather than be developed separately for different situations. Such methodologies are being developed and applied. The risk-based corrective action approach and a state risk reduction program illustrate methodologies that are being considered for broad application.

Risk-Based Corrective Action

The risk-based corrective action (RBCA) approach takes the risk assessment methodology and applies it to many other situations. The initial RBCA guide (ASTM, 1995) was developed for decision making at sites containing subsurface petroleum hydrocarbons. RBCA is a standardized approach for developing remediation strategies, and it has gained wide acceptance from the EPA and state regulatory agencies. It identifies the types of risks to human health and the environment at the sites and allows the types of corrective actions needed to be commensurate with those risks.

Sites with subsurface contamination vary greatly in terms of complexity, physical and chemical characteristics, and in the risk that they may pose to human health and environmental resources. The RBCA process recognizes this diversity, and utilizes a tiered approach involving increasingly sophisticated levels of data collection and analysis. The conservative assumptions of earlier tiers are replaced with site-specific assumptions in later tiers. Upon completion of each tier, the user reviews the results and recommendations, and decides if more site-specific analysis is required.

In tier 1, sites are classified by the urgency of need for initial corrective action, based on information collected from historical records, a visual inspection, and minimal site assessment data. The user is required to identify contaminant sources, obvious environmental impacts, if any, the presence of potentially impacted humans and environmental resources (workers, residents, water bodies, etc.), and potential significant transport pathways (groundwater flow, atmospheric dispersion, etc.). Associated with site classifications are prescribed initial response actions that are to be implemented prior to proceeding further with the RBCA process.

In addition, as part of tier 1, conservative corrective action goals are based on a list of non-site-specific, risk-based screening levels (RBSLs), aesthetic criteria, and other appropriate standards such as Maximum Contaminant Levels (MCLs) for potable groundwater use. Tier 1 RBSLs are typically derived for standard exposure scenarios using current reasonable maximum exposure (RME), toxicological parameters as recommended by the EPA, and conservative contaminant migration models. These values will change as new methodologies and parameters are developed. Tier 1 RBSLs may be presented as a range of values, corresponding to a range of risks, and a risk management decision is made to select the screening levels to be used. This evaluation may include a cost–benefit analysis, where the user considers the costs associated with achieving various levels of risk reduction.

Tier 2 provides the user with an option for determining site-specific target levels (SSTLs) and appropriate points of compliance when it is judged that tier 1 corrective action goals are not appropriate. This decision is typically based on comparing the cost of achieving tier 1 corrective action goals with the cost for tier 2 analyses, considering the probability that the tier 2 site-specific goals will be significantly less costly to achieve than tier 1 goals.

Both tier 1 and tier 2 screening levels are based on achieving similar levels of human health and environmental resource protection (e.g. 10^{-4} to 10^{-6} risk levels). However, in moving to higher tiers, the user is able to develop more cost-effective corrective action plans because the conservative assumptions of earlier tiers are replaced with more realistic site-specific assumptions. Additional site assessment data may be required, but minimal incremental effort is usually required relative to tier 1.

In some cases the tier 2 SSTLs are derived from the same equations used to calculate tier 1 RBSLs, except that site-specific parameters are used in the calculations. At other sites the tier 2 analysis may involve applying tier 1 RBSLs at more probable points of exposure, such as property boundaries and negotiated points of compliance, and then deriving tier 2 corrective action goals for the contaminant source areas based on demonstrated and predicted attenuation of hydrocarbon compounds with distance. Tier 2 corrective action goals are considered conservative and are consistent with USEPA-recommended practices.

Tier 3 provides the user with an option for determining SSTLs and appropriate points of compliance when it is judged that tier 2 corrective action goals are not appropriate. This decision is typically based on comparing the cost of achieving tier 2 corrective action goals with the cost for tier 3 analyses, considering the probability that the tier 3 site-specific goals will be significantly less costly to achieve than tier 2 goals. The major distinction between tier 2 and tier 3 analyses is that a tier 3 analysis is generally a substantial incremental effort relative to tiers 1 and 2, since the analysis is much more complex and may include detailed site assessment, probabilistic evaluations, and sophisticated chemical fate/transport models.

If the selected target levels are exceeded and corrective action is necessary, the user develops a corrective action plan in order to reduce the potential for adverse impacts. One option is to utilize traditional remediation processes to reduce contaminant concentrations below the target levels. Another option is to achieve exposure reduction (or elimination) through the institutional controls or through the use of containment measures, such as capping and hydraulic control.

The RBCA process integrates components of the site assessment, risk assessment, risk management, and remediation into a holistic site-specific approach that is consistent and technically defensible while still being practical and cost effective. The details of the process and examples are available in the ASTM Guide (ASTM, 1995).

In the RBCA process, remedial action is determined to be appropriate based on the comparison of representative concentrations to the target levels determined under the tier evaluation. This allows the project to focus only on those areas or media posing a potential threat to human health or the environment. Monitoring is conducted during or following a remedial action to demonstrate that target levels are met and continue to be met, and to verify the assumptions and predictions using tier 2 and tier 3.

There are some who view RBCA as an approach to avoid remediating a contaminated site. Based on experience with the use of RBCA and with the overview provided by regulatory agencies, that is not the case. Rather, RBCA provides the following to facilitate effective and protective risk-based and site-specific remediations: (1) flexible framework, (2) procedure consistency, (3) a classification scheme that helps focus efforts and direct the type and urgency of response, and (4) a tiered approach that provides an increasingly site-specific assessment where site conditions warrant. It also is resource effective and focuses resources toward assessment and remedial measures on sites, exposure pathways, and substances of significant concern, with remedial goals based on reducing risk to acceptable levels.

The original RBCA effort (ASTM, 1995) focused on sites containing chemicals resulting from petroleum releases. Additional efforts are underway to provide a similar

RBCA approach for sites containing other chemicals. This additional guide will feature the tiered methods of the original RBCA process but will cover a large number of organic and metallic chemicals.

Not included in the original ASTM guide was an emphasis on ecological risk. Such risks are of growing importance in state and federal regulations. The broader RBCA guide for other chemicals and metals will call for determining whether a pathway to ecological exposure is present at a site. If it is, a site-specific ecological risk assessment can be recommended.

Texas Risk Reduction Program Overview

The Texas Risk Reduction Rules were initiated in 1993 by the state agency responsible for environmental matters, the Texas Natural Resources Conservation Commission (TNRCC). These rules represent the broad implementation and policy improvements for closures and remediations regulated under the state petroleum storage tank, hazardous / industrial solid waste, Superfund, spill and voluntary cleanup programs. The rules adopt a risk-based approach for determining the extent and type of closures or remediations necessary at a site to be protective of human health and the environment. They represent a move away from the previous approach of requiring removal of all contaminants to background levels or to contain the materials and perform proper postclosure activities. The Risk Reduction Rules use quantitative health-based risk assessment procedures, recognizing that limited quantities of contaminants may remain in soil or groundwater at a site and not pose an unacceptable threat to human health or the environment. Reasons identifying the value and logic of these rules are noted in Table 28-10.

These rules were developed to have a consistent risk management policy applied uniformly across all affected programs to define the necessary cleanup actions that are protective of human health and the environment. The intent is to have consistent application of these rules to the various TNRCC programs in order to prevent a fragmented regulatory system that does not have a consistent approach for managing public health and environmental risks. The value of the program is that it uses sound and most recent scientific knowledge, it involves supportable and protective risk assessments, and it involves common sense.

The rules require cleanups to levels that are protective of human health and the environment using remedies that are permanent or that have a high degree of long-term effectiveness. *Long-term effectiveness* is defined as the ability of a remedy to maintain its required level of protection over time. A permanent remedy is one that will endure indefinitely without posing the threat of any future release that would increase the risk above levels established for the facility or area.

As indicated, the Texas Risk Reduction Rules are designed to protect human health and the environment. However, the rules also balance these fundamental goals with the economic welfare of the citizens of Texas. A key purpose in development of these rules was to encourage remedial actions that serve to preserve or enhance the economic vitality of the affected property and surrounding community. To this end, the rules set forth a risk management program targeted toward preservation of active and productive land use. This risk reduction process is structured around three optional "remedy standards" which, based upon the desired future land use of the affected property, establish specific procedures for site investigation, exposure assessment, remedial action, and postclosure care that must be implemented to ensure adequate protection of public health and the environment. Within this framework, the responsible person is given flexibility for development of site-specific remediation goals and performance-based remedial action plans. These procedures are intended to streamline the application and review process and to expedite implementation of appropriate and cost-effective remedial actions. As a result

TABLE 28-10   Texas Risk Reduction Rules: Reasons for use of a Risk-Based Program

- Protects public and environment
- Takes rational approach
- Stays consistent and defensible
- Encourages voluntary and proactive cleanups
- Uses sound scientific knowledge
- Provides for better use of public and private sector resources
- Focuses on available resources at sites that pose the greatest risk to human health and the environment

the paperwork burden on both regulated parties and the TNRCC should be reduced. Responsible parties are required to submit information and reports that are commensurate with the level of risk posed by a site and the type of remedy/Risk Reduction Standard selected.

Tiered Approach   The Texas rules take into consideration threats to both human health and ecological systems and consist of two interrelated tiered processes (Figure 28-6). The tiered system for determining risk-based concentration levels for human health is modeled after the RBCA process (ASTM, 1995) (Table 28-11). Each successive tier represents an increase in the degree of sophistication used in the site evaluation and a more site-specific and less conservative evaluation of the residual contaminant concentration levels which will protect human health.

A tiered approach also is used to protect ecological receptors. These tiers help identify those sites where little or no ecological risk is present and develop numerical risk-based concentration levels only for those sites where it is warranted. The TNRCC seeks to maximize efficiency and cost-effectiveness in this tiered system by ensuring that the scope of the assessment is consistent with the specific degree of ecological concern.

Tier 1 of the ecological evaluation consists of a simple checklist to evaluate all sites for possible environmental impacts. The purpose of this checklist is to provide a general picture of the ecological setting of the site and to identify potential exposure pathways between contaminated media and ecological receptors. Tier 2 is a screening-level risk assessment and is conducted when the tier 1 evaluation indicates that there are one or more complete exposure pathways. Tier 3 is a quantitative assessment, that results in the

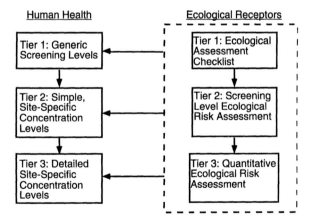

Figure 28-6   Texas risk reduction rules: Tiered processes for determining risk-based concentration levels.

TABLE 28-11   Texas Risk Reduction Rules: Tiered Process for Determining Human Health Risk-Based Concentration Levels

---

Tier 1

- Provides generic screening levels based on direct human exposure to source area materials
- Requires source area delineation and receptor identification
- Includes lookup tables

Tier 2

- Provides simple, site-specific concentration levels to protect human health due to exposure at source area or at specific points of exposure
- Determines cross-media and lateral contaminant transport via default and conservative analytical models
- Requires source delineation and receptor data
- Can involve site-specific parameter data in place of default values

Tier 3

- Provides detailed, site-specific concentration levels to protect human health due to exposure at source area or at separate points of exposure
- Can use alternative numerical models to analyze cross-media and lateral contaminant transport
- Requires detailed site-specific data on source materials, transport mechanisms, and receptors

---

development of a site-specific contaminant concentration that will ensure protection of ecological receptors.

The human health and ecological evaluations are interrelated as follows. Initially, a responsible person would proceed as far down the human health tiered process as desired. Once human health risk-based concentration levels have been determined, the person must evaluate whether protection of the environment will require lower concentrations by proceeding as far through the ecological receptor tiered process as is required. The risk-based concentration level determined for human health considerations is used as the final value unless a lower concentration is required to adequately protect ecological receptors.

Remedy Standards   The Texas Risk Reduction Program is constructed around a series of closure/remediation performance standards, referred to as *remedy standards*. These standards are used to fulfill cleanup responsibilities at contaminated facilities and areas. These remedy standards identify the available risk management options that may be selected. Each remedy standard is protective of human health and the environment in different ways. The rules allow the responsible person to choose the remedy standard to be attained unless an alternative approach is required by another regulation, permit, or regulatory order.

Each standard specifies types of actions allowed, future land use assumed, whether control measures are allowed, and the performance required to attain the standard. Long-term protective care requirements, depending on the standard, may include notification to future owners of the land of limitations on property or resource use; the type, extent, and duration of inspections, monitoring, and maintenance; and financial assurance to perform the necessary maintenance or to respond to the failure of engineering or institutional controls.

The site evaluation remedy selection, and site closure steps represent a phased process for identification and control of both active (i.e., *immediate*) and chronic (i.e., *long-term*) hazards to public health and the environment. Acute hazards, involving high concentrations sufficient to pose an immediate risk of fire, exposure, or health impairment, are identified and abated per the emergency response provisions of the applicable waste management regulations. Following proper control of any acute hazards associated with the site, the risk management process addresses media cleanup goals that will protect against *chronic* health or environmental impacts, such as carcinogenic or toxic effects caused by long-term exposure to lower levels of contaminants. In some cases, even after constituent concentrations have been reduced to levels posing no further acute or chronic health concern, further adjustment of protective concentration levels may be required to address aesthetic or ecological considerations that may affect the future use of the property or resource.

Based on this site evaluation, subsequent steps of the risk reduction process involve development and implementation of remedial measures targeted toward preservation of the desired future land use, in accordance with the selected remedy standard. Following completion of the remedy, site monitoring is conducted for an appropriate time period to verify compliance with applicable response objectives. Following TNRCC review and approval of the site remediation / closure effort, the site may then be closed, subject to relevant postclosure care requirements. The end product of this risk reduction process is a site that is restored for its intended property use in a manner that is protective of public health and the environment.

To develop risk-based concentration limits and associated remedial action plans, the responsible person, in cooperation with the property owner(s), first identifies the type of future land use for which the impacted area is to be restored. Under these Rules, three optional remedy standards, involving varying degrees of on-site land use restrictions, may be considered:

- *Type A*: Unrestricted land use / permanent remedies
- *Type B*: Restricted land use / remedy with controls
- *Type C*: No Active land use / remedy with controls

Each of these remedy standards is protective of unrestricted land use and environmental resources on surrounding off-site properties. However, the degree of land use flexibility to be restored on the affected site itself dictates the degree of site remediation and/or post-closure care requirements that will apply. For example, to restore conditions suitable for unrestricted on-site land use (either residential or commercial), the responsible person must implement a type A remedy standard to reduce constituent concentrations to applicable protective concentration levels (PCLs) in all affected media. Should moderate restrictions on the on-site land use be acceptable (e.g., prohibition on on-site groundwater development), a type B remedy may be selected, allowing constituent concentrations to exceed relevant PCL values in on-site media but requiring long-term control measures to achieve protection of public health and the environment. Under a type C remedy standard, no on-site active land use is restored. Rather, future property access is restricted, and remedial actions are implemented as needed to protect surrounding off-site properties.

The selected remedy standard serves as a template for the evaluation and design of necessary remedial measures. Each remedy standard dictates (1) the applicable exposure assumptions to be used in development of PCL values, (2) the response objectives to be achieved by the remedial action program, and (3) the postclosure care measures to be maintained at the site. In practice, the steps involved can be conducted in an iterative manner, with the selected remedy standard and associated PCL values adjusted to develop a cost-effective remedial action plan that is consistent with future land use plans.

Summary The above material identifies the key components of the Texas Risk Reduction Rules and indicates the media and regulatory programs to which the Rules apply. The Risk Reduction Program is active and being implemented successfully. Additional information can be obtained from the Texas Natural Resources Conservation Commission, Office of Waste Management, 12100 Park 35 Circle, Austin, Texas 78753.

CONCLUSIONS

The concept of environmental risk and its use for environmental decision making and site remediation selection has emerged as an important aspect of environmental engineering in the past ten years. Before that time the emphasis in the regulatory agencies was on determining technology based release or discharge standards. Environmental engineers then would develop or use treatment technologies that could be used to meet such standards.

This technology driven, command-and-control approach to environmental problems has been effective in remediating past environmental problems and minimizing new environmental problems. For some environmental problems, such conventional approaches as end-of-pipe performance standards, design standards, and product specifications will continue to be needed. Together with strict enforcement of existing environmental regulations, these approaches provide a strong incentive to look for cheaper, innovative ways to achieve environmental goals. Strict enforcement of existing regulations will continue, but to reduce continuing and future risks to human health and the environment, the EPA, and the nation as a whole, must have a broader range of tools.

The use of environmental risk for decision making and treatment or remedy selection has resulted from the recognition that (1) not all environmental problems are equally serious, (2) the resources for environmental protection are not limitless, and (3) the focus should be on sites and situations that pose the greatest risk to human health and the environment. Using relative risk to determine the sites and situations of greater risk is protective and is a rational approach. However, it must be based on sound scientific information and supportable risk assessments.

Practical applications of the risk assessment paradigm for environmental engineering purposes include situations as diverse as Superfund, biosolids management, and contaminated sediments. In addition generic risk-based protocols, such as RBCA and state risk reduction rules, are now available and are being used for broad applications.

The determination of site-specific risks will require knowledge from medical doctors, as well as toxicologists and other scientists. Environmental engineers increasingly will use the RBCA type framework and knowledge about site-specific human health and ecological risks to determine the degree of treatment or remediation necessary and the appropriate environmental technologies that should be used at a site. Overall, the concept of environmental risk can help the nation consistently and systematically develop policies to deal with these problems and to choose more wisely among the policy options for reducing environmental risks.

REFERENCES

American Society for Testing Materials. 1995. *Guide for Risk-Based Corrective Action Applied at Petroleum Release Sites*. Philadelphia: E-1739-95.

Code of Federal Regulations. 1993. *Part 503—Standards for the Use or Disposal of Sewage Sludge*. Title 40, Protection of the Environment. Washington, DC: Office of the Federal Register, National Archives and Records Administration.

Federal Register. 1985. *Executive Order* 12498: *Regulatory Planning Process*. Washington, DC: Government Printing Office, 50:1036.

Federal Register. 1993. *Executive Order* 12866: *Regulatory Planning and Review*. Washington, DC: Government Printing Office, 58: 51735.

Fuhrman, R. E. 1984. History of water pollution control. *J. Water Poll. Control Fed.* 56: 306–313.

Graham, J. D. 1994. *A Historical Perspective on Risk Assessment in the Federal Government.* Boston: Center for Risk Analysis, Harvard School of Public Health.

Habicht, F. H. 1992. Guidance on Risk Characterization for Risk Managers and Risk Assessors, *Memo of February 26, 1992 to Assistant and Regional Administrators.* Washington, DC: U.S. Environmental Protection Agency.

Lowrance, W. W. 1976. *Of Acceptable Risk: Science and the Determination of Safety.* Los Altos, CA: Kaufmann.

Minard, R. W. 1995. RCRA and the states: History, politics, and results. In *Comparing Environmental Risks–Tools for Setting Government Priorities*, ed. J. C. Davies. Washington, DC: Resources for the Future.

National Academy of Sciences. 1994. *Science and Judgment in Risk Assessment.* Washington, DC: National Academy Press.

National Research Council. 1983. *Risk Assessment in the Federal Government: Managing the Process.* Washington, DC: National Academy Press.

National Research Council. 1997. *Contaminated Sediments in Ports and Waterways—Cleanup Strategies and Technologies.* Washington, DC: National Academy Press.

Paustenbach, D. J. 1989. *The Risk Assessment of Environmental and Human Health Hazards: A Textbook of Case Studies.* New York: Wiley.

Presidential/Congressional Commission on Risk Assessment and Risk Management. 1997. *Framework for Environmental Health Risk Management: Final Report*, vol. 1. Washington, DC: Government Printing Office.

Reilly, W. K. 1990. Aiming before we shoot: The quiet revolution in environmental policy. Presentation at the National Press Club, September 26, 1990, Washington, DC. Washington, DC: U.S. Environmental Protection Agency, 20Z–1011.

U.S. Environmental Protection Agency. 1984. *Risk Assessment and Management: Framework for Decision Making.* Washington, DC: EPA 600/9-85-002.

U.S. Environmental Protection Agency. 1987. *Risk Assessment and Management: Framework for Decision Making.* Washington, DC: EPA 600/8–87/085.

U.S. Environmental Protection Agency. 1988. *Guidance for Conducting Remedial Investigations and Feasibility Studies under CERCLA.* Washington, DC: Office of Solid Waste and Emergency Response, EPA/540/6–89/004.

U.S. Environmental Protection Agency. 1989a. *Risk Assessment Guidance for Superfund. Volume 1: Human Health Evaluation Manual.* Washington, DC: Office of Emergency and Remedial Response, EPA/540/1-89/002.

U.S. Environmental Protection Agency. 1989b. *Risk Assessment Guidance for Superfund. Volume 2: Environmental Evaluation Manual.* Washington, DC: Office of Emergency and Remedial Response, EPA/540/1-89/001.

U.S. Environmental Protection Agency. 1989c. *Ecological Assessments of Hazardous Waste Sites: A Field and Laboratory Reference Manual.* Washington, DC: Office of Research and Development, EPA/600/3–89/013.

U.S. Environmental Protection Agency. 1990. *Reducing Risk: Setting Priorities and Strategies for Environmental Protection.* Washington, DC: Science Advisory Board SAB-EC-90-021.

U.S. Environmental Protection Agency. 1991a. *Risk Assessment Guidance for Superfund. Volume 1: Human Health Evaluation Manual (Part B, Development of Risk-Based Preliminary Remediation Goals).* Washington, DC: EPA/540/R–92/003.

U.S. Environmental Protection Agency. 1991b. *Risk Assessment in Superfund: A Primer.* Washington, DC: Office of Emergency and Remedial Response, EPA/540/X91/002.

U.S. Environmental Protection Agency. 1992. *Comparative Risk Projects.* Washington, DC: Office of Policy, Planning and Evaluation, Regional and State Planning Branch.

U.S. General Accounting Office. 1991. *Environmental Protection: Meeting Public Expectations with Limited Resources*, Washington, DC.

29 Clinical Perspective on Respiratory Toxicology

MARK J. UTELL, M.D.
JONATHAN M. SAMET, M.D.

The chapters in this volume have described the adverse effects of diverse agents on the lung and other target organs. These effects have been characterized through multidisciplinary approaches, typically involving in vitro and in vivo laboratory studies and often controlled human exposures and epidemiological investigations. The resulting evidence on adverse effects may have substantial societal impact through regulatory and nonregulatory pathways. However, exposed individuals sustain the associated risk and disease burden. In this chapter we address the extension of this information to the diagnosis and management of environmentally related disease in individual patients and in exposed groups.

The care of individuals falls to the practicing physician or other health care providers. Often the physician addresses the fears a patient raises about the consequences of exposure or manages the disease that may have resulted from or was exacerbated by exposure. The physician may also become enmeshed in legal questions as to the causation of disease and to compensation. In this chapter we consider the clinical approach to the individual who has been exposed to a respiratory hazard. We review the tools available to the health care provider with the purpose of describing clinical methods and their strengths and limits in answering the frequently complex questions that arise around environmental exposures.

The evaluation of exposed populations, such as specific worker groups, may also fall to health care providers. However, to address the effects of exposure on populations, the approach must extend beyond simply evaluating individuals to provide measures of impact on groups. Epidemiological studies, typically cross-sectional surveys, are often conducted to evaluate potential adverse respiratory effects. In this review we consider the tools used to conduct such surveys. Although a survey might be performed in response to recognition of a perceived hazard, persons exposed to potential or known hazards may be subject to ongoing surveillance, often required in the workplace. We also review surveillance methodology. Of necessity our treatment of these subjects is limited. Textbooks on environmental medicine are available (Rom, 1998; Rosenstock and Cullen, 1994). Additionally a series of case studies has been published by the Institute of Medicine (1996).

Environmental Toxicants: Human Exposures and Their Health Effects, 2/e. Edited by Morton Lippmann.
ISBN: 0-471-29298-2 © 2000 John Wiley & Sons, Inc.

CONCEPTS OF EXPOSURE

Patterns of time use and activity place people in diverse indoor and outdoor environments throughout the day, each environment possibly having its own unique set of air contaminants. The characteristics of these environments and the time spent in them varies with age, sex, and other sociodemographic factors. Personal exposure to air pollutants represents the time-weighted average of pollutant concentrations in microenvironments, environments having relatively homogeneous air quality (Sexton and Ryan, 1988). Diverse microenvironments that may be relevant for health include the home, the workplace, schools, outdoors, transportation environments, and locations where recreational time is spent.

The clinician's approach to assessing exposure in these microenvironments primarily involves interviewing the patient. Standardized instruments for collecting information on environmental and occupational exposures have been published (Occupational and Environmental Health Committee, 1983), but clinicians generally take exposure histories in idiosyncratic ways, the completeness of the history reflecting the clinician's training, fund of knowledge, and familiarity with the environments of concern to specific patients. The clinical history of exposures may touch on a few widely know hazards, such as asbestos, but rarely inventories the duties of specific jobs, the materials handled, or the use of respiratory protection. Most physicians have limited knowledge of the exposures associated with specific occupations.

Biological markers of exposure are available on a routine clinical basis for only a few inhaled pollutants, including, for example, carboxyhemoglobin for carbon monoxide and blood or urine lead level for inhaled lead (National Research Council, 1989). Levels of other metals can be measured in blood or other samples, if needed.

Serum antibodies or skin test reactivity to intradermal antigen injection can be measured to provide an indication of past exposure and the development of sensitivity to selected antigens; tests are available for some common biological antigens, such as the house dust mite, but for only a few inhaled chemicals. Routine clinical tests for adducts and antibodies to adducts are not yet available, nor are tests readily available for most intermediate endpoints that may be relevant from a toxicological perspective.

Thus the routine clinical evaluation does not usually provide comprehensive information concerning environmental exposure. In fact the routine history taken by a primary care provider usually addresses only tobacco smoking and the current or usual employment; some common exposures with well-known consequences, such as asbestos, may also be covered. Often, however, it is the identification of a disease known to be caused by a specific agent that prompts full questioning of the patient concerning relevant exposures and thus routine medical records do not usually offer any more than a superficial assessment of inhaled exposures.

A physician trained in environmental or occupational medicine routinely obtains more detailed and disease-relevant information; this type of physician should be consulted in cases involving possible effects of complex environmental exposures. Physicians trained in pulmonary medicine may also have special expertise related to environmental lung disease, and allergists may be appropriate for addressing workplace-related allergic disorders. In evaluating the chest X ray for the pneumoconioses, fibrotic disorders of the lung, the chest X ray may be interpreted according to a standard system, the International Labour Office (ILO) classification (International Labour Office, 1980). The "B Reader" certification uses this system and is given by the National Institute for Occupational Safety and Health (NIOSH) to persons who have taken a two day course and successfully passed an examination involving standardized interpretation of chest roentgenographs showing various occupational lung diseases. This certification demonstrates competency in interpreting patterns of radiographic abnormality, but does not specifically establish expertise in occupational lung disease.

TOOLS FOR STUDYING INDIVIDUALS

Environmental diseases frequently masquerade as common medical disorders. From a clinical perspective, primary care physicians underdiagnose environmentally and occupationally related disorders and far too infrequently enter them into their differential diagnosis. For example, more than 80% of occupational or environmental disease diagnoses had not been correctly recognized prior to evaluation in an occupational medicine clinic, although most patients had consulted one or more physicians (Cullen and Cherniack, 1989). The inadequate knowledge base of primary care physicians in environmental medicine (Institute of Medicine, 1988) and the physician shortages in these specialized disciplines have been emphasized (Castorina and Rosenstock, 1990). Unfortunately, there has been little progress since the 1988 Institute of Medicine report on environmental and occupational medicine.

In considering environmentally induced lung diseases, it is important to recognize that symptoms and signs of lung damage are seldom indicative of the specific injuring agent. For the clinician, the recognition of occupational or environmental respiratory illness may be obscured by the nonspecificity of symptoms, findings on physical examination, alterations of pulmonary function, or radiographic changes. Lung biopsy is rarely indicated to confirm a diagnosis of environmentally related disease, and even when tissue is available, pathological findings may be nonspecific and not indicate a specific etiologic agent. For example, airways inflammation may reflect the consequence of a myriad of inhaled agents. Specific links between exposure and disease, such as beryllium exposure and noncaseating granulomas, are few. Rarely, specific diagnostic fibers or dusts may be identified in lung tissue. In addition, exposures are often multiple or mixed, symptoms may be minimal until disease is advanced or more severe than anticipated for the extent of physiological and radiographic abnormality, and latency periods between onset of exposure and disease development may be long. Identifying occupationally related lung disease is further complicated by the frequent overlay of cigarette smoking and the possibility of additive or even synergistic effects acting in combination with other agents, (e.g., asbestos-related lung tumors); thus the association between lung disease and occupational exposure is often neither obvious nor simple.

The clinician is now called on to deal not only with the more classical occupational diseases, like the pneumoconioses, but also the more problematic "environmental" illnesses of the 1980s and 1990s. For example, as new construction techniques and ventilation practices were directed at conserving energy, and sealed buildings began to age, outbreaks of illnesses characterized by persistent respiratory symptoms, headaches, lassitude, and other symptoms were reported for building occupants (Samet et al., 1988). This problem is widely referred to as *sick-building syndrome.* Even more perplexing is the appearance of illness in previously healthy individuals who, following accidental exposure to solvents, gases, or irritating fumes, develop unrelenting respiratory complaints, lethargy, and central nervous system dysfunction when subsequently exposed to trace amounts of the material or other irritants such as fumes or cigarette smoke. This symptom complex has been labeled *multiple chemical sensitivities* (Cullen, 1987); it poses substantial diagnostic and therapeutic difficulty. Finally the clinician is not infrequently called on to assess the individual exposed on one or more occasions to "low-level" asbestos in a public building, a work site, or the home.

TABLE 29-1 Tools for Evaluating Individuals with Suspected Occupational or Environmental Lung Disease

General evaluation

    Medical and respiratory history
    Detailed occupational history
    Identification of materials
    Identification of toxic responses
    Chest X ray

Special studies

    Immunologic and skin tests
    Airway hyperreactivity testing
    CT scan
    Fiberoptic bronchoscopy with bronchoalveolar lavage
Industrial hygiene information
Site or plant visit
Epidemiological investigation

In this section we focus on the tools available to the clinician for evaluating the individual patient suspected of having an environmentally related pulmonary disorder. The emphasis on respiratory disorders is highly relevant: Respiratory diseases are the most frequently diagnosed work-related conditions in industrial regions, and the best-established medical consequences of mining and farming involve the lower respiratory tract and the airway is most important portal of entry for toxic agents from the environment. The tools commonly available for evaluating the individual are shown in Table 29-1; the general principles also apply to the evaluation of environmentally related nonrespiratory disorders.

Clinical Approaches

For the physician the central problem in environmental lung medicine is determining that a respiratory symptom or particular structural or functional derangement of the lung is caused by a certain inhaled agent. Table 29-2 lists examples of the pathophysiological responses of the respiratory tract to environmental particles and gases. As with all disorders associated with the environment, a careful and thorough history is mandatory. Both the work and home environments need to be considered for exposure to known

TABLE 29-2 Pathophysiological Responses of Respiratory Tract to Occupational and Environmental Particles and Gases

Site	Agent	Potential Response
Nose	Pollen	Hay fever, rhinitis
	Formaldehyde	Nasal cancer
Airways	Sulfur dioxide, nitrogen dioxide	Bronchoconstriction
	High- and low-molecular weight chemicals	Asthma
	Aeroallergens	Asthma
	Formaldehyde, wood smoke	Irritation, cough
	Radon, asbestos	Cancer
Parenchyma	Inorganic dusts	Pneumoconiosis
	Thermophilic actinomycetes, fungi	Hypersensitivity pneumonitis

allergens, irritants, chemicals, or organic dust. Careful inquiry is necessary concerning not only the materials the individual is working with, but also those being used by coworkers. The occurrence of similar problems in coworkers also should be assessed. Other clues in the history are useful. With occupational asthma, these is often a latent period between the first exposure to the offending agent and the onset of asthma (Chan-Yeung, 1990). This period may vary from a few weeks to over 20 years. Therefore the physician must attempt to correlate temporally respiratory and/or systemic symptoms with exposure to a particular environment, although varying temporal relationships between exposure and outcome may cloud interpretation of the clinical history. Thus, in some instances, the causal relationship between exposure and symptoms may not be readily recognized. Correlation of symptom occurrence with exposure may be difficult in cases of late-onset, delayed, or repetitive patterns of response or in those responses in which cough, chest tightness, or malaise predominates. This contrasts with the clinical picture of a worker who develops symptoms immediately and repeatedly when working with a particular substance.

The initial care of individual patients exposed to potentially toxic materials usually falls to the practicing primary care physician or other health care providers. Typically the exposure history obtained by such practitioners is insufficient and characterizes the workplace qualitatively, as "dusty" or "extensive smoke and fumes." Major effort should be extended to accurately identify the specific toxic agent or agents involved in each work site. This may require direct contact with employers and/or assistance from governmental agencies (NIOSH or OSHA) for information. Some efforts have been focused on development of occupational/environmental history forms to assist the clinician in collecting the data base (Occupational and Environmental Health Committee, 1983; Kilbourne and Weiner, 1990).

The newer problems of sick building syndrome and multiple chemical sensitivity may be readily recognized if the patient presents with an unmistakable clinical picture. The clinician is faced with an individual with a myriad of complaints, often including intractable upper respiratory symptoms, ill-defined central nervous system dysfunction, headache, fatigue, and low productivity that are attributed to odors, poor ventilation, or other aspects of a sealed building. Despite a careful physical evaluation, there may be no physical signs revealed on examination. In outbreaks with an identified etiology, a spectrum of causative agents has been identified: infectious agents, specific air contaminants, and environmental conditions such as temperature and humidity (Finnegan and Pickering, 1986; American Thoracic Society, 1997). Outbreaks without an identifiable etiology have frequently occurred in tight buildings and have given rise to the sick building syndrome. However, these outbreaks are by no means limited to tight buildings; they may occur because of maintenance problems, changing uses, and other factors.

An even more puzzling syndrome is the so-called multiple chemical sensitivities (MCS) in which the individual becomes "sensitized" to almost all organic and synthetic chemicals (Cullen, 1987). The history is typically that of a healthy individual who after accidental exposure to a solvent or irritant gas or fumes develops progressive symptoms with exposure to traces of the original agent or a variety of nonspecific agents. The assessment lies in the historical data, since the remainder of the evaluation is quite unremarkable. Many hypotheses have now been examined, and there are few known, extrinsic causes of MCS supported by research. Immunologic abnormalities now appear to be a less plausible cause (Simon et al., 1993). It has been suggested that the clinician is dealing with a variant of a posttraumatic stress disorder (Schottenfeld and Cullen, 1986), and case reports have revealed a probable role of conditioned response, especially to odor. Although no well-controlled studies establish a clear mechanism, the MCS patient often requires comprehensive evaluation and compassionate support. Several major medical societies, including the American College of Physicians (1989), the American Medical Association (1992), and the American College of Occupational and Environmental

Medicine (1991), have concluded that the existence of MCS is an unproved hypothesis and that credible scientific research is needed.

Physical examination is often unrevealing in cases of environmental lung disease. There should be a full evaluation of the nose, oropharynx, and chest and lungs. Abnormal lung sounds such as bibasilar rales (cracking sounds) are heard with interstitial lung disease, as in asbestosis which results from asbestos exposure. Signs of airway disease such as wheezing and cough are typically associated with environmental asthma. However, neither a normal examination nor one in which wheezing persists even after avoidance of the work environment, excludes environmental airway disease from the diagnostic possibilities. There may be a need to systematically correlate symptoms and lung function levels with activities and exposure in the work environment and at home. There are no pathognomonic findings with sick building syndrome or multiple chemical sensitivities.

Imaging Studies

Since the clinician is likely to obtain a chest X ray in the evaluation of any individual with respiratory complaints, it is worth emphasizing that radiological examination remains a major diagnostic tool for revealing occupationally induced interstitial lung disease. The principle disorders, the pneumoconioses, include asbestosis, coal workers' pneumoconiosis, silicosis, and berylliosis.

The chest X ray in asbestos exposure may serve to identify biological markers of exposure or evidence of disease providing documentation of fiber exposure of the parenchyma and/or pleural reactions. Workers exposed to asbestos fibers may develop a variety of pleural processes including effusions, plaques, or diffuse thickening; the pleural changes serve as markers of asbestos exposure and rarely are associated with symptoms or functional changes (Craighead and Mossman, 1982). In contrast, workers exposed to high concentrations of asbestos fibers may develop interstitial infiltrates primarily in the lower lung fields, characterized by an irregular, linear pattern. Persons with this pattern typically have reduced lung function.

Workers exposed to other dusts such as silica and/or coal dust typically demonstrate bilateral upper lobe interstitial infiltrates (Fraser et al., 1990). These infiltrates characteristically are nodular in appearance; the nodules range in size from 1 to 10 mm, may coalesce, and eventually distort or cause retraction in the hilar region. It should be emphasized that the diagnosis of pneumoconiosis in the absence of an abnormal chest radiograph is highly unusual. The rare patient in this category, symptomatic but with a normal chest X ray, would require additional supportive data to substantiate the diagnosis.

For the clinician evaluating the patient with suspected environmental or occupational asthma, the chest X ray may not be of great diagnostic help. Often it is normal or reveals only minimal hyperinflation. The patient with hypersensitivity pneumonitis will often demonstrate diffuse infiltrates on the radiograph. Finally occupationally related pulmonary malignancies present with the various X ray patterns of lung cancers associated with smoking. The radiographic changes in various occupational lung diseases have been described in detail (Fraser et al., 1990).

More sophisticated imaging techniques used in clinical practice, such as computed tomography (CT), are not currently applicable in large surveys, but they may be useful in the evaluation of specific chest X ray abnormalities. In environmental medicine, the CT scan is an important modality in locating and characterizing small lesions that could represent early lung tumors. The CT scan has been useful in assessing the location, extent, and potential for surgical resection of small lung lesions and masses. In addition the CT scan has been useful in confirming the presence of pleural plaques noted on chest X ray; it also raises the possibility that there are large groups of persons with pleural disease undetectable on standard radiographs (Friedman et al., 1988). High-resolution chest CT (HRCT) can detect pneumoconiotic small opacities or abnormal lung tissue associated with diffuse forms of interstitial fibrosis not visible on plain chest X ray (Aberle et al., 1988). Schwartz et al. (1990) observed that among asbestos-exposed patients with normal parenchyma on plain chest X ray, patients with pleural disease are more likely than those with normal pleura to have interstitial abnormalities on the HRCT. Clearly, prospective, controlled evaluations are required to determine the prognostic significance of these abnormalities on HRCT among exposed persons with normal-looking parenchyma by chest X ray.

Pulmonary Function Testing

Tests of pulmonary function are useful tools for evaluating the physiologic consequences of lung damage caused by inhaled materials. In evaluating individual patients with respiratory complaints or with potentially toxic exposures, physicians obtain pulmonary function tests. In fact failure to obtain such studies almost invariably represents inadequate clinical evaluation. Guidelines for characteristics of pulmonary function equipment, test interpretation, and quality assurance are available (Clausen, 1982; American Thoracic Society, 1995).

The clinical utility of physiological function testing in individual patients lies in finding evidence of response to inhaled toxic agents. The tests can show the functional manifestations of structural changes in the respiratory system, whether the changes are transient (e.g., bronchoconstriction) or permanent (e.g., fibrosis). However, these tests have little specificity for effects of specific environmental agents. The lung responds to injury in a limited number of ways, and the physiological manifestation of various types of injury are often the same, regardless of the causative agent. Thus abnormal lung function tests are a general, rather than a specific, indication of injury. One type of testing, inhalation challenge with specific agents may lead to more specific findings.

The real workhorse in the evaluation of the individual patient is simple spirometry, a test that can be readily performed in the field or office setting. The spirometric tracing, which describes the rate of forced exhalation, distinguishes the obstructive pattern from restrictive patterns of physiologic impairment. Detailed reviews of the use of pulmonary function testing in evaluation of the patient with occupational lung disease are available (Miller, 1985). In brief, the restrictive pattern, typical of interstitial lung disease, is suggested by a forced vital capacity (FVC) $< 80\%$ predicted and $FEV_1/FVC > 75\%$. In contrast, the obstructive pattern, typical of airways disease, includes an FVC $> 80\%$ predicted, $FEV_1 < 80\%$ predicted, and $FEV_1/FVC < 75\%$. In addition the maximum voluntary ventilation (MVV) is usually reduced below 80% predicted. Although the MVV is a valuable test when properly performed, it requires considerable patient cooperation and effort. A reduction in the forced expiratory flow from 25% to 75% of FVC, $FEF_{25-75\%}$, below 70% predicted with otherwise normal flow rates is a marker of early but mild airway obstruction. Predicted values take into account patient age, height, and sex.

The restrictive pattern is the hallmark of interstitial lung diseases such as asbestosis, but it is not specific and can result from such diverse processes as large pleural effusions, muscle weakness, and even marked obesity. In the presence of significant obstructive airway disease, as in smoking-caused chronic obstructive pulmonary disease, it is difficult to interpret the spirogram for restrictive changes unless these are extremely severe, since obstructive disease may also reduce the forced vital capacity. In this case more sophisticated measurements of lung volumes, using body plethysmography or helium dilution techniques, may be necessary. Restrictive disease is classically defined by a reduced total lung capacity below 80% predicted. A reduction in the diffusing capacity for carbon monoxide may be valuable in supporting a diagnosis of interstitial lung disease.

Although cigarette smoking is the most common cause of the obstructive pattern, a history of smoking should not preclude careful investigation into occupational exposures as contributing if not causal factors for physiological impairment. All too often an abnormality in lung function is attributed to cigarettes to the exclusion of other potential agents. On the other hand, some of the impairment in persons with occupational lung disease may be due to smoking. Smokers are usually diagnosed with chronic obstructive respiratory diseases when the level of airflow limitation interferes with activities that they would otherwise be able to perform (Speizer and Tager, 1979). There is a continuum between health and respiratory disease. Disability typically occurs when the FEV_1 approaches 40% to 50% of the predicted value. Pulmonary clinicians consider the reduction of FEV_1 below 80% of the predicted value as indicative of obstructive disease; as the reduction in the FEV_1 progresses, the severity of disease increases.

In the evaluation of potential occupational or environmental asthma, it is important to establish objectively the relationship of exposure with symptom occurrence and reduction of lung function. The recording of peak expiratory flow rates (PEFR) with a mini-peak-flow meter by the patient at work or at home may be a valuable method of establishing a causal relationship. These devices are inexpensive and sufficiently accurate if used properly. The serial measurement of lung function generally provides stronger information on the effect of exposure than one or two spirometric measurements spaced over time. In following the PEFR, the individual typically measures and records the value every 2 to 4 hours from waking to sleeping (Chan-Yeung, 1990). A record is maintained for several work weeks, often followed by at least one week away from any work exposure. Although criteria for a positive response have not been well established, the clinician is seeking to find a pattern of exposure followed by symptoms and a change in PEFR. Improvement in lung function and reduction in symptoms during the week away from work are also helpful in confirming a diagnosis. A major concern with PEFR measurement is the effort dependence of the test such that inadequate respiratory effort can lead to misleading data.

Specialized testing, including an assessment of airway hyperreactivity, may be needed to evaluate environmental asthma. Nonspecific airway hyperreactivity is defined as an exaggerated bronchoconstrictor response to a variety of chemical, physical, and pharmacological stimuli. There is now nearly a consensus that nonspecific airway hyperreactivity is a characteristic shared by virtually all asthmatics (Boushey et al., 1980; National Institutes of Health, 1997); that is, the asthmatic develops bronchoconstriction after inhaling a lower concentration of a provoking agent than is needed to cause a similar degree of change in airway tone in a healthy subject.

In the laboratory, airway reactivity testing is divided into two general categories, depending on the choice of nonspecific versus specific agents. In both, the increased bronchoconstrictor response is assessed with pulmonary function tests. Nonspecific stimuli include pharmacological agents such as methacholine, carbachol, and histamine; exercise; hyperpnea with cold or dry air; and inhalation of hypertonic or hypotonic aerosols. Although pharmacological challenge is used most often in the clinical laboratory, it is less suitable for population studies, especially those involving children because of safety considerations. Cold-air challenge with hyperventilation has been used effectively, and response to cold air is generally correlated closely with methacholine responses (O'Byrne et al., 1982). Challenge with specific agents, common antigens, chemicals such as isocyanates, and organic materials such as plicatic acid (from western red cedar) can be used to identify specific sensitizing agents. These approaches can be particularly powerful in incriminating occupational chemicals and confirming the diagnosis of occupation-related airway disease; the challenge may provoke immediate and/or late pulmonary responses that do not resolve spontaneously. Even with specific agents, the interpretation of responses can be difficult and confounded by a variety of factors such as dose and irritant effects (McKay, 1986).

In the assessment of asthma induced by occupational agents, airway reactivity testing with nonspecific and specific agents serves a diagnostic function. Chan-Yeung (1995) and Chan-Yeung and Lam (1986) have published comprehensive reviews on the subject of occupational asthma and the role of airway reactivity testing. Nonspecific airway hyperreactivity occurs in most workers with occupationally induced asthma despite their not having the usual factors such as atopy. Furthermore Lam and coworkers (1983) found a good correlation between the degree of nonspecific bronchial hyperreactivity and the severity of response to the provoking agent, plicatic acid in workers with red cedar asthma. Measurement of hyperreactivity also assists in providing objective evidence of sensitization (Chan-Yeung and Lam, 1986). The demonstration of an increase in bronchial reactivity on returning to the workplace and a decrease away from work, with appropriate changes in lung function, is evidence for a causal relationship between symptoms and the work environment. To pinpoint the etiological agent in the workplace responsible for asthma, a specific challenge may be necessary. Chan-Yeung and Lam (1986) emphasize that such testing can be dangerous and should be performed only by experienced persons in a hospital setting for the following conditions: studying previously unrecognized occupational asthma, determining the precise etiological agent in a complex industrial environment, and confirming a diagnosis for medicolegal purposes. Detailed guidelines and testing procedures have been developed and published (Pepys and Hutchcroft, 1975; Salvaggio and Hendrick, 1989).

Special Laboratory Investigations

In a vast majority of patients, a diagnosis of environmental or occupationally related lung disease will be made through careful history and physical exam performed in conjunction with pulmonary function tests and a chest X ray. The clinician rarely proceeds to specialized laboratory testing. In selected cases, however, additional supportive information can be obtained from skin testing with appropriate extracts, particularly of high-molecular-weight compounds for specific agents responsible for occupational asthma. Skin tests are generally accepted for IgE-mediated protein allergens. For example, extracts from flour (Block et al., 1983) and animal products produce immediate positive reaction on skin testing in sensitized subjects. Unfortunately, these skin tests are not always available. There is no established value for skin tests against chemicals, such as formaldehyde, or cigarette smoke. This contrasts with more routine allergy skin tests with common inhalants and food allergens that are used to define the atopic status of the individual.

Antigen-specific IgE antibody testing can be done with RAST or by ELISA for occupational asthma. Specific IgE antibodies against low-molecular-weight compounds conjugated to a protein (e.g., isocyanate) have been demonstrated in some exposed individuals (Butcher et al., 1980). Again, such tests are not readily available, and a positive response may occur in exposed workers without asthma. It is not appropriate to obtain antibodies to evaluate symptoms resulting from a single exposure.

Serum precipitin testing can be done for hypersensitivity pneumonitis. The precipitins can be detected in farmer's lung disease with antibodies to the thermophilic actinomyces, especially *Micropolyspora faeni*, or in pigeon breeders with antibodies to various proteins contained in pigeon serum or pigeon-dropping extracts. Office workers may develop hypersensitivity from fungal contaminants in ventilation systems; exposures have been reported to thermophilic actinomyces and penicillium species.

Several studies have examined the role of bronchoalveolar lavage (BAL) in occupational lung diseases (Rom et al., 1987). Workers with farmer's lung demonstrate a predominantly suppressor T-cell lymphocytic alveolitis (Cormier et al., 1986), and worker with chronic beryllium disease show a T-helper-cell lymphocytosis (Epstein et al.,

1982), whereas workers with asbestosis demonstrate an increase in alveolar macrophages with or without a modest increase in neutrophils (depending on the smoking status) (Rom et al., 1987). Not only can the cellular differentials provide a clue to the underlying disorder, but also the asbestos fibers in the lavage fluid can be quantified. Although the utility of these research techniques in patient evaluation and diagnosis remains largely investigational, BAL may have diagnostic and prognostic implications in chronic beryllium disease. The extent of BAL cellularity, lymphocytosis, and beryllium lymphocyte proliferation test response correlate with disease severity (Newman et al., 1994), suggesting that the magnitude of the inflammatory and antigenic response in the lung may help predict disease progression or response to therapy.

Exposure Assessments

For the clinician insufficient information on exposure data often limits establishing a causal relationship between exposure and disease. Especially in large industries, industrial hygiene information may be available that provides a quantitative estimate of dusts, vapors, or aerosols in the work environment. An understanding of the pathophysiology of environmentally induced lung disorders requires a working knowledge of the mechanisms involved in the uptake of gases, the deposition of dusts, and their subsequent retention. For example, in relating clinical disease to specific exposures, the clinician must recognize that penetration into and retention within the respiratory tract of toxic gases can vary widely depend on a number of factors: the physical properties of the gas (e.g., solubility), the concentration of the gas in the expired air, the rate of depth of ventilation, and the extent to which the material is reactive (Utell and Samet, 1990). Likewise, the aerodynamic properties of particles, airway anatomy, and breathing pattern largely determine the site of deposition of particles and fibers in the airways. Thus the identification and characterization of the inhaled materials are essential in linking inhaled materials with specific types of lung damage.

Patterns of time use and activity place individuals in diverse indoor and outdoor environments throughout the day, each environment having its own unique set of air contaminants. Perhaps because of the distinct sources contaminating outdoor air and indoor air and the separate regulatory mechanisms for outdoor air, the workplace, and the home, the health effects of inhaled toxicants have often been addressed separately for outdoor and indoor air.

However, the concept of total personal exposure is most relevant for health; personal exposure to air pollution represents the time-weighted average of pollutant concentrations in microenvironments which are environments having relatively homogeneous air quality. Thus, for an office worker, relevant microenvironments might include home, office, car, outdoors at work, and a movie theater. For some pollutants, such as ozone or acid aerosols, outdoor environments make the predominant contribution to total personal exposure; for others, such as radon and formaldehyde, indoor locations are most important. In considering the health consequences of environmental toxicants, the physician should recognize the potential contributions of various pollution sources.

In the workplace the safety officer or industrial hygienist can be very helpful in reviewing exposures and assisting in interpreting the results. In the investigation of building-related illnesses, indoor contaminants such as formaldehyde, smoke, and microorganisms as well as the adequacy of the ventilation system need to be assessed. In special situations a visit to the work or environmental site may be crucial in assisting the physician to better understand the potential exposure or even the ventilation system. Occasionally intensive investigation of the individual will lead to a recommendation for a population study as a result of introduction of new materials or issues of "safe" levels in the workplace.

TOOLS FOR STUDYING POPULATIONS

Persons may be exposed to inhaled pollutants in a variety of locations, including outdoors, workplaces, and other indoor environments. Typically epidemiological investigations of health effects are initiated because of concern about the consequences of exposure in a particular location, such as the outdoors or the workplace. For example, many studies of asbestos-exposed workers were undertaken after adverse consequences of exposure to this agent first became apparent. Studies of outdoor air pollution have been implemented in areas with unusual localized patterns of exposure, such as petrochemical or other manufacturing plants, or with regional patterns of pollution, such as photochemical or acid aerosol pollution. Similarly groups have been targeted because of particular exposures indoors.

Epidemiological studies may also be implemented because of concern about the contribution of inhaled pollutants to particular diseases, both malignant and nonmalignant. For example, lung cancer increased in epidemic fashion among males in many countries beginning in the 1940s. Many of the initial investigations focused on exposure to outdoor air pollution in addition to cigarette smoking, which was subsequently found to be the cause of most cases. At present, the contribution of indoor air pollutants, particularly environmental tobacco smoke and radon, to lung cancer remains an area of active investigation.

Although some individuals may be sufficiently affected by inhaled pollutants to have clinically evident effects, the anticipated effects of most current exposures of concern are likely to be more subtle and not detectable by routine clinical assessment. However, epidemiological assessment of populations may provide evidence for adverse effects and the finding of such effects may become a basis for regulating or legal action. Comparisons of exposed with nonexposed populations or of more highly exposed with less-exposed populations are made to find evidence of adverse effects that may not be manifest on evaluation of single individuals. Epidemiology comprises the methods used to study the effect of exposure on the population. Of the complementary approaches used to study inhaled pollutants, laboratory studies, clinical studies, and epidemiological studies, only the results of epidemiological studies provide evidence of the effects of agents as exposures occur in the community. Epidemiologic data may span the full range of susceptibility and inherently incorporate the interaction among agents.

Surveillance refers to ongoing, systematic collection of data on health and disease (Baker et al., 1989). Programs for surveillance may be implemented to monitor the consequences of intervention programs or to identify "sentinel" cases signaling unacceptable exposures (Rutstein et al., 1983). Exposures to hazards can also be monitored (Froines et al., 1989). Surveillance approaches have been most widely used for monitoring the occurrence of occupational diseases; surveillance may be implemented within populations or within exposed work forces. Data sources on populations include reporting by clinicians, death certificates, cancer registries, workers' compensation systems, hospital discharge records, employer reports, and special surveys (Baker et al., 1989; Melius et al., 1989; Freund et al., 1989). Large industries have implemented their own surveillance systems.

A report on silicosis illustrates the application of a surveillance system in a defined population. Valiante and Rosenman (1989) implemented a surveillance system for silicosis in the state of New Jersey; death certificates, hospital discharge data, and physicians were the principal sources for case ascertainment. For the period 1979 through 1987, 401 cases were identified, primarily by screening of hospital discharge data. Only one case was reported by a physician, and most hospitals did not voluntarily report their cases despite state requirements. Follow-up inspections at industries where cases had occurred identified inadequate control of exposure at most. This system had the purpose of finding all cases of this fully preventable disease.

TABLE 29-3   Epidemiological Study Designs Used to Investigate the Effects of Inhaled Pollutants

Case-control study

An analytical design involving selection of diseased cases and nondiseased controls
    followed by assessment of past exposures.

Cohort study

An analytical design involving selection of exposed and nonexposed subjects with
    subsequent observation for disease occurrence. Short-term cohort studies of the health
    status of susceptible groups are often called *panel studies.*

Cross-sectional study

Subjects are identified, and exposure and disease status determined, at one point in time.

Epidemiological Approaches

Conventional epidemiological approaches used to study the adverse effects of inhaled
pollutants on the lung are the cross-sectional study, the cohort study, and the case-control
study (Table 29-3). These designs have the exposed individual as the unit of observation.
Ecological designs, also used to study the environment and health, have groups of
individuals, such as communities or even countries, as one unit of observation. Multi-level
designs incorporate elements of both the ecologic studies and the individual-level designs.
Each design has advantages and disadvantages for examining the effects of environmental
exposures.

Ecological study designs have long been used to investigate the health effects of air
pollution. Cross-sectional studies have compared the health characteristics or rates of
disease occurrence in communities having differing levels of exposure to air pollution
(Lave and Seskin, 1977). Time-series designs have also received widespread application.
In these ecological studies temporal associations between air pollution levels and disease
measures are evaluated. For example, a series of recent studies have assessed daily
concentrations of air pollution levels with mortality counts and morbidity measures (Pope
et al., 1995; Bascom et al., 1996). A principal limitation of the ecologic design is the
assumption that associations observed at the group level reflect effects at the individual
level, the so-called ecologic fallacy. Nonetheless, the time-series studies have raised
concern that current levels of air pollution in the United States and other developed
countries may be adversely affecting public health.

The cross-sectional study is a generally economical and feasible approach, often used
to investigate indoor and outdoor air pollution and occupational lung diseases. When this
design is used to study indoor or outdoor air pollution, populations of children or adults are
typically surveyed, and health status is assessed. Exposure to outdoor air pollution may be
inferred from geographic location or the results of area and limited personal monitoring; in
studies of indoor air pollution, exposure may be categorized by the presence of sources or
by monitoring the indoors. For example, in the Harvard Six-Cities Study of air pollution,
outdoor exposures have been inferred from the city of residence and centrally sited
monitors, and indoor exposures have been classified by sources and monitoring for some
specific pollutants (Ware et al., 1984; Dockery et al., 1989; Neas et al., 1991). Personal
monitoring has been used to assess the contributions of indoor and outdoor pollutants to
total personal exposures of the subjects (Spengler et al., 1985)

The cross-sectional design is also widely used to evaluate the effects of occupational
agents on the lung. In a typical cross-sectional study or survey, employed workers receive
an assessment that includes a standardized respiratory symptom questionnaire, spirometry,

chest radiograph, and often a limited physical examination. Exposure classification may be based on job title or duties, length of employment, reported duration of exposure to materials of interest, or a cumulative exposure measure calculated from measured or presumed concentrations of an agent and length of time at each level of exposure. For example, Samet and colleagues (1984) conducted a respiratory survey of long-term underground uranium miners. The study population was recruited by sampling from employed miners at two large companies. Increasing duration of underground employment, used as an index of exposure to potentially hazardous agents underground, such as silica, radon, and blasting fumes, was associated with lower level of midmaximum expiratory flow. The prevalence of an abnormal chest radiograph compatible with silicosis increased with longer duration worked underground.

The cross-sectional study, although one of the most economical and feasible designs, is subject to potentially significant methodological limitations. Estimates of the effects of exposure may be biased by the tendency of more susceptible or more affected persons to reduce their level of exposure, for example, by leaving an industry or polluted area. In the survey of uranium miners reported by Samet et al., (1984), long-term miners who had already developed disease may have retired or even died, leaving a population less susceptible to develop silicosis or lung cancer. This type of selection bias is likely to be most prominent for agents with immediate effects on susceptible persons; thus asthmatic persons are likely to leave jobs involving exposures that worsen their disease. The temporal relationship between exposure and disease may be obscured or misrepresented in cross-sectional data because exposure and disease are assessed at only one point in time.

Cohort and case-control studies, which establish the proper sequence between exposure and disease, are also used to investigate the effects of inhaled pollutants on the lung. Cohort studies represent the optimal approach for assessing the effects of rare and special exposures, such as inhalation of toxic gases or exposure to asbestos. Cohort studies are termed "prospective" if the disease events will occur in the future, after the study population is established, and "retrospective" if disease events have already occurred when the cohort is assembled. The cohort design has the advantages of permitting direct estimation of disease incidence or mortality rates for exposed and nonexposed persons and of prospectively accumulating comprehensive data on exposure. The retrospective cohort design, often applied to occupational groups, can be used to quickly assess the effects of a pollutant, since exposure and disease have already taken place when the investigation is initiated. The principal disadvantages of the cohort design include potentially high costs and losses to follow-up.

Use of the cohort design is well illustrated by the many studies of mortality from cancer, asbestosis, and other causes of death in asbestos-exposed workers. For example, Selikoff and colleagues have described the mortality experience of 17,800 members of the insulation workers' union in the United States (Selikoff et al., 1979). The cohort members were active in the union on January 1, 1967; follow-up of mortality was described through 1976 in the 1979 publication. Mortality in the cohort was compared to U.S. death rates for white males. Overall, 2271 deaths were observed with 1659 expected; cancer of the lung occurred with a fivefold excess, and 49 deaths from mesothelioma were identified. In this study, comparison of the mortality of the exposed population (asbestos workers) with the unexposed population (U.S. white males) provided strong evidence for associations of asbestos exposure with excess mortality from several causes of death.

The case-control study, like the cohort study, provides a measure of association between exposure and disease. This design has been widely used for studying lung cancer and occupational and environmental agents but infrequently for nonmalignant respiratory diseases. In comparison with the cohort study, the case-control study has the advantages of generally lower cost, greater feasibility, and usually a shorter time frame. The case-control study is the optimum approach for studying uncommon diseases. The results of this design may be limited by bias in assessing exposure or by bias in the method used to select cases and controls.

The application of the case-control approach can also be illustrated by studies of the effects of asbestos. Analyses of geographic patterns of lung cancer mortality for the United States showed the highest rates along the coastal regions, particularly in the southeast (Blot and Fraumeni, 1976). A series of case-control studies were conducted to assess occupational and other factors potentially contributing to the excess lung cancer (Blot et al., 1978; Vineis et al., 1988). Cases were identified through hospitals and death certificates, and controls were sampled from persons admitted to the same hospitals with diseases other than lung cancer, from death certificate files, or from the general population. Significant associations were found between employment in coastal shipyards, where asbestos was used for insulating ships, and lung cancer risk. For example, in a study conducted in coastal Georgia, employment in area shipyards was associated with a 60% increase in lung cancer risk after adjustment for smoking (Blot et al., 1978). These case-control studies provided a relatively rapid and informative evaluation of the excess mortality from lung cancer documented by mortality rates.

The results of each type of study may be affected by biases, which alter the relationship between exposure to an inhaled agent and the health effect of concern; bias may increase or decrease the strength of an association. The three principal types of bias are selection bias, misclassification bias, and confounding bias.

Selection bias refers to distortion of the exposure–outcome relationship by differential patterns of subject participation depending on exposure and disease status. For example, subjects with airway hyperresponsiveness might be more likely to withdraw from occupational cohorts exposed to respiratory irritants.

Error in measuring either pollutant exposure or the health outcome results in misclassification. If the error equally affects cases and controls in a case-control study or exposed and nonexposed subjects in a cohort study, the bias reduces associations toward the null value, namely no effect of exposure. Such nondifferential or random misclassification is of concern in most studies of inhaled pollutants and the lung; pollutant exposures are generally estimated using limited measurements or surrogates, such as presence of sources or duration of employment. Statistical power, the ability of a study to detect exposure-disease associations, declines as the degree of random misclassification increases (Gladen and Rogan, 1979; Shy et al., 1979). For example, Lubin et al., (1990) estimated sample sizes needed for case-control studies of indoor radon and lung cancer. As the degree of measurement error increased from the implausible level of 0% to more plausible levels above 50%, statistical power declined well below the desired level of 80% to 90%.

If misclassification is differential (varying with case or control status in a case-control study or with exposure status in a cohort study), then the bias may increase or decrease the strength of association. Differential misclassification is of particular concern in case-control studies using interview to assess exposure. Information obtained from persons with and without a disease may not have comparable validity. For example, in comparison with controls, persons with lung cancer might minimize the extent of prior smoking or better recall occupational exposures such as asbestos.

Bias from confounding results when the effect of the exposure of interest is altered by another risk factor. For example, confounding by cigarette smoking would occur in a cohort study of asbestos workers if smoking differed between exposed and nonexposed subjects. In fact, in studies of inhaled pollutants, particularly those with weak effects, confounding can be controlled through matching exposed and nonexposed subjects on potential confounding factors or through collection of data on potential confounding factors and use of appropriate data analysis methods.

TABLE 29-4   Assessment of Inhaled Pollutant Exposure in Epidemiological Studies

Occupational Agents	Outdoor Air Pollutants	Indoor Air Pollutants
Job title and industry	Residence location	Source inventory
Length of employment	Proximity to sources	Indoor monitoring
Self-reported exposure	Self-reported exposure	Personal monitoring
Job-exposure matrices	Central site monitoring	Biological monitoring
Area monitoring	Small-area monitoring	
Personal monitoring	Personal monitoring	
Biological monitoring	Biological monitoring	

Exposure Assessment

A wide range of approaches are used in epidemiological studies to assess exposure to inhaled agents (Table 29-4). Some approaches can be used feasibly and at low cost in large populations, whereas others require intensive and costly personal or biological monitoring. The simplest approaches, such as using job title in an occupational study or residence location in a study of outdoor air pollution, are likely to be subject to the greatest degree of misclassification. Misclassification is least if personal exposures are directly monitored. However, personal monitoring is not possible for all pollutants, and small passive monitors are only available for a few pollutants of concern (Wallace and Ott, 1982; McCarthy et al., 1991). Moreover current exposures may not be relevant to many chronic diseases with risks reflecting cumulative rather than immediate exposures. Biological monitoring is feasible in large populations for only a few pollutants, such as carbon monoxide, lead, and nicotine, with exposure markers that can be measured inexpensively and noninvasively.

Tiered approaches for exposure assessment have been proposed (Leaderer et al., 1986). Nesting more intensive monitoring approaches for small numbers of subjects selected from a larger study population permits estimation of the misclassification resulting from use of less intense but feasible approaches.

Outcome Assessment

The range of adverse health effects caused by inhaled pollutants is wide, extending from excess mortality to subtle effects on function or symptom occurrence (Table 29-5). Studies of morbidity most often examine symptom and disease occurrence and level of lung function. Standardized methods have been developed for collecting data on symptoms and for assessing lung function and airway responsiveness (Ferris, 1978; Samet, 1989;

TABLE 29-5   Health Outcomes in Epidemiological Studies of Inhaled Pollutants

Occupational Agents	Outdoor and Indoor Air Pollutants
Mortality, specific or all causes	Mortality, specific or all causes
Occurrence of specific diseases	Hospitalization
Respiratory symptoms	Emergency room or other outpatient visit
Reduced lung function	Absenteeism
Abnormality on chest radiograph	Disease occurrence
Increased airway responsiveness	Respiratory symptoms
Immunologic sensitization	Reduced lung function
	Increased airway responsiveness
	Immunologic sensitization

Sparrow and Weiss, 1989). The American Thoracic Society has published standardized respiratory symptoms questionnaires for children and for adults (Ferris, 1978). The questionnaires emphasize chronic respiratory symptoms and conditions; they are not appropriate instruments for investigations of acute responses to inhaled pollutants. Questionnaires specific to the investigation of asthma are available (Burney and Chinn, 1987; Asher et al., 1995). Recommendations for spirometric testing cover the characteristics of the equipment, procedures for testing, and data acceptability and interpretation (American Thoracic Society, 1994).

In studying the pneumoconioses, occupational lung diseases caused by inhalation of inorganic dusts, chest radiographs are usually classified according to the system of the International Labour Office, most recently revised in 1980 (International Labour Office, 1980). This system classifies abnormalities of the lung parenchyma on the basis of size and extent and changes in the pleura. The system was designed to provide a uniform method for coding changes on chest radiographs and thereby to facilitate comparisons across regions and over time. In the United States, training is offered in the use of this system by the American College of Radiology; those successfully passing an examination in its use are designated as "B readers" by the National Institute for Occupational Safety and Health. Even the use of a standardized classification and trained film readers may not eliminate strong observer bias in X ray interpretation (Ducatman et al., 1988; Parker et al., 1989).

LIMITATIONS OF CLINICAL AND EPIDEMIOLOGICAL ASSESMENTS OF THE EFFECTS OF THE INHALED AGENTS

As the twentieth century ends, many respiratory hazards have been recognized and controlled in the United States and other developed countries. Concern remains, however, about the safety provided by standards for workplace and environmental exposures and the risks of new and unevaluated agents. Large segments of the population are exposed to indoor and outdoor pollutants with adverse effects, and workers expect that their jobs will not carry unacceptable risks. In response to individual and societal fears, clinicians and epidemiologists are asked to assess the effects of inhaled pollutants: the clinician to evaluate the health of exposed individuals and the epidemiologist to address the effects on exposed groups. Both types of assessments have limitations, particularly for answering concerns about safety.

Few clinicians have the proper training to evaluate patients with toxic occupational and environmental exposures. About 10 years ago, an assessment identified a supply of 1200 to 1500 appropriately trained physicians while there was a need for 4600 to 6700 (Castorina and Rosenstock, 1990). This gap remains. Most primary care providers (internists and family practitioners) lack training in toxicology and in occupational and environmental medicine. They do not have skills for characterizing exposures and making links between exposures and health outcomes; they are also unlikely to have an understanding of such key concepts as individual susceptibility, interactions among agents, and exposure–response relationships. Their skills in counseling patients concerning risks may also be limited. Furthermore clinical methods for assessing respiratory effects may be insensitive if applied in the conventional, clinical fashion. For example, pulmonary function testing may be unstandardized, and the chest radiograph may only be interpreted for gross clinical abnormalities and not for subtle changes reflective of early disease.

Epidemiology has been an extremely effective tool for investigating inhaled pollutants with either very strong (e.g., cigarette smoking and lung cancer) or very specific (e.g., asbestos and mesothelioma) effects. In investigating agents that may have effects that are not strong but of public health concern, the epidemiological studies may be limited by misclassification of exposure and disease, confounding, and other methodological problems. Large sample sizes may be needed to test for the anticipated effects, particularly if exposure estimates are subject to substantial misclassification (Lubin et al., 1990). The results of an epidemiological study cannot provide sufficient precision to exclude the possibility of some increased risk of exposure to an agent. Thus the findings of epidemiological studies of inhaled pollutants often leave uncertainty concerning the risks posed and do not fully address the concerns and questions of exposed persons and those involved in policy and regulation.

ADVICE AND COUNSELING OF PATIENTS

Patient-Oriented

Although often called on to advise on control strategies for minimizing exposure to occupational and environmental exposure, the primary care physician may have little training or experience in this arena. Approaches for limiting the health risks of breathing polluted ambient air have received little investigation and dissemination to primary care practitioners. Present understanding of the determinants of exposure suggest that modifying time-activity patterns to limit time outside during episodes of pollution represents the most effective strategy. The levels of some reactive pollutants tend to be lower indoors than outdoors. Ozone levels in buildings are lower than outdoor levels but can be driven upward by increasing the rate of exchange of indoor with outdoor air. Fine acid aerosols can penetrate indoors, but neutralization by ammonia produced by occupants, household products, and pets may reduce concentrations. Other types of particles in outdoor air may also enter indoor air. Nevertheless, health care providers can reasonably advise patients to stay indoors during pollution episodes. Vigorous exercise outdoors, which increases the dose of pollution delivered to the respiratory tract, should also be avoided at such times.

Susceptible patients should be counseled concerning the nature and degree of their susceptibility. The use of medications should follow the usual clinical indications, and therapeutic regimens should not be adjusted because of the occurrence of a pollution episode without evidence of an adverse effect on symptoms or function. In the laboratory, inhalation of cromolyn sodium and bronchodilating agents may block the response to some pollutants, but use of these drugs solely because of exposure to air pollution cannot be advised.

Respiratory protective equipment has been developed for use in the workplace in order to minimize exposure to toxic gases and particles. Many of these devices, particularly those likely to be most effective, add to the work of breathing and cannot be tolerated by persons with respiratory disease. Respirators can provide effective personal protection only when they are properly selected and when they are used in the context of a comprehensive respiratory protection program. OSHA has specified the minimum requirements for an acceptable program. In order for respirators to provide adequate worker protection, both the proper selection and the correct use of respirators are essential. Respirators are the least preferred method of protection from respiratory hazards, and they should be used only when engineering controls are not technically feasible, while controls are being installed or repaired, or in emergency or other temporary situations. Under most circumstances health care providers should not suggest respiratory protection as a method of reducing the risks of ambient air pollution. Similarly air cleaners have not been shown to have health benefits, whether directed at indoor pollutants generated by indoor sources or those brought in with outside air.

A variety of federal agencies are active in the area of environmental health and have services of some degree of value to practicing physicians. Unfortunately, the responsibilities among the agencies are often fragmented, and no one source is targeted for providing assistance to the practicing physician. If the clinician wishes further information or consultation, the following agencies may be of value:

1. Agency for Toxic Substances and Disease Registry. Funded via Superfund legislation, this agency is part of the U.S. Public Health Service and affiliated with the Center for Disease Control. Among its mandates are the education of physicians concerning toxic hazards associated with hazardous wastes.

2. Centers for Disease Control. This agency is available to investigate illnesses that may be linked to environmental hazards.

3. Environmental Protection Agency. This federal agency has the responsibility of protecting humans and the environment from the unwanted effects of chemicals and physical agents. It has focused primarily on providing the public with information on environmental risks and has not been a major resource for the practicing physician.

4. National Institute for Occupational Safety and Health. This agency has responsibilities for issues related to worker health. It can provide information about specific workplace hazards and has the authority to enter workplaces to evaluate health and safety problems.

5. Other important resources may include medical school faculty with expertise in areas of environmental and occupational medicine, poison control centers, and occupational and environmental medicine clinics.

As a result, the Occupational Safety and Health Administrations Hazard Communication Standard; industries that use chemicals in the workplace have a Material Safety Data Sheet (MSDS) for each hazardous chemical. The companies should have these available on request of the physician or the worker. Goldstein and Gochfeld (1990) present additional discussion of resource agencies for clinicians and mechanisms for making professional contacts.

Community-Oriented

Frequently communities become concerned about the impact of particular local sources, perhaps a power plant or manufacturing facility. Concern about the health risks may quickly lead to controversy and litigation. Thus understanding the health risks posed by local sources may be difficult and require skills in community health as well as in epidemiology and toxicology. Local physicians may become involved through concerns about the health of their patients or as advocates for the community's environment or for the polluting facility. Often the dimensions of such complex problems exceed the skills of local physicians. Nevertheless, involvement may be appropriate, but guidance should be obtained from appropriate public health and environmental agencies.

In the United States no regulatory agency has authority over indoor air quality. Workplaces are regulated by the Occupational Safety and Health Administration, although standards do not directly address the new problem of building-related illnesses. Good practice guidelines that often are adopted as standards for ventilation in nonresidential buildings are set by the American Society of Heating, Refrigerating and Air Conditioning Engineers.

The interplay of factors that must be manipulated to prevent environmentally induced disease is complex, but standards are considered to be objective indicators of success preventive measures or strategies. In 1976 the Environmental Protection Agency proposed cautionary statements for public reporting of outdoor air quality, the Pollutant Standards Index (PSI) for criteria pollutants. The actions taken when "alert levels" are reached or expected to be reached include the issuance of health advisories (or cautionary statements) to the public. The Environmental Protection Agency's advice is intended to be applied by local air pollution agencies in preparing daily air quality summaries, which are disseminated to the media. Although the cautionary statements require some revisions, especially as related to ozone exposures, useful guidelines are offered for physicians and public health officials.

Finally there are important impacts to the community and workplace resulting from changes in health care insurance and the delivery of health care. Nearly 75% of employees in the United States are enrolled in health plans through health maintenance organizations (HMOs) and their provider networks. Both physicians and employees are subject to managed care's efforts to hold health care professionals more accountable for the medical and financial aspects of care. This often results in managing occupational health care demands and workers" compensation according to established guidelines. Although the original goal of all of these programs was to provide high-quality care, the focus of many stakeholders has been cost containment. With the introduction of workers' compensation managed care, many businesses have developed and implemented transitional work programs, developed alliances with Occupational Medicine clinics, retained the services of case managers, requested more independent medical examinations, and contested more claims, all in an effort to contain costs.

Although it is premature to assess the impact of managed care, it certainly has the potential to negatively affect health care of the injured worker. However, the Managed Care Pilot Project in Washington State (Sparks and Feldstein, 1997) studied the effect of experienced-based capitation on medical and disability costs, quality of care, worker satisfaction with medical care, and employer satisfaction. Much of the care, and all of the treatment coordination, was provided by physicians specialized in occupational medicine and oriented toward timely return to work. The study revealed that "medical costs were reduced by approximately 27%, functional outcomes remained the same, workers were less satisfied with their treatment and access to care initially, and employers were much more satisfied with the quality and speed of the information received from the providers." As the effort to contain costs extend into occupational health, it will be important to carefully track injury outcomes and worker satisfaction.

SUMMARY

Environmental medicine very likely requires a greater interdisciplinary approach than any other medical specialty. For the primary care physician tackling an occupational or environmental medicine problem, there is a necessity not only to work closely with nonmedical personnel such as industrial hygienists, ergonomists, toxicologists, epidemiologists, lawyers, regulators, and union representatives but also to become knowledgeable about these various disciplines. The diseases of individuals may provide indications of unacceptable exposures in the environment or workplace; health care providers should be able to recognize such "sentinel" disease and respond appropriately by contacting employers and regulatory or public health agencies. Ultimately it may be necessary to visit a workplace or environmental site, request industrial hygiene data, and consider screening the exposed population of individuals in order to determine whether an environmental pulmonary hazard exists. In the final analysis, an inquisitive mind and a bit of detective work are often prerequisites for establishing causation between an environmental exposure and a pulmonary disorder.

REFERENCES

Aberle, D. R., G. Gamsu, C. S. Ray, and I. M. Feuerstein. 1988. Asbestos-related parenchymal fibrosis: Detection with high-resolution CT. *Radiology* 166: 729–734.

American College of Occupational and Environmental Medicine. 1991. ACOEM Statement on multiple chemical hypersensitivity syndrome, multiple chemical sensitivities, environmental tobacco smoke, and indoor air quality. May 2, 1991. Multiple Chemical Sensitivities (Addendum, 1993). (Available from the College).

American College of Physicians. 1989. American College of Physicians position statement: Clinical ecology. *Ann. Intern. Med.* 111: 168–178.

American Medical Association, Council on Scientific Affairs. 1992. Clinical ecology. *JAMA* 268: 3465–3467.

American Thoracic Society. 1997. Achieving healthy indoor air. *Am. J. Respir. Crit. Care Med.* 156 (suppl.): 533–544.

American Thoracic Society. 1995. Standardization of spirometry— 1994 update. *Am. J. Respir. Crit. Care Med.* 152: 1107–1136.

Asher, M. I., U. Keil, H. R. Anderson, R. Beasley, J. Crane, F. Martinez, E. A. Mitchell, N. Pearce, B. Sibbald, A. W. Stewart, D. Strachan, S. K. Weiland, and H. C. Williams. 1995. International study of asthma and allergies in childhood (ISAAC): Rationale and methods. *Eur. Respir. J.* 8: 483–491.

Baker, E. L., E. A. Honchar, and L. J. Fine. 1989. I. Surveillance in occupational illness and injury: Concepts and content. *Am. J. Public Health* 79 (suppl.): 9–11.

Bascom, R., P. A. Bromberg, D. A. Costa, R. Devlin, D. W. Dockery, M. W. Frampton, W. Lambert, J. M. Samet, F. E. Speizer, and M. J. Utell. 1996. Health effects of outdoor air pollution. *Am. J. Respir. Crit. Care Med.* 153: 3–50, 477–498.

Block, G., K. S. Tse, K. Kijek, H. Chan, and M. Chan-Yeung. 1983. Baker's asthma: Clinical and immunological studies. *Clin. Allergy* 13: 359–370.

Blot, W. J., and J. E. Fraumeni Jr. 1976. Geographical patterns of lung cancer: Industrial correlations. *Am. J. Epidemiol.* 103: 539–550.

Blot, W. J., J. H. Harrington, A. Tolego, R. Hoover, C. W. Health, and J. E. Fraumeni Jr. 1978. Lung cancer after employment in shipyards during World War II. *N. Engl. J. Med.* 299: 620–624.

Boushey, H. A., M. J. Holtzman, J. R. Sheller, and J. A. Nadel. 1980. Bronchial hyperreactivity. *Am. Rev. Respir. Dis.* 121: 389–413.

Burney, P., and S. Chinn. 1987. Developing a new questionnaire for measuring the prevalence and distribution of asthma. *Chest.* 91(suppl.): 79S–83S.

Butcher, B. T., C. E. O'Neil, M. A. Reed, and J. E. Salvaggio. 1980. Radioallergosorbent testing of toluene diisocyanate-reactive individuals using p-tolyl isocyanate antigen. *J. Allergy Clin. Immunol.* 66: 213–216.

Castorina, J. S., and L. Rosenstock. 1990. Physician shortage in occupational and environmental medicine. *Ann. Intern. Med.* 113: 983–986.

Chan-Yeung, M. 1995. American College of Physicians consensus statement: Assessment of asthma in the workplace. *Chest.* 108: 1084–1117.

Chan-Yeung, M. 1986. Occupational asthma. *Chest* 98: 148SL161S.

Chan-Yeung, M., and S. Lam. 1986. Occupational asthma. *Am. Rev. Respir. Dis.* 133: 686–703.

Clausen, J. L., ed.. 1982. *Pulmonary Function Testing Guidelines and Controversies: Equipment, Methods, and Normal Values.* New York: Academic Press.

Cormier, Y. J., Belanger, P. LeBlanc, and M. Laviolette. 1986. Bronchoalveolar lavage in farmer's lung disease: Diagnostic and Physiologic significance. *Br. J. Ind. Med.* 43: 401–405.

Craighead, J. E., and B. T. Mossman. 1982. The pathogenesis of asbestos-associated diseases. *N. Engl. J. Med.* 306: 1446–1455.

Cullen, M. R., 1987. The worker with multiple chemical sensitivities: An overview. *State Art Rev. Occup. Med.* 2: 655–661.

Cullen, M. R., and M. G. Cherniack. 1989. Spectrum of occupational disease in an academic hospital-based referral center in Connecticut from 1979 to 1987. *Arch. Intern. Med.* 149: 1621–1626.

Dockery, D. W., F. E. Speizer, D. O. Stram, J. H. Ware, J. D. Spengler, and B. G. Ferris Jr. 1989. Effects of inhalable particles on respiratory health of children. *Am. Rev. Respir. Dis.* 139: 587–594.

Ducatman, A. M., W. N. Yang, and S. A. Forman. 1988. "B-readers" and asbestos medical surveillance. *J. Occup. Med.* 30: 644–647.

Epstein, P. E., J. H. Dauber, M. D. Rossman, and R. P. Danick. 1988. Bronchoalveolar lavage in a patient with chronic berylliosis: Evidence for hypersensitivity pneumonitis. *Ann. Intern. Med.* 108: 687–693.

Ferris, B. G. 1978. Epidemiology standardization project. *Am. Rev. Respir. Dis.* 118: 1–120.

Finnegan, M. J., and C. A. C. Pickering. 1986. Building related illness. *Clin. Allergy* 16: 389–405.

Fraser, R. G., J. A. Pare, P. D. Pare, R. S. Fraser, and G. P. Genereux, eds. 1990. Pleuropulmonary disease caused by inhalation of inorganic dust. In: *Diagnosis of Diseases of the Chest*, 3rd edition, vol. 3, pp. 2276–2282. Philadelphia: Saunders.

Freund, E., P. J. Seligman, T. L. Chorba, S. K. Safford, J. G. Drachman, and H. F. Hull. 1989. Mandatory reporting of occupational diseases by clinicians. *JAMA* 262: 3041–3044.

Friedman, A. C., S. B. Fiel, M. S. Fisher, P. D. Radecki, A. S. Ler-Toaft, and D. F. Caroline. 1988. Asbestos-related pleural diseases and asbestosis: A comparison of CT and chest radiography. *Am. J. Roentgenol.* 150: 269–275.

Froines, J., D. Wegman, and E. Eisen. 1989. VI. Hazard surveillance in occupational disease. *Am. J. Public Health* 79 (suppl): 26–31.

Gladen, B., and W. J. Rogan. 1979. Misclassification and the design of environmental studies. *Am. J. Epidemiol.* 109: 607–616.

Goldstein, B. D., and M. Gochfeld. 1990. Role of the physician in environmental medicine. *Med. Clin. North Am.* 74: 245–261.

Institute of Medicine. 1995. *Environmental Medicine*, eds. A.M. Pope and D. R. Rall. Washington, DC: National Academy Press.

Institute of Medicine. 1989. Role of the Primary Care Physician in Occupational and Environmental Medicine. Washington, DC: National Academy Press.

International Labour Office. 1980. *Guidelines for the Use of International Labour Office Classification of Radiographs of Pneumoconioses.* Occupational Safety and Health Sciences 22. Geneva: International Labour Office.

Kilbourne, E. M., and J. Weiner. 1990. Occupational and environmental medicine: The internist's role. *Ann. Intern. Med.* 113: 974–982.

Lam, S., F. Tan, H. Chan, and M. Chan-Yeung. 1983. Relationship between types of asthmatic reaction, nonspecific bronchial reactivity, and specific IgE antibodies in patients with red cedar asthma. *J. Allergy Clin. Immunol.* 72: 134–139.

Lave, L. B., and E. P. Seskin. 1997. *Air Pollution and Human Health.* Baltimore: Johns Hopkins University Press.

Leaderer, B. P., R. T. Zagraniski, M. Berwick, and J. A. J. Stolwijk. 1986. Assessment of exposure to indoor air contaminants from combustion sources: Methodology and application. *Am. J. Epidemiol.* 124: 275–289.

Lubin, J. H., J. M. Samet, and C. Weinberg. 1990. Design issues in epidemiologic studies of indoor exposure to Rn and risk of lung cancer. *Health Phys.* 59: 807–817.

McCarthy, J. F., D. W. Bearg, and J. D. Spengler. 1991. Assessment of indoor quality. In *Indoor Air Pollution: A Health Perspective*, eds. J. M. Samet and J. D. Spengler. Baltimore: Johns Hopkins University Press.

McKay, R. T. 1986. Bronchoprovocation challenge testing in occupational airways disorders. *Semin. Respir. Med.* 7: 297–306.

Melius, J. M., J. P. Sestito, and P. J. Seligman. 1989. Occupational disease surveillance with existing data sources. *Am. J. Public Health* 79 (suppl.): 46–52.

Miller, A. 1985. *Pulmonary Function Tests in Clinical and Occupational Lung Disease.* Orlando: Grune and Straton.

National Institutes of Health, National Heart, Lung, and Blood Institute. 1997. *National Asthma Education and Prevention Program: Guidelines for the Diagnosis and Management of Asthma*, pp. 6–11. NIH Publication #97-4051. Bethesda, MD.

National Research Council, Subcommittee on Pulmonary Toxicology, Committee on Biologic Markers. 1989. *Biologic Markers in Pulmonary Toxicology*. Washington, DC: National Academy Press.

Neas, L. M., J. G. Ware, D. W. Dockery, J. D. Spengler, F. E. Speizer, and B. G. Ferris Jr. 1991. Association of indoor nitrogen dioxide with respiratory symptoms and pulmonary function in children. *Am. J. Epidemiol.* 134: 204–219.

Newman, L. S., C. Bobka, B. Schumacher, E. Daniloff, B. Zhen, M. M. Mroz, and T. E. King Jr. 1994. Compartmentalized immune response reflects clinical severity of beryllium disease. *Am. J. Respir. Crit. Care Med. 150: 135–142.*

O'Byrne, P. M., G. Ryan, M. Morris, D. McCormack, N. L. Jones, J. L. C. Morse, and F. E. Hargreave. 1982. Asthma induced by cold air and its relationship to nonspecific bronchial responsiveness to methacholine. *Am. Rev. Respir. Dis.* 125: 281–285.

Occupational and Environmental Health Committee of the American Lung Association of San Diego and Imperial Counties. 1983. Taking the occupational history. *Ann. Intern. Med.* 99: 641–651.

Parker, D. L., A. P. Bender, S. Hankinson, and D. Aeppli, 1989. Public health implication of the variability in the interpretation of "B" readings for pleural changes. *J. Occup. Med.* 31: 775–780.

Pepys, J., and B. J. Hutchcroft. 1975. Bronchial provocation tests in etiologic diagnosis and analysis of asthma. *Am. Rev. Respir. Dis.* 112: 829–859.

Pope, C. A. III, D. W. Dockery, and J. Schwartz. 1995. Review of epidemiological evidence of health effects of particulate air pollution. *Inhal. Toxicol.* 7: 1–18.

Rom, W. N. 1998. *Environmental and Occupational Medicine*. Philadelphia: Lippincott-Raven.

Rom, W. N., P. B. Bitterman, S. I. Rennard, A. Catin, and R. G. Crystal. 1987. Characterization of the lower respiratory tract inflammation of non-smoking individuals with interstitial lung disease associated with chronic inhalation of inorganic dusts. *Am. Rev. Respir. Dis.* 136: 1429–1434.

Rosenstock, L., and M. R. Cullen. 1994. *Textbook of Clinical Occupational and Environmental Medicine*. Philadelphia: Saunders.

Rutstein, D. D., R. J. Mullan, M. Todd, T. M. Frazier, W. E. Halperin, J. M. Melius, and J. P. Sestito. 1983. Sentinel health events (occupational): A basis for physician recognition and public health surveillance. *Am. J. Public Health* 73: 1054–1062.

Salvaggio, J. E.; and D. J. Hendrick. 1989. The use of bronchial inhalation challenge in the investigation of occupational diseases. In *Provocative Challenge Procedures: Background and Methodology*, ed. S. Spector. Mount Kisco, NY: Futura.

Samet, J. M. 1989. Definitions and methodology in COPD research. In *Clinical Epidemiology of Chronic Obstructive Pulmonary Disease*, eds. M. J. Hensley and N. A. Saunders, pp. 1–22. New York: Marcel Dekker.

Samet, J. M., M. D. Marbury, and J. D. Spengler. 1988. Health effects and sources of indoor air pollution. *Am. Rev. Respir. Dis.* 137: 221–242.

Samet, J. M., R. A. Young, M. V. Morgan, C. G. Humble, G. R. Epler, and T. C. McCloud. 1984. Prevalence survey of respiratory abnormalities in New Mexico uranium miners. *Health Phys.* 46: 361–370.

Schottenfeld, R. W., and M. R. Cullen. 1986. Recognition of occupation-induced post traumatic stress disorders. *J. Occup. Med.* 28: 365–369.

Schwartz, D. A., J. R. Galvin, and C. S. Dayton. 1990. Determinants of restrictive lung function in asbestos-induced pleural fibrosis. *J. Appl. Physiol.* 68: 1932–1937.

Selikoff, I. J., E. C. Hammond, and H. Seidman. 1979. Mortality experience of insulation workers in the United States and Canada, 1943–1976. *Ann. NY Acad. Sci.* 330: 91–116.

Sexton, K., and P. B. Ryan. 1988. Assessment of human exposure to air pollution: Methods, measurements, and models. In *Air Pollution, the Automobile, and Public Health*, eds. A. Y. Watson, R. R. Bates, and D. Kennedy. Washington, DC: National Academy Press.

Shy, C. M., D. G. Kleinbaum, and H. Morgenstern. 1978. The effect of misclassification of exposure status in epidemiological studies of air pollution health effects. *Bull. NY Acad. Med.* 54: 1155–1165.

Simon, G. W., Daniell, H. Stockbridge, K. Claypool, and L. Rosenstock. 1993. Immunologic, psychological, and neuropsychological factors in multiple chemical sensitivity: A controlled study. *Ann. Intern. Med.* 119: 97–103.

Sparks, P. J., and A. Feldstein. 1997. The success of the Washington Department of Labor and industries managed care pilot project: the occupational medicine-based delivery model. *J. Occup. Environ. Med.* 39: 1068–1073.

Sparrow, D., and S. T. Weiss. 1989. Methodological issues in airway responsiveness testing. In *Airway Responsiveness and Atopy in the Development of Chronic Lung Disease*, eds. S. T. Weiss and D. Sparrow, pp. 121–155. New York: Raven Press.

Speizer, F. E., and I. B. Tager. 1979. Epidemiology of chronic mucus hypersecretion and obstructive airways disease. *Epidmiol. Rev.* 1: 124–142.

Spengler, J. D., R. D. Treitmen, T. D. Tosteson, D. T. Mage, and M. L. Soczek, 1985. Personal exposure to respirable particulate and implications for air pollution epidemiology. *Environ. Sci. Technol.* 19: 700–706.

Utell, M. J. and J. M. Samet. 1990. Environmentally mediated disorders of the respiratory tract. *Med. Clin. North Am.* 74: 291–306.

Valiante, D. J., and K. D. Rosenman. 1989. Does silicosis still occur? *JAMA* 262: 3003–3007.

Vineis, P., T. Thomas, R. B. Hayes, W. M. Blot, T. J. Mason, L. W. Pickle, P. Corvia, E. T. H. Fontham, and J. Schoenberg. 1988. Proportion of lung cancers in males, due to occupation, in different areas of the USA. *Int. J. Cancer* 42: 851–856.

Wallace, L. A., and W. R. Ott. 1982. Personal monitors: A state-of-the-art survey. *J. Air Pollut. Control Assoc.* 32: 601–610.

Ware, J. H., D. W. Dockery, A. Spiro III, F. E. Speizer, and B.G. Ferris Jr. 1984. Passive smoking, gas cooking, and respiratory health of children living in six cities. *Am. Rev. Respir. Dis.* 129: 366–374.

30 Industrial Perspectives: Translating the Knowledge Base into Corporate Policies, Programs, and Practices for Health Protection

FRED D. HOERGER, Ph.D., LARRY W. RAMPY, Ph.D.
DOUGLAS A. RAUSCH, Ph.D., JAMES S. BUS, Ph.D.

This chapter presents an overview of the important considerations involved in establishing policies, programs, and practices for the manufacture, use, and disposal of commercial chemicals in ways that are reflective of the available knowledge of potential hazards. From the standpoint of a manufacturer of a broad and diversified product line of basic chemicals, plastics, and specialty products, such as The Dow Chemical Company, extensive industrial hygiene, occupational health, and product stewardship programs are essential. From the standpoint of the chemical industry, increasingly attention is being focused on a program of Responsible Care® embodying a set of codes relating to process safety, emissions reduction, and product stewardship.

Knowledge of the health effects of environmental toxicants is an essential background for establishing corporate or industrywide programs that provide adequate protection for workers and the community. From an industry perspective, health-protective operating and marketing practices depend on critical reviews, such as those published in this book. They are extremely useful to industrial scientists, physicians, and engineers as a basis for reviewing the literature and current practices on specific chemicals. Equally important are critical reviews published on chemicals that have received much investigation, since the reviews provide useful background education for these disciplines. By analogy, critical reviews provide insight for the design of operating practices and research and monitoring programs for other chemicals. Now a days many corporations recruiting new industrial hygienists, occupational physicians, and toxicologists seek candidates who have a thorough background in the health effects of the environmental toxicants covered in this book.

The chemical industry employs a spectrum of practices that provide human health protection. These policies and programs address not only human health and environmental concerns, but also include issues such as process safety and chemical reactivity.

LIFE CYCLE OF A CHEMICAL

Design of appropriate health protection policies, programs, and practices for environmental toxicants requires consideration of the entire life cycle of the substance.

Environmental Toxicants: Human Exposures and Their Health Effects, 2/e. Edited by Morton Lippmann.
ISBN: 0-471-29298-2   © 2000 John Wiley & Sons, Inc.

969

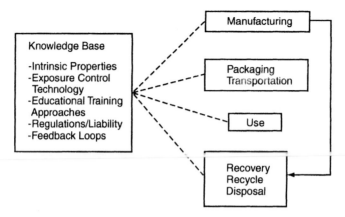

Figure 30-1   Knowledge base relevant to all phases of the life cycle of a chemical.

A generalized description of a typical life cycle for a commercial chemical is shown in Figure 30-1, it involves the sequence of manufacture, transportation, use, and ultimate disposition. The life cycle of a specific chemical may include divergent patterns of use. For example, benzene used as a component of gasoline becomes widely dispersed in the environment, whereas benzene as a chemical intermediate in manufacture of styrene is released in only relatively small quantities to the environment. As another example, formaldehyde has many uses; some uses have the potential for exposure at low concentration levels to large numbers of people; some chemical intermediate uses have only limited potential for exposure, and only to the work force involved in processing.

Many of the environmental toxicants reviewed in this book are exclusively or largely unintentional by-products of manufacturing, processing, or energy production, such as carbon monoxide, diesel exhaust, dioxin, disinfection byproducts, nitrogen oxides, ozone, and sulfur oxides. The theoretician may wish to consider the life-cycle sequence of environmental toxicant generation, environmental transport, and environmental fate. However, even for unintentional by-products, the life-cycle sequence shown in Figure. 30-1 is useful in the design of control and stewardship practices, since it highlights the points at which intervention practices can be considered.

KNOWLEDGE BASE FOR THE IDENTIFICATION OF HAZARD CONTROL STRATEGIES

The previous chapters have indicated the complexity of the health effects data base for many environmental toxicants. Extensive judgmental considerations are involved in interpreting the data to determine the toxicological endpoint(s) used in establishing regulatory or risk-reduction controls. Strategies for the protection of human health become chemical specific because of the multiplicity of health effects that might be of concern from one substance to another, such as pulmonary effects from asbestos, neurotoxicity from lead, and leukemia from benzene. Added to these complexities in designing appropriate controls is the fact that environmental and process safety considerations need to be integrated into the overall risk control strategies. Thus it is important to consider briefly some additional features that are essential to the design of protective measures during the life cycle of a chemical.

General knowledge of options for exposure control and education/training can be tailored to the specific substance and to specific points in the life cycle. Shown in

TABLE 30-1   Components of the Knowledge Base for Establishing Hazard Control Strategies

Intrinsic properties

Toxicological and clinical information
Flammability and chemical reactivity
measurements
Other physical and chemical property
information
Ecological and environmental fate
characteristics
Product use characteristics

Exposure control technology

Restriction of use
Engineering controls
Process efficiency, waste reduction
Emission / discharge treatment or destruction

Educational and training approaches

Labels
Material safety data sheets
Technical brochures
Work force training
Public availability

Regulatory requirements' liability potential

Feedback loops
Industrial hygiene and environmental monitoring
Health surveillance programs

Table 30-1 are the important components of this knowledge base: They include the intrinsic properties of the substance, the current knowledge of exposure control technology, the educational and training approaches that are available, and information feedback loops.

Several intrinsic properties of a substance may be critical in considering hazard control strategies. Certain flammability and chemical reactivity properties may be critical for process safety and selection of containers and packaging. Knowledge of downstream product use and disposal practices is essential for evaluating points of environmental release. Basic ecological properties such as phytotoxicity and information on toxicity for typical aquatic and mammalian species and environmental bioconcentration potential, fate, and transport may be essential to evaluate potential ecological hazards.

Once one has identified the intrinsic properties that are of concern at various stages in the life cycle of a chemical, possible exposure control and monitoring technologies can be considered for application. In a few instances, decisions may be made to restrict use of a substance, such as has been done by manufacturers and regulatory agencies in the cases of asbestos, PCBs, DDT, flame retardants in children's sleepwear, or cyclamates as a food additive. Significantly a wide array of engineering controls and operating practices have evolved over the years to minimize environmental release—a few examples include vapor recovery systems for tanks and vents, enclosed systems, designs to improve processing efficiency, waste reduction programs, and biological or chemical treatment or incineration of emissions and discharges.

Education and training, and other means of information transfer, are an important aspect of control strategies. Over the years, there have evolved various modes of information transfer, including product labeling, use of material safety data sheets (MSDS), product brochures containing summaries of hazard information, precautionary approaches, and frequently recommendations for storage or operation. Increasingly there has been attention to the implementation of training programs for the work force; these have evolved to include operations of leak control, cleanup of spills, and sophisticated technology that minimizes process perturbations leading to unanticipated releases.

The fields of industrial hygiene and environmental monitoring have standardized some analytical methods and techniques for detecting environmental toxicants. These standardized measures ensure the effectiveness of control strategies. Occupational health programs can provide both exposure control and knowledge of the intrinsic properties of toxicants. Health surveillance and epidemiological programs help identify a cause-and-effect relationship between an adverse health effect and an exposure, and they enable adjustments to be made in exposure and health protection strategies.

In addition regulations, public perceptions, and potentials for liability influence corporate policies and programs. Many regulations require extensive record keeping and prescribe emission control standards. The risk of litigation and public perceptions of hazard and risk also influence the types of controls that are decided upon.

The need for feedback on manufacturing operations in establishing a knowledge base and the need to ensure compliance with company or regulatory emission or ambient standards have prompted the introduction of industrial hygiene and occupational health programs in many companies.

INDUSTRIAL HYGIENE AND OCCUPATIONAL HEALTH PROGRAMS

Exposure Estimation

Many scholarly articles have been written on the subject of measuring exposure to chemicals and other stresses in the occupational setting. The sampling and analytical points are beyond the scope of this chapter, but we try to make a few observations about the strategies that lead to good estimates of actual exposures while providing a reasonable basis for evaluating and controlling hazards.

There are three main objectives of monitoring:

1. To ensure that untoward health effects are not encountered.
2. To describe an actual exposure for future use in exposure–response (epidemiology) studies.
3. To ensure that exposures are within legal requirements (e.g., OSHA's permissible exposure limits) or consistent with other guidelines (e.g., ACGIH TLVs).

These three objectives are not mutually exclusive, but they may require different approaches.

Knowledge of the potential effect a chemical may exhibit and an estimate of its toxicokinetic properties are important to meet the first two monitoring objectives. For example, for gases or vapors that are believed to cause only respiratory irritation, a method should be chosen that will measure peak exposures, since the toxic effect is likely to be closest to the highest concentration reached than to the total dose received. Hydrogen chloride and other acid gases are examples of chemicals in this category.

In contrast, the toxic effects of some substances like vinyl chloride are closest to the total dose received than to the concentration seen over any short period of time. Vinyl chloride has been linked to hemangiosarcomas of the liver, and it appears that exposures over relatively long periods (years) are required to produce this effect. This finding suggests that exposure during a given short period is relatively unimportant compared with cumulative exposures over time. Thus the exposure measurement strategy should give an estimate of the time-weighted average over lengthy periods. This is also the European Economic Community (EEC) directive for vinyl chloride. The United Kingdom has adopted a standard with the same requirements as the EEC directive. It requires that exposure to vinyl chloride be controlled to 3 ppm averaged over a 1 year period. Additionally exposures must be controlled to no more than 5 ppm for 1 month, 6 ppm for 1 week, 7 ppm for 8 hours and 8 ppm for 1 hour. Although this perspective has not been widely adopted, it does appear to correspond to our knowledge of the properties of vinyl chloride, and other chemicals should, no doubt, be considered similarly.

For the second monitoring objective, measurements taken to be useful for epidemiology studies must reflect as much as is known about the exposure. In other words, the objective must be to estimate the actual dose to the person(s) as accurately as possible. When much is known about the biological properties of a chemical, it is easier to design a sampling strategy, but it must be borne in mind that new effects may be discovered in the future. In any case, as complete a description of exposure should be obtained as is feasible. For example, even though it may be thought that exposure over relatively long periods of time is the most important concern for a hazardous substance, it is best to estimate both long-term and excursion (short-term) exposures.

How the chemical is being used should also be a factor in deciding when, where, and how long to take samples. It is necessary to know what the probability will be of a person actually encountering a given concentration before deciding whether to take a measurement under those conditions. For example, if an in-line filter in a chemical process is periodically changed, it would be sensible to measure the level of chemical encountered over the range(s) of time it takes to change the filter. On the other hand, if a chemical is likely to be present in the general work area, either continually or for major portions of a work shift, a full shift-length sample would probably be the best type of sample to take. Other sampling strategies should be considered depending on the way people will encounter the exposure.

In designing sampling approaches, it is necessary to consider each situation in the light of the chemical or chemicals to be encountered, their toxic properties, and how they are used. In judging the seriousness or acceptability of an exposure, permissible exposure limits or guidelines would certainly be taken into account, but the toxicokinetic properties that might be dependent on the pattern of exposure should be considered as well as potential future use of the data for epidemiological studies. This is in contrast to merely characterizing full-shift time-weighted averages just because the exposure standard or guidelines happen to be written in the most common form, an 8 hour time-weighted average.

Biomonitoring

Biomonitoring is defined, for the purpose of this discussion, as the evaluation of the internal exposure of a human to a chemical agent as determined by an analysis of biological specimens. Depending on the chemical agent and biological specimen collected, the internal exposure reflects the amount of the chemical recently absorbed, the amount of chemical in the body, or, less frequently, the amount of the chemical at its action site(s).

Biological monitoring techniques potentially offer better estimates of internal exposure than environmental monitoring because biological parameters related to internal exposure are more directly associated with potential systemic adverse health effects than environmental measurements. Biological monitoring takes into consideration absorption by all routes of exposure and measures occupational as well as nonoccupational exposures. Biological monitoring may also allow a better estimate of an individual worker's exposure than environmental measurements, since there are always individual differences in work habits and individual differences in the way chemicals are handled in the body.

However, it is important to distinguish between measuring the amount of the substance and the actual exposure or the risk to the person because of that amount. For example, it is often possible to measure quantitatively the amount of a chemical present in a urine sample. If the duration of exposure cannot be inferred from the urine concentration, then correlations to acceptable or unacceptable limits may be impossible.

In order to make the best use of biological monitoring, it is necessary to know how the level to be measured is related to exposure so that judgments can be made about risk. Ideally controlled experiments in humans will have been done to determine the quantitative relationship between exposure and concentration of the chemical or metabolite in the medium to be measured. When this is not available, it may be possible to arrive at concentration ranges of acceptability by referring to animal studies if a model can be constructed with confidence that relates how the chemical is handled in the animal species with how the chemical is handled by humans. Similarly biological monitoring techniques may not be appropriate if the primary adverse response involves acute exposure to the respiratory tract, skin, or eyes. Biological monitoring has little value in detecting peak chemical exposure levels unless one knows the time interval between an acute exposure and sample collection as well as the metabolic fate of the chemical in the body.

Over the past decade there has been much research interest in identifying biological markers of exposure. Systematic monitoring of population groups, however, has been somewhat limited. In the design of applied biomonitoring programs, a number of points need to be considered. Sampling times must be carefully selected and controlled with respect to when exposure occurred, when a chemical is rapidly excreted, and when individual variability is great. Programs of biological monitoring should be undertaken only when the relationship between exposure and the parameter to be measured is known. Sufficient pharmacokinetic information should be available when a chemical or metabolite is to be measured. Finally appropriate evaluation criteria such as biological limit values should be established before these ongoing programs are undertaken.

Health Surveillance

The goal of all effective monitoring and exposure control strategies should be to achieve exposure results that do not result in adverse changes in health parameters. Health surveillance programs can provide insight on the effectiveness of control strategies in addition to their other purposes, such as the early detection of nonoccupationally related disease. At Dow and a number of other companies in the manufacturing and processing industries, a standard physical examination is offered to employees on a periodic basis. This is a general screening approach, and it is followed up with physician–employee consultation when further diagnosis and treatment is indicated.

Some might consider the measurement of such health screening parameters as enzyme counts related to liver function, pulmonary function testing, and chest X rays to be types of biomonitoring. However, it should be kept in mind that these programs are not a substitute for environmental and/or biological monitoring as discussed above.

To be useful in epidemiological studies, health surveillance programs should be designed to gather information from related groups in a fashion that will permit valid statistical analysis of the data and comparison with appropriate control groups. Epidemiological experts should be consulted when data of this type are to be used in evaluating population or subpopulation groups.

In a sense the health surveillance program may be regarded as providing feedback to the monitoring/exposure control strategy and the toxicological/epidemiological knowledge base. Under ideal circumstances it offers a degree of support and assurance that an exposure control strategy and its knowledge base on potential health effects are appropriate. Infrequently, the feedback may suggest modification in the control strategy or suggest further toxicological or epidemiological studies.

PRODUCT STEWARDSHIP

Knowledge of the potential health and environmental effects of chemicals has been advanced by increases in the amount and sophistication of toxicological and epidemiological literature, in the number of professionals in the field, and in the proliferation of industrial hygiene, environmental health, and environmental medicine curricula and postgraduate research programs. Industrial approaches to expanding the knowledge base and its application to product stewardship have also been evolving. The Dow Chemical Company, a pioneer and leader in many aspects of environmental health and product safety, established one of the first toxicology research laboratories for study of industrial chemicals in the early 1930s. Industrial hygiene and occupational medicine departments were established in the 1940s, and epidemiology and environmental science groups in the early 1970s.

Over the years Dow has increasingly recognized that the knowledge base had to be transferred to its customers, many of whom further processed or formulated the chemicals into other products. For example, safety and material-handling information began to be supplied to customers some 40 years ago. This recognition led to the development at Dow of product stewardship — an ethic associated with its practice to promote a partnership of knowledge between manufacturer and customer. Product stewardship, or product safety as it is referred to in some companies, is now practiced by a number of chemical companies. The remainder of this chapter reflects the relatively advanced product stewardship programs of Dow and a few other major chemical suppliers and then briefly describes the current development of an industrywide program called Responsible Care®, which is based on these advanced company programs.

In 1972, Dow adopted the following product stewardship philosophy:

> The Dow Chemical Company has a fundamental concern for all who make, distribute, and use its products, and for the environment in which we live. This concern is the basis for our product stewardship philosophy by which we assess the safety, health, and environmental information on our products and then take appropriate steps to protect employee and public health and the environment. Our product stewardship program rests with each and every individual involved with Dow products—from the initial concept and research to the manufacture, sale, distribution, use, and disposal of each product.

In short, product stewardship is a commitment to action—To do the right things. This commitment must permeate all levels and functions of an organization, from top management policy, to planning, to day-to-day decisions and work site practices.

The purpose of product stewardship is fivefold:

- Protect employees, public health, and the environment.
- Protect products from the environment.
- Reduce liability.
- Prevent adverse publicity.
- Build the trust of employees and customers.

Each of these objectives is self-explanatory. Although the protection of people and the environment is most important, it is also important that the products be protected from the environment and not be misused, abused, and disposed of improperly. Such practice could lead to calls for a product ban, product restrictions, and tighter regulations.

Product stewardship must be the responsibility of all employees. It cannot just be the responsibility of a safety coordinator or a single department. It ranges from the chemist experimenting on a substance for future application to the salesperson taking orders for large quantities of an established product such as caustic soda. Industrial health and environmental scientists have the responsibility for generating safety data that evaluate a product's impact on potential or existing applications, and ultimately communicating this information in understandable terms to all concerned. Manufacturing people must inform all employees of the potential health effects, proper safety practices, and other product related facts and ensure that necessary equipment is available and used. It is also their responsibility to adhere to pollution control and industrial hygiene standards and practices.

Stewardship does not end when a product leaves the plant. Distribution people must select carriers, warehouses, and terminals that will perform consistently within guidelines and ensure that products reach the customer in a safe manner. Marketing people must furnish customers and distributors with appropriate handling and application information, and be on the lookout for potential misuse, mishandling, or improper disposal of products. They should form a supplier–customer partnership that promotes safe uses and applications of chemicals.

Another key person to a product safety program is what at Dow Chemical is called the product steward—the person responsible for recommendation of needed health and environmental studies and safety assessments for each product. The product stewards help evaluate the appropriateness of a customer's use and disposal of a product, and they facilitate preparation of safety training tools. Each Dow product has an assigned steward who maintains contact with sales representatives, customers, health and environmental scientists, and government regulators in order to maintain appropriate health and environmental information and address concerns at all stages of product development and use.

A number of considerations are central to a product evaluation: How is the product manufactured? What are its raw materials? What is the manufacturing process? What impurities does a product contain, and what problems can be expected if changes are made in the process? In addition product distribution must be evaluated: Is the product transported by road, rail, or water? Does it go through terminals? Is it handled by distributors? How is it packaged?

Other considerations may include how the product will be used and how, potentially, it can be misused: Can it be ingested? Inhaled? Touched? What are recommended disposal practices? Will it be burned? Land filled? What would happen if the product is spilled?

Additional considerations may include evaluation of the probability and extent of human exposure. Two or three decades ago, only worker exposures to healthy males between the ages of 18 and 65 were considered. Today the unborn fetus of a pregnant employee must be considered. And if the product leaves a plant site, the potential for adverse effects on sick people, children, the elderly—every demographic group—must be considered.

Furthermore the probability and amount of environmental release to the air, water, and land must be evaluated along with the toxicity and persistence of the product in the environment.

In more recent years health and environmental concerns have often dominated product stewardship evaluations. However, safety concerns involving fire, explosion, and reactivity cannot be underestimated—or overlooked. It should not be forgotten that the Bhopal, India, incident in 1984 was caused by a reaction of methyl isocyanate with water and that the tragic accident earlier the same year in Mexico City was the result of a fire and explosion of a hydrocarbon.

How much health and environmental data are needed on a new product is a question always asked during the developmental cycle. Range-finding toxicological data are obtained for early-stage research work. These studies include acute oral, eye irritation, and skin irritation studies. In addition it is at this point that reactive chemical data should be obtained to determine if a product is shock sensitive, is flammable, undergoes exothermic decomposition, and so on. Its reactivity with other chemicals and construction materials should also be determined or anticipated. When a potential new product reaches pilot plant stage, range-finding studies may suffice, depending on the results and the applications considered for the material.

Finally, when a material is sent to potential customers for applications development, a review must be conducted to determine the need for more acute and subchronic toxicological and environmental testing. It is at this point that long-range studies must be considered and, if needed, planned for the future.

An important link in the product stewardship philosophy is to establish a supplier–customer partnership in health, safety, and environmental matters. Experience has shown that in addition to having a high-quality product at a competitive price, the supplier must be the buyer's expert in avoiding injury or environmental damage from downstream use of its products—a trend that is in the supplier's own interest. The time when a company could sell a product merely on the basis of a competitive price is past. Today the key to successful marketing is to reduce the knowledge gap between seller and buyer.

The supplier has to focus attention on the buyer's needs and experience in handling chemicals. Regulation is only one factor influencing these needs; the most essential factors are product knowledge and an attitude of commitment to developing and carrying out sound practices. Knowledge about health, safety, and the environment is a specialty the supplier must offer with its products. This knowledge is essential for customer success. Only if customers are successful will the supplier be successful. The amount of time and effort required for product stewardship depends on both the properties of the product and the resources and expertise of the customer. Some of the approaches to supplier–customer interchange are shown in Table 30-2. Obviously more supplier resources are required for a highly toxic product such as chlorine being used by a customer with limited resources than for a polystyrene resin sold to another large manufacturing company. In both cases,

TABLE 30-2   Product Stewardship: Types of Information and Consultation Provided to Customers

Material safety data sheets

Technical literature and summary brochures
Label instructions
Posters and video or audio tapes for training
Phone consultation
Presentations at safety meetings by experts
Seminars on regulatory compliance
Plant visitations and information exchange
Industrial hygiene surveys at customer's site
Vent stack monitoring
"How-to" presentations at professional and trade association meetings

Note: These materials depend on the nature of the product, its intended use, and the resources of the customer.

however, it is important that a safety partnership be developed between the supplier and the customer.

The challenge for the future is to build supplier–customer relationships on an industrywide basis with emphasis on all areas of stewardship—manufacturing, transportation, storage, use, and disposal. This challenge is being addressed by the Chemical Manufacturers Association, a trade association representing about 200 companies that produce approximately 90% of U.S. industrial chemicals. In 1988 the Association began an industrywide initiative to enhance operational performance on all these matters. Adherence to Responsible Care® is condition for membership in the CMA.

RESPONSIBLE CARE

Responsible Care® has two critical program elements. The first is intended to guide companies toward continually improving their health, safety, and environmental performance; a second is designed to assist companies to do a better job of understanding and responding to public concerns about safely managing the use of chemicals. The framework to accomplish these objectives consists of 10 Guiding Principles, which serve as the operational philosophy of the program, and 6 Codes of Management Practices, which describe the key activities companies must undertake to manage chemicals as safely as possible while constantly improving performance.

The purpose of the Guiding Principles is to provide the foundation for instituting cultural change within the chemical industry, in order to improve openness with the public, and to make a commitment to continue performance improvements. The Guiding Principles are described as:

- Recognize and respond to community concerns about chemicals and production operations
- Develop and produce chemicals that can be manufactured, transported, used and disposed of safely
- Make health, safety and environment considerations a priority in planning for all existing and new products and processes
- Report promptly to officials, employees, customers and the public, information on chemical-related health or environmental hazards and recommend protective measures
- Counsel customers on the safe use, transportation and disposal of chemical products
- Operate plants and facilities in a manner that protects the environment and the health and safety of employees and the public
- Extend knowledge by conducting or supporting research on the health, safety and environmental effects of products processes and waste materials
- Work with others to resolve problems created by past handling and disposal of hazardous substances
- Participate with government and others in creating responsible laws, regulations and standards to safeguard the community, workplace and environment
- Promote the principles and practices of Responsible Care® by sharing experiences and offering assistance to others who produce, handle, use, transport or dispose of chemicals

The first code of management or practice, community awareness and emergency response (CAER), was approved by CMA in 1989. This program element had its beginnings prior to 1989 when the CMA realized that, following the 1984 chemical release incident in Bhopal, India, few of its members had emergency plans that addressed what responses needed to be implemented and coordinated with local emergency services should an accidental release occur. The CAER program' Action Steps, many of which are incorporated into the 1986 Superfund Amendment Reauthorization Act (SARA), required formation of State Emergency Response Commissions and Local Emergency Planning Committees (LEPCs). Importantly this code element also mandated companies to implement community outreach through formation of Community Advisory Panels (CAPs). CAP members are citizens who provide perspectives of issues and questions arising from chemical manufacturing facilities located within their communities. As of 1998, over 300 CAPs have been established in communities where chemicals are manufactured across the United States. The CAER program also provides an important mechanism for the chemical industry to facilitate the development of community communication plans consistent with the EPA-mandated Risk Management Planning (RMP) rule, which requires disclosure of worst-case release scenarios to public emergency response teams.

The second management practice code, pollution prevention, was adopted in 1990. It requires both reporting and a commitment to reduction of emissions. EPA annually publishes emission information as the Toxics Release Inventory (TRI). The combination of these programs has had significant impact on pollution prevention; from 1988 through 1996, TRI emissions decreased overall by 51%, while CMA members achieved over a 60% reduction from 1988 to 1994. Public reporting of emission data is intended to encourage continued improvement, coupled with trackable public progress, in future emission reduction programs. For example, the Dow Chemical Company has announced year 2005 goals of achieving reductions in air and water emissions of 75% for priority chemicals (e.g., carcinogens, persistent, toxic and bioaccumulative chemicals) and 50% for other chemical emissions. These targeted reductions are to be accompanied by a 50% reduction in waste and wastewater, and a 20% reduction in energy, generated per pound of chemical production.

The employee health and safety management code requires Occupational Injury and Illness Reports (OIIR) be submitted semiannually to CMA. These are the same data that must be recorded under the OSHA record-keeping standards and provide a publicly visible measurement of industry progress. For example, in 1995 CMA members improved performance by 11% over 1994, and the overall rate of 2.5 incidents per 200,000 exposure hours compared to 10.4 incidents per 200,000 exposure hours for all manufacturing.

The fourth and fifth safety management codes are distribution and process safety. Beginning in 1995 the CMA developed a DOT Hazardous Materials Incident Report data base for measuring performance against distribution-related incidents. The reports provide improved reporting and investigation of incidents and strengthen implementation of preventative measures. The process safety code identifies improved processes for prevention of fires, explosions, and accidental releases, and it is aligned with regulatory mandates such as the OSHA process safety rule and the EPA risk management planning rule.

The sixth and last management code is product stewardship. This process, as described earlier in this chapter, supports management of environmental health, and safety risks through the entire life cycle of a product design, manufacture, marketing, distribution, use, recycling and disposal. An important element of this code is collection and communication of safety data to customers. Another critical code element is a commitment to conduct of research that contributes to knowledge necessary for evaluating chemical risks. In 1998 the CMA announced a plan, in cooperation with the EPA, to initiate a voluntary testing program to develop expanded health and environmental safety information on a spectrum of high-production volume (HPV) chemicals. The information obtained from these studies will be shared with the EPA and the public through a readily available data base. The CMA also initiated a research program intended to improve the generic science-based understanding of potential chemical risks to humans and the environment. This program included assuming governance and partial financial support for the Chemical Industry Institute of Toxicology, a not-for-profit research institute committed to independent research into mechanisms of chemical toxicity.

An issue fundamental to the credibility of Responsible Care is external verification of performance. To facilitate this objective, CMA has implemented a Management Systems Verification (MSV) program. This process includes reviews of compliance with the management codes conducted by CMA member company peers and community representatives of individual companies and it supports the integrity of the initiative for employees, local communities, public officials, and the public at large.

CONCLUDING PRESPECTIVE

From an industry perspective, meeting health, safety, and environmental concerns will remain a top priority. However, there is often a gap between public perceptions of risk and realities of risk as evaluated by scientific methods. Sometimes perceived concerns have been without scientific foundation; in other instances, there has been a failure to recognize hazards or to respond in a timely manner. Critical reviews of the literature, like those in this book assist professionals in prioritizing health and environment resources more effectively.

INDEX